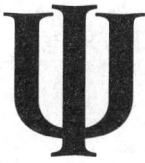

GRADUATE STUDY IN PSYCHOLOGY

— 2011 —

American Psychological Association

American Psychological Association
Washington, DC

Copyright © 2011 by the American Psychological Association. All rights reserved. Except as permitted under the United States Copyright Act of 1976, no part of this publication may be reproduced or distributed in any form or by any means, including, but not limited to, the process of scanning and digitization, or stored in a database or retrieval system, without the prior written permission of the publisher.

Published by
American Psychological Association
750 First Street, NE
Washington, DC 20002

www.apa.org

Typeset by Cadmus Communications, Baltimore, MD

Printer: United Book Press, Inc., Baltimore, MD
Cover Designer: Naylor Design, Washington, DC

ISBN-13: 978-1-4338-0902-6
ISBN-10: 1-4338-0902-8
ISSN: 0742-7220
44th edition

To order
APA Order Department
P.O. Box 92984
Washington, DC 20090-2984
Tel: (800) 374-2721, Direct: (202) 336-5510
Fax: (202) 336-5502, TDD/TTY: (202) 336-6123
Online: www.apa.org/pubs/books/
E-mail: order@apa.org

Printed in the United States of America

Contents

Foreword	v	Contact Information	xii
Considering Graduate Study	vii	Department Information	xii
Programs, Degrees, and Employment	vii	Programs and Degrees Offered	xii
Accreditation in Professional Psychology	viii	APA Accreditation Status	xii
Doctoral Internship Training in Professional		Student Applications/Admissions	xii
Psychology	viii	Financial Information/Assistance	xii
Admission Requirements	ix	Employment of Department Graduates	xii
Application Information	x	Additional Information	xii
Time to Degree	x	Application Information	xii
Tuition and Financial Assistance	x		
Rules for Acceptance of Offers for Admission		**Department Listings by State**	1
and Financial Aid	xi	Index of Programs by Area of Study Offered	885
Explanation of Program Listings	xii	Alphabetical Index	899

Foreword

This is the 44th edition of a book prepared to assist individuals interested in graduate study in psychology. The current edition provides information for more than 600 graduate departments, programs, and schools of psychology in the United States and Canada. The information was obtained from questionnaires sent to graduate departments and schools of psychology and was provided voluntarily. The American Psychological Association (APA) is not responsible for the accuracy of the information reported.

The purpose of this publication is to provide an information service, offering in one book information about the majority of graduate programs in psychology. Inclusion in this publication does not signify APA approval or endorsement of a graduate program, nor should it be assumed that a listing of a program in *Graduate Study in Psychology* means that its graduates are automatically qualified to sit for licensure as psychologists or are eligible for positions requiring a psychology degree.

However, programs listed in this publication have agreed to the following quality assurance provisions:

1. They have agreed to honor April 15 as the date allowed for graduate applicants to accept or reject an offer of admission and financial assistance for fall matriculation. This date adheres to national policy guidelines as stated by the Council of Graduate Schools and the Council of Graduate Departments of Psychology.

2. They have satisfied the following criteria: The program offers a graduate degree and is sponsored by a public or private higher education institution accredited by one of six regional accrediting bodies recognized by the U.S. Secretary of Education or, in the case of Canadian programs, the institution is publicly recognized by the Association of Universities and Colleges of Canada as a member in good standing, or the program indicates that it meets *all* of the following criteria:
   A. The graduate program, wherever it may be administratively housed, is publicly labeled as a psychology program in pertinent institutional catalogs and brochures.
   B. The psychology program stands as a recognizable, coherent organizational entity within the institution.
   C. There is an identifiable core of full-time psychology faculty.
   D. Psychologists have clear authority and primary responsibility for the academic core and specialty preparation, whether or not the program involves multiple administrative lines.
   E. There is an identifiable body of graduate students who are enrolled in the program for the attainment of the graduate degree offered.
   F. The program is an organized, integrated sequence of study designed by the psychology faculty responsible for the program.
   G. Programs leading to a doctoral degree require at least the equivalent of 3 full-time academic years of graduate study.
   H. Doctoral programs ensure appropriate breadth and depth of education and training in psychology as follows:
   1) Methodology and history, including systematic preparation in scientific standards and responsibilities, research design and methodology, quantitative methods (e.g., statistics, psychometric methods), and historical foundations in psychology.
   2) Foundations in psychology, including
      a. biological bases of behavior (e.g., physiological psychology, comparative psychology, neuropsychology, psychopharmacology);
      b. cognitive–affective bases of behavior (e.g., learning, memory, perception, cognition, thinking, motivation, emotion);
      c. social bases of behavior (e.g., social psychology; cultural, ethnic, and group processes; sex roles; organizational behavior); and
      d. individual differences (e.g., personality theory, human development, individual differences, abnormal psychology, psychology of women, psychology of persons with disabilities, psychology of the minority experience).
   3) Additional preparation in the program's area of specialization, to include
      a. knowledge and application of ethical principles and guidelines and standards as may apply to scientific and professional practice activities;
      b. supervised practicum and/or laboratory experiences appropriate to the area of practice, teaching, or research in psychology; and
      c. advanced preparation appropriate to the area of specialization.

This publication may not answer all questions you have about graduate education in psychology. Some questions you may want to direct to particular graduate departments, programs, or schools of psychology. *For more information about general policies and information related to graduate education, visit the APA Education Web site (http://www.apa.org/ed).*

Producing this annual publication involves the cooperation of many individuals each year. We wish to express appreciation to all graduate departments, programs, and schools that contributed information. We also wish to acknowledge the support and contributions by individuals in the Education Directorate, Internet Services, Publications and Databases, and the Center for Psychology Workforce Analysis and Research.

Caroline Cope, MA
Research Officer
Office of Graduate and Postgraduate Education and Training
Education Directorate
American Psychological Association

Considering Graduate Study

Psychology is a broad scientific discipline bridging the social and biological sciences. Psychology's applications include education and human development, health and human resilience, family and community relations, organizations and other work environments, engineering and technology, the arts and architecture, communications, and political and judiciary systems.

There are many types of graduate programs in psychology. Selecting a graduate program that is best for you requires thoughtful consideration. The American Psychological Association (APA) does not rank graduate programs in psychology. Rather, APA encourages selecting graduate programs based on the best match for you. Some programs focus on preparing students for an academic research career, while others focus on preparing students for applied research outside the university. Other programs prepare students to provide psychological services as licensed professional psychologists. Some programs offer professional development, in addition to a focus in psychology, to prepare students for a college teaching career. Psychology subfields of recent master's and doctoral graduates are illustrated in Figures 1 and 2.

Figure 1. Master's Degrees Awarded by Psychology Subfield: 2007–2008

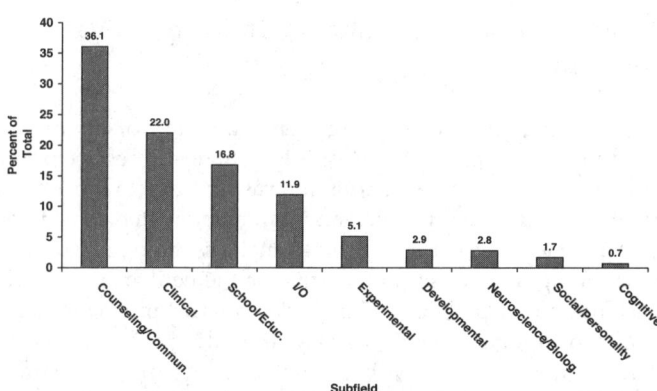

Source: *Graduate Study in Psychology 2011 Edition* data. Prepared by APA Office of Graduate and Postgraduate Education and Training.

Figure 2. Doctoral Degrees Awarded by Psychology Subfield: 2007–2008

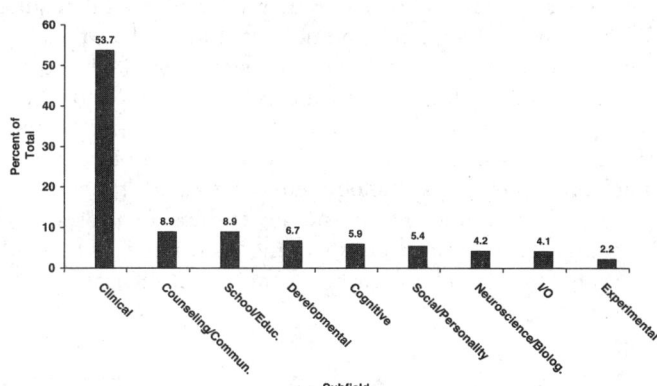

Source: *Graduate Study in Psychology 2011 Edition* data. Prepared by APA Office of Graduate and Postgraduate Education and Training.

Programs, Degrees, and Employment

Although employment in research, teaching, and human service positions is possible for those with a master's degree in psychology, the doctoral degree is generally considered the entry-level degree in psychology for the independent, licensed practice of psychology as a profession. The doctoral degree is the preferred degree for college and university faculty, and it has long been a requirement for faculty positions in research universities. For specific information about employment outcomes of a program's graduates, review the section entitled "Employment of Department Graduates" in each listing in this publication.

Figures 3 and 4 summarize the types of postdegree outcomes of graduates of master's and doctoral degree programs. About one fourth of those awarded a baccalaureate degree in psychology

Figure 3. Employment and Outcomes of Master's Recipients: 2007–2008

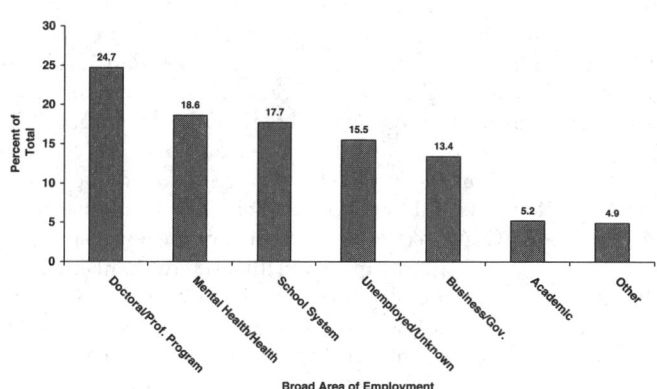

Source: *Graduate Study in Psychology 2011 Edition* data. Prepared by APA Office of Graduate and Postgraduate Education and Training.

Figure 4. Employment and Outcomes of Doctoral Recipients: 2007–2008

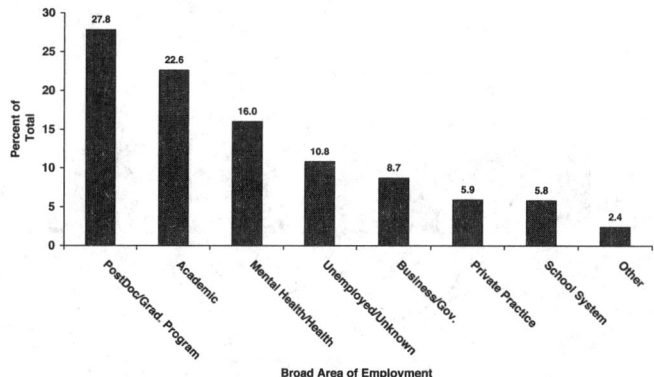

Source: *Graduate Study in Psychology 2011 Edition* data. Prepared by APA Office of Graduate and Postgraduate Education and Training.

continue in graduate or professional education in psychology or other fields.

Doctoral programs differ in the type of doctoral degree awarded. The two most common doctoral degrees are the PhD (Doctor of Philosophy) and the PsyD (Doctor of Psychology). Programs in colleges of education may offer the EdD (Doctor of Education) degree. The PhD is generally regarded as a research degree. Although many professional psychology programs award the PhD degree, especially those in university academic departments, these programs typically have an emphasis on research training integrated with applied or practice training. The PsyD is a professional degree in psychology (similar to the MD in medicine). Programs awarding the PsyD typically emphasize preparing their graduates for professional practice with less training in the production of scientific knowledge. About 70% of all doctoral degrees in psychology are PhDs; of the degrees awarded in clinical psychology, about the same percentage receive PhDs as PsyDs. Figure 5 gives a profile of initial employment outcomes for PhD and PsyD program graduates. For more information about degrees, employment, and salaries in psychology, visit the APA Center for Workforce Studies Web site (http://www.apa.org/workforce).

Accreditation in Professional Psychology

Accreditation is the mechanism by which students and the public are assured the general quality of the education provided has met a set of educational and professional standards. Accreditation bodies include those that review and accredit at the institutional level and those that accredit at the program or area level. Institutions that confer advanced degrees (i.e., colleges, universities, and professional schools) are eligible for accreditation by regional accrediting bodies. The APA Commission on Accreditation (CoA) accredits at the program level and only reviews doctoral programs in regionally accredited institutions. The CoA accredits doctoral programs in professional psychology (e.g., clinical, counseling, school, and combinations of these areas), as well as internship and postdoctoral residency programs. The APA CoA does not accredit master's degree programs. Accreditation by the APA CoA applies to educational programs (i.e., doctoral programs in professional psychology), not to individuals. Doctoral programs accredited by the APA or the Canadian Psychological Association are required to make publicly available information about the education and training outcomes of their students so that prospective students can make informed decisions. Please refer to the section entitled "APA Accreditation Status" for the URL to locate the information for a specific program.

Graduation from an accredited institution or program does not guarantee employment or licensure for individuals, although being a graduate of an accredited program may facilitate such achievement and is required in some jurisdictions.

All programs listed in this publication are, at a minimum, situated in regionally accredited institutions. The doctoral programs that are APA-accredited are identified as such. For more information and the most current lists of accredited programs, see the APA Office of Program Consultation and Accreditation Web site (http://www.apa.org/ed/accreditation).

Doctoral Internship Training in Professional Psychology

Doctoral programs that prepare their graduates for the professional practice of psychology, especially in health service provision, typically require a doctoral internship prior to the awarding of the doctorate. The doctoral internship is often considered the capstone experience in professional psychology education and training and consists of 1 year (or the equivalent) of full-time supervised practice training. The internship is completed in a professional service agency training program that is typically not affiliated with the students' graduate program. Internship programs vary widely in terms of the settings and populations served as well as their models of training. Students sometimes relocate geographically to complete their internships. All accredited internship programs (and some nonaccredited) select students through a nationwide computerized matching process that has a standardized application and fixed deadlines. For many years the number of available internships has not grown at the rate the number of students has, resulting in an imbalance in which large numbers of students do not successfully match to an internship (e.g., 23% in 2010). While efforts are underway by APA and the education and training community to address this, the imbalance is a significant issue facing professional psychology education and training. To learn more about the match and internships in professional psychology, refer to the Web site of the Association of Psychology Postdoctoral and Internship Centers (APPIC) at http://www.appic.org.

Figure 5. Employment of PhD and PsyD Recipients: 2006–2007

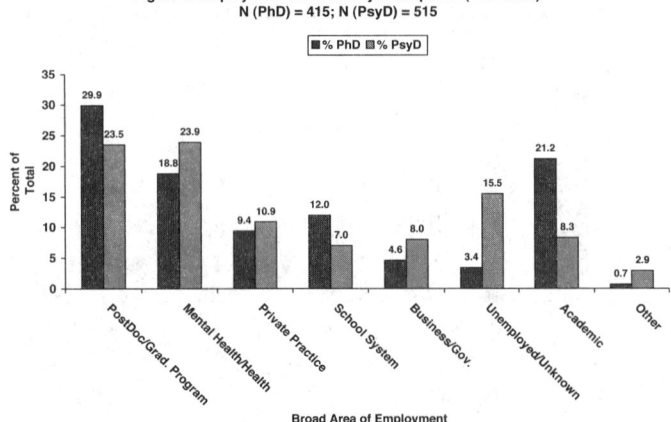

Source: *Graduate Study in Psychology 2011 Edition* data. Prepared by APA Office of Graduate and Postgraduate Education and Training.

Internship match rates for professional psychology doctoral programs can be found under the specific institution listing in this book. Figure 6 shows the percentage of graduate students who were matched to an internship and the internship placement type for APA-accredited doctoral programs and nonaccredited programs.

Admission Requirements

Requirements for admission vary from program to program. Some psychology programs may require significant undergraduate coursework in psychology, often the equivalent of a major or minor, while others do not. Sixty-five percent of recent psychology PhD recipients have also received a bachelor's degree in psychology.

Of the graduate departments listed in this publication that offer master's degrees, 52% require the Graduate Record Examination (GRE) Verbal and Quantitative sections and 11% require the GRE-Subject (Psychology). Sixty-one percent of the doctoral programs listed require the GRE-Verbal and Quantitative sections, 23% require the GRE-Subject (Psychology). If the programs in which you are interested require these standardized tests, you should take the GRE-V, GRE-Q, and GRE-Subject (Psychology) in time for the scores to be included with your application materials. The overall median GRE scores reported for applicants admitted to master's degree programs listed in this publication are 516 (GRE-V), 585 (GRE-Q), and 625 (GRE-Subject). The overall median GRE scores reported for applicants admitted to doctoral degree programs listed in this publication are 584 (GRE-V), 654 (GRE-Q), and 685 (GRE-Subject).

Other criteria considered as admission factors may include previous research activities, work experience, relevant public service, extracurricular activities, letters of recommendation, statement of goals and objectives, an interview, a major or minor in psychology or a record of specific courses in psychology, and undergraduate GPA. Figure 7 shows the ratings of importance of these other admissions criteria by master's and doctoral programs listed in this publication. A rating of 3 indicates that the individual admissions criterion is considered to be of high importance, while a rating of 0 indicates that the admissions criterion holds no importance in a program's admissions process. The three admissions criteria rated as of highest importance for both master's and doctoral programs are undergraduate GPA, letters of recommendation, and a statement of goals and interests. The overall median undergraduate GPA reported for applicants admitted to master's degree programs listed in this publication is 3.40, while that for doctoral programs is 3.6.

The number of graduate school applicants typically exceeds the number of student openings. The number of applications received by a program and the number of students accepted provide a sense of the expected competition when applying to a particular department, program, or school. Figure 8 shows the percentage of students admitted in relationship to the number of applications for psychology programs in different areas. For more information, review the section entitled "Student Applications/Admissions" for each of the programs of interest to you listed in this publication.

Figure 6. Internship Placement by Program Type: 2007–2008

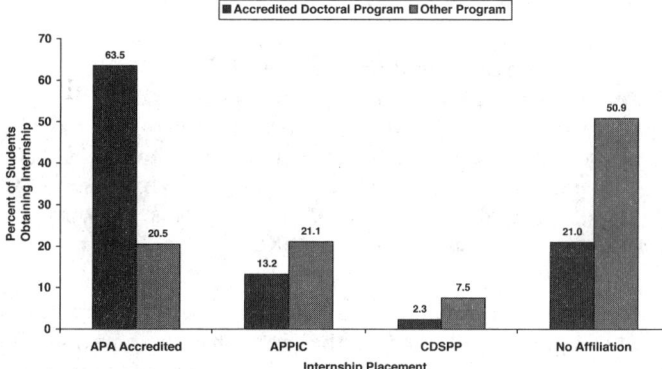

Source: *Graduate Study in Psychology 2011 Edition* data. Prepared by APA Office of Graduate and Postgraduate Education and Training.

Figure 7. Mean Rating of Importance of Various Admissions Criteria

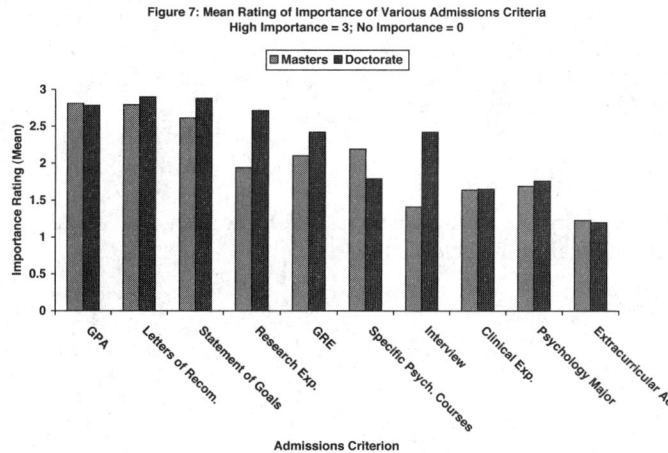

Source: *Graduate Study in Psychology 2011 Edition* data. Prepared by APA Office of Graduate and Postgraduate Education and Training.

Figure 8. Percent of Applicants Admitted to Graduate Programs by Selected Psychology Subfield: 2007–2008

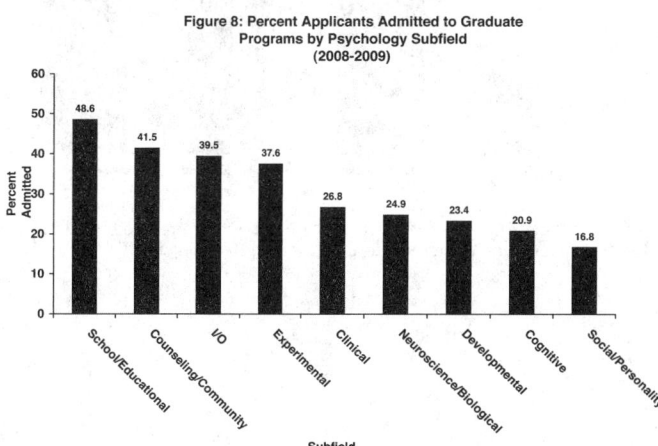

Source: *Graduate Study in Psychology 2011 Edition* data. Prepared by APA Office of Graduate and Postgraduate Education and Training.

Application Information

An application to a department or program of study is a very important document. Always confirm (a) the deadline for filing the application, (b) what documents are required, and (c) who should receive the application. Include the required application fee.

Most graduate programs in psychology accept students only for fall admission. However, if you are interested in winter, spring, or summer admission, check the application information listed in this publication for the program to which you are applying. Information about application deadlines in this publication is listed in the section entitled "Application Information."

Time to Degree

Programs should be clear about the average number of years in full-time study (or part-time equivalent) required to complete the degree requirements. On average, graduate students take 7 years from entrance into a graduate program to complete the doctoral degree. Eighty percent of recent psychology PhD recipients also have master's degrees.

Tuition and Financial Assistance

Graduate education can be expensive. Figure 9 shows the average in-state and out-of-state public university and private university tuition rates for master's and doctoral level programs in psychology.

Financial assistance in various forms is available to students. You can apply for a fellowship, scholarship, assistantship, or another type of financial assistance. Many fellowships and scholarships are grants that do not require service to the department or university. Of departments and programs listed in this publication, 68% indicate that they offer some form of fellowship or scholarship to 1st-year students, and 65% indicate that they offer some form of fellowship or scholarship to advanced students. Assistantships in teaching and research are also available in many programs. These are forms of employment for services in a department. Teaching assistantships may require teaching a class or assisting a professor by grading papers, acting as a laboratory assistant, or performing other such supporting work. Research assistants ordinarily work on research projects being conducted by program faculty. Among departments and programs reporting for this publication, 75% indicate that they offer teaching and research assistantships to 1st-year students and 80% report offering teaching and research assistantships to advanced students.

The amount of work required for fellowships, assistantships, and traineeships is expressed in hours per week. Stipends are expressed in terms of total stipend for an academic year of 9 months. Students should inquire, when receiving an offer of financial assistance, as to the amount to be given in terms of tuition remission (not requiring the student to pay tuition) versus a stipend (actual cash in hand).

For information about tuition costs and the types of assistance offered by departments and programs, review the section entitled "Financial Information/Assistance" for the programs of interest listed in this publication. You can review information listed on the APA Education Web site (http://www.apa.org/ed/graduate) for information about scholarships, fellowships, grants, and other funding opportunities.

The summary information presented in this introduction is based on the responses provided by the graduate programs listed in this publication. This information is not exhaustive in that a number of graduate programs in the United States and Canada are not listed in this publication and not all programs listed provide complete information to all questions. For this reason, you should look closely at the information provided by a specific program of interest to you and not rely exclusively on the group averages presented in this introduction.

Clare Porac, PhD
Catherine Grus, PhD
Associate Executive Directors

Caroline Cope, MA
Research Officer
Office of Graduate and Postgraduate Education and Training
APA Education Directorate

Figure 9. Median Tuition by Type of Institution/Residency: 2007–2008

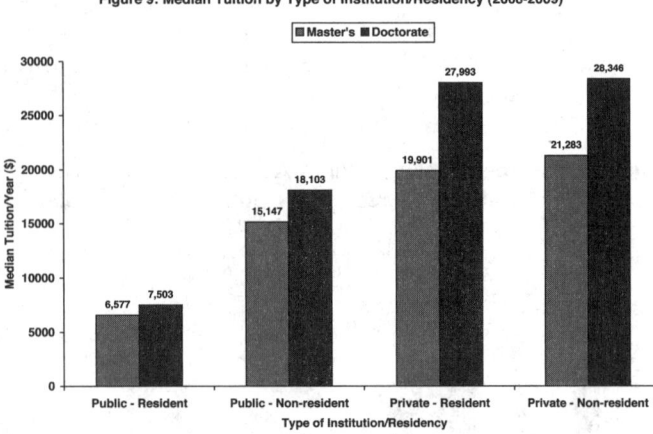

Source: *Graduate Study in Psychology 2011 Edition* data. Prepared by APA Office of Graduate and Postgraduate Education and Training.

Rules for Acceptance of Offers for Admission and Financial Aid

The Council of Graduate Schools has adopted the following policy that provides guidance to students and graduate programs regarding offers of financial support. The policy was adopted by the Council of Graduate Schools in 1965 and reaffirmed in 1992. It was endorsed by the Council of Graduate Departments of Psychology in 1981 and reaffirmed in 2000. Graduate programs and schools currently listed in the book have agreed to honor the policy. The policy reads as follows:

> Acceptance of an offer of financial support (such as graduate scholarship, fellowship, traineeship, or assistantship) for the next academic year by a prospective or enrolled graduate student completes an agreement that both student and graduate school expect to honor. In that context, the conditions affecting such offers and their acceptance must be defined carefully and understood by all parties.

Students are under no obligation to respond to offers of financial support prior to April 15; earlier deadlines for acceptance of such offers violate the intent of this Resolution. In those instances in which the student accepts the offer before April 15 and subsequently desires to withdraw that acceptance, the student may submit in writing a resignation of the appointment at any time through April 15. However, an acceptance given or left in force after April 15 commits the student not to accept another offer without first obtaining a written release from the institution to which a commitment has been made. Similarly, an offer by an institution after April 15 is conditional on presentation by the student of the written release from any previously accepted offer. It is further agreed by the institutions and organizations subscribing to the above Resolution that a copy of this Resolution should accompany every scholarship, fellowship, traineeship, and assistantship offer.

Explanation of Program Listings

The following summarizes the information solicited from each program:

Contact Information

The name of the university or school, address, telephone number, fax number, e-mail, and World Wide Web address are provided. There may be more than one department in an institution that offers degrees in psychology, and if so, each department is listed separately.

Department Information

The year the department was established is provided, including the name of the department chairperson, and the number of full-time and part-time faculty members including information on the number of minority faculty employees.

Programs and Degrees Offered

This heading highlights the program areas in which degrees are offered by the department or school and includes the type of degree awarded and the number of degrees awarded.

APA Accreditation Status

Whether a department or school has a program accredited in clinical psychology, counseling psychology, school psychology, or combined professional–scientific psychology is noted. Because changes in accreditation status may occur after publication, please contact the APA Office of Program Consultation and Accreditation, or review the Web site (http://www.apa.org/ed/accreditation).

Student Applications/Admissions

This section includes information about the number of applications received by the individual program areas of departments and schools. Also listed are the number of applicants accepted into the program and the number of openings anticipated in the next year. In addition, the information reflects the median number of years required for a degree and the number of students enrolled who were dismissed or voluntarily withdrew from the program before completing their degree requirements.

Information on standardized test scores and other criteria considered during admission decisions are rated according to their importance.

This section also includes characteristics of students enrolled in the department or psychology program.

Financial Information/Assistance

Tuition figures per year and per academic unit are indicated. Note that some schools and institutions have different fee structures for doctoral and master's students. The words *non-state residents* are used by state universities that charge more for out-of-state residents than students who reside in the state. These fees should be used as rough guidelines and are subject to change.

Teaching assistantships, research assistantships, traineeships, or fellowships and scholarships are reported. The data for each type of assistance are listed for 1st-year and advanced students. The average amount awarded to each student and the average number of hours that must be worked each week are included in the listing. Contact information for financial assistance is also listed.

Information has been added by departments on those programs that require a professional internship of doctoral students prior to graduation. Information is included on the number of students who applied for an internship, the number who obtained an internship, and if the internship was paid or unpaid. In addition, the department was asked to indicate whether the student achieved an APA- or CPA-accredited internship, and if the internship was listed by the Association of Psychology Postdoctoral Internship Centers or by the Council of Directors of School Psychology Programs. Lastly, many departments provided additional information about the types of settings where students were located, the number of hours spent weekly at the internship site, and other information.

Employment of Department Graduates

This section provides information about employment activities of graduates. Data presented by departments or schools include information about master's and doctoral degree graduates, such as enrollment in psychology doctoral programs, and employment in academic positions, business, and government.

Additional Information

This section provides an opportunity for the department or school to present the orientation, objectives, and emphasis of the department or school. Information is also presented about the special facilities or resources offered by the school or institution.

Also included in this section are statements related to personal behavior and religious beliefs statements that are considered a condition for admission and retention with the program. All information in *Graduate Study in Psychology* is self-reported. In the interest of full disclosure to prospective students, therefore, departments, programs, or institutions by which they are governed that have a statement to this effect are requested to cite the statement or provide a Web site or address at which it can be found.

Application Information

This last section provides the addresses, deadlines, and fees for the submission of applications for each department or school.

2011

Graduate Study in Psychology

ALABAMA

Alabama, University of
Department of Psychology
College of Arts and Sciences
Box 870348
Tuscaloosa, AL 35487-0348
Telephone: (205) 348-1919
Fax: (205) 348-8648
E-mail: *mbhubbard@as.ua.edu*
Web: *http://psychology.ua.edu*

Department Information:
1937. Chairperson: Beverly E. Thorn. Number of faculty: total—full-time 29, part-time 1; women—full-time 14; total—minority—full-time 4; women minority—full-time 4; faculty subject to the Americans With Disabilities Act 1.

Programs and Degrees Offered:
Listed in the following order: Program area, degree type (T if terminal Master's), number awarded 7/08–6/09. Clinical Psychology PhD (Doctor of Philosophy) 6, Cognitive Psychology PhD (Doctor of Philosophy) 0, Social Psychology PhD (Doctor of Philosophy) 1, Developmental Science PhD (Doctor of Philosophy) 0.

APA Accreditation: Clinical PhD (Doctor of Philosophy). Student Outcome Data Website: http://psychology.ua.edu/academics/graduate/clinical/clinical.html.

Student Applications/Admissions:
Student Applications
Clinical Psychology PhD (Doctor of Philosophy)—Applications 2009–2010, 191. Total applicants accepted 2009–2010, 19. Number full-time enrolled (new admits only) 2009–2010, 10. Total enrolled 2009–2010 full-time, 73, part-time, 1. Openings 2010–2011, 14. The median number of years required for completion of a degree in 2008–2009 were 6. The number of students enrolled full- and part-time who were dismissed or voluntarily withdrew from this program area in 2008–2009 were 2. *Cognitive Psychology PhD (Doctor of Philosophy)*—Applications 2009–2010, 15. Total applicants accepted 2009–2010, 4. Number full-time enrolled (new admits only) 2009–2010, 2. Total enrolled 2009–2010 full-time, 8, part-time, 1. Openings 2010–2011, 3. The number of students enrolled full- and part-time who were dismissed or voluntarily withdrew from this program area in 2008–2009 were 0. *Social Psychology PhD (Doctor of Philosophy)*—Applications 2009–2010, 23. Total applicants accepted 2009–2010, 1. Number full-time enrolled (new admits only) 2009–2010, 1. Number part-time enrolled (new admits only) 2009–2010, 0. Total enrolled 2009–2010 full-time, 8, part-time, 1. Openings 2010–2011, 4. The median number of years required for completion of a degree in 2008–2009 were 6. The number of students enrolled full- and part-time who were dismissed or voluntarily withdrew from this program area in 2008–2009 were 1. *Developmental Science PhD (Doctor of Philosophy)*—Applications 2009–2010, 13. Total applicants accepted 2009–2010, 4. Number full-time enrolled (new admits only) 2009–2010, 3. Number part-time enrolled (new admits only) 2009–2010, 0. Openings 2010–2011, 4. The number of students enrolled full- and part-time who were dismissed or voluntarily withdrew from this program area in 2008–2009 were 1.

Scores: Entries appear in this order: required test or GPA, minimum score (if required), median score of students entering in 2009–2010. *Clinical Psychology PhD (Doctor of Philosophy)*: GRE-V no minimum stated, 640, GRE-Q no minimum stated, 645, GRE-Analytical no minimum stated, 5.0, overall undergraduate GPA no minimum stated, 3.8; *Cognitive Psychology PhD (Doctor of Philosophy)*: GRE-V no minimum stated, 570, GRE-Q no minimum stated, 555, GRE-Analytical no minimum stated, 4.75, overall undergraduate GPA no minimum stated, 3.45; *Social Psychology PhD (Doctor of Philosophy)*: GRE-V no minimum stated, 700, GRE-Q no minimum stated, 720, GRE-Analytical no minimum stated, 5.0, overall undergraduate GPA no minimum stated, 3.6; *Developmental Science PhD (Doctor of Philosophy)*: GRE-V no minimum stated, 520, GRE-Q no minimum stated, 540, GRE-Analytical no minimum stated, 4.5, overall undergraduate GPA no minimum stated, 3.2.

Other Criteria: (importance of criteria rated low, medium, or high): GRE scores—high, research experience—high, work experience—low, extracurricular activity—low, clinically related public service—low, GPA—medium, letters of recommendation—high, interview—medium, statement of goals and objectives—high, undergraduate major in psychology—medium, specific undergraduate psychology courses taken—high, Interview typical only for clinical program. For additional information on admission requirements, go to http://psychology.ua.edu/academics/graduate/prospective.html.

Student Characteristics: The following represents characteristics of students in 2009–2010 in all graduate psychology programs in the department: Female—full-time 76, part-time 1; Male—full-time 22, part-time 2; African American/Black—full-time 7, part-time 0; Hispanic/Latino(a)—full-time 6, part-time 0; Asian/Pacific Islander—full-time 4, part-time 0; American Indian/Alaska Native—full-time 0, part-time 0; Caucasian/White—full-time 81, part-time 3; Multi-ethnic—full-time 0, part-time 0; students subject to the Americans With Disabilities Act—full-time 0, part-time 0; Unknown ethnicity—full-time 0, part-time 0; International students who hold an F-1 or J-1 Visa—full-time 4, part-time 0.

Financial Information/Assistance:
Tuition for Full-Time Study: *Doctoral:* State residents: per academic year $7,000; Nonstate residents: per academic year $19,200. Tuition is subject to change. Additional fees are assessed to students beyond the costs of tuition for the following: Course fee - $10.00 per hour; facility/technology fee - $7.00 per hour. See the following Web site for updates and changes in tuition costs: http://cost.ua.edu.

Financial Assistance:
First-Year Students: Teaching assistantships available for first year. Average amount paid per academic year: $11,142. Aver-

age number of hours worked per week: 20. Research assistantships available for first year. Average amount paid per academic year: $11,142. Average number of hours worked per week: 20. Fellowships and scholarships available for first year. Average amount paid per academic year: $15,000.

Advanced Students: Teaching assistantships available for advanced students. Average amount paid per academic year: $11,142. Average number of hours worked per week: 20. Research assistantships available for advanced students. Average amount paid per academic year: $11,142. Average number of hours worked per week: 20. Traineeships available for advanced students. Average amount paid per academic year: $11,142. Average number of hours worked per week: 20. Fellowships and scholarships available for advanced students. Average amount paid per academic year: $15,000.

Additional Information: Of all students currently enrolled full time, 99% benefited from one or more of the listed financial assistance programs. Application and information available online at: http://graduate.ua.edu/financial/.

Internships/Practica: Doctoral Degree (PhD Clinical Psychology): For those doctoral students for whom a professional internship was required in this program prior to graduation, (11) students applied for an internship in 2008–2009, with (10) students obtaining an internship. Of those students who obtained an internship, (10) were paid internships. Of those students who obtained an internship, (10) students placed in APA/CPA accredited internships, (0) students placed in internships not APA/CPA accredited, but listed with the Association of Psychology Postdoctoral and Internship Programs (APPIC), (0) students placed in internships conforming to guidelines of the Council of Directors of School Psychology Programs (CDSPP), (0) students placed in internships that were not APA/CPA accredited, APPIC or CDSPP listed. There are a number of practica available to graduate students. Most doctoral students take PY695/696, a teaching internship, in which the student teaches an introductory psychology class under the supervision of a faculty member. Two semesters of basic psychotherapy practicum are required of every doctoral student in clinical psychology. In this practicum, students conduct psychotherapy with four to six clients in the Department's Psychological Clinic. Students complete approximately 100 hours of direct client contact to fulfill this requirement. After basic psychotherapy practicum, doctoral clinical psychology students take either one or two (depending on specialty area) advanced practica in their area of specialization. Many of these practica are housed in community service agencies (e.g., state psychiatric hospital, community mental health center, University-operated treatment center for disturbed children). In addition to these formal practica, most doctoral students in the clinical program are financially supported at some time during their graduate school years through field placements in various community agencies. These students are supervised by either licensed psychologists employed by these agencies or by Department of Psychology clinical faculty. In addition to the intervention practica discussed above, all clinical doctoral students must take two of the three graduate psychological assessment courses offered. These courses have a significant practicum component, requiring approximately 5 administrations of commonly used psychological assessment instruments with Psychological Clinic clients.

Housing and Day Care: On-campus housing is available. See the following Web site for more information: http://housing.ua.edu/. On-campus day care facilities are available. See the following Web site for more information: http://www.ches.ua.edu/departments/hd/childrensprogram/.

Employment of Department Graduates:
Master's Degree Graduates: Of those who graduated in the academic year 2008–2009, the following categories and numbers represent the postgraduate activities and employment of master's degree graduates: Enrolled in a postdoctoral residency/fellowship (n/a), employed in independent practice (n/a), total from the above (master's) (0).

Doctoral Degree Graduates: Of those who graduated in the academic year 2008–2009, the following categories and numbers represent the postgraduate activities and employment of doctoral degree graduates: Enrolled in a psychology doctoral program (n/a), employed in independent practice (1), employed in an academic position at a university (1), employed in a community mental health/counseling center (1), employed in a hospital/medical center (5), still seeking employment (1), total from the above (doctoral) (9).

Additional Information:
Orientation, Objectives, and Emphasis of Department: The University of Alabama doctoral program in psychology was founded in 1957 and trains students in clinical and experimental psychology. The clinical program has been continually accredited by the American Psychological Association since 1959. The department trains scientists and scientist–practitioners for a variety of roles: research, teaching, and applied practice. Both the clinical and the experimental programs strongly emphasize furthering psychology as a science. The clinical program has specialty areas in psychology-law, clinical-child, gerontology, and health and the experimental program has specialty areas in cognitive, social, and developmental. The social and developmental training areas involve exciting collaborations with other units on campus. The doctoral programs emphasize core knowledge in the social, cognitive, developmental, and biological aspects of behavior as well as methodological/statistical foundations. All students take additional courses designed to prepare them with the necessary knowledge and skills in their chosen specialty area. A further objective of the department is to promote independent scholarship and professional development. Coursework is supplemented by the active collaboration of faculty and students in ongoing research projects and clinical activities. The department maintains access to a wide range of settings in which students can refine their research and applied skills.

Special Facilities or Resources: The department is housed in a four-story building that it shares with the Department of Mathematics. It is directly connected to the department's Psychological Clinic and the University's Seebeck Computer Center. Facilities include faculty offices, student offices, classroom and seminar space, and research laboratories. Graduate students have access to microcomputers for research and word processing and videotaping capabilities for instruction and training. A major resource is the Psychological Clinic, which provides psychological assessment, referral, treatment planning, and direct intervention for a variety of clinical populations. The department's Child and Family Research Clinic serves as a specialized training and research laboratory. Both clinics include observation facilities. Also affiliated with the department is the brand new Child Development Research Center, which has research, office, and training space, and runs a state-of-the-art preschool. Other affiliations on campus include the Center for Mental Health and Aging, the Institute for Social Science Research, the Brewer-Porch Childrens Center, the Student Counseling Center, and the University Medical Center. In the community, the department maintains research and clinical relationships with DCH Regional Medical Center, VA Medical Center, Bryce Hospital, Family Counseling Services, city and county school systems, Indian Rivers Mental Health Center, Partlow Developmental Center, and the Taylor Hardin Forensic Medical Facility.

Information for Students With Physical Disabilities: See the following Web site for more information: http://ods.ua.edu.

Application Information:
Send to Office of the Graduate School, University of Alabama, Box 870118, Tuscaloosa, AL 35487-0118. Application available online. URL of online application: http://graduate.ua.edu/application/index.html. Students are admitted in the Fall, application deadline December 1. Deadline for the applications to the clinical program is December 1; January 15 is the deadline for the cognitive, social, and developmental programs. *Fee:* $50. Application fee is waived for McNair Scholars.

Alabama, University of, at Birmingham
Department of Psychology
Arts and Sciences
415 Campbell Hall
Birmingham, AL 35294-1170
Telephone: (205) 934-3850
Fax: (205) 975-6110
E-mail: *kball@uab.edu*
Web: *http://www.psy.uab.edu*

Department Information:
1969. Chairperson: Karlene Ball, PhD. Number of faculty: total—full-time 30, part-time 58; women—full-time 9, part-time 16; total—minority—full-time 5, part-time 5; women minority—full-time 1, part-time 2.

Programs and Degrees Offered:
Listed in the following order: Program area, degree type (T if terminal Master's), number awarded 7/08–6/09. Behavioral Neuroscience PhD (Doctor of Philosophy) 1, Developmental Psychology PhD (Doctor of Philosophy) 4, Medical/Clinical Psychology PhD (Doctor of Philosophy) 12.

APA Accreditation: Clinical PhD (Doctor of Philosophy). Student Outcome Data Website: http://www.psy.uab.edu/medpsych.htm.

Student Applications/Admissions:
Student Applications
Behavioral Neuroscience PhD (Doctor of Philosophy)—Applications 2009–2010, 19. Total applicants accepted 2009–2010, 2. Number full-time enrolled (new admits only) 2009–2010, 2. Openings 2010–2011, 2. The median number of years required for completion of a degree in 2008–2009 were 7. The number of students enrolled full- and part-time who were dismissed or voluntarily withdrew from this program area in 2008–2009 were 0. *Developmental Psychology PhD (Doctor of Philosophy)*—Applications 2009–2010, 13. Total applicants accepted 2009–2010, 5. Number full-time enrolled (new admits only) 2009–2010, 5. Number part-time enrolled (new admits only) 2009–2010, 0. Openings 2010–2011, 4. The median number of years required for completion of a degree in 2008–2009 were 4. The number of students enrolled full- and part-time who were dismissed or voluntarily withdrew from this program area in 2008–2009 were 0. *Medical/Clinical Psychology PhD (Doctor of Philosophy)*—Applications 2009–2010, 86. Total applicants accepted 2009–2010, 7. Number full-time enrolled (new admits only) 2009–2010, 6. Number part-time enrolled (new admits only) 2009–2010, 0. Openings 2010–2011, 7. The median number of years required for completion of a degree in 2008–2009 were 6. The number of students enrolled full- and part-time who were dismissed or voluntarily withdrew from this program area in 2008–2009 were 1.

Other Criteria: (importance of criteria rated low, medium, or high): GRE scores—high, research experience—high, work experience—low, extracurricular activity—low, clinically related public service—medium, GPA—high, letters of recommendation—medium, interview—medium, statement of goals and objectives—medium. For additional information on admission requirements, go to http://www.psy.uab.edu.

Student Characteristics: The following represents characteristics of students in 2009–2010 in all graduate psychology programs in the department: Female—full-time 59, part-time 0; Male—full-time 10, part-time 0; African American/Black—full-time 8, part-time 0; Hispanic/Latino(a)—full-time 2, part-time 0; Asian/Pacific Islander—full-time 4, part-time 0; American Indian/Alaska Native—full-time 0, part-time 0; Caucasian/White—full-time 55, part-time 0; Multi-ethnic—full-time 0, part-time 0; students subject to the Americans With Disabilities Act—full-time 1, part-time 0; Unknown ethnicity—full-time 0, part-time 0; International students who hold an F-1 or J-1 Visa—full-time 2, part-time 0.

Financial Information/Assistance:
Tuition for Full-Time Study: Doctoral: State residents: per academic year $8,172, $227 per credit hour; Nonstate residents: per academic year $20,448, $568 per credit hour. Tuition is subject to change.

Financial Assistance:
First-Year Students: Fellowships and scholarships available for first year. Average amount paid per academic year: $16,590. Average number of hours worked per week: 20. Apply by February 1.

Advanced Students: Teaching assistantships available for advanced students. Average amount paid per academic year: $18,500. Average number of hours worked per week: 20. Research assistantships available for advanced students. Average amount paid per academic year: $17,500. Average number of hours worked per week: 20. Traineeships available for advanced students. Average amount paid per academic year: $20,770. Average number of hours worked per week: 20. Fellowships and scholarships available for advanced students. Average amount paid per academic year: $17,500. Average number of hours worked per week: 20.

Additional Information: Of all students currently enrolled full time, 100% benefited from one or more of the listed financial assistance programs.

Internships/Practica: Doctoral Degree (PhD Medical/Clinical Psychology): For those doctoral students for whom a professional internship was required in this program prior to graduation, (5) students applied for an internship in 2008–2009, with (5) students obtaining an internship. Of those students who obtained an internship, (5) were paid internships. Of those students who obtained an internship, (5) students placed in APA/CPA accredited internships, (0) students placed in internships not APA/CPA accredited, but listed with the Association of Psychology Postdoctoral and Internship Programs (APPIC), (0) students placed in internships conforming to guidelines of the Council of Directors of School Psychology Programs (CDSPP), (0) students placed in internships that were not APA/CPA accredited, APPIC or CDSPP listed. Students in the Medical/Clinical Psychology program have opportunities for clinical/research practica at multiple sites across the UAB campus as well as off-campus sites, including Departments of Psychology, Anesthesiology, Neurology, Pediatrics, Psychiatry, Rehabilitation Medicine, Center for Aging, Sparks Center for Developmental and Learning Disorders, VA Medical Center, Hill Crest Hospital, and several private practices.

Housing and Day Care: On-campus housing is available. On-campus day care facilities are available.

Employment of Department Graduates:
Master's Degree Graduates: Of those who graduated in the academic year 2008–2009, the following categories and numbers represent the postgraduate activities and employment of master's degree graduates: Enrolled in a postdoctoral residency/fellowship (n/a), employed in independent practice (n/a), total from the above (master's) (0).
Doctoral Degree Graduates: Of those who graduated in the academic year 2008–2009, the following categories and numbers represent the postgraduate activities and employment of doctoral degree graduates: Enrolled in a psychology doctoral program (n/a), enrolled in a postdoctoral residency/fellowship (3), employed in a hospital/medical center (1), total from the above (doctoral) (4).

Additional Information:
Orientation, Objectives, and Emphasis of Department: The Department offers three doctoral programs: Clinical/Medical Psychology, Behavioral Neuroscience, and Developmental Psychology. Each program promotes rigorous scientific training for students pursuing basic or applied research careers. The programs are designed to produce scholars who will engage in independent research, practice, and teaching. Medical Psychology is a specialty within clinical psychology that focuses on psychological factors in health care. It is cosponsored by the UAB School of Medicine. The Behavioral Neuroscience program provides individualized, interdisciplinary training for research on the biological bases of behavior. The Developmental program trains students to conduct research to discover and apply basic principles of developmental psychology across the lifespan in an interdisciplinary context. Students are exposed to the issues of development in its natural and social contexts, as well as in laboratories. Faculty research interests include: health psychology, substance abuse, clinical neuropsychology, psychopharmacology, human psychophysiology, brain imaging, sensation and perception, spinal cord injury, control of movement, aging, mental retardation/developmental disabilities, motivation, pediatric psychology, social ecology, cognitive development, developmental psychopathology, psychosocial influences on cancer, pain, and clinical outcomes evaluation.

Special Facilities or Resources: The University of Alabama at Birmingham is a comprehensive, urban research university, recently ranked by U.S. News and World Report as the number one up-and-coming university in the country. The UAB Psychology Department, in the College of Arts and Sciences, ranks among the top 100 psychology departments in the U.S. by NSF in federal/research funding and the Clinical Psychology doctoral program was recognized as 10th in the nation for scholarly productivity. The UAB campus encompasses a 75-block area on Birmingham's Southside, offering all of the advantages of a university within a highly supportive city. Resources are available from the School of Medicine, Department of Physiological Optics, School of Public Health, Civitan International Research Center, Sparks Center for Developmental and Learning Disorders, Center for Aging, Department of Pediatrics, Department of Psychiatry and Behavioral Neurobiology, Neurobiology Research Center, School of Education, School of Nursing, Department of Computer and Information Sciences, Department of Biocommunications, University Hospital, a psychiatric hospital, and Children's Hospital. The Department boasts two faculty at the rank of University Professor as recognized by The University of Alabama Board of Trustees.

Application Information:
Send to The Graduate School, University of Alabama at Birmingham, Birmingham, AL 35294. Application available online. URL of online application: http://main.uab.edu/Sites/gradschool/. Students are admitted in the Fall, application deadline; Medical/Clinical - November 30, BNS - January 15, Developmental - November 30. *Fee:* $35.

Alabama, University of, at Huntsville
Department of Psychology
Liberal Arts
Morton Hall 335, University of Alabama in Huntsville
Huntsville, AL 35899
Telephone: (256) 824-6191
Fax: (256) 824-6949
E-mail: *carpens@email.uah.edu*
Web: *http://www.uah.edu/colleges/liberal/psychology/*

Department Information:
1968. Chairperson: Jeffrey Neuschatz. Number of faculty: total—full-time 6, part-time 1; women—full-time 4, part-time 1; total—minority—full-time 1; women minority—full-time 1.

Programs and Degrees Offered:
Listed in the following order: Program area, degree type (T if terminal Master's), number awarded 7/08–6/09. General Experimental Psychology MA/MS (Master of Arts/Science) (T) 4.

Student Applications/Admissions:
Student Applications
General Experimental Psychology MA/MS (*Master of Arts/Science*)—Applications 2009–2010, 9. Total applicants accepted 2009–2010, 6. Number full-time enrolled (new admits only) 2009–2010, 3. Number part-time enrolled (new admits only) 2009–2010, 3. Total enrolled 2009–2010 full-time, 5, part-time, 6. Openings 2010–2011, 10. The median number of years required for completion of a degree in 2008–2009 were 2. The number of students enrolled full- and part-time who

were dismissed or voluntarily withdrew from this program area in 2008–2009 were 0.

Scores: Entries appear in this order: required test or GPA, minimum score (if required), median score of students entering in 2009–2010. *General Experimental Psychology MA/MS (Master of Arts/Science):* GRE-V no minimum stated, GRE-Q no minimum stated, overall undergraduate GPA 3.25.

Other Criteria: (importance of criteria rated low, medium, or high): GRE scores—high, research experience—high, work experience—low, clinically related public service—low, GPA—high, letters of recommendation—high, interview—low, statement of goals and objectives—high, empirical paper—high, undergraduate major in psychology—low, specific undergraduate psychology courses taken—high.

Student Characteristics: The following represents characteristics of students in 2009–2010 in all graduate psychology programs in the department: Female—full-time 7, part-time 1; Male—full-time 2, part-time 1; African American/Black—full-time 1, part-time 0; Hispanic/Latino(a)—full-time 0, part-time 0; Asian/Pacific Islander—full-time 0, part-time 0; American Indian/Alaska Native—full-time 0, part-time 0; Caucasian/White—full-time 8, part-time 2; Multi-ethnic—full-time 0, part-time 0; students subject to the Americans With Disabilities Act—full-time 0, part-time 0; Unknown ethnicity—full-time 0, part-time 0; International students who hold an F-1 or J-1 Visa—full-time 0, part-time 0.

Financial Information/Assistance:
Tuition for Full-Time Study: *Master's:* State residents: per academic year $5,132, $285 per credit hour; Nonstate residents: per academic year $10,532, $585 per credit hour. Tuition is subject to change.

Financial Assistance:
First-Year Students: Fellowships and scholarships available for first year. Average number of hours worked per week: 0. Apply by June 1.

Advanced Students: Teaching assistantships available for advanced students. Average amount paid per academic year: $8,400. Average number of hours worked per week: 20. Apply by June 1. Research assistantships available for advanced students. Average amount paid per academic year: $8,400. Average number of hours worked per week: 20. Apply by June 1. Traineeships available for advanced students. Average amount paid per academic year: $4,000. Average number of hours worked per week: 10. Apply by June 1. Fellowships and scholarships available for advanced students. Average amount paid per academic year: $4,000. Average number of hours worked per week: 0. Apply by June 1.

Additional Information: Of all students currently enrolled full time, 75% benefited from one or more of the listed financial assistance programs.

Internships/Practica: Internships in academic student advising and in psychological test administration may be available for some students.

Housing and Day Care: On-campus housing is available. On-campus day care facilities are available.

Employment of Department Graduates:
Master's Degree Graduates: Of those who graduated in the academic year 2008–2009, the following categories and numbers represent the postgraduate activities and employment of master's degree graduates: Enrolled in a psychology doctoral program (2), enrolled in a postdoctoral residency/fellowship (n/a), employed in independent practice (n/a), employed in an academic position at a university (1), employed in other positions at a higher education institution (1), total from the above (master's) (4).

Doctoral Degree Graduates: Of those who graduated in the academic year 2008–2009, the following categories and numbers represent the postgraduate activities and employment of doctoral degree graduates: Enrolled in a psychology doctoral program (n/a), total from the above (doctoral) (0).

Additional Information:
Orientation, Objectives, and Emphasis of Department: The content of our program is directed toward the study of psychology as an intellectual and scientific pursuit, as contrasted with training directly applicable to counselor or psychologist licensure and practice. Specialization areas include applied psychology, social/personality, cognitive, developmental and biopsychological psychology. The program is designed for a small number of students who will work in close interaction with individual faculty members and with each other. Although there are a few structured courses that are required of all students, a substantial portion of the student's program focuses on individual readings, research, and a thesis.

Special Facilities or Resources: Access to research facilities at NASA's-Marshall Space Flight Center is available via an existing Space Act Agreement. Students also have access to archives at the National Children's Advocacy Center. Some students work collaboratively with the scientists in the Center for Simulation and Modeling on the UAH campus.

Application Information:
Send to Department Chair, Department of Psychology, Morton Hall 335, University of Alabama in Huntsville, Huntsville, AL 35899. Application available online. URL of online application: http://www.uah.edu/gradschool/. Students are admitted in the Fall, application deadline July 1; Spring, application deadline December 1; Summer, application deadline May 1. *Fee:* $35.

Auburn University
Department of Psychology
College of Liberal Arts
226 Thach Hall
Auburn University, AL 36849-5214
Telephone: (334) 844-4412
Fax: (334) 844-4447
E-mail: *bryangt@auburn.edu*
Web: *http://www.auburn.edu/psychology*

Department Information:
1948. Chairperson: Daniel Svyantek. Number of faculty: total—full-time 25, part-time 2; women—full-time 7, part-time 2; total—minority—full-time 4; women minority—full-time 2.

GRADUATE STUDY IN PSYCHOLOGY

Programs and Degrees Offered:
Listed in the following order: Program area, degree type (T if terminal Master's), number awarded 7/08–6/09. Clinical Psychology PhD (Doctor of Philosophy) 8, Experimental Psychology PhD (Doctor of Philosophy) 3, Industrial/Organizational Psychology PhD (Doctor of Philosophy) 0, ABA in Developmental Disabilities MA/MS (Master of Arts/Science) (T) 16.

APA Accreditation: Clinical PhD (Doctor of Philosophy). Student Outcome Data Website: http://media.cla.auburn.edu/psychology/gs/clinical/full_disclosure.cfm.

Student Applications/Admissions:

Student Applications

Clinical Psychology PhD (Doctor of Philosophy)—Applications 2009–2010, 161. Total applicants accepted 2009–2010, 11. Number full-time enrolled (new admits only) 2009–2010, 7. Number part-time enrolled (new admits only) 2009–2010, 0. Openings 2010–2011, 7. The median number of years required for completion of a degree in 2008–2009 were 6. The number of students enrolled full- and part-time who were dismissed or voluntarily withdrew from this program area in 2008–2009 were 1. *Experimental Psychology PhD (Doctor of Philosophy)*—Applications 2009–2010, 37. Total applicants accepted 2009–2010, 6. Number full-time enrolled (new admits only) 2009–2010, 3. Number part-time enrolled (new admits only) 2009–2010, 0. Openings 2010–2011, 3. The median number of years required for completion of a degree in 2008–2009 were 6. The number of students enrolled full- and part-time who were dismissed or voluntarily withdrew from this program area in 2008–2009 were 0. *Industrial/Organizational Psychology PhD (Doctor of Philosophy)*—Applications 2009–2010, 52. Total applicants accepted 2009–2010, 7. Number full-time enrolled (new admits only) 2009–2010, 3. Number part-time enrolled (new admits only) 2009–2010, 0. Openings 2010–2011, 3. The number of students enrolled full- and part-time who were dismissed or voluntarily withdrew from this program area in 2008–2009 were 0. *ABA in Developmental Disabilities MA/MS (Master of Arts/Science)*—Applications 2009–2010, 50. Total applicants accepted 2009–2010, 13. Number full-time enrolled (new admits only) 2009–2010, 13. Number part-time enrolled (new admits only) 2009–2010, 0. Openings 2010–2011, 14. The median number of years required for completion of a degree in 2008–2009 was 1. The number of students enrolled full- and part-time who were dismissed or voluntarily withdrew from this program area in 2008–2009 were 2.

Scores: Entries appear in this order: required test or GPA, minimum score (if required), median score of students entering in 2009–2010. *Clinical Psychology PhD (Doctor of Philosophy)*: GRE-V no minimum stated, 560, GRE-Q no minimum stated, 600, GRE-Analytical no minimum stated, 4.5, overall undergraduate GPA no minimum stated, 3.8; *Experimental Psychology PhD (Doctor of Philosophy)*: GRE-V no minimum stated, 630, GRE-Q no minimum stated, 620, GRE-Analytical no minimum stated, 5.0, overall undergraduate GPA no minimum stated, 3.8; *Industrial/Organizational Psychology PhD (Doctor of Philosophy)*: GRE-V no minimum stated, 590, GRE-Q no minimum stated, 600, GRE-Analytical no minimum stated, 4, overall undergraduate GPA no minimum stated, 3.8; *ABA in Developmental Disabilities MA/MS (Master of Arts/Science)*: GRE-V no minimum stated, 480, GRE-Q no minimum stated, 610, GRE-Analytical no minimum stated, 4.0, overall undergraduate GPA no minimum stated, 3.7.

Other Criteria: (importance of criteria rated low, medium, or high): GRE scores—medium, research experience—high, work experience—medium, extracurricular activity—low, clinically related public service—medium, GPA—high, letters of recommendation—high, interview—high, statement of goals and objectives—medium. For I/O and EXP programs, clinically related public service has less significance. For additional information on admission requirements, go to http://www.auburn.edu/psychology.

Student Characteristics: The following represents characteristics of students in 2009–2010 in all graduate psychology programs in the department: Female—full-time 77, part-time 0; Male—full-time 40, part-time 0; African American/Black—full-time 8, part-time 0; Hispanic/Latino(a)—full-time 6, part-time 0; Asian/Pacific Islander—full-time 4, part-time 0; American Indian/Alaska Native—full-time 0, part-time 0; Caucasian/White—full-time 97, part-time 0; Multi-ethnic—full-time 2, part-time 0; students subject to the Americans With Disabilities Act—full-time 1, part-time 0; Unknown ethnicity—full-time 0, part-time 0; International students who hold an F-1 or J-1 Visa—full-time 0, part-time 0.

Financial Information/Assistance:

Tuition for Full-Time Study: *Master's:* State residents: per academic year $10,098, $258 per credit hour; Nonstate residents: per academic year $28,818, $774 per credit hour. *Doctoral:* State residents: per academic year $10,098, $258 per credit hour; Nonstate residents: per academic year $28,818, $774 per credit hour. Tuition is subject to change. See the following Web site for updates and changes in tuition costs: http://www.auburn.edu/administration/business_office/finaid/.

Financial Assistance:

First-Year Students: Teaching assistantships available for first year. Average amount paid per academic year: $12,600. Average number of hours worked per week: 13.

Advanced Students: Teaching assistantships available for advanced students. Average number of hours worked per week: 13. Research assistantships available for advanced students. Average amount paid per academic year: $14,600. Average number of hours worked per week: 13.

Additional Information: Of all students currently enrolled full time, 80% benefited from one or more of the listed financial assistance programs.

Internships/Practica: Doctoral Degree (PhD Clinical Psychology): For those doctoral students for whom a professional internship was required in this program prior to graduation, (7) students applied for an internship in 2008–2009, with (6) students obtaining an internship. Of those students who obtained an internship, (6) were paid internships. Of those students who obtained an internship, (6) students placed in APA/CPA accredited internships, (0) students placed in internships not APA/CPA accredited, but listed with the Association of Psychology Postdoctoral and Internship Programs (APPIC), (0) students placed in internships conforming to guidelines of the Council of Directors of School Psychology Programs (CDSPP), (0) students placed in internships that were not APA/CPA accredited, APPIC or CDSPP listed. Master's Degree (MA/MS ABA in Developmental

Disabilities): An internship experience, such as a final research project or "capstone" experience is required of graduates. Current practicum sites that offer assistantships for clinical graduate students are Auburn University Psychological Services Center, Auburn University Student Counseling Services, Mt. Meigs Adolescent Correctional Facility (Mt. Meigs, AL), Lee County Youth Development Center (Opelika, AL), Head Start Program of Lee County (Auburn and Opelika, AL), the Auburn University School of Pharmacy, the Auburn University College of Veterinary Medicine, UAB/Montgomery Internal Medicine/Family Medicine Residency Program (Montgomery, AL) and the Central Alabama Veterans Health Care System. Industrial/organizational psychology students receive paid practicum training at a number of area organizations, including Auburn University's Center for Governmental Services, Auburn University at Montgomery's Center for Business and Economic Development, and the Fort Benning Field Station of the Army Research Institute. I/O students participate in consulting internship work before completing their doctoral work. Experimental students have participated in practica at the Army Research Institute (GA). Students in the Master's Program in Applied Behavior Analysis in Developmental Disabilities participate in an intensive practicum program that involves various sites serving individuals with developmental disabilities, including Opelika City Schools, the Little Tree Preschool, the Learning Tree Tallassee Campus, and Lee Co. Dept. of Human Resources.

Housing and Day Care: On-campus housing is available. See the following Web site for more information: http://www.auburn.edu/housing/. No on-campus day care facilities are available.

Employment of Department Graduates:

Master's Degree Graduates: Of those who graduated in the academic year 2008–2009, the following categories and numbers represent the postgraduate activities and employment of master's degree graduates: Enrolled in a postdoctoral residency/fellowship (n/a), employed in independent practice (n/a), employed in other positions at a higher education institution (1), employed in a professional position in a school system (1), employed in government agency (2), employed in a community mental health/counseling center (12), total from the above (master's) (16).

Doctoral Degree Graduates: Of those who graduated in the academic year 2008–2009, the following categories and numbers represent the postgraduate activities and employment of doctoral degree graduates: Enrolled in a psychology doctoral program (n/a), enrolled in a postdoctoral residency/fellowship (4), employed in independent practice (0), employed in an academic position at a university (4), employed in an academic position at a 2-year/4-year college (1), employed in a community mental health/counseling center (1), employed in a hospital/medical center (1), total from the above (doctoral) (11).

Additional Information:

Orientation, Objectives, and Emphasis of Department: Graduate education in Auburn's psychology program offers training in basic research and in the application of knowledge and theory to societal problems. Faculty are committed to the premise that inquiry, breadth, and respect for the research process and the application of behavioral science knowledge are valued elements in graduate education. Students work closely in laboratories with fellow students and faculty mentors. Students interested in applied work are provided with direct experience and supervision within community agencies and organizations where theory and technique can be practiced and refined. The Clinical Psychology training program applies a scientist–practitioner model that blends an empirical approach to knowledge within an experiential context. The Experimental program provides training opportunities in Cognitive and Behavioral Sciences. Excellent animal and human laboratories are available in a number of settings. The Industrial/Organizational program emphasizes a scientist–practitioner approach in which research is used to improve both organizational effectiveness and the quality of work life of individual employees. The Applied Behavior Analysis in Developmental Disabilities program (Master's) trains students to provide evidence-based behavioral services to individuals with developmental disabilities and prepares students to qualify for certification by the Behavior Analyst Certification Board. This one-year program integrates foundational and specialized coursework with carefully designed practicum experiences.

Special Facilities or Resources: A substantial clinical psychology training grant from the State of Alabama, university teaching assistantships, a wide variety of contracts with community agencies, and faculty research contracts and grants have typically provided all doctoral psychology graduate students with financial support throughout their graduate careers. The department administers a multipurpose psychological services center in a renovated and newly furnished building. Relationships with extra-university agencies and organizations facilitate training in applied research.

Information for Students With Physical Disabilities: See the following Web site for more information: http://www.auburn.edu/academic/disabilities/.

Application Information:
Send to Thane Bryant, Department of Psychology, 226 Thach Hall, Auburn University, AL 36849-5214. Application available online. URL of online application: http://www.auburn.edu/psychology. Students are admitted in the Fall, application deadline December 1. Clinical PhD: December 1; I/O and Experimental PhD: January 15; Master's Concentration in Applied Behavior Analysis in Developmental Disabilities: February 15. *Fee:* $50.

Auburn University
Special Education, Rehabilitation, Counseling/School Psychology
College of Education
2084 Haley Center
Auburn University, AL 36849-5222
Telephone: (334) 844-7676
Fax: (334) 844-7677
E-mail: *pipesrb@auburn.edu*
Web: *http://www.auburn.edu/coun*

Department Information:
1965. Chairperson: Everett D. Martin. Number of faculty: total—full-time 20; women—full-time 12; total—minority—full-time 3; women minority—full-time 3; faculty subject to the Americans With Disabilities Act 1.

GRADUATE STUDY IN PSYCHOLOGY

Programs and Degrees Offered:
Listed in the following order: Program area, degree type (T if terminal Master's), number awarded 7/08–6/09. Counseling Psychology PhD (Doctor of Philosophy) 8.

APA Accreditation: Counseling PhD (Doctor of Philosophy). Student Outcome Data Website: http://education.auburn.edu/academic_departments/serc/academicprograms/counpsych.html.

Student Applications/Admissions:
Student Applications
Counseling Psychology PhD (Doctor of Philosophy)—Applications 2009–2010, 60. Total applicants accepted 2009–2010, 6. Number full-time enrolled (new admits only) 2009–2010, 7. Number part-time enrolled (new admits only) 2009–2010, 0. Openings 2010–2011, 6. The median number of years required for completion of a degree in 2008–2009 were 6. The number of students enrolled full- and part-time who were dismissed or voluntarily withdrew from this program area in 2008–2009 were 0.

Scores: Entries appear in this order: required test or GPA, minimum score (if required), median score of students entering in 2009–2010. *Counseling Psychology PhD (Doctor of Philosophy)*: GRE-V no minimum stated, 570, GRE-Q no minimum stated, 610, GRE-Analytical no minimum stated, overall undergraduate GPA no minimum stated, 3.7, last 2 years GPA no minimum stated, psychology GPA no minimum stated.

Other Criteria: (importance of criteria rated low, medium, or high): GRE scores—medium, research experience—high, work experience—medium, extracurricular activity—low, clinically related public service—medium, GPA—high, letters of recommendation—high, interview—high, statement of goals and objectives—high, clinical experience—medium, undergraduate major in psychology—medium, specific undergraduate psychology courses taken—medium. For additional information on admission requirements, go to http://www.auburn.edu/serc/academicprograms/counpsych.html.

Student Characteristics: The following represents characteristics of students in 2009–2010 in all graduate psychology programs in the department: Female—full-time 25, part-time 0; Male—full-time 7, part-time 0; African American/Black—full-time 7, part-time 0; Hispanic/Latino(a)—full-time 0, part-time 0; Asian/Pacific Islander—full-time 0, part-time 0; American Indian/Alaska Native—full-time 0, part-time 0; Caucasian/White—full-time 24, part-time 0; Multi-ethnic—full-time 1, part-time 0; students subject to the Americans With Disabilities Act—full-time 0, part-time 0; Unknown ethnicity—full-time 0, part-time 0; International students who hold an F-1 or J-1 Visa—full-time 1, part-time 0.

Financial Information/Assistance:
Tuition for Full-Time Study: *Doctoral:* State residents: per academic year $6,240; Nonstate residents: per academic year $18,720. Tuition is subject to change. Additional fees are assessed to students beyond the costs of tuition for the following: Approximately $600/yr. See the following Web site for updates and changes in tuition costs: http://www.auburn.edu/administration/business_office/sfs/.

Financial Assistance:
First-Year Students: Research assistantships available for first year. Average amount paid per academic year: $5,508. Average number of hours worked per week: 10. Apply by April 1. Fellowships and scholarships available for first year. Average amount paid per academic year: $15,000. Average number of hours worked per week: 10.

Advanced Students: Teaching assistantships available for advanced students. Average amount paid per academic year: $5,508. Average number of hours worked per week: 10. Apply by April 1. Research assistantships available for advanced students. Average amount paid per academic year: $5,508. Average number of hours worked per week: 10. Apply by April 1. Traineeships available for advanced students. Average amount paid per academic year: $5,508. Average number of hours worked per week: 12. Apply by April 1. Fellowships and scholarships available for advanced students. Average amount paid per academic year: $5,508. Average number of hours worked per week: 10.

Additional Information: Of all students currently enrolled full time, 100% benefited from one or more of the listed financial assistance programs. Application and information available online at: http://www.auburn.edu/administration/business_office/finaid/.

Internships/Practica: Doctoral Degree (PhD Counseling Psychology): For those doctoral students for whom a professional internship was required in this program prior to graduation, (2) students applied for an internship in 2008–2009, with (2) students obtaining an internship. Of those students who obtained an internship, (2) were paid internships. Of those students who obtained an internship, (2) students placed in APA/CPA accredited internships, (0) students placed in internships not APA/CPA accredited, but listed with the Association of Psychology Postdoctoral and Internship Programs (APPIC), (0) students placed in internships conforming to guidelines of the Council of Directors of School Psychology Programs (CDSPP), (0) students placed in internships that were not APA/CPA accredited, APPIC or CDSPP listed. University counseling centers; community mental health centers; VAs, hospitals, community counseling agencies.

Housing and Day Care: On-campus housing is available. See the following Web site for more information: https://fp.auburn.edu/housing/. No on-campus day care facilities are available.

Employment of Department Graduates:
Master's Degree Graduates: Of those who graduated in the academic year 2008–2009, the following categories and numbers represent the postgraduate activities and employment of master's degree graduates: Enrolled in a postdoctoral residency/fellowship (n/a), employed in independent practice (n/a), total from the above (master's) (0).

Doctoral Degree Graduates: Of those who graduated in the academic year 2008–2009, the following categories and numbers represent the postgraduate activities and employment of doctoral degree graduates: Enrolled in a psychology doctoral program (n/a), employed in other positions at a higher education institution (4), employed in government agency (2), total from the above (doctoral) (6).

Additional Information:
Orientation, Objectives, and Emphasis of Department: The Department offers the PhD in Counseling Psychology with masters and doctoral degrees in several other areas. The department values teaching, research, and outreach that contribute to the missions of the College and University. Further, the department seeks to foster a culture in which individual creativity and scholarship is

reinforced and nurtured. Diversity is considered a core value in all that we do.

Special Facilities or Resources: Interdisciplinary community. University partnership serving underserved, rural minority communities devoted to education, research and service. We also partner with University Student Affairs, Career Services, Housing, and the Athletic Department.

Information for Students With Physical Disabilities: See the following Web site for more information: http://www.auburn.edu/academic/disabilities/.

Application Information:
Send to Counseling Psychology, Special Education, Rehabilitation, Counseling/School Psychology, 2084 Haley Center, Auburn University, AL 36849-5222. Application available online. URL of online application: http://www.grad.auburn.edu/. Students are admitted in the Fall, application deadline December 10. *Fee:* $50.

Jacksonville State University
Department of Psychology
College of Graduate Studies
700 Pelham Road, N.
Jacksonville, AL 36265-1602
Telephone: (256) 782-5402
Fax: (256) 782-5637
E-mail: *pmkerchar@jsu.edu*
Web: *http://www.jsu.edu/psychology/*

Department Information:
1971. Interim Department Head: Ted Klimasewski, PhD. Number of faculty: total—full-time 6; women—full-time 2.

Programs and Degrees Offered:
Listed in the following order: Program area, degree type (T if terminal Master's), number awarded 7/08–6/09. Applied Behavior Analysis MA/MS (Master of Arts/Science) (T) 12.

Student Applications/Admissions:
Student Applications
Applied Behavior Analysis MA/MS (Master of Arts/Science)—Applications 2009–2010, 30. Total applicants accepted 2009–2010, 15. Number full-time enrolled (new admits only) 2009–2010, 11. Number part-time enrolled (new admits only) 2009–2010, 2. Total enrolled 2009–2010 full-time, 19, part-time, 17. Openings 2010–2011, 15. The median number of years required for completion of a degree in 2008–2009 were 2. The number of students enrolled full- and part-time who were dismissed or voluntarily withdrew from this program area in 2008–2009 were 1.
Scores: Entries appear in this order: required test or GPA, minimum score (if required), median score of students entering in 2009–2010. *Applied Behavior Analysis MA/MS (Master of Arts/Science):* GRE-V no minimum stated, GRE-Q no minimum stated, GRE-Analytical no minimum stated, overall undergraduate GPA no minimum stated.
Other Criteria: (importance of criteria rated low, medium, or high): GRE scores—medium, research experience—low, GPA—medium, letters of recommendation—high, statement of goals and objectives—high, undergraduate major in psychology—low, specific undergraduate psychology courses taken—low. For additional information on admission requirements, go to http://www.jsu.edu/psychology/gradfaq.html.

Student Characteristics: The following represents characteristics of students in 2009–2010 in all graduate psychology programs in the department: Female—full-time 14, part-time 13; Male—full-time 5, part-time 4; African American/Black—full-time 3, part-time 4; Hispanic/Latino(a)—full-time 1, part-time 0; Asian/Pacific Islander—full-time 0, part-time 0; American Indian/Alaska Native—full-time 0, part-time 0; Caucasian/White—full-time 12, part-time 11; Multi-ethnic—full-time 1, part-time 0; students subject to the Americans With Disabilities Act—full-time 0, part-time 0; Unknown ethnicity—full-time 2, part-time 2; International students who hold an F-1 or J-1 Visa—full-time 1, part-time 3.

Financial Information/Assistance:
Tuition for Full-Time Study: Master's: State residents: per academic year $4,932, $274 per credit hour; Nonstate residents: per academic year $9,864, $548 per credit hour. Tuition is subject to change. See the following Web site for updates and changes in tuition costs: http://www.jsu.edu/bursar/tuition.html.

Financial Assistance:
First-Year Students: No information provided.
Advanced Students: No information provided.
Additional Information: Of all students currently enrolled full time, 0% benefited from one or more of the listed financial assistance programs.

Internships/Practica: Applied Behavior Analysis Practica are available in a variety of settings in which behavioral principles are used to improve human behavior. Currently, these opportunities include The Little Tree Preschool (a preschool for children with developmental disabilities and their typically developing peers), The Learning Tree (a residential program for individuals with developmental disabilities and challenging behavior), The Bridge (a substance abuse treatment center), Anniston Middle School, and the ExSEL summer skill-building program in the Department of Learning Services. An Instructional Practicum is also available and allows students to gain teaching experience assisting a psychology professor.

Housing and Day Care: On-campus housing is available. See the following Web site for more information: http://www.jsu.edu/housing/index.html. On-campus day care facilities are available. See the following Web site for more information: http://www.jsu.edu/edprof/fcs/cdc.html.

Employment of Department Graduates:
Master's Degree Graduates: Of those who graduated in the academic year 2008–2009, the following categories and numbers represent the postgraduate activities and employment of master's degree graduates: Enrolled in a postdoctoral residency/fellowship (n/a), employed in independent practice (n/a), do not know (12), total from the above (master's) (12).
Doctoral Degree Graduates: Of those who graduated in the academic year 2008–2009, the following categories and numbers represent the postgraduate activities and employment of doctoral

degree graduates: Enrolled in a psychology doctoral program (n/a), total from the above (doctoral) (0).

Additional Information:
Orientation, Objectives, and Emphasis of Department: JSU's master's program in psychology offers instruction and training in the analysis of behavior. Students complete courses in the experimental analysis of behavior and applied behavior analysis. Courses in the experimental analysis of behavior teach students about basic functional relations between environmental events and behavior, whereas courses in applied behavior analysis train students in the application of those basic behavioral principles to human populations. Hands-on experience is available in our animal and human research facilities and local practicum sites. The program has a Behavior Analyst Certified Board (BACB)-approved course sequence.

Special Facilities or Resources: Special facilities include an animal room, a running room with 15 chambers, student offices, and a seminar computer room. A network of control computers (which were developed at JSU and used in many other universities) runs experiments and provides interactive graphical analyses. Students can work under the supervision of Board Certified Behavior Analysts in an inclusive preschool for children with developmental disabilities, a residential/education facility for individuals with developmental disabilities and challenging behavior, a local middle school, and a nearby substance abuse treatment center. The Department of Learning Services works with the Psychology Department to offer students opportunities to apply psychological principles in an instructional setting for incoming college freshmen using precision teaching techniques.

Information for Students With Physical Disabilities: See the following Web site for more information: http://www.jsu.edu/depart/dss/.

Application Information:
Send to Jacksonville State University, College of Graduate Studies, 700 Pelham Road N., Jacksonville, AL 36265-1602. Application available online. URL of online application: http://www.jsu.edu/graduate/grad_app.html. Students are admitted in the Fall, application deadline August 15. *Fee:* $30.

South Alabama, University of
Department of Psychology
Arts and Sciences
LSCB Room 326
Mobile, AL 36688
Telephone: (251) 460-6371
Fax: (251) 460-6320
E-mail: lchriste@usouthal.edu
Web: http://www.southalabama.edu/psychology/

Department Information:
1964. Chairperson: Larry Christensen. Number of faculty: total—full-time 13, part-time 14; women—full-time 5, part-time 6; total—minority—full-time 1, part-time 2; women minority—full-time 1.

Programs and Degrees Offered:
Listed in the following order: Program area, degree type (T if terminal Master's), number awarded 7/08–6/09. Clinical Psychology MA/MS (Master of Arts/Science) (T) 6, Experimental Psychology MA/MS (Master of Arts/Science) (T) 1, Clinical/Counseling Psychology PhD (Doctor of Philosophy) 0.

Student Applications/Admissions:
Student Applications

Clinical Psychology MA/MS (Master of Arts/Science)—Applications 2009–2010, 27. Total applicants accepted 2009–2010, 10. Number full-time enrolled (new admits only) 2009–2010, 5. Openings 2010–2011, 6. The median number of years required for completion of a degree in 2008–2009 were 2. The number of students enrolled full- and part-time who were dismissed or voluntarily withdrew from this program area in 2008–2009 were 0. *Experimental Psychology MA/MS (Master of Arts/Science)*—Applications 2009–2010, 6. Total applicants accepted 2009–2010, 2. Number full-time enrolled (new admits only) 2009–2010, 0. Number part-time enrolled (new admits only) 2009–2010, 0. Openings 2010–2011, 2. The median number of years required for completion of a degree in 2008–2009 were 2. The number of students enrolled full- and part-time who were dismissed or voluntarily withdrew from this program area in 2008–2009 were 0. *Clinical/Counseling Psychology PhD (Doctor of Philosophy)*—Applications 2009–2010, 19. Total applicants accepted 2009–2010, 6. Number full-time enrolled (new admits only) 2009–2010, 6. Number part-time enrolled (new admits only) 2009–2010, 0. Openings 2010–2011, 6. The number of students enrolled full- and part-time who were dismissed or voluntarily withdrew from this program area in 2008–2009 were 0.

Scores: Entries appear in this order: required test or GPA, minimum score (if required), median score of students entering in 2009–2010. *Clinical Psychology MA/MS (Master of Arts/Science)*: GRE-V 500, 500, GRE-Q 500, 590, overall undergraduate GPA 3.11, 3.69; *Experimental Psychology MA/MS (Master of Arts/Science)*: GRE-V 500, 510, GRE-Q 500, 520, overall undergraduate GPA 2.9, 3.27, psychology GPA 3.13, 3.57; *Clinical/Counseling Psychology PhD (Doctor of Philosophy)*: GRE-V 550, 560, GRE-Q 580, 595, GRE-Analytical 4, 4.25, Masters GPA 3.91, 4.0.

Other Criteria: (importance of criteria rated low, medium, or high): GRE scores—high, research experience—medium, work experience—low, extracurricular activity—low, clinically related public service—medium, GPA—high, letters of recommendation—high, interview—high, statement of goals and objectives—medium, undergraduate major in psychology—high, specific undergraduate psychology courses taken—high, Admission to the doctoral program requires a Master's degree in psychology, counseling or related mental health field.

Student Characteristics: The following represents characteristics of students in 2009–2010 in all graduate psychology programs in the department: Female—full-time 19, part-time 0; Male—full-time 7, part-time 0; African American/Black—full-time 1, part-time 0; Hispanic/Latino(a)—full-time 1, part-time 0; Asian/Pacific Islander—part-time 0; American Indian/Alaska Native—full-time 0, part-time 0; Caucasian/White—full-time 24, part-time 0; Multi-ethnic—full-time 0, part-time 0; students subject to the Americans With Disabilities Act—full-time 0, part-time

0; Unknown ethnicity—full-time 0, part-time 0; International students who hold an F-1 or J-1 Visa—full-time 0, part-time 0.

Financial Information/Assistance:
Tuition for Full-Time Study: *Master's:* State residents: $218 per credit hour; Nonstate residents: $460 per credit hour. *Doctoral:* State residents: $218 per credit hour; Nonstate residents: $460 per credit hour. Tuition is subject to change. Additional fees are assessed to students beyond the costs of tuition for the following: Registration, student health, building, library, activity/athletic fee. See the following Web site for updates and changes in tuition costs: http://www.southalabama.edu/studentaccounting/tuition.html.

Financial Assistance:
First-Year Students: Research assistantships available for first year. Average amount paid per academic year: $9,000. Average number of hours worked per week: 20. Apply by February 15.

Advanced Students: Teaching assistantships available for advanced students. Average amount paid per academic year: $11,000. Average number of hours worked per week: 20. Apply by February 15. Research assistantships available for advanced students. Average amount paid per academic year: $11,000. Average number of hours worked per week: 20. Apply by February 15.

Additional Information: Of all students currently enrolled full time, 75% benefited from one or more of the listed financial assistance programs. Application and information available online at: http://www.southalabama.edu/psychology/index.html.

Internships/Practica: Doctoral Degree (PhD Clinical/Counseling Psychology): For those doctoral students for whom a professional internship was required in this program prior to graduation, (0) students applied for an internship in 2008–2009, with (0) students obtaining an internship. Of those students who obtained an internship, (0) were paid internships. Of those students who obtained an internship, (0) students placed in APA/CPA accredited internships, (0) students placed in internships not APA/CPA accredited, but listed with the Association of Psychology Postdoctoral and Internship Programs (APPIC), (0) students placed in internships conforming to guidelines of the Council of Directors of School Psychology Programs (CDSPP), (0) students placed in internships that were not APA/CPA accredited, APPIC or CDSPP listed. Graduate students receive practical experience in the application of psychological assessment and treatment procedures in a variety of clinical settings. Emphasis is given to ethical and professional issues with intensive individual and group supervision. The Department of Psychology operates an outpatient teaching clinic where a variety of children and adults are seen for short-term assessment and treatment. External practicum placements are also available in a variety of community settings including a state mental hospital, a mental retardation facility and community substance abuse programs.

Housing and Day Care: On-campus housing is available. See the following Web site for more information: http://www.southalabama.edu/housing/. No on-campus day care facilities are available.

Employment of Department Graduates:
Master's Degree Graduates: Of those who graduated in the academic year 2008–2009, the following categories and numbers represent the postgraduate activities and employment of master's degree graduates: Enrolled in a psychology doctoral program (5), enrolled in a postdoctoral residency/fellowship (n/a), employed in independent practice (n/a), employed in government agency (1), employed in a community mental health/counseling center (3), do not know (2), total from the above (master's) (11).

Doctoral Degree Graduates: Of those who graduated in the academic year 2008–2009, the following categories and numbers represent the postgraduate activities and employment of doctoral degree graduates: Enrolled in a psychology doctoral program (n/a), total from the above (doctoral) (0).

Additional Information:
Orientation, Objectives, and Emphasis of Department: The University of South Alabama offers a combined Clinical/Counseling Psychology (CCP) doctoral program of studies integrating the missions and philosophies of clinical and counseling psychology. The CCP program will train students to provide the most effective types of psychological treatment and, upon completion of the program of studies, students will have a set of competencies enabling them to work successfully with a variety of professionals for the purpose of health promotion and treatment of mental illness. Students will be trained in the asset-strength model traditionally associated with counseling psychology and to conduct research and provide treatment for serious psychopathology traditionally associated with clinical psychology. The University of South Alabama also offers a master's program in general psychology that allows the student to choose either an applied or experimental focus. All students complete a core curriculum designed to provide them with knowledge of current theories, principles, and methods of experimental and applied psychology. This is followed by courses in either clinical or experimental areas. The clinical courses are designed to equip students with basic psychological assessment and treatment skills that will enable them to function later in an applied employment setting under supervision of a licensed psychologist. Courses for the experimental student are designed to provide more extensive information in research design and experimental methods as well as theoretical background related to the student's thesis research. Both programs, as well as the core curriculum, are designed to provide students with the necessary theoretical and research background to pursue further graduate study, if they so choose. Graduate students in both areas receive individual attention and close supervision by departmental faculty.

Special Facilities or Resources: The Comparative Hearing Laboratory maintains exceptional sound room, computer, and animal facilities. Through the comparison of human, monkey, gerbil, and computer simulations of perception, the laboratory seeks to study how the brain has become specialized for language, and what has gone wrong with particular classes of communication and learning disorders. In addition to the Psychological Clinic and the Comparative Hearing Laboratory, the Department has laboratory facilities for neuropsychological and behavioral research, and has access to both mainframe and personal computer facilities. An EEG/ERP laboratory exists that is used for conducting research requiring the utilization of a dense array electrode cap. This laboratory is available for both faculty and graduate student research. A family interaction laboratory exists for studying parent-child interactions with the goal of enhancing parenting skills. A cognitive laboratory exists with the capability of studying linguistic enhancement. This laboratory also has an eye-tracking apparatus capable of being integrated into a variety of research projects. A social interaction and a sound attenuation laboratory have recently been constructed to provide a laboratory for research into the dynamics of phenomena such as echolocation and social interactions. A biofeedback laboratory exists for research into the treatment of issues such as headaches.

Information for Students With Physical Disabilities: See the following Web site for more information: http://www.southalabama.edu/dss/.

Application Information:
Send to Director of Admission, Meisler Hall Suite 2500, University of South Alabama, Mobile, AL 36688-0002. URL of online application: http://www.southalabama.edu/psychology/application.html. Students are admitted in the Fall, application deadline February 15. *Fee:* $35.

ALASKA

Alaska, University of, Fairbanks/Anchorage
Department of Psychology/Joint PhD Program in Clinical-Community Psychology
UAF College of Liberal Arts/UAA College of Arts & Sciences
P.O. Box 756480/3211 Providence Drive
Fairbanks, AK 99775
Telephone: (907) 474-7012/786-1640
Fax: (907) 474-5781
E-mail: *anaeh@uaa.alaska.edu*
Web: *http://psyphd.alaska.edu*

Department Information:
1984. Co-Directors of Clinical Training: UAF Dr. William Connor and UAA Dr. Christiane Brems. Number of faculty: total—full-time 9, part-time 7; women—full-time 4, part-time 5; total—minority—full-time 2; women minority—full-time 1.

Programs and Degrees Offered:
Listed in the following order: Program area, degree type (T if terminal Master's), number awarded 7/08–6/09. Clinical-Community Psychology PhD (Doctor of Philosophy) 0.

Student Applications/Admissions:
Student Applications
Clinical-Community Psychology PhD (Doctor of Philosophy)—Applications 2009–2010, 50. Total applicants accepted 2009–2010, 8. Number full-time enrolled (new admits only) 2009–2010, 8. Number part-time enrolled (new admits only) 2009–2010, 0. Total enrolled 2009–2010 full-time, 28, part-time, 1. Openings 2010–2011, 8. The number of students enrolled full- and part-time who were dismissed or voluntarily withdrew from this program area in 2008–2009 were 1.
Scores: Entries appear in this order: required test or GPA, minimum score (if required), median score of students entering in 2009–2010. Clinical-Community Psychology PhD (Doctor of Philosophy): overall undergraduate GPA 3.0.
Other Criteria: (importance of criteria rated low, medium, or high): GRE scores—low, research experience—medium, work experience—medium, extracurricular activity—medium, clinically related public service—medium, GPA—medium, letters of recommendation—high, interview—high, statement of goals and objectives—high, rural/indigenous interest—medium, undergraduate major in psychology—low, specific undergraduate psychology courses taken—high. For additional information on admission requirements, go to http://psyphd.alaska.edu.

Student Characteristics: The following represents characteristics of students in 2009–2010 in all graduate psychology programs in the department: Female—full-time 20, part-time 1; Male—full-time 8, part-time 0; African American/Black—full-time 1, part-time 0; Hispanic/Latino(a)—full-time 3, part-time 0; Asian/Pacific Islander—full-time 2, part-time 0; American Indian/Alaska Native—full-time 5, part-time 0; Caucasian/White—full-time 15, part-time 1; Multi-ethnic—full-time 2, part-time 0; students subject to the Americans With Disabilities Act—full-time 0, part-time 0; Unknown ethnicity—full-time 0, part-time 0; International students who hold an F-1 or J-1 Visa—full-time 0, part-time 0.

Financial Information/Assistance:
Tuition for Full-Time Study: *Doctoral:* State residents: $316 per credit hour; Nonstate residents: $646 per credit hour. Tuition is subject to change. See the following Web site for updates and changes in tuition costs: http://www.uaf.edu/uaf/costs/.

Financial Assistance:
First-Year Students: Teaching assistantships available for first year. Average amount paid per academic year: $26,322. Average number of hours worked per week: 20. Apply by February 1. Research assistantships available for first year. Average amount paid per academic year: $26,322. Average number of hours worked per week: 20. Apply by February 1.
Advanced Students: Teaching assistantships available for advanced students. Average amount paid per academic year: $28,900. Average number of hours worked per week: 20. Apply by February 1. Research assistantships available for advanced students. Average amount paid per academic year: $28,900. Average number of hours worked per week: 20. Apply by February 1.
Additional Information: Of all students currently enrolled full time, 100% benefited from one or more of the listed financial assistance programs. Application and information available online at: http://psyphd.alaska.edu.

Internships/Practica: Doctoral Degree (PhD Clinical-Community Psychology): For those doctoral students for whom a professional internship was required in this program prior to graduation, (2) students applied for an internship in 2008–2009, with (2) students obtaining an internship. Of those students who obtained an internship, (2) were paid internships. Of those students who obtained an internship, (1) students placed in APA/CPA accredited internships, (0) students placed in internships not APA/CPA accredited, but listed with the Association of Psychology Postdoctoral and Internship Programs (APPIC), (0) students placed in internships conforming to guidelines of the Council of Directors of School Psychology Programs (CDSPP), (1) students placed in internships that were not APA/CPA accredited, APPIC or CDSPP listed. Both campuses provide clinical practica through on-campus clinics and placements in local behavioral health centers. Community practica in a variety of community settings are also provided to all students. Internship placements in Alaska will also be available to students.

Housing and Day Care: On-campus housing is available. See the following Web site for more information: UAA on-campus housing: http://www.uaa.alaska.edu/housing/ UAF on-campus housing: http://www.uaf.edu/reslife/. On-campus day care facilities are available. See the following Web site for more information: UAA child care center: http://www.tanainachildren.org/ UAF child care center: http://www.tvc.uaf.edu/programs/Bunnell House/.

Employment of Department Graduates:
Master's Degree Graduates: Of those who graduated in the academic year 2008–2009, the following categories and numbers

represent the postgraduate activities and employment of master's degree graduates: Enrolled in a postdoctoral residency/fellowship (n/a), employed in independent practice (n/a), total from the above (master's) (0).

Doctoral Degree Graduates: Of those who graduated in the academic year 2008–2009, the following categories and numbers represent the postgraduate activities and employment of doctoral degree graduates: Enrolled in a psychology doctoral program (n/a), total from the above (doctoral) (0).

Additional Information:
Orientation, Objectives, and Emphasis of Department: The PhD Program in Clinical-Community Psychology is a program jointly delivered and administered by the Departments of Psychology at the University of Alaska Fairbanks and the University of Alaska Anchorage. All program courses are co-taught across campuses via video conference and all program components are delivered by faculty at both campuses. The student experience is identical regardless of students' city of residence (Fairbanks or Anchorage). The PhD Program integrates clinical and community psychology and focuses on rural, indigenous, and cultural psychology with an applied emphasis. The program uniquely combines the spirit of clinical and community psychology. As such, it places strong emphasis on non-traditional service delivery and social action, as well as clinical service delivery to individuals, groups, families, and communities. The program is on the forefront of creative and enriching knowledge dissemination that is locally relevant; focused on public service; sensitive to the unique environments of Alaska; and concerned with acknowledging, fostering, and celebrating diversity. The program has many unique features that combine to make for a rigorous training experience that requires a student's full-time commitment. Prior to admission, students must submit a disclosure statement and a criminal background check. The disclosure statement is located by clicking on the Disclosure Form link at this site: http://psyphd.alaska.edu/app-procedures.htm.

Special Facilities or Resources: In Fairbanks, the program is housed in the Gruening Building on the UAF campus, a seven-story structure complete in 1970. Facilities available to graduate students include two high definition video classrooms, individual study areas, and a newly renovated clinic with individual therapy rooms, a family/group therapy room, a child therapy room, and a telehealth therapy room. Other facilities available to graduate students include a departmental lab and several university labs with PCs and Macs. UAF is an international center for research in the Arctic and the North. At UAA, the academic facilities available to graduate students include two high definition video classrooms, individual study areas, clinical space in the Psychological Service Center, consisting of individual, family/group, child, and telehealth therapy rooms, and the Consortium Library, the major research library for southcentral Alaska. Research facilities available to graduate students include the Center for Behavioral Health Research and Services, a departmental laboratory and several university computer labs with PCs and Macs.

Information for Students With Physical Disabilities: See the following Web site for more information: http://www.uaa.alaska.edu/dss/ and http://www.uaf.edu/chc/disabilityr.html.

Application Information:
Send to William Connor, UAF Co-Director of Clinical Training, University of Alaska Fairbanks, P.O. Box 756480, Fairbanks, AK 99775-6480; Christiane Brems, UAA Co-Director of Clinical Training, University of Alaska Anchorage, 3211 Providence Drive, Anchorage, AK 99508. Application available online. URL of online application: http://psyphd.alaska.edu/admissions.htm. Students are admitted in the Fall, application deadline February 1. *Fee:* $120.

ARIZONA

Arizona State University (2009 data)
Applied Psychology
College of Technology and Innovation
Santa Catalina Hall, 7291 East Sonoran Arroyo Mall
Mesa, AZ 85212
Telephone: (480) 727-1177
Fax: (480) 727-1538
E-mail: vaughn.becker@asu.edu
Web: http://poly.asu.edu/saas/appliedpsych/

Department Information:
2000. Chairperson: Rob Gray. Number of faculty: total—full-time 6, part-time 4; women—full-time 1, part-time 3; total—minority—full-time 1.

Programs and Degrees Offered:
Listed in the following order: Program area, degree type (T if terminal Master's), number awarded 7/08–6/09. Applied Psychology MA/MS (Master of Arts/Science) (T) 6.

Student Applications/Admissions:
Student Applications
Applied Psychology MA/MS (Master of Arts/Science)—Applications 2009–2010, 16. Total applicants accepted 2009–2010, 7. Number full-time enrolled (new admits only) 2009–2010, 5. Number part-time enrolled (new admits only) 2009–2010, 0. Openings 2010–2011, 5. The median number of years required for completion of a degree in 2008–2009 were 2. The number of students enrolled full- and part-time who were dismissed or voluntarily withdrew from this program area in 2008–2009 were 0.
Other Criteria: (importance of criteria rated low, medium, or high): GRE scores—high, research experience—high, work experience—medium, extracurricular activity—low, GPA—high, letters of recommendation—medium, interview—low, statement of goals and objectives—high.

Student Characteristics: The following represents characteristics of students in 2009–2010 in all graduate psychology programs in the department: Female—full-time 0, part-time 0; Male—full-time 0, part-time 0; African American/Black—full-time 0, part-time 0; Hispanic/Latino(a)—full-time 0, part-time 0; Asian/Pacific Islander—full-time 0, part-time 0; American Indian/Alaska Native—full-time 0, part-time 0; Caucasian/White—full-time 0, part-time 0; Multi-ethnic—full-time 0, part-time 0; students subject to the Americans With Disabilities Act—full-time 0, part-time 0; Unknown ethnicity—full-time 0, part-time 0; International students who hold an F-1 or J-1 Visa—full-time 0, part-time 0.

Financial Information/Assistance:
Tuition for Full-Time Study: *Master's:* State residents: per academic year $6,028, $335 per credit hour; Nonstate residents: per academic year $16,074, $713 per credit hour. Tuition is subject to change. See the following Web site for updates and changes in tuition costs: http://www.asu.edu/sbs/fees.html.

Financial Assistance:
First-Year Students: Research assistantships available for first year. Average amount paid per academic year: $16,000. Average number of hours worked per week: 20.
Advanced Students: Research assistantships available for advanced students. Average amount paid per academic year: $17,000.
Additional Information: Of all students currently enrolled full time, 100% benefited from one or more of the listed financial assistance programs.

Internships/Practica: Master's Degree (MA/MS Applied Psychology): An internship experience, such as a final research project or "capstone" experience is required of graduates. Students currently work on projects at the Air Force Research Laboratory, at Boeing, at Intel, and at Motorola. Other opportunities are continually being sought as the program develops.

Housing and Day Care: On-campus housing is available. See the following Web site for more information: http://www.poly.asu.edu/housing/. On-campus day care facilities are available.

Employment of Department Graduates:
Master's Degree Graduates: Of those who graduated in the academic year 2008–2009, the following categories and numbers represent the postgraduate activities and employment of master's degree graduates: Enrolled in a psychology doctoral program (2), enrolled in a postdoctoral residency/fellowship (n/a), employed in independent practice (n/a), employed in business or industry (4), employed in government agency (2), total from the above (master's) (8).
Doctoral Degree Graduates: Of those who graduated in the academic year 2008–2009, the following categories and numbers represent the postgraduate activities and employment of doctoral degree graduates: Enrolled in a psychology doctoral program (n/a), total from the above (doctoral) (0).

Additional Information:
Orientation, Objectives, and Emphasis of Department: The Applied Psychology Department has adopted a strong research emphasis as a major goal in addition to providing a first-rate education for both graduate and undergraduate students. Research in the unit is motivated by applied issues, but our goal is to seek answers to fundamental issues within the applied framework. Some research appears in the best journals publishing basic empirical and theoretical research. Other projects will find more appropriate audiences in the best applied journals. Students studying for the MS degree are prepared both for further graduate study and for employment in government and industry.

Special Facilities or Resources: Excellent research facilities in a newly completed laboratory building, including a driving simulator, an eyetracker, 4-channel psychophysiological recording equipment, sports simulations with motion tracking, and state of the art computing resources. The affiliated Cognitve Engineering Research Institute, under the direction of faculty member Nancy Cooke, houses two Synthetic Task Environments (STE) for studying team cognition, in the context of Uninhabited Air Vehicle (UAV) Ground Control operations and collaborative planning.

Application Information:
Send to Admissions Secretary. Application available online. URL of online application: http://www.asu.edu/graduate. Students are admitted in the Fall, application deadline January 31; Spring, application deadline September 15. *Fee:* $50.

Arizona State University
Department of Psychology
College of Liberal Arts and Sciences
Box 871104
Tempe, AZ 85287-1104
Telephone: (480) 965-7598
Fax: (480) 965-8544
E-mail: *laurie.chassin@asu.edu*
Web: *http://www.asu.edu/clas/psych*

Department Information:
1932. Chairperson: Keith Crnic. Number of faculty: total—full-time 46; women—full-time 16; total—minority—full-time 9; women minority—full-time 4; faculty subject to the Americans With Disabilities Act 1.

Programs and Degrees Offered:
Listed in the following order: Program area, degree type (T if terminal Master's), number awarded 7/08–6/09. Clinical Psychology PhD (Doctor of Philosophy) 4, Developmental Psychology PhD (Doctor of Philosophy) 5, Quantitative Psychology PhD (Doctor of Philosophy) 2, Social Psychology PhD (Doctor of Philosophy) 1, Behavioral Neuroscience PhD (Doctor of Philosophy) 2, Cognition and Behavior PhD (Doctor of Philosophy) 3, Law/Psychology PhD (Doctor of Philosophy) 0.

APA Accreditation: Clinical PhD (Doctor of Philosophy). Student Outcome Data Website: http://psychology.clas.asu.edu/graduate/clinical/disclosuredata.

Student Applications/Admissions:
Student Applications
Clinical Psychology PhD (Doctor of Philosophy)—Applications 2009–2010, 163. Total applicants accepted 2009–2010, 13. Number full-time enrolled (new admits only) 2009–2010, 6. Openings 2010–2011, 8. The median number of years required for completion of a degree in 2008–2009 were 6. The number of students enrolled full- and part-time who were dismissed or voluntarily withdrew from this program area in 2008–2009 were 0. *Developmental Psychology PhD (Doctor of Philosophy)*—Applications 2009–2010, 37. Total applicants accepted 2009–2010, 4. Number full-time enrolled (new admits only) 2009–2010, 2. Number part-time enrolled (new admits only) 2009–2010, 0. Openings 2010–2011, 4. The median number of years required for completion of a degree in 2008–2009 were 6. The number of students enrolled full- and part-time who were dismissed or voluntarily withdrew from this program area in 2008–2009 were 0. *Quantitative Psychology PhD (Doctor of Philosophy)*—Applications 2009–2010, 39. Total applicants accepted 2009–2010, 3. Number full-time enrolled (new admits only) 2009–2010, 1. Number part-time enrolled (new admits only) 2009–2010, 0. Openings 2010–2011, 4. The median number of years required for completion of a degree in 2008–2009 were 6. The number of students enrolled full- and part-time who were dismissed or voluntarily withdrew from this program area in 2008–2009 were 0. *Social Psychology PhD (Doctor of Philosophy)*—Applications 2009–2010, 107. Total applicants accepted 2009–2010, 7. Number full-time enrolled (new admits only) 2009–2010, 4. Number part-time enrolled (new admits only) 2009–2010, 0. Openings 2010–2011, 5. The median number of years required for completion of a degree in 2008–2009 were 7. The number of students enrolled full- and part-time who were dismissed or voluntarily withdrew from this program area in 2008–2009 were 0. *Behavioral Neuroscience PhD (Doctor of Philosophy)*—Applications 2009–2010, 43. Total applicants accepted 2009–2010, 6. Number full-time enrolled (new admits only) 2009–2010, 3. Total enrolled 2009–2010 full-time, 15. Openings 2010–2011, 4. The median number of years required for completion of a degree in 2008–2009 were 8. The number of students enrolled full- and part-time who were dismissed or voluntarily withdrew from this program area in 2008–2009 were 0. *Cognition and Behavior PhD (Doctor of Philosophy)*—Applications 2009–2010, 17. Total applicants accepted 2009–2010, 4. Number full-time enrolled (new admits only) 2009–2010, 2. Total enrolled 2009–2010 full-time, 16. Openings 2010–2011, 4. The median number of years required for completion of a degree in 2008–2009 were 6. The number of students enrolled full- and part-time who were dismissed or voluntarily withdrew from this program area in 2008–2009 were 3. *Law/Psychology PhD (Doctor of Philosophy)*—Applications 2009–2010, 19. Total applicants accepted 2009–2010, 2. Number full-time enrolled (new admits only) 2009–2010, 1. Total enrolled 2009–2010 full-time, 1. Openings 2010–2011, 1. The number of students enrolled full- and part-time who were dismissed or voluntarily withdrew from this program area in 2008–2009 were 0.

Other Criteria: (importance of criteria rated low, medium, or high): GRE scores—medium, research experience—high, work experience—low, extracurricular activity—low, clinically related public service—medium, GPA—medium, letters of recommendation—high, interview—high, statement of goals and objectives—high. For additional information on admission requirements, go to http://www.asu.edu/clas/psych/.

Student Characteristics: The following represents characteristics of students in 2009–2010 in all graduate psychology programs in the department: Female—full-time 86, part-time 0; Male—full-time 39, part-time 0; African American/Black—full-time 1, part-time 0; Hispanic/Latino(a)—full-time 14, part-time 0; Asian/Pacific Islander—full-time 12, part-time 0; American Indian/Alaska Native—part-time 0; Caucasian/White—full-time 98, part-time 0; Multi-ethnic—full-time 0, part-time 0; students subject to the Americans With Disabilities Act—full-time 0, part-time 0; Unknown ethnicity—full-time 0, part-time 0; International students who hold an F-1 or J-1 Visa—full-time 10, part-time 0.

Financial Information/Assistance:
Tuition for Full-Time Study: Doctoral: State residents: per academic year $7,976, $509 per credit hour; Nonstate residents: per academic year $21,370, $847 per credit hour. Tuition is subject to change. See the following Web site for updates and changes in tuition costs: http://students/asu.edu/tuitionandbilling.

Financial Assistance:
First-Year Students: Teaching assistantships available for first year. Average amount paid per academic year: $14,300. Average number of hours worked per week: 20. Research assistantships available for first year. Average amount paid per academic year: $14,300. Average number of hours worked per week: 20. Fellowships and scholarships available for first year.
Advanced Students: Teaching assistantships available for advanced students. Average amount paid per academic year: $15,300. Average number of hours worked per week: 20. Research assistantships available for advanced students. Average amount paid per academic year: $15,300. Average number of hours worked per week: 20. Traineeships available for advanced students. Fellowships and scholarships available for advanced students.
Additional Information: Of all students currently enrolled full time, 100% benefited from one or more of the listed financial assistance programs.

Internships/Practica: Doctoral Degree (PhD Clinical Psychology): For those doctoral students for whom a professional internship was required in this program prior to graduation, (10) students applied for an internship in 2008–2009, with (10) students obtaining an internship. Of those students who obtained an internship, (10) were paid internships. Of those students who obtained an internship, (10) students placed in APA/CPA accredited internships, (0) students placed in internships not APA/CPA accredited, but listed with the Association of Psychology Postdoctoral and Internship Programs (APPIC), (0) students placed in internships conforming to guidelines of the Council of Directors of School Psychology Programs (CDSPP), (0) students placed in internships that were not APA/CPA accredited, APPIC or CDSPP listed. Doctoral clinical students complete practica in community agencies and in our in-house training clinic.

Housing and Day Care: On-campus housing is available. On-campus day care facilities are available.

Employment of Department Graduates:
Master's Degree Graduates: Of those who graduated in the academic year 2008–2009, the following categories and numbers represent the postgraduate activities and employment of master's degree graduates: Enrolled in a postdoctoral residency/fellowship (n/a), employed in independent practice (n/a), total from the above (master's) (0).
Doctoral Degree Graduates: Of those who graduated in the academic year 2008–2009, the following categories and numbers represent the postgraduate activities and employment of doctoral degree graduates: Enrolled in a psychology doctoral program (n/a), employed in an academic position at a university (5), employed in government agency (1), employed in a hospital/medical center (1), total from the above (doctoral) (7).

Additional Information:
Orientation, Objectives, and Emphasis of Department: The department seeks to instill in students knowledge, skills, and an appreciation of psychology as a science and as a profession. To do so, it offers undergraduate and graduate programs emphasizing theory, research, and applied practice. The department encourages a multiplicity of theoretical viewpoints and research interests. The behavioral neuroscience area emphasizes the neural bases of motor disorders, drug abuse and recovery of function following brain damage. The clinical program includes areas of emphasis in health psychology, child-clinical psychology, and community-prevention. Also offered are classes in psychopathology, prevention, assessment and psychotherapy. The cognitive systems area includes cognitive psychology, adaptive systems, learning, sensation and perception, and cognitive development. The developmental area includes coursework and research experience in the core areas of cognitive and social development. The environmental area emphasizes the application of psychological research to environmental and population problems, including architectural design, urban planning, and human ecology. The quantitative area focuses on design, measurement, and statistical analysis issues that arise in diverse areas of psychological research. The social area emphasizes theoretical and laboratory skills combined with program evaluation and applied social psychology. New interdisciplinary training opportunities are in Arts, Media, and Engineering and Law and Psychology

Special Facilities or Resources: The department has the Child Study Laboratory for training and research in developmental psychology, including both normal and clinical groups, particularly of preschool age; the Clinical Psychology Center, whose clients represent a wide range of psychological disorders and are not limited to the university community; and the experimental laboratories, with exceptional computer facilities for the study of speech perception, neural networks, categorization, memory, sensory processes and learning. The clinical and social programs maintain continuing liaisons with a wide range of off-campus agencies for research applications of psychological theory and research. Our NIMH-funded Preventive Intervention Research Center provides a site for training in the design, implementation, and evaluation of preventative interventions. Quantitatively oriented students receive methodological experience in large-scale research programs and in our statistical laboratory.

Application Information:
Send to Admissions Secretary, Department of Psychology, Arizona State University, PO Box 871104, Tempe, AZ 85287-1104. Application available online. URL of online application: http://www.asu.edu/clas/psych. Students are admitted in the Fall, application deadline December 15 for Clinical, January 5 for all other programs. *Fee:* $70. $90 for international students.

Arizona State University (2009 data)
Division of Psychology in Education
Mary Lou Fulton College of Education
Payne Hall 302, P.O. Box 870611
Tempe, AZ 85287-0611
Telephone: (480) 965-3384
Fax: (480) 965-0300
E-mail: *james.klein@asu.edu*
Web: *http://education.asu.edu*

Department Information:
1968. Division Director: James D. Klein. Number of faculty: total—full-time 30, part-time 5; women—full-time 14, part-time 2; total—minority—full-time 6; women minority—full-time 3.

GRADUATE STUDY IN PSYCHOLOGY

Programs and Degrees Offered:
Listed in the following order: Program area, degree type (T if terminal Master's), number awarded 7/08–6/09. Educational Psychology MEd (Education) 11, Educational Psychology: Lifespan Development PhD (Doctor of Philosophy) 3, Educational Technology MEd (Education) 12, School Psychology PhD (Doctor of Philosophy) 3, Educational Technology PhD (Doctor of Philosophy) 3, Educational Psychology: Learning PhD (Doctor of Philosophy) 3, Counseling Psychology PhD (Doctor of Philosophy) 8, Master Of Counseling MA/MS (Master of Arts/Science) (T) 40, Counselor Education MEd (Education) 5, Educational Psychology: Measurement and Statistics PhD (Doctor of Philosophy) 3.

APA Accreditation: School PhD (Doctor of Philosophy). Counseling PhD (Doctor of Philosophy).

Student Applications/Admissions:
Student Applications
Educational Psychology MEd (Education)—Applications 2009–2010, 27. Total applicants accepted 2009–2010, 21. Number full-time enrolled (new admits only) 2009–2010, 7. Number part-time enrolled (new admits only) 2009–2010, 5. Total enrolled 2009–2010 full-time, 13, part-time, 17. Openings 2010–2011, 10. The median number of years required for completion of a degree in 2008–2009 were 2. The number of students enrolled full- and part-time who were dismissed or voluntarily withdrew from this program area in 2008–2009 were 2. *Educational Psychology: Lifespan Development PhD (Doctor of Philosophy)*—Applications 2009–2010, 9. Total applicants accepted 2009–2010, 7. Number full-time enrolled (new admits only) 2009–2010, 2. Number part-time enrolled (new admits only) 2009–2010, 4. Total enrolled 2009–2010 full-time, 5, part-time, 13. Openings 2010–2011, 5. The median number of years required for completion of a degree in 2008–2009 were 4. The number of students enrolled full- and part-time who were dismissed or voluntarily withdrew from this program area in 2008–2009 were 0. *Educational Technology MEd (Education)*—Applications 2009–2010, 60. Total applicants accepted 2009–2010, 46. Number full-time enrolled (new admits only) 2009–2010, 3. Number part-time enrolled (new admits only) 2009–2010, 31. Total enrolled 2009–2010 full-time, 9, part-time, 49. Openings 2010–2011, 25. The median number of years required for completion of a degree in 2008–2009 were 2. The number of students enrolled full- and part-time who were dismissed or voluntarily withdrew from this program area in 2008–2009 were 3. *School Psychology PhD (Doctor of Philosophy)*—Applications 2009–2010, 54. Total applicants accepted 2009–2010, 11. Number full-time enrolled (new admits only) 2009–2010, 8. Number part-time enrolled (new admits only) 2009–2010, 0. Total enrolled 2009–2010 full-time, 29, part-time, 16. Openings 2010–2011, 6. The median number of years required for completion of a degree in 2008–2009 were 5. The number of students enrolled full- and part-time who were dismissed or voluntarily withdrew from this program area in 2008–2009 were 3. *Educational Technology PhD (Doctor of Philosophy)*—Applications 2009–2010, 23. Total applicants accepted 2009–2010, 12. Number full-time enrolled (new admits only) 2009–2010, 11. Number part-time enrolled (new admits only) 2009–2010, 0. Total enrolled 2009–2010 full-time, 17, part-time, 12. Openings 2010–2011, 10. The median number of years required for completion of a degree in 2008–2009 were 4. The number of students enrolled full- and part-time who were dismissed or voluntarily withdrew from this program area in 2008–2009 were 1. *Educational Psychology: Learning PhD (Doctor of Philosophy)*—Applications 2009–2010, 4. Total applicants accepted 2009–2010, 1. Number full-time enrolled (new admits only) 2009–2010, 0. Number part-time enrolled (new admits only) 2009–2010, 0. Total enrolled 2009–2010 full-time, 5, part-time, 9. Openings 2010–2011, 6. The median number of years required for completion of a degree in 2008–2009 were 4. The number of students enrolled full- and part-time who were dismissed or voluntarily withdrew from this program area in 2008–2009 were 0. *Counseling Psychology PhD (Doctor of Philosophy)*—Applications 2009–2010, 119. Total applicants accepted 2009–2010, 9. Number full-time enrolled (new admits only) 2009–2010, 7. Number part-time enrolled (new admits only) 2009–2010, 1. Total enrolled 2009–2010 full-time, 27, part-time, 17. Openings 2010–2011, 9. The median number of years required for completion of a degree in 2008–2009 were 6. The number of students enrolled full- and part-time who were dismissed or voluntarily withdrew from this program area in 2008–2009 were 0. *Master Of Counseling MA/MS (Master of Arts/Science)*—Applications 2009–2010, 120. Total applicants accepted 2009–2010, 77. Number full-time enrolled (new admits only) 2009–2010, 33. Number part-time enrolled (new admits only) 2009–2010, 1. Total enrolled 2009–2010 full-time, 71, part-time, 33. Openings 2010–2011, 40. The median number of years required for completion of a degree in 2008–2009 were 3. The number of students enrolled full- and part-time who were dismissed or voluntarily withdrew from this program area in 2008–2009 were 4. *Counselor Education MEd (Education)*—Applications 2009–2010, 1. Total applicants accepted 2009–2010, 1. Number full-time enrolled (new admits only) 2009–2010, 0. Number part-time enrolled (new admits only) 2009–2010, 1. Total enrolled 2009–2010 full-time, 1, part-time, 1. Openings 2010–2011, 4. The median number of years required for completion of a degree in 2008–2009 were 2. The number of students enrolled full- and part-time who were dismissed or voluntarily withdrew from this program area in 2008–2009 were 0. *Educational Psychology: Measurement and Statistics PhD (Doctor of Philosophy)*—Applications 2009–2010, 12. Total applicants accepted 2009–2010, 4. Number full-time enrolled (new admits only) 2009–2010, 3. Number part-time enrolled (new admits only) 2009–2010, 0. Total enrolled 2009–2010 full-time, 6, part-time, 11. Openings 2010–2011, 6. The median number of years required for completion of a degree in 2008–2009 were 4. The number of students enrolled full- and part-time who were dismissed or voluntarily withdrew from this program area in 2008–2009 were 1.

Other Criteria: (importance of criteria rated low, medium, or high): GRE scores—medium, research experience—high, work experience—medium, extracurricular activity—low, clinically related public service—medium, GPA—medium, letters of recommendation—low, interview—medium, statement of goals and objectives—medium. Programs use the FRK index which combines GRE V+Q with undergraduate GPA. Minimum FRKs are set by faculty admissions committees. For additional information on admission requirements, go to http://education.asu.edu.

Student Characteristics: The following represents characteristics of students in 2009–2010 in all graduate psychology programs in the department: Female—full-time 155, part-time 135; Male—

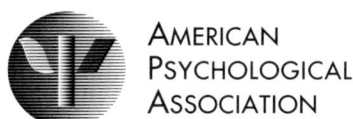

AMERICAN PSYCHOLOGICAL ASSOCIATION

Affiliate Membership Application

Students | High School Teachers | Community College Teachers | International

Please complete the required information below. Return your completed application with payment to:
American Psychological Association, Service Center/Membership, 750 First Street, NE, Washington, DC 20002-4242

Applicant Information

Please print clearly or type.

Name (First/Middle/Last) _____

Contact Address _____

_____

City _____

State/Province/Country _____ Zip/Postal/Country Code _____

Phone (_____) _____ Fax (_____) _____

Add phone (include area/country code), e-mail and school or institution.

▶ E-mail _____

▶ Name of School or Institution _____

▶ ☐ Your contact information will be listed in the APA Membership Directory. If you wish to publish <u>only your name</u> in the directory, please check here.

Membership Category

Please check the affiliate type that best describes you. See reverse side for requirements.

Student: ☐ Graduate $53.00*   Undergraduate ☐ $27.00 or ☐ $53.00*   ☐ High School $27.00
☐ Please check here if you attend a community college
*Includes membership in the American Psychological Association of Graduate Students (APAGS) and a subscription to *gradPSYCH*

Teacher: ☐ High School $40.00   ☐ Community College $40.00

International: ☐ Psychologists residing outside the U.S. or Canada $27.00
Name of the psychological association of the country of which you are a member; or give highest degree in psychology, date, institution and major field of study (required) _____

For Students Only

All U.S. graduate and undergraduate student applicants must complete sections A, B, and C.

A **Licensure/Ethics**
If the graduate degree for which you are currently enrolled is a health service provider subfield (i.e., clinical, child clinical, counseling, school, geropsychology, or health), do you intend to seek licensure/certification by a state or provincial board of psychologist examiners for the independent practice of psychology?
☐ Yes, within the next year   ☐ Yes, eventually   ☐ No
☐ N/A, already licensed for the independent practice of psychology

B Have you at any time been convicted of a felony, sanctioned by any professional ethics body, licensing board, or other regulatory body or by any professional or scientific organization?   ☐ Yes *If yes, please provide an explanation on a separate sheet of paper.*   ☐ No

In submitting this application, I subscribe to and will support the objectives of the American Psychological Association as set forth in Article 1 of the Bylaws, and the Ethical Principles of Psychologists and Code of Conduct, as adopted by the Association, and I affirm that the statements made in this application correctly represent my qualifications for election, and understand that if they do not, my affiliation may be voided.
The Ethical Principles of Psychologists and Code of Conduct is available on APA's Web site at http://www.apa.org/ethics/. The Bylaws are available at http://www.apa.org/about/governance/. Copies of these documents are also available to me upon request.

All students must sign the ethics statement (section C).

C Signature _____   Date _____

Additional Information

The following items are voluntary and are used for research purposes only.

☐ Male   ☐ Female   ☐ Transgender   Date of birth (MM/DD/YY) _____

What is your race/ethnicity? *(U.S. residents, mark all that apply)*
☐ American Indian or Alaska Native   ☐ Hispanic/Latino(a)   ☐ African American/Black
☐ Caucasian/White   ☐ Asian or Pacific Islander   ☐ Other (Specify) _____

Payment Method

Applications will not be processed without payment. All payments must be drawn on a U.S. bank in U.S. dollars.

APA membership is based on the calendar year (January–December).

I am paying my total of $ _____ by:
☐ Check or money order Check # _____ payable to the American Psychological Association
☐ American Express   ☐ MasterCard   ☐ Visa

Account Number _____   Expiration Date _____

Cardholder Name _____

Credit Card Billing Address _____

City/State/ZIP Code/Country _____

Daytime Telephone Number **(include area code)** _____

Signature of Credit Card Holder **(Required)** _____

GS11

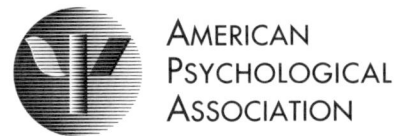

Affiliate Membership Requirements Summary

Student requirements: High school, undergraduate, and graduate students taking psychology courses can become APA student affiliates. Graduate student affiliates are automatically enrolled in the American Psychological Association of Graduate Students (APAGS). Undergraduate affiliates may choose to join APAGS by paying the same rate as graduate students.

Teacher requirements: Teachers of psychology in high schools, junior colleges, and community colleges qualify as APA teacher affiliates. High school teacher affiliates are automatically members of Teachers of Psychology in Secondary Schools (TOPSS), an APA organization. Community college teacher affiliates receive membership in Psychology Teachers at Community Colleges (PT@CC), an APA organization.

Psychologists residing in countries other than the United States or Canada: May become APA international affiliates by providing required documentation indicating membership in your country's national psychology organization or evidence of appropriate qualifications.

Complete membership requirements: Requirements are available from APA's Service Center/Membership (see below for contact information).

Dues: Payment must accompany application. Applications without payment can not be processed. Payment must be made in U.S. dollars, drawn on a U.S. bank. APA affiliate dues (stated on the front of this application) are substantially discounted, over 75% off full member rates.

Membership term: APA membership is based on the calendar year (January–December). If your application is approved in September through December of the current year, your membership (including your subscriptions to the *Monitor on Psychology* and the *American Psychologist*) will automatically be extended to the end of the following year.

Standard inclusions: All APA affiliates receive a subscription to the *Monitor on Psychology* (11 issues*). Undergraduate and graduate students receive a subscription to *American Psychologist* (9 issues*). APAGS members receive a subscription to *gradPSYCH* (4 issues*).

Membership also includes substantial discounts (up to 60%) on various APA publications and electronic products. A detailed list of publications will be sent to you upon acceptance of your application.

Delivery of products and services: Allow 3–4 weeks for the processing of your application and 6–8 weeks for the initial delivery of your APA publications. International orders are sent via surface mail and may take longer.

APA Member and Affiliate Directory: Upon acceptance, your contact information will automatically be included in the official directory, which is a main source of member-to-member communication. To publish <u>only your name</u> in the directory, please check the appropriate box on the front of this application.

For questions or additional information:

Service Center/Membership: (202) 336-5580 or (800) 374-2721 or TDD/TTY: (202) 336-6123; Fax: (202) 336-5568; E-mail: membership@apa.org; Web: http://www.apa.org

Return your completed application to: American Psychological Association, Service Center/Membership, 750 First Street, NE, Washington, DC 20002-4242

*$6.00 of APA dues is allocated towards the *Monitor on Psychology* subscription and $12.00 of APA dues is allocated towards the *American Psychologist* subscription. If you receive *gradPSYCH*, $3.00 of APA dues is allocated towards the subscription.

full-time 57, part-time 44; African American/Black—full-time 10, part-time 4; Hispanic/Latino(a)—full-time 24, part-time 12; Asian/Pacific Islander—full-time 10, part-time 6; American Indian/Alaska Native—full-time 2, part-time 1; Caucasian/White—full-time 166, part-time 156; Multi-ethnic—full-time 0, part-time 0; students subject to the Americans With Disabilities Act—full-time 0, part-time 1; Unknown ethnicity—full-time 0, part-time 0; International students who hold an F-1 or J-1 Visa—full-time 0, part-time 0.

Financial Information/Assistance:
Tuition for Full-Time Study: *Master's:* State residents: per academic year $7,128, $509 per credit hour; Nonstate residents: per academic year $20,322, $847 per credit hour. *Doctoral:* State residents: per academic year $7,128, $509 per credit hour; Nonstate residents: per academic year $20,322, $847 per credit hour. Tuition is subject to change. See the following Web site for updates and changes in tuition costs: http://www.asu.edu/sbs/GraduateFees.html.

Financial Assistance:
First-Year Students: Teaching assistantships available for first year. Average amount paid per academic year: $6,342. Average number of hours worked per week: 10. Apply by April 15. Research assistantships available for first year. Average amount paid per academic year: $6,342. Average number of hours worked per week: 10. Apply by April 15.
Advanced Students: Teaching assistantships available for advanced students. Average amount paid per academic year: $6,342. Average number of hours worked per week: 10. Apply by April 15. Research assistantships available for advanced students. Average amount paid per academic year: $6,342. Average number of hours worked per week: 10. Apply by April 15.
Additional Information: Of all students currently enrolled full time, 26% benefited from one or more of the listed financial assistance programs.

Internships/Practica: Doctoral Degree (PhD School Psychology): For those doctoral students for whom a professional internship was required in this program prior to graduation, (6) students applied for an internship in 2008–2009, with (6) students obtaining an internship. Of those students who obtained an internship, (6) were paid internships. Of those students who obtained an internship, (1) students placed in APA/CPA accredited internships, (1) students placed in internships not APA/CPA accredited, but listed with the Association of Psychology Postdoctoral and Internship Programs (APPIC), (4) students placed in internships conforming to guidelines of the Council of Directors of School Psychology Programs (CDSPP), (0) students placed in internships that were not APA/CPA accredited, APPIC or CDSPP listed. Doctoral Degree (PhD Counseling Psychology): For those doctoral students for whom a professional internship was required in this program prior to graduation, (4) students applied for an internship in 2008–2009, with (4) students obtaining an internship. Of those students who obtained an internship, (4) were paid internships. Of those students who obtained an internship, (4) students placed in APA/CPA accredited internships, (0) students placed in internships not APA/CPA accredited, but listed with the Association of Psychology Postdoctoral and Internship Programs (APPIC), (0) students placed in internships conforming to guidelines of the Council of Directors of School Psychology Programs (CDSPP), (0) students placed in internships that were not APA/CPA accredited, APPIC or CDSPP listed. Our doctoral internships include APA-approved sites throughout the nation. Sites include university counseling centers, community mental health clinics, and hospitals. Practica for doctoral and master's students typically are local (the greater Phoenix area) and include university counseling centers, community mental health clinics, and hospitals.

Housing and Day Care: No on-campus housing is available. No on-campus day care facilities are available.

Employment of Department Graduates:
Master's Degree Graduates: Of those who graduated in the academic year 2008–2009, the following categories and numbers represent the postgraduate activities and employment of master's degree graduates: Enrolled in a postdoctoral residency/fellowship (n/a), employed in independent practice (n/a), total from the above (master's) (0).
Doctoral Degree Graduates: Of those who graduated in the academic year 2008–2009, the following categories and numbers represent the postgraduate activities and employment of doctoral degree graduates: Enrolled in a psychology doctoral program (n/a), total from the above (doctoral) (0).

Additional Information:
Orientation, Objectives, and Emphasis of Department: The Division adheres to a scientist–practitioner model across all areas. The Counseling Psychology and School Psychology doctoral programs are APA accredited. Less than half of the doctoral graduates accept positions in colleges and universities, the remainder function in applied settings.

Special Facilities or Resources: The department staffs and operates a large-scale psychological assessment laboratory, and most students are currently assigned research and study space. Strong research relations exist with local schools, agencies, and private industry. The Counseling Training Center is a training facility for Master's and PhD level counseling students. The center serves clients from both the university and the general public.

Information for Students With Physical Disabilities: See the following Web site for more information: http://www.asu.edu/drc.

Application Information:
Supplemental materials should be sent to: Admissions Secretary, Psychology in Education, Arizona State University, Payne Hall 302, P.O. Box 870611, Tempe, AZ 85287-0611. Application available online. URL of online application: http://www.asu.edu/graduate/admissions. Students are admitted in the Fall, application deadline; Spring, application deadline. Counseling Psychology - December 1; School Psychology- January 1; Master of Counseling - January 15; Educational Psychology, Learning, Lifespan, Measurement, and Educational Technology - February 15 for fall & October 15 for spring. *Fee:* $65. Application fee for international students is $80.

GRADUATE STUDY IN PSYCHOLOGY

Arizona, The University of
Department of Psychology
College of Sciences
P.O. Box 210068
Tucson, AZ 85721
Telephone: (520) 621-7447
Fax: (520) 621-9306
E-mail: *kaszniak@u.arizona.edu*
Web: *http://psychology.arizona.edu/*

Department Information:
1914. Head: Alfred W. Kaszniak. Number of faculty: total—full-time 36, part-time 8; women—full-time 13, part-time 3; total—minority—full-time 3; women minority—full-time 2.

Programs and Degrees Offered:
Listed in the following order: Program area, degree type (T if terminal Master's), number awarded 7/08–6/09. Clinical Psychology PhD (Doctor of Philosophy) 4, Cognition and Neural Systems PhD (Doctor of Philosophy) 1, Ethology and Evolutionary Psychology PhD (Doctor of Philosophy) 0, Psychology, Policy, and Law PhD (Doctor of Philosophy) 0, Social Psychology PhD (Doctor of Philosophy) 1, Undeclared/General PhD (Doctor of Philosophy) 1.

APA Accreditation: Clinical PhD (Doctor of Philosophy). Student Outcome Data Website: http://psychology.arizona.edu/programs/g_each/studentdata.php.

Student Applications/Admissions:
Student Applications
Clinical Psychology PhD (Doctor of Philosophy)—Applications 2009–2010, 180. Total applicants accepted 2009–2010, 5. Number full-time enrolled (new admits only) 2009–2010, 5. Number part-time enrolled (new admits only) 2009–2010, 0. Openings 2010–2011, 7. The median number of years required for completion of a degree in 2008–2009 were 6. The number of students enrolled full- and part-time who were dismissed or voluntarily withdrew from this program area in 2008–2009 were 0. *Cognition and Neural Systems PhD (Doctor of Philosophy)*—Applications 2009–2010, 81. Total applicants accepted 2009–2010, 5. Number full-time enrolled (new admits only) 2009–2010, 5. Openings 2010–2011, 5. The median number of years required for completion of a degree in 2008–2009 were 7. The number of students enrolled full- and part-time who were dismissed or voluntarily withdrew from this program area in 2008–2009 were 0. *Ethology and Evolutionary Psychology PhD (Doctor of Philosophy)*—Applications 2009–2010, 0. Total applicants accepted 2009–2010, 0. Number full-time enrolled (new admits only) 2009–2010, 0. Openings 2010–2011, 2. The number of students enrolled full- and part-time who were dismissed or voluntarily withdrew from this program area in 2008–2009 were 0. *Psychology, Policy, and Law PhD (Doctor of Philosophy)*—Applications 2009–2010, 39. Total applicants accepted 2009–2010, 0. Number full-time enrolled (new admits only) 2009–2010, 0. Number part-time enrolled (new admits only) 2009–2010, 0. Openings 2010–2011, 1. The number of students enrolled full- and part-time who were dismissed or voluntarily withdrew from this program area in 2008–2009 were 0. *Social Psychology PhD (Doctor of Philosophy)*—Applications 2009–2010, 78. Total applicants accepted 2009–2010, 1. Number full-time enrolled (new admits only) 2009–2010, 1. Openings 2010–2011, 1. The median number of years required for completion of a degree in 2008–2009 were 4. The number of students enrolled full- and part-time who were dismissed or voluntarily withdrew from this program area in 2008–2009 were 0. *Undeclared/General PhD (Doctor of Philosophy)*—Applications 2009–2010, 0. Total applicants accepted 2009–2010, 0. Number full-time enrolled (new admits only) 2009–2010, 0. Number part-time enrolled (new admits only) 2009–2010, 0. The median number of years required for completion of a degree in 2008–2009 were 4. The number of students enrolled full- and part-time who were dismissed or voluntarily withdrew from this program area in 2008–2009 were 0.

Scores: Entries appear in this order: required test or GPA, minimum score (if required), median score of students entering in 2009–2010. *Clinical Psychology PhD (Doctor of Philosophy)*: GRE-V no minimum stated, 542, GRE-Q no minimum stated, 684, GRE-Analytical no minimum stated, 4.4, GRE-Subject (Psychology) no minimum stated, 648, overall undergraduate GPA 3.0; *Cognition and Neural Systems PhD (Doctor of Philosophy)*: GRE-V no minimum stated, 533, GRE-Q no minimum stated, 647, GRE-Analytical no minimum stated, 4.3; *Ethology and Evolutionary Psychology PhD (Doctor of Philosophy)*: GRE-V no minimum stated, 595, GRE-Q no minimum stated, 740.

Other Criteria: (importance of criteria rated low, medium, or high): GRE scores—medium, research experience—high, work experience—low, extracurricular activity—low, clinically related public service—low, GPA—medium, letters of recommendation—high, interview—medium, statement of goals and objectives—high, undergraduate major in psychology—medium, specific undergraduate psychology courses taken—medium. For additional information on admission requirements, go to http://psychology.arizona.edu/programs/g_each.php?option=12.

Student Characteristics: The following represents characteristics of students in 2009–2010 in all graduate psychology programs in the department: Female—full-time 60, part-time 0; Male—full-time 34, part-time 0; African American/Black—full-time 1, part-time 0; Hispanic/Latino(a)—full-time 10, part-time 0; Asian/Pacific Islander—full-time 8, part-time 0; American Indian/Alaska Native—full-time 2, part-time 0; Caucasian/White—full-time 59, part-time 0; Multi-ethnic—full-time 0, part-time 0; students subject to the Americans With Disabilities Act—full-time 1, part-time 0; Unknown ethnicity—full-time 14, part-time 0; International students who hold an F-1 or J-1 Visa—full-time 10, part-time 0.

Financial Information/Assistance:
Tuition for Full-Time Study: Doctoral: State residents: $343 per credit hour; Nonstate residents: $839 per credit hour. Tuition is subject to change. Additional fees are assessed to students beyond the costs of tuition for the following: We have a surcharge fee ranging from $55–$483. See the following Web site for updates and changes in tuition costs: http://www.bursar.arizona.edu/students/fees/index.asp.

Financial Assistance:
First-Year Students: Teaching assistantships available for first year. Average amount paid per academic year: $13,710. Aver-

age number of hours worked per week: 20. Research assistantships available for first year. Average amount paid per academic year: $13,710. Average number of hours worked per week: 20. Traineeships available for first year. Average amount paid per academic year: $13,710. Average number of hours worked per week: 20. Fellowships and scholarships available for first year. Average amount paid per academic year: $13,428. Average number of hours worked per week: 10.

Advanced Students: Teaching assistantships available for advanced students. Average amount paid per academic year: $13,710. Average number of hours worked per week: 20. Research assistantships available for advanced students. Average amount paid per academic year: $13,710. Average number of hours worked per week: 20. Traineeships available for advanced students. Average amount paid per academic year: $13,710. Average number of hours worked per week: 20. Fellowships and scholarships available for advanced students. Average amount paid per academic year: $13,428. Average number of hours worked per week: 10.

Additional Information: Of all students currently enrolled full time, 95% benefited from one or more of the listed financial assistance programs. Application and information available online at: http://financialaid.arizona.edu/.

Internships/Practica: Doctoral Degree (PhD Clinical Psychology): For those doctoral students for whom a professional internship was required in this program prior to graduation, (6) students applied for an internship in 2008–2009, with (6) students obtaining an internship. Of those students who obtained an internship, (6) were paid internships. Of those students who obtained an internship, (6) students placed in APA/CPA accredited internships, (0) students placed in internships not APA/CPA accredited, but listed with the Association of Psychology Postdoctoral and Internship Programs (APPIC), (0) students placed in internships conforming to guidelines of the Council of Directors of School Psychology Programs (CDSPP), (0) students placed in internships that were not APA/CPA accredited, APPIC or CDSPP listed. Clinical students are required to do a 1-year internship. UMC medical school does offer internship positions, although most of our students leave campus for the internship. All of the clinical students are placed in APA-accredited internships. There are also various clinical externships and practica available within the department as well as throughout the community.

Housing and Day Care: On-campus housing is available. See the following Web site for more information: http://www.life.arizona.edu/graduate/cl/index.asp. On-campus day care facilities are available. See the following Web site for more information: http://lifework.arizona.edu/cc/.

Employment of Department Graduates:

Master's Degree Graduates: Of those who graduated in the academic year 2008–2009, the following categories and numbers represent the postgraduate activities and employment of master's degree graduates: Enrolled in a postdoctoral residency/fellowship (n/a), employed in independent practice (n/a), total from the above (master's) (0).

Doctoral Degree Graduates: Of those who graduated in the academic year 2008–2009, the following categories and numbers represent the postgraduate activities and employment of doctoral degree graduates: Enrolled in a psychology doctoral program (n/a), enrolled in a postdoctoral residency/fellowship (2), employed in an academic position at a university (2), employed in an academic position at a 2-year/4-year college (0), employed in other positions at a higher education institution (1), employed in government agency (1), employed in a community mental health/counseling center (0), employed in a hospital/medical center (1), other employment position (1), total from the above (doctoral) (8).

Additional Information:

Orientation, Objectives, and Emphasis of Department: Our objectives as a department include contributing to the growth of knowledge about the mind and its workings, and the training of students to participate in this pursuit, as well as using this knowledge to benefit society. The department emphasizes research and training students headed toward both academic and applied careers. Required courses provide breadth of coverage, but emphasis is on research within the area of specialization, relying on independent work with individual faculty members. The interdisciplinary nature of the department fosters specialization in areas that cut across program boundaries and permits work with faculty members in various programs. The cognition and neural systems area emphasizes language, perception, attention, memory, aging, ensemble recording of neural activity, and human neuroimaging; the clinical area emphasizes clinical neuropsychology, psychotherapy research, sleep disorders, psychophysiology, and assessment; the social area emphasizes prejudice and stereotyping, cognitive dissonance, self-esteem, and motivational factors in thought and behavior; the psychology, policy and law area emphasizes the contributions of psychological science to legal and policy decisions; and the ethology and evolutionary area emphasizes quantitative ethology, invertebrate behavior and human behavioral ecology. In addition to these formal programs, the department also offers specialization in evaluation and research methods. The department is the administrative home for the Center for Consciousness Studies, and the Cognition and Neuroimaging Laboratory.

Special Facilities or Resources: The department has modern laboratories devoted to research in various areas of cognitive, clinical, neuroscientific, social, and comparative research. The department employs 5 technicians available for assistance with computers and other equipment. There are a number of clinics within the department, bringing in patients associated with research projects on aging, sleep disorders, memory disorders, depression, and others. The department has ties with a number of other programs on campus, including the departments of Anatomy, Family and Community Medicine, Neurology, Ophthalmology, Pediatrics, Pharmacology, Physiology and Psychiatry in the College of Medicine, and the departments of Ecology and Evolutionary Biology, Family Studies, Linguistics, Management and Policy, Mathematics, Philosophy, Renewable and Natural Resources, Speech and Hearing Sciences, and Physics on the main campus. Ties also exist with various interdisciplinary programs, including Cognitive Science (many of whose laboratories are located in the Psychology Building), Applied Mathematics, and Neuroscience. Most of the department's faculty members are holders of research grants, permitting a significant proportion of the graduate students to serve as research assistants at various times during their training.

Information for Students With Physical Disabilities: See the following Web site for more information: http://drc.arizona.edu/.

Application Information:
Send to The University of Arizona, Department of Psychology, Graduate Admissions, 1503 E University Blvd., Room 312, PO Box 210068,

Tucson, AZ 85721-0068. Application available online. URL of online application: https://sbs.arizona.edu/project/admission/psych/login.php. Students are admitted in the Fall, application deadline December 15. *Fee*: $75.

Midwestern University
Clinical Psychology
College of Health Sciences
19555 North 59th Avenue
Glendale, AZ 85308
Telephone: (623) 572-3860
Fax: (623) 572-3830
E-mail: *phutch@midwestern.edu*
Web: *http://www.midwestern.edu*

Department Information:
2006. Program Director: Philinda Smith Hutchings, PhD, ABPP. Number of faculty: total—full-time 6, part-time 1; women—full-time 4, part-time 1; total—minority—full-time 2, part-time 1; women minority—full-time 1, part-time 1.

Programs and Degrees Offered:
Listed in the following order: Program area, degree type (T if terminal Master's), number awarded 7/08–6/09. Clinical Psychology PsyD (Doctor of Psychology) 0.

Student Applications/Admissions:
Student Applications
Clinical Psychology PsyD (Doctor of Psychology)—Applications 2009–2010, 30. Total applicants accepted 2009–2010, 15. Number full-time enrolled (new admits only) 2009–2010, 11. Number part-time enrolled (new admits only) 2009–2010, 0. Openings 2010–2011, 15. The number of students enrolled full- and part-time who were dismissed or voluntarily withdrew from this program area in 2008–2009 were 0.
Scores: Entries appear in this order: required test or GPA, minimum score (if required), median score of students entering in 2009–2010. *Clinical Psychology PsyD (Doctor of Psychology):* GRE-V no minimum stated, 465, GRE-Q no minimum stated, 490, overall undergraduate GPA 3.0, 3.26.
Other Criteria: (importance of criteria rated low, medium, or high): GRE scores—medium, research experience—low, work experience—medium, extracurricular activity—medium, clinically related public service—high, GPA—high, letters of recommendation—high, interview—high, statement of goals and objectives—high, undergraduate major in psychology—medium, specific undergraduate psychology courses taken—high. For additional information on admission requirements, go to http://www.midwestern.edu/Programs_and_Admission/AZ_Clinical_Psychology.html.

Student Characteristics: The following represents characteristics of students in 2009–2010 in all graduate psychology programs in the department: Female—full-time 17, part-time 0; Male—full-time 6, part-time 0; African American/Black—full-time 1, part-time 0; Hispanic/Latino(a)—full-time 1, part-time 0; Asian/Pacific Islander—full-time 0, part-time 0; American Indian/Alaska Native—full-time 0, part-time 0; Caucasian/White—full-time 19, part-time 0; Multi-ethnic—full-time 2, part-time 0; students subject to the Americans With Disabilities Act—full-time 0, part-time 0; Unknown ethnicity—full-time 0, part-time 0; International students who hold an F-1 or J-1 Visa—full-time 2, part-time 0.

Financial Information/Assistance:
Tuition for Full-Time Study: *Doctoral:* State residents: per academic year $23,662; Nonstate residents: per academic year $23,662. Additional fees are assessed to students beyond the costs of tuition for the following: Student services, disability insurance. See the following Web site for updates and changes in tuition costs: http://www.midwestern.edu/Programs_and_Admission/AZ_Clinical_Psychology.html.

Financial Assistance:
First-Year Students: Fellowships and scholarships available for first year.
Advanced Students: Teaching assistantships available for advanced students. Fellowships and scholarships available for advanced students.
Additional Information: Of all students currently enrolled full time, 4% benefited from one or more of the listed financial assistance programs. Application and information available online at: http://www.midwestern.edu/Programs_and_Admission/Financial_Aid.html.

Internships/Practica: Students begin their clinical experiences with a clerkship in the first year of the program, which exposes them to clinical practice. The specific clinical focus of the experience varies according to the student's needs, interests, and availability of sites. Students complete a minimum of eight quarters of practicum in the second and third years, approximately 16 to 20 hours per week in a clinical setting. The practicum experiences in psychodiagnostics and psychotherapy total a minimum of 1,000 hours over two years. A variety of practicum sites are available, including Midwestern University's Clinic on campus. Internship is completed in the fourth year of the program, and may be completed at any APPIC-member internship site in the U.S. or Canada.

Housing and Day Care: On-campus housing is available. See the following Web site for more information: http://www.midwestern.edu/x731.xml. No on-campus day care facilities are available.

Employment of Department Graduates:
Master's Degree Graduates: Of those who graduated in the academic year 2008–2009, the following categories and numbers represent the postgraduate activities and employment of master's degree graduates: Enrolled in a postdoctoral residency/fellowship (n/a), employed in independent practice (n/a), total from the above (master's) (0).
Doctoral Degree Graduates: Of those who graduated in the academic year 2008–2009, the following categories and numbers represent the postgraduate activities and employment of doctoral degree graduates: Enrolled in a psychology doctoral program (n/a), enrolled in another graduate/professional program (0), enrolled in a postdoctoral residency/fellowship (0), employed in independent practice (0), employed in an academic position at a university (0), employed in an academic position at a 2-year/4-year college (0), employed in other positions at a higher education institution (0), employed in a professional position in a school system (0), employed in business or industry (0), employed in government

agency (0), employed in a community mental health/counseling center (0), employed in a hospital/medical center (0), still seeking employment (0), not seeking employment (0), other employment position (0), do not know (0), total from the above (doctoral) (0).

Additional Information:
Orientation, Objectives, and Emphasis of Department: The clinical psychology program at Midwestern University offers generalist training in clinical psychology, with an emphasis on integrated healthcare, offering psychological services in primary care settings. Midwestern University provides an environment of collaborative training in the healthcare professions, so that as you pursue your studies, you will be surrounded by students of osteopathic medicine, pharmacy, podiatry, physician's assistance, nurse-anesthesia, occupational therapy, cardiovascular science/perfusion, dentistry, physical therapy, optometry and biomedical sciences. The program curriculum includes the foundations of psychological science and emphasizes professional skills in relationship, assessment, intervention, research and evaluation, consultation and education, management and supervision, and diversity. In three years of full-time academic coursework and practicum experiences, and one year of internship, students gain the knowledge, skill, and values to practice clinical psychology in primary care settings, hospitals, outpatient clinics, schools, and private practice. The knowledgeable and dedicated faculty members are accessible and available to students in small classes, seminars, and individually.

Special Facilities or Resources: MWU Clinic provides training for all clinical psychology students in integrated healthcare, consulting and training with medicine, pharmacy, optometry, podiatry, dentistry and other healthcare professions students.

Information for Students With Physical Disabilities: See the following Web site for more information: http://www.midwestern.edu/Glendale_AZ_Campus/Student_Services.html.

Application Information:
Send to Office of Admissions, Midwestern University, 19555 N. 59th Avenue, Glendale, AZ 85308. Application available online. URL of online application: http://www.midwestern.edu/Programs_and_Admission/AZ_Clinical_Psychology/AdmissionApply.html. Students are admitted in the Fall, application deadline August 1; Programs have rolling admissions. *Fee:* $50.

Northcentral University
School of Psychology
10000 East University Drive
Prescott Valley, AZ 86314
Telephone: (888) 327-2877
Fax: (928) 541-7817
E-mail: *hfrederick@ncu.edu*
Web: *http://www.ncu.edu*

Department Information:
1999. Dean: Heather R. Frederick. Number of faculty: total—full-time 4, part-time 78; women—full-time 2, part-time 40; minority—part-time 6; women minority—part-time 12.

Programs and Degrees Offered:
Listed in the following order: Program area, degree type (T if terminal Master's), number awarded 7/08–6/09. Marriage and Family Therapy MA/MS (Master of Arts/Science) 3, Psychology MA/MS (Master of Arts/Science) 59, Marriage and Family Therapy PhD (Doctor of Philosophy) 0, Psychology PhD (Doctor of Philosophy) 33.

Student Applications/Admissions:
Student Applications
Marriage and Family Therapy MA/MS (Master of Arts/Science)—Applications 2009–2010, 65. Total applicants accepted 2009–2010, 57. Number full-time enrolled (new admits only) 2009–2010, 1. Number part-time enrolled (new admits only) 2009–2010, 62. Total enrolled 2009–2010 full-time, 2, part-time, 130. The median number of years required for completion of a degree in 2008–2009 were 2. The number of students enrolled full- and part-time who were dismissed or voluntarily withdrew from this program area in 2008–2009 were 21. *Psychology MA/MS (Master of Arts/Science)*—Applications 2009–2010, 216. Total applicants accepted 2009–2010, 190. Number full-time enrolled (new admits only) 2009–2010, 1. Number part-time enrolled (new admits only) 2009–2010, 166. Total enrolled 2009–2010 full-time, 11, part-time, 528. The median number of years required for completion of a degree in 2008–2009 were 2. The number of students enrolled full- and part-time who were dismissed or voluntarily withdrew from this program area in 2008–2009 were 152. *Marriage and Family Therapy PhD (Doctor of Philosophy)*—Applications 2009–2010, 31. Total applicants accepted 2009–2010, 24. Number full-time enrolled (new admits only) 2009–2010, 0. Number part-time enrolled (new admits only) 2009–2010, 28. The number of students enrolled full- and part-time who were dismissed or voluntarily withdrew from this program area in 2008–2009 were 7. *Psychology PhD (Doctor of Philosophy)*—Applications 2009–2010, 468. Total applicants accepted 2009–2010, 395. Number full-time enrolled (new admits only) 2009–2010, 4. Number part-time enrolled (new admits only) 2009–2010, 382. Total enrolled 2009–2010 full-time, 8, part-time, 1305. The median number of years required for completion of a degree in 2008–2009 were 5. The number of students enrolled full- and part-time who were dismissed or voluntarily withdrew from this program area in 2008–2009 were 251.

Other Criteria: (importance of criteria rated low, medium, or high): research experience—low, work experience—medium, extracurricular activity—low, clinically related public service—medium, GPA—low, letters of recommendation—low, interview—low, statement of goals and objectives—medium.

Student Characteristics: The following represents characteristics of students in 2009–2010 in all graduate psychology programs in the department: Female—full-time 12, part-time 1334; Male—full-time 9, part-time 704; African American/Black—full-time 0, part-time 92; Hispanic/Latino(a)—full-time 0, part-time 36; Asian/Pacific Islander—full-time 0, part-time 19; American Indian/Alaska Native—full-time 0, part-time 17; Caucasian/White—full-time 4, part-time 488; Multi-ethnic—full-time 17, part-time 4; students subject to the Americans With Disabilities Act—full-time 0, part-time 0; Unknown ethnicity—full-time 0, part-time 1382; International students who hold an F-1 or J-1 Visa—full-time 0, part-time 0.

GRADUATE STUDY IN PSYCHOLOGY

Financial Information/Assistance:
Tuition for Full-Time Study: *Master's:* State residents: $560 per credit hour; Nonstate residents: $560 per credit hour. *Doctoral:* State residents: $600 per credit hour; Nonstate residents: $600 per credit hour. Tuition is subject to change. See the following Web site for updates and changes in tuition costs: http://www2.ncu.edu/northcentral-global/tuition.

Financial Assistance:
First-Year Students: No information provided.
Advanced Students: No information provided.
Additional Information: Application and information available online at: http://www.ncu.edu/northcentral-admissions/financing.

Internships/Practica: Learners may enroll in supervised practica.

Housing and Day Care: No on-campus housing is available. No on-campus day care facilities are available.

Employment of Department Graduates:
Master's Degree Graduates: Of those who graduated in the academic year 2008–2009, the following categories and numbers represent the postgraduate activities and employment of master's degree graduates: Enrolled in a postdoctoral residency/fellowship (n/a), employed in independent practice (n/a), total from the above (master's) (0).
Doctoral Degree Graduates: Of those who graduated in the academic year 2008–2009, the following categories and numbers represent the postgraduate activities and employment of doctoral degree graduates: Enrolled in a psychology doctoral program (n/a), total from the above (doctoral) (0).

Additional Information:
Orientation, Objectives, and Emphasis of Department: The department emphasizes applications of psychology. All instruction is carried out via distance learning in which learners and mentors work together in a one-on-one relationship. Learners need to be highly motivated, independent, and conscientious.

Application Information:
Application available online. URL of online application: http://www.ncu.edu/application/. Students are admitted in the Programs have rolling admissions. *Fee:* $50.

Northern Arizona University
Department of Psychology
Social and Behavioral Sciences
NAU Box 15106
Flagstaff, AZ 86011
Telephone: (928) 523-3063
Fax: (928) 523-6777
E-mail: laurie.dickson@nau.edu
Web: http://www.nau.edu/~psych/index.html

Department Information:
1967. Chairperson: K. Laurie Dickson. Number of faculty: total—full-time 19, part-time 6; women—full-time 9, part-time 4; total—minority—full-time 2, part-time 1; women minority—part-time 1.

Programs and Degrees Offered:
Listed in the following order: Program area, degree type (T if terminal Master's), number awarded 7/08–6/09. Clinical Health Psychology MA/MS (Master of Arts/Science) (T) 0, Pre-Doctoral General Psychology MA/MS (Master of Arts/Science) (T) 3, Teaching Of Psychology MA/MS (Master of Arts/Science) (T) 0, Pre-Doctoral Clinical Health Psychology MA/MS (Master of Arts/Science) (T) 0.

Student Applications/Admissions:
Student Applications
Clinical Health Psychology MA/MS (Master of Arts/Science)—Applications 2009–2010, 15. Total applicants accepted 2009–2010, 5. Number full-time enrolled (new admits only) 2009–2010, 2. Total enrolled 2009–2010 full-time, 4. Openings 2010–2011, 2. The number of students enrolled full- and part-time who were dismissed or voluntarily withdrew from this program area in 2008–2009 were 0. *Pre-Doctoral General Psychology MA/MS (Master of Arts/Science)*—Applications 2009–2010, 26. Total applicants accepted 2009–2010, 10. Number full-time enrolled (new admits only) 2009–2010, 7. Total enrolled 2009–2010 full-time, 14. Openings 2010–2011, 8. The median number of years required for completion of a degree in 2008–2009 were 2. The number of students enrolled full- and part-time who were dismissed or voluntarily withdrew from this program area in 2008–2009 were 1. *Teaching Of Psychology MA/MS (Master of Arts/Science)*—Applications 2009–2010, 3. Total applicants accepted 2009–2010, 0. Number full-time enrolled (new admits only) 2009–2010, 0. Openings 2010–2011, 2. The median number of years required for completion of a degree in 2008–2009 were 2. The number of students enrolled full- and part-time who were dismissed or voluntarily withdrew from this program area in 2008–2009 were 0. *Pre-Doctoral Clinical Health Psychology MA/MS (Master of Arts/Science)*—Applications 2009–2010, 30. Total applicants accepted 2009–2010, 11. Number full-time enrolled (new admits only) 2009–2010, 7. Total enrolled 2009–2010 full-time, 9. Openings 2010–2011, 6. The number of students enrolled full- and part-time who were dismissed or voluntarily withdrew from this program area in 2008–2009 were 2.

Scores: Entries appear in this order: required test or GPA, minimum score (if required), median score of students entering in 2009–2010. *Clinical Health Psychology MA/MS (Master of Arts/Science):* GRE-V no minimum stated, 600, GRE-Q no minimum stated, 500, overall undergraduate GPA no minimum stated, 3.5, psychology GPA no minimum stated, 3.7; *Pre-doctoral General Psychology MA/MS (Master of Arts/Science):* GRE-V no minimum stated, 600, GRE-Q no minimum stated, 500, overall undergraduate GPA no minimum stated, 3.5, psychology GPA no minimum stated, 3.7; *Teaching of Psychology MA/MS (Master of Arts/Science):* GRE-V no minimum stated, 600, GRE-Q no minimum stated, 500, overall undergraduate GPA no minimum stated, 3.5, psychology GPA no minimum stated, 3.7; *Pre-doctoral Clinical Health Psychology MA/MS (Master of Arts/Science):* GRE-V no minimum stated, 600, GRE-Q no minimum stated, 500, overall undergraduate GPA no minimum stated, 3.5, last 2 years GPA no minimum stated, psychology GPA no minimum stated, 3.7.

Other Criteria: (importance of criteria rated low, medium, or high): GRE scores—high, research experience—high, work experience—low, extracurricular activity—low, clinically related public service—low, GPA—high, letters of recommendation—high, interview—medium, statement of goals and objectives—high, undergraduate major in psychology—low, specific undergraduate psychology courses taken—high. Clinically related public service used only for Clinical Health Psychology program. Work experience and extracurricular activity given somewhat higher importance for Clinical Health Psychology program. Phone interviews are conducted for selected applicants for the Clinical Health and Predoctoral training in Clinical Health Psychology. For additional information on admission requirements, go to http://www.nau.edu/~psych/grad.html.

Student Characteristics: The following represents characteristics of students in 2009–2010 in all graduate psychology programs in the department: Female—full-time 13, part-time 7; Male—full-time 10, part-time 1; African American/Black—full-time 0, part-time 0; Hispanic/Latino(a)—full-time 2, part-time 0; Asian/Pacific Islander—full-time 0, part-time 1; American Indian/Alaska Native—full-time 1, part-time 1; Caucasian/White—full-time 20, part-time 6; Multi-ethnic—full-time 0, part-time 0; students subject to the Americans With Disabilities Act—full-time 0, part-time 0; Unknown ethnicity—full-time 0, part-time 0; International students who hold an F-1 or J-1 Visa—full-time 0, part-time 1.

Financial Information/Assistance:
Tuition for Full-Time Study: *Master's:* State residents: per academic year $6,948, $386 per credit hour; Nonstate residents: per academic year $11,754, $653 per credit hour. Tuition is subject to change. See the following Web site for updates and changes in tuition costs: http://home.nau.edu/bursar/tuition_fees.asp.

Financial Assistance:
First-Year Students: Teaching assistantships available for first year. Average number of hours worked per week: 10. Apply by February 15. Research assistantships available for first year. Average number of hours worked per week: 10. Apply by February 15.
Advanced Students: Teaching assistantships available for advanced students. Average number of hours worked per week: 10. Research assistantships available for advanced students. Average number of hours worked per week: 10.
Additional Information: Of all students currently enrolled full time, 80% benefited from one or more of the listed financial assistance programs.

Internships/Practica: Master's Degree (MA/MS Clinical Health Psychology): An internship experience, such as a final research project or "capstone" experience is required of graduates. Master's Degree (MA/MS Pre-doctoral General Psychology): An internship experience, such as a final research project or "capstone" experience is required of graduates. Master's Degree (MA/MS Teaching of Psychology): An internship experience, such as a final research project or "capstone" experience is required of graduates. Master's Degree (MA/MS Pre-doctoral Clinical Health Psychology): An internship experience, such as, a final research project or "capstone" experience is required of graduates. Clinical Health and Pre-doctoral Clinical Health Psychology students are required to take two or three semesters of practicum in the department's Health Psychology Center. Our multipurpose training and service facility serves NAU students, faculty, and staff as well as community residents. In the Center, supervised graduate students in applied health psychology work to promote wellness and healthy lifestyles in adults and children through a variety of educational and treatment modalities. The Center offers programs on such topics as stress management, healthy eating and weight control, exercise, and smoking cessation, as well as group and individual interventions for these topics. The Center also provides psychological evaluation and behavioral management for health-related problems such as headaches, high blood pressure, cardiovascular disease, obesity, premenstrual syndrome, ulcers, diabetes, asthma, smoking, cancer, and chronic pain. Health Psychology students also are encouraged to take one or more semesters of fieldwork placement at a variety of agencies in the surrounding communities (including ethnic and rural communities). Pre-doctoral General Psychology students also may enroll in fieldwork placement. Teaching of Psychology students are required to enroll in a teaching practicum and teaching fieldwork.

Housing and Day Care: On-campus housing is available. See the following Web site for more information: http://home.nau.edu/reslife/. No on-campus day care facilities are available.

Employment of Department Graduates:
Master's Degree Graduates: Of those who graduated in the academic year 2008–2009, the following categories and numbers represent the postgraduate activities and employment of master's degree graduates: Enrolled in a psychology doctoral program (0), enrolled in another graduate/professional program (2), enrolled in a postdoctoral residency/fellowship (n/a), employed in independent practice (n/a), employed in an academic position at a university (1), employed in an academic position at a 2-year/4-year college (1), employed in business or industry (2), total from the above (master's) (6).
Doctoral Degree Graduates: Of those who graduated in the academic year 2008–2009, the following categories and numbers represent the postgraduate activities and employment of doctoral degree graduates: Enrolled in a psychology doctoral program (n/a), total from the above (doctoral) (0).

Additional Information:
Orientation, Objectives, and Emphasis of Department: The Psychology Department is committed to excellence in education at the graduate level, emphasizing teaching, scholarship, and service to the university and to the larger community. The department emphasizes theoretical foundations, empirical research, innovative curriculum, and practical hands-on applications of psychological knowledge. Four graduate programs are offered. First, the Pre-doctoral General Psychology Training program, which involves study of the theoretical and methodological foundations of general (clinical, cognitive, developmental, experimental, industrial/organizational, social, personality, neurosciences) psychology, is appropriate if you plan to pursue a doctoral degree or to conduct research and data management in a variety of settings. Second, the Pre-doctoral Clinical Health Psychology Training program, which involves study of the theoretical and methodological foundations of Clinical Health psychology, is appropriate if you plan to pursue a doctoral degree or to conduct research and data management in a variety of settings. Third, the Teaching of Psychology graduate program provides extensive training in the theoretical and methodological foundations of psychology and affords students a variety of teaching experiences and skills in face-to-face, web, and hybrid settings. This program prepares students to pursue a teaching career at the high school or community college level.

GRADUATE STUDY IN PSYCHOLOGY

Fourth, the Clinical Health Psychology program is appropriate if you plan to work in a master's-level position using skills related to the promotion of health and wellness and the prevention and treatment of illness.

Special Facilities or Resources: The Department of Psychology has over 1,500 square feet of clinic space dedicated to training in Health Psychology and a state-of-the-art psychophysiology/biofeedback laboratory. Other well-equipped research facilities are available in an adjunct building, and are assigned to faculty members engaged in research. A computer laboratory used for teaching purposes is also available for data collection. The department is housed in a modern building at the south end of the Flagstaff Mountain Campus. All teaching rooms are equipped with up-to-date technology. NAU is located in the city of Flagstaff, a four-season community of approximately 50,000 residents at the base of the majestic, 12,670-foot-high San Francisco Peaks. Flagstaff and the surrounding area offer excellent hiking and mountain-biking trails as well as cross-country and downhill skiing. Students enjoy the nearby diversity of Arizona's climate and attractions, from Grand Canyon National Park to metropolitan Phoenix in the Sonoran desert.

Information for Students With Physical Disabilities: See the following Web site for more information: http://www4.nau.edu/dr/.

Application Information:
Send to Departmental Application: Department of Psychology, Graduate Programs, Northern Arizona University, Box 15106, Flagstaff, AZ 86011. Graduate Application: NAU Graduate College, P.O. Box 4125, Flagstaff, AZ 86011-4125. Application available online. URL of online application: http://www.nau.edu/gradcol/. Students are admitted in the Fall, application deadline February 15. *Fee:* $50.

Northern Arizona University
Educational Psychology
College of Education
COE 5774
Flagstaff, AZ 86011
Telephone: (928) 523-7103
Fax: (928) 523-9284
E-mail: *kathy.bohan@nau.edu*
Web: *http://coe.nau.edu/academics/eps*

Department Information:
1962. Chairperson: Kathy Bohan. Number of faculty: total—full-time 20, part-time 1; women—full-time 10, part-time 1; total—minority—full-time 2; women minority—full-time 1.

Programs and Degrees Offered:
Listed in the following order: Program area, degree type (T if terminal Master's), number awarded 7/08–6/09. Community Counseling MA/MS (Master of Arts/Science) (T) 19, School Psychology Certification 8, School Counseling MEd (Education) 11, Student Affairs MEd (Education) 4, Counseling Psychology PhD (Doctor of Philosophy) 3, School Psychology PhD (Doctor of Philosophy) 3, Learning and Instruction PhD (Doctor of Philosophy) 0, Human Relations MEd (Education) 7.

Student Applications/Admissions:
Student Applications

Community Counseling MA/MS (Master of Arts/Science)—Applications 2009–2010, 74. Total applicants accepted 2009–2010, 40. Number full-time enrolled (new admits only) 2009–2010, 28. Number part-time enrolled (new admits only) 2009–2010, 4. Total enrolled 2009–2010 full-time, 62, part-time, 38. Openings 2010–2011, 35. The median number of years required for completion of a degree in 2008–2009 were 2. The number of students enrolled full- and part-time who were dismissed or voluntarily withdrew from this program area in 2008–2009 were 1. *School Psychology Certification*—Applications 2009–2010, 33. Total applicants accepted 2009–2010, 12. Number full-time enrolled (new admits only) 2009–2010, 6. Number part-time enrolled (new admits only) 2009–2010, 0. Total enrolled 2009–2010 full-time, 12, part-time, 10. Openings 2010–2011, 12. The median number of years required for completion of a degree in 2008–2009 were 3. The number of students enrolled full- and part-time who were dismissed or voluntarily withdrew from this program area in 2008–2009 were 0. *School Counseling MEd (Education)*—Applications 2009–2010, 50. Total applicants accepted 2009–2010, 35. Number full-time enrolled (new admits only) 2009–2010, 30. Number part-time enrolled (new admits only) 2009–2010, 6. Total enrolled 2009–2010 full-time, 40, part-time, 5. Openings 2010–2011, 40. The median number of years required for completion of a degree in 2008–2009 were 2. The number of students enrolled full- and part-time who were dismissed or voluntarily withdrew from this program area in 2008–2009 were 1. *Student Affairs MEd (Education)*—Applications 2009–2010, 11. Total applicants accepted 2009–2010, 6. Number full-time enrolled (new admits only) 2009–2010, 4. Number part-time enrolled (new admits only) 2009–2010, 2. Total enrolled 2009–2010 full-time, 12, part-time, 4. Openings 2010–2011, 10. The median number of years required for completion of a degree in 2008–2009 were 2. The number of students enrolled full- and part-time who were dismissed or voluntarily withdrew from this program area in 2008–2009 were 1. *Counseling Psychology PhD (Doctor of Philosophy)*—Applications 2009–2010, 6. Total applicants accepted 2009–2010, 2. Number full-time enrolled (new admits only) 2009–2010, 8. Number part-time enrolled (new admits only) 2009–2010, 1. Total enrolled 2009–2010 full-time, 14, part-time, 2. Openings 2010–2011, 6. The median number of years required for completion of a degree in 2008–2009 were 5. The number of students enrolled full- and part-time who were dismissed or voluntarily withdrew from this program area in 2008–2009 were 0. *School Psychology PhD (Doctor of Philosophy)*—Applications 2009–2010, 4. Total applicants accepted 2009–2010, 0. Number full-time enrolled (new admits only) 2009–2010, 0. Number part-time enrolled (new admits only) 2009–2010, 0. Total enrolled 2009–2010 full-time, 8, part-time, 1. Openings 2010–2011, 5. The median number of years required for completion of a degree in 2008–2009 were 4. The number of students enrolled full- and part-time who were dismissed or voluntarily withdrew from this program area in 2008–2009 were 0. *Learning and Instruction PhD (Doctor of Philosophy)*—Applications 2009–2010, 0. Total applicants accepted 2009–2010, 0. Number full-time enrolled (new admits only) 2009–2010, 2. Number part-time enrolled (new admits only) 2009–2010, 0. Openings 2010–2011, 3. The median number of years required for completion of a degree in 2008–2009 were 5. The number of students enrolled full- and part-time who were dismissed or voluntarily withdrew from this program area in 2008–2009 were 1. *Human Relations MEd (Education)*—Applications 2009–2010, 20. Total applicants accepted 2009–2010, 15. Number full-time enrolled (new admits only) 2009–2010, 8. Number part-time enrolled (new admits only) 2009–2010, 6. Total enrolled 2009–2010 full-time, 12, part-time, 4. Openings 2010–2011, 10. The median number of years required for completion of a degree in 2008–2009 were 2. The number of students enrolled full- and part-time who were dismissed or voluntarily withdrew from this program area in 2008–2009 were 0.

Scores: Entries appear in this order: required test or GPA, minimum score (if required), median score of students entering in 2009–2010. *Community Counseling MA/MS (Master of Arts/Science):* GRE-V no minimum stated, GRE-Q no minimum stated, overall undergraduate GPA no minimum stated; *School Psychology Certification:* GRE-V no minimum stated, GRE-Q no minimum stated, overall undergraduate GPA no minimum stated; *School Counseling MEd (Education):* GRE-V no minimum stated, GRE-Q no minimum stated, overall undergraduate GPA no minimum stated; *Student Affairs MEd (Education):* GRE-V no minimum stated, GRE-Q no minimum stated, overall undergraduate GPA no minimum stated; *Counseling Psychology PhD (Doctor of Philosophy):* GRE-V no minimum stated, GRE-Q no minimum stated, overall undergraduate GPA no minimum stated; *School Psychology PhD (Doctor of Philosophy):* GRE-V no minimum stated, GRE-Q no minimum stated, overall undergraduate GPA no minimum stated; *Human Relations MEd (Education):* overall undergraduate GPA 3.0, last 2 years GPA 3.0.

Other Criteria: (importance of criteria rated low, medium, or high): GRE scores—medium, research experience—low, work experience—medium, extracurricular activity—low, clinically related public service—low, GPA—medium, letters of recommendation—medium, interview—low, statement of goals and objectives—high. For additional information on admission requirements, go to http://coe.nau.edu/academics/eps.

Student Characteristics: The following represents characteristics of students in 2009–2010 in all graduate psychology programs in the department: Female—full-time 94, part-time 48; Male—full-time 33, part-time 18; African American/Black—full-time 9, part-time 5; Hispanic/Latino(a)—full-time 12, part-time 5; Asian/Pacific Islander—full-time 2, part-time 1; American Indian/Alaska Native—full-time 9, part-time 5; Caucasian/White—full-time 93, part-time 50; Multi-ethnic—full-time 2, part-time 0; students subject to the Americans With Disabilities Act—full-time 1, part-time 0; Unknown ethnicity—full-time 0, part-time 0; International students who hold an F-1 or J-1 Visa—full-time 0, part-time 0.

Financial Information/Assistance:
Tuition for Full-Time Study: *Master's:* State residents: per academic year $6,726, $332 per credit hour; Nonstate residents: per academic year $17,500, $972 per credit hour. *Doctoral:* State residents: per academic year $6,726, $332 per credit hour; Nonstate residents: per academic year $17,500, $972 per credit hour. Tuition is subject to change. Additional fees are assessed to students beyond the costs of tuition for the following: practicum and internship. See the following Web site for updates and changes in tuition costs: http://home.nau.edu/bursar/tuition_fees.asp.

Financial Assistance:
First-Year Students: Teaching assistantships available for first year. Average amount paid per academic year: $8,910. Average number of hours worked per week: 20. Apply by April 15.
Advanced Students: Teaching assistantships available for advanced students. Average amount paid per academic year: $9,900. Average number of hours worked per week: 20. Apply by April 15. Research assistantships available for advanced students. Average amount paid per academic year: $9,575. Average number of hours worked per week: 20. Apply by April 15.
Additional Information: Of all students currently enrolled full time, 25% benefited from one or more of the listed financial assistance programs. Application and information available online at: http://www4.nau.edu/finaid/.

Internships/Practica: Doctoral Degree (PhD Counseling Psychology): For those doctoral students for whom a professional internship was required in this program prior to graduation, (4) students applied for an internship in 2008–2009, with (4) students obtaining an internship. Of those students who obtained an internship, (4) were paid internships. Of those students who obtained an internship, (1) students placed in APA/CPA accredited internships, (3) students placed in internships not APA/CPA accredited, but listed with the Association of Psychology Postdoctoral and Internship Programs (APPIC), (0) students placed in internships conforming to guidelines of the Council of Directors of School Psychology Programs (CDSPP), (0) students placed in internships that were not APA/CPA accredited, APPIC or CDSPP listed. Doctoral Degree (PhD School Psychology): For those doctoral students for whom a professional internship was required in this program prior to graduation, (3) students applied for an internship in 2008–2009, with (3) students obtaining an internship. Of those students who obtained an internship, (3) were paid internships. Of those students who obtained an internship, (0) students placed in APA/CPA accredited internships, (0) students placed in internships not APA/CPA accredited, but listed with the Association of Psychology Postdoctoral and Internship Programs (APPIC), (3) students placed in internships conforming to guidelines of the Council of Directors of School Psychology Programs (CDSPP), (0) students placed in internships that were not APA/CPA accredited, APPIC or CDSPP listed. Master's Degree (MA/MS Community Counseling): An internship experience, such as, a final research project or "capstone" experience is required of graduates. Master's Degree (School Psychology Certification): An internship experience, such as a final research project or "capstone" experience is required of graduates. Master's Degree (MEd Student Affairs): An internship experience, such as a final research project or "capstone" experience is required of graduates. Our programs are built on competency-based models and include closely supervised experiential practica and internship components. Many of these experiences are offered in NAU's Counseling and Testing Center and the Institute for Human Development; student service facilities; public-school settings; reservation schools and communities; rural settings; and community agencies. In addition, the College of Education houses a Skills Lab Network that includes comprehensive testing and curriculum libraries and a practicum facility that uses both videotape and direct live feedback in the supervision of students working with clients.

Housing and Day Care: On-campus housing is available. See the following Web site for more information: http://www.nau.edu/reslife/. On-campus day care facilities are available.

Employment of Department Graduates:
Master's Degree Graduates: Of those who graduated in the academic year 2008–2009, the following categories and numbers represent the postgraduate activities and employment of master's degree graduates: Enrolled in a psychology doctoral program (2), enrolled in a postdoctoral residency/fellowship (n/a), employed in independent practice (n/a), total from the above (master's) (2).
Doctoral Degree Graduates: Of those who graduated in the academic year 2008–2009, the following categories and numbers represent the postgraduate activities and employment of doctoral degree graduates: Enrolled in a psychology doctoral program (n/a), enrolled in a postdoctoral residency/fellowship (0), employed in an academic position at a university (2), employed in an academic position at a 2-year/4-year college (0), total from the above (doctoral) (2).

Additional Information:
Orientation, Objectives, and Emphasis of Department: Because of the barriers to learning and living in our society, there is an increasing need for professionally trained counseling and school psychology personnel. Our graduate programs are based on a developmental, experiential training model that includes understanding theory, learning assessment and intervention skills, practicing skills in a supervised clinical setting, and performing skills in like settings. Integrated throughout our programs is a scientist–practitioner orientation that prepares students to ascertain the efficacy of assessment and intervention techniques.

Special Facilities or Resources: Students in School Psychology programs complete portions of their practicum at sites located on the Indian reservations and work with children and schools affiliated with the Navajo, Hopi and Supai tribes. The MA Community Counseling and the MEd School Counseling programs are also available at select sites in Arizona (i.e., Phoenix, Tucson and Yuma).

Information for Students With Physical Disabilities: See the following Web site for more information: http://www.nau.edu/dr/.

Application Information:
Application available online. URL of online application: http://www.applyweb.com/apply/northazg/. Students are admitted in the Spring, application deadline September 15; Fall application deadline February 15. PhD - Counseling Psychology and School Psychology - January 15. PhD-Learning and Instruction - Rolling deadline, MA + Certification in School Psychology - February 15. MA Community Counseling, MEd School Counseling - Dates above for Fall and Spring apply. MA Student Affairs-September 15 & April 1.

ARKANSAS

Arkansas, University of
Department of Psychology
J. William Fulbright College of Arts and Science
216 Memorial Hall
Fayetteville, AR 72701
Telephone: (479) 575-4256
Fax: (479) 575-3219
E-mail: *psycapp@uark.edu*
Web: *http://www.uark.edu/depts/psyc*

Department Information:
1926. Chairperson: Douglas A. Behrend. Number of faculty: total—full-time 17; women—full-time 6; total—minority—full-time 1; women minority—full-time 1; faculty subject to the Americans With Disabilities Act 1.

Programs and Degrees Offered:
Listed in the following order: Program area, degree type (T if terminal Master's), number awarded 7/08–6/09. Clinical PhD (Doctor of Philosophy) 6, Experimental PhD (Doctor of Philosophy) 4.

APA Accreditation: Clinical PhD (Doctor of Philosophy). Student Outcome Data Website: http://www.uark.edu/depts/psyc/statistical.pdf.

Student Applications/Admissions:
Student Applications
Clinical PhD (Doctor of Philosophy)—Applications 2009–2010, 89. Total applicants accepted 2009–2010, 6. Number full-time enrolled (new admits only) 2009–2010, 6. Openings 2010–2011, 6. The median number of years required for completion of a degree in 2008–2009 were 5. The number of students enrolled full- and part-time who were dismissed or voluntarily withdrew from this program area in 2008–2009 were 2. *Experimental PhD (Doctor of Philosophy)*—Applications 2009–2010, 28. Total applicants accepted 2009–2010, 3. Number full-time enrolled (new admits only) 2009–2010, 2. Openings 2010–2011, 3. The median number of years required for completion of a degree in 2008–2009 were 5. The number of students enrolled full- and part-time who were dismissed or voluntarily withdrew from this program area in 2008–2009 were 1.
Scores: Entries appear in this order: required test or GPA, minimum score (if required), median score of students entering in 2009–2010. *Clinical PhD (Doctor of Philosophy)*: GRE-V no minimum stated, 586, GRE-Q no minimum stated, 631, overall undergraduate GPA no minimum stated, 3.61; *Experimental PhD (Doctor of Philosophy)*: GRE-V no minimum stated, 570, GRE-Q no minimum stated, 650, GRE-Analytical no minimum stated, 5.0, overall undergraduate GPA no minimum stated, 3.6.
Other Criteria: (importance of criteria rated low, medium, or high): GRE scores—high, research experience—high, work experience—low, extracurricular activity—low, clinically related public service—medium, GPA—high, letters of recommendation—high, interview—high, statement of goals and objectives—high, fit with faculty research—high, undergraduate major in psychology—medium, specific undergraduate psychology courses taken—low, Clinically relevant service only considered for clinical applicants.

Student Characteristics: The following represents characteristics of students in 2009–2010 in all graduate psychology programs in the department: Female—full-time 29, part-time 0; Male—full-time 17, part-time 0; African American/Black—full-time 0, part-time 0; Hispanic/Latino(a)—full-time 2, part-time 0; Asian/Pacific Islander—full-time 0, part-time 0; American Indian/Alaska Native—full-time 1, part-time 0; Caucasian/White—full-time 40, part-time 0; Multi-ethnic—full-time 1, part-time 0; students subject to the Americans With Disabilities Act—full-time 0, part-time 0; Unknown ethnicity—full-time 2, part-time 0; International students who hold an F-1 or J-1 Visa—full-time 2, part-time 0.

Financial Information/Assistance:
Tuition for Full-Time Study: *Doctoral*: State residents: per academic year $4,070, $294 per credit hour; Nonstate residents: per academic year $8,900, $697 per credit hour. Tuition is subject to change. Additional fees are assessed to students beyond the costs of tuition for the following: health insurance (optional), student activity fees, technology fees. See the following Web site for updates and changes in tuition costs: http://grad.uark.edu/.

Financial Assistance:
First-Year Students: Teaching assistantships available for first year. Average amount paid per academic year: $9,500. Average number of hours worked per week: 20. Apply by December 1. Research assistantships available for first year. Average amount paid per academic year: $9,500. Average number of hours worked per week: 20. Apply by December 1. Fellowships and scholarships available for first year. Average amount paid per academic year: $20,000. Average number of hours worked per week: 20. Apply by December 1.
Advanced Students: Teaching assistantships available for advanced students. Average amount paid per academic year: $9,500. Average number of hours worked per week: 20. Research assistantships available for advanced students. Average amount paid per academic year: $9,500. Average number of hours worked per week: 20. Fellowships and scholarships available for advanced students. Average amount paid per academic year: $20,000. Average number of hours worked per week: 20.
Additional Information: Of all students currently enrolled full time, 100% benefited from one or more of the listed financial assistance programs. Application and information available online at: http://www.uark.edu/depts/psyc.

Internships/Practica: Doctoral Degree (PhD Clinical): For those doctoral students for whom a professional internship was required in this program prior to graduation, (4) students applied for an internship in 2008–2009, with (4) students obtaining an internship. Of those students who obtained an internship, (4) were paid internships. Of those students who obtained an internship, (4) students placed in APA/CPA accredited internships, (0) students placed in internships not APA/CPA accredited, but listed with the Association of Psychology Postdoctoral and Internship Programs (APPIC), (0) students placed in internships conforming to guidelines of the Council of Directors of School Psychology Programs (CDSPP), (0) students placed in internships that were not APA/CPA accredited, APPIC or CDSPP listed. Doctoral students in the Clinical Training Program have always been able to obtain high-quality, APA-accredited predoctoral internships. Additionally, our students have numerous mental health agency placement opportunities throughout their tenure with us. These clerkship placements include local community mental health centers, the University Health Service, inpatient psychiatric hospitals, and several facilities dealing with disabilities, neuropsychology, and other clinical specialties.

Housing and Day Care: On-campus housing is available. See the following Web site for more information: http://housing.uark.edu/. On-campus day care facilities are available. See the following Web site for more information: Infant Development Center: http://hesc.uark.edu/2662.htm. University Nursery School: http://hesc.uark.edu/2660.htm.

Employment of Department Graduates:
Master's Degree Graduates: Of those who graduated in the academic year 2008–2009, the following categories and numbers represent the postgraduate activities and employment of master's degree graduates: Enrolled in a postdoctoral residency/fellowship (n/a), employed in independent practice (n/a), total from the above (master's) (0).
Doctoral Degree Graduates: Of those who graduated in the academic year 2008–2009, the following categories and numbers represent the postgraduate activities and employment of doctoral degree graduates: Enrolled in a psychology doctoral program (n/a), enrolled in a postdoctoral residency/fellowship (2), employed in independent practice (2), employed in an academic position at a 2-year/4-year college (1), employed in a hospital/medical center (1), total from the above (doctoral) (6).

Additional Information:
Orientation, Objectives, and Emphasis of Department: The PhD program in clinical psychology follows the scientist/practitioner model of training. Although some of our graduates obtain applied, direct service provision positions, our training curriculum is such that those students whose career aspirations have been directed toward academic and research positions also have been successful. The clinical training program is based on the premise that clinical psychologists should be skilled practitioners and mental health service providers as well as competent researchers. To facilitate these goals, we strive to maximize the match between the clinical and research interests of the faculty with those of the graduate students. The academic courses and clinical experiences are designed to promote development in both areas. The objective of the Clinical Training Program is to graduate clinical psychologists capable of applying psychological theory, research methodology, and clinical skills to complex clinical problems and diverse populations. The program is fully accredited by the American Psychological Association. The PhD program in experimental psychology provides students with a broad knowledge of psychology via a core curriculum, with a specialized training emphasis in our social and cognitive processes focus area via research team meetings, colloquia, and advanced seminars. Training in social, developmental and cognitive psychology within the focus area includes independent research experience and extensive, supervised classroom teaching experience. The program provides students with a thorough understanding of psychological principles and prepares them for careers as academics and researchers.

Special Facilities or Resources: The Department of Psychology is housed in Memorial Hall, a multilevel building with 58,000 square feet of office and research space for faculty and students. The building contains modern facilities for both human and small animal research, including specialized space for use with individuals and small groups of children and adults. The on-site Psychological Clinic is a state-of-the-art training and research facility dedicated to providing practicum and applied research experiences for clinical students. The clinic's treatment, testing, and research rooms are equipped with a closed-circuit videotaping system. Memorial Hall has comprehensive data analysis facilities, including personal computers networked to the University and internet. Finally, the department is the beneficiary of a generous bequest that established the Marie Wilson Howells Fund, which provides funding for thesis and dissertation research, numerous research assistantships, student travel, and departmental colloquia. The department also nominates qualified students for supplemental Doctoral Fellowships available through the Graduate School.

Information for Students With Physical Disabilities: See the following Web site for more information: http://www.uark.edu/ua/csd/.

Application Information:
Send to Graduate Studies Secretary, Department of Psychology, 216 Memorial Hall, University of Arkansas, Fayetteville, AR 72701. Application available online. URL of online application: http://www.uark.edu/depts/psyc/application.html. Students are admitted in the Fall, application deadline December 1. The deadline for the Clinical Program is December 1. The deadline for the Experimental Program is January 1. *Fee:* $0. The Department will pay the Graduate School application fees for admitted students. International applicants must apply to the Graduate School and pay a $50 application fee.

Central Arkansas, University of
Department of Psychology and Counseling
Health and Behavioral Sciences
201 Donaghey Avenue
Conway, AR 72035-0001
Telephone: (501) 450-3193
Fax: (501) 450-5424
E-mail: *DavidS@uca.edu*
Web: *http://www.uca.edu/psychology*

Department Information:
1967. Chairperson: David Skotko. Number of faculty: total—full-time 21, part-time 5; women—full-time 6, part-time 4; total—minority—full-time 2, part-time 2; women minority—full-time 1, part-time 1.

Programs and Degrees Offered:
Listed in the following order: Program area, degree type (T if terminal Master's), number awarded 7/08–6/09. School Psychology PhD (Doctor of Philosophy) 3, School Psychology MA/MS (Master of Arts/Science) (T) 6, Counseling Psychology MA/MS (Master of Arts/Science) (T) 13, Community Counseling MA/MS

(Master of Arts/Science) (T) 9, Counseling Psychology Emphasis PhD (Doctor of Philosophy) 0.

APA Accreditation: School PhD (Doctor of Philosophy). Student Outcome Data Website: http://www.uca.edu/psychology/programs/documents/graduate/phdschoolpsyc.php.

Student Applications/Admissions:
Student Applications
School Psychology PhD (Doctor of Philosophy)—Applications 2009–2010, 7. Total applicants accepted 2009–2010, 2. Number full-time enrolled (new admits only) 2009–2010, 2. Number part-time enrolled (new admits only) 2009–2010, 0. Total enrolled 2009–2010 full-time, 13, part-time, 7. Openings 2010–2011, 5. The median number of years required for completion of a degree in 2008–2009 were 5. The number of students enrolled full- and part-time who were dismissed or voluntarily withdrew from this program area in 2008–2009 were 3. *School Psychology MA/MS (Master of Arts/Science)*—Applications 2009–2010, 6. Total applicants accepted 2009–2010, 5. Number full-time enrolled (new admits only) 2009–2010, 5. Number part-time enrolled (new admits only) 2009–2010, 0. Openings 2010–2011, 8. The median number of years required for completion of a degree in 2008–2009 were 3. The number of students enrolled full- and part-time who were dismissed or voluntarily withdrew from this program area in 2008–2009 were 0. *Counseling Psychology MA/MS (Master of Arts/Science)*—Applications 2009–2010, 24. Total applicants accepted 2009–2010, 14. Number full-time enrolled (new admits only) 2009–2010, 11. Number part-time enrolled (new admits only) 2009–2010, 0. Openings 2010–2011, 15. The median number of years required for completion of a degree in 2008–2009 were 2. The number of students enrolled full- and part-time who were dismissed or voluntarily withdrew from this program area in 2008–2009 were 1. *Community Counseling MA/MS (Master of Arts/Science)*—Applications 2009–2010, 20. Total applicants accepted 2009–2010, 14. Number full-time enrolled (new admits only) 2009–2010, 11. Total enrolled 2009–2010 full-time, 28. Openings 2010–2011, 15. The median number of years required for completion of a degree in 2008–2009 were 2. The number of students enrolled full- and part-time who were dismissed or voluntarily withdrew from this program area in 2008–2009 were 1. *Counseling Psychology Emphasis PhD (Doctor of Philosophy)*—Applications 2009–2010, 6. Total applicants accepted 2009–2010, 3. Number full-time enrolled (new admits only) 2009–2010, 3. Number part-time enrolled (new admits only) 2009–2010, 0. Openings 2010–2011, 5. The median number of years required for completion of a degree in 2008–2009 were 5. The number of students enrolled full- and part-time who were dismissed or voluntarily withdrew from this program area in 2008–2009 were 1.

Scores: Entries appear in this order: required test or GPA, minimum score (if required), median score of students entering in 2009–2010. *School Psychology PhD (Doctor of Philosophy)*: GRE-V no minimum stated, 500, GRE-Q no minimum stated, 700, overall undergraduate GPA no minimum stated, 3.8; *School Psychology MA/MS (Master of Arts/Science)*: GRE-V no minimum stated, 440, GRE-Q no minimum stated, 500, overall undergraduate GPA no minimum stated, 3.4; *Counseling Psychology MA/MS (Master of Arts/Science)*: GRE-V no minimum stated, 455, GRE-Q no minimum stated, 555, overall undergraduate GPA no minimum stated, 3.6; *Community Counseling MA/MS (Master of Arts/Science)*: GRE-V no minimum stated, 490, GRE-Q no minimum stated, 450, overall undergraduate GPA no minimum stated, 3.5; *Counseling Psychology Emphasis PhD (Doctor of Philosophy)*: GRE-V no minimum stated, 500, GRE-Q no minimum stated, 640, overall undergraduate GPA no minimum stated, 3.8.

Other Criteria: (importance of criteria rated low, medium, or high): GRE scores—medium, research experience—medium, work experience—low, extracurricular activity—low, clinically related public service—medium, GPA—high, letters of recommendation—medium, interview—high, statement of goals and objectives—high, undergraduate major in psychology—low, specific undergraduate psychology courses taken—low. Doctoral programs place greater emphasis on research experience.

Student Characteristics: The following represents characteristics of students in 2009–2010 in all graduate psychology programs in the department: Female—full-time 79, part-time 7; Male—full-time 10, part-time 0; African American/Black—full-time 9, part-time 0; Hispanic/Latino(a)—full-time 2, part-time 0; Asian/Pacific Islander—full-time 1, part-time 0; American Indian/Alaska Native—part-time 0; Caucasian/White—full-time 77, part-time 7; Multi-ethnic—full-time 0, part-time 0; students subject to the Americans With Disabilities Act—full-time 0, part-time 0; Unknown ethnicity—full-time 0, part-time 0; International students who hold an F-1 or J-1 Visa—full-time 1, part-time 0.

Financial Information/Assistance:
Tuition for Full-Time Study: *Master's:* State residents: $250 per credit hour; Nonstate residents: $460 per credit hour. *Doctoral:* State residents: $250 per credit hour; Nonstate residents: $460 per credit hour. Tuition is subject to change. See the following Web site for updates and changes in tuition costs: http://www.uca.edu/financialaid/index.php.

Financial Assistance:
First-Year Students: Research assistantships available for first year. Average amount paid per academic year: $7,000. Average number of hours worked per week: 20.

Advanced Students: Teaching assistantships available for advanced students. Average amount paid per academic year: $8,000. Average number of hours worked per week: 20. Research assistantships available for advanced students. Average amount paid per academic year: $8,000. Average number of hours worked per week: 20.

Additional Information: Of all students currently enrolled full time, 40% benefited from one or more of the listed financial assistance programs. Application and information available online at: http://www.uca.edu/graduateschool/assistantshipsandotheraid/.

Internships/Practica: Doctoral Degree (PhD School Psychology): For those doctoral students for whom a professional internship was required in this program prior to graduation, (3) students applied for an internship in 2008–2009, with (3) students obtaining an internship. Of those students who obtained an internship, (3) were paid internships. Of those students who obtained an internship, (2) students placed in APA/CPA accredited internships, (0) students placed in internships not APA/CPA accredited, but listed with the Association of Psychology Postdoctoral and Internship Programs (APPIC), (1) students placed in internships conforming to guidelines of the Council of Directors of School Psychology Programs (CDSPP), (0) students placed in internships that were not APA/CPA accredited, APPIC or CDSPP listed. Master's Degree (MA/MS Counseling Psychology): An internship experience, such as a final research project or "capstone" experience is required of graduates. Master's Degree (MA/MS Community Counseling): An internship experience, such as a final research project or "capstone" experience is required of graduates. Students are placed in a wide range of practica and internships depending on their program of study, career aspirations, and match between the practicum/internship site and our program objectives. Examples of placements include schools, community agencies, hospitals, and clinics.

Housing and Day Care: On-campus housing is available. See the following Web site for more information: http://www.uca.edu/housing/. On-campus day care facilities are available. See the following Web site for more information: http://www.uca.edu/ecse/childstudy.php.

Employment of Department Graduates:
Master's Degree Graduates: Of those who graduated in the academic year 2008–2009, the following categories and numbers represent the postgraduate activities and employment of master's degree graduates: Enrolled in a psychology doctoral program (0), enrolled in another graduate/professional program (0), enrolled in a postdoctoral residency/fellowship (n/a), employed in independent practice (n/a), employed in an academic position at a university (0), employed in an academic position at a 2-year/4-year college (0), employed in other positions at a higher education institution (0), employed in a professional position in a school system (6), employed in business or industry (0), employed in government agency (0), employed in a community mental health/counseling center (19), employed in a hospital/medical center (3), still seeking employment (0), not seeking employment (0), other employment position (0), do not know (0), total from the above (master's) (28).
Doctoral Degree Graduates: Of those who graduated in the academic year 2008–2009, the following categories and numbers represent the postgraduate activities and employment of doctoral degree graduates: Enrolled in a psychology doctoral program (n/a), enrolled in another graduate/professional program (0), employed in independent practice (0), employed in an academic position at a university (1), employed in an academic position at a 2-year/4-year college (0), employed in other positions at a higher education institution (0), employed in a professional position in a school system (1), employed in business or industry (0), employed in government agency (0), employed in a community mental health/counseling center (1), employed in a hospital/medical center (0), still seeking employment (0), not seeking employment (0), other employment position (0), do not know (0), total from the above (doctoral) (3).

Additional Information:
Orientation, Objectives, and Emphasis of Department: The MS programs in Counseling Psychology, Community Counseling, and School Psychology are designed to serve as terminal degrees with professional employment opportunities or as a firm foundation for prospective doctoral candidates. Broad training is offered in understanding of psychological theories, assessment, and mental health interventions to enable graduates to function successfully in a variety of mental health and educational settings. The PhD in School Psychology is grounded in the scientist–practitioner model of training. Strong emphasis is placed on child mental health promotion, primary prevention, and intervention with a broad range of community related problems involving children, families, and schools. The program is responsive to ongoing societal concerns and issues pertaining to children, families, and schools. It prepares its graduates to function in schools, clinics, community agencies, and hospitals. The Counseling Psychology Emphasis (leading to a PhD in School Psychology, Emphasis in Counseling Psychology) is structured as a counseling psychology program. The program of study is based on the scientist–practitioner model of training and emphasizes community mental health intervention and prevention services for clients with a wide variety of mental health problems. Graduates will be prepared to provide evidence-based assessment and treatment services and to conduct research in clinical and university settings. The department plans to seek APA accreditation of the Counseling Psychology Emphasis as a Counseling Psychology program at the earliest possible time.

Special Facilities or Resources: The department has (a) a fully operational computer instruction/research room that can be used for onsite research purposes; (b) human and animal research labs; (c) a multi-media computer system for research-related editing (e.g., self-modeling, therapy tapes).

Information for Students With Physical Disabilities: See the following Web site for more information: http://www.uca.edu/disability/.

Application Information:
Send to Department Chair, Dept. of Psychology & Counseling, Box 4915, UCA, Conway, AR 72035. Application available online. URL of online application: http://www.uca.edu/psychology/. Students are admitted in the Fall, application deadline March 15; July 15. School Psychology PhD Program Deadline: February 10. Counseling Psychology Emphasis Deadline: February 10. *Fee:* $25.

CALIFORNIA

Alliant International University: Fresno
Forensic Psychology Programs
California School of Forensic Studies
5130 East Clinton Way
Fresno, CA 93727-2014
Telephone: (559) 456-2777
Fax: (559) 253-2267
E-mail: brianevans@alliant.edu
Web: http://www.alliant.edu/

Department Information:
1996. Program Director: William Holcomb, PhD. Number of faculty: total—full-time 8, part-time 16; women—full-time 5, part-time 9; total—minority—full-time 1, part-time 3; women minority—full-time 1, part-time 2.

Programs and Degrees Offered:
Listed in the following order: Program area, degree type (T if terminal Master's), number awarded 7/08–6/09. Forensic Psychology PhD (Doctor of Philosophy) 8, Forensic Psychology PsyD (Doctor of Psychology) 5.

Student Applications/Admissions:
Student Applications
Forensic Psychology PhD (Doctor of Philosophy)—Applications 2009–2010, 35. Total applicants accepted 2009–2010, 28. Number full-time enrolled (new admits only) 2009–2010, 20. Number part-time enrolled (new admits only) 2009–2010, 0. Total enrolled 2009–2010 full-time, 84, part-time, 9. Openings 2010–2011, 20. The median number of years required for completion of a degree in 2008–2009 were 4. The number of students enrolled full- and part-time who were dismissed or voluntarily withdrew from this program area in 2008–2009 were 5. Forensic Psychology PsyD (Doctor of Psychology)—Applications 2009–2010, 22. Total applicants accepted 2009–2010, 19. Number full-time enrolled (new admits only) 2009–2010, 13. Number part-time enrolled (new admits only) 2009–2010, 2. Total enrolled 2009–2010 full-time, 33, part-time, 11. Openings 2010–2011, 15. The median number of years required for completion of a degree in 2008–2009 were 4. The number of students enrolled full- and part-time who were dismissed or voluntarily withdrew from this program area in 2008–2009 were 2.
Scores: Entries appear in this order: required test or GPA, minimum score (if required), median score of students entering in 2009–2010. Forensic Psychology PhD (Doctor of Philosophy): overall undergraduate GPA 3.0, 3.16, psychology GPA 3.0; Forensic Psychology PsyD (Doctor of Psychology): overall undergraduate GPA 3.0, 3.21, psychology GPA 3.0.
Other Criteria: (importance of criteria rated low, medium, or high): research experience—high, work experience—high, extracurricular activity—low, clinically related public service—medium, GPA—high, letters of recommendation—high, interview—high, statement of goals and objectives—high, Requirements vary by program. The PhD program puts more emphasis on prior research experience; the PsyD program on prior clinically-related experience. For additional information on admission requirements, go to http://www.alliant.edu/wps/wcm/connect/website/Home/Admissions/.

Student Characteristics: The following represents characteristics of students in 2009–2010 in all graduate psychology programs in the department: Female—full-time 90, part-time 16; Male—full-time 27, part-time 4; African American/Black—full-time 8, part-time 1; Hispanic/Latino(a)—full-time 21, part-time 1; Asian/Pacific Islander—full-time 7, part-time 1; American Indian/Alaska Native—full-time 1, part-time 0; Caucasian/White—full-time 63, part-time 13; Multi-ethnic—full-time 3, part-time 0; students subject to the Americans With Disabilities Act—full-time 3, part-time 0; Unknown ethnicity—full-time 14, part-time 4; International students who hold an F-1 or J-1 Visa—full-time 2, part-time 0.

Financial Information/Assistance:
Tuition for Full-Time Study: Doctoral: State residents: $950 per credit hour; Nonstate residents: $950 per credit hour. Tuition is subject to change. Tuition costs vary by program. See the following Web site for updates and changes in tuition costs: http://www.alliant.edu/wps/wcm/connect/website/Home/Admissions/Tuition+and+Fees/.

Financial Assistance:
First-Year Students: Research assistantships available for first year. Average amount paid per academic year: $1,000. Average number of hours worked per week: 10. Apply by see dept. Fellowships and scholarships available for first year. Average amount paid per academic year: $1,500. Apply by January 2.
Advanced Students: Teaching assistantships available for advanced students. Average amount paid per academic year: $3,000. Average number of hours worked per week: 20. Apply by see dept. Research assistantships available for advanced students. Average amount paid per academic year: $1,000. Average number of hours worked per week: 10. Apply by see dept. Fellowships and scholarships available for advanced students. Average amount paid per academic year: $1,500. Apply by April 15.
Additional Information: Of all students currently enrolled full time, 51% benefited from one or more of the listed financial assistance programs.

Internships/Practica: Doctoral Degree (PhD Forensic Psychology): For those doctoral students for whom a professional internship was required in this program prior to graduation, (1) students applied for an internship in 2008–2009, with (0) students obtaining an internship. Of those students who obtained an internship, (0) were paid internships. Of those students who obtained an internship, (0) students placed in APA/CPA accredited internships, (0) students placed in internships not APA/CPA accredited, but listed with the Association of Psychology Postdoctoral and Internship Programs (APPIC), (0) students placed in internships conforming to guidelines of the Council of Directors of School Psychology Programs (CDSPP), (0) students placed in internships that were not APA/CPA accredited, APPIC or CDSPP listed. Doctoral Degree (PsyD Forensic Psychology): For those doctoral students for whom a professional internship was required in this program prior to graduation, (3) students applied for an internship in 2008–2009, with (2) students obtaining an internship. Of those students who obtained an internship, (2) were paid internships. Of those students who obtained an internship, (0) students placed in APA/CPA accredited internships, (2) students placed in internships not APA/CPA accredited, but listed with the Association of Psychology Postdoctoral and Internship Programs (APPIC), (0) students placed in internships conforming to guidelines of the Council of Directors of School Psychology Programs (CDSPP), (0) students placed in internships that were not APA/CPA accredited, APPIC or CDSPP listed. Students in the PhD program complete a research internship in a law enforcement or other forensic setting. Students in the PsyD program complete a predoctoral internship. For full-time students, these internships typically occur in the fourth year and involve full-time or close to full-time activity.

Housing and Day Care: No on-campus housing is available. No on-campus day care facilities are available.

Employment of Department Graduates:
Master's Degree Graduates: Of those who graduated in the academic year 2008–2009, the following categories and numbers represent the postgraduate activities and employment of master's degree graduates: Enrolled in a postdoctoral residency/fellowship (n/a), employed in independent practice (n/a), total from the above (master's) (0).
Doctoral Degree Graduates: Of those who graduated in the academic year 2008–2009, the following categories and numbers represent the postgraduate activities and employment of doctoral degree graduates: Enrolled in a psychology doctoral program (n/a), total from the above (doctoral) (0).

Additional Information:
Orientation, Objectives, and Emphasis of Department: The forensic psychology PhD program prepares students for roles in administration in a variety of mental health agencies, correctional facilities and organizations, and law enforcement departments. Students are prepared to conduct research in both academic and government institutions; examine policy initiatives; and provide advocacy, lobbying and mediation skills to agencies and organizations. The PsyD program has an applied psychology orientation. This curriculum prepares students to conduct assessments for the courts, to serve as expert witnesses, or to work as mental health treatment providers in a variety of forensic settings, including prisons, jails, offender treatment groups, youth facilities, among many others. Core areas in both programs include forensic psychology, theories of crime and justice, industrial and organizational psychology, legal research, psychopathology, research design and data analysis, forensic mediation and dispute resolution, ethics, and substance abuse theory and treatment. While the programs are not specifically designed to train licensed psychologists, some students who enter the program may wish to seek clinical licensure after graduation. Arrangements can be made to take additional psychology courses required for licensing exams, and both PsyD and PhD students have become licensed.

Application Information:
Send to Alliant International University, Admissions Processing Center, 10455 Pomerado Road, San Diego CA 92131-1799. Application available online. URL of online application: http://www.alliant.edu/applyonline/. Students are admitted in the Fall, application deadline varies; Spring, application deadline varies; Programs have rolling admissions. Applicants wishing notification by April 1 should submit their applications in January. however, applications are welcomed on a rolling basis and will be processed on a space available basis. *Fee:* $70. A limited number of fee waivers are available for those with significant financial need.

Alliant International University: Fresno/Sacramento
Programs in Clinical Psychology
California School of Professional Psychology
5130 East Clinton Way
Fresno, CA 93727
Telephone: (559) 253-2256
Fax: (559) 253-2267
E-mail: *jkulbeck@alliant.edu*
Web: *http://www.alliant.edu/cspp/*

Department Information:
1973. Dean, California School of Professional Psychology: Morgan T. Sammons, PhD, ABPP. Number of faculty: total—full-time 12, part-time 38; women—full-time 6, part-time 23; total—minority—full-time 2, part-time 3; women minority—part-time 3.

Programs and Degrees Offered:
Listed in the following order: Program area, degree type (T if terminal Master's), number awarded 7/08–6/09. Clinical Psychology PsyD (Doctor of Psychology) 21, Clinical Psychology PhD (Doctor of Philosophy) 2.

APA Accreditation: Clinical PsyD (Doctor of Psychology). Clinical PhD (Doctor of Philosophy).

Student Applications/Admissions:
Student Applications
Clinical Psychology PsyD (Doctor of Psychology)—Applications 2009–2010, 90. Total applicants accepted 2009–2010, 57. Number full-time enrolled (new admits only) 2009–2010, 40. Number part-time enrolled (new admits only) 2009–2010, 0. Total enrolled 2009–2010 full-time, 130, part-time, 9. Openings 2010–2011, 30. The median number of years required for completion of a degree in 2008–2009 were 4. The number of students enrolled full- and part-time who were dismissed or voluntarily withdrew from this program area in 2008–2009 were 4. *Clinical Psychology PhD (Doctor of Philosophy)*—Applications 2009–2010, 22. Total applicants accepted 2009–2010, 14. Number full-time enrolled (new admits only) 2009–2010, 7. Number part-time enrolled (new admits only) 2009–2010, 1. Total enrolled 2009–2010 full-time, 35, part-time, 5. Openings 2010–2011, 10. The median number of years required for completion of a degree in 2008–2009 were 7. The number of students enrolled full- and part-time who were dismissed or voluntarily withdrew from this program area in 2008–2009 were 0.

Scores: Entries appear in this order: required test or GPA, minimum score (if required), median score of students entering in 2009–2010. *Clinical Psychology PsyD (Doctor of Psychology):* overall undergraduate GPA 3.0, 3.25, psychology GPA 3.0; *Clinical Psychology PhD (Doctor of Philosophy):* overall undergraduate GPA 3.0, 3.24, psychology GPA 3.0.

Other Criteria: (importance of criteria rated low, medium, or high): research experience—medium, work experience—medium, extracurricular activity—low, clinically related public service—medium, GPA—high, letters of recommendation—high, interview—high, statement of goals and objectives—high, undergraduate major in psychology—medium, specific undergraduate psychology courses taken—medium. For additional information on admission requirements, go to http://www.alliant.edu/wps/wcm/connect/website/Home/Admissions/Graduate+Student+Admissions/.

Student Characteristics: The following represents characteristics of students in 2009–2010 in all graduate psychology programs in the department: Female—full-time 132, part-time 10; Male—full-time 33, part-time 4; African American/Black—full-time 12, part-time 1; Hispanic/Latino(a)—full-time 13, part-time 1; Asian/Pacific Islander—full-time 18, part-time 1; American Indian/Alaska Native—full-time 2, part-time 0; Caucasian/White—full-time 88, part-time 8; Multi-ethnic—full-time 7, part-time 0; students subject to the Americans With Disabilities Act—full-time 6, part-time 0; Unknown ethnicity—full-time 25, part-time 3; International students who hold an F-1 or J-1 Visa—full-time 3, part-time 0.

Financial Information/Assistance:
Tuition for Full-Time Study: *Doctoral:* State residents: $950 per credit hour; Nonstate residents: $950 per credit hour. Tuition is subject to change. See the following Web site for updates and changes in tuition costs: http://www.alliant.edu/wps/wcm/connect/website/Home/Admissions/Tuition+and+Fees/.

Financial Assistance:
First-Year Students: Research assistantships available for first year. Average amount paid per academic year: $1,000. Average number of hours worked per week: 10. Apply by see dept. Fellowships and scholarships available for first year. Average amount paid per academic year: $1,500. Apply by January 15.

Advanced Students: Teaching assistantships available for advanced students. Average amount paid per academic year: $3,000. Average number of hours worked per week: 10. Apply by see dept. Research assistantships available for advanced students. Average amount paid per academic year: $1,000. Average number of hours worked per week: 10. Apply by see dept. Fellowships and scholarships available for advanced students. Average amount paid per academic year: $1,500. Apply by April 15.

Additional Information: Of all students currently enrolled full time, 56% benefited from one or more of the listed financial assistance programs.

Internships/Practica: Doctoral Degree (PsyD Clinical Psychology): For those doctoral students for whom a professional internship was required in this program prior to graduation, (20) students applied for an internship in 2008–2009, with (19) students obtaining an internship. Of those students who obtained an internship, (16) were paid internships. Of those students who obtained an internship, (9) students placed in APA/CPA accredited internships, (5) students placed in internships not APA/CPA accredited, but listed with the Association of Psychology Postdoctoral and Internship Programs (APPIC), (0) students placed in internships conforming to guidelines of the Council of Directors of School Psychology Programs (CDSPP), (5) students placed in internships that were not APA/CPA accredited, APPIC or CDSPP listed. Doctoral Degree (PhD Clinical Psychology): For those doctoral students for whom a professional internship was required in this program prior to graduation, (6) students applied for an internship in 2008–2009, with (6) students obtaining an internship. Of those students who obtained an internship, (6) were paid internships. Of those students who obtained an internship, (2) students placed in APA/CPA accredited internships, (3) students placed in internships not APA/CPA accredited, but listed with the Association of Psychology Postdoctoral and Internship Programs (APPIC), (0) students placed in internships conforming to guidelines of the Council of Directors of School Psychology Programs (CDSPP), (1) students placed in internships that were not APA/CPA accredited, APPIC or CDSPP listed. The clinical psychology programs at Fresno and Sacramento emphasize the integration of academic coursework and research with clinical practice. In order to integrate appropriate skills with material learned in the classroom, students participate in a professional training placement experience beginning in the first year. The settings where students complete the professional training requirements include community mental health centers, clinics, inpatient mental health facilities, medical settings, specialized service centers, rehabilitation programs, residential/day care programs, forensic/correctional facilities, and educational programs. Third year students will spend fifteen hours per week in a practicum either at CSPP's Psychological Service Center or at some other CSPP-approved agency. During their final year, clinical students complete a full year internship at an appropriate APA or APPIC internship. PhD students must also complete teaching practica.

Housing and Day Care: No on-campus housing is available. No on-campus day care facilities are available.

Employment of Department Graduates:
Master's Degree Graduates: Of those who graduated in the academic year 2008–2009, the following categories and numbers represent the postgraduate activities and employment of master's degree graduates: Enrolled in a postdoctoral residency/fellowship (n/a), employed in independent practice (n/a), total from the above (master's) (0).

Doctoral Degree Graduates: Of those who graduated in the academic year 2008–2009, the following categories and numbers represent the postgraduate activities and employment of doctoral degree graduates: Enrolled in a psychology doctoral program (n/a), total from the above (doctoral) (0).

Additional Information:
Orientation, Objectives, and Emphasis of Department: The clinical psychology PsyD program emphasizes training in clinical skills and clinical application of research knowledge and is designed for students who are interested in careers as practitioners but it also includes a research component. The program is multisystemically or ecosystemically oriented and trains students to consider the role of diverse systems in creating and/or remedying individual and social problems. An empirical PsyD dissertation is required and may focus on program development and/or evaluation, test development, survey research or therapeutic outcomes. The program is offered in an evening/weekend format for working professionals at the Sacramento site. The clinical psychology PhD program puts equal weight on training in clinical, research, and teaching skills. The program is for students whose goal is a teaching career in psychology. Emphasis areas offered are: ecosystemic

clinical child emphasis — trains students to work with infants, children, and adolescents, as well as with the adults in these clients' lives; health psychology emphasis — provides students with exposure to the expanding field of health psychology and behavioral medicine; forensic clinical psychology emphasis — prepares students to practice clinical psychology in a forensic environment. All courses required for an emphasis may not be available at the Sacramento site; students interested in an emphasis may need to travel to Fresno for courses.

Special Facilities or Resources: The Psychological Service Center serves the dual purpose of offering high quality psychological services to the community, particularly underserved segments, and continuing the tradition of education, training and service. The facility consists of eight therapy and two play therapy rooms, large conference room, student work room, TV/monitor, and staff offices. The campus is also home to the Association for Play Therapy.

Application Information:
Send to Alliant International University Admissions Processing Center, 10455 Pomerado Road, San Diego, CA 92131-1799. Application available online. URL of online application: http://www.alliant.edu/applyonline/. Students are admitted in the Fall, application deadline January 15. The programs have a January 15 priority deadline in order to provide a response by April 1 for applicants who need a decision by that date. Programs accept and admit applicants on a space available basis after any stated deadlines. *Fee:* $70. A limited number of application fee waivers are available for students with significant financial need.

Alliant International University: Fresno/Sacramento
Programs in Organizational Psychology
Marshall Goldsmith School of Management
5130 East Clinton Way
Fresno, CA 93727-2014
Telephone: (559) 253-2262
Fax: (559) 253-2267
E-mail: lpyle@alliant.edu
Web: http://mgsm.alliant.edu

Department Information:
1995. Program Director: Carl Mack, PhD. Number of faculty: total—full-time 3, part-time 15; women—full-time 2, part-time 6; total—minority—full-time 1, part-time 2; women minority—part-time 1.

Programs and Degrees Offered:
Listed in the following order: Program area, degree type (T if terminal Master's), number awarded 7/08–6/09. Organizational Behavior MA/MS (Master of Arts/Science) (T) 9, Organization Development PsyD (Doctor of Psychology) 6.

Student Applications/Admissions:
Student Applications
 Organizational Behavior MA/MS (Master of Arts/Science)—Applications 2009–2010, 7. Total applicants accepted 2009–2010, 7. Number full-time enrolled (new admits only) 2009–2010, 5. Number part-time enrolled (new admits only) 2009–2010, 0. Openings 2010–2011, 18. The median number of years required for completion of a degree in 2008–2009 was 1. The number of students enrolled full- and part-time who were dismissed or voluntarily withdrew from this program area in 2008–2009 were 0. *Organization Development PsyD (Doctor of Psychology)*—Applications 2009–2010, 5. Total applicants accepted 2009–2010, 4. Number full-time enrolled (new admits only) 2009–2010, 0. Number part-time enrolled (new admits only) 2009–2010, 2. Total enrolled 2009–2010 full-time, 23, part-time, 14. Openings 2010–2011, 10. The median number of years required for completion of a degree in 2008–2009 were 4. The number of students enrolled full- and part-time who were dismissed or voluntarily withdrew from this program area in 2008–2009 were 0.

Scores: Entries appear in this order: required test or GPA, minimum score (if required), median score of students entering in 2009–2010. *Organizational Behavior MA/MS (Master of Arts/Science)*: overall undergraduate GPA 3.0, 2.8, psychology GPA 3.0; *Organization Development PsyD (Doctor of Psychology)*: overall undergraduate GPA 3.0, 2.71, psychology GPA 3.0.

Other Criteria: (importance of criteria rated low, medium, or high): research experience—low, work experience—high, extracurricular activity—medium, GPA—high, letters of recommendation—high, interview—high, statement of goals and objectives—high. For additional information on admission requirements, go to http://www.alliant.edu/wps/wcm/connect/website/Home/Admissions/.

Student Characteristics: The following represents characteristics of students in 2009–2010 in all graduate psychology programs in the department: Female—full-time 18, part-time 7; Male—full-time 15, part-time 7; African American/Black—full-time 5, part-time 2; Hispanic/Latino(a)—full-time 4, part-time 1; Asian/Pacific Islander—full-time 2, part-time 2; American Indian/Alaska Native—full-time 0, part-time 0; Caucasian/White—full-time 16, part-time 4; Multi-ethnic—full-time 1, part-time 0; students subject to the Americans With Disabilities Act—full-time 0, part-time 2; Unknown ethnicity—full-time 5, part-time 5; International students who hold an F-1 or J-1 Visa—full-time 0, part-time 0.

Financial Information/Assistance:
Tuition for Full-Time Study: *Master's:* State residents: $700 per credit hour; Nonstate residents: $700 per credit hour. *Doctoral:* State residents: $950 per credit hour; Nonstate residents: $950 per credit hour. Tuition is subject to change. Tuition costs vary by program. See the following Web site for updates and changes in tuition costs: http://www.alliant.edu/wps/wcm/connect/website/Home/Admissions/Tuition+and+Fees/.

Financial Assistance:
 First-Year Students: Research assistantships available for first year. Average amount paid per academic year: $1,000. Average number of hours worked per week: 10. Fellowships and scholarships available for first year. Average amount paid per academic year: $1,500. Apply by February 1.
 Advanced Students: Teaching assistantships available for advanced students. Average amount paid per academic year: $3,000. Average number of hours worked per week: 10. Research assistantships available for advanced students. Average amount paid per academic year: $1,000. Average number of hours worked per week: 10. Fellowships and scholarships available for advanced

students. Average amount paid per academic year: $1,500. Apply by April 15.

Additional Information: Of all students currently enrolled full time, 51% benefited from one or more of the listed financial assistance programs.

Internships/Practica: The second and third years of the doctoral program involves a professional placement in organizational studies.

Housing and Day Care: No on-campus housing is available. No on-campus day care facilities are available.

Employment of Department Graduates:
Master's Degree Graduates: Of those who graduated in the academic year 2008–2009, the following categories and numbers represent the postgraduate activities and employment of master's degree graduates: Enrolled in a psychology doctoral program (0), enrolled in a postdoctoral residency/fellowship (n/a), employed in independent practice (n/a), employed in an academic position at a university (0), employed in an academic position at a 2-year/4-year college (0), employed in other positions at a higher education institution (0), employed in a professional position in a school system (0), employed in business or industry (0), employed in government agency (0), employed in a community mental health/counseling center (0), employed in a hospital/medical center (0), still seeking employment (0), not seeking employment (0), other employment position (0), do not know (0), total from the above (master's) (0).
Doctoral Degree Graduates: Of those who graduated in the academic year 2008–2009, the following categories and numbers represent the postgraduate activities and employment of doctoral degree graduates: Enrolled in a psychology doctoral program (n/a), enrolled in another graduate/professional program (0), enrolled in a postdoctoral residency/fellowship (0), employed in independent practice (0), employed in an academic position at a university (0), employed in an academic position at a 2-year/4-year college (0), employed in other positions at a higher education institution (0), employed in a professional position in a school system (0), employed in business or industry (0), employed in government agency (0), employed in a community mental health/counseling center (0), employed in a hospital/medical center (0), still seeking employment (0), not seeking employment (0), other employment position (0), do not know (0), total from the above (doctoral) (0).

Additional Information:
Orientation, Objectives, and Emphasis of Department: The doctoral program prepares students for careers as consultants, leaders/managers, or faculty in community-college or other academic institutions. The program is three-years post-masters and accessible to working adults. Students focus on the individual as a scholar-practitioner, themes and cultures of organizations, and practice in the global community. During the program they learn about managing change in complex organizations, examine and assess organizational procedures and processes, design interventions at the system/group/individual levels, and learn skills for OD consulting and conducting applied research. A PsyD project is a required part of the program. The master's program is a two year program for working professionals and may be taken jointly with another doctoral program at Alliant in Fresno. The program has a practical curriculum related to management issues involving people and organizational processes. The PsyD program is accredited by the Organization Development Institute.

Special Facilities or Resources: The Marshall Goldsmith School of Management operates the Organizational Consulting Center (OCC). Students may have opportunities to participate with faculty and OCC associates on consulting projects during their programs.

Application Information:
Send to Alliant International University, Admissions Processing Center, 10455 Pomerado Road, San Diego, CA 92131-1799. Application available online. URL of online application: http://www.alliant.edu/applyonline/. Students are admitted in the Fall, application deadline February 1; Winter, application deadline November 1; Spring, application deadline varies; Programs have rolling admissions. Doctoral program has a February 1 deadline in order to provide a response by April 1 for applicants who need a decsion by that date. The program accepts applications and admits students on a space available basis after any stated deadlines. *Fee:* $70. A limited number of fee waivers are available to those with significant financial need.

Alliant International University: Irvine
Forensic Psychology Program
California School of Forensic Studies
2500 Michelson Drive, Building 400
Irvine, CA 92612-1548
Telephone: (949) 833-2651
Fax: (949) 833-3507
E-mail: *rpettay@alliant.edu*
Web: *http://www.alliant.edu*

Department Information:
2007. Program Director: Sean Sterling, PhD. Number of faculty: total—full-time 3, part-time 7; women—full-time 1, part-time 5; minority—part-time 1; women minority—part-time 1.

Programs and Degrees Offered:
Listed in the following order: Program area, degree type (T if terminal Master's), number awarded 7/08–6/09. Forensic Psychology PsyD (Doctor of Psychology) 0.

Student Applications/Admissions:
Student Applications
Forensic Psychology PsyD (Doctor of Psychology)—Applications 2009–2010, 30. Total applicants accepted 2009–2010, 26. Number full-time enrolled (new admits only) 2009–2010, 15. Number part-time enrolled (new admits only) 2009–2010, 4. Total enrolled 2009–2010 full-time, 39, part-time, 6. Openings 2010–2011, 15. The number of students enrolled full- and part-time who were dismissed or voluntarily withdrew from this program area in 2008–2009 were 0.
Scores: Entries appear in this order: required test or GPA, minimum score (if required), median score of students entering in 2009–2010. *Forensic Psychology PsyD (Doctor of Psychology):* overall undergraduate GPA 3.0, 3.1, psychology GPA 3.0.
Other Criteria: (importance of criteria rated low, medium, or high): research experience—medium, work experience—high, extracurricular activity—low, clinically related public ser-

vice—high, GPA—high, letters of recommendation—high, interview—high, statement of goals and objectives—high. For additional information on admission requirements, go to http://www.alliant.edu/wps/wcm/connect/website/Home/Admissions/.

Student Characteristics: The following represents characteristics of students in 2009–2010 in all graduate psychology programs in the department: Female—full-time 33, part-time 4; Male—full-time 6, part-time 2; African American/Black—full-time 5, part-time 0; Hispanic/Latino(a)—full-time 6, part-time 1; Asian/Pacific Islander—full-time 4, part-time 1; American Indian/Alaska Native—full-time 0, part-time 0; Caucasian/White—full-time 18, part-time 2; Multi-ethnic—full-time 2, part-time 0; students subject to the Americans With Disabilities Act—full-time 1, part-time 0; Unknown ethnicity—full-time 4, part-time 2; International students who hold an F-1 or J-1 Visa—full-time 0, part-time 0.

Financial Information/Assistance:
Tuition for Full-Time Study: *Doctoral:* State residents: $950 per credit hour; Nonstate residents: $950 per credit hour. Tuition is subject to change. See the following Web site for updates and changes in tuition costs: http://www.alliant.edu/wps/wcm/connect/website/Home/Admissions/Tuition+and+Fees/.

Financial Assistance:
First-Year Students: Research assistantships available for first year. Average amount paid per academic year: $1,000. Average number of hours worked per week: 10. Fellowships and scholarships available for first year. Average amount paid per academic year: $1,500. Apply by February 15.
Advanced Students: Teaching assistantships available for advanced students. Average amount paid per academic year: $3,000. Research assistantships available for advanced students. Average amount paid per academic year: $1,000. Fellowships and scholarships available for advanced students. Average amount paid per academic year: $1,500. Apply by February 15.
Additional Information: Application and information available online at: https://www.e-fao.com/efao_site.html?OEID=011117&ViewID={10EF815B-422E-4C55-B8CD-BDBD3063BA18}.

Internships/Practica: A one year predoctoral internship is part of the program; this occurs in the fourth/fifth year, depending on the student's pace through the program.

Housing and Day Care: No on-campus housing is available. No on-campus day care facilities are available.

Employment of Department Graduates:
Master's Degree Graduates: Of those who graduated in the academic year 2008–2009, the following categories and numbers represent the postgraduate activities and employment of master's degree graduates: Enrolled in a postdoctoral residency/fellowship (n/a), employed in independent practice (n/a), total from the above (master's) (0).
Doctoral Degree Graduates: Of those who graduated in the academic year 2008–2009, the following categories and numbers represent the postgraduate activities and employment of doctoral degree graduates: Enrolled in a psychology doctoral program (n/a), total from the above (doctoral) (0).

Additional Information:
Orientation, Objectives, and Emphasis of Department: The PsyD program has an applied psychology orientation and is offered in a part-time five-year curriculum. This format attracts students with prior work experience from a variety of fields. The curriculum prepares students to conduct assessments for the courts, to serve as expert witnesses, or to work as mental health treatment providers in a variety of forensic settings, including prisons, jails, offender treatment groups, and youth facilities, among many others. Core areas include forensic psychology, theories of crime and justice, industrial and organizational psychology, legal research, psychopathology, research design and data analysis, forensic mediation and dispute resolution, ethics, and substance abuse theory and treatment. While licensure is not required for most forensic careers, some students who enter the program may choose to seek clinical licensure after graduating from the program. These students take additional courses in psychology that are required in order to be eligible to sit for the psychology licensing exam.

Application Information:
Send to Alliant International University, Admissions Processing Center, 10455 Pomerado Road, San Diego CA 92131-1799. Application available online. URL of online application: https://www.alliant.edu/applyonline/. Students are admitted in the Fall, application deadline varies; Spring, application deadline varies; Programs have rolling admissions. Applicants wishing notification by April 1 should submit their applications in January. however, applications are welcomed on a rolling basis and will be processed on a space available basis. *Fee:* $70. A limited number of fee waivers are available for those with significant financial need.

Alliant International University: Irvine
Marital and Family Therapy Program
California School of Professional Psychology
2500 Michelson Drive, Building 400
Irvine, CA 92612-1548
Telephone: (949) 812-7469
Fax: (949) 833-3507
E-mail: *jkulbeck@alliant.edu*
Web: *http://www.alliant.edu/cspp*

Department Information:
1973. Program Director: Scott Woolley, PhD. Number of faculty: total—full-time 6, part-time 23; women—full-time 4, part-time 16; total—minority—full-time 2, part-time 5; women minority—full-time 2, part-time 3.

Programs and Degrees Offered:
Listed in the following order: Program area, degree type (T if terminal Master's), number awarded 7/08–6/09. Marital and Family Therapy MA/MS (Master of Arts/Science) (T) 11, Marital and Family Therapy PsyD (Doctor of Psychology) 9.

Student Applications/Admissions:
Student Applications
Marital and Family Therapy MA/MS (Master of Arts/Science)—Applications 2009–2010, 57. Total applicants accepted 2009–2010, 34. Number full-time enrolled (new admits only) 2009–2010, 23. Number part-time enrolled (new admits only) 2009–

2010, 0. Total enrolled 2009–2010 full-time, 48, part-time, 7. Openings 2010–2011, 15. The median number of years required for completion of a degree in 2008–2009 were 2. The number of students enrolled full- and part-time who were dismissed or voluntarily withdrew from this program area in 2008–2009 were 4. *Marital and Family Therapy PsyD (Doctor of Psychology)*—Applications 2009–2010, 25. Total applicants accepted 2009–2010, 15. Number full-time enrolled (new admits only) 2009–2010, 9. Number part-time enrolled (new admits only) 2009–2010, 1. Total enrolled 2009–2010 full-time, 38, part-time, 50. Openings 2010–2011, 15. The median number of years required for completion of a degree in 2008–2009 were 4. The number of students enrolled full- and part-time who were dismissed or voluntarily withdrew from this program area in 2008–2009 were 4.

Scores: Entries appear in this order: required test or GPA, minimum score (if required), median score of students entering in 2009–2010. *Marital and Family Therapy MA/MS (Master of Arts/Science):* overall undergraduate GPA 3.0, 3.04, psychology GPA 3.0; *Marital and Family Therapy PsyD (Doctor of Psychology):* overall undergraduate GPA 3.0, 3.58, psychology GPA 3.0.

Other Criteria: (importance of criteria rated low, medium, or high): research experience—medium, work experience—medium, extracurricular activity—low, clinically related public service—medium, GPA—high, letters of recommendation—medium, interview—high, statement of goals and objectives—high, undergraduate major in psychology—medium, specific undergraduate psychology courses taken—medium. For additional information on admission requirements, go to http://www.alliant.edu/wps/wcm/connect/website/Home/Admissions/Graduate+Student+Admissions/.

Student Characteristics: The following represents characteristics of students in 2009–2010 in all graduate psychology programs in the department: Female—full-time 73, part-time 49; Male—full-time 13, part-time 8; African American/Black—full-time 1, part-time 2; Hispanic/Latino(a)—full-time 11, part-time 8; Asian/Pacific Islander—full-time 13, part-time 8; American Indian/Alaska Native—full-time 2, part-time 2; Caucasian/White—full-time 39, part-time 25; Multi-ethnic—full-time 6, part-time 1; students subject to the Americans With Disabilities Act—full-time 1, part-time 1; Unknown ethnicity—full-time 14, part-time 11; International students who hold an F-1 or J-1 Visa—full-time 1, part-time 0.

Financial Information/Assistance:
Tuition for Full-Time Study: *Master's:* State residents: $950 per credit hour; Nonstate residents: $950 per credit hour. *Doctoral:* State residents: $950 per credit hour; Nonstate residents: $950 per credit hour. Tuition is subject to change. Tuition costs vary by program. See the following Web site for updates and changes in tuition costs: http://www.alliant.edu/wps/wcm/connect/website/Home/Admissions/Tuition+and+Fees/.

Financial Assistance:
First-Year Students: Research assistantships available for first year. Average amount paid per academic year: $1,000. Average number of hours worked per week: 10. Fellowships and scholarships available for first year. Average amount paid per academic year: $750. Apply by January 15.

Advanced Students: Teaching assistantships available for advanced students. Average amount paid per academic year: $3,000. Average number of hours worked per week: 10. Research assistantships available for advanced students. Average amount paid per academic year: $1,000. Average number of hours worked per week: 10. Fellowships and scholarships available for advanced students. Average amount paid per academic year: $750.

Additional Information: Of all students currently enrolled full time, 58% benefited from one or more of the listed financial assistance programs. Application and information available online at: https://www.e-fao.com/eFAO_site.html?OEID=011117&ViewID={10EF815B-422E-4C55-B8CD-BDBD3063BA18}.

Internships/Practica: As part of the practicum experience, students complete 500 client contact hours, 250 of which must be with couples and families. Students receive at least 100 hours of individual and group supervision, 50 hours of which are based on direct observation, videotape, or audiotape. At least 25 of those hours must be videotape or direct observation. When students are ready to begin practicum, experienced faculty and staff assist students through each step in obtaining a field placement site approved by Alliant. While students are doing practicum training they are required to perform marriage and family therapy under a California state licensed, AAMFT-approved supervisor or the equivalent.

Housing and Day Care: No on-campus housing is available. No on-campus day care facilities are available.

Employment of Department Graduates:
Master's Degree Graduates: Of those who graduated in the academic year 2008–2009, the following categories and numbers represent the postgraduate activities and employment of master's degree graduates: Enrolled in a postdoctoral residency/fellowship (n/a), employed in independent practice (n/a), total from the above (master's) (0).

Doctoral Degree Graduates: Of those who graduated in the academic year 2008–2009, the following categories and numbers represent the postgraduate activities and employment of doctoral degree graduates: Enrolled in a psychology doctoral program (n/a), total from the above (doctoral) (0).

Additional Information:
Orientation, Objectives, and Emphasis of Department: The mission of the Marital and Family Therapy Program is to prepare graduate students who are skilled in the theory, research, and clinical practice of the field of Marriage and Family Therapy and can integrate individual and systemic therapeutic models in an international, multicultural environment. The Marital and Family Therapy (MFT) programs provide students with the essential training needed to pursue a career as a professional marriage and family therapist. The Master of Arts in MFT allows students to be licensed as a marital and family therapist (MFT) and the Doctor of Psychology in MFT allows a student to be licensed as a marital and family therapist and/or as a psychologist. Students who complete the MFT Masters at Alliant can apply all of their masters degree coursework and practicum hours toward the doctoral program. The programs are accredited by COAMFTE.

Application Information:
Send to Alliant International University Admissions Processing Center, 10455 Pomerado Road, San Diego CA 92131-1799. Application

available online. URL of online application: http://www.alliant.edu/applyonline/. Students are admitted in the Fall, application deadline January 15; Programs have rolling admissions. Applications for the Fall semester are due January 15 (priority deadline), March 1, and April 16. Applications received after the priority deadline are considered on a space-available basis. *Fee:* $70. A limited number of fee waivers are available for those with significant financial need.

Alliant International University: Irvine
Programs in Educational and School Psychology
Hufstedler School of Education
2500 Michelson Drive, Building 400
Irvine, CA 92612-1548
Telephone: (949) 833-2651
Fax: (949) 833-3507
E-mail: *kjanowsky@alliant.edu*
Web: *http://www.alliant.edu*

Department Information:
2002. Program Director: Donald Wofford, PsyD. Number of faculty: total—full-time 1, part-time 24; women—part-time 15; minority—part-time 3; women minority—part-time 2.

Programs and Degrees Offered:
Listed in the following order: Program area, degree type (T if terminal Master's), number awarded 7/08–6/09. Educational Psychology PsyD (Doctor of Psychology) 6, School Psychology MA/MS (Master of Arts/Science) (T) 6.

Student Applications/Admissions:
Student Applications
Educational Psychology PsyD (Doctor of Psychology)—Applications 2009–2010, 7. Total applicants accepted 2009–2010, 7. Number full-time enrolled (new admits only) 2009–2010, 0. Number part-time enrolled (new admits only) 2009–2010, 4. Openings 2010–2011, 15. The median number of years required for completion of a degree in 2008–2009 were 3. The number of students enrolled full- and part-time who were dismissed or voluntarily withdrew from this program area in 2008–2009 were 0. *School Psychology MA/MS (Master of Arts/Science)*—Applications 2009–2010, 16. Total applicants accepted 2009–2010, 13. Number full-time enrolled (new admits only) 2009–2010, 10. Number part-time enrolled (new admits only) 2009–2010, 0. Total enrolled 2009–2010 full-time, 19, part-time, 8. Openings 2010–2011, 18. The median number of years required for completion of a degree in 2008–2009 were 2. The number of students enrolled full- and part-time who were dismissed or voluntarily withdrew from this program area in 2008–2009 were 2.
Scores: Entries appear in this order: required test or GPA, minimum score (if required), median score of students entering in 2009–2010. *Educational Psychology PsyD (Doctor of Psychology)*: overall undergraduate GPA 3.0, psychology GPA 3.0; *School Psychology MA/MS (Master of Arts/Science)*: overall undergraduate GPA 2.5, 2.98, psychology GPA 2.5.
Other Criteria: (importance of criteria rated low, medium, or high): research experience—medium, work experience—medium, extracurricular activity—low, clinically related public service—high, GPA—high, letters of recommendation—high, interview—high, statement of goals and objectives—high. For additional information on admission requirements, go to http://www.alliant.edu/wps/wcm/connect/website/Home/Admissions/.

Student Characteristics: The following represents characteristics of students in 2009–2010 in all graduate psychology programs in the department: Female—full-time 16, part-time 24; Male—full-time 3, part-time 2; African American/Black—full-time 1, part-time 1; Hispanic/Latino(a)—full-time 1, part-time 5; Asian/Pacific Islander—full-time 5, part-time 2; American Indian/Alaska Native—full-time 0, part-time 0; Caucasian/White—full-time 9, part-time 16; Multi-ethnic—full-time 0, part-time 0; students subject to the Americans With Disabilities Act—full-time 0, part-time 0; Unknown ethnicity—full-time 3, part-time 2; International students who hold an F-1 or J-1 Visa—full-time 0, part-time 0.

Financial Information/Assistance:
Tuition for Full-Time Study: *Master's:* State residents: $540 per credit hour; Nonstate residents: $540 per credit hour. *Doctoral:* State residents: $880 per credit hour; Nonstate residents: $880 per credit hour. Tuition is subject to change. Tuition costs vary by program. See the following Web site for updates and changes in tuition costs: http://www.alliant.edu/wps/wcm/connect/website/Home/Admissions/Tuition+and+Fees/.

Financial Assistance:
First-Year Students: Research assistantships available for first year. Average amount paid per academic year: $1,000. Average number of hours worked per week: 10. Fellowships and scholarships available for first year. Average amount paid per academic year: $750. Apply by June 1.
Advanced Students: Teaching assistantships available for advanced students. Average amount paid per academic year: $3,000. Average number of hours worked per week: 10. Research assistantships available for advanced students. Average amount paid per academic year: $1,000. Average number of hours worked per week: 10. Fellowships and scholarships available for advanced students. Average amount paid per academic year: $750. Apply by April 1.
Additional Information: Of all students currently enrolled full time, 40% benefited from one or more of the listed financial assistance programs. Application and information available online at: https://www.e-fao.com/efao_site.html?OEID=011117&ViewID={10EF815B-422E-4C55-B8CD-BDBD3063BA18}.

Internships/Practica: Students in the master's program have practica tied to their coursework beginning in the first semester of their programs. Internships are required of students seeking a Pupil Personnel Services (PPS) credential post-masters or as part of the doctoral program in educational psychology. The 1200 required internship hours are completed at a public school district. Students interested in seeking clinical licensure must complete a separate psychology internship.

Housing and Day Care: No on-campus housing is available. No on-campus day care facilities are available.

Employment of Department Graduates:
Master's Degree Graduates: Of those who graduated in the academic year 2008–2009, the following categories and numbers

represent the postgraduate activities and employment of master's degree graduates: Enrolled in a postdoctoral residency/fellowship (n/a), employed in independent practice (n/a), total from the above (master's) (0).

Doctoral Degree Graduates: Of those who graduated in the academic year 2008–2009, the following categories and numbers represent the postgraduate activities and employment of doctoral degree graduates: Enrolled in a psychology doctoral program (n/a), total from the above (doctoral) (0).

Additional Information:
Orientation, Objectives, and Emphasis of Department: Programs train students with the skills necessary to work with students, teachers, parents, and other professionals in today's school environments. Curriculum includes professional skills, professional roles courses, applied research, and professional concepts. The master's degree program prepares students to gain the PPS (Pupil Personnel Services) credential that allows them to practice in California's schools. Students take afternoon, evening, and weekend classes and engage in fieldwork. At the doctoral level, students complete special focus area courses, examples of which include adolescent stress and coping, school culture and administration, pediatric psychology, infant and preschool mental health, child neuropsychology, and provision of services for children in alternative placement. Students also complete a PsyD project.

Application Information:
Send to Alliant International University, Admissions Processing Center, 10455 Pomerado Road, San Diego CA 92131-1799. Application available online. URL of online application: http://www.alliant.edu/applyonline/. Students are admitted in the Fall, application deadline June 1; Spring, application deadline varies; Summer, application deadline varies. *Fee:* $55. A limited number of fee waivers are available to those with significant financial need.

Alliant International University: Los Angeles
Forensic Psychology Programs
California School of Forensic Studies
1000 South Fremont Avenue
Alhambra, CA 91803-1360
Telephone: (626) 284-2777
Fax: (626) 284-0550
E-mail: *rpettay@alliant.edu*
Web: *http://www.alliant.edu/*

Department Information:
1999. Program Director: Deborah Miora, PhD. Number of faculty: total—full-time 7, part-time 8; women—full-time 6, part-time 3.

Programs and Degrees Offered:
Listed in the following order: Program area, degree type (T if terminal Master's), number awarded 7/08–6/09. Forensic Psychology PsyD (Doctor of Psychology) 6.

Student Applications/Admissions:
Student Applications
Forensic Psychology PsyD (Doctor of Psychology)—Applications 2009–2010, 45. Total applicants accepted 2009–2010, 33. Number full-time enrolled (new admits only) 2009–2010, 24. Number part-time enrolled (new admits only) 2009–2010, 0. Total enrolled 2009–2010 full-time, 85, part-time, 6. Openings 2010–2011, 25. The median number of years required for completion of a degree in 2008–2009 were 6. The number of students enrolled full- and part-time who were dismissed or voluntarily withdrew from this program area in 2008–2009 were 6.

Scores: Entries appear in this order: required test or GPA, minimum score (if required), median score of students entering in 2009–2010. *Forensic Psychology PsyD (Doctor of Psychology):* overall undergraduate GPA 3.0, 3.16, psychology GPA 3.0.

Other Criteria: (importance of criteria rated low, medium, or high): research experience—medium, work experience—high, extracurricular activity—low, clinically related public service—high, GPA—high, letters of recommendation—high, interview—high, statement of goals and objectives—high. For additional information on admission requirements, go to http://www.alliant.edu/wps/wcm/connect/website/Home/Admissions/.

Student Characteristics: The following represents characteristics of students in 2009–2010 in all graduate psychology programs in the department: Female—full-time 72, part-time 3; Male—full-time 13, part-time 3; African American/Black—full-time 8, part-time 1; Hispanic/Latino(a)—full-time 14, part-time 1; Asian/Pacific Islander—full-time 6, part-time 0; American Indian/Alaska Native—full-time 0, part-time 0; Caucasian/White—full-time 37, part-time 3; Multi-ethnic—full-time 4, part-time 1; students subject to the Americans With Disabilities Act—full-time 0, part-time 0; Unknown ethnicity—full-time 16, part-time 0; International students who hold an F-1 or J-1 Visa—full-time 0, part-time 0.

Financial Information/Assistance:
Tuition for Full-Time Study: Doctoral: State residents: $950 per credit hour; Nonstate residents: $950 per credit hour. Tuition is subject to change. See the following Web site for updates and changes in tuition costs: http://www.alliant.edu/wps/wcm/connect/website/Home/Admissions/Tuition+and+Fees/.

Financial Assistance:
First-Year Students: Research assistantships available for first year. Average amount paid per academic year: $1,000. Average number of hours worked per week: 10. Fellowships and scholarships available for first year. Average amount paid per academic year: $1,500. Apply by February 15.

Advanced Students: Teaching assistantships available for advanced students. Average amount paid per academic year: $3,000. Average number of hours worked per week: 20. Research assistantships available for advanced students. Average amount paid per academic year: $1,000. Average number of hours worked per week: 10. Fellowships and scholarships available for advanced students. Average amount paid per academic year: $1,500. Apply by February 15.

Additional Information: Of all students currently enrolled full time, 52% benefited from one or more of the listed financial assistance programs. Application and information available online at: https://www.e-fao.com/efao_site.html?OEID=011117&ViewID={10EF815B-422E-4C55-B8CD-BDBD3063BA18}.

Internships/Practica: Doctoral Degree (PsyD Forensic Psychology): For those doctoral students for whom a professional internship was required in this program prior to graduation, (17) students applied for an internship in 2008–2009, with (17) students obtaining an internship. Of those students who obtained an internship, (7) were paid internships. Of those students who obtained an internship, (0) students placed in APA/CPA accredited internships, (4) students placed in internships not APA/CPA accredited, but listed with the Association of Psychology Postdoctoral and Internship Programs (APPIC), (0) students placed in internships conforming to guidelines of the Council of Directors of School Psychology Programs (CDSPP), (13) students placed in internships that were not APA/CPA accredited, APPIC or CDSPP listed. A one year predoctoral internship is part of the program; this occurs in the fifth year of the program.

Housing and Day Care: No on-campus housing is available. No on-campus day care facilities are available.

Employment of Department Graduates:
Master's Degree Graduates: Of those who graduated in the academic year 2008–2009, the following categories and numbers represent the postgraduate activities and employment of master's degree graduates: Enrolled in a postdoctoral residency/fellowship (n/a), employed in independent practice (n/a), total from the above (master's) (0).
Doctoral Degree Graduates: Of those who graduated in the academic year 2008–2009, the following categories and numbers represent the postgraduate activities and employment of doctoral degree graduates: Enrolled in a psychology doctoral program (n/a), total from the above (doctoral) (0).

Additional Information:
Orientation, Objectives, and Emphasis of Department: The PsyD program has an applied psychology orientation and is offered in a part-time five-year curriculum. This format attracts students with prior work experience from a variety of fields. The curriculum prepares students to conduct assessments for the courts, to serve as expert witnesses, or to work as mental health treatment providers in a variety of forensic settings, including prisons, jails, offender treatment groups, youth facilities, among many others. Core areas include forensic psychology, theories of crime and justice, industrial and organizational psychology, legal research, psychopathology, research design and data analysis, forensic mediation and dispute resolution, ethics, and substance abuse theory and treatment. While licensure is not required for most forensic careers, some students who enter the program may choose to seek clinical licensure after graduating from the program. These students take additional courses in psychology that are required in order to be eligible to sit for the psychology licensing exam.

Application Information:
Send to Alliant International University, Admissions Processing Center, 10455 Pomerado Road, San Diego CA 92131-1799. Application available online. URL of online application: http://www.alliant.edu/applyonline/. Students are admitted in the Fall, application deadline varies; Spring, application deadline varies; Programs have rolling admissions. Applicants wishing notification by April 1 should submit their applications in January. However, applications are welcomed on a rolling basis and will be processed on a space available basis. *Fee:* $70. A limited number of fee waivers are available for those with significant financial need.

Alliant International University: Los Angeles
Programs in Clinical Psychology and Marital and Family Therapy
California School of Professional Psychology
1000 South Fremont Avenue, Unit 5
Alhambra, CA 91803-1360
Telephone: (626) 270-3315
Fax: (626) 284-0550
E-mail: *jkulbeck@alliant.edu*
Web: *http://www.alliant.edu/cspp/*

Department Information:
1970. Dean, California School of Professional Psychology: Morgan T. Sammons, PhD, ABPP. Number of faculty: total—full-time 31, part-time 58; women—full-time 15, part-time 33; total—minority—full-time 11, part-time 18; women minority—full-time 8, part-time 10; faculty subject to the Americans With Disabilities Act 1.

Programs and Degrees Offered:
Listed in the following order: Program area, degree type (T if terminal Master's), number awarded 7/08–6/09. Clinical Psychology PsyD (Doctor of Psychology) 73, Clinical Psychology PhD (Doctor of Philosophy) 26, Marital and Family Therapy MA/MS (Master of Arts/Science) (T) 0.

APA Accreditation: Clinical PsyD (Doctor of Psychology). Clinical PhD (Doctor of Philosophy).

Student Applications/Admissions:
Student Applications
Clinical Psychology PsyD (Doctor of Psychology)—Applications 2009–2010, 193. Total applicants accepted 2009–2010, 98. Number full-time enrolled (new admits only) 2009–2010, 68. Number part-time enrolled (new admits only) 2009–2010, 0. Total enrolled 2009–2010 full-time, 262, part-time, 16. Openings 2010–2011, 65. The median number of years required for completion of a degree in 2008–2009 were 4. The number of students enrolled full- and part-time who were dismissed or voluntarily withdrew from this program area in 2008–2009 were 4. *Clinical Psychology PhD (Doctor of Philosophy)*—Applications 2009–2010, 74. Total applicants accepted 2009–2010, 37. Number full-time enrolled (new admits only) 2009–2010, 25. Number part-time enrolled (new admits only) 2009–2010, 0. Total enrolled 2009–2010 full-time, 141, part-time, 5. Openings 2010–2011, 25. The median number of years required for completion of a degree in 2008–2009 were 5. The number of students enrolled full- and part-time who were dismissed or voluntarily withdrew from this program area in 2008–2009 were 1. *Marital and Family Therapy MA/MS (Master of Arts/Science)*—Applications 2009–2010, 48. Total applicants accepted 2009–2010, 30. Number full-time enrolled (new admits only) 2009–2010, 13. Number part-time enrolled (new admits only) 2009–2010, 0. Total enrolled 2009–2010 full-time, 21, part-time, 1. Openings 2010–2011, 15. The number of students enrolled full- and part-time who were dismissed or voluntarily withdrew from this program area in 2008–2009 were 0.

Scores: Entries appear in this order: required test or GPA, minimum score (if required), median score of students entering

in 2009–2010. *Clinical Psychology PsyD (Doctor of Psychology)*: overall undergraduate GPA 3.0, 3.32, psychology GPA 3.0; *Clinical Psychology PhD (Doctor of Philosophy)*: overall undergraduate GPA 3.0, 3.23, psychology GPA 3.0; *Marital and Family Therapy MA/MS (Master of Arts/Science)*: overall undergraduate GPA 3.0, 3.17, psychology GPA 3.0.

Other Criteria: (importance of criteria rated low, medium, or high): research experience—medium, work experience—medium, extracurricular activity—low, clinically related public service—medium, GPA—high, letters of recommendation—medium, interview—high, statement of goals and objectives—high, undergraduate major in psychology—medium, specific undergraduate psychology courses taken—medium. For additional information on admission requirements, go to http://www.alliant.edu/wps/wcm/connect/website/Home/Admissions/Graduate+Student+Admissions/.

Student Characteristics: The following represents characteristics of students in 2009–2010 in all graduate psychology programs in the department: Female—full-time 347, part-time 17; Male—full-time 77, part-time 5; African American/Black—full-time 17, part-time 1; Hispanic/Latino(a)—full-time 61, part-time 5; Asian/Pacific Islander—full-time 66, part-time 2; American Indian/Alaska Native—full-time 2, part-time 0; Caucasian/White—full-time 172, part-time 11; Multi-ethnic—full-time 10, part-time 1; students subject to the Americans With Disabilities Act—full-time 3, part-time 1; Unknown ethnicity—full-time 96, part-time 2; International students who hold an F-1 or J-1 Visa—full-time 10, part-time 0.

Financial Information/Assistance:
Tuition for Full-Time Study: *Master's:* State residents: $950 per credit hour; Nonstate residents: $950 per credit hour. *Doctoral:* State residents: $950 per credit hour; Nonstate residents: $950 per credit hour. Tuition is subject to change. See the following Web site for updates and changes in tuition costs: http://www.alliant.edu/wps/wcm/connect/website/Home/Admissions/Tuition+and+Fees/.

Financial Assistance:
First-Year Students: Research assistantships available for first year. Average amount paid per academic year: $1,000. Average number of hours worked per week: 10. Fellowships and scholarships available for first year. Average amount paid per academic year: $1,500. Apply by January 15.

Advanced Students: Teaching assistantships available for advanced students. Average amount paid per academic year: $3,000. Average number of hours worked per week: 10. Research assistantships available for advanced students. Average amount paid per academic year: $1,000. Average number of hours worked per week: 10. Traineeships available for advanced students. Average number of hours worked per week: 25. Apply by variable. Fellowships and scholarships available for advanced students. Average amount paid per academic year: $1,500. Apply by April 15.

Additional Information: Of all students currently enrolled full time, 57% benefited from one or more of the listed financial assistance programs. Application and information available online at: https://www.e-fao.com/eFAO_site.html?OEID=011117&ViewID={10EF815B-422E-4C55-B8CD-BDBD3063BA18}.

Internships/Practica: Doctoral Degree (PsyD Clinical Psychology): For those doctoral students for whom a professional internship was required in this program prior to graduation, (166) students applied for an internship in 2008–2009, with (166) students obtaining an internship. Of those students who obtained an internship, (25) were paid internships. Of those students who obtained an internship, (3) students placed in APA/CPA accredited internships, (6) students placed in internships not APA/CPA accredited, but listed with the Association of Psychology Postdoctoral and Internship Programs (APPIC), (0) students placed in internships conforming to guidelines of the Council of Directors of School Psychology Programs (CDSPP), (157) students placed in internships that were not APA/CPA accredited, APPIC or CDSPP listed. Doctoral Degree (PhD Clinical Psychology): For those doctoral students for whom a professional internship was required in this program prior to graduation, (58) students applied for an internship in 2008–2009, with (57) students obtaining an internship. Of those students who obtained an internship, (12) were paid internships. Of those students who obtained an internship, (4) students placed in APA/CPA accredited internships, (3) students placed in internships not APA/CPA accredited, but listed with the Association of Psychology Postdoctoral and Internship Programs (APPIC), (0) students placed in internships conforming to guidelines of the Council of Directors of School Psychology Programs (CDSPP), (50) students placed in internships that were not APA/CPA accredited, APPIC or CDSPP listed. All students engage in practica and internships. Clinical psychology students complete 2000 predoctoral internship hours as part of their programs. The majority of the professional training sites are within 40 miles of the campus. These agencies serve a diverse range of individuals across ethnicity, culture, religion, and sexual orientation. These sites provide excellent training, offering a variety of theoretical orientations related to children, adolescents, adults, families and the elderly. Students who wish to pursue full-time internships are encouraged to make applications throughout the country. Marital and Family Therapy students complete 500 client contact hours, 250 of which must be with couples and families. Students receive at least 100 hours of individual and group supervision, 50 hours of which are based on direct observation, videotape, or audiotape. At least 25 of those hours must be videotape or direct observation. When students are ready to begin practicum, experienced faculty and staff assist students through each step in obtaining a field placement site approved by Alliant. While students are doing practicum training they are required to perform marriage and family therapy under a California state licensed, AAMFT-approved supervisor or the equivalent.

Housing and Day Care: No on-campus housing is available. No on-campus day care facilities are available.

Employment of Department Graduates:
Master's Degree Graduates: Of those who graduated in the academic year 2008–2009, the following categories and numbers represent the postgraduate activities and employment of master's degree graduates: Enrolled in a postdoctoral residency/fellowship (n/a), employed in independent practice (n/a), total from the above (master's) (0).

Doctoral Degree Graduates: Of those who graduated in the academic year 2008–2009, the following categories and numbers represent the postgraduate activities and employment of doctoral degree graduates: Enrolled in a psychology doctoral program (n/a), total from the above (doctoral) (0).

GRADUATE STUDY IN PSYCHOLOGY

Additional Information:
Orientation, Objectives, and Emphasis of Department: The clinical psychology PsyD and PhD programs at the California School of Professional Psychology prepare students to function as multifaceted clinical psychologists through a curriculum based on an integration of psychological theory, research, and practice. Students develop competencies in seven areas: clinical health psychology; interpersonal/relationship; assessment; multifaceted multimodal intervention; research and evaluation; consultation/teaching; management/supervision/training; and quality assurance. The PsyD program is a practitioner program where candidates gain relatively greater mastery in assessment, intervention, and management/supervision. The PhD program is a based on a scholar-practitioner model where practice and scholarship receive equal emphasis and includes the following guiding principles: the generation and application of knowledge must occur with an awareness of the sociocultural and sociopolitical contexts of mental health and mental illness; scholarship and practice must not only build upon existing literature but also maintain relevance to the diverse elements in our society and assume the challenges of attending to the complex social issues associated with psychological functioning; and methods of research and intervention must be appropriate to the culture in which they are conducted. Practicum and internship experiences are integrated throughout the programs. Students have the opportunity to choose a curricular emphasis in clinical health psychology, multicultural community clinical, or family and couple clinical psychology. The mission of the Marital and Family Therapy program is to prepare graduate students who are skilled in the theory, research, and clinical practice of the field of Marriage and Family Therapy and can integrate individual and systemic therapeutic models in an international, multicultural environment. The Marital and Family Therapy (MFT) program provides students with the essential training needed to pursue a career as a professional marriage and family therapist. The Master of Arts in MFT allows students to be licensed as a marital and family therapist (MFT). The program is accredited by COAMFTE.

Special Facilities or Resources: The Psychological Services Center (PSC) is charged with the mission of developing professional training, research, and consultation opportunities for CSPP faculty and students, while providing services to a variety of public/private agencies. It is committed to developing effective and innovative service strategies and resources that address the needs of a wide range of clients; with a particular focus on ethnically diverse, underserved populations. As a center "without walls," the PSC is the administrative umbrella for two major community-based programs: the Children, Youth, and Family Consortium and the School Court Accountability Project. These projects are designed to provide hands-on research, consulting, and clinical experience for students and to enhance the critically needed services to school-aged youth within the court system and school-aged populations. These programs enable participating CSPP faculty, staff, students, alumni/ae, and external consultant associates to provide services few other institutions can offer. Students also receive unique training and supervision that prepares them for critically needed roles as community advocates and leaders.

Application Information:
Send to Alliant International University, Admissions Processing Center, 10455 Pomerado Road, San Diego, CA 92131-1799. Application available online. URL of online application: http://www.alliant.edu/applyonline/. Students are admitted in the Fall, application deadline January 15; Programs have rolling admissions. The programs have a January 15 priority deadline in order to provide a response by April 1 for applicants who need a decision by that date. Programs accept applications and admit students on a space-available basis after any stated deadlines. *Fee:* $70. A limited number of application fee waivers are available for students with significant financial need.

Alliant International University: Los Angeles
Programs in Educational and School Psychology
Hufstedler School of Education
1000 South Fremont Avenue
Alhambra, CA 91803-1360
Telephone: (626) 284-2777
Fax: (626) 284-0550
E-mail: *kjanowsky@alliant.edu*
Web: *http://www.alliant.edu*

Department Information:
1999. Systemwide Program Director: Donald Wofford, PsyD. Number of faculty: total—full-time 2, part-time 24; women—part-time 18; total—minority—full-time 1, part-time 8; women minority—part-time 7.

Programs and Degrees Offered:
Listed in the following order: Program area, degree type (T if terminal Master's), number awarded 7/08–6/09. School Psychology MA/MS (Master of Arts/Science) (T) 9, Educational Psychology PsyD (Doctor of Psychology) 1.

Student Applications/Admissions:
Student Applications
School Psychology MA/MS (*Master of Arts/Science*)—Applications 2009–2010, 12. Total applicants accepted 2009–2010, 7. Number full-time enrolled (new admits only) 2009–2010, 3. Number part-time enrolled (new admits only) 2009–2010, 0. Total enrolled 2009–2010 full-time, 12, part-time, 10. Openings 2010–2011, 18. The median number of years required for completion of a degree in 2008–2009 were 2. The number of students enrolled full- and part-time who were dismissed or voluntarily withdrew from this program area in 2008–2009 were 0. *Educational Psychology PsyD (Doctor of Psychology)*—Applications 2009–2010, 11. Total applicants accepted 2009–2010, 11. Number full-time enrolled (new admits only) 2009–2010, 1. Number part-time enrolled (new admits only) 2009–2010, 7. Total enrolled 2009–2010 full-time, 2, part-time, 22. Openings 2010–2011, 10. The median number of years required for completion of a degree in 2008–2009 were 5. The number of students enrolled full- and part-time who were dismissed or voluntarily withdrew from this program area in 2008–2009 were 0.
Scores: Entries appear in this order: required test or GPA, minimum score (if required), median score of students entering in 2009–2010. *School Psychology MA/MS (Master of Arts/Science):* overall undergraduate GPA 2.5, 2.79, psychology GPA 2.5; *Educational Psychology PsyD (Doctor of Psychology):* overall undergraduate GPA 3.0, psychology GPA 3.0.
Other Criteria: (importance of criteria rated low, medium, or high): research experience—medium, work experience—high,

extracurricular activity—low, clinically related public service—high, GPA—high, letters of recommendation—high, interview—high, statement of goals and objectives—high. For additional information on admission requirements, go to http://www.alliant.edu/wps/wcm/connect/website/Home/Admissions/.

Student Characteristics: The following represents characteristics of students in 2009–2010 in all graduate psychology programs in the department: Female—full-time 13, part-time 22; Male—full-time 1, part-time 10; African American/Black—full-time 2, part-time 6; Hispanic/Latino(a)—full-time 8, part-time 9; Asian/Pacific Islander—full-time 0, part-time 3; American Indian/Alaska Native—full-time 0, part-time 0; Caucasian/White—full-time 1, part-time 7; Multi-ethnic—full-time 1, part-time 1; students subject to the Americans With Disabilities Act—full-time 0, part-time 0; Unknown ethnicity—full-time 2, part-time 6; International students who hold an F-1 or J-1 Visa—full-time 0, part-time 0.

Financial Information/Assistance:
Tuition for Full-Time Study: *Master's:* State residents: $540 per credit hour; Nonstate residents: $540 per credit hour. *Doctoral:* State residents: $880 per credit hour; Nonstate residents: $880 per credit hour. Tuition is subject to change. Tuition costs vary by program. See the following Web site for updates and changes in tuition costs: http://www.alliant.edu/wps/wcm/connect/website/Home/Admissions/Tuition+and+Fees/.

Financial Assistance:
First-Year Students: Research assistantships available for first year. Average amount paid per academic year: $1,000. Average number of hours worked per week: 10. Fellowships and scholarships available for first year. Average amount paid per academic year: $1,500. Apply by June 1.

Advanced Students: Teaching assistantships available for advanced students. Average amount paid per academic year: $3,000. Average number of hours worked per week: 10. Research assistantships available for advanced students. Average amount paid per academic year: $1,000. Average number of hours worked per week: 10. Fellowships and scholarships available for advanced students. Average amount paid per academic year: $1,500. Apply by April 1.

Additional Information: Of all students currently enrolled full time, 40% benefited from one or more of the listed financial assistance programs. Application and information available online at: https://www.e-fao.com/efao_site.html?OEID=011117&ViewID={10EF815B-422E-4C55-B8CD-BDBD3063BA18}.

Internships/Practica: Students in the master's program have practica tied to their coursework beginning in the first semester of their programs. Internships are required of any students seeking the Pupil Personnel Services (PPS) credential post-masters or as part of the doctoral program in educational psychology. The 1200 internship hours are completed at a public school district. Those in the doctoral program who are interested in clinical licensure must complete a separate psychology internship.

Housing and Day Care: No on-campus housing is available. No on-campus day care facilities are available.

Employment of Department Graduates:
Master's Degree Graduates: Of those who graduated in the academic year 2008–2009, the following categories and numbers represent the postgraduate activities and employment of master's degree graduates: Enrolled in a postdoctoral residency/fellowship (n/a), employed in independent practice (n/a), total from the above (master's) (0).

Doctoral Degree Graduates: Of those who graduated in the academic year 2008–2009, the following categories and numbers represent the postgraduate activities and employment of doctoral degree graduates: Enrolled in a psychology doctoral program (n/a), total from the above (doctoral) (0).

Additional Information:
Orientation, Objectives, and Emphasis of Department: Programs train students with the skills necessary to work with students, teachers, parents, and other school professionals in today's school environments. The curriculum includes professional skills, professional roles courses, applied research, and professional concepts. The master's degree program prepares students to gain the PPS (Pupil Personnel Services) credential that allow them to practice in California's schools. Students take afternoon, evening and weekend classes and engage in fieldwork. At the doctoral level students complete special focus area courses, examples of which include adolescent stress and coping, school culture and administration, pediatric psychology, infant and preschool mental health, child neuropsychology, and provision of services for children in alternative placement. Students also complete a PsyD project.

Application Information:
Send to Alliant International University, Admissions Processing Center, 10455 Pomerado Road, San Diego CA 93121-1799. Application available online. URL of online application: http://www.alliant.edu/applyonline/. Students are admitted in the Fall, application deadline June 1; Spring, application deadline varies; Programs have rolling admissions. Fee: $70. A limited number of fee waivers are available for those with significant financial need.

Alliant International University: Los Angeles
Programs in Organizational Psychology
Marshall Goldsmith School of Management
1000 South Fremont Avenue
Alhambra, CA 91803-1360
Telephone: (626) 284-2777
Fax: (626) 284-0550
E-mail: *hmcbride@alliant.edu*
Web: *http://mgsm.alliant.edu*

Department Information:
1981. Systemwide Associate Dean and Program Director: Jay M. Finkelman, PhD. Number of faculty: total—full-time 5, part-time 7; women—full-time 1, part-time 3; total—minority—full-time 2, part-time 3; women minority—full-time 1, part-time 1.

Programs and Degrees Offered:
Listed in the following order: Program area, degree type (T if terminal Master's), number awarded 7/08–6/09. Industrial/Organizational Psychology MA/MS (Master of Arts/Science) (T) 8, Industrial/Organizational Psychology Respecialization Diploma 0,

GRADUATE STUDY IN PSYCHOLOGY

Industrial/Organizational Psychology PhD (Doctor of Philosophy) 1.

Student Applications/Admissions:
Student Applications
Industrial/Organizational Psychology MA/MS (Master of Arts/Science)—Applications 2009–2010, 13. Total applicants accepted 2009–2010, 9. Number full-time enrolled (new admits only) 2009–2010, 6. Number part-time enrolled (new admits only) 2009–2010, 1. Total enrolled 2009–2010 full-time, 17, part-time, 3. Openings 2010–2011, 15. The median number of years required for completion of a degree in 2008–2009 were 2. The number of students enrolled full- and part-time who were dismissed or voluntarily withdrew from this program area in 2008–2009 were 0. *Industrial/Organizational Psychology Respecialization Diploma*—Applications 2009–2010, 0. Total applicants accepted 2009–2010, 0. Number full-time enrolled (new admits only) 2009–2010, 0. Number part-time enrolled (new admits only) 2009–2010, 0. Openings 2010–2011, 2. The number of students enrolled full- and part-time who were dismissed or voluntarily withdrew from this program area in 2008–2009 were 0. *Industrial/Organizational Psychology PhD (Doctor of Philosophy)*—Applications 2009–2010, 12. Total applicants accepted 2009–2010, 10. Number full-time enrolled (new admits only) 2009–2010, 5. Number part-time enrolled (new admits only) 2009–2010, 2. Total enrolled 2009–2010 full-time, 42, part-time, 14. Openings 2010–2011, 12. The median number of years required for completion of a degree in 2008–2009 were 6. The number of students enrolled full- and part-time who were dismissed or voluntarily withdrew from this program area in 2008–2009 were 0.
Scores: Entries appear in this order: required test or GPA, minimum score (if required), median score of students entering in 2009–2010. *Industrial/Organizational Psychology MA/MS (Master of Arts/Science)*: overall undergraduate GPA 3.0, 3.2, psychology GPA 3.0; *Industrial/Organizational Psychology Respecialization Diploma*: overall undergraduate GPA 3.0, psychology GPA 3.0; *Industrial/Organizational Psychology PhD (Doctor of Philosophy)*: overall undergraduate GPA 3.0, 3.42, psychology GPA 3.0.
Other Criteria: (importance of criteria rated low, medium, or high): research experience—high, work experience—high, extracurricular activity—low, clinically related public service—low, GPA—high, letters of recommendation—high, interview—high, statement of goals and objectives—high. For additional information on admission requirements, go to http://www.alliant.edu/wps/wcm/connect/website/Home/Admissions/.

Student Characteristics: The following represents characteristics of students in 2009–2010 in all graduate psychology programs in the department: Female—full-time 38, part-time 8; Male—full-time 21, part-time 9; African American/Black—full-time 4, part-time 2; Hispanic/Latino(a)—full-time 5, part-time 1; Asian/Pacific Islander—full-time 7, part-time 1; American Indian/Alaska Native—full-time 0, part-time 0; Caucasian/White—full-time 26, part-time 9; Multi-ethnic—full-time 1, part-time 0; students subject to the Americans With Disabilities Act—full-time 0, part-time 1; Unknown ethnicity—full-time 16, part-time 4; International students who hold an F-1 or J-1 Visa—full-time 2, part-time 2.

Financial Information/Assistance:
Tuition for Full-Time Study: Master's: State residents: $950 per credit hour; Nonstate residents: $950 per credit hour. *Doctoral:* State residents: $950 per credit hour; Nonstate residents: $950 per credit hour. Tuition is subject to change. Tuition costs vary by program. See the following Web site for updates and changes in tuition costs: http://www.alliant.edu/wps/wcm/connect/website/Home/Admissions/Tuition+and+Fees/.

Financial Assistance:
First-Year Students: Research assistantships available for first year. Average amount paid per academic year: $1,000. Average number of hours worked per week: 10. Fellowships and scholarships available for first year. Average amount paid per academic year: $1,500.
Advanced Students: Teaching assistantships available for advanced students. Average amount paid per academic year: $3,000. Average number of hours worked per week: 10. Research assistantships available for advanced students. Average amount paid per academic year: $1,000. Average number of hours worked per week: 10. Fellowships and scholarships available for advanced students. Average amount paid per academic year: $1,500. Apply by April 15.
Additional Information: Of all students currently enrolled full time, 53% benefited from one or more of the listed financial assistance programs. Application and information available online at: https://www.e-fao.com/efao_site.html?OEID=011117&ViewID={10EF815B-422E-4C55-B8CD-BDBD3063BA18}.

Internships/Practica: Doctoral students may begin their practical training though the Center for Innovation and Change, working with faculty on pro bono consulting projects. A doctoral level field placement/internship is completed typically in the fourth year. Students spend 8-40 hours per week in a corporate, business, governmental, or non-profit setting. The majority of these are local to the student's campus; a few are outside the area, and are usually identified as part of a student's own career development interests. Students in the organizational psychology master's program have a one semester practicum in organizational studies.

Housing and Day Care: No on-campus housing is available. No on-campus day care facilities are available.

Employment of Department Graduates:
Master's Degree Graduates: Of those who graduated in the academic year 2008–2009, the following categories and numbers represent the postgraduate activities and employment of master's degree graduates: Enrolled in a postdoctoral residency/fellowship (n/a), employed in independent practice (n/a), total from the above (master's) (0).
Doctoral Degree Graduates: Of those who graduated in the academic year 2008–2009, the following categories and numbers represent the postgraduate activities and employment of doctoral degree graduates: Enrolled in a psychology doctoral program (n/a), total from the above (doctoral) (0).

Additional Information:
Orientation, Objectives, and Emphasis of Department: The doctoral program is based on the philosophy that the foundations of effective organizational change are science-based, especially the

science of human behavior in work settings. The program is designed to address both sides of the consultant/client relationship. The program integrates a strong foundation in the behavioral and organizational sciences; an understanding of intrapersonal and self-reflective approaches for examining human behavior; knowledge of interpersonal dynamics and political processes in professional practice, organizational interventions and consultant-client relations; and professional experiential training. Graduates are prepared for careers in a wide variety of practice areas including management consulting, organizational assessment and design, human resources development, organizational development, diversity training and change management. The master's degree program is for those seeking preparation to begin or continue careers in organizational leadership and management. Some master's students are seeking an academic foundation for future doctoral work. Students in the programs are hired in the field as early as the first year of the program. Doctoral students find employment in such companies as Disney, JPL, City of Hope, IBM Business Consulting Services, and Korn Ferry International.

Special Facilities or Resources: At the Center for Innovation and Change in Los Angeles, graduate students apply what they are learning in the classroom by providing consulting services to non-profit organizations. Through the Center first and second year students form consulting teams that provide pro bono service to clients in the Los Angeles area. Each consulting team works with a faculty supervisor. Thus students get practical training beginning early on in their programs.

Application Information:
Send to Alliant International University, Admissions Processing Center, 10455 Pomerado Road, San Diego CA 92131-1799. Application available online. URL of online application: http://www.alliant.edu/applyonline/. Students are admitted in the Fall, application deadline varies; Spring, application deadline varies; Programs have rolling admissions. The doctoral program has a February 1 priority deadline in order to provide a response by April 1 for applicants who need a decision by that date. Master's programs have later deadlines. Programs accept and admit applicants on a space available basis after any stated deadlines. *Fee:* $70. A limited number of fee waivers are available to those with significant financial need.

Alliant International University: Sacramento
Forensic Psychology Program
California School of Forensic Studies
2030 West El Camino Avenue, Suite 200
Sacramento, CA 95833
Telephone: (916) 565-2955
Fax: (916) 565-2959
E-mail: *brianevans@alliant.edu*
Web: *http://www.alliant.edu*

Department Information:
2008. Program Director: William Holbomb, PhD. Number of faculty: total—full-time 3, part-time 4; women—full-time 2, part-time 1; total—minority—full-time 1, part-time 2; women minority—full-time 1.

Programs and Degrees Offered:
Listed in the following order: Program area, degree type (T if terminal Master's), number awarded 7/08–6/09. Forensic Psychology PsyD (Doctor of Psychology) 0.

Student Applications/Admissions:
Student Applications
Forensic Psychology PsyD (Doctor of Psychology)—Applications 2009–2010, 21. Total applicants accepted 2009–2010, 15. Number full-time enrolled (new admits only) 2009–2010, 9. Number part-time enrolled (new admits only) 2009–2010, 0. Total enrolled 2009–2010 full-time, 25, part-time, 4. Openings 2010–2011, 15. The number of students enrolled full- and part-time who were dismissed or voluntarily withdrew from this program area in 2008–2009 were 1.
Scores: Entries appear in this order: required test or GPA, minimum score (if required), median score of students entering in 2009–2010. *Forensic Psychology PsyD (Doctor of Psychology):* overall undergraduate GPA 3.0, 3.47, psychology GPA 3.0.
Other Criteria: (importance of criteria rated low, medium, or high): research experience—medium, work experience—high, extracurricular activity—low, clinically related public service—high, GPA—high, letters of recommendation—high, interview—high, statement of goals and objectives—high. For additional information on admission requirements, go to http://www.alliant.edu/wps/wcm/connect/website/Home/Admissions/.

Student Characteristics: The following represents characteristics of students in 2009–2010 in all graduate psychology programs in the department: Female—full-time 19, part-time 3; Male—full-time 6, part-time 1; African American/Black—full-time 1, part-time 1; Hispanic/Latino(a)—full-time 9, part-time 1; Asian/Pacific Islander—full-time 1, part-time 0; American Indian/Alaska Native—full-time 0, part-time 0; Caucasian/White—full-time 13, part-time 1; Multi-ethnic—full-time 0, part-time 0; students subject to the Americans With Disabilities Act—full-time 0, part-time 0; Unknown ethnicity—full-time 1, part-time 1; International students who hold an F-1 or J-1 Visa—full-time 0, part-time 0.

Financial Information/Assistance:
Tuition for Full-Time Study: Doctoral: State residents: $950 per credit hour; Nonstate residents: $950 per credit hour. Tuition is subject to change. See the following Web site for updates and changes in tuition costs: http://www.alliant.edu/wps/wcm/connect/website/Home/Admissions/Tuition+and+Fees/.

Financial Assistance:
   First-Year Students: Research assistantships available for first year. Average amount paid per academic year: $1,000. Average number of hours worked per week: 10. Fellowships and scholarships available for first year. Average amount paid per academic year: $1,500. Apply by February 15.
   Advanced Students: Teaching assistantships available for advanced students. Average amount paid per academic year: $3,000. Average number of hours worked per week: 20. Research assistantships available for advanced students. Average amount paid per academic year: $1,000. Average number of hours worked per week: 10. Fellowships and scholarships available for advanced students. Average amount paid per academic year: $1,500. Apply by February 15.

Additional Information: Application and information available online at: https://www.e-fao.com/efao_site.html?OEID=011117&ViewID={10EF815B-422E-4C55-B8CD-BDBD3063BA18}.

Internships/Practica: A one year predoctoral internship is part of the program; this occurs in the fourth or fifth year of the program, depending on student pace thorugh the curriculum.

Housing and Day Care: No on-campus housing is available. No on-campus day care facilities are available.

Employment of Department Graduates:
Master's Degree Graduates: Of those who graduated in the academic year 2008–2009, the following categories and numbers represent the postgraduate activities and employment of master's degree graduates: Enrolled in a postdoctoral residency/fellowship (n/a), employed in independent practice (n/a), total from the above (master's) (0).
Doctoral Degree Graduates: Of those who graduated in the academic year 2008–2009, the following categories and numbers represent the postgraduate activities and employment of doctoral degree graduates: Enrolled in a psychology doctoral program (n/a), total from the above (doctoral) (0).

Additional Information:
Orientation, Objectives, and Emphasis of Department: The PsyD program has an applied psychology orientation and is offered in a part-time five-year curriculum. This format attracts students with prior work experience from a variety of fields. The curriculum prepares students to conduct assessments for the courts, to serve as expert witnesses, or to work as mental health treatment providers in a variety of forensic settings, including prisons, jails, offender treatment groups, and youth facilities, among many others. Core areas include forensic psychology, theories of crime and justice, industrial and organizational psychology, legal research, psychopathology, research design and data analysis, forensic mediation and dispute resolution, ethics, and substance abuse theory and treatment. While licensure is not required for most forensic careers, some students who enter the program may choose to seek clinical licensure after graduating from the program. These students take additional courses in psychology that are required in order to be eligible to sit for the psychology licensing exam.

Application Information:
Send to Alliant International University, Admissions Processing Center, 10455 Pomerado Road, San Diego CA 92131-1799. Application available online. URL of online application: https://www.alliant.edu/applyonline. Students are admitted in the Fall, application deadline varies; Spring, application deadline varies; Programs have rolling admissions. Applicants wishing notification by April 1 should submit their applications in January. However, applications are welcomed on a rolling basis and will be processed on a space available basis. *Fee:* $70. A limited number of fee waivers are available for those with significant financial need. Please contact the Director of Admissions for details.

Alliant International University: Sacramento
Marital and Family Therapy Program
California School of Professional Psychology
2030 West El Camino Avenue, Suite 200
Sacramento, CA 95833
Telephone: (916) 561-3206
Fax: (916) 565-2959
E-mail: jkulbeck@alliant.edu
Web: http://www.alliant.edu/cspp

Department Information:
2005. Program Director: Scott Woolley, PhD. Number of faculty: total—full-time 3, part-time 18; women—full-time 2, part-time 13; minority—part-time 3; women minority—part-time 3.

Programs and Degrees Offered:
Listed in the following order: Program area, degree type (T if terminal Master's), number awarded 7/08–6/09. Marital and Family Therapy MA/MS (Master of Arts/Science) (T) 11, Marital and Family Therapy PsyD (Doctor of Psychology) 0.

Student Applications/Admissions:
Student Applications
Marital and Family Therapy MA/MS (Master of Arts/Science)—Applications 2009–2010, 31. Total applicants accepted 2009–2010, 23. Number full-time enrolled (new admits only) 2009–2010, 16. Number part-time enrolled (new admits only) 2009–2010, 0. Total enrolled 2009–2010 full-time, 27, part-time, 5. Openings 2010–2011, 15. The median number of years required for completion of a degree in 2008–2009 were 2. The number of students enrolled full- and part-time who were dismissed or voluntarily withdrew from this program area in 2008–2009 were 1. *Marital and Family Therapy PsyD (Doctor of Psychology)*—Applications 2009–2010, 15. Total applicants accepted 2009–2010, 10. Number full-time enrolled (new admits only) 2009–2010, 7. Number part-time enrolled (new admits only) 2009–2010, 1. Total enrolled 2009–2010 full-time, 15, part-time, 2. Openings 2010–2011, 10. The number of students enrolled full- and part-time who were dismissed or voluntarily withdrew from this program area in 2008–2009 were 0.
Scores: Entries appear in this order: required test or GPA, minimum score (if required), median score of students entering in 2009–2010. *Marital and Family Therapy MA/MS (Master of Arts/Science):* overall undergraduate GPA 3.0, 3.22, psychology GPA 3.0; *Marital and Family Therapy PsyD (Doctor of Psychology):* overall undergraduate GPA 3.0, 3.05, psychology GPA 3.0.
Other Criteria: (importance of criteria rated low, medium, or high): research experience—medium, work experience—medium, extracurricular activity—low, clinically related public service—medium, GPA—high, letters of recommendation—medium, interview—high, statement of goals and objectives—high, undergraduate major in psychology—medium, specific undergraduate psychology courses taken—medium. For additional information on admission requirements, go to http://www.alliant.edu/wps/wcm/connect/website/Home/Admissions/Graduate+Student+Admissions/.

Student Characteristics: The following represents characteristics of students in 2009–2010 in all graduate psychology programs in the department: Female—full-time 35, part-time 4; Male—full-time 7, part-time 3; African American/Black—full-time 0, part-time 1; Hispanic/Latino(a)—full-time 4, part-time 1; Asian/Pacific Islander—full-time 6, part-time 1; American Indian/Alaska Native—full-time 1, part-time 0; Caucasian/White—full-time 22, part-time 3; Multi-ethnic—full-time 4, part-time 0; students subject to the Americans With Disabilities Act—full-time 1, part-time 0; Unknown ethnicity—full-time 5, part-time 1; International students who hold an F-1 or J-1 Visa—full-time 0, part-time 0.

Financial Information/Assistance:
Tuition for Full-Time Study: *Master's:* State residents: $950 per credit hour; Nonstate residents: $950 per credit hour. *Doctoral:* State residents: $950 per credit hour; Nonstate residents: $950 per credit hour. Tuition is subject to change. Tuition costs vary by program. See the following Web site for updates and changes in tuition costs: http://www.alliant.edu/wps/wcm/connect/website/Home/Admissions/Tuition+and+Fees/.

Financial Assistance:
First-Year Students: Fellowships and scholarships available for first year. Average amount paid per academic year: $1,500. Apply by January 15.
Advanced Students: Fellowships and scholarships available for advanced students. Average amount paid per academic year: $1,500.
Additional Information: Of all students currently enrolled full time, 65% benefited from one or more of the listed financial assistance programs. Application and information available online at: https://www.e-fao.com/eFAO_site.html?OEID=011117&ViewID={10EF815B-422E-4C55-B8CD-BDBD3063BA18}.

Internships/Practica: As part of the practicum experience, students complete 500 client contact hours, 250 of which must be with couples and families. Students recieve at least 100 hours of individual and group supervision, 50 hours of which are based on direct observation, videotape, or audiotape. At least 25 of those hours must be videotaped or direct observation. When students are ready to begin practicum, experienced faculty and staff assist students through each step in obtaining a field placement site approved by Alliant. While students are doing practicum training they are required to perform marriage and family therapy under a California state licensed, AAMFT-approved supervisor or the equivalent.

Housing and Day Care: No on-campus housing is available. No on-campus day care facilities are available.

Employment of Department Graduates:
Master's Degree Graduates: Of those who graduated in the academic year 2008–2009, the following categories and numbers represent the postgraduate activities and employment of master's degree graduates: Enrolled in a postdoctoral residency/fellowship (n/a), employed in independent practice (n/a), total from the above (master's) (0).
Doctoral Degree Graduates: Of those who graduated in the academic year 2008–2009, the following categories and numbers represent the postgraduate activities and employment of doctoral degree graduates: Enrolled in a psychology doctoral program (n/a), total from the above (doctoral) (0).

Additional Information:
Orientation, Objectives, and Emphasis of Department: The mission of the Marital and Family Therapy program is to prepare graduate students who are skilled in the theory, research, and clinical practice of the field of Marriage and Family Therapy and can integrate individual and systemic therapeutic models in an international, multicultural environment. The Marital and Family Therapy (MFT) programs provide students with the essential training needed to pursue a career as a professional marriage and family therapist. The Master of Arts in MFT allows students to be licensed as a marital and family therapist (MFT) and the Doctor of Psychology in MFT allows a student to be licensed as a marital and family therapist and as a psychologist. Students who complete the MFT masters at Alliant can apply all of their masters degree coursework and practicum hours toward the doctoral program. The programs are accredited by COAMFTE.

Application Information:
Send to Alliant International University Admissions Processing Center, 10455 Pomerado Road, San Diego CA 92131-1799. Application available online. URL of online application: http://www.alliant.edu/applyonline/. Students are admitted in the Fall, application deadline January 15; Spring, application deadline varies; Programs have rolling admissions. Applications for the Fall semester are due January 15 (priority deadline), March 15, and April 16. Applications received after the priority deadline will be accepted on a space-available basis. *Fee:* $70. A limited number of fee waivers are available for those with significant financial need.

Alliant International University: San Diego
Forensic Psychology Programs
California School of Forensic Studies
10455 Pomerado Road
San Diego, CA 92131
Telephone: (858) 635-4772
Fax: (858) 635-4739
E-mail: *rpettay@alliant.edu*
Web: *http://www.alliant.edu*

Department Information:
2008. Progam Director: Robert Lark. Number of faculty: total—full-time 3, part-time 4; women—part-time 1; minority—part-time 1.

Programs and Degrees Offered:
Listed in the following order: Program area, degree type (T if terminal Master's), number awarded 7/08–6/09. Forensic Psychology PsyD (Doctor of Psychology) 0.

Student Applications/Admissions:
Student Applications
Forensic Psychology PsyD (Doctor of Psychology)—Applications 2009–2010, 38. Total applicants accepted 2009–2010, 27. Number full-time enrolled (new admits only) 2009–2010, 19. Number part-time enrolled (new admits only) 2009–2010, 0. Openings 2010–2011, 25. The number of students enrolled

full- and part-time who were dismissed or voluntarily withdrew from this program area in 2008–2009 were 0.

Scores: Entries appear in this order: required test or GPA, minimum score (if required), median score of students entering in 2009–2010. *Forensic Psychology PsyD (Doctor of Psychology):* overall undergraduate GPA 3.0, 3.28, psychology GPA 3.0, Masters GPA 3.0, 3.71.

Other Criteria: (importance of criteria rated low, medium, or high): research experience—medium, work experience—high, extracurricular activity—low, clinically related public service—high, GPA—high, letters of recommendation—high, interview—high, statement of goals and objectives—high. For additional information on admission requirements, go to http://www.alliant.edu/wps/wcm/connect/website/Home/Admissions/.

Student Characteristics: The following represents characteristics of students in 2009–2010 in all graduate psychology programs in the department: Female—full-time 26, part-time 0; Male—full-time 9, part-time 0; African American/Black—full-time 2, part-time 0; Hispanic/Latino(a)—full-time 4, part-time 0; Asian/Pacific Islander—full-time 2, part-time 0; American Indian/Alaska Native—full-time 0, part-time 0; Caucasian/White—full-time 23, part-time 0; Multi-ethnic—full-time 1, part-time 0; students subject to the Americans With Disabilities Act—full-time 0, part-time 0; Unknown ethnicity—full-time 3, part-time 0; International students who hold an F-1 or J-1 Visa—full-time 0, part-time 0.

Financial Information/Assistance:
Tuition for Full-Time Study: *Doctoral:* State residents: $950 per credit hour; Nonstate residents: $950 per credit hour. Tuition is subject to change. See the following Web site for updates and changes in tuition costs: http://www.alliant.edu/wps/wcm/connect/website/Home/Admissions/Tuition+and+Fees/.

Financial Assistance:
First-Year Students: Research assistantships available for first year. Average amount paid per academic year: $1,000. Average number of hours worked per week: 10. Fellowships and scholarships available for first year. Average amount paid per academic year: $1,500. Apply by February 15.

Advanced Students: Teaching assistantships available for advanced students. Average amount paid per academic year: $3,000. Average number of hours worked per week: 20. Research assistantships available for advanced students. Average amount paid per academic year: $1,000. Average number of hours worked per week: 10. Fellowships and scholarships available for advanced students. Average amount paid per academic year: $1,500. Apply by February 15.

Additional Information: Application and information available online at: https://www.e-fao.com/efao_site.aspx?OEID=011117&ViewID={10EF815B-422E-4C55-B8CD-BDBD3063BA18}.

Internships/Practica: A one year predoctoral internship is part of the program; this occurs in the fourth or fifth year of the program, depending on student pace through the curriculum.

Housing and Day Care: No on-campus housing is available. No on-campus day care facilities are available.

Employment of Department Graduates:
Master's Degree Graduates: Of those who graduated in the academic year 2008–2009, the following categories and numbers represent the postgraduate activities and employment of master's degree graduates: Enrolled in a postdoctoral residency/fellowship (n/a), employed in independent practice (n/a), total from the above (master's) (0).

Doctoral Degree Graduates: Of those who graduated in the academic year 2008–2009, the following categories and numbers represent the postgraduate activities and employment of doctoral degree graduates: Enrolled in a psychology doctoral program (n/a), total from the above (doctoral) (0).

Additional Information:
Orientation, Objectives, and Emphasis of Department: The PsyD program has an applied psychology orientation and is offered in a part-time five-year curriculum. This format attracts students with prior work experience from a variety of fields. The curriculum prepares students to conduct assessments for the courts, to serve as expert witnesses, or to work as mental health treatment providers in a variety of forensic settings, including prisons, jails, offender treatment groups, and youth facilities, among many others. Core areas include forensic psychology, theories of crime and justice, industrial and organizational psychology, legal research, psychopathology, research design and data analysis, forensic mediation and dispute resolution, ethics, and substance abuse theory and treatment. While licensure is not required for most forensic careers, some students who enter the program may choose to seek clinical licensure after graduating from the program. These students take additional courses in psychology that are required in order to be eligible to sit for the psychology licensing exam.

Application Information:
Send to Alliant International University, Admissions Processing Center, 10455 Pomerado Road, San Diego, CA 92131-1799. Application available online. URL of online application: http://www.alliant.edu/applyonline/. Students are admitted in the Fall, application deadline varies; Spring, application deadline varies; Programs have rolling admissions. Applicants wishing notification by April 1 should submit their applications in January, however, applications are welcomed on a rolling basis and will be processed on a space available basis. *Fee:* $70. A limited number of fee waivers are available for those with significant financial need.

Alliant International University: San Diego
Programs in Clinical Psychology and Marital and Family Therapy
California School of Professional Psychology
10455 Pomerado Road
San Diego, CA 92131-1799
Telephone: (858) 635-4820
Fax: (858) 635-4739
E-mail: *jkulbeck@alliant.edu*
Web: *http://www.alliant.edu/cspp/*

Department Information:
1972. Dean, California School of Professional Psychology: Morgan Sammons, PhD, ABPP. Number of faculty: total—full-time 30, part-time 96; women—full-time 12, part-time 56; total—minor-

ity—full-time 7, part-time 17; women minority—full-time 4, part-time 14.

Programs and Degrees Offered:
Listed in the following order: Program area, degree type (T if terminal Master's), number awarded 7/08–6/09. Clinical Psychology PhD (Doctor of Philosophy) 27, Marital and Family Therapy MA/MS (Master of Arts/Science) (T) 27, Marital and Family Therapy PsyD (Doctor of Psychology) 5, Clinical Psychology PsyD (Doctor of Psychology) 42, Clinical Psychology Respecialization Diploma 0.

APA Accreditation: Clinical PhD (Doctor of Philosophy). Clinical PsyD (Doctor of Psychology).

Student Applications/Admissions:
Student Applications

Clinical Psychology PhD (Doctor of Philosophy)—Applications 2009–2010, 103. Total applicants accepted 2009–2010, 61. Number full-time enrolled (new admits only) 2009–2010, 29. Number part-time enrolled (new admits only) 2009–2010, 1. Total enrolled 2009–2010 full-time, 197, part-time, 43. Openings 2010–2011, 30. The median number of years required for completion of a degree in 2008–2009 were 7. The number of students enrolled full- and part-time who were dismissed or voluntarily withdrew from this program area in 2008–2009 were 2. *Marital and Family Therapy MA/MS (Master of Arts/Science)*—Applications 2009–2010, 107. Total applicants accepted 2009–2010, 66. Number full-time enrolled (new admits only) 2009–2010, 39. Number part-time enrolled (new admits only) 2009–2010, 1. Total enrolled 2009–2010 full-time, 66, part-time, 15. Openings 2010–2011, 35. The median number of years required for completion of a degree in 2008–2009 were 2. The number of students enrolled full- and part-time who were dismissed or voluntarily withdrew from this program area in 2008–2009 were 1. *Marital and Family Therapy PsyD (Doctor of Psychology)*—Applications 2009–2010, 31. Total applicants accepted 2009–2010, 18. Number full-time enrolled (new admits only) 2009–2010, 12. Number part-time enrolled (new admits only) 2009–2010, 2. Total enrolled 2009–2010 full-time, 41, part-time, 38. Openings 2010–2011, 15. The median number of years required for completion of a degree in 2008–2009 were 6. The number of students enrolled full- and part-time who were dismissed or voluntarily withdrew from this program area in 2008–2009 were 0. *Clinical Psychology PsyD (Doctor of Psychology)*—Applications 2009–2010, 156. Total applicants accepted 2009–2010, 67. Number full-time enrolled (new admits only) 2009–2010, 44. Number part-time enrolled (new admits only) 2009–2010, 1. Total enrolled 2009–2010 full-time, 194, part-time, 39. Openings 2010–2011, 42. The median number of years required for completion of a degree in 2008–2009 were 5. The number of students enrolled full- and part-time who were dismissed or voluntarily withdrew from this program area in 2008–2009 were 1. *Clinical Psychology Respecialization Diploma*—Applications 2009–2010, 3. Total applicants accepted 2009–2010, 3. Number full-time enrolled (new admits only) 2009–2010, 0. Number part-time enrolled (new admits only) 2009–2010, 1. Openings 2010–2011, 2. The number of students enrolled full- and part-time who were dismissed or voluntarily withdrew from this program area in 2008–2009 were 0.

Scores: Entries appear in this order: required test or GPA, minimum score (if required), median score of students entering in 2009–2010. *Clinical Psychology PhD (Doctor of Philosophy)*: overall undergraduate GPA 3.0, 3.38, psychology GPA 3.0; *Marital and Family Therapy MA/MS (Master of Arts/Science)*: overall undergraduate GPA 3.0, 3.2, psychology GPA 3.0; *Marital and Family Therapy PsyD (Doctor of Psychology)*: overall undergraduate GPA 3.0, 3.27, psychology GPA 3.0; *Clinical Psychology PsyD (Doctor of Psychology)*: overall undergraduate GPA 3.0, 3.37, psychology GPA 3.0, Masters GPA 3.0, 3.82; *Clinical Psychology Respecialization Diploma*: overall undergraduate GPA 3.0, 3.2, psychology GPA 3.0.

Other Criteria: (importance of criteria rated low, medium, or high): research experience—medium, work experience—medium, extracurricular activity—low, clinically related public service—medium, GPA—high, letters of recommendation—medium, interview—high, statement of goals and objectives—high, undergraduate major in psychology—medium, specific undergraduate psychology courses taken—medium. For additional information on admission requirements, go to http://www.alliant.edu/wps/wcm/connect/website/Home/Admissions/Graduate+Student+Admissions/.

Student Characteristics: The following represents characteristics of students in 2009–2010 in all graduate psychology programs in the department: Female—full-time 423, part-time 113; Male—full-time 90, part-time 30; African American/Black—full-time 20, part-time 6; Hispanic/Latino(a)—full-time 53, part-time 16; Asian/Pacific Islander—full-time 39, part-time 9; American Indian/Alaska Native—full-time 6, part-time 1; Caucasian/White—full-time 312, part-time 91; Multi-ethnic—full-time 10, part-time 1; students subject to the Americans With Disabilities Act—full-time 7, part-time 6; Unknown ethnicity—full-time 73, part-time 19; International students who hold an F-1 or J-1 Visa—full-time 3, part-time 3.

Financial Information/Assistance:
Tuition for Full-Time Study: *Master's:* State residents: $950 per credit hour; Nonstate residents: $950 per credit hour. *Doctoral:* State residents: $950 per credit hour; Nonstate residents: $950 per credit hour. Tuition is subject to change. Tuition costs vary by program. See the following Web site for updates and changes in tuition costs: http://www.alliant.edu/wps/wcm/connect/website/Home/Admissions/Tuition+and+Fees/.

Financial Assistance:
First-Year Students: Research assistantships available for first year. Average amount paid per academic year: $1,000. Average number of hours worked per week: 10. Fellowships and scholarships available for first year. Average amount paid per academic year: $1,500. Apply by January 15.

Advanced Students: Teaching assistantships available for advanced students. Average amount paid per academic year: $3,000. Average number of hours worked per week: 10. Research assistantships available for advanced students. Average amount paid per academic year: $1,000. Average number of hours worked per week: 10. Fellowships and scholarships available for advanced students. Average amount paid per academic year: $1,500. Apply by April 15.

Additional Information: Of all students currently enrolled full time, 62% benefited from one or more of the listed financial assistance programs. Application and information available online at: https://www.e-fao.com/eFAO_site.html?OEID=011117&ViewID={10EF815B-422E-4C55-B8CD-BDBD3063BA18}.

Internships/Practica: Doctoral Degree (PhD Clinical Psychology): For those doctoral students for whom a professional internship was required in this program prior to graduation, (58) students applied for an internship in 2008–2009, with (57) students obtaining an internship. Of those students who obtained an internship, (40) were paid internships. Of those students who obtained an internship, (8) students placed in APA/CPA accredited internships, (0) students placed in internships not APA/CPA accredited, but listed with the Association of Psychology Postdoctoral and Internship Programs (APPIC), (0) students placed in internships conforming to guidelines of the Council of Directors of School Psychology Programs (CDSPP), (49) students placed in internships that were not APA/CPA accredited, APPIC or CDSPP listed. Doctoral Degree (PsyD Clinical Psychology): For those doctoral students for whom a professional internship was required in this program prior to graduation, (61) students applied for an internship in 2008–2009, with (59) students obtaining an internship. Of those students who obtained an internship, (42) were paid internships. Of those students who obtained an internship, (0) students placed in APA/CPA accredited internships, (0) students placed in internships not APA/CPA accredited, but listed with the Association of Psychology Postdoctoral and Internship Programs (APPIC), (0) students placed in internships conforming to guidelines of the Council of Directors of School Psychology Programs (CDSPP), (59) students placed in internships that were not APA/CPA accredited, APPIC or CDSPP listed. Clinical psychology doctoral students receive practicum and internship experience at more than 80 agencies which meet the requirements for licensure set by the California Board of Psychology. Assignments to these agencies result from an application process conducted by year level, with third, fourth, and fifth year students receiving priority for licensable placements. The option of doing an APA-accredited full-time internship in the fourth or fifth years (depending on the program and year level requirements) is available and encouraged. Marital and family therapy students complete a required practicum including 500 client contact hours, 250 of which must be with couples and families. Students receive at least 100 hours of individual and group supervision, 50 hours of which are based on direct observation, videotape, or audiotape. At least 25 of those hours must be videotape or direct observation. While students are doing practicum training, they are required to perform marriage and family therapy under a California state licensed AAMFT-approved supervisor or the equivalent. MFT doctoral students complete a predoctoral internship.

Housing and Day Care: On-campus housing is available. See the following Web site for more information: http://www.alliant.edu/wps/wcm/connect/website/Home/Campuses/San+Diego+Campus/. No on-campus day care facilities are available.

Employment of Department Graduates:
Master's Degree Graduates: Of those who graduated in the academic year 2008–2009, the following categories and numbers represent the postgraduate activities and employment of master's degree graduates: Enrolled in a postdoctoral residency/fellowship (n/a), employed in independent practice (n/a), total from the above (master's) (0).
Doctoral Degree Graduates: Of those who graduated in the academic year 2008–2009, the following categories and numbers represent the postgraduate activities and employment of doctoral degree graduates: Enrolled in a psychology doctoral program (n/a), employed in independent practice (0), employed in an academic position at a university (0), employed in an academic position at a 2-year/4-year college (0), employed in a professional position in a school system (0), employed in a community mental health/counseling center (0), employed in a hospital/medical center (0), total from the above (doctoral) (0).

Additional Information:
Orientation, Objectives, and Emphasis of Department: The California School of Professional Psychology (CSPP) at Alliant International University offers comprehensive PhD and PsyD program of instruction in professional psychology with an emphasis on doctoral training in clinical psychology in which academic requirements are integrated with supervised field experience. Students are evaluated by instructors and field supervisors on the basis of their performance and participation throughout the year. Theory, personal growth, professional skill, humanities, investigatory skills courses, and field experience are designed to stimulate the graduate toward a scholarly as well as a professional contribution to society. Elective areas of emphasis in health psychology (PhD only), family and child psychology, clinical forensic psychology, psychodynamic, multicultural and international, and integrative psychology (PsyD only) are available within the clinical programs. Students in CSPP's Marital and Family Therapy MA and PsyD are trained to treat individuals, couples, and families with relational mental health issues from a systemic perspective. Skills are developed in mental health assessment, diagnosis, and treatment of individuals and relationship systems. The PsyD is based on the scholar-practitioner model; both degrees are offered in a format for working professionals. The MFT programs are accredited by COAMFTE. The dual clinical/industrial-organizational psychology PhD program is offered jointly with the Marshall Goldsmith School of Management; students fulfill the requirements of both specialties.

Special Facilities or Resources: The Center for Applied Behavioral Services (CABS) is a multi-service and training center. The Center incorporates the expertise of CSPP faculty in the delivery of direct services and in modeling specific techniques of treatment and service for practicum and internships. This is currently accomplished through an array of clinical and community services which are directed by faculty members.

Application Information:
Send to Alliant International University Admissions Processing Center, 10455 Pomerado Road, San Diego, CA 92131-1799. Application available online. URL of online application: http://www.alliant.edu/applyonline/. Students are admitted in the Fall, application deadline January 15; Programs have rolling admissions. Deadlines vary by program. Most doctoral programs have priority deadlines in January in order to provide a response by April 1 to applicants who need a decision by that date. Some doctoral programs and most master's programs have later deadlines. Programs accept applications and admit students on a space available basis after any stated deadlines. *Fee:* $70. A limited number of fee waivers are available for those with significant financial need.

Alliant International University: San Diego
Programs in Educational and School Psychology
Hufstedler School of Education
10455 Pomerado Road
San Diego, CA 92131-1799
Telephone: (858) 635-4772
Fax: (858) 635-4555
E-mail: kjanowsky@alliant.edu
Web: http://www.alliant.edu/

Department Information:
2002. Program Director: Steven Fisher. Number of faculty: total—full-time 1, part-time 25; women—part-time 16; minority—part-time 6; women minority—part-time 4.

Programs and Degrees Offered:
Listed in the following order: Program area, degree type (T if terminal Master's), number awarded 7/08–6/09. Educational Psychology PsyD (Doctor of Psychology) 3, School Psychology MA/MS (Master of Arts/Science) (T) 13.

Student Applications/Admissions:
Student Applications
Educational Psychology PsyD (Doctor of Psychology)—Applications 2009–2010, 11. Total applicants accepted 2009–2010, 9. Number full-time enrolled (new admits only) 2009–2010, 1. Number part-time enrolled (new admits only) 2009–2010, 7. Total enrolled 2009–2010 full-time, 1, part-time, 19. Openings 2010–2011, 15. The median number of years required for completion of a degree in 2008–2009 were 3. The number of students enrolled full- and part-time who were dismissed or voluntarily withdrew from this program area in 2008–2009 were 0. *School Psychology MA/MS (Master of Arts/Science)*—Applications 2009–2010, 17. Total applicants accepted 2009–2010, 16. Number full-time enrolled (new admits only) 2009–2010, 12. Number part-time enrolled (new admits only) 2009–2010, 1. Total enrolled 2009–2010 full-time, 29, part-time, 13. Openings 2010–2011, 18. The median number of years required for completion of a degree in 2008–2009 were 2. The number of students enrolled full- and part-time who were dismissed or voluntarily withdrew from this program area in 2008–2009 were 2.
Scores: Entries appear in this order: required test or GPA, minimum score (if required), median score of students entering in 2009–2010. *Educational Psychology PsyD (Doctor of Psychology):* overall undergraduate GPA 3.0, psychology GPA 3.0; *School Psychology MA/MS (Master of Arts/Science):* overall undergraduate GPA 2.5, 3.07, psychology GPA 2.5.
Other Criteria: (importance of criteria rated low, medium, or high): research experience—medium, work experience—medium, extracurricular activity—low, clinically related public service—high, GPA—high, letters of recommendation—high, interview—high, statement of goals and objectives—high. For additional information on admission requirements, go to http://www.alliant.edu/wps/wcm/connect/website/Home/Admissions/.

Student Characteristics: The following represents characteristics of students in 2009–2010 in all graduate psychology programs in the department: Female—full-time 23, part-time 24; Male—full-time 7, part-time 8; African American/Black—full-time 1, part-time 2; Hispanic/Latino(a)—full-time 7, part-time 5; Asian/Pacific Islander—full-time 2, part-time 1; American Indian/Alaska Native—full-time 0, part-time 0; Caucasian/White—full-time 13, part-time 19; Multi-ethnic—full-time 0, part-time 1; students subject to the Americans With Disabilities Act—full-time 0, part-time 0; Unknown ethnicity—full-time 7, part-time 4; International students who hold an F-1 or J-1 Visa—full-time 1, part-time 0.

Financial Information/Assistance:
Tuition for Full-Time Study: *Master's:* State residents: $540 per credit hour; Nonstate residents: $540 per credit hour. *Doctoral:* State residents: $880 per credit hour; Nonstate residents: $880 per credit hour. Tuition is subject to change. Tuition costs vary by program. See the following Web site for updates and changes in tuition costs: http://www.alliant.edu/wps/wcm/connect/website/Home/Admissions/Tuition+and+Fees/.

Financial Assistance:
First-Year Students: Research assistantships available for first year. Average amount paid per academic year: $1,000. Average number of hours worked per week: 10. Fellowships and scholarships available for first year. Average amount paid per academic year: $750. Apply by June 1.
Advanced Students: Teaching assistantships available for advanced students. Average amount paid per academic year: $3,000. Average number of hours worked per week: 10. Research assistantships available for advanced students. Average amount paid per academic year: $1,000. Average number of hours worked per week: 10. Fellowships and scholarships available for advanced students. Average amount paid per academic year: $750. Apply by April 1.
Additional Information: Of all students currently enrolled full time, 40% benefited from one or more of the listed financial assistance programs. Application and information available online at: https://www.e-fao.com/efao_site.html?OEID=011117&ViewID={10EF815B-422E-4C55-B8CD-BDBD3063BA18}.

Internships/Practica: Students in the master's program have practica tied to their coursework beginning in the first semester of their programs. Internships are required of students seeking a Pupil Personnel Services (PPS) credential post-masters or as part of the doctoral program in educational psychology. The 1,200 required internship hours are completed at a public school district. Students interested in seeking clinical licensure must complete a separate psychology internship.

Housing and Day Care: On-campus housing is available. See the following Web site for more information: http://www.alliant.edu/wps/wcm/connect/website/Home/Campuses/San+Diego+Campuses. No on-campus day care facilities are available.

Employment of Department Graduates:
Master's Degree Graduates: Of those who graduated in the academic year 2008–2009, the following categories and numbers represent the postgraduate activities and employment of master's degree graduates: Enrolled in a postdoctoral residency/fellowship (n/a), employed in independent practice (n/a), total from the above (master's) (0).
Doctoral Degree Graduates: Of those who graduated in the academic year 2008–2009, the following categories and numbers

GRADUATE STUDY IN PSYCHOLOGY

represent the postgraduate activities and employment of doctoral degree graduates: Enrolled in a psychology doctoral program (n/a), total from the above (doctoral) (0).

Additional Information:
Orientation, Objectives, and Emphasis of Department: Programs train students with the skills necessary to work with students, teachers, parents, and other school professionals in today's school environments. Curriculum includes professional skills, professional roles courses, applied research, and professional concepts. The master's degree program prepares students to gain the PPS (Pupil Personnel Services) credential that allows them to practice in California's schools. Students take afternoon, evening, and weekend classes and engage in fieldwork. At the doctoral level, students complete special focus area courses, examples of which include adolescent stress and coping, school culture and administration, pediatric psychology, infant and preschool mental health, child neuropsychology, and provision of services for children in alternative placement. Students also complete a PsyD project.

Special Facilities or Resources: The Graduate School of Education at the San Diego campus houses the World Council of Curriculum and Instruction.

Application Information:
Send to Alliant International University, Admissions Processing Center, 10455 Pomerado Road, San Diego, CA 92131-1799. Application available online. URL of online application: http://www.alliant.edu/applyonline/. Students are admitted in the Fall, application deadline June 1; Spring, application deadline varies; Summer, application deadline varies; Programs have rolling admissions. *Fee:* $70. A limited number of fee waivers are available for those with significant financial need.

Alliant International University: San Diego
Programs in Organizational Psychology
Marshall Goldsmith School of Management
10455 Pomerado Road
San Diego, CA 92121-1799
Telephone: (858) 635-4772
Fax: (858) 635-4739
E-mail: *hmcbride@alliant.edu*
Web: *http://mgsm.alliant.edu*

Department Information:
1981. Program Director: Jay M Finkelman, PhD. Number of faculty: total—full-time 8, part-time 14; women—full-time 1, part-time 3; total—minority—full-time 2, part-time 1.

Programs and Degrees Offered:
Listed in the following order: Program area, degree type (T if terminal Master's), number awarded 7/08–6/09. Consulting Psychology PhD (Doctor of Philosophy) 3, Industrial/Organizational Psychology MA/MS (Master of Arts/Science) (T) 7, Industrial/Organizational Psychology Respecialization Diploma 0, Dual Clinical-Industrial/Organizational Psychology PhD (Doctor of Philosophy) 3, Industrial/Organizational Psychology PhD (Doctor of Philosophy) 5.

Student Applications/Admissions:
Student Applications
Consulting Psychology PhD (Doctor of Philosophy)—Applications 2009–2010, 7. Total applicants accepted 2009–2010, 6. Number full-time enrolled (new admits only) 2009–2010, 4. Number part-time enrolled (new admits only) 2009–2010, 0. Total enrolled 2009–2010 full-time, 21, part-time, 12. Openings 2010–2011, 12. The median number of years required for completion of a degree in 2008–2009 were 6. The number of students enrolled full- and part-time who were dismissed or voluntarily withdrew from this program area in 2008–2009 were 1. Industrial/Organizational Psychology MA/MS (Master of Arts/Science)—Applications 2009–2010, 8. Total applicants accepted 2009–2010, 7. Number full-time enrolled (new admits only) 2009–2010, 4. Number part-time enrolled (new admits only) 2009–2010, 2. Total enrolled 2009–2010 full-time, 16, part-time, 6. Openings 2010–2011, 15. The median number of years required for completion of a degree in 2008–2009 were 2. The number of students enrolled full- and part-time who were dismissed or voluntarily withdrew from this program area in 2008–2009 were 1. Industrial/Organizational Psychology Respecialization Diploma—Applications 2009–2010, 0. Total applicants accepted 2009–2010, 0. Number full-time enrolled (new admits only) 2009–2010, 0. Number part-time enrolled (new admits only) 2009–2010, 0. Openings 2010–2011, 2. The number of students enrolled full- and part-time who were dismissed or voluntarily withdrew from this program area in 2008–2009 were 0. Dual Clinical-Industrial/Organizational Psychology PhD (Doctor of Philosophy)—Applications 2009–2010, 10. Total applicants accepted 2009–2010, 8. Number full-time enrolled (new admits only) 2009–2010, 2. Number part-time enrolled (new admits only) 2009–2010, 1. Total enrolled 2009–2010 full-time, 15, part-time, 7. Openings 2010–2011, 6. The median number of years required for completion of a degree in 2008–2009 were 7. The number of students enrolled full- and part-time who were dismissed or voluntarily withdrew from this program area in 2008–2009 were 0. Industrial/Organizational Psychology PhD (Doctor of Philosophy)—Applications 2009–2010, 18. Total applicants accepted 2009–2010, 12. Number full-time enrolled (new admits only) 2009–2010, 8. Number part-time enrolled (new admits only) 2009–2010, 0. Total enrolled 2009–2010 full-time, 31, part-time, 18. Openings 2010–2011, 12. The median number of years required for completion of a degree in 2008–2009 were 7. The number of students enrolled full- and part-time who were dismissed or voluntarily withdrew from this program area in 2008–2009 were 0.

Scores: Entries appear in this order: required test or GPA, minimum score (if required), median score of students entering in 2009–2010. Consulting Psychology PhD (Doctor of Philosophy): overall undergraduate GPA 3.0, 2.88, psychology GPA 3.0; Industrial/Organizational Psychology MA/MS (Master of Arts/Science): overall undergraduate GPA 3.0, 3.56, psychology GPA 3.0; Industrial/Organizational Psychology Respecialization Diploma: overall undergraduate GPA 3.0, psychology GPA 3.0; Dual Clinical-Industrial/Organizational Psychology PhD (Doctor of Philosophy): overall undergraduate GPA 3.0, 3.66, psychology GPA 3.0; Industrial/Organizational Psychology PhD (Doctor of Philosophy): overall undergraduate GPA 3.0, 3.14, psychology GPA 3.0.

Other Criteria: (importance of criteria rated low, medium, or high): research experience—high, work experience—medium, extracurricular activity—low, clinically related public service—low, GPA—high, letters of recommendation—high, interview—high, statement of goals and objectives—high. Research experience is more important for doctoral applicants; work experience is more important for some master's programs. For additional information on admission requirements, go to http://www.alliant.edu/wps/wcm/connect/website/Home/Admissions/.

Student Characteristics: The following represents characteristics of students in 2009–2010 in all graduate psychology programs in the department: Female—full-time 53, part-time 23; Male—full-time 30, part-time 20; African American/Black—full-time 6, part-time 1; Hispanic/Latino(a)—full-time 5, part-time 7; Asian/Pacific Islander—full-time 11, part-time 4; American Indian/Alaska Native—full-time 1, part-time 0; Caucasian/White—full-time 40, part-time 18; Multi-ethnic—full-time 2, part-time 1; students subject to the Americans With Disabilities Act—full-time 2, part-time 0; Unknown ethnicity—full-time 18, part-time 12; International students who hold an F-1 or J-1 Visa—full-time 1, part-time 1.

Financial Information/Assistance:
Tuition for Full-Time Study: *Master's:* State residents: $950 per credit hour; Nonstate residents: $950 per credit hour. *Doctoral:* State residents: $950 per credit hour; Nonstate residents: $950 per credit hour. Tuition is subject to change. Tuition costs vary by program. See the following Web site for updates and changes in tuition costs: http://www.alliant.edu/wps/wcm/connect/website/Home/Admissions/Tuition+and+Fees/.

Financial Assistance:
First-Year Students: Research assistantships available for first year. Average amount paid per academic year: $1,000. Average number of hours worked per week: 10. Fellowships and scholarships available for first year. Average amount paid per academic year: $1,500. Apply by April 1.

Advanced Students: Teaching assistantships available for advanced students. Average amount paid per academic year: $3,000. Average number of hours worked per week: 10. Research assistantships available for advanced students. Average amount paid per academic year: $1,000. Average number of hours worked per week: 10. Fellowships and scholarships available for advanced students. Average amount paid per academic year: $1,500. Apply by April 15.

Additional Information: Of all students currently enrolled full time, 51% benefited from one or more of the listed financial assistance programs. Application and information available online at: https://www.e-fao.com/efao_site.html?OEID=011117&ViewID={10EF815B-422E-4C55-B8CD-BDBD3063BA18}.

Internships/Practica: Doctoral students participate in two half-time internships in the third and fourth years of the program; this allows for the integration of professional training with courses, seminars and research. Consulting psychology doctoral students' internships have an individual/group focus in the third year and systemwide interventions focus in the fourth year. Master's students in I/O psychology have a one-semester practicum in the last term of their programs. The majority of these internships are local to the students' campus.

Housing and Day Care: On-campus housing is available. See the following Web site for more information: http://www.alliant.edu/wps/wcm/connect/website/Home/Campuses/San+Diego+Campus. No on-campus day care facilities are available.

Employment of Department Graduates:
Master's Degree Graduates: Of those who graduated in the academic year 2008–2009, the following categories and numbers represent the postgraduate activities and employment of master's degree graduates: Enrolled in a postdoctoral residency/fellowship (n/a), employed in independent practice (n/a), total from the above (master's) (0).

Doctoral Degree Graduates: Of those who graduated in the academic year 2008–2009, the following categories and numbers represent the postgraduate activities and employment of doctoral degree graduates: Enrolled in a psychology doctoral program (n/a), total from the above (doctoral) (0).

Additional Information:
Orientation, Objectives, and Emphasis of Department: The consulting psychology doctoral program combines individual, group, organization and systemic consultation skills to produce specialists in the psychological aspects of organizational consulting. The individual focus includes career assessment and executive coaching; the group focus includes team building and assisting dysfunctional work groups; the organizational/systemic focus includes the understanding, diagnosis and intervention with organizational systems. The industrial-organizational doctoral program is patterned after the doctoral level training guidelines prepared by the Educational and Training Committee of the Society for Industrial and Organizational Psychology (Division 14 of the APA). The programs emphasize personnel selections, work motivation, design of compensation systems, measurement and productivity. Master's programs lead to careers as internal consultants within organizations or other master's-level or entry-level careers in organizations and provide foundations for further study if desired. These programs stress leadership, management, and organizational skills. Some master's programs are structured specifically for working professionals.

Special Facilities or Resources: The Marshall Goldsmith School of Management houses an Organizational Consulting Center (OCC). Some students may have opportunities to work with faculty or consultant associates from the Center during their programs.

Application Information:
Send to Alliant International University, Admissions Processing Center, 10455 Pomerado Road, San Diego, CA 92121-1799. Application available online. URL of online application: http://www.alliant.edu/applyonline/. Students are admitted in the Fall, application deadline February 1; Spring, application deadline varies; Summer, application deadline varies; Programs have rolling admissions. Doctoral programs have a February 1 priority deadline in order to provide a response by April 1 for applicants who need a decision by that date. Master's programs have later deadlines. Programs accept and admit applicants on a space available basis after any stated deadlines. *Fee:* $70. A limited number of fee waivers are available to those with significant financial need.

Alliant International University: San Francisco
Programs in Clinical Psychology and Clinical Psychopharmacology
California School of Professional Psychology
One Beach Street
San Francisco, CA 94133-1221
Telephone: (415) 955-2146
Fax: (415) 955-2179
E-mail: *jkulbeck@alliant.edu*
Web: *http://www.alliant.edu/cspp*

Department Information:
1969. Dean, California School of Professional Psychology: Morgan T. Sammons, PhD, ABPP. Number of faculty: total—full-time 31, part-time 97; women—full-time 13, part-time 54; total—minority—full-time 13, part-time 17; women minority—full-time 7, part-time 11; faculty subject to the Americans With Disabilities Act 2.

Programs and Degrees Offered:
Listed in the following order: Program area, degree type (T if terminal Master's), number awarded 7/08–6/09. Clinical Psychology PsyD (Doctor of Psychology) 59, Clinical Psychology PhD (Doctor of Philosophy) 22, Clinical Psychology Respecialization Diploma 0, Clinical Psychopharmacology MA/MS (Master of Arts/Science) (T) 67.

APA Accreditation: Clinical PsyD (Doctor of Psychology). Clinical PhD (Doctor of Philosophy).

Student Applications/Admissions:
Student Applications
Clinical Psychology PsyD (Doctor of Psychology)—Applications 2009–2010, 172. Total applicants accepted 2009–2010, 111. Number full-time enrolled (new admits only) 2009–2010, 63. Number part-time enrolled (new admits only) 2009–2010, 0. Total enrolled 2009–2010 full-time, 266, part-time, 77. Openings 2010–2011, 55. The median number of years required for completion of a degree in 2008–2009 were 5. The number of students enrolled full- and part-time who were dismissed or voluntarily withdrew from this program area in 2008–2009 were 4. Clinical Psychology PhD (Doctor of Philosophy)—Applications 2009–2010, 68. Total applicants accepted 2009–2010, 40. Number full-time enrolled (new admits only) 2009–2010, 21. Number part-time enrolled (new admits only) 2009–2010, 0. Total enrolled 2009–2010 full-time, 120, part-time, 32. Openings 2010–2011, 24. The median number of years required for completion of a degree in 2008–2009 were 6. The number of students enrolled full- and part-time who were dismissed or voluntarily withdrew from this program area in 2008–2009 were 1. Clinical Psychology Respecialization Diploma—Applications 2009–2010, 3. Total applicants accepted 2009–2010, 3. Number full-time enrolled (new admits only) 2009–2010, 0. Number part-time enrolled (new admits only) 2009–2010, 1. Total enrolled 2009–2010 full-time, 2, part-time, 2. Openings 2010–2011, 1. The number of students enrolled full- and part-time who were dismissed or voluntarily withdrew from this program area in 2008–2009 were 0. Clinical Psychopharmacology MA/MS (Master of Arts/Science)—Applications 2009–2010, 15. Total applicants accepted 2009–2010, 15. Number full-time enrolled (new admits only) 2009–2010, 1. Number part-time enrolled (new admits only) 2009–2010, 11. Total enrolled 2009–2010 full-time, 2, part-time, 102. Openings 2010–2011, 10. The median number of years required for completion of a degree in 2008–2009 were 2. The number of students enrolled full- and part-time who were dismissed or voluntarily withdrew from this program area in 2008–2009 were 2.

Scores: Entries appear in this order: required test or GPA, minimum score (if required), median score of students entering in 2009–2010. Clinical Psychology PsyD (Doctor of Psychology): overall undergraduate GPA 3.0, 3.37, psychology GPA 3.0; Clinical Psychology PhD (Doctor of Philosophy): overall undergraduate GPA 3.0, 3.54, psychology GPA 3.0; Clinical Psychology Respecialization Diploma: overall undergraduate GPA 3.0, 3.67, psychology GPA no minimum stated.

Other Criteria: (importance of criteria rated low, medium, or high): research experience—high, work experience—high, extracurricular activity—low, clinically related public service—high, GPA—high, letters of recommendation—high, interview—high, statement of goals and objectives—high, undergraduate major in psychology—medium, specific undergraduate psychology courses taken—medium. For additional information on admission requirements, go to http://www.alliant.edu/wps/wcm/connect/website/Home/Admissions/Graduate+Student+Admissions/.

Student Characteristics: The following represents characteristics of students in 2009–2010 in all graduate psychology programs in the department: Female—full-time 289, part-time 151; Male—full-time 101, part-time 62; African American/Black—full-time 25, part-time 10; Hispanic/Latino(a)—full-time 53, part-time 17; Asian/Pacific Islander—full-time 47, part-time 26; American Indian/Alaska Native—full-time 0, part-time 3; Caucasian/White—full-time 219, part-time 128; Multi-ethnic—full-time 13, part-time 7; students subject to the Americans With Disabilities Act—full-time 16, part-time 2; Unknown ethnicity—full-time 33, part-time 22; International students who hold an F-1 or J-1 Visa—full-time 16, part-time 0.

Financial Information/Assistance:
Tuition for Full-Time Study: *Master's:* State residents: per academic year $5,192; Nonstate residents: per academic year $5,192. *Doctoral:* State residents: $950 per credit hour; Nonstate residents: $950 per credit hour. Tuition is subject to change. Tuition costs vary by program. See the following Web site for updates and changes in tuition costs: http://www.alliant.edu/wps/wcm/connect/website/Home/Admissions/Tuition+and+Fees/.

Financial Assistance:
First-Year Students: Research assistantships available for first year. Average amount paid per academic year: $1,500. Average number of hours worked per week: 10. Fellowships and scholarships available for first year. Average amount paid per academic year: $1,500. Apply by January 15.

Advanced Students: Teaching assistantships available for advanced students. Average amount paid per academic year: $3,000. Average number of hours worked per week: 10. Research assistantships available for advanced students. Average amount paid per academic year: $1,000. Average number of hours worked per week: 10. Fellowships and scholarships available for advanced

students. Average amount paid per academic year: $1,500. Apply by April 15.

Additional Information: Of all students currently enrolled full time, 58% benefited from one or more of the listed financial assistance programs. Application and information available online at: https://www.e-fao.com/eFAO_site.html?OEID=011117&ViewID ={10EF815B-422E-4C55-B8CD-BDBD3063BA18}.

Internships/Practica: Doctoral Degree (PsyD Clinical Psychology): For those doctoral students for whom a professional internship was required in this program prior to graduation, (60) students applied for an internship in 2008–2009, with (60) students obtaining an internship. Of those students who obtained an internship, (45) were paid internships. Of those students who obtained an internship, (10) students placed in APA/CPA accredited internships, (13) students placed in internships not APA/CPA accredited, but listed with the Association of Psychology Postdoctoral and Internship Programs (APPIC), (0) students placed in internships conforming to guidelines of the Council of Directors of School Psychology Programs (CDSPP), (37) students placed in internships that were not APA/CPA accredited, APPIC or CDSPP listed. Doctoral Degree (PhD Clinical Psychology): For those doctoral students for whom a professional internship was required in this program prior to graduation, (16) students applied for an internship in 2008–2009, with (16) students obtaining an internship. Of those students who obtained an internship, (14) were paid internships. Of those students who obtained an internship, (8) students placed in APA/CPA accredited internships, (3) students placed in internships not APA/CPA accredited, but listed with the Association of Psychology Postdoctoral and Internship Programs (APPIC), (0) students placed in internships conforming to guidelines of the Council of Directors of School Psychology Programs (CDSPP), (5) students placed in internships that were not APA/CPA accredited, APPIC or CDSPP listed. During the first three years of the PsyD program and during the second and third years of the PhD program, students are engaged in field practica 8-16 hours per week. All students get experience working with adults, children/adolescents, and persons with severe mental illness as well as more moderate forms of dysfunction. The tremendous ethnic/racial diversity of the San Francisco Bay Area insures that all students get exposure to working with clients from a variety of cultural groups. Practica are selected and approved by CSPP based on the quality of training and supervision provided for the students. They include community mental health centers, neuropsychology clinics, hospitals, child guidance clinics, college counseling centers, forensic settings, couple and family therapy agencies, residential treatment centers, infant/toddler mental health programs, corporate settings, and school programs for children and adolescents. Students begin the required internship in the fourth year (PsyD program) or the fifth year (PhD program). Full-time internship options include APA-accredited or APPIC-member training programs pursued through the national selection process, or local internship programs approved by the California Psychology Internship Council (CAPIC). Students have the option of completing the internship requirement in two years of half-time experience.

Housing and Day Care: No on-campus housing is available. No on-campus day care facilities are available.

Employment of Department Graduates:
Master's Degree Graduates: Of those who graduated in the academic year 2008–2009, the following categories and numbers represent the postgraduate activities and employment of master's degree graduates: Enrolled in a postdoctoral residency/fellowship (n/a), employed in independent practice (n/a), total from the above (master's) (0).

Doctoral Degree Graduates: Of those who graduated in the academic year 2008–2009, the following categories and numbers represent the postgraduate activities and employment of doctoral degree graduates: Enrolled in a psychology doctoral program (n/a), total from the above (doctoral) (0).

Additional Information:
Orientation, Objectives, and Emphasis of Department: CSPP's clinical psychology programs combine supervised field experiences with study of psychological theory, clinical techniques, and applied research. The PsyD is a practitioner-oriented program. The PhD provides a balance of clinical and research training and is intended for students who expect independent research, teaching, and scholarship to be a significant part of their professional careers in addition to clinical work. In addition to the usual offerings, special training opportunities are available in five areas: family-child-adolescent psychology, health psychology, multicultural-community psychology, psychodynamic psychology, and gender studies (which includes psychology of women and men, and lesbian, gay, bisexual and transgender issues). The PsyD program also offers an intensive Child and Family Track (which focuses on child assessment, child therapy, and family therapy) and a Forensic Family/Child Track (which focuses on child abuse, child custody, delinquency, and family court services). Students in the PsyD tracks are required to complete a specific sequence of courses, a dissertation, and an internship related to their track's focus. Other students in the PhD and PsyD programs can take many of these same training experiences on an elective basis. Multicultural/diversity issues are infused throughout the entire curriculum. Three major theoretical orientations are strongly represented in the program: cognitive-behavioral, family systems, and psychodynamic.

Special Facilities or Resources: Students can elect to receive supervised clinical experience through CSPP's Psychological Services Center (PSC)—a community mental health clinic that serves children, adults, couples, and families. The PSC enables faculty to model professional service delivery and to directly supervise and evaluate students' clinical work. Clinical services provided at the PSC include psychodiagnostic assessment and individual, couple, family, and group psychotherapy. The PSC has both Adult-Clinical and Child/Family-Clinical training programs. The Rockway Institute works to counter antigay prejudice and inform public policies affecting lesbian, gay, bisexual, and transgender (LGBT) people. Primary goals of the Institute are to convey accurate scientific and professional information about LGBT issues to the media, legislatures and the courts, and conduct research relevant to LGBT public policy questions in the areas of family relations, education, healthcare, social services, and the workplace. Computer labs are available to students and are fully equipped with SPSS and other statistical programs for research purposes. Designated space is available on campus for research activities (such as data collection), and the library is equipped with the major searchable databases for the research literature in psychology and related areas. The campus occupies approximately 31,000 square feet of space in an historic building near the San Francisco waterfront across from Pier 39.

GRADUATE STUDY IN PSYCHOLOGY

Application Information:
Send to Alliant International University, Admissions Processing Center, 10455 Pomerado Road, San Diego CA 92131. Application available online. URL of online application: http://www.alliant.edu/applyonline/. Students are admitted in the Fall, application deadline January 15; Programs have rolling admissions. The priority deadline for doctoral programs is January 15; applicants who complete an application by that date are guaranteed notification by April 1. Applications submitted after that date will be reviewed on a space-available basis. Applications to the clinical psychopharmacology master's programs vary by location and cohort start date. *Fee:* $70. A limited number of fee waivers are available for those with significant financial need.

Alliant International University: San Francisco
Programs in Educational and School Psychology
Hufstedler School of Education
One Beach Street
San Francisco, CA 94133-1221
Telephone: (415) 955-2146
Fax: (415) 955-2179
E-mail: *jaquino@alliant.edu*
Web: *http://www.alliant.edu*

Department Information:
2002. Program Director: James Hiramoto, PhD. Number of faculty: total—full-time 1, part-time 13; women—part-time 8; total—minority—full-time 1, part-time 2; women minority—part-time 2.

Programs and Degrees Offered:
Listed in the following order: Program area, degree type (T if terminal Master's), number awarded 7/08–6/09. School Psychology MA/MS (Master of Arts/Science) (T) 2, Educational Psychology PsyD (Doctor of Psychology) 0.

Student Applications/Admissions:
Student Applications
School Psychology MA/MS (Master of Arts/Science)—Applications 2009–2010, 15. Total applicants accepted 2009–2010, 12. Number full-time enrolled (new admits only) 2009–2010, 5. Number part-time enrolled (new admits only) 2009–2010, 1. Total enrolled 2009–2010 full-time, 16, part-time, 4. Openings 2010–2011, 15. The median number of years required for completion of a degree in 2008–2009 were 2. The number of students enrolled full- and part-time who were dismissed or voluntarily withdrew from this program area in 2008–2009 were 2. *Educational Psychology PsyD (Doctor of Psychology)*—Applications 2009–2010, 6. Total applicants accepted 2009–2010, 4. Number full-time enrolled (new admits only) 2009–2010, 0. Number part-time enrolled (new admits only) 2009–2010, 4. Openings 2010–2011, 5. The number of students enrolled full- and part-time who were dismissed or voluntarily withdrew from this program area in 2008–2009 were 0.
Scores: Entries appear in this order: required test or GPA, minimum score (if required), median score of students entering in 2009–2010. *School Psychology MA/MS (Master of Arts/Science):* overall undergraduate GPA 2.5, 2.96, psychology GPA 2.5; *Educational Psychology PsyD (Doctor of Psychology):* overall undergraduate GPA 3.0, psychology GPA 3.0.

Other Criteria: (importance of criteria rated low, medium, or high): research experience—medium, work experience—high, extracurricular activity—low, clinically related public service—high, GPA—high, letters of recommendation—high, interview—high, statement of goals and objectives—high. For additional information on admission requirements, go to http://www.alliant.edu/wps/wcm/connect/website/Home/Admissions/.

Student Characteristics: The following represents characteristics of students in 2009–2010 in all graduate psychology programs in the department: Female—full-time 14, part-time 18; Male—full-time 2, part-time 1; African American/Black—full-time 3, part-time 1; Hispanic/Latino(a)—full-time 1, part-time 2; Asian/Pacific Islander—full-time 2, part-time 1; American Indian/Alaska Native—full-time 0, part-time 0; Caucasian/White—full-time 7, part-time 9; Multi-ethnic—full-time 1, part-time 0; students subject to the Americans With Disabilities Act—full-time 0, part-time 0; Unknown ethnicity—full-time 2, part-time 6; International students who hold an F-1 or J-1 Visa—full-time 1, part-time 0.

Financial Information/Assistance:
Tuition for Full-Time Study: Master's: State residents: $540 per credit hour; Nonstate residents: $540 per credit hour. *Doctoral:* State residents: $880 per credit hour; Nonstate residents: $880 per credit hour. Tuition is subject to change. See the following Web site for updates and changes in tuition costs: http://www.alliant.edu/wps/wcm/connect/website/Home/Admissions/Tuition+and+Fees/.

Financial Assistance:
First-Year Students: Research assistantships available for first year. Average amount paid per academic year: $1,000. Average number of hours worked per week: 10. Fellowships and scholarships available for first year. Average amount paid per academic year: $750. Apply by June 1.
Advanced Students: Teaching assistantships available for advanced students. Average amount paid per academic year: $3,000. Average number of hours worked per week: 10. Research assistantships available for advanced students. Average amount paid per academic year: $1,000. Average number of hours worked per week: 10. Fellowships and scholarships available for advanced students. Average amount paid per academic year: $750. Apply by April 1.
Additional Information: Of all students currently enrolled full time, 40% benefited from one or more of the listed financial assistance programs. Application and information available online at: https://www.e-fao.com/efao_site.html?OEID=011117&ViewID={10EF815B-422E-4C55-B8CD-BDBD3063BA18}.

Internships/Practica: Students in the master's program have practica tied to their coursework beginning in the first semester of their programs. Internships are required of any students seeking a Pupil Personnel Services (PPS) credential post-masters or as part of the doctoral program in educational psychology. The 1200 internships hours are completed at a public school district. Those in the doctoral program who are interested in clinical licensure must complete a separate psychology internship.

Housing and Day Care: No on-campus housing is available. No on-campus day care facilities are available.

Employment of Department Graduates:
Master's Degree Graduates: Of those who graduated in the academic year 2008–2009, the following categories and numbers represent the postgraduate activities and employment of master's degree graduates: Enrolled in a postdoctoral residency/fellowship (n/a), employed in independent practice (n/a), total from the above (master's) (0).
Doctoral Degree Graduates: Of those who graduated in the academic year 2008–2009, the following categories and numbers represent the postgraduate activities and employment of doctoral degree graduates: Enrolled in a psychology doctoral program (n/a), total from the above (doctoral) (0).

Additional Information:
Orientation, Objectives, and Emphasis of Department: Programs train students with the skills necessary to work with students, teachers, parents, and other school professionals in today's school environments. The curriculum includes professional skills, professional roles courses, applied research, and professional concepts. The master's degree program prepares students to gain the PPS (Pupil Personnel Services) credential that allows them to practice in California's schools. Students take afternoon, evening and weekend classes and engage in fieldwork. At the doctoral level, students complete special focus area courses, examples of which include adolescent stress and coping, school culture and administration, pediatric psychology, infant and preschool mental health, child neuropsychology, and provision of services for children in alternative placement. Students also complete a PsyD project.

Application Information:
Send to Alliant International University, Admissions Processing Center, 10455 Pomerado Road, San Diego, CA 92131-1799. Application available online. URL of online application: http://www.alliant.edu/applyonline/. Students are admitted in the Fall, application deadline June 1; Spring, application deadline varies; Summer, application deadline varies; Programs have rolling admissions. *Fee:* $70. A limited number of fee waivers are available for those with significant financial need.

Alliant International University: San Francisco
Programs in Organizational Psychology
Marshall Goldsmith School of Management
One Beach Street
San Francisco, CA 94133-1221
Telephone: (415) 955-2146
Fax: (415) 955-2179
E-mail: *lpyle@alliant.edu*
Web: *http://mgsm.alliant.edu/*

Department Information:
1983. Program Director: Ira Levin, PhD. Number of faculty: total—full-time 6, part-time 10; women—full-time 4, part-time 8; total—minority—full-time 1, part-time 1; women minority—full-time 1.

Programs and Degrees Offered:
Listed in the following order: Program area, degree type (T if terminal Master's), number awarded 7/08–6/09. Organizational Psychology PhD (Doctor of Philosophy) 9, Organizational Psychology MA/MS (Master of Arts/Science) (T) 0, Organizational Development MA/MS (Master of Arts/Science) (T) 0, Organizational Psychology Respecialization Diploma 0.

Student Applications/Admissions:
Student Applications
Organizational Psychology PhD (Doctor of Philosophy)—Applications 2009–2010, 13. Total applicants accepted 2009–2010, 13. Number full-time enrolled (new admits only) 2009–2010, 7. Number part-time enrolled (new admits only) 2009–2010, 2. Total enrolled 2009–2010 full-time, 21, part-time, 30. Openings 2010–2011, 12. The median number of years required for completion of a degree in 2008–2009 were 7. The number of students enrolled full- and part-time who were dismissed or voluntarily withdrew from this program area in 2008–2009 were 2. *Organizational Psychology MA/MS (Master of Arts/Science)*—Applications 2009–2010, 5. Total applicants accepted 2009–2010, 5. Number full-time enrolled (new admits only) 2009–2010, 1. Number part-time enrolled (new admits only) 2009–2010, 2. Total enrolled 2009–2010 full-time, 5, part-time, 6. Openings 2010–2011, 15. The number of students enrolled full- and part-time who were dismissed or voluntarily withdrew from this program area in 2008–2009 were 0. *Organizational Development MA/MS (Master of Arts/Science)*—Applications 2009–2010, 0. Total applicants accepted 2009–2010, 0. Number full-time enrolled (new admits only) 2009–2010, 0. Number part-time enrolled (new admits only) 2009–2010, 0. Total enrolled 2009–2010 full-time, 1, part-time, 2. Openings 2010–2011, 5. The number of students enrolled full- and part-time who were dismissed or voluntarily withdrew from this program area in 2008–2009 were 1. *Organizational Psychology Respecialization Diploma*—Applications 2009–2010, 1. Total applicants accepted 2009–2010, 1. Number full-time enrolled (new admits only) 2009–2010, 0. Number part-time enrolled (new admits only) 2009–2010, 1. Openings 2010–2011, 2. The number of students enrolled full- and part-time who were dismissed or voluntarily withdrew from this program area in 2008–2009 were 0.
Scores: Entries appear in this order: required test or GPA, minimum score (if required), median score of students entering in 2009–2010. *Organizational Psychology PhD (Doctor of Philosophy):* overall undergraduate GPA 3.0, 3.14, psychology GPA 3.0; *Organizational Psychology MA/MS (Master of Arts/Science):* overall undergraduate GPA 3.0, 3.42, psychology GPA 3.0; *Organizational Development MA/MS (Master of Arts/Science):* overall undergraduate GPA 3.0, psychology GPA 3.0; *Organizational Psychology Respecialization Diploma:* overall undergraduate GPA 3.0, 3.61, psychology GPA 3.0.
Other Criteria: (importance of criteria rated low, medium, or high): research experience—high, work experience—high, extracurricular activity—low, clinically related public service—low, GPA—high, letters of recommendation—high, interview—high, statement of goals and objectives—high. For additional information on admission requirements, go to http://www.alliant.edu/wps/wcm/connect/website/Home/Admissions/.

Student Characteristics: The following represents characteristics of students in 2009–2010 in all graduate psychology programs in the department: Female—full-time 19, part-time 24; Male—full-time 8, part-time 16; African American/Black—full-time 5, part-time 3; Hispanic/Latino(a)—full-time 2, part-time 3; Asian/Pa-

cific Islander—full-time 3, part-time 8; American Indian/Alaska Native—full-time 0, part-time 0; Caucasian/White—full-time 15, part-time 20; Multi-ethnic—full-time 1, part-time 0; students subject to the Americans With Disabilities Act—full-time 0, part-time 1; Unknown ethnicity—full-time 1, part-time 6; International students who hold an F-1 or J-1 Visa—full-time 1, part-time 0.

Financial Information/Assistance:
Tuition for Full-Time Study: *Master's:* State residents: $950 per credit hour; Nonstate residents: $950 per credit hour. *Doctoral:* State residents: $950 per credit hour; Nonstate residents: $950 per credit hour. Tuition is subject to change. Tuition costs vary by program. See the following Web site for updates and changes in tuition costs: http://www.alliant.edu/wps/wcm/connect/website/Home/Admissions/Tuition+and+Fees/.

Financial Assistance:
First-Year Students: Research assistantships available for first year. Average amount paid per academic year: $1,000. Average number of hours worked per week: 10. Fellowships and scholarships available for first year. Average amount paid per academic year: $1,500. Apply by February 15.

Advanced Students: Teaching assistantships available for advanced students. Average amount paid per academic year: $3,000. Average number of hours worked per week: 10. Research assistantships available for advanced students. Average amount paid per academic year: $1,000. Average number of hours worked per week: 10. Fellowships and scholarships available for advanced students. Average amount paid per academic year: $1,500. Apply by April 15.

Additional Information: Of all students currently enrolled full time, 53% benefited from one or more of the listed financial assistance programs. Application and information available online at: https://www.e-fao.com/efao_site.html?OEID=011117&ViewID={10EF815B-422E-4C55-B8CD-BDBD3063BA18}.

Internships/Practica: Organizational doctoral students develop skills through practical training experiences during the third and fourth years of the program. Students usually devote 8-40 hours per week to field placement assignments. Some training sites are local to the student's campus location; occasionally students find internships at out-of-area or out-of-state sites that meet their professional training needs. Placements are available in a variety of settings including consulting firms, major corporations, government agencies, healthcare organizations, and non-profit agencies. Students in the master's programs have a one semester applied experience with supervision.

Housing and Day Care: No on-campus housing is available. No on-campus day care facilities are available.

Employment of Department Graduates:
Master's Degree Graduates: Of those who graduated in the academic year 2008–2009, the following categories and numbers represent the postgraduate activities and employment of master's degree graduates: Enrolled in a postdoctoral residency/fellowship (n/a), employed in independent practice (n/a), total from the above (master's) (0).
Doctoral Degree Graduates: Of those who graduated in the academic year 2008–2009, the following categories and numbers represent the postgraduate activities and employment of doctoral degree graduates: Enrolled in a psychology doctoral program (n/a), total from the above (doctoral) (0).

Additional Information:
Orientation, Objectives, and Emphasis of Department: Doctoral students gain exposure to three core areas of study: organizational theory, grounded in the behavioral sciences; quantitative and qualitative research methods; and professional practice skill development. The program focuses on research and practice in organizational consulting at the individual, team, and system levels; collaborative strategic change; organizational culture and leadership; multicultural competence; executive coaching and mentoring; organizational innovation, creativity and knowledge management. Programs are structured so students can attend at a moderated pace—this allows students to continue working while in their programs. Master's level programs provide solid education in organizational psychology and behavior; they are suitable for students who may wish to continue on to doctoral education. The Master's in organization development is primarily for those who have backgrounds in other fields and wish to move into managerial or OD position; three concentrations are offered in systemic change in a global context, building healthy organizations and applied research. The Master's in organizational psychology provides a stronger research foundation.

Special Facilities or Resources: Marshall Goldsmith School of Management offers the Organizational Consulting Center (OCC). Students may have opportunities to participate with faculty and OCC associates on consulting projects during their programs.

Application Information:
Send to Alliant International University, Admissions Processing Center, 10455 Pomerado Road, San Diego CA 92131-1799. Application available online. URL of online application: http://www.alliant.edu/applyonline/. Students are admitted in the Fall, application deadline February 1; Spring, application deadline varies; Programs have rolling admissions. Doctoral program has a February 1 deadline in order to provide a response by April 1 for applicants who need a decision by that date. Master's programs have later deadlines. Programs accept applications and admit students on a space available basis after any stated deadlines. *Fee:* $70. A limited number of fee waivers are available for those with significant financial need.

Antioch University, Santa Barbara
Graduate Psychology Programs
801 Garden Street, Suite 101
Santa Barbara, CA 93101
Telephone: (805) 962-8179
Fax: (805) 962-4786
E-mail: *mharway@antioch.edu*
Web: *http://www.antiochsb.edu*

Department Information:
1977. Chairperson: Michele Harway, PhD. Number of faculty: total—full-time 6, part-time 24; women—full-time 4, part-time 13; total—minority—full-time 1, part-time 7; women minority—part-time 3; faculty subject to the Americans With Disabilities Act 1.

Programs and Degrees Offered:
Listed in the following order: Program area, degree type (T if terminal Master's), number awarded 7/08–6/09. Clinical Psychology PsyD (Doctor of Psychology) 4.

Student Applications/Admissions:
Student Applications
Clinical Psychology PsyD (Doctor of Psychology)—Applications 2009–2010, 47. Total applicants accepted 2009–2010, 26. Number full-time enrolled (new admits only) 2009–2010, 12. Number part-time enrolled (new admits only) 2009–2010, 0. Total enrolled 2009–2010 full-time, 58, part-time, 2. Openings 2010–2011, 16. The median number of years required for completion of a degree in 2008–2009 were 4. The number of students enrolled full- and part-time who were dismissed or voluntarily withdrew from this program area in 2008–2009 were 2.

Other Criteria: (importance of criteria rated low, medium, or high): research experience—low, work experience—medium, extracurricular activity—low, clinically related public service—medium, GPA—high, letters of recommendation—medium, interview—high, statement of goals and objectives—high, writing sample—high, undergraduate major in psychology—medium, specific undergraduate psychology courses taken—low. The doctoral program requires two essays in lieu of GREs that are used to assess analytic and critical thinking. These are heavily weighted. For additional information on admission requirements, go to http://www.antiochsb.edu/admissions-financial/doctoral-program.

Student Characteristics: The following represents characteristics of students in 2009–2010 in all graduate psychology programs in the department: Female—full-time 42, part-time 1; Male—full-time 16, part-time 1; African American/Black—full-time 6, part-time 0; Hispanic/Latino(a)—full-time 7, part-time 1; Asian/Pacific Islander—full-time 1, part-time 1; American Indian/Alaska Native—full-time 0, part-time 0; Caucasian/White—full-time 42, part-time 0; Multi-ethnic—full-time 2, part-time 0; students subject to the Americans With Disabilities Act—full-time 2, part-time 0; Unknown ethnicity—full-time 0, part-time 0; International students who hold an F-1 or J-1 Visa—full-time 1, part-time 0.

Financial Information/Assistance:
Tuition for Full-Time Study: Doctoral: State residents: per academic year $20,655, $690 per credit hour; Nonstate residents: per academic year $20,655, $690 per credit hour. Tuition is subject to change. Additional fees are assessed to students beyond the costs of tuition for the following: Testing supplies, malpractice insurance. Tuition costs vary by program. See the following Web site for updates and changes in tuition costs: http://www.antiochsb.edu/admissions-financial/tuition.

Financial Assistance:
First-Year Students: No information provided.
Advanced Students: Teaching assistantships available for advanced students. Research assistantships available for advanced students. Fellowships and scholarships available for advanced students.
Additional Information: Of all students currently enrolled full time, 10% benefited from one or more of the listed financial assistance programs. Application and information available online at: http://www.antiochsb.edu/admissions-financial/financial-aid.

Internships/Practica: Doctoral Degree (PsyD Clinical Psychology): For those doctoral students for whom a professional internship was required in this program prior to graduation, (7) students applied for an internship in 2008–2009, with (7) students obtaining an internship. Of those students who obtained an internship, (2) were paid internships. Of those students who obtained an internship, (0) students placed in APA/CPA accredited internships, (1) students placed in internships not APA/CPA accredited, but listed with the Association of Psychology Postdoctoral and Internship Programs (APPIC), (0) students placed in internships conforming to guidelines of the Council of Directors of School Psychology Programs (CDSPP), (6) students placed in internships that were not APA/CPA accredited, APPIC or CDSPP listed. Practica are available in community agencies, schools, and clinics, in Santa Barbara, San Luis Obispo, Los Angeles and Ventura Counties. Students apply for internships through the national APPIC Match and also through the CAPIC (California Psychology Internship Council) Match. Applicants for internship have typically obtained either APPIC or CAPIC internships.

Housing and Day Care: No on-campus housing is available. No on-campus day care facilities are available.

Employment of Department Graduates:
Master's Degree Graduates: Of those who graduated in the academic year 2008–2009, the following categories and numbers represent the postgraduate activities and employment of master's degree graduates: Enrolled in a postdoctoral residency/fellowship (n/a), employed in independent practice (n/a), total from the above (master's) (0).
Doctoral Degree Graduates: Of those who graduated in the academic year 2008–2009, the following categories and numbers represent the postgraduate activities and employment of doctoral degree graduates: Enrolled in a psychology doctoral program (n/a), enrolled in a postdoctoral residency/fellowship (1), employed in independent practice (1), employed in government agency (2), total from the above (doctoral) (4).

Additional Information:
Orientation, Objectives, and Emphasis of Department: The doctoral program is a PsyD degree in Clinical Psychology with a Family Psychology emphasis and a Family Forensic Concentration. Students enroll either post bachelor's or are given Year 2 advanced standing with an earned master's in psychology and with equivalent courses.

Special Facilities or Resources: Faculty are all practicing professionals in their respective areas of expertise. Core faculty are engaged in a variety of research projects (according to their professional interests) which provide an opportunity for research assistantships for financial aid-eligible students. We are seeking funds for a training clinic to serve a primarily Spanish-speaking clientele with training to be done in Spanish.

Application Information:
Send to Admissions Office, Antioch University Santa Barbara, 801 Garden Street, Santa Barbara, CA 93101. Application available online. URL of online application: http://www.antiochsb.edu/admissions-

financial/doctoral-program. Students are admitted in the Fall, application deadline January 31. *Fee:* $60. Fee may be waived in circumstances of financial need.

Argosy University/Orange County
Psychology
School of Psychology and Behavioral Sciences
601 South Lewis
Orange, CA 92868
Telephone: (714) 620-3701
Fax: (714) 620-3804
E-mail: *gbruss@argosy.edu*
Web: *http://www.argosy.edu*

Department Information:
2001. Program Chair, Clinical Psychology: Gary Bruss, PhD. Number of faculty: total—full-time 11, part-time 8; women—full-time 5, part-time 3; total—minority—full-time 5, part-time 3; women minority—full-time 3, part-time 1.

Programs and Degrees Offered:
Listed in the following order: Program area, degree type (T if terminal Master's), number awarded 7/08–6/09. Clinical Psychology PsyD (Doctor of Psychology) 9, Counseling Psychology EdD (Doctor of Education), Counseling Psychology MA/MS (Master of Arts/Science) (T), Forensic Psychology MA/MS (Master of Arts/Science) (T) 0, Clinical Psychology MA/MS (Master of Arts/Science) (T) 19.

APA Accreditation: Clinical PsyD (Doctor of Psychology). Student Outcome Data Website: http://www.argosy.edu/colleges/ProgramDetail.aspx?ID=679&section=outcomes.

Student Applications/Admissions:
Student Applications
Clinical Psychology PsyD (Doctor of Psychology)—Applications 2009–2010, 123. Total applicants accepted 2009–2010, 61. Number full-time enrolled (new admits only) 2009–2010, 23. Number part-time enrolled (new admits only) 2009–2010, 0. Openings 2010–2011, 35. The median number of years required for completion of a degree in 2008–2009 were 5. The number of students enrolled full- and part-time who were dismissed or voluntarily withdrew from this program area in 2008–2009 were 6. *Counseling Psychology EdD (Doctor of Education)*—The median number of years required for completion of a degree in 2008–2009 were 4. *Counseling Psychology MA/MS (Master of Arts/Science)—Forensic Psychology MA/MS (Master of Arts/Science)*—The median number of years required for completion of a degree in 2008–2009 were 2. *Clinical Psychology MA/MS (Master of Arts/Science)*—Applications 2009–2010, 42. Total applicants accepted 2009–2010, 30. Number full-time enrolled (new admits only) 2009–2010, 9. Total enrolled 2009–2010 full-time, 36. Openings 2010–2011, 30. The median number of years required for completion of a degree in 2008–2009 were 2. The number of students enrolled full- and part-time who were dismissed or voluntarily withdrew from this program area in 2008–2009 were 1.

Scores: Entries appear in this order: required test or GPA, minimum score (if required), median score of students entering in 2009–2010. *Clinical Psychology PsyD (Doctor of Psychology):* overall undergraduate GPA 3.25, 3.56, Masters GPA 3.25, 3.88; *Clinical Psychology MA/MS (Master of Arts/Science):* overall undergraduate GPA 3.00, last 2 years GPA 3.00.

Other Criteria: (importance of criteria rated low, medium, or high): research experience—low, work experience—medium, extracurricular activity—medium, clinically related public service—medium, GPA—high, letters of recommendation—high, interview—high, statement of goals and objectives—high, undergraduate major in psychology—medium, specific undergraduate psychology courses taken—high. High emphasis on work experience for doctoral programs, although outstanding presentation in areas related to GPA, recommendation letters, interview, and personal statement can offset a deficit in work experience. Letters of recommendation from work, prior training, and/or academic references are expected for all programs. Emphasis on both clinical and academic references for doctoral applicants.

Student Characteristics: The following represents characteristics of students in 2009–2010 in all graduate psychology programs in the department: Female—full-time 136, part-time 4; Male—full-time 37, part-time 1; African American/Black—full-time 20, part-time 2; Hispanic/Latino(a)—full-time 33, part-time 1; Asian/Pacific Islander—full-time 26, part-time 0; American Indian/Alaska Native—full-time 0, part-time 0; Caucasian/White—full-time 94, part-time 2; Multi-ethnic—full-time 0, part-time 0; students subject to the Americans With Disabilities Act—full-time 2, part-time 0; Unknown ethnicity—full-time 0, part-time 0; International students who hold an F-1 or J-1 Visa—full-time 3, part-time 0.

Financial Information/Assistance:
Financial Assistance:
First-Year Students: Teaching assistantships available for first year. Fellowships and scholarships available for first year. Average amount paid per academic year: $2,000. Average number of hours worked per week: 3. Apply by June 30.

Advanced Students: Teaching assistantships available for advanced students. Average amount paid per academic year: $1,000. Average number of hours worked per week: 6. Apply by June 30. Research assistantships available for advanced students. Average amount paid per academic year: $2,000. Average number of hours worked per week: 3. Apply by June 30. Fellowships and scholarships available for advanced students. Average amount paid per academic year: $3,000. Average number of hours worked per week: 5. Apply by June 30.

Additional Information: Of all students currently enrolled full time, 8% benefited from one or more of the listed financial assistance programs.

Internships/Practica: Doctoral Degree (PsyD Clinical Psychology): For those doctoral students for whom a professional internship was required in this program prior to graduation, (16) students applied for an internship in 2008–2009, with (16) students obtaining an internship. Of those students who obtained an internship, (11) were paid internships. Of those students who obtained an internship, (2) students placed in APA/CPA accredited internships, (9) students placed in internships not APA/CPA accredited, but listed with the Association of Psychology Postdoctoral and Internship Programs (APPIC), (0) students placed in internships conforming to guidelines of the Council of Directors of School Psychology Programs (CDSPP), (5) students placed in internships that were not APA/CPA accredited, APPIC or CDSPP listed. Master's Degree (MA/MS Clinical Psychology): An internship experience, such as a final research project or "capstone" experience is required of graduates. The specific clinical focus of the practicum varies according to the student's program, training needs, professional interests and goals, and the availability of practicum sites. MA Counseling and Clinical practica focus on training students in couples/family counseling and therapy skills. The PsyD Clinical Psychology practica provide one year of psychodiagnostic assessment training and one year of therapy training. The program is committed to finding a wide range of practicum sites to provide many options for student professional exposure and development.

Housing and Day Care: No on-campus housing is available. No on-campus day care facilities are available.

Employment of Department Graduates:
Master's Degree Graduates: Of those who graduated in the academic year 2008–2009, the following categories and numbers represent the postgraduate activities and employment of master's degree graduates: Enrolled in a psychology doctoral program (0), enrolled in another graduate/professional program (0), enrolled in a postdoctoral residency/fellowship (n/a), employed in independent practice (n/a), employed in an academic position at a university (0), employed in an academic position at a 2-year/4-year college (0), employed in other positions at a higher education institution (0), employed in a professional position in a school system (0), employed in business or industry (0), employed in government agency (0), employed in a community mental health/counseling center (0), employed in a hospital/medical center (0), still seeking employment (0), other employment position (0), total from the above (master's) (0).
Doctoral Degree Graduates: Of those who graduated in the academic year 2008–2009, the following categories and numbers represent the postgraduate activities and employment of doctoral degree graduates: Enrolled in a psychology doctoral program (n/a), enrolled in a postdoctoral residency/fellowship (1), employed in independent practice (3), employed in an academic position at a university (0), employed in an academic position at a 2-year/4-year college (0), employed in other positions at a higher education institution (0), employed in a professional position in a school system (0), employed in business or industry (0), employed in government agency (0), employed in a community mental health/counseling center (6), employed in a hospital/medical center (2), still seeking employment (2), other employment position (0), total from the above (doctoral) (14).

Additional Information:
Orientation, Objectives, and Emphasis of Department: The graduate programs in psychology are designed to educate and train practitioners, with an additional emphasis on scholarly training in the doctoral programs. Courses and fieldwork experiences embrace multiple theoretical and intervention approaches, and a range of psychodiagnostic techniques (in the clinical programs), all of which are designed to serve a wide and diverse range of populations. PsyD concentrations are available in Forensic Psychology and in Child/Adolescent Psychology. Students are taught by faculty with strong teaching and practitioner skills, with a strong focus on developing students with the fundamental clinical, counseling and relevant scholarly competencies required to pursue careers in psychology. Courses in applied and academic areas are considered to be critical in the development of practitioners with the skills to develop, innovate, implement, and assess delivery of services to clientele in clinical, counseling, and educational types of settings.

Application Information:
Send to Director of Admissions, c/o Argosy University/Orange County 601, South Lewis Street, Orange, CA 92868. Application available online. URL of online application: http://www.argosy.edu. Students are admitted in the Fall, application deadline May 15; Spring, application deadline October 15; Summer, application deadline March 30. We offer a year around rolling admissions process for both the EdD-CP and MACP programs, with admissions points for Fall, Spring, and Summer semesters. PsyD and MA Clinical applicant deadlines are January 15 for fall, with a May 15 deadline if spaces available, and October 15 for Spring term with a November 15 deadline if spaces are still available. *Fee:* $50.

Argosy University/San Francisco Bay Area
Clinical Psychology
College of Psychology and Behavioral Sciences
1005 Atlantic Avenue
Alameda, CA 94501
Telephone: (510) 217-4700
Fax: (510) 217-4800
E-mail: *plytle@argosy.edu*
Web: *http://www.argosy.edu*

Department Information:
1999. Program Chair: Pauline Lytle, PhD. Number of faculty: total—full-time 11, part-time 4; women—full-time 8, part-time 1; total—minority—full-time 2, part-time 2; women minority—full-time 1; faculty subject to the Americans With Disabilities Act 1.

Programs and Degrees Offered:
Listed in the following order: Program area, degree type (T if terminal Master's), number awarded 7/08–6/09. Clinical Psychology MA/MS (Master of Arts/Science) (T) 0, Clinical Psychology PsyD (Doctor of Psychology) 25.

APA Accreditation: Clinical PsyD (Doctor of Psychology).

Student Applications/Admissions:
Student Applications
Clinical Psychology MA/MS (*Master of Arts/Science*)—Applications 2009–2010, 43. Total applicants accepted 2009–2010, 41. Number full-time enrolled (new admits only) 2009–2010, 9. Number part-time enrolled (new admits only) 2009–2010, 1. Total enrolled 2009–2010 full-time, 9, part-time, 4. Openings

2010–2011, 10. The number of students enrolled full- and part-time who were dismissed or voluntarily withdrew from this program area in 2008–2009 were 0. *Clinical Psychology PsyD (Doctor of Psychology)*—Applications 2009–2010, 178. Total applicants accepted 2009–2010, 173. Number full-time enrolled (new admits only) 2009–2010, 39. Number part-time enrolled (new admits only) 2009–2010, 1. Total enrolled 2009–2010 full-time, 249, part-time, 11. Openings 2010–2011, 48. The median number of years required for completion of a degree in 2008–2009 were 5. The number of students enrolled full- and part-time who were dismissed or voluntarily withdrew from this program area in 2008–2009 were 4.

Scores: Entries appear in this order: required test or GPA, minimum score (if required), median score of students entering in 2009–2010. *Clinical Psychology MA/MS (Master of Arts/Science)*: overall undergraduate GPA 3.00; *Clinical Psychology PsyD (Doctor of Psychology)*: overall undergraduate GPA 3.25.

Other Criteria: (importance of criteria rated low, medium, or high): research experience—medium, work experience—medium, extracurricular activity—medium, clinically related public service—medium, GPA—high, letters of recommendation—high, interview—high, statement of goals and objectives—high, TOEFL as needed—high, undergraduate major in psychology—medium, specific undergraduate psychology courses taken—medium. For the PsyD Program, a GPA of at least 3.25 (on a 4.0 scale) in work leading to the bachelor's degree OR any subsequent graduate study (one year) is required. For the MA Program, a GPA of at least 3.25 (on a 4.0 scale) in work leading to the bachelor's degree is required. For additional information on admission requirements, go to http://www.argosy.edu/colleges/ProgramDetail.aspx?ID=732&section=admissions-requirements.

Student Characteristics: The following represents characteristics of students in 2009–2010 in all graduate psychology programs in the department: Caucasian/White—full-time 0, part-time 0; students subject to the Americans With Disabilities Act—full-time 10, part-time 0; Unknown ethnicity—full-time 0, part-time 0; International students who hold an F-1 or J-1 Visa—full-time 0, part-time 0.

Financial Information/Assistance:
Tuition for Full-Time Study: *Master's:* State residents: $998 per credit hour; Nonstate residents: $998 per credit hour. *Doctoral:* State residents: $998 per credit hour; Nonstate residents: $998 per credit hour. Tuition is subject to change. Additional fees are assessed to students beyond the costs of tuition for the following: child abuse reporting class, professional liability insurance, student activity fee, technology fee. See the following Web site for updates and changes in tuition costs: http://www.argosy.edu/admissions/tuition-fees.aspx.

Financial Assistance:
First-Year Students: Fellowships and scholarships available for first year. Average amount paid per academic year: $1,000.
Advanced Students: Teaching assistantships available for advanced students. Average amount paid per academic year: $800. Average number of hours worked per week: 5. Research assistantships available for advanced students. Traineeships available for advanced students. Fellowships and scholarships available for advanced students. Average amount paid per academic year: $1,000.

Additional Information: Of all students currently enrolled full time, 90% benefited from one or more of the listed financial assistance programs. Application and information available online at: http://www.argosy.edu/admissions/scholarships-financial-aid/Default.aspx.

Internships/Practica: Doctoral Degree (PsyD Clinical Psychology): For those doctoral students for whom a professional internship was required in this program prior to graduation, (66) students applied for an internship in 2008–2009, with (66) students obtaining an internship. Of those students who obtained an internship, (41) were paid internships. Of those students who obtained an internship, (3) students placed in APA/CPA accredited internships, (18) students placed in internships not APA/CPA accredited, but listed with the Association of Psychology Postdoctoral and Internship Programs (APPIC), (0) students placed in internships conforming to guidelines of the Council of Directors of School Psychology Programs (CDSPP), (45) students placed in internships that were not APA/CPA accredited, APPIC or CDSPP listed. Master's Degree (MA/MS Clinical Psychology): An internship experience, such as a final research project or "capstone" experience is required of graduates. Argosy University SFBA students are encouraged to choose the internship experience that best meets their long term training goals. Students from our program are able to apply to both APPIC (including APA internships) and CAPIC (California Psychology Internship Council) internship agencies. CAPIC is a collaboration between professional psychology graduate programs and internship programs in California. This allows students to have the option of applying to either a full-time or a half-time internship. Argosy University SFBA's database of approved San Francisco Bay Area practicum sites includes community mental health centers, consortiums, state, community and private psychiatric hospitals, medical and trauma centers, university counseling centers, schools, correctional facilities, residential treatment programs, independent and group practices, and corporate settings. Some sites serve the general population while others service specific populations (e.g., children, adolescents, geriatrics, particular ethnic or racial groups, criminal offenders, etc.) or clinical problems (e.g., chemical dependency, eating disorders, medical and psychiatric rehabilitation, etc.). Students are required to seek a combination of practicum placements that will provide a breadth of experience including working with severely disordered clients, children or adolescents, and adults. The Training Department works throughout the year to maintain positive relationships with existing sites and to affiliate itself with new sites throughout the Bay Area. Argosy University SFBA strongly encourages students to complete their training in settings that provide opportunities to work with diverse populations. It is essential that students learn to work with people who are different from themselves (e.g. race, ethnicity, disability, sexual orientation, etc.) in a supervised setting where they can learn the skills, knowledge and attitudes necessary to practice as a competent clinician.

Housing and Day Care: No on-campus housing is available. No on-campus day care facilities are available.

Employment of Department Graduates:
Master's Degree Graduates: Of those who graduated in the academic year 2008–2009, the following categories and numbers represent the postgraduate activities and employment of master's degree graduates: Enrolled in a psychology doctoral program (0),

enrolled in another graduate/professional program (0), enrolled in a postdoctoral residency/fellowship (n/a), employed in independent practice (n/a), do not know (0), total from the above (master's) (0).

Doctoral Degree Graduates: Of those who graduated in the academic year 2008–2009, the following categories and numbers represent the postgraduate activities and employment of doctoral degree graduates: Enrolled in a psychology doctoral program (n/a), enrolled in another graduate/professional program (0), total from the above (doctoral) (0).

Additional Information:

Orientation, Objectives, and Emphasis of Department: The Clinical Psychology program is focused on providing students with a general theoretical basis from which they will choose which orientation(s) best fit who they are. All major theoretical orientations are presented including psychodynamic, family systems, developmental, cognitive and person centered or humanistic and evidence based practice is emphasized in all courses. The general goals of the program are to prepare professionals who are capable of delivering effective and ethical diagnostic and assessment services and a wide range of therapeutic interventions to a diverse set of clients and to prepare professionals who are able to understand and use the scientific bases of psychology to inform their practice of professional psychology and to evaluate the methods of assessment and intervention they use in practice. Given the location of our campus in the San Francisco Bay Area, students obtain practicum experience with a wide range of diverse populations.

Special Facilities or Resources: Argosy University San Francisco Bay Area campus emphasizes specialized hands-on clinical training through our Intensive Clinical Training facility. Through the Intensive Clinical Training series, students work directly with clients referred from the community while being observed by a team through a one-way mirror. The team consists of the instructor and/or clinical assistant and fellow students who participate in pre and post-therapy sessions in which they provide input and feedback about the therapeutic process. Each client session is guided by the instructor/assistant who, through the use of a microphone, provides clinical guidance and interventions directly to the student therapist through an earpiece worn by the student. As the session progresses, the instructor/assistant educates the team about the dynamics of the therapist/client interaction and the treatment approach. Students may participate on three levels: 1) as a clinical observer and a member of the team; 2) as a student therapist working directly with clients, and 3) as a clinical assistant in concert with our Supervision/Consultation course.

Application Information:
Send to Admissions Department, Argosy University, San Francisco Bay Area, 1005 Atlantic Avenue, Alameda, CA 94501. Application available online. URL of online application: https://portal.argosy.edu/Applicant/ApplyOnline_Login.aspx. Students are admitted in the Fall, application deadline January 15; Spring, application deadline October 15. Programs have rolling admissions. January 15 priority deadline for Fall. May 15 final deadline depending on space availability. Rolling admissions depending on availability. *Fee:* $50.

Azusa Pacific University
Department of Graduate Psychology
901 East Alosta, P.O. Box 7000
Azusa, CA 91702-7000
Telephone: (626) 815-5008
Fax: (626) 815-5015
E-mail: *rwelsh@apu.edu*
Web: *http://www.apu.edu/bas/graduatepsychology*

Department Information:
1976. Chairperson: Robert K. Welsh, PhD, ABPP. Number of faculty: total—full-time 14, part-time 1; women—full-time 8; total—minority—full-time 1, part-time 1.

Programs and Degrees Offered:
Listed in the following order: Program area, degree type (T if terminal Master's), number awarded 7/08–6/09. Clinical Psychology MA/MS (Master of Arts/Science) (T) 54, Clinical Psychology MA/MS (Master of Arts/Science) 26, Clinical Psychology PsyD (Doctor of Psychology) 11.

APA Accreditation: Clinical PsyD (Doctor of Psychology). Student Outcome Data Website: http://www.apu.edu/bas/graduatepsychology/psyd/.

Student Applications/Admissions:
Student Applications
Clinical Psychology MA/MS (Master of Arts/Science)—Applications 2009–2010, 228. Total applicants accepted 2009–2010, 130. Number full-time enrolled (new admits only) 2009–2010, 76. Number part-time enrolled (new admits only) 2009–2010, 7. Total enrolled 2009–2010 full-time, 157, part-time, 45. Openings 2010–2011, 95. The median number of years required for completion of a degree in 2008–2009 were 3. The number of students enrolled full- and part-time who were dismissed or voluntarily withdrew from this program area in 2008–2009 were 10. *Clinical Psychology MA/MS (Master of Arts/Science)*—Applications 2009–2010, 110. Total applicants accepted 2009–2010, 42. Number full-time enrolled (new admits only) 2009–2010, 23. Number part-time enrolled (new admits only) 2009–2010, 0. Openings 2010–2011, 25. The median number of years required for completion of a degree in 2008–2009 were 2. The number of students enrolled full- and part-time who were dismissed or voluntarily withdrew from this program area in 2008–2009 were 2. *Clinical Psychology PsyD (Doctor of Psychology)*—Applications 2009–2010, 138. Total applicants accepted 2009–2010, 48. Number full-time enrolled (new admits only) 2009–2010, 27. Number part-time enrolled (new admits only) 2009–2010, 0. Total enrolled 2009–2010 full-time, 78, part-time, 36. Openings 2010–2011, 28. The median number of years required for completion of a degree in 2008–2009 were 5. The number of students enrolled full- and part-time who were dismissed or voluntarily withdrew from this program area in 2008–2009 were 2.

Scores: Entries appear in this order: required test or GPA, minimum score (if required), median score of students entering in 2009–2010. *Clinical Psychology MA/MS (Master of Arts/Science)*: overall undergraduate GPA 2.7, 3.2; *Clinical Psychology MA/MS (Master of Arts/Science)*: GRE-V 500, 550, GRE-Q 500, 550, GRE-Analytical 4.0, 4.5, overall undergraduate

GPA 3.0, 3.6, last 2 years GPA no minimum stated, psychology GPA no minimum stated; *Clinical Psychology PsyD (Doctor of Psychology)*: GRE-V 500, 550, GRE-Q 500, 550, GRE-Analytical 4.0, 4.5, overall undergraduate GPA 3.0, 3.5, last 2 years GPA no minimum stated, psychology GPA no minimum stated, Masters GPA 3.5, 3.7.

Other Criteria: (importance of criteria rated low, medium, or high): GRE scores—medium, research experience—medium, work experience—medium, extracurricular activity—medium, clinically related public service—medium, GPA—high, letters of recommendation—high, interview—high, statement of goals and objectives—high. No GRE scores required for MA; Work experience of medium importance for MA; Research experience of medium importance for MA; Clinically Related Public Service low for MA. For additional information on admission requirements, go to http://www.apu.edu/bas/graduatepsychology/.

Student Characteristics: The following represents characteristics of students in 2009–2010 in all graduate psychology programs in the department: Female—full-time 200, part-time 62; Male—full-time 58, part-time 19; African American/Black—full-time 16, part-time 4; Hispanic/Latino(a)—full-time 39, part-time 13; Asian/Pacific Islander—full-time 33, part-time 10; American Indian/Alaska Native—full-time 1, part-time 2; Caucasian/White—full-time 124, part-time 46; Multi-ethnic—full-time 0, part-time 0; students subject to the Americans With Disabilities Act—full-time 1, part-time 0; Unknown ethnicity—full-time 38, part-time 6; International students who hold an F-1 or J-1 Visa—full-time 7, part-time 0.

Financial Information/Assistance:
Tuition for Full-Time Study: *Master's:* State residents: $540 per credit hour; Nonstate residents: $540 per credit hour. *Doctoral:* State residents: $760 per credit hour; Nonstate residents: $760 per credit hour. Tuition is subject to change. Tuition costs vary by program. See the following Web site for updates and changes in tuition costs: http://www.apu.edu/graduatecenter/sfs/costs/.

Financial Assistance:
First-Year Students: Teaching assistantships available for first year. Average amount paid per academic year: $6,250. Average number of hours worked per week: 15. Apply by April 15. Research assistantships available for first year. Average amount paid per academic year: $6,250. Average number of hours worked per week: 15. Apply by April 15.
Advanced Students: No information provided.
Additional Information: Of all students currently enrolled full time, 5% benefited from one or more of the listed financial assistance programs.

Internships/Practica: Doctoral Degree (PsyD Clinical Psychology): For those doctoral students for whom a professional internship was required in this program prior to graduation, (22) students applied for an internship in 2008–2009, with (22) students obtaining an internship. Of those students who obtained an internship, (20) were paid internships. Of those students who obtained an internship, (15) students placed in APA/CPA accredited internships, (4) students placed in internships not APA/CPA accredited, but listed with the Association of Psychology Postdoctoral and Internship Programs (APPIC), (0) students placed in internships conforming to guidelines of the Council of Directors of School Psychology Programs (CDSPP), (3) students placed in internships that were not APA/CPA accredited, APPIC or CDSPP listed. PsyD students are required to complete 6 semesters of practicum experience. These experiences are gained in placements throughout Los Angeles, Orange, and San Bernardino Counties which provide diverse clinical and multicultural experiences. A Counseling Center on the Azusa Pacific University campus also serves as a practicum site for doctoral students. A sequence of clinical practicum courses is offered simultaneously with the field placement experience. All doctoral students are required to complete one full year of psychology internship. APU places interns in a variety of sites (must be APA approved or those meeting APPIC standards) across the country. Students enrolled in the MA Program in Clinical Psychology complete a clinical training sequence that meets all requirements for future licensure as a Marriage and Family Therapist (MFT) in the state of California. Students complete 150 hours of direct client contact in diverse, multi-cultural settings, such as community counseling centers, domestic violence clinics, and schools. Students receive training in individual, marital, and group therapy and exposure to treatments that have been demonstrated to be effective with specific problems.

Housing and Day Care: No on-campus housing is available. No on-campus day care facilities are available.

Employment of Department Graduates:
Master's Degree Graduates: Of those who graduated in the academic year 2008–2009, the following categories and numbers represent the postgraduate activities and employment of master's degree graduates: Enrolled in a postdoctoral residency/fellowship (n/a), employed in independent practice (n/a), employed in other positions at a higher education institution (1), employed in government agency (2), employed in a community mental health/counseling center (6), still seeking employment (2), not seeking employment (1), other employment position (1), do not know (41), total from the above (master's) (54).
Doctoral Degree Graduates: Of those who graduated in the academic year 2008–2009, the following categories and numbers represent the postgraduate activities and employment of doctoral degree graduates: Enrolled in a psychology doctoral program (n/a), employed in independent practice (2), employed in government agency (1), employed in a community mental health/counseling center (2), employed in a hospital/medical center (4), do not know (2), total from the above (doctoral) (11).

Additional Information:
Orientation, Objectives, and Emphasis of Department: The PsyD in Clinical Psychology with an emphasis in Family Psychology (APA accredited) prepares students for the practice of professional psychology. The program adheres to a practitioner-scholar model of training and emphasizes development of the core competencies in clinical psychology adopted by the National Council of Schools and Programs of Professional Psychology. The program requires completion of a rigorous sequence of courses in the science and practice of psychology. Requirements include three years of clinical training, successful demonstration of clinical competency through examination, completion of a clinical dissertation, and a predoctoral internship. Prespecialty education in family psychology and an emphasis in interdisciplinary studies, relating psychology to ethics, theology, and philosophy, are included. The program was designed to be consistent with the requirements of the Guide-

lines and Principles for Accreditation of Programs in Professional Psychology. The MA in Clinical Psychology with an emphasis in Marriage and Family Therapy meets requirements for California MFT licensure. Concepts of individual psychology are integrated with interpersonal and ecological concepts of systems theory. Goals include cultivating the examined life, fostering theoretical mastery, developing practical clinical skills, encouraging clinically integrative strategies, and preparing psychotherapists to work in a culturally diverse world.

Special Facilities or Resources: All students have access to the APA PsycINFO database and all APA journals full-text online as part of their student library privileges. The Darling Library provides an attractive and functional set of resources for the APU PsyD and MA. The library is technology-friendly and includes the Ahmanson Information Technology Center, an area with 75 computer desks. Each computer is wired into the university system for Internet and library catalog system searches. PsycINFO, as well as over 100 additional licensed databases, are available for student literature and subject searches. Eight "scholar rooms" were designed as a part of the Darling Graduate Library to be used for conducting research and writing. Doctoral students in the dissertation phase of their program are given priority in the reservation of these rooms. There are also several conference rooms in the Darling Library that may be reserved for student study groups or research teams. The Department of Graduate Psychology runs the Community Counseling Center (CCC), which offers psychological services to the surrounding community as well as to faculty, staff and university students. The CCC also contracts to provide services to the surrounding 12 schools in the Azusa Unified School District. The CCC currently trains 50 MA and PsyD graduate students and has provided data for two doctoral dissertations.

Information for Students With Physical Disabilities: See the following Web site for more information: http://www.apu.edu/lec/language/.

Application Information:
Send to Azusa Pacific University, Graduate Admissions, 901 E. Alosta, P.O. Box 7000, Azusa, CA 91702-7000. Application available online. URL of online application: http://www.apu.edu/apply/. Students are admitted in the Fall, application deadline January 15; Spring, application deadline October 15. Application deadlines for MA are as follows: Fall deadline is March 15 and Spring deadline is October 15. *Fee:* $45. $65 International.

California Institute of Integral Studies (2009 data)
PsyD Program
School of Professional Psychology
1453 Mission Street
San Francisco, CA 94103
Telephone: (415) 575-6100
Fax: (415) 575-1266
E-mail: *kmcgovern@ciis.edu*
Web: *http://www.ciis.edu*

Department Information:
1979. Program Chair: Katie McGovern. Number of faculty: total—full-time 12, part-time 30; women—full-time 7, part-time 20; total—minority—full-time 3; women minority—full-time 2; faculty subject to the Americans With Disabilities Act 1.

Programs and Degrees Offered:
Listed in the following order: Program area, degree type (T if terminal Master's), number awarded 7/08–6/09. Clinical Psychology PsyD (Doctor of Psychology) 16, Counseling Psychology MA/MS (Master of Arts/Science) (T) 58.

APA Accreditation: Clinical PsyD (Doctor of Psychology).

Student Applications/Admissions:
Student Applications
Clinical Psychology PsyD (Doctor of Psychology)—Applications 2009–2010, 141. Total applicants accepted 2009–2010, 63. Number full-time enrolled (new admits only) 2009–2010, 38. Number part-time enrolled (new admits only) 2009–2010, 0. Total enrolled 2009–2010 full-time, 139, part-time, 35. Openings 2010–2011, 32. The number of students enrolled full- and part-time who were dismissed or voluntarily withdrew from this program area in 2008–2009 were 4. *Counseling Psychology MA/MS (Master of Arts/Science)*—Applications 2009–2010, 274. Total applicants accepted 2009–2010, 124. Number full-time enrolled (new admits only) 2009–2010, 100. Number part-time enrolled (new admits only) 2009–2010, 24. Total enrolled 2009–2010 full-time, 287, part-time, 70. Openings 2010–2011, 125. The median number of years required for completion of a degree in 2008–2009 were 3. The number of students enrolled full- and part-time who were dismissed or voluntarily withdrew from this program area in 2008–2009 were 6.

Other Criteria: (importance of criteria rated low, medium, or high): research experience—low, work experience—medium, extracurricular activity—medium, clinically related public service—high, GPA—high, letters of recommendation—high, interview—high, statement of goals and objectives—high, written work sample—high, undergraduate major in psychology—medium, specific undergraduate psychology courses taken—low. Admissions criteria listed above apply to PsyD program. For the MA program GRE is not required. For additional information on admission requirements, go to http://www.ciis.edu.

Student Characteristics: The following represents characteristics of students in 2009–2010 in all graduate psychology programs in the department: Female—full-time 185, part-time 70; Male—full-time 45, part-time 20; African American/Black—full-time 14, part-time 0; Hispanic/Latino(a)—full-time 15, part-time 0; Asian/Pacific Islander—full-time 14, part-time 0; American Indian/Alaska Native—full-time 1, part-time 0; Caucasian/White—full-time 183, part-time 0; Multi-ethnic—full-time 3, part-time 3; students subject to the Americans With Disabilities Act—full-time 2, part-time 0; Unknown ethnicity—full-time 0, part-time 0; International students who hold an F-1 or J-1 Visa—full-time 0, part-time 0.

Financial Information/Assistance:
Tuition for Full-Time Study: *Master's:* State residents: per academic year $15,270, $725 per credit hour; Nonstate residents: per academic year $15,270, $725 per credit hour. *Doctoral:* State residents: per academic year $24,700, $955 per credit hour; Nonstate residents: per academic year $24,700, $955 per credit hour.

Tuition is subject to change. See the following Web site for updates and changes in tuition costs: http://www.ciis.edu.

Financial Assistance:
First-Year Students: Teaching assistantships available for first year. Fellowships and scholarships available for first year. Average amount paid per academic year: $5,000. Apply by May 1.
Advanced Students: Teaching assistantships available for advanced students. Apply by varies. Fellowships and scholarships available for advanced students. Average amount paid per academic year: $5,000. Apply by May 1.
Additional Information: Of all students currently enrolled full time, 15% benefited from one or more of the listed financial assistance programs.

Internships/Practica: Doctoral Degree (PsyD Clinical Psychology): For those doctoral students for whom a professional internship was required in this program prior to graduation, (31) students applied for an internship in 2008–2009, with (31) students obtaining an internship. Of those students who obtained an internship, (14) were paid internships. Of those students who obtained an internship, (2) students placed in APA/CPA accredited internships, (7) students placed in internships not APA/CPA accredited, but listed with the Association of Psychology Postdoctoral and Internship Programs (APPIC), (0) students placed in internships conforming to guidelines of the Council of Directors of School Psychology Programs (CDSPP), (22) students placed in internships that were not APA/CPA accredited, APPIC or CDSPP listed. Internship and practicum placements are available throughout the greater San Francisco Bay Area at a broad variety of mental health service agencies. All doctoral internship sites are approved by APPIC or CAPIC. Not all internship positions are funded.

Housing and Day Care: No on-campus housing is available. No on-campus day care facilities are available.

Employment of Department Graduates:
Master's Degree Graduates: Of those who graduated in the academic year 2008–2009, the following categories and numbers represent the postgraduate activities and employment of master's degree graduates: Enrolled in a postdoctoral residency/fellowship (n/a), employed in independent practice (n/a), total from the above (master's) (0).
Doctoral Degree Graduates: Of those who graduated in the academic year 2008–2009, the following categories and numbers represent the postgraduate activities and employment of doctoral degree graduates: Enrolled in a psychology doctoral program (n/a), total from the above (doctoral) (0).

Additional Information:
Orientation, Objectives, and Emphasis of Department: The Institute offers a unique program of education and training, broadening the usual conceptual framework for graduate training in psychology by including in the curriculum some exposure to Asian philosophic, humanistic, and transpersonal approaches to understanding human experience. The educational philosophy simultaneously values scholarly knowledge, inner development, applied research, and human service. Psychology programs at CIIS flourish within a fertile and broadening climate provided by other social science graduate programs in philosophy/religion, anthropology, and women's spirituality, along with online degree programs.

Within the practitioner-scholar training model, the APA-accredited PsyD program provides knowledge of the foundations of scientific and professional psychology while emphasizing the understanding of consciousness, self-knowledge, and human evolution embodied in the philosophical and psychological traditions of both East and West. The clinical specialization prepares students for work with the broad range of clientele and systems found across the range of multidisciplinary service settings and the spectrum of populations served by the clinical psychologist. Experiential growth work is required in all programs. Several clinical concentrations are available. CIIS has a 35,000-volume library and a well-developed Placement Office to support academic studies.

Special Facilities or Resources: CIIS operates four separate community-based counseling centers: the on-campus Psychological Services Center operated by the PsyD Clinical Psychology program, and three counseling centers operated by the MA Counseling program. All counseling centers serve as primary training sites for the MA and PsyD programs.

Application Information:
Send to Office of Admissions. Students are admitted in the Fall, application deadline January 15. MA programs: April 15 for Fall, September 15 for Spring. *Fee:* $65.

California Lutheran University
Psychology Department
60 West Olsen Road
Thousand Oaks, CA 91360-2787
Telephone: (805) 493-3528
Fax: (805) 493-3479
E-mail: *mpuopolo@clunet.edu*
Web: *http://www.callutheran.edu/schools/cas/*

Department Information:
1959. Director, Graduate Programs in Psychology: Mindy Puopolo, PsyD. Number of faculty: total—full-time 4, part-time 20; women—full-time 1, part-time 14; total—minority—full-time 1, part-time 4; women minority—part-time 2.

Programs and Degrees Offered:
Listed in the following order: Program area, degree type (T if terminal Master's), number awarded 7/08–6/09. Clinical MA/MS (Master of Arts/Science) (T) 8, Marital and Family Therapy MA/MS (Master of Arts/Science) (T) 19, Clinical Psychology PsyD (Doctor of Psychology).

Student Applications/Admissions:
Student Applications
Clinical MA/MS (Master of Arts/Science)—Applications 2009–2010, 70. Total applicants accepted 2009–2010, 24. Number full-time enrolled (new admits only) 2009–2010, 23. Number part-time enrolled (new admits only) 2009–2010, 1. Total enrolled 2009–2010 full-time, 52, part-time, 1. Openings 2010–2011, 18. The median number of years required for completion of a degree in 2008–2009 were 2. The number of students enrolled full- and part-time who were dismissed or voluntarily withdrew from this program area in 2008–2009

were 0. *Marital and Family Therapy MA/MS (Master of Arts/Science)*—Applications 2009–2010, 108. Total applicants accepted 2009–2010, 55. Number full-time enrolled (new admits only) 2009–2010, 64. Number part-time enrolled (new admits only) 2009–2010, 2. Total enrolled 2009–2010 full-time, 117, part-time, 2. Openings 2010–2011, 56. The median number of years required for completion of a degree in 2008–2009 were 2. The number of students enrolled full- and part-time who were dismissed or voluntarily withdrew from this program area in 2008–2009 were 0. *Clinical Psychology PsyD (Doctor of Psychology)*—Total applicants accepted 2009–2010, 17. Openings 2010–2011, 17.

Scores: Entries appear in this order: required test or GPA, minimum score (if required), median score of students entering in 2009–2010. *Clinical MA/MS (Master of Arts/Science)*: last 2 years GPA 3.0; *Marital and Family Therapy MA/MS (Master of Arts/Science)*: last 2 years GPA 3.0; *Clinical Psychology PsyD (Doctor of Psychology)*: GRE-V no minimum stated, GRE-Q no minimum stated, GRE-Analytical no minimum stated, GRE-Subject (Psychology) no minimum stated, overall undergraduate GPA 3.0.

Other Criteria: (importance of criteria rated low, medium, or high): GRE scores—medium, research experience—medium, work experience—medium, extracurricular activity—low, clinically related public service—medium, GPA—high, letters of recommendation—medium, interview—high, statement of goals and objectives—high, undergraduate major in psychology—medium, specific undergraduate psychology courses taken—high. The PsyD in Clinical Psychology requires GRE scores as well as statements regarding previous research and practice experience. The Masters programs require either a minimum 3.0 GPA in upper division courses or GRE scores. For additional information on admission requirements, go to http://www.callutheran.edu/admission/graduate/downloads/documents/psych_checklist.pdf.

Student Characteristics: The following represents characteristics of students in 2009–2010 in all graduate psychology programs in the department: Female—full-time 136, part-time 3; Male—full-time 32, part-time 1; African American/Black—full-time 2, part-time 0; Hispanic/Latino(a)—full-time 45, part-time 1; Asian/Pacific Islander—full-time 11, part-time 0; American Indian/Alaska Native—full-time 4, part-time 0; Caucasian/White—full-time 99, part-time 3; Multi-ethnic—full-time 1, part-time 0; students subject to the Americans With Disabilities Act—full-time 4, part-time 0; Unknown ethnicity—full-time 6, part-time 0; International students who hold an F-1 or J-1 Visa—full-time 1, part-time 0.

Financial Information/Assistance:
  Tuition for Full-Time Study: *Master's:* State residents: $595 per credit hour; Nonstate residents: $595 per credit hour. *Doctoral:* State residents: $875 per credit hour; Nonstate residents: $875 per credit hour. Tuition is subject to change. Additional fees are assessed to students beyond the costs of tuition for the following: practicum fee; assessment lab fee; competency exam fee. See the following Web site for updates and changes in tuition costs: http://www.callutheran.edu/financial_aid/graduate/.

Financial Assistance:
  First-Year Students: Teaching assistantships available for first year. Average amount paid per academic year: $1,200. Average number of hours worked per week: 5. Apply by August 15. Research assistantships available for first year. Average amount paid per academic year: $1,200. Average number of hours worked per week: 5. Apply by August 15.
  Advanced Students: Teaching assistantships available for advanced students. Average amount paid per academic year: $1,750. Average number of hours worked per week: 5. Apply by May 1. Research assistantships available for advanced students. Average amount paid per academic year: $1,750. Average number of hours worked per week: 5. Apply by May 1. Fellowships and scholarships available for advanced students. Average amount paid per academic year: $2,000. Average number of hours worked per week: 0.
  Additional Information: Of all students currently enrolled full time, 25% benefited from one or more of the listed financial assistance programs. Application and information available online at: http://www.callutheran.edu/financial_aid/graduate/grants.php.

Internships/Practica: Master's Degree (MA/MS Marital and Family Therapy): An internship experience, such as a final research project or "capstone" experience is required of graduates. The Graduate Psychology Programs at CLU provide training through two Community Counseling and Parent Child Study Centers. Both centers offer low cost therapy services to the community. In addition, each center provides state-of-the-art counseling facilities including video and audio recording capabilities, two-way observation windows, play therapy rooms and a professional staff. Individual supervision, group supervision, case conference, staff training, peer support, and sharing of learning experiences in an atmosphere designed to facilitate growth as a therapist create exceptional training opportunities. The PsyD Program in Clinical Psychology requires three years of practicum experience and a one year full-time internship. The first year of practicum experience is completed at one of CLU's Counseling Centers. Practicum students have opportunities to work with individuals, couples, families and groups. A special feature of the Counseling Psychology Marital and Family Therapy Program is a 12-month practicum placement in the University's Community Counseling Services Center. Students may also choose an external practicum in a local community agency. Approximately 500 hours applicable to the California licensing requirement can be obtained through the MFT practicum experience.

Housing and Day Care: On-campus housing is available. See the following Web site for more information: http://www.callutheran.edu/student_life/res_life/graduate_housing.php. No on-campus day care facilities are available.

Employment of Department Graduates:
  Master's Degree Graduates: Of those who graduated in the academic year 2008–2009, the following categories and numbers represent the postgraduate activities and employment of master's degree graduates: Enrolled in a postdoctoral residency/fellowship (n/a), employed in independent practice (n/a), total from the above (master's) (0).
  Doctoral Degree Graduates: Of those who graduated in the academic year 2008–2009, the following categories and numbers represent the postgraduate activities and employment of doctoral degree graduates: Enrolled in a psychology doctoral program (n/a), total from the above (doctoral) (0).

GRADUATE STUDY IN PSYCHOLOGY

Additional Information:

Orientation, Objectives, and Emphasis of Department: California Lutheran University's Doctor of Psychology (PsyD) degree in Clinical Psychology is a five-year program that integrates theoretical and practical approaches to prepare graduates for careers as licensed clinical psychologists. The program provides students with a broad perspective of psychology and explores the role of research in clinical practice. The program is accredited by the Western Association of Schools and Colleges (WASC), one of six regional accrediting associations in the United States. The curriculum includes six core courses that provide an in-depth developmental examination of major diagnostic categories, as well as areas of emphasis in research and practical skill development. The Master of Science degree in Clinical Psychology provides both a scientific and practitioner foundation in addition to providing excellent preparation for application to doctoral programs. The Master of Science Degree in Counseling Psychology prepares the student to become a professional Marital and Family Therapist (MFT). The program is designed to meet all academic requirements for the state license in marriage and family therapy, administered by the California Board of Behavioral Sciences.

Special Facilities or Resources: In addition to the two Community Counseling and Parent Child Study Centers, CLU is in the process of completing a new Social and Behavioral Science Building complete with lab space and research facilities. The graduate programs in psychology also benefit from close relationships with local mental health agencies, both private and public.

Information for Students With Physical Disabilities: See the following Web site for more information: http://www.callutheran.edu/car/.

Application Information:
Send to Julius Munyantwali, Graduate Admission Counselor, 60 W Olsen Road, Thousand Oaks, CA 91360. Application available online. URL of online application: http://www.callutheran.edu/admission/graduate/apply/. Students are admitted in the Fall, application deadline January 15. Fee: $75. Candidates who attend the regularly scheduled Information Meetings are eligible for an application fee waiver.

California Polytechnic State University
Psychology and Child Development
Liberal Arts
1 Grand Avenue Building 47-24
San Luis Obispo, CA 93407
Telephone: (805) 756-2805
Fax: (805) 756-1134
E-mail: *kmoreno@calpoly.edu*
Web: *http://psycd.calpoly.edu/*

Department Information:
1969. Chairperson: Gary D. Laver. Number of faculty: total—full-time 20, part-time 11; women—full-time 14, part-time 6; total—minority—full-time 7, part-time 1; women minority—full-time 5; faculty subject to the Americans With Disabilities Act 1.

Programs and Degrees Offered:
Listed in the following order: Program area, degree type (T if terminal Master's), number awarded 7/08–6/09. Counseling Marriage and Family MA/MS (Master of Arts/Science) (T) 11.

Student Applications/Admissions:
Student Applications
Counseling Marriage and Family MA/MS (Master of Arts/Science)—Applications 2009–2010, 65. Total applicants accepted 2009–2010, 27. Number full-time enrolled (new admits only) 2009–2010, 18. Number part-time enrolled (new admits only) 2009–2010, 1. Total enrolled 2009–2010 full-time, 33, part-time, 13. Openings 2010–2011, 20. The median number of years required for completion of a degree in 2008–2009 were 3. The number of students enrolled full- and part-time who were dismissed or voluntarily withdrew from this program area in 2008–2009 were 3.

Scores: Entries appear in this order: required test or GPA, minimum score (if required), median score of students entering in 2009–2010. *Counseling Marriage and Family MA/MS (Master of Arts/Science)*: GRE-V no minimum stated, 497, GRE-Q no minimum stated, 598, GRE-Analytical no minimum stated, 4.5, last 2 years GPA no minimum stated, 3.59.

Other Criteria: (importance of criteria rated low, medium, or high): GRE scores—high, research experience—low, work experience—medium, extracurricular activity—medium, clinically related public service—medium, GPA—high, letters of recommendation—high, interview—high, statement of goals and objectives—high, undergraduate major in psychology—low, specific undergraduate psychology courses taken—low. For additional information on admission requirements, go to http://psycd.calpoly.edu/graduate/psychology.asp?pid=3.

Student Characteristics: The following represents characteristics of students in 2009–2010 in all graduate psychology programs in the department: Female—full-time 29, part-time 12; Male—full-time 4, part-time 1; African American/Black—full-time 0, part-time 0; Hispanic/Latino(a)—full-time 5, part-time 1; Asian/Pacific Islander—full-time 0, part-time 0; American Indian/Alaska Native—full-time 0, part-time 0; Caucasian/White—full-time 21, part-time 9; Multi-ethnic—full-time 2, part-time 0; students subject to the Americans With Disabilities Act—full-time 0, part-time 0; Unknown ethnicity—full-time 5, part-time 3; International students who hold an F-1 or J-1 Visa—full-time 0, part-time 1.

Financial Information/Assistance:
Tuition for Full-Time Study: Master's: State residents: per academic year $7,134; Nonstate residents: per academic year $16,062. Tuition is subject to change. See the following Web site for updates and changes in tuition costs: http://www.afd.calpoly.edu/fees/index.asp.

Financial Assistance:
First-Year Students: No information provided.
Advanced Students: No information provided.
Additional Information: Of all students currently enrolled full time, 0% benefited from one or more of the listed financial assistance programs. Application and information available online at: http://www.ess.calpoly.edu/_finaid/.

Internships/Practica: Master's Degree (MA/MS Counseling Marriage and Family): An internship experience, such as a final research project or "capstone" experience is required of graduates. The Central Coast of California offers numerous well-supervised clinical internships in public and private non-profit agencies with a variety of client populations. Internships are selected based on their ability to provide: 1) quality supervision by a state-qualified licensed clinician; 2) clients with a wide variety of psychological disorders; 3) a variety of treatment modalities, i.e., individual, couple, family, and group therapy; 4) a wide variety of clients that represent the diversity of the community. Most internship students are placed at public agency sites which serve the country's entire range of ethnic and minority populations.

Housing and Day Care: On-campus housing is available. See the following Web site for more information: http://www.housing.calpoly.edu/. On-campus day care facilities are available. See the following Web site for more information: http://www.asi.calpoly.edu/childrens_center.

Employment of Department Graduates:
Master's Degree Graduates: Of those who graduated in the academic year 2008–2009, the following categories and numbers represent the postgraduate activities and employment of master's degree graduates: Enrolled in a postdoctoral residency/fellowship (n/a), employed in independent practice (n/a), total from the above (master's) (0).
Doctoral Degree Graduates: Of those who graduated in the academic year 2008–2009, the following categories and numbers represent the postgraduate activities and employment of doctoral degree graduates: Enrolled in a psychology doctoral program (n/a), total from the above (doctoral) (0).

Additional Information:
Orientation, Objectives, and Emphasis of Department: The M.S. in Psychology is designed for persons who desire to practice in the field of clinical/counseling psychology. The program's mission is to provide the state of California with highly competent master's-level clinicians who are academically prepared for the Marriage and Family therapist (MFT) license and counseling with individuals, couples, families, and groups in a multicultural society. The program fulfills the educational requirements for the state of California's Marriage and Family Therapist (MFT) License. Its mission is also to provide students who want to proceed on to doctoral programs in clinical or counseling psychology with sound research skills, thesis experience and clinical intervention training. Graduates find career opportunities in public social service agencies such as Mental Health and Departments of Social Services as well as in private non-profit and private practice counseling centers. Ten to twenty percent of graduates go on to doctoral programs in clinical or counseling psychology.

Special Facilities or Resources: Closely supervised, on-campus practicum experiences leading to challenging internships in community agencies are the cornerstone of Cal Poly's preparation for the future clinician. The program runs a community counseling services clinic with three counseling offices and an observation room that provides direct viewing through one-way mirrors and remotely controlled video equipment. Closely supervised experience in Cal Poly's practicum clinic serving clients from the community provides trainees with the opportunity to develop skills and confidence before undertaking an internship.

Information for Students With Physical Disabilities: See the following Web site for more information: http://drc.calpoly.edu/.

Application Information:
Send to Admissions Office, California Polytechnic State University, San Luis Obispo, CA 93407. Application available online. URL of online application: http://www.csumentor.edu/AdmissionApp/grad_apply.asp. Students are admitted in the Fall, application deadline December 1. Portfolio deadline is February 15. *Fee:* $55.

California State University, Dominguez Hills
Department of Psychology
Natural and Behavioral Sciences
1000 East Victoria Street
Carson, CA 90747
Telephone: (310) 243-3427
Fax: (310) 516-3642
E-mail: kmason@csudh.edu
Web: *http://www.nbs.csudh.edu/psychology*

Department Information:
1969. Coordinator, M.A in Psychology Program: Karen I. Mason, PhD. Number of faculty: total—full-time 10, part-time 20; women—full-time 6, part-time 6; total—minority—full-time 6, part-time 10; women minority—full-time 5, part-time 2.

Programs and Degrees Offered:
Listed in the following order: Program area, degree type (T if terminal Master's), number awarded 7/08–6/09. Psychology (Clinical Emphasis) MA/MS (Master of Arts/Science) (T) 8.

Student Applications/Admissions:
Student Applications
Psychology (Clinical Emphasis) MA/MS *(Master of Arts/Science)*—Applications 2009–2010, 54. Total applicants accepted 2009–2010, 25. Number full-time enrolled (new admits only) 2009–2010, 16. Number part-time enrolled (new admits only) 2009–2010, 2. Total enrolled 2009–2010 full-time, 44, part-time, 5. Openings 2010–2011, 20. The median number of years required for completion of a degree in 2008–2009 were 2. The number of students enrolled full- and part-time who were dismissed or voluntarily withdrew from this program area in 2008–2009 were 0.
Scores: Entries appear in this order: required test or GPA, minimum score (if required), median score of students entering in 2009–2010. *Psychology (Clinical Emphasis) MA/MS (Master of Arts/Science)*: GRE-V no minimum stated, GRE-Q no minimum stated, last 2 years GPA 3.0.
Other Criteria: (importance of criteria rated low, medium, or high): GRE scores—medium, research experience—medium, work experience—low, clinically related public service—medium, GPA—high, letters of recommendation—high, interview—low, statement of goals and objectives—high. For additional information on admission requirements, go to http://www.nbs.csudh.edu/psychology/ma.htm.

Student Characteristics: The following represents characteristics of students in 2009–2010 in all graduate psychology programs in the department: Female—full-time 38, part-time 3; Male—full-time 6, part-time 2; African American/Black—full-time 8, part-time 1; Hispanic/Latino(a)—full-time 16, part-time 2; Asian/Pacific Islander—full-time 1, part-time 0; American Indian/Alaska

Native—full-time 0, part-time 0; Caucasian/White—full-time 18, part-time 2; Multi-ethnic—full-time 0, part-time 0; students subject to the Americans With Disabilities Act—full-time 0, part-time 0; Unknown ethnicity—full-time 1, part-time 0; International students who hold an F-1 or J-1 Visa—full-time 0, part-time 0.

Financial Information/Assistance:
Tuition for Full-Time Study: *Master's:* State residents: per academic year $5,576; Nonstate residents: $372 per credit hour. Tuition is subject to change. See the following Web site for updates and changes in tuition costs: http://www.csudh.edu/admfin/accounting_services_sfs.shtml.

Financial Assistance:
First-Year Students: Fellowships and scholarships available for first year. Average amount paid per academic year: $2,000. Apply by March.
Advanced Students: Teaching assistantships available for advanced students. Research assistantships available for advanced students. Average amount paid per academic year: $10,000. Average number of hours worked per week: 15. Fellowships and scholarships available for advanced students. Average amount paid per academic year: $2,000. Apply by March.
Additional Information: Of all students currently enrolled full time, 12% benefited from one or more of the listed financial assistance programs.

Internships/Practica: Master's Degree (MA/MS Psychology (Clinical Emphasis)): An internship experience, such as a final research project or "capstone" experience is required of graduates. The Master of Arts in Psychology offers 550 supervised hours of practicum experience in a variety of settings.

Housing and Day Care: On-campus housing is available. See the following Web site for more information: http://www.csudh.edu/studentaffairs/housing/. On-campus day care facilities are available. See the following Web site for more information: http://www.csudh.edu/asi/pages/cdc.html.

Employment of Department Graduates:
Master's Degree Graduates: Of those who graduated in the academic year 2008–2009, the following categories and numbers represent the postgraduate activities and employment of master's degree graduates: Enrolled in a psychology doctoral program (1), enrolled in another graduate/professional program (0), enrolled in a postdoctoral residency/fellowship (n/a), employed in independent practice (n/a), employed in an academic position at a 2-year/4-year college (4), employed in a community mental health/counseling center (3), other employment position (0), do not know (0), total from the above (master's) (8).
Doctoral Degree Graduates: Of those who graduated in the academic year 2008–2009, the following categories and numbers represent the postgraduate activities and employment of doctoral degree graduates: Enrolled in a psychology doctoral program (n/a), total from the above (doctoral) (0).

Additional Information:
Orientation, Objectives, and Emphasis of Department: The Clinical Psychology Master of Arts Program provides you with a solid academic background in clinical psychology as it is applied within a community mental health framework. This program prepares you for a career in counseling, teaching and research in community settings, which includes public or private agencies. Eighteen units of additional coursework prepare you for practice as a marriage and family therapist. Our graduates are successful in gaining admission to and graduating from the doctoral programs of their choice.

Special Facilities or Resources: Special resources include laboratory facilities.

Information for Students With Physical Disabilities: See the following Web site for more information: http://www.csudh.edu/studentaffairs/disabledstudentservices/.

Application Information:
Send to Department of Psychology, California State University, Dominguez Hills, 1000 E. Victoria Street, Carson, CA 90747. Application available online. URL of online application: http://www.nbs.csudh.edu/psychology/ma.htm. Students are admitted in the Fall, application deadline March 1. *Fee:* $55.

California State University, Fullerton
Department of Psychology
Humanities and Social Sciences
P.O. Box 6846
Fullerton, CA 92834-6846
Telephone: (714) 278-3589
Fax: (714) 278-7134
E-mail: kkarlson@fullerton.edu
Web: http://hss.fullerton.edu/psychology/graduate.asp

Department Information:
1957. Chairperson: Jack Mearns. Number of faculty: total—full-time 26, part-time 32; women—full-time 15, part-time 26; total—minority—full-time 6, part-time 7; women minority—full-time 3, part-time 4.

Programs and Degrees Offered:
Listed in the following order: Program area, degree type (T if terminal Master's), number awarded 7/08–6/09. Clinical Psychology MA/MS (Master of Arts/Science) (T) 16, Psychological Research MA/MS (Master of Arts/Science) (T) 13.

Student Applications/Admissions:
Student Applications
Clinical Psychology MA/MS (*Master of Arts/Science*)—Applications 2009–2010, 55. Total applicants accepted 2009–2010, 22. Number full-time enrolled (new admits only) 2009–2010, 19. Number part-time enrolled (new admits only) 2009–2010, 0. Openings 2010–2011, 20. The median number of years required for completion of a degree in 2008–2009 were 2. The number of students enrolled full- and part-time who were dismissed or voluntarily withdrew from this program area in 2008–2009 were 1. *Psychological Research MA/MS (Master of Arts/Science)*—Applications 2009–2010, 70. Total applicants accepted 2009–2010, 20. Number full-time enrolled (new admits only) 2009–2010, 18. Number part-time enrolled (new admits only) 2009–2010, 0. Openings 2010–2011, 20. The

median number of years required for completion of a degree in 2008–2009 were 2.

Other Criteria: (importance of criteria rated low, medium, or high): GRE scores—high, research experience—high, clinically related public service—high, GPA—high, letters of recommendation—high, interview—high, statement of goals and objectives—high, specific undergraduate psychology courses taken—high. The Master of Science program requires an interview. There is no interview required for the Master of Arts program. For additional information on admission requirements, go to http://hss.fullerton.edu/psychology/graduate.asp.

Student Characteristics: The following represents characteristics of students in 2009–2010 in all graduate psychology programs in the department: Female—full-time 40, part-time 12; Male—full-time 5, part-time 8; African American/Black—full-time 1, part-time 0; Hispanic/Latino(a)—full-time 9, part-time 3; Asian/Pacific Islander—full-time 3, part-time 2; American Indian/Alaska Native—full-time 0, part-time 0; Caucasian/White—full-time 30, part-time 15; Multi-ethnic—full-time 2, part-time 0; students subject to the Americans With Disabilities Act—full-time 0, part-time 0; Unknown ethnicity—full-time 0, part-time 0; International students who hold an F-1 or J-1 Visa—full-time 0, part-time 0.

Financial Information/Assistance:
Financial Assistance:
First-Year Students: No information provided.
Advanced Students: No information provided.
Additional Information: Of all students currently enrolled full time, 0% benefited from one or more of the listed financial assistance programs.

Internships/Practica: Master's Degree (MA/MS Clinical Psychology): An internship experience, such as a final research project or "capstone" experience is required of graduates. Master's Degree (MA/MS Psychological Research): An internship experience, such as a final research project or "capstone" experience is required of graduates. A majority of the internships are done in agencies which do family therapy and substance abuse prevention and training. Most internships have live and videotape supervision. Students have done internships in policy psychology, county clinics, and inpatient settings as well. Most agencies combine clinical and community work and serve low income and minority populations.

Housing and Day Care: On-campus housing is available. See the following Web site for more information: http://www.fullerton.edu/housing. On-campus day care facilities are available. See the following Web site for more information: http://asi.fullerton.edu/cc/.

Employment of Department Graduates:
Master's Degree Graduates: Of those who graduated in the academic year 2008–2009, the following categories and numbers represent the postgraduate activities and employment of master's degree graduates: Enrolled in a psychology doctoral program (6), enrolled in another graduate/professional program (1), enrolled in a postdoctoral residency/fellowship (n/a), employed in independent practice (n/a), employed in an academic position at a 2-year/4-year college (1), employed in business or industry (7), employed in a community mental health/counseling center (9), total from the above (master's) (24).
Doctoral Degree Graduates: Of those who graduated in the academic year 2008–2009, the following categories and numbers represent the postgraduate activities and employment of doctoral degree graduates: Enrolled in a psychology doctoral program (n/a), total from the above (doctoral) (0).

Additional Information:
Orientation, Objectives, and Emphasis of Department: The MA program provides advanced coursework and research training in core areas of psychology. Completion of the MA can facilitate application to PhD programs in psychology and provides skills important to careers in education, the health professions, and industry. The MS program in clinical psychology is intended to prepare students for work in a variety of mental health settings, and the program contains coursework relevant for the MFT license in California. The program is also designed to prepare students for PhD work in both academic and professional schools of clinical psychology.

Special Facilities or Resources: The department has laboratories for research in cognitive psychology, conditioning, perception, biopsychology, social psychology, psychological testing, and developmental psychology. The department also has extensive computer facilities.

Application Information:
Send to Graduate Office, Department of Psychology, California State Fullerton, P.O. Box 6846, Fullerton CA 92834-6846. Application available online. URL of online application: http://hss.fullerton.edu/psychology/graduate.asp. Students are admitted in the Fall, application deadline March 1. *Fee:* $55. The fee waiver process is built in CSU Mentor (on line application) so you will not need to file a separate Request for an Application Fee Waiver. Only California residents are eligible.

California State University, Long Beach
Department of Psychology
1250 Bellflower Boulevard
Long Beach, CA 90840-0901
Telephone: (562) 985-5000
E-mail: *psygrad@csulb.edu*
Web: *http://www.csulb.edu/psychology*

Department Information:
1949. Chairperson: Kenneth F. Green. Number of faculty: total—full-time 26, part-time 27; women—full-time 9, part-time 20; total—minority—full-time 7, part-time 5; women minority—full-time 5, part-time 4.

Programs and Degrees Offered:
Listed in the following order: Program area, degree type (T if terminal Master's), number awarded 7/08–6/09. Psychological Research MA/MS (Master of Arts/Science) (T) 9, Industrial/Organizational Psychology MA/MS (Master of Arts/Science) (T) 7, Human Factors MA/MS (Master of Arts/Science) (T) 4.

GRADUATE STUDY IN PSYCHOLOGY

Student Applications/Admissions:

Student Applications

Psychological Research MA/MS (Master of Arts/Science)—Applications 2009–2010, 81. Total applicants accepted 2009–2010, 32. Number full-time enrolled (new admits only) 2009–2010, 15. Number part-time enrolled (new admits only) 2009–2010, 0. Total enrolled 2009–2010 full-time, 27, part-time, 4. Openings 2010–2011, 25. The median number of years required for completion of a degree in 2008–2009 were 2. The number of students enrolled full- and part-time who were dismissed or voluntarily withdrew from this program area in 2008–2009 were 1. *Industrial/Organizational Psychology MA/MS (Master of Arts/Science)*—Applications 2009–2010, 62. Total applicants accepted 2009–2010, 12. Number full-time enrolled (new admits only) 2009–2010, 5. Number part-time enrolled (new admits only) 2009–2010, 0. Total enrolled 2009–2010 full-time, 15, part-time, 1. Openings 2010–2011, 12. The median number of years required for completion of a degree in 2008–2009 were 2. The number of students enrolled full- and part-time who were dismissed or voluntarily withdrew from this program area in 2008–2009 were 0. *Human Factors MA/MS (Master of Arts/Science)*—Applications 2009–2010, 16. Total applicants accepted 2009–2010, 11. Number full-time enrolled (new admits only) 2009–2010, 2. Number part-time enrolled (new admits only) 2009–2010, 1. Total enrolled 2009–2010 full-time, 3, part-time, 11. Openings 2010–2011, 10. The median number of years required for completion of a degree in 2008–2009 were 2.

Scores: Entries appear in this order: required test or GPA, minimum score (if required), median score of students entering in 2009–2010. *Psychological Research MA/MS (Master of Arts/Science):* GRE-V no minimum stated, 508, GRE-Q no minimum stated, 613, GRE-Analytical no minimum stated, 4.48, last 2 years GPA no minimum stated, 3.70, psychology GPA no minimum stated, 3.69; *Industrial/Organizational Psychology MA/MS (Master of Arts/Science):* GRE-V no minimum stated, 540, GRE-Q no minimum stated, 636., GRE-Analytical no minimum stated, 4.93, last 2 years GPA no minimum stated, 3.82, psychology GPA no minimum stated, 3.83; *Human Factors MA/MS (Master of Arts/Science):* GRE-V no minimum stated, 472, GRE-Q no minimum stated, 630, GRE-Analytical no minimum stated, 4.6, last 2 years GPA no minimum stated, 3.63, psychology GPA no minimum stated, 3.78.

Other Criteria: (importance of criteria rated low, medium, or high): GRE scores—high, research experience—high, work experience—low, extracurricular activity—low, GPA—high, letters of recommendation—high, statement of goals and objectives—high, undergraduate major in psychology—medium, specific undergraduate psychology courses taken—high. For additional information on admission requirements, go to http://www.csulb.edu/psychology.

Student Characteristics: The following represents characteristics of students in 2009–2010 in all graduate psychology programs in the department: Female—full-time 33, part-time 8; Male—full-time 12, part-time 8; African American/Black—full-time 2, part-time 2; Hispanic/Latino(a)—full-time 4, part-time 0; Asian/Pacific Islander—full-time 6, part-time 5; American Indian/Alaska Native—full-time 0, part-time 0; Caucasian/White—full-time 30, part-time 9; Multi-ethnic—full-time 3, part-time 0; students subject to the Americans With Disabilities Act—full-time 0, part-time 0; Unknown ethnicity—full-time 0, part-time 0; International students who hold an F-1 or J-1 Visa—full-time 1, part-time 0.

Financial Information/Assistance:

Tuition for Full-Time Study: *Master's:* State residents: per academic year $5,840; Nonstate residents: per academic year $5,840, $339 per credit hour. Tuition is subject to change. See the following Web site for updates and changes in tuition costs: http://www.csulb.edu/depts/enrollment/registration/fees_basics.html.

Financial Assistance:

First-Year Students: Research assistantships available for first year. Average amount paid per academic year: $5,500. Average number of hours worked per week: 10. Apply by April 15. Fellowships and scholarships available for first year. Average amount paid per academic year: $3,500. Apply by March 1.

Advanced Students: Research assistantships available for advanced students. Average amount paid per academic year: $5,500. Average number of hours worked per week: 10. Apply by April 15. Fellowships and scholarships available for advanced students. Average amount paid per academic year: $3,500. Apply by March 1.

Additional Information: Of all students currently enrolled full time, 29% benefited from one or more of the listed financial assistance programs. Application and information available online at: http://www.csulb.edu/depts/enrollment/financial_aid/.

Internships/Practica: Master's Degree (MA/MS Psychological Research): An internship experience, such as a final research project or "capstone" experience is required of graduates. Master's Degree (MA/MS Industrial/Organizational Psychology): An internship experience, such as a final research project or "capstone" experience is required of graduates. Master's Degree (MA/MS Human Factors): An internship experience, such as a final research project or "capstone" experience is required of graduates. Graduate assistantship positions provide teaching, computer, and internship experiences to selected students in all the master's programs. Applications for graduate assistantships are available through the Graduate Office and are included in the application packet and online. Graduate assistantship assignments are based upon the pairing of each applicant's academic background, interests, and experience with current department needs. Specific assignments are geared toward providing educational experiences most appropriate for students in each program. Appointments are for ten hours per week. Available teaching assignments include assistance to the introductory and intermediate statistics, psychological assessment, critical thinking, program evaluation, computer applications, and research methods courses. In addition to the aforementioned paid departmental positions, volunteer and/or externally funded research positions can be arranged with individual faculty members. Such research opportunities are often available in the physiological, cognition, language, human factors, language acquisition, and social psychology laboratories. Various internships in outside industrial and organizational settings are options for second-year MSIO students. Internships are available through Boeing and CUDA for MSHF students.

Housing and Day Care: On-campus housing is available. See the following Web site for more information: http://www.csulb.edu/divisions/students/housing/. On-campus day care facilities are available. See the following Web site for more information: http://www.csulb.edu/divisions/students2/child_dev_ctr/index.html.

Employment of Department Graduates:
Master's Degree Graduates: Of those who graduated in the academic year 2008–2009, the following categories and numbers represent the postgraduate activities and employment of master's degree graduates: Enrolled in a postdoctoral residency/fellowship (n/a), employed in independent practice (n/a), total from the above (master's) (0).
Doctoral Degree Graduates: Of those who graduated in the academic year 2008–2009, the following categories and numbers represent the postgraduate activities and employment of doctoral degree graduates: Enrolled in a psychology doctoral program (n/a), total from the above (doctoral) (0).

Additional Information:
Orientation, Objectives, and Emphasis of Department: California State University Long Beach has three master's programs in psychology. The Master of Science in Human Factors prepares students to apply knowledge of psychology to the design of jobs, information systems, consumer products, workplaces and equipment in order to improve user performance, safety and comfort. Students acquire a background in the core areas of experimental psychology, research design and methodology, human factors, computer applications and applied research methods. The Master of Arts, Psychological Research Option (MAPR) prepares students for doctoral work in any psychology field or for master's-level research or teaching positions. Core seminars include cognition, learning, physiological and sensory psychology, social, personality, and developmental psychology, and quantitative methods. MAPR graduates who apply to doctoral programs have high acceptance rates with financial support. The Master of Science, Industrial and Organizational option (MSIO) offers preparation for careers for which a background in industrial/organizational psychology is essential. These fields include personnel, organizational development, industrial relations, employee training, and marketing research.

Special Facilities or Resources: The psychology building has extensive facilities available without charge. Computer facilities, with microcomputers and mainframe stations include many current software packages. The physiological research lab, with a staffed animal compound, is used to study conditioned analgesia and neurotransmission. For research in stress and coping, interpersonal relations, social influence, gender psychology, and the biopsychology of mood, there are many research suites and a test materials center. These facilities, located in the psychology building, are for research and training in interviewing and case studies, forensic psychology, program and treatment evaluation, assessment of social support and family systems, self-management, and intervention strategies for hard-to-reach populations. Computer facilities are central to research in decision analysis, human-computer interface, statistical theory, assessment, and computer-aided instruction. A computerized human-factors lab is used to study auditory and visual perception. Our diversified facilities also accommodate a large AIDS-education project, research in managing diversity in the workplace, and other topics in industrial/organizational psychology. Outstanding CSULB Library facilities are available.

Information for Students With Physical Disabilities: See the following Web site for more information: http://www.csulb.edu/divisions/students/dss.

Application Information:
Send to Psychology Graduate Office, 1250 Bellflower Blvd., Long Beach, CA 90840-0901. Application available online. URL of online application: http://www.csulb.edu/psychology. Students are admitted in the Fall, application deadline February 7-March 1; Spring, application deadline October 15-November 1. Spring admission deadline for MAR/MSHF: October 15/November 1, Fall admission deadline for MSIO: February 7; MAPR: February 21; MSHF: March 1. *Fee:* $55. Fee for University application only.

California State University, Northridge
Department of Psychology
Social and Behavioral Sciences
18111 Nordhoff Street
Northridge, CA 91330-8255
Telephone: (818) 677-2827
Fax: (818) 677-2829
E-mail: *carrie.saetermoe@csun.edu*
Web: *http://www.csun.edu/psychology*

Department Information:
1958. Chair: Carrie Saetermoe. Number of faculty: total—full-time 32, part-time 23; women—full-time 18, part-time 8; total—minority—full-time 5, part-time 6; women minority—full-time 5; faculty subject to the Americans With Disabilities Act 2.

Programs and Degrees Offered:
Listed in the following order: Program area, degree type (T if terminal Master's), number awarded 7/08–6/09. Clinical Psychology MA/MS (Master of Arts/Science) (T) 6, General Psychology MA/MS (Master of Arts/Science) 4, Human Factors MA/MS (Master of Arts/Science) (T) 3.

Student Applications/Admissions:
Student Applications
Clinical Psychology MA/MS *(Master of Arts/Science)*—Applications 2009–2010, 64. Total applicants accepted 2009–2010, 18. Number full-time enrolled (new admits only) 2009–2010, 16. Number part-time enrolled (new admits only) 2009–2010, 0. Openings 2010–2011, 15. The median number of years required for completion of a degree in 2008–2009 were 2. The number of students enrolled full- and part-time who were dismissed or voluntarily withdrew from this program area in 2008–2009 were 0. General Psychology MA/MS *(Master of Arts/Science)*—Applications 2009–2010, 45. Total applicants accepted 2009–2010, 12. Number full-time enrolled (new admits only) 2009–2010, 9. Number part-time enrolled (new admits only) 2009–2010, 0. Openings 2010–2011, 12. The median number of years required for completion of a degree in 2008–2009 were 2. The number of students enrolled full- and part-time who were dismissed or voluntarily withdrew from this program area in 2008–2009 were 0. Human Factors MA/MS *(Master of Arts/Science)*—Applications 2009–2010, 26. Total applicants accepted 2009–2010, 11. Number full-time enrolled (new admits only) 2009–2010, 10. Number part-time enrolled (new admits only) 2009–2010, 0. Openings 2010–2011, 12. The median number of years required for completion of a degree in 2008–2009 were 2. The number of students enrolled

full- and part-time who were dismissed or voluntarily withdrew from this program area in 2008–2009 were 1.

Scores: Entries appear in this order: required test or GPA, minimum score (if required), median score of students entering in 2009–2010. *Clinical Psychology MA/MS (Master of Arts/Science):* GRE-V no minimum stated, GRE-Q no minimum stated, GRE-Analytical no minimum stated, GRE-Subject (Psychology) no minimum stated; *General Psychology MA/MS (Master of Arts/Science):* GRE-V no minimum stated, GRE-Q no minimum stated, GRE-Analytical no minimum stated; *Human Factors MA/MS (Master of Arts/Science):* GRE-V no minimum stated, GRE-Q no minimum stated, GRE-Analytical no minimum stated.

Other Criteria: (importance of criteria rated low, medium, or high): GRE scores—low, research experience—high, work experience—medium, extracurricular activity—medium, clinically related public service—high, GPA—medium, letters of recommendation—high, interview—low, statement of goals and objectives—high, undergraduate major in psychology—medium, specific undergraduate psychology courses taken—medium. Clinically Related Public Services is rated high by the Clinical option; low relevance for the General Experimental and Human Factors options. Interviews are required by the Clinical option, either in-person (preferred) or via telephone (if necessary due to geographical restrictions). For additional information on admission requirements, go to http://www.csun.edu/psychology.

Student Characteristics: The following represents characteristics of students in 2009–2010 in all graduate psychology programs in the department: Female—full-time 56, part-time 0; Male—full-time 38, part-time 0; African American/Black—full-time 3, part-time 0; Hispanic/Latino(a)—full-time 7, part-time 0; Asian/Pacific Islander—full-time 5, part-time 0; American Indian/Alaska Native—full-time 0, part-time 0; Caucasian/White—full-time 20, part-time 0; Multi-ethnic—full-time 20, part-time 0; students subject to the Americans With Disabilities Act—full-time 0, part-time 0; Unknown ethnicity—full-time 39, part-time 0; International students who hold an F-1 or J-1 Visa—full-time 0, part-time 0.

Financial Information/Assistance:
Tuition for Full-Time Study: *Master's:* State residents: per academic year $4,460; Nonstate residents: $339 per credit hour. Tuition is subject to change. See the following Web site for updates and changes in tuition costs: http://www-admn.csun.edu/ucs/.

Financial Assistance:
First-Year Students: Research assistantships available for first year. Fellowships and scholarships available for first year.
Advanced Students: Teaching assistantships available for advanced students. Apply by March 13. Research assistantships available for advanced students. Fellowships and scholarships available for advanced students.
Additional Information: Application and information available online at: http://www.csun.edu/grip/graduatestudies/sfo/index.html.

Internships/Practica: Graduate students in applied fields have available an array of practicum experiences in the area. Direct clinical practicum experience is required of the Clinical students, who receive supervised training in three campus clinics specializing in Parent Child Interaction Training, Child and Adolescent Diagnostic Assessment, and Cognitive-Behavioral Psychotherapy. In addition, clinical internships are available in many community sites including the University Counseling Services and local mental health care facilities. Human Factors students are connected with research and applications positions in the region. General Experimental students work with departmental faculty as well as with those at neighboring universities.

Housing and Day Care: On-campus housing is available. See the following Web site for more information: http://housing.csun.edu. On-campus day care facilities are available.

Employment of Department Graduates:
Master's Degree Graduates: Of those who graduated in the academic year 2008–2009, the following categories and numbers represent the postgraduate activities and employment of master's degree graduates: Enrolled in a postdoctoral residency/fellowship (n/a), employed in independent practice (n/a), total from the above (master's) (0).
Doctoral Degree Graduates: Of those who graduated in the academic year 2008–2009, the following categories and numbers represent the postgraduate activities and employment of doctoral degree graduates: Enrolled in a psychology doctoral program (n/a), total from the above (doctoral) (0).

Additional Information:
Orientation, Objectives, and Emphasis of Department: The Department of Psychology has, as a primary goal, the assurance that students receive a strong theoretical foundation as well as rigorous methodological and statistical coursework. In addition, all students must complete a project or a thesis in order to display their knowledge of their content area and their methodological sophistication. The applied Human Factors program emphasizes both job-related skills and general skills should students desire to continue their education at the doctoral level (and many do). The General Experimental and Clinical programs emphasize the basic research and content knowledge required to enhance students' opportunities for entry into doctoral programs.

Special Facilities or Resources: Some professors have federal or private grants that employ graduate students as research assistants. In addition, we have laboratories in Physiological Psychology (NeuroScan, BioPac), computer applications for Cognitive and Human Factors Psychology, multiple childcare sites for observation of children, and extensive research space. In addition, we also have a state-of-the-art Statistics Laboratory that can be used for data analysis for theses or projects.

Information for Students With Physical Disabilities: See the following Web site for more information: http://www.csun.edu/cod/index.htm.

Application Information:
Send to Psychology Graduate Office, California State University Northridge, 18111 Nordhoff Street, Northridge, CA 91330-8255. Students are admitted in the Fall, application deadline February 15; Spring, application deadline November 15. The Clinical Psychology Program accepts Fall applications only. General-Experimental and Human Factors will accept Spring and Fall applications, space permitting. Fee: $55. Contact Admissions and Records Office for details (818) 677-3700.

California State University, Sacramento
Department of Psychology
6000 J Street
Sacramento, CA 95819-6007
Telephone: (916) 278-6254
Fax: (916) 278-6820
E-mail: youngl@csus.edu
Web: http://www.csus.edu/psyc/

Department Information:
1947. Chairperson: Bruce Behrman. Number of faculty: total—full-time 22, part-time 23; women—full-time 10, part-time 13; total—minority—full-time 7, part-time 5; women minority—full-time 3, part-time 4; faculty subject to the Americans With Disabilities Act 1.

Programs and Degrees Offered:
Listed in the following order: Program area, degree type (T if terminal Master's), number awarded 7/08–6/09. Counseling Psychology MA/MS (Master of Arts/Science) (T), Doctoral Preparation MA/MS (Master of Arts/Science) (T), Industrial/Organizational Psychology MA/MS (Master of Arts/Science) (T), General Psychology MA/MS (Master of Arts/Science) (T), Applied Behavior Analysis MA/MS (Master of Arts/Science) (T).

Student Applications/Admissions:
Student Applications
Counseling Psychology MA/MS (Master of Arts/Science)—Applications 2009–2010, 60. Total applicants accepted 2009–2010, 0. Number full-time enrolled (new admits only) 2009–2010, 0. The median number of years required for completion of a degree in 2008–2009 were 4. Doctoral Preparation MA/MS (Master of Arts/Science)—Applications 2009–2010, 60. Total applicants accepted 2009–2010, 12. Number full-time enrolled (new admits only) 2009–2010, 8. Total enrolled 2009–2010 full-time, 8. Openings 2010–2011, 7. The median number of years required for completion of a degree in 2008–2009 were 3. The number of students enrolled full- and part-time who were dismissed or voluntarily withdrew from this program area in 2008–2009 were 4. Industrial/Organizational Psychology MA/MS (Master of Arts/Science)—Applications 2009–2010, 25. Total applicants accepted 2009–2010, 8. Number full-time enrolled (new admits only) 2009–2010, 5. Openings 2010–2011, 6. The median number of years required for completion of a degree in 2008–2009 were 3. The number of students enrolled full- and part-time who were dismissed or voluntarily withdrew from this program area in 2008–2009 were 3. General Psychology MA/MS (Master of Arts/Science)—Applications 2009–2010, 20. Total applicants accepted 2009–2010, 2. Number full-time enrolled (new admits only) 2009–2010, 2. Total enrolled 2009–2010 full-time, 2. Openings 2010–2011, 5. The median number of years required for completion of a degree in 2008–2009 were 2. Applied Behavior Analysis MA/MS (Master of Arts/Science)—Applications 2009–2010, 38. Total applicants accepted 2009–2010, 10. Number full-time enrolled (new admits only) 2009–2010, 6. Openings 2010–2011, 7. The number of students enrolled full- and part-time who were dismissed or voluntarily withdrew from this program area in 2008–2009 were 4.

Scores: Entries appear in this order: required test or GPA, minimum score (if required), median score of students entering in 2009–2010. Counseling Psychology MA/MS (Master of Arts/Science): GRE-V no minimum stated, 550, GRE-Q no minimum stated, 550, overall undergraduate GPA 3.0, 3.4; Doctoral Preparation MA/MS (Master of Arts/Science): GRE-V no minimum stated, 550, GRE-Q no minimum stated, 550, GRE-Analytical no minimum stated, 4.0, GRE-Subject (Psychology) no minimum stated, 550, overall undergraduate GPA 3.0, 3.4; Industrial/Organizational Psychology MA/MS (Master of Arts/Science): GRE-V no minimum stated, 550, GRE-Q no minimum stated, 550, GRE-Subject (Psychology) no minimum stated, 550, overall undergraduate GPA 3.0, 3.4; General Psychology MA/MS (Master of Arts/Science): GRE-V no minimum stated, 550, GRE-Q no minimum stated, 550, GRE-Analytical no minimum stated, 4.0, GRE-Subject (Psychology) no minimum stated, 550, overall undergraduate GPA 3.0, 3.4; Applied Behavior Analysis MA/MS (Master of Arts/Science): GRE-V no minimum stated, GRE-Q no minimum stated, overall undergraduate GPA 3.0.

Other Criteria: (importance of criteria rated low, medium, or high): GRE scores—high, research experience—medium, work experience—medium, extracurricular activity—low, clinically related public service—medium, GPA—high, letters of recommendation—high, statement of goals and objectives—high, undergraduate major in psychology—high. For additional information on admission requirements, go to http://www.csus.edu/psyc/programs/graduate/index.htm.

Student Characteristics: The following represents characteristics of students in 2009–2010 in all graduate psychology programs in the department: Female—full-time 20, part-time 21; Male—full-time 20, part-time 15; African American/Black—full-time 3, part-time 1; Hispanic/Latino(a)—full-time 8, part-time 2; Asian/Pacific Islander—full-time 10, part-time 3; American Indian/Alaska Native—full-time 0, part-time 0; Caucasian/White—full-time 20, part-time 20; Multi-ethnic—full-time 0, part-time 0; students subject to the Americans With Disabilities Act—full-time 0, part-time 0; Unknown ethnicity—full-time 0, part-time 0; International students who hold an F-1 or J-1 Visa—full-time 3, part-time 0.

Financial Information/Assistance:
Tuition for Full-Time Study: Master's: State residents: per academic year $4,818; Nonstate residents: per academic year $11,514. Tuition is subject to change. See the following Web site for updates and changes in tuition costs: http://www.csus.edu/schedule/Fall2009Spring2010/fees.stm.

Financial Assistance:
First-Year Students: No information provided.
Advanced Students: Teaching assistantships available for advanced students. Fellowships and scholarships available for advanced students.

Additional Information: Of all students currently enrolled full time, 10% benefited from one or more of the listed financial assistance programs.

Internships/Practica: Master's Degree (MA/MS Counseling Psychology): An internship experience, such as a final research project or "capstone" experience is required of graduates. Master's Degree (MA/MS Doctoral Preparation): An internship experience, such as a final research project or "capstone" experience is required of graduates. Master's Degree (MA/MS Industrial/Organizational Psychology): An internship experience, such as, a final research project or "capstone" experience is required of graduates. Master's Degree (MA/MS General Psychology): An internship experience, such as a final research project or "capstone" experience is required of graduates. Master's Degree (MA/MS Applied Behavior Analysis): An internship experience, such as a final research project or "capstone" experience is required of graduates. Students following the Industrial-Organizational (I/O), Applied Behavior Analysis (ABA), and the Counseling Psychology programs will gain supervised on-site experience. I/O students typically enroll for several semesters of internship supervised by one of our faculty members. Opportunities are available in public sector organizations (e.g., state, county, and city personnel departments; public utilities) as well as private sector consulting firms, small businesses, and large corporations. Admisson to the Counseling Psychology program has been suspended for the years 2010 and 2011 pending program modifications. Counseling Psychology students normally would enroll for additional fieldwork in a community mental health setting with an on-site supervisor. Students may choose from more than a hundred sites in the Sacramento metropolitan area. These community sites must enter into a formal arrangement with the department, and the student's supervision hours must be officially logged. Applied Behavior Analysis students have numerous options for funded internships and job opportunities in both private and public sector agencies and schools throughout the Sacramento region.

Housing and Day Care: On-campus housing is available. See the following Web site for more information: http://www.csus.edu/housing/. On-campus day care facilities are available. See the following Web site for more information: http://www.asi.csus.edu/children/.

Employment of Department Graduates:
Master's Degree Graduates: Of those who graduated in the academic year 2008–2009, the following categories and numbers represent the postgraduate activities and employment of master's degree graduates: Enrolled in a psychology doctoral program (15), enrolled in a postdoctoral residency/fellowship (n/a), employed in independent practice (n/a), employed in an academic position at a university (2), employed in an academic position at a 2-year/4-year college (8), employed in business or industry (8), employed in government agency (12), employed in a community mental health/counseling center (20), total from the above (master's) (65).
Doctoral Degree Graduates: Of those who graduated in the academic year 2008–2009, the following categories and numbers represent the postgraduate activities and employment of doctoral degree graduates: Enrolled in a psychology doctoral program (n/a), total from the above (doctoral) (0).

Additional Information:
Orientation, Objectives, and Emphasis of Department: Our major programs are Doctoral Preparation, Industrial/Organizational (I/O), and Applied Behavior Analysis (ABA). Admission to the Counseling Psychology program has been suspended for the years 2010 and 2011 pending program modifications. Doctoral preparation students take a strong research methods and quantitative course sequence in addition to content coursework in their interest area. They also engage in research during most of their program, and are encouraged to become teaching assistants. Our I/O program has been designed to meet the competencies specified by SIOP and involves both classroom and fieldwork experience. Students take both general survey and current literature I/O courses in addition to their research, statistics, and measurement/testing courses, and are also expected to gain job experience as an intern. The Counseling Psychology program is suspended for 2010 and 2011. It otherwise meets the state licensing requirements for Marriage and Family Therapy; students are exposed to a variety of therapeutic orientations and must participate in multiple practicum courses. In addition, graduate students can supplement their program with a Teaching of Psychology mini-program in which they enroll in a formal teaching course and are then eligible to team teach an introductory psychology course in a subsequent semester. Those oriented toward a teaching career in a community college are advised to supplement their main course of study with this mini-program. We also have a program in Behavior Analysis which partially fulfills the requirements to become a Board Certified Behavior Analyst.

Special Facilities or Resources: The department occupies much of a relatively large building. Extensive facilities for human and animal research are available. We have a modern surgery room, animal colony, small group rooms with capabilities for audiovisual monitoring and recording, and a perception lab. A multi-room counseling suite within the building also has audiovisual capabilities; students enrolled in our practicum course provide services in this suite (under supervision) to clients from the community. One room in the building (maintained by the computer center) contains thirty workstations. Our ABA facilities include operant laboratories and research rooms for data collection with children and adults. ABA students may assist in our on-campus, after-school ABA Clinic for assessment and treatment of behavior problems, the UCP Autism Center of Excellence, and the Children's Hospital at UC Davis.

Information for Students With Physical Disabilities: See the following Web site for more information: http://www.csus.edu/SSWD/.

Application Information:
Send to Graduate Coordinator, Psychology Department, California State University Sacramento, 6000 J Street, Sacramento, CA 95819-6007. Application available online. URL of online application: http://www.csus.edu/gradstudies/appinfo_general.htm. Students are admitted in the Fall, application deadline February 1; Spring, application deadline October 1. Spring admission cycle available only if all openings were not filled during the prior fall admission cycle. Counseling Psychology admissions have been suspended for 2010 and 2011. *Fee:* $55.

California, University of, Berkeley
Psychology Department
Letters and Sciences
3210 Tolman Hall MC 1650
Berkeley, CA 94720-1650
Telephone: (510) 642-1382
Fax: (510) 642-5293
E-mail: *psychgradinfo@berkeley.edu*
Web: *http://psychology.berkeley.edu/*

Department Information:
1921. Acting Chair: Richard Ivry. Number of faculty: total—full-time 41; women—full-time 19; total—minority—full-time 8; women minority—full-time 4; faculty subject to the Americans With Disabilities Act 1.

Programs and Degrees Offered:
Listed in the following order: Program area, degree type (T if terminal Master's), number awarded 7/08–6/09. Cognition, Brain, and Behavior PhD (Doctor of Philosophy) 5, Social/Personality Psychology PhD (Doctor of Philosophy) 6, Change, Plasticity, and Development PhD (Doctor of Philosophy) 2, Behavioral Neuroscience PhD (Doctor of Philosophy) 0, Clinical Science PhD (Doctor of Philosophy) 2.

APA Accreditation: Clinical PhD (Doctor of Philosophy). Student Outcome Data Website: http://psychology.berkeley.edu/graduate/cl_program.html.

Student Applications/Admissions:

Student Applications

Cognition, Brain, and Behavior PhD (Doctor of Philosophy)—Applications 2009–2010, 125. Total applicants accepted 2009–2010, 10. Number full-time enrolled (new admits only) 2009–2010, 5. Number part-time enrolled (new admits only) 2009–2010, 0. Openings 2010–2011, 12. The median number of years required for completion of a degree in 2008–2009 were 5. The number of students enrolled full- and part-time who were dismissed or voluntarily withdrew from this program area in 2008–2009 were 1. *Social/Personality Psychology PhD (Doctor of Philosophy)*—Applications 2009–2010, 185. Total applicants accepted 2009–2010, 8. Number full-time enrolled (new admits only) 2009–2010, 4. Number part-time enrolled (new admits only) 2009–2010, 0. Openings 2010–2011, 6. The median number of years required for completion of a degree in 2008–2009 were 6. The number of students enrolled full- and part-time who were dismissed or voluntarily withdrew from this program area in 2008–2009 were 0. *Change, Plasticity, and Development PhD (Doctor of Philosophy)*—Applications 2009–2010, 41. Total applicants accepted 2009–2010, 3. Number full-time enrolled (new admits only) 2009–2010, 2. Total enrolled 2009–2010 full-time, 20. Openings 2010–2011, 5. The median number of years required for completion of a degree in 2008–2009 were 6. The number of students enrolled full- and part-time who were dismissed or voluntarily withdrew from this program area in 2008–2009 were 1. *Behavioral Neuroscience PhD (Doctor of Philosophy)*—Applications 2009–2010, 13. Total applicants accepted 2009–2010, 0. Number full-time enrolled (new admits only) 2009–2010, 0. Number part-time enrolled (new admits only) 2009–2010, 0. Openings 2010–2011, 2. The number of students enrolled full- and part-time who were dismissed or voluntarily withdrew from this program area in 2008–2009 were 0. *Clinical Science PhD (Doctor of Philosophy)*—Applications 2009–2010, 245. Total applicants accepted 2009–2010, 7. Number full-time enrolled (new admits only) 2009–2010, 7. Number part-time enrolled (new admits only) 2009–2010, 0. Openings 2010–2011, 8. The median number of years required for completion of a degree in 2008–2009 were 6. The number of students enrolled full- and part-time who were dismissed or voluntarily withdrew from this program area in 2008–2009 were 0.

Scores: Entries appear in this order: required test or GPA, minimum score (if required), median score of students entering in 2009–2010. *Cognition, Brain, and Behavior PhD (Doctor of Philosophy)*: GRE-V no minimum stated, 680, GRE-Q no minimum stated, 760, GRE-Analytical no minimum stated, 5.25, overall undergraduate GPA 3.0, 3.75, last 2 years GPA 3.0, 3.67; *Social/Personality Psychology PhD (Doctor of Philosophy)*: GRE-V no minimum stated, 660, GRE-Q no minimum stated, 730, GRE-Analytical no minimum stated, 5.5, overall undergraduate GPA 3.0, 3.84, last 2 years GPA 3.0, 3.87; *Change, Plasticity, and Development PhD (Doctor of Philosophy)*: GRE-V no minimum stated, 660, GRE-Q no minimum stated, 695, GRE-Analytical no minimum stated, 5.0, overall undergraduate GPA 3.0, 3.95, last 2 years GPA 3.0, 3.70; *Behavioral Neuroscience PhD (Doctor of Philosophy)*: GRE-V no minimum stated, GRE-Q no minimum stated, GRE-Analytical no minimum stated, overall undergraduate GPA 3.0, last 2 years GPA 3.0; *Clinical Science PhD (Doctor of Philosophy)*: GRE-V no minimum stated, 730, GRE-Q no minimum stated, 720, GRE-Analytical no minimum stated, 5.0, overall undergraduate GPA 3.0, 3.55, last 2 years GPA 3.0, 3.70.

Other Criteria: (importance of criteria rated low, medium, or high): GRE scores—medium, research experience—high, work experience—high, extracurricular activity—medium, clinically related public service—high, GPA—medium, letters of recommendation—high, interview—high, statement of goals and objectives—high, interest in faculty research—high. For additional information on admission requirements, go to http://psychology.berkeley.edu/graduate/grad_application.html.

Student Characteristics: The following represents characteristics of students in 2009–2010 in all graduate psychology programs in the department: Female—full-time 74, part-time 0; Male—full-time 51, part-time 0; African American/Black—full-time 2, part-time 0; Hispanic/Latino(a)—full-time 9, part-time 0; Asian/Pacific Islander—full-time 15, part-time 0; American Indian/Alaska Native—full-time 0, part-time 0; Caucasian/White—full-time 67, part-time 0; Multi-ethnic—full-time 8, part-time 0; students subject to the Americans With Disabilities Act—full-time 0, part-time 0; Unknown ethnicity—full-time 24, part-time 0; International students who hold an F-1 or J-1 Visa—full-time 10, part-time 0.

GRADUATE STUDY IN PSYCHOLOGY

Financial Information/Assistance:
  Tuition for Full-Time Study: *Doctoral:* State residents: per academic year $11,454; Nonstate residents: per academic year $26,502. Tuition is subject to change. See the following Web site for updates and changes in tuition costs: http://registrar.berkeley.edu/.

Financial Assistance:
  First-Year Students: Teaching assistantships available for first year. Average amount paid per academic year: $16,637. Research assistantships available for first year. Average amount paid per academic year: $18,600. Fellowships and scholarships available for first year. Average amount paid per academic year: $19,500. Apply by November 30.
  Advanced Students: Teaching assistantships available for advanced students. Average amount paid per academic year: $16,637. Research assistantships available for advanced students. Average amount paid per academic year: $18,600. Fellowships and scholarships available for advanced students. Average amount paid per academic year: $24,000.
  Additional Information: Of all students currently enrolled full time, 90% benefited from one or more of the listed financial assistance programs. Application and information available online at: http://students.berkeley.edu/finaid/graduates/index.htm.

Internships/Practica: Doctoral Degree (PhD Clinical Science): For those doctoral students for whom a professional internship was required in this program prior to graduation, (5) students applied for an internship in 2008–2009, with (5) students obtaining an internship. Of those students who obtained an internship, (5) were paid internships. Of those students who obtained an internship, (5) students placed in APA/CPA accredited internships, (0) students placed in internships not APA/CPA accredited, but listed with the Association of Psychology Postdoctoral and Internship Programs (APPIC), (0) students placed in internships conforming to guidelines of the Council of Directors of School Psychology Programs (CDSPP), (0) students placed in internships that were not APA/CPA accredited, APPIC or CDSPP listed. The sole practicum experience on-site is the Psychology Clinic, a pre-internship site for 2nd and 3rd year students in the Clinical Science program. A community clinic, operating on a sliding scale basis, for individuals and families in the Bay Area, the Clinic offers assessment, individual therapy, couples therapy, child/family therapy, and consultations.

Housing and Day Care: On-campus housing is available. See the following Web site for more information: http://www.housing.berkeley.edu/. On-campus day care facilities are available. See the following Web site for more information: http://www.housing.berkeley.edu/child/families/.

Employment of Department Graduates:
  Master's Degree Graduates: Of those who graduated in the academic year 2008–2009, the following categories and numbers represent the postgraduate activities and employment of master's degree graduates: Enrolled in a postdoctoral residency/fellowship (n/a), employed in independent practice (n/a), total from the above (master's) (0).

  Doctoral Degree Graduates: Of those who graduated in the academic year 2008–2009, the following categories and numbers represent the postgraduate activities and employment of doctoral degree graduates: Enrolled in a psychology doctoral program (n/a), enrolled in another graduate/professional program (0), enrolled in a postdoctoral residency/fellowship (9), employed in independent practice (1), employed in an academic position at a university (3), employed in an academic position at a 2-year/4-year college (0), employed in other positions at a higher education institution (3), employed in a professional position in a school system (0), employed in business or industry (1), employed in government agency (1), employed in a community mental health/counseling center (0), employed in a hospital/medical center (0), still seeking employment (0), not seeking employment (0), other employment position (0), do not know (2), total from the above (doctoral) (20).

Additional Information:
  Orientation, Objectives, and Emphasis of Department: The goal of the graduate program in Psychology at Berkeley is to produce scholar-researchers with sufficient breadth to retain perspective on the field of psychology and sufficient depth to permit successful independent and significant research. The members of the Department have organized themselves into four graduate training areas. These areas reflect a sense of intellectual community among the faculty and correspond, in general, with traditional designations in the field. However, each graduate training area has a distinctive stamp placed upon it by the faculty and students that make up the program. The majority of our students enter graduate training and fulfill the requirements established by the existent training areas listed below. These requirements vary from area to area but always involve a combination of courses, seminars, and supervised independent research. Students are also encouraged to take courses outside the Psychology Department, using the unique faculty strengths found on the Berkeley campus to enrich their graduate training.

  Special Facilities or Resources: The Department of Psychology is housed in Tolman Hall, a building shared with the Graduate School of Education. A library devoted to books and journals in psychology and education is maintained on the second floor of this building. The main office of the Psychology Department, as well as faculty and teaching assistant offices are on the third floor of Tolman Hall. Research rooms for carrying out a variety of studies with human subjects are on the basement, ground, fourth, and fifth floors. The basement also houses a human audition laboratory and an electronics shop. The Institute of Human Development is housed on the first floor of Tolman Hall, the Psychology Clinic on the second floor, and the Institute of Personality and Social Research on the fourth floor. The remaining research units—the Institute for Cognitive and Brain Sciences, the Field Station for the Study of Behavior, Ecology and Reproduction, the Institute of Business and Employee Relations, the Helen Wills Neuroscience Institute, the Henry H. Wheeler Center for Brain Imaging, and the Northwest Animal Facility—are located elsewhere on campus and in the adjacent areas.

  Information for Students With Physical Disabilities: See the following Web site for more information: http://dsp.berkeley.edu/.

Application Information:
Send to University of California, Berkeley, Department of Psychology, Graduate Admissions, 3210 Tolman Hall, Berkeley, CA 94720-1652. Application available online. URL of online application: http://www.grad.berkeley.edu/prospective/index.shtml. Students are admitted in the Fall, application deadline November 30. *Fee:* $70. Fee is $90 for international applicants.

California, University of, Berkeley
School Psychology Program
Graduate School of Education
4511 Tolman Hall
Berkeley, CA 94720-1670
Telephone: (510) 642-7581
Fax: (510) 642-3555
E-mail: *frankc@berkeley.edu*
Web: *http://www-gse.berkeley.edu/program/sp/sp.html*

Department Information:
1966. Program Director: Frank C. Worrell. Number of faculty: total—full-time 2, part-time 7; women—full-time 1, part-time 5; total—minority—full-time 1.

Programs and Degrees Offered:
Listed in the following order: Program area, degree type (T if terminal Master's), number awarded 7/08–6/09. School Psychology PhD (Doctor of Philosophy) 4.

APA Accreditation: School PhD (Doctor of Philosophy). Student Outcome Data Website: http://www-gse.berkeley.edu/program/sp/html/admissions.html.

Student Applications/Admissions:
Student Applications
School Psychology PhD (Doctor of Philosophy)—Applications 2009–2010, 47. Total applicants accepted 2009–2010, 6. Number full-time enrolled (new admits only) 2009–2010, 6. Total enrolled 2009–2010 full-time, 37. Openings 2010–2011, 6. The median number of years required for completion of a degree in 2008–2009 were 6. The number of students enrolled full- and part-time who were dismissed or voluntarily withdrew from this program area in 2008–2009 were 3.
Scores: Entries appear in this order: required test or GPA, minimum score (if required), median score of students entering in 2009–2010. School Psychology PhD (Doctor of Philosophy): GRE-V no minimum stated, 650, GRE-Q no minimum stated, 650, overall undergraduate GPA 3.5, 3.5.
Other Criteria: (importance of criteria rated low, medium, or high): GRE scores—high, research experience—high, work experience—medium, extracurricular activity—medium, clinically related public service—medium, GPA—high, letters of recommendation—high, interview—high, statement of goals and objectives—high, undergraduate major in psychology—medium, specific undergraduate psychology courses taken—medium. For additional information on admission requirements, go to http://www-gse.berkeley.edu/program/SP/html/admissions.html.

Student Characteristics: The following represents characteristics of students in 2009–2010 in all graduate psychology programs in the department: Female—full-time 31, part-time 0; Male—full-time 6, part-time 0; African American/Black—full-time 5, part-time 0; Hispanic/Latino(a)—full-time 3, part-time 0; Asian/Pacific Islander—full-time 5, part-time 0; American Indian/Alaska Native—full-time 1, part-time 0; Caucasian/White—full-time 22, part-time 0; Multi-ethnic—full-time 1, part-time 0; students subject to the Americans With Disabilities Act—full-time 0, part-time 0; Unknown ethnicity—full-time 0, part-time 0; International students who hold an F-1 or J-1 Visa—full-time 2, part-time 0.

Financial Information/Assistance:
Tuition for Full-Time Study: Doctoral: State residents: per academic year $11,343; Nonstate residents: per academic year $26,037. Tuition is subject to change. See the following Web site for updates and changes in tuition costs: http://registrar.berkeley.edu/Registration/feesched.html.

Financial Assistance:
First-Year Students: Teaching assistantships available for first year. Average amount paid per academic year: $16,637. Average number of hours worked per week: 20. Research assistantships available for first year. Average amount paid per academic year: $16,212. Average number of hours worked per week: 20. Fellowships and scholarships available for first year. Average amount paid per academic year: $15,000. Apply by December 1.
Advanced Students: Teaching assistantships available for advanced students. Average amount paid per academic year: $18,408. Average number of hours worked per week: 20. Research assistantships available for advanced students. Average amount paid per academic year: $20,928. Average number of hours worked per week: 20. Fellowships and scholarships available for advanced students. Average amount paid per academic year: $10,000. Apply by March 1.
Additional Information: Of all students currently enrolled full time, 80% benefited from one or more of the listed financial assistance programs. Application and information available online at: http://gse.berkeley.edu/admin/sas/admissions/req_aid.html.

Internships/Practica: Doctoral Degree (PhD School Psychology): For those doctoral students for whom a professional internship was required in this program prior to graduation, (12) students applied for an internship in 2008–2009, with (12) students obtaining an internship. Of those students who obtained an internship, (8) were paid internships. Of those students who obtained an internship, (0) students placed in APA/CPA accredited internships, (0) students placed in internships not APA/CPA accredited, but listed with the Association of Psychology Postdoctoral and Internship Programs (APPIC), (12) students placed in internships conforming to guidelines of the Council of Directors of School Psychology Programs (CDSPP), (0) students placed in internships that were not APA/CPA accredited, APPIC or CDSPP listed. Students on school-based internships are usually paid on the basis of school-district schedule for half to three quarter time, usually from $13,000–$17,000/school year.

Housing and Day Care: On-campus housing is available. See the following Web site for more information: http://www.housing.berkeley.edu/livingatcal/graduatestudents.html. On-campus day care facilities are available. See the following Web site for more information: http://berkeley.edu/work/child.shtml.

Employment of Department Graduates:
Master's Degree Graduates: Of those who graduated in the academic year 2008–2009, the following categories and numbers represent the postgraduate activities and employment of master's degree graduates: Enrolled in a postdoctoral residency/fellowship (n/a), employed in independent practice (n/a), total from the above (master's) (0).
Doctoral Degree Graduates: Of those who graduated in the academic year 2008–2009, the following categories and numbers represent the postgraduate activities and employment of doctoral degree graduates: Enrolled in a psychology doctoral program (n/a), employed in an academic position at a university (2), employed in a professional position in a school system (2), total from the above (doctoral) (4).

Additional Information:
Orientation, Objectives, and Emphasis of Department: The school psychology program is a doctoral program within the cognition and development area. The program emphasizes the scientist-professional model of school psychological services, linking strong preparation in theory and research to applications in the professional context of schools and school systems. Through the thoughtful application of knowledge and skills, school psychologists work together with teachers and other school professionals to clarify and resolve problems regarding the educational and mental health needs of children in classrooms. Working as consultants and collaborators, school psychologists help others to accommodate the social systems of schools to the individual differences of students, with the ultimate goal of promoting academic and social development. Graduate work within the program is supervised by professors from the Departments of Education and Psychology. Students fulfill all requirements for the academic PhD in human development, with additional coursework representing professional preparation for the specialty practice of school psychology. The program is accredited by APA.

Special Facilities or Resources: The school psychology program is based at the University of California, Berkeley, which is a major research university in a large metropolitan area of the country. Students have access to faculty research and university resources in countless topics and areas of specialization. The university and department sponsor numerous colloquia, speakers, and visiting lecturers from around the world throughout the year. Both intellectual and cultural resources abound. Ongoing research programs of faculty offer students opportunities to engage in applications of psychology to educational problems during their first three years of the program and in their dissertation research.

Information for Students With Physical Disabilities: See the following Web site for more information: http://dsp.berkeley.edu.

Application Information:
Send to Admission Office, Graduate School of Education. Application available online. URL of online application: http://gse.berkeley.edu/admin/sas/requirements.html. Students are admitted in the Fall, application deadline December 1. *Fee:* $70.

California, University of, Davis
Department of Psychology
College of Letters and Science
One Shields Avenue
Davis, CA 95616-8686
Telephone: (530) 752-9362
Fax: (530) 752-2087
E-mail: *lmoakes@ucdavis.edu*
Web: *http://www.psychology.ucdavis.edu*

Department Information:
1957. Chairperson: Debra Long. Number of faculty: total—full-time 42; women—full-time 15; total—minority—full-time 10; women minority—full-time 3.

Programs and Degrees Offered:
Listed in the following order: Program area, degree type (T if terminal Master's), number awarded 7/08–6/09. Cognition and Cognitive Neuroscience PhD (Doctor of Philosophy) 2, Psychobiology PhD (Doctor of Philosophy) 2, Developmental Psychology PhD (Doctor of Philosophy) 3, Quantitative Psychology PhD (Doctor of Philosophy) 0, Social/Personality Psychology PhD (Doctor of Philosophy) 1.

Student Applications/Admissions:
Student Applications
Cognition and Cognitive Neuroscience PhD (Doctor of Philosophy)—Applications 2009–2010, 103. Total applicants accepted 2009–2010, 13. Number full-time enrolled (new admits only) 2009–2010, 6. Number part-time enrolled (new admits only) 2009–2010, 0. Openings 2010–2011, 6. The median number of years required for completion of a degree in 2008–2009 were 5. The number of students enrolled full- and part-time who were dismissed or voluntarily withdrew from this program area in 2008–2009 were 1. *Psychobiology PhD (Doctor of Philosophy)*—Applications 2009–2010, 25. Total applicants accepted 2009–2010, 5. Number full-time enrolled (new admits only) 2009–2010, 1. Openings 2010–2011, 2. The median number of years required for completion of a degree in 2008–2009 were 5. The number of students enrolled full- and part-time who were dismissed or voluntarily withdrew from this program area in 2008–2009 were 0. *Developmental Psychology PhD (Doctor of Philosophy)*—Applications 2009–2010, 56. Total applicants accepted 2009–2010, 7. Number full-time enrolled (new admits only) 2009–2010, 4. Number part-time enrolled (new admits only) 2009–2010, 0. Openings 2010–2011, 4. The median number of years required for completion of a degree in 2008–2009 were 5. The number of students enrolled full- and part-time who were dismissed or voluntarily withdrew from this program area in 2008–2009 were 0. *Quantitative Psychology PhD (Doctor of Philosophy)*—Applications 2009–2010, 13. Total applicants accepted 2009–2010, 4. Number full-time enrolled (new admits only) 2009–2010, 1. Total enrolled 2009–2010 full-time, 6. Openings 2010–2011, 2. The median number of years required for completion of a degree in 2008–2009 were 5. The number of students enrolled full- and part-time who were dismissed or voluntarily withdrew from this program area in 2008–2009 were 0. *Social/Personality Psychology PhD (Doctor of Philosophy)*—Applications 2009–2010, 153. Total applicants accepted 2009–2010, 7. Number

full-time enrolled (new admits only) 2009–2010, 4. Number part-time enrolled (new admits only) 2009–2010, 0. Openings 2010–2011, 4. The median number of years required for completion of a degree in 2008–2009 were 5. The number of students enrolled full- and part-time who were dismissed or voluntarily withdrew from this program area in 2008–2009 were 1.

Scores: Entries appear in this order: required test or GPA, minimum score (if required), median score of students entering in 2009–2010. *Cognition and Cognitive Neuroscience PhD (Doctor of Philosophy):* GRE-V no minimum stated, GRE-Q no minimum stated, GRE-Analytical no minimum stated, overall undergraduate GPA 3.0; *Psychobiology PhD (Doctor of Philosophy):* GRE-V no minimum stated, GRE-Q no minimum stated, GRE-Analytical no minimum stated, overall undergraduate GPA 3.0; *Developmental Psychology PhD (Doctor of Philosophy):* GRE-V no minimum stated, GRE-Q no minimum stated, GRE-Analytical no minimum stated, overall undergraduate GPA 3.0; *Quantitative Psychology PhD (Doctor of Philosophy):* GRE-V no minimum stated, GRE-Q no minimum stated, GRE-Analytical no minimum stated, overall undergraduate GPA 3.0; *Social/Personality Psychology PhD (Doctor of Philosophy):* GRE-V no minimum stated, GRE-Q no minimum stated, GRE-Analytical no minimum stated, overall undergraduate GPA 3.0.

Other Criteria: (importance of criteria rated low, medium, or high): GRE scores—high, research experience—high, work experience—low, extracurricular activity—low, GPA—high, letters of recommendation—high, interview—high, statement of goals and objectives—high, undergraduate major in psychology—low, specific undergraduate psychology courses taken—low. For additional information on admission requirements, go to http://psychology.ucdavis.edu/graduate/.

Student Characteristics: The following represents characteristics of students in 2009–2010 in all graduate psychology programs in the department: Female—full-time 56, part-time 0; Male—full-time 36, part-time 0; African American/Black—full-time 2, part-time 0; Hispanic/Latino(a)—full-time 3, part-time 0; Asian/Pacific Islander—full-time 10, part-time 0; American Indian/Alaska Native—full-time 0, part-time 0; Caucasian/White—full-time 58, part-time 0; Multi-ethnic—full-time 0, part-time 0; students subject to the Americans With Disabilities Act—full-time 1, part-time 0; Unknown ethnicity—full-time 19, part-time 0; International students who hold an F-1 or J-1 Visa—full-time 5, part-time 0.

Financial Information/Assistance:

Tuition for Full-Time Study: *Doctoral:* State residents: per academic year $11,631; Nonstate residents: per academic year $26,556. Tuition is subject to change. See the following Web site for updates and changes in tuition costs: http://budget.ucdavis.edu/studentfees.

Financial Assistance:

First-Year Students: Teaching assistantships available for first year. Average amount paid per academic year: $16,641. Average number of hours worked per week: 20. Research assistantships available for first year. Average amount paid per academic year: $15,696. Average number of hours worked per week: 20. Fellowships and scholarships available for first year. Average amount paid per academic year: $5,000. Apply by January 15.

Advanced Students: Teaching assistantships available for advanced students. Average amount paid per academic year: $16,641. Average number of hours worked per week: 20. Research assistantships available for advanced students. Average amount paid per academic year: $16,740. Average number of hours worked per week: 20. Fellowships and scholarships available for advanced students. Average amount paid per academic year: $5,000. Apply by January 15.

Additional Information: Of all students currently enrolled full time, 100% benefited from one or more of the listed financial assistance programs. Application and information available online at: http://psychology.ucdavis.edu/graduate/.

Housing and Day Care: On-campus housing is available. See the following Web site for more information: http://www.housing.ucdavis.edu. On-campus day care facilities are available. See the following Web site for more information: http://www.hr.ucdavis.edu/worklife-wellness/Life/childcare.

Employment of Department Graduates:

Master's Degree Graduates: Of those who graduated in the academic year 2008–2009, the following categories and numbers represent the postgraduate activities and employment of master's degree graduates: Enrolled in a postdoctoral residency/fellowship (n/a), employed in independent practice (n/a), total from the above (master's) (0).

Doctoral Degree Graduates: Of those who graduated in the academic year 2008–2009, the following categories and numbers represent the postgraduate activities and employment of doctoral degree graduates: Enrolled in a psychology doctoral program (n/a), enrolled in a postdoctoral residency/fellowship (4), employed in an academic position at a university (5), employed in other positions at a higher education institution (1), employed in government agency (1), total from the above (doctoral) (11).

Additional Information:

Orientation, Objectives, and Emphasis of Department: The department places strong emphasis on empirical research in five broad areas: (1) psychobiology (e.g., animal behavior, primatology, hormones and behavior, brain bases of social attachments, eating and obesity); (2) perception, cognition, and cognitive neuroscience (e.g., memory, attention, language, consciousness); (3) personality, social psychology, and social neuroscience (e.g., emotions, attitudes, prejudice, close relationships, cultural psychology, psychology of religion, brain bases of personality traits); (4) developmental psychology (cognitive, affective, and social development, personality development, effects of child abuse, brain bases of developmental disorders); and (5) quantitative psychology (e.g., psychometrics, multivariate statistics, hierarchical linear models, statistical models used in areas as diverse as neuroscience and longitudinal developmental research). Weekly colloquia in these five areas provide students with opportunities to hear about new research and present their own ideas and findings. Each student selects a three-person faculty advisory committee, which guides and evaluates the student's progress through the program. Major exams are tailored to each student by his or her advisory committee. Every faculty member has an active lab, permitting students to learn about anything from cellular recording and brain imaging to behavioral studies of development, perception, cognition, language, emotion, and both individual and social behavior, in both humans and nonhuman animals.

Special Facilities or Resources: The Psychology Department, which contains numerous state-of-the art laboratories, computer facilities, and a survey research facility, overlaps with several other major research centers on campus: a regional Primate Research Center, a Center for Neuroscience, a Center for Mind and Brain, and the M.I.N.D. Institute for research on developmental disorders. Departmental faculty members participate in campus-wide graduate groups in psychology, human development, animal behavior, neuroscience, and other fields, and in a cross-university Bay Area Affective Sciences Training Program. The university includes a medical school, a veterinary school, a business school, and a law school, as well as exceptionally strong programs in all of the biological and social sciences. The Department of Psychology offers graduate students an education that is intellectually exciting, personally challenging, and very forward-looking, one that prepares new teacher-scientist-scholars to advance the study of mind, brain, and behavior.

Information for Students With Physical Disabilities: See the following Web site for more information: http://sdc.ucdavis.edu/.

Application Information:
Send to Graduate Program Coordinator, Psychology Department, University of California, One Shields Avenue, Davis, CA 95616-8686. Application available online. URL of online application: http://gradstudies.ucdavis.edu/prospective/apply_online.cfm. Students are admitted in the Fall, application deadline December 15. *Fee:* $70.

California, University of, Davis
Human Development
Agricultural and Environmental Sciences
One Shields Avenue
Davis, CA 95616-8523
Telephone: (530) 754-4109
Fax: (530) 752-5660
E-mail: *dmbesser@ucdavis.edu*
Web: *http://humandevelopment.ucdavis.edu*

Department Information:
1971. Chair, Human & Child Development Graduate Groups: Larry V. Harper. Number of faculty: total—full-time 29; women—full-time 23; faculty subject to the Americans With Disabilities Act 1.

Programs and Degrees Offered:
Listed in the following order: Program area, degree type (T if terminal Master's), number awarded 7/08–6/09. Child Development MA/MS (Master of Arts/Science) (T) 6, Human Development PhD (Doctor of Philosophy) 6.

Student Applications/Admissions:
Student Applications
Child Development MA/MS (*Master of Arts/Science*)—Applications 2009–2010, 22. Total applicants accepted 2009–2010, 4. Number full-time enrolled (new admits only) 2009–2010, 2. Openings 2010–2011, 2. The median number of years required for completion of a degree in 2008–2009 were 2. The number of students enrolled full- and part-time who were dismissed or voluntarily withdrew from this program area in 2008–2009 were 0. Human Development PhD (*Doctor of Philosophy*)—Applications 2009–2010, 30. Total applicants accepted 2009–2010, 6. Number full-time enrolled (new admits only) 2009–2010, 6. Total enrolled 2009–2010 full-time, 31. Openings 2010–2011, 4. The median number of years required for completion of a degree in 2008–2009 were 7. The number of students enrolled full- and part-time who were dismissed or voluntarily withdrew from this program area in 2008–2009 were 2.

Other Criteria: (importance of criteria rated low, medium, or high): GRE scores—high, research experience—high, work experience—high, extracurricular activity—low, clinically related public service—low, GPA—high, letters of recommendation—high, interview—high, statement of goals and objectives—high, undergraduate major in psychology—medium, specific undergraduate psychology courses taken—high. For the Human Development PhD, we require a writing sample/paper. This can be a MS Thesis but more often it is a past publication where the applicant is considered a major author. For additional information on admission requirements, go to http://humandevelopment.ucdavis.edu/.

Student Characteristics: The following represents characteristics of students in 2009–2010 in all graduate psychology programs in the department: Female—full-time 33, part-time 1; Male—full-time 5, part-time 1; African American/Black—full-time 4, part-time 0; Hispanic/Latino(a)—full-time 5, part-time 0; Asian/Pacific Islander—full-time 9, part-time 0; American Indian/Alaska Native—full-time 0, part-time 0; Caucasian/White—full-time 0, part-time 0; Multi-ethnic—full-time 1, part-time 0; students subject to the Americans With Disabilities Act—full-time 1, part-time 0; Unknown ethnicity—full-time 0, part-time 0; International students who hold an F-1 or J-1 Visa—full-time 0, part-time 0.

Financial Information/Assistance:
Tuition for Full-Time Study: Master's: State residents: per academic year $11,632; Nonstate residents: per academic year $26,674. Doctoral: State residents: per academic year $11,632; Nonstate residents: per academic year $26,674. Tuition is subject to change. See the following Web site for updates and changes in tuition costs: http://budget.ucdavis.edu/studentfees.

Financial Assistance:
First-Year Students: Teaching assistantships available for first year. Average number of hours worked per week: 20. Research assistantships available for first year. Average number of hours worked per week: 20. Fellowships and scholarships available for first year. Apply by January 15.

Advanced Students: Teaching assistantships available for advanced students. Average number of hours worked per week: 20. Research assistantships available for advanced students. Average number of hours worked per week: 20. Fellowships and scholarships available for advanced students. Apply by January 15.

Additional Information: Of all students currently enrolled full time, 90% benefited from one or more of the listed financial assistance programs. Application and information available online at: http://humandevelopment.ucdavis.edu/.

Internships/Practica: Master's Degree (MA/MS Child Development): An internship experience, such as a final research project or "capstone" experience is required of graduates. For Child Development MS students application of theories of learning and development to interaction with children six months to five years at the Center for Child and Family Studies and field studies with children and adolescents. Study of children's affective, cognitive and social development within the context of family/school environments, hospitals, and foster group homes. Child Life internships through the University of California Davis Medical Center. Internships through the 4-H Center for Youth Development, includng 4-H and CE-sponsored out-of-school childcare, and the M.I.N.D. Institute, etc.

Housing and Day Care: No on-campus housing is available. On-campus day care facilities are available.

Employment of Department Graduates:
Master's Degree Graduates: Of those who graduated in the academic year 2008–2009, the following categories and numbers represent the postgraduate activities and employment of master's degree graduates: Enrolled in a psychology doctoral program (3), enrolled in a postdoctoral residency/fellowship (n/a), employed in independent practice (n/a), do not know (1), total from the above (master's) (4).
Doctoral Degree Graduates: Of those who graduated in the academic year 2008–2009, the following categories and numbers represent the postgraduate activities and employment of doctoral degree graduates: Enrolled in a psychology doctoral program (n/a), enrolled in a postdoctoral residency/fellowship (1), employed in an academic position at a university (1), employed in business or industry (2), employed in a community mental health/counseling center (1), do not know (1), total from the above (doctoral) (6).

Additional Information:
Orientation, Objectives, and Emphasis of Department: Both the Child Development Master of Science and Human Development PhD are offered by a graduate group which is interdisciplinary in nature, with a core faculty housed in the Department of Human and Community Development, and other graduate group faculty housed in education, law, medicine, psychiatry, M.I.N.D. Institute and psychology. Child Development MS students will be prepared to teach at the community college level in developmental and to do applied/evaluation research, or pursue higher degrees. The Human Development PhD students will be prepared to teach at the University level and to do basic or applied research in lifespan, cognitive, and social-emotional development from an interdisciplinary perspective with an appreciation of the contexts of development (family, school, health, social-cultural, and social policy). There are extensive student research opportunities within all the departments from which faculty are drawn, as well as the Center for Child and Family Studies, the 4-H Extension Program's Center for Youth Development, the M.I.N.D. Institute, and the Center for Neuroscience.

Special Facilities or Resources: Center for Child and Family Studies, Infant Sleep Lab, Parent and Child Lab, Center for Neuroscience, Center for Youth Development, Cooperative Research and Extension Services for Schools, M.I.N.D. Institute. Extensive community placements in education and social welfare.

Information for Students With Physical Disabilities: See the following Web site for more information: http://sdc.ucdavis.edu.

Application Information:
Send to Graduate Advisor, Human Development Graduate Group, University of California Davis, One Shields Avenue, Davis, CA 65616-8523. Application available online. URL of online application: https://apply.embark.com/grad/UCDavis/30/. Students are admitted in the Fall, application deadline December 15.

California, University of, Irvine
Department of Cognitive Sciences
2201 Social & Behavioral Sciences Gateway Building
Irvine, CA 92697-5100
Telephone: (949) 824-3771
Fax: (949) 824-2307
E-mail: *cogsci@uci.edu*
Web: *http://www.cogsci.uci.edu/*

Department Information:
1986. Chairperson: Michael D'Zmura. Number of faculty: total—full-time 29, part-time 7; women—full-time 8, part-time 3; total—minority—full-time 1, part-time 1; faculty subject to the Americans With Disabilities Act 1.

Programs and Degrees Offered:
Listed in the following order: Program area, degree type (T if terminal Master's), number awarded 7/08–6/09. Cognitive Science PhD (Doctor of Philosophy) 8.

Student Applications/Admissions:
Student Applications
Cognitive Science PhD (Doctor of Philosophy)—Applications 2009–2010, 86. Total applicants accepted 2009–2010, 18. Number full-time enrolled (new admits only) 2009–2010, 9. Openings 2010–2011, 15. The median number of years required for completion of a degree in 2008–2009 were 5. The number of students enrolled full- and part-time who were dismissed or voluntarily withdrew from this program area in 2008–2009 were 1.
Scores: Entries appear in this order: required test or GPA, minimum score (if required), median score of students entering in 2009–2010. Cognitive Science PhD (Doctor of Philosophy): GRE-V no minimum stated, GRE-Q no minimum stated.
Other Criteria: (importance of criteria rated low, medium, or high): GRE scores—high, research experience—high, work experience—low, GPA—medium, letters of recommendation—high, interview—high, statement of goals and objectives—high. For additional information on admission requirements, go to http://www.cogsci.uci.edu/gradProgram.php.

Student Characteristics: The following represents characteristics of students in 2009–2010 in all graduate psychology programs in the department: Female—full-time 24, part-time 0; Male—full-time 40, part-time 0; African American/Black—full-time 0, part-time 0; Hispanic/Latino(a)—full-time 8, part-time 0; Asian/Pacific Islander—full-time 14, part-time 0; American Indian/Alaska Native—full-time 0, part-time 0; Caucasian/White—full-time 28, part-time 0; Multi-ethnic—full-time 1, part-time 0; students subject to the Americans With Disabilities Act—full-time 0, part-time 0; Unknown ethnicity—full-time 13, part-time 0; Interna-

tional students who hold an F-1 or J-1 Visa—full-time 5, part-time 0.

Financial Information/Assistance:
Tuition for Full-Time Study: Doctoral: State residents: per academic year $13,415; Nonstate residents: per academic year $28,517. Tuition is subject to change. See the following Web site for updates and changes in tuition costs: http://www.reg.uci.edu/fees/.

Financial Assistance:
First-Year Students: Teaching assistantships available for first year. Average amount paid per academic year: $16,637. Average number of hours worked per week: 20. Apply by April 15. Research assistantships available for first year. Average amount paid per academic year: $12,159. Average number of hours worked per week: 20. Apply by April 15. Fellowships and scholarships available for first year. Apply by April 15.

Advanced Students: Teaching assistantships available for advanced students. Average amount paid per academic year: $16,637. Average number of hours worked per week: 20. Research assistantships available for advanced students. Average amount paid per academic year: $15,696. Average number of hours worked per week: 20. Fellowships and scholarships available for advanced students.

Additional Information: Of all students currently enrolled full time, 99% benefited from one or more of the listed financial assistance programs. Application and information available online at: http://www.ofas.uci.edu/content/.

Housing and Day Care: On-campus housing is available. See the following Web site for more information: http://www.housing.uci.edu. On-campus day care facilities are available. See the following Web site for more information: http://www.childcare.uci.edu.

Employment of Department Graduates:
Master's Degree Graduates: Of those who graduated in the academic year 2008–2009, the following categories and numbers represent the postgraduate activities and employment of master's degree graduates: Enrolled in a postdoctoral residency/fellowship (n/a), employed in independent practice (n/a), total from the above (master's) (0).
Doctoral Degree Graduates: Of those who graduated in the academic year 2008–2009, the following categories and numbers represent the postgraduate activities and employment of doctoral degree graduates: Enrolled in a psychology doctoral program (n/a), enrolled in a postdoctoral residency/fellowship (3), employed in an academic position at a university (1), employed in business or industry (4), total from the above (doctoral) (8).

Additional Information:
Orientation, Objectives, and Emphasis of Department: The Department of Cognitive Sciences offers a PhD degree program in Psychology, with a specialization in cognitive science, to prepare students for research and teaching careers in academia, industry, and government. The emphasis is on modern techniques of experimentation and theory construction. Special attention is given to providing hands-on research experience and equipping students with sophisticated mathematical and computing skills. Of the Department faculty, two are members of the National Academy of Sciences, and many have served as editors or editorial board members of leading professional journals and as members of NSF and NIH study panels. Many Cognitive Sciences faculty are also members of UCI's Institute of Mathematical Behavioral Sciences, and the Department is generally regarded as one of the world's leading centers for mathematically-oriented research in cognitive psychology. The Department is also allied closely to the School's Center for Cognitive Neuroscience.

Special Facilities or Resources: The facilities of the Department of Cognitive Sciences are housed in four buildings with teaching labs, lecture rooms, and instructional computing equipment. Its research laboratories are on the technological forefront and highly computerized. A research-dedicated 4.0T whole body MR Imaging/Spectroscopy System supports research in cognitive neuroscience.

Information for Students With Physical Disabilities: See the following Web site for more information: http://www.disability.uci.edu/.

Application Information:
Send to Graduate Program, Department of Cognitive Sciences, 3151 Social Science Plaza, University of California, Irvine, CA 92697-5100. Application available online. URL of online application: http://www.grad.uci.edu/prospective/. Students are admitted in the Fall, application deadline December 15. *Fee:* $70.

California, University of, Irvine (2009 data)
Department of Psychology and Social Behavior
3340 Social Ecology II, University of California, Irvine
Irvine, CA 92697-7085
Telephone: (949) 824-5574
Fax: (949) 824-3002
E-mail: *samorris@uci.edu*
Web: *http://www.seweb.uci.edu/psb/*

Department Information:
1992. Chairperson: Pete Ditto, PhD. Number of faculty: total—full-time 25, part-time 8; women—full-time 19, part-time 2; total—minority—full-time 1, part-time 3; women minority—part-time 1.

Programs and Degrees Offered:
Listed in the following order: Program area, degree type (T if terminal Master's), number awarded 7/08–6/09. Psychology and Social Behavior PhD (Doctor of Philosophy) 9.

Student Applications/Admissions:
Student Applications
Psychology and Social Behavior PhD (Doctor of Philosophy)— Applications 2009–2010, 205. Total applicants accepted 2009–2010, 30. Number full-time enrolled (new admits only) 2009–2010, 13. Openings 2010–2011, 8. The median number of years required for completion of a degree in 2008–2009 were 5. The number of students enrolled full- and part-time who were dismissed or voluntarily withdrew from this program area in 2008–2009 were 0.
Other Criteria: (importance of criteria rated low, medium, or high): GRE scores—high, research experience—high, work

experience—low, extracurricular activity—low, GPA—high, letters of recommendation—high, interview—high, statement of goals and objectives—high. For additional information on admission requirements, go to http://www.seweb.uci.edu/psb/gradprog.uci.

Student Characteristics: The following represents characteristics of students in 2009–2010 in all graduate psychology programs in the department: Female—full-time 43, part-time 0; Male—full-time 11, part-time 1; African American/Black—full-time 1, part-time 0; Hispanic/Latino(a)—full-time 4, part-time 0; Asian/Pacific Islander—full-time 5, part-time 1; American Indian/Alaska Native—full-time 0, part-time 0; Caucasian/White—full-time 43, part-time 0; Multi-ethnic—full-time 1, part-time 0; students subject to the Americans With Disabilities Act—full-time 0, part-time 1; Unknown ethnicity—full-time 0, part-time 0; International students who hold an F-1 or J-1 Visa—full-time 0, part-time 0.

Financial Information/Assistance:

Tuition for Full-Time Study: *Doctoral:* State residents: per academic year $11,262; Nonstate residents: per academic year $26,268. Tuition is subject to change. See the following Web site for updates and changes in tuition costs: http://www.reg.uci.edu/registrar/soc/fees.html.

Financial Assistance:

First-Year Students: Teaching assistantships available for first year. Average amount paid per academic year: $16,637. Average number of hours worked per week: 20. Research assistantships available for first year. Average amount paid per academic year: $12,459. Average number of hours worked per week: 20. Fellowships and scholarships available for first year. Average amount paid per academic year: $18,500. Average number of hours worked per week: 20.

Advanced Students: Teaching assistantships available for advanced students. Average amount paid per academic year: $16,637. Average number of hours worked per week: 20. Research assistantships available for advanced students. Average amount paid per academic year: $12,459. Average number of hours worked per week: 20. Fellowships and scholarships available for advanced students. Average amount paid per academic year: $18,500. Average number of hours worked per week: 20.

Additional Information: Of all students currently enrolled full time, 100% benefited from one or more of the listed financial assistance programs. Application and information available online at: http://www.rgs.uci.edu/grad/prospective/finance_edu.htm.

Internships/Practica: The school places a strong emphasis on training in conducting research that has both theoretical and practical applications. The school maintains a list of community agencies where students may seek various forms of research involvement. All students are required to take the course "Applied Psychological Research."

Housing and Day Care: On-campus housing is available. See the following Web site for more information: http://www.housing.uci.edu/. On-campus day care facilities are available. See the following Web site for more information: http://www.childcare.uci.edu/.

Employment of Department Graduates:

Master's Degree Graduates: Of those who graduated in the academic year 2008–2009, the following categories and numbers represent the postgraduate activities and employment of master's degree graduates: Enrolled in a postdoctoral residency/fellowship (n/a), employed in independent practice (n/a), total from the above (master's) (0).

Doctoral Degree Graduates: Of those who graduated in the academic year 2008–2009, the following categories and numbers represent the postgraduate activities and employment of doctoral degree graduates: Enrolled in a psychology doctoral program (n/a), enrolled in a postdoctoral residency/fellowship (1), employed in an academic position at a university (3), employed in an academic position at a 2-year/4-year college (2), still seeking employment (2), not seeking employment (1), total from the above (doctoral) (9).

Additional Information:

Orientation, Objectives, and Emphasis of Department: The Department of Psychology and Social Behavior is united by an overarching interest in human adaptation in various sociocultural and developmental contexts. The department has emphases in four areas (Health Psychology, Developmental Psychology, Social and Personality Psychology, and Psychopathology and Behavioral Disorders). The multidisciplinary faculty, whose training is mainly in social, developmental, clinical, and community psychology, examines human health, well-being, and the ways in which individuals respond and adjust to changing circumstances over the life span. Faculty interests include stress and coping, cognitive and biobehavioral processes in health behavior, subjective well-being, cognition and emotion, social development and developmental transitions across the life span, cultural influences on cognition and behavior, psychology and law, aging and health, and societal problems such as violence and unemployment.

Special Facilities or Resources: In-house laboratories, including the Consortium for Integrative Health Studies, the Family Studies Lab, the Development in Cultural Contexts Lab, and the Health Psychology Lab, provide graduate students with direct access to state-of-the-art facilities and opportunities for research training. In addition, the department maintains strong ties with psychologists at other campuses in the area, including UC Los Angeles, UC Riverside, and UC San Diego (each approximately one hour away), and the UCI College of Medicine. For example, we participate in the Consortium on Families and Human Development, a joint undertaking of faculty members and graduate students at UCLA, UCR, UCI, and the University of Southern California. Selected students participate as predoctoral fellows in the Department's NIMH Training Program, and opportunities continually arise for all students to become involved in many ongoing faculty research projects.

Information for Students With Physical Disabilities: See the following Web site for more information: http://www.disability.uci.edu/.

Application Information:

Send to Suzy Morrison, Graduate Coordinator, 3340 Social Ecology II, Psychology and Social Behavior, School of Social Ecology UCI, Irvine, CA 92697-7085. Application available online. URL of online application: http://www.grad.uci.edu/prospective. Students are admitted in the Fall, application deadline December 15. *Fee:* $60.

California, University of, Los Angeles
Department of Psychology
Letters and Science
405 Hilgard Avenue
Los Angeles, CA 90095-1563
Telephone: (310) 825-2617
Fax: (310) 206-5895
E-mail: gradadm@psych.ucla.edu
Web: http://www.psych.ucla.edu

Department Information:
1937. Chairperson: Bruce Baker. Number of faculty: total—full-time 69; women—full-time 29; total—minority—full-time 17; women minority—full-time 10.

Programs and Degrees Offered:
Listed in the following order: Program area, degree type (T if terminal Master's), number awarded 7/08–6/09. Clinical Psychology PhD (Doctor of Philosophy) 15, Cognitive Psychology PhD (Doctor of Philosophy) 2, Developmental Psychology PhD (Doctor of Philosophy) 2, Learning and Behavior PhD (Doctor of Philosophy) 0, Quantitative Psychology PhD (Doctor of Philosophy) 2, Social Psychology PhD (Doctor of Philosophy) 5, Behavioral Neuroscience PhD (Doctor of Philosophy) 2, Health Psychology PhD (Doctor of Philosophy) 0.

APA Accreditation: Clinical PhD (Doctor of Philosophy). Student Outcome Data Website: http://www.psych.ucla.edu/graduate/prospective-students/clinical-student-data.

Student Applications/Admissions:

Student Applications

Clinical Psychology PhD (Doctor of Philosophy)—Applications 2009–2010, 399. Total applicants accepted 2009–2010, 18. Number full-time enrolled (new admits only) 2009–2010, 10. Number part-time enrolled (new admits only) 2009–2010, 0. Openings 2010–2011, 12. The median number of years required for completion of a degree in 2008–2009 were 6. The number of students enrolled full- and part-time who were dismissed or voluntarily withdrew from this program area in 2008–2009 were 0. *Cognitive Psychology PhD (Doctor of Philosophy)*—Applications 2009–2010, 55. Total applicants accepted 2009–2010, 6. Number full-time enrolled (new admits only) 2009–2010, 6. Openings 2010–2011, 6. The median number of years required for completion of a degree in 2008–2009 were 6. The number of students enrolled full- and part-time who were dismissed or voluntarily withdrew from this program area in 2008–2009 were 0. *Developmental Psychology PhD (Doctor of Philosophy)*—Applications 2009–2010, 57. Total applicants accepted 2009–2010, 6. Number full-time enrolled (new admits only) 2009–2010, 7. Openings 2010–2011, 6. The median number of years required for completion of a degree in 2008–2009 were 6. The number of students enrolled full- and part-time who were dismissed or voluntarily withdrew from this program area in 2008–2009 were 0. *Learning and Behavior PhD (Doctor of Philosophy)*—Applications 2009–2010, 12. Total applicants accepted 2009–2010, 2. Number full-time enrolled (new admits only) 2009–2010, 0. Openings 2010–2011, 2. The number of students enrolled full- and part-time who were dismissed or voluntarily withdrew from this program area in 2008–2009 were 0. *Quantitative Psychology PhD (Doctor of Philosophy)*—Applications 2009–2010, 11. Total applicants accepted 2009–2010, 2. Number full-time enrolled (new admits only) 2009–2010, 4. Openings 2010–2011, 2. The median number of years required for completion of a degree in 2008–2009 were 6. The number of students enrolled full- and part-time who were dismissed or voluntarily withdrew from this program area in 2008–2009 were 0. *Social Psychology PhD (Doctor of Philosophy)*—Applications 2009–2010, 90. Total applicants accepted 2009–2010, 6. Number full-time enrolled (new admits only) 2009–2010, 4. Openings 2010–2011, 6. The median number of years required for completion of a degree in 2008–2009 were 6. The number of students enrolled full- and part-time who were dismissed or voluntarily withdrew from this program area in 2008–2009 were 0. *Behavioral Neuroscience PhD (Doctor of Philosophy)*—Applications 2009–2010, 17. Total applicants accepted 2009–2010, 3. Number full-time enrolled (new admits only) 2009–2010, 5. Number part-time enrolled (new admits only) 2009–2010, 0. Openings 2010–2011, 3. The median number of years required for completion of a degree in 2008–2009 were 6. The number of students enrolled full- and part-time who were dismissed or voluntarily withdrew from this program area in 2008–2009 were 0. *Health Psychology PhD (Doctor of Philosophy)*—Applications 2009–2010, 34. Total applicants accepted 2009–2010, 5. Number full-time enrolled (new admits only) 2009–2010, 0. Number part-time enrolled (new admits only) 2009–2010, 0. Openings 2010–2011, 5. The number of students enrolled full- and part-time who were dismissed or voluntarily withdrew from this program area in 2008–2009 were 0.

Scores: Entries appear in this order: required test or GPA, minimum score (if required), median score of students entering in 2009–2010. *Clinical Psychology PhD (Doctor of Philosophy):* GRE-V no minimum stated, 655, GRE-Q no minimum stated, 770, GRE-Analytical no minimum stated, 5.0, overall undergraduate GPA no minimum stated, 3.77; *Cognitive Psychology PhD (Doctor of Philosophy):* GRE-V no minimum stated, GRE-Q no minimum stated.

Other Criteria: (importance of criteria rated low, medium, or high): GRE scores—high, research experience—high, work experience—medium, extracurricular activity—medium, clinically related public service—medium, GPA—high, letters of recommendation—high, interview—high, statement of goals and objectives—high. The Clinical, Developmental, Health, and Social areas require an interview as part of their admissions process. After an initial screening of applications, the areas invites selected candidates to an on-campus interview. For additional information on admission requirements, go to http://www.psych.ucla.edu/graduate/prospective-students.

Student Characteristics: The following represents characteristics of students in 2009–2010 in all graduate psychology programs in the department: Female—full-time 131, part-time 0; Male—full-time 58, part-time 0; African American/Black—full-time 7, part-time 0; Hispanic/Latino(a)—full-time 12, part-time 0; Asian/Pacific Islander—full-time 22, part-time 0; American Indian/Alaska Native—full-time 0, part-time 0; Caucasian/White—full-time 148, part-time 0; Multi-ethnic—full-time 0, part-time 0; students subject to the Americans With Disabilities Act—full-time 0, part-time 0; Unknown ethnicity—full-time 0, part-time 0; International students who hold an F-1 or J-1 Visa—full-time 1, part-time 0.

Financial Information/Assistance:

Tuition for Full-Time Study: *Doctoral:* State residents: per academic year $10,767; Nonstate residents: per academic year $25,809. Tuition is subject to change. See the following Web site for updates and changes in tuition costs: http://www.registrar.ucla.edu/fees/.

Financial Assistance:

First-Year Students: Teaching assistantships available for first year. Average amount paid per academic year: $16,637. Average number of hours worked per week: 20. Research assistantships available for first year. Average amount paid per academic year: $13,104. Average number of hours worked per week: 20. Traineeships available for first year. Average amount paid per academic year: $20,000. Average number of hours worked per week: 0. Fellowships and scholarships available for first year. Average amount paid per academic year: $20,000. Average number of hours worked per week: 0. Apply by December 15.

Advanced Students: Teaching assistantships available for advanced students. Average amount paid per academic year: $18,569. Average number of hours worked per week: 20. Research assistantships available for advanced students. Average amount paid per academic year: $16,740. Average number of hours worked per week: 20. Traineeships available for advanced students. Average amount paid per academic year: $20,000. Average number of hours worked per week: 0. Fellowships and scholarships available for advanced students. Average amount paid per academic year: $20,000. Average number of hours worked per week: 0.

Additional Information: Of all students currently enrolled full time, 100% benefited from one or more of the listed financial assistance programs. Application and information available online at: http://www.gdnet.ucla.edu/prospective.html.

Internships/Practica: Doctoral Degree (PhD Clinical Psychology): For those doctoral students for whom a professional internship was required in this program prior to graduation, (9) students applied for an internship in 2008–2009, with (9) students obtaining an internship. Of those students who obtained an internship, (9) were paid internships. Of those students who obtained an internship, (9) students placed in APA/CPA accredited internships, (0) students placed in internships not APA/CPA accredited, but listed with the Association of Psychology Postdoctoral and Internship Programs (APPIC), (0) students placed in internships conforming to guidelines of the Council of Directors of School Psychology Programs (CDSPP), (0) students placed in internships that were not APA/CPA accredited, APPIC or CDSPP listed. VA Hospitals; San Fernando Valley Child Guidance Center; St. John's Child Development Center; Neuropsychiatric Institute/UCLA; UCLA Student Psych Services.

Housing and Day Care: On-campus housing is available. See the following Web site for more information: http://www.housing.ucla.edu. On-campus day care facilities are available.

Employment of Department Graduates:

Master's Degree Graduates: Of those who graduated in the academic year 2008–2009, the following categories and numbers represent the postgraduate activities and employment of master's degree graduates: Enrolled in a postdoctoral residency/fellowship (n/a), employed in independent practice (n/a), total from the above (master's) (0).

Doctoral Degree Graduates: Of those who graduated in the academic year 2008–2009, the following categories and numbers represent the postgraduate activities and employment of doctoral degree graduates: Enrolled in a psychology doctoral program (n/a), enrolled in another graduate/professional program (0), enrolled in a postdoctoral residency/fellowship (12), employed in independent practice (0), employed in an academic position at a university (1), employed in an academic position at a 2-year/4-year college (0), employed in other positions at a higher education institution (2), employed in a professional position in a school system (0), employed in business or industry (0), employed in government agency (0), employed in a community mental health/counseling center (0), employed in a hospital/medical center (0), still seeking employment (5), not seeking employment (0), other employment position (0), do not know (0), total from the above (doctoral) (20).

Additional Information:

Orientation, Objectives, and Emphasis of Department: Rigorous scientific training is the foundation of the PhD program. The graduate curriculum focuses on the usage of systematic methods of investigation to understand and quantify general principles of human behavior, pathology, cognition and emotion. More specifically, the department includes such research clusters as psychobiology and the brain; child-clinical and developmental psychology; adult psychopathology and family dynamics; cognition and memory; health, community, and political psychology; minority mental health; social cognition and intergroup relations; quantitative; and learning and behavior. In all these areas, the department's central aim is to train researchers dedicated to expanding the scientific knowledge upon which the discipline of psychology rests. This orientation also applies to the clinical program; while it offers excellent clinical training, its emphasis is on training researchers rather than private practitioners. In sum, the graduate training is designed to prepare research psychologists for careers in academic and applied settings—as college and university instructors; for leadership roles in community, government, and business organizations; and as professional research psychologists.

Special Facilities or Resources: The department is one of the largest on campus. Our three connected buildings (known collectively as Franz Hall) provide ample space (over 120,000 square feet) for psychological research. Laboratory facilities are of the highest quality. Precision equipment is available for electro-physiological stimulation and recording, magnetic resonance imaging (MRI), and for all major areas of sensory study. Specially designed laboratories exist for studies of group behavior and naturalistic observation. An extensive vivarium contains facilities for physiological animal studies. Computing facilities are leading-edge at all levels, from microcomputers to supercomputer clusters. The department also houses the Psychology Clinic, a training and research center for psychotherapy and diagnostics. Other resources include the Fernald Child Study Center (a research facility committed to investigating childhood behavioral disorders); the National Research Center for Asian American Mental Health; the California Self-Help Center; and the Center for Computer-Based Behavioral Studies. Departmental affiliations with the Brain Research Institute, the University Elementary School, the Neuropsychiatric Institute, and the local Veterans Administration also provide year-round research opportunities.

GRADUATE STUDY IN PSYCHOLOGY

Application Information:
Send to Graduate Admissions Advisor, Psychology Department, 405 Hilgard Avenue, 1285 Franz Hall, Los Angeles, CA 90095-1563. Application available online. URL of online application: http://www.psych.ucla.edu/graduate/prospective-students. Students are admitted in the Fall, application deadline December 1. *Fee:* $70.

California, University of, Merced
Psychological Sciences
Social Sciences, Humanities, and Arts
5200 North Lake Road
Merced, CA 95343
Telephone: (209) 228-4372
Fax: (209) 228-4390
E-mail: *wshadish@ucmerced.edu*
Web: *http://psychology.ucmerced.edu*

Department Information:
2007. Chairperson: William R. Shadish. Number of faculty: total—full-time 7, part-time 4; women—full-time 2, part-time 1; total—minority—full-time 1; women minority—full-time 1.

Programs and Degrees Offered:
Listed in the following order: Program area, degree type (T if terminal Master's), number awarded 7/08–6/09. Developmental Psychology PhD (Doctor of Philosophy) 0, Health Psychology PhD (Doctor of Philosophy) 0, Quantitative Psychology PhD (Doctor of Philosophy) 0.

Student Applications/Admissions:
Student Applications
Developmental Psychology PhD (Doctor of Philosophy)—Applications 2009–2010, 6. Total applicants accepted 2009–2010, 0. Number full-time enrolled (new admits only) 2009–2010, 0. Number part-time enrolled (new admits only) 2009–2010, 0. Openings 2010–2011, 2. The number of students enrolled full- and part-time who were dismissed or voluntarily withdrew from this program area in 2008–2009 were 1. Health Psychology PhD (Doctor of Philosophy)—Applications 2009–2010, 5. Total applicants accepted 2009–2010, 1. Number full-time enrolled (new admits only) 2009–2010, 1. Number part-time enrolled (new admits only) 2009–2010, 0. Openings 2010–2011, 4. The number of students enrolled full- and part-time who were dismissed or voluntarily withdrew from this program area in 2008–2009 were 0. Quantitative Psychology PhD (Doctor of Philosophy)—Applications 2009–2010, 3. Total applicants accepted 2009–2010, 2. Number full-time enrolled (new admits only) 2009–2010, 2. Number part-time enrolled (new admits only) 2009–2010, 0. Openings 2010–2011, 2. The number of students enrolled full- and part-time who were dismissed or voluntarily withdrew from this program area in 2008–2009 were 1.
Other Criteria: (importance of criteria rated low, medium, or high): GRE scores—medium, research experience—medium, work experience—low, extracurricular activity—low, clinically related public service—low, GPA—medium, letters of recommendation—medium, statement of goals and objectives—medium, undergraduate major in psychology—medium, specific undergraduate psychology courses taken—low. Admission decisions are based on a combination of factors, including academic degrees and records, the statement of purpose, letters of recommendation, test scores, and relevant work experience. We also consider the appropriateness of your goals to the degree program in which you are interested and to the research interests of the program's faculty. In addition, consideration may be given to how your background and life experience would contribute significantly to an educationally beneficial blend of students. For additional information on admission requirements, go to http://psychology.ucmerced.edu/.

Student Characteristics: The following represents characteristics of students in 2009–2010 in all graduate psychology programs in the department: Female—full-time 8, part-time 0; Male—full-time 3, part-time 0; African American/Black—full-time 0, part-time 0; Hispanic/Latino(a)—full-time 1, part-time 0; Asian/Pacific Islander—full-time 0, part-time 0; American Indian/Alaska Native—full-time 0, part-time 0; Caucasian/White—full-time 10, part-time 0; Multi-ethnic—full-time 0, part-time 0; students subject to the Americans With Disabilities Act—full-time 0, part-time 0; Unknown ethnicity—full-time 0, part-time 0; International students who hold an F-1 or J-1 Visa—full-time 2, part-time 0.

Financial Information/Assistance:
Tuition for Full-Time Study: *Doctoral:* State residents: per academic year $11,163; Nonstate residents: per academic year $26,205. Tuition is subject to change. See the following Web site for updates and changes in tuition costs: http://registrar.ucmerced.edu/policies/fees.

Financial Assistance:
First-Year Students: Teaching assistantships available for first year. Average amount paid per academic year: $18,000. Average number of hours worked per week: 20. Apply by March 2. Research assistantships available for first year. Average amount paid per academic year: $18,000. Average number of hours worked per week: 20. Apply by March 2. Fellowships and scholarships available for first year. Average amount paid per academic year: $18,000. Average number of hours worked per week: 20. Apply by March 2.

Advanced Students: Teaching assistantships available for advanced students. Average amount paid per academic year: $19,000. Average number of hours worked per week: 20. Apply by March 2. Research assistantships available for advanced students. Average amount paid per academic year: $19,000. Average number of hours worked per week: 20. Apply by March 2. Fellowships and scholarships available for advanced students. Average amount paid per academic year: $19,000. Average number of hours worked per week: 20. Apply by March 2.

Additional Information: Of all students currently enrolled full time, 100% benefited from one or more of the listed financial assistance programs. Application and information available online at: http://graduatedivision.ucmerced.edu/financial-support.

Housing and Day Care: No on-campus housing is available. On-campus day care facilities are available. See the following Web site for more information: http://ecec.ucmerced.edu/welcome/.

Employment of Department Graduates:
Master's Degree Graduates: Of those who graduated in the academic year 2008–2009, the following categories and numbers

represent the postgraduate activities and employment of master's degree graduates: Enrolled in a postdoctoral residency/fellowship (n/a), employed in independent practice (n/a), total from the above (master's) (0).

Doctoral Degree Graduates: Of those who graduated in the academic year 2008–2009, the following categories and numbers represent the postgraduate activities and employment of doctoral degree graduates: Enrolled in a psychology doctoral program (n/a), total from the above (doctoral) (0).

Additional Information:
Orientation, Objectives, and Emphasis of Department: UC Merced is the first research university built in the U.S. this century. Our graduate training started in 2006, and is growing very rapidly in developmental, health, and quantitative psychology. We are highly research-oriented, and do not offer any clinical training. We place priority on graduate students who desire a research career, but welcome applications from students with other aspirations as well. Applicants should review UC Merced psychology faculty research interests before applying, and then indicate when applying how their interests fit within our faculty's interests.

Special Facilities or Resources: We are housed in a general office building, but will be housed in a new Social Sciences and Management building to be completed in May 2011.

Information for Students With Physical Disabilities: See the following Web site for more information: http://disability.ucmerced.edu/.

Application Information:
Send to University of California, Merced, Attn: Graduate Division Application, 5200 N. Lake Road, Ste. KL 227, Merced, CA 95343. Application available online. URL of online application: http://graduatedivision.ucmerced.edu/prospective-students/how-apply. Students are admitted in the Fall, application deadline January 15. We will accept late applications. *Fee:* $70. International student application fee is $90.

California, University of, Riverside
Department of Psychology
College of Humanities, Arts & Social Sciences
Olmsted Hall
Riverside, CA 92521-0426
Telephone: (951) 827-6306
Fax: (951) 827-3985
E-mail: *dianne.fewkes@ucr.edu*
Web: *http://www.psych.ucr.edu*

Department Information:
1962. Chairperson: Glenn Stanley. Number of faculty: total—full-time 31; women—full-time 15; total—minority—full-time 6; women minority—full-time 4.

Programs and Degrees Offered:
Listed in the following order: Program area, degree type (T if terminal Master's), number awarded 7/08–6/09. Cognitive Psychology PhD (Doctor of Philosophy) 1, Developmental Psychology PhD (Doctor of Philosophy) 1, Social/Personality Psychology PhD (Doctor of Philosophy) 5, Systems Neuroscience PhD (Doctor of Philosophy) 0.

Student Applications/Admissions:
Student Applications
Cognitive Psychology PhD (Doctor of Philosophy)—Applications 2009–2010, 37. Total applicants accepted 2009–2010, 8. Number full-time enrolled (new admits only) 2009–2010, 5. Openings 2010–2011, 3. The median number of years required for completion of a degree in 2008–2009 were 5. The number of students enrolled full- and part-time who were dismissed or voluntarily withdrew from this program area in 2008–2009 were 2. *Developmental Psychology PhD (Doctor of Philosophy)*—Applications 2009–2010, 45. Total applicants accepted 2009–2010, 9. Number full-time enrolled (new admits only) 2009–2010, 3. Openings 2010–2011, 3. The median number of years required for completion of a degree in 2008–2009 were 5. The number of students enrolled full- and part-time who were dismissed or voluntarily withdrew from this program area in 2008–2009 were 1. *Social/Personality Psychology PhD (Doctor of Philosophy)*—Applications 2009–2010, 122. Total applicants accepted 2009–2010, 16. Number full-time enrolled (new admits only) 2009–2010, 11. Openings 2010–2011, 8. The median number of years required for completion of a degree in 2008–2009 were 5. The number of students enrolled full- and part-time who were dismissed or voluntarily withdrew from this program area in 2008–2009 were 0. *Systems Neuroscience PhD (Doctor of Philosophy)*—Applications 2009–2010, 8. Total applicants accepted 2009–2010, 7. Number full-time enrolled (new admits only) 2009–2010, 4. Openings 2010–2011, 2. The number of students enrolled full- and part-time who were dismissed or voluntarily withdrew from this program area in 2008–2009 were 0.

Other Criteria: (importance of criteria rated low, medium, or high): GRE scores—medium, research experience—high, work experience—low, extracurricular activity—low, GPA—medium, letters of recommendation—high, interview—high, statement of goals and objectives—high. For additional information on admission requirements, go to http://www.psych.ucr.edu/grad/admissions.html.

Student Characteristics: The following represents characteristics of students in 2009–2010 in all graduate psychology programs in the department: Female—full-time 54, part-time 0; Male—full-time 34, part-time 0; African American/Black—full-time 1, part-time 0; Hispanic/Latino(a)—full-time 8, part-time 0; Asian/Pacific Islander—full-time 8, part-time 0; American Indian/Alaska Native—full-time 0, part-time 0; Caucasian/White—full-time 68, part-time 0; Multi-ethnic—full-time 3, part-time 0; students subject to the Americans With Disabilities Act—full-time 0, part-time 0; Unknown ethnicity—full-time 0, part-time 0; International students who hold an F-1 or J-1 Visa—full-time 0, part-time 0.

Financial Information/Assistance:
Tuition for Full-Time Study: *Doctoral:* State residents: per academic year $12,111; Nonstate residents: per academic year $27,810. Tuition is subject to change. See the following Web site for updates and changes in tuition costs: http://www.graduate.ucr.edu/Admiss/FinSupportFM.html.

Financial Assistance:
First-Year Students: Teaching assistantships available for first year. Average amount paid per academic year: $16,637. Average number of hours worked per week: 20. Apply by January 2. Research assistantships available for first year. Average amount paid per academic year: $16,314. Average number of hours worked per week: 20. Apply by January 2. Fellowships and scholarships available for first year. Average amount paid per academic year: $17,000. Average number of hours worked per week: 0. Apply by January 2.
Advanced Students: Teaching assistantships available for advanced students. Average amount paid per academic year: $16,637. Average number of hours worked per week: 20. Apply by January 2. Research assistantships available for advanced students. Average amount paid per academic year: $19,542. Average number of hours worked per week: 20. Apply by January 2.
Additional Information: Of all students currently enrolled full time, 100% benefited from one or more of the listed financial assistance programs. Application and information available online at: http://www.psych.ucr.edu/grad/admissions.html.

Housing and Day Care: On-campus housing is available. See the following Web site for more information: http://housing.ucr.edu/. On-campus day care facilities are available. See the following Web site for more information: http://www.childrenservices.ucr.edu.

Employment of Department Graduates:
Master's Degree Graduates: Of those who graduated in the academic year 2008–2009, the following categories and numbers represent the postgraduate activities and employment of master's degree graduates: Enrolled in a postdoctoral residency/fellowship (n/a), employed in independent practice (n/a), total from the above (master's) (0).
Doctoral Degree Graduates: Of those who graduated in the academic year 2008–2009, the following categories and numbers represent the postgraduate activities and employment of doctoral degree graduates: Enrolled in a psychology doctoral program (n/a), enrolled in a postdoctoral residency/fellowship (7), employed in an academic position at a university (2), employed in business or industry (3), total from the above (doctoral) (12).

Additional Information:
Orientation, Objectives, and Emphasis of Department: The orientation is toward theoretical and research training. Objectives are to provide the appropriate theoretical, quantitative, and methodological background to enable graduates of the program to engage in high-quality research. Additionally, training and experience in university-level teaching are provided. We also offer a minor in quantitative psychology which may be completed by any student in the PhD program in Psychology regardless of main area of interest. A concentration in health psychology is also offered in the social and developmental areas. The cognitive area has a strong concentration in cognitive modeling.

Special Facilities or Resources: The Psychology Department has recently moved into a new building built specifically for the department. The department has equipment and support systems to help students conduct research in all aspects of behavior. The neuroscience laboratories are equipped with the latest instrumentation for hormonal assays, extracellular and intracellular electrophysiology, and microscopic analysis of neuronal morphology. Research in the cognitive area incorporates computer-assisted experimental control for most any kind of reaction time experiment and has facilities for video and speech digitization and infrared eye-tracking. The developmental faculty have laboratory facilities to study parents and children, have access to the campus day-care center for studies that involve toddlers and preschool children, and have been very successful in conducting research in a culturally diverse local school system. The developmental faculty all participate in the Center for Family Studies, an interdisciplinary center. The social/personality psychology labs support research in social perception, nonverbal communication, health psychology, emotional expression, and attribution processes using audiovisual laboratories and observation rooms. Direct, free access is available to PsycInfo, PubMed, and many other online journals and databases.

Information for Students With Physical Disabilities: See the following Web site for more information: http://specialservices.ucr.edu/.

Application Information:
Send to Graduate Admissions Psychology Department, University of California, Riverside, Riverside, CA 92521. Application available online. URL of online application: http://www.graduate.ucr.edu/Admtoc.html. Students are admitted in the Fall, application deadline January 2. *Fee:* $80.

California, University of, San Diego
Department of Psychology
9500 Gilman Drive #0109
La Jolla, CA 92093-0109
Telephone: (858) 534-3002
Fax: (858) 534-7190
E-mail: *chermosillo@ucsd.edu*
Web: *http://psy.ucsd.edu/*

Department Information:
1965. Chairperson: John T. Wixted. Number of faculty: total—full-time 32; women—full-time 6.

Programs and Degrees Offered:
Listed in the following order: Program area, degree type (T if terminal Master's), number awarded 7/08–6/09. Experimental Psychology PhD (Doctor of Philosophy) 7.

Student Applications/Admissions:
Student Applications
Experimental Psychology PhD (Doctor of Philosophy)—Applications 2009–2010, 372. Total applicants accepted 2009–2010, 21. Number full-time enrolled (new admits only) 2009–2010, 13. Openings 2010–2011, 10. The median number of years required for completion of a degree in 2008–2009 were 6. The number of students enrolled full- and part-time who were dismissed or voluntarily withdrew from this program area in 2008–2009 were 1.
Scores: Entries appear in this order: required test or GPA, minimum score (if required), median score of students entering in 2009–2010. Experimental Psychology PhD (Doctor of Philosophy): GRE-V 450, 654, GRE-Q 610, 753, overall undergraduate GPA 3.0, 3.7.

Other Criteria: (importance of criteria rated low, medium, or high): GRE scores—high, research experience—high, work experience—medium, extracurricular activity—low, clinically related public service—low, GPA—high, letters of recommendation—high, interview—high, statement of goals and objectives—high, undergraduate major in psychology—medium, specific undergraduate psychology courses taken—high. For additional information on admission requirements, go to http://psy.ucsd.edu/graduate_program/prospective_students/admissions.php.

Student Characteristics: The following represents characteristics of students in 2009–2010 in all graduate psychology programs in the department: Female—full-time 44, part-time 0; Male—full-time 21, part-time 0; African American/Black—full-time 0, part-time 0; Hispanic/Latino(a)—full-time 1, part-time 0; Asian/Pacific Islander—full-time 5, part-time 0; American Indian/Alaska Native—full-time 0, part-time 0; Caucasian/White—full-time 57, part-time 0; Multi-ethnic—full-time 2, part-time 0; students subject to the Americans With Disabilities Act—full-time 1, part-time 0; Unknown ethnicity—full-time 0, part-time 0; International students who hold an F-1 or J-1 Visa—full-time 2, part-time 0.

Financial Information/Assistance:
Tuition for Full-Time Study: *Doctoral:* State residents: per academic year $12,631; Nonstate residents: per academic year $27,733. Tuition is subject to change. See the following Web site for updates and changes in tuition costs: http://ogs.ucsd.edu/FinancialSupport/Pages/Tuition_Fees.aspx.

Financial Assistance:
First-Year Students: Teaching assistantships available for first year. Average amount paid per academic year: $16,637. Average number of hours worked per week: 20.
Advanced Students: Teaching assistantships available for advanced students. Average amount paid per academic year: $16,637. Average number of hours worked per week: 20. Research assistantships available for advanced students. Average amount paid per academic year: $16,740. Average number of hours worked per week: 20.
Additional Information: Of all students currently enrolled full time, 97% benefited from one or more of the listed financial assistance programs. Application and information available online at: http://psy.ucsd.edu/graduate_program/prospective_students/financialSupport.php.

Housing and Day Care: On-campus housing is available. See the following Web site for more information: http://hdh.ucsd.edu/arch/gradhousing.html. On-campus day care facilities are available. See the following Web site for more information: http://blink.ucsd.edu/go/ecec.

Employment of Department Graduates:
Master's Degree Graduates: Of those who graduated in the academic year 2008–2009, the following categories and numbers represent the postgraduate activities and employment of master's degree graduates: Enrolled in a postdoctoral residency/fellowship (n/a), employed in independent practice (n/a), total from the above (master's) (0).
Doctoral Degree Graduates: Of those who graduated in the academic year 2008–2009, the following categories and numbers represent the postgraduate activities and employment of doctoral degree graduates: Enrolled in a psychology doctoral program (n/a), enrolled in another graduate/professional program (1), enrolled in a postdoctoral residency/fellowship (6), employed in an academic position at a 2-year/4-year college (1), other employment position (1), total from the above (doctoral) (9).

Additional Information:
Orientation, Objectives, and Emphasis of Department: The Department of Psychology at the University of California San Diego provides advanced training in research on most aspects of experimental psychology. Modern laboratories and an attractive physical setting combine with a distinguished faculty, both within the Department of Psychology and in supporting disciplines, to provide research opportunities and training at the frontiers of psychological science. The graduate training program emphasizes and supports individual research, starting with the first year of study. The Department offers the following emphases: behavior analysis, cognitive psychology, developmental psychology, sensation and perception, neuroscience and behavior and social psychology.

Special Facilities or Resources: The Department shares research space and facilities with the Center for Brain and Cognition. Within the joint facilities, there are two computing facilities, a computational laboratory, visual and auditory laboratories, social psychology laboratories, cognitive laboratories, developmental laboratories, a clinic for autistic children, animal facilities, and extensive contacts with hospitals, industry, and the legal system. In addition to the numerous impressive libraries on campus, the Department also keeps a large selection of literature within our Mandler Library. Collaborative research is carried on with members of the Departments of Linguistics, Cognitive Science, Computer Science and Engineering, Sociology, Music, Ophthalmology, Neurosciences, members of the UCSD School of Medicine, Scripps Clinic and Research Foundation, and with the Salk Institute for Biological Studies. The Scripps Institution of Oceanography, located on campus, provides facilities in neurosciences as does the School of Medicine.

Information for Students With Physical Disabilities: See the following Web site for more information: http://www.ucsd.edu/current-students/_organizations/osd/index.html.

Application Information:
Send to Graduate Admission, Dept. of Psychology-0109, University of California-San Diego, La Jolla, CA 92093. Application available online. URL of online application: http://graduateapp.ucsd.edu/. Students are admitted in the Fall, application deadline December 15. *Fee:* $70. U.S. citizens and permanent residents only may request a waiver of the application fee. All fee waivers are granted provisionally. Applicants must provide supporting information and documentation to finalize the waiver. Waivers are provided to applicants in the following situations: applicants who are currently receiving need-based financial assistance from an undergraduate or graduate institution; applicants who are able to demonstrate financial hardship; applicants who are participating in selected federal, state and private graduate school preparation programs.

GRADUATE STUDY IN PSYCHOLOGY

California, University of, Santa Barbara
Counseling, Clinical, and School Psychology
Gevirtz Graduate School of Education
Education Building 275, University of California, Santa Barbara
Santa Barbara, CA 93106-9490
Telephone: (805) 893-3375
Fax: (805) 893-3375
E-mail: *ccspapp@education.ucsb.edu*
Web: *http://education.ucsb.edu/Graduate-Studies/CCSP/CCSP-home.html*

Department Information:
1965. Chairperson: Merith Cosden. Number of faculty: total—full-time 14; women—full-time 7; total—minority—full-time 3; women minority—full-time 2.

Programs and Degrees Offered:
Listed in the following order: Program area, degree type (T if terminal Master's), number awarded 7/08–6/09. Counseling/Clinical/School PhD (Doctor of Philosophy) 8, School Psychology MEd (Education) 3.

APA Accreditation: Combination PhD (Doctor of Philosophy). Student Outcome Data Website: http://education.ucsb.edu/Graduate-Studies/CCSP/programofstudy/combined_doctoral/candidates.htm.

Student Applications/Admissions:
Student Applications
Counseling/Clinical/School PhD (Doctor of Philosophy)—Applications 2009–2010, 191. Total applicants accepted 2009–2010, 29. Number full-time enrolled (new admits only) 2009–2010, 14. Number part-time enrolled (new admits only) 2009–2010, 0. Openings 2010–2011, 20. The median number of years required for completion of a degree in 2008–2009 were 5. The number of students enrolled full- and part-time who were dismissed or voluntarily withdrew from this program area in 2008–2009 were 0. *School Psychology MEd (Education)*—Applications 2009–2010, 37. Total applicants accepted 2009–2010, 8. Number full-time enrolled (new admits only) 2009–2010, 5. Number part-time enrolled (new admits only) 2009–2010, 0. Openings 2010–2011, 6. The median number of years required for completion of a degree in 2008–2009 were 2. The number of students enrolled full- and part-time who were dismissed or voluntarily withdrew from this program area in 2008–2009 were 0.
Scores: Entries appear in this order: required test or GPA, minimum score (if required), median score of students entering in 2009–2010. *Counseling/Clinical/School PhD (Doctor of Philosophy)*: GRE-V no minimum stated, 570, GRE-Q no minimum stated, 650, GRE-Analytical no minimum stated, 5.0, last 2 years GPA 3.0, 3.81; *School Psychology MEd (Education)*: GRE-V no minimum stated, 570, GRE-Q no minimum stated, 595, GRE-Analytical no minimum stated, 4.5, last 2 years GPA 3.0, 3.84.
Other Criteria: (importance of criteria rated low, medium, or high): GRE scores—medium, research experience—high, work experience—high, extracurricular activity—medium, clinically related public service—high, GPA—high, letters of recommendation—high, interview—high, statement of goals and objectives—high, undergraduate major in psychology—medium, specific undergraduate psychology courses taken—medium. For additional information on admission requirements, go to http://education.ucsb.edu/Graduate-Studies/CCSP/prospective-students/how-to-apply-checklist.htm.

Student Characteristics: The following represents characteristics of students in 2009–2010 in all graduate psychology programs in the department: Female—full-time 72, part-time 0; Male—full-time 13, part-time 0; African American/Black—full-time 3, part-time 0; Hispanic/Latino(a)—full-time 16, part-time 0; Asian/Pacific Islander—full-time 15, part-time 0; American Indian/Alaska Native—full-time 1, part-time 0; Caucasian/White—full-time 36, part-time 0; Multi-ethnic—full-time 8, part-time 0; students subject to the Americans With Disabilities Act—full-time 2, part-time 0; Unknown ethnicity—full-time 6, part-time 0; International students who hold an F-1 or J-1 Visa—full-time 2, part-time 0.

Financial Information/Assistance:
Tuition for Full-Time Study: *Master's:* State residents: per academic year $11,665; Nonstate residents: per academic year $26,707. *Doctoral:* State residents: per academic year $11,665; Nonstate residents: per academic year $26,707. Tuition is subject to change. See the following Web site for updates and changes in tuition costs: http://www.registrar.ucsb.edu/feechart-grad.htm.

Financial Assistance:
First-Year Students: Research assistantships available for first year. Average amount paid per academic year: $15,000. Average number of hours worked per week: 10. Fellowships and scholarships available for first year. Average amount paid per academic year: $20,200. Average number of hours worked per week: 0. Apply by November 15.
Advanced Students: Teaching assistantships available for advanced students. Average amount paid per academic year: $16,000. Average number of hours worked per week: 10. Research assistantships available for advanced students. Average amount paid per academic year: $17,000. Average number of hours worked per week: 10. Fellowships and scholarships available for advanced students. Average amount paid per academic year: $22,500. Average number of hours worked per week: 0.
Additional Information: Of all students currently enrolled full time, 70% benefited from one or more of the listed financial assistance programs. Application and information available online at: http://education.ucsb.edu/Graduate-Studies/Student-Services/prospective-students/financial-aid.htm.

Internships/Practica: Doctoral Degree (PhD Counseling/Clinical/School): For those doctoral students for whom a professional internship was required in this program prior to graduation, (11) students applied for an internship in 2008–2009, with (11) students obtaining an internship. Of those students who obtained an internship, (11) were paid internships. Of those students who obtained an internship, (11) students placed in APA/CPA accredited internships, (0) students placed in internships not APA/CPA accredited, but listed with the Association of Psychology Postdoctoral and Internship Programs (APPIC), (0) students placed in internships conforming to guidelines of the Council of Directors of School Psychology Programs (CDSPP), (0) students placed in internships that were not APA/CPA accredited, APPIC or CDSPP listed. During their first years in the program, students receive practicum experience in the Hosford Psychological Services Clinic on campus, a sliding scale agency which serves adults, children, and families from the community. Advanced students receive experience as supervisors in the clinic. Students in the clinical emphasis have external practica in community-based settings, including an agency that serves families and children exposed to violence, a local hospital, and programs associated with county alcohol, drug and mental health services. Students in the counseling emphasis have external practica at UCSB's Counseling and Career Services centers. Students in the school emphasis have external practica in the schools. All doctoral students apply for predoctoral internships at APA-accredited sites across the country and participate in the APPIC match. The school psychology MEd students receive their degree in two years and have a third year of school internship for their credential.

Housing and Day Care: On-campus housing is available. See the following Web site for more information: http://www.housing.ucsb.edu/. On-campus day care facilities are available. See the following Web site for more information: http://childrenscenter.sa.ucsb.edu/.

Employment of Department Graduates:
Master's Degree Graduates: Of those who graduated in the academic year 2008–2009, the following categories and numbers represent the postgraduate activities and employment of master's degree graduates: Enrolled in a postdoctoral residency/fellowship (n/a), employed in independent practice (n/a), employed in a professional position in a school system (1), do not know (1), total from the above (master's) (2).
Doctoral Degree Graduates: Of those who graduated in the academic year 2008–2009, the following categories and numbers represent the postgraduate activities and employment of doctoral degree graduates: Enrolled in a psychology doctoral program (n/a), employed in an academic position at a university (2), employed in other positions at a higher education institution (4), employed in a community mental health/counseling center (2), employed in a hospital/medical center (3), do not know (1), total from the above (doctoral) (12).

Additional Information:
Orientation, Objectives, and Emphasis of Department: The primary goal of the combined psychology program is to prepare graduates who will (a) conduct research and teach in university settings and (b) assume leadership roles in the academic community and in the helping professions. The program has a secondary goal of training students to provide psychological services in university, school, and community agency settings. The Department recently moved to the new Education Building on campus with state-of-the-art instructional equipment and technologically-enhanced clinics.

Special Facilities or Resources: The UCSB Combined Psychology Program houses several training clinics: the Hosford Clinic serves community clients and is equipped with state-of-the-art equipment for recording, reviewing, editing, and live monitoring of assessment and counseling sessions; the Psychology Assessment Center provides psychological assessment services for the measurement of disorders that affect psychological, emotional, academic, and occupational functioning; and the Koegel Autism Center provides training in evidence-based practices for children with an autism spectrum disorder. Faculty have research labs in their areas of interest.

Information for Students With Physical Disabilities: See the following Web site for more information: http://dsp.sa.ucsb.edu/.

Application Information:
Send to Student Affairs Office, Gevirtz Graduate School of Education, University of California, Santa Barbara CA 93106-9490. Application available online. URL of online application: http://education.ucsb.edu/Graduate-Studies/CCSP/prospective-students/how-to-apply-checklist.htm. Students are admitted in the Fall, application deadline November 15. *Fee:* $70. $90 for international students.

California, University of, Santa Cruz
Psychology Department
273 Social Sciences 2
Santa Cruz, CA 95064
Telephone: (831) 459-4932
Fax: (831) 459-3519
E-mail: *allison@ucsc.edu*
Web: *http://psych.ucsc.edu/*

Department Information:
1965. Chairperson: Avril Thorne. Number of faculty: total—full-time 24; women—full-time 16; total—minority—full-time 8; women minority—full-time 6.

Programs and Degrees Offered:
Listed in the following order: Program area, degree type (T if terminal Master's), number awarded 7/08–6/09. Developmental Psychology PhD (Doctor of Philosophy) 4, Social Psychology PhD (Doctor of Philosophy) 2, Cognitive Psychology PhD (Doctor of Philosophy) 3.

Student Applications/Admissions:
Student Applications
Developmental Psychology PhD (Doctor of Philosophy)—Applications 2009–2010, 35. Total applicants accepted 2009–2010, 8. Number full-time enrolled (new admits only) 2009–2010, 4. Total enrolled 2009–2010 full-time, 21. Openings 2010–2011, 5. The median number of years required for completion of a degree in 2008–2009 were 6. The number of students enrolled full- and part-time who were dismissed or voluntarily withdrew from this program area in 2008–2009 were 0. *Social Psychology PhD (Doctor of Philosophy)*—Applications 2009–2010, 90. Total applicants accepted 2009–2010, 5. Number full-time enrolled (new admits only) 2009–2010, 5. Total enrolled 2009–2010 full-time, 19, part-time, 1. Openings 2010–2011, 5. The median number of years required for completion of a degree in 2008–2009 were 8. The number of students enrolled full- and part-time who were dismissed or voluntarily withdrew from this program area in 2008–2009 were 1. *Cognitive Psychology PhD (Doctor of Philosophy)*—Applications 2009–2010, 31. Total applicants accepted 2009–2010, 7. Number full-time enrolled (new admits only) 2009–2010, 2. Total enrolled 2009–2010 full-time, 16, part-time, 1. Openings 2010–2011, 5. The median number of years required for completion of a degree in 2008–2009 were 5. The number of students enrolled full- and part-time who were dismissed or voluntarily withdrew from this program area in 2008–2009 were 0.

Scores: Entries appear in this order: required test or GPA, minimum score (if required), median score of students entering in 2009–2010. *Developmental Psychology PhD (Doctor of Philosophy):* GRE-V no minimum stated, 560, GRE-Q no minimum stated, 600, GRE-Analytical no minimum stated, 4.75, overall undergraduate GPA no minimum stated, 3.69; *Social Psychology PhD (Doctor of Philosophy):* GRE-V no minimum stated, 650, GRE-Q no minimum stated, 720, GRE-Analytical no minimum stated, 5, overall undergraduate GPA no minimum stated, 3.87; *Cognitive Psychology PhD (Doctor of Philosophy):* GRE-V no minimum stated, 670, GRE-Q no minimum stated, 710, GRE-Analytical no minimum stated, 5, overall undergraduate GPA no minimum stated, 3.79.

Other Criteria: (importance of criteria rated low, medium, or high): GRE scores—high, research experience—high, work experience—medium, extracurricular activity—medium, GPA—high, letters of recommendation—high, statement of goals and objectives—high. For additional information on admission requirements, go to http://psych.ucsc.edu/graduate/admission_requirements.php.

Student Characteristics: The following represents characteristics of students in 2009–2010 in all graduate psychology programs in the department: Female—full-time 41, part-time 2; Male—full-time 15, part-time 0; African American/Black—full-time 3, part-time 0; Hispanic/Latino(a)—full-time 10, part-time 1; Asian/Pacific Islander—full-time 8, part-time 0; American Indian/Alaska Native—full-time 0, part-time 0; Caucasian/White—full-time 24, part-time 1; Multi-ethnic—full-time 2, part-time 0; students subject to the Americans With Disabilities Act—full-time 0, part-time 0; Unknown ethnicity—full-time 9, part-time 0; International students who hold an F-1 or J-1 Visa—full-time 0, part-time 0.

Financial Information/Assistance:
Tuition for Full-Time Study: *Doctoral:* State residents: per academic year $12,692; Nonstate residents: per academic year $27,734. Tuition is subject to change. See the following Web site for updates and changes in tuition costs: http://reg.ucsc.edu/Fees/fees.html.

Financial Assistance:
First-Year Students: Teaching assistantships available for first year. Average number of hours worked per week: 20. Research assistantships available for first year. Average number of hours worked per week: 20. Traineeships available for first year. Fellowships and scholarships available for first year. Apply by December 15.

Advanced Students: Teaching assistantships available for advanced students. Average number of hours worked per week: 20. Research assistantships available for advanced students. Average number of hours worked per week: 20. Traineeships available for advanced students. Average number of hours worked per week: 20.

Additional Information: Of all students currently enrolled full time, 95% benefited from one or more of the listed financial assistance programs. Application and information available online at: http://www2.ucsc.edu/fin-aid/graduate_students.shtml.

Housing and Day Care: On-campus housing is available. See the following Web site for more information: http://housing.ucsc.edu/sponsored-housing/grad-index.html. On-campus day care facilities are available. See the following Web site for more information: http://housing.ucsc.edu/childcare/index.html.

Employment of Department Graduates:
Master's Degree Graduates: Of those who graduated in the academic year 2008–2009, the following categories and numbers represent the postgraduate activities and employment of master's degree graduates: Enrolled in a postdoctoral residency/fellowship (n/a), employed in independent practice (n/a), total from the above (master's) (0).

Doctoral Degree Graduates: Of those who graduated in the academic year 2008–2009, the following categories and numbers represent the postgraduate activities and employment of doctoral degree graduates: Enrolled in a psychology doctoral program (n/a), employed in an academic position at a university (4), employed in other positions at a higher education institution (2), employed in business or industry (1), do not know (2), total from the above (doctoral) (9).

Additional Information:
Orientation, Objectives, and Emphasis of Department: The Psychology Department at UC Santa Cruz offers a PhD degree with areas of specialization in cognitive, developmental, and social psychology. The program does not offer courses, training, or supervision in counseling or clinical psychology. Students are not admitted to pursue only a Master's degree. However, students may be awarded a Master's degree as part of their studies for the PhD Students are prepared for research, teaching, and administrative positions in colleges and universities, as well as positions in schools, government, and other public and private organizations. The PhD is a research degree. Students are required to demonstrate the ability to carry through to completion rigorous empirical research and to be active in research throughout their graduate career. Course requirements establish a foundation for critical evaluation of research literature and the design of conceptually important empirical research. To support students in achieving these goals, each student must be associated with one of the faculty, who serves as academic advisor and research sponsor. The program requires full-time enrollment.

Special Facilities or Resources: The department provides training to prepare the student for academic and applied settings. Graduate students have the use of a variety of research facilities, including a number of computer-controlled experimental laboratories. Electronic equipment is available to allow the generation of sophisticated written and pictorial vision displays, musical sequences, and synthesized and visual speech patterns. There are observational facilities for developmental psychological research and a discourse analysis lab. A bilingual survey unit is under development which will utilize public opinion survey technology to study significant public policy, legal, and political issues that are critical to California's emerging majority population. Research opportunities exist with diverse sample groups in both laboratory and natural settings. The department has collaborative relationships with the National Center for Research on Cultural Diversity, Second Language Learning, and the Bilingual Research Center.

Information for Students With Physical Disabilities: See the following Web site for more information: http://drc.ucsc.edu/.

Application Information:
Send to Psychology Department, Graduate Program, 1156 High Street, University of California, Santa Cruz, CA 95064-1077. Application available online. URL of online application: http://graddiv.ucsc.edu/prospective/. Students are admitted in the Fall, application deadline December 15. *Fee:* $70. Fee waivers for cases of hardship are available to U.S. citizens and permanent residents only.

Claremont Graduate University
Graduate Department of Psychology
School of Behavioral and Organizational Sciences
123 East Eighth Street
Claremont, CA 91711-3955
Telephone: (909) 621-8084
Fax: (909) 621-8905
E-mail: *Stewart.Donaldson@cgu.edu*
Web: *http://www.cgu.edu/sbos*

Department Information:
1926. Dean: Stewart I. Donaldson. Number of faculty: total—full-time 17, part-time 59; women—full-time 7, part-time 29; total—minority—full-time 2, part-time 14; women minority—full-time 1, part-time 7.

Programs and Degrees Offered:
Listed in the following order: Program area, degree type (T if terminal Master's), number awarded 7/08–6/09. Applied Social Psych/Evaluation Co-Concentration MA/MS (Master of Arts/Science) (T) 6, Cognitive Psychology/Evaluation Co-Concentration MA/MS (Master of Arts/Science) (T) 0, Organizational/Evaluation Co-Concentration MA/MS (Master of Arts/Science) (T) 15, Developmental Psych/Evaluation Co-Concentration MA/MS (Master of Arts/Science) (T) 0, Human Resources Design MA/MS (Master of Arts/Science) (T) 8, Applied Cognitive Psychology PhD (Doctor of Philosophy) 2, Applied Developmental Psychology PhD (Doctor of Philosophy) 3, Applied Social Psychology PhD (Doctor of Philosophy) 3, Evaluation and Applied Research Methods PhD (Doctor of Philosophy) 3, Organizational Behavior, Industrial/Organizational PhD (Doctor of Philosophy) 4, Positive Developmental Psychology PhD (Doctor of Philosophy), Positive Organizational Psychology PhD (Doctor of Philosophy), Positive Developmental Psych/Evaluation Co-Concen MA/MS (Master of Arts/Science) (T), Positive Organizational Psych/Evaluation Co-Concen MA/MS (Master of Arts/Science) (T), Health Behavior Research/Evaluation MA/MS (Master of Arts/Science) (T) 0.

Student Applications/Admissions:
Student Applications
Applied Social Psych/Evaluation Co-Concentration MA/MS (Master of Arts/Science)—Applications 2009–2010, 53. Number full-time enrolled (new admits only) 2009–2010, 8. Total enrolled 2009–2010 full-time, 18, part-time, 1. Openings 2010–2011, 9. The median number of years required for completion of a degree in 2008–2009 were 2. The number of students enrolled full- and part-time who were dismissed or voluntarily withdrew from this program area in 2008–2009 were 0. Cognitive Psychology/Evaluation Co-Concentration MA/MS (Master of Arts/Science)—Applications 2009–2010, 15. Number full-time enrolled (new admits only) 2009–2010, 1. Total enrolled 2009–2010 full-time, 1, part-time, 1. Openings 2010–2011, 3. The median number of years required for completion of a degree in 2008–2009 were 2. The number of students enrolled full- and part-time who were dismissed or voluntarily withdrew from this program area in 2008–2009 were 0. *Organizational/Evaluation Co-Concentration MA/MS (Master of Arts/Science)*—Applications 2009–2010, 86. Number full-time enrolled (new admits only) 2009–2010, 11. Total enrolled 2009–2010 full-time, 29, part-time, 2. Openings 2010–2011, 10. The median number of years required for completion of a degree in 2008–2009 were 2. The number of students enrolled full- and part-time who were dismissed or voluntarily withdrew from this program area in 2008–2009 were 0. *Developmental Psych/Evaluation Co-Concentration MA/MS (Master of Arts/Science)*—Applications 2009–2010, 14. Number full-time enrolled (new admits only) 2009–2010, 3. Total enrolled 2009–2010 full-time, 4, part-time, 1. Openings 2010–2011, 6. The median number of years required for completion of a degree in 2008–2009 were 2. The number of students enrolled full- and part-time who were dismissed or voluntarily withdrew from this program area in 2008–2009 were 0. *Human Resources Design MA/MS (Master of Arts/Science)*—Applications 2009–2010, 51. Total applicants accepted 2009–2010, 22. Number full-time enrolled (new admits only) 2009–2010, 20. Number part-time enrolled (new admits only) 2009–2010, 0. Total enrolled 2009–2010 full-time, 22, part-time, 8. Openings 2010–2011, 20. The median number of years required for completion of a degree in 2008–2009 were 2. The number of students enrolled full- and part-time who were dismissed or voluntarily withdrew from this program area in 2008–2009 were 0. *Applied Cognitive Psychology PhD (Doctor of Philosophy)*—Applications 2009–2010, 20. Number full-time enrolled (new admits only) 2009–2010, 8. Total enrolled 2009–2010 full-time, 26, part-time, 2. Openings 2010–2011, 6. The median number of years required for completion of a degree in 2008–2009 were 7. The number of students enrolled full- and part-time who were dismissed or voluntarily withdrew from this program area in 2008–2009 were 0. *Applied Developmental Psychology PhD (Doctor of Philosophy)*—Applications 2009–2010, 15. Number full-time enrolled (new admits only) 2009–2010, 1. Total enrolled 2009–2010 full-time, 19, part-time, 1. Openings 2010–2011, 8. The median number of years required for completion of a degree in 2008–2009 were 6. The number of students enrolled full- and part-time who were dismissed or voluntarily withdrew from this program area in 2008–2009 were 0. *Applied Social Psychology PhD (Doctor of Philosophy)*—Applications 2009–2010, 47. Number full-time enrolled (new admits only) 2009–2010, 9. Total enrolled 2009–2010 full-time, 53, part-time, 7. Openings 2010–2011, 9. The median number of years required for completion of a degree in 2008–2009 were 6. The number of students enrolled full- and part-time who were dismissed or voluntarily withdrew from this program area in 2008–2009 were 0. *Evaluation and Applied Research Methods PhD (Doctor of Philosophy)*—Applications 2009–2010, 7. Number full-time enrolled (new admits only) 2009–2010, 4. Number part-time enrolled (new admits only) 2009–2010, 1. Total enrolled 2009–2010 full-time, 14, part-time, 5. Openings 2010–2011, 6. The median number of years required for completion of a degree in 2008–2009 were 6. The number of students enrolled full- and part-time who were dismissed or voluntarily withdrew from this program area

in 2008–2009 were 1. *Organizational Behavior, Industrial/Organizational PhD (Doctor of Philosophy)*—Applications 2009–2010, 27. Number full-time enrolled (new admits only) 2009–2010, 2. Total enrolled 2009–2010 full-time, 27, part-time, 2. Openings 2010–2011, 4. The median number of years required for completion of a degree in 2008–2009 were 7. The number of students enrolled full- and part-time who were dismissed or voluntarily withdrew from this program area in 2008–2009 were 0. *Positive Developmental Psychology PhD (Doctor of Philosophy)*—Applications 2009–2010, 21. Number full-time enrolled (new admits only) 2009–2010, 4. Total enrolled 2009–2010 full-time, 10. Openings 2010–2011, 3. *Positive Organizational Psychology PhD (Doctor of Philosophy)*—Applications 2009–2010, 20. Number full-time enrolled (new admits only) 2009–2010, 2. Total enrolled 2009–2010 full-time, 5, part-time, 1. Openings 2010–2011, 3. *Positive Developmental Psych/Evaluation Co-Concen MA/MS (Master of Arts/Science)*—Applications 2009–2010, 28. Number full-time enrolled (new admits only) 2009–2010, 3. Total enrolled 2009–2010 full-time, 9. Openings 2010–2011, 3. *Positive Organizational Psych/Evaluation Co-Concen MA/MS (Master of Arts/Science)*—Applications 2009–2010, 33. Number full-time enrolled (new admits only) 2009–2010, 12. Total enrolled 2009–2010 full-time, 18. Openings 2010–2011, 3. *Health Behavior Research/Evaluation MA/MS (Master of Arts/Science)*—Applications 2009–2010, 6. Number full-time enrolled (new admits only) 2009–2010, 3. Total enrolled 2009–2010 full-time, 5, part-time, 1. Openings 2010–2011, 5. The number of students enrolled full- and part-time who were dismissed or voluntarily withdrew from this program area in 2008–2009 were 0.

Scores: Entries appear in this order: required test or GPA, minimum score (if required), median score of students entering in 2009–2010. *Applied Social Psych/Evaluation Co-Concentration MA/MS (Master of Arts/Science)*: GRE-V no minimum stated, 513, GRE-Q no minimum stated, 602, GRE-Analytical no minimum stated, 4.47, overall undergraduate GPA no minimum stated; *Cognitive Psychology/Evaluation Co-Concentration MA/MS (Master of Arts/Science)*: GRE-V no minimum stated, 513, GRE-Q no minimum stated, 602, GRE-Analytical no minimum stated, 4.47, overall undergraduate GPA no minimum stated; *Organizational/Evaluation Co-Concentration MA/MS (Master of Arts/Science)*: GRE-V no minimum stated, 513, GRE-Q no minimum stated, 602, GRE-Analytical no minimum stated, 4.47, overall undergraduate GPA no minimum stated; *Developmental Psych/Evaluation Co-Concentration MA/MS (Master of Arts/Science)*: GRE-V no minimum stated, 513, GRE-Q no minimum stated, 602, GRE-Analytical no minimum stated, 4.47, overall undergraduate GPA no minimum stated; *Applied Cognitive Psychology PhD (Doctor of Philosophy)*: GRE-V no minimum stated, 572, GRE-Q no minimum stated, 692, GRE-Analytical no minimum stated, 4.92, overall undergraduate GPA no minimum stated; *Applied Developmental Psychology PhD (Doctor of Philosophy)*: GRE-V no minimum stated, 525, GRE-Q no minimum stated, 700, GRE-Analytical no minimum stated, 4, overall undergraduate GPA no minimum stated; *Applied Social Psychology PhD (Doctor of Philosophy)*: GRE-V no minimum stated, 578, GRE-Q no minimum stated, 612, GRE-Analytical no minimum stated, 4.67, overall undergraduate GPA no minimum stated; *Evaluation and Applied Research Methods PhD (Doctor of Philosophy)*: GRE-V no minimum stated, 510, GRE-Q no minimum stated, 710, GRE-Analytical no minimum stated, 4.5, overall undergraduate GPA no minimum stated; *Organizational Behavior, Industrial/Organizational PhD (Doctor of Philosophy)*: GRE-V no minimum stated, 645, GRE-Q no minimum stated, 690, GRE-Analytical no minimum stated, 4.75, overall undergraduate GPA no minimum stated; *Positive Developmental Psychology PhD (Doctor of Philosophy)*: GRE-V no minimum stated, 553, GRE-Q no minimum stated, 720, GRE-Analytical no minimum stated, 4.5, overall undergraduate GPA no minimum stated; *Positive Organizational Psychology PhD (Doctor of Philosophy)*: GRE-V no minimum stated, 645, GRE-Q no minimum stated, 690, GRE-Analytical no minimum stated, 4.75, overall undergraduate GPA no minimum stated; *Positive Developmental Psych/Evaluation Co-Concen MA/MS (Master of Arts/Science)*: GRE-V no minimum stated, 513, GRE-Q no minimum stated, 602, GRE-Analytical no minimum stated, 4.47, overall undergraduate GPA no minimum stated; *Positive Organizational Psych/Evaluation Co-Concen MA/MS (Master of Arts/Science)*: GRE-V no minimum stated, 513, GRE-Q no minimum stated, 602, GRE-Analytical no minimum stated, 4.47, overall undergraduate GPA no minimum stated; *Health Behavior Research/Evaluation MA/MS (Master of Arts/Science)*: GRE-V no minimum stated, 513, GRE-Q no minimum stated, 602, GRE-Analytical no minimum stated, 4.47, overall undergraduate GPA no minimum stated.

Other Criteria: (importance of criteria rated low, medium, or high): GRE scores—high, research experience—medium, work experience—medium, extracurricular activity—medium, GPA—high, letters of recommendation—high, statement of goals and objectives—high, undergraduate major in psychology—medium, specific undergraduate psychology courses taken—medium, HRD program does not require research experience but emphasizes work experience more strongly. For additional information on admission requirements, go to http://www.cgu.edu/sbos.

Student Characteristics: The following represents characteristics of students in 2009–2010 in all graduate psychology programs in the department: Female—full-time 172, part-time 25; Male—full-time 88, part-time 7; African American/Black—full-time 16, part-time 1; Hispanic/Latino(a)—full-time 19, part-time 6; Asian/Pacific Islander—full-time 31, part-time 2; American Indian/Alaska Native—full-time 1, part-time 0; Caucasian/White—full-time 102, part-time 13; Multi-ethnic—full-time 6, part-time 0; students subject to the Americans With Disabilities Act—full-time 0, part-time 0; Unknown ethnicity—full-time 85, part-time 10; International students who hold an F-1 or J-1 Visa—full-time 0, part-time 0.

Financial Information/Assistance:

Tuition for Full-Time Study: *Master's:* State residents: per academic year $30,490, $1,524 per credit hour; Nonstate residents: per academic year $30,490, $1,524 per credit hour. *Doctoral:* State residents: per academic year $26,284, $1,524 per credit hour; Nonstate residents: per academic year $26,284, $1,524 per credit hour. Tuition is subject to change. See the following Web site for updates and changes in tuition costs: http://www.cgu.edu/new_tuition.

Financial Assistance:

First-Year Students: Teaching assistantships available for first year. Average amount paid per academic year: $5,200. Average number of hours worked per week: 10. Research assistantships available for first year. Average amount paid per academic year: $5,200. Average number of hours worked per week: 12. Fellowships and scholarships available for first year. Average amount paid per academic year: $8,761. Apply by January 15.

Advanced Students: Teaching assistantships available for advanced students. Average amount paid per academic year: $5,200. Average number of hours worked per week: 10. Research assistantships available for advanced students. Average amount paid per academic year: $5,200. Average number of hours worked per week: 12. Fellowships and scholarships available for advanced students. Average amount paid per academic year: $8,761. Apply by January 15.

Additional Information: Of all students currently enrolled full time, 100% benefited from one or more of the listed financial assistance programs. Application and information available online at: http://www.cgu.edu/pages/102.asp.

Internships/Practica: Research and consulting internships are available and encouraged for all students. Appropriate settings and roles are arranged according to the interests of individual students within the wide range of opportunities available in a large urban area. Typical settings include social service agencies; business and industrial organizations; hospitals, clinics, and mental health agencies; schools; governmental and regulatory agencies; and nonacademic research institutions, as well as numerous onsite research institutes.

Housing and Day Care: On-campus housing is available. See the following Web site for more information: http://www.cgu.edu/pages/1156.asp. On-campus day care facilities are available.

Employment of Department Graduates:
Master's Degree Graduates: Of those who graduated in the academic year 2008–2009, the following categories and numbers represent the postgraduate activities and employment of master's degree graduates: Enrolled in another graduate/professional program (1), enrolled in a postdoctoral residency/fellowship (n/a), employed in independent practice (n/a), employed in an academic position at a university (1), employed in an academic position at a 2-year/4-year college (1), employed in other positions at a higher education institution (1), employed in a professional position in a school system (3), employed in business or industry (2), employed in a community mental health/counseling center (2), employed in a hospital/medical center (1), other employment position (1), total from the above (master's) (13).

Doctoral Degree Graduates: Of those who graduated in the academic year 2008–2009, the following categories and numbers represent the postgraduate activities and employment of doctoral degree graduates: Enrolled in a psychology doctoral program (n/a), enrolled in a postdoctoral residency/fellowship (4), employed in an academic position at a university (2), employed in an academic position at a 2-year/4-year college (3), employed in other positions at a higher education institution (2), employed in a professional position in a school system (1), employed in business or industry (3), employed in a community mental health/counseling center (2), employed in a hospital/medical center (2), other employment position (3), total from the above (doctoral) (22).

Additional Information:
Orientation, Objectives, and Emphasis of Department: The program emphasizes contemporary human problems and social issues, and the organizations and systems involved in such issues, as well as on basic substantive research in social, organizational, developmental, and cognitive psychology and health behavior. Unusual specialty opportunities are available in positive psychology, organizational behavior, applied cognitive psychology, applied social psychology, health psychology, and program evaluation research. The program offers preparation for careers in public service and business and industry as well as teaching and research. Research, theory, and practice are stressed in such policy and program areas as organizations and work; human social and physical environments; social service systems; psychological effects of educational computer technology; health and mental health systems; crime, delinquency, and law; and aging and life span education. Many opportunities are available for research, consulting, and field experiences in these and related areas. Strong emphasis is given to training in a broad range of research methodologies, from naturalistic observation to experimental design, with special attention to field research methods. Seminars, tutorials, independent research, individualized student program plans, practical field experience, and close advisory and collaborative relations with the faculty are designed to foster clarifications of individual goals, intellectual and professional growth, self-pacing, and attractive career opportunities.

Special Facilities or Resources: The school is equipped with labs for social, developmental, identity, health, positive psychology, and cognitive research, supplies and equipment for field research, a student lounge, and department library. The computer facilities are excellent, conveniently located, and include a wide variety of application programs. The department cooperates in overseeing research institutes for student-faculty grant or contract research, focusing on major problems of organizational and program evaluation research as well as research on social issues. Claremont Graduate University is a free-standing graduate institution within the context of the Claremont University Consortium of five colleges, the Graduate University, and the Keck Graduate Institute. This context allows the department to concentrate exclusively on graduate education in a relaxed, intimate context while enjoying the resources of a major university. In addition to the full-time graduate psychology faculty, there are more than 40 full-time faculty members from the undergraduate Claremont Colleges who participate in the graduate program and who are available to students for research, advising, and instruction. Resources from other programs within the Graduate University are also available to psychology students, in such areas as public policy, education, information sciences, business administration, executive management, economics, and government. The nearby Los Angeles basin is a major urban area that offers rich and varied opportunities for interesting research, field placements and internships, part-time employment, and career development.

Application Information:
Send to Admissions Office, McManus Hall 131, Claremont Graduate University, Claremont, CA 91711. Application available online. URL of online application: http://www.cgu.edu/pages/102.asp. Students are admitted in the Fall, application deadline January 15; Spring, application deadline November 15. The Human Resources Design MS program accepts applications throughout the year on a space-available basis. *Fee:* $60. Fee waived or deferred if need is certified.

Fielding Graduate University (2009 data)

School of Psychology
2112 Santa Barbara Street
Santa Barbara, CA 93105
Telephone: (805) 687-1099
Fax: (805) 687-9793
E-mail: psyadmissions@fielding.edu
Web: http://www.fielding.edu

Department Information:
1974. Dean, School of Psychology: Raymond J. Trybus. Number of faculty: total—full-time 40; women—full-time 17; total—minority—full-time 4; faculty subject to the Americans With Disabilities Act 1.

Programs and Degrees Offered:
Listed in the following order: Program area, degree type (T if terminal Master's), number awarded 7/08–6/09. Clinical Psychology Respecialization Diploma 2, Clinical PhD (Doctor of Philosophy) 41, Media Psychology PhD (Doctor of Philosophy) 1, Post Doctorate Neuropsychology Certificate 22, Media Psychology & Social Change MA/MS (Master of Arts/Science) (T).

APA Accreditation: Clinical PhD (Doctor of Philosophy).

Student Applications/Admissions:

Student Applications

Clinical Psychology Respecialization Diploma—Applications 2009–2010, 14. Total applicants accepted 2009–2010, 9. Number full-time enrolled (new admits only) 2009–2010, 6. Total enrolled 2009–2010 full-time, 25. Openings 2010–2011, 6. The median number of years required for completion of a degree in 2008–2009 were 5. The number of students enrolled full- and part-time who were dismissed or voluntarily withdrew from this program area in 2008–2009 were 2. *Clinical PhD (Doctor of Philosophy)*—Applications 2009–2010, 391. Total applicants accepted 2009–2010, 129. Number full-time enrolled (new admits only) 2009–2010, 96. Number part-time enrolled (new admits only) 2009–2010, 0. Openings 2010–2011, 80. The median number of years required for completion of a degree in 2008–2009 were 8. The number of students enrolled full- and part-time who were dismissed or voluntarily withdrew from this program area in 2008–2009 were 27. *Media Psychology PhD (Doctor of Philosophy)*—Applications 2009–2010, 43. Total applicants accepted 2009–2010, 43. Number full-time enrolled (new admits only) 2009–2010, 28. Number part-time enrolled (new admits only) 2009–2010, 0. Openings 2010–2011, 30. The median number of years required for completion of a degree in 2008–2009 were 4. The number of students enrolled full- and part-time who were dismissed or voluntarily withdrew from this program area in 2008–2009 were 5. *Post Doctorate Neuropsychology Certificate*—Applications 2009–2010, 30. Total applicants accepted 2009–2010, 29. Number full-time enrolled (new admits only) 2009–2010, 0. Number part-time enrolled (new admits only) 2009–2010, 23. Openings 2010–2011, 25. The median number of years required for completion of a degree in 2008–2009 were 2. The number of students enrolled full- and part-time who were dismissed or voluntarily withdrew from this program area in 2008–2009 were 8. *Media Psychology & Social Change MA/MS (Master of Arts/Science)*—

Other Criteria: (importance of criteria rated low, medium, or high): research experience—high, work experience—high, extracurricular activity—medium, clinically related public service—high, GPA—medium, letters of recommendation—high, interview—high, statement of goals and objectives—high, autobio & writing sample—medium, undergraduate major in psychology—medium, specific undergraduate psychology courses taken—medium, Watson-Glaser for Clinical program only. For additional information on admission requirements, go to http://www.fielding.edu/admission.

Student Characteristics: The following represents characteristics of students in 2009–2010 in all graduate psychology programs in the department: Female—full-time 420, part-time 0; Male—full-time 157, part-time 0; African American/Black—full-time 44, part-time 0; Hispanic/Latino(a)—full-time 36, part-time 0; Asian/Pacific Islander—full-time 17, part-time 0; American Indian/Alaska Native—full-time 8, part-time 0; Caucasian/White—full-time 442, part-time 0; Multi-ethnic—full-time 29, part-time 0; students subject to the Americans With Disabilities Act—full-time 2, part-time 0; Unknown ethnicity—full-time 0, part-time 0; International students who hold an F-1 or J-1 Visa—full-time 0, part-time 0.

Financial Information/Assistance:

Tuition for Full-Time Study: *Doctoral:* State residents: per academic year $19,695; Nonstate residents: per academic year $19,695. Tuition is subject to change. See the following Web site for updates and changes in tuition costs: http://www.fielding.edu/financialaid/tuition.aspx.

Financial Assistance:

First-Year Students: No information provided.

Advanced Students: Fellowships and scholarships available for advanced students. Average amount paid per academic year: $5,000.

Additional Information: Of all students currently enrolled full time, 10% benefited from one or more of the listed financial assistance programs. Application and information available online at: http://www.fielding.edu/financialaid/.

Internships/Practica: Doctoral Degree (PhD Clinical): For those doctoral students for whom a professional internship was required in this program prior to graduation, (35) students applied for an internship in 2008–2009, with (32) students obtaining an internship. Of those students who obtained an internship, (23) were paid internships. Of those students who obtained an internship, (18) students placed in APA/CPA accredited internships, (8) students placed in internships not APA/CPA accredited, but listed with the Association of Psychology Postdoctoral and Internship Programs (APPIC), (0) students placed in internships conforming to guidelines of the Council of Directors of School Psychology Programs (CDSPP), (6) students placed in internships that were not APA/CPA accredited, APPIC or CDSPP listed. Master's Degree (MA/MS Media Psychology & Social Change): An internship experience, such as a final research project or "capstone" experience is required of graduates. Students apply to APA or APPIC approved or comparable internship sites that offer organized training programs lasting one year full-time or two consecutive years half-time. Such internships provide a planned, integrated sequence of clinical and didactic experiences with the goal of providing sufficient training and supervision so that upon completion our graduates can function responsibly as postdoctoral psychologists.

Housing and Day Care: No on-campus housing is available. No on-campus day care facilities are available.

Employment of Department Graduates:
Master's Degree Graduates: Of those who graduated in the academic year 2008–2009, the following categories and numbers represent the postgraduate activities and employment of master's degree graduates: Enrolled in a postdoctoral residency/fellowship (n/a), employed in independent practice (n/a), total from the above (master's) (0).
Doctoral Degree Graduates: Of those who graduated in the academic year 2008–2009, the following categories and numbers represent the postgraduate activities and employment of doctoral degree graduates: Enrolled in a psychology doctoral program (n/a), enrolled in a postdoctoral residency/fellowship (7), employed in independent practice (6), employed in an academic position at a university (1), employed in other positions at a higher education institution (2), employed in a professional position in a school system (1), employed in business or industry (1), employed in government agency (1), employed in a community mental health/counseling center (4), employed in a hospital/medical center (4), still seeking employment (1), other employment position (2), do not know (14), total from the above (doctoral) (44).

Additional Information:
Orientation, Objectives, and Emphasis of Department: Fielding Graduate University's School of Psychology enables mid-career adults with mental health and human service experience to earn the PhD in clinical or media psychology as well as postdoctoral certificates in neuropsychology or respecialization in clinical psychology. Our students bring a sense of autonomy and extensive personal and professional experience to their studies. The programs' scholar-practitioner model accommodates the special characteristics of adult students. Through seminars and guided study, the adult learner pursues study at whatever location life circumstances permit.

Special Facilities or Resources: Students become members of a "cluster" in their geographical area consisting of a Regional Faculty member and other students. Meetings are held regularly and consist of a variety of learning activities including seminars, clinical and research training, faculty supervision consultation, as well as peer contact and support. Each student is assigned to an Associate Dean who is located in Santa Barbara, CA, and who oversees the student's academic program. Two intensive week-long residential sessions are offered each year that bring together students, faculty, and other scholars who offer seminars and other educational and training events. Two residential research sessions are held each year. These include research training, dissertation seminars, instruction in the use of research libraries and electronic databases, and lectures by invited research scholars. Psychological assessment laboratories are offered several times each year to provide training in conducting comprehensive psychodiagnostic evaluations.

Application Information:
Send to Psychology Admission Counselor, Fielding Graduate University, 2112 Santa Barbara Street, Santa Barbara, CA 93105. Application available online. URL of online application: http://www.fielding.edu/admission. Students are admitted in the Fall, application deadline February 27; Spring, application deadline August 22. Clinical and Respecialization - February 27 and August 22; Media - April 25 and October 25. *Fee:* $75.

Fuller Theological Seminary
Department of Clinical Psychology
School of Psychology
180 North Oakland Avenue
Pasadena, CA 91101
Telephone: (626) 584-5500
Fax: (626) 584-9630
E-mail: *clements@fuller.edu*
Web: *http://www.fuller.edu/academics/school-of-psychology/about-sop.aspx*

Department Information:
1965. Chairperson: Mari L. Clements, PhD. Number of faculty: total—full-time 11, part-time 3; women—full-time 3, part-time 3; total—minority—full-time 3, part-time 1; women minority—full-time 1.

Programs and Degrees Offered:
Listed in the following order: Program area, degree type (T if terminal Master's), number awarded 7/08–6/09. Clinical Psychology PhD (Doctor of Philosophy) 26, Clinical Psychology PsyD (Doctor of Psychology) 12.

APA Accreditation: Clinical PhD (Doctor of Philosophy). Student Outcome Data Website: http://www.fuller.edu/academics/school-of-psychology/department-of-clinical-psychology/department-of-clinical-psychology/program-statistics.aspx. Clinical PsyD (Doctor of Psychology). Student Outcome Data Website: http://www.fuller.edu/academics/school-of-psychology/department-of-clinical-psychology/department-of-clinical-psychology/program-statistics.aspx.

Student Applications/Admissions:
Student Applications
Clinical Psychology PhD (Doctor of Philosophy)—Applications 2009–2010, 58. Total applicants accepted 2009–2010, 44. Number full-time enrolled (new admits only) 2009–2010, 26. Number part-time enrolled (new admits only) 2009–2010, 0. Openings 2010–2011, 25. The median number of years required for completion of a degree in 2008–2009 were 6. The number of students enrolled full- and part-time who were dismissed or voluntarily withdrew from this program area in 2008–2009 were 1. *Clinical Psychology PsyD (Doctor of Psychology)*—Applications 2009–2010, 50. Total applicants accepted 2009–2010, 31. Number full-time enrolled (new admits only) 2009–2010, 9. Number part-time enrolled (new admits only) 2009–2010, 0. Openings 2010–2011, 20. The median number of years required for completion of a degree in 2008–2009 were 6. The number of students enrolled full- and part-time who were dismissed or voluntarily withdrew from this program area in 2008–2009 were 2.
Scores: Entries appear in this order: required test or GPA, minimum score (if required), median score of students entering in 2009–2010. *Clinical Psychology PhD (Doctor of Philosophy):*

GRE-V no minimum stated, 510, GRE-Q no minimum stated, 640, psychology GPA no minimum stated, 3.75; *Clinical Psychology PsyD (Doctor of Psychology)*: GRE-V no minimum stated, 510, GRE-Q no minimum stated, 600, psychology GPA no minimum stated, 3.67.

Other Criteria: (importance of criteria rated low, medium, or high): GRE scores—high, research experience—high, work experience—medium, extracurricular activity—low, clinically related public service—medium, GPA—high, letters of recommendation—high, interview—high, statement of goals and objectives—high. Research experience is less important for PsyD candidates than for PhD candidates. For additional information on admission requirements, go to http://www.fuller.edu/admissions/apply/admission-requirements-sopclinical.aspx.

Student Characteristics: The following represents characteristics of students in 2009–2010 in all graduate psychology programs in the department: Female—full-time 195, part-time 0; Male—full-time 98, part-time 0; African American/Black—full-time 23, part-time 0; Hispanic/Latino(a)—full-time 17, part-time 0; Asian/Pacific Islander—full-time 47, part-time 0; American Indian/Alaska Native—full-time 1, part-time 0; Caucasian/White—full-time 186, part-time 0; Multi-ethnic—full-time 2, part-time 0; students subject to the Americans With Disabilities Act—full-time 9, part-time 0; Unknown ethnicity—full-time 17, part-time 0; International students who hold an F-1 or J-1 Visa—full-time 0, part-time 0.

Financial Information/Assistance:
  Tuition for Full-Time Study: *Doctoral:* State residents: per academic year $32,100, $575 per credit hour; Nonstate residents: per academic year $32,100, $575 per credit hour. Tuition is subject to change. Tuition costs vary by program. See the following Web site for updates and changes in tuition costs: http://www.fuller.edu/admissions/tuition-and-fees.aspx.

  Financial Assistance:
    First-Year Students: Research assistantships available for first year. Average amount paid per academic year: $8,100. Average number of hours worked per week: 15. Fellowships and scholarships available for first year. Average amount paid per academic year: $9,500. Average number of hours worked per week: 0.
    Advanced Students: Teaching assistantships available for advanced students. Average amount paid per academic year: $10,000. Average number of hours worked per week: 10. Research assistantships available for advanced students. Average amount paid per academic year: $8,100. Average number of hours worked per week: 15. Traineeships available for advanced students. Average amount paid per academic year: $10,000. Average number of hours worked per week: 10. Fellowships and scholarships available for advanced students. Average amount paid per academic year: $13,000. Average number of hours worked per week: 15. Apply by March 31.
    Additional Information: Of all students currently enrolled full time, 60% benefited from one or more of the listed financial assistance programs. Application and information available online at: http://www.fuller.edu/admission/financial-aid/financial-aid.aspx.

Internships/Practica: Doctoral Degree (PhD Clinical Psychology): For those doctoral students for whom a professional internship was required in this program prior to graduation, (16) students applied for an internship in 2008–2009, with (11) students obtaining an internship. Of those students who obtained an internship, (11) were paid internships. Of those students who obtained an internship, (4) students placed in APA/CPA accredited internships, (7) students placed in internships not APA/CPA accredited, but listed with the Association of Psychology Postdoctoral and Internship Programs (APPIC), (0) students placed in internships conforming to guidelines of the Council of Directors of School Psychology Programs (CDSPP), (0) students placed in internships that were not APA/CPA accredited, APPIC or CDSPP listed. Doctoral Degree (PsyD Clinical Psychology): For those doctoral students for whom a professional internship was required in this program prior to graduation, (16) students applied for an internship in 2008–2009, with (11) students obtaining an internship. Of those students who obtained an internship, (11) were paid internships. Of those students who obtained an internship, (6) students placed in APA/CPA accredited internships, (5) students placed in internships not APA/CPA accredited, but listed with the Association of Psychology Postdoctoral and Internship Programs (APPIC), (0) students placed in internships conforming to guidelines of the Council of Directors of School Psychology Programs (CDSPP), (0) students placed in internships that were not APA/CPA accredited, APPIC or CDSPP listed. Students are placed in field training sites throughout their program including 2 years of practicum, 1 year of assessment clerkship, 1 year of pre-internship (PhD only) and a 1-year full-time clinical internship. Students are placed at Fuller Psychological and Family Services clinic as well as in over 50 sites throughout the L.A. metropolitan area. Because of our location, students are exposed to multiple methods of service delivery as well as to diverse ethnic, clinical, and age populations. Students obtain internships throughout the U.S. and Canada.

Housing and Day Care: On-campus housing is available. See the following Web site for more information: http://www.fuller.edu/admissions/housing.aspx. No on-campus day care facilities are available.

Employment of Department Graduates:
  Master's Degree Graduates: Of those who graduated in the academic year 2008–2009, the following categories and numbers represent the postgraduate activities and employment of master's degree graduates: Enrolled in a postdoctoral residency/fellowship (n/a), employed in independent practice (n/a), total from the above (master's) (0).
  Doctoral Degree Graduates: Of those who graduated in the academic year 2008–2009, the following categories and numbers represent the postgraduate activities and employment of doctoral degree graduates: Enrolled in a psychology doctoral program (n/a), do not know (38), total from the above (doctoral) (38).

Additional Information:
  Orientation, Objectives, and Emphasis of Department: The purpose of the Graduate School of Psychology is to prepare a distinctive kind of clinical psychologist: men and women whose understanding and action are deeply informed by both psychology and the Christian faith. It is based on the conviction that the coupling of Christian understanding with refined clinical and research skills will produce a psychologist with a special ability to help persons of faith on their journeys to wholeness. The school has adopted

the scientist–practitioner model for its PhD program and the clinical scientist model for its PsyD program.

Special Facilities or Resources: The Lee Edward Travis Research Institute (TRI) in the School of Psychology at Fuller Theological Seminary is committed to fostering interdisciplinary research into the relationships between social systems, environmental situations, personality, mental and affective states, biological processes, and spiritual and religious states and practices. Fuller Psychological & Family Services clinic provides assistance to individuals, couples, and families, including services to children and adolescents. Psychological interventions are offered for adjustment disorders, anxiety, depression, stress management, abuse and domestic violence, and physical conditions affected by psychological factors. Student trainees may be placed in the clinic for practicum, clerkship or pre-internship.

Information for Students With Physical Disabilities: See the following Web site for more information: http://www.fuller.edu/current-students/current-students.aspx.

Application Information:
Send to Office of Admissions, Fuller Theological Seminary, 135 N. Oakland Avenue, Pasadena, CA 91182. Application available online. URL of online application: https://www.applyweb.com/apply/fuller/menu.html. Students are admitted in the Fall, application deadline December 15. We have three application deadlines. Early admissions is November 5, Regular is December 15, Final is January 10. *Fee:* $100. Fee is waived for early admission. On line application fee is $50 for regular admissions deadline and $75 for final admissions deadline.

Humboldt State University
Department of Psychology
College of Natural Resources & Sciences
1 Harpst Street
Arcata, CA 95521
Telephone: (707) 826-3755
Fax: (707) 826-4993
E-mail: *bbd1@humboldt.edu*
Web: *http://www.humboldt.edu/psychology*

Department Information:
1964. Chairperson: Brent Duncan, PhD Number of faculty: total—full-time 13, part-time 13; women—full-time 5, part-time 9; total—minority—full-time 3, part-time 1; women minority—full-time 2, part-time 1.

Programs and Degrees Offered:
Listed in the following order: Program area, degree type (T if terminal Master's), number awarded 7/08–6/09. Academic Research MA/MS (Master of Arts/Science) (T) 5, Counseling MA/MS (Master of Arts/Science) (T) 4, School Psychology MA/MS (Master of Arts/Science) (T) 10.

Student Applications/Admissions:
Student Applications
Academic Research MA/MS (Master of Arts/Science)—Applications 2009–2010, 15. Total applicants accepted 2009–2010, 12. Number full-time enrolled (new admits only) 2009–2010, 12. Number part-time enrolled (new admits only) 2009–2010, 0. Openings 2010–2011, 14. The median number of years required for completion of a degree in 2008–2009 were 2. The number of students enrolled full- and part-time who were dismissed or voluntarily withdrew from this program area in 2008–2009 were 0. *Counseling MA/MS (Master of Arts/Science)*—Applications 2009–2010, 25. Total applicants accepted 2009–2010, 7. Number full-time enrolled (new admits only) 2009–2010, 7. Number part-time enrolled (new admits only) 2009–2010, 0. Total enrolled 2009–2010 full-time, 13, part-time, 1. The median number of years required for completion of a degree in 2008–2009 were 3. The number of students enrolled full- and part-time who were dismissed or voluntarily withdrew from this program area in 2008–2009 were 0. *School Psychology MA/MS (Master of Arts/Science)*—Applications 2009–2010, 13. Total applicants accepted 2009–2010, 8. Number full-time enrolled (new admits only) 2009–2010, 8. Number part-time enrolled (new admits only) 2009–2010, 0. The median number of years required for completion of a degree in 2008–2009 were 3. The number of students enrolled full- and part-time who were dismissed or voluntarily withdrew from this program area in 2008–2009 were 0.

Other Criteria: (importance of criteria rated low, medium, or high): GRE scores—low, research experience—medium, work experience—medium, extracurricular activity—medium, clinically related public service—medium, GPA—high, letters of recommendation—high, interview—medium, statement of goals and objectives—high, undergraduate major in psychology—low. An interview is required for Counseling and School Psychology; research experience is important for Academic Research; clinically related public service or work experience is highly important for Counseling and School Psychology; school/child related work experience highly important for School Psychology. For additional information on admission requirements, go to http://www.humboldt.edu/psychology/grad/gradhome.htm.

Student Characteristics: The following represents characteristics of students in 2009–2010 in all graduate psychology programs in the department: Female—full-time 49, part-time 0; Male—full-time 19, part-time 1; African American/Black—full-time 0, part-time 0; Hispanic/Latino(a)—full-time 6, part-time 1; Asian/Pacific Islander—full-time 2, part-time 2; American Indian/Alaska Native—full-time 0, part-time 0; Caucasian/White—full-time 53, part-time 10; Multi-ethnic—full-time 1, part-time 1; students subject to the Americans With Disabilities Act—full-time 0, part-time 0; Unknown ethnicity—full-time 0, part-time 0; International students who hold an F-1 or J-1 Visa—full-time 0, part-time 0.

Financial Information/Assistance:
Tuition for Full-Time Study: *Master's:* State residents: per academic year $4,962; Nonstate residents: per academic year $4,962, $372 per credit hour. Tuition is subject to change. See the following Web site for updates and changes in tuition costs: http://www.humboldt.edu/~fiscal/topics/cashiers/regfees.html.

Financial Assistance:
First-Year Students: Fellowships and scholarships available for first year. Average amount paid per academic year: $4,000.

Advanced Students: Fellowships and scholarships available for advanced students.

Additional Information: Of all students currently enrolled full time, 0% benefited from one or more of the listed financial assistance programs.

Internships/Practica: Master's Degree (MA/MS Academic Research): An internship experience, such as a final research project or "capstone" experience is required of graduates. Master's Degree (MA/MS Counseling): An internship experience, such as a final research project or "capstone" experience is required of graduates. Master's Degree (MA/MS School Psychology): An internship experience, such as a final research project or "capstone" experience is required of graduates. School Psychology internships (paid) are required of all students seeking the School Psychology credential. Counseling MA students are provided the opportunity to do fieldwork/practica in the department's psychology clinic, as well as in several local mental heath agencies.

Housing and Day Care: On-campus housing is available. On-campus day care facilities are available.

Employment of Department Graduates:
Master's Degree Graduates: Of those who graduated in the academic year 2008–2009, the following categories and numbers represent the postgraduate activities and employment of master's degree graduates: Enrolled in a psychology doctoral program (2), enrolled in a postdoctoral residency/fellowship (n/a), employed in independent practice (n/a), employed in an academic position at a 2-year/4-year college (1), employed in a professional position in a school system (10), employed in business or industry (2), employed in government agency (1), employed in a community mental health/counseling center (6), total from the above (master's) (22).

Doctoral Degree Graduates: Of those who graduated in the academic year 2008–2009, the following categories and numbers represent the postgraduate activities and employment of doctoral degree graduates: Enrolled in a psychology doctoral program (n/a), total from the above (doctoral) (0).

Additional Information:
Orientation, Objectives, and Emphasis of Department: The objectives of our department of psychology are to provide students with an understanding of principles and theories concerning human behavior and to the processes by which such information is obtained; to provide a sound academic education for those working for degrees in psychology with a future goal of professional work in psychology; to offer a liberal arts major and minor in psychology for students seeking a quality liberal education; to provide quality professional graduate education for students working toward California School Psychologist credentials, Marriage and Family Therapist licenses and other specialized occupational fields; and to provide a flexibility in our offerings that responds to changing societal agenda and student needs. Our Academic Research Masters Program provides specializations in the following areas: Developmental Psychopathology, Biological Psychology, and Social and Environmental Psychology. Students should select one of these areas when they apply to the AR program.

Special Facilities or Resources: The department has an on-campus clinic staffed by MA counseling students, an electronic equipment shop, a lab with biofeedback and EEG equipment, a lab equipped for research on motion sickness, observation and research access to an on-campus demonstration nursery school, a test library, and a computer laboratory. Our new Behavioral and Social Sciences Building provides exceptional research, instruction, faculty and student space for the Department of Psychology.

Information for Students With Physical Disabilities: See the following Web site for more information: http://www.humboldt.edu/~sdrc/.

Application Information:
Send to Department of Psychology, Humboldt State University, Arcata, CA 95521. Application available online. URL of online application: http://www.csumentor.edu/AdmissionApp/. Students are admitted in the Fall. Deadline for Academic Research MA program is March 1. Deadline for Counseling MA program is February 1. Deadline for School Psychology MA program is January 15. However, we will accept applications until August 1 or we accept a full cohort. *Fee:* $55.

John F. Kennedy University
College of Professional Studies
100 Ellinwood Way
Pleasant Hill, CA 94523
Telephone: (925) 969-3400
Fax: (925) 969-3401
E-mail: *smagraw@jfku.edu*
Web: *http://www.jfku.edu/Programs-and-Courses/College-of-Professional-Studies.html*

Department Information:
1965. Number of faculty: total—full-time 10, part-time 89; women—full-time 8, part-time 76; total—minority—full-time 3, part-time 8; women minority—full-time 2, part-time 4; faculty subject to the Americans With Disabilities Act 2.

Programs and Degrees Offered:
Listed in the following order: Program area, degree type (T if terminal Master's), number awarded 7/08–6/09. Counseling Psychology MA/MS (Master of Arts/Science) (T) 78, Clinical Psychology PsyD (Doctor of Psychology) 19, Sport Psychology MA/MS (Master of Arts/Science) (T) 12.

APA Accreditation: Clinical PsyD (Doctor of Psychology). Student Outcome Data Website: http://www.jfku.edu/Programs-and-Courses/College-of-Professional-Studies/Department-of-Clinical-Psychology.html.

Student Applications/Admissions:
Student Applications
Counseling Psychology MA/MS (Master of Arts/Science)—Applications 2009–2010, 175. Total applicants accepted 2009–2010, 130. Number full-time enrolled (new admits only) 2009–2010, 27. Number part-time enrolled (new admits only) 2009–2010, 48. Total enrolled 2009–2010 full-time, 126, part-time, 146. Openings 2010–2011, 75. The median number of years required for completion of a degree in 2008–2009 were 2. The number of students enrolled full- and part-time who were dismissed or voluntarily withdrew from this program area in

2008–2009 were 8. *Clinical Psychology PsyD (Doctor of Psychology)*—Applications 2009–2010, 158. Total applicants accepted 2009–2010, 77. Number full-time enrolled (new admits only) 2009–2010, 25. Number part-time enrolled (new admits only) 2009–2010, 4. Total enrolled 2009–2010 full-time, 88, part-time, 47. Openings 2010–2011, 30. The median number of years required for completion of a degree in 2008–2009 were 5. The number of students enrolled full- and part-time who were dismissed or voluntarily withdrew from this program area in 2008–2009 were 1. *Sport Psychology MA/MS (Master of Arts/Science)*—Applications 2009–2010, 33. Total applicants accepted 2009–2010, 28. Number full-time enrolled (new admits only) 2009–2010, 8. Number part-time enrolled (new admits only) 2009–2010, 10. Total enrolled 2009–2010 full-time, 16, part-time, 35. Openings 2010–2011, 20. The median number of years required for completion of a degree in 2008–2009 were 2.

Other Criteria: (importance of criteria rated low, medium, or high): research experience—medium, work experience—high, extracurricular activity—high, clinically related public service—high, GPA—high, letters of recommendation—high, interview—high, statement of goals and objectives—high, undergraduate major in psychology—medium, specific undergraduate psychology courses taken—low. The PsyD program puts more emphasis on the GPA than do the MA Programs.

Student Characteristics: The following represents characteristics of students in 2009–2010 in all graduate psychology programs in the department: Female—full-time 159, part-time 172; Male—full-time 71, part-time 56; African American/Black—full-time 17, part-time 25; Hispanic/Latino(a)—full-time 14, part-time 18; Asian/Pacific Islander—full-time 13, part-time 16; American Indian/Alaska Native—full-time 2, part-time 3; Caucasian/White—full-time 123, part-time 121; Multi-ethnic—full-time 21, part-time 11; students subject to the Americans With Disabilities Act—full-time 4, part-time 2; Unknown ethnicity—full-time 40, part-time 34; International students who hold an F-1 or J-1 Visa—full-time 0, part-time 0.

Financial Information/Assistance:
Tuition for Full-Time Study: *Master's:* State residents: $475 per credit hour; Nonstate residents: $475 per credit hour. *Doctoral:* State residents: $610 per credit hour; Nonstate residents: $610 per credit hour. Tuition is subject to change. Additional fees are assessed to students beyond the costs of tuition for the following: comprehensive exams, petition to graduate, student services, and technology fees. Tuition costs vary by program. See the following Web site for updates and changes in tuition costs: http://www.jfku.edu.

Financial Assistance:
First-Year Students: No information provided.
Advanced Students: No information provided.
Additional Information: Of all students currently enrolled full time, 0% benefited from one or more of the listed financial assistance programs. Application and information available online at: http://www.jfku.edu/Admissions/Financial-Aid.html.

Internships/Practica: Doctoral Degree (PsyD Clinical Psychology): For those doctoral students for whom a professional internship was required in this program prior to graduation, (24) students applied for an internship in 2008–2009, with (23) students obtaining an internship. Of those students who obtained an internship, (17) were paid internships. Of those students who obtained an internship, (2) students placed in APA/CPA accredited internships, (7) students placed in internships not APA/CPA accredited, but listed with the Association of Psychology Postdoctoral and Internship Programs (APPIC), (0) students placed in internships conforming to guidelines of the Council of Directors of School Psychology Programs (CDSPP), (14) students placed in internships that were not APA/CPA accredited, APPIC or CDSPP listed. The Graduate School of Professional Psychology has three community counseling centers, located near one of our two campuses, which provide state-of-the-art supervision for students and provide thousands of hours of low-fee counseling each year. Additionally, approximately 150 external fieldwork sites, monitored by our faculty, are available in the surrounding counties. Students in the Counseling MA program and the PsyD program accumulate hours toward their respective licenses at both the community counseling centers and the external sites. The MA in Sport Psychology and Expressive Art programs offer summer camps for children which also serve as additional field placement sites for graduate students.

Housing and Day Care: No on-campus housing is available. No on-campus day care facilities are available.

Employment of Department Graduates:
Master's Degree Graduates: Of those who graduated in the academic year 2008–2009, the following categories and numbers represent the postgraduate activities and employment of master's degree graduates: Enrolled in a postdoctoral residency/fellowship (n/a), employed in independent practice (n/a), total from the above (master's) (0).
Doctoral Degree Graduates: Of those who graduated in the academic year 2008–2009, the following categories and numbers represent the postgraduate activities and employment of doctoral degree graduates: Enrolled in a psychology doctoral program (n/a), total from the above (doctoral) (0).

Additional Information:
Orientation, Objectives, and Emphasis of Department: The mission of the Graduate School of Professional Psychology is to create an innovative, diverse, and responsive environment for students that supports personal and professional learning. We are committed to active learning and community service, and are guided by a commitment to traditionally underserved populations. Students acquire excellence in both traditional and emerging competencies and are taught by faculty who are practicing professionals in their field. The MA in Counseling Psychology program offers specializations in Child and Adolescent Therapy, Addiction Studies, Cross-Cultural Issues, Expressive Arts, Couples and Families, and Sport Psychology. In addition to the MA degree, the Organizational Psychology program offers certificates in Coaching and Conflict Management. Students may also enroll in the Link Program and receive both the MA in Sports Psychology and the PsyD in Clinical Psychology.

Special Facilities or Resources: As noted, the Graduate School of Professional Psychology community counseling centers serve a broad-based clientele throughout the surrounding communities. The programs in the school are actively engaged in community service. For example, the Sports Psychology program is an active participant in the Life Enhancement Through Athletic and Academic Participation (LEAP) in numerous Bay Area schools. The Expressive Arts specialization in the Counseling Psychology MA program works with elementary school children from a variety of sites.

Application Information:
Send to Office of Admissions, John F. Kennedy University, 100 Ellinwood Way, Pleasant Hill, CA 94523. Application available online. URL of online application: http://www.jfku.edu/Admissions.html. Students are admitted in the Fall, application deadline January 2; Programs have rolling admissions. January 2 for PsyD (Fall admissions only). MA Counseling Program takes new students in Fall and Spring. MA in Sport Psychology take new students each quarter. *Fee:* $60. $85 application fee for PsyD Program.

La Verne, University of
Psychology Department
Arts and Sciences
1950 Third Street
La Verne, CA 91750
Telephone: (909) 593-3511, ext. 4414
Fax: (909) 392-2745
E-mail: *jkernes@laverne.edu*
Web: *http://www.laverne.edu/academics/arts-sciences/psychology/doctoral/*

Department Information:
1968. PsyD Program Chair: Jerry L. Kernes, PhD. Number of faculty: total—full-time 12, part-time 5; women—full-time 7, part-time 2; total—minority—full-time 5, part-time 2; women minority—full-time 4.

Programs and Degrees Offered:
Listed in the following order: Program area, degree type (T if terminal Master's), number awarded 7/08–6/09. Clinical-Community Psychology PsyD (Doctor of Psychology) 4.

APA Accreditation: Clinical PsyD (Doctor of Psychology). Student Outcome Data Website: http://laverne.edu/academics/arts-sciences/psychology/doctoral/.

Student Applications/Admissions:
Student Applications
Clinical-Community Psychology PsyD (Doctor of Psychology)—Applications 2009–2010, 81. Total applicants accepted 2009–2010, 23. Number full-time enrolled (new admits only) 2009–2010, 21. Number part-time enrolled (new admits only) 2009–2010, 0. Total enrolled 2009–2010 full-time, 99. Openings 2010–2011, 25. The median number of years required for completion of a degree in 2008–2009 were 5. The number of students enrolled full- and part-time who were dismissed or voluntarily withdrew from this program area in 2008–2009 were 1.
Other Criteria: (importance of criteria rated low, medium, or high): research experience—medium, work experience—high, extracurricular activity—low, clinically related public service—high, GPA—high, letters of recommendation—high, interview—high, statement of goals and objectives—high, undergraduate major in psychology—medium, specific undergraduate psychology courses taken—medium. For additional information on admission requirements, go to http://laverne.edu/academics/arts-sciences/psychology/doctoral/admissions/.

Student Characteristics: The following represents characteristics of students in 2009–2010 in all graduate psychology programs in the department: Female—full-time 52, part-time 0; Male—full-time 8, part-time 0; African American/Black—full-time 6, part-time 0; Hispanic/Latino(a)—full-time 23, part-time 0; Asian/Pacific Islander—full-time 5, part-time 0; American Indian/Alaska Native—full-time 0, part-time 0; Caucasian/White—full-time 28, part-time 0; Multi-ethnic—full-time 2, part-time 0; students subject to the Americans With Disabilities Act—full-time 0, part-time 0; Unknown ethnicity—full-time 0, part-time 0; International students who hold an F-1 or J-1 Visa—full-time 0, part-time 0.

Financial Information/Assistance:
Tuition for Full-Time Study: *Doctoral:* State residents: $820 per credit hour; Nonstate residents: $820 per credit hour. Tuition is subject to change. See the following Web site for updates and changes in tuition costs: http://laverne.edu/catalog/current/tuition-and-fees/.

Financial Assistance:
First-Year Students: Teaching assistantships available for first year. Average amount paid per academic year: $2,000. Average number of hours worked per week: 8. Apply by June. Research assistantships available for first year. Average amount paid per academic year: $2,000. Average number of hours worked per week: 8. Apply by June.
Advanced Students: Teaching assistantships available for advanced students. Average amount paid per academic year: $2,000. Average number of hours worked per week: 8. Apply by June. Research assistantships available for advanced students. Average amount paid per academic year: $2,000. Average number of hours worked per week: 8. Apply by June. Traineeships available for advanced students. Average amount paid per academic year: $4,000. Average number of hours worked per week: 20. Apply by March.
Additional Information: Of all students currently enrolled full time, 20% benefited from one or more of the listed financial assistance programs.

Internships/Practica: Doctoral Degree (PsyD Clinical-Community Psychology): For those doctoral students for whom a professional internship was required in this program prior to graduation, (19) students applied for an internship in 2008–2009, with (19) students obtaining an internship. Of those students who obtained an internship, (18) were paid internships. Of those students who obtained an internship, (11) students placed in APA/CPA accredited internships, (7) students placed in internships not APA/CPA accredited, but listed with the Association of Psychology Postdoctoral and Internship Programs (APPIC), (0) students placed in internships conforming to guidelines of the Council of Directors of School Psychology Programs (CDSPP), (1) students placed in internships that were not APA/CPA accredited, APPIC or CDSPP listed. The PsyD program includes required supervised practica in the second and third years of the program, with an optional fourth year practicum available. A minimum of 1500 hours of clinical-community practicum activities is required for the PsyD The culminating predoctoral internship in the fifth and final year of the program consists of an additional 1500 clinical hours, which is typically completed as a one-year full-time internship. While most students follow this track, a two-year half-time internship option is available. The PsyD program participates in a regional consortium of program and training site directors for doctoral programs, and is a doctoral program member of CAPIC and NCSPP. The Psychology department has an extensive network of practica, fieldwork, and internship sites with mental health and educational settings throughout the San Gabriel and Pomona valleys and the Inland Empire region. The on-campus Counseling Center is part of the Psychology department, is staffed by PsyD and Master's students, and is one of the largest practicum training sites.

Housing and Day Care: On-campus housing is available. No on-campus day care facilities are available.

Employment of Department Graduates:
Master's Degree Graduates: Of those who graduated in the academic year 2008–2009, the following categories and numbers represent the postgraduate activities and employment of master's degree graduates: Enrolled in a psychology doctoral program (0), enrolled in another graduate/professional program (0), enrolled in a postdoctoral residency/fellowship (n/a), employed in independent practice (n/a), employed in an academic position at a university (0), employed in an academic position at a 2-year/4-year college (0), employed in other positions at a higher education institution (0), employed in a professional position in a school system (0), employed in business or industry (0), employed in government agency (0), still seeking employment (0), not seeking employment (0), other employment position (0), do not know (0), total from the above (master's) (0).
Doctoral Degree Graduates: Of those who graduated in the academic year 2008–2009, the following categories and numbers represent the postgraduate activities and employment of doctoral degree graduates: Enrolled in a psychology doctoral program (n/a), enrolled in another graduate/professional program (0), enrolled in a postdoctoral residency/fellowship (3), employed in independent practice (0), employed in an academic position at a university (0), employed in an academic position at a 2-year/4-year college (0), employed in other positions at a higher education institution (0), employed in a professional position in a school system (0), employed in business or industry (0), employed in government agency (0), employed in a community mental health/counseling center (0), employed in a hospital/medical center (0), still seeking employment (0), not seeking employment (0), other employment position (0), do not know (1), total from the above (doctoral) (4).

Additional Information:
Orientation, Objectives, and Emphasis of Department: The clinical faculty consists of psychologists whose theoretical orientations include psychodynamic, humanist, cognitive-behavioral, family systems, and community psychology, and who are clinically active in a range of settings and populations. Faculty research interests include topics such as multi-culturalism, psychotherapy outcome research, racial identity and acculturation, professional violations of mental health professionals, child and family development, positive psychology, moral development and decision making, and violence and victimization. The curriculum of the PsyD program in Clinical-Community psychology is anchored in an ecological and multi-cultural perspective, and involves a multi-disciplinary faculty who are actively involved in clinical and research activities. The PsyD program meets all predoctoral requirements for California psychology licensure. The program received APA accreditation in 2003 and reaccreditation in 2008. Students proceed through the program in a cohort model, taking all but elective courses together with their entering group. This fosters a high level of cooperation among students. Student-faculty ratios are relatively small, resulting in multiple opportunities for mentoring by faculty, and for student-faculty collaboration.

Special Facilities or Resources: Students have access to a wide network of local and regional clinical, research and library facilities in the metropolitan Los Angeles and Southern California area. The campus University Counseling Center is directed by the Psychology department and provides counseling services to university students and staff. The Center is equipped with videotape and biofeedback equipment. ULV's Wilson Library contains 200,000 volumes and over 2,000 current journal subscriptions. Access to library resources is available through reciprocal borrowing privileges at many academic libraries in the Southern California area, as well as through online catalogs and CD-ROM databases.

Information for Students With Physical Disabilities: See the following Web site for more information: http://laverne.edu/students/students-with-disabilities.

Application Information:
Send to Graduate Admissions, 1950 Third Street, University of La Verne, La Verne, CA 91750. Students are admitted in the Fall, application deadline January 15. Students will be considered for the PsyD program after the deadline if space is available. *Fee:* $75. The application fee is waived for current ULV students.

Loma Linda University
Department of Psychology
School of Science and Technology
11130 Anderson Street, Suite 106
Loma Linda, CA 92350
Telephone: (909) 558-8577
Fax: (909) 558-0971
E-mail: *sLane@llu.edu*
Web: *http://www.llu.edu/llu/grad/psychology*

Department Information:
1994. Chairperson: Louis E Jenkins, PhD, ABPP. Number of faculty: total—full-time 10, part-time 2; women—full-time 2, part-time 1; total—minority—full-time 3.

Programs and Degrees Offered:
Listed in the following order: Program area, degree type (T if terminal Master's), number awarded 7/08–6/09. Clinical Psychology PhD (Doctor of Philosophy) 9, Clinical Psychology PsyD (Doctor of Psychology) 14.

APA Accreditation: Clinical PhD (Doctor of Philosophy). Clinical PsyD (Doctor of Psychology).

Student Applications/Admissions:

Student Applications

Clinical Psychology PhD (Doctor of Philosophy)—Applications 2009–2010, 38. Total applicants accepted 2009–2010, 10. Number full-time enrolled (new admits only) 2009–2010, 9. Number part-time enrolled (new admits only) 2009–2010, 0. The median number of years required for completion of a degree in 2008–2009 were 7. The number of students enrolled full- and part-time who were dismissed or voluntarily withdrew from this program area in 2008–2009 were 1. *Clinical Psychology PsyD (Doctor of Psychology)*—Applications 2009–2010, 21. Total applicants accepted 2009–2010, 9. Number full-time enrolled (new admits only) 2009–2010, 9. Number part-time enrolled (new admits only) 2009–2010, 0. The median number of years required for completion of a degree in 2008–2009 were 5. The number of students enrolled full- and part-time who were dismissed or voluntarily withdrew from this program area in 2008–2009 were 0.

Scores: Entries appear in this order: required test or GPA, minimum score (if required), median score of students entering in 2009–2010. *Clinical Psychology PhD (Doctor of Philosophy)*: GRE-V 500, 580, GRE-Q 580, 650, GRE-Analytical 4.0, 5.0, overall undergraduate GPA 3.0, 3.5; *Clinical Psychology PsyD (Doctor of Psychology)*: GRE-V 410, 500, GRE-Q 670, 590, GRE-Analytical 4.0, 4.8, overall undergraduate GPA 3.0, 3.50, last 2 years GPA 3.0, 3.45.

Other Criteria: (importance of criteria rated low, medium, or high): GRE scores—high, research experience—high, work experience—medium, extracurricular activity—medium, clinically related public service—high, GPA—high, letters of recommendation—high, interview—high, statement of goals and objectives—high, undergraduate major in psychology—high, specific undergraduate psychology courses taken—high, For PhD applicants, research experience is highly desirable. For PsyD applicants, clinical related experience is highly desirable.

Student Characteristics: The following represents characteristics of students in 2009–2010 in all graduate psychology programs in the department: Female—full-time 109, part-time 0; Male—full-time 36, part-time 0; African American/Black—full-time 11, part-time 0; Hispanic/Latino(a)—full-time 14, part-time 0; Asian/Pacific Islander—full-time 22, part-time 0; American Indian/Alaska Native—full-time 0, part-time 0; Caucasian/White—full-time 92, part-time 0; Multi-ethnic—full-time 6, part-time 0; students subject to the Americans With Disabilities Act—full-time 5, part-time 0; Unknown ethnicity—full-time 0, part-time 0; International students who hold an F-1 or J-1 Visa—full-time 0, part-time 0.

Financial Information/Assistance:

Tuition for Full-Time Study: Doctoral: State residents: per academic year $27,100; Nonstate residents: per academic year $27,100. Tuition is subject to change. Tuition costs vary by program.

Financial Assistance:

First-Year Students: Research assistantships available for first year. Average amount paid per academic year: $3,280. Average number of hours worked per week: 5. Fellowships and scholarships available for first year. Average amount paid per academic year: $3,000. Apply by August 15.

Advanced Students: Teaching assistantships available for advanced students. Average amount paid per academic year: $1,950. Average number of hours worked per week: 7. Research assistantships available for advanced students. Average amount paid per academic year: $6,560. Average number of hours worked per week: 10. Fellowships and scholarships available for advanced students. Average amount paid per academic year: $3,000. Apply by August 15.

Additional Information: Of all students currently enrolled full time, 40% benefited from one or more of the listed financial assistance programs.

Internships/Practica: Doctoral Degree (PhD Clinical Psychology): For those doctoral students for whom a professional internship was required in this program prior to graduation, (14) students applied for an internship in 2008–2009, with (12) students obtaining an internship. Of those students who obtained an internship, (12) were paid internships. Of those students who obtained an internship, (9) students placed in APA/CPA accredited internships, (3) students placed in internships not APA/CPA accredited, but listed with the Association of Psychology Postdoctoral and Internship Programs (APPIC), (0) students placed in internships conforming to guidelines of the Council of Directors of School Psychology Programs (CDSPP), (0) students placed in internships that were not APA/CPA accredited, APPIC or CDSPP listed. Doctoral Degree (PsyD Clinical Psychology): For those doctoral students for whom a professional internship was required in this program prior to graduation, (9) students applied for an internship in 2008–2009, with (7) students obtaining an internship. Of those students who obtained an internship, (7) were paid internships. Of those students who obtained an internship, (5) students placed in APA/CPA accredited internships, (2) students placed in internships not APA/CPA accredited, but listed with the Association of Psychology Postdoctoral and Internship Programs (APPIC), (0) students placed in internships conforming to guidelines of the Council of Directors of School Psychology Programs (CDSPP), (0) students placed in internships that were not APA/CPA accredited, APPIC or CDSPP listed. Second-year practicum experiences are obtained in the departmental clinic and in a satellite clinic which reaches a previously underserved area of the City of San Bernardino. Other department training experiences include the LLU Pediatrics Department population. Second-year practicum students may also receive some supervised clinical training in area public and private school settings. The external practicum (20 hours per week, normally in the third year of the program) is entirely off the departmental campus. Students are expected to accumulate 950 to 1000 hours of supervised experience while on external practicum, with an absolute minimum of 250 hours being spent in direct service experiences with patients. External practicum students are presently placed in six settings: 1) The Rehabilitation Unit of the Loma Linda University Medical Center; 2) the California Youth Authority; 3) The San Bernardino County Department of Mental Health; 4) the Casa Colina Hospital for Rehabilitative Medicine; 5) LLU Dept of Family Medicine-Primary Care; and 6) Local Indian Reservation. A full-year (40 hours per week) internship is required with sites available across the country. All acceptable internship sites must meet the criteria for membership in the Association of Psychology Postdoctoral and Internship Centers.

Housing and Day Care: On-campus housing is available. See the following Web site for more information: http://www.llu.edu/central/housing. On-campus day care facilities are available.

Employment of Department Graduates:

Master's Degree Graduates: Of those who graduated in the academic year 2008–2009, the following categories and numbers represent the postgraduate activities and employment of master's degree graduates: Enrolled in a postdoctoral residency/fellowship (n/a), employed in independent practice (n/a), employed in an academic position at a university (0), employed in an academic position at a 2-year/4-year college (0), employed in other positions at a higher education institution (0), employed in a professional position in a school system (0), employed in business or industry (0), employed in government agency (0), employed in a community mental health/counseling center (0), employed in a hospital/medical center (0), still seeking employment (0), other employment position (0), total from the above (master's) (0).

Doctoral Degree Graduates: Of those who graduated in the academic year 2008–2009, the following categories and numbers represent the postgraduate activities and employment of doctoral degree graduates: Enrolled in a psychology doctoral program (n/a), enrolled in a postdoctoral residency/fellowship (13), employed in independent practice (0), employed in an academic position at a university (0), employed in an academic position at a 2-year/4-year college (0), employed in other positions at a higher education institution (0), employed in a professional position in a school system (0), employed in business or industry (0), employed in government agency (0), employed in a community mental health/counseling center (13), employed in a hospital/medical center (6), still seeking employment (0), other employment position (2), total from the above (doctoral) (34).

Additional Information:

Orientation, Objectives, and Emphasis of Department: Doctoral training at Loma Linda University takes place within the context of a holistic approach to human health and welfare. The university motto to make man whole takes in every aspect of being human—the physical, psychological, spiritual, and social. Building on a university tradition of health sciences research, training, and service, the doctoral programs in the department offer a combination of traditional and innovative training opportunities. The PhD in clinical psychology follows the traditional scientist–practitioner model and emphasizes research and clinical training. The PsyD is oriented toward clinical practice with emphasis on the understanding and application of the principles and research of psychological science. The PsyD/DrPH dual degree program offers an innovative combination of education in psychology and the health sciences to train practitioners who are highly qualified in the application of psychology to health promotion, preventive medicine, and health care as well as clinical practice and research.

Special Facilities or Resources: As a health sciences university, Loma Linda provides an ideal environment with resources for research and clinical training in such areas as health psychology/behavioral medicine and the delivery of health services. LLU Medical Center has nearly 900 beds, is staffed by more than 5000 people, and is the "flagship" of a system including hundreds of health care institutions around the world. In addition, a number of institutions in the area, such as the LLU Behavioral Medicine Center, Jerry L. Pettis VA Hospital, Patton State Hospital, and the San Bernardino County Mental Health Department represent numerous opportunities for research and clinical training in psychology. In the area of teaching and research the department has an arrangement with the department of psychology at California State University, San Bernardino. By this agreement, students at a post-master's level have TA opportunities to get experience teaching undergraduate courses. At the same time, a select group of graduate faculty members at CSUSB have appointments at LLU, significantly enhancing advanced seminar offerings and opportunities for research training in a number of areas, and strengthening and complementing those available at LLU.

Application Information:
Send to Loma Linda University, School of Science and Technology, Office of Admissions, 11065 Campus Street, Suite 103 (Griggs Hall), Loma Linda, CA 92350. Application available online. URL of online application: http://www.llu.edu/apply. Students are admitted in the Fall, application deadline December 31. Applicants to our dual-degree program, PsyD/DrPH must apply to our School of Public Health concurrently with their application to our PsyD program in the Department of Psychology. *Fee:* $60.

Pacific Graduate School of Psychology & Stanford University School of Medicine, Department of Psychiatry and Behavioral Sciences
PGSP - STANFORD PsyD CONSORTIUM
1791 Arastradero Road
Palo Alto, CA 94304
Telephone: (650) 433-3836
Fax: (650) 433-3890
E-mail: *acastrillo@paloaltou.edu*
Web: *http://www.pgsp.edu/program_stanford_psyd_home.php*

Department Information:
2002. Directors of Clinical Training: James N. Breckenridge, PhD & Bruce Arnow, PhD. Number of faculty: total—full-time 8, part-time 27; women—full-time 5, part-time 13; minority—part-time 4; women minority—part-time 3.

Programs and Degrees Offered:
Listed in the following order: Program area, degree type (T if terminal Master's), number awarded 7/08–6/09. Clinical Psychology PsyD (Doctor of Psychology) 19.

APA Accreditation: Clinical PsyD (Doctor of Psychology).

Student Applications/Admissions:

Student Applications

Clinical Psychology PsyD (Doctor of Psychology)—Applications 2009–2010, 205. Total applicants accepted 2009–2010, 38. Number full-time enrolled (new admits only) 2009–2010, 30. Number part-time enrolled (new admits only) 2009–2010, 0. Openings 2010–2011, 30. The median number of years required for completion of a degree in 2008–2009 were 5. The number of students enrolled full- and part-time who were dismissed or voluntarily withdrew from this program area in 2008–2009 were 4.

Other Criteria: (importance of criteria rated low, medium, or high): GRE scores—medium, research experience—low, work experience—high, extracurricular activity—medium, clinically related public service—high, GPA—high, letters of recommendation—high, interview—high, statement of goals and objectives—high, undergraduate major in psychology—medium, specific undergraduate psychology courses taken—medium. For additional information on admission requirements, go to http://www.pgsp.edu/program_stanford_psyd_home.php.

Student Characteristics: The following represents characteristics of students in 2009–2010 in all graduate psychology programs in the department: Female—full-time 114, part-time 0; Male—full-time 25, part-time 0; African American/Black—full-time 1, part-time 0; Hispanic/Latino(a)—full-time 8, part-time 0; Asian/Pacific Islander—full-time 23, part-time 0; American Indian/Alaska Native—full-time 1, part-time 0; Caucasian/White—full-time 80, part-time 0; Multi-ethnic—full-time 0, part-time 0; students subject to the Americans With Disabilities Act—full-time 6, part-time 0; Unknown ethnicity—full-time 26, part-time 0; International students who hold an F-1 or J-1 Visa—full-time 6, part-time 0.

Financial Information/Assistance:
Tuition for Full-Time Study: *Doctoral:* State residents: per academic year $39,048; Nonstate residents: per academic year $39,048. Tuition is subject to change. See the following Web site for updates and changes in tuition costs: http://www.pgsp.edu/program_stanford_psyd_home.php.

Financial Assistance:
First-Year Students: Research assistantships available for first year. Average amount paid per academic year: $1,000. Average number of hours worked per week: 5. Fellowships and scholarships available for first year. Average amount paid per academic year: $3,000. Average number of hours worked per week: 8. Apply by April 1.

Advanced Students: Teaching assistantships available for advanced students. Average amount paid per academic year: $750. Average number of hours worked per week: 6. Research assistantships available for advanced students. Average amount paid per academic year: $1,000. Average number of hours worked per week: 5. Fellowships and scholarships available for advanced students. Average amount paid per academic year: $3,000. Average number of hours worked per week: 8. Apply by March 31.

Additional Information: Of all students currently enrolled full time, 77% benefited from one or more of the listed financial assistance programs.

Internships/Practica: Doctoral Degree (PsyD Clinical Psychology): For those doctoral students for whom a professional internship was required in this program prior to graduation, (22) students applied for an internship in 2008–2009, with (20) students obtaining an internship. Of those students who obtained an internship, (18) were paid internships. Of those students who obtained an internship, (15) students placed in APA/CPA accredited internships, (3) students placed in internships not APA/CPA accredited, but listed with the Association of Psychology Postdoctoral and Internship Programs (APPIC), (0) students placed in internships conforming to guidelines of the Council of Directors of School Psychology Programs (CDSPP), (2) students placed in internships that were not APA/CPA accredited, APPIC or CDSPP listed. The PGSP-Stanford Consortium training program provides students with experiences that are sequenced with increasing amounts of time spent in clinical work during each year of graduate training, with a total of approximately 2,000 clinical hours obtained prior to internship. Graduate students begin working in clinical settings as a volunteer during their first year; during their second and third years, students enroll in field practica that may take place in a variety of settings, such as Stanford and UCSF medical school hospitals and programs, community mental health centers, the Palo Alto V.A. Health Care System medical centers, county mental health systems, AIDS prevention project, and child/family psychiatric clinics. In the fourth year students will work on a clinical dissertation, and a fourth year practicum is optional but highly recommended. In the fifth year, following advancement to the candidacy for the Doctor of Psychology (PsyD) degree, the student is required to complete a 2,000-hour external predoctoral internship that provides high quality professional supervision and experience.

Housing and Day Care: No on-campus housing is available. No on-campus day care facilities are available.

Employment of Department Graduates:
Master's Degree Graduates: Of those who graduated in the academic year 2008–2009, the following categories and numbers represent the postgraduate activities and employment of master's degree graduates: Enrolled in a postdoctoral residency/fellowship (n/a), employed in independent practice (n/a), total from the above (master's) (0).

Doctoral Degree Graduates: Of those who graduated in the academic year 2008–2009, the following categories and numbers represent the postgraduate activities and employment of doctoral degree graduates: Enrolled in a psychology doctoral program (n/a), total from the above (doctoral) (0).

Additional Information:
Orientation, Objectives, and Emphasis of Department: This training program emphasizes a biopsychosocial understanding of psychological disorders (i.e., a model that conceptualizes psychological disorders and problems as having biological, psychological and social components). In addition, the program provides "cutting edge" training for student psychologist-practitioners in the use of empirically supported treatments for a wide variety of psychiatric illnesses and behavioral disorders. There are four primary training goals for the PGSP - Stanford Consortium: 1. To develop psychologists who can effectively evaluate sophisticated social research and apply empirically supported psychological intervention in their practice of psychology. 2. To educate highly trained psychologists who can contribute to the advancement of clinical psychology. 3. To produce clinical psychologists who are competent in psychological assessment, consultation, and supervision. 4. To provide theory, skills, and supervision necessary to enable students to confidentially and effectively engage in treatment interventions in response to societal needs.

Special Facilities or Resources: The PGSP-Stanford Doctor of Psychology program draws upon nationally renowned faculty and resources from the Pacific Graduate School and the Stanford University School of Medicine's Department of Psychiatry and Behavioral Sciences. The five-year Doctor of Psychology degree program consists of three years of graduate coursework, a year spent working on a clinical dissertation, followed by a year-long internship in clinical psychology. As a practitioner-oriented graduate program, the focus is on intensive clinical training and will utilize the rich resources of the San Francisco Bay area mental health community for pre-internship basic and advanced supervised clinical experiences. The program strives for the earliest possible full recognition of the first year class (entering in 2002-2003) for licensure in all 50 states, as well as interstate mobility through the "Certificate of Professional Qualification in Psychology" from the Association of State and Provincial Psychology Boards.

Application Information:
Send to PGSP-Stanford PsyD Consortium, Palo Alto University, Admissions Office, 1791 Arastradero Road, Palo Alto, CA 94304. Application available online. Students are admitted in the Fall, application deadline January 2. *Fee:* $50.

Pacific, University of the
Department of Psychology
3601 Pacific Avenue
Stockton, CA 95211
Telephone: (209) 946-2133
Fax: (209) 946-2454
E-mail: *mnormand@pacific.edu*
Web: *http://www.pacific.edu/x13811.xml*

Department Information:
1960. Chairperson: Carolynn Kohn, PhD. Number of faculty: total—full-time 6, part-time 1; women—full-time 3, part-time 1; minority—part-time 1; women minority—part-time 1.

Programs and Degrees Offered:
Listed in the following order: Program area, degree type (T if terminal Master's), number awarded 7/08–6/09. Doctoral Preparation MA/MS (Master of Arts/Science) (T) 0, Applied Behavior Analysis MA/MS (Master of Arts/Science) (T) 3.

Student Applications/Admissions:
Student Applications
Doctoral Preparation MA/MS (Master of Arts/Science)—Applications 2009–2010, 5. Total applicants accepted 2009–2010, 2. Number full-time enrolled (new admits only) 2009–2010, 2. Number part-time enrolled (new admits only) 2009–2010, 0. Openings 2010–2011, 5. The median number of years required for completion of a degree in 2008–2009 were 2. The number of students enrolled full- and part-time who were dismissed or voluntarily withdrew from this program area in 2008–2009 were 0. *Applied Behavior Analysis MA/MS (Master of Arts/Science)*—Applications 2009–2010, 15. Total applicants accepted 2009–2010, 5. Number full-time enrolled (new admits only) 2009–2010, 3. Number part-time enrolled (new admits only) 2009–2010, 0. Openings 2010–2011, 4. The median number of years required for completion of a degree in 2008–2009 were 3. The number of students enrolled full- and part-time who were dismissed or voluntarily withdrew from this program area in 2008–2009 were 0.
Scores: Entries appear in this order: required test or GPA, minimum score (if required), median score of students entering in 2009–2010. *Doctoral Preparation MA/MS (Master of Arts/Science):* GRE-V 450, GRE-Q 450, GRE-Analytical 3.5, overall undergraduate GPA 3.0, last 2 years GPA 3.0, psychology GPA 3.0; *Applied Behavior Analysis MA/MS (Master of Arts/Science):* GRE-V 450, GRE-Q 450, GRE-Analytical 3.5, overall undergraduate GPA 3.0, last 2 years GPA 3.0, psychology GPA 3,0.

Other Criteria: (importance of criteria rated low, medium, or high): GRE scores—medium, research experience—high, work experience—low, clinically related public service—low, GPA—high, letters of recommendation—high, statement of goals and objectives—high, Applied experience—medium, undergraduate major in psychology—medium, specific undergraduate psychology courses taken—medium. Those applying to the Behavior Analysis track should have some relevant course work and research in behavior analysis. For additional information on admission requirements, go to http://web.pacific.edu/x17688.xml.

Student Characteristics: The following represents characteristics of students in 2009–2010 in all graduate psychology programs in the department: Female—full-time 9, part-time 0; Male—full-time 6, part-time 0; African American/Black—full-time 0, part-time 0; Hispanic/Latino(a)—full-time 3, part-time 0; Asian/Pacific Islander—full-time 3, part-time 0; American Indian/Alaska Native—full-time 0, part-time 0; Caucasian/White—full-time 9, part-time 0; Multi-ethnic—full-time 0, part-time 0; students subject to the Americans With Disabilities Act—full-time 0, part-time 0; Unknown ethnicity—full-time 0, part-time 0; International students who hold an F-1 or J-1 Visa—full-time 1, part-time 0.

Financial Information/Assistance:
Tuition for Full-Time Study: *Master's:* State residents: per academic year $15,872, $992 per credit hour; Nonstate residents: per academic year $15,872, $992 per credit hour. See the following Web site for updates and changes in tuition costs: http://www.pacific.edu/x8056.xml.

Financial Assistance:
First-Year Students: Teaching assistantships available for first year. Average amount paid per academic year: $9,802. Average number of hours worked per week: 20. Apply by February 15. Traineeships available for first year. Average amount paid per academic year: $12,400. Average number of hours worked per week: 20. Apply by February 15.
Advanced Students: Teaching assistantships available for advanced students. Average amount paid per academic year: $9,802. Average number of hours worked per week: 20. Apply by February 15. Traineeships available for advanced students. Average amount paid per academic year: $12,400. Average number of hours worked per week: 20. Apply by February 15.
Additional Information: Of all students currently enrolled full time, 100% benefited from one or more of the listed financial assistance programs. Application and information available online at: http://web.pacific.edu/x17681.xml.

Internships/Practica: Master's Degree (MA/MS Doctoral Preparation): An internship experience, such as a final research project or "capstone" experience is required of graduates. Master's Degree (MA/MS Applied Behavior Analysis): An internship experience, such as a final research project or "capstone" experience is required of graduates. The department directs the Community Re-entry Program (contracted directly with the local county), which provides a wide range of behaviorally-based programs to assist the mentally disabled/ill in becoming independent. This program provides half-time employment for eight graduate students per year. Students interested in developmental disabilities can work with the Behavioral Instructional Service (in cooperation with Valley

Mountain Regional Center, which serves these clients), and part-time employment is available with this program. We also have contracts with several outside agencies at which students can obtain practicum experience, including the Stockton Unified School District (ABA assessment and interventions for school problem behaviors) and BEST (early ABA interventions with children diagnosed with autism).

Housing and Day Care: On-campus housing is available. See the following Web site for more information: http://web.pacific.edu/x19961.xml. No on-campus day care facilities are available.

Employment of Department Graduates:
Master's Degree Graduates: Of those who graduated in the academic year 2008–2009, the following categories and numbers represent the postgraduate activities and employment of master's degree graduates: Enrolled in a psychology doctoral program (2), enrolled in a postdoctoral residency/fellowship (n/a), employed in independent practice (n/a), employed in a professional position in a school system (1), employed in business or industry (0), employed in a community mental health/counseling center (1), other employment position (1), total from the above (master's) (5).
Doctoral Degree Graduates: Of those who graduated in the academic year 2008–2009, the following categories and numbers represent the postgraduate activities and employment of doctoral degree graduates: Enrolled in a psychology doctoral program (n/a), total from the above (doctoral) (0).

Additional Information:
Orientation, Objectives, and Emphasis of Department: The Psychology Department offers a program of graduate study leading to the MA degree in Psychology. We offer two tracks: (1) Behavior Analysis track (MA or doctoral preparation); and (2) Doctoral Preparation track (Clinical/Counseling, Behavioral, Developmental, Biological, Social, and Cognitive, and School psychology). Students wishing to pursue a doctorate in applied behavior analysis should apply under the applied behavior analysis track, but indicate in a cover letter that they ultimately wish to apply to a doctoral program in ABA. We do not offer an MFT or a Counseling MA. The overall program focus for both tracks includes: a wide variety of applied experience in a number of different settings; intensive involvement in designing, conducting, and evaluating research; coursework in theoretical and research foundations of applied behavior analysis and cognitive behavior theory; and commitment to the development of student potential by active, supportive, involved faculty. As a potential applicant to a private university, you may be concerned about high tuition rates and decide that it is too expensive for you. This note is written to reassure you that it is not. First, and most important, in a typical year almost all graduate students in Psychology receive a substantial amount of financial aid, which includes the remission of a substantial portion of your tuition costs plus a stipend for performing a job (e.g., teaching assistant, traineeship in departmental treatment programs for the mentally disabled or the developmentally disabled). In the 2008-09 academic year, 100% of students (both first and second year) are receiving substantial amounts of tuition remission (covering approximately 80-90% of their total tuition costs) and 100% of our students received stipends. Therefore, if you feel the nature of the program meets your needs and goals, we encourage you to apply. Second, you may be assuming that graduate students take 15–16 units a semester, as undergraduates do. However, graduate students in Psychology take only 8-10 units a semester during their first year of study. Thus, for the 2008-09 academic year, the total tuition cost for first year students taking 16 units ($992/unit), with tuition remission covering approximately 85% of the tuition costs. During the second year of study, graduate students take fewer units, typically 6 units in the Fall and 8 units in the Spring. Tuition remission will reduce these costs by 75% or more for most students.

Special Facilities or Resources: The department provides office space for faculty and graduate students, computing equipment, and video equipment for research projects. Applied research projects are also conducted in community settings (e.g. schools, medical settings). The Community Re-entry Program and Valley Mountain Regional Center (described above) also provide rich opportunities for research in community settings.

Information for Students With Physical Disabilities: See the following Web site for more information: http://web.pacific.edu/x10591.xml.

Application Information:
Send to Dean of the Graduate School, University of the Pacific, 3601 Pacific Avenue, Stockton, CA 95211. Application available online. URL of online application: https://www.applyweb.com/apply/uopg/menu.html. Students are admitted in the Fall, application deadline February 15. Although the deadline for applications is February 15, on occasion we accept late applications. However, applying after the deadline decreases an applicant's chances to receive funding. *Fee:* $75.

Pacifica Graduate Institute
PhD in Clinical Psychology with emphasis in Depth Psychology
Department of Psychology
249 Lambert Road
Carpinteria, CA 93013
Telephone: (805) 969-3626 ext. 305
Fax: (805) 879-7391
E-mail: *admissions@pacifica.edu*
Web: *http://www.pacifica.edu/*

Department Information:
1989. Chairperson: James L. Broderick, PhD. Number of faculty: total—full-time 12, part-time 37; women—full-time 2, part-time 21; total—minority—full-time 1, part-time 3; women minority—part-time 2.

Programs and Degrees Offered:
Listed in the following order: Program area, degree type (T if terminal Master's), number awarded 7/08–6/09. Clinical Psychology PhD (Doctor of Philosophy).

Student Applications/Admissions:
Student Applications
Clinical Psychology PhD (Doctor of Philosophy)
Other Criteria: (importance of criteria rated low, medium, or high): research experience—medium, work experience—medium, extracurricular activity—medium, clinically related

public service—medium, GPA—high, letters of recommendation—high, interview—high, statement of goals and objectives—high, Writing ability—high, undergraduate major in psychology—high, specific undergraduate psychology courses taken—high. For additional information on admission requirements, go to http://www.pacifica.edu/admissions.aspx.

Student Characteristics: The following represents characteristics of students in 2009–2010 in all graduate psychology programs in the department: Female—full-time 0, part-time 0; Male—full-time 0, part-time 0; African American/Black—full-time 0, part-time 0; Hispanic/Latino(a)—full-time 0, part-time 0; Asian/Pacific Islander—full-time 0, part-time 0; American Indian/Alaska Native—full-time 0, part-time 0; Caucasian/White—full-time 0, part-time 0; Multi-ethnic—full-time 0, part-time 0; students subject to the Americans With Disabilities Act—full-time 0, part-time 0; Unknown ethnicity—full-time 0, part-time 0; International students who hold an F-1 or J-1 Visa—full-time 0, part-time 0.

Financial Information/Assistance:
Tuition for Full-Time Study: Doctoral: State residents: per academic year $24,100. Tuition is subject to change. Additional fees are assessed to students beyond the costs of tuition for the following: residential fees for on-site meals and accommodations. Tuition costs vary by program. See the following Web site for updates and changes in tuition costs: http://www.pacifica.edu/fee.aspx.

Financial Assistance:
First-Year Students: No information provided.
Advanced Students: No information provided.
Additional Information: Application and information available online at: http://www.pacifica.edu/financial_aid.aspx.

Internships/Practica: The practicum sites are to serve as laboratory settings that allow students the opportunity for mastering the fundamental skills and knowledge being taught in the introductory courses in psychopathology, assessment, and intervention. The internship experience follows from both this practicum experience and the successful completion of three core practicum courses. Internship training requires more responsibility on the part of the students, with interns viewed as junior colleagues who perform, under supervision, all the duties of staff psychologists. The internship years are designed to prepare the students for the assumption of an autonomous professional role by allowing for the participation in the full repertoire of activities in which psychologists engage. Interns are expected to refine and to coordinate the skills acquired in the first three years of practica, as well as to acquire new skills that are specifically related to supervision, care management, decision making, and treatment team leadership.

Housing and Day Care: On-campus housing is available. No on-campus day care facilities are available.

Employment of Department Graduates:
Master's Degree Graduates: Of those who graduated in the academic year 2008–2009, the following categories and numbers represent the postgraduate activities and employment of master's degree graduates: Enrolled in a postdoctoral residency/fellowship (n/a), employed in independent practice (n/a), total from the above (master's) (0).

Doctoral Degree Graduates: Of those who graduated in the academic year 2008–2009, the following categories and numbers represent the postgraduate activities and employment of doctoral degree graduates: Enrolled in a psychology doctoral program (n/a), total from the above (doctoral) (0).

Additional Information:
Orientation, Objectives, and Emphasis of Department: Pacifica Graduate Institute's doctoral program in Clinical Psychology offers a course of study situated within the depth psychological traditions.

Application Information:
Send to Department of Admissions. Application available online. URL of online application: http://www.pacifica.edu/innercontent-m.aspx?id=3834. Students are admitted in the Fall, application deadline Rolling. *Fee:* $60.

Palo Alto University
Clinical Psychology Program
1791 Arastradero Road
Palo Alto, CA 94304
Telephone: (800) 818-6136
Fax: (650) 433-3888
E-mail: *dsims@paloaltou.edu*
Web: *http://www.paloaltou.edu*

Department Information:
1975. Director of Admissions: Dacien Sims. Number of faculty: total—full-time 22, part-time 25; women—full-time 10, part-time 15; total—minority—full-time 6, part-time 3; women minority—full-time 5, part-time 1.

Programs and Degrees Offered:
Listed in the following order: Program area, degree type (T if terminal Master's), number awarded 7/08–6/09. MBA/PhD Other 2, Clinical Psychology PhD (Doctor of Philosophy) 28, Psychology and Law Other 2, Psychology MA/MS (Master of Arts/Science) (T) 14.

APA Accreditation: Clinical PhD (Doctor of Philosophy). Student Outcome Data Website: http://www.paloaltou.edu/content/clone-full-disclosure-information.

Student Applications/Admissions:
Student Applications
MBA/PhD Other—Applications 2009–2010, 0. Total applicants accepted 2009–2010, 0. Number full-time enrolled (new admits only) 2009–2010, 0. Number part-time enrolled (new admits only) 2009–2010, 0. Openings 2010–2011, 5. The median number of years required for completion of a degree in 2008–2009 were 5. The number of students enrolled full- and part-time who were dismissed or voluntarily withdrew from this program area in 2008–2009 were 0. *Clinical Psychology PhD (Doctor of Philosophy)*—Applications 2009–2010, 227. Total applicants accepted 2009–2010, 209. Number full-time enrolled (new admits only) 2009–2010, 82. Number part-time enrolled (new admits only) 2009–2010, 0. Openings 2010–

2011, 90. The median number of years required for completion of a degree in 2008–2009 were 6. The number of students enrolled full- and part-time who were dismissed or voluntarily withdrew from this program area in 2008–2009 were 11. *Psychology and Law Other*—Applications 2009–2010, 0. Total applicants accepted 2009–2010, 0. Number full-time enrolled (new admits only) 2009–2010, 1. Number part-time enrolled (new admits only) 2009–2010, 0. Openings 2010–2011, 4. The median number of years required for completion of a degree in 2008–2009 were 6. The number of students enrolled full- and part-time who were dismissed or voluntarily withdrew from this program area in 2008–2009 were 0. *Psychology MA/MS (Master of Arts/Science)*—Applications 2009–2010, 18. Total applicants accepted 2009–2010, 18. Number full-time enrolled (new admits only) 2009–2010, 0. Number part-time enrolled (new admits only) 2009–2010, 17. Openings 2010–2011, 30. The median number of years required for completion of a degree in 2008–2009 were 2. The number of students enrolled full- and part-time who were dismissed or voluntarily withdrew from this program area in 2008–2009 were 4.

Scores: Entries appear in this order: required test or GPA, minimum score (if required), median score of students entering in 2009–2010. MBA/PhD Other: GRE-V no minimum stated, GRE-Q no minimum stated, GRE-Analytical no minimum stated, overall undergraduate GPA no minimum stated, last 2 years GPA no minimum stated, psychology GPA no minimum stated; *Clinical Psychology PhD (Doctor of Philosophy)*: GRE-V no minimum stated, 535, GRE-Q no minimum stated, 580, GRE-Analytical no minimum stated, overall undergraduate GPA no minimum stated, last 2 years GPA no minimum stated, psychology GPA no minimum stated, Masters GPA no minimum stated; *Psychology and Law Other*: GRE-V no minimum stated, GRE-Q no minimum stated, GRE-Analytical no minimum stated, overall undergraduate GPA no minimum stated, last 2 years GPA no minimum stated, psychology GPA no minimum stated; *Psychology MA/MS (Master of Arts/Science)*: GRE-V no minimum stated, GRE-Q no minimum stated, GRE-Analytical no minimum stated, overall undergraduate GPA no minimum stated, last 2 years GPA no minimum stated, psychology GPA no minimum stated.

Other Criteria: (importance of criteria rated low, medium, or high): GRE scores—high, research experience—medium, work experience—medium, extracurricular activity—medium, clinically related public service—medium, GPA—high, letters of recommendation—high, interview—medium, statement of goals and objectives—medium. Interview required for the following programs: PhD Program, PGSP - STANFORD PsyD CONSORTIUM, JD/PhD Program, and MBA/PhD Programs. For additional information on admission requirements, go to http://www.paloaltou.edu.

Student Characteristics: The following represents characteristics of students in 2009–2010 in all graduate psychology programs in the department: Female—full-time 418, part-time 23; Male—full-time 105, part-time 4; African American/Black—full-time 16, part-time 1; Hispanic/Latino(a)—full-time 34, part-time 3; Asian/Pacific Islander—full-time 91, part-time 3; American Indian/Alaska Native—full-time 3, part-time 0; Caucasian/White—full-time 293, part-time 13; Multi-ethnic—full-time 0, part-time 0; students subject to the Americans With Disabilities Act—full-time 0, part-time 0; Unknown ethnicity—full-time 86, part-time 7; International students who hold an F-1 or J-1 Visa—full-time 26, part-time 0.

Financial Information/Assistance:
Tuition for Full-Time Study: *Master's:* State residents: per academic year $17,844; Nonstate residents: per academic year $17,844. *Doctoral:* State residents: per academic year $38,391; Nonstate residents: per academic year $38,391. Tuition is subject to change. Additional fees are assessed to students beyond the costs of tuition for the following: medical insurance - unless opt out. Tuition costs vary by program. See the following Web site for updates and changes in tuition costs: http://www.paloaltou.edu. Higher tuition cost for this program: PGSP-Stanford PsyD Consortium.

Financial Assistance:
 First-Year Students: Fellowships and scholarships available for first year. Average amount paid per academic year: $5,000. Average number of hours worked per week: 0. Apply by January 15.

 Advanced Students: Teaching assistantships available for advanced students. Average amount paid per academic year: $3,000. Average number of hours worked per week: 25. Research assistantships available for advanced students. Average amount paid per academic year: $4,000. Average number of hours worked per week: 30.

 Additional Information: Of all students currently enrolled full time, 25% benefited from one or more of the listed financial assistance programs. Application and information available online at: http://www.paloaltou.edu.

Internships/Practica: Doctoral Degree (PhD Clinical Psychology): For those doctoral students for whom a professional internship was required in this program prior to graduation, (36) students applied for an internship in 2008–2009, with (25) students obtaining an internship. Of those students who obtained an internship, (25) were paid internships. Of those students who obtained an internship, (17) students placed in APA/CPA accredited internships, (5) students placed in internships not APA/CPA accredited, but listed with the Association of Psychology Postdoctoral and Internship Programs (APPIC), (0) students placed in internships conforming to guidelines of the Council of Directors of School Psychology Programs (CDSPP), (3) students placed in internships that were not APA/CPA accredited, APPIC or CDSPP listed. All students take their second year of practicum in our Kurt and Barbara Gronowski Clinic and the third and fourth years in local agencies. All students are expected to complete an APA-accredited, APPIC or CAPIC-approved internship.

Housing and Day Care: No on-campus housing is available. No on-campus day care facilities are available.

Employment of Department Graduates:
 Master's Degree Graduates: Of those who graduated in the academic year 2008–2009, the following categories and numbers represent the postgraduate activities and employment of master's degree graduates: Enrolled in a postdoctoral residency/fellowship (n/a), employed in independent practice (n/a), total from the above (master's) (0).

 Doctoral Degree Graduates: Of those who graduated in the academic year 2008–2009, the following categories and numbers represent the postgraduate activities and employment of doctoral

degree graduates: Enrolled in a psychology doctoral program (n/a), enrolled in a postdoctoral residency/fellowship (47), employed in a community mental health/counseling center (0), employed in a hospital/medical center (0), other employment position (0), do not know (0), total from the above (doctoral) (47).

Additional Information:
Orientation, Objectives, and Emphasis of Department: Palo Alto University, formerly Pacific Graduate School of Psychology, is a university offering doctoral degrees in clinical psychology to students from diverse backgrounds. The program is designed to integrate academic work, research, and clinical experiences at every level of the student's training. All students must develop a thorough understanding of a systematic body of knowledge that comprises the current field of psychology. They are expected to carry out an independent investigation that makes an original contribution to scientific knowledge in psychology and to demonstrate excellence in the application of specific clinical skills. PAU considers this integration of scholarship, research, and practical experience the best training model for preparing psychologists to meet the highest standards of scholarly research and community service. Graduates are expected to enter the community at large prepared to do research, practice, and teach in culturally and professionally diverse settings.

Special Facilities or Resources: PAU's setting as a free-standing graduate school of psychology is much enhanced by our San Francisco Bay Area location. We provide students with access to local university libraries (e.g., Stanford, UC Berkeley). The range of clinical experience available to students is inexhaustible. All faculty have active research programs in which students participate. Furthermore, PAU has a close relationship with local VA hospitals.

Application Information:
Send to Office of Admissions, Pacific Graduate School of Psychology, 405 Broadway Street, Redwood City, CA. 94063. Application available online. Programs have rolling admissions, however application is due January 15 for those who want to be considered for a PGSP fellowship. *Fee:* $50.

Phillips Graduate Institute
Clinical Psychology Doctoral Program
5445 Balboa Boulevard
Encino, CA 91316
Telephone: (818) 386-5600
Fax: (818) 386-5699
E-mail: *albustamante@pgi.edu*
Web: *http://www.pgi.edu*

Department Information:
2001. Chairperson: Ana Luisa Bustamante, PhD. Number of faculty: total—full-time 6, part-time 15; women—full-time 5, part-time 8; total—minority—full-time 2, part-time 1; women minority—full-time 1; faculty subject to the Americans With Disabilities Act 3.

Programs and Degrees Offered:
Listed in the following order: Program area, degree type (T if terminal Master's), number awarded 7/08–6/09. Clinical Psychology PsyD (Doctor of Psychology) 13.

Student Applications/Admissions:
Student Applications
Clinical Psychology PsyD (Doctor of Psychology)—Applications 2009–2010, 61. Total applicants accepted 2009–2010, 46. Number full-time enrolled (new admits only) 2009–2010, 23. Number part-time enrolled (new admits only) 2009–2010, 0. Total enrolled 2009–2010 full-time, 71, part-time, 19. Openings 2010–2011, 20. The median number of years required for completion of a degree in 2008–2009 were 5. The number of students enrolled full- and part-time who were dismissed or voluntarily withdrew from this program area in 2008–2009 were 6.

Other Criteria: (importance of criteria rated low, medium, or high): research experience—low, work experience—medium, extracurricular activity—medium, clinically related public service—high, GPA—high, letters of recommendation—high, interview—high, statement of goals and objectives—high, undergraduate major in psychology—medium, specific undergraduate psychology courses taken—low.

Student Characteristics: The following represents characteristics of students in 2009–2010 in all graduate psychology programs in the department: Female—full-time 33, part-time 22; Male—full-time 7, part-time 8; African American/Black—full-time 2, part-time 2; Hispanic/Latino(a)—full-time 6, part-time 6; Asian/Pacific Islander—full-time 1, part-time 1; American Indian/Alaska Native—full-time 1, part-time 0; Caucasian/White—full-time 29, part-time 21; Multi-ethnic—full-time 0, part-time 0; students subject to the Americans With Disabilities Act—full-time 0, part-time 0; Unknown ethnicity—full-time 0, part-time 0; International students who hold an F-1 or J-1 Visa—full-time 0, part-time 0.

Financial Information/Assistance:
Tuition for Full-Time Study: Doctoral: State residents: per academic year $20,592, $858 per credit hour; Nonstate residents: per academic year $20,592, $858 per credit hour. Tuition is subject to change. Additional fees are assessed to students beyond the costs of tuition for the following: administrative fee: $300 per semester.

Financial Assistance:
First-Year Students: No information provided.
Advanced Students: Teaching assistantships available for advanced students. Average amount paid per academic year: $5,000. Average number of hours worked per week: 10. Apply by May 30.
Additional Information: Of all students currently enrolled full time, 5% benefited from one or more of the listed financial assistance programs.

Internships/Practica: Doctoral Degree (PsyD Clinical Psychology): For those doctoral students for whom a professional internship was required in this program prior to graduation, (22) students applied for an internship in 2008–2009, with (22) students obtaining an internship. Of those students who obtained an internship, (16) were paid internships. Of those students who obtained an internship, (3) students placed in APA/CPA accredited internships, (4) students placed in internships not APA/CPA accredited, but listed with the Association of Psychology Postdoctoral and Internship Programs (APPIC), (0) students placed in internships conforming to guidelines of the Council of Directors of School Psychology Programs (CDSPP), (15) students placed in internships that were not APA/CPA accredited, APPIC or CDSPP listed. The Clinical Placement Office provides students information and guidance in the choice of practicum and internship experiences.

Housing and Day Care: No on-campus housing is available. No on-campus day care facilities are available.

Employment of Department Graduates:
Master's Degree Graduates: Of those who graduated in the academic year 2008–2009, the following categories and numbers represent the postgraduate activities and employment of master's degree graduates: Enrolled in a postdoctoral residency/fellowship (n/a), employed in independent practice (n/a), total from the above (master's) (0).
Doctoral Degree Graduates: Of those who graduated in the academic year 2008–2009, the following categories and numbers represent the postgraduate activities and employment of doctoral degree graduates: Enrolled in a psychology doctoral program (n/a), enrolled in a postdoctoral residency/fellowship (5), employed in an academic position at a university (1), employed in a community mental health/counseling center (5), still seeking employment (3), not seeking employment (1), other employment position (2), total from the above (doctoral) (17).

Additional Information:
Orientation, Objectives, and Emphasis of Department: The Doctor of Psychology in Clinical Psychology provides the education and training to be eligible to apply for licensure in the state of California. The program integrates ecosystemic and family systems theory throughout the curriculum. In addition, students select advanced coursework in either diversity or forensic psychology to fulfill concentration area requirements.

Application Information:
Send to Phillips Graduate Institute, Office of Admissions, 5445 Balboa Blvd., Encino, CA 91316. Students are admitted in the Fall, application deadline January 31; *Fee:* $75.

San Diego State University (2009 data)
Department of Psychology
College of Sciences
5500 Campanile Drive
San Diego, CA 92182-4611
Telephone: (619) 594-5359
Fax: (619) 594-1332
E-mail: *mcrawfor@sciences.sdsu.edu*
Web: *http://www.psychology.sdsu.edu/new-web/gradprograms.htm*

Department Information:
1947. Chair: Georg Matt. Number of faculty: total—full-time 42, part-time 18; women—full-time 23, part-time 10; total—minority—full-time 5, part-time 2; women minority—full-time 3, part-time 2.

Programs and Degrees Offered:
Listed in the following order: Program area, degree type (T if terminal Master's), number awarded 7/08–6/09. Psychology MA/MS (Master of Arts/Science) 29, Applied Psychology MA/MS (Master of Arts/Science) (T) 9.

Student Applications/Admissions:
Student Applications
Psychology MA/MS (*Master of Arts/Science*)—Applications 2009–2010, 105. Total applicants accepted 2009–2010, 54. Number full-time enrolled (new admits only) 2009–2010, 33. Number part-time enrolled (new admits only) 2009–2010, 0. Openings 2010–2011, 28. The median number of years required for completion of a degree in 2008–2009 were 2. The number of students enrolled full- and part-time who were dismissed or voluntarily withdrew from this program area in 2008–2009 were 0. *Applied Psychology MA/MS (Master of Arts/Science)*—Applications 2009–2010, 36. Total applicants accepted 2009–2010, 8. Number full-time enrolled (new admits only) 2009–2010, 5. Number part-time enrolled (new admits only) 2009–2010, 0. Total enrolled 2009–2010 full-time, 12. Openings 2010–2011, 7. The median number of years required for completion of a degree in 2008–2009 were 3. The number of students enrolled full- and part-time who were dismissed or voluntarily withdrew from this program area in 2008–2009 were 0.
Other Criteria: (importance of criteria rated low, medium, or high): GRE scores—medium, research experience—high, work experience—medium, extracurricular activity—medium, clinically related public service—low, GPA—high, letters of recommendation—high, statement of goals and objectives—high, undergraduate major in psychology—low, specific undergraduate psychology courses taken—medium. Work experience is viewed more closely by the Applied Psychology (MS) faculty than by the MA faculty. Research experience is particularly important in the MA program as this is a predoctoral program. For additional information on admission requirements, go to http://www.psychology.sdsu.edu/admisReq.html.

Student Characteristics: The following represents characteristics of students in 2009–2010 in all graduate psychology programs in the department: Female—full-time 80, part-time 0; Male—full-time 30, part-time 0; African American/Black—full-time 1, part-time 0; Hispanic/Latino(a)—full-time 8, part-time 0; Asian/Pacific Islander—full-time 10, part-time 0; American Indian/Alaska Native—full-time 2, part-time 0; Caucasian/White—full-time 86, part-time 0; Multi-ethnic—full-time 5, part-time 0; students subject to the Americans With Disabilities Act—full-time 0, part-time 0; Unknown ethnicity—full-time 0, part-time 0; International students who hold an F-1 or J-1 Visa—full-time 0, part-time 0.

Financial Information/Assistance:
Tuition for Full-Time Study: Master's: State residents: per academic year $4,462; Nonstate residents: per academic year $4,462. Tuition is subject to change. Additional fees are assessed to students beyond the costs of tuition for the following: out of state and int'l students pay $339/unit unless awarded a waiver. See the

following Web site for updates and changes in tuition costs: http://bfa.sdsu.edu/fm/co/sfs/registration.html.

Financial Assistance:

First-Year Students: Teaching assistantships available for first year. Average amount paid per academic year: $10,126. Average number of hours worked per week: 20. Apply by February 1. Research assistantships available for first year. Average amount paid per academic year: $11,042. Average number of hours worked per week: 20. Apply by February 1.

Advanced Students: Teaching assistantships available for advanced students. Average amount paid per academic year: $12,198. Average number of hours worked per week: 20. Apply by January 15. Research assistantships available for advanced students. Average amount paid per academic year: $11,085. Average number of hours worked per week: 20. Apply by January 15.

Additional Information: Of all students currently enrolled full time, 80% benefited from one or more of the listed financial assistance programs.

Internships/Practica: An essential component of graduate training in Applied Psychology is an internship experience that provides students with an opportunity to apply their classroom training and acquire new skills in a field setting. Interns are placed in a variety of settings, such as community-based organizations, consulting firms, city and county organizations, education, hospitality, high tech and private industry. Through the internship experience students also develop close contacts with other psychologists and practitioners working in their field. Internships are normally undertaken during the summer following the first year in the program and during the fall semester of the second year.

Housing and Day Care: On-campus housing is available. See the following Web site for more information: http://www.sa.sdsu.edu/housing/grad.html. On-campus day care facilities are available. See the following Web site for more information: http://edweb.sdsu.edu/cfd/childstudy.htm.

Employment of Department Graduates:

Master's Degree Graduates: Of those who graduated in the academic year 2008–2009, the following categories and numbers represent the postgraduate activities and employment of master's degree graduates: Enrolled in a psychology doctoral program (10), enrolled in another graduate/professional program (3), enrolled in a postdoctoral residency/fellowship (n/a), employed in independent practice (n/a), employed in an academic position at a university (0), employed in an academic position at a 2-year/4-year college (4), employed in other positions at a higher education institution (0), employed in a professional position in a school system (0), employed in business or industry (7), employed in government agency (0), employed in a community mental health/counseling center (1), employed in a hospital/medical center (2), still seeking employment (0), not seeking employment (1), other employment position (4), do not know (3), total from the above (master's) (35).

Doctoral Degree Graduates: Of those who graduated in the academic year 2008–2009, the following categories and numbers represent the postgraduate activities and employment of doctoral degree graduates: Enrolled in a psychology doctoral program (n/a), total from the above (doctoral) (0).

Additional Information:

Orientation, Objectives, and Emphasis of Department: The MA degree program provides graduate level studies and preparation for PhD programs in several areas. It is particularly appropriate for students who need advanced work to strengthen their profiles for application to PhD programs, or for those wishing to explore graduate-level work before committing to PhD training. Areas of emphasis within the MA are: Behavioral Psychology, Social Psychology, Physical and/or Mental Health Psychology, Developmental Psychology, and Learning/Cognition Psychology. Our research-oriented program does not offer instruction in technical skills (e.g., intelligence testing) and does not have a counseling practicum or provide opportunities for development of clinical skills. Students gain valuable research experience, which may involve working with humans in non-clinical areas. Upon admission to the program students are assigned a faculty research mentor who guides them through the research process leading to the thesis. Students take core classes in the major areas of psychology and electives in their areas of specialization. The MS Degree program in Applied Psychology has emphases in Program Evaluation and Industrial/Organizational Psychology. Students are prepared for professional careers in the public and private sectors or for doctoral-level training in Applied Psychology. All MS students take core courses in statistics and measurement and complete an internship.

Special Facilities or Resources: The following research labs welcome master's students: Anxiety and Depression in Children/Adolescents; Stereotype Threat, Aging/Dementia, Active Living/Healthy Eating; Alcohol Research; Behavioral Teratology; Brain Development Imaging; Categorical Distortions; Child Language/Emotion; Child and Adolescent Mental Health; Cognitive Development; Culture, Work Values/Organizational Behavior; Generational Differences; Child Abuse/Neglect; Health Outcomes; Intergroup Relations; Life-Span Human Senses; Measurement and Evaluation; Minority Community Health Intervention; Organizational Leadership/Citizenship; Organizational Research; Personality Assessment/Psychometrics; Personality Measurement Binge Drinking/Intervention; Family Library Use/Lifelong Learning; Social Support and Education on Health/Well Being of People with Chronic Diseases; Psychosocial Factors in Coronary Disease; Language/Cognitive Studies; Psychosocial, Chronic Illness Adjustment; Smoking; Social Development; Social Influence and Group Dynamics; Social Rejection; Stress/Coping; and Activity for Adolescent Girls. Students may conduct research at Children's Hospital, where several faculty members have their offices. Other resources include a community psychology clinic, the Center for Behavioral and Community Health Studies, Center for Behavioral Teratology, and the Center for Research in Mathematics and Science Education. Also available is an exchange program with the University of Mannheim, Germany. Students can choose to spend a semester or a year attending classes in Mannheim, and graduate students from Mannheim can spend a semester or a year taking classes here.

Information for Students With Physical Disabilities: See the following Web site for more information: http://www.sa.sdsu.edu/sds/index.html.

Application Information:
Send to Master's Programs Admissions Coordinator Department of Psychology San Diego State University, 5500 Campanile Drive, San

Diego, CA 92182-4611. Application available online. URL of online application: http://arweb.sdsu.edu/es/admissions/apply. *Fee:* $55.

San Diego State University/University of California, San Diego Joint Doctoral Program in Clinical Psychology

SDSU Department of Psychology/UCSD Department of Psychiatry
SDSU: College of Sciences UCSD: School of Medicine
San Diego State University, 6363 Alvarado Court, Suite #103
San Diego, CA 92120-4913
Telephone: (619) 594-2246
Fax: (619) 594-6780
E-mail: *sscott@sciences.sdsu.edu*
Web: *http://www.psychology.sdsu.edu/doctoral*

Department Information:
1985. Co-Directors: Elizabeth Klonoff, PhD, Robert Heaton, PhD. Number of faculty: total—full-time 58, part-time 58; women—full-time 25, part-time 28; total—minority—full-time 5, part-time 2; women minority—full-time 2.

Programs and Degrees Offered:
Listed in the following order: Program area, degree type (T if terminal Master's), number awarded 7/08–6/09. Clinical Psychology PhD (Doctor of Philosophy) 13.

APA Accreditation: Clinical PhD (Doctor of Philosophy). Student Outcome Data Website: http://www.psychology.sdsu.edu/doctoral/Demographics.html.

Student Applications/Admissions:
Student Applications
Clinical Psychology PhD (Doctor of Philosophy)—Applications 2009–2010, 351. Total applicants accepted 2009–2010, 14. Number full-time enrolled (new admits only) 2009–2010, 14. Number part-time enrolled (new admits only) 2009–2010, 0. Openings 2010–2011, 15. The median number of years required for completion of a degree in 2008–2009 were 6. The number of students enrolled full- and part-time who were dismissed or voluntarily withdrew from this program area in 2008–2009 were 0.
Scores: Entries appear in this order: required test or GPA, minimum score (if required), median score of students entering in 2009–2010. *Clinical Psychology PhD (Doctor of Philosophy):* GRE-V no minimum stated, GRE-Q no minimum stated, GRE-Subject (Psychology) no minimum stated, overall undergraduate GPA no minimum stated, psychology GPA no minimum stated, Masters GPA no minimum stated.
Other Criteria: (importance of criteria rated low, medium, or high): GRE scores—medium, research experience—high, work experience—low, clinically related public service—medium, GPA—high, letters of recommendation—high, interview—high, statement of goals and objectives—high, undergraduate major in psychology—medium, specific undergraduate psychology courses taken—medium. For additional information on admission requirements, go to http://www.psychology.sdsu.edu/doctoral.

Student Characteristics: The following represents characteristics of students in 2009–2010 in all graduate psychology programs in the department: Female—full-time 61, part-time 0; Male—full-time 11, part-time 0; African American/Black—full-time 1, part-time 0; Hispanic/Latino(a)—full-time 11, part-time 0; Asian/Pacific Islander—full-time 9, part-time 0; American Indian/Alaska Native—full-time 1, part-time 0; Caucasian/White—full-time 48, part-time 0; Multi-ethnic—full-time 0, part-time 0; students subject to the Americans With Disabilities Act—full-time 0, part-time 0; Unknown ethnicity—full-time 2, part-time 0; International students who hold an F-1 or J-1 Visa—full-time 0, part-time 0.

Financial Information/Assistance:
Tuition for Full-Time Study: Doctoral: State residents: per academic year $4,821; Nonstate residents: per academic year $4,821, $372 per credit hour. Tuition is subject to change. See the following Web site for updates and changes in tuition costs: Go to SDSU home page and click on cashiers office link. http://bfa.sdsu.edu/fm/co/sfs/registration.html.

Financial Assistance:
First-Year Students: Research assistantships available for first year. Average amount paid per academic year: $14,000. Average number of hours worked per week: 20. Fellowships and scholarships available for first year. Average amount paid per academic year: $14,000. Average number of hours worked per week: 20.
Advanced Students: Teaching assistantships available for advanced students. Average amount paid per academic year: $15,954. Average number of hours worked per week: 20. Research assistantships available for advanced students. Average amount paid per academic year: $16,000. Average number of hours worked per week: 20.
Additional Information: Of all students currently enrolled full time, 100% benefited from one or more of the listed financial assistance programs. Application and information available online at: http://www.psychology.sdsu.edu/doctoral.

Internships/Practica: Doctoral Degree (PhD Clinical Psychology): For those doctoral students for whom a professional internship was required in this program prior to graduation, (14) students applied for an internship in 2008–2009, with (13) students obtaining an internship. Of those students who obtained an internship, (13) were paid internships. Of those students who obtained an internship, (13) students placed in APA/CPA accredited internships, (0) students placed in internships not APA/CPA accredited, but listed with the Association of Psychology Postdoctoral and Internship Programs (APPIC), (0) students placed in internships conforming to guidelines of the Council of Directors of School Psychology Programs (CDSPP), (0) students placed in internships that were not APA/CPA accredited, APPIC or CDSPP listed. SDSU: Primary placement for all students in their second year is the Psychology Clinic. Students are taught general clinical skills. Therapy sessions are routinely videotaped for review in intensive weekly supervision sessions. UCSD: VA Outpatient Clinic: psychiatric outpatients—assessment and individual and group therapy. VA Medical Center: psychiatric inpatients—assessment, individual and group therapy. UCSD Outpatient Psychiatric Clinic: psychiatric outpatients—neuropsychological assessment and individual and group therapy. UCSD Medical Center: assessment and therapy of all types. All practicum placements are assigned for one full year beginning in the student's second year.

Housing and Day Care: On-campus housing is available. On-campus day care facilities are available.

Employment of Department Graduates:
Master's Degree Graduates: Of those who graduated in the academic year 2008–2009, the following categories and numbers represent the postgraduate activities and employment of master's degree graduates: Enrolled in a postdoctoral residency/fellowship (n/a), employed in independent practice (n/a), total from the above (master's) (0).
Doctoral Degree Graduates: Of those who graduated in the academic year 2008–2009, the following categories and numbers represent the postgraduate activities and employment of doctoral degree graduates: Enrolled in a psychology doctoral program (n/a), enrolled in a postdoctoral residency/fellowship (12), total from the above (doctoral) (12).

Additional Information:
Orientation, Objectives, and Emphasis of Department: Our PhD program is a cooperative venture of an academic Department of Psychology (SDSU) and a medical school Department of Psychiatry (UCSD). This partnership between two different departments in two universities provides unusual opportunities for interdisciplinary research. We currently offer concentrations in behavioral medicine, neuropsychology, and experimental psychopathology. The scientist–practitioner model on which the program is based involves a strong commitment to research as well as clinical training. The program aims to prepare students for leadership roles in academic and research settings. Our program is designed as a 5-year curriculum with a core of classroom instruction followed by apprenticeship training in specialty areas with appropriate seminars and tutorials. Clinical experiences are integrated with formal instruction throughout.

Special Facilities or Resources: The UCSD Department of Psychiatry, through the medical school, UCSD hospitals, and the VA Medical Center, has available all of the modern research and clinical facilities consistent with the School of Medicine's ranking among the top ten in the country in biomedical research. These include specialty laboratories (e.g., sleep labs), access to clinical trials, supercomputing facilities, and state-of-the-art neurochemical and biochemical laboratory facilities. Qualified students interested in MRI studies have access to a number of fully-supported imagers. At SDSU, the Department of Psychology has a state-of-the-art video-equipped therapy training complex, as well as experiment rooms, equipment (e.g. computerized test administration capabilities), and supplies available for research, including computerized physiological assessment and biofeedback laboratories. Animal research can be conducted on campus, where small animals are housed in a modern vivarium staffed with a veterinarian. SDSU faculty also supervise research on more exotic species at Sea World and the San Diego Zoo. The College of Sciences maintains a completely equipped electronics shop, a wood shop, a metal shop, and computer support facilities with several high end Unix servers, all staffed with full-time technicians. Collaborative relationships with faculty in the Graduate School of Public Health allow access to resources there as well.

Application Information:
Send to Student Selection Committee, 6363 Alvarado Ct. #103, San Diego, CA 92120-4913. Application available online. URL of online application: http://www.psychology.sdsu.edu/doctoral. Students are admitted in the Fall, application deadline December 1.

San Jose State University
Department of Psychology
Social Sciences
One Washington Square
San Jose, CA 95192-0120
Telephone: (408) 924-5600
Fax: (408) 924-5605
E-mail: *daan.giron@sjsu.edu*
Web: *http://www.sjsu.edu/psych/*

Department Information:
44. Chairperson: Dr. Sheila Bienenfeld. Number of faculty: total—full-time 21, part-time 31; women—full-time 12, part-time 17; total—minority—full-time 6, part-time 11; women minority—full-time 4, part-time 8; faculty subject to the Americans With Disabilities Act 1.

Programs and Degrees Offered:
Listed in the following order: Program area, degree type (T if terminal Master's), number awarded 7/08–6/09. Clinical Psychology MA/MS (Master of Arts/Science) (T) 13, Experimental Psychology MA/MS (Master of Arts/Science) (T) 5, Industrial/Organizational MA/MS (Master of Arts/Science) (T) 7.

Student Applications/Admissions:
Student Applications
Clinical Psychology MA/MS (Master of Arts/Science)—Applications 2009–2010, 71. Total applicants accepted 2009–2010, 12. Number full-time enrolled (new admits only) 2009–2010, 10. Number part-time enrolled (new admits only) 2009–2010, 0. Openings 2010–2011, 12. The median number of years required for completion of a degree in 2008–2009 were 2. The number of students enrolled full- and part-time who were dismissed or voluntarily withdrew from this program area in 2008–2009 were 0. *Experimental Psychology MA/MS (Master of Arts/Science)*—Applications 2009–2010, 32. Total applicants accepted 2009–2010, 17. Number full-time enrolled (new admits only) 2009–2010, 12. Number part-time enrolled (new admits only) 2009–2010, 0. Openings 2010–2011, 11. The median number of years required for completion of a degree in 2008–2009 were 2. The number of students enrolled full- and part-time who were dismissed or voluntarily withdrew from this program area in 2008–2009 were 1. *Industrial/Organizational MA/MS (Master of Arts/Science)*—Applications 2009–2010, 45. Total applicants accepted 2009–2010, 13. Number full-time enrolled (new admits only) 2009–2010, 12. Number part-time enrolled (new admits only) 2009–2010, 0. Openings 2010–2011, 15. The median number of years required for completion of a degree in 2008–2009 were 3. The number of students enrolled full- and part-time who were dismissed or voluntarily withdrew from this program area in 2008–2009 were 1.

Scores: Entries appear in this order: required test or GPA, minimum score (if required), median score of students entering in 2009–2010. *Experimental Psychology MA/MS (Master of Arts/Science):* GRE-V no minimum stated, GRE-Q no minimum stated, last 2 years GPA 3.0, psychology GPA 3.0.

Other Criteria: (importance of criteria rated low, medium, or high): Clinical Program has specific course requirements for admission and requires minimum 1 year of applied clinical experience and 100 hours. For additional information on admission requirements, go to http://www.sjsu.edu/psych/GraduatePrograms/.

Student Characteristics: The following represents characteristics of students in 2009–2010 in all graduate psychology programs in the department: Female—full-time 47, part-time 0; Male—full-time 16, part-time 0; African American/Black—full-time 1, part-time 0; Hispanic/Latino(a)—full-time 3, part-time 0; Asian/Pacific Islander—full-time 5, part-time 0; American Indian/Alaska Native—full-time 0, part-time 0; Caucasian/White—full-time 0, part-time 0; Multi-ethnic—full-time 2, part-time 0; students subject to the Americans With Disabilities Act—full-time 0, part-time 0; Unknown ethnicity—full-time 0, part-time 0; International students who hold an F-1 or J-1 Visa—full-time 0, part-time 0.

Financial Information/Assistance:
Tuition for Full-Time Study: *Master's:* State residents: per academic year $9,770; Nonstate residents: per academic year $12,686. Tuition is subject to change. See the following Web site for updates and changes in tuition costs: http://www.sjsu.edu/bursar/.

Financial Assistance:
First-Year Students: Teaching assistantships available for first year. Research assistantships available for first year. Fellowships and scholarships available for first year.
Advanced Students: Teaching assistantships available for advanced students. Research assistantships available for advanced students. Fellowships and scholarships available for advanced students.
Additional Information: Of all students currently enrolled full time, 50% benefited from one or more of the listed financial assistance programs. Application and information available online at: http://www.sjsu.edu/faso/.

Internships/Practica: An internship is required for students in the Industrial/Organizational Psychology program. The program coordinator works with each student to determine the student's interests and helps find a placement site for each student. Some students in the Experimental Program are offered internships at NASA/Ames Research Center.

Housing and Day Care: On-campus housing is available. See the following Web site for more information: http://housing.sjsu.edu/. On-campus day care facilities are available. See the following Web site for more information: http://as.sjsu.edu/ascdc/.

Employment of Department Graduates:
Master's Degree Graduates: Of those who graduated in the academic year 2008–2009, the following categories and numbers represent the postgraduate activities and employment of master's degree graduates: Enrolled in a psychology doctoral program (4), enrolled in a postdoctoral residency/fellowship (n/a), employed in independent practice (n/a), employed in business or industry (3), employed in government agency (4), employed in a community mental health/counseling center (10), total from the above (master's) (21).
Doctoral Degree Graduates: Of those who graduated in the academic year 2008–2009, the following categories and numbers represent the postgraduate activities and employment of doctoral degree graduates: Enrolled in a psychology doctoral program (n/a), total from the above (doctoral) (0).

Additional Information:
Orientation, Objectives, and Emphasis of Department: The mission of the University is to enrich the lives of its students, to transmit knowledge to its students along with the necessary skills for applying it in the service of our society, and to expand the base of knowledge through research and scholarship. It emphasizes the following goals for both undergraduate and graduate students: in-depth knowledge of a major field of study; broad understanding of the sciences, social sciences, humanities, and the arts; skills in communication and in critical inquiry; multi-cultural and global perspectives gained through intellectual and social exchange with people of diverse economic and ethnic backgrounds; and active participation in professional, artistic, and ethnic communities, responsible citizenship and an understanding of ethical choices inherent in human development.

Special Facilities or Resources: The department maintains a variety of facilities and support staff to enhance instruction and research. For biological and cognitive research and instruction, the department has a number of laboratories and specialized laboratory equipment on campus, and lab technicians are available to construct additional equipment. For work in clinical and counseling psychology, the department has a Psychology Clinic consisting of therapy rooms and adjoining observation rooms equipped with audio and video equipment. These rooms are also available to individuals working in other areas, such as developmental, personality, and social psychology. In addition, students interested in counseling-related activities have access to a number of off-campus organizations. Three computer laboratories containing microcomputers and terminals hooked up to minicomputers and mainframes are available for students. These labs have extensive software, and computer consultants are on call to help with software and hardware problems, design and interpretation of statistical analyses, and computer exercises. There is a child care center on campus.

Information for Students With Physical Disabilities: See the following Web site for more information: http://www.drc.sjsu.edu/.

Application Information:
Send to Program Coordinator. Application available online. URL of online application: http://www.sjsu.edu/psych/GraduatePrograms/. Students are admitted in the Fall, application deadline January 15. Deadline for Clinical program is January 15; for the Experimental Psychology Program and the Industrial/Organizational Psychology program it is February 1. *Fee:* $55.

Santa Clara University (2009 data)
Department of Counseling Psychology
Counseling Psychology, Education, and Pastoral Ministries
500 El Camino Real - Bannan Hall 243
Santa Clara, CA 95053-0201
Telephone: (408) 551-1603
Fax: (408) 554-2392
E-mail: *sbabbel@scu.edu*
Web: *http://www.scu.edu/ecppm/*

Department Information:
1970. Chairperson: Teri Quatman, PhD. Number of faculty: total—full-time 5, part-time 22; women—full-time 4, part-time 10; women minority—full-time 1, part-time 2.

Programs and Degrees Offered:
Listed in the following order: Program area, degree type (T if terminal Master's), number awarded 7/08–6/09. Counseling Psychology MA/MS (Master of Arts/Science) (T) 75, Counseling MA/MS (Master of Arts/Science) 9.

Student Applications/Admissions:
Student Applications
Counseling Psychology MA/MS (Master of Arts/Science)—Applications 2009–2010, 120. Total applicants accepted 2009–2010, 100. Number full-time enrolled (new admits only) 2009–2010, 38. Number part-time enrolled (new admits only) 2009–2010, 42. Total enrolled 2009–2010 full-time, 140, part-time, 160. Openings 2010–2011, 100. The median number of years required for completion of a degree in 2008–2009 were 3. The number of students enrolled full- and part-time who were dismissed or voluntarily withdrew from this program area in 2008–2009 were 10. *Counseling MA/MS (Master of Arts/Science)*—Applications 2009–2010, 25. Total applicants accepted 2009–2010, 15. Number full-time enrolled (new admits only) 2009–2010, 7. Number part-time enrolled (new admits only) 2009–2010, 8. Total enrolled 2009–2010 full-time, 15, part-time, 10. Openings 2010–2011, 15. The median number of years required for completion of a degree in 2008–2009 were 2. The number of students enrolled full- and part-time who were dismissed or voluntarily withdrew from this program area in 2008–2009 were 4.
Other Criteria: (importance of criteria rated low, medium, or high): GRE scores—low, research experience—low, work experience—medium, extracurricular activity—medium, clinically related public service—high, GPA—medium, letters of recommendation—high, statement of goals and objectives—high. For additional information on admission requirements, go to http://www.scu.edu/cp/.

Student Characteristics: The following represents characteristics of students in 2009–2010 in all graduate psychology programs in the department: Female—full-time 29, part-time 185; Male—full-time 4, part-time 31; African American/Black—full-time 2, part-time 3; Hispanic/Latino(a)—full-time 6, part-time 35; Asian/Pacific Islander—full-time 4, part-time 38; American Indian/Alaska Native—full-time 0, part-time 1; Caucasian/White—full-time 21, part-time 77; Multi-ethnic—full-time 0, part-time 2; students subject to the Americans With Disabilities Act—full-time 2, part-time 3; Unknown ethnicity—full-time 0, part-time 0; International students who hold an F-1 or J-1 Visa—full-time 0, part-time 0.

Financial Information/Assistance:
Tuition for Full-Time Study: Master's: State residents: $438 per credit hour; Nonstate residents: $438 per credit hour. Tuition is subject to change. See the following Web site for updates and changes in tuition costs: http://www.scu.edu/ecppm/studentservices/financialaid.cfm.

Financial Assistance:
First-Year Students: Teaching assistantships available for first year. Average amount paid per academic year: $1,200. Average number of hours worked per week: 3. Research assistantships available for first year. Average amount paid per academic year: $600. Average number of hours worked per week: 6. Fellowships and scholarships available for first year. Average amount paid per academic year: $1,400. Average number of hours worked per week: 0.

Advanced Students: Teaching assistantships available for advanced students. Average amount paid per academic year: $1,200. Average number of hours worked per week: 3. Research assistantships available for advanced students. Average amount paid per academic year: $600. Average number of hours worked per week: 6. Fellowships and scholarships available for advanced students. Average amount paid per academic year: $1,400. Average number of hours worked per week: 0.

Additional Information: Of all students currently enrolled full time, 26% benefited from one or more of the listed financial assistance programs. Application and information available online at: http://www.scu.edu/ecppm/about/financialinformation.

Internships/Practica: Master's Degree (MA/MS Counseling Psychology): An internship experience, such as a final research project or "capstone" experience is required of graduates. Counseling Practicum: Marriage and Family Therapy. Supervised counseling experience designed specifically to meet California MFT licensing requirements. Weekly seminars for consultation and discussion with a licensed supervisor on such topics as case management and evaluation, referral procedures, ethical practices, professional and client interaction, confidential communication, and interprofessional ethical considerations.

Housing and Day Care: No on-campus housing is available. On-campus day care facilities are available. See the following Web site for more information: http://www.scu.edu/koc/.

Employment of Department Graduates:
Master's Degree Graduates: Of those who graduated in the academic year 2008–2009, the following categories and numbers represent the postgraduate activities and employment of master's degree graduates: Enrolled in a psychology doctoral program (7), enrolled in another graduate/professional program (1), enrolled in a postdoctoral residency/fellowship (n/a), employed in independent practice (n/a), employed in an academic position at a 2-year/4-year college (2), employed in other positions at a higher education institution (4), employed in a professional position in a school system (4), employed in a community mental health/counseling center (8), employed in a hospital/medical center (1), other employment position (6), do not know (47), total from the above (master's) (80).

GRADUATE STUDY IN PSYCHOLOGY

Doctoral Degree Graduates: Of those who graduated in the academic year 2008–2009, the following categories and numbers represent the postgraduate activities and employment of doctoral degree graduates: Enrolled in a psychology doctoral program (n/a), total from the above (doctoral) (0).

Additional Information:
Orientation, Objectives, and Emphasis of Department: Santa Clara University's graduate programs in counseling and counseling psychology are offered through the School of Education, Counseling Psychology, and Pastoral Ministries. Programs lead to the Master of Arts in Counseling or the Master of Arts in Counseling Psychology, with the option of an emphasis in Health Psychology, Career Counseling, Latino Counseling and Correctional Psychology. All of the Counseling Psychology (78-unit) programs prepares students for MFT licensure through the California Board of Behavioral Sciences (BBS). Santa Clara is accredited by the Western Association of Schools and Colleges and is approved by the Board of Behavioral Science, Department of Consumer Affairs (California) to prepare students for MFT licensure. The faculty represent a diverse set of clinical theories and perspectives, and students gain a broad exposure to a range of theories and practical applications in counseling.

Special Facilities or Resources: Santa Clara University is located in the heart of Silicon Valley, with close connection to major business and academic resources in this area. The University has a complete complement of facilities including an excellent library, theatre, museum and state of the art physical fitness center. The University has a dedication to educating the whole person and includes Centers of Distinction which explore diversity, ethics and the interface of Technology and Society.

Information for Students With Physical Disabilities: See the following Web site for more information: http://www.scu.edu/advising/learning/disabilities/index.cfm.

Application Information:
Send to Graduate Admissions, School of ECPPM, Bannan Hall, 243, Santa Clara University, 500 El Camino Real, Santa Clara, CA 95053-0201. Application available online. URL of online application: https://www.scu.edu/apply/edcp/handler.cfm?event=home. Students are admitted in the Fall, application deadline April 15; Winter, application deadline October 15; Spring, application deadline February 15; Summer, application deadline April 15. *Fee:* $50.

Saybrook University
Graduate School
747 Front Street, Third Floor
San Francisco, CA 94111-1920
Telephone: (415) 433-9200
Fax: (415) 433-9271
E-mail: *sseligman@saybrook.edu*
Web: *http://www.saybrook.edu*

Department Information:
1971. Vice President for Academic Affairs: Vincent Pelligrino. Number of faculty: total—full-time 24, part-time 71; women—full-time 8, part-time 28; total—minority—full-time 3, part-time 13; women minority—full-time 2, part-time 6; faculty subject to the Americans With Disabilities Act 6.

Programs and Degrees Offered:
Listed in the following order: Program area, degree type (T if terminal Master's), number awarded 7/08–6/09. Human Science MA/MS (Master of Arts/Science) 1, Organizational Systems PhD (Doctor of Philosophy) 3, Clinical Psychology PhD (Doctor of Philosophy) 8, Human Science PhD (Doctor of Philosophy) 1, Organizational Systems MA/MS (Master of Arts/Science) 0, Psychology MA/MS (Master of Arts/Science) 17, Psychology PhD (Doctor of Philosophy) 17, Clinical Psychology PsyD (Doctor of Psychology) 0, Systems Counseling MA/MS (Master of Arts/Science), Mind-Body Medicine MA/MS (Master of Arts/Science) 0.

Student Applications/Admissions:
Student Applications
Human Science MA/MS (Master of Arts/Science)—Applications 2009–2010, 13. Total applicants accepted 2009–2010, 8. Number full-time enrolled (new admits only) 2009–2010, 5. Number part-time enrolled (new admits only) 2009–2010, 0. Total enrolled 2009–2010 full-time, 8, part-time, 1. Openings 2010–2011, 10. The median number of years required for completion of a degree in 2008–2009 were 3. The number of students enrolled full- and part-time who were dismissed or voluntarily withdrew from this program area in 2008–2009 were 2. *Organizational Systems PhD (Doctor of Philosophy)*—Applications 2009–2010, 38. Total applicants accepted 2009–2010, 16. Number full-time enrolled (new admits only) 2009–2010, 9. Number part-time enrolled (new admits only) 2009–2010, 0. Total enrolled 2009–2010 full-time, 40, part-time, 6. Openings 2010–2011, 30. The median number of years required for completion of a degree in 2008–2009 were 6. The number of students enrolled full- and part-time who were dismissed or voluntarily withdrew from this program area in 2008–2009 were 9. *Clinical Psychology PhD (Doctor of Philosophy)*—Applications 2009–2010, 90. Total applicants accepted 2009–2010, 57. Number full-time enrolled (new admits only) 2009–2010, 10. Number part-time enrolled (new admits only) 2009–2010, 3. Total enrolled 2009–2010 full-time, 65, part-time, 11. Openings 2010–2011, 30. The median number of years required for completion of a degree in 2008–2009 were 6. The number of students enrolled full- and part-time who were dismissed or voluntarily withdrew from this program area in 2008–2009 were 12. *Human Science PhD (Doctor of Philosophy)*—Applications 2009–2010, 35. Total applicants accepted 2009–2010, 19. Number full-time enrolled (new admits only) 2009–2010, 7. Total enrolled 2009–2010 full-time, 23, part-time, 4. Openings 2010–2011, 20. The median number of years required for completion of a degree in 2008–2009 were 3. The number of students enrolled full- and part-time who were dismissed or voluntarily withdrew from this program area in 2008–2009 were 5. *Organizational Systems MA/MS (Master of Arts/Science)*—Applications 2009–2010, 19. Total applicants accepted 2009–2010, 9. Number full-time enrolled (new admits only) 2009–2010, 6. Total enrolled 2009–2010 full-time, 11, part-time, 2. Openings 2010–2011, 20. The number of students enrolled full- and part-time who were dismissed or voluntarily withdrew from this program area in 2008–2009 were 0. *Psychology MA/MS (Master of Arts/Science)*—Applications 2009–2010, 191. Total applicants accepted 2009–2010,

97. Number full-time enrolled (new admits only) 2009–2010, 45. Number part-time enrolled (new admits only) 2009–2010, 0. Total enrolled 2009–2010 full-time, 71, part-time, 23. Openings 2010–2011, 50. The median number of years required for completion of a degree in 2008–2009 were 2. The number of students enrolled full- and part-time who were dismissed or voluntarily withdrew from this program area in 2008–2009 were 14. *Psychology PhD (Doctor of Philosophy)*—Applications 2009–2010, 92. Total applicants accepted 2009–2010, 62. Number full-time enrolled (new admits only) 2009–2010, 24. Number part-time enrolled (new admits only) 2009–2010, 14. Total enrolled 2009–2010 full-time, 99, part-time, 35. Openings 2010–2011, 50. The median number of years required for completion of a degree in 2008–2009 were 6. The number of students enrolled full- and part-time who were dismissed or voluntarily withdrew from this program area in 2008–2009 were 23. *Clinical Psychology PsyD (Doctor of Psychology)*—Applications 2009–2010, 58. Total applicants accepted 2009–2010, 38. Number full-time enrolled (new admits only) 2009–2010, 19. Number part-time enrolled (new admits only) 2009–2010, 0. Total enrolled 2009–2010 full-time, 30, part-time, 3. Openings 2010–2011, 25. The number of students enrolled full- and part-time who were dismissed or voluntarily withdrew from this program area in 2008–2009 were 2. *Systems Counseling MA/MS (Master of Arts/Science)*—The number of students enrolled full- and part-time who were dismissed or voluntarily withdrew from this program area in 2008–2009 were 4. *Mind-Body Medicine MA/MS (Master of Arts/Science)*—Applications 2009–2010, 76. Total applicants accepted 2009–2010, 50. Number full-time enrolled (new admits only) 2009–2010, 21. Number part-time enrolled (new admits only) 2009–2010, 2. Total enrolled 2009–2010 full-time, 23, part-time, 9. Openings 2010–2011, 35. The number of students enrolled full- and part-time who were dismissed or voluntarily withdrew from this program area in 2008–2009 were 5.

Scores: Entries appear in this order: required test or GPA, minimum score (if required), median score of students entering in 2009–2010. *Clinical Psychology PsyD (Doctor of Psychology):* overall undergraduate GPA 3.00.

Other Criteria: (importance of criteria rated low, medium, or high): GRE scores—low, research experience—high, work experience—high, extracurricular activity—medium, clinically related public service—medium, GPA—high, letters of recommendation—high, interview—low, statement of goals and objectives—high, undergraduate major in psychology—medium, specific undergraduate psychology courses taken—medium, GRE score is only required for admission to Saybrook's clinical PsyD degree program. Saybrook does not require the GRE for other MA or PhD degrees.

Student Characteristics: The following represents characteristics of students in 2009–2010 in all graduate psychology programs in the department: Female—full-time 317, part-time 63; Male—full-time 124, part-time 30; African American/Black—full-time 27, part-time 3; Hispanic/Latino(a)—full-time 19, part-time 2; Asian/Pacific Islander—full-time 10, part-time 0; American Indian/Alaska Native—full-time 3, part-time 0; Caucasian/White—full-time 275, part-time 32; Multi-ethnic—full-time 0, part-time 0; students subject to the Americans With Disabilities Act—full-time 4, part-time 0; Unknown ethnicity—full-time 82, part-time 16; International students who hold an F-1 or J-1 Visa—full-time 0, part-time 0.

Financial Information/Assistance:
  Tuition for Full-Time Study: *Master's:* State residents: per academic year $19,990; Nonstate residents: per academic year $19,990. *Doctoral:* State residents: per academic year $19,990; Nonstate residents: per academic year $19,900. Additional fees are assessed to students beyond the costs of tuition for the following: residential conferences for food and lodging.

Financial Assistance:
  First-Year Students: Fellowships and scholarships available for first year. Average amount paid per academic year: $2,000.
  Advanced Students: Research assistantships available for advanced students. Average amount paid per academic year: $7,300. Fellowships and scholarships available for advanced students. Average amount paid per academic year: $2,000.
  Additional Information: Of all students currently enrolled full time, 43% benefited from one or more of the listed financial assistance programs.

Internships/Practica: Saybrook University students are distributed throughout the United States and the world. Because of the distance learning format, it is impractical for Saybrook to offer internship and practica training based at Saybrook. Saybrook graduate students are often successful midlife professionals who are accomplished in their first careers. The Clinical Training Coordinator works with doctoral students to find training experiences that will provide solid clinical training while drawing upon the strengths and clinical interests of these mature students.

Housing and Day Care: No on-campus housing is available. No on-campus day care facilities are available.

Employment of Department Graduates:
  Master's Degree Graduates: Of those who graduated in the academic year 2008–2009, the following categories and numbers represent the postgraduate activities and employment of master's degree graduates: Enrolled in a psychology doctoral program (0), enrolled in another graduate/professional program (0), enrolled in a postdoctoral residency/fellowship (n/a), employed in independent practice (n/a), employed in an academic position at a university (0), employed in an academic position at a 2-year/4-year college (1), employed in other positions at a higher education institution (0), employed in a professional position in a school system (1), employed in a community mental health/counseling center (2), employed in a hospital/medical center (0), other employment position (1), total from the above (master's) (5).
  Doctoral Degree Graduates: Of those who graduated in the academic year 2008–2009, the following categories and numbers represent the postgraduate activities and employment of doctoral degree graduates: Enrolled in a psychology doctoral program (n/a), employed in independent practice (2), employed in an academic position at a university (1), employed in an academic position at a 2-year/4-year college (1), employed in business or industry (1), employed in a community mental health/counseling center (1), total from the above (doctoral) (6).

Additional Information:
  Orientation, Objectives, and Emphasis of Department: The mission of Saybrook University is to provide a unique and creative environment for graduate study, research, and communication in humanistic psychology, focused on understanding the human experience, in a distance learning format. Applying the highest

standards of scholarship, Saybrook is dedicated to fostering the full expression of the human spirit and humanistic values in society.

Application Information:
Send to Saybrook University, Admissions Department, 747 Front Street, 3rd floor, San Francisco, CA 94111-1920. Application available online. URL of online application: https://mars.saybrook.edu/SMS/MainAdmissionsLogin.jsp. Students are admitted in the Fall, application deadline May 1; Spring, application deadline October 1; Programs have rolling admissions. *Fee:* $50.

Sonoma State University (2009 data)
Department of Psychology
1801 East Cotati Avenue
Rohnert Park, CA 94928
Telephone: (707) 664-2682
Fax: (707) 664-3113
E-mail: *karen.fischer@sonoma.edu*
Web: *http://www.sonoma.edu/exed*

Department Information:
1961. Chairperson: Laurel McCabe, PhD. Number of faculty: total—full-time 12, part-time 10; women—full-time 9, part-time 9.

Programs and Degrees Offered:
Listed in the following order: Program area, degree type (T if terminal Master's), number awarded 7/08–6/09. Depth Psychology MA/MS (Master of Arts/Science) 8, Organization Development MA/MS (Master of Arts/Science) 10.

Student Applications/Admissions:
Student Applications
Depth Psychology MA/MS (Master of Arts/Science)—Applications 2009–2010, 25. Total applicants accepted 2009–2010, 12. Number full-time enrolled (new admits only) 2009–2010, 8. Number part-time enrolled (new admits only) 2009–2010, 0. Total enrolled 2009–2010 full-time, 20, part-time, 10. Openings 2010–2011, 15. The median number of years required for completion of a degree in 2008–2009 were 3. The number of students enrolled full- and part-time who were dismissed or voluntarily withdrew from this program area in 2008–2009 were 2. *Organization Development MA/MS (Master of Arts/Science)*—Applications 2009–2010, 27. Total applicants accepted 2009–2010, 18. Number full-time enrolled (new admits only) 2009–2010, 16. Total enrolled 2009–2010 full-time, 30, part-time, 8. Openings 2010–2011, 16. The median number of years required for completion of a degree in 2008–2009 were 3. The number of students enrolled full- and part-time who were dismissed or voluntarily withdrew from this program area in 2008–2009 were 1.
Other Criteria: (importance of criteria rated low, medium, or high): research experience—low, work experience—medium, extracurricular activity—medium, clinically related public service—medium, GPA—high, letters of recommendation—high, interview—high, statement of goals and objectives—high, emotional maturity—high, specific undergraduate psychology courses taken—high. Demonstrated graduate level writing ability in all programs. For additional information on admission requirements, go to http://www.sonoma.edu/psychology/depth/admissions or http://www.sonoma.edu/programs/od.

Student Characteristics: The following represents characteristics of students in 2009–2010 in all graduate psychology programs in the department: Female—full-time 60, part-time 5; Male—full-time 12, part-time 0; African American/Black—full-time 0, part-time 0; Hispanic/Latino(a)—full-time 0, part-time 0; Asian/Pacific Islander—full-time 0, part-time 0; American Indian/Alaska Native—full-time 0, part-time 1; Caucasian/White—full-time 50, part-time 5; Multi-ethnic—full-time 0, part-time 0; students subject to the Americans With Disabilities Act—full-time 0, part-time 0; Unknown ethnicity—full-time 0, part-time 0; International students who hold an F-1 or J-1 Visa—full-time 0, part-time 0.

Financial Information/Assistance:
Financial Assistance:
First-Year Students: Teaching assistantships available for first year. Research assistantships available for first year. Fellowships and scholarships available for first year. Average amount paid per academic year: $700. Apply by January 15.
Advanced Students: Teaching assistantships available for advanced students. Research assistantships available for advanced students. Fellowships and scholarships available for advanced students. Apply by January 15.
Additional Information: Of all students currently enrolled full time, 90% benefited from one or more of the listed financial assistance programs. Application and information available online at: http://www.sonoma.edu/finaid/.

Internships/Practica: Internships are optional in the Depth Psychology program. About half of the students engage in a supervised teaching internship teaching an undergraduate psychology class at SSU. Field projects working as a team of two or three students studying an organization are required in the Organization Development program.

Housing and Day Care: On-campus housing is available. On-campus day care facilities are available.

Employment of Department Graduates:
Master's Degree Graduates: Of those who graduated in the academic year 2008–2009, the following categories and numbers represent the postgraduate activities and employment of master's degree graduates: Enrolled in a psychology doctoral program (5), enrolled in another graduate/professional program (1), enrolled in a postdoctoral residency/fellowship (n/a), employed in independent practice (n/a), employed in an academic position at a university (4), employed in an academic position at a 2-year/4-year college (4), employed in other positions at a higher education institution (2), employed in a professional position in a school system (2), employed in business or industry (20), employed in government agency (0), employed in a community mental health/counseling center (10), employed in a hospital/medical center (0), still seeking employment (10), not seeking employment (10), other employment position (10), total from the above (master's) (78).
Doctoral Degree Graduates: Of those who graduated in the academic year 2008–2009, the following categories and numbers

represent the postgraduate activities and employment of doctoral degree graduates: Enrolled in a psychology doctoral program (n/a), total from the above (doctoral) (0).

Additional Information:
Orientation, Objectives, and Emphasis of Department: Depth Psychology: An embodied 36-unit curriculum which integrates intensive personal process work in Jungian and archetypal psychology with conceptual learning and practical skills development. A small group environment enables students to develop skills in process work, group facilitation, arts expressions, dream work, personal growth facilitation and cross-cultural awareness. Organization Development: Provides professional preparation for mid-career individuals interested in learning how to develop more effective and humane organizations. A 36-unit program of seminar discussions, skill-building activities, and extensive field projects under faculty guidance. Participants gain the practical skills, conceptual knowledge, and field-tested experience to successfully lead organization improvement efforts.

Special Facilities or Resources: Facilities include a biofeedback lab and computer lab. The faculty are open to investigations in depth psychology and organization development. The department has excellent interdisciplinary cooperation with sociology, gerontology, business and other related programs. Sonoma State University has a "state of the art" new library and information center.

Information for Students With Physical Disabilities: See the following Web site for more information: http://www.sonoma.edu/dss/.

Application Information:
Send to MA Programs in Psychology, Department of Psychology, Sonoma State University, 1801 E. Cotati Avenue, Rohnert Park, CA 94928. Application available online. URL of online application: http://www.sonoma.edu/psychology/depth/admissions and http://www.sonoma.edu/programs/od/. Students are admitted in the Fall; programs have rolling admissions. Applications accepted on a rolling basis until quota reached. *Fee:* $55.

Southern California, University of
Department of Psychology
College of Letters, Arts and Sciences
University Park - SGM 501
Los Angeles, CA 90089-1061
Telephone: (213) 740-2203
Fax: (213) 746-9082
E-mail: *itakarag@usc.edu*
Web: *http://college.usc.edu/psyc/home/*

Department Information:
1929. Chairperson: Margaret Gatz. Number of faculty: total—full-time 34; women—full-time 10; total—minority—full-time 5.

Programs and Degrees Offered:
Listed in the following order: Program area, degree type (T if terminal Master's), number awarded 7/08–6/09. Brain and Cognitive Sciences PhD (Doctor of Philosophy) 4, Clinical Science PhD (Doctor of Philosophy) 3, Developmental Psychology PhD (Doctor of Philosophy) 3, Quantitative Methods PhD (Doctor of Philosophy) 3, Social Psychology PhD (Doctor of Philosophy) 3.

APA Accreditation: Clinical PhD (Doctor of Philosophy). Student Outcome Data Website: http://college.usc.edu/psyc/doctoral/areas-clinical-outcome-data.cfm.

Student Applications/Admissions:
Student Applications
Brain and Cognitive Sciences PhD (Doctor of Philosophy)—Applications 2009–2010, 63. Total applicants accepted 2009–2010, 7. Number full-time enrolled (new admits only) 2009–2010, 5. Openings 2010–2011, 5. The median number of years required for completion of a degree in 2008–2009 were 6. The number of students enrolled full- and part-time who were dismissed or voluntarily withdrew from this program area in 2008–2009 were 0. *Clinical Science PhD (Doctor of Philosophy)*—Applications 2009–2010, 271. Total applicants accepted 2009–2010, 8. Number full-time enrolled (new admits only) 2009–2010, 5. Openings 2010–2011, 6. The median number of years required for completion of a degree in 2008–2009 were 6. The number of students enrolled full- and part-time who were dismissed or voluntarily withdrew from this program area in 2008–2009 were 1. *Developmental Psychology PhD (Doctor of Philosophy)*—Applications 2009–2010, 25. Total applicants accepted 2009–2010, 1. Number full-time enrolled (new admits only) 2009–2010, 0. Openings 2010–2011, 1. The median number of years required for completion of a degree in 2008–2009 were 6. The number of students enrolled full- and part-time who were dismissed or voluntarily withdrew from this program area in 2008–2009 were 0. *Quantitative Methods PhD (Doctor of Philosophy)*—Applications 2009–2010, 8. Total applicants accepted 2009–2010, 3. Number full-time enrolled (new admits only) 2009–2010, 1. Openings 2010–2011, 2. The median number of years required for completion of a degree in 2008–2009 were 9. The number of students enrolled full- and part-time who were dismissed or voluntarily withdrew from this program area in 2008–2009 were 0. *Social Psychology PhD (Doctor of Philosophy)*—Applications 2009–2010, 61. Total applicants accepted 2009–2010, 6. Number full-time enrolled (new admits only) 2009–2010, 2. Openings 2010–2011, 2. The median number of years required for completion of a degree in 2008–2009 were 7. The number of students enrolled full- and part-time who were dismissed or voluntarily withdrew from this program area in 2008–2009 were 0.

Scores: Entries appear in this order: required test or GPA, minimum score (if required), median score of students entering in 2009–2010. *Brain and Cognitive Sciences PhD (Doctor of Philosophy):* GRE-V no minimum stated, 680, GRE-Q 550, 750, GRE-Analytical no minimum stated, 4.5; *Clinical Science PhD (Doctor of Philosophy):* GRE-V no minimum stated, 690, GRE-Q 550, 770, GRE-Analytical no minimum stated, 5.0; *Developmental Psychology PhD (Doctor of Philosophy):* GRE-V no minimum stated, GRE-Q 550, GRE-Analytical no minimum stated; *Quantitative Methods PhD (Doctor of Philosophy):* GRE-V no minimum stated, GRE-Q 550, GRE-Analytical no minimum stated; *Social Psychology PhD (Doctor of Philosophy):* GRE-V no minimum stated, 625, GRE-Q 550, 720, GRE-Analytical no minimum stated, 5.75.

Other Criteria: (importance of criteria rated low, medium, or high): GRE scores—high, research experience—high, work experience—medium, extracurricular activity—low, clinically related public service—medium, GPA—high, letters of recommendation—high, statement of goals and objectives—high. Interview and clinically related public service are very important for the Clinical Science program but less so for other areas. For additional information on admission requirements, go to http://college.usc.edu/psyc/doctoral/.

Student Characteristics: The following represents characteristics of students in 2009–2010 in all graduate psychology programs in the department: Female—full-time 63, part-time 0; Male—full-time 32, part-time 0; African American/Black—full-time 7, part-time 0; Hispanic/Latino(a)—full-time 9, part-time 0; Asian/Pacific Islander—full-time 16, part-time 0; American Indian/Alaska Native—full-time 0, part-time 0; Caucasian/White—full-time 42, part-time 0; Multi-ethnic—full-time 0, part-time 0; students subject to the Americans With Disabilities Act—full-time 0, part-time 0; Unknown ethnicity—full-time 0, part-time 0; International students who hold an F-1 or J-1 Visa—full-time 21, part-time 0.

Financial Information/Assistance:
Tuition for Full-Time Study: *Doctoral:* State residents: per academic year $31,176, $1,299 per credit hour; Nonstate residents: per academic year $31,176, $1,299 per credit hour. Tuition is subject to change. Additional fees are assessed to students beyond the costs of tuition for the following: orientation fee (entering semester only) plus additional nominal fees (~$50) per semester. See the following Web site for updates and changes in tuition costs: http://fbs.usc.edu/depts/sfs.

Financial Assistance:
First-Year Students: Teaching assistantships available for first year. Average amount paid per academic year: $19,000. Average number of hours worked per week: 20. Research assistantships available for first year. Average amount paid per academic year: $19,000. Average number of hours worked per week: 20. Traineeships available for first year. Average amount paid per academic year: $20,976. Average number of hours worked per week: 0. Fellowships and scholarships available for first year. Average amount paid per academic year: $22,500. Average number of hours worked per week: 0.

Advanced Students: Teaching assistantships available for advanced students. Average amount paid per academic year: $19,000. Average number of hours worked per week: 20. Research assistantships available for advanced students. Average amount paid per academic year: $19,000. Average number of hours worked per week: 20. Traineeships available for advanced students. Average amount paid per academic year: $29,760. Average number of hours worked per week: 0. Fellowships and scholarships available for advanced students. Average amount paid per academic year: $19,000. Average number of hours worked per week: 0.

Additional Information: Of all students currently enrolled full time, 84% benefited from one or more of the listed financial assistance programs. Application and information available online at: http://college.usc.edu/psyc/doctoral/.

Internships/Practica: Doctoral Degree (PhD Clinical Science): For those doctoral students for whom a professional internship was required in this program prior to graduation, (7) students applied for an internship in 2008–2009, with (7) students obtaining an internship. Of those students who obtained an internship, (7) were paid internships. Of those students who obtained an internship, (7) students placed in APA/CPA accredited internships, (0) students placed in internships not APA/CPA accredited, but listed with the Association of Psychology Postdoctoral and Internship Programs (APPIC), (0) students placed in internships conforming to guidelines of the Council of Directors of School Psychology Programs (CDSPP), (0) students placed in internships that were not APA/CPA accredited, APPIC or CDSPP listed. Students in the clinical psychology area take at least six semesters of clinical didactic-practica, each of which involves instruction and supervised clinical service provision. Students receive both group and individual supervision of their cases. The first year practica focus on clinical interviewing and formal assessment. In the second and third year, students take practica based on their interests and specialty track. Practica are offered in general adult psychotherapy, psychotherapy with older adults, and child/family psychotherapy. After admission to doctoral candidacy, all students must complete a one-year, APA approved clinical internship for which students separately apply at the time.

Housing and Day Care: On-campus housing is available. See the following Web site for more information: http://housing.usc.edu/. On-campus day care facilities are available. See the following Web site for more information: http://www.usc.edu/dept/adminops/childcare/.

Employment of Department Graduates:
Master's Degree Graduates: Of those who graduated in the academic year 2008–2009, the following categories and numbers represent the postgraduate activities and employment of master's degree graduates: Enrolled in a postdoctoral residency/fellowship (n/a), employed in independent practice (n/a), total from the above (master's) (0).
Doctoral Degree Graduates: Of those who graduated in the academic year 2008–2009, the following categories and numbers represent the postgraduate activities and employment of doctoral degree graduates: Enrolled in a psychology doctoral program (n/a), enrolled in a postdoctoral residency/fellowship (8), employed in an academic position at a university (4), employed in business or industry (4), total from the above (doctoral) (16).

Additional Information:
Orientation, Objectives, and Emphasis of Department: Though oriented toward research and teaching, graduate training in psychology also shows concern for the applications of psychology. In addition to completing the required coursework, students in all specialty areas are expected to engage in empirical research throughout graduate study. Areas of specialization include clinical psychology, child development, adult development and aging, cognitive psychology, behavioral neuroscience, quantitative methods, and social psychology. Within the clinical science program, there are formal tracks in clinical-aging and child and family. The APA-approved clinical program incorporates the scientist–practitioner model and prepares students for careers in teaching and research, as well as in empirically-oriented applied settings.

Special Facilities or Resources: We are housed in the upper six floors of a 10-story building. Ample laboratory and office space are supplemented by facilities in the Hedco Neurosciences building that is adjacent to the main Psychology building. The Dornsife Cognitive Neuroscience Imaging Center, attached to the Psychology building, makes available a state-of-the-art fMRI imaging facility for faculty and student research.

Information for Students With Physical Disabilities: See the following Web site for more information: http://sait.usc.edu/academicsupport/centerprograms/dsp/home_index.html.

Application Information:
Send to Irene Takaragawa, Graduate Advisor, Department of Psychology/SGM 508, University of Southern California, Los Angeles, CA 90089-1061. Application available online. URL of online application: http://www.usc.edu/admission/graduate/apply/. Students are admitted in the Fall, application deadline December 1. *Fee:* $85. Indicate in online application that financial hardship waiver is requested. Applicant must also submit to the Office of Graduate and International Admissions, University of Southern California, Los Angeles, CA, 90089-0911, the most current financial aid statement from current/last school of enrollment.

Southern California, University of, Keck School of Medicine
Department of Preventive Medicine, Division of Health Behavior Research
USC/IPR, 1000 South Fremont Avenue, Unit 8
Alhambra, CA 91803
Telephone: (626) 457-6648
Fax: (626) 457-4012
E-mail: *barovich@usc.edu*
Web: *http://www.usc.edu/medicine/hbrphd*

Department Information:
1984. Director: Mary Ann Pentz. Number of faculty: total—full-time 19; women—full-time 11; total—minority—full-time 3; women minority—full-time 1.

Programs and Degrees Offered:
Listed in the following order: Program area, degree type (T if terminal Master's), number awarded 7/08–6/09. Health Behavior Research PhD (Doctor of Philosophy) 7.

Student Applications/Admissions:
Student Applications
Health Behavior Research PhD (Doctor of Philosophy)—Applications 2009–2010, 35. Total applicants accepted 2009–2010, 6. Number full-time enrolled (new admits only) 2009–2010, 7. Number part-time enrolled (new admits only) 2009–2010, 0. Openings 2010–2011, 4. The median number of years required for completion of a degree in 2008–2009 were 5. The number of students enrolled full- and part-time who were dismissed or voluntarily withdrew from this program area in 2008–2009 were 0.
Scores: Entries appear in this order: required test or GPA, minimum score (if required), median score of students entering in 2009–2010. Health Behavior Research PhD (Doctor of Philosophy): GRE-V 470, 580, GRE-Q 660, 710, overall undergraduate GPA 3.15, 3.25, Masters GPA 3.5, 3.81.

Other Criteria: (importance of criteria rated low, medium, or high): GRE scores—high, research experience—medium, work experience—low, extracurricular activity—low, GPA—high, letters of recommendation—high, interview—low, statement of goals and objectives—high, undergraduate major in psychology—low. Students are invited to interview, but interviews are not required. For additional information on admission requirements, go to http://www.usc.edu/medicine/hbrphd.

Student Characteristics: The following represents characteristics of students in 2009–2010 in all graduate psychology programs in the department: Female—full-time 28, part-time 0; Male—full-time 4, part-time 0; African American/Black—full-time 1, part-time 0; Hispanic/Latino(a)—full-time 2, part-time 0; Asian/Pacific Islander—full-time 7, part-time 0; American Indian/Alaska Native—full-time 1, part-time 0; Caucasian/White—full-time 19, part-time 0; Multi-ethnic—full-time 2, part-time 0; students subject to the Americans With Disabilities Act—full-time 0, part-time 0; Unknown ethnicity—full-time 0, part-time 0; International students who hold an F-1 or J-1 Visa—full-time 3, part-time 0.

Financial Information/Assistance:
Tuition for Full-Time Study: *Doctoral:* State residents: per academic year $21,808, $1,363 per credit hour; Nonstate residents: per academic year $21,808, $1,363 per credit hour. Tuition is subject to change.

Financial Assistance:
First-Year Students: Teaching assistantships available for first year. Average amount paid per academic year: $20,700. Average number of hours worked per week: 20. Apply by February 1. Research assistantships available for first year. Average amount paid per academic year: $20,700. Average number of hours worked per week: 20. Apply by February 1. Traineeships available for first year. Average amount paid per academic year: $20,700. Average number of hours worked per week: 20. Fellowships and scholarships available for first year. Average amount paid per academic year: $20,700. Average number of hours worked per week: 20. Apply by December 1.
Advanced Students: Teaching assistantships available for advanced students. Average amount paid per academic year: $20,700. Average number of hours worked per week: 20. Research assistantships available for advanced students. Average amount paid per academic year: $20,700. Average number of hours worked per week: 20. Traineeships available for advanced students. Average amount paid per academic year: $20,700. Average number of hours worked per week: 20. Fellowships and scholarships available for advanced students. Average amount paid per academic year: $20,700. Average number of hours worked per week: 20.
Additional Information: Of all students currently enrolled full time, 96% benefited from one or more of the listed financial assistance programs. Application and information available online at: http://www.usc.edu/admission/fa/.

Internships/Practica: Three practica in health behavior are available to doctoral students: a) prevention, b) compliance, and c) health behavior topics. Through the practica, students gain practical experience in a variety of field settings to gain a certain type of skill such as curriculum development, media production, and patient education.

Housing and Day Care: On-campus housing is available. See the following Web site for more information: http://housing.usc.edu. On-campus day care facilities are available. See the following Web site for more information: http://www.usc.edu/dept/adminops/childcare/.

Employment of Department Graduates:
  Master's Degree Graduates: Of those who graduated in the academic year 2008–2009, the following categories and numbers represent the postgraduate activities and employment of master's degree graduates: Enrolled in a postdoctoral residency/fellowship (n/a), employed in independent practice (n/a), total from the above (master's) (0).
  Doctoral Degree Graduates: Of those who graduated in the academic year 2008–2009, the following categories and numbers represent the postgraduate activities and employment of doctoral degree graduates: Enrolled in a psychology doctoral program (n/a), enrolled in a postdoctoral residency/fellowship (4), employed in independent practice (1), employed in government agency (1), employed in a hospital/medical center (1), total from the above (doctoral) (7).

Additional Information:
  Orientation, Objectives, and Emphasis of Department: The University of Southern California (USC) School of Medicine, Department of Preventive Medicine, Division of Health Behavior Research, offers a doctorate in health behavior research (HBR), providing academic and research training for students interested in pursuing career opportunities in the field of health promotion and disease prevention research. The specific objective of the program is to train exceptional researchers and scholars in the multidisciplinary field of health behavior research who will apply this knowledge creatively to the goal of primary and secondary prevention of disease. Students receive well-rounded training that encompasses theory and methods from many allied fields, including communication, psychology, preventive medicine, statistics, public health, and epidemiology. Students receive research experience participating in projects conducted through the USC Institute for Health Promotion and Disease Prevention Research (IPR). Required core courses: foundations of health behavior, data analysis, behavioral epidemiology, biological basis of disease, basic theory and strategies in prevention, basic theories and strategies for compliance/adaptation, health behavior research methods, and research seminar in health behavior. In addition to core course requirements, the curriculum includes content courses from the Department of Preventive Medicine, Divisions of Biostatistics, Epidemiology, or Occupational Medicine.

  Special Facilities or Resources: Faculty and other researchers at IPR are recognized leaders in community-based approaches to health promotion and disease prevention. The research at IPR integrates the scientific perspectives of epidemiology, the behavioral sciences, biology, communication, and policy research in disease etiology and prevention. IPR enjoys research collaborations in 10 schools and 35 departments within USC and with noted researchers and public health leaders in leading universities across the U.S., Europe, Latin America, and Asia. IPR's faculty and researchers are world leaders in school- and community-based prevention, cancer epidemiology, tobacco control, drug abuse, childhood obesity, nutrition, physical activity, cardiovascular disease, diabetes, health disparities, and health communication campaigns for chronic disease prevention. IPR has two National Institutes of Health (NIH) funded transdisciplinary research centers that integrate theories and methods across multiple disciplines to approach the complex problems of tobacco use, drug abuse, and obesity prevention within diverse communities. The USC Center for Transdisciplinary Research on Energetics and Cancer, funded by NIDDK, addresses the physiological, metabolic, behavioral, genetic, and environmental influences on obesity, metabolic health and cancer risk with a focus on minority children. And the new Comprehensive Center of Excellence in Minority Health, funded by MCMHD, focuses on understanding why obesity and associated factors increase the risk for type-2 diabetes and cardiovascular disease within minority populations. All centers also train students and faculty in transdisciplinary approaches to research.

  Information for Students With Physical Disabilities: See the following Web site for more information: http://sait.usc.edu/academicsupport/centerprograms/dsp/home_index.html.

Application Information:
Send to Doctoral Program Admissions (attn: Marny Barovich) USC/IPR, 1000 S. Fremont Avenue, Unit 8 Alhambra, CA 91803. Application available online. URL of online application: http://www.usc.edu/admission/graduate/apply/index.html. Students are admitted in the Fall, application deadline February 1. *Fee:* $85. Waivers are granted under these conditions: You are a full-time USC employee, or dependent of a full-time USC employee; You are a U.S. citizen/permanent resident, and paying the fee would cause financial hardship; You are a USC student or alumnus/alumna; You are a McNair Scholar.

Stanford University
Department of Psychology
Humanities & Sciences
450 Serra Mall, Jordan Hall, Building 420
Stanford, CA 94305-2130
Telephone: (650) 725-2400
Fax: (650) 725-5699
E-mail: *psych-info@lists.stanford.edu*
Web: *https://www.stanford.edu/dept/psychology/*

Department Information:
  1892. Chairperson: James L. McClelland. Number of faculty: total—full-time 28; women—full-time 10; total—minority—full-time 4; women minority—full-time 2.

Programs and Degrees Offered:
  Listed in the following order: Program area, degree type (T if terminal Master's), number awarded 7/08–6/09. Cognitive Psychology PhD (Doctor of Philosophy) 4, Social Psychology PhD (Doctor of Philosophy) 2, Neuroscience PhD (Doctor of Philosophy) 2, Personality Psychology PhD (Doctor of Philosophy) 3, Developmental Psychology PhD (Doctor of Philosophy) 2.

Student Applications/Admissions:
  Student Applications
    Cognitive Psychology PhD (Doctor of Philosophy)—Applications 2009–2010, 70. Total applicants accepted 2009–2010, 0. Number full-time enrolled (new admits only) 2009–2010, 0. Number part-time enrolled (new admits only) 2009–2010, 0. Openings 2010–2011, 3. The median number of years required for

completion of a degree in 2008–2009 were 5. The number of students enrolled full- and part-time who were dismissed or voluntarily withdrew from this program area in 2008–2009 were 0. *Social Psychology PhD (Doctor of Philosophy)*—Applications 2009–2010, 130. Total applicants accepted 2009–2010, 4. Number full-time enrolled (new admits only) 2009–2010, 3. Number part-time enrolled (new admits only) 2009–2010, 0. Openings 2010–2011, 3. The median number of years required for completion of a degree in 2008–2009 were 5. The number of students enrolled full- and part-time who were dismissed or voluntarily withdrew from this program area in 2008–2009 were 0. *Neuroscience PhD (Doctor of Philosophy)*—Applications 2009–2010, 50. Total applicants accepted 2009–2010, 3. Number full-time enrolled (new admits only) 2009–2010, 3. Number part-time enrolled (new admits only) 2009–2010, 0. Openings 2010–2011, 3. The median number of years required for completion of a degree in 2008–2009 were 5. The number of students enrolled full- and part-time who were dismissed or voluntarily withdrew from this program area in 2008–2009 were 0. *Personality Psychology PhD (Doctor of Philosophy)*—Applications 2009–2010, 72. Total applicants accepted 2009–2010, 3. Number full-time enrolled (new admits only) 2009–2010, 3. Number part-time enrolled (new admits only) 2009–2010, 0. Openings 2010–2011, 4. The median number of years required for completion of a degree in 2008–2009 were 5. The number of students enrolled full- and part-time who were dismissed or voluntarily withdrew from this program area in 2008–2009 were 0. *Developmental Psychology PhD (Doctor of Philosophy)*—Applications 2009–2010, 31. Total applicants accepted 2009–2010, 2. Number full-time enrolled (new admits only) 2009–2010, 2. Number part-time enrolled (new admits only) 2009–2010, 0. Openings 2010–2011, 3. The median number of years required for completion of a degree in 2008–2009 were 5. The number of students enrolled full- and part-time who were dismissed or voluntarily withdrew from this program area in 2008–2009 were 0.

Other Criteria: (importance of criteria rated low, medium, or high): GRE scores—medium, research experience—high, work experience—low, extracurricular activity—low, clinically related public service—low, GPA—high, letters of recommendation—high, interview—high, statement of goals and objectives—high, undergraduate major in psychology—low, specific undergraduate psychology courses taken—low. For additional information on admission requirements, go to http://gradadmissions.stanford.edu.

Student Characteristics: The following represents characteristics of students in 2009–2010 in all graduate psychology programs in the department: Female—full-time 52, part-time 0; Male—full-time 27, part-time 0; African American/Black—full-time 4, part-time 0; Hispanic/Latino(a)—full-time 7, part-time 0; Asian/Pacific Islander—full-time 10, part-time 0; American Indian/Alaska Native—full-time 0, part-time 0; Caucasian/White—full-time 30, part-time 0; Multi-ethnic—full-time 0, part-time 0; students subject to the Americans With Disabilities Act—full-time 0, part-time 0; Unknown ethnicity—full-time 28, part-time 0; International students who hold an F-1 or J-1 Visa—full-time 12, part-time 0.

Financial Information/Assistance:

Financial Assistance:

First-Year Students: Teaching assistantships available for first year. Average amount paid per academic year: $30,000. Average number of hours worked per week: 20. Research assistantships available for first year. Average amount paid per academic year: $30,000. Average number of hours worked per week: 20. Traineeships available for first year. Average amount paid per academic year: $30,000. Average number of hours worked per week: 20. Fellowships and scholarships available for first year. Average amount paid per academic year: $30,000. Average number of hours worked per week: 20.

Advanced Students: Teaching assistantships available for advanced students. Average amount paid per academic year: $30,000. Average number of hours worked per week: 20. Research assistantships available for advanced students. Average amount paid per academic year: $30,000. Average number of hours worked per week: 20. Traineeships available for advanced students. Average amount paid per academic year: $30,000. Average number of hours worked per week: 20. Fellowships and scholarships available for advanced students. Average amount paid per academic year: $30,000. Average number of hours worked per week: 20.

Additional Information: Of all students currently enrolled full time, 90% benefited from one or more of the listed financial assistance programs. Application and information available online at: https://www.stanford.edu/dept/psychology/.

Housing and Day Care: On-campus housing is available. See the following Web site for more information: http://studenthousing.stanford.edu/. On-campus day care facilities are available. See the following Web site for more information: http://worklife.stanford.edu/child_resource.html.

Employment of Department Graduates:

Master's Degree Graduates: Of those who graduated in the academic year 2008–2009, the following categories and numbers represent the postgraduate activities and employment of master's degree graduates: Enrolled in a postdoctoral residency/fellowship (n/a), employed in independent practice (n/a), total from the above (master's) (0).

Doctoral Degree Graduates: Of those who graduated in the academic year 2008–2009, the following categories and numbers represent the postgraduate activities and employment of doctoral degree graduates: Enrolled in a psychology doctoral program (n/a), total from the above (doctoral) (0).

Special Facilities or Resources: The department comprises facilities and personnel housed in Jordan Hall, where it maintains an extensive laboratory and shop facilities, supervised by specialized technical assistants. These facilities include laboratories for behavioral and neural (fMRI, EEG, and TMS) research. Most of the laboratories are equipped with computer terminals linked directly to the university's computer center. Others are equipped with their own computers. In addition, the department has its own computer and a computer programmer on the psychology staff. The department maintains a nursery school close to the married students' housing area. This provides a laboratory for child observation, for training in nursery school practice, and for research.

Information for Students With Physical Disabilities: See the following Web site for more information: http://www.stanford.edu/group/ORC/.

GRADUATE STUDY IN PSYCHOLOGY

Application Information:
Application available online. URL of online application: http://gradadmissions.stanford.edu. Students are admitted in the Fall, application deadline November.

Vanguard University of Southern California (2009 data)
Graduate Program in Clinical Psychology
55 Fair Drive
Costa Mesa, CA 92626
Telephone: (714) 556-3610
Fax: (714) 662-5226
E-mail: gradpsych@vanguard.edu
Web: http://www.vanguard.edu/gradpsych/

Department Information:
1998. Director: Jerre White. Number of faculty: total—full-time 2, part-time 3; women—full-time 2, part-time 1.

Programs and Degrees Offered:
Listed in the following order: Program area, degree type (T if terminal Master's), number awarded 7/08–6/09. Clinical Psychology MA/MS (Master of Arts/Science) (T) 17.

Student Applications/Admissions:
Student Applications
Clinical Psychology MA/MS (*Master of Arts/Science*)—Applications 2009–2010, 95. Total applicants accepted 2009–2010, 46. Number full-time enrolled (new admits only) 2009–2010, 18. Number part-time enrolled (new admits only) 2009–2010, 9. Total enrolled 2009–2010 full-time, 45, part-time, 21. Openings 2010–2011, 25. The median number of years required for completion of a degree in 2008–2009 were 3. The number of students enrolled full- and part-time who were dismissed or voluntarily withdrew from this program area in 2008–2009 were 5.
Other Criteria: (importance of criteria rated low, medium, or high): research experience—low, work experience—medium, extracurricular activity—low, clinically related public service—medium, GPA—high, letters of recommendation—high, interview—high, statement of goals and objectives—high, undergraduate major in psychology—low, specific undergraduate psychology courses taken—low. For additional information on admission requirements, go to http://www.vanguard.edu/GradPsych/.

Student Characteristics: The following represents characteristics of students in 2009–2010 in all graduate psychology programs in the department: Female—full-time 34, part-time 18; Male—full-time 8, part-time 8; African American/Black—full-time 2, part-time 3; Hispanic/Latino(a)—full-time 8, part-time 7; Asian/Pacific Islander—full-time 2, part-time 1; American Indian/Alaska Native—full-time 1, part-time 0; Caucasian/White—full-time 28, part-time 15; Multi-ethnic—full-time 1, part-time 0; students subject to the Americans With Disabilities Act—full-time 0, part-time 0; Unknown ethnicity—full-time 0, part-time 0; International students who hold an F-1 or J-1 Visa—full-time 0, part-time 0.

Financial Information/Assistance:
Tuition for Full-Time Study: Master's: State residents: $674 per credit hour; Nonstate residents: $674 per credit hour. Tuition is subject to change. See the following Web site for updates and changes in tuition costs: http://www.vanguard.edu/gradadmissions/.

Financial Assistance:
First-Year Students: Fellowships and scholarships available for first year. Average amount paid per academic year: $1,200. Average number of hours worked per week: 0.
Advanced Students: Teaching assistantships available for advanced students. Average amount paid per academic year: $2,400. Average number of hours worked per week: 5. Research assistantships available for advanced students. Average amount paid per academic year: $2,400. Average number of hours worked per week: 5. Fellowships and scholarships available for advanced students. Average amount paid per academic year: $2,400. Average number of hours worked per week: 5.
Additional Information: Of all students currently enrolled full time, 65% benefited from one or more of the listed financial assistance programs. Application and information available online at: http://www.vanguard.edu/gradadmissions/.

Internships/Practica: Master's Degree (MA/MS Clinical Psychology): An internship experience, such as a final research project or "capstone" experience is required of graduates. Each student is required to complete a minimum of 150 client contact hours at approved practicum sites. These sites currently include domestic violence shelters, county agencies, community clinics, and student counseling centers serving a variety of populations.

Housing and Day Care: No on-campus housing is available. No on-campus day care facilities are available.

Employment of Department Graduates:
Master's Degree Graduates: Of those who graduated in the academic year 2008–2009, the following categories and numbers represent the postgraduate activities and employment of master's degree graduates: Enrolled in a psychology doctoral program (2), enrolled in another graduate/professional program (0), enrolled in a postdoctoral residency/fellowship (n/a), employed in independent practice (n/a), employed in an academic position at a university (0), employed in an academic position at a 2-year/4-year college (0), employed in other positions at a higher education institution (1), employed in a professional position in a school system (0), employed in business or industry (2), employed in government agency (0), employed in a community mental health/counseling center (12), employed in a hospital/medical center (2), still seeking employment (0), other employment position (0), do not know (0), total from the above (master's) (19).
Doctoral Degree Graduates: Of those who graduated in the academic year 2008–2009, the following categories and numbers represent the postgraduate activities and employment of doctoral degree graduates: Enrolled in a psychology doctoral program (n/a), total from the above (doctoral) (0).

Additional Information:
Orientation, Objectives, and Emphasis of Department: Vanguard University of Southern California is a university of Christian liberal arts and sciences. It is within this faith-based context that we offer a Master of Science in Clinical Psychology degree, which

meets the educational requirements for licensure as a Marriage and Family Therapist in the state of California. The goal of the Graduate Program in Clinical Psychology is to equip its students to serve with excellence as Christian mental health professionals. Our goal is met by providing the highest quality of rigorous academic training, guided professional development, and integrative faith based learning in a collaborative and supportive environment.

Application Information:
Send to Graduate Admissions, 55 Fair Drive, Costa Mesa, CA 92626. Application available online. URL of online application: http://www.vanguard.edu/gradpsych/application/. Students are admitted in the Fall, application deadline March 1. *Fee:* $45.

Wright Institute
Graduate School of Psychology
2728 Durant Avenue
Berkeley, CA 94704
Telephone: (510) 841-9230
Fax: (510) 841-0167
E-mail: *info@wi.edu*
Web: *http://www.wi.edu*

Department Information:
1969. Dean: Charles Alexander, PhD. Number of faculty: total—full-time 13, part-time 48; women—full-time 10, part-time 23; total—minority—full-time 5, part-time 5; women minority—full-time 5, part-time 4; faculty subject to the Americans With Disabilities Act 5.

Programs and Degrees Offered:
Listed in the following order: Program area, degree type (T if terminal Master's), number awarded 7/08–6/09. Clinical Psychology PsyD (Doctor of Psychology) 48.

APA Accreditation: Clinical PsyD (Doctor of Psychology).

Student Applications/Admissions:
Student Applications
Clinical Psychology PsyD (Doctor of Psychology)—Applications 2009–2010, 308. Total applicants accepted 2009–2010, 120. Number full-time enrolled (new admits only) 2009–2010, 59. Number part-time enrolled (new admits only) 2009–2010, 0. Openings 2010–2011, 58. The median number of years required for completion of a degree in 2008–2009 were 5. The number of students enrolled full- and part-time who were dismissed or voluntarily withdrew from this program area in 2008–2009 were 4.
Other Criteria: (importance of criteria rated low, medium, or high): GRE scores—medium, research experience—medium, work experience—medium, extracurricular activity—medium, clinically related public service—high, GPA—high, letters of recommendation—high, interview—high, statement of goals and objectives—high, specific undergraduate psychology courses taken—high. For additional information on admission requirements, go to http://www.wi.edu/admissions_faqs.html.

Student Characteristics: The following represents characteristics of students in 2009–2010 in all graduate psychology programs in the department: Female—full-time 232, part-time 0; Male—full-time 99, part-time 0; African American/Black—full-time 12, part-time 0; Hispanic/Latino(a)—full-time 25, part-time 0; Asian/Pacific Islander—full-time 28, part-time 0; American Indian/Alaska Native—full-time 2, part-time 0; Caucasian/White—full-time 244, part-time 0; Multi-ethnic—full-time 18, part-time 0; students subject to the Americans With Disabilities Act—full-time 4, part-time 0; Unknown ethnicity—full-time 2, part-time 0; International students who hold an F-1 or J-1 Visa—full-time 5, part-time 0.

Financial Information/Assistance:
Tuition for Full-Time Study: *Doctoral:* State residents: per academic year $25,550; Nonstate residents: per academic year $25,550. Tuition is subject to change. See the following Web site for updates and changes in tuition costs: http://www.wi.edu/admissions_tuition.html.

Financial Assistance:
First-Year Students: Research assistantships available for first year. Average amount paid per academic year: $1,700. Average number of hours worked per week: 4.
Advanced Students: Teaching assistantships available for advanced students. Average amount paid per academic year: $2,200. Average number of hours worked per week: 5. Research assistantships available for advanced students. Average amount paid per academic year: $2,200. Average number of hours worked per week: 5. Fellowships and scholarships available for advanced students. Average amount paid per academic year: $2,000. Apply by December 4.
Additional Information: Of all students currently enrolled full time, 44% benefited from one or more of the listed financial assistance programs. Application and information available online at: http://www.wi.edu/admissions_aid.html.

Internships/Practica: Doctoral Degree (PsyD Clinical Psychology): For those doctoral students for whom a professional internship was required in this program prior to graduation, (63) students applied for an internship in 2008–2009, with (59) students obtaining an internship. Of those students who obtained an internship, (39) were paid internships. Of those students who obtained an internship, (17) students placed in APA/CPA accredited internships, (8) students placed in internships not APA/CPA accredited, but listed with the Association of Psychology Postdoctoral and Internship Programs (APPIC), (0) students placed in internships conforming to guidelines of the Council of Directors of School Psychology Programs (CDSPP), (34) students placed in internships that were not APA/CPA accredited, APPIC or CDSPP listed. Through three years of practicum plus the internship, the Institute's field training program prepares students to integrate the knowledge base of psychology with clinical experience while working in a variety of roles. Beginning with the first-year practicum, students work with a range of clinical populations, treatment modalities, and train in a variety of clinical settings serving the ethno-culturally diverse populations of the San Francisco Bay Area. The Field Placement Office furnishes information and support to students in the practicum and internship application process, and students are encouraged to attend APA-approved internships. The Bay Area has an established community of internship agencies, which are members of the California Psychology Internship Council (CAPIC). California licensing recognizes as a formal internship a program that is accredited by the APA or that is a member of APPIC or CAPIC. Because many students are established residents of the Bay Area, the Wright Institute approves internships at APPIC and CAPIC member programs. Our internship match rate is comparable to the national rate for students applying throughout the nation for APA internships, and Wright Institute students are valued by the nation's most well-regarded internship sites and local Bay Area hospitals, clinics, and community health and mental health centers.

Housing and Day Care: No on-campus housing is available. No on-campus day care facilities are available.

Employment of Department Graduates:
Master's Degree Graduates: Of those who graduated in the academic year 2008–2009, the following categories and numbers represent the postgraduate activities and employment of master's degree graduates: Enrolled in a psychology doctoral program (0), enrolled in a postdoctoral residency/fellowship (n/a), employed in independent practice (n/a), total from the above (master's) (0).
Doctoral Degree Graduates: Of those who graduated in the academic year 2008–2009, the following categories and numbers represent the postgraduate activities and employment of doctoral degree graduates: Enrolled in a psychology doctoral program (n/a), enrolled in another graduate/professional program (0), enrolled in a postdoctoral residency/fellowship (19), employed in independent practice (4), employed in an academic position at a university (2), employed in an academic position at a 2-year/4-year college (0), employed in other positions at a higher education institution (3), employed in a professional position in a school system (0), employed in business or industry (1), employed in government agency (0), employed in a community mental health/counseling center (5), employed in a hospital/medical center (2), still seeking employment (5), not seeking employment (3), other employment position (0), do not know (5), total from the above (doctoral) (49).

Additional Information:
Orientation, Objectives, and Emphasis of Department: The Wright Institute teaches the scientific knowledge base of clinical psychology, preparing students to think rigorously and critically. Students learn to apply critical thinking skills to three fundamental areas: clinical theory and research, understanding of the self in social context, and appreciation of the interaction between clinician and client. Students are exposed to a number of clinical orientations while learning to explore the meanings of their experiences and actions with clients. This unique learning method enables students to formulate and address clinical problems by examining the lenses through which they filter experience. Coursework is integrated with rigorous practical experience, providing for the systematic, progressive acquisition of skills and knowledge. Students actively participate in case conferences/professional development seminars over the full three years of residency. The weekly, three-hour small-group seminars provide a rich forum for developing and integrating theory, technique, and reflective judgment. Practica and internship experiences consolidate the applied aspects of scientific knowledge. Education about the multiple roles of the modern psychologist clinician, supervisor, consultant and advocate prepares students for working in fulfilling ways amid the changing realities of the healthcare field. We expect our graduates not only to become excellent clinicians but also to assume roles in which they can exhibit clinical leadership.

Special Facilities or Resources: The Wright Institute has traditional low fee psychotherapy clinics as well as innovative programs in schools and primary care facilities. The Institute's psychodynamically oriented clinic has been in operation for over 35 years, and the Institute recently opened clinics focusing on 1) CBT treatment, and 2) addiction recovery. The Wright Institute's School-Based Collaboration program enables students to work with students, teachers and parents in communities challenged by violence, discrimination and poverty. Our approach is to tackle the severe non-academic barriers to learning by viewing the school community as a whole, and collaborating to identify key needs and deliver relevant services. In the Institute's Integrated Health Psychology Training Program students learn primary care health psychology and perform as part of a multidisciplinary team, addressing the lifestyle and behavioral components contributing to poor health, and treating the co-occurring psychological disorders many patients experience. Through these clinics and programs, the Institute educates students to apply psychological knowledge and skills, not just to work with the problems and dysfunctions of underserved populations, but also to appreciate and cultivate those populations' strengths and aspirations. In so doing our students build a deeper multicultural perspective grounded in their own developing experience.

Application Information:
Send to Admissions Director, The Wright Institute, 2728 Durant Avenue, Berkeley, CA 94704. Application available online. URL of online application: http://www.wi.edu/admissions.html. Students are admitted in the Fall, application deadline January 15. *Fee:* $50.

COLORADO

Colorado State University
Department of Psychology
Natural Sciences
200 West Lake Street, 1876 Campus Delivery
Fort Collins, CO 80523-1876
Telephone: (970) 491-6363
Fax: (970) 491-1032
E-mail: *ernest.chavez@colostate.edu*
Web: *http://www.colostate.edu/Depts/Psychology/*

Department Information:
1962. Chairperson: Ernest L. Chavez. Number of faculty: total—full-time 32, part-time 3; women—full-time 17, part-time 2; total—minority—full-time 3; women minority—full-time 1.

Programs and Degrees Offered:
Listed in the following order: Program area, degree type (T if terminal Master's), number awarded 7/08–6/09. Counseling Psychology PhD (Doctor of Philosophy) 6, Industrial/Organizational Psychology PhD (Doctor of Philosophy) 5, Cognitive Psychology PhD (Doctor of Philosophy) 0, Applied Social Psychology PhD (Doctor of Philosophy) 5, Perceptual and Brain Science PhD (Doctor of Philosophy) 0.

APA Accreditation: Counseling PhD (Doctor of Philosophy). Student Outcome Data Website: http://www.colostate.edu/Depts/Psychology/counseling/FAQ.shtml.

Student Applications/Admissions:

Student Applications

Counseling Psychology PhD (Doctor of Philosophy)—Applications 2009–2010, 192. Total applicants accepted 2009–2010, 9. Number full-time enrolled (new admits only) 2009–2010, 5. Number part-time enrolled (new admits only) 2009–2010, 0. Total enrolled 2009–2010 full-time, 31, part-time, 12. Openings 2010–2011, 5. The median number of years required for completion of a degree in 2008–2009 were 6. The number of students enrolled full- and part-time who were dismissed or voluntarily withdrew from this program area in 2008–2009 were 0. *Industrial/Organizational Psychology PhD (Doctor of Philosophy)*—Applications 2009–2010, 58. Total applicants accepted 2009–2010, 10. Number full-time enrolled (new admits only) 2009–2010, 5. Number part-time enrolled (new admits only) 2009–2010, 0. Total enrolled 2009–2010 full-time, 17, part-time, 5. Openings 2010–2011, 5. The median number of years required for completion of a degree in 2008–2009 were 5. The number of students enrolled full- and part-time who were dismissed or voluntarily withdrew from this program area in 2008–2009 were 0. *Cognitive Psychology PhD (Doctor of Philosophy)*—Applications 2009–2010, 32. Total applicants accepted 2009–2010, 4. Number full-time enrolled (new admits only) 2009–2010, 1. Number part-time enrolled (new admits only) 2009–2010, 0. Openings 2010–2011, 2. The median number of years required for completion of a degree in 2008–2009 were 5. The number of students enrolled full- and part-time who were dismissed or voluntarily withdrew from this program area in 2008–2009 were 0. *Applied Social Psychology PhD (Doctor of Philosophy)*—Applications 2009–2010, 61. Total applicants accepted 2009–2010, 1. Number full-time enrolled (new admits only) 2009–2010, 1. Number part-time enrolled (new admits only) 2009–2010, 0. Total enrolled 2009–2010 full-time, 9, part-time, 7. Openings 2010–2011, 2. The median number of years required for completion of a degree in 2008–2009 were 5. The number of students enrolled full- and part-time who were dismissed or voluntarily withdrew from this program area in 2008–2009 were 0. *Perceptual and Brain Science PhD (Doctor of Philosophy)*—Applications 2009–2010, 29. Total applicants accepted 2009–2010, 1. Number full-time enrolled (new admits only) 2009–2010, 1. Number part-time enrolled (new admits only) 2009–2010, 0. Total enrolled 2009–2010 full-time, 6, part-time, 1. Openings 2010–2011, 2. The median number of years required for completion of a degree in 2008–2009 were 5. The number of students enrolled full- and part-time who were dismissed or voluntarily withdrew from this program area in 2008–2009 were 0.

Scores: Entries appear in this order: required test or GPA, minimum score (if required), median score of students entering in 2009–2010. *Counseling Psychology PhD (Doctor of Philosophy)*: GRE-V 500, GRE-Q 560, overall undergraduate GPA 3.6; *Industrial/Organizational Psychology PhD (Doctor of Philosophy)*: GRE-V 500, GRE-Q 560, overall undergraduate GPA 3.6; *Cognitive Psychology PhD (Doctor of Philosophy)*: GRE-V 500, GRE-Q 560, overall undergraduate GPA 3.6; *Applied Social Psychology PhD (Doctor of Philosophy)*: GRE-V 500, GRE-Q 560, overall undergraduate GPA 3.6; *Perceptual and Brain Science PhD (Doctor of Philosophy)*: GRE-V 500, GRE-Q 560, overall undergraduate GPA 3.6.

Other Criteria: (importance of criteria rated low, medium, or high): GRE scores—medium, research experience—high, work experience—medium, extracurricular activity—medium, clinically related public service—medium, GPA—high, letters of recommendation—high, statement of goals and objectives—high, undergraduate major in psychology—low, specific undergraduate psychology courses taken—medium. Scientific writing sample required by Applied Social and Industrial/Organizational Programs; optional for Cognitive. For additional information on admission requirements, go to http://www.colostate.edu/Depts/Psychology/students/grad_apply.shtml.

Student Characteristics: The following represents characteristics of students in 2009–2010 in all graduate psychology programs in the department: Female—full-time 53, part-time 18; Male—full-time 26, part-time 7; African American/Black—full-time 1, part-time 0; Hispanic/Latino(a)—full-time 4, part-time 2; Asian/Pacific Islander—full-time 6, part-time 1; American Indian/Alaska Native—full-time 4, part-time 2; Caucasian/White—full-time 58, part-time 20; Multi-ethnic—full-time 5, part-time 2; students subject to the Americans With Disabilities Act—full-time 0, part-time 0; Unknown ethnicity—full-time 0, part-time 0; International students who hold an F-1 or J-1 Visa—full-time 1, part-time 1.

Financial Information/Assistance:
Tuition for Full-Time Study: *Doctoral:* State residents: per academic year $6,464, $442 per credit hour; Nonstate residents: per

academic year $18,116, $1,089 per credit hour. Tuition is subject to change. Additional fees are assessed to students beyond the costs of tuition for the following: general fees - $718, university technology fee - $20, university facility fee - $10/credit hour. See the following Web site for updates and changes in tuition costs: http://registrar.colostate.edu/students/tuitionfees/index.aspx.

Financial Assistance:
First-Year Students: Teaching assistantships available for first year. Average amount paid per academic year: $12,330. Average number of hours worked per week: 20. Apply by January 15. Research assistantships available for first year. Average amount paid per academic year: $12,330. Average number of hours worked per week: 20. Apply by January 15. Fellowships and scholarships available for first year. Average amount paid per academic year: $1,600. Average number of hours worked per week: 0. Apply by January 15.

Advanced Students: Teaching assistantships available for advanced students. Average amount paid per academic year: $12,650. Average number of hours worked per week: 20. Apply by January 15. Research assistantships available for advanced students. Average amount paid per academic year: $12,650. Average number of hours worked per week: 20. Apply by January 15. Traineeships available for advanced students. Fellowships and scholarships available for advanced students. Average amount paid per academic year: $0. Average number of hours worked per week: 0. Apply by January 15.

Additional Information: Of all students currently enrolled full time, 98% benefited from one or more of the listed financial assistance programs. Application and information available online at: http://graduateschool.colostate.edu/financial-resources/.

Internships/Practica: Doctoral Degree (PhD Counseling Psychology): For those doctoral students for whom a professional internship was required in this program prior to graduation, (10) students applied for an internship in 2008–2009, with (10) students obtaining an internship. Of those students who obtained an internship, (10) were paid internships. Of those students who obtained an internship, (10) students placed in APA/CPA accredited internships, (0) students placed in internships not APA/CPA accredited, but listed with the Association of Psychology Postdoctoral and Internship Programs (APPIC), (0) students placed in internships conforming to guidelines of the Council of Directors of School Psychology Programs (CDSPP), (0) students placed in internships that were not APA/CPA accredited, APPIC or CDSPP listed. There are a number of related practica for counseling students throughout Northern Colorado. The following are examples: neuropsychology, local community college, primary health care, and school districts. Industrial/Organizational students consult with a variety of businesses throughout the state including: United Airlines, HP, Sun Systems, IBM, microbreweries and hospitals. The Tri Ethnic Center for Prevention Research (TEC) and the Colorado Injury Control Research Center (CICRC) are a part of the department. The Institute of Applied Prevention Research was designated a Center of Research and Scholarly Excellence by the University in 2008.

Housing and Day Care: On-campus housing is available. See the following Web site for more information: http://www.housing.colostate.edu/. On-campus day care facilities are available. See the following Web site for more information: http://www.csukids.colostate.edu/.

Employment of Department Graduates:
Master's Degree Graduates: Of those who graduated in the academic year 2008–2009, the following categories and numbers represent the postgraduate activities and employment of master's degree graduates: Enrolled in a psychology doctoral program (0), enrolled in another graduate/professional program (0), enrolled in a postdoctoral residency/fellowship (n/a), employed in independent practice (n/a), employed in an academic position at a university (0), employed in an academic position at a 2-year/4-year college (0), employed in other positions at a higher education institution (0), employed in a professional position in a school system (0), employed in business or industry (0), employed in government agency (0), employed in a community mental health/counseling center (0), employed in a hospital/medical center (0), still seeking employment (0), not seeking employment (0), other employment position (0), do not know (0), total from the above (master's) (0).

Doctoral Degree Graduates: Of those who graduated in the academic year 2008–2009, the following categories and numbers represent the postgraduate activities and employment of doctoral degree graduates: Enrolled in a psychology doctoral program (n/a), enrolled in another graduate/professional program (0), enrolled in a postdoctoral residency/fellowship (2), employed in independent practice (0), employed in an academic position at a university (2), employed in an academic position at a 2-year/4-year college (1), employed in other positions at a higher education institution (0), employed in a professional position in a school system (1), employed in business or industry (4), employed in government agency (0), employed in a community mental health/counseling center (1), employed in a hospital/medical center (5), still seeking employment (0), not seeking employment (0), other employment position (0), do not know (1), total from the above (doctoral) (17).

Additional Information:
Orientation, Objectives, and Emphasis of Department: Colorado State University offers graduate training leading to the MS and PhD degrees in applied social, cognitive, counseling, industrial/organizational psychology and perceptual and brain science. A core program of study is required of all students in the first years of graduate work to insure a broad and thorough grounding in psychology. Graduate students in applied social, cognitive and behavioral neuroscience areas take positions in academic, research, or government agencies. Industrial/Organizational has opportunities for students to have experiences in selection techniques, occupational health psychology, assessment centers, organizational climate and structure, and consultation. Counseling students are trained in academic and applied skills with opportunities in behavior therapy, group techniques, assessment, outreach, consultation, and supervision. Emphasis is on diversity and breadth. In addition to the adult specialty, a program is available that will lead to a PhD in counseling psychology with advanced courses that deal with children and adolescents.

Special Facilities or Resources: Tri Ethnic Center for Prevention research, a NIDA, CDC and Justice Department funded research center, focuses on adolescent issues such as substance use, violence, rural issues, and culturally appropriate prevention strategies. The CICR is currently in year 2 of a 5 year second cycle of funding by the CDC and the National Center for Injury Prevention and Control. CICR's focus is to address the prevention and control of injuries among rural and under-served populations. The Institute for Applied Prevention Research (IAPR), which is a Diversity Program of Research and Scholarly Excellence, is the umbrella group for a number of centers including Tri-Ethnic, CICRC, CFERT and CoAMP.

Information for Students With Physical Disabilities: See the following Web site for more information: http://www.rds.colostate.edu/.

Application Information:
Send to Graduate Admissions Committee, Department of Psychology, Colorado State University 1876 Campus Delivery Fort Collins, CO 80526-1876. Application available online. URL of online application: http://www.colostate.edu/Depts/Psychology/students/grad_apply.shtml. Students are admitted in the Fall, application deadline December 15. Counseling - December 15 application deadline. Industrial/Organizational - January 1 application deadline. Applied Social, Cognitive, Perceptual and Brain Sciences - January 15 application deadline. *Fee:* $50. Fee is waived for McNair, Fulbright, Peace Corps, Project 1000.

Colorado, University of, at Colorado Springs
Department of Psychology
Letters, Arts, and Sciences
1420 Austin Bluffs Parkway, P.O. Box 7150
Colorado Springs, CO 80933-7150
Telephone: (719) 255-4500
Fax: (719) 255-4166
E-mail: *kklebe@uccs.edu*
Web: *http://www.uccs.edu/psych*

Department Information:
1965. Chairperson: Dr. Kelli Klebe. Number of faculty: total—full-time 16, part-time 13; women—full-time 8, part-time 8; minority—part-time 1; women minority—full-time 1, part-time 1.

Programs and Degrees Offered:
Listed in the following order: Program area, degree type (T if terminal Master's), number awarded 7/08–6/09. Clinical Psychology MA/MS (Master of Arts/Science) (T) 5, General Experimental Psychology MA/MS (Master of Arts/Science) (T) 3, Clinical Psychology PhD (Doctor of Philosophy) 1.

APA Accreditation: Clinical PhD (Doctor of Philosophy).

Student Applications/Admissions:
Student Applications
Clinical Psychology MA/MS (*Master of Arts/Science*)—Applications 2009–2010, 44. Total applicants accepted 2009–2010, 16. Number full-time enrolled (new admits only) 2009–2010, 7. Number part-time enrolled (new admits only) 2009–2010, 0. Openings 2010–2011, 12. The median number of years required for completion of a degree in 2008–2009 were 2. The number of students enrolled full- and part-time who were dismissed or voluntarily withdrew from this program area in 2008–2009 were 0. General Experimental Psychology MA/MS (*Master of Arts/Science*)—Applications 2009–2010, 17. Total applicants accepted 2009–2010, 11. Number full-time enrolled (new admits only) 2009–2010, 5. Total enrolled 2009–2010 full-time, 12. Openings 2010–2011, 5. The median number of years required for completion of a degree in 2008–2009 were 2. The number of students enrolled full- and part-time who were dismissed or voluntarily withdrew from this program area in 2008–2009 were 0. Clinical Psychology PhD (*Doctor of Philosophy*)—Applications 2009–2010, 31. Total applicants accepted 2009–2010, 4. Number full-time enrolled (new admits only) 2009–2010, 3. Openings 2010–2011, 3. The number of students enrolled full- and part-time who were dismissed or voluntarily withdrew from this program area in 2008–2009 were 0.

Scores: Entries appear in this order: required test or GPA, minimum score (if required), median score of students entering in 2009–2010. Clinical Psychology MA/MS (*Master of Arts/Science*): GRE-V no minimum stated, 547, GRE-Q no minimum stated, 598, GRE-Analytical no minimum stated, overall undergraduate GPA no minimum stated, 3.54, psychology GPA no minimum stated; General Experimental Psychology MA/MS (*Master of Arts/Science*): GRE-V no minimum stated, 547, GRE-Q no minimum stated, 598, GRE-Analytical no minimum stated, overall undergraduate GPA no minimum stated, 3.54; Clinical Psychology PhD (*Doctor of Philosophy*): GRE-V no minimum stated, GRE-Q no minimum stated, GRE-Analytical no minimum stated, overall undergraduate GPA no minimum stated.

Other Criteria: (importance of criteria rated low, medium, or high): GRE scores—medium, research experience—high, work experience—low, extracurricular activity—medium, clinically related public service—high, GPA—medium, letters of recommendation—high, interview—high, statement of goals and objectives—high, undergraduate major in psychology—low, specific undergraduate psychology courses taken—high. For the experimental MA program, clinically related public service is not required. Interviews are only for applicants to the doctoral program. MA students do not need to complete an interview as part of the application process. For additional information on admission requirements, go to http://www.uccs.edu/psych.

Student Characteristics: The following represents characteristics of students in 2009–2010 in all graduate psychology programs in the department: Female—full-time 40, part-time 0; Male—full-time 11, part-time 0; African American/Black—full-time 2, part-time 0; Hispanic/Latino(a)—full-time 1, part-time 0; Asian/Pacific Islander—full-time 2, part-time 0; American Indian/Alaska Native—full-time 0, part-time 0; Caucasian/White—full-time 46, part-time 0; Multi-ethnic—full-time 0, part-time 0; students subject to the Americans With Disabilities Act—full-time 0, part-time 0; Unknown ethnicity—full-time 0, part-time 0; International students who hold an F-1 or J-1 Visa—full-time 0, part-time 0.

Financial Information/Assistance:
Tuition for Full-Time Study: *Master's:* State residents: $601 per credit hour; Nonstate residents: $1,093 per credit hour. *Doctoral:* State residents: $601 per credit hour; Nonstate residents: $1,093 per credit hour. Tuition is subject to change. Additional fees are assessed to students beyond the costs of tuition for the following: university set fees; psychology program fee. Tuition costs vary by program. See the following Web site for updates and changes in tuition costs: http://www.uccs.edu/~burgan/pages/tuition.shtml.

Financial Assistance:

First-Year Students: Teaching assistantships available for first year. Research assistantships available for first year. Fellowships and scholarships available for first year.

Advanced Students: Teaching assistantships available for advanced students. Research assistantships available for advanced students. Fellowships and scholarships available for advanced students.

Additional Information: Of all students currently enrolled full time, 65% benefited from one or more of the listed financial assistance programs. Application and information available online at: http://www.uccs.edu/~finaid/.

Internships/Practica: Doctoral Degree (PhD Clinical Psychology): For those doctoral students for whom a professional internship was required in this program prior to graduation, (4) students applied for an internship in 2008–2009, with (4) students obtaining an internship. Of those students who obtained an internship, (4) were paid internships. Of those students who obtained an internship, (4) students placed in APA/CPA accredited internships, (0) students placed in internships not APA/CPA accredited, but listed with the Association of Psychology Postdoctoral and Internship Programs (APPIC), (0) students placed in internships conforming to guidelines of the Council of Directors of School Psychology Programs (CDSPP), (0) students placed in internships that were not APA/CPA accredited, APPIC or CDSPP listed. Master's Degree (MA/MS Clinical Psychology): An internship experience, such as a final research project or "capstone" experience is required of graduates. Master's Degree (MA/MS General Experimental Psychology): An internship experience, such as a final research project or "capstone" experience is required of graduates. Required practicum experiences for MA and PhD students are completed at the departmental CU Aging Center, the CU Counseling Center, or in community placements under licensed supervision (e.g., school settings, community health centers, state mental health facility, domestic violence center, inpatient psychiatric hospital). The goal of these experiences is to expose students to clinical settings, to roles of clinical psychologists, and to begin the development of clinical skills.

Housing and Day Care: On-campus housing is available. See the following Web site for more information: http://www.uccs.edu/~residence/. On-campus day care facilities are available. See the following Web site for more information: http://www.uccs.edu/~fdc/.

Employment of Department Graduates:

Master's Degree Graduates: Of those who graduated in the academic year 2008–2009, the following categories and numbers represent the postgraduate activities and employment of master's degree graduates: Enrolled in a postdoctoral residency/fellowship (n/a), employed in independent practice (n/a), total from the above (master's) (0).

Doctoral Degree Graduates: Of those who graduated in the academic year 2008–2009, the following categories and numbers represent the postgraduate activities and employment of doctoral degree graduates: Enrolled in a psychology doctoral program (n/a), total from the above (doctoral) (0).

Additional Information:

Orientation, Objectives, and Emphasis of Department: The MA program places special emphasis in general areas of applied clinical practice and general experimental psychology. The MA training will enable a student to prepare for a doctoral program, teach in community colleges, work under a licensed psychologist in private and public agencies, work in university counseling centers, or work as a researcher in a variety of organizations. A research thesis is required of all students. There is a broad range of faculty research interests including: aging (e.g., psychopathology and psychological treatment of older adults, family dynamics, self-concept development, memory, cognition, and personality), social psychology, psychology and the law, personality, program evaluation, prevention of child abuse, adolescent psychology and psychological trauma. There are optional tracks for Psychology and Law, Trauma Psychology, Cognitive Psychology, or Developmental Psychology for Masters students. The accredited clinical PhD program has an emphasis in parapsychology.

Special Facilities or Resources: Research facilities include clinical training laboratories with observational capabilities, laboratories for individual and small group research, and a psychophysiological laboratory. Columbine Hall houses a 50-station computer lab that is available for general use. The CU Aging Center, administered through the Psychology Department, is a community-based nonprofit mental health clinic designed to serve the mental health needs of older adults and their families. The mission of the Center is to provide state-of-the-art psychological assessment and treatment services to older persons and their families, to study psychological aging processes, and to train students in clinical psychology and related disciplines.

Application Information:
Send to Dr. Michael Kisley, Director of Graduate Studies/Psychology Department. Application available online. URL of online application: http://www.uccs.edu/gradschl/app/. Students are admitted in the Fall, application deadline January 1. *Fee:* $60. International Application Fee: $75.

Colorado, University of, Boulder
Department of Psychology and Neuroscience
Arts and Sciences
Muenzinger D244, UCB 345
Boulder, CO 80309-0345
Telephone: (303) 492-8662
Fax: (303) 492-2967
E-mail: *asst.to.chair@psych.Colorado.EDU*
Web: *http://psych.colorado.edu*

Department Information:
1910. Chairperson: Lewis O. Harvey, Jr. Number of faculty: total—full-time 45; women—full-time 16; total—minority—full-time 7; women minority—full-time 5.

Programs and Degrees Offered:
Listed in the following order: Program area, degree type (T if terminal Master's), number awarded 7/08–6/09. Social Psychology PhD (Doctor of Philosophy) 3, Behavioral Genetics PhD (Doctor of Philosophy) 1, Behavioral Neuroscience PhD (Doctor of Philosophy) 5, Clinical Psychology PhD (Doctor of Philosophy) 7, Cognitive Psychology PhD (Doctor of Philosophy) 2.

APA Accreditation: Clinical PhD (Doctor of Philosophy). Student Outcome Data Website: http://psych.colorado.edu/~clinical/disclosure-descending.html.

Student Applications/Admissions:
Student Applications
Social Psychology PhD (Doctor of Philosophy)—Number full-time enrolled (new admits only) 2009–2010, 5. Openings 2010–2011, 1. The median number of years required for completion of a degree in 2008–2009 were 5. The number of students enrolled full- and part-time who were dismissed or voluntarily withdrew from this program area in 2008–2009 were 0. *Behavioral Genetics PhD (Doctor of Philosophy)*—Number full-time enrolled (new admits only) 2009–2010, 3. Openings 2010–2011, 1. The median number of years required for completion of a degree in 2008–2009 were 5. *Behavioral Neuroscience PhD (Doctor of Philosophy)*—Number full-time enrolled (new admits only) 2009–2010, 4. The median number of years required for completion of a degree in 2008–2009 were 5. The number of students enrolled full- and part-time who were dismissed or voluntarily withdrew from this program area in 2008–2009 were 0. *Clinical Psychology PhD (Doctor of Philosophy)*—Applications 2009–2010, 198. Total applicants accepted 2009–2010, 6. Number full-time enrolled (new admits only) 2009–2010, 4. The median number of years required for completion of a degree in 2008–2009 were 6. The number of students enrolled full- and part-time who were dismissed or voluntarily withdrew from this program area in 2008–2009 were 0. *Cognitive Psychology PhD (Doctor of Philosophy)*—Number full-time enrolled (new admits only) 2009–2010, 3. Total enrolled 2009–2010 full-time, 24. Openings 2010–2011, 4. The median number of years required for completion of a degree in 2008–2009 were 5. The number of students enrolled full- and part-time who were dismissed or voluntarily withdrew from this program area in 2008–2009 were 0.

Other Criteria: (importance of criteria rated low, medium, or high): GRE scores—high, research experience—high, work experience—medium, extracurricular activity—medium, clinically related public service—medium, GPA—high, letters of recommendation—high, interview—high, statement of goals and objectives—high. Clinical work experience is only relevant in clinical program. Research experience is critical to admissions to all programs. For additional information on admission requirements, go to http://psych.colorado.edu.

Student Characteristics: The following represents characteristics of students in 2009–2010 in all graduate psychology programs in the department: Female—full-time 58, part-time 0; Male—full-time 40, part-time 0; African American/Black—full-time 1, part-time 0; Hispanic/Latino(a)—full-time 3, part-time 0; Asian/Pacific Islander—full-time 1, part-time 0; American Indian/Alaska Native—full-time 2, part-time 0; Caucasian/White—full-time 89, part-time 0; Multi-ethnic—full-time 2, part-time 0; students subject to the Americans With Disabilities Act—full-time 1, part-time 0; Unknown ethnicity—full-time 0, part-time 0; International students who hold an F-1 or J-1 Visa—full-time 0, part-time 0.

Financial Information/Assistance:
Financial Assistance:
First-Year Students: Teaching assistantships available for first year. Average amount paid per academic year: $15,284. Average number of hours worked per week: 20. Research assistantships available for first year. Average amount paid per academic year: $15,284. Average number of hours worked per week: 20. Traineeships available for first year. Average amount paid per academic year: $20,000. Average number of hours worked per week: 20. Fellowships and scholarships available for first year.

Advanced Students: Teaching assistantships available for advanced students. Average amount paid per academic year: $15,284. Average number of hours worked per week: 20. Research assistantships available for advanced students. Average amount paid per academic year: $15,284. Average number of hours worked per week: 20. Traineeships available for advanced students. Average amount paid per academic year: $20,000. Average number of hours worked per week: 20. Fellowships and scholarships available for advanced students.

Additional Information: Of all students currently enrolled full time, 98% benefited from one or more of the listed financial assistance programs.

Internships/Practica: Doctoral Degree (PhD Clinical Psychology): For those doctoral students for whom a professional internship was required in this program prior to graduation, (4) students applied for an internship in 2008–2009, with (4) students obtaining an internship. Of those students who obtained an internship, (4) were paid internships. Of those students who obtained an internship, (4) students placed in APA/CPA accredited internships, (0) students placed in internships not APA/CPA accredited, but listed with the Association of Psychology Postdoctoral and Internship Programs (APPIC), (0) students placed in internships conforming to guidelines of the Council of Directors of School Psychology Programs (CDSPP), (0) students placed in internships that were not APA/CPA accredited, APPIC or CDSPP listed.

Housing and Day Care: On-campus housing is available. See the following Web site for more information: http://housing.colorado.edu. On-campus day care facilities are available. See the following Web site for more information: http://housing.colorado.edu/fh/fh_childrens_center.cfm.

Employment of Department Graduates:
Master's Degree Graduates: Of those who graduated in the academic year 2008–2009, the following categories and numbers represent the postgraduate activities and employment of master's degree graduates: Enrolled in a psychology doctoral program (3), enrolled in a postdoctoral residency/fellowship (n/a), employed in independent practice (n/a), total from the above (master's) (3).
Doctoral Degree Graduates: Of those who graduated in the academic year 2008–2009, the following categories and numbers represent the postgraduate activities and employment of doctoral degree graduates: Enrolled in a psychology doctoral program (n/a), enrolled in a postdoctoral residency/fellowship (4), employed in an academic position at a university (0), employed in an academic position at a 2-year/4-year college (1), employed in other positions at a higher education institution (5), employed in a community mental health/counseling center (1), do not know (2), total from the above (doctoral) (13).

Additional Information:
Orientation, Objectives, and Emphasis of Department: Our emphasis is on training graduate students who have the capability to advance knowledge in the field, and who are committed to

applying their knowledge. We emphasize rigorous training in both the theory and methods of psychological research.

Special Facilities or Resources: The department is housed in a large and modern four-story building that contains ample space for offices, a clinic, and research laboratories. There are extensive research facilities available to students, both in individual laboratories and from the department generally. The department maintains its own network of Macintosh, Linux, and Windows computers used for data collection, data analysis, and manuscript preparation. There is also a departmental laboratory of Macintosh and DOS personal computers for real-time data collection. In addition, numerous laboratories in the department have their own computing capabilities. The facilities of the Institute of Behavioral Genetics, the Institute of Behavioral Science, the Institute of Cognitive Science and the Center for Neuroscience are available to students. Each of these institutes has its own laboratory space and specialized computer facilities. In addition, they attract a number of scholars from other disciplines on the campus.

Information for Students With Physical Disabilities: See the following Web site for more information: http://www.colorado.edu/disabilityservices/.

Application Information:
Send to Department of Psychology and Neuroscience, Muenzinger Psychology Building, UCB 345, Boulder, CO 80309-0345. Application available online. URL of online application: http://psych.colorado.edu/grad-appinfo.html. Students are admitted in the Fall, application deadline December 15*. *Clinical and Social areas only; Behavioral Neuroscience, Behavioral Genetics and Cognitive areas have a deadline of January 1. *Fee:* $50. $70 Foreign Students.

Colorado, University of, Denver
Department of Psychology
College of Liberal Arts and Sciences
Campus Box 173, P.O. Box 173364
Denver, CO 80217-3364
Telephone: (303) 556-8565
Fax: (303) 556-3520
E-mail: *gay.freebern@ucdenver.edu*
Web: *http://thunder1.cudenver.edu/clas/psychology/index.html*

Department Information:
1960. Chairperson: Peter Kaplan, PhD. Number of faculty: total—full-time 15, part-time 2; women—full-time 8, part-time 1; total—minority—full-time 2; women minority—full-time 1.

Programs and Degrees Offered:
Listed in the following order: Program area, degree type (T if terminal Master's), number awarded 7/08–6/09. Clinical Psychology MA/MS (Master of Arts/Science) (T) 11, Clinical Health Psychology PhD (Doctor of Philosophy).

Student Applications/Admissions:
Student Applications
Clinical Psychology MA/MS (Master of Arts/Science)—Applications 2009–2010, 115. Total applicants accepted 2009–2010, 12. Number full-time enrolled (new admits only) 2009–2010, 8. Number part-time enrolled (new admits only) 2009–2010, 0. Total enrolled 2009–2010 full-time, 16, part-time, 3. Openings 2010–2011, 5. The median number of years required for completion of a degree in 2008–2009 were 2. The number of students enrolled full- and part-time who were dismissed or voluntarily withdrew from this program area in 2008–2009 were 1. *Clinical Health Psychology PhD (Doctor of Philosophy)*—Applications 2009–2010, 35. Total applicants accepted 2009–2010, 5. Number full-time enrolled (new admits only) 2009–2010, 4. Total enrolled 2009–2010 full-time, 9. Openings 2010–2011, 5.

Scores: Entries appear in this order: required test or GPA, minimum score (if required), median score of students entering in 2009–2010. *Clinical Health Psychology PhD (Doctor of Philosophy):* GRE-V no minimum stated, 590, GRE-Q no minimum stated, 665, GRE-Subject (Psychology) no minimum stated, 690, overall undergraduate GPA no minimum stated, 3.64, last 2 years GPA no minimum stated, 3.73.

Other Criteria: (importance of criteria rated low, medium, or high): GRE scores—medium, research experience—high, work experience—medium, extracurricular activity—low, clinically related public service—low, GPA—high, letters of recommendation—high, interview—high, statement of goals and objectives—high, undergraduate major in psychology—low, specific undergraduate psychology courses taken—medium. For additional information on admission requirements, go to http://thunder1.cudenver.edu/clas/psychology/gradPrograms.html.

Student Characteristics: The following represents characteristics of students in 2009–2010 in all graduate psychology programs in the department: Female—full-time 20, part-time 0; Male—full-time 5, part-time 3; African American/Black—full-time 1, part-time 0; Hispanic/Latino(a)—full-time 0, part-time 0; Asian/Pacific Islander—full-time 4, part-time 0; American Indian/Alaska Native—full-time 0, part-time 0; Caucasian/White—full-time 18, part-time 2; Multi-ethnic—full-time 1, part-time 1; students subject to the Americans With Disabilities Act—full-time 0, part-time 0; Unknown ethnicity—full-time 1, part-time 0; International students who hold an F-1 or J-1 Visa—full-time 1, part-time 0.

Financial Information/Assistance:
Tuition for Full-Time Study: Master's: State residents: per academic year $6,430, $345 per credit hour; Nonstate residents: per academic year $17,622, $1,055 per credit hour. *Doctoral:* State residents: per academic year $6,430, $345 per credit hour; Nonstate residents: per academic year $14,622, $1,055 per credit hour. Tuition is subject to change. Additional fees are assessed to students beyond the costs of tuition for the following: Transportation, technology, student services, etc. Tuition costs vary by program. See the following Web site for updates and changes in tuition costs: http://www.ucdenver.edu/student-services/resources/CostsAndFinancing.

Financial Assistance:
First-Year Students: Teaching assistantships available for first year. Average amount paid per academic year: $6,138. Average number of hours worked per week: 10. Research assistantships available for first year. Average amount paid per academic year: $6,000. Average number of hours worked per week: 10. Fellow-

ships and scholarships available for first year. Average amount paid per academic year: $15,000.

Advanced Students: Teaching assistantships available for advanced students. Average amount paid per academic year: $6,138. Average number of hours worked per week: 10. Research assistantships available for advanced students. Average amount paid per academic year: $6,000. Average number of hours worked per week: 10. Fellowships and scholarships available for advanced students. Average amount paid per academic year: $15,000.

Additional Information: Of all students currently enrolled full time, 100% benefited from one or more of the listed financial assistance programs. Application and information available online at: http://www.cudenver.edu/Admissions/Financial+Aid/default.htm.

Internships/Practica: Master's Degree (MA/MS Clinical Psychology): An internship experience, such as a final research project or "capstone" experience is required of graduates. Internships and practica are widely available at several community agencies. Past students have completed internships at local hospitals, mental health centers, residential treatment centers, and the division of corrections. MA students may elect to complete both an internship and a thesis. Students electing the internship option may begin internships after completing the first year of courses. A total of 800 hours of supervised field experience is required for the full-time internship, and students may elect to do 200-, 400-, or 600-hour internships in addition to a thesis. All field placements must be approved by the program director in advance.

Housing and Day Care: On-campus housing is available. See the following Web site for more information: http://thunder1.cudenver.edu/housing/. On-campus day care facilities are available. See the following Web site for more information: http://www.tivoli.org/earlylearning/index.html.

Employment of Department Graduates:
Master's Degree Graduates: Of those who graduated in the academic year 2008–2009, the following categories and numbers represent the postgraduate activities and employment of master's degree graduates: Enrolled in a psychology doctoral program (5), enrolled in a postdoctoral residency/fellowship (n/a), employed in independent practice (n/a), employed in other positions at a higher education institution (1), employed in government agency (2), employed in a community mental health/counseling center (5), total from the above (master's) (13).
Doctoral Degree Graduates: Of those who graduated in the academic year 2008–2009, the following categories and numbers represent the postgraduate activities and employment of doctoral degree graduates: Enrolled in a psychology doctoral program (n/a), total from the above (doctoral) (0).

Additional Information:
Orientation, Objectives, and Emphasis of Department: Both programs adhere to the scientist–practitioner model, and training emphasizes the contribution of research to the understanding, treatment, and prevention of human problems, and the application of knowledge that is grounded in scientific evidence. Students in our clinical health PhD program will be trained to work within the community to use psychological tools and techniques to promote health, prevent and treat illness, and improve the health care system. In addition to coursework, students acquire expertise in research by completing a master's thesis and doctoral dissertation, and demonstrate competence in clinical assessment and intervention through several applied practicum experiences and a predoctoral internship. We will be seeking accreditation by the APA as a Clinical PhD. The principal objective of the clinical MA program is to prepare graduates for doctoral-level work. The program offers rigorous training in diagnostic evaluation, psychological assessment, and empirically-based psychotherapy. After one year of coursework, students have the option of completing a thesis and/or an internship. Applied practicum and internship experiences can be completed with a wide variety of populations in the area.

Special Facilities or Resources: In July 2004, the University of Colorado, Downtown Denver Campus (our campus) merged with the University of Colorado Health Sciences Center. There are numerous possibilities for research collaborations with faculty at the Health Sciences Center (renamed Anschutz Medical Campus) in addition to the faculty members in our own department. There are also several affiliated institutions (e.g., AMC Cancer Research Center, The Children's Hospital and Kempe Center, Denver Health Medical Center, National Jewish Health, and the VA) in the area that provide additional opportunities for research collaborations and applied clinical work.

Information for Students With Physical Disabilities: See the following Web site for more information: http://www.ucdenver.edu/disabilityresources.

Application Information:
Send to Gay Freebern, Program Assistant, Department of Psychology, University of Colorado Denver, Campus Box 173, PO Box 173364, Denver, CO 80217-3364. Application available online. URL of online application: http://www.ucdenver.edu/admissions/Pages/index.aspx. Students are admitted in the Fall, application deadline December 1. PhD application deadline is December 1; MA application deadline for fall enrollment is February 1. *Fee:* $50. International student application fee: $75.

Denver, University of
Child, Family, and School Psychology Program
Morgridge College of Education
2450 South Vine Street
Denver, CO 80208
Telephone: (303) 871-2509
Fax: (303) 871-4456
E-mail: smondrag@du.edu
Web: http://www.du.edu/education/programs/cfsp/index.html

Department Information:
2003. Program Chair: Gloria Miller, PhD. Number of faculty: total—full-time 5, part-time 1; women—full-time 5, part-time 1.

Programs and Degrees Offered:
Listed in the following order: Program area, degree type (T if terminal Master's), number awarded 7/08–6/09. Child, Family and School Psychology EdS (School Psychology) 7, Child, Family and School Psychology PhD (Doctor of Philosophy) 0, Child, Family and School Psychology MA/MS (Master of Arts/Science) 3.

GRADUATE STUDY IN PSYCHOLOGY

Student Applications/Admissions:
Student Applications
Child, Family and School Psychology EdS (School Psychology)—Applications 2009–2010, 36. Total applicants accepted 2009–2010, 31. Number full-time enrolled (new admits only) 2009–2010, 10. Number part-time enrolled (new admits only) 2009–2010, 0. Openings 2010–2011, 12. The median number of years required for completion of a degree in 2008–2009 were 4. The number of students enrolled full- and part-time who were dismissed or voluntarily withdrew from this program area in 2008–2009 were 0. *Child, Family and School Psychology PhD (Doctor of Philosophy)*—Applications 2009–2010, 20. Total applicants accepted 2009–2010, 7. Number full-time enrolled (new admits only) 2009–2010, 3. Number part-time enrolled (new admits only) 2009–2010, 2. Total enrolled 2009–2010 full-time, 14, part-time, 10. Openings 2010–2011, 8. The median number of years required for completion of a degree in 2008–2009 were 4. The number of students enrolled full- and part-time who were dismissed or voluntarily withdrew from this program area in 2008–2009 were 0. *Child, Family and School Psychology MA/MS (Master of Arts/Science)*—Applications 2009–2010, 10. Total applicants accepted 2009–2010, 4. Number full-time enrolled (new admits only) 2009–2010, 2. Number part-time enrolled (new admits only) 2009–2010, 0. The median number of years required for completion of a degree in 2008–2009 were 2. The number of students enrolled full- and part-time who were dismissed or voluntarily withdrew from this program area in 2008–2009 were 0.

Other Criteria: (importance of criteria rated low, medium, or high): GRE scores—medium, research experience—medium, work experience—medium, extracurricular activity—medium, clinically related public service—medium, GPA—medium, letters of recommendation—medium, interview—high, statement of goals and objectives—medium. For additional information on admission requirements, go to http://www.du.edu/education/calls/admission.html.

Student Characteristics: The following represents characteristics of students in 2009–2010 in all graduate psychology programs in the department: Female—full-time 0, part-time 0; Male—full-time 0, part-time 0; African American/Black—full-time 0, part-time 0; Hispanic/Latino(a)—full-time 0, part-time 0; Asian/Pacific Islander—full-time 0, part-time 0; American Indian/Alaska Native—full-time 0, part-time 0; Caucasian/White—full-time 0, part-time 0; Multi-ethnic—full-time 0, part-time 0; students subject to the Americans With Disabilities Act—full-time 0, part-time 0; Unknown ethnicity—full-time 0, part-time 0; International students who hold an F-1 or J-1 Visa—full-time 0, part-time 0.

Financial Information/Assistance:
Tuition for Full-Time Study: *Master's:* State residents: $974 per credit hour; Nonstate residents: $974 per credit hour. *Doctoral:* State residents: $974 per credit hour; Nonstate residents: $974 per credit hour. Tuition is subject to change. Additional fees are assessed to students beyond the costs of tuition for the following: technology fee of $4 per credit hour. See the following Web site for updates and changes in tuition costs: http://www.du.edu/registrar.

Financial Assistance:
First-Year Students: Teaching assistantships available for first year. Research assistantships available for first year. Traineeships available for first year. Fellowships and scholarships available for first year.

Advanced Students: Teaching assistantships available for advanced students. Research assistantships available for advanced students. Traineeships available for advanced students. Fellowships and scholarships available for advanced students.

Additional Information: Of all students currently enrolled full time, 90% benefited from one or more of the listed financial assistance programs. Application and information available online at: http://www.du.edu/education/calls/financial-aid/index.html.

Internships/Practica: Integrated and well supervised field experiences taken during coursework and as independent placement courses are an integral part of the training of future school psychologists and child and family professionals. Such experiences in total provide opportunities for students to build and reflect upon professional roles and competencies and to master critical professional skills. Field coursework experiences are designed as a developmental Chain of Relevant Experiences (CoRE) where students progress from being Critical Observers, to Directed Participants, to Active Contributors, and ultimately to become Independent Practitioners in professional practice. Although the structure and content of our field courses differ across degree programs, all students complete a required Mentorship, a Clinic Practicum, and a Field Practicum. EdS and PhD School Psychology Licensure track students also complete a 1200-hour (EdS) or 1500-hour (PhD) internship, which can occur over one full year or two consecutive years. Our programmatic field-based coursework includes training and practice in the following: comprehensive assessment of developmental strengths and weaknesses; direct and preventative interventions within home, school, and community settings; communication and collaboration with families and children with diverse life experiences; individual, group, and family crisis counseling; interdisciplinary and transdisciplinary team collaboration in school and community settings; delivery of in-service trainings and presentations; system-wide program evaluation, research, and intervention; and applications of emergent technology.

Housing and Day Care: On-campus housing is available. See the following Web site for more information: http://www.du.edu/housing/. On-campus day care facilities are available. See the following Web site for more information: http://www.du.edu/felc/.

Employment of Department Graduates:
Master's Degree Graduates: Of those who graduated in the academic year 2008–2009, the following categories and numbers represent the postgraduate activities and employment of master's degree graduates: Enrolled in a postdoctoral residency/fellowship (n/a), employed in independent practice (n/a), employed in government agency (1), not seeking employment (1), do not know (1), total from the above (master's) (3).

Doctoral Degree Graduates: Of those who graduated in the academic year 2008–2009, the following categories and numbers represent the postgraduate activities and employment of doctoral degree graduates: Enrolled in a psychology doctoral program (n/a), total from the above (doctoral) (0).

Additional Information:
Orientation, Objectives, and Emphasis of Department: The Child, Family, & School Psychology program, which stresses serving children in the context of their families and communities,

teaches students about psychological factors that influence human development and learning. Students can be prepared for licensure as school psychologists through the National Association of School Psychologists (NASP) approved EdS degree program, or for professional careers in a broad range of educational, medical, research, or treatment-oriented service systems serving children from birth through age 21. The program offers a distinctive opportunity for interested students to develop a specialization in early childhood education. The curriculum emphasizes strategies for supporting and intervening with children and families with diverse needs, as well as policy development, research, and program development and evaluation. The CFSP program provides students expanded career options in schools and the community. As a student in this program, you will have the opportunity to work in a broad range of educational, medical, research, or treatment-oriented service systems at the local, state and national levels. You will also acquire a broad base of information about normal and atypical development, learning, and biological and environmental contexts that affect these areas. You'll gain expertise in a wide array of diagnostic, assessment, prevention, intervention, consultation, evaluation and research methods that reinforce expertise within a concentrated area of study.

Special Facilities or Resources: Doctoral students are supervised at the Child and Family Clinic (CFC) located in the Fisher Early Learning Center and most EdS and School Psychology Licensure track Doctoral students are supervised at the Counseling and Educational Services Clinic (CESC) located in the Ammi Hyde Building.

Information for Students With Physical Disabilities: See the following Web site for more information: http://www.du.edu/disability/.

Application Information:
Send to Morgridge College of Education, Child, Family, & School Psychology, 2450 S. Vine Street, Denver, CO 80208. Application available online. URL of online application: http://www.du.edu/education/calls/admission.html. Students are admitted in the Fall, application deadline December 15. *Fee:* $60.

Denver, University of (2009 data)
Counseling Psychology
Morgridge College of Education
2450 South Vine Street
Denver, CO 80208
Telephone: (303) 871-2509
Fax: (303) 871-4456
E-mail: *psherry@du.edu*
Web: *http://www.du.edu/education*

Department Information:
1980. Program Chair: Jesse Valdez. Number of faculty: total—full-time 6; women—full-time 4; total—minority—full-time 2; women minority—full-time 1.

Programs and Degrees Offered:
Listed in the following order: Program area, degree type (T if terminal Master's), number awarded 7/08–6/09. Counseling MA/MS (Master of Arts/Science) (T) 23, Counseling Psychology PhD (Doctor of Philosophy) 5.

APA Accreditation: Counseling PhD (Doctor of Philosophy).

Student Applications/Admissions:
Student Applications
Counseling MA/MS *(Master of Arts/Science)*—Applications 2009–2010, 125. Number full-time enrolled (new admits only) 2009–2010, 27. Number part-time enrolled (new admits only) 2009–2010, 1. Total enrolled 2009–2010 full-time, 46, part-time, 6. Openings 2010–2011, 26. The median number of years required for completion of a degree in 2008–2009 were 2. The number of students enrolled full- and part-time who were dismissed or voluntarily withdrew from this program area in 2008–2009 were 1. *Counseling Psychology PhD (Doctor of Philosophy)*—Applications 2009–2010, 75. Number full-time enrolled (new admits only) 2009–2010, 8. Number part-time enrolled (new admits only) 2009–2010, 0. Total enrolled 2009–2010 full-time, 27, part-time, 9. Openings 2010–2011, 7. The median number of years required for completion of a degree in 2008–2009 were 5. The number of students enrolled full- and part-time who were dismissed or voluntarily withdrew from this program area in 2008–2009 were 0.

Other Criteria: (importance of criteria rated low, medium, or high): GRE scores—medium, research experience—high, work experience—high, extracurricular activity—low, clinically related public service—medium, GPA—medium, letters of recommendation—high, interview—high, statement of goals and objectives—high, undergraduate major in psychology—medium, specific undergraduate psychology courses taken—low.

Student Characteristics: The following represents characteristics of students in 2009–2010 in all graduate psychology programs in the department: Female—full-time 26, part-time 2; Male—full-time 7, part-time 0; African American/Black—full-time 0, part-time 0; Hispanic/Latino(a)—full-time 5, part-time 0; Asian/Pacific Islander—full-time 6, part-time 0; American Indian/Alaska Native—full-time 3, part-time 0; Caucasian/White—full-time 0, part-time 0; Multi-ethnic—full-time 2, part-time 0; students subject to the Americans With Disabilities Act—full-time 0, part-time 0; Unknown ethnicity—full-time 0, part-time 0; International students who hold an F-1 or J-1 Visa—full-time 0, part-time 0.

Financial Information/Assistance:
Tuition for Full-Time Study: *Master's:* State residents: $874 per credit hour; Nonstate residents: $874 per credit hour. *Doctoral:* State residents: $874 per credit hour; Nonstate residents: $874 per credit hour. Tuition is subject to change. Additional fees are assessed to students beyond the costs of tuition for the following: Technology Fee of $4 per credit hour. See the following Web site for updates and changes in tuition costs: http://www.du.edu/registrar/.

Financial Assistance:
First-Year Students: Teaching assistantships available for first year. Average amount paid per academic year: $5,000. Average number of hours worked per week: 10. Apply by April 1. Research assistantships available for first year. Average amount paid per academic year: $5,000. Average number of hours worked

per week: 10. Apply by April 1. Fellowships and scholarships available for first year. Average number of hours worked per week: 0.

Advanced Students: Teaching assistantships available for advanced students. Average amount paid per academic year: $5,000. Average number of hours worked per week: 10. Apply by April 1. Research assistantships available for advanced students. Average number of hours worked per week: 10. Apply by April 1. Fellowships and scholarships available for advanced students. Average amount paid per academic year: $5,000. Average number of hours worked per week: 0. Apply by April 1.

Additional Information: Of all students currently enrolled full time, 90% benefited from one or more of the listed financial assistance programs.

Internships/Practica: Doctoral Degree (PhD Counseling Psychology): For those doctoral students for whom a professional internship was required in this program prior to graduation, (5) students applied for an internship in 2008–2009, with (5) students obtaining an internship. Of those students who obtained an internship, (5) were paid internships. Of those students who obtained an internship, (5) students placed in APA/CPA accredited internships, (0) students placed in internships not APA/CPA accredited, but listed with the Association of Psychology Postdoctoral and Internship Programs (APPIC), (0) students placed in internships conforming to guidelines of the Council of Directors of School Psychology Programs (CDSPP), (0) students placed in internships that were not APA/CPA accredited, APPIC or CDSPP listed. Master's Degree (MA/MS Counseling): An internship experience, such as a final research project or "capstone" experience is required of graduates. Both Doctoral and Master's students complete practica and internships as well as hours in a campus clinic. Most practica and internships are off campus. Doctoral students must complete APA approved internships (exceptions made in unusual circumstances). Doctoral students have opportunities to complete advanced practica in variety of settings including college counseling centers, hospitals and mental health agencies. MA students complete practica and internships in the Denver area, including at adolescent treatment facilities, mental health centers, women's crisis centers, schools, etc.

Housing and Day Care: On-campus housing is available. On-campus day care facilities are available.

Employment of Department Graduates:
Master's Degree Graduates: Of those who graduated in the academic year 2008–2009, the following categories and numbers represent the postgraduate activities and employment of master's degree graduates: Enrolled in a psychology doctoral program (1), enrolled in a postdoctoral residency/fellowship (n/a), employed in independent practice (n/a), employed in other positions at a higher education institution (1), employed in a community mental health/counseling center (4), still seeking employment (1), do not know (16), total from the above (master's) (23).
Doctoral Degree Graduates: Of those who graduated in the academic year 2008–2009, the following categories and numbers represent the postgraduate activities and employment of doctoral degree graduates: Enrolled in a psychology doctoral program (n/a), enrolled in a postdoctoral residency/fellowship (2), employed in an academic position at a university (1), employed in government agency (1), employed in a community mental health/counseling center (1), total from the above (doctoral) (5).

Additional Information:
Orientation, Objectives, and Emphasis of Department: As a graduate student in the Counseling Psychology program, you'll develop the skills necessary to become an effective practitioner, researcher, and/or leader in your field. Our goal is to develop professionals who are insightful and self-reflective, who are innovative risk takers and superior critical thinkers. Our highly selective doctoral program is accredited by the American Psychological Association and is well known for providing access to high quality internships for our students. We want our students not only to demonstrate accurate and current knowledge, but to have expertise related to the many issues confronting society and to have the skills to create effective strategies and approaches to address these challenges. To work professionally in counseling psychology at the master's or doctoral level, you will need a strong background in the practice of counseling and psychotherapy, as well as a knowledge of the scientific foundations of psychology in order to evaluate and think critically about your practice.

Special Facilities or Resources: PhD students are required to complete a minor in one of two APA-approved clinical psychology programs on campus. Microcomputers and video equipment are available for use in conjunction with coursework. In-house clinic is available. Students are required to spend one evening a week for two quarters in clinic. Intensive supervision provided.

Application Information:
Send to Graduate Studies, Office of Admission, 2199 South University Boulevard, Denver, CO 80208-0302. Application available online. URL of online application: http://www.du.edu/education/calls/admission.html. Students are admitted in the Fall, application deadline December 15. Master's Degree in Counseling applcation deadline is January 15. *Fee:* $60.

Denver, University of
Department of Psychology
Frontier Hall, 2155 South Race Street
Denver, CO 80208
Telephone: (303) 871-3803
Fax: (303) 871-4747
E-mail: *rroberts@du.edu*
Web: *http://www.du.edu/psychology*

Department Information:
1952. Chairperson: Ralph J. Roberts. Number of faculty: total—full-time 19, part-time 1; women—full-time 9, part-time 1; total—minority—full-time 1.

Programs and Degrees Offered:
Listed in the following order: Program area, degree type (T if terminal Master's), number awarded 7/08–6/09. Clinical Child Psychology PhD (Doctor of Philosophy) 5, Developmental Psychology PhD (Doctor of Philosophy) 1, Psychology and The Law MA/MS (Master of Arts/Science) (T) 0, Social Psychology PhD (Doctor of Philosophy) 0, Developmental Cognitive Neuroscience PhD (Doctor of Philosophy) 5, Cognitive Psychology PhD (Doctor of Philosophy) 1, Affective Science PhD (Doctor of Philosophy) 0.

COLORADO

APA Accreditation: Clinical PhD (Doctor of Philosophy). Student Outcome Data Website: http://www.du.edu/psychology/research/child_clinical_breakdown.htm.

Student Applications/Admissions:
Student Applications
Clinical Child Psychology PhD (Doctor of Philosophy)—Applications 2009–2010, 240. Total applicants accepted 2009–2010, 10. Number full-time enrolled (new admits only) 2009–2010, 5. Openings 2010–2011, 6. The median number of years required for completion of a degree in 2008–2009 were 6. The number of students enrolled full- and part-time who were dismissed or voluntarily withdrew from this program area in 2008–2009 were 1. *Developmental Psychology PhD (Doctor of Philosophy)*—Applications 2009–2010, 21. Total applicants accepted 2009–2010, 2. Number full-time enrolled (new admits only) 2009–2010, 1. Openings 2010–2011, 2. The median number of years required for completion of a degree in 2008–2009 were 7. The number of students enrolled full- and part-time who were dismissed or voluntarily withdrew from this program area in 2008–2009 were 0. *Psychology and The Law MA/MS (Master of Arts/Science)*—Applications 2009–2010, 0. Total applicants accepted 2009–2010, 0. Number full-time enrolled (new admits only) 2009–2010, 0. Openings 2010–2011, 1. The number of students enrolled full- and part-time who were dismissed or voluntarily withdrew from this program area in 2008–2009 were 0. *Social Psychology PhD (Doctor of Philosophy)*—Applications 2009–2010, 32. Total applicants accepted 2009–2010, 2. Number full-time enrolled (new admits only) 2009–2010, 0. Total enrolled 2009–2010 full-time, 1. Openings 2010–2011, 2. The number of students enrolled full- and part-time who were dismissed or voluntarily withdrew from this program area in 2008–2009 were 0. *Developmental Cognitive Neuroscience PhD (Doctor of Philosophy)*—Applications 2009–2010, 75. Total applicants accepted 2009–2010, 9. Number full-time enrolled (new admits only) 2009–2010, 3. Total enrolled 2009–2010 full-time, 13. Openings 2010–2011, 6. The median number of years required for completion of a degree in 2008–2009 were 6. The number of students enrolled full- and part-time who were dismissed or voluntarily withdrew from this program area in 2008–2009 were 0. *Cognitive Psychology PhD (Doctor of Philosophy)*—Applications 2009–2010, 9. Total applicants accepted 2009–2010, 2. Number full-time enrolled (new admits only) 2009–2010, 2. Total enrolled 2009–2010 full-time, 5. Openings 2010–2011, 2. The median number of years required for completion of a degree in 2008–2009 were 6. The number of students enrolled full- and part-time who were dismissed or voluntarily withdrew from this program area in 2008–2009 were 0. *Affective Science PhD (Doctor of Philosophy)*—Applications 2009–2010, 32. Total applicants accepted 2009–2010, 3. Number full-time enrolled (new admits only) 2009–2010, 0. Total enrolled 2009–2010 full-time, 3. Openings 2010–2011, 4. The number of students enrolled full- and part-time who were dismissed or voluntarily withdrew from this program area in 2008–2009 were 0.
Scores: Entries appear in this order: required test or GPA, minimum score (if required), median score of students entering in 2009–2010. Clinical Child Psychology PhD (Doctor of Philosophy): GRE-V no minimum stated, 670, GRE-Q no minimum stated, 770, GRE-Analytical no minimum stated, 5.0; *Developmental Psychology PhD (Doctor of Philosophy)*: GRE-V no minimum stated, 540, GRE-Q no minimum stated, 670, GRE-Analytical no minimum stated, 5.0, overall undergraduate GPA no minimum stated, 3.81; *Psychology and the Law MA/MS (Master of Arts/Science)*: GRE-V no minimum stated, GRE-Q no minimum stated, GRE-Analytical no minimum stated; *Social Psychology PhD (Doctor of Philosophy)*: GRE-V no minimum stated, 630, GRE-Q no minimum stated, 700, GRE-Analytical no minimum stated, 5; *Developmental Cognitive Neuroscience PhD (Doctor of Philosophy)*: GRE-V no minimum stated, 670, GRE-Q no minimum stated, 740, GRE-Analytical no minimum stated, 5.5; *Cognitive Psychology PhD (Doctor of Philosophy)*: GRE-V no minimum stated, 670, GRE-Q no minimum stated, 685, GRE-Analytical no minimum stated, 5.25; *Affective Science PhD (Doctor of Philosophy)*: GRE-V no minimum stated, 630, GRE-Q no minimum stated, 700, GRE-Analytical no minimum stated, 5, overall undergraduate GPA no minimum stated, 3.6.
Other Criteria: (importance of criteria rated low, medium, or high): GRE scores—high, research experience—high, work experience—medium, extracurricular activity—medium, clinically related public service—high, GPA—high, letters of recommendation—high, interview—high, statement of goals and objectives—high. For additional information on admission requirements, go to http://www.du.edu/psychology/index.htm.

Student Characteristics: The following represents characteristics of students in 2009–2010 in all graduate psychology programs in the department: Female—full-time 40, part-time 0; Male—full-time 6, part-time 0; African American/Black—full-time 0, part-time 0; Hispanic/Latino(a)—full-time 5, part-time 0; Asian/Pacific Islander—full-time 6, part-time 0; American Indian/Alaska Native—full-time 0, part-time 0; Caucasian/White—full-time 34, part-time 0; Multi-ethnic—full-time 1, part-time 0; students subject to the Americans With Disabilities Act—full-time 0, part-time 0; Unknown ethnicity—full-time 0, part-time 0; International students who hold an F-1 or J-1 Visa—full-time 3, part-time 0.

Financial Information/Assistance:
Tuition for Full-Time Study: *Master's:* State residents: per academic year $29,670, $989 per credit hour; Nonstate residents: per academic year $29,670, $989 per credit hour. *Doctoral:* State residents: per academic year $29,670, $989 per credit hour; Nonstate residents: per academic year $29,670, $989 per credit hour. See the following Web site for updates and changes in tuition costs: http://www.du.edu/registrar/.

Financial Assistance:
First-Year Students: Teaching assistantships available for first year. Average amount paid per academic year: $18,000. Average number of hours worked per week: 20. Research assistantships available for first year. Average amount paid per academic year: $18,000. Average number of hours worked per week: 20.
Advanced Students: Teaching assistantships available for advanced students. Average amount paid per academic year: $18,000. Average number of hours worked per week: 20. Research assistantships available for advanced students. Average amount paid per academic year: $18,000. Average number of hours worked per week: 20.
Additional Information: Of all students currently enrolled full time, 100% benefited from one or more of the listed financial assistance programs. Application and information available online at: http://www.du.edu/psychology.

Internships/Practica: Doctoral Degree (PhD Clinical Child Psychology): For those doctoral students for whom a professional internship was required in this program prior to graduation, (8) students applied for an internship in 2008–2009, with (8) students obtaining an internship. Of those students who obtained an internship, (8) were paid internships. Of those students who obtained an internship, (8) students placed in APA/CPA accredited internships, (0) students placed in internships not APA/CPA accredited, but listed with the Association of Psychology Postdoctoral and Internship Programs (APPIC), (0) students placed in internships conforming to guidelines of the Council of Directors of School Psychology Programs (CDSPP), (0) students placed in internships that were not APA/CPA accredited, APPIC or CDSPP listed. The department offers two clinical training facilities: the Child and Family Clinic and the Developmental Neuropsychology Clinic. The Child and Family Clinic provides training in assessment and psychotherapy with children, families, and adults. The Neuropsychology Clinic provides specialized training in assessment of learning disorders, mainly in school-age children. Thus, a considerable amount of clinical training is provided within our Department by faculty supervisors, ensuring that each clinical student is solidly grounded in both assessment and treatment. Clinical students also typically do externships in the community, such as local hospitals, day treatment programs, and other community agencies. Graduate students who are not in clinical can also get experience with patient populations either by internships in the neuropsychology clinic or through research in labs that study developmental disorders.

Housing and Day Care: On-campus housing is available. See the following Web site for more information: http://www.du.edu/housing/grad/. On-campus day care facilities are available. See the following Web site for more information: http://www.du.edu/fisher/index.html.

Employment of Department Graduates:
Master's Degree Graduates: Of those who graduated in the academic year 2008–2009, the following categories and numbers represent the postgraduate activities and employment of master's degree graduates: Enrolled in a postdoctoral residency/fellowship (n/a), employed in independent practice (n/a), total from the above (master's) (0).
Doctoral Degree Graduates: Of those who graduated in the academic year 2008–2009, the following categories and numbers represent the postgraduate activities and employment of doctoral degree graduates: Enrolled in a psychology doctoral program (n/a), enrolled in a postdoctoral residency/fellowship (5), employed in a professional position in a school system (1), total from the above (doctoral) (6).

Additional Information:
Orientation, Objectives, and Emphasis of Department: Programs are oriented toward training students to pursue careers in research, teaching, and professional practice. They include a new program in Affective Science, and established programs in Clinical Child, Cognitive, Developmental, and Social, as well as Developmental Cognitive Neuroscience, a program open to students in any of the other programs, and that fosters an interdisciplinary approach to cognitive, affective, and social neuroscience. The department has one of the few APA-accredited child clinical programs, and has been ranked very highly in past rankings by the American Psychological Society for publication impact. The department offers close collaborative relationships between faculty and students, with an emphasis on individualized tutorial relationships. The atmosphere encourages and offers students the freedom to seek out and work with multiple faculty members as fits the student's evolving interests. Our students are successful in publishing in prestigious journals, in winning predoctoral grants, and obtaining their first choice for clinical internships. Situated at the foot of the Rocky Mountains, Denver combines urban culture with readily accessible skiing, hiking, and biking in a climate that has over 300 days of sunshine.

Special Facilities or Resources: Our labs are custom-designed for the kinds of research conducted in our department. They include the Center for Marital and Family Studies, the Relationship Center, the Developmental Neuropsychology Center, the Cognitive Neuroscience Lab, the Reading & Language Lab, the Emotion Regulation Lab, the Center for Infant Development, the Center for Research on Family Stress, the Perception/Action Lab, the Emotion and Coping Lab, the Traumatic Stress Studies Lab, the Mechanisms of Cognitive Control Lab, the Affective Neuroscience Lab and the Child Health and Development Lab. Labs are equipped with computers for controlling the presentation of stimuli and the collection of data. Some labs include equipment to measure EDA, ECG, and EMG. The Perception-Action Lab employs eye movement recording methods in children and adults. The Child Health and Development Lab is equipped with a modified wet lab for processing saliva samples including a -80 freezer for storage. In addition, we have a host of conventional laboratory rooms with one-way observation windows and up-to-date audio and video recording equipment. Finally, we are closely partnered with the neuroimaging facilities at the University of Colorado Health Sciences Center and a genotyping facility at the Institute for Behavioral Genetics at UC-Boulder. The neuroimaging facilities allow us to conduct fMRI and MEG studies. Genotype data allow us to test directly genetic effects on behavior. In addition to research laboratories, the department also maintains its own clinical training facility, the Child Study Center, and houses the Neuropsychology Clinic. The department enjoys excellent computer facilities. It maintains a local area computer network (LAN) that interconnects over 100 departmental PCs. Many graduate student offices are equipped with computers, and there is also a graduate student computer lab with PCs, printers, and scanners. Research subjects are available from undergraduate classes, and from nearby schools and the university daycare center, and local hospitals and rehab centers for patients with neuropsychological disorders. Classrooms are smart-to-the-seat, allowing Internet access for students' laptops.

Information for Students With Physical Disabilities: See the following Web site for more information: http://www.du.edu/studentlife/disability/dsp/index.html.

Application Information:
Send to Graduate Studies Office, University of Denver, 2199 S. University Blvd, Denver, CO 80208. Application available online. URL of online application: http://www.du.edu/grad/appinfo/info.html. Students are admitted in the Fall, application deadline December 1. Fee: $60.

Denver, University of
Graduate School of Professional Psychology
2460 South Vine Street, MSC 4101
Denver, CO 80208-3626
Telephone: (303) 871-3736
Fax: (303) 871-7656
E-mail: *gsppinfo@du.edu*
Web: *http://www.du.edu/gspp/*

Department Information:
1976. Dean: Dr. Peter Buirski. Number of faculty: total—full-time 14, part-time 5; women—full-time 7, part-time 3; total—minority—full-time 3, part-time 1; women minority—full-time 1, part-time 1.

Programs and Degrees Offered:
Listed in the following order: Program area, degree type (T if terminal Master's), number awarded 7/08–6/09. Clinical Psychology PsyD (Doctor of Psychology) 40, Forensic Psychology MA/MS (Master of Arts/Science) (T) 33, Sport and Performance Psychology MA/MS (Master of Arts/Science) (T) 14, International Disaster Psychology MA/MS (Master of Arts/Science) (T) 15.

APA Accreditation: Clinical PsyD (Doctor of Psychology). Student Outcome Data Website: http://www.du.edu/gspp/degree-programs/clinical-psychology/overview/program-statistics.html.

Student Applications/Admissions:
Student Applications

Clinical Psychology PsyD (Doctor of Psychology)—Applications 2009–2010, 360. Total applicants accepted 2009–2010, 72. Number full-time enrolled (new admits only) 2009–2010, 37. Openings 2010–2011, 35. The median number of years required for completion of a degree in 2008–2009 were 4. The number of students enrolled full- and part-time who were dismissed or voluntarily withdrew from this program area in 2008–2009 were 5. *Forensic Psychology MA/MS (Master of Arts/Science)*—Applications 2009–2010, 73. Total applicants accepted 2009–2010, 44. Number full-time enrolled (new admits only) 2009–2010, 24. Openings 2010–2011, 25. The median number of years required for completion of a degree in 2008–2009 were 2. The number of students enrolled full- and part-time who were dismissed or voluntarily withdrew from this program area in 2008–2009 were 0. *Sport and Performance Psychology MA/MS (Master of Arts/Science)*—Applications 2009–2010, 64. Total applicants accepted 2009–2010, 44. Number full-time enrolled (new admits only) 2009–2010, 24. Total enrolled 2009–2010 full-time, 43. Openings 2010–2011, 25. The median number of years required for completion of a degree in 2008–2009 were 2. The number of students enrolled full- and part-time who were dismissed or voluntarily withdrew from this program area in 2008–2009 were 0. *International Disaster Psychology MA/MS (Master of Arts/Science)*—Applications 2009–2010, 48. Total applicants accepted 2009–2010, 27. Number full-time enrolled (new admits only) 2009–2010, 18. Total enrolled 2009–2010 full-time, 31. Openings 2010–2011, 15. The median number of years required for completion of a degree in 2008–2009 were 2. The number of students enrolled full- and part-time who were dismissed or voluntarily withdrew from this program area in 2008–2009 were 1.

Scores: Entries appear in this order: required test or GPA, minimum score (if required), median score of students entering in 2009–2010. *Clinical Psychology PsyD (Doctor of Psychology):* GRE-V no minimum stated, GRE-Q no minimum stated.

Other Criteria: (importance of criteria rated low, medium, or high): GRE scores—high, research experience—medium, work experience—high, extracurricular activity—high, clinically related public service—high, GPA—high, letters of recommendation—high, interview—high, statement of goals and objectives—high, required essay responses—high. For additional information on admission requirements, go to http://www.du.edu/gspp/degree-programs/clinical-psychology/application.html.

Student Characteristics: The following represents characteristics of students in 2009–2010 in all graduate psychology programs in the department: Female—full-time 208, part-time 0; Male—full-time 54, part-time 0; African American/Black—full-time 9, part-time 0; Hispanic/Latino(a)—full-time 6, part-time 0; Asian/Pacific Islander—full-time 9, part-time 0; American Indian/Alaska Native—full-time 2, part-time 0; Caucasian/White—full-time 207, part-time 0; Multi-ethnic—full-time 1, part-time 0; students subject to the Americans With Disabilities Act—full-time 0, part-time 0; Unknown ethnicity—full-time 28, part-time 0; International students who hold an F-1 or J-1 Visa—full-time 0, part-time 0.

Financial Information/Assistance:
Tuition for Full-Time Study: *Master's:* State residents: per academic year $35,604, $989 per credit hour; Nonstate residents: per academic year $35,604, $989 per credit hour. *Doctoral:* State residents: per academic year $47,472, $989 per credit hour; Nonstate residents: per academic year $47,472, $989 per credit hour. Tuition is subject to change. See the following Web site for updates and changes in tuition costs: http://www.du.edu/registrar/regbill/reg_tuitionfees.html.

Financial Assistance:
First-Year Students: Research assistantships available for first year. Average amount paid per academic year: $5,000. Fellowships and scholarships available for first year. Average amount paid per academic year: $5,000.

Advanced Students: Research assistantships available for advanced students. Average amount paid per academic year: $2,500.

Additional Information: Of all students currently enrolled full time, 45% benefited from one or more of the listed financial assistance programs. Application and information available online at: http://www.du.edu/finaid/grad.htm.

Internships/Practica: Doctoral Degree (PsyD Clinical Psychology): For those doctoral students for whom a professional internship was required in this program prior to graduation, (29) students applied for an internship in 2008–2009, with (27) students obtaining an internship. Of those students who obtained an internship, (27) were paid internships. Of those students who obtained an internship, (27) students placed in APA/CPA accredited internships, (0) students placed in internships not APA/CPA accredited, but listed with the Association of Psychology Postdoctoral and Internship Programs (APPIC), (0) students placed in internships conforming to guidelines of the Council of Directors of School Psychology Programs (CDSPP), (0) students placed in internships that were not APA/CPA accredited, APPIC or CDSPP listed. In addition to participation in the APPIC internship match, the GSPP offers an exclusive consortium of APA-accredited internship sites for which appropriate students may apply.

Housing and Day Care: On-campus housing is available. See the following Web site for more information: http://www.du.edu/live/housing.html. On-campus day care facilities are available. See the following Web site for more information: http://www.du.edu/childcare/.

Employment of Department Graduates:
Master's Degree Graduates: Of those who graduated in the academic year 2008–2009, the following categories and numbers represent the postgraduate activities and employment of master's degree graduates: Enrolled in a postdoctoral residency/fellowship (n/a), employed in independent practice (n/a), total from the above (master's) (0).
Doctoral Degree Graduates: Of those who graduated in the academic year 2008–2009, the following categories and numbers represent the postgraduate activities and employment of doctoral degree graduates: Enrolled in a psychology doctoral program (n/a), total from the above (doctoral) (0).

Additional Information:
Orientation, Objectives, and Emphasis of Department: The Graduate School of Professional Psychology focuses on scientifically-based training for applied professional work rather than on the more traditional academic-scientific approach to clinical training. In addition to the basic clinical curriculum, special emphases are available in several areas. Our students should have a probing, questioning stance toward human problems and, therefore, should be: (1) knowledgeable about intra- and interpersonal theories, including assessment and intervention; (2) conversant with relevant issues and techniques in research; (3) sensitive to self and to interpersonal interactions as primary clinical tools; (4) skilled in assessing and effectively intervening in human problems; (5) able to assess effectiveness of outcomes; and (6) aware of current professional and ethical issues. To these ends the programs focus on major social and psychological theories; research training directed toward the consumer rather than the producer of research; technical knowledge of assessment; and intervention in problems involving individuals, families, groups, and institutional systems. Strong emphasis is placed on practicum training. There are no requirements for empirical research output. The Master's degree in Forensic Psychology supplements graduate-level clinical training with course work and practicum experiences in the legal, criminal justice, and law enforcement systems. The Master's degree in International Disaster Psychology supplements graduate-level clinical training with coursework and practicum experiences in trauma, community building, and international field experience.

Special Facilities or Resources: The program offers its own in-house community psychological services center, and varied opportunities are available in many community facilities for the required practicum experiences.

Information for Students With Physical Disabilities: See the following Web site for more information: http://www.du.edu/studentlife/disability/.

Application Information:
Application available online. URL of online application: http://www.du.edu/gspp/admissions/apply-now.html. Students are admitted in the Fall, application deadline December 5. Priority deadline is December 5; final application deadline is January 5. *Fee:* $60.

Northern Colorado, University of
School of Applied Psychology and Counselor Education
College of Education and Behavioral Sciences
501 20th Street, Box 131
Greeley, CO 80639
Telephone: (970) 351-2731
Fax: (970) 351-2625
E-mail: *diane.greenshields@unco.edu*
Web: *http://www.unco.edu/cebs/ppsy/*

Department Information:
1911. School Director: Fred Hanna. Number of faculty: total—full-time 15; women—full-time 10; total—minority—full-time 3; women minority—full-time 2.

Programs and Degrees Offered:
Listed in the following order: Program area, degree type (T if terminal Master's), number awarded 7/08–6/09. School Psychology EdS (School Psychology) 5, Counseling Psychology PhD (Doctor of Philosophy) 5, School Psychology PhD (Doctor of Philosophy) 11, School Psychology Endorsement 0.

APA Accreditation: Counseling PhD (Doctor of Philosophy). Student Outcome Data Website: http://www.unco.edu/cebs/counspsych/prospective.html. School PhD (Doctor of Philosophy). Student Outcome Data Website: http://www.unco.edu/cebs/SchoolPsych/phd_psychology/phd_prospective.html.

Student Applications/Admissions:
Student Applications
School Psychology EdS (School Psychology)—Applications 2009–2010, 21. Total applicants accepted 2009–2010, 15. Number full-time enrolled (new admits only) 2009–2010, 8. Total enrolled 2009–2010 full-time, 26. Openings 2010–2011, 15. The median number of years required for completion of a degree in 2008–2009 were 3. The number of students enrolled full- and part-time who were dismissed or voluntarily withdrew from this program area in 2008–2009 were 0. *Counseling Psychology PhD (Doctor of Philosophy)*—Applications 2009–2010, 103. Total applicants accepted 2009–2010, 8. Number full-time enrolled (new admits only) 2009–2010, 8. Number part-time enrolled (new admits only) 2009–2010, 0. Openings 2010–2011, 7. The median number of years required for completion of a degree in 2008–2009 were 4. The number of

students enrolled full- and part-time who were dismissed or voluntarily withdrew from this program area in 2008–2009 were 0. *School Psychology PhD (Doctor of Philosophy)*—Applications 2009–2010, 28. Total applicants accepted 2009–2010, 10. Number full-time enrolled (new admits only) 2009–2010, 8. Total enrolled 2009–2010 full-time, 40. Openings 2010–2011, 8. The median number of years required for completion of a degree in 2008–2009 were 4. The number of students enrolled full- and part-time who were dismissed or voluntarily withdrew from this program area in 2008–2009 were 1. *School Psychology Endorsement*—Applications 2009–2010, 12. Total applicants accepted 2009–2010, 10. Number full-time enrolled (new admits only) 2009–2010, 0. Number part-time enrolled (new admits only) 2009–2010, 9. The median number of years required for completion of a degree in 2008–2009 were 2. The number of students enrolled full- and part-time who were dismissed or voluntarily withdrew from this program area in 2008–2009 were 0.

Scores: Entries appear in this order: required test or GPA, minimum score (if required), median score of students entering in 2009–2010. *School Psychology EdS (School Psychology)*: GRE-V 450, GRE-Q 450, GRE-Analytical 3.5, overall undergraduate GPA 3.0, last 2 years GPA no minimum stated; *Counseling Psychology PhD (Doctor of Philosophy)*: GRE-V 450, 550, GRE-Q 450, 575, GRE-Analytical 3.5, 4.5; *School Psychology PhD (Doctor of Philosophy)*: GRE-V 450, GRE-Q 450, GRE-Analytical 3.5.

Other Criteria: (importance of criteria rated low, medium, or high): GRE scores—high, research experience—medium, work experience—medium, extracurricular activity—medium, clinically related public service—medium, GPA—high, letters of recommendation—high, interview—high, statement of goals and objectives—high, undergraduate major in psychology—medium, specific undergraduate psychology courses taken—low. Research experience is of low importance for the master's degree programs, but of medium importance for the other programs. For additional information on admission requirements, go to http://www.unco.edu/cebs/ppsy/.

Student Characteristics: The following represents characteristics of students in 2009–2010 in all graduate psychology programs in the department: Female—full-time 195, part-time 12; Male—full-time 50, part-time 3; African American/Black—full-time 4, part-time 0; Hispanic/Latino(a)—full-time 7, part-time 0; Asian/Pacific Islander—full-time 7, part-time 0; American Indian/Alaska Native—full-time 0, part-time 0; Caucasian/White—full-time 227, part-time 15; Multi-ethnic—full-time 0, part-time 0; students subject to the Americans With Disabilities Act—full-time 0, part-time 0; Unknown ethnicity—full-time 0, part-time 0; International students who hold an F-1 or J-1 Visa—full-time 5, part-time 0.

Financial Information/Assistance:
Financial Assistance:
First-Year Students: Research assistantships available for first year. Average amount paid per academic year: $6,000. Average number of hours worked per week: 8. Apply by April 15. Fellowships and scholarships available for first year. Average amount paid per academic year: $1,500. Apply by April 15.

Advanced Students: Teaching assistantships available for advanced students. Average amount paid per academic year: $6,000. Average number of hours worked per week: 8. Research assistantships available for advanced students. Average amount paid per academic year: $6,000. Average number of hours worked per week: 8. Apply by April 15. Fellowships and scholarships available for advanced students. Average amount paid per academic year: $1,500.

Additional Information: Of all students currently enrolled full time, 80% benefited from one or more of the listed financial assistance programs. Application and information available online at: http://www.unco.edu/cebs/ppsy/.

Internships/Practica: Doctoral Degree (PhD Counseling Psychology): For those doctoral students for whom a professional internship was required in this program prior to graduation, (5) students applied for an internship in 2008–2009, with (5) students obtaining an internship. Of those students who obtained an internship, (5) were paid internships. Of those students who obtained an internship, (5) students placed in APA/CPA accredited internships, (0) students placed in internships not APA/CPA accredited, but listed with the Association of Psychology Postdoctoral and Internship Programs (APPIC), (0) students placed in internships conforming to guidelines of the Council of Directors of School Psychology Programs (CDSPP), (0) students placed in internships that were not APA/CPA accredited, APPIC or CDSPP listed. Doctoral Degree (PhD School Psychology): For those doctoral students for whom a professional internship was required in this program prior to graduation, (2) students applied for an internship in 2008–2009, with (2) students obtaining an internship. Of those students who obtained an internship, (2) were paid internships. Of those students who obtained an internship, (2) students placed in APA/CPA accredited internships, (0) students placed in internships not APA/CPA accredited, but listed with the Association of Psychology Postdoctoral and Internship Programs (APPIC), (0) students placed in internships conforming to guidelines of the Council of Directors of School Psychology Programs (CDSPP), (0) students placed in internships that were not APA/CPA accredited, APPIC or CDSPP listed. Master's and doctoral practica take place within our in-house clinic. Master's internships are in mental health agencies or schools. Doctoral internships are APPIC and/or APA accredited.

Housing and Day Care: On-campus housing is available. See the following Web site for more information: http://www.unco.edu/housing. No on-campus day care facilities are available.

Employment of Department Graduates:
Master's Degree Graduates: Of those who graduated in the academic year 2008–2009, the following categories and numbers represent the postgraduate activities and employment of master's degree graduates: Enrolled in a postdoctoral residency/fellowship (n/a), employed in independent practice (n/a), total from the above (master's) (0).

Doctoral Degree Graduates: Of those who graduated in the academic year 2008–2009, the following categories and numbers represent the postgraduate activities and employment of doctoral degree graduates: Enrolled in a psychology doctoral program (n/a), enrolled in a postdoctoral residency/fellowship (2), employed in independent practice (6), employed in an academic position at a university (2), employed in a professional position in a school system (8), employed in a community mental health/counseling center (4), total from the above (doctoral) (22).

Additional Information:
Orientation, Objectives, and Emphasis of Department: The School of Applied Psychology and Counselor Education offers graduate programs in the fields of Counseling and School Psychology that prepare students for careers in schools, community agencies, industry, higher education, and private practice. The school offers professional psychological services to the university and the local community through its departmental clinic, a research and training facility. The School Psychology program is based on the scientist–practitioner model of training and focuses on the interaction of content knowledge, process and assessment skills, the educational and community context, and research. The Counseling Psychology program is based on the scientist–practitioner model with a greater emphasis on practice. Its training focuses on content knowledge, the educational and community context, therapeutic/assessment skills and their interaction. Students can be part of a cluster of outstanding psychology training programs. All programs are nestled within the School of Applied Psychology and Counselor Education with training in Counseling Psychology, School Psychology, Counselor Education, School Counseling, Community Counseling, and Family Therapy. Students have the opportunity to pursue elective course work in any or all of these areas.

Special Facilities or Resources: The school maintains a laboratory facility for use by the counseling and school psychology programs. This facility is built around a central observation area, from which eight counseling rooms, one testing room, two family therapy, one group therapy, one neuropsychology lab and three play therapy rooms can be observed and videotaped through one-way windows. All are furnished appropriately for the specific functions of each. All rooms are equipped with ceiling-mounted microphones with the observation area for each room supplied with an amplifier and earphone jacks. Several observation areas are also equipped with speakers. The main university library has provided excellent support for the professional psychology programs. Sufficient funding is provided annually for the purchase of relevant journals, books and digital media. Many journals can be retrieved online and from the student's home. Additionally, funding is available for purchasing tests listed in the Mental Measurements Yearbook.

Information for Students With Physical Disabilities: See the following Web site for more information: http://www.unco.edu/dss/geninfo.asp.

Application Information:
Send to Admissions Secretary, School of Applied Psychology and Counselor Education, University of Northern Colorado, Greeley, CO 80639. Application available online. URL of online application: http://www.unco.edu/grad/admissions/home.htm. Students are admitted in the Fall, application deadline (see below); Counseling Psychology, PhD - December 1; School Psychology, EdS & PhD - December 15; Counselor Education PhD - January 1; Clinical Counseling & Marriage/Family, School Counseling, MA degrees - December 15. *Fee:* $50.

Northern Colorado, University of (2009 data)
School of Psychological Sciences
Education and Behavioral Sciences
501 20th Street
Greeley, CO 80639-0001
Telephone: (970) 351-2957
Fax: (970) 351-1103
E-mail: *Roberta.ochsner@unco.edu*
Web: *http://www.unco.edu/psychology/*

Department Information:
1982. Director: Mark Alcorn. Number of faculty: total—full-time 19; women—full-time 7.

Programs and Degrees Offered:
Listed in the following order: Program area, degree type (T if terminal Master's), number awarded 7/08–6/09. Educational Psychology PhD (Doctor of Philosophy) 2, Educational Psychology MA/MS (Master of Arts/Science) (T) 3.

Student Applications/Admissions:
Student Applications
Educational Psychology PhD (Doctor of Philosophy)—Applications 2009–2010, 10. Total applicants accepted 2009–2010, 6. Number full-time enrolled (new admits only) 2009–2010, 3. Total enrolled 2009–2010 full-time, 21. Openings 2010–2011, 6. The median number of years required for completion of a degree in 2008–2009 were 4. The number of students enrolled full- and part-time who were dismissed or voluntarily withdrew from this program area in 2008–2009 were 0. *Educational Psychology MA/MS (Master of Arts/Science)*—Applications 2009–2010, 28. Total applicants accepted 2009–2010, 17. Number full-time enrolled (new admits only) 2009–2010, 7. Total enrolled 2009–2010 full-time, 12. Openings 2010–2011, 10. The median number of years required for completion of a degree in 2008–2009 was 1. The number of students enrolled full- and part-time who were dismissed or voluntarily withdrew from this program area in 2008–2009 were 0.

Other Criteria: (importance of criteria rated low, medium, or high): GRE scores—medium, research experience—medium, work experience—medium, extracurricular activity—medium, clinically related public service—low, GPA—high, letters of recommendation—high, statement of goals and objectives—high.

Student Characteristics: The following represents characteristics of students in 2009–2010 in all graduate psychology programs in the department: Female—full-time 11, part-time 0; Male—full-time 7, part-time 0; African American/Black—full-time 1, part-time 0; Hispanic/Latino(a)—full-time 0, part-time 0; Asian/Pacific Islander—full-time 1, part-time 0; American Indian/Alaska Native—full-time 0, part-time 0; Caucasian/White—full-time 14, part-time 0; Multi-ethnic—full-time 0, part-time 0; students subject to the Americans With Disabilities Act—full-time 0, part-time 0; Unknown ethnicity—full-time 0, part-time 0; International students who hold an F-1 or J-1 Visa—full-time 0, part-time 0.

Financial Information/Assistance:
Tuition for Full-Time Study: *Master's:* State residents: per academic year $4,704; Nonstate residents: per academic year $11,989.

Doctoral: State residents: per academic year $4,704; Nonstate residents: per academic year $11,989. Tuition is subject to change. See the following Web site for updates and changes in tuition costs: http://www.unco.edu/costs.

Financial Assistance:
First-Year Students: Research assistantships available for first year. Average amount paid per academic year: $5,532. Average number of hours worked per week: 9. Apply by March 15. Fellowships and scholarships available for first year. Average amount paid per academic year: $1,200. Average number of hours worked per week: 0. Apply by March 1.
Advanced Students: Teaching assistantships available for advanced students. Average amount paid per academic year: $7,554. Average number of hours worked per week: 11. Research assistantships available for advanced students. Average amount paid per academic year: $6,536. Average number of hours worked per week: 9.
Additional Information: Application and information available online at: http://www.unco.edu/grad/financial.

Internships/Practica: Doctoral students in Educational Psychology are given priority by the School in hiring Teaching Assistants. TAs are instructors of record, administering their own undergraduate classes, such as introductory psychology, human growth and development, and educational psychology. Our practicum experiences for both MA and PhD students include a seminar in college teaching, individually-scheduled directed studies, apprenticeships in teaching or research, as well as research practica that are closely supervised by faculty members.

Housing and Day Care: On-campus housing is available. See the following Web site for more information: http://housing.unco.edu/. No on-campus day care facilities are available.

Employment of Department Graduates:
Master's Degree Graduates: Of those who graduated in the academic year 2008–2009, the following categories and numbers represent the postgraduate activities and employment of master's degree graduates: Enrolled in a psychology doctoral program (5), enrolled in another graduate/professional program (1), enrolled in a postdoctoral residency/fellowship (n/a), employed in independent practice (n/a), employed in an academic position at a university (0), employed in an academic position at a 2-year/4-year college (0), employed in other positions at a higher education institution (0), employed in a professional position in a school system (0), employed in business or industry (2), employed in government agency (1), employed in a community mental health/counseling center (0), employed in a hospital/medical center (0), still seeking employment (0), other employment position (0), total from the above (master's) (9).
Doctoral Degree Graduates: Of those who graduated in the academic year 2008–2009, the following categories and numbers represent the postgraduate activities and employment of doctoral degree graduates: Enrolled in a psychology doctoral program (n/a), enrolled in a postdoctoral residency/fellowship (0), employed in independent practice (0), employed in an academic position at a university (2), employed in an academic position at a 2-year/4-year college (0), employed in other positions at a higher education institution (0), employed in a professional position in a school system (2), employed in business or industry (0), employed in government agency (0), employed in a community mental health/counseling center (0), employed in a hospital/medical center (0), still seeking employment (0), other employment position (0), total from the above (doctoral) (4).

Additional Information:
Orientation, Objectives, and Emphasis of Department: Our society faces many critical educational issues, such as how to make learning meaningful and authentic, develop critical thinking skills and creativity in individuals of various ages, and effectively educate special populations, including minorities and gifted students. These issue fall under the purview of Educational Psychology, which is the study of human learning and motivation. It encompasses investigations of cognition and the brain, the influence of affect, goals, and interest on learning; the role of assessment in learning, the psychology of teaching, the effectiveness of instructional interventions, the relationship between cognition and technology, the social psychology of learning organizations, and methods for conducting educational research. It addresses such issues in school contexts, work contexts, and everyday contexts such as the home or museums. The MA and PhD program at UNC prepares individuals to become leaders in addressing these issues. Students are trained in the art of reading, writing, and empirically researching such issues through course work and collaboration on research projects with faculty members. Our program is flexible and we help students design a course of study that best suits their needs. Faculty members take pride in mentoring students and building lasting professional relationships as both scholars and teachers.

Special Facilities or Resources: The University of Northern Colorado is accredited by the North Central Association of Colleges and Schools (NCA), the National Council for Accreditation of Teacher Education (NCATE) and the Colorado Department of Education (CDE). The Michener Library, a 150,000 sq ft facility is named for and endowed by James A. Michener. It houses almost 1.5 million hardbound volumes, periodicals, monographs, government documents, filmstrips, slides, and software programs. The university's Research Consulting Laboratory is located in the College of Education and Behavioral Sciences (CEBS) and supports faculty, students, and community agencies by offering consultation on research design and statistical analyses. The university also has several computer labs, both Mac and PC, available for student use, and the School of Psychological Sciences has its own laboratory with computers equipped with a software program to construct experimental paradigms. The School also has a fully-equipped physiological and experimental psychology laboratory, and access to the University Animal Facility. The Sponsored Program and Academic Research Center (SPARC) administers and oversees the Internal Review Board (IRB) of the university and employs grants and contracts specialists who have expertise in grant development, as well as monitoring the day-to-day financial aspects of grant administration.

Information for Students With Physical Disabilities: See the following Web site for more information: http://www.unco.edu/dss/.

Application Information:
Send to Graduate School, University of Northern Colorado, Greeley, CO 80639. Application available online. Students are admitted in the Fall, deadline March 15: *Fee:* $50.

GRADUATE STUDY IN PSYCHOLOGY

University of the Rockies
Psychology
School of Professional Psychology
555 East Pikes Peak Avenue, #108
Colorado Springs, CO 80903-3612
Telephone: (719) 442-0505
Fax: (719) 442-6999
E-mail: *info@Rockies.edu*
Web: *http://www.Rockies.edu*

Department Information:
1998. Dean, School of Professional Psychology: David C. Solly. Number of faculty: total—full-time 12, part-time 26; women—full-time 3, part-time 16; total—minority—full-time 2, part-time 5; women minority—full-time 1, part-time 3; faculty subject to the Americans With Disabilities Act 1.

Programs and Degrees Offered:
Listed in the following order: Program area, degree type (T if terminal Master's), number awarded 7/08–6/09. Clinical Psychology PsyD (Doctor of Psychology) 12, Professional Counseling MA/MS (Master of Arts/Science) (T) 14, Marriage and Family Therapy MA/MS (Master of Arts/Science) (T) 12, General Psychology MA/MS (Master of Arts/Science) 2, Sport & Performance Psychology MA/MS (Master of Arts/Science) 2, Sport & Performance Psychology PsyD (Doctor of Psychology) 2.

Student Applications/Admissions:
Student Applications
Clinical Psychology PsyD (Doctor of Psychology)—Applications 2009–2010, 58. Total applicants accepted 2009–2010, 22. Number full-time enrolled (new admits only) 2009–2010, 20. Number part-time enrolled (new admits only) 2009–2010, 2. Total enrolled 2009–2010 full-time, 56, part-time, 19. Openings 2010–2011, 20. The median number of years required for completion of a degree in 2008–2009 were 4. The number of students enrolled full- and part-time who were dismissed or voluntarily withdrew from this program area in 2008–2009 were 0. *Professional Counseling MA/MS (Master of Arts/Science)*—Applications 2009–2010, 30. Total applicants accepted 2009–2010, 11. Number full-time enrolled (new admits only) 2009–2010, 9. Number part-time enrolled (new admits only) 2009–2010, 0. Total enrolled 2009–2010 full-time, 26, part-time, 4. Openings 2010–2011, 10. The median number of years required for completion of a degree in 2008–2009 were 2. The number of students enrolled full- and part-time who were dismissed or voluntarily withdrew from this program area in 2008–2009 were 0. *Marriage and Family Therapy MA/MS (Master of Arts/Science)*—Applications 2009–2010, 27. Total applicants accepted 2009–2010, 14. Number full-time enrolled (new admits only) 2009–2010, 9. Number part-time enrolled (new admits only) 2009–2010, 4. Total enrolled 2009–2010 full-time, 23, part-time, 5. Openings 2010–2011, 10. The median number of years required for completion of a degree in 2008–2009 were 2. The number of students enrolled full- and part-time who were dismissed or voluntarily withdrew from this program area in 2008–2009 were 0. *General Psychology MA/MS (Master of Arts/Science)*—Applications 2009–2010, 157. Total applicants accepted 2009–2010, 45. Number full-time enrolled (new admits only) 2009–2010, 40. Number part-time enrolled (new admits only) 2009–2010, 5. Total enrolled 2009–2010 full-time, 38, part-time, 3. Openings 2010–2011, 25. The median number of years required for completion of a degree in 2008–2009 were 2. The number of students enrolled full- and part-time who were dismissed or voluntarily withdrew from this program area in 2008–2009 were 0. *Sport & Performance Psychology MA/MS (Master of Arts/Science)*—Applications 2009–2010, 37. Total applicants accepted 2009–2010, 10. Number full-time enrolled (new admits only) 2009–2010, 4. Number part-time enrolled (new admits only) 2009–2010, 6. Total enrolled 2009–2010 full-time, 11, part-time, 12. Openings 2010–2011, 10. The median number of years required for completion of a degree in 2008–2009 were 2. The number of students enrolled full- and part-time who were dismissed or voluntarily withdrew from this program area in 2008–2009 were 0. *Sport & Performance Psychology PsyD (Doctor of Psychology)*—Applications 2009–2010, 123. Total applicants accepted 2009–2010, 9. Number full-time enrolled (new admits only) 2009–2010, 5. Number part-time enrolled (new admits only) 2009–2010, 3. Total enrolled 2009–2010 full-time, 7, part-time, 15. Openings 2010–2011, 10. The median number of years required for completion of a degree in 2008–2009 were 3. The number of students enrolled full- and part-time who were dismissed or voluntarily withdrew from this program area in 2008–2009 were 0.

Scores: Entries appear in this order: required test or GPA, minimum score (if required), median score of students entering in 2009–2010. *Clinical Psychology PsyD (Doctor of Psychology)*: overall undergraduate GPA 3.0, 3.57, last 2 years GPA 3.0, 3.62, psychology GPA 3.0, 3.75, Masters GPA 3.0, 3.76; *Professional Counseling MA/MS (Master of Arts/Science)*: overall undergraduate GPA 3.0, 3.39, last 2 years GPA 3.0, 3.41, psychology GPA 3.0, 3.62; *Marriage and Family Therapy MA/MS (Master of Arts/Science)*: overall undergraduate GPA 3.0, 3.25, last 2 years GPA 3.0, 3.30, psychology GPA 3.0, 3.28; *General Psychology MA/MS (Master of Arts/Science)*: overall undergraduate GPA 2.75, 3.20, last 2 years GPA 2.75, 3.33, psychology GPA 3.0, 3.44; *Sport & Performance Psychology MA/MS (Master of Arts/Science)*: overall undergraduate GPA 2.75, 3.21, last 2 years GPA 2.75, 3.28; *Sport & Performance Psychology PsyD (Doctor of Psychology)*: overall undergraduate GPA 3.0, 3.35, last 2 years GPA 3.0, 3.39, Masters GPA 3.0, 3.63.

Other Criteria: (importance of criteria rated low, medium, or high): research experience—low, work experience—high, extracurricular activity—low, clinically related public service—medium, GPA—high, letters of recommendation—high, interview—high, statement of goals and objectives—high, MAT scores—high, specific undergraduate psychology courses taken—low. For additional information on admission requirements, go to http://www.rockies.edu/campus/admissions.php.

Student Characteristics: The following represents characteristics of students in 2009–2010 in all graduate psychology programs in the department: Female—full-time 117, part-time 31; Male—full-time 16, part-time 12; African American/Black—full-time 4, part-time 2; Hispanic/Latino(a)—full-time 26, part-time 15; Asian/Pacific Islander—full-time 6, part-time 1; American Indian/Alaska Native—full-time 2, part-time 4; Caucasian/White—full-time 94, part-time 15; Multi-ethnic—full-time 94, part-time 0; students subject to the Americans With Disabilities Act—full-time 2, part-time 0; Unknown ethnicity—full-time 0, part-time

0; International students who hold an F-1 or J-1 Visa—full-time 3, part-time 0.

Financial Information/Assistance:
Tuition for Full-Time Study: *Master's:* State residents: $665 per credit hour; Nonstate residents: $665 per credit hour. *Doctoral:* State residents: $800 per credit hour; Nonstate residents: $800 per credit hour. Tuition is subject to change. Additional fees are assessed to students beyond the costs of tuition for the following: specialized program area and course fees. See the following Web site for updates and changes in tuition costs: http://www.rockies.edu/campus/finaidinfo.php.

Financial Assistance:
First-Year Students: Teaching assistantships available for first year. Average amount paid per academic year: $5,000. Average number of hours worked per week: 20. Apply by March 1. Fellowships and scholarships available for first year. Average amount paid per academic year: $1,500. Average number of hours worked per week: 0. Apply by March 1.

Advanced Students: Teaching assistantships available for advanced students. Average amount paid per academic year: $5,000. Average number of hours worked per week: 20. Apply by March 1. Fellowships and scholarships available for advanced students. Average amount paid per academic year: $1,500. Average number of hours worked per week: 0. Apply by March 1.

Additional Information: Of all students currently enrolled full time, 10% benefited from one or more of the listed financial assistance programs.

Internships/Practica: Doctoral Degree (PsyD Clinical Psychology): For those doctoral students for whom a professional internship was required in this program prior to graduation, (16) students applied for an internship in 2008–2009, with (16) students obtaining an internship. Of those students who obtained an internship, (15) were paid internships. Of those students who obtained an internship, (1) students placed in APA/CPA accredited internships, (14) students placed in internships not APA/CPA accredited, but listed with the Association of Psychology Postdoctoral and Internship Programs (APPIC), (0) students placed in internships conforming to guidelines of the Council of Directors of School Psychology Programs (CDSPP), (1) students placed in internships that were not APA/CPA accredited, APPIC or CDSPP listed. Master's Degree (MA/MS Professional Counseling): An internship experience, such as a final research project or "capstone" experience is required of graduates. Master's Degree (MA/MS Marriage and Family Therapy): An internship experience, such as a final research project or "capstone" experience is required of graduates. The Switzer Behavioral Center is a campus based mental health center serving a broad range of clientele from greater Colorado Springs. Most of our students begin their practica in the Switzer Center. Two internships are available in the Switzer Center, and approximately 15 are available through a regional internship consortium. A postdoctoral residency positon is also available.

Housing and Day Care: No on-campus housing is available. No on-campus day care facilities are available.

Employment of Department Graduates:
Master's Degree Graduates: Of those who graduated in the academic year 2008–2009, the following categories and numbers represent the postgraduate activities and employment of master's degree graduates: Enrolled in a psychology doctoral program (12), enrolled in another graduate/professional program (0), enrolled in a postdoctoral residency/fellowship (n/a), employed in independent practice (n/a), employed in an academic position at a university (0), employed in an academic position at a 2-year/4-year college (2), employed in other positions at a higher education institution (0), employed in a professional position in a school system (0), employed in business or industry (0), employed in government agency (8), employed in a community mental health/counseling center (5), employed in a hospital/medical center (0), still seeking employment (0), not seeking employment (0), other employment position (3), do not know (0), total from the above (master's) (30).

Doctoral Degree Graduates: Of those who graduated in the academic year 2008–2009, the following categories and numbers represent the postgraduate activities and employment of doctoral degree graduates: Enrolled in a psychology doctoral program (n/a), enrolled in another graduate/professional program (0), enrolled in a postdoctoral residency/fellowship (12), employed in independent practice (0), employed in an academic position at a university (3), employed in an academic position at a 2-year/4-year college (3), employed in other positions at a higher education institution (1), employed in a professional position in a school system (2), employed in business or industry (4), employed in government agency (5), employed in a community mental health/counseling center (6), employed in a hospital/medical center (1), still seeking employment (0), not seeking employment (0), other employment position (1), do not know (0), total from the above (doctoral) (38).

Additional Information:
Orientation, Objectives, and Emphasis of Department: We are a department that embraces a strong practitioner-scholar orientation. Our objective is to prepare psychological practitioners who are strong scholars and outstanding resources to the agencies and communities in which they work. We practice, demonstrate, follow, and advocate a strong collegial model, and offer broad-based training across theoretical models, respecting each.

Special Facilities or Resources: The University of the Rockies Health and Neuropsychology Center offers opportunities for pre- and postdoctoral training in neuropsychological assessment and treatment, and research opportunities in both neuropsychology and health promotion. Relationships with local military facilities (Ft. Carson, Peterson Air Force Base, NORAD, and the U.S. Air Force Academy) and amateur sports organizations, including the U.S. Olympic Training Center, provide many opportunities to our students.

Information for Students With Physical Disabilities: See the following Web site for more information: http://www.rockies.edu/campus/disabilityservices.php.

Application Information:
Send to Office of Admissions University of the Rockies 555 E. Pikes Peak Avenue, # 108 Colorado Springs, CO 80903-3612. Application available online. URL of online application: http://www.rockies.edu/campus/admissions.php. Students are admitted in the Fall, application deadline July 1; Winter, application deadline November 1; Spring, application deadline February 15; Summer, application deadline May 1. *Fee:* $50.

CONNECTICUT

Central Connecticut State University
Department of Psychology
1615 Stanley Street
New Britain, CT 06050-4010
Telephone: (860) 832-3100
Fax: (860) 832-3123
E-mail: bowman@ccsu.edu
Web: http://www.ccsu.edu/psychology/

Department Information:
1967. Chairperson: Dr. Laura Bowman. Number of faculty: total—full-time 20, part-time 20; women—full-time 13, part-time 6; total—minority—full-time 2, part-time 2; women minority—part-time 1.

Programs and Degrees Offered:
Listed in the following order: Program area, degree type (T if terminal Master's), number awarded 7/08–6/09. Community Psychology MA/MS (Master of Arts/Science) (T) 1, General Psychology MA/MS (Master of Arts/Science) (T) 5, Health Psychology MA/MS (Master of Arts/Science) (T) 2.

Student Applications/Admissions:
Student Applications
Community Psychology MA/MS (Master of Arts/Science)—Applications 2009–2010, 12. Total applicants accepted 2009–2010, 4. Number full-time enrolled (new admits only) 2009–2010, 1. Number part-time enrolled (new admits only) 2009–2010, 2. Total enrolled 2009–2010 full-time, 2, part-time, 8. Openings 2010–2011, 5. The median number of years required for completion of a degree in 2008–2009 were 8. The number of students enrolled full- and part-time who were dismissed or voluntarily withdrew from this program area in 2008–2009 were 0. *General Psychology MA/MS (Master of Arts/Science)*—Applications 2009–2010, 25. Total applicants accepted 2009–2010, 10. Number full-time enrolled (new admits only) 2009–2010, 6. Number part-time enrolled (new admits only) 2009–2010, 3. Total enrolled 2009–2010 full-time, 12, part-time, 15. Openings 2010–2011, 10. The median number of years required for completion of a degree in 2008–2009 were 8. *Health Psychology MA/MS (Master of Arts/Science)*—Applications 2009–2010, 12. Total applicants accepted 2009–2010, 7. Number full-time enrolled (new admits only) 2009–2010, 3. Number part-time enrolled (new admits only) 2009–2010, 2. Total enrolled 2009–2010 full-time, 7, part-time, 8. Openings 2010–2011, 7. The median number of years required for completion of a degree in 2008–2009 were 6.
Scores: Entries appear in this order: required test or GPA, minimum score (if required), median score of students entering in 2009–2010. *Community Psychology MA/MS (Master of Arts/Science)*: overall undergraduate GPA 2.75, psychology GPA 3.0; *General Psychology MA/MS (Master of Arts/Science)*: overall undergraduate GPA 2.75, psychology GPA 3.0; *Health Psychology MA/MS (Master of Arts/Science)*: overall undergraduate GPA 2.75, psychology GPA 3.0.
Other Criteria: (importance of criteria rated low, medium, or high): research experience—medium, work experience—medium, extracurricular activity—low, clinically related public service—medium, GPA—high, letters of recommendation—high, statement of goals and objectives—high, 18 credits in psychology—medium, undergraduate major in psychology—low, specific undergraduate psychology courses taken—medium. For additional information on admission requirements, go to http://www.ccsu.edu/page.cfm?p=1969.

Student Characteristics: The following represents characteristics of students in 2009–2010 in all graduate psychology programs in the department: Female—full-time 19, part-time 27; Male—full-time 2, part-time 4; African American/Black—full-time 2, part-time 2; Hispanic/Latino(a)—full-time 2, part-time 3; Asian/Pacific Islander—full-time 0, part-time 0; American Indian/Alaska Native—full-time 0, part-time 0; Caucasian/White—full-time 16, part-time 23; Multi-ethnic—full-time 0, part-time 0; students subject to the Americans With Disabilities Act—full-time 0, part-time 0; Unknown ethnicity—full-time 1, part-time 4; International students who hold an F-1 or J-1 Visa—full-time 0, part-time 0.

Financial Information/Assistance:
Tuition for Full-Time Study: *Master's:* State residents: per academic year $8,268, $502 per credit hour; Nonstate residents: per academic year $17,916, $502 per credit hour. Tuition is subject to change. See the following Web site for updates and changes in tuition costs: http://www.ccsu.edu/page.cfm?p=1991.

Financial Assistance:
First-Year Students: Teaching assistantships available for first year. Average amount paid per academic year: $2,700. Average number of hours worked per week: 10. Apply by April 25.
Advanced Students: Teaching assistantships available for advanced students. Average amount paid per academic year: $2,700. Average number of hours worked per week: 10. Apply by April 25.
Additional Information: Of all students currently enrolled full time, 7% benefited from one or more of the listed financial assistance programs. Application and information available online at: http://www.ccsu.edu/page.cfm?p=2307.

Internships/Practica: Master's Degree (MA/MS Community Psychology): An internship experience, such as a final research project or "capstone" experience is required of graduates. Master's Degree (MA/MS Health Psychology): An internship experience, such as a final research project or "capstone" experience is required of graduates. We offer a variety of internships. For students in the community specialization, there are internships in prevention-oriented community programs dealing with substance abuse, teen pregnancy, etc. We also offer internships in developmental and counseling areas.

Housing and Day Care: On-campus housing is available. See the following Web site for more information: http://www.ccsu.edu/page.cfm?p=2595. On-campus day care facilities are available. See the following Web site for more information: http://www.ccsu.edu/page.cfm?p=403.

Employment of Department Graduates:
Master's Degree Graduates: Of those who graduated in the academic year 2008–2009, the following categories and numbers represent the postgraduate activities and employment of master's degree graduates: Enrolled in a postdoctoral residency/fellowship (n/a), employed in independent practice (n/a), total from the above (master's) (0).
Doctoral Degree Graduates: Of those who graduated in the academic year 2008–2009, the following categories and numbers represent the postgraduate activities and employment of doctoral degree graduates: Enrolled in a psychology doctoral program (n/a), total from the above (doctoral) (0).

Additional Information:
Orientation, Objectives, and Emphasis of Department: The psychology department includes 20 faculty members whose interests cover a wide range of psychological areas. Collectively, the orientation of the department is toward applied areas (clinical, community, health, applied, developmental), with generally little emphasis on animal learning/behavior. The specialization in community psychology focuses heavily on primary prevention. The general specialization is intended to expose students to a broad range of applied areas in psychology, while the one in health psychology prepares students for careers in the field of health psychology. The three specializations have a strong research emphasis.

Special Facilities or Resources: The psychology department has limited space available for human experimental research. The department has a computer laboratory, and the university has very good computer facilities available for student use. Students may also work on applied research projects with faculty through the Institute for Municipal and Regional Policy at the University.

Information for Students With Physical Disabilities: See the following Web site for more information: http://www.ccsu.edu/page.cfm?p=3639.

Application Information:
Send to Office of Graduate Admissions, Central Connecticut State University, 1615 Stanley Street, New Britain, CT 06050-4010. Application available online. URL of online application: http://www.ccsu.edu/grad/admissionprocess.htm. Students are admitted in the Fall, application deadline April 25; Spring, application deadline December 1. *Fee:* $50.

Connecticut, University of
Department of Psychology
College of Liberal Arts and Sciences
406 Babbidge Road, Unit 1020
Storrs, CT 06269-1020
Telephone: (860) 486-3515
Fax: (860) 486-2760
E-mail: *judith.jansen@uconn.edu*
Web: *http://web.uconn.edu/psychology/*

Department Information:
1939. Head: Charles A. Lowe. Number of faculty: total—full-time 51, part-time 2; women—full-time 26, part-time 2; total—minority—full-time 3, part-time 1; women minority—full-time 2, part-time 1.

Programs and Degrees Offered:
Listed in the following order: Program area, degree type (T if terminal Master's), number awarded 7/08–6/09. Behavioral Neuroscience PhD (Doctor of Philosophy) 4, Developmental Psychology PhD (Doctor of Philosophy) 2, Clinical Psychology PhD (Doctor of Philosophy) 12, Perception, Action, Cognition PhD (Doctor of Philosophy) 1, Industrial/Organizational Psychology PhD (Doctor of Philosophy) 1, Social Psychology PhD (Doctor of Philosophy) 4.

APA Accreditation: Clinical PhD (Doctor of Philosophy).

Student Applications/Admissions:
Student Applications
Behavioral Neuroscience PhD (Doctor of Philosophy)—Applications 2009–2010, 29. Total applicants accepted 2009–2010, 1. Number full-time enrolled (new admits only) 2009–2010, 1. Number part-time enrolled (new admits only) 2009–2010, 0. Openings 2010–2011, 3. The median number of years required for completion of a degree in 2008–2009 were 4. The number of students enrolled full- and part-time who were dismissed or voluntarily withdrew from this program area in 2008–2009 were 0. *Developmental Psychology PhD (Doctor of Philosophy)*—Applications 2009–2010, 21. Total applicants accepted 2009–2010, 1. Number full-time enrolled (new admits only) 2009–2010, 1. Number part-time enrolled (new admits only) 2009–2010, 0. Openings 2010–2011, 3. The median number of years required for completion of a degree in 2008–2009 were 5. The number of students enrolled full- and part-time who were dismissed or voluntarily withdrew from this program area in 2008–2009 were 0. *Clinical Psychology PhD (Doctor of Philosophy)*—Applications 2009–2010, 360. Total applicants accepted 2009–2010, 10. Number full-time enrolled (new admits only) 2009–2010, 6. Number part-time enrolled (new admits only) 2009–2010, 0. Openings 2010–2011, 7. The median number of years required for completion of a degree in 2008–2009 were 6. The number of students enrolled full- and part-time who were dismissed or voluntarily withdrew from this program area in 2008–2009 were 0. *Perception, Action, Cognition PhD (Doctor of Philosophy)*—Applications 2009–2010, 24. Total applicants accepted 2009–2010, 6. Number full-time enrolled (new admits only) 2009–2010, 4. Number part-time enrolled (new admits only) 2009–2010, 0. Total enrolled 2009–2010 full-time, 29, part-time, 2. Openings

2010–2011, 4. The median number of years required for completion of a degree in 2008–2009 were 7. The number of students enrolled full- and part-time who were dismissed or voluntarily withdrew from this program area in 2008–2009 were 1. *Industrial/Organizational Psychology PhD (Doctor of Philosophy)*—Applications 2009–2010, 57. Total applicants accepted 2009–2010, 6. Number full-time enrolled (new admits only) 2009–2010, 3. Number part-time enrolled (new admits only) 2009–2010, 0. Openings 2010–2011, 4. The median number of years required for completion of a degree in 2008–2009 were 4. The number of students enrolled full- and part-time who were dismissed or voluntarily withdrew from this program area in 2008–2009 were 0. *Social Psychology PhD (Doctor of Philosophy)*—Applications 2009–2010, 71. Total applicants accepted 2009–2010, 6. Number full-time enrolled (new admits only) 2009–2010, 5. Number part-time enrolled (new admits only) 2009–2010, 0. Openings 2010–2011, 5. The median number of years required for completion of a degree in 2008–2009 were 5. The number of students enrolled full- and part-time who were dismissed or voluntarily withdrew from this program area in 2008–2009 were 0.

Other Criteria: (importance of criteria rated low, medium, or high): GRE scores—medium, research experience—high, work experience—low, clinically related public service—low, GPA—medium, letters of recommendation—high, interview—medium, statement of goals and objectives—high. The Clinical Division interviews applicants by invitation only. The clinical interviews are considered to be high in importance of criteria used for offering admission. The Behavioral Neuroscience Division may interview by invitation or by applicant request, however interviews are not required. The Developmental, Experimental, Industrial/Organizational, and Social divisions do not interview applicants as part of the admissions process. For additional information on admission requirements, go to http://web2.uconn.edu/psychology/academics/graduate/graduate_program.html.

Student Characteristics: The following represents characteristics of students in 2009–2010 in all graduate psychology programs in the department: Female—full-time 110, part-time 0; Male—full-time 51, part-time 2; African American/Black—full-time 8, part-time 1; Hispanic/Latino(a)—full-time 10, part-time 0; Asian/Pacific Islander—full-time 23, part-time 0; American Indian/Alaska Native—full-time 0, part-time 0; Caucasian/White—full-time 110, part-time 1; Multi-ethnic—full-time 0, part-time 0; students subject to the Americans With Disabilities Act—full-time 0, part-time 0; Unknown ethnicity—full-time 10, part-time 0; International students who hold an F-1 or J-1 Visa—full-time 22, part-time 0.

Financial Information/Assistance:
  Tuition for Full-Time Study: *Doctoral:* State residents: per academic year $9,972, $554 per credit hour; Nonstate residents: per academic year $25,884, $1,438 per credit hour. Tuition is subject to change. Additional fees are assessed to students beyond the costs of tuition for the following: general university, infrastructure, graduate matriculation, activity, transit and student union. See the following Web site for updates and changes in tuition costs: http://www.grad.uconn.edu/tuition.html.

Financial Assistance:
  First-Year Students: Teaching assistantships available for first year. Average amount paid per academic year: $14,324. Average number of hours worked per week: 15. Research assistantships available for first year. Average amount paid per academic year: $14,324. Average number of hours worked per week: 15. Fellowships and scholarships available for first year. Average amount paid per academic year: $2,133. Average number of hours worked per week: 0.

  Advanced Students: Teaching assistantships available for advanced students. Average amount paid per academic year: $16,757. Average number of hours worked per week: 15. Research assistantships available for advanced students. Average amount paid per academic year: $16,757. Average number of hours worked per week: 15. Fellowships and scholarships available for advanced students. Average amount paid per academic year: $2,133. Average number of hours worked per week: 0.

  Additional Information: Of all students currently enrolled full time, 84% benefited from one or more of the listed financial assistance programs. Application and information available online at: http://www.financialaid.uconn.edu.

Internships/Practica: Doctoral Degree (PhD Clinical Psychology): For those doctoral students for whom a professional internship was required in this program prior to graduation, (5) students applied for an internship in 2008–2009, with (5) students obtaining an internship. Of those students who obtained an internship, (5) were paid internships. Of those students who obtained an internship, (5) students placed in APA/CPA accredited internships, (0) students placed in internships not APA/CPA accredited, but listed with the Association of Psychology Postdoctoral and Internship Programs (APPIC), (0) students placed in internships conforming to guidelines of the Council of Directors of School Psychology Programs (CDSPP), (0) students placed in internships that were not APA/CPA accredited, APPIC or CDSPP listed.

Housing and Day Care: On-campus housing is available. See the following Web site for more information: http://www.reslife.uconn.edu/graduate_housing.html and http://www.grad.uconn.edu/housing.html. On-campus day care facilities are available. See the following Web site for more information: http://www.childlabs.uconn.edu.

Employment of Department Graduates:
  Master's Degree Graduates: Of those who graduated in the academic year 2008–2009, the following categories and numbers represent the postgraduate activities and employment of master's degree graduates: Enrolled in a postdoctoral residency/fellowship (n/a), employed in independent practice (n/a), total from the above (master's) (0).
  Doctoral Degree Graduates: Of those who graduated in the academic year 2008–2009, the following categories and numbers represent the postgraduate activities and employment of doctoral degree graduates: Enrolled in a psychology doctoral program (n/a), enrolled in a postdoctoral residency/fellowship (18), employed in an academic position at a university (2), employed in business or industry (2), employed in a community mental health/counseling center (1), other employment position (1), total from the above (doctoral) (24).

Additional Information:

Orientation, Objectives, and Emphasis of Department: The department is focused on a dual mission of pursuing excellence in both research and teaching, while not losing sight of its broader mission to engage in meaningful outreach. The department is comprised of six divisions, each of which offers doctoral training in one or more areas of concentration as follows: (1) Behavioral Neuroscience (biopsychology, neuroscience); (2) Clinical Psychology; (3) Developmental Psychology; (4) Perception, Action, Cognition (ecological psychology, language and cognition); (5) Industrial/Organizational Psychology; and (6) Social Psychology. Interdivisional areas of strength, and targets for future growth, include (a) quantitative research methods, (b) health psychology, (c) cognitive science, (d) neuropsychology, and (e) developmental psychopathology. The pursuit of new knowledge (i.e., discovery through research) is the dominant emphasis of the department. This emphasis relies heavily on the interactive contributions from faculty, graduate students, and undergraduate students. In addition, the department's Graduate Student Teacher Training Program provides multiple, mentored teaching experiences for graduate students interested in pursuing a teaching/research career. Despite these varied emphases and endeavors, the department continues to maintain a collegial and supportive atmosphere where individual contributions are both recognized and rewarded.

Special Facilities or Resources: Multiple facilities, resources, and opportunities for research and training endeavors are not only available, but also are encouraged, fostered, and strongly supported by the department. These opportunities include existing and strong research collaborations with the University of Connecticut Health Center, with Haskins Laboratories in New Haven, with the Olin Neuropsychiatry Research Center at the Institute of Living in Hartford, and with a wide variety of research and internship opportunities available at multiple industries, hospitals, mental institutions, and school systems located in Connecticut. In addition, the department makes available and encourages research and training opportunities with units located within the department and/or within the University, including the Center for Health Intervention and Prevention, the Psychological Services Clinic (PSC), the Industrial Psychology Applications Center (IPAC), and the Center for the Ecological Study of Perception and Action (CESPA). Collectively, these collaborative relationships provide graduate students with myriad opportunities to pursue their research and training experience objectives.

Information for Students With Physical Disabilities: See the following Web site for more information: http://www.csd.uconn.edu.

Application Information:
Send to University of Connecticut Graduate School, 438 Whitney Road Ext., Unit 1006, Storrs, CT 06269-1006. Application available online. URL of online application: http://www.grad.uconn.edu/apply.html. Students are admitted in the Fall, application deadline January 1. Clinical Psychology program: December 1; Social Psychology and Industrial/Organizational Psychology programs: December 15; all other programs: January 1. *Fee:* $75. $55 fee for applications submitted using online application system.

Connecticut, University of
School Psychology Program
NEAG School of Education
249 Glenbrook Road, Unit 2064
Storrs, CT 06269-2064
Telephone: (860) 486-4031
Fax: (860) 486-0180
E-mail: *thomas.kehle@uconn.edu*
Web: *http://education.uconn.edu/departments/epsy/*

Department Information:
1960. Director, School Psychology Program: Thomas J. Kehle. Number of faculty: total—full-time 4, part-time 1; women—full-time 3, part-time 1.

Programs and Degrees Offered:
Listed in the following order: Program area, degree type (T if terminal Master's), number awarded 7/08–6/09. School Psychology PhD (Doctor of Philosophy) 1, School Psychology MA/MS (Master of Arts/Science) 1.

APA Accreditation: School PhD (Doctor of Philosophy).

Student Applications/Admissions:
Student Applications

School Psychology PhD (Doctor of Philosophy)—Applications 2009–2010, 38. Total applicants accepted 2009–2010, 12. Number full-time enrolled (new admits only) 2009–2010, 7. Number part-time enrolled (new admits only) 2009–2010, 0. Total enrolled 2009–2010 full-time, 17, part-time, 2. Openings 2010–2011, 6. The median number of years required for completion of a degree in 2008–2009 were 5. The number of students enrolled full- and part-time who were dismissed or voluntarily withdrew from this program area in 2008–2009 were 0. School Psychology MA/MS (Master of Arts/Science)—Applications 2009–2010, 57. Total applicants accepted 2009–2010, 11. Number full-time enrolled (new admits only) 2009–2010, 6. Number part-time enrolled (new admits only) 2009–2010, 0. Openings 2010–2011, 6. The median number of years required for completion of a degree in 2008–2009 were 3. The number of students enrolled full- and part-time who were dismissed or voluntarily withdrew from this program area in 2008–2009 were 0.

Scores: Entries appear in this order: required test or GPA, minimum score (if required), median score of students entering in 2009–2010. School Psychology PhD (Doctor of Philosophy): GRE-V 500, 608, GRE-Q 500, 644, overall undergraduate GPA 3.0, 3.68; School Psychology MA/MS (Master of Arts/Science): GRE-V 500, 577, GRE-Q 500, 642, overall undergraduate GPA 3.0, 3.68.

Other Criteria: (importance of criteria rated low, medium, or high): GRE scores—high, research experience—medium, work experience—medium, extracurricular activity—low, clinically related public service—low, GPA—medium, letters of recommendation—high, interview—high, statement of goals and objectives—high, undergraduate major in psychology—low, specific undergraduate psychology courses taken—low. For additional information on admission requirements, go to http://grad.uconn.edu/apply.html.

Student Characteristics: The following represents characteristics of students in 2009–2010 in all graduate psychology programs in the department: Female—full-time 28, part-time 1; Male—full-time 5, part-time 1; African American/Black—full-time 1, part-time 0; Hispanic/Latino(a)—full-time 1, part-time 0; Asian/Pacific Islander—full-time 0, part-time 0; American Indian/Alaska Native—full-time 0, part-time 0; Caucasian/White—full-time 31, part-time 2; Multi-ethnic—full-time 0, part-time 0; students subject to the Americans With Disabilities Act—full-time 0, part-time 0; Unknown ethnicity—full-time 0, part-time 0; International students who hold an F-1 or J-1 Visa—full-time 1, part-time 0.

Financial Information/Assistance:
Tuition for Full-Time Study: *Master's:* State residents: per academic year $9,950, $525 per credit hour; Nonstate residents: per academic year $24,534, $1,363 per credit hour. *Doctoral:* State residents: per academic year $9,950, $525 per credit hour; Nonstate residents: per academic year $24,534, $1,363 per credit hour. Additional fees are assessed to students beyond the costs of tuition for the following: general university, infrastructure/maintenance, graduate matriculation, activity, transit. See the following Web site for updates and changes in tuition costs: http://bursar.uconn.edu/tuit_grad_current.html.

Financial Assistance:
First-Year Students: Research assistantships available for first year. Average amount paid per academic year: $19,098. Average number of hours worked per week: 20. Apply by September 1.
Advanced Students: Research assistantships available for advanced students. Average amount paid per academic year: $22,342. Average number of hours worked per week: 20. Apply by September 1.
Additional Information: Of all students currently enrolled full time, 95% benefited from one or more of the listed financial assistance programs. Application and information available online at: http://grad.uconn.edu/funding_resources.html.

Internships/Practica: Doctoral Degree (PhD School Psychology): For those doctoral students for whom a professional internship was required in this program prior to graduation, (2) students applied for an internship in 2008–2009, with (2) students obtaining an internship. Of those students who obtained an internship, (2) were paid internships. Of those students who obtained an internship, (0) students placed in APA/CPA accredited internships, (0) students placed in internships not APA/CPA accredited, but listed with the Association of Psychology Postdoctoral and Internship Programs (APPIC), (2) students placed in internships conforming to guidelines of the Council of Directors of School Psychology Programs (CDSPP), (0) students placed in internships that were not APA/CPA accredited, APPIC or CDSPP listed. There are a number of practicum and internship placement opportunities for school psychology students at the University of Connecticut, affiliated sites, and school districts. The overwhelming majority of internship placements are paid, as are many of the practicum placements.

Housing and Day Care: On-campus housing is available. See the following Web site for more information: http://www.reslife.uconn.edu/. On-campus day care facilities are available. See the following Web site for more information: http://childlabs.uconn.edu/.

Employment of Department Graduates:
Master's Degree Graduates: Of those who graduated in the academic year 2008–2009, the following categories and numbers represent the postgraduate activities and employment of master's degree graduates: Enrolled in a psychology doctoral program (2), enrolled in a postdoctoral residency/fellowship (n/a), employed in independent practice (n/a), employed in a professional position in a school system (1), total from the above (master's) (3).
Doctoral Degree Graduates: Of those who graduated in the academic year 2008–2009, the following categories and numbers represent the postgraduate activities and employment of doctoral degree graduates: Enrolled in a psychology doctoral program (n/a), employed in a professional position in a school system (1), total from the above (doctoral) (1).

Additional Information:
Orientation, Objectives, and Emphasis of Department: The Department of Educational Psychology sponsors master of arts/sixth-year and doctor of philosophy programs in school psychology. The programs are an integrated and organized preparation of psychologists whose primary professional interests involve children, families, and the educational process. The programs adhere to the scientist–practitioner model of training that assumes the effective practice of school psychology is based on knowledge gained from established methods of scientific inquiry. The faculty are committed to a learning environment that stresses an organized and explicit curriculum with clear expectations. In addition, the programs are designed to acquaint students with the diversity of theories and practices of school psychology, allowing students sufficient intellectual freedom to experiment with different delivery systems and various theoretical bases. The atmosphere is intended to foster informal student-faculty interactions, critical debate, and respect for theoretical diversity of practice, thus creating a more intense and exciting learning experience. It is believed that such a philosophy encourages and reinforces students' creativity and intellectual risk taking that are fundamental in the further development of the professional practice of school psychology.

Special Facilities or Resources: Research space, equipment and/or opportunities exist in the following center/labs: Center for Behavioral and Educational Research; The National Research Center for Gifted and Talented; The Pappanikou Special Education Center; University Program for Students with Learning Disabilities; The University of Connecticut Educational Microcomputing Laboratory; and The Hartford Professional Development Academy.

Information for Students With Physical Disabilities: See the following Web site for more information: http://www.csd.uconn.edu/index.html.

Application Information:
Send to Graduate Admissions, Room 108, Whetten Center Box U-6A, 438 Whitney Road Ext, Storrs, CT 06269-1006. Application available online. URL of online application: http://grad.uconn.edu/online.html. Students are admitted in the Fall, application deadline December 1. *Fee:* $55 for electronic application; $75 for paper application.

Hartford, University of
Department of Psychology
Arts and Sciences
200 Bloomfield Avenue, East Hall
West Hartford, CT 06117
Telephone: (860) 768-4544
Fax: (860) 768-5292
E-mail: kablack@hartford.edu
Web: http://uhaweb.hartford.edu/PSYCH/

Department Information:
1957. Chairperson: Katherine A. Black, PhD. Number of faculty: total—full-time 20, part-time 23; women—full-time 12, part-time 10; total—minority—full-time 1, part-time 4; women minority—full-time 1, part-time 1.

Programs and Degrees Offered:
Listed in the following order: Program area, degree type (T if terminal Master's), number awarded 7/08–6/09. Clinical Practices in Psychology MA/MS (Master of Arts/Science) (T) 9, General Psychology MA/MS (Master of Arts/Science) (T) 5, School Psychology MA/MS (Master of Arts/Science) (T) 11, Organizational Psychology MA/MS (Master of Arts/Science) (T) 13.

Student Applications/Admissions:
Student Applications
Clinical Practices in Psychology MA/MS (Master of Arts/Science)—Applications 2009–2010, 37. Total applicants accepted 2009–2010, 23. Number full-time enrolled (new admits only) 2009–2010, 11. Number part-time enrolled (new admits only) 2009–2010, 0. Total enrolled 2009–2010 full-time, 22, part-time, 1. Openings 2010–2011, 11. The median number of years required for completion of a degree in 2008–2009 were 2. The number of students enrolled full- and part-time who were dismissed or voluntarily withdrew from this program area in 2008–2009 were 0. *General Psychology MA/MS (Master of Arts/Science)*—Applications 2009–2010, 17. Total applicants accepted 2009–2010, 12. Number full-time enrolled (new admits only) 2009–2010, 4. Number part-time enrolled (new admits only) 2009–2010, 4. Total enrolled 2009–2010 full-time, 7, part-time, 5. Openings 2010–2011, 5. The median number of years required for completion of a degree in 2008–2009 were 4. The number of students enrolled full- and part-time who were dismissed or voluntarily withdrew from this program area in 2008–2009 were 1. *School Psychology MA/MS (Master of Arts/Science)*—Applications 2009–2010, 26. Total applicants accepted 2009–2010, 14. Number full-time enrolled (new admits only) 2009–2010, 11. Number part-time enrolled (new admits only) 2009–2010, 0. Total enrolled 2009–2010 full-time, 32, part-time, 2. Openings 2010–2011, 12. The median number of years required for completion of a degree in 2008–2009 were 2. The number of students enrolled full- and part-time who were dismissed or voluntarily withdrew from this program area in 2008–2009 were 0. *Organizational Psychology MA/MS (Master of Arts/Science)*—Applications 2009–2010, 47. Total applicants accepted 2009–2010, 20. Number full-time enrolled (new admits only) 2009–2010, 4. Number part-time enrolled (new admits only) 2009–2010, 8. Total enrolled 2009–2010 full-time, 6, part-time, 20. Openings 2010–2011, 12. The median number of years required for completion of a degree in 2008–2009 were 2. The number of students enrolled full- and part-time who were dismissed or voluntarily withdrew from this program area in 2008–2009 were 0.

Scores: Entries appear in this order: required test or GPA, minimum score (if required), median score of students entering in 2009–2010. *Clinical Practices in Psychology MA/MS (Master of Arts/Science)*: GRE-V no minimum stated, 535, GRE-Q no minimum stated, 525, GRE-Analytical no minimum stated, 4.25, GRE-Subject (Psychology) no minimum stated, 610; *General Psychology MA/MS (Master of Arts/Science)*: GRE-V no minimum stated, GRE-Q no minimum stated, GRE-Analytical no minimum stated, overall undergraduate GPA no minimum stated; *School Psychology MA/MS (Master of Arts/Science)*: GRE-V no minimum stated, 435, GRE-Q no minimum stated, 520, GRE-Analytical no minimum stated, 4.25, GRE-Subject (Psychology) no minimum stated, 570; *Organizational Psychology MA/MS (Master of Arts/Science)*: GRE-V no minimum stated, 450, GRE-Q no minimum stated, 480, GRE-Analytical no minimum stated, 4.25.

Other Criteria: (importance of criteria rated low, medium, or high): GRE scores—medium, research experience—medium, work experience—medium, extracurricular activity—low, clinically related public service—medium, GPA—high, letters of recommendation—high, interview—high. Only the school psychology program requires an interview. For additional information on admission requirements, go to http://uhaweb.hartford.edu/PSYCH/PsyDeptPrograms.htm.

Student Characteristics: The following represents characteristics of students in 2009–2010 in all graduate psychology programs in the department: Female—full-time 55, part-time 21; Male—full-time 12, part-time 9; African American/Black—full-time 4, part-time 3; Hispanic/Latino(a)—full-time 4, part-time 3; Asian/Pacific Islander—full-time 0, part-time 0; American Indian/Alaska Native—full-time 0, part-time 0; Caucasian/White—full-time 47, part-time 19; Multi-ethnic—full-time 0, part-time 0; students subject to the Americans With Disabilities Act—full-time 0, part-time 0; Unknown ethnicity—full-time 12, part-time 2; International students who hold an F-1 or J-1 Visa—full-time 2, part-time 1.

Financial Information/Assistance:
Tuition for Full-Time Study: *Master's:* State residents: $415 per credit hour; Nonstate residents: $415 per credit hour. Tuition is subject to change. Additional fees are assessed to students beyond the costs of tuition for the following: registration fee, technology fee, thesis continuance fee, graduation fee. See the following Web site for updates and changes in tuition costs: http://uhaweb.hartford.edu/bursar/Tuition.htm.

Financial Assistance:
First-Year Students: Teaching assistantships available for first year. Average amount paid per academic year: $2,550. Average number of hours worked per week: 8. Research assistantships available for first year. Average amount paid per academic year: $2,550. Average number of hours worked per week: 8.
Advanced Students: Teaching assistantships available for advanced students. Average amount paid per academic year: $2,550. Average number of hours worked per week: 8. Research assistantships available for advanced students. Average amount

paid per academic year: $2,550. Average number of hours worked per week: 8.

Additional Information: Of all students currently enrolled full time, 26% benefited from one or more of the listed financial assistance programs. Application and information available online at: http://admission.hartford.edu/financial_aid/.

Internships/Practica: Master's Degree (MA/MS Clinical Practices in Psychology): An internship experience, such as a final research project or "capstone" experience is required of graduates. Master's Degree (MA/MS General Psychology): An internship experience, such as a final research project or "capstone" experience is required of graduates. Master's Degree (MA/MS School Psychology): An internship experience, such as a final research project or "capstone" experience is required of graduates. Master's Degree (MA/MS Organizational Psychology): An internship experience, such as a final research project or "capstone" experience is required of graduates. All Clinical Practices in Psychology students are assigned a half-time practicum in the second year of their academic program. The assignments for practica include mental health clinics, in- and out-patient services in hospitals, community centers, schools, and correctional institutions. Students are supervised both on-site by professional psychologists and at the University by the faculty. All School Psychology students are assigned a half-time practicum in their second year in a school setting and a full-time internship in their third year. Students are supervised by school psychologists on site and at the University by the faculty. Organizational Psychology students have an option of a one-semester practicum or capstone project, and General Psychology students have an option of a two-semester, half-time practicum at a facility in an area relevant to the student's training or a thesis.

Housing and Day Care: On-campus housing is available. See the following Web site for more information: http://uhaweb.hartford.edu/RESLIFE/. No on-campus day care facilities are available.

Employment of Department Graduates:
Master's Degree Graduates: Of those who graduated in the academic year 2008–2009, the following categories and numbers represent the postgraduate activities and employment of master's degree graduates: Enrolled in a postdoctoral residency/fellowship (n/a), employed in independent practice (n/a), total from the above (master's) (0).
Doctoral Degree Graduates: Of those who graduated in the academic year 2008–2009, the following categories and numbers represent the postgraduate activities and employment of doctoral degree graduates: Enrolled in a psychology doctoral program (n/a), total from the above (doctoral) (0).

Additional Information:
Orientation, Objectives, and Emphasis of Department: The Department of Psychology at the University of Hartford is strongly student-centered and committed to engaging students in the understanding of behavior, cognition, emotion, and social interaction. Major emphasis is placed on the development of critical thinking and analytical skills so students become adept at formulating meaningful questions, implementing strategies to enhance growth and development, and solving problems of individual and group behavior. Students are encouraged to understand, appreciate, and embrace diversity and the need for community involvement. The Department promotes self-awareness and life-long learning aimed at developing well-rounded, resourceful, ethical, competent, and compassionate graduates at all levels of education.

Special Facilities or Resources: In addition to mock therapy observational studios, located within the Department of Psychology, there are research labs dedicated to the study of stress management, pain management, and attachment. Numerous on-campus and community organizations are available for student internships and practica.

Application Information:
Send to Center for Graduate and Adult Academic Services, University of Hartford, 200 Bloomfield Avenue, West Hartford, CT 06117. Application available online. URL of online application: https://banweb8.hartford.edu/. Students are admitted in the Fall, application deadline February 15; Spring, application deadline November 1. Only the General Psychology program admits students in the spring. *Fee:* $45.

Hartford, University of
Department of Psychology: Graduate Institute of Professional Psychology
Arts and Sciences
200 Bloomfield Avenue
West Hartford, CT 06117-1599
Telephone: (860) 768-4778
Fax: (860) 768-4814
E-mail: *viereck@hartford.edu*
Web: *http://uhaweb.hartford.edu/gipppsyd/*

Department Information:
1957. Chairperson: Katherine Black, PhD. Number of faculty: total—full-time 20, part-time 23; women—full-time 12, part-time 10; total—minority—full-time 1, part-time 4; women minority—full-time 1, part-time 1.

Programs and Degrees Offered:
Listed in the following order: Program area, degree type (T if terminal Master's), number awarded 7/08–6/09. Clinical Psychology PsyD (Doctor of Psychology) 21.

APA Accreditation: Clinical PsyD (Doctor of Psychology). Student Outcome Data Website: http://uhaweb.hartford.edu/gipppsyd/PROGRAM-DATA.html.

Student Applications/Admissions:
Student Applications
Clinical Psychology PsyD (Doctor of Psychology)—Applications 2009–2010, 218. Total applicants accepted 2009–2010, 35. Number full-time enrolled (new admits only) 2009–2010, 24. Number part-time enrolled (new admits only) 2009–2010, 0. Openings 2010–2011, 24. The median number of years required for completion of a degree in 2008–2009 were 7. The number of students enrolled full- and part-time who were dismissed or voluntarily withdrew from this program area in 2008–2009 were 3.
Scores: Entries appear in this order: required test or GPA, minimum score (if required), median score of students entering in 2009–2010. *Clinical Psychology PsyD (Doctor of Psychology):*

GRE-V no minimum stated, 530, GRE-Q no minimum stated, 605, GRE-Analytical no minimum stated, 4.33, GRE-Subject (Psychology) no minimum stated, 610.

Other Criteria: (importance of criteria rated low, medium, or high): GRE scores—medium, research experience—medium, work experience—medium, extracurricular activity—low, clinically related public service—medium, GPA—high, letters of recommendation—high, interview—high, statement of goals and objectives—high, undergraduate major in psychology—medium, specific undergraduate psychology courses taken—medium. For additional information on admission requirements, go to http://uhaweb.hartford.edu/gipppsyd/AdmissionReq.html.

Student Characteristics: The following represents characteristics of students in 2009–2010 in all graduate psychology programs in the department: Female—full-time 131, part-time 0; Male—full-time 24, part-time 0; African American/Black—full-time 5, part-time 0; Hispanic/Latino(a)—full-time 9, part-time 0; Asian/Pacific Islander—full-time 13, part-time 0; American Indian/Alaska Native—full-time 0, part-time 0; Caucasian/White—full-time 112, part-time 0; Multi-ethnic—full-time 6, part-time 0; students subject to the Americans With Disabilities Act—full-time 1, part-time 0; Unknown ethnicity—full-time 10, part-time 0; International students who hold an F-1 or J-1 Visa—full-time 2, part-time 0.

Financial Information/Assistance:
Tuition for Full-Time Study: *Doctoral:* State residents: per academic year $22,500, $900 per credit hour; Nonstate residents: per academic year $22,500, $900 per credit hour. Tuition is subject to change. Additional fees are assessed to students beyond the costs of tuition for the following: registration fee, technology fee, graduation fee. See the following Web site for updates and changes in tuition costs: http://uhaweb.hartford.edu/bursar/Tuition.htm.

Financial Assistance:
First-Year Students: Research assistantships available for first year. Average amount paid per academic year: $3,100. Average number of hours worked per week: 6. Fellowships and scholarships available for first year. Average amount paid per academic year: $4,000. Average number of hours worked per week: 0.

Advanced Students: Teaching assistantships available for advanced students. Average amount paid per academic year: $6,200. Average number of hours worked per week: 12. Research assistantships available for advanced students. Average amount paid per academic year: $3,100. Average number of hours worked per week: 6. Fellowships and scholarships available for advanced students. Average amount paid per academic year: $3,100.

Additional Information: Of all students currently enrolled full time, 59% benefited from one or more of the listed financial assistance programs. Application and information available online at: http://www.hartford.edu/graduate/resources/financialaid.html.

Internships/Practica: Doctoral Degree (PsyD Clinical Psychology): For those doctoral students for whom a professional internship was required in this program prior to graduation, (20) students applied for an internship in 2008–2009, with (17) students obtaining an internship. Of those students who obtained an internship, (17) were paid internships. Of those students who obtained an internship, (16) students placed in APA/CPA accredited internships, (1) students placed in internships not APA/CPA accredited, but listed with the Association of Psychology Postdoctoral and Internship Programs (APPIC), (0) students placed in internships conforming to guidelines of the Council of Directors of School Psychology Programs (CDSPP), (0) students placed in internships that were not APA/CPA accredited, APPIC or CDSPP listed. Our practicum network is extensive (approximately 75 sites in 4 states) and includes child, adolescent, and adult placements. Students generally get their first or second choice of sites. Practicum placement is coordinated with Professional Practice Seminar (2nd year) and Case Conference Seminar (3rd year) to insure student's clinical training needs are being met. Emphasis is placed upon the concept of "self-in-role" learning.

Housing and Day Care: On-campus housing is available. See the following Web site for more information: http://uhaweb.hartford.edu/reslife/. No on-campus day care facilities are available.

Employment of Department Graduates:
Master's Degree Graduates: Of those who graduated in the academic year 2008–2009, the following categories and numbers represent the postgraduate activities and employment of master's degree graduates: Enrolled in a postdoctoral residency/fellowship (n/a), employed in independent practice (n/a), total from the above (master's) (0).

Doctoral Degree Graduates: Of those who graduated in the academic year 2008–2009, the following categories and numbers represent the postgraduate activities and employment of doctoral degree graduates: Enrolled in a psychology doctoral program (n/a), total from the above (doctoral) (0).

Additional Information:
Orientation, Objectives, and Emphasis of Department: The primary mission of the program is to prepare students for effective functioning in the multiple roles they will need to fill as practicing psychologists in these rapidly changing times. The program also espouses the principle of affirmative diversity, defined as upholding the fundamental values of human differences and the belief that respect for individual and cultural differences enhances and increases the quality of educational and interpersonal experiences.

Special Facilities or Resources: The Graduate Institute added a Child and Adolescent Proficiency Track in the Fall of 2003. The goal of the track is to allow students to develop not only broad clinical skills, but also strong therapeutic, assessment, and program development skills in working specifically with children, adolescents, and families.

Information for Students With Physical Disabilities: See the following Web site for more information: http://www.hartford.edu/support/.

Application Information:
Send to Center for Graduate and Adult Services, University of Hartford, 200 Bloomfield Avenue, Hartford, CT 06107. Application available online. URL of online application: http://uhaweb.hartford.edu/gipppsyd/Application.html. Students are admitted in the Fall, application deadline December 15. *Fee:* $45.

New Haven, University of
Graduate Psychology
College of Arts and Sciences, University of New Haven
300 Boston Post Road
West Haven, CT 06516
Telephone: (203) 932-7339
Fax: (203) 931-6032
E-mail: *ssidle@newhaven.edu*
Web: *http://www.newhaven.edu*

Department Information:
1972. Chairperson: Stuart Sidle PhD. Number of faculty: total—full-time 15, part-time 11; women—full-time 6, part-time 6; total—minority—full-time 2, part-time 3; women minority—full-time 1, part-time 2.

Programs and Degrees Offered:
Listed in the following order: Program area, degree type (T if terminal Master's), number awarded 7/08–6/09. Industrial/Organizational Psychology MA/MS (Master of Arts/Science) (T) 56, Community Psychology MA/MS (Master of Arts/Science) 11.

Student Applications/Admissions:
Student Applications
Industrial/Organizational Psychology MA/MS (Master of Arts/Science)—Applications 2009–2010, 140. Total applicants accepted 2009–2010, 112. Number full-time enrolled (new admits only) 2009–2010, 47. Number part-time enrolled (new admits only) 2009–2010, 26. Total enrolled 2009–2010 full-time, 88, part-time, 38. Openings 2010–2011, 35. The median number of years required for completion of a degree in 2008–2009 were 2. The number of students enrolled full- and part-time who were dismissed or voluntarily withdrew from this program area in 2008–2009 were 3. *Community Psychology MA/MS (Master of Arts/Science)*—Applications 2009–2010, 30. Total applicants accepted 2009–2010, 22. Number full-time enrolled (new admits only) 2009–2010, 11. Number part-time enrolled (new admits only) 2009–2010, 6. Total enrolled 2009–2010 full-time, 17, part-time, 6. Openings 2010–2011, 25. The median number of years required for completion of a degree in 2008–2009 were 2.
Scores: Entries appear in this order: required test or GPA, minimum score (if required), median score of students entering in 2009–2010. *Industrial/Organizational Psychology MA/MS (Master of Arts/Science):* overall undergraduate GPA 2.8, 3.4, last 2 years GPA 3.0, 3.5; *Community Psychology MA/MS (Master of Arts/Science):* overall undergraduate GPA 2.8, 3.3, last 2 years GPA 3.0, 3.4.
Other Criteria: (importance of criteria rated low, medium, or high): research experience—medium, work experience—medium, extracurricular activity—medium, clinically related public service—low, GPA—high, letters of recommendation—high, statement of goals and objectives—high.

Student Characteristics: The following represents characteristics of students in 2009–2010 in all graduate psychology programs in the department: Female—full-time 78, part-time 27; Male—full-time 27, part-time 17; African American/Black—full-time 8, part-time 11; Hispanic/Latino(a)—full-time 4, part-time 6; Asian/Pacific Islander—full-time 8, part-time 0; American Indian/Alaska Native—full-time 1, part-time 0; Caucasian/White—full-time 84, part-time 27; Multi-ethnic—full-time 0, part-time 0; students subject to the Americans With Disabilities Act—full-time 0, part-time 0; Unknown ethnicity—full-time 0, part-time 0; International students who hold an F-1 or J-1 Visa—full-time 11, part-time 0.

Financial Information/Assistance:
Tuition for Full-Time Study: *Master's:* State residents: $630 per credit hour; Nonstate residents: $630 per credit hour.

Financial Assistance:
First-Year Students: Teaching assistantships available for first year. Average number of hours worked per week: 15. Research assistantships available for first year. Average number of hours worked per week: 15.
Advanced Students: Teaching assistantships available for advanced students. Research assistantships available for advanced students.
Additional Information: Of all students currently enrolled full time, 90% benefited from one or more of the listed financial assistance programs.

Internships/Practica: Most of the full time students complete an internship which allows the student to acquire special skills through coordinating formal coursework with an internship or practicum in an organizational setting. The internship gives the student with limited work experience the opportunity to work in cooperating organizations or consulting firms. We have longstanding relationships with a wide variety of business organizations that seek our students as interns.

Housing and Day Care: No on-campus housing is available. No on-campus day care facilities are available.

Employment of Department Graduates:
Master's Degree Graduates: Of those who graduated in the academic year 2008–2009, the following categories and numbers represent the postgraduate activities and employment of master's degree graduates: Enrolled in a psychology doctoral program (2), enrolled in another graduate/professional program (1), enrolled in a postdoctoral residency/fellowship (n/a), employed in independent practice (n/a), employed in an academic position at a university (0), employed in an academic position at a 2-year/4-year college (0), employed in other positions at a higher education institution (2), employed in a professional position in a school system (0), employed in business or industry (44), employed in government agency (8), employed in a community mental health/counseling center (6), employed in a hospital/medical center (2), do not know (1), total from the above (master's) (66).
Doctoral Degree Graduates: Of those who graduated in the academic year 2008–2009, the following categories and numbers represent the postgraduate activities and employment of doctoral degree graduates: Enrolled in a psychology doctoral program (n/a), total from the above (doctoral) (0).

Additional Information:
Orientation, Objectives, and Emphasis of Department: The primary goal of the Master of Arts in Industrial and Organizational Psychology program is to provide students with the knowledge and experience necessary to improve the satisfaction and productivity of people at work. Graduates obtain challenging and re-

warding positions in public and private corporations, consulting firms, and government agencies. Even though our program has a strong applied/career orientation, we have been quite successful in providing those students who wish to pursue doctoral study with a strong research foundation.

Application Information:
Send to Graduate Admissions, 300 Boston Post Road, University of New Haven, West Haven, CT 06516. Application available online. URL of online application: http://www.newhaven.edu/admissions/gradadmissions. Programs have rolling admissions. *Fee:* $50.

Southern Connecticut State University
Department of Psychology
501 Crescent Street
New Haven, CT 06515
Telephone: (203) 392-6868
Fax: (203) 392-6805
E-mail: *hauseltw1@southernct.edu*
Web: *http://www.southernct.edu/departments/psychology/*

Department Information:
1893. Graduate Coordinator: W. J. Hauselt. Number of faculty: total—full-time 20, part-time 4; women—full-time 13, part-time 2.

Programs and Degrees Offered:
Listed in the following order: Program area, degree type (T if terminal Master's), number awarded 7/08–6/09. General Psychology MA/MS (Master of Arts/Science) (T) 16.

Student Applications/Admissions:
Student Applications
General Psychology MA/MS (Master of Arts/Science)—Applications 2009–2010, 76. Total applicants accepted 2009–2010, 32. Number full-time enrolled (new admits only) 2009–2010, 13. Number part-time enrolled (new admits only) 2009–2010, 7. Total enrolled 2009–2010 full-time, 29, part-time, 25. Openings 2010–2011, 18. The number of students enrolled full- and part-time who were dismissed or voluntarily withdrew from this program area in 2008–2009 were 2.
Scores: Entries appear in this order: required test or GPA, minimum score (if required), median score of students entering in 2009–2010. *General Psychology MA/MS (Master of Arts/Science):* GRE-V no minimum stated, GRE-Q no minimum stated, GRE-Analytical no minimum stated, overall undergraduate GPA 2.7, psychology GPA 3.0.
Other Criteria: (importance of criteria rated low, medium, or high): GRE scores—medium, research experience—low, work experience—low, extracurricular activity—low, GPA—high, letters of recommendation—high, statement of goals and objectives—high, undergraduate major in psychology—low, specific undergraduate psychology courses taken—high. For additional information on admission requirements, go to http://www.southernct.edu/psychology/graduate/.

Student Characteristics: The following represents characteristics of students in 2009–2010 in all graduate psychology programs in the department: Female—full-time 13, part-time 21; Male—full-time 3, part-time 6; African American/Black—full-time 0, part-time 0; Hispanic/Latino(a)—full-time 0, part-time 0; Asian/Pacific Islander—full-time 0, part-time 0; American Indian/Alaska Native—full-time 0, part-time 0; Caucasian/White—full-time 0, part-time 0; Multi-ethnic—full-time 0, part-time 0; students subject to the Americans With Disabilities Act—full-time 0, part-time 0; Unknown ethnicity—full-time 0, part-time 0; International students who hold an F-1 or J-1 Visa—full-time 0, part-time 0.

Financial Information/Assistance:
Tuition for Full-Time Study: *Master's:* State residents: per academic year $8,402; Nonstate residents: per academic year $18,050. Tuition is subject to change. See the following Web site for updates and changes in tuition costs: http://www.southernct.edu/bursar/tuitionfees/.

Financial Assistance:
First-Year Students: Teaching assistantships available for first year. Average amount paid per academic year: $4,400. Average number of hours worked per week: 20. Apply by May 1.
Advanced Students: Teaching assistantships available for advanced students. Average amount paid per academic year: $4,400. Average number of hours worked per week: 20. Apply by May 1.
Additional Information: Of all students currently enrolled full time, 20% benefited from one or more of the listed financial assistance programs. Application and information available online at: http://www.southernct.edu/financialaid/.

Internships/Practica: Master's Degree (MA/MS General Psychology): An internship experience, such as a final research project or "capstone" experience is required of graduates. With departmental permission, MA students may arrange a one- or two-semester clinical internship (3 credits for one semester; 6 credits for two semesters).

Housing and Day Care: On-campus housing is available. See the following Web site for more information: http://www.southernct.edu/residencelife/. No on-campus day care facilities are available.

Employment of Department Graduates:
Master's Degree Graduates: Of those who graduated in the academic year 2008–2009, the following categories and numbers represent the postgraduate activities and employment of master's degree graduates: Enrolled in a psychology doctoral program (1), enrolled in another graduate/professional program (2), enrolled in a postdoctoral residency/fellowship (n/a), employed in independent practice (n/a), employed in other positions at a higher education institution (2), employed in a professional position in a school system (1), employed in business or industry (3), employed in a community mental health/counseling center (4), do not know (4), total from the above (master's) (17).
Doctoral Degree Graduates: Of those who graduated in the academic year 2008–2009, the following categories and numbers represent the postgraduate activities and employment of doctoral degree graduates: Enrolled in a psychology doctoral program (n/a), total from the above (doctoral) (0).

Additional Information:
Orientation, Objectives, and Emphasis of Department: This rigorous, research-based program is designed to develop creative,

problem-solving skills that graduates can apply to a variety of clinical, industrial, and educational settings. Leading to a Master of Arts degree, this program is flexible enough to be completed on either a full-or part-time basis, meeting the needs of a wide range of candidates. For potential doctoral candidates who can enter neither a PhD nor a PsyD program at the present time, this program may provide the basis for later acceptance into a doctoral program. For those who are already working in clinical, educational, or industrial settings, it offers updating and credentials. In addition, this program provides ideal training for people who want to explore their personal interest in careers related to psychology. High school teachers may use the program to prepare themselves to teach psychology in addition to their current certification. The program emphasizes faculty advisement to help tailor the program to the needs of each individual student.

Information for Students With Physical Disabilities: See the following Web site for more information: http://www.southernct.edu/drc/.

Application Information:
Send to School of Graduate Studies, Southern Connecticut State University, New Haven, CT 06515. Application available online. URL of online application: http://www.southernct.edu/grad/admissions/. Students are admitted in the Fall, application deadline June 1; Spring, application deadline November 1. *Fee:* $50.

Yale University
Department of Psychology
P.O. Box 208205
New Haven, CT 06520-8205
Telephone: (203) 432-4518
Fax: (203) 432-7172
E-mail: *lauretta.olivi@yale.edu*
Web: *http://www.yale.edu/psychology*

Department Information:
1928. Chairperson: Marcia Johnson. Number of faculty: total—full-time 28; women—full-time 13; total—minority—full-time 1; women minority—full-time 1.

Programs and Degrees Offered:
Listed in the following order: Program area, degree type (T if terminal Master's), number awarded 7/08–6/09. Behavioral Neuroscience PhD (Doctor of Philosophy) 3, Clinical Psychology PhD (Doctor of Philosophy) 3, Cognitive Psychology PhD (Doctor of Philosophy) 6, Developmental Psychology PhD (Doctor of Philosophy) 4, Social/Personality Psychology PhD (Doctor of Philosophy) 1.

APA Accreditation: Clinical PhD (Doctor of Philosophy). Student Outcome Data Website: http://www.yale.edu/psychology/clinical_perfdata.html.

Student Applications/Admissions:
Student Applications
Behavioral Neuroscience PhD (Doctor of Philosophy)—Applications 2009–2010, 27. Total applicants accepted 2009–2010, 3. Number full-time enrolled (new admits only) 2009–2010, 2. Number part-time enrolled (new admits only) 2009–2010, 0. Openings 2010–2011, 3. The median number of years required for completion of a degree in 2008–2009 were 6. The number of students enrolled full- and part-time who were dismissed or voluntarily withdrew from this program area in 2008–2009 were 0. *Clinical Psychology PhD (Doctor of Philosophy)*—Applications 2009–2010, 326. Total applicants accepted 2009–2010, 4. Number full-time enrolled (new admits only) 2009–2010, 3. Number part-time enrolled (new admits only) 2009–2010, 0. Openings 2010–2011, 4. The median number of years required for completion of a degree in 2008–2009 were 6. The number of students enrolled full- and part-time who were dismissed or voluntarily withdrew from this program area in 2008–2009 were 0. *Cognitive Psychology PhD (Doctor of Philosophy)*—Applications 2009–2010, 87. Total applicants accepted 2009–2010, 3. Number full-time enrolled (new admits only) 2009–2010, 3. Number part-time enrolled (new admits only) 2009–2010, 0. Openings 2010–2011, 4. The median number of years required for completion of a degree in 2008–2009 were 6. The number of students enrolled full- and part-time who were dismissed or voluntarily withdrew from this program area in 2008–2009 were 0. *Developmental Psychology PhD (Doctor of Philosophy)*—Applications 2009–2010, 57. Total applicants accepted 2009–2010, 6. Number full-time enrolled (new admits only) 2009–2010, 4. Number part-time enrolled (new admits only) 2009–2010, 0. Openings 2010–2011, 3. The median number of years required for completion of a degree in 2008–2009 were 6. The number of students enrolled full- and part-time who were dismissed or voluntarily withdrew from this program area in 2008–2009 were 0. *Social/Personality Psychology PhD (Doctor of Philosophy)*—Applications 2009–2010, 156. Total applicants accepted 2009–2010, 5. Number full-time enrolled (new admits only) 2009–2010, 4. Number part-time enrolled (new admits only) 2009–2010, 0. Openings 2010–2011, 3. The median number of years required for completion of a degree in 2008–2009 were 6. The number of students enrolled full- and part-time who were dismissed or voluntarily withdrew from this program area in 2008–2009 were 0.

Scores: Entries appear in this order: required test or GPA, minimum score (if required), median score of students entering in 2009–2010. *Behavioral Neuroscience PhD (Doctor of Philosophy)*: GRE-V no minimum stated, GRE-Q no minimum stated, GRE-Analytical no minimum stated, overall undergraduate GPA no minimum stated, last 2 years GPA no minimum stated, psychology GPA no minimum stated, Masters GPA no minimum stated; *Clinical Psychology PhD (Doctor of Philosophy)*: GRE-V no minimum stated, GRE-Q no minimum stated, GRE-Analytical no minimum stated, overall undergraduate GPA no minimum stated, last 2 years GPA no minimum stated, psychology GPA no minimum stated, Masters GPA no minimum stated; *Cognitive Psychology PhD (Doctor of Philosophy)*: GRE-V no minimum stated, GRE-Q no minimum stated, GRE-Analytical no minimum stated, overall undergraduate GPA no minimum stated, last 2 years GPA no minimum stated, psychology GPA no minimum stated, Masters GPA no minimum stated; *Developmental Psychology PhD (Doctor of Philosophy)*: GRE-V no minimum stated, GRE-Q no minimum stated, GRE-Analytical no minimum stated, overall undergraduate GPA no minimum stated, last 2 years GPA no minimum stated, psychology GPA no minimum stated, Mas-

ters GPA no minimum stated; *Social/Personality Psychology PhD (Doctor of Philosophy)*: GRE-V no minimum stated, GRE-Q no minimum stated, GRE-Analytical no minimum stated, overall undergraduate GPA no minimum stated, last 2 years GPA no minimum stated, psychology GPA no minimum stated, Masters GPA no minimum stated.
Other Criteria: (importance of criteria rated low, medium, or high): GRE scores—high, research experience—high, work experience—low, extracurricular activity—low, clinically related public service—low, GPA—high, letters of recommendation—high, interview—medium, statement of goals and objectives—high, undergraduate major in psychology—medium, specific undergraduate psychology courses taken—medium. For additional information on admission requirements, go to http://www.yale.edu/graduateschool/admissions/.

Student Characteristics: The following represents characteristics of students in 2009–2010 in all graduate psychology programs in the department: Female—full-time 52, part-time 0; Male—full-time 19, part-time 0; African American/Black—full-time 2, part-time 0; Hispanic/Latino(a)—full-time 9, part-time 0; Asian/Pacific Islander—full-time 10, part-time 0; American Indian/Alaska Native—full-time 0, part-time 0; Caucasian/White—full-time 40, part-time 0; Multi-ethnic—full-time 10, part-time 0; students subject to the Americans With Disabilities Act—full-time 1, part-time 0; Unknown ethnicity—full-time 0, part-time 0; International students who hold an F-1 or J-1 Visa—full-time 3, part-time 0.

Financial Information/Assistance:
Tuition for Full-Time Study: *Doctoral:* State residents: per academic year $32,500; Nonstate residents: per academic year $32,500. Tuition is subject to change. See the following Web site for updates and changes in tuition costs: http://www.yale.edu/graduateschool/financial/costs.html.

Financial Assistance:
First-Year Students: No information provided.
Advanced Students: Teaching assistantships available for advanced students. Average amount paid per academic year: $16,000. Average number of hours worked per week: 15. Apply by June 30. Research assistantships available for advanced students. Average number of hours worked per week: 10. Traineeships available for advanced students. Fellowships and scholarships available for advanced students.
Additional Information: Of all students currently enrolled full time, 100% benefited from one or more of the listed financial assistance programs. Application and information available online at: http://www.yale.edu/graduateschool/financial/.

Internships/Practica: Doctoral Degree (PhD Clinical Psychology): For those doctoral students for whom a professional internship was required in this program prior to graduation, (3) students applied for an internship in 2008–2009, with (3) students obtaining an internship. Of those students who obtained an internship, (3) were paid internships. Of those students who obtained an internship, (3) students placed in APA/CPA accredited internships, (0) students placed in internships not APA/CPA accredited, but listed with the Association of Psychology Postdoctoral and Internship Programs (APPIC), (0) students placed in internships conforming to guidelines of the Council of Directors of School Psychology Programs (CDSPP), (0) students placed in internships that were not APA/CPA accredited, APPIC or CDSPP listed. Students are required to assist in teaching an average of 10-15 hours per week in their second, third, and fourth years as part of their educational program. Local facilities for predoctoral internships are the Veterans Administration Center in West Haven, Yale Psychological Services Clinic, the Yale Child Study Center, and Yale Department of Psychiatry, with placement in the Connecticut Mental Health Center, Yale-New Haven Hospital, or the Yale Psychiatric Institute. Also, internships are arranged in accredited facilities throughout the United States.

Housing and Day Care: On-campus housing is available. See the following Web site for more information: http://www.yale.edu/gradhousing/. On-campus day care facilities are available. See the following Web site for more information: http://www.yale.edu/hronline/worklife/ccd.html.

Employment of Department Graduates:
Master's Degree Graduates: Of those who graduated in the academic year 2008–2009, the following categories and numbers represent the postgraduate activities and employment of master's degree graduates: Enrolled in a postdoctoral residency/fellowship (n/a), employed in independent practice (n/a), total from the above (master's) (0).
Doctoral Degree Graduates: Of those who graduated in the academic year 2008–2009, the following categories and numbers represent the postgraduate activities and employment of doctoral degree graduates: Enrolled in a psychology doctoral program (n/a), enrolled in a postdoctoral residency/fellowship (8), employed in an academic position at a university (8), other employment position (1), total from the above (doctoral) (17).

Additional Information:
Orientation, Objectives, and Emphasis of Department: The chief goal of graduate education in psychology at Yale University is the training of research workers in academic and other settings who will broaden the basic scientific knowledge on which the discipline of psychology rests. Major emphasis is given to preparation for research; a definite effort is made to give students a background for teaching. The concentration of doctoral training on research and teaching is consistent with a variety of career objectives in addition to traditional academics. The department believes that rigorous and balanced exposure to basic psychology is the best preparation for research careers. The first important aspect of graduate training is advanced study of general psychology, including method and psychological theory. The second is specialized training within a subfield. Third, the student is encouraged to take advantage of opportunities for wider training emphasizing research rather than practice. For the clinical area, research and practica are strongly integrated. Training is geared to the expectation that the majority of students will have research careers.

Special Facilities or Resources: Facilities available as adjuncts to research and teaching include The Yale Capuchin Cognition Lab, The Yale Parenting Center and Child Conduct Clinic, The Rudd Center for Food Policy and Obesity, and the Yale Anxiety and Mood Disorders Clinic. Other facilities include special rooms equipped for observation, intercommunication, and recording as required for clinical supervision or testing or for interview training and research. Also available to our students is an fMRI facility in the Yale University School of Medicine.

Information for Students With Physical Disabilities: See the following Web site for more information: http://www.yale.edu/rod/.

Application Information:
Send to Graduate School, Yale University, Office of Admissions, P.O. Box 208323, New Haven, CT 06520-8323. Application available online. URL of online application: http://www.yale.edu/graduateschool/admissions/. Students are admitted in the Fall, application deadline December 15. *Fee:* $95.

DELAWARE

Delaware, University of
Department of Psychology
College of Arts and Science
108 Wolf Hall
Newark, DE 19716
Telephone: (302) 831-2271
Fax: (302) 831-3645
E-mail: *mchermol@psych.udel.edu*
Web: *http://www.psych.udel.edu/graduate/index.asp*

Department Information:
1946. Chairperson: Thomas DiLorenzo. Number of faculty: total—full-time 27; women—full-time 10; total—minority—full-time 3; women minority—full-time 1.

Programs and Degrees Offered:
Listed in the following order: Program area, degree type (T if terminal Master's), number awarded 7/08–6/09. Clinical Science PhD (Doctor of Philosophy) 3, Behavioral Neuroscience PhD (Doctor of Philosophy) 1, Social Psychology PhD (Doctor of Philosophy) 1, Cognitive Psychology PhD (Doctor of Philosophy) 0.

APA Accreditation: Clinical PhD (Doctor of Philosophy). Student Outcome Data Website: http://www.psych.udel.edu/graduate/detail/admission_and_student_outcome_data_disclosure_data/.

Student Applications/Admissions:
Student Applications
Clinical Science PhD (Doctor of Philosophy)—Applications 2009–2010, 194. Total applicants accepted 2009–2010, 5. Number full-time enrolled (new admits only) 2009–2010, 3. Number part-time enrolled (new admits only) 2009–2010, 0. The number of students enrolled full- and part-time who were dismissed or voluntarily withdrew from this program area in 2008–2009 were 0. Behavioral Neuroscience PhD (Doctor of Philosophy)—Applications 2009–2010, 32. Total applicants accepted 2009–2010, 2. Number full-time enrolled (new admits only) 2009–2010, 0. Number part-time enrolled (new admits only) 2009–2010, 0. The number of students enrolled full- and part-time who were dismissed or voluntarily withdrew from this program area in 2008–2009 were 0. Social Psychology PhD (Doctor of Philosophy)—Applications 2009–2010, 55. Total applicants accepted 2009–2010, 3. Number full-time enrolled (new admits only) 2009–2010, 3. Number part-time enrolled (new admits only) 2009–2010, 0. The number of students enrolled full- and part-time who were dismissed or voluntarily withdrew from this program area in 2008–2009 were 1. Cognitive Psychology PhD (Doctor of Philosophy)—Applications 2009–2010, 37. Total applicants accepted 2009–2010, 4. Number full-time enrolled (new admits only) 2009–2010, 1. Number part-time enrolled (new admits only) 2009–2010, 0. The number of students enrolled full- and part-time who were dismissed or voluntarily withdrew from this program area in 2008–2009 were 0.

Scores: Entries appear in this order: required test or GPA, minimum score (if required), median score of students entering in 2009–2010. *Clinical Science PhD (Doctor of Philosophy):* GRE-V no minimum stated, 650, GRE-Q no minimum stated, 715, GRE-Analytical no minimum stated, 5.0, overall undergraduate GPA no minimum stated, 3.89.

Other Criteria: (importance of criteria rated low, medium, or high): GRE scores—high, research experience—medium, work experience—low, extracurricular activity—low, clinically related public service—medium, GPA—high, letters of recommendation—high, interview—high, statement of goals and objectives—high. In the behavioral neuroscience, cognitive and social areas, GRE scores are emphasized less and research experience is emphasized more relative to the clinical area. For additional information on admission requirements, go to http://www.psych.udel.edu/graduate/detail/category/prospective_graduate_students/.

Student Characteristics: The following represents characteristics of students in 2009–2010 in all graduate psychology programs in the department: Female—full-time 33, part-time 0; Male—full-time 12, part-time 0; African American/Black—full-time 4, part-time 0; Hispanic/Latino(a)—full-time 0, part-time 0; Asian/Pacific Islander—full-time 4, part-time 0; American Indian/Alaska Native—full-time 0, part-time 0; Caucasian/White—full-time 35, part-time 0; Multi-ethnic—full-time 1, part-time 0; students subject to the Americans With Disabilities Act—full-time 0, part-time 0; Unknown ethnicity—full-time 1, part-time 0; International students who hold an F-1 or J-1 Visa—full-time 5, part-time 0.

Financial Information/Assistance:
Tuition for Full-Time Study: *Doctoral:* State residents: per academic year $11,120, $1,236 per credit hour; Nonstate residents: per academic year $11,120, $1,236 per credit hour. Additional fees are assessed to students beyond the costs of tuition for the following: student health fees and student health center fees. See the following Web site for updates and changes in tuition costs: http://www.udel.edu/bill_coll/fees.html.

Financial Assistance:
First-Year Students: Teaching assistantships available for first year. Average amount paid per academic year: $15,579. Average number of hours worked per week: 20. Apply by January 7. Research assistantships available for first year. Average amount paid per academic year: $15,579. Average number of hours worked per week: 20. Apply by January 7. Fellowships and scholarships available for first year. Average amount paid per academic year: $15,579. Apply by January 7.

Advanced Students: Teaching assistantships available for advanced students. Average amount paid per academic year: $16,158. Average number of hours worked per week: 20. Research assistantships available for advanced students. Average amount paid per academic year: $15,996. Average number of hours worked per week: 20. Fellowships and scholarships available for advanced students. Average amount paid per academic year: $16,329.

Additional Information: Of all students currently enrolled full time, 100% benefited from one or more of the listed financial

assistance programs. Application and information available online at: http://www.udel.edu/gradoffice/financial/index.html.

Internships/Practica: Doctoral Degree (PhD Clinical Science): For those doctoral students for whom a professional internship was required in this program prior to graduation, (4) students applied for an internship in 2008–2009, with (4) students obtaining an internship. Of those students who obtained an internship, (4) were paid internships. Of those students who obtained an internship, (4) students placed in APA/CPA accredited internships, (0) students placed in internships not APA/CPA accredited, but listed with the Association of Psychology Postdoctoral and Internship Programs (APPIC), (0) students placed in internships conforming to guidelines of the Council of Directors of School Psychology Programs (CDSPP), (0) students placed in internships that were not APA/CPA accredited, APPIC or CDSPP listed. A wide range of practica are available for clinical graduate students.

Housing and Day Care: On-campus housing is available. See the following Web site for more information: http://www.udel.edu/housing/. On-campus day care facilities are available. See the following Web site for more information: http://www.udel.edu/hr/childcare.html.

Employment of Department Graduates:
Master's Degree Graduates: Of those who graduated in the academic year 2008–2009, the following categories and numbers represent the postgraduate activities and employment of master's degree graduates: Enrolled in a postdoctoral residency/fellowship (n/a), employed in independent practice (n/a), total from the above (master's) (0).
Doctoral Degree Graduates: Of those who graduated in the academic year 2008–2009, the following categories and numbers represent the postgraduate activities and employment of doctoral degree graduates: Enrolled in a psychology doctoral program (n/a), total from the above (doctoral) (0).

Additional Information:
Orientation, Objectives, and Emphasis of Department: The department fosters a scientific approach to all areas of psychology. The training is organized around clinical, cognitive, behavioral neuroscience, and social areas, as well as an integrative developmental focus that cuts across areas. All first-year students are required to complete first and second year research projects as well as take seminars in their program area of study. In the third and fourth year, students take additional seminars, take a comprehensive qualifying exam or prepare a comprehensive paper and prepare dissertation proposals. Clinical students also participate in the training of practice skills. Beyond the first year, students work out their own research programs with faculty advisors. The goal of this training is to prepare students to function as scientists and teachers in academic, applied, and clinical settings. Major current research interests in these areas are as follows: (1) clinical: evaluation of therapy, social development of children, community mental health, theory of emotions, communication of emotions, organic brain syndromes, family therapy, sex roles, sensation seeking, and sexuality; (2) cognitive: attention, pattern recognition, psycholinguistics, visual information processing, memory, and cognitive development; (3) behavioral neuroscience: neuroanatomy, developmental psychobiology, psychopharmacology, and neurobiology of learning; and (4) social: interpersonal conflict, racism, helping behavior, nonverbal communications, social power and influence, and decision-making. The program is flexible and encourages each student to develop his or her unique interests. The clinical program emphasizes empirically supported intervention and prevention techniques. A particular strength of the program is in child-clinical research, intervention and prevention, but students with interests in adult psychopathology and intervention would be equally at home and well served. The department has strengths in early experience and developmental processes, visual cognition, and brain plasticity during development and learning.

Special Facilities or Resources: The University's mainframe computing needs are met by several Unix timesharing systems. These systems are used primarily for administrative purposes, some special statistical analysis applications and for cognitive model simulations. The Department of Psychology is well equipped to handle department computing needs with a large assortment of Windows and Macintosh microcomputers and several department servers that bear the brunt of department computing needs. Graduate students will find generous laboratory resources aimed to meet their scientific and computing needs individually. There is also a state-of-the-art computer classroom used for instructional purposes and available to graduate students around the clock for data reduction, statistical analysis and general word processing. The department laboratories are well equipped for the online control of experiments for human and animal subjects as well as for data analysis and modeling. Laboratories are generously equipped with videotape, acoustic, behavioral and physiological recording systems. The department also operates the Psychological Services Training Center for practicum training in clinical psychology.

Information for Students With Physical Disabilities: See the following Web site for more information: http://www.udel.edu/DSS/.

Application Information:
Send to The Office of Graduate Studies, 234 Hullihen Hall, University of Delaware, Newark, DE 19716. Application available online. URL of online application: http://www.udel.edu/gradoffice/apply/. Students are admitted in the Fall, application deadline January 7. *Fee:* $60. The fee may be waived or deferred by the Department of Psychology.

DISTRICT OF COLUMBIA

American University
Department of Psychology
College of Arts and Sciences
321 Asbury, 4400 Massachusetts Avenue, NW
Washington, DC 20016-8062
Telephone: (202) 885-1710
Fax: (202) 885-1023
E-mail: *psychology@american.edu*
Web: *http://www.american.edu/cas/psychology*

Department Information:
1929. Chairperson: Anthony L. Riley. Number of faculty: total—full-time 20; women—full-time 8; total—minority—full-time 4; women minority—full-time 3.

Programs and Degrees Offered:
Listed in the following order: Program area, degree type (T if terminal Master's), number awarded 7/08–6/09. Behavior, Cognition and Neuroscience (BCAN) PhD (Doctor of Philosophy) 5, Clinical Psychology PhD (Doctor of Philosophy) 7, General Psychology MA/MS (Master of Arts/Science) (T) 25.

APA Accreditation: Clinical PhD (Doctor of Philosophy). Student Outcome Data Website: http://www.american.edu/cas/psychology/clinical.cfm.

Student Applications/Admissions:
Student Applications

Behavior, Cognition and Neuroscience (BCAN) PhD (Doctor of Philosophy)—Applications 2009–2010, 43. Total applicants accepted 2009–2010, 8. Number full-time enrolled (new admits only) 2009–2010, 5. Number part-time enrolled (new admits only) 2009–2010, 0. Openings 2010–2011, 5. The median number of years required for completion of a degree in 2008–2009 were 5. The number of students enrolled full- and part-time who were dismissed or voluntarily withdrew from this program area in 2008–2009 were 0. *Clinical Psychology PhD (Doctor of Philosophy)*—Applications 2009–2010, 247. Total applicants accepted 2009–2010, 6. Number full-time enrolled (new admits only) 2009–2010, 5. Number part-time enrolled (new admits only) 2009–2010, 0. Openings 2010–2011, 6. The median number of years required for completion of a degree in 2008–2009 were 6. The number of students enrolled full- and part-time who were dismissed or voluntarily withdrew from this program area in 2008–2009 were 0. *General Psychology MA/MS (Master of Arts/Science)*—Applications 2009–2010, 154. Total applicants accepted 2009–2010, 66. Number full-time enrolled (new admits only) 2009–2010, 16. Number part-time enrolled (new admits only) 2009–2010, 0. Total enrolled 2009–2010 full-time, 18, part-time, 22. Openings 2010–2011, 20. The median number of years required for completion of a degree in 2008–2009 were 2. The number of students enrolled full- and part-time who were dismissed or voluntarily withdrew from this program area in 2008–2009 were 4.

Scores: Entries appear in this order: required test or GPA, minimum score (if required), median score of students entering in 2009–2010. *Behavior, Cognition and Neuroscience (BCAN) PhD (Doctor of Philosophy):* GRE-V 650, 560, GRE-Q 700, 640, GRE-Analytical 5, 4.5, GRE-Subject (Psychology) no minimum stated, 630, overall undergraduate GPA 3.59, 3.66; *Clinical Psychology PhD (Doctor of Philosophy):* GRE-V 648, 640, GRE-Q 658, 650, GRE-Analytical 4.8, 5, GRE-Subject (Psychology) 698, 700, overall undergraduate GPA 3.35, 3.51; *General Psychology MA/MS (Master of Arts/Science):* GRE-V 570, GRE-Q 581, GRE-Analytical no minimum stated, overall undergraduate GPA 3.41.

Other Criteria: (importance of criteria rated low, medium, or high): GRE scores—high, research experience—high, work experience—medium, clinically related public service—medium, GPA—high, letters of recommendation—high, interview—high, statement of goals and objectives—high, undergraduate major in psychology—medium, specific undergraduate psychology courses taken—medium. Interview, clinically related public service not required for Behavior, Cognition, and Neuroscience program. For additional information on admission requirements, go to http://www.american.edu/cas/.

Student Characteristics: The following represents characteristics of students in 2009–2010 in all graduate psychology programs in the department: Female—full-time 41, part-time 50; Male—full-time 11, part-time 8; African American/Black—full-time 6, part-time 3; Hispanic/Latino(a)—full-time 4, part-time 2; Asian/Pacific Islander—full-time 2, part-time 3; American Indian/Alaska Native—full-time 0, part-time 0; Caucasian/White—full-time 39, part-time 46; Multi-ethnic—full-time 1, part-time 4; students subject to the Americans With Disabilities Act—full-time 0, part-time 0; Unknown ethnicity—full-time 0, part-time 0; International students who hold an F-1 or J-1 Visa—full-time 0, part-time 4.

Financial Information/Assistance:
Tuition for Full-Time Study: *Master's:* State residents: $1,299 per credit hour; Nonstate residents: $1,299 per credit hour. *Doctoral:* State residents: $1,299 per credit hour; Nonstate residents: $1,299 per credit hour. Tuition is subject to change. See the following Web site for updates and changes in tuition costs: http://www.american.edu/provost/registrar/registration/tuition.cfm.

Financial Assistance:
First-Year Students: Teaching assistantships available for first year. Average amount paid per academic year: $19,200. Average number of hours worked per week: 20. Apply by January 1. Fellowships and scholarships available for first year. Average amount paid per academic year: $23,382.

Advanced Students: Teaching assistantships available for advanced students. Average amount paid per academic year: $19,200. Average number of hours worked per week: 20. Apply by January 1. Fellowships and scholarships available for advanced students. Average amount paid per academic year: $23,382.

Additional Information: Of all students currently enrolled full time, 75% benefited from one or more of the listed financial

assistance programs. Application and information available online at: http://www.american.edu/cas/admissions/finance.cfm.

Internships/Practica: Doctoral Degree (PhD Clinical Psychology): For those doctoral students for whom a professional internship was required in this program prior to graduation, (5) students applied for an internship in 2008–2009, with (4) students obtaining an internship. Of those students who obtained an internship, (4) were paid internships. Of those students who obtained an internship, (4) students placed in APA/CPA accredited internships, (0) students placed in internships not APA/CPA accredited, but listed with the Association of Psychology Postdoctoral and Internship Programs (APPIC), (0) students placed in internships conforming to guidelines of the Council of Directors of School Psychology Programs (CDSPP), (0) students placed in internships that were not APA/CPA accredited, APPIC or CDSPP listed. The greater Washington, DC metropolitan area provides a wealth of applied and research resources to complement our students' work in the classroom and faculty laboratories. These include the university's Counseling Center, local hospitals (Children's, St. Elizabeth's, Walter Reed, Georgetown University, National Rehabilitation), the Kennedy Institute, Gallaudet University, the NIH (NIMH, NINDS, NIA, NCI), the National Zoo, and the national offices of many agencies (e.g., APA, APS, NAMI). Field work and short-term externships are available in many city, county, and private organizations, such as the Alexandria, VA Community Mental Health Center, the Montgomery County, MD Department of Addiction, Victim, and Mental Health Services, and the DC Rape Crisis Center. MA and PhD students can also earn degree credit while obtaining practical experience working in the private sector with autistic children, teaching self-management skills, or volunteering at shelters for battered women or the homeless. Many of these positions sometimes can provide funding. Clinical students participate in Rogerian, cognitive-behavioral, and psychodynamic therapy practica.

Housing and Day Care: On-campus housing is available. See the following Web site for more information: http://www.american.edu/ocl/housing/aboutHDP.cfm. On-campus day care facilities are available. See the following Web site for more information: http://www.american.edu/hr/cdc.cfm.

Employment of Department Graduates:
Master's Degree Graduates: Of those who graduated in the academic year 2008–2009, the following categories and numbers represent the postgraduate activities and employment of master's degree graduates: Enrolled in a psychology doctoral program (12), enrolled in another graduate/professional program (2), enrolled in a postdoctoral residency/fellowship (n/a), employed in independent practice (n/a), employed in a community mental health/counseling center (8), total from the above (master's) (22).
Doctoral Degree Graduates: Of those who graduated in the academic year 2008–2009, the following categories and numbers represent the postgraduate activities and employment of doctoral degree graduates: Enrolled in a psychology doctoral program (n/a), enrolled in a postdoctoral residency/fellowship (4), employed in an academic position at a university (4), employed in a professional position in a school system (1), employed in a community mental health/counseling center (2), employed in a hospital/medical center (2), total from the above (doctoral) (13).

Additional Information:
Orientation, Objectives, and Emphasis of Department: The psychology department of American University offers two graduate programs. The PhD program has separate tracks in clinical psychology and behavior, cognition and neuroscience. The MA program has tracks in general, personality/social, and biological/experimental psychology. The doctoral program in clinical psychology trains psychologists to do therapy, assessment, research, university teaching, and consultation. The theoretical orientation is eclectic and follows the Boulder scientist–practitioner model. The doctoral program in behavioral neuroscience/experimental psychology involves intensive training in both pure and applied research settings. Students can work in laboratories exploring conditioning and learning, the experimental analysis of behavior, cognition and memory, physiological psychology, neuropsychology, and neuropharmacology. Study at the master's level provides the basis for further doctoral-level work and prepares students for immediate employment in a variety of careers including clinical-medical research, teaching, counseling and policy formulation, law enforcement, and government work. Our graduate students are expected to be professional, ethical, committed, full-time members of our psychology community. This concept of community implies an atmosphere of mutual support rather than competition, communication rather than isolation, and stimulation rather than disinterest.

Special Facilities or Resources: Nine well-equipped laboratories investigate conditioning and learning, clinical and experimental neuropsychology, human cognition and memory, neuropharmacology, physiological psychology, rodent olfaction, social behavior, psychopathology, depression, anxiety disorders, emotion, eating disorders, parent-child interaction, addictive behavior, child development, and various other issues in applied and experimental psychology. In addition, students train in the Department's cognitive behavioral training clinic. Close working relationships with laboratories at the National Institutes of Health, the Walter Reed Army Institutes of Research, and Georgetown University's Hospital and School of Medicine allow additional training opportunities. The Washington Research Library Consortium (WRLC) provides access to six local college and university libraries in addition to AU's Bender Library, the National Library of Medicine, and the Library of Congress. AU's computing center supports IBM, Macintosh, and Unix systems, has dial-in access, and maintains fifteen computing labs. EagleNet, a campus-wide network service runs on Novell Netware 4.x and 5.0. Applications include WordPerfect, Quattro Pro, Presentations, Paradox, SAS, SPSS, Photoshop, Netscape, and e-mail as well as many Internet applications and services.

Information for Students With Physical Disabilities: See the following Web site for more information: http://www.american.edu/ocl/dss/.

Application Information:
Send to College of Arts and Sciences, Graduate Admissions, McKinley Building, 4400 Massachusetts Avenue, NW, Washington, DC 20016-8107. Application available online. URL of online application: http://

american.edu/cas/admissions. Students are admitted in the Fall, application deadline — Clinical, January 1; Behavior, Cognition and Neuroscience, January 1; MA, March 1. *Fee:* $50. Application fee is $80 if a paper application is used.

Gallaudet University
Department of Psychology
College of Liberal Arts, Sciences and Technologies
800 Florida Avenue, Northeast
Washington, DC 20002
Telephone: (202) 651-5540
Fax: (202) 651-5747
E-mail: *irene.leigh@gallaudet.edu*
Web: *http://psychology.gallaudet.edu/*

Department Information:
1955. Chairperson: Irene W. Leigh, PhD. Number of faculty: total—full-time 14, part-time 6; women—full-time 9, part-time 4; total—minority—full-time 3, part-time 1; women minority—full-time 2; faculty subject to the Americans With Disabilities Act 5.

Programs and Degrees Offered:
Listed in the following order: Program area, degree type (T if terminal Master's), number awarded 7/08–6/09. Clinical Psychology PhD (Doctor of Philosophy) 5, School Psychology Other 5.

APA Accreditation: Clinical PhD (Doctor of Philosophy). Student Outcome Data Website: http://aaweb.gallaudet.edu/graduate_programs/PhD_Clinical_Psychology/Student_Summary_Data.html.

Student Applications/Admissions:
Student Applications
Clinical Psychology PhD (Doctor of Philosophy)—Applications 2009–2010, 25. Total applicants accepted 2009–2010, 7. Number full-time enrolled (new admits only) 2009–2010, 7. Number part-time enrolled (new admits only) 2009–2010, 0. Total enrolled 2009–2010 full-time, 33, part-time, 10. Openings 2010–2011, 7. The median number of years required for completion of a degree in 2008–2009 were 6. The number of students enrolled full- and part-time who were dismissed or voluntarily withdrew from this program area in 2008–2009 were 0. *School Psychology Other*—Applications 2009–2010, 8. Total applicants accepted 2009–2010, 7. Number full-time enrolled (new admits only) 2009–2010, 6. Number part-time enrolled (new admits only) 2009–2010, 0. Openings 2010–2011, 8. The median number of years required for completion of a degree in 2008–2009 were 3. The number of students enrolled full- and part-time who were dismissed or voluntarily withdrew from this program area in 2008–2009 were 1.
Other Criteria: (importance of criteria rated low, medium, or high): GRE scores—medium, research experience—high, work experience—medium, extracurricular activity—medium, clinically related public service—high, GPA—medium, letters of recommendation—medium, interview—high, statement of goals and objectives—medium, psychology courses—high, undergraduate major in psychology—medium, specific undergraduate psychology courses taken—medium. Students with little experience with deaf people or sign language may be required to take sign language (ASL) courses prior to enrolling. Prior research experience is highly valued in doctoral program admissions, but has a medium weight for the Specialist program.

Student Characteristics: The following represents characteristics of students in 2009–2010 in all graduate psychology programs in the department: Female—full-time 36, part-time 8; Male—full-time 13, part-time 2; African American/Black—full-time 5, part-time 1; Hispanic/Latino(a)—full-time 4, part-time 3; Asian/Pacific Islander—full-time 1, part-time 0; American Indian/Alaska Native—full-time 0, part-time 0; Caucasian/White—full-time 38, part-time 6; Multi-ethnic—full-time 1, part-time 0; students subject to the Americans With Disabilities Act—full-time 15, part-time 0; Unknown ethnicity—full-time 0, part-time 0; International students who hold an F-1 or J-1 Visa—full-time 3, part-time 2.

Financial Information/Assistance:
Tuition for Full-Time Study: *Master's:* State residents: per academic year $5,965, $663 per credit hour; Nonstate residents: per academic year $5,965, $663 per credit hour. *Doctoral:* State residents: per academic year $5,965, $663 per credit hour; Nonstate residents: per academic year $5,965, $663 per credit hour. Tuition is subject to change. Additional fees are assessed to students beyond the costs of tuition for the following: unit fee, health insurance and services. See the following Web site for updates and changes in tuition costs: http://gallaudet.edu/af/financeoffice_tuitionandfees.xml. Higher tuition cost for this program: International students pay higher tuition.

Financial Assistance:
First-Year Students: Teaching assistantships available for first year. Average amount paid per academic year: $4,500. Average number of hours worked per week: 8. Research assistantships available for first year. Average amount paid per academic year: $4,500. Average number of hours worked per week: 8. Fellowships and scholarships available for first year. Average amount paid per academic year: $7,000. Average number of hours worked per week: 10.
Advanced Students: Teaching assistantships available for advanced students. Average amount paid per academic year: $4,500. Average number of hours worked per week: 8. Research assistantships available for advanced students. Average amount paid per academic year: $4,500. Average number of hours worked per week: 8. Fellowships and scholarships available for advanced students. Average amount paid per academic year: $7,000. Average number of hours worked per week: 10.
Additional Information: Of all students currently enrolled full time, 90% benefited from one or more of the listed financial assistance programs.

Internships/Practica: Doctoral Degree (PhD Clinical Psychology): For those doctoral students for whom a professional internship was required in this program prior to graduation, (6) students applied for an internship in 2008–2009, with (6) students obtaining an internship. Of those students who obtained an internship, (6) were paid internships. Of those students who obtained

an internship, (6) students placed in APA/CPA accredited internships, (0) students placed in internships not APA/CPA accredited, but listed with the Association of Psychology Postdoctoral and Internship Programs (APPIC), (0) students placed in internships conforming to guidelines of the Council of Directors of School Psychology Programs (CDSPP), (0) students placed in internships that were not APA/CPA accredited, APPIC or CDSPP listed. Students in the School Psychology Specialist Program (which includes the MA as a non-terminal degree) begin with a practicum experience in their first semester, visiting and observing school programs as part of their Introduction to School Psychology course. During their second semester they are involved in Practicum I (3 credit course), which involves closely supervised practicum doing cognitive assessments of deaf and hearing children (if appropriate) at laboratory schools on campus and a D.C. neighborhood school. Practicum II (3 credits) is taken the third semester and requires two full days per week for a minimum of 14 weeks in which they work with a school psychologist in the Washington Metropolitan area doing comprehensive assessments, and some counseling if opportunities are available, and observation on a limited basis during their fourth semester (an option). The third year (semesters 5 and 6) are spent in a full-time internship in a school approved by the program. These internships are typically located in both residential schools for the deaf as well as public school systems serving mainstreamed deaf youngsters. Internship sites are located in all parts of the United States. Students in the Clinical Psychology doctoral program begin practicum in their second year, conducting psychological assessments and psychotherapy at the Gallaudet University Mental Health Center. Advanced students can apply for any of the more than 80 externships available in the Washington, DC area. These externships allow students to work with a wide variety of settings and populations in assessment, psychotherapy, and other psychological interventions. Experiences with both deaf and hearing clients are available. A full-time, one-year doctoral level internship (typically in an APA-accredited internship program) is required.

Housing and Day Care: On-campus housing is available. See the following Web site for more information: http://sa.gallaudet.edu/Student_Affairs/Residence_Life.html. On-campus day care facilities are available. See the following Web site for more information: http://www.gallaudet.edu/af/cdc.xml.

Employment of Department Graduates:
Master's Degree Graduates: Of those who graduated in the academic year 2008–2009, the following categories and numbers represent the postgraduate activities and employment of master's degree graduates: Enrolled in a psychology doctoral program (0), enrolled in another graduate/professional program (0), enrolled in a postdoctoral residency/fellowship (n/a), employed in independent practice (n/a), employed in a professional position in a school system (5), total from the above (master's) (5).
Doctoral Degree Graduates: Of those who graduated in the academic year 2008–2009, the following categories and numbers represent the postgraduate activities and employment of doctoral degree graduates: Enrolled in a psychology doctoral program (n/a), enrolled in a postdoctoral residency/fellowship (2), employed in independent practice (1), employed in an academic position at a university (1), employed in government agency (1), total from the above (doctoral) (5).

Additional Information:
Orientation, Objectives, and Emphasis of Department: The Psychology department at Gallaudet University offers graduate programs in school psychology and clinical psychology. The school psychology program awards a nonterminal Master of Arts degree in developmental psychology plus a Specialist in School Psychology degree with specialization in deafness. The clinical psychology program is a scholar-practitioner model PhD program, and trains generalist clinical psychologists to work with deaf, hard-of-hearing, and hearing populations. The school psychology program is both NCATE/NASP and NASDTEC-approved, and leads to certification as a school psychologist in the District of Columbia and approximately 24 states with reciprocity of certification. The full-time, three-year program requires completion of at least 72 graduate semester hours, including a one-year internship. The APA accredited clinical psychology doctoral program is a five-year program providing balanced training in research and clinical skills with a variety of age groups, including deaf and hard-of-hearing children, adults, and older adults. The fifth year is designed as a full-time clinical psychology internship. A research-based dissertation is required.

Special Facilities or Resources: Gallaudet University is an internationally recognized center for research and training in areas related to deafness. With a diverse student body of approximately 1600, the university trains deaf, hard of hearing, and hearing students in a variety of fields at the bachelor, master's, and doctoral levels. Gallaudet programs are located on historic Kendall Green, in northeast Washington, DC near the U.S. Capitol, the Library of Congress, and the Smithsonian Institute. Also located on the campus are the Gallaudet University Mental Health Center, the Kendall Demonstration Elementary School, the Model Secondary School for the Deaf, the Gallaudet Research Institute, the Kellogg Conference Center, and the Gallaudet Library, which contains the largest collection of references on deafness in the world. Gallaudet faculty, including both deaf and hearing individuals, possess a unique combination of scholarly activity in their respective disciplines and experience with deaf clients and research on deafness. The University is committed to a working model of a bilingual (American Sign Language and English), multicultural community, where deaf, hard of hearing, and hearing people can work together without communication barriers. Gallaudet University is a member of the Consortium of Universities of the Washington Metropolitan Area and the Washington Research Library Consortium.

Information for Students With Physical Disabilities: See the following Web site for more information: http://sa.gallaudet.edu.

Application Information:
Send to Office of Graduate Admissions, Gallaudet University, 800 Florida Avenue N.E., Washington, DC 20002. Application available online. URL of online application: http://aaweb.gallaudet.edu/GradAdmissions.xml. Students are admitted in the Fall, application deadline February 1. *Fee:* $50. Waived for McNair Scholars.

George Washington University
Department of Psychology
Columbian College of Arts and Sciences
2125 G Street, Northwest
Washington, DC 20052
Telephone: (202) 994-6320
Fax: (202) 994-1602
E-mail: pjp@gwu.edu
Web: http://www.gwu.edu/~psycdept

Department Information:
1922. Chairperson: Paul Poppen. Number of faculty: total—full-time 20, part-time 2; women—full-time 11, part-time 2; total—minority—full-time 7; women minority—full-time 6.

Programs and Degrees Offered:
Listed in the following order: Program area, degree type (T if terminal Master's), number awarded 7/08–6/09. Applied Social Psychology PhD (Doctor of Philosophy) 2, Clinical Psychology PhD (Doctor of Philosophy) 5, Cognitive Neuroscience PhD (Doctor of Philosophy) 2.

APA Accreditation: Clinical PhD (Doctor of Philosophy). Student Outcome Data Website: http://www.gwu.edu/~psycdept/graduate_studies/clinical/index.cfm.

Student Applications/Admissions:
Student Applications
Applied Social Psychology PhD (Doctor of Philosophy)—Applications 2009–2010, 65. Total applicants accepted 2009–2010, 1. Number full-time enrolled (new admits only) 2009–2010, 1. Number part-time enrolled (new admits only) 2009–2010, 0. Openings 2010–2011, 2. The median number of years required for completion of a degree in 2008–2009 were 5. *Clinical Psychology PhD (Doctor of Philosophy)*—Applications 2009–2010, 300. Total applicants accepted 2009–2010, 4. Number full-time enrolled (new admits only) 2009–2010, 4. Number part-time enrolled (new admits only) 2009–2010, 0. Openings 2010–2011, 5. The median number of years required for completion of a degree in 2008–2009 were 6. The number of students enrolled full- and part-time who were dismissed or voluntarily withdrew from this program area in 2008–2009 were 0. *Cognitive Neuroscience PhD (Doctor of Philosophy)*—Applications 2009–2010, 45. Total applicants accepted 2009–2010, 1. Number full-time enrolled (new admits only) 2009–2010, 1. Openings 2010–2011, 2. The median number of years required for completion of a degree in 2008–2009 were 5.
Scores: Entries appear in this order: required test or GPA, minimum score (if required), median score of students entering in 2009–2010. *Applied Social Psychology PhD (Doctor of Philosophy):* GRE-V no minimum stated, 600, GRE-Q no minimum stated, 650, GRE-Analytical no minimum stated, 650, overall undergraduate GPA no minimum stated, 3.65; *Clinical Psychology PhD (Doctor of Philosophy):* GRE-V no minimum stated, 600, GRE-Q no minimum stated, 650, GRE-Analytical no minimum stated, overall undergraduate GPA no minimum stated, 3.70; *Cognitive Neuroscience PhD (Doctor of Philosophy):* GRE-V no minimum stated, 660, GRE-Q no minimum stated, 680, GRE-Analytical no minimum stated, overall undergraduate GPA no minimum stated, 3.50.

Other Criteria: (importance of criteria rated low, medium, or high): GRE scores—medium, research experience—high, work experience—medium, extracurricular activity—medium, clinically related public service—medium, GPA—high, letters of recommendation—medium, interview—high, statement of goals and objectives—high, undergraduate major in psychology—low, specific undergraduate psychology courses taken—medium. Interview and clinical public service apply to Clinical program.

Student Characteristics: The following represents characteristics of students in 2009–2010 in all graduate psychology programs in the department: Female—full-time 45, part-time 0; Male—full-time 11, part-time 0; African American/Black—full-time 3, part-time 0; Hispanic/Latino(a)—full-time 7, part-time 0; Asian/Pacific Islander—full-time 6, part-time 0; American Indian/Alaska Native—full-time 0, part-time 0; Caucasian/White—full-time 40, part-time 0; Multi-ethnic—full-time 0, part-time 0; students subject to the Americans With Disabilities Act—full-time 0, part-time 0; Unknown ethnicity—full-time 0, part-time 0; International students who hold an F-1 or J-1 Visa—full-time 2, part-time 0.

Financial Information/Assistance:
Tuition for Full-Time Study: *Doctoral:* State residents: per academic year $21,000, $1,116 per credit hour; Nonstate residents: per academic year $21,000, $1,116 per credit hour. Tuition is subject to change. See the following Web site for updates and changes in tuition costs: http://www.gwu.edu/apply/costsfinancialplanning/graduate/tuitionfees.

Financial Assistance:
First-Year Students: Teaching assistantships available for first year. Average amount paid per academic year: $18,000. Research assistantships available for first year. Average amount paid per academic year: $18,000. Fellowships and scholarships available for first year. Average amount paid per academic year: $21,000.
Advanced Students: Teaching assistantships available for advanced students. Average amount paid per academic year: $18,000. Research assistantships available for advanced students. Average amount paid per academic year: $18,000. Fellowships and scholarships available for advanced students. Average amount paid per academic year: $21,000.
Additional Information: Of all students currently enrolled full time, 100% benefited from one or more of the listed financial assistance programs. Application and information available online at: http://www.gwu.edu/~psycdept/graduate_studies/financial_aid.cfm.

Internships/Practica: Doctoral Degree (PhD Clinical Psychology): For those doctoral students for whom a professional internship was required in this program prior to graduation, (3) students applied for an internship in 2008–2009, with (3) students obtaining an internship. Of those students who obtained an internship, (3) were paid internships. Of those students who obtained an internship, (3) students placed in APA/CPA accredited internships, (0) students placed in internships not APA/CPA accredited, but listed with the Association of Psychology Postdoctoral and Internship Programs (APPIC), (0) students placed in internships conforming to guidelines of the Council of Directors of School Psychology Programs (CDSPP), (0) students placed in internships that were not APA/CPA accredited, APPIC or

CDSPP listed. There is a wide variety of placements available in the DC Metro area. Placements are a required part of training in the clinical programs.

Housing and Day Care: On-campus housing is available. See the following Web site for more information: http://living.gwu.edu/halls/graduatehousing. On-campus day care facilities are available. See the following Web site for more information: http://gradlife.gwu.edu/gradlife/information2/WashingtonDCResourcesandInformation/Family/Daycare/.

Employment of Department Graduates:
Master's Degree Graduates: Of those who graduated in the academic year 2008–2009, the following categories and numbers represent the postgraduate activities and employment of master's degree graduates: Enrolled in a postdoctoral residency/fellowship (n/a), employed in independent practice (n/a), total from the above (master's) (0).
Doctoral Degree Graduates: Of those who graduated in the academic year 2008–2009, the following categories and numbers represent the postgraduate activities and employment of doctoral degree graduates: Enrolled in a psychology doctoral program (n/a), enrolled in a postdoctoral residency/fellowship (5), total from the above (doctoral) (5).

Additional Information:
Orientation, Objectives, and Emphasis of Department: The department provides training in the basic science of psychology for each of its graduate programs. Specialized training is offered in three program areas: applied social, clinical, and cognitive neuropsychology. The applied social program focuses on theory and methods of addressing current social problems such as in health care, education, and the prevention of high risk social behaviors. The clinical program is an APA-approved program emphasizing both the basic science and applied aspects of clinical psychology. The focus of the program is health promotion and disease prevention in diverse urban communities. The cognitive neuroscience program focuses on cognition, learning, and memory with emphasis on the psychobiological determinants of these functions. The training in each program addresses both scientific and professional objectives. Students are trained for careers in academic institutions, applied research, and professional practice.

Special Facilities or Resources: Excellent on-campus computer facilities; laboratories for child study, group studies, cognitive testing and small animal research. Convenient access to staff, libraries, and facilities at national health and mental health institutes (NIH); mental health training centers for clinical students.

Information for Students With Physical Disabilities: See the following Web site for more information: http://gwired.gwu.edu/dss.

Application Information:
Send to Graduate School, CCAS, George Washington University, Washington, DC 20052. Application available online. URL of online application: http://www.gwu.edu/apply/graduateprofessional. Students are admitted in the Fall, application deadline December 1. Cognitive Neuroscience and Applied Social Psychology deadline is January 15. *Fee:* $65.

FLORIDA

Barry University
Department of Psychology
School of Arts and Sciences
11300 NE 2nd Avenue
Miami Shores, FL 33161
Telephone: (305) 899-3270
Fax: (305) 899-3279
E-mail: *lszuchman@mail.barry.edu*
Web: *http://www.barry.edu/psychologyclinical/*

Department Information:
1978. Chairperson: Lenore T. Szuchman. Number of faculty: total—full-time 8, part-time 5; women—full-time 3, part-time 3; total—minority—full-time 2, part-time 1; women minority—full-time 1.

Programs and Degrees Offered:
Listed in the following order: Program area, degree type (T if terminal Master's), number awarded 7/08–6/09. Clinical Psychology MA/MS (Master of Arts/Science) (T) 14.

Student Applications/Admissions:
Student Applications
Clinical Psychology MA/MS (Master of Arts/Science)—Applications 2009–2010, 57. Total applicants accepted 2009–2010, 28. Number full-time enrolled (new admits only) 2009–2010, 10. Total enrolled 2009–2010 full-time, 19. Openings 2010–2011, 15. The median number of years required for completion of a degree in 2008–2009 were 2. The number of students enrolled full- and part-time who were dismissed or voluntarily withdrew from this program area in 2008–2009 were 1.
Other Criteria: (importance of criteria rated low, medium, or high): GRE scores—medium, research experience—medium, work experience—medium, extracurricular activity—low, clinically related public service—medium, GPA—high, letters of recommendation—high, statement of goals and objectives—high, undergraduate major in psychology—medium, specific undergraduate psychology courses taken—high. For additional information on admission requirements, go to http://www.barry.edu/psychologyclinical/admissions/requirements.asp.

Student Characteristics: The following represents characteristics of students in 2009–2010 in all graduate psychology programs in the department: Female—full-time 15, part-time 0; Male—full-time 4, part-time 0; African American/Black—full-time 2, part-time 0; Hispanic/Latino(a)—full-time 8, part-time 0; Asian/Pacific Islander—full-time 1, part-time 0; American Indian/Alaska Native—full-time 0, part-time 0; Caucasian/White—full-time 6, part-time 0; Multi-ethnic—full-time 0, part-time 0; students subject to the Americans With Disabilities Act—full-time 2, part-time 0; Unknown ethnicity—full-time 2, part-time 0; International students who hold an F-1 or J-1 Visa—full-time 0, part-time 0.

Financial Information/Assistance:
Tuition for Full-Time Study: Master's: State residents: $845 per credit hour; Nonstate residents: $845 per credit hour. Tuition is subject to change. See the following Web site for updates and changes in tuition costs: http://www.barry.edu/psychologyclinical/admissions/tuitionFees.asp.

Financial Assistance:
First-Year Students: Teaching assistantships available for first year. Average amount paid per academic year: $3,675. Average number of hours worked per week: 14. Apply by April 30.
Advanced Students: Teaching assistantships available for advanced students. Average amount paid per academic year: $3,675. Average number of hours worked per week: 14. Apply by April 30.
Additional Information: Of all students currently enrolled full time, 26% benefited from one or more of the listed financial assistance programs.

Internships/Practica: Master's Degree (MA/MS Clinical Psychology): An internship experience, such as a final research project or "capstone" experience is required of graduates. All students enrolled in the M.S. in Clinical Psychology program must complete a one-semester practicum. Students in the 60-credit program must also complete a two-semester full-time clinical internship. Because Barry University is located in a large, multi-cultural metropolitan area, the program is able to offer more than the usual number and variety of settings for the internship experience. Sites include but are not limited to community mental health centers, assessment centers (primarily for the assessment of children), psychiatric hospitals, addiction treatment programs, nursing homes, and prison settings. Supervision is provided both at the site and by a clinical supervisor on campus.

Housing and Day Care: No on-campus housing is available. No on-campus day care facilities are available.

Employment of Department Graduates:
Master's Degree Graduates: Of those who graduated in the academic year 2008–2009, the following categories and numbers represent the postgraduate activities and employment of master's degree graduates: Enrolled in a postdoctoral residency/fellowship (n/a), employed in independent practice (n/a), total from the above (master's) (0).
Doctoral Degree Graduates: Of those who graduated in the academic year 2008–2009, the following categories and numbers represent the postgraduate activities and employment of doctoral degree graduates: Enrolled in a psychology doctoral program (n/a), total from the above (doctoral) (0).

Additional Information:
Orientation, Objectives, and Emphasis of Department: In the M.S. Program in Clinical Psychology, students are expected to achieve competence in theory, assessment, therapy, and research. All clinical psychology students complete a thesis and a practicum. The 36-credit option, a 2-year program, is designed for students who want to go directly into a doctoral program. Students who complete the 3-year, 60-credit program meet licensure require-

ments for the Mental Health Counselor in Florida. In the third year these students complete a full-time internship.

Special Facilities or Resources: The psychology department is normally composed of 8 full-time faculty members. Classes are small, and the students are given individual attention and supervision.

Information for Students With Physical Disabilities: See the following Web site for more information: http://www.barry.edu/DisabilityServices/default.htm.

Application Information:
Send to Office of Enrollment Services, Barry University, 11300 NE 2nd Avenue, Miami, FL 33161. Application available online. URL of online application: http://www.barry.edu/gradadmissions/default.htm. Students are admitted in the Fall, application deadline February 15. Deadline is February 15 with review continuing as long as space is available. *Fee:* $30.

Central Florida, University of (2009 data)
Department of Psychology
College of Sciences
P.O. Box 161390
Orlando, FL 32816-1390
Telephone: (407) 823-4344
Fax: (407) 823-5862
E-mail: *psychinfo@mail.ucf.edu*
Web: *http://www.psych.ucf.edu/*

Department Information:
1968. Chairperson: Robert L. Dipboye. Number of faculty: total—full-time 41; women—full-time 19; total—minority—full-time 5; women minority—full-time 2; faculty subject to the Americans With Disabilities Act 1.

Programs and Degrees Offered:
Listed in the following order: Program area, degree type (T if terminal Master's), number awarded 7/08–6/09. Clinical MA/MS (Master of Arts/Science) (T) 11, Industrial/Organizational MA/MS (Master of Arts/Science) (T) 15, Applied Experimental and Human Factors PhD (Doctor of Philosophy) 8, Clinical Psychology PhD (Doctor of Philosophy) 1, Industrial/Organizational Psychology PhD (Doctor of Philosophy) 6.

APA Accreditation: Clinical PhD (Doctor of Philosophy).

Student Applications/Admissions:
Student Applications
Clinical MA/MS (Master of Arts/Science)—Applications 2009–2010, 94. Total applicants accepted 2009–2010, 24. Number full-time enrolled (new admits only) 2009–2010, 15. Total enrolled 2009–2010 full-time, 23. Openings 2010–2011, 15. The median number of years required for completion of a degree in 2008–2009 were 2. The number of students enrolled full- and part-time who were dismissed or voluntarily withdrew from this program area in 2008–2009 were 0. *Industrial/Organizational MA/MS (Master of Arts/Science)*—Applications 2009–2010, 85. Total applicants accepted 2009–2010, 27. Number full-time enrolled (new admits only) 2009–2010, 12. Total enrolled 2009–2010 full-time, 28, part-time, 1. Openings 2010–2011, 16. The median number of years required for completion of a degree in 2008–2009 were 2. The number of students enrolled full- and part-time who were dismissed or voluntarily withdrew from this program area in 2008–2009 were 0. *Applied Experimental and Human Factors PhD (Doctor of Philosophy)*—Applications 2009–2010, 42. Total applicants accepted 2009–2010, 9. Number full-time enrolled (new admits only) 2009–2010, 8. Number part-time enrolled (new admits only) 2009–2010, 0. Openings 2010–2011, 12. The median number of years required for completion of a degree in 2008–2009 were 5. The number of students enrolled full- and part-time who were dismissed or voluntarily withdrew from this program area in 2008–2009 were 1. *Clinical Psychology PhD (Doctor of Philosophy)*—Applications 2009–2010, 157. Total applicants accepted 2009–2010, 7. Number full-time enrolled (new admits only) 2009–2010, 7. Openings 2010–2011, 7. The median number of years required for completion of a degree in 2008–2009 were 7. The number of students enrolled full- and part-time who were dismissed or voluntarily withdrew from this program area in 2008–2009 were 1. *Industrial/Organizational Psychology PhD (Doctor of Philosophy)*—Applications 2009–2010, 69. Total applicants accepted 2009–2010, 18. Number full-time enrolled (new admits only) 2009–2010, 9. Number part-time enrolled (new admits only) 2009–2010, 0. Openings 2010–2011, 7. The median number of years required for completion of a degree in 2008–2009 were 5. The number of students enrolled full- and part-time who were dismissed or voluntarily withdrew from this program area in 2008–2009 were 0.

Other Criteria: (importance of criteria rated low, medium, or high): GRE scores—high, research experience—high, work experience—low, extracurricular activity—medium, clinically related public service—medium, GPA—high, letters of recommendation—high, interview—high, statement of goals and objectives—high, undergraduate major in psychology—low, specific undergraduate psychology courses taken—medium. Criteria vary by program.

Student Characteristics: The following represents characteristics of students in 2009–2010 in all graduate psychology programs in the department: Female—full-time 102, part-time 7; Male—full-time 53, part-time 4; African American/Black—full-time 5, part-time 0; Hispanic/Latino(a)—full-time 6, part-time 0; Asian/Pacific Islander—full-time 2, part-time 0; American Indian/Alaska Native—full-time 0, part-time 0; Caucasian/White—full-time 142, part-time 11; Multi-ethnic—full-time 0, part-time 0; students subject to the Americans With Disabilities Act—full-time 0, part-time 0; Unknown ethnicity—full-time 0, part-time 0; International students who hold an F-1 or J-1 Visa—full-time 0, part-time 0.

Financial Information/Assistance:
Tuition for Full-Time Study: Master's: State residents: per academic year $4,276, $237 per credit hour; Nonstate residents: per academic year $17,865, $992 per credit hour. *Doctoral:* State residents: per academic year $4,276, $237 per credit hour; Nonstate residents: per academic year $17,865, $992 per credit hour. Tuition is subject to change. Additional fees are assessed to students beyond the costs of tuition for the following: for state

resident, $55.00 per credit hour; for nonresident, $92.74 per credit hour. See the following Web site for updates and changes in tuition costs: http://www.graduate.ucf.edu.

Financial Assistance:

First-Year Students: Teaching assistantships available for first year. Average amount paid per academic year: $10,000. Average number of hours worked per week: 20. Research assistantships available for first year. Average amount paid per academic year: $15,000. Average number of hours worked per week: 20. Fellowships and scholarships available for first year. Average amount paid per academic year: $13,500. Average number of hours worked per week: 20.

Advanced Students: Teaching assistantships available for advanced students. Average amount paid per academic year: $10,000. Average number of hours worked per week: 20. Research assistantships available for advanced students. Average amount paid per academic year: $15,000. Average number of hours worked per week: 20. Fellowships and scholarships available for advanced students. Average amount paid per academic year: $13,500. Average number of hours worked per week: 20.

Additional Information: Of all students currently enrolled full time, 90% benefited from one or more of the listed financial assistance programs. Application and information available online at: http://www.graduate.ucf.edu.

Internships/Practica: Doctoral Degree (PhD Clinical Psychology): For those doctoral students for whom a professional internship was required in this program prior to graduation, (1) students applied for an internship in 2008–2009, with (0) students obtaining an internship. Of those students who obtained an internship, (0) were paid internships. Of those students who obtained an internship, (0) students placed in APA/CPA accredited internships, (0) students placed in internships not APA/CPA accredited, but listed with the Association of Psychology Postdoctoral and Internship Programs (APPIC), (0) students placed in internships conforming to guidelines of the Council of Directors of School Psychology Programs (CDSPP), (0) students placed in internships that were not APA/CPA accredited, APPIC or CDSPP listed. Master's Degree (MA/MS Industrial/Organizational): An internship experience, such as a final research project or "capstone" experience is required of graduates. Internships for clinical masters students exist in community mental health centers and other agencies throughout Central Florida. Doctoral students complete their practica in our on-campus clinic as well as in a variety of community based clinical agencies. Human Factors students complete internships in a variety of government, business, and industry settings. I/O master's students complete practicum placements in a variety of government, business and industry settings. Doctoral students complete an internship in a variety of business, industry and government settings.

Housing and Day Care: On-campus housing is available. See the following Web site for more information: http://www.housing.ucf.edu/. On-campus day care facilities are available. See the following Web site for more information: http://www.csc.sdes.ucf.edu/.

Employment of Department Graduates:

Master's Degree Graduates: Of those who graduated in the academic year 2008–2009, the following categories and numbers represent the postgraduate activities and employment of master's degree graduates: Enrolled in a psychology doctoral program (2), enrolled in another graduate/professional program (1), enrolled in a postdoctoral residency/fellowship (n/a), employed in independent practice (n/a), employed in business or industry (6), employed in government agency (4), employed in a community mental health/counseling center (8), still seeking employment (1), do not know (3), total from the above (master's) (25).

Doctoral Degree Graduates: Of those who graduated in the academic year 2008–2009, the following categories and numbers represent the postgraduate activities and employment of doctoral degree graduates: Enrolled in a psychology doctoral program (n/a), employed in an academic position at a university (2), employed in business or industry (13), employed in government agency (1), employed in a hospital/medical center (1), total from the above (doctoral) (17).

Additional Information:

Orientation, Objectives, and Emphasis of Department: The PhD program in clinical psychology is an APA accredited program, designed for individuals seeking a research oriented career in the field of clinical psychology. The program also emphasizes training in consultation, teaching, supervision, and the design/evaluation of mental health programs. The MA program in clinical psychology has major emphases in assessment and evaluation skills; intervention, counseling, and psychotherapy skills; and an academic foundation in research methods. The program is designed to provide training and preparation for persons desiring to deliver clinical services at the master's level through community agencies. Graduates of this program meet the educational requirements for the mental health counselor state license. The MS program in Industrial/Organizational psychology has major emphases in selection and training of employees, applied theories of organizational behavior, job satisfaction, test theory and construction; assessment center technology, statistics and experimental design. As of Fall 2000 a PhD in Industrial/Organizational was approved and admitted an initial class of 10 students. I/O students receive training in the 21 competence areas detailed by Division 14 of the APA. The PhD program in applied experimental/human factors is patterned on the scientist–practitioner model of the APA. It adheres to the guidelines for education and training established by the committee for Education and Training of APA's Division 21 (Applied Experimental and Engineering Psychology). The Applied Experimental and Human Factors program is accredited by the Educational Committee of the Human Factors and Ergonomics Society. Concentration areas include human-computer interaction, human performance, and human factors in simulation and training.

Special Facilities or Resources: The department's facilities and resources include extensive videotape capability, an intelligence and personality testing library, a statistics library, computer facilities within the department and in the computer center, a counseling and testing center, a creative school for children, and a communicative disorders clinic. Doctoral students have use of specialized equipment in the department-based Human Visual Performance Laboratory and Team Performance Laboratory. The clinical program has extensive ties to a number of community agencies for practica and assistantship as well as an on-site clinic.

Information for Students With Physical Disabilities: See the following Web site for more information: http://www.sds.sdes.ucf.edu/.

GRADUATE STUDY IN PSYCHOLOGY

Application Information:
Send to University of Central Florida, Department of Psychology-ATTN: Graduate Admissions, P. O. Box 161390, Orlando, FL 32816-1390. Application available online. URL of online application: http://www.graduate.ucf.edu/gradonlineapp/. Students are admitted in the Fall, application deadline December 15. *Fee:* $30.

Florida Atlantic University
Psychology
Charles E. Schmidt College of Science
777 Glades Road, P.O. Box 3091
Boca Raton, FL 33431-0991
Telephone: (561) 297-3360
Fax: (561) 297-2160
E-mail: *laursen@fau.edu*
Web: *http://www.psy.fau.edu*

Department Information:
1965. Chairperson: David L. Wolgin. Number of faculty: total—full-time 30; women—full-time 9; total—minority—full-time 1; women minority—full-time 1.

Programs and Degrees Offered:
Listed in the following order: Program area, degree type (T if terminal Master's), number awarded 7/08–6/09. Psychology MA/MS (Master of Arts/Science) (T) 8, Psychology PhD (Doctor of Philosophy) 4.

Student Applications/Admissions:
Student Applications
Psychology MA/MS (Master of Arts/Science)—Applications 2009–2010, 68. Total applicants accepted 2009–2010, 28. Number full-time enrolled (new admits only) 2009–2010, 12. Number part-time enrolled (new admits only) 2009–2010, 0. Openings 2010–2011, 20. The median number of years required for completion of a degree in 2008–2009 were 2. The number of students enrolled full- and part-time who were dismissed or voluntarily withdrew from this program area in 2008–2009 were 5. Psychology PhD (Doctor of Philosophy)—Applications 2009–2010, 75. Total applicants accepted 2009–2010, 6. Number full-time enrolled (new admits only) 2009–2010, 4. Number part-time enrolled (new admits only) 2009–2010, 0. Total enrolled 2009–2010 full-time, 39, part-time, 1. Openings 2010–2011, 10. The median number of years required for completion of a degree in 2008–2009 were 5. The number of students enrolled full- and part-time who were dismissed or voluntarily withdrew from this program area in 2008–2009 were 0.
Scores: Entries appear in this order: required test or GPA, minimum score (if required), median score of students entering in 2009–2010. Psychology MA/MS (Master of Arts/Science): GRE-V 550, GRE-Q 550, last 2 years GPA 3.0; Psychology PhD (Doctor of Philosophy): GRE-V 550, 600, GRE-Q 550, 690, last 2 years GPA 3.0.
Other Criteria: (importance of criteria rated low, medium, or high): GRE scores—high, research experience—high, clinically related public service—low, GPA—high, letters of recommendation—high, statement of goals and objectives—high, undergraduate major in psychology—medium.

Student Characteristics: The following represents characteristics of students in 2009–2010 in all graduate psychology programs in the department: Female—full-time 23, part-time 3; Male—full-time 17, part-time 0; African American/Black—full-time 0, part-time 1; Hispanic/Latino(a)—full-time 2, part-time 0; Asian/Pacific Islander—full-time 5, part-time 0; American Indian/Alaska Native—full-time 1, part-time 0; Caucasian/White—full-time 0, part-time 0; Multi-ethnic—full-time 0, part-time 0; students subject to the Americans With Disabilities Act—full-time 1, part-time 0; Unknown ethnicity—full-time 0, part-time 0; International students who hold an F-1 or J-1 Visa—full-time 0, part-time 0.

Financial Information/Assistance:
Tuition for Full-Time Study: *Master's:* State residents: $294 per credit hour; Nonstate residents: $921 per credit hour. *Doctoral:* State residents: $294 per credit hour; Nonstate residents: $921 per credit hour. Tuition is subject to change. Additional fees are assessed to students beyond the costs of tuition for the following: see website for details. See the following Web site for updates and changes in tuition costs: http://www.fau.edu/controller/student_information/tuition_breakdown.php.

Financial Assistance:
First-Year Students: Teaching assistantships available for first year. Average amount paid per academic year: $20,000. Average number of hours worked per week: 20. Apply by August 1. Research assistantships available for first year. Average amount paid per academic year: $20,000. Average number of hours worked per week: 20. Apply by August 1. Fellowships and scholarships available for first year. Average amount paid per academic year: $25,000. Average number of hours worked per week: 20. Apply by January 1.
Advanced Students: Teaching assistantships available for advanced students. Average amount paid per academic year: $20,000. Average number of hours worked per week: 20. Apply by August 1. Research assistantships available for advanced students. Average amount paid per academic year: $20,000. Average number of hours worked per week: 20. Apply by August 1. Fellowships and scholarships available for advanced students. Average amount paid per academic year: $25,000. Average number of hours worked per week: 20. Apply by January 1.
Additional Information: Of all students currently enrolled full time, 100% benefited from one or more of the listed financial assistance programs.

Housing and Day Care: On-campus housing is available. See the following Web site for more information: http://www.fau.edu/housing/. On-campus day care facilities are available. See the following Web site for more information: http://www.coe.fau.edu/erccd/.

Employment of Department Graduates:
Master's Degree Graduates: Of those who graduated in the academic year 2008–2009, the following categories and numbers represent the postgraduate activities and employment of master's degree graduates: Enrolled in a psychology doctoral program (8), enrolled in another graduate/professional program (4), enrolled in a postdoctoral residency/fellowship (n/a), employed in independent practice (n/a), employed in business or industry (2), employed in a community mental health/counseling center (2), do not know (3), total from the above (master's) (19).

Doctoral Degree Graduates: Of those who graduated in the academic year 2008–2009, the following categories and numbers represent the postgraduate activities and employment of doctoral degree graduates: Enrolled in a psychology doctoral program (n/a), enrolled in a postdoctoral residency/fellowship (2), employed in an academic position at a university (0), employed in an academic position at a 2-year/4-year college (2), employed in a professional position in a school system (1), do not know (1), total from the above (doctoral) (6).

Additional Information:
Orientation, Objectives, and Emphasis of Department: The PhD program emphasizes research in several areas of experimental psychology. Students may select courses and conduct research in five areas: cognitive psychology, developmental psychology, evolutionary psychology, psychobiology/neuroscience, and social/personality psychology. Current research by faculty includes psycholinguistics, sentence processing, visual perception, and speech production and perception; conflict in married couples, the relationship between tool use and style of play in preschool children, psychological adaptations to sperm competition in humans, and mental synchronization in social interaction; neural mechanisms in recovery of function from brain damage, psychopharmacology, and nonlinear dynamics of brain and behavior; the use of traits to predict behavior, sex differences in mating, domestic violence, and the dynamics of social influence. The MA program is designed to prepare students for entry into doctoral-level programs in all areas of psychology. Research in developmental psychology uses a campus laboratory school for children in kindergarten through the eighth grade. Research in social/personality psychology uses laboratories with video and online computer facilities. The cognitive psychology laboratories include testing rooms with a network of PCs for online control of experiments in perception, learning, language, and cognition. The EEG laboratory includes an acoustic isolation chamber and a variety of amplifying and recording systems.

Information for Students With Physical Disabilities: See the following Web site for more information: http://www.osd.fav.edu.

Application Information:
Application available online. URL of online application: http://psy.fau.edu/graduate_programs/. Students are admitted in the Fall, application deadline January 15. PhD application deadline January 15; MA application deadline May 1. *Fee:* $30.

Florida Institute of Technology
School of Psychology
College of Psychology and Liberal Arts
150 West University Boulevard
Melbourne, FL 32901-6988
Telephone: (321) 674-8104
Fax: (321) 674-7105
E-mail: *mkenkel@fit.edu*
Web: *http://cpla.fit.edu/psych/*

Department Information:
1978. Dean: Mary Beth Kenkel. Number of faculty: total—full-time 28, part-time 3; women—full-time 12; total—minority—full-time 4; women minority—full-time 3; faculty subject to the Americans With Disabilities Act 2.

Programs and Degrees Offered:
Listed in the following order: Program area, degree type (T if terminal Master's), number awarded 7/08–6/09. Applied Behavior Analysis MA/MS (Master of Arts/Science) (T) 15, Clinical Psychology PsyD (Doctor of Psychology) 15, Organizational Behavior Management MA/MS (Master of Arts/Science) 10, Industrial/Organizational Psychology MA/MS (Master of Arts/Science) (T) 8, Industrial/Organizational Psychology PhD (Doctor of Philosophy) 3, Applied Behavior Analysis PhD (Doctor of Philosophy) 0.

APA Accreditation: Clinical PsyD (Doctor of Psychology). Student Outcome Data Website: http://cpla.fit.edu/clinical/outcomes.php.

Student Applications/Admissions:
Student Applications

Applied Behavior Analysis MA/MS (Master of Arts/Science)—Applications 2009–2010, 61. Total applicants accepted 2009–2010, 42. Number full-time enrolled (new admits only) 2009–2010, 26. Number part-time enrolled (new admits only) 2009–2010, 0. Total enrolled 2009–2010 full-time, 57, part-time, 6. Openings 2010–2011, 30. The median number of years required for completion of a degree in 2008–2009 were 2. The number of students enrolled full- and part-time who were dismissed or voluntarily withdrew from this program area in 2008–2009 were 0. *Clinical Psychology PsyD (Doctor of Psychology)*—Applications 2009–2010, 148. Total applicants accepted 2009–2010, 47. Number full-time enrolled (new admits only) 2009–2010, 18. Number part-time enrolled (new admits only) 2009–2010, 0. Openings 2010–2011, 25. The median number of years required for completion of a degree in 2008–2009 were 5. The number of students enrolled full- and part-time who were dismissed or voluntarily withdrew from this program area in 2008–2009 were 0. *Organizational Behavior Management MA/MS (Master of Arts/Science)*—Applications 2009–2010, 10. Total applicants accepted 2009–2010, 8. Number full-time enrolled (new admits only) 2009–2010, 2. Number part-time enrolled (new admits only) 2009–2010, 0. Openings 2010–2011, 15. The median number of years required for completion of a degree in 2008–2009 were 2. The number of students enrolled full- and part-time who were dismissed or voluntarily withdrew from this program area in 2008–2009 were 0. *Industrial/Organizational Psychology MA/MS (Master of Arts/Science)*—Applications 2009–2010, 69. Total applicants accepted 2009–2010, 31. Number full-time enrolled (new admits only) 2009–2010, 12. Number part-time enrolled (new admits only) 2009–2010, 0. Openings 2010–2011, 6. The median number of years required for completion of a degree in 2008–2009 were 2. The number of students enrolled full- and part-time who were dismissed or voluntarily withdrew from this program area in 2008–2009 were 0. *Industrial/Organizational Psychology PhD (Doctor of Philosophy)*—Applications 2009–2010, 36. Total applicants accepted 2009–2010, 17. Number full-time enrolled (new admits only) 2009–2010, 10. Number part-time enrolled (new admits only) 2009–2010, 0. Total enrolled 2009–2010 full-time, 23, part-time, 6. Openings 2010–2011, 6. The median number of years required for completion of a degree in 2008–2009 were 4. The number of students enrolled full- and part-time who were dismissed or voluntarily withdrew from this program area in 2008–2009 were 0. *Applied Behavior Analysis PhD (Doctor of Philosophy)*—Applications 2009–2010, 15. Total applicants accepted 2009–2010, 3. Number full-time enrolled (new admits only) 2009–2010, 1. Number part-time enrolled (new admits only) 2009–2010, 0. Openings 2010–2011, 3. The median number of years required for completion of a degree in 2008–2009 were 2. The number of students enrolled full- and part-time who were dismissed or voluntarily withdrew from this program area in 2008–2009 were 0.

Scores: Entries appear in this order: required test or GPA, minimum score (if required), median score of students entering in 2009–2010. *Applied Behavior Analysis MA/MS (Master of Arts/Science):* GRE-V no minimum stated, 450, GRE-Q no minimum stated, 550, GRE-Analytical no minimum stated, 4.0, overall undergraduate GPA 3.0, 3.48, last 2 years GPA no minimum stated, 3.58, psychology GPA no minimum stated, 3.58; *Clinical Psychology PsyD (Doctor of Psychology):* GRE-V no minimum stated, 540, GRE-Q no minimum stated, 610, GRE-Analytical no minimum stated, 4.0, overall undergraduate GPA 3.0, 3.62, last 2 years GPA no minimum stated, 3.74, psychology GPA no minimum stated, 3.76, Masters GPA 3.2, 3.94; *Organizational Behavior Management MA/MS (Master of Arts/Science):* GRE-V no minimum stated, 420, GRE-Q no minimum stated, 580, GRE-Analytical no minimum stated, 4.0, overall undergraduate GPA 3.0, 3.44, last 2 years GPA no minimum stated, 3.8, psychology GPA no minimum stated, 3.66; *Industrial/Organizational Psychology MA/MS (Master of Arts/Science):* GRE-V no minimum stated, 510, GRE-Q no minimum stated, 630, GRE-Analytical no minimum stated, 4.3, overall undergraduate GPA 3.0, 3.45, last 2 years GPA no minimum stated, 3.72, psychology GPA no minimum stated, 3.6; *Industrial/Organizational Psychology PhD (Doctor of Philosophy):* GRE-V no minimum stated, 610, GRE-Q no minimum stated, 690, GRE-Analytical no minimum stated, 4.5, overall undergraduate GPA 3.0, 3.65, last 2 years GPA no minimum stated, 3.85, psychology GPA no minimum stated, 3.77, Masters GPA 3.26, 3.9; *Applied Behavior Analysis PhD (Doctor of Philosophy):* GRE-V no minimum stated, 550, GRE-Q no minimum stated, 580, GRE-Analytical no minimum stated, 4.5, overall undergraduate GPA 3.0, 3.3, last 2 years GPA no minimum stated, 3.7, psychology GPA no minimum stated, 3.8, Masters GPA 3.2, 4.0.

Other Criteria: (importance of criteria rated low, medium, or high): GRE scores—medium, research experience—medium, work experience—high, extracurricular activity—medium, clinically related public service—high, GPA—high, letters of recommendation—high, interview—medium, statement of goals and objectives—medium.

Student Characteristics: The following represents characteristics of students in 2009–2010 in all graduate psychology programs in the department: Female—full-time 175, part-time 5; Male—full-time 38, part-time 7; African American/Black—full-time 10, part-time 2; Hispanic/Latino(a)—full-time 18, part-time 1; Asian/Pacific Islander—full-time 16, part-time 1; American Indian/Alaska Native—full-time 0, part-time 0; Caucasian/White—full-time 157, part-time 7; Multi-ethnic—full-time 6, part-time 0; students subject to the Americans With Disabilities Act—full-time 1, part-time 0; Unknown ethnicity—full-time 6, part-time 1; International students who hold an F-1 or J-1 Visa—full-time 21, part-time 1.

Financial Information/Assistance:
Tuition for Full-Time Study: *Master's:* State residents: per academic year $18,720, $1,040 per credit hour; Nonstate residents: per academic year $18,720, $1,040 per credit hour. *Doctoral:* State residents: per academic year $28,665, $1,040 per credit hour; Nonstate residents: per academic year $28,665, $1,040 per credit hour. Tuition is subject to change. Tuition costs vary by program.

Financial Assistance:
First-Year Students: Fellowships and scholarships available for first year. Average amount paid per academic year: $5,000. Apply by June 1.

Advanced Students: Teaching assistantships available for advanced students. Average amount paid per academic year: $8,000. Average number of hours worked per week: 15. Apply by March 15. Research assistantships available for advanced students. Average amount paid per academic year: $4,000. Average number of hours worked per week: 5. Apply by March 15. Fellowships and scholarships available for advanced students. Average amount paid per academic year: $6,477. Average number of hours worked per week: 10. Apply by June 1.

Additional Information: Of all students currently enrolled full time, 43% benefited from one or more of the listed financial assistance programs. Application and information available online at: http://www.fit.edu/grad/financial_aid.php.

Internships/Practica: Doctoral Degree (PsyD Clinical Psychology): For those doctoral students for whom a professional internship was required in this program prior to graduation, (10) students applied for an internship in 2008–2009, with (9) students obtaining an internship. Of those students who obtained an internship, (9) were paid internships. Of those students who obtained an internship, (9) students placed in APA/CPA accredited internships, (0) students placed in internships not APA/CPA accredited, but listed with the Association of Psychology Postdoctoral and Internship Programs (APPIC), (0) students placed in internships conforming to guidelines of the Council of Directors of School Psychology Programs (CDSPP), (0) students placed in internships that were not APA/CPA accredited, APPIC or CDSPP listed. Students in the PsyD program complete a sequence of three or more separate practicum placements prior to internship. These include the Florida Tech's Community Psychological Services Center, and then options at other outpatient and inpatient facilities. Inpatient sites include adult psychiatric hospitals, rehabilitation hospitals, child and adolescent inpatient units, behavioral medicine practica within a medical hospital and a prison setting. Outpatient sites include mental health centers, private practice settings, VA outpatient clinics, and neuropsychological practices. Students gain experience in assessment and treatment of individuals, groups, couples and families, consultation and psychoeducational presentations. Treatment specialties include neuropsychology, aging, sexual abuse, domestic violence, PTSD, and drug and alcohol abuse. The I/O program has strong ties to local businesses in Brevard County. Students have been placed in a wide range of practicum sites including county and federal departments, aerospace and electronics industries, financial institutions, health care organizations, and management consulting firms. The Applied Behavior Analysis program has practicum sites with private and public agencies working with children with developmental disabilities, serious emotional and behavioral disorders and autism. Students receive on-site supervision as well as ancillary supervision by program faculty. The Organizational Behavior Management (OBM) program has internships with local businesses as well as with national consulting firms. Florida Tech's Scott Center for Autism Treatment provides training in early intervention, social skills training and treatment of challenging problem behaviors.

Housing and Day Care: On-campus housing is available: http://www.fit.edu/housing. No on-campus day care facilities are available.

Employment of Department Graduates:
Master's Degree Graduates: Of those who graduated in the academic year 2008–2009, the following categories and numbers represent the postgraduate activities and employment of master's degree graduates: Enrolled in a psychology doctoral program (8), enrolled in another graduate/professional program (1), enrolled in a postdoctoral residency/fellowship (n/a), employed in independent practice (n/a), employed in an academic position at a university (0), employed in an academic position at a 2-year/4-year college (0), employed in other positions at a higher education institution (0), employed in a professional position in a school system (2), employed in business or industry (4), employed in government agency (0), employed in a community mental health/counseling center (12), employed in a hospital/medical center (0), still seeking employment (0), not seeking employment (0), other employment position (2), do not know (1), total from the above (master's) (30).
Doctoral Degree Graduates: Of those who graduated in the academic year 2008–2009, the following categories and numbers represent the postgraduate activities and employment of doctoral degree graduates: Enrolled in a psychology doctoral program (n/a), enrolled in another graduate/professional program (0), enrolled in a postdoctoral residency/fellowship (4), employed in independent practice (0), employed in an academic position at a university (0), employed in an academic position at a 2-year/4-year college (2), employed in other positions at a higher education institution (2), employed in a professional position in a school system (0), employed in business or industry (1), employed in government agency (1), employed in a community mental health/counseling center (4), employed in a hospital/medical center (3), still seeking employment (0), not seeking employment (0), other employment position (0), do not know (1), total from the above (doctoral) (18).

Additional Information:
Orientation, Objectives, and Emphasis of Department: The School of Psychology at Florida Institute of Technology offers the MS and PhD in Industrial/Organizational Psychology, the MS and PhD in Behavior Analysis and the MS in Organizational Behavior Management, and the PsyD in Clinical Psychology. The clinical PsyD program trains students based on a practitioner/scientist model focused on development of clinical skills. The program incorporates multiple theoretical orientations and has emphases in neuropsychology and health psychology, child and family therapy, and forensic psychology. In the Industrial/Organizational Psychology program, students are trained in advanced statistics, organizational research, industrial training and development, personnel selection, performance appraisal, group and team development and organizational research methodology. The program prepares graduates for a wide variety of careers in academics, management, human resources and consulting. The master's program in Behavioral Psychology offers two degrees: one in Applied Behavior Analysis (ABA) and one in Organizational Behavior Management (OBM). The program prepares graduates for employment as Board Certified Behavior Analysts and/or as internal or external consultants in business and industry. Students from the ABA program upon graduation meet all the educational and supervised practicum requirements to seek certification as a BCBA. The ABA PhD prepares students for teaching, research, and management/supervision careers.

Special Facilities or Resources: The facilities of the School of Psychology include the Psychology building, the Scott Center which includes autism treatment facilities and general psychological services, the Neuropsychology Lab, the Industrial/Organizational Psychology Lab, and the Applied Research Lab. The academic building contains offices, classrooms, and computer facilities. The University's Academic Computing Services-Microcenter provides computers and software, media conversion, digital graphic assistance, and professional editing of theses and papers for publication. The Scott Center includes early intervention rooms, observation rooms, group and individual treatment rooms. Additionally students receive training and conduct research in several community service programs operated by the School of Psychology. These include: Center for Professional Services, a campus based consulting and research organization; East Central Florida Memory Clinic, through a contract with Holmes Regional Medical Center, serves individuals with memory disorders by providing memory screenings, case management, education, wellness and support groups; Family Learning Program offers psychological assessment and treatment to child victims of sexual abuse and their family members.

Information for Students With Physical Disabilities: See the following Web site for more information: http://www.fit.edu/asc/disabilities.php.

Application Information:
Send to Florida Institute of Technology, Office of Graduate Admissions, 150 W. University Boulevard, Melbourne, FL 32901. Application available online. URL of online application: http://www.fit.edu/apply. Students are admitted in the Fall. PsyD deadline is January 15. Industrial/Organizational Psychology deadline is February 1. ABA-PhD deadline is February 1 and the ABA-MS February 15. *Fee:* PsyD $60; PhD $60; MS $50.

Florida International University
Psychology
Arts and Sciences
11200 SW 8th Street
Miami, FL 33199
Telephone: (305) 348-2881
Fax: (305) 348-3879
E-mail: *levittmj@fiu.edu*
Web: *http://psych.fiu.edu/*

Department Information:
1972. Chairperson: Mary J Levitt. Number of faculty: total—full-time 27; women—full-time 12; total—minority—full-time 3; women minority—full-time 2.

GRADUATE STUDY IN PSYCHOLOGY

Programs and Degrees Offered:
Listed in the following order: Program area, degree type (T if terminal Master's), number awarded 7/08–6/09. Life Span Developmental Science PhD (Doctor of Philosophy) 1, Industrial/Organizational Psychology PhD (Doctor of Philosophy) 2, Legal Psychology PhD (Doctor of Philosophy) 2, Counseling MA/MS (Master of Arts/Science) (T) 6, Behavior Analysis MA/MS (Master of Arts/Science) (T) 2, Clinical Science PhD (Doctor of Philosophy) 0.

Student Applications/Admissions:
Student Applications
Life Span Developmental Science PhD (Doctor of Philosophy)—Applications 2009–2010, 16. Total applicants accepted 2009–2010, 10. Number full-time enrolled (new admits only) 2009–2010, 9. Total enrolled 2009–2010 full-time, 39, part-time, 2. The median number of years required for completion of a degree in 2008–2009 were 5. The number of students enrolled full- and part-time who were dismissed or voluntarily withdrew from this program area in 2008–2009 were 0. *Industrial/Organizational Psychology PhD (Doctor of Philosophy)*—Applications 2009–2010, 31. Total applicants accepted 2009–2010, 8. Number full-time enrolled (new admits only) 2009–2010, 4. Total enrolled 2009–2010 full-time, 16. Openings 2010–2011, 7. The median number of years required for completion of a degree in 2008–2009 were 5. The number of students enrolled full- and part-time who were dismissed or voluntarily withdrew from this program area in 2008–2009 were 0. *Legal Psychology PhD (Doctor of Philosophy)*—Applications 2009–2010, 21. Total applicants accepted 2009–2010, 4. Number full-time enrolled (new admits only) 2009–2010, 4. Total enrolled 2009–2010 full-time, 16. The median number of years required for completion of a degree in 2008–2009 were 4. The number of students enrolled full- and part-time who were dismissed or voluntarily withdrew from this program area in 2008–2009 were 0. *Counseling MA/MS (Master of Arts/Science)*—Applications 2009–2010, 33. Total applicants accepted 2009–2010, 14. Number full-time enrolled (new admits only) 2009–2010, 8. Number part-time enrolled (new admits only) 2009–2010, 1. Total enrolled 2009–2010 full-time, 30, part-time, 1. Openings 2010–2011, 15. The median number of years required for completion of a degree in 2008–2009 were 4. The number of students enrolled full- and part-time who were dismissed or voluntarily withdrew from this program area in 2008–2009 were 2. *Behavior Analysis MA/MS (Master of Arts/Science)*—Applications 2009–2010, 8. Total applicants accepted 2009–2010, 6. Number full-time enrolled (new admits only) 2009–2010, 2. Total enrolled 2009–2010 full-time, 9. The median number of years required for completion of a degree in 2008–2009 were 2. The number of students enrolled full- and part-time who were dismissed or voluntarily withdrew from this program area in 2008–2009 were 0. *Clinical Science PhD (Doctor of Philosophy)*—Applications 2009–2010, 25. Number full-time enrolled (new admits only) 2009–2010, 0. Openings 2010–2011, 4. The number of students enrolled full- and part-time who were dismissed or voluntarily withdrew from this program area in 2008–2009 were 0.

Scores: Entries appear in this order: required test or GPA, minimum score (if required), median score of students entering in 2009–2010. *Life Span Developmental Science PhD (Doctor of Philosophy)*: GRE-V no minimum stated, 517, GRE-Q no minimum stated, 614, last 2 years GPA 3.0, 3.67; *Industrial/Organizational Psychology PhD (Doctor of Philosophy)*: GRE-V no minimum stated, 549, GRE-Q no minimum stated, 650, last 2 years GPA 3.0, 3.5; *Legal Psychology PhD (Doctor of Philosophy)*: GRE-V no minimum stated, 520, GRE-Q no minimum stated, 595, last 2 years GPA 3.0, 3.52; *Counseling MA/MS (Master of Arts/Science)*: GRE-V no minimum stated, 539, GRE-Q no minimum stated, 597, last 2 years GPA 3.0, 3.61; *Behavior Analysis MA/MS (Master of Arts/Science)*: GRE-V no minimum stated, 509, GRE-Q no minimum stated, 601, last 2 years GPA 3.0, 3.43; *Clinical Science PhD (Doctor of Philosophy)*: GRE-V no minimum stated, GRE-Q no minimum stated, last 2 years GPA 3.0.

Other Criteria: (importance of criteria rated low, medium, or high): GRE scores—high, research experience—high, work experience—medium, extracurricular activity—low, GPA—high, letters of recommendation—high, interview—medium, statement of goals and objectives—high, undergraduate major in psychology—medium, specific undergraduate psychology courses taken—low. For additional information on admission requirements, go to http://psych.fiu.edu/.

Student Characteristics: The following represents characteristics of students in 2009–2010 in all graduate psychology programs in the department: Female—full-time 93, part-time 4; Male—full-time 27, part-time 2; African American/Black—full-time 0, part-time 0; Hispanic/Latino(a)—full-time 5, part-time 1; Asian/Pacific Islander—full-time 0, part-time 0; American Indian/Alaska Native—full-time 0, part-time 0; Caucasian/White—full-time 0, part-time 0; Multi-ethnic—full-time 0, part-time 0; students subject to the Americans With Disabilities Act—full-time 0, part-time 0; Unknown ethnicity—full-time 0, part-time 0; International students who hold an F-1 or J-1 Visa—full-time 0, part-time 0.

Financial Information/Assistance:
Tuition for Full-Time Study: *Master's:* State residents: per academic year $8,160, $340 per credit hour; Nonstate residents: per academic year $20,280, $845 per credit hour. *Doctoral:* State residents: per academic year $8,160, $340 per credit hour; Nonstate residents: per academic year $20,280, $845 per credit hour. Tuition is subject to change. Additional fees are assessed to students beyond the costs of tuition for the following: athletic, health, photo ID, and parking fees. See the following Web site for updates and changes in tuition costs: http://www.fiu.edu/orgs/controller/UG Calculator.htm.

Financial Assistance:
First-Year Students: Teaching assistantships available for first year. Average amount paid per academic year: $18,540. Average number of hours worked per week: 20. Apply by December 15. Research assistantships available for first year. Average amount paid per academic year: $18,540. Average number of hours worked per week: 20. Apply by December 15.

Advanced Students: Teaching assistantships available for advanced students. Average amount paid per academic year: $18,540. Average number of hours worked per week: 20. Apply by December 15. Research assistantships available for advanced students. Average amount paid per academic year: $18,540. Average number of hours worked per week: 20. Apply by December 15.

Additional Information: Of all students currently enrolled full time, 50% benefited from one or more of the listed financial assistance programs.

Housing and Day Care: On-campus housing is available. See the following Web site for more information: http://www.housing.fiu.edu/. On-campus day care facilities are available. See the following Web site for more information: http://www.fiu.edu/~children/info.htm.

Employment of Department Graduates:
Master's Degree Graduates: Of those who graduated in the academic year 2008–2009, the following categories and numbers represent the postgraduate activities and employment of master's degree graduates: Enrolled in a psychology doctoral program (1), enrolled in a postdoctoral residency/fellowship (n/a), employed in independent practice (n/a), employed in a community mental health/counseling center (1), do not know (6), total from the above (master's) (8).
Doctoral Degree Graduates: Of those who graduated in the academic year 2008–2009, the following categories and numbers represent the postgraduate activities and employment of doctoral degree graduates: Enrolled in a psychology doctoral program (n/a), employed in an academic position at a university (2), do not know (3), total from the above (doctoral) (5).

Additional Information:
Orientation, Objectives, and Emphasis of Department: The mission of the Department of Psychology at Florida International University is to create new knowledge about human behavior, apply what is known to improve the human condition, and educate and train students. Our graduate programs are designed to foster a commitment both to basic research and application as an integral part of the student's specialty area.

Information for Students With Physical Disabilities: See the following Web site for more information: http://drc.fiu.edu/.

Application Information:
Send to Graduate Studies Admissions Committee, Department of Psychology, Florida International University DM 256, Miami, FL 33199. Application available online. URL of online application: http://gradschool.fiu.edu/admissions.html. Students are admitted in the Fall, application deadline December 15. *Fee:* $30.

Florida State University
Department of Psychology
Arts and Sciences
1107 West Call Street, P.O. Box 3064301
Tallahassee, FL 32306-4301
Telephone: (850) 644-2499
Fax: (850) 644-7739
E-mail: *plant@psy.fsu.edu*
Web: *http://www.psy.fsu.edu*

Department Information:
1918. Chairperson: Janet A. Kistner. Number of faculty: total—full-time 43; women—full-time 18; total—minority—full-time 3; women minority—full-time 1.

Programs and Degrees Offered:
Listed in the following order: Program area, degree type (T if terminal Master's), number awarded 7/08–6/09. Cognitive Psychology PhD (Doctor of Philosophy) 3, Clinical Psychology PhD (Doctor of Philosophy) 9, Neuroscience PhD (Doctor of Philosophy) 4, Applied Behavior Analysis MA/MS (Master of Arts/Science) (T) 12, Social Psychology PhD (Doctor of Philosophy) 0, Developmental Psychology PhD (Doctor of Philosophy) 2.

APA Accreditation: Clinical PhD (Doctor of Philosophy).

Student Applications/Admissions:
Student Applications
Cognitive Psychology PhD (Doctor of Philosophy)—Applications 2009–2010, 46. Total applicants accepted 2009–2010, 8. Number full-time enrolled (new admits only) 2009–2010, 6. Openings 2010–2011, 6. The median number of years required for completion of a degree in 2008–2009 were 5. The number of students enrolled full- and part-time who were dismissed or voluntarily withdrew from this program area in 2008–2009 were 2. *Clinical Psychology PhD (Doctor of Philosophy)*—Applications 2009–2010, 176. Total applicants accepted 2009-2010, 19. Number full-time enrolled (new admits only) 2009–2010, 14. Number part-time enrolled (new admits only) 2009–2010, 0. Openings 2010–2011, 10. The median number of years required for completion of a degree in 2008–2009 were 6. The number of students enrolled full- and part-time who were dismissed or voluntarily withdrew from this program area in 2008–2009 were 0. *Neuroscience PhD (Doctor of Philosophy)*—Applications 2009–2010, 45. Total applicants accepted 2009–2010, 14. Number full-time enrolled (new admits only) 2009–2010, 9. Openings 2010–2011, 6. The median number of years required for completion of a degree in 2008–2009 were 5. The number of students enrolled full- and part-time who were dismissed or voluntarily withdrew from this program area in 2008–2009 were 3. *Applied Behavior Analysis MA/MS (Master of Arts/Science)*—Applications 2009–2010, 51. Total applicants accepted 2009–2010, 22. Number full-time enrolled (new admits only) 2009–2010, 12. Openings 2010–2011, 16. The median number of years required for completion of a degree in 2008–2009 were 2. The number of students enrolled full- and part-time who were dismissed or voluntarily withdrew from this program area in 2008–2009 were 0. *Social Psychology PhD (Doctor of Philosophy)*—Applications 2009–2010, 102. Total applicants accepted 2009–2010, 3. Number full-time enrolled (new admits only) 2009–2010, 3. Total enrolled 2009–2010 full-time, 21. Openings 2010–2011, 6. The number of students enrolled full- and part-time who were dismissed or voluntarily withdrew from this program area in 2008–2009 were 1. *Developmental Psychology PhD (Doctor of Philosophy)*—Applications 2009–2010, 20. Total applicants accepted 2009–2010, 2. Number full-time enrolled (new admits only) 2009–2010, 2. Total enrolled 2009–2010 full-time, 10. Openings 2010–2011, 4. The median number of years required for completion of a degree in 2008–2009 were 4. The number of students enrolled full- and part-time who were dismissed or voluntarily withdrew from this program area in 2008–2009 were 0.

Scores: Entries appear in this order: required test or GPA, minimum score (if required), median score of students entering in 2009–2010. *Neuroscience PhD (Doctor of Philosophy):* GRE-V 500, 520, GRE-Q 500, 630, last 2 years GPA 3.0, 3.45; *Social Psychology PhD (Doctor of Philosophy):* GRE-V 550, 610, GRE-Q 550, 750, last 2 years GPA 3.0, 3.88; *Developmental*

Psychology PhD (Doctor of Philosophy): GRE-V 500, 520, GRE-Q 500, 600, last 2 years GPA 3.0, 3.76.

Other Criteria: (importance of criteria rated low, medium, or high): GRE scores—high, research experience—high, work experience—low, extracurricular activity—low, clinically related public service—low, GPA—high, letters of recommendation—high, interview—medium, statement of goals and objectives—high, match w/ fac res interest—high, undergraduate major in psychology—medium, specific undergraduate psychology courses taken—medium. Research experience is not an important factor for admission to the Applied Behavior Analysis master's program; work or volunteer experience in behavior analysis is of high importance for this program. For additional information on admission requirements, go to http://www.psy.fsu.edu.

Student Characteristics: The following represents characteristics of students in 2009–2010 in all graduate psychology programs in the department: Female—full-time 113, part-time 4; Male—full-time 57, part-time 2; African American/Black—full-time 8, part-time 0; Hispanic/Latino(a)—full-time 9, part-time 2; Asian/Pacific Islander—full-time 6, part-time 0; American Indian/Alaska Native—full-time 1, part-time 0; Caucasian/White—full-time 142, part-time 4; Multi-ethnic—full-time 0, part-time 0; students subject to the Americans With Disabilities Act—full-time 0, part-time 0; Unknown ethnicity—full-time 2, part-time 0; International students who hold an F-1 or J-1 Visa—full-time 2, part-time 0.

Financial Information/Assistance:

Tuition for Full-Time Study: *Master's:* State residents: per academic year $5,796, $322 per credit hour; Nonstate residents: per academic year $17,172, $954 per credit hour. *Doctoral:* State residents: per academic year $5,796, $322 per credit hour; Nonstate residents: per academic year $17,172, $954 per credit hour. Tuition is subject to change. See the following Web site for updates and changes in tuition costs: http://www.sfs.fsu.edu/tuition.html.

Financial Assistance:

First-Year Students: Teaching assistantships available for first year. Average amount paid per academic year: $15,000. Average number of hours worked per week: 16. Research assistantships available for first year. Average amount paid per academic year: $18,000. Average number of hours worked per week: 20. Traineeships available for first year. Average amount paid per academic year: $20,000. Average number of hours worked per week: 20. Fellowships and scholarships available for first year. Average amount paid per academic year: $20,000. Average number of hours worked per week: 0.

Advanced Students: Teaching assistantships available for advanced students. Average amount paid per academic year: $15,000. Average number of hours worked per week: 16. Research assistantships available for advanced students. Average amount paid per academic year: $18,000. Average number of hours worked per week: 20. Traineeships available for advanced students. Average amount paid per academic year: $20,000. Average number of hours worked per week: 20. Fellowships and scholarships available for advanced students. Average amount paid per academic year: $20,000. Average number of hours worked per week: 0.

Additional Information: Of all students currently enrolled full time, 100% benefited from one or more of the listed financial assistance programs.

Internships/Practica: Doctoral Degree (PhD Clinical Psychology): For those doctoral students for whom a professional internship was required in this program prior to graduation, (8) students applied for an internship in 2008–2009, with (8) students obtaining an internship. Of those students who obtained an internship, (8) were paid internships. Of those students who obtained an internship, (8) students placed in APA/CPA accredited internships, (0) students placed in internships not APA/CPA accredited, but listed with the Association of Psychology Postdoctoral and Internship Programs (APPIC), (0) students placed in internships conforming to guidelines of the Council of Directors of School Psychology Programs (CDSPP), (0) students placed in internships that were not APA/CPA accredited, APPIC or CDSPP listed. Master's Degree (MA/MS Applied Behavior Analysis): An internship experience, such as a final research project or "capstone" experience is required of graduates. Community facilities provide a multitude of settings for practicum placements for clinical students and for master's students in applied behavior analysis. Clinical students receive a stipend and tuition waivers for their practicum work in the community as well as excellent supervised experience and opportunities for research. Practicum settings for clinical students include an inpatient psychiatric hospital, a comprehensive evaluation center for children, a juvenile treatment program, forensic facilities, and other agencies in the community. Clinical psychology students complete a required unpaid practicum at our nationally recognized on-campus Psychology Clinic during the second and typically third year of study. The clinic provides empirically based assessment and therapy services to adults, children, and families in the north Florida region. Psychology faculty provide supervision. The clinical program culminates in a required one-year internship in an APA-approved facility. Clinical students from the FSU program have, over the years, been highly successful in obtaining excellent internships throughout the country. Applied Behavior Analysis master's students have diverse practicum sites from which to choose, including public schools, family homes, residential treatment facilities, businesses, consulting firms, and state agencies. Stipends and tuition waivers are available for many of the applied behavior analysis practicum settings.

Housing and Day Care: On-campus housing is available. See the following Web site for more information: http://www.housing.fsu.edu/. On-campus day care facilities are available. See the following Web site for more information: http://www.childcare.fsu.edu/.

Employment of Department Graduates:

Master's Degree Graduates: Of those who graduated in the academic year 2008–2009, the following categories and numbers represent the postgraduate activities and employment of master's degree graduates: Enrolled in a postdoctoral residency/fellowship (n/a), employed in independent practice (n/a), employed in other positions at a higher education institution (1), employed in a professional position in a school system (1), employed in business or industry (13), do not know (2), total from the above (master's) (17).

Doctoral Degree Graduates: Of those who graduated in the academic year 2008–2009, the following categories and numbers represent the postgraduate activities and employment of doctoral degree graduates: Enrolled in a psychology doctoral program (n/a), enrolled in a postdoctoral residency/fellowship (2), employed in an academic position at a university (2), employed in a community mental health/counseling center (2), employed in a hospital/medical center (5), total from the above (doctoral) (11).

Additional Information:
Orientation, Objectives, and Emphasis of Department: This is a scientifically-oriented department with over $6 million in annual grant funding. The Clinical Psychology program promotes a scientifically based approach to understanding, assessing, and ameliorating cognitive, emotional, behavioral, and health problems. Integrative training in clinical science and clinical service delivery is provided. Cognitive Psychology students develop research and analytical skills while learning to coordinate basic research with theory development and application. Current research includes expert performance, skill acquisition, reading, memory, attention, language processing, and cognitive aging. Students in the Developmental Psychology program conduct basic and applied research. A developmental perspective is interdisciplinary; consequently, members of the developmental faculty routinely hold appointments in one of our other doctoral programs. The Social Psychology program provides students with in-depth training in personality and social psychology, focusing on basic and applied research. Current research areas include the self, prejudice and stereotyping, social cognition, and evolutionary perspectives on various topics. The interdisciplinary Neuroscience program offers students broad training in brain and behavior research. Areas of emphasis include sensory processes, neural development and plasticity, behavioral and molecular genetics, regulation of energy balance and hormonal control of behavior. The terminal master's program in Applied Behavior Analysis focuses on analyzing and modifying behavior using well-established principles of learning.

Special Facilities or Resources: The department's technical staff and support facilities are some of the best in the country. Fully staffed and equipped electronic and machine shops support faculty and graduate student research. Highly trained staff provides assistance in graphic arts, photography, instrument and computer software design, and electronic communication services. A neurosurgical operating room and a neurohistological laboratory are available. Faculty and students have available to them a supercomputer and workstations offering human eyetracking and brain wave and psychophysiological recording, among others. A molecular neuroscience laboratory provides equipment and training for studies of gene cloning and gene expression, as well as techniques to measure levels of hormones and neurotransmitters. The Clinical program administers an in department outpatient clinic that offers empirically based assessment and therapy services to members of the Tallahassee and surrounding communities. The department was one of four in the U.S. recognized in 2003 by APA for innovative practices in graduate education in psychology. This recognition was for the in-department clinic, which is a full-fledged clinical research laboratory. Based on research and case studies conducted at the clinic, faculty and students have published many books and peer-reviewed articles. The department and clinic are housed in a new, state-of-the-art building.

Information for Students With Physical Disabilities: See the following Web site for more information: http://www.disabilitycenter.fsu.edu.

Application Information:
Send to Graduate Program, Department of Psychology, Florida State University, 1107 West Call Street, P.O. Box 3064301, Tallahassee, FL 32306-4301. Application available online. URL of online application: http://www.psy.fsu.edu. Students are admitted in the Fall, application deadline December 1 for Clinical Psychology; December 15 for Social Psychology and Neuroscience; January 11 for Cognitive; and January 15 Developmental Psychology. The Applied Behavior Analysis application deadline is February 1. *Fee:* $30.

Florida State University
Psychological Services in Education: PhD Combined Counseling/School Psychology
Education
306 Stone Building
Tallahassee, FL 32306-4453
Telephone: (850) 644-4592
Fax: (850) 644-8776
E-mail: *spfeiffer@fsu.edu*
Web: *http://www.epls.fsu.edu/psych_services/*

Department Information:
2002. Director of Clinical Training: Steven Pfeiffer. Number of faculty: total—full-time 9; women—full-time 6; total—minority—full-time 1; faculty subject to the Americans With Disabilities Act 1.

Programs and Degrees Offered:
Listed in the following order: Program area, degree type (T if terminal Master's), number awarded 7/08–6/09. Combined Counseling and School Psychology PhD (Doctor of Philosophy) 10, Mental Health Counseling MA/MS (Master of Arts/Science) (T) 12, School Psychology EdS (School Psychology) 15, Career Counseling MA/MS (Master of Arts/Science) 4, Rehab Counseling MA/MS (Master of Arts/Science) (T) 10.

APA Accreditation: Combination PhD (Doctor of Philosophy).

Student Applications/Admissions:
Student Applications

Combined Counseling and School Psychology PhD (Doctor of Philosophy)—Applications 2009–2010, 70. Total applicants accepted 2009–2010, 9. Number full-time enrolled (new admits only) 2009–2010, 9. Number part-time enrolled (new admits only) 2009–2010, 0. Openings 2010–2011, 9. The median number of years required for completion of a degree in 2008–2009 were 6. The number of students enrolled full- and part-time who were dismissed or voluntarily withdrew from this program area in 2008–2009 were 1. *Mental Health Counseling MA/MS (Master of Arts/Science)*—Applications 2009–2010, 40. Total applicants accepted 2009–2010, 14. Number full-time enrolled (new admits only) 2009–2010, 14. Number part-time enrolled (new admits only) 2009–2010, 0. Openings 2010–2011, 15. The median number of years required for completion of a degree in 2008–2009 were 2. The number of students enrolled full- and part-time who were dismissed or voluntarily withdrew from this program area in 2008–2009 were 0. *School Psychology EdS (School Psychology)*—Applications 2009–2010, 75. Total applicants accepted 2009–2010, 14. Number full-time enrolled (new admits only) 2009–2010, 14. Number part-time enrolled (new admits only) 2009–2010, 0. Openings 2010–2011, 16. The median number of years required for completion of a degree in 2008–2009 were 3. The number of students enrolled full- and part-time who were dismissed or voluntarily withdrew from this program area in 2008–2009 were 2. *Career Counseling MA/MS (Master of Arts/Science)*—Applications 2009–2010, 15. Total applicants accepted 2009–2010, 4. Number full-time enrolled (new admits only) 2009–2010, 3. Total enrolled 2009–2010 full-time, 6. Openings 2010–2011, 5. The median number of years required for completion of a degree in 2008–2009 were 2. The number of students enrolled full- and part-time who were dismissed or voluntarily withdrew from this program area in 2008–2009 were 0. *Rehab Counseling MA/MS (Master of Arts/Science)*—Applications 2009–2010, 30. Total applicants accepted 2009–2010, 10. Number full-time enrolled (new admits only) 2009–2010, 10. Total enrolled 2009–2010 full-time, 20. Openings 2010–2011, 14. The median number of years required for completion of a degree in 2008–2009 were 2. The number of students enrolled full- and part-time who were dismissed or voluntarily withdrew from this program area in 2008–2009 were 0.

Scores: Entries appear in this order: required test or GPA, minimum score (if required), median score of students entering in 2009–2010. *Combined Counseling and School Psychology PhD (Doctor of Philosophy)*: GRE-V 500, 575, GRE-Q 500, 575, overall undergraduate GPA 3.0, 3.4, last 2 years GPA 3.2, 3.5; *Mental Health Counseling MA/MS (Master of Arts/Science)*: GRE-V 500, 540, GRE-Q 500, 540, overall undergraduate GPA 3.0, 3.25, last 2 years GPA 3.0, 3.4; *School Psychology EdS (School Psychology)*: GRE-V 500, 550, GRE-Q 500, 550, overall undergraduate GPA 3.0, 3.4, last 2 years GPA 3.0, 3.5; *Career Counseling MA/MS (Master of Arts/Science)*: GRE-V 500, 550, GRE-Q 500, 550, overall undergraduate GPA 3.0, 3.4, last 2 years GPA 3.2, 3.5; *Rehab Counseling MA/MS (Master of Arts/Science)*: GRE-V 500, 500, GRE-Q 500, 500, overall undergraduate GPA 3.0, 3.0, last 2 years GPA 3.0, 3.2.

Other Criteria: (importance of criteria rated low, medium, or high): GRE scores—high, research experience—medium, work experience—medium, extracurricular activity—low, clinically related public service—medium, GPA—high, letters of recommendation—high, interview—high, statement of goals and objectives—high, undergraduate major in psychology—low, specific undergraduate psychology courses taken—low. Research experience emphasized for the doctoral program.

Student Characteristics: The following represents characteristics of students in 2009–2010 in all graduate psychology programs in the department: Female—full-time 98, part-time 0; Male—full-time 43, part-time 0; African American/Black—full-time 10, part-time 0; Hispanic/Latino(a)—full-time 8, part-time 0; Asian/Pacific Islander—full-time 6, part-time 0; American Indian/Alaska Native—full-time 0, part-time 0; Caucasian/White—full-time 117, part-time 0; Multi-ethnic—full-time 0, part-time 0; students subject to the Americans With Disabilities Act—full-time 4, part-time 0; Unknown ethnicity—full-time 0, part-time 0; International students who hold an F-1 or J-1 Visa—full-time 3, part-time 0.

Financial Information/Assistance:
  Tuition for Full-Time Study: Master's: State residents: per academic year $6,900, $230 per credit hour; Nonstate residents: per academic year $25,830, $861 per credit hour. *Doctoral:* State residents: per academic year $6,900, $230 per credit hour; Non-state residents: per academic year $25,830, $861 per credit hour. Tuition is subject to change.

Financial Assistance:
  First-Year Students: Teaching assistantships available for first year. Average amount paid per academic year: $3,200. Average number of hours worked per week: 10. Research assistantships available for first year. Average amount paid per academic year: $3,600. Average number of hours worked per week: 10. Fellowships and scholarships available for first year. Average amount paid per academic year: $6,300. Average number of hours worked per week: 10. Apply by January 3.

  Advanced Students: Teaching assistantships available for advanced students. Average amount paid per academic year: $3,400. Average number of hours worked per week: 10. Research assistantships available for advanced students. Average amount paid per academic year: $3,800. Average number of hours worked per week: 10. Fellowships and scholarships available for advanced students. Average amount paid per academic year: $6,400. Average number of hours worked per week: 10. Apply by January 3.

  Additional Information: Of all students currently enrolled full time, 60% benefited from one or more of the listed financial assistance programs.

Internships/Practica: Doctoral Degree (PhD Combined Counseling and School Psychology): For those doctoral students for whom a professional internship was required in this program prior to graduation, (8) students applied for an internship in 2008–2009, with (7) students obtaining an internship. Of those students who obtained an internship, (7) were paid internships. Of those students who obtained an internship, (6) students placed in APA/CPA accredited internships, (1) students placed in internships not APA/CPA accredited, but listed with the Association of Psychology Postdoctoral and Internship Programs (APPIC), (0) students placed in internships conforming to guidelines of the Council of Directors of School Psychology Programs (CDSPP), (0) students placed in internships that were not APA/CPA accredited, APPIC or CDSPP listed. Master's Degree (MA/MS Mental Health Counseling): An internship experience, such as a final research project or "capstone" experience is required of graduates. Master's Degree (MA/MS Rehab Counseling): An internship experience, such as a final research project or "capstone" experience is required of graduates. The program offers both on-campus and off-campus practicum experiences; on-campus clinical practica include a mental health clinic serving clients from the community; adult learning disability clinic serving college students and the community; student career counseling center; multidisciplinary center serving K-12 students from a number of school districts; university student counseling center. Off-campus practica include a wide range of mental health, psychiatric, educational, and behavioral healthcare agencies and private practices.

Housing and Day Care: On-campus housing is available. See the following Web site for more information: http://www.housing.fsu.edu/. On-campus day care facilities are available. See the following Web site for more information: http://www.childcare.fsu.edu/.

Employment of Department Graduates:
  Master's Degree Graduates: Of those who graduated in the academic year 2008–2009, the following categories and numbers represent the postgraduate activities and employment of master's degree graduates: Enrolled in a psychology doctoral program (3),

enrolled in another graduate/professional program (2), enrolled in a postdoctoral residency/fellowship (n/a), employed in independent practice (n/a), employed in a professional position in a school system (12), employed in business or industry (1), employed in government agency (4), other employment position (6), do not know (5), total from the above (master's) (33).

Doctoral Degree Graduates: Of those who graduated in the academic year 2008–2009, the following categories and numbers represent the postgraduate activities and employment of doctoral degree graduates: Enrolled in a psychology doctoral program (n/a), enrolled in a postdoctoral residency/fellowship (2), employed in independent practice (1), employed in an academic position at a university (2), employed in a professional position in a school system (1), employed in government agency (1), employed in a community mental health/counseling center (1), employed in a hospital/medical center (1), total from the above (doctoral) (9).

Additional Information:
Orientation, Objectives, and Emphasis of Department: The Combined Doctoral Program in Counseling Psychology and School Psychology is fully accredited by the American Psychological Association. This unique program allows students to acquire knowledge and skills necessary for leadership positions in the practice of counseling psychology and school psychology in a variety of academic and applied settings. Students acquire basic competency in counseling psychology and school psychology, and advanced expertise in either counseling psychology or school psychology. The program prepares graduates for national certification and state licensure. Within the combined program, all students share a common core of experience in research and practice in counseling psychology and school psychology (70% shared coursework/practica); students also are afforded the opportunity to concentrate in counseling psychology or school psychology (a few students decide to concentrate in both). The Combined program embraces a scientist–practitioner model consistent with the mission of Florida State, a Research I University. The program faculty enjoy diverse research and clinical interests, providing students with a range of opportunities for professional development in the areas of mental health counseling, school psychology, career counseling, rehabilitation counseling, addictions counseling, prevention and early intervention, wellness, and psychology of the gifted.

Special Facilities or Resources: The program uses the following clinic facilities for the development of assessment, counseling and consultation skills: (1) The Human Services Center is a mental health training clinic that provides counseling services at no cost to residents of Tallahassee and surrounding communities. This center offers counseling for a wide range of mental health and psychiatric problems, social skill training, anger management, relationship counseling, family counseling, and personal growth and development. The center works with the juvenile justice system in providing services to court referred cases. (2) The Adult Learning and Evaluation Center is a referral source for FSU, our other two local colleges, FAMU and TCC, and the community. It serves to assist adults in identifying learning disabilities and related problems that may compromise the attainment of educational and career progress. It offers students practica and assistantships in psychological assessment and consultation. (3) The Career Center is located in the Student Services Center and provides one of the most technologically-advanced career facilities in the nation. The Career Center provides opportunities for practica and internships as well as for student employment opportunities as career advisors. This Center serves as many as 6000 students per year with a variety of career concerns from choice of major to job placement. The philosophy is one of a full-service career center that is able to address not only presenting career concerns but related mental health issues as well.

Information for Students With Physical Disabilities: See the following Web site for more information: http://www.disabilitycenter.fsu.edu/.

Application Information:
Send to Admissions Committee, Psychological Services in Education, Florida State University, Stone Building, Tallahassee, FL 32306-4453. Application available online. URL of online application: http://www.epls.fsu.edu/psych_services/index.htm. Students are admitted in the Fall, application deadline January 15. *Fee:* $30.

Florida, University of
Department of Clinical and Health Psychology
Public Health and Health Professions
Box 100165 HSC
Gainesville, FL 32610-0165
Telephone: (352) 273-6455
Fax: (352) 273-6530
E-mail: *soltvl@phhp.ufl.edu*
Web: *http://chp.phhp.ufl.edu/*

Department Information:
1959. Chairperson: Russell M Bauer. Number of faculty: total—full-time 27; women—full-time 11; total—minority—full-time 2; faculty subject to the Americans With Disabilities Act 1.

Programs and Degrees Offered:
Listed in the following order: Program area, degree type (T if terminal Master's), number awarded 7/08–6/09. Clinical Psychology PhD (Doctor of Philosophy) 15.

APA Accreditation: Clinical PhD (Doctor of Philosophy). Student Outcome Data Website: http://chp.phhp.ufl.edu/programs/doctoral/data/.

Student Applications/Admissions:
Student Applications

Clinical Psychology PhD (Doctor of Philosophy)—Applications 2009–2010, 330. Total applicants accepted 2009–2010, 25. Number full-time enrolled (new admits only) 2009–2010, 13. Number part-time enrolled (new admits only) 2009–2010, 0. Total enrolled 2009–2010 full-time, 77, part-time, 1. Openings 2010–2011, 15. The median number of years required for completion of a degree in 2008–2009 were 6. The number of students enrolled full- and part-time who were dismissed or voluntarily withdrew from this program area in 2008–2009 were 1.

Scores: Entries appear in this order: required test or GPA, minimum score (if required), median score of students entering in 2009–2010. *Clinical Psychology PhD (Doctor of Philosophy):* GRE-V no minimum stated, 610, GRE-Q no minimum stated,

700, overall undergraduate GPA no minimum stated, 3.78, last 2 years GPA no minimum stated.
Other Criteria: (importance of criteria rated low, medium, or high): GRE scores—medium, research experience—high, work experience—medium, extracurricular activity—medium, clinically related public service—high, GPA—medium, letters of recommendation—high, interview—high, statement of goals and objectives—high, undergraduate major in psychology—medium, specific undergraduate psychology courses taken—medium. For additional information on admission requirements, go to http://chp.phhp.ufl.edu/programs/doctoral/.

Student Characteristics: The following represents characteristics of students in 2009–2010 in all graduate psychology programs in the department: Female—full-time 60, part-time 1; Male—full-time 17, part-time 0; African American/Black—full-time 4, part-time 0; Hispanic/Latino(a)—full-time 5, part-time 0; Asian/Pacific Islander—full-time 5, part-time 0; American Indian/Alaska Native—full-time 0, part-time 0; Caucasian/White—full-time 63, part-time 1; Multi-ethnic—full-time 0, part-time 0; students subject to the Americans With Disabilities Act—full-time 1, part-time 0; Unknown ethnicity—full-time 0, part-time 0; International students who hold an F-1 or J-1 Visa—full-time 0, part-time 0.

Financial Information/Assistance:
Tuition for Full-Time Study: *Doctoral:* State residents: per academic year $8,190, $395 per credit hour; Nonstate residents: per academic year $23,315, $1,200 per credit hour. Tuition is subject to change. See the following Web site for updates and changes in tuition costs: http://fa.ufl.edu/ufs/cashiers/feecalc.asp.

Financial Assistance:
First-Year Students: Research assistantships available for first year. Average amount paid per academic year: $15,000. Average number of hours worked per week: 20. Apply by December 1. Fellowships and scholarships available for first year. Average amount paid per academic year: $20,000. Average number of hours worked per week: 20. Apply by December 1.
Advanced Students: Teaching assistantships available for advanced students. Average amount paid per academic year: $15,000. Average number of hours worked per week: 20. Research assistantships available for advanced students. Average amount paid per academic year: $15,000. Average number of hours worked per week: 20. Fellowships and scholarships available for advanced students. Average amount paid per academic year: $20,000.
Additional Information: Of all students currently enrolled full time, 99% benefited from one or more of the listed financial assistance programs. Application and information available online at: http://chp.phhp.ufl.edu/programs/doctoral/.

Internships/Practica: Doctoral Degree (PhD Clinical Psychology): For those doctoral students for whom a professional internship was required in this program prior to graduation, (13) students applied for an internship in 2008–2009, with (13) students obtaining an internship. Of those students who obtained an internship, (13) were paid internships. Of those students who obtained an internship, (13) students placed in APA/CPA accredited internships, (0) students placed in internships not APA/CPA accredited, but listed with the Association of Psychology Postdoctoral and Internship Programs (APPIC), (0) students placed in internships conforming to guidelines of the Council of Directors of School Psychology Programs (CDSPP), (0) students placed in internships that were not APA/CPA accredited, APPIC or CDSPP listed. The Department of Clinical and Health Psychology operates a Psychology Clinic which is part of Shands Hospital within the University of Florida Health Science Center. This clinic provides consultation, assessment, and intervention services to medical-surgical inpatients and outpatients, as well as community patients with emotional and behavioral problems. Major services include clinical health psychology, child/pediatric psychology and clinical neuropsychology.

Housing and Day Care: On-campus housing is available. See the following Web site for more information: http://www.housing.ufl.edu/. On-campus day care facilities are available. See the following Web site for more information: http://www.babygator.ufl.edu/default.htm.

Employment of Department Graduates:
Master's Degree Graduates: Of those who graduated in the academic year 2008–2009, the following categories and numbers represent the postgraduate activities and employment of master's degree graduates: Enrolled in a postdoctoral residency/fellowship (n/a), employed in independent practice (n/a), total from the above (master's) (0).
Doctoral Degree Graduates: Of those who graduated in the academic year 2008–2009, the following categories and numbers represent the postgraduate activities and employment of doctoral degree graduates: Enrolled in a psychology doctoral program (n/a), enrolled in a postdoctoral residency/fellowship (12), employed in an academic position at a university (2), other employment position (1), total from the above (doctoral) (15).

Additional Information:
Orientation, Objectives, and Emphasis of Department: The program is designed to train doctoral-level professional psychologists in the scientist–practitioner model through the development of broad clinical skills and competencies, through mastery of broad areas of knowledge in psychology and clinical psychology, and through demonstrated competencies in contributing to that knowledge by research. Within these program objectives particular emphases can be identified: clinical health psychology, clinical neuropsychology and clinical child/pediatric psychology. Courses, practica, conferences, committees, supervision, and settings are designed to augment each emphasis.

Special Facilities or Resources: The Department and its parent College, the College of Public Health and Health Professions, is housed in a new building that contains faculty offices, student work spaces, and state-of-the-art classroom facilities. In addition, department faculty currently occupy several thousand square feet of laboratory space for clinical and basic research. The Department is particularly strong in instrumentation and methodology for clinical research in pediatric psychology, health psychology, and neuropsychology. Psychophysiological and neuroimaging capabilities are present and utilized by many faculty. The clinical psychology program uses the extensive resources of the campus and community. Sites utilized for clinical training include the department's Psychology Clinic, university student health services, the university counseling center; and the VA Medical Center in Gainesville. Agencies and centers throughout the state and nation are also available, principally for internship training for students. The use of these varied resources is consonant with the program objectives.

The trainee is directly involved with a broad range of clinical and health problems, professionals, agencies, and settings.

Information for Students With Physical Disabilities: See the following Web site for more information: http://www.dso.ufl.edu/drc/.

Application Information:
Send to Graduate Admissions, Department of Clinical and Health Psychology, Box 100165 HSC, University of Florida, Gainesville, FL 32610-0165. Application available online. URL of online application: http://chp.phhp.ufl.edu/admissions/. Students are admitted in the Fall, application deadline December 1. *Fee:* $30.

Florida, University of
Department of Psychology
Liberal Arts and Sciences
P.O. Box 112250
Gainesville, FL 32611-2250
Telephone: (352) 392-0601
Fax: (352) 392-7985
E-mail: *west51@ufl.edu*
Web: *http://www.psych.ufl.edu*

Department Information:
1947. Chairperson: Neil Rowland. Number of faculty: total—full-time 35, part-time 1; women—full-time 10, part-time 1; total—minority—full-time 3; women minority—full-time 2.

Programs and Degrees Offered:
Listed in the following order: Program area, degree type (T if terminal Master's), number awarded 7/08–6/09. Behavior Analysis PhD (Doctor of Philosophy) 8, Counseling Psychology PhD (Doctor of Philosophy) 7, Developmental Psychology PhD (Doctor of Philosophy) 1, Social Psychology PhD (Doctor of Philosophy) 6, Behavioral and Cognitive Neuroscience PhD (Doctor of Philosophy) 3.

APA Accreditation: Counseling PhD (Doctor of Philosophy).

Student Applications/Admissions:
Student Applications
Behavior Analysis PhD (Doctor of Philosophy)—Applications 2009–2010, 35. Total applicants accepted 2009–2010, 6. Number full-time enrolled (new admits only) 2009–2010, 3. Number part-time enrolled (new admits only) 2009–2010, 0. Openings 2010–2011, 5. The median number of years required for completion of a degree in 2008–2009 were 6. The number of students enrolled full- and part-time who were dismissed or voluntarily withdrew from this program area in 2008–2009 were 1. *Counseling Psychology PhD (Doctor of Philosophy)*—Applications 2009–2010, 125. Total applicants accepted 2009–2010, 9. Number full-time enrolled (new admits only) 2009–2010, 5. Number part-time enrolled (new admits only) 2009–2010, 0. Total enrolled 2009–2010 full-time, 37, part-time, 1. Openings 2010–2011, 9. The median number of years required for completion of a degree in 2008–2009 were 6. The number of students enrolled full- and part-time who were dismissed or voluntarily withdrew from this program area in 2008–2009 were 1. *Developmental Psychology PhD (Doctor of Philosophy)*—Applications 2009–2010, 30. Total applicants accepted 2009–2010, 6. Number full-time enrolled (new admits only) 2009–2010, 5. Number part-time enrolled (new admits only) 2009–2010, 0. Openings 2010–2011, 5. The median number of years required for completion of a degree in 2008–2009 were 5. The number of students enrolled full- and part-time who were dismissed or voluntarily withdrew from this program area in 2008–2009 were 1. *Social Psychology PhD (Doctor of Philosophy)*—Applications 2009–2010, 50. Total applicants accepted 2009–2010, 6. Number full-time enrolled (new admits only) 2009–2010, 4. Number part-time enrolled (new admits only) 2009–2010, 0. Openings 2010–2011, 5. The median number of years required for completion of a degree in 2008–2009 were 4. The number of students enrolled full- and part-time who were dismissed or voluntarily withdrew from this program area in 2008–2009 were 1. *Behavioral and Cognitive Neuroscience PhD (Doctor of Philosophy)*—Applications 2009–2010, 27. Total applicants accepted 2009–2010, 3. Number full-time enrolled (new admits only) 2009–2010, 1. Number part-time enrolled (new admits only) 2009–2010, 0. Openings 2010–2011, 6. The median number of years required for completion of a degree in 2008–2009 were 6. The number of students enrolled full- and part-time who were dismissed or voluntarily withdrew from this program area in 2008–2009 were 2.

Other Criteria: (importance of criteria rated low, medium, or high): GRE scores—medium, research experience—high, work experience—low, extracurricular activity—medium, clinically related public service—high, GPA—high, letters of recommendation—high, interview—medium, statement of goals and objectives—medium, match w/ faculty interest—high, undergraduate major in psychology—medium, specific undergraduate psychology courses taken—medium, Only the Counseling Psychology program requires clinically related experience. Weight given to these criteria varies from program to program. Some programs do not conduct interviews every year. For additional information on admission requirements, go to http://www.psych.ufl.edu/Graduate/Prospective/admissions.htm.

Student Characteristics: The following represents characteristics of students in 2009–2010 in all graduate psychology programs in the department: Female—full-time 75, part-time 0; Male—full-time 27, part-time 1; African American/Black—full-time 0, part-time 1; Hispanic/Latino(a)—full-time 6, part-time 0; Asian/Pacific Islander—full-time 9, part-time 0; American Indian/Alaska Native—full-time 1, part-time 0; Caucasian/White—full-time 79, part-time 0; Multi-ethnic—full-time 5, part-time 0; students subject to the Americans With Disabilities Act—full-time 0, part-time 0; Unknown ethnicity—full-time 2, part-time 0; International students who hold an F-1 or J-1 Visa—full-time 8, part-time 0.

Financial Information/Assistance:
Tuition for Full-Time Study: *Doctoral:* State residents: per academic year $7,400, $350 per credit hour; Nonstate residents: per academic year $20,000, $1,000 per credit hour. Tuition is subject to change. See the following Web site for updates and changes in tuition costs: http://fa.ufl.edu/ufs/cashiers/feecalc.asp.

Financial Assistance:
First-Year Students: Teaching assistantships available for first year. Average amount paid per academic year: $15,000. Average number of hours worked per week: 14. Apply by December 10. Research assistantships available for first year. Average amount paid per academic year: $15,000. Average number of hours worked per week: 14. Apply by December 10. Fellowships and scholarships available for first year. Average amount paid per academic year: $20,000. Average number of hours worked per week: 14. Apply by December 10.

Advanced Students: Teaching assistantships available for advanced students. Average amount paid per academic year: $15,000. Average number of hours worked per week: 14. Research assistantships available for advanced students. Average amount paid per academic year: $14,000. Average number of hours worked per week: 14. Fellowships and scholarships available for advanced students. Average amount paid per academic year: $20,000. Average number of hours worked per week: 14.

Additional Information: Of all students currently enrolled full time, 98% benefited from one or more of the listed financial assistance programs. Application and information available online at: http://www.psych.ufl.edu/Graduate/Prospective/financial.htm.

Internships/Practica: Doctoral Degree (PhD Counseling Psychology): For those doctoral students for whom a professional internship was required in this program prior to graduation, (7) students applied for an internship in 2008–2009, with (7) students obtaining an internship. Of those students who obtained an internship, (7) were paid internships. Of those students who obtained an internship, (6) students placed in APA/CPA accredited internships, (1) students placed in internships not APA/CPA accredited, but listed with the Association of Psychology Postdoctoral and Internship Programs (APPIC), (0) students placed in internships conforming to guidelines of the Council of Directors of School Psychology Programs (CDSPP), (0) students placed in internships that were not APA/CPA accredited, APPIC or CDSPP listed. University Counseling Center, University of Florida Student Health Service, Family Practice Medical Group, Meridian Behavioral Healthcare, Alachua County Crisis Center, VA Medical Center, North Florida Treatment and Evaluation Center, and Northeast Florida State Hospital.

Housing and Day Care: On-campus housing is available. See the following Web site for more information: http://www.housing.ufl.edu/villages/. On-campus day care facilities are available. See the following Web site for more information: http://www.babygator.ufl.edu/default.htm.

Employment of Department Graduates:
Master's Degree Graduates: Of those who graduated in the academic year 2008–2009, the following categories and numbers represent the postgraduate activities and employment of master's degree graduates: Enrolled in a postdoctoral residency/fellowship (n/a), employed in independent practice (n/a), total from the above (master's) (0).

Doctoral Degree Graduates: Of those who graduated in the academic year 2008–2009, the following categories and numbers represent the postgraduate activities and employment of doctoral degree graduates: Enrolled in a psychology doctoral program (n/a), enrolled in a postdoctoral residency/fellowship (7), employed in independent practice (2), employed in an academic position at a university (2), employed in an academic position at a 2-year/4-year college (1), employed in other positions at a higher education institution (1), employed in business or industry (1), employed in government agency (1), employed in a community mental health/counseling center (2), employed in a hospital/medical center (2), still seeking employment (2), other employment position (2), do not know (4), total from the above (doctoral) (27).

Additional Information:
Orientation, Objectives, and Emphasis of Department: The graduate program in Psychology at the University of Florida is designed for those planning careers as researchers, teacher-scholars, and scientist–practitioners in psychology. In addition to specialized training in one or more areas, a core program of theories, methods, and research in general psychology insures that each student will be well prepared in the basic areas of psychology. The primary goal of the Department is educating scientists who will help advance psychology as a science through teaching, research, and professional practice. Because the University of Florida is a broad spectrum university, including almost all the major academic departments as well as professional schools on a single campus, a unique atmosphere exists for the evolution of the general program and the development of personal programs of study. Each student also receives specialized training in at least one of the areas of specialization including counseling psychology, developmental, behavior analysis, behavioral and cognitive neuroscience, and social. One of the fundamental goals of the doctoral program is to engage the student as early as possible in the area of interest while ensuring a sound background of knowledge of theory, methodology, and major content areas so that maximum integration may be achieved. All students participate in ongoing aspects of the academic community such as teaching, research, field experience, and professional activities. Seminars are offered in techniques of teaching accompanied by supervised undergraduate teaching. Continuous research experience is required. The Department participates in a number of interdisciplinary programs including sensory studies, neurobiological sciences, and aging training.

Special Facilities or Resources: Special facilities in the department include laboratories in developmental (child, adolescent, aging), experimental analysis of behavior, cognitive and information processing, perception, psychobiology, and social; an animal colony; a statistical computation laboratory; a laboratory in neuropsychology and developmental learning disabilities; and the Computing Center.

Information for Students With Physical Disabilities: See the following Web site for more information: http://www.dso.ufl.edu/drc/.

Application Information:
Send to Graduate Program Assistant, P.O. Box 112250 - Psychology, University of Florida, Gainesville, FL 32611-2250. Application available online. URL of online application: http://gradschool.ufl.edu/students/application-and-admission.html. Students are admitted in the Fall, application deadline December 10. *Fee:* $30.

Miami, University of
Department of Educational & Psychological Studies/Area of Counseling Psychology
Education
P.O. Box 248065
Coral Gables, FL 33124-2040
Telephone: (305) 284-3001
Fax: (305) 284-3003
E-mail: blewis@miami.edu
Web: http://education.miami.edu/eps

Department Information:
1967. Director of Training, Counseling Psychology Program: Brian L. Lewis. Number of faculty: total—full-time 7, part-time 2; women—full-time 2, part-time 2; total—minority—full-time 3; women minority—full-time 2.

Programs and Degrees Offered:
Listed in the following order: Program area, degree type (T if terminal Master's), number awarded 7/08–6/09. Counseling Psychology PhD (Doctor of Philosophy) 5, Marriage and Family Therapy MA/MS (Master of Arts/Science) (T) 3, Mental Health Counseling MA/MS (Master of Arts/Science) (T) 6, Counseling and Research MA/MS (Master of Arts/Science) (T) 0.

APA Accreditation: Counseling PhD (Doctor of Philosophy).

Student Applications/Admissions:
Student Applications
Counseling Psychology PhD (Doctor of Philosophy)—Applications 2009–2010, 158. Total applicants accepted 2009–2010, 7. Number full-time enrolled (new admits only) 2009–2010, 7. Total enrolled 2009–2010 full-time, 26, part-time, 7. Openings 2010–2011, 6. The median number of years required for completion of a degree in 2008–2009 were 5. The number of students enrolled full- and part-time who were dismissed or voluntarily withdrew from this program area in 2008–2009 were 0. Marriage and Family Therapy MA/MS (Master of Arts/Science)—Applications 2009–2010, 25. Total applicants accepted 2009–2010, 16. Number full-time enrolled (new admits only) 2009–2010, 9. Number part-time enrolled (new admits only) 2009–2010, 1. Total enrolled 2009–2010 full-time, 11, part-time, 15. Openings 2010–2011, 15. The median number of years required for completion of a degree in 2008–2009 were 2. The number of students enrolled full- and part-time who were dismissed or voluntarily withdrew from this program area in 2008–2009 were 2. Mental Health Counseling MA/MS (Master of Arts/Science)—Applications 2009–2010, 40. Total applicants accepted 2009–2010, 19. Number full-time enrolled (new admits only) 2009–2010, 9. Number part-time enrolled (new admits only) 2009–2010, 2. Total enrolled 2009–2010 full-time, 19, part-time, 14. Openings 2010–2011, 15. The median number of years required for completion of a degree in 2008–2009 were 4. The number of students enrolled full- and part-time who were dismissed or voluntarily withdrew from this program area in 2008–2009 were 3. Counseling and Research MA/MS (Master of Arts/Science)—Applications 2009–2010, 11. Total applicants accepted 2009–2010, 7. Number full-time enrolled (new admits only) 2009–2010, 3. Number part-time enrolled (new admits only) 2009–2010, 1. Total enrolled 2009–2010 full-time, 3, part-time, 2. Openings 2010–2011, 10. The number of students enrolled full- and part-time who were dismissed or voluntarily withdrew from this program area in 2008–2009 were 3.

Scores: Entries appear in this order: required test or GPA, minimum score (if required), median score of students entering in 2009–2010. *Counseling Psychology PhD (Doctor of Philosophy):* GRE-V 480, 540, GRE-Q 480, 640, GRE-Analytical 4.0, 5.0, overall undergraduate GPA 2.64, 3.59, last 2 years GPA no minimum stated, psychology GPA no minimum stated, Masters GPA 3.48, 3.91; *Marriage and Family Therapy MA/MS (Master of Arts/Science):* GRE-V 400, 508, GRE-Q 400, 586, GRE-Analytical 4, overall undergraduate GPA no minimum stated; *Mental Health Counseling MA/MS (Master of Arts/Science):* GRE-V 400, 501, GRE-Q 400, 606, GRE-Analytical 4, overall undergraduate GPA no minimum stated; *Counseling and Research MA/MS (Master of Arts/Science):* GRE-V 400, 518, GRE-Q 400, 646, GRE-Analytical no minimum stated, overall undergraduate GPA no minimum stated.

Other Criteria: (importance of criteria rated low, medium, or high): GRE scores—high, research experience—high, work experience—medium, extracurricular activity—low, clinically related public service—medium, GPA—high, letters of recommendation—high, interview—high, statement of goals and objectives—high, undergraduate major in psychology—medium, specific undergraduate psychology courses taken—low.

Student Characteristics: The following represents characteristics of students in 2009–2010 in all graduate psychology programs in the department: Female—full-time 20, part-time 6; Male—full-time 6, part-time 1; African American/Black—full-time 3, part-time 1; Hispanic/Latino(a)—full-time 6, part-time 2; Asian/Pacific Islander—full-time 0, part-time 0; American Indian/Alaska Native—full-time 0, part-time 0; Caucasian/White—full-time 16, part-time 3; Multi-ethnic—full-time 1, part-time 1; students subject to the Americans With Disabilities Act—full-time 0, part-time 1; Unknown ethnicity—full-time 0, part-time 0; International students who hold an F-1 or J-1 Visa—full-time 0, part-time 0.

Financial Information/Assistance:
Tuition for Full-Time Study: *Master's:* State residents: $1,480 per credit hour; Nonstate residents: $1,480 per credit hour. *Doctoral:* State residents: $1,480 per credit hour; Nonstate residents: $1,480 per credit hour.

Financial Assistance:
First-Year Students: Teaching assistantships available for first year. Average amount paid per academic year: $18,900. Average number of hours worked per week: 20. Apply by January 2. Research assistantships available for first year. Average amount paid per academic year: $18,900. Average number of hours worked per week: 20. Apply by January 2. Fellowships and scholarships available for first year. Average amount paid per academic year: $25,000. Average number of hours worked per week: 0. Apply by January 2.

Advanced Students: Teaching assistantships available for advanced students. Average amount paid per academic year: $18,900. Average number of hours worked per week: 20. Apply by April 15. Research assistantships available for advanced students. Average amount paid per academic year: $18,900. Average number of hours worked per week: 20. Apply by April 15. Fellowships and scholarships available for advanced students. Average amount paid per academic year: $28,900. Average number of hours worked per week: 0. Apply by February 1.

Additional Information: Of all students currently enrolled full time, 100% benefited from one or more of the listed financial assistance programs.

Internships/Practica: Doctoral Degree (PhD Counseling Psychology): For those doctoral students for whom a professional internship was required in this program prior to graduation, (4) students applied for an internship in 2008–2009, with (4) students obtaining an internship. Of those students who obtained an internship, (4) were paid internships. Of those students who obtained an internship, (4) students placed in APA/CPA accredited internships, (0) students placed in internships not APA/CPA accredited, but listed with the Association of Psychology Postdoctoral and Internship Programs (APPIC), (0) students placed in internships conforming to guidelines of the Council of Directors of School Psychology Programs (CDSPP), (0) students placed in internships that were not APA/CPA accredited, APPIC or CDSPP listed. Students complete two academic years of practicum: the first year in our on-campus training clinic and the second year in an agency or hospital setting located in the community. Program faculty supervise the practicum through weekly one-to-one meetings and group supervision meetings. Therapeutic modalities in these placements include individual, couple, and group therapies. The off-campus placement is tailored to the student's career goals. Many students also complete an optional advanced practicum in their third year with placements tailored to their career goals. Placements include university counseling centers, psychiatric facilities, VA hospitals, behavioral medicine settings, correctional facilities, and schools, among others.

Housing and Day Care: On-campus housing is available. See the following Web site for more information: http://www.miami.edu/housing. On-campus day care facilities are available.

Employment of Department Graduates:
Master's Degree Graduates: Of those who graduated in the academic year 2008–2009, the following categories and numbers represent the postgraduate activities and employment of master's degree graduates: Enrolled in a postdoctoral residency/fellowship (n/a), employed in independent practice (n/a), total from the above (master's) (0).
Doctoral Degree Graduates: Of those who graduated in the academic year 2008–2009, the following categories and numbers represent the postgraduate activities and employment of doctoral degree graduates: Enrolled in a psychology doctoral program (n/a), enrolled in a postdoctoral residency/fellowship (2), employed in independent practice (0), employed in an academic position at a university (2), employed in other positions at a higher education institution (1), employed in a community mental health/counseling center (0), employed in a hospital/medical center (0), total from the above (doctoral) (5).

Additional Information:
Orientation, Objectives, and Emphasis of Department: The multicultural, health psychology, and family areas are foci in the doctoral program that is designed to educate counseling psychologists following the scientist–practitioner model to prepare individuals who will contribute to knowledge in psychology and who will be exemplary practitioners of psychological science. A sequence of research experiences is required as well as at least four semesters of supervised practicum and a full-year internship. In addition to coursework in the psychological foundations, requirements include the study of human development and personality (including career development), theories of therapy and the change process, therapeutic methodologies, and psychological assessment. We offer a 5 course sequence leading to a certificate in bilingual counseling (Spanish/English).

Special Facilities or Resources: The Institute for Individual and Family Counseling, an on-campus clinic, is used as the primary practicum site. It is equipped with facilities for audio, video, and live supervision. The multi-cultural clientele of the Institute and the other agencies and schools in the Miami area are available for practica and fieldwork. Computer laboratories are available to students in the department. A microcomputer laboratory is available to all students in the department. In addition, an assessment laboratory is an integral part of assessment training in the program.

Information for Students With Physical Disabilities: See the following Web site for more information: http://www.umarc.miami.edu.

Application Information:
Send to Coordinator of Graduate Studies, School of Education, (312 Merrick Building), University of Miami, P.O. Box 248065, Coral Gables, FL 33124. Application available online. URL of online application: https://www.applyweb.com/aw?mgred/. Students are admitted in the Fall, application deadline January 2; January 2 deadline is for Doctoral program applicants. August 1 deadline is for master's degree applicants. *Fee:* $50.

Miami, University of
Department of Psychology
College of Arts and Sciences
P.O. Box 248185
Coral Gables, FL 33124
Telephone: (305) 284-2814
Fax: (305) 284-8469
E-mail: *rwellens@miami.edu*
Web: *http://www.psy.miami.edu*

Department Information:
1937. Chairperson: A. Rodney Wellens. Number of faculty: total—full-time 39; women—full-time 22; total—minority—full-time 7; women minority—full-time 6.

Programs and Degrees Offered:
Listed in the following order: Program area, degree type (T if terminal Master's), number awarded 7/08–6/09. Developmental Psychology PhD (Doctor of Philosophy) 4, Behavioral Neuroscience PhD (Doctor of Philosophy) 0, Clinical Psychology PhD (Doctor of Philosophy) 12.

APA Accreditation: Clinical PhD (Doctor of Philosophy). Student Outcome Data Website: http://www.psy.miami.edu/graduate/clinical_training/.

Student Applications/Admissions:
Student Applications
Developmental Psychology PhD (Doctor of Philosophy)—Applications 2009–2010, 19. Total applicants accepted 2009–2010, 3. Number full-time enrolled (new admits only) 2009–2010, 3. Number part-time enrolled (new admits only) 2009–2010, 0. Openings 2010–2011, 4. The median number of years required for completion of a degree in 2008–2009 were 6. The number of students enrolled full- and part-time who were dismissed or voluntarily withdrew from this program area in 2008–2009 were 0. *Behavioral Neuroscience PhD (Doctor of Philosophy)*—Applications 2009–2010, 6. Total applicants accepted 2009–2010, 0. Number full-time enrolled (new admits only) 2009–2010, 0. Number part-time enrolled (new admits only) 2009–2010, 0. Openings 2010–2011, 1. The number of students enrolled full- and part-time who were dismissed or voluntarily withdrew from this program area in 2008–2009 were 0. *Clinical Psychology PhD (Doctor of Philosophy)*—Applications 2009–2010, 343. Total applicants accepted 2009–2010, 21. Number full-time enrolled (new admits only) 2009–2010, 13. Number part-time enrolled (new admits only) 2009–2010, 0. Openings 2010–2011, 14. The median number of years required for completion of a degree in 2008–2009 were 6. The number of students enrolled full- and part-time who were dismissed or voluntarily withdrew from this program area in 2008–2009 were 2.

Other Criteria: (importance of criteria rated low, medium, or high): GRE scores—high, research experience—high, work experience—medium, extracurricular activity—medium, clinically related public service—medium, GPA—high, letters of recommendation—high, interview—high, statement of goals and objectives—high, undergraduate major in psychology—medium, specific undergraduate psychology courses taken—medium. Clinically related public service not weighted for non-clinical programs. For additional information on admission requirements, go to http://www.psy.miami.edu/graduate/admissions.phtml.

Student Characteristics: The following represents characteristics of students in 2009–2010 in all graduate psychology programs in the department: Female—full-time 71, part-time 0; Male—full-time 17, part-time 0; African American/Black—full-time 4, part-time 0; Hispanic/Latino(a)—full-time 14, part-time 0; Asian/Pacific Islander—full-time 9, part-time 0; American Indian/Alaska Native—full-time 1, part-time 0; Caucasian/White—full-time 58, part-time 0; Multi-ethnic—full-time 2, part-time 0; students subject to the Americans With Disabilities Act—full-time 0, part-time 0; Unknown ethnicity—full-time 0, part-time 0; International students who hold an F-1 or J-1 Visa—full-time 3, part-time 0.

Financial Information/Assistance:
Tuition for Full-Time Study: Doctoral: State residents: per academic year $32,560, $1,480 per credit hour; Nonstate residents: per academic year $32,560, $1,480 per credit hour. Additional fees are assessed to students beyond the costs of tuition for the following: Student Activity Fee. See the following Web site for updates and changes in tuition costs: http://www.miami.edu/index.php/graduate_school/costs_and_financial_aid/tuition_and_fee_rates/.

Financial Assistance:
First-Year Students: Teaching assistantships available for first year. Average amount paid per academic year: $20,000. Average number of hours worked per week: 15. Apply by December 1. Research assistantships available for first year. Average amount paid per academic year: $22,660. Average number of hours worked per week: 20. Apply by December 1. Traineeships available for first year. Average amount paid per academic year: $22,660. Average number of hours worked per week: 15. Apply by December 1. Fellowships and scholarships available for first year. Average amount paid per academic year: $22,660. Average number of hours worked per week: 0. Apply by December 1.

Advanced Students: Teaching assistantships available for advanced students. Average amount paid per academic year: $20,000. Average number of hours worked per week: 15. Research assistantships available for advanced students. Average amount paid per academic year: $22,660. Average number of hours worked per week: 20. Traineeships available for advanced students. Average amount paid per academic year: $22,660. Average number of hours worked per week: 15. Fellowships and scholarships available for advanced students. Average amount paid per academic year: $22,660. Average number of hours worked per week: 0.

Additional Information: Of all students currently enrolled full time, 100% benefited from one or more of the listed financial assistance programs. Application and information available online at: http://www.psy.miami.edu/graduate/financing.phtml.

Internships/Practica: Doctoral Degree (PhD Clinical Psychology): For those doctoral students for whom a professional internship was required in this program prior to graduation, (8) students applied for an internship in 2008–2009, with (8) students obtaining an internship. Of those students who obtained an internship, (8) were paid internships. Of those students who obtained an internship, (8) students placed in APA/CPA accredited internships, (0) students placed in internships not APA/CPA accredited, but listed with the Association of Psychology Postdoctoral and Internship Programs (APPIC), (0) students placed in internships conforming to guidelines of the Council of Directors of School Psychology Programs (CDSPP), (0) students placed in internships that were not APA/CPA accredited, APPIC or CDSPP listed. Practicum sites are available for students enrolled in our APA-approved clinical program on the Coral Gables campus, Medical School campus and throughout Miami-Dade County. The department's Psychological Services Center represents a primary site for students developing skills in psychological assessment and empirically-based interventions. Additional specialty practica are located in the Department of Pediatrics at the Medical School, the Veterans Administration Medical Center and various clinics throughout Miami-Dade County.

Housing and Day Care: No on-campus housing is available. On-campus day care facilities are available. See the following Web site for more information: http://www.umcanterbury.com/.

Employment of Department Graduates:
Master's Degree Graduates: Of those who graduated in the academic year 2008–2009, the following categories and numbers represent the postgraduate activities and employment of master's degree graduates: Enrolled in a postdoctoral residency/fellowship (n/a), employed in independent practice (n/a), total from the above (master's) (0).

Doctoral Degree Graduates: Of those who graduated in the academic year 2008–2009, the following categories and numbers represent the postgraduate activities and employment of doctoral degree graduates: Enrolled in a psychology doctoral program (n/a), enrolled in a postdoctoral residency/fellowship (3), employed in an academic position at a university (5), employed in other positions at a higher education institution (1), employed in business or industry (2), employed in a community mental health/counseling center (2), employed in a hospital/medical center (1), other employment position (1), total from the above (doctoral) (15).

Additional Information:
Orientation, Objectives, and Emphasis of Department: The Department of Psychology's mission is to acquire, advance, and disseminate knowledge within the psychological and biobehavioral sciences. The Department seeks a balance among several academic endeavors including: basic scientific research, applied research, undergraduate teaching, graduate teaching, professional training, and community service. The department offers courses leading to the degree of Doctor of Philosophy. The Clinical Psychology Program, with tracks in adult, child, pediatric health, and health, uses a scientist–practitioner model of training with somewhat greater emphasis on the clinical science component. A mentor-model method of research training is employed. Prospective students in Psychology are admitted to graduate study within the Adult, Child, or Health Divisions. The Adult Division houses the adult clinical track that includes a focus on personality-social psychology in addition to adult psychopathology and treatment. The Child Division houses the clinical child and pediatric heath tracks of the clinical program and also the developmental program. The Health Division houses the health clinical track and the behavioral neuroscience program. All students teach at least one undergraduate course as part of their graduate training. Students are supported via training grants, fellowships, teaching assistantships and research assistantships.

Special Facilities or Resources: The Psychological Services Center serves as a community-based mental health training clinic for clinical students. The Behavioral Medicine Research Building provides excellent research facilities for students in behavioral neuroscience and health psychology. The Behavioral Medicine Research Center located at the UM Miller School of Medicine Clinical Research Building provides state-of-the-art facilities for research in psychoneuroimmunology. The Linda Ray Intervention Center and the Center for Autism and Related Disabilities provide excellent research opportunities for students in our child programs. Faculty research is supported by more than $15 million yearly in federal and state funding. The department resides in a new state-of-the-art research and teaching facility constructed for its use in 2003.

Information for Students With Physical Disabilities: See the following Web site for more information: http://www.miami.edu/index.php/academic_resource_center/disability_services.

Application Information:
Send to Graduate Admissions, Department of Psychology, P.O. Box 248185, Coral Gables, FL 33124. Application available online. URL of online application: http://www.psy.miami.edu/graduate/admissions.phtml. Students are admitted in the Fall, application deadline December 1. *Fee:* $65.

North Florida, University of
Department of Psychology
College of Arts and Sciences
1 UNF Drive
Jacksonville, FL 32224-2673
Telephone: (904) 620-1624
Fax: (904) 620-3814
E-mail: m.toglia@unf.edu
Web: http://www.unf.edu/coas/psychology/

Department Information:
1972. Chairperson: Michael P. Toglia. Number of faculty: total—full-time 21, part-time 18; women—full-time 8, part-time 9; total—minority—full-time 6; women minority—full-time 4; faculty subject to the Americans With Disabilities Act 2.

Programs and Degrees Offered:
Listed in the following order: Program area, degree type (T if terminal Master's), number awarded 7/08–6/09. General Psychology MA/MS (Master of Arts/Science) (T) 4, Counseling Psychology MA/MS (Master of Arts/Science) (T) 18.

Student Applications/Admissions:
Student Applications
General Psychology MA/MS (Master of Arts/Science)—Applications 2009–2010, 39. Total applicants accepted 2009–2010, 17. Number full-time enrolled (new admits only) 2009–2010, 16. Number part-time enrolled (new admits only) 2009–2010, 0. Openings 2010–2011, 12. The median number of years required for completion of a degree in 2008–2009 were 2. The number of students enrolled full- and part-time who were dismissed or voluntarily withdrew from this program area in 2008–2009 were 1. *Counseling Psychology MA/MS (Master of Arts/Science)*—Applications 2009–2010, 87. Total applicants accepted 2009–2010, 18. Number full-time enrolled (new admits only) 2009–2010, 18. Number part-time enrolled (new admits only) 2009–2010, 0. Total enrolled 2009–2010 full-time, 38, part-time, 3. Openings 2010–2011, 18. The median number of years required for completion of a degree in 2008–2009 were 2. The number of students enrolled full- and part-time who were dismissed or voluntarily withdrew from this program area in 2008–2009 were 1.
Other Criteria: (importance of criteria rated low, medium, or high): GRE scores—high, research experience—high, work experience—medium, extracurricular activity—low, clinically related public service—medium, GPA—high, letters of recommendation—medium, interview—high, statement of goals and objectives—high, volunteerism—low. Research experience weighted more heavily for MAGP. Interview and clinically-related public service for MACP. For additional information on admission requirements, go to http://www.unf.edu/coas/psychology.

Student Characteristics: The following represents characteristics of students in 2009–2010 in all graduate psychology programs in the department: Female—full-time 41, part-time 2; Male—full-time 20, part-time 0; African American/Black—full-time 4, part-time 0; Hispanic/Latino(a)—full-time 3, part-time 0; Asian/Pacific Islander—full-time 1, part-time 0; American Indian/Alaska Native—full-time 0, part-time 0; Caucasian/White—full-time 49,

part-time 3; Multi-ethnic—full-time 0, part-time 0; students subject to the Americans With Disabilities Act—full-time 1, part-time 0; Unknown ethnicity—full-time 0, part-time 0; International students who hold an F-1 or J-1 Visa—full-time 0, part-time 0.

Financial Information/Assistance:
Tuition for Full-Time Study: *Master's:* State residents: $206 per credit hour; Nonstate residents: $966 per credit hour.

Financial Assistance:
First-Year Students: Teaching assistantships available for first year. Research assistantships available for first year. Traineeships available for first year. Average amount paid per academic year: $5,000. Apply by September 30. Fellowships and scholarships available for first year. Average amount paid per academic year: $2,000. Apply by September 30.
Advanced Students: Teaching assistantships available for advanced students. Average amount paid per academic year: $1,800. Apply by June 1. Research assistantships available for advanced students. Traineeships available for advanced students. Average amount paid per academic year: $10,000. Apply by April 1. Fellowships and scholarships available for advanced students.
Additional Information: Of all students currently enrolled full time, 15% benefited from one or more of the listed financial assistance programs.

Internships/Practica: MACP students take part in a required 1,000 hour practicum/internship that provides application experience. The greater Jacksonville area allows for a great variety of internship placements with a diverse set of clientele and clinical/contextual issues.

Housing and Day Care: On-campus housing is available. On-campus day care facilities are available.

Employment of Department Graduates:
Master's Degree Graduates: Of those who graduated in the academic year 2008–2009, the following categories and numbers represent the postgraduate activities and employment of master's degree graduates: Enrolled in a psychology doctoral program (3), enrolled in another graduate/professional program (1), enrolled in a postdoctoral residency/fellowship (n/a), employed in independent practice (n/a), employed in an academic position at a university (1), employed in an academic position at a 2-year/4-year college (1), employed in other positions at a higher education institution (2), employed in a professional position in a school system (1), employed in business or industry (0), employed in government agency (1), employed in a community mental health/counseling center (10), do not know (3), total from the above (master's) (23).
Doctoral Degree Graduates: Of those who graduated in the academic year 2008–2009, the following categories and numbers represent the postgraduate activities and employment of doctoral degree graduates: Enrolled in a psychology doctoral program (n/a), total from the above (doctoral) (0).

Additional Information:
Orientation, Objectives, and Emphasis of Department: The Master of Arts in Counseling Psychology program is designed to prepare students for emerging professional roles as Florida licensed master's level practitioners. The program consists of 60 semester hours of course work, including a two-semester practicum in a community mental health agency. The program balances theory and practice and is designed to provide the prospective practitioner with a firm theoretical foundation for developing counseling strategies as well as the ability to apply particular goal-oriented intervention tactics. The Master of Arts in General Psychology program is a broad-based, research-oriented program intended to equip students with the critical skills and knowledge necessary for continued occupation and educational advancement in fields related to psychology. The program consists of 37 semester hours of course work designed around a core curriculum of statistics, research design, substantive areas of psychology, and a research-based thesis.

Special Facilities or Resources: The Department of Psychology moved into an aesthetically-pleasing facility in Fall 2006, located on the edge of scenic wetlands and hosting cutting-edge technology, including closed-circuit digital recording capabilities for research and counselor training purposes and student response technology for an interactional classroom environment. Several teaching laboratories are housed within the psychology department. The counseling lab and the psychometric lab each consist of a large observation room, three small rooms for individual counseling/testing and one large seminar/classroom. A computer applications lab has 24 individual computer work stations and an instructor's server, with a local area network and connections to the university mainframe, with hardware updated frequently. An animal lab allows for research with rodents. Finally, a department conference room serves as a comfortable gathering place for graduate training. In addition to these teaching laboratories, individual faculty research labs also are housed within the Department. Laboratory emphases include preschool education, cognitive development, child-father interactions, adolescent psychopathology, psychometrics, psychophysiology, human performance, human factors, social cognition, social interaction, and psychology and law.

Application Information:
Send to Gabriel J. Ybarra, PhD, Coordinator, Master of Arts in Counseling Psychology; Randall Russac, PhD, Coordinator, Master of Arts in General Psychology. Application available online. URL of online application: http://www.unf.edu/graduatestudies/prospective/applying. Students are admitted in the Fall, application deadline March 1. Application deadlines: MACP March 1; MAGP March 1. *Fee:* $20. $20 online; $30 paper.

Nova Southeastern University
Center for Psychological Studies
3301 College Avenue
Fort Lauderdale, FL 33314
Telephone: (954) 262-5700
Fax: (954) 262-3859
E-mail: *karol@nsu.nova.edu*
Web: *http://www.cps.nova.edu*

Department Information:
1967. Dean: Karen S. Grosby. Number of faculty: total—full-time 39, part-time 115; women—full-time 14, part-time 50; total—minority—full-time 7, part-time 11; women minority—full-time

4, part-time 5; faculty subject to the Americans With Disabilities Act 1.

Programs and Degrees Offered:
Listed in the following order: Program area, degree type (T if terminal Master's), number awarded 7/08–6/09. Mental Health Counseling MA/MS (Master of Arts/Science) (T) 136, Clinical Psychology PhD (Doctor of Philosophy) 14, Clinical Psychology PsyD (Doctor of Psychology) 66, Clinical Psychopharmacology MA/MS (Master of Arts/Science) (T) 8, School Counseling MA/MS (Master of Arts/Science) (T) 50, School Psychology Other 26, Counseling MA/MS (Master of Arts/Science) (T) 50.

APA Accreditation: Clinical PhD (Doctor of Philosophy). Clinical PsyD (Doctor of Psychology).

Student Applications/Admissions:
Student Applications
Mental Health Counseling MA/MS (Master of Arts/Science)—Applications 2009–2010, 472. Total applicants accepted 2009–2010, 291. Number full-time enrolled (new admits only) 2009–2010, 154. Total enrolled 2009–2010 full-time, 498. Openings 2010–2011, 175. The median number of years required for completion of a degree in 2008–2009 were 3. The number of students enrolled full- and part-time who were dismissed or voluntarily withdrew from this program area in 2008–2009 were 15. Clinical Psychology PhD (Doctor of Philosophy)—Applications 2009–2010, 142. Total applicants accepted 2009–2010, 25. Number full-time enrolled (new admits only) 2009–2010, 14. Number part-time enrolled (new admits only) 2009–2010, 0. Openings 2010–2011, 8. The median number of years required for completion of a degree in 2008–2009 were 6. The number of students enrolled full- and part-time who were dismissed or voluntarily withdrew from this program area in 2008–2009 were 2. Clinical Psychology PsyD (Doctor of Psychology)—Applications 2009–2010, 264. Total applicants accepted 2009–2010, 141. Number full-time enrolled (new admits only) 2009–2010, 86. Number part-time enrolled (new admits only) 2009–2010, 0. Openings 2010–2011, 82. The median number of years required for completion of a degree in 2008–2009 were 5. The number of students enrolled full- and part-time who were dismissed or voluntarily withdrew from this program area in 2008–2009 were 5. Clinical Psychopharmacology MA/MS (Master of Arts/Science)—Applications 2009–2010, 12. Total applicants accepted 2009–2010, 10. Number part-time enrolled (new admits only) 2009–2010, 0. Openings 2010–2011, 10. The median number of years required for completion of a degree in 2008–2009 were 2. The number of students enrolled full- and part-time who were dismissed or voluntarily withdrew from this program area in 2008–2009 were 0. School Counseling MA/MS (Master of Arts/Science)—Applications 2009–2010, 163. Total applicants accepted 2009–2010, 75. Number full-time enrolled (new admits only) 2009–2010, 25. Number part-time enrolled (new admits only) 2009–2010, 0. Total enrolled 2009–2010 full-time, 166. Openings 2010–2011, 75. The median number of years required for completion of a degree in 2008–2009 were 2. The number of students enrolled full- and part-time who were dismissed or voluntarily withdrew from this program area in 2008–2009 were 1. School Psychology Other—Applications 2009–2010, 102. Total applicants accepted 2009–2010, 37. Number full-time enrolled (new admits only) 2009–2010, 30. Number part-time enrolled (new admits only) 2009–2010, 0. Openings 2010–2011, 30. The median number of years required for completion of a degree in 2008–2009 were 4. The number of students enrolled full- and part-time who were dismissed or voluntarily withdrew from this program area in 2008–2009 were 7. Counseling MA/MS (Master of Arts/Science)—Applications 2009–2010, 245. Total applicants accepted 2009–2010, 161. Number full-time enrolled (new admits only) 2009–2010, 150. Number part-time enrolled (new admits only) 2009–2010, 0. Openings 2010–2011, 150. The median number of years required for completion of a degree in 2008–2009 were 2. The number of students enrolled full- and part-time who were dismissed or voluntarily withdrew from this program area in 2008–2009 were 25.

Scores: Entries appear in this order: required test or GPA, minimum score (if required), median score of students entering in 2009–2010. Clinical Psychology PhD (Doctor of Philosophy): GRE-V no minimum stated, 555, GRE-Q no minimum stated, 625, GRE-Analytical no minimum stated, 4.5, overall undergraduate GPA no minimum stated, 3.58; Clinical Psychology PsyD (Doctor of Psychology): GRE-V no minimum stated, 470, GRE-Q no minimum stated, 562, GRE-Analytical no minimum stated, 4.1, overall undergraduate GPA no minimum stated, 3.5.

Other Criteria: (importance of criteria rated low, medium, or high): GRE scores—high, work experience—medium, extracurricular activity—low, clinically related public service—medium, GPA—high, letters of recommendation—high, interview—high, statement of goals and objectives—high. The importance of research is high for the PhD program; Undergraduate major in psychology is highly recommended for the PhD and PsyD programs. For additional information on admission requirements, go to http://cps.nova.edu/.

Student Characteristics: The following represents characteristics of students in 2009–2010 in all graduate psychology programs in the department: Female—full-time 1487, part-time 0; Male—full-time 214, part-time 0; African American/Black—full-time 268, part-time 0; Hispanic/Latino(a)—full-time 343, part-time 0; Asian/Pacific Islander—full-time 40, part-time 0; American Indian/Alaska Native—full-time 2, part-time 0; Caucasian/White—full-time 985, part-time 0; Multi-ethnic—full-time 0, part-time 0; students subject to the Americans With Disabilities Act—full-time 8, part-time 0; Unknown ethnicity—full-time 63, part-time 0; International students who hold an F-1 or J-1 Visa—full-time 22, part-time 0.

Financial Information/Assistance:
Tuition for Full-Time Study: *Master's:* State residents: per academic year $570, $545 per credit hour; Nonstate residents: per academic year $570, $545 per credit hour. *Doctoral:* State residents: per academic year $875, $830 per credit hour; Nonstate residents: per academic year $875, $830 per credit hour. Tuition is subject to change. Additional fees are assessed to students beyond the costs of tuition for the following: online counseling program: one-time fee $750 for practicum. Tuition costs vary by program. See the following Web site for updates and changes in tuition costs: http://www.cps.nova.edu/admissions/tuition.html. Higher tuition cost for this program: Specialist in School Psychology - $625 per credit hour.

Financial Assistance:

First-Year Students: Research assistantships available for first year. Average amount paid per academic year: $5,600. Average number of hours worked per week: 15.

Advanced Students: Teaching assistantships available for advanced students. Average amount paid per academic year: $2,000. Average number of hours worked per week: 6. Research assistantships available for advanced students. Average amount paid per academic year: $5,600. Average number of hours worked per week: 15. Traineeships available for advanced students. Average amount paid per academic year: $5,800. Average number of hours worked per week: 15. Fellowships and scholarships available for advanced students.

Additional Information: Of all students currently enrolled full time, 12% benefited from one or more of the listed financial assistance programs.

Internships/Practica: Doctoral Degree (PhD Clinical Psychology): For those doctoral students for whom a professional internship was required in this program prior to graduation, (27) students applied for an internship in 2008–2009, with (25) students obtaining an internship. Of those students who obtained an internship, (25) were paid internships. Of those students who obtained an internship, (20) students placed in APA/CPA accredited internships, (5) students placed in internships not APA/CPA accredited, but listed with the Association of Psychology Postdoctoral and Internship Programs (APPIC), (0) students placed in internships conforming to guidelines of the Council of Directors of School Psychology Programs (CDSPP), (0) students placed in internships that were not APA/CPA accredited, APPIC or CDSPP listed. Doctoral Degree (PsyD Clinical Psychology): For those doctoral students for whom a professional internship was required in this program prior to graduation, (64) students applied for an internship in 2008–2009, with (60) students obtaining an internship. Of those students who obtained an internship, (59) were paid internships. Of those students who obtained an internship, (38) students placed in APA/CPA accredited internships, (22) students placed in internships not APA/CPA accredited, but listed with the Association of Psychology Postdoctoral and Internship Programs (APPIC), (0) students placed in internships conforming to guidelines of the Council of Directors of School Psychology Programs (CDSPP), (0) students placed in internships that were not APA/CPA accredited, APPIC or CDSPP listed. Accredited by the American Psychological Association, the Psychology Services Center Internship Program offers doctoral candidates in psychology the opportunity to develop professionally, to enhance their ability to use scholarly research for informed practice, to develop proficiency in psychological assessment and psychotherapeutic intervention, and to acquire basic competence in the provision of supervision and consultation. In addition, the Center for Psychological Studies sponsors the Consortium Internship Program (APPIC member) that provides internship experiences in hospital and other settings within the South Florida Community. In addition to the extensive practicum placements available in the community, practicum opportunities for more than 100 students are provided through various CPS faculty supervised applied-research clinical programs located within the NSU Psychology Services Center. Areas of research include ADHD, alcohol and substance abuse, anxiety treatment, child and adolescent traumatic stress, clinical biofeedback, interpersonal violence, neuropsychological assessment, older adults, school psychology assessment and testing, the seriously emotionally disturbed, and trauma resolution integration.

Housing and Day Care: No On-campus housing is available. On-campus day care facilities are available. See the following Web site for more information: http://www.nova.edu/msi.

Employment of Department Graduates:

Master's Degree Graduates: Of those who graduated in the academic year 2008–2009, the following categories and numbers represent the postgraduate activities and employment of master's degree graduates: Enrolled in a psychology doctoral program (1), enrolled in a postdoctoral residency/fellowship (n/a), employed in independent practice (n/a), employed in a professional position in a school system (76), employed in government agency (1), employed in a community mental health/counseling center (9), still seeking employment (11), not seeking employment (1), other employment position (86), do not know (85), total from the above (master's) (270).

Doctoral Degree Graduates: Of those who graduated in the academic year 2008–2009, the following categories and numbers represent the postgraduate activities and employment of doctoral degree graduates: Enrolled in a psychology doctoral program (n/a), enrolled in a postdoctoral residency/fellowship (51), employed in independent practice (3), employed in government agency (5), employed in a community mental health/counseling center (3), employed in a hospital/medical center (1), not seeking employment (2), do not know (8), total from the above (doctoral) (73).

Additional Information:

Orientation, Objectives, and Emphasis of Department: The Center for Psychological Studies (CPS) is committed to providing the highest quality educational experience to future psychologists and counseling professionals. These training experiences provide individuals with a sophisticated understanding of psychological research and the delivery of the highest-quality mental health care. Through the intimate interplay between CPS academic programs and the Nova Southeastern University (NSU) Psychology Services Center, learning becomes rooted in real problems, and research activities attempt to find answers to extant concerns. The center offers master's programs in counseling, mental health counseling, school guidance and counseling, clinical psychopharmacology, a specialist program (PsyS) in school psychology, and two APA-accredited doctoral programs in clinical psychology. The doctor of psychology (PsyD) program provides emphasis on training professionals to do service while the doctor of philosophy (PhD) program provides greater emphasis on applied research. In response to changes in health care delivery and the profession of psychology, the center developed concentrations at the doctoral level. Concentrations/tracks based on the existing PsyD and PhD curriculum are available in the areas of clinical neuropsychology, clinical health psychology, forensic psychology, psychodynamic psychology, psychology of long-term mental illness, multicultural/diversity, and child, adolescent and family.

Special Facilities or Resources: The Center for Psychological Studies is housed in the Maltz Psychology Building, a 65,000 square-foot facility that includes classrooms with state-of-the-art computer technology, a microcomputer lab with 30 multimedia computers connected to major databases and the Internet, study carrels, lounges and meeting rooms, and the Psychology Services Center where there are therapy rooms with audio and video monitoring capability, play-therapy rooms, and workstations for practicum students assigned to faculty specialty clinical programs. As a university-based professional school, CPS provides access to the NSU 325,000 square-foot Library, Research and Information Technology Center, as well as NSU's Schools of Law, Business and Systemic Studies, the colleges of its Health Professions Division (Medicine, Dentistry, Pharmacy, Allied Health, and Optometry), and its Family and School Center. Also included on NSU's 232-acre campus are five residence halls, recreation facilities, and the Miami Dolphins Training Center.

Information for Students With Physical Disabilities: See the following Web site for more information: http://www.nova.edu/disabilityservices/.

Application Information:
Send to Enrollment Processing Services, Attn: Center for Psychological Studies, P.O. Box 299000, Fort Lauderdale, FL 33329-9905. URL of online application: http://www.cps.nova.edu/. Students are admitted in the Fall, application deadline January 8. Applications for the doctoral programs are accepted only for the fall; the deadline is January 8. Application deadlines for master's and school psychology programs vary by site. *Fee:* $50.

South Florida, University of
Department of Psychological and Social Foundations
College of Education
EDU 105
Tampa, FL 33620-7750
Telephone: (813) 974-4614
Fax: (813) 974-5814
E-mail: *kbradley@tempest.coedu.usf.edu*
Web: *http://www.coedu.usf.edu/schoolpsych*

Department Information:
1970. Chairperson: Herbert Exum, PhD. Number of faculty: total—full-time 23; women—full-time 18; total—minority—full-time 6; women minority—full-time 4.

Programs and Degrees Offered:
Listed in the following order: Program area, degree type (T if terminal Master's), number awarded 7/08–6/09. School Psychology PhD (Doctor of Philosophy) 9, School Psychology EdS (School Psychology) 6.

APA Accreditation: School PhD (Doctor of Philosophy).

Student Applications/Admissions:
Student Applications
School Psychology PhD *(Doctor of Philosophy)*—Applications 2009–2010, 42. Total applicants accepted 2009–2010, 11. Number full-time enrolled (new admits only) 2009–2010, 5. Number part-time enrolled (new admits only) 2009–2010, 0. Openings 2010–2011, 6. The median number of years required for completion of a degree in 2008–2009 were 7. The number of students enrolled full- and part-time who were dismissed or voluntarily withdrew from this program area in 2008–2009 were 2. *School Psychology EdS (School Psychology)*—Applications 2009–2010, 39. Total applicants accepted 2009–2010, 3. Number full-time enrolled (new admits only) 2009–2010, 3. Number part-time enrolled (new admits only) 2009–2010, 0. Openings 2010–2011, 3. The median number of years required for completion of a degree in 2008–2009 were 5. The number of students enrolled full- and part-time who were dismissed or voluntarily withdrew from this program area in 2008–2009 were 0.

Other Criteria: (importance of criteria rated low, medium, or high): GRE scores—medium, research experience—high, work experience—medium, extracurricular activity—low, clinically related public service—medium, GPA—high, letters of recommendation—high, interview—high, statement of goals and objectives—high, writing sample—high, undergraduate major in psychology—medium, specific undergraduate psychology courses taken—high. For additional information on admission requirements, go to http://www.coedu.usf.edu/schoolpsych/Program/program_admissions.htm.

Student Characteristics: The following represents characteristics of students in 2009–2010 in all graduate psychology programs in the department: Female—full-time 39, part-time 0; Male—full-time 10, part-time 0; African American/Black—full-time 6, part-time 0; Hispanic/Latino(a)—full-time 6, part-time 0; Asian/Pacific Islander—full-time 2, part-time 0; American Indian/Alaska Native—full-time 1, part-time 0; Caucasian/White—full-time 33, part-time 0; Multi-ethnic—full-time 1, part-time 0; students subject to the Americans With Disabilities Act—full-time 0, part-time 0; Unknown ethnicity—full-time 0, part-time 0; International students who hold an F-1 or J-1 Visa—full-time 3, part-time 0.

Financial Information/Assistance:
Tuition for Full-Time Study: *Master's:* State residents: per academic year $10,923, $331 per credit hour; Nonstate residents: per academic year $26,994, $818 per credit hour. *Doctoral:* State residents: per academic year $10,923, $331 per credit hour; Nonstate residents: per academic year $26,994, $818 per credit hour. Tuition is subject to change. Additional fees are assessed to students beyond the costs of tuition for the following: Athletic fees, service fees, technology fees, and student union fees. See the following Web site for updates and changes in tuition costs: http://www.registrar.usf.edu.

Financial Assistance:
First-Year Students: Research assistantships available for first year. Average amount paid per academic year: $10,250. Average number of hours worked per week: 20. Apply by May 1. Fellowships and scholarships available for first year. Average amount paid per academic year: $10,250. Average number of hours worked per week: 0. Apply by February 15.

Advanced Students: Teaching assistantships available for advanced students. Average amount paid per academic year:

$10,250. Average number of hours worked per week: 20. Apply by May 1. Research assistantships available for advanced students. Average amount paid per academic year: $10,250. Average number of hours worked per week: 20. Apply by May 1. Fellowships and scholarships available for advanced students. Average amount paid per academic year: $10,000. Average number of hours worked per week: 0. Apply by February 15.

Additional Information: Of all students currently enrolled full time, 97% benefited from one or more of the listed financial assistance programs.

Internships/Practica: Doctoral Degree (PhD School Psychology): For those doctoral students for whom a professional internship was required in this program prior to graduation, (3) students applied for an internship in 2008–2009, with (3) students obtaining an internship. Of those students who obtained an internship, (3) were paid internships. Of those students who obtained an internship, (3) students placed in APA/CPA accredited internships, (0) students placed in internships not APA/CPA accredited, but listed with the Association of Psychology Postdoctoral and Internship Programs (APPIC), (0) students placed in internships conforming to guidelines of the Council of Directors of School Psychology Programs (CDSPP), (0) students placed in internships that were not APA/CPA accredited, APPIC or CDSPP listed. Our practica and internships integrate home, school, and community service programs for students at risk for educational failure and their families, including students with disabilities. We focus especially on the priorities of researching and promoting effective educational and mental health practices for all children, youth and their families. All doctoral students participate in practica during the first three years of the program. Practicum settings include schools (public, charter, alternative), hospital settings, research settings, university-affiliated agencies (e.g., USF Dept. of Pediatrics, Florida Mental Health Institute) and special programs (e.g., Early Intervention Program). Doctoral students participate in approximately 1,000 hours of practicum prior to internship. All doctoral students complete a 2,000-hour predoctoral internship in an APA-accredited/APPIC site or one that meets the APA/APPIC criteria.

Housing and Day Care: On-campus housing is available. See the following Web site for more information: http://www.housing.usf.edu/. On-campus day care facilities are available. See the following Web site for more information: http://www.usf.edu/about-usf/child-care.asp.

Employment of Department Graduates:
Master's Degree Graduates: Of those who graduated in the academic year 2008–2009, the following categories and numbers represent the postgraduate activities and employment of master's degree graduates: Enrolled in a psychology doctoral program (6), enrolled in another graduate/professional program (1), enrolled in a postdoctoral residency/fellowship (n/a), employed in independent practice (n/a), total from the above (master's) (7).
Doctoral Degree Graduates: Of those who graduated in the academic year 2008–2009, the following categories and numbers represent the postgraduate activities and employment of doctoral degree graduates: Enrolled in a psychology doctoral program (n/a), enrolled in another graduate/professional program (0), enrolled in a postdoctoral residency/fellowship (0), employed in independent practice (1), employed in an academic position at a university (0), employed in an academic position at a 2-year/4-year college (0), employed in other positions at a higher education institution (1), employed in a professional position in a school system (6), employed in business or industry (0), employed in government agency (0), employed in a community mental health/counseling center (0), employed in a hospital/medical center (1), still seeking employment (0), not seeking employment (0), other employment position (0), do not know (0), total from the above (doctoral) (9).

Additional Information:
Orientation, Objectives, and Emphasis of Department: Thorough admissions procedures result in the selection of outstanding students. This makes possible a faculty commitment to do everything possible to guide each student to a high level of professional competence. The curriculum is well organized and explicit such that students are always aware of program expectations and their progress in relation to these expectations. The student body is kept small, resulting in greater student-faculty contact than would otherwise be possible. Skills of practice are developed through non-threatening apprenticeship networks established with local school systems. This model encourages students to assist several professors and practicing school psychologists throughout their training. The notion here is to provide positive environments, containing rich feedback, in which competent psychological skills develop. We emphasize a scientist–practitioner model representing primarily a cognitive-behavioral orientation. Further, we support comprehensive school psychology, including consultation, prevention, intervention, and program evaluation.

Special Facilities or Resources: The University of South Florida is a comprehensive Research I (FL) and Doctoral/Research Universities-Extensive (Carnegie) university that has over 45,000 students on a 1,700 acre campus 10 miles northeast of downtown Tampa, a city of over 350,000 people. Amongst its faculty, the School Psychology program has one APA Fellow, two past presidents of the National Association of School Psychologists, the current president of the Council of Directors of School Psychology Programs, the 2009 recipient of the APA Division 16 Lightner Witmer Award, and faculty who have received over $35 million in federal and state grants over the past years. Students collaborate with professors and researchers in the program, the College of Education, Departments of Psychology and Psychiatry, the Florida Mental Health Institute, the Department of Pediatrics, Shriner's Hospital, Tampa General and St. Joseph's hospitals, the Florida Department of Education and other settings. The program is housed in a new College of Education physical plant that has the latest fiber optic based technology, clinical and research observation areas, and strong technology support. Strong links exist with community schools and agencies.

Information for Students With Physical Disabilities: See the following Web site for more information: http://www.usf.edu/sds.

Application Information:
Send to Linda Raffaele Mendez, Coordinator of Admissions, School Psychology Program, EDU 105, University of South Florida, Tampa, FL 33620-7750. Application available online. URL of online application: http://www.grad.usf.edu. Students are admitted in the Fall, application deadline January 1.

South Florida, University of
Department of Psychology
Arts and Sciences
4202 East Fowler Avenue, PCD 4118G
Tampa, FL 33620-7200
Telephone: (813) 974-2492
Fax: (813) 974-4617
E-mail: *lpierce@cas.usf.edu*
Web: *http://psychology.usf.edu/*

Department Information:
1964. Interim Chairperson: Michael Brannick. Number of faculty: total—full-time 39; women—full-time 14; total—minority—full-time 2; women minority—full-time 1.

Programs and Degrees Offered:
Listed in the following order: Program area, degree type (T if terminal Master's), number awarded 7/08–6/09. Clinical PhD (Doctor of Philosophy) 8, Cognition, Neuroscience, and Social Psychology PhD (Doctor of Philosophy) 6, Industrial/Organizational PhD (Doctor of Philosophy) 10.

APA Accreditation: Clinical PhD (Doctor of Philosophy). Student Outcome Data Website: http://psychology.usf.edu/grad/studentstat/.

Student Applications/Admissions:
Student Applications
Clinical PhD (Doctor of Philosophy)—Applications 2009–2010, 240. Total applicants accepted 2009–2010, 17. Number full-time enrolled (new admits only) 2009–2010, 11. Number part-time enrolled (new admits only) 2009–2010, 0. Openings 2010–2011, 8. The median number of years required for completion of a degree in 2008–2009 were 7. The number of students enrolled full- and part-time who were dismissed or voluntarily withdrew from this program area in 2008–2009 were 0. Cognition, Neuroscience, and Social Psychology PhD (Doctor of Philosophy)—Applications 2009–2010, 75. Total applicants accepted 2009–2010, 9. Number full-time enrolled (new admits only) 2009–2010, 6. Number part-time enrolled (new admits only) 2009–2010, 0. Openings 2010–2011, 7. The median number of years required for completion of a degree in 2008–2009 were 6. The number of students enrolled full- and part-time who were dismissed or voluntarily withdrew from this program area in 2008–2009 were 0. Industrial/Organizational PhD (Doctor of Philosophy)—Applications 2009–2010, 119. Total applicants accepted 2009–2010, 17. Number full-time enrolled (new admits only) 2009–2010, 7. Number part-time enrolled (new admits only) 2009–2010, 0. Openings 2010–2011, 8. The median number of years required for completion of a degree in 2008–2009 were 6. The number of students enrolled full- and part-time who were dismissed or voluntarily withdrew from this program area in 2008–2009 were 0.

Scores: Entries appear in this order: required test or GPA, minimum score (if required), median score of students entering in 2009–2010. Clinical PhD (Doctor of Philosophy): GRE-V 500, 607, GRE-Q 600, 691, GRE-Analytical no minimum stated, last 2 years GPA 3.40, 3.79; Cognition, Neuroscience, and Social Psychology PhD (Doctor of Philosophy): GRE-V 500, 558, GRE-Q 600, 715, GRE-Analytical no minimum stated, last 2 years GPA 3.4, 3.73; Industrial/Organizational PhD (Doctor of Philosophy): GRE-V 500, 581, GRE-Q 600, 750, GRE-Analytical no minimum stated, last 2 years GPA 3.4, 3.76.

Other Criteria: (importance of criteria rated low, medium, or high): GRE scores—high, research experience—high, work experience—low, clinically related public service—low, GPA—high, letters of recommendation—high, interview—medium, statement of goals and objectives—high. For additional information on admission requirements, go to http://psychology.usf.edu/grad/admission/adminreq/.

Student Characteristics: The following represents characteristics of students in 2009–2010 in all graduate psychology programs in the department: Female—full-time 69, part-time 0; Male—full-time 52, part-time 0; African American/Black—full-time 4, part-time 0; Hispanic/Latino(a)—full-time 6, part-time 0; Asian/Pacific Islander—full-time 11, part-time 0; American Indian/Alaska Native—full-time 0, part-time 0; Caucasian/White—full-time 100, part-time 0; Multi-ethnic—full-time 0, part-time 0; students subject to the Americans With Disabilities Act—full-time 1, part-time 0; Unknown ethnicity—full-time 0, part-time 0; International students who hold an F-1 or J-1 Visa—full-time 14, part-time 0.

Financial Information/Assistance:
Tuition for Full-Time Study: Master's: State residents: per academic year $7,962, $331 per credit hour; Nonstate residents: per academic year $19,647, $818 per credit hour. Doctoral: State residents: per academic year $5,972, $331 per credit hour; Nonstate residents: per academic year $14,735, $818 per credit hour. Tuition is subject to change. Additional fees are assessed to students beyond the costs of tuition for the following: $37 flat fees, $4.42 per credit hour technology fee, $35 one-time orientation fee. See the following Web site for updates and changes in tuition costs: http://usfweb.usf.edu/controller/cashaccounting/tuition.

Financial Assistance:
First-Year Students: Teaching assistantships available for first year. Average amount paid per academic year: $13,500. Average number of hours worked per week: 20. Research assistantships available for first year. Average amount paid per academic year: $13,500. Average number of hours worked per week: 20. Fellowships and scholarships available for first year. Average amount paid per academic year: $20,600. Average number of hours worked per week: 10.

Advanced Students: Teaching assistantships available for advanced students. Average amount paid per academic year: $13,500. Average number of hours worked per week: 20. Research assistantships available for advanced students. Average amount paid per academic year: $13,500. Average number of hours worked per week: 20. Fellowships and scholarships available for advanced students. Average amount paid per academic year: $20,600. Average number of hours worked per week: 10.

Additional Information: Of all students currently enrolled full time, 83% benefited from one or more of the listed financial assistance programs. Application and information available online at: http://usfweb2.usf.edu/finaid/.

Internships/Practica: Doctoral Degree (PhD Clinical): For those doctoral students for whom a professional internship was required in this program prior to graduation, (6) students applied for an internship in 2008–2009, with (6) students obtaining an internship. Of those students who obtained an internship, (6) were paid internships. Of those students who obtained an internship, (6) students placed in APA/CPA accredited internships, (0) students placed in internships not APA/CPA accredited, but listed with the Association of Psychology Postdoctoral and Internship Programs (APPIC), (0) students placed in internships conforming to guidelines of the Council of Directors of School Psychology Programs (CDSPP), (0) students placed in internships that were not APA/CPA accredited, APPIC or CDSPP listed. The Clinical Program operates its own Psychology Clinic within the Psychology Department, providing opportunities for practical training in clinical assessment and clinical psychological interventions. Students are active in the Psychology Clinic throughout their training. Clinical core faculty provide most of the supervision of Clinic cases. The Clinical Psychology Program is fortunate to have a unique cluster of campus and community training facilities available for student placement. For example, we have student placements at or near such campus facilities as the USF Florida Mental Health Research Institute, the USF Counseling Center for Human Development, the Moffitt Cancer Center and Research Institute and the Tampa Veterans Administration Hospital as well as carefully selected community agencies. Students in the Industrial/Organizational Program are required to complete a predoctoral internship. Placements are made in numerous governmental, corporate and consulting firms both locally and nationally. Recent placements have included the cities of Tampa and Clearwater, GTE, Tampa Electric Company, Personnel Decisions Research Institute, Personnel Decisions, Inc., Florida Power and USF&G.

Housing and Day Care: On-campus housing is available. See the following Web site for more information: http://www.housing.usf.edu/. On-campus day care facilities are available. See the following Web site for more information: http://www.usf.edu/About-USF/child-care.asp.

Employment of Department Graduates:
Master's Degree Graduates: Of those who graduated in the academic year 2008–2009, the following categories and numbers represent the postgraduate activities and employment of master's degree graduates: Enrolled in a postdoctoral residency/fellowship (n/a), employed in independent practice (n/a), total from the above (master's) (0).
Doctoral Degree Graduates: Of those who graduated in the academic year 2008–2009, the following categories and numbers represent the postgraduate activities and employment of doctoral degree graduates: Enrolled in a psychology doctoral program (n/a), enrolled in another graduate/professional program (0), enrolled in a postdoctoral residency/fellowship (1), employed in independent practice (0), employed in an academic position at a university (6), employed in an academic position at a 2-year/4-year college (0), employed in other positions at a higher education institution (0), employed in a professional position in a school system (0), employed in business or industry (6), employed in government agency (1), employed in a community mental health/counseling center (2), employed in a hospital/medical center (4), still seeking employment (0), not seeking employment (0), other employment position (0), do not know (0), total from the above (doctoral) (20).

Additional Information:
Orientation, Objectives, and Emphasis of Department: The department attempts to educate graduate students to a high level of proficiency in research and in practice. The department expects its doctoral students to be of such quality as to take their place at major institutions of learning if they choose academic careers and to assume roles of responsibility and importance if they choose professional careers. The doctoral program in clinical psychology provides broad-based professional and research training to prepare students for careers in a variety of applied, research, and teaching settings. The doctoral program in cognition, neuroscience, and social psychology prepares students for research careers in both applied and academic environments. This program also offers an interdisciplinary degree in Speech, Language, and Hearing Science in conjunction with the Department of Communication Sciences and Disorders. The doctoral program in industrial/organizational psychology provides professional and research training to prepare students for careers in industrial, governmental, academic, and related organizational settings.

Special Facilities or Resources: State-of-the-art facilities and equipment houses the Psychology Department. There is ample research space for faculty, graduate, and advanced undergraduate students, including a large vivarium. An open-use lab has been equipped with computer terminals that access the mainframe computer on campus. The University Computer Center is available. The Psychological Services Center is operated as the department's facility for clinical practicum work. A state-of-the-art video system permits supervisory capabilities for clinical practica.

Information for Students With Physical Disabilities: See the following Web site for more information: http://www.sds.usf.edu/.

Application Information:
Send to Department of Psychology, University of South Florida, 4202 East Fowler Avenue, PCD4118G, Attn: Graduate Admissions Coordinator, Tampa, FL 33620-7200. Application available online. URL of online application: http://www.grad.usf.edu/graduate-admissions.asp. Students are admitted in the Fall, application deadline December 1. Clinical deadline is December 1. Industrial/Organizational deadline is January 2. CNS deadline for International applicants is January 2 and for U.S. Residents is January 15. *Fee:* $30. Waiver available for McNair Scholars Program, FAMU Feeder Program, RISE Program, USTAR-MARC Program. Application Fee Waiver Verification Request Form submission required prior to application submission.

West Florida, The University of
Department of Psychology
College of Arts and Sciences
11000 University Parkway
Pensacola, FL 32514-5751
Telephone: (850) 474-2363
Fax: (850) 857-6060
E-mail: *psych@uwf.edu*
Web: *http://www.uwf.edu/psychology*

Department Information:
1967. Chairperson: Laura L. Koppes. Number of faculty: total—full-time 14, part-time 1; women—full-time 5.

Programs and Degrees Offered:
Listed in the following order: Program area, degree type (T if terminal Master's), number awarded 7/08–6/09. General Psychol-

ogy MA/MS (Master of Arts/Science) (T) 7, Industrial/Organizational Psychology MA/MS (Master of Arts/Science) (T) 13, Counseling Psychology MA/MS (Master of Arts/Science) (T) 10.

Student Applications/Admissions:
Student Applications
General Psychology MA/MS (Master of Arts/Science)—Applications 2009–2010, 22. Total applicants accepted 2009–2010, 10. Number full-time enrolled (new admits only) 2009–2010, 10. Openings 2010–2011, 15. The median number of years required for completion of a degree in 2008–2009 were 2. The number of students enrolled full- and part-time who were dismissed or voluntarily withdrew from this program area in 2008–2009 were 0. Industrial/Organizational Psychology MA/MS (Master of Arts/Science)—Applications 2009–2010, 40. Total applicants accepted 2009–2010, 13. Number full-time enrolled (new admits only) 2009–2010, 13. Openings 2010–2011, 18. The median number of years required for completion of a degree in 2008–2009 were 2. The number of students enrolled full- and part-time who were dismissed or voluntarily withdrew from this program area in 2008–2009 were 1. Counseling Psychology MA/MS (Master of Arts/Science)—Applications 2009–2010, 45. Total applicants accepted 2009–2010, 14. Number full-time enrolled (new admits only) 2009–2010, 14. Openings 2010–2011, 18. The median number of years required for completion of a degree in 2008–2009 were 3. The number of students enrolled full- and part-time who were dismissed or voluntarily withdrew from this program area in 2008–2009 were 2.
Scores: Entries appear in this order: required test or GPA, minimum score (if required), median score of students entering in 2009–2010. General Psychology MA/MS (Master of Arts/Science): GRE-V no minimum stated, GRE-Q no minimum stated, last 2 years GPA 3.0; Industrial/Organizational Psychology MA/MS (Master of Arts/Science): GRE-V no minimum stated, GRE-Q no minimum stated, last 2 years GPA 3.0; Counseling Psychology MA/MS (Master of Arts/Science): GRE-V no minimum stated, GRE-Q no minimum stated, last 2 years GPA 3.0.
Other Criteria: (importance of criteria rated low, medium, or high): GRE scores—high, research experience—medium, work experience—medium, extracurricular activity—medium, clinically related public service—medium, GPA—high, letters of recommendation—high, interview—high, statement of goals and objectives—high, undergraduate major in psychology—high, specific undergraduate psychology courses taken—high. Counseling applicants are required to complete an interview. For additional information on admission requirements, go to http://uwf.edu/psychology/grad-admissions/.

Student Characteristics: The following represents characteristics of students in 2009–2010 in all graduate psychology programs in the department: Female—full-time 69, part-time 12; Male—full-time 18, part-time 7; African American/Black—full-time 6, part-time 3; Hispanic/Latino(a)—full-time 2, part-time 1; Asian/Pacific Islander—full-time 7, part-time 0; American Indian/Alaska Native—full-time 3, part-time 0; Caucasian/White—full-time 68, part-time 14; Multi-ethnic—full-time 1, part-time 1; students subject to the Americans With Disabilities Act—full-time 0, part-time 0; Unknown ethnicity—full-time 0, part-time 0; International students who hold an F-1 or J-1 Visa—full-time 0, part-time 0.

Financial Information/Assistance:
Tuition for Full-Time Study: *Master's:* State residents: $252 per credit hour; Nonstate residents: $912 per credit hour. Tuition is subject to change. See the following Web site for updates and changes in tuition costs: http://uwf.edu/enrserv/tuition.cfm.

Financial Assistance:
First-Year Students: Teaching assistantships available for first year. Average amount paid per academic year: $3,280. Average number of hours worked per week: 10. Apply by April 15. Research assistantships available for first year. Average amount paid per academic year: $3,760. Average number of hours worked per week: 10. Apply by April 15. Fellowships and scholarships available for first year. Average amount paid per academic year: $2,000. Apply by April 15.
Advanced Students: Teaching assistantships available for advanced students. Average amount paid per academic year: $3,760. Average number of hours worked per week: 10. Apply by April 15. Fellowships and scholarships available for advanced students. Average amount paid per academic year: $750. Apply by April 15.
Additional Information: Of all students currently enrolled full time, 65% benefited from one or more of the listed financial assistance programs. Application and information available online at: http://uwf.edu/finaid/.

Internships/Practica: Master's Degree (MA/MS General Psychology): An internship experience, such as a final research project or "capstone" experience is required of graduates. Master's Degree (MA/MS Industrial/Organizational Psychology): An internship experience, such as a final research project or "capstone" experience is required of graduates. Master's Degree (MA/MS Counseling Psychology): An internship experience, such as a final research project or "capstone" experience is required of graduates. Master's students may elect either thesis or 600-hour internship (850-hour for mental health counseling licensure option). Faculty assist in finding suitable placements in field settings under qualified supervision. The student also prepares a portfolio demonstrating mastery of several specific competencies and includes an integrative paper reflecting on professional development. Practica (required for counseling students, optional for other students) are completed earlier in the program and involve more limited applied experience and closer supervision by faculty. Internship placements for counseling students include a variety of local mental health agencies providing inpatient, outpatient and community outreach services. Internship placements for industrial/organizational students include a variety of business and healthcare settings.

Housing and Day Care: On-campus housing is available. See the following Web site for more information: http://uwf.edu/housing/. On-campus day care facilities are available. See the following Web site for more information: http://uwf.edu/childdev.

Employment of Department Graduates:
Master's Degree Graduates: Of those who graduated in the academic year 2008–2009, the following categories and numbers represent the postgraduate activities and employment of master's degree graduates: Enrolled in a psychology doctoral program (4), enrolled in a postdoctoral residency/fellowship (n/a), employed in independent practice (n/a), employed in business or industry (9), employed in government agency (1), employed in a commu-

nity mental health/counseling center (7), total from the above (master's) (21).

Doctoral Degree Graduates: Of those who graduated in the academic year 2008–2009, the following categories and numbers represent the postgraduate activities and employment of doctoral degree graduates: Enrolled in a psychology doctoral program (n/a), total from the above (doctoral) (0).

Additional Information:
Orientation, Objectives, and Emphasis of Department: The department is a member of the Council of Applied Master's Programs in Psychology and is committed to the philosophy of training with a foundation in general psychology (individual, social, biological, and learned bases of behavior) as the basis for training in application of psychology. Applied students receive significant supervised field experience. The departmental mission is preparation of master's level practitioners and preparation of students for doctoral work as well. The programs in Counseling Psychology and Industrial/Organizational Psychology are accredited by the Master's in Psychology Accreditation Council (MPAC). The department also offers a certificate in Health Psychology and Cognitive Psychology. The Counseling Psychology program offers a 60-hour option with coursework comparable to requirements for licensure as a Mental Health Counselor in Florida.

Special Facilities or Resources: The department is housed in a modern, 22,000 sq. ft. building with excellent research facilities, including a Neurocognition lab with a 128 channel Neuroscan ESI System. The University of West Florida Center for Applied Psychology (CAP) is a consulting group within the Department of Psychology aimed at optimizing human performance across the lifespan in educational, health, and workplace contexts. Other University resources include Institute for Business and Economic Research and the Institute for Human and Machine Cognition. We have links with CMHCs and local health/mental health professionals and organizations. Community resources include three major hospitals and a large Naval training facility. The department hosts student chapters of Psi Chi, Society for Human Resource Management (SHRM), and Student Psychological Association.

Information for Students With Physical Disabilities: See the following Web site for more information: http://uwf.edu/sdrc/.

Application Information:
Send to Department of Psychology-Graduate Admissions, University of West Florida, 11000 University Parkway, Pensacola FL 32514-5751. Application available online. URL of online application: http://www.uwf.edu/admissions/gap.cfm. Students are admitted in the Fall, application deadline February 1. *Fee:* $30.

GEORGIA

Argosy University/Atlanta
Clinical Psychology
980 Hammond Drive, Building 2, Suite 100
Atlanta, GA 30328
Telephone: (888) 671-4777
Fax: (770) 671-0476
E-mail: tcbrown@argosy.edu
Web: http://www.argosy.edu

Department Information:
1990. Chairperson: Timothy C. Brown, PhD. Number of faculty: total—full-time 14, part-time 2; women—full-time 9, part-time 1; total—minority—full-time 2; women minority—full-time 2.

Programs and Degrees Offered:
Listed in the following order: Program area, degree type (T if terminal Master's), number awarded 7/08–6/09. Clinical Psychology MA/MS (Master of Arts/Science) (T) 9, Clinical Psychology PsyD (Doctor of Psychology) 42.

APA Accreditation: Clinical PsyD (Doctor of Psychology). Student Outcome Data Website: http://www.argosy.edu/colleges/ProgramDetail.aspx?ID=577&section=outcomes.

Student Applications/Admissions:
Student Applications
Clinical Psychology MA/MS (Master of Arts/Science)—Applications 2009–2010, 32. Total applicants accepted 2009–2010, 23. Number full-time enrolled (new admits only) 2009–2010, 17. Number part-time enrolled (new admits only) 2009–2010, 0. Openings 2010–2011, 15. The median number of years required for completion of a degree in 2008–2009 were 2. The number of students enrolled full- and part-time who were dismissed or voluntarily withdrew from this program area in 2008–2009 were 1. Clinical Psychology PsyD (Doctor of Psychology)—Applications 2009–2010, 129. Total applicants accepted 2009–2010, 48. Number full-time enrolled (new admits only) 2009–2010, 31. Number part-time enrolled (new admits only) 2009–2010, 0. Openings 2010–2011, 25. The median number of years required for completion of a degree in 2008–2009 were 6. The number of students enrolled full- and part-time who were dismissed or voluntarily withdrew from this program area in 2008–2009 were 5.
Scores: Entries appear in this order: required test or GPA, minimum score (if required), median score of students entering in 2009–2010. Clinical Psychology PsyD (Doctor of Psychology): overall undergraduate GPA 3.25, 3.47.
Other Criteria: (importance of criteria rated low, medium, or high): GRE scores—low, research experience—low, work experience—high, extracurricular activity—low, clinically related public service—high, GPA—high, letters of recommendation—high, interview—high, statement of goals and objectives—high, undergraduate major in psychology—medium, specific undergraduate psychology courses taken—medium. For additional information on admission requirements, go to http://www.argosy.edu.

Student Characteristics: The following represents characteristics of students in 2009–2010 in all graduate psychology programs in the department: Female—full-time 189, part-time 0; Male—full-time 47, part-time 0; African American/Black—full-time 49, part-time 0; Hispanic/Latino(a)—full-time 7, part-time 0; Asian/Pacific Islander—full-time 6, part-time 0; American Indian/Alaska Native—full-time 0, part-time 0; Caucasian/White—full-time 168, part-time 0; Multi-ethnic—full-time 6, part-time 0; students subject to the Americans With Disabilities Act—full-time 12, part-time 0; Unknown ethnicity—full-time 0, part-time 0; International students who hold an F-1 or J-1 Visa—full-time 2, part-time 0.

Financial Information/Assistance:
Tuition for Full-Time Study: *Master's:* State residents: $998 per credit hour; Nonstate residents: $998 per credit hour. *Doctoral:* State residents: $998 per credit hour; Nonstate residents: $998 per credit hour. Tuition is subject to change. Additional fees are assessed to students beyond the costs of tuition for the following: Technology fee $10 per credit. See the following Web site for updates and changes in tuition costs: http://www.argosy.edu.

Financial Assistance:
First-Year Students: Research assistantships available for first year. Average amount paid per academic year: $1,000. Average number of hours worked per week: 5. Fellowships and scholarships available for first year. Average amount paid per academic year: $3,000. Average number of hours worked per week: 0. Apply by June 30.
Advanced Students: Teaching assistantships available for advanced students. Average amount paid per academic year: $1,500. Average number of hours worked per week: 7. Apply by September 1. Research assistantships available for advanced students. Average amount paid per academic year: $1,000. Average number of hours worked per week: 5. Fellowships and scholarships available for advanced students. Average amount paid per academic year: $3,000. Average number of hours worked per week: 0. Apply by June 30.
Additional Information: Of all students currently enrolled full time, 30% benefited from one or more of the listed financial assistance programs. Application and information available online at: http://www.argosy.edu.

Internships/Practica: Doctoral Degree (PsyD Clinical Psychology): For those doctoral students for whom a professional internship was required in this program prior to graduation, (50) students applied for an internship in 2008–2009, with (48) students obtaining an internship. Of those students who obtained an internship, (48) were paid internships. Of those students who obtained an internship, (40) students placed in APA/CPA accredited internships, (8) students placed in internships not APA/CPA accredited, but listed with the Association of Psychology Postdoctoral and Internship Programs (APPIC), (0) students placed in internships conforming to guidelines of the Council of Directors of School Psychology Programs (CDSPP), (0) students placed in internships that were not APA/CPA accredited, APPIC or CDSPP listed. Master's Degree (MA/MS Clinical Psychology): An internship experience, such as a final research project or "capstone" experience is required of graduates. Practica and internships involve supervised clinical field training in which students work with clinical populations in health delivery settings. Practica offer opportunities to apply classroom knowledge, increase assessment and therapeutic skills, and develop professional and personal attitudes important to the identity of a professional psychologist. While all doctoral students complete a minimum of two years of practicum training, many elect to complete an additional one-year advanced practicum to gain further experience before internship. Students are placed at a diverse set of training sites formally affiliated with the MA and PsyD programs. The specific content and training vary according to the setting and expertise of supervisors. Training sites include state mental health facilities, outpatient clinics, private psychiatric hospitals, psychiatric units in community hospitals, university counseling centers, and private practice settings, as well as treatment facilities for developmentally disabled, behavior disordered and/or emotionally disturbed adults and children. In addition, a variety of specialized placements are available in facilities such as children's/pediatric hospitals, treatment centers for eating disorders, and neuropsychiatric rehabilitation programs.

Housing and Day Care: No on-campus housing is available. No on-campus day care facilities are available.

Employment of Department Graduates:
Master's Degree Graduates: Of those who graduated in the academic year 2008–2009, the following categories and numbers represent the postgraduate activities and employment of master's degree graduates: Enrolled in a postdoctoral residency/fellowship (n/a), employed in independent practice (n/a), do not know (9), total from the above (master's) (9).
Doctoral Degree Graduates: Of those who graduated in the academic year 2008–2009, the following categories and numbers represent the postgraduate activities and employment of doctoral degree graduates: Enrolled in a psychology doctoral program (n/a), do not know (42), total from the above (doctoral) (42).

Additional Information:
Orientation, Objectives, and Emphasis of Department: The primary purpose of the Clinical Psychology doctoral program is to educate and train students in the major aspects of clinical practice. The curriculum integrates theory, training, research, and practice, preparing graduates to work in a broad range of roles and to work with a wide range of populations in need of psychological services. Students who graduate from the doctoral program earn a Doctor of Psychology degree, indicating that the recipient has completed academic and training experiences essential to pursuing professional endeavors in the field of clinical psychology.

Application Information:
Send to Office of Admissions, Argosy University, 980 Hammond Drive, Building 2, Suite 100, Atlanta, GA 30328. Application available online. URL of online application: http://www.argosy.edu. Students are admitted in the Fall, application deadline January 15. *Fee:* $50.

Augusta State University
Department of Psychology
2500 Walton Way
Augusta, GA 30904-2200
Telephone: (706) 737-1694
Fax: (706) 737-1538
E-mail: *kscott4@aug.edu*
Web: *http://www.aug.edu/psychology/*

Department Information:
1963. Chairperson: Dr. Sabina Widner. Number of faculty: total—full-time 11, part-time 13; women—full-time 6, part-time 8.

Programs and Degrees Offered:
Listed in the following order: Program area, degree type (T if terminal Master's), number awarded 7/08–6/09. Clinical/Counseling Psychology MA/MS (Master of Arts/Science) (T) 6, Experimental Psychology MA/MS (Master of Arts/Science) (T) 2.

Student Applications/Admissions:
Student Applications
Counseling Psychology MA/MS (Master of Arts/Science)—Applications 2009–2010, 87. Total applicants accepted 2009–2010, 15. Number full-time enrolled (new admits only) 2009–2010, 15. Number part-time enrolled (new admits only) 2009–2010, 0. Openings 2010–2011, 20. The median number of years required for completion of a degree in 2008–2009 were 2. The number of students enrolled full- and part-time who were dismissed or voluntarily withdrew from this program area in 2008–2009 were 1. *Experimental Psychology MA/MS (Master of Arts/Science)*—Applications 2009–2010, 7. Total applicants accepted 2009–2010, 5. Number full-time enrolled (new admits only) 2009–2010, 5. Number part-time enrolled (new admits only) 2009–2010, 0. Openings 2010–2011, 8. The median number of years required for completion of a degree in 2008–2009 were 2. The number of students enrolled full- and part-time who were dismissed or voluntarily withdrew from this program area in 2008–2009 were 0.
Scores: Entries appear in this order: required test or GPA, minimum score (if required), median score of students entering in 2009–2010. *Counseling Psychology MA/MS (Master of Arts/Science)*: GRE-V 400, GRE-Q 400, GRE-Analytical 3.5, overall undergraduate GPA 2.5; *Experimental Psychology MA/MS (Master of Arts/Science)*: GRE-V 400, GRE-Q 400, GRE-Analytical 3.5, overall undergraduate GPA 2.5.
Other Criteria: (importance of criteria rated low, medium, or high): GRE scores—high, research experience—medium, work experience—medium, extracurricular activity—low, clinically related public service—low, GPA—high, letters of recommendation—high, statement of goals and objectives—medium, undergraduate major in psychology—medium, specific undergraduate psychology courses taken—high.

Student Characteristics: The following represents characteristics of students in 2009–2010 in all graduate psychology programs in the department: Female—full-time 25, part-time 0; Male—full-time 5, part-time 0; African American/Black—full-time 5, part-time 0; Hispanic/Latino(a)—full-time 2, part-time 0; Asian/Pacific Islander—full-time 1, part-time 0; American Indian/Alaska Native—full-time 0, part-time 0; Caucasian/White—full-time 21,

part-time 0; Multi-ethnic—full-time 1, part-time 0; students subject to the Americans With Disabilities Act—full-time 1, part-time 0; Unknown ethnicity—full-time 0, part-time 0; International students who hold an F-1 or J-1 Visa—full-time 1, part-time 0.

Financial Information/Assistance:
Tuition for Full-Time Study: *Master's:* State residents: per academic year $4,500, $150 per credit hour; Nonstate residents: per academic year $10,800, $600 per credit hour. Tuition is subject to change. See the following Web site for updates and changes in tuition costs: http://www.aug.edu.

Financial Assistance:
First-Year Students: Traineeships available for first year. Average amount paid per academic year: $7,500. Average number of hours worked per week: 10.
Advanced Students: Teaching assistantships available for advanced students. Average amount paid per academic year: $7,500. Average number of hours worked per week: 10. Apply by May 1. Research assistantships available for advanced students. Average amount paid per academic year: $7,500. Average number of hours worked per week: 10. Apply by May 1. Traineeships available for advanced students.
Additional Information: Of all students currently enrolled full time, 80% benefited from one or more of the listed financial assistance programs. Application and information available online at: http://www.aug.edu/psychology/Graduate_Info/assistantships.htm.

Internships/Practica: Master's Degree (MA/MS Counseling Psychology): An internship experience, such as a final research project or "capstone" experience is required of graduates. Institutions that provide unique opportunities for fieldwork and internship experiences include two Veterans Administration hospitals, a regional psychiatric hospital, the Medical College of Georgia, Gracewood State School and Hospital, Dwight David Eisenhower Medical Center, and various other agencies. Internships are also available in business, education and private practice settings.

Housing and Day Care: On-campus housing is available. No on-campus day care facilities are available.

Employment of Department Graduates:
Master's Degree Graduates: Of those who graduated in the academic year 2008–2009, the following categories and numbers represent the postgraduate activities and employment of master's degree graduates: Enrolled in a psychology doctoral program (1), enrolled in another graduate/professional program (0), enrolled in a postdoctoral residency/fellowship (n/a), employed in independent practice (n/a), employed in an academic position at a university (2), employed in a professional position in a school system (1), employed in business or industry (0), employed in government agency (0), employed in a community mental health/counseling center (2), employed in a hospital/medical center (2), still seeking employment (1), do not know (1), total from the above (master's) (10).
Doctoral Degree Graduates: Of those who graduated in the academic year 2008–2009, the following categories and numbers represent the postgraduate activities and employment of doctoral degree graduates: Enrolled in a psychology doctoral program (n/a), total from the above (doctoral) (0).

Additional Information:
Orientation, Objectives, and Emphasis of Department: Augusta State University offers three tracks at the masters level: clinical/counseling, general experimental, and applied experimental. The clinical/counseling track is MPAC accredited and meets the educational requirements for the LPC license in Georgia. Coursework is offered in psychological assessments, individual and group psychotherapies, research methods, and foundation psychology courses. The Augusta area provides a wealth of clinical and research internship experiences including placements at the Augusta VAMC, the Medical College of Georgia, and Eisenhower Army Hospital. The general experimental track is geared toward preparing students for doctoral level work. A thesis is required. Those who pursue the applied experimental track seek to work after the master's degree in a research, teaching, or business field. The applied experimental track requires internship experiences in lieu of a thesis. Most students finish the degree in 5 semesters or two years.

Special Facilities or Resources: The department maintains an active human and animal research laboratory and a clinical facility with videotaping and closed circuit television capabilities, and the university provides easy access to advanced computer resources. Students and faculty additionally engage in collaborative research at the Medical College of Georgia and Veterans Medical Center. Social and developmental labs are available for teaching and research.

Information for Students With Physical Disabilities: See the following Web site for more information: http://www.aug.edu/testing_and_disability_services/.

Application Information:
Send to Director of Graduate Studies, Department of Psychology, 2500 Walton Way, Augusta State University, Augusta, GA 30904-2200. Application available online. URL of online application: http://www.aug.edu/psychology/Graduate_Info/applicant.htm. Students are admitted in the Fall, application deadline May 1. *Fee:* $30.

Brenau University
Psychology/ M.S. in Clinical Counseling Psychology
School of Health and Science
500 Washington Street
Gainesville, GA 30501
Telephone: (770) 534-6225
E-mail: *gbauman@brenau.edu*
Web: *http://www.brenau.edu/shs/psychology*

Department Information:
1999. Chairperson: Dr. Julie Battle. Number of faculty: total—full-time 5, part-time 1; women—full-time 4; total—minority—full-time 1; women minority—full-time 1.

Programs and Degrees Offered:
Listed in the following order: Program area, degree type (T if terminal Master's), number awarded 7/08–6/09. Clinical Counseling Psychology MA/MS (Master of Arts/Science) (T) 6, Applied Gerontology MA/MS (Master of Arts/Science) (T).

Student Applications/Admissions:

Student Applications

Clinical Counseling Psychology MA/MS (Master of Arts/Science)—Applications 2009–2010, 28. Total applicants accepted 2009–2010, 16. Number full-time enrolled (new admits only) 2009–2010, 13. Number part-time enrolled (new admits only) 2009–2010, 3. Total enrolled 2009–2010 full-time, 20, part-time, 14. Openings 2010–2011, 16. The median number of years required for completion of a degree in 2008–2009 were 2. The number of students enrolled full- and part-time who were dismissed or voluntarily withdrew from this program area in 2008–2009 were 4. *Applied Gerontology MA/MS (Master of Arts/Science)*—

Scores: Entries appear in this order: required test or GPA, minimum score (if required), median score of students entering in 2009–2010. *Clinical Counseling Psychology MA/MS (Master of Arts/Science)*: GRE-V 400, 500, GRE-Q 400, 500, overall undergraduate GPA 2.50, 3.00.

Other Criteria: (importance of criteria rated low, medium, or high): GRE scores—medium, research experience—medium, work experience—medium, extracurricular activity—medium, clinically related public service—medium, GPA—medium, letters of recommendation—medium, interview—medium, statement of goals and objectives—medium, undergraduate major in psychology—medium, specific undergraduate psychology courses taken—medium.

Student Characteristics: The following represents characteristics of students in 2009–2010 in all graduate psychology programs in the department: Female—full-time 19, part-time 11; Male—full-time 1, part-time 3; African American/Black—full-time 2, part-time 2; Hispanic/Latino(a)—full-time 1, part-time 0; Asian/Pacific Islander—full-time 0, part-time 0; American Indian/Alaska Native—full-time 0, part-time 0; Caucasian/White—full-time 17, part-time 12; Multi-ethnic—full-time 0, part-time 0; students subject to the Americans With Disabilities Act—full-time 0, part-time 0; Unknown ethnicity—full-time 0, part-time 0; International students who hold an F-1 or J-1 Visa—full-time 0, part-time 0.

Financial Information/Assistance:

Tuition for Full-Time Study: *Master's:* State residents: per academic year $13,000, $490 per credit hour; Nonstate residents: per academic year $13,000, $490 per credit hour.

Financial Assistance:

First-Year Students: No information provided.

Advanced Students: Teaching assistantships available for advanced students. Average amount paid per academic year: $10,000. Average number of hours worked per week: 20.

Additional Information: Of all students currently enrolled full time, 15% benefited from one or more of the listed financial assistance programs.

Internships/Practica: Master's Degree (MA/MS Clinical Counseling Psychology): An internship experience, such as a final research project or "capstone" experience is required of graduates. Master's Degree (MA/MS Applied Gerontology): An internship experience, such as a final research project or "capstone" experience is required of graduates. Faculty and students will work together to set up practicum site placements. It is the student's responsibility to research available sites and determine his/her top three choices for placement. If a student wishes to receive practicum experience at a placement that has not been approved by the faculty, the student is responsible for providing faculty with the needed information for the approval of that site. The student must turn in his/her top three choices for placement, using the practicum pre-registration approval form, by the end of the semester preceding placement. The faculty member overseeing practicum placement will review student preferences, contact potential placement sites, and attempt to match students to placement sites. In the case that there are more students interested in a practicum site than there are openings at that practicum site, the students may be required to set up interviews with their potential supervisors at the site. Following the interviews, the site supervisor will report back to the faculty member who will make the final decision about placement.

Housing and Day Care: No on-campus housing is available. On-campus day care facilities are available.

Employment of Department Graduates:

Master's Degree Graduates: Of those who graduated in the academic year 2008–2009, the following categories and numbers represent the postgraduate activities and employment of master's degree graduates: Enrolled in a postdoctoral residency/fellowship (n/a), employed in independent practice (n/a), employed in an academic position at a university (1), employed in a community mental health/counseling center (5), total from the above (master's) (6).

Doctoral Degree Graduates: Of those who graduated in the academic year 2008–2009, the following categories and numbers represent the postgraduate activities and employment of doctoral degree graduates: Enrolled in a psychology doctoral program (n/a), total from the above (doctoral) (0).

Additional Information:

Orientation, Objectives, and Emphasis of Department: The MS program in Clinical Counseling Psychology is committed to excellence in preparing students for work in a wide variety of clinical, counseling, assessment, and research settings. Our mission is to provide an education founded in the scientist–practitioner model, which will lead to competency in applied clinical/counseling work as well as to an understanding of the importance of ongoing research into the effectiveness of our work and an ability to competently carry out research. Furthermore, the mission of the program is to provide an education that fosters personal growth, promotes reflection about practice, cultivates compassion and sensitivity in the therapeutic approach, encourages community responsibility and global understanding, and leads to intellectual and professional competence. The program provides coursework and practicum/internship experiences which emphasize the application of theories of human development, psychopathology, and behavior change to psychosocial problems of a diverse clientele seeking mental health services. The program provides a base in general psychological principles, therapeutic principles, a framework of research methodology, evaluation and statistics as well as applied work with these skills through the thesis requirement, and applied work in the area of clinical counseling psychology including the theory and practice of therapy, psychological assessment, ethics and professional identity, and social and cultural diversity. The program includes 57 hours of coursework with the option of completing an additional 6 hours of coursework in a specialty area. Part of the coursework involves completing an applied research thesis, and part of the coursework involves gaining 700 hours of applied practica and internship experiences. Graduates are eligible to sit for the National Counselor's Exam (NCE). Passing of the exam in conjunction with program requirements and additional supervised experience support eligibility for licensure as Licensed Professional Counselor (LPC).

Application Information:
Send to Admissions, Brenau University, 500 Washington Street, Gainesville, GA 30501 Attention: Michelle Leavell. Application available online. URL of online application: http://www.brenau.edu/admissions/default.cfm. Students are admitted in the Fall, application deadline April. *Fee:* $35.

Emory University
Department of Psychology
36 Eagle Row
Atlanta, GA 30322
Telephone: (404) 727-7438
Fax: (404) 727-0372
E-mail: *paula.mitchell@emory.edu*
Web: *http://www.psychology.emory.edu/*

Department Information:
1945. Chairperson: Robyn Fivush. Number of faculty: total—full-time 37; women—full-time 16; total—minority—full-time 1.

Programs and Degrees Offered:
Listed in the following order: Program area, degree type (T if terminal Master's), number awarded 7/08–6/09. Clinical Psychology PhD (Doctor of Philosophy) 5, Cognition & Development PhD (Doctor of Philosophy) 2, Neuroscience & Animal Behavior PhD (Doctor of Philosophy) 1.

APA Accreditation: Clinical PhD (Doctor of Philosophy). Student Outcome Data Website: http://www.psychology.emory.edu/clinical/admission.html.

Student Applications/Admissions:
Student Applications
Clinical Psychology PhD (Doctor of Philosophy)—Applications 2009–2010, 230. Total applicants accepted 2009–2010, 5. Number full-time enrolled (new admits only) 2009–2010, 5. Number part-time enrolled (new admits only) 2009–2010, 0. Openings 2010–2011, 6. The median number of years required for completion of a degree in 2008–2009 were 6. The number of students enrolled full- and part-time who were dismissed or voluntarily withdrew from this program area in 2008–2009 were 2. Cognition & Development PhD (Doctor of Philosophy)—Applications 2009–2010, 48. Total applicants accepted 2009–2010, 2. Number full-time enrolled (new admits only) 2009–2010, 2. Openings 2010–2011, 4. The median number of years required for completion of a degree in 2008–2009 were 6. The number of students enrolled full- and part-time who were dismissed or voluntarily withdrew from this program area in 2008–2009 were 1. Neuroscience & Animal Behavior PhD (Doctor of Philosophy)—Applications 2009–2010, 49. Total applicants accepted 2009–2010, 2. Number full-time enrolled (new admits only) 2009–2010, 2. Number part-time enrolled (new admits only) 2009–2010, 0. Openings 2010–2011, 4. The median number of years required for completion of a degree in 2008–2009 were 6. The number of students enrolled full- and part-time who were dismissed or voluntarily withdrew from this program area in 2008–2009 were 1.

Scores: Entries appear in this order: required test or GPA, minimum score (if required), median score of students entering in 2009–2010. Clinical Psychology PhD (Doctor of Philosophy): GRE-V 600, GRE-Q 600, GRE-Analytical 5.0, overall undergraduate GPA 3.5, Masters GPA no minimum stated; Cognition & Development PhD (Doctor of Philosophy): GRE-V 550, GRE-Q 650, GRE-Analytical 5.0, overall undergraduate GPA 3.5, Masters GPA no minimum stated; Neuroscience & Animal Behavior PhD (Doctor of Philosophy): GRE-V 600, GRE-Q 600, GRE-Analytical 5.0, overall undergraduate GPA 3.5, Masters GPA no minimum stated.

Other Criteria: (importance of criteria rated low, medium, or high): GRE scores—high, research experience—high, work experience—medium, extracurricular activity—low, clinically related public service—medium, GPA—high, letters of recommendation—high, interview—high, statement of goals and objectives—high, fit w/ faculty research—high, undergraduate major in psychology—medium, specific undergraduate psychology courses taken—medium. Clinically related public service is less pertinent to the Cognition & Development and the Neuroscience & Animal Behavior programs. For additional information on admission requirements, go to http://www.psychology.emory.edu/graduate/admission.html.

Student Characteristics: The following represents characteristics of students in 2009–2010 in all graduate psychology programs in the department: Female—full-time 57, part-time 0; Male—full-time 19, part-time 0; African American/Black—full-time 8, part-time 0; Hispanic/Latino(a)—full-time 0, part-time 0; Asian/Pacific Islander—full-time 5, part-time 0; American Indian/Alaska Native—full-time 0, part-time 0; Caucasian/White—full-time 63, part-time 0; Multi-ethnic—full-time 0, part-time 0; students subject to the Americans With Disabilities Act—full-time 0, part-time 0; Unknown ethnicity—full-time 0, part-time 0; International students who hold an F-1 or J-1 Visa—full-time 2, part-time 0.

Financial Information/Assistance:
Tuition for Full-Time Study: Doctoral: State residents: per academic year $37,286, $1,367 per credit hour; Nonstate residents: per academic year $37,286, $1,367 per credit hour. Tuition is subject to change. See the following Web site for updates and changes in tuition costs: http://www.emory.edu/studentfinancials/Student_Tuition.htm.

Financial Assistance:
First-Year Students: Fellowships and scholarships available for first year. Average amount paid per academic year: $22,000. Average number of hours worked per week: 10. Apply by February 9.

Advanced Students: Teaching assistantships available for advanced students. Average amount paid per academic year: $23,000. Average number of hours worked per week: 10. Apply by December 15. Fellowships and scholarships available for advanced students. Average amount paid per academic year: $23,000. Average number of hours worked per week: 10.

Additional Information: Of all students currently enrolled full time, 100% benefited from one or more of the listed financial assistance programs. Application and information available online at: http://www.gs.emory.edu/admissions/assistance.php.

Internships/Practica: Doctoral Degree (PhD Clinical Psychology): For those doctoral students for whom a professional internship was required in this program prior to graduation, (6) students applied for an internship in 2008–2009, with (6) students obtaining an internship. Of those students who obtained an internship, (6) were paid internships. Of those students who obtained an internship, (6) students placed in APA/CPA accredited internships, (0) students placed in internships not APA/CPA accredited, but listed with the Association of Psychology Postdoctoral and Internship Programs (APPIC), (0) students placed in internships conforming to guidelines of the Council of Directors of School Psychology Programs (CDSPP), (0) students placed in internships that were not APA/CPA accredited, APPIC or CDSPP listed. Clinical students generally go through a series of interviews to find the best match for their internships.

Housing and Day Care: No on-campus housing is available. On-campus day care facilities are available. See the following Web site for more information: http://www.emory.edu/HOUSING/CLAIRMONT/child.html.

Employment of Department Graduates:
Master's Degree Graduates: Of those who graduated in the academic year 2008–2009, the following categories and numbers represent the postgraduate activities and employment of master's degree graduates: Enrolled in a postdoctoral residency/fellowship (n/a), employed in independent practice (n/a), total from the above (master's) (0).
Doctoral Degree Graduates: Of those who graduated in the academic year 2008–2009, the following categories and numbers represent the postgraduate activities and employment of doctoral degree graduates: Enrolled in a psychology doctoral program (n/a), enrolled in a postdoctoral residency/fellowship (5), employed in an academic position at a university (2), other employment position (1), total from the above (doctoral) (8).

Additional Information:
Orientation, Objectives, and Emphasis of Department: The primary emphasis of our clinical curriculum is to provide students with the knowledge and skills they need to function as productive clinical researchers in psychology. This requires a basic understanding of the determinants of human behavior, including biological, psychological, and social factors, and a strong background in research design and quantitative methods. The program in cognition and development at Emory is committed to the principle that cognition and its development are best studied together. The research interests of the faculty span a wide range, and are reflected in our graduate courses, which include memory, emotion, language, perception, and concepts and categories. The program in neuroscience and animal behavior approaches topics within the areas of neuroscience, physiological psychology, acquired behavior, and ethology as a unified entity. Thus, the emphasis is on behavior as a biological phenomenon. Research in neuroscience and physiological psychology explores brain-behavior relationships; research on acquired behavior studies the ongoing and evolutionary factors influenced in individual adaptations; and ethological studies are concerned with understanding how animals function in their natural environment.

Special Facilities or Resources: The department has affiliations with the Emory Medical School, Yerkes National Primate Center, and the Center for Behavioral Neuroscience. In addition, faculty and students from many of the universities in the Atlanta area meet formally and informally to discuss common research interests.

Information for Students With Physical Disabilities: See the following Web site for more information: http://www.ods.emory.edu/.

Application Information:
Send to Mrs. Paula Mitchell, Graduate Program Specialist, Department of Psychology, Emory University, 532 Kilgo Circle, Atlanta, GA 30322. Application available online. URL of online application: http://www.gs.emory.edu/admissions/application.php. Students are admitted in the Fall, application deadline December 1. Clinical: December 1; Cognition and Development: January 2; Neuroscience and Animal Behavior: January 2. Fee: $50.

Georgia Southern University
Department of Psychology
College of Liberal Arts and Social Sciences
P.O. Box 8041
Statesboro, GA 30460-8041
Telephone: (912) 478-5539
Fax: (912) 478-0751
E-mail: JMurray@georgiasouthern.edu
Web: http://class.georgiasouthern.edu/psychology/

Department Information:
1967. Chairperson: Dr. John Murray. Number of faculty: total—full-time 16; women—full-time 7.

Programs and Degrees Offered:
Listed in the following order: Program area, degree type (T if terminal Master's), number awarded 7/08–6/09. Psychology MA/MS (Master of Arts/Science) (T) 4, Clinical Psychology PsyD (Doctor of Psychology) 0.

Student Applications/Admissions:
Student Applications
Psychology MA/MS (Master of Arts/Science)—Applications 2009–2010, 18. Total applicants accepted 2009–2010, 13. Number full-time enrolled (new admits only) 2009–2010, 10. Number part-time enrolled (new admits only) 2009–2010, 0. Openings 2010–2011, 12. The median number of years required for completion of a degree in 2008–2009 were 2. The number of students enrolled full- and part-time who were dismissed or voluntarily withdrew from this program area in 2008–2009 were 2. Clinical Psychology PsyD (Doctor of Psychology)—Applications 2009–2010, 25. Total applicants accepted 2009–2010, 9. Number full-time enrolled (new admits only) 2009–2010, 4. Number part-time enrolled (new admits only) 2009–2010, 1. Total enrolled 2009–2010 full-time, 13, part-

time, 1. Openings 2010–2011, 8. The number of students enrolled full- and part-time who were dismissed or voluntarily withdrew from this program area in 2008–2009 were 2.

Scores: Entries appear in this order: required test or GPA, minimum score (if required), median score of students entering in 2009–2010. *Psychology MA/MS (Master of Arts/Science):* GRE-V 450, GRE-Q 450, overall undergraduate GPA 3.0; *Clinical Psychology PsyD (Doctor of Psychology):* GRE-V no minimum stated, 518, GRE-Q no minimum stated, 630, overall undergraduate GPA no minimum stated, 3.65.

Other Criteria: (importance of criteria rated low, medium, or high): GRE scores—high, research experience—medium, clinically related public service—medium, GPA—high, letters of recommendation—medium, interview—medium, statement of goals and objectives—high, undergraduate major in psychology—low, specific undergraduate psychology courses taken—high. MS: GRE, grades, research experience all important. PsyD: GRE, grades, statement most important. For additional information on admission requirements, go to http://class.georgiasouthern.edu/psychology/.

Student Characteristics: The following represents characteristics of students in 2009–2010 in all graduate psychology programs in the department: Female—full-time 18, part-time 1; Male—full-time 14, part-time 0; African American/Black—full-time 2, part-time 0; Hispanic/Latino(a)—part-time 0; Asian/Pacific Islander—full-time 1, part-time 0; American Indian/Alaska Native—full-time 0, part-time 0; Caucasian/White—full-time 29, part-time 1; Multi-ethnic—full-time 0, part-time 0; students subject to the Americans With Disabilities Act—full-time 0, part-time 0; Unknown ethnicity—full-time 0, part-time 0; International students who hold an F-1 or J-1 Visa—full-time 0, part-time 0.

Financial Information/Assistance:
Tuition for Full-Time Study: Master's: State residents: per academic year $5,040, $210 per credit hour; Nonstate residents: per academic year $20,136, $839 per credit hour. *Doctoral:* State residents: per academic year $5,040, $210 per credit hour; Nonstate residents: per academic year $20,136, $839 per credit hour. Tuition is subject to change. Additional fees are assessed to students beyond the costs of tuition for the following: technology, health insurance. See the following Web site for updates and changes in tuition costs: http://services.georgiasouthern.edu/bursar/tuitionandfees/main.htm.

Financial Assistance:
First-Year Students: Research assistantships available for first year. Average amount paid per academic year: $6,850. Average number of hours worked per week: 20. Apply by April 15.
Advanced Students: Teaching assistantships available for advanced students. Average amount paid per academic year: $14,000. Average number of hours worked per week: 20. Research assistantships available for advanced students. Average amount paid per academic year: $7,200. Average number of hours worked per week: 20. Apply by April 15.
Additional Information: Of all students currently enrolled full time, 75% benefited from one or more of the listed financial assistance programs. Application and information available online at: http://cogs.georgiasouthern.edu/appsforms.htm.

Internships/Practica: Master's Degree (MA/MS Psychology): An internship experience, such as, a final research project or "capstone" experience is required of graduates.

Housing and Day Care: On-campus housing is available. See the following Web site for more information: http://students.georgiasouthern.edu/housing/. On-campus day care facilities are available. See the following Web site for more information: http://www.georgiasouthernhealthscience.com/departments/htfcs/resources/centers_cdc_overview.html.

Employment of Department Graduates:
Master's Degree Graduates: Of those who graduated in the academic year 2008–2009, the following categories and numbers represent the postgraduate activities and employment of master's degree graduates: Enrolled in a psychology doctoral program (1), enrolled in a postdoctoral residency/fellowship (n/a), employed in independent practice (n/a), employed in an academic position at a 2-year/4-year college (1), employed in government agency (1), do not know (1), total from the above (master's) (4).
Doctoral Degree Graduates: Of those who graduated in the academic year 2008–2009, the following categories and numbers represent the postgraduate activities and employment of doctoral degree graduates: Enrolled in a psychology doctoral program (n/a), total from the above (doctoral) (0).

Additional Information:
Orientation, Objectives, and Emphasis of Department: The MS program focuses on general psychology and prepares students for doctoral study in any area of psychology. The program consists of coursework and supervised research in traditional areas of interest such as social, developmental, learning, cognitive, physiological, and industrial/organizational and has a thesis requirement. The PsyD program in clinical psychology is new (beginning Fall 2007) and follows the practitioner/scholar model of training. The program is 5 years (including internship) and is consistent with the guidelines for accreditation set forth by the APA (although is not yet accredited). It has been granted 'designated' status by the National Register of Health Care Providers. The program emphasizes training in psychotherapy and assessment with individuals in rural settings.

Special Facilities or Resources: The department houses faculty research laboratories in a variety of subdisciplines in psychology (social, cognitive, physiological). The department also houses a community psychology clinic, where students in the clinical program are supervised in seeing adults from the Statesboro community and surrounding rural areas.

Information for Students With Physical Disabilities: See the following Web site for more information: http://students.georgiasouthern.edu/disability/.

Application Information:
Send to Office of Graduate Admissions, Georgia Southern University, P.O. Box 8113, Statesboro, GA 30460-8113. Application available online. URL of online application: http://cogs.georgiasouthern.edu/future_students/grad_application.html. Students are admitted in the Fall, application deadline January 15. PsyD applications are due January 15. MS: priority deadline: March 1, final deadline: July 1. *Fee:* $50.

Georgia State University
Department of Psychology
College of Arts and Sciences
P.O. Box 5010
Atlanta, GA 30302-5010
Telephone: (404) 413-6200
Fax: (404) 413-6207
E-mail: kdhill@gsu.edu
Web: http://www2.gsu.edu/~wwwpsy/

Department Information:
1955. Chairperson: David Washburn. Number of faculty: total—full-time 36; women—full-time 28; total—minority—full-time 7; women minority—full-time 5.

Programs and Degrees Offered:
Listed in the following order: Program area, degree type (T if terminal Master's), number awarded 7/08–6/09. Clinical Psychology PhD (Doctor of Philosophy) 3, Community Psychology PhD (Doctor of Philosophy) 2, Developmental Psychology PhD (Doctor of Philosophy) 0, Neuropsychology and Behavioral Neurosciences PhD (Doctor of Philosophy) 0, Social/Cognitive Psychology PhD (Doctor of Philosophy) 0.

APA Accreditation: Clinical PhD (Doctor of Philosophy).

Student Applications/Admissions:
Student Applications

Clinical Psychology PhD (Doctor of Philosophy)—Applications 2009–2010, 372. Total applicants accepted 2009–2010, 18. Number full-time enrolled (new admits only) 2009–2010, 10. Number part-time enrolled (new admits only) 2009–2010, 0. Openings 2010–2011, 10. The median number of years required for completion of a degree in 2008–2009 were 8. The number of students enrolled full- and part-time who were dismissed or voluntarily withdrew from this program area in 2008–2009 were 0. Community Psychology PhD (Doctor of Philosophy)—Applications 2009–2010, 53. Total applicants accepted 2009–2010, 7. Number full-time enrolled (new admits only) 2009–2010, 3. Number part-time enrolled (new admits only) 2009–2010, 0. Openings 2010–2011, 4. The median number of years required for completion of a degree in 2008–2009 were 6. The number of students enrolled full- and part-time who were dismissed or voluntarily withdrew from this program area in 2008–2009 were 0. Developmental Psychology PhD (Doctor of Philosophy)—Applications 2009–2010, 31. Total applicants accepted 2009–2010, 7. Number full-time enrolled (new admits only) 2009–2010, 5. Number part-time enrolled (new admits only) 2009–2010, 0. Openings 2010–2011, 4. The number of students enrolled full- and part-time who were dismissed or voluntarily withdrew from this program area in 2008–2009 were 0. Neuropsychology and Behavioral Neurosciences PhD (Doctor of Philosophy)—Applications 2009–2010, 34. Total applicants accepted 2009–2010, 2. Number full-time enrolled (new admits only) 2009–2010, 1. Number part-time enrolled (new admits only) 2009–2010, 0. The number of students enrolled full- and part-time who were dismissed or voluntarily withdrew from this program area in 2008–2009 were 10. Social/Cognitive Psychology PhD (Doctor of Philosophy)—Applications 2009–2010, 36. Total applicants accepted 2009–2010, 4. Number full-time enrolled (new admits only) 2009–2010, 4. Number part-time enrolled (new admits only) 2009–2010, 0. Openings 2010–2011, 4. The number of students enrolled full- and part-time who were dismissed or voluntarily withdrew from this program area in 2008–2009 were 0.

Other Criteria: (importance of criteria rated low, medium, or high): GRE scores—high, research experience—high, work experience—medium, extracurricular activity—low, clinically related public service—medium, GPA—high, letters of recommendation—high, interview—high, statement of goals and objectives—high, undergraduate major in psychology—medium, specific undergraduate psychology courses taken—high. For additional information on admission requirements, go to http://www2.gsu.edu/~wwwpsy/2693.html.

Student Characteristics: The following represents characteristics of students in 2009–2010 in all graduate psychology programs in the department: Female—full-time 84, part-time 0; Male—full-time 27, part-time 0; African American/Black—full-time 14, part-time 0; Hispanic/Latino(a)—full-time 7, part-time 0; Asian/Pacific Islander—full-time 3, part-time 0; American Indian/Alaska Native—full-time 0, part-time 0; Caucasian/White—full-time 75, part-time 0; Multi-ethnic—full-time 6, part-time 0; students subject to the Americans With Disabilities Act—full-time 0, part-time 0; Unknown ethnicity—full-time 1, part-time 0; International students who hold an F-1 or J-1 Visa—full-time 5, part-time 0.

Financial Information/Assistance:
Tuition for Full-Time Study: *Doctoral:* State residents: $267 per credit hour; Nonstate residents: $1,068 per credit hour. Tuition is subject to change. See the following Web site for updates and changes in tuition costs: http://www.gsu.edu/es/tuition.html.

Financial Assistance:
First-Year Students: Teaching assistantships available for first year. Average amount paid per academic year: $15,054. Average number of hours worked per week: 20. Research assistantships available for first year. Average amount paid per academic year: $15,054. Average number of hours worked per week: 20. Fellowships and scholarships available for first year. Average amount paid per academic year: $21,000.

Advanced Students: Teaching assistantships available for advanced students. Average amount paid per academic year: $15,614. Average number of hours worked per week: 20. Research assistantships available for advanced students. Average amount paid per academic year: $15,614. Average number of hours worked per week: 20. Fellowships and scholarships available for advanced students. Average amount paid per academic year: $21,000.

Additional Information: Of all students currently enrolled full time, 95% benefited from one or more of the listed financial assistance programs. Application and information available online at: http://www.gsu.edu/financialaid.

Internships/Practica: Doctoral Degree (PhD Clinical Psychology): For those doctoral students for whom a professional internship was required in this program prior to graduation, (6) students applied for an internship in 2008–2009, with (5) students obtaining an internship. Of those students who obtained an internship, (5) were paid internships. Of those students who obtained an internship, (5) students placed in APA/CPA accredited internships, (0) students placed in internships not APA/CPA accredited, but listed with the Association of Psychology Postdoctoral and Internship Programs (APPIC), (0) students placed in internships conforming to guidelines of the Council of Directors of School Psychology Programs (CDSPP), (0) students placed in internships that were not APA/CPA accredited, APPIC or CDSPP listed. Practicum experiences are an important component of the clinical training program. Supervised therapy and assessment practica are available in a variety of settings. For clinical students, one source of training is the Psychology Clinic which is located within the department. It provides services to students and members of the community in a variety of modalities, including assessment, individual therapy, group therapy, and family therapy. Another facility within the department is the Regent's Center for Learning Disorders, which offers comprehensive psychoeducational assessments to students and members of the community. Student clinicians are the primary providers of services in both of these clinics. In addition, there are numerous off-campus settings that offer supervised practicum experiences in a variety of areas including health psychology, neuropsychological assessment, personality assessment, psychiatric emergency room services, day treatment programs, etc. Many of these practica are available at Grady Memorial Hospital, a major metropolitan full-service facility located two blocks from the center of campus. Community students likewise do practica at various community based organizations. Often this research takes the form of needs assessment, program development, and program evaluation.

Housing and Day Care: On-campus housing is available. See the following Web site for more information: http://www.gsu.edu/housing/. On-campus day care facilities are available. See the following Web site for more information: http://education.gsu.edu/cdc/.

Employment of Department Graduates:
Master's Degree Graduates: Of those who graduated in the academic year 2008–2009, the following categories and numbers represent the postgraduate activities and employment of master's degree graduates: Enrolled in a postdoctoral residency/fellowship (n/a), employed in independent practice (n/a), total from the above (master's) (0).
Doctoral Degree Graduates: Of those who graduated in the academic year 2008–2009, the following categories and numbers represent the postgraduate activities and employment of doctoral degree graduates: Enrolled in a psychology doctoral program (n/a), total from the above (doctoral) (0).

Additional Information:
Orientation, Objectives, and Emphasis of Department: The department is eclectic, and many philosophical perspectives and research interests are represented. The policy of the department is to promote the personal and professional development of students. This includes the discovery of individual interests and goals, the growth of independent scholarship and research skills, the mastery of fundamental psychological knowledge and methodology, and the development of various professional skills (e.g., clinical skills, community intervention).

Special Facilities or Resources: The facilities of the department permit work in cognition, development, neuroscience + neuropsychology, learning, infant behavior, sensation and perception, motivation, aging, social psychology, assessment, individual, group and family therapy, behavior therapy, and community psychology.

Students may work with both human and nonhuman populations. Human populations include all age ranges and a variety of ethnic and socioeconomic backgrounds. Nonhuman populations include a variety of rodent and nonhuman primates.

Information for Students With Physical Disabilities: See the following Web site for more information: http://www.gsu.edu/~wwwods/.

Application Information:
Send to Office of Graduate Studies - College of Arts and Sciences, Georgia State University, P.O. Box 3993, Atlanta, GA 30302-3993. Application available online. URL of online application: https://apply.embark.com/grad/gastate/55/. Students are admitted in the Fall, application deadline December 1. The following programs have an application deadline of December 1: CLG (General Clinical) CLN (Joint Clinical and Neuropsychology) CLC (Joint Clinical and Community) NBN (Neuropsychology and Behavioral Neuroscience) SCG (Social/Cogntive). The following programs have an application deadline of January 5: COR (Community) DEV (Developmental). *Fee:* $50.

Georgia, University of
Department of Counseling and Human Development Services
College of Education
402 Aderhold Hall
Athens, GA 30602
Telephone: (706) 542-1812
Fax: (706) 542-4130
E-mail: *edelgado@uga.edu*
Web: *http://www.coe.uga.edu/chds/counselingpsych/index.html*

Department Information:
1946. Department Head: Rosemary E. Phelps. Number of faculty: total—full-time 25, part-time 2; women—full-time 15, part-time 1; total—minority—full-time 6, part-time 2; women minority—full-time 2, part-time 1.

Programs and Degrees Offered:
Listed in the following order: Program area, degree type (T if terminal Master's), number awarded 7/08–6/09. Counseling Psychology PhD (Doctor of Philosophy) 10.

APA Accreditation: Counseling PhD (Doctor of Philosophy). Student Outcome Data Website: http://www.coe.uga.edu/chds/counselingpsych/overview.html.

Student Applications/Admissions:
Student Applications
Counseling Psychology PhD (Doctor of Philosophy)—Applications 2009–2010, 82. Total applicants accepted 2009–2010, 21. Number full-time enrolled (new admits only) 2009–2010, 9. Number part-time enrolled (new admits only) 2009–2010, 0. Openings 2010–2011, 10. The median number of years required for completion of a degree in 2008–2009 were 4. The number of students enrolled full- and part-time who were dismissed or voluntarily withdrew from this program area in 2008–2009 were 1.
Scores: Entries appear in this order: required test or GPA, minimum score (if required), median score of students entering

in 2009–2010. *Counseling Psychology PhD (Doctor of Philosophy)*: GRE-V no minimum stated, GRE-Q no minimum stated, GRE-Analytical no minimum stated.

Other Criteria: (importance of criteria rated low, medium, or high): GRE scores—medium, research experience—high, work experience—high, extracurricular activity—low, clinically related public service—medium, GPA—medium, letters of recommendation—high, interview—high, statement of goals and objectives—high, undergraduate major in psychology—low. For additional information on admission requirements, go to http://www.coe.uga.edu/chds/counselingpsych/admissions.html.

Student Characteristics: The following represents characteristics of students in 2009–2010 in all graduate psychology programs in the department: Female—full-time 37, part-time 1; Male—full-time 13, part-time 1; African American/Black—full-time 16, part-time 1; Hispanic/Latino(a)—full-time 2, part-time 0; Asian/Pacific Islander—full-time 3, part-time 0; American Indian/Alaska Native—full-time 0, part-time 0; Caucasian/White—full-time 26, part-time 1; Multi-ethnic—full-time 1, part-time 0; students subject to the Americans With Disabilities Act—full-time 1, part-time 0; Unknown ethnicity—full-time 2, part-time 0; International students who hold an F-1 or J-1 Visa—full-time 1, part-time 0.

Financial Information/Assistance:

Tuition for Full-Time Study: *Master's:* State residents: per academic year $6,000, $250 per credit hour; Nonstate residents: per academic year $20,904, $871 per credit hour. *Doctoral:* State residents: per academic year $6,000, $250 per credit hour; Nonstate residents: per academic year $20,904, $871 per credit hour. Tuition is subject to change. See the following Web site for updates and changes in tuition costs: https://busfin1.busfin.uga.edu/bursar/schedule.cfm.

Financial Assistance:

First-Year Students: Teaching assistantships available for first year. Average amount paid per academic year: $11,515. Average number of hours worked per week: 13. Apply by December 1. Research assistantships available for first year. Average amount paid per academic year: $11,515. Average number of hours worked per week: 13. Apply by December 1.

Advanced Students: Teaching assistantships available for advanced students. Average amount paid per academic year: $11,515. Average number of hours worked per week: 13. Apply by December 1. Research assistantships available for advanced students. Average amount paid per academic year: $11,515. Average number of hours worked per week: 13. Apply by December 1.

Additional Information: Of all students currently enrolled full time, 100% benefited from one or more of the listed financial assistance programs. Application and information available online at: http://www.coe.uga.edu/chds/.

Internships/Practica: Doctoral Degree (PhD Counseling Psychology): For those doctoral students for whom a professional internship was required in this program prior to graduation, (10) students applied for an internship in 2008–2009, with (10) students obtaining an internship. Of those students who obtained an internship, (10) were paid internships. Of those students who obtained an internship, (7) students placed in APA/CPA accredited internships, (2) students placed in internships not APA/CPA accredited, but listed with the Association of Psychology Postdoctoral and Internship Programs (APPIC), (0) students placed in internships conforming to guidelines of the Council of Directors of School Psychology Programs (CDSPP), (1) students placed in internships that were not APA/CPA accredited, APPIC or CDSPP listed. Practicum opportunities are provided at one of three sites: the Juvenile Counseling and Assessment Program (JCAP), the Counseling and Personal Evaluation Center (department clinic) and Counseling Psychological Services (the university counseling center). Advanced practica are available in the area and in Atlanta.

Housing and Day Care: On-campus housing is available. See the following Web site for more information: http://www.uga.edu/housing/. On-campus day care facilities are available. See the following Web site for more information: http://www.fcs.uga.edu/cfd/cdl/.

Employment of Department Graduates:

Master's Degree Graduates: Of those who graduated in the academic year 2008–2009, the following categories and numbers represent the postgraduate activities and employment of master's degree graduates: Enrolled in a postdoctoral residency/fellowship (n/a), employed in independent practice (n/a), total from the above (master's) (0).

Doctoral Degree Graduates: Of those who graduated in the academic year 2008–2009, the following categories and numbers represent the postgraduate activities and employment of doctoral degree graduates: Enrolled in a psychology doctoral program (n/a), enrolled in a postdoctoral residency/fellowship (7), employed in independent practice (1), employed in a hospital/medical center (2), total from the above (doctoral) (10).

Additional Information:

Orientation, Objectives, and Emphasis of Department: The goal of the program is to educate students in the scientist–practitioner model of training in professional counseling psychology. The program focuses on professional competency development in three areas: teaching, research, and clinical service. The theoretical orientations of faculty members vary widely including representatives of most major schools of thought. The broad emphases of the program include developmental perspectives, cultural diversity perspectives, cognitive-behavioral approaches, and psychodynamic therapies.

Special Facilities or Resources: The University, the College, and the Department separately and collectively offer a number of services and fully-equipped facilities to assist students in conducting academic inquiry, including special computer labs, research assistance centers, and major libraries.

Information for Students With Physical Disabilities: See the following Web site for more information: http://drc.uga.edu/.

Application Information:

Send to Admissions Committee, Department of Counseling and Human Development Services, University of Georgia, 402 Aderhold Hall, Athens, GA 30602. Application available online. URL of online application: http://www.coe.uga.edu/chds/. Students are admitted in the Fall, application deadline December 1. *Fee:* $75.

GRADUATE STUDY IN PSYCHOLOGY

Georgia, University of
Department of Psychology
Franklin College of Arts and Sciences
Athens, GA 30602-3013
Telephone: (706) 542-2174
Fax: (706) 542-3275
E-mail: bhammond@uga.edu
Web: http://psychology.uga.edu/

Department Information:
1921. Chairperson: W. Keith Campbell. Number of faculty: total—full-time 45, part-time 3; women—full-time 20; total—minority—full-time 3; women minority—full-time 3.

Programs and Degrees Offered:
Listed in the following order: Program area, degree type (T if terminal Master's), number awarded 7/08–6/09. Applied Psychology PhD (Doctor of Philosophy) 1, Clinical Psychology PhD (Doctor of Philosophy) 6, Cognitive Experimental Psychology PhD (Doctor of Philosophy) 6, Lifespan Developmental Psychology PhD (Doctor of Philosophy) 0, Social Psychology PhD (Doctor of Philosophy) 1, Neuroscience and Behavior PhD (Doctor of Philosophy) 1.

APA Accreditation: Clinical PhD (Doctor of Philosophy).

Student Applications/Admissions:
Student Applications
Applied Psychology PhD (Doctor of Philosophy)—Applications 2009–2010, 52. Total applicants accepted 2009–2010, 8. Number full-time enrolled (new admits only) 2009–2010, 5. Total enrolled 2009–2010 full-time, 23, part-time, 4. Openings 2010–2011, 5. The median number of years required for completion of a degree in 2008–2009 were 5. The number of students enrolled full- and part-time who were dismissed or voluntarily withdrew from this program area in 2008–2009 were 1. Clinical Psychology PhD (Doctor of Philosophy)—Applications 2009–2010, 242. Total applicants accepted 2009–2010, 9. Number full-time enrolled (new admits only) 2009–2010, 7. Openings 2010–2011, 6. The median number of years required for completion of a degree in 2008–2009 were 5. The number of students enrolled full- and part-time who were dismissed or voluntarily withdrew from this program area in 2008–2009 were 1. Cognitive Experimental Psychology PhD (Doctor of Philosophy)—Applications 2009–2010, 25. Total applicants accepted 2009–2010, 10. Number full-time enrolled (new admits only) 2009–2010, 5. Openings 2010–2011, 5. The median number of years required for completion of a degree in 2008–2009 were 5. The number of students enrolled full- and part-time who were dismissed or voluntarily withdrew from this program area in 2008–2009 were 0. Lifespan Developmental Psychology PhD (Doctor of Philosophy)—Applications 2009–2010, 14. Total applicants accepted 2009–2010, 2. Number full-time enrolled (new admits only) 2009–2010, 1. Total enrolled 2009–2010 full-time, 8, part-time, 2. Openings 2010–2011, 2. The median number of years required for completion of a degree in 2008–2009 were 6. The number of students enrolled full- and part-time who were dismissed or voluntarily withdrew from this program area in 2008–2009 were 0. Social Psychology PhD (Doctor of Philosophy)—Applications 2009–2010, 38. Total applicants accepted 2009–2010, 1. Number full-time enrolled (new admits only) 2009–2010, 0. Openings 2010–2011, 3. The median number of years required for completion of a degree in 2008–2009 were 5. The number of students enrolled full- and part-time who were dismissed or voluntarily withdrew from this program area in 2008–2009 were 0. Neuroscience and Behavior PhD (Doctor of Philosophy)—Applications 2009–2010, 20. Total applicants accepted 2009–2010, 2. Number full-time enrolled (new admits only) 2009–2010, 0. Openings 2010–2011, 5. The median number of years required for completion of a degree in 2008–2009 were 5.

Scores: Entries appear in this order: required test or GPA, minimum score (if required), median score of students entering in 2009–2010. *Applied Psychology PhD (Doctor of Philosophy):* GRE-V no minimum stated, GRE-Q no minimum stated, GRE-Analytical no minimum stated, overall undergraduate GPA 3.25; *Clinical Psychology PhD (Doctor of Philosophy):* GRE-V 550, 620, GRE-Q 550, 700, GRE-Analytical no minimum stated, overall undergraduate GPA 3.0, 3.71; *Cognitive Experimental Psychology PhD (Doctor of Philosophy):* GRE-V no minimum stated, GRE-Q no minimum stated, GRE-Analytical no minimum stated; *Lifespan Developmental Psychology PhD (Doctor of Philosophy):* GRE-V no minimum stated, GRE-Q no minimum stated, GRE-Analytical no minimum stated; *Social Psychology PhD (Doctor of Philosophy):* GRE-V no minimum stated, GRE-Q no minimum stated, GRE-Analytical no minimum stated; *Neuroscience and Behavior PhD (Doctor of Philosophy):* GRE-V no minimum stated, GRE-Q no minimum stated, GRE-Analytical no minimum stated.

Other Criteria: (importance of criteria rated low, medium, or high): GRE scores—medium, research experience—high, work experience—high, extracurricular activity—medium, clinically related public service—medium, GPA—medium, letters of recommendation—medium, interview—medium, statement of goals and objectives—high. Each program weighs according to its own criteria. Interviews are only required by Clinical. For additional information on admission requirements, go to http://psychology.uga.edu/.

Student Characteristics: The following represents characteristics of students in 2009–2010 in all graduate psychology programs in the department: Female—full-time 72, part-time 6; Male—full-time 31, part-time 0; African American/Black—full-time 7, part-time 1; Hispanic/Latino(a)—full-time 4, part-time 0; Asian/Pacific Islander—full-time 11, part-time 0; American Indian/Alaska Native—full-time 0, part-time 0; Caucasian/White—full-time 79, part-time 5; Multi-ethnic—full-time 2, part-time 0; students subject to the Americans With Disabilities Act—full-time 0, part-time 0; Unknown ethnicity—full-time 0, part-time 0; International students who hold an F-1 or J-1 Visa—full-time 10, part-time 0.

Financial Information/Assistance:
Tuition for Full-Time Study: *Master's:* State residents: per academic year $6,000, $250 per credit hour; Nonstate residents: per academic year $20,904, $871 per credit hour. *Doctoral:* State residents: per academic year $6,000, $250 per credit hour; Nonstate residents: per academic year $20,904, $871 per credit hour.

Tuition is subject to change. Additional fees are assessed to students beyond the costs of tuition for the following: transportation, activity, athletic, health, student facilities, tech (total: $830/sem). See the following Web site for updates and changes in tuition costs: http://www.bursar.uga.edu/.

Financial Assistance:
First-Year Students: Teaching assistantships available for first year. Average amount paid per academic year: $14,270. Average number of hours worked per week: 17. Research assistantships available for first year. Average amount paid per academic year: $14,270. Average number of hours worked per week: 17. Fellowships and scholarships available for first year. Average amount paid per academic year: $15,383. Average number of hours worked per week: 16.
Advanced Students: Teaching assistantships available for advanced students. Average amount paid per academic year: $15,226. Average number of hours worked per week: 17. Research assistantships available for advanced students. Average amount paid per academic year: $15,226. Average number of hours worked per week: 17. Fellowships and scholarships available for advanced students. Average amount paid per academic year: $15,383. Average number of hours worked per week: 16.
Additional Information: Of all students currently enrolled full time, 98% benefited from one or more of the listed financial assistance programs. Application and information available online at: http://www.grad.uga.edu.

Housing and Day Care: On-campus housing is available. See the following Web site for more information: http://www.uga.edu/housing. On-campus day care facilities are available. See the following Web site for more information: http://www.fcs.uga.edu/cfd/cdl/.

Employment of Department Graduates:
Master's Degree Graduates: Of those who graduated in the academic year 2008–2009, the following categories and numbers represent the postgraduate activities and employment of master's degree graduates: Enrolled in a postdoctoral residency/fellowship (n/a), employed in independent practice (n/a), total from the above (master's) (0).
Doctoral Degree Graduates: Of those who graduated in the academic year 2008–2009, the following categories and numbers represent the postgraduate activities and employment of doctoral degree graduates: Enrolled in a psychology doctoral program (n/a), enrolled in a postdoctoral residency/fellowship (8), employed in an academic position at a university (4), employed in an academic position at a 2-year/4-year college (3), total from the above (doctoral) (15).

Additional Information:
Orientation, Objectives, and Emphasis of Department: Our emphasis is on research and the basic science aspects of psychology with a focus on doctoral education. A few state and private facilities provide internships. We have a cooperative liaison with several mental health facilities in the region as well as other universities.

Special Facilities or Resources: Facilities include a research and Regents Center for Learning Disabilities and the Institute for Behavioral Research, Psychology Clinic and the Vision Sciences Laboratory. We recently opened a new center (9,000 square feet) for Bioimaging which contains equipment for high-density EEG, MEG, MRI and fMRI. We are also part of the Biomedical and Health Sciences Institute which focuses on the neurosciences and biomedical applications.

Information for Students With Physical Disabilities: See the following Web site for more information: http://drc.uga.edu/.

Application Information:
Send to Department of Psychology c/o Graduate Coordinator, University of Georgia, Athens, GA 30602-3013. Application available online. URL of online application: http://www.grad.uga.edu. Students are admitted in the Fall, application deadline December 1. *Fee:* $75. Fee for international applicants is $100. Participation in certain programs may qualify an applicant to waive the application fee.

Georgia, University of
School Psychology Program
Education
630 Aderhold Hall
Athens, GA 30602-7143
Telephone: (706) 542-4110
Fax: (706) 542-4240
E-mail: *jmcmpbll@uga.edu*
Web: *http://www.coe.uga.edu/epit/spy/*

Department Information:
1968. Program Coordinator: Jonathan M. Campbell. Number of faculty: total—full-time 4, part-time 2; women—full-time 2, part-time 2.

Programs and Degrees Offered:
Listed in the following order: Program area, degree type (T if terminal Master's), number awarded 7/08–6/09. School Psychology PhD (Doctor of Philosophy) 10.

APA Accreditation: School PhD (Doctor of Philosophy). Student Outcome Data Website: http://www.coe.uga.edu/epit/spy/table2008.pdf.

Student Applications/Admissions:
Student Applications
School Psychology PhD (Doctor of Philosophy)—Applications 2009–2010, 50. Total applicants accepted 2009–2010, 8. Number full-time enrolled (new admits only) 2009–2010, 5. Number part-time enrolled (new admits only) 2009–2010, 0. Openings 2010–2011, 5. The median number of years required for completion of a degree in 2008–2009 were 5. The number of students enrolled full- and part-time who were dismissed or voluntarily withdrew from this program area in 2008–2009 were 0.
Scores: Entries appear in this order: required test or GPA, minimum score (if required), median score of students entering in 2009–2010. School Psychology PhD (Doctor of Philosophy):

GRE-V 500, GRE-Q 500, overall undergraduate GPA 3.0, Masters GPA 3.5.

Other Criteria: (importance of criteria rated low, medium, or high): GRE scores—medium, research experience—high, work experience—low, extracurricular activity—low, clinically related public service—medium, GPA—high, letters of recommendation—high, interview—medium, statement of goals and objectives—medium, undergraduate major in psychology—low, specific undergraduate psychology courses taken—low.

Student Characteristics: The following represents characteristics of students in 2009–2010 in all graduate psychology programs in the department: Female—full-time 29, part-time 0; Male—full-time 7, part-time 0; African American/Black—full-time 3, part-time 0; Hispanic/Latino(a)—full-time 1, part-time 0; Asian/Pacific Islander—full-time 2, part-time 0; American Indian/Alaska Native—full-time 0, part-time 0; Caucasian/White—full-time 13, part-time 0; Multi-ethnic—full-time 1, part-time 0; students subject to the Americans With Disabilities Act—full-time 0, part-time 0; Unknown ethnicity—full-time 0, part-time 0; International students who hold an F-1 or J-1 Visa—full-time 0, part-time 0.

Financial Information/Assistance:
Tuition for Full-Time Study: *Doctoral:* State residents: per academic year $5,044; Nonstate residents: per academic year $20,300. Tuition is subject to change. See the following Web site for updates and changes in tuition costs: https://busfin1.busfin.uga.edu/bursar/semester_program.cfm.

Financial Assistance:
First-Year Students: Teaching assistantships available for first year. Average amount paid per academic year: $12,623. Average number of hours worked per week: 13. Apply by February 1. Research assistantships available for first year. Average amount paid per academic year: $12,623. Average number of hours worked per week: 13. Apply by February 1. Fellowships and scholarships available for first year. Average amount paid per academic year: $12,623. Average number of hours worked per week: 13.

Advanced Students: Teaching assistantships available for advanced students. Average amount paid per academic year: $13,643. Average number of hours worked per week: 13. Apply by February 1. Research assistantships available for advanced students. Average amount paid per academic year: $13,643. Average number of hours worked per week: 13. Apply by February 1. Fellowships and scholarships available for advanced students. Average amount paid per academic year: $13,643.

Additional Information: Of all students currently enrolled full time, 73% benefited from one or more of the listed financial assistance programs.

Internships/Practica: Doctoral Degree (PhD School Psychology): For those doctoral students for whom a professional internship was required in this program prior to graduation, (9) students applied for an internship in 2008–2009, with (9) students obtaining an internship. Of those students who obtained an internship, (9) were paid internships. Of those students who obtained an internship, (5) students placed in APA/CPA accredited internships, (0) students placed in internships not APA/CPA accredited, but listed with the Association of Psychology Postdoctoral and Internship Programs (APPIC), (4) students placed in internships conforming to guidelines of the Council of Directors of School Psychology Programs (CDSPP), (0) students placed in internships that were not APA/CPA accredited, APPIC or CDSPP listed.

Housing and Day Care: On-campus housing is available. On-campus day care facilities are available.

Employment of Department Graduates:
Master's Degree Graduates: Of those who graduated in the academic year 2008–2009, the following categories and numbers represent the postgraduate activities and employment of master's degree graduates: Enrolled in a postdoctoral residency/fellowship (n/a), employed in independent practice (n/a), total from the above (master's) (0).

Doctoral Degree Graduates: Of those who graduated in the academic year 2008–2009, the following categories and numbers represent the postgraduate activities and employment of doctoral degree graduates: Enrolled in a psychology doctoral program (n/a), enrolled in a postdoctoral residency/fellowship (5), employed in independent practice (0), employed in an academic position at a university (0), employed in an academic position at a 2-year/4-year college (0), employed in other positions at a higher education institution (0), employed in a professional position in a school system (6), employed in business or industry (0), employed in government agency (0), employed in a community mental health/counseling center (0), employed in a hospital/medical center (0), still seeking employment (0), other employment position (0), total from the above (doctoral) (11).

Additional Information:
Orientation, Objectives, and Emphasis of Department: The PhD program in school psychology trains research-oriented school psychologists for work in educational settings, hospitals, clinics, and universities in which they can provide leadership in applied practice, research and teaching. The school psychology program follows the scientist–practitioner model, and emphasizes human development and developmental psychopathology and the central core elements of training.

Special Facilities or Resources: Special facilities and resources include access to a superior computer center, decentralized computational equipment, a major research library, and faculty members who are extraordinarily accessible to students. The department is strongly committed to affirmative action and fair treatment. Despite the suburban setting (a small urban area of 75,000 over an hour from Atlanta), we attract ethnic minority as well as out-of-state and out-of-region students and faculty. NASP and APA requirements and full accreditation from APA and NCATE form the foundation of our programs.

Application Information:
Send to Graduate Admissions Office, Graduate Studies Building, The University of Georgia, Athens, GA 30602. Students are admitted in the Fall, application deadline December 15. *Fee:* $75.

West Georgia, University of
Department of Psychology
Arts and Sciences
1600 Maple Street
Carrollton, GA 30118
Telephone: (678) 839-6510
Fax: (678) 839-0611
E-mail: drice@westga.edu
Web: http://www.westga.edu/psydept

Department Information:
1967. Professor and Chair: Donadrian L. Rice. Number of faculty: total—full-time 16, part-time 1; women—full-time 3, part-time 1; total—minority—full-time 2; women minority—full-time 1.

Programs and Degrees Offered:
Listed in the following order: Program area, degree type (T if terminal Master's), number awarded 7/08–6/09. Humanistic/Transpersonal Psychology MA/MS (Master of Arts/Science) (T) 18, Individual, Organizational and Community Trans PsyD (Doctor of Psychology) 0.

Student Applications/Admissions:
Student Applications
Humanistic/Transpersonal Psychology MA/MS (Master of Arts/Science)—Applications 2009–2010, 71. Total applicants accepted 2009–2010, 38. Number full-time enrolled (new admits only) 2009–2010, 32. Number part-time enrolled (new admits only) 2009–2010, 8. Total enrolled 2009–2010 full-time, 76, part-time, 11. Openings 2010–2011, 35. The median number of years required for completion of a degree in 2008–2009 were 3. The number of students enrolled full- and part-time who were dismissed or voluntarily withdrew from this program area in 2008–2009 were 0. *Individual, Organizational and Community Trans PsyD (Doctor of Psychology)*—Applications 2009–2010, 30. Total applicants accepted 2009–2010, 8. Number full-time enrolled (new admits only) 2009–2010, 8. Number part-time enrolled (new admits only) 2009–2010, 0. Openings 2010–2011, 10. The number of students enrolled full- and part-time who were dismissed or voluntarily withdrew from this program area in 2008–2009 were 0.
Scores: Entries appear in this order: required test or GPA, minimum score (if required), median score of students entering in 2009–2010. *Humanistic/Transpersonal Psychology MA/MS (Master of Arts/Science):* GRE-V 400, GRE-Q 400, overall undergraduate GPA 2.5; *Individual, Organizational and Community Trans PsyD (Doctor of Psychology):* GRE-V 500, GRE-Q 500.
Other Criteria: (importance of criteria rated low, medium, or high): GRE scores—medium, research experience—high, work experience—high, extracurricular activity—medium, clinically related public service—high, GPA—high, letters of recommendation—high, interview—high, statement of goals and objectives—high, undergraduate major in psychology—medium, specific undergraduate psychology courses taken—medium. For additional information on admission requirements, go to http://www.westga.edu/~psydept/.

Student Characteristics: The following represents characteristics of students in 2009–2010 in all graduate psychology programs in the department: Female—full-time 49, part-time 5; Male—full-time 27, part-time 3; African American/Black—full-time 5, part-time 0; Hispanic/Latino(a)—full-time 4, part-time 0; Asian/Pacific Islander—full-time 2, part-time 0; American Indian/Alaska Native—full-time 0, part-time 0; Caucasian/White—full-time 65, part-time 0; Multi-ethnic—full-time 0, part-time 0; students subject to the Americans With Disabilities Act—full-time 1, part-time 0; Unknown ethnicity—full-time 0, part-time 0; International students who hold an F-1 or J-1 Visa—full-time 2, part-time 0.

Financial Information/Assistance:
Tuition for Full-Time Study: Master's: State residents: per academic year $3,370, $117 per credit hour; Nonstate residents: per academic year $11,730, $465 per credit hour. *Doctoral:* State residents: per academic year $3,370, $117 per credit hour; Nonstate residents: per academic year $11,730, $465 per credit hour. Tuition is subject to change. Tuition costs vary by program. See the following Web site for updates and changes in tuition costs: http://www.westga.edu/bursar.

Financial Assistance:
First-Year Students: Teaching assistantships available for first year. Research assistantships available for first year. Average amount paid per academic year: $3,000. Average number of hours worked per week: 13.
Advanced Students: No information provided.
Additional Information: Of all students currently enrolled full time, 25% benefited from one or more of the listed financial assistance programs. Application and information available online at: http://www.westga.edu/~gradsch/finaid.php.

Internships/Practica: Master's Degree (MA/MS Humanistic/Transpersonal Psychology): An internship experience, such as a final research project or "capstone" experience is required of graduates. Internships are available at local facilities.

Housing and Day Care: On-campus housing is available. No on-campus day care facilities are available.

Employment of Department Graduates:
Master's Degree Graduates: Of those who graduated in the academic year 2008–2009, the following categories and numbers represent the postgraduate activities and employment of master's degree graduates: Enrolled in a psychology doctoral program (4), enrolled in another graduate/professional program (3), enrolled in a postdoctoral residency/fellowship (n/a), employed in independent practice (n/a), employed in an academic position at a university (1), employed in an academic position at a 2-year/4-year college (3), employed in other positions at a higher education institution (1), employed in a professional position in a school system (2), employed in business or industry (2), employed in a community mental health/counseling center (5), total from the above (master's) (21).
Doctoral Degree Graduates: Of those who graduated in the academic year 2008–2009, the following categories and numbers represent the postgraduate activities and employment of doctoral degree graduates: Enrolled in a psychology doctoral program (n/a), total from the above (doctoral) (0).

Additional Information:
Orientation, Objectives, and Emphasis of Department: The department is a pioneer of humanistic-transpersonal psychology. It

differs from other programs in that it goes beyond conventional subjects and approaches a holistic and integrative understanding of human experience. Alongside demanding academic work, student growth and personal awareness are inherent to this venture since such reflection is considered an important factor in human understanding. Individual programs are designed according to personal needs and interests; the overall atmosphere is communal, encouraging personal and intellectual dialogue and encounter. Most conventional topic areas are taught. Beyond these are areas almost uniquely explorable in a program such as this: the horizons of consciousness through such vantages as Eastern and transpersonal psychologies, hermeneutics, existential and phenomenological psychologies, and critical psychology. Specific areas include women's studies; aesthetic and sacred experience; myths, dreams, and symbols; and creativity. Areas of applied interest are viewed as correlates of the learning process: skill courses related to human services, prevention and community psychology, counseling psychology, cross-cultural psychology, organizational development, and growth therapies. The department offers training in qualitative and traditional methodologies of research. Practicum and internship experience along with individual research and reading are highly encouraged for those who can profit from these. Interest areas include human science research; parapsychology; transpersonal and Eastern psychologies; counseling, clinical, community, and organizational development; and psychology in the classroom.

Special Facilities or Resources: Special resources include large library holdings in the areas of humanistic, parapsychology, transpersonal, philosophical, and Asian psychology. The library holds papers of Sidney M. Jourard, Edith Weiskoff-Joelsen and the Psychical Research Foundation Library. The department hosts major conferences, and faculty are associated with several journals and newsletters exploring orientation areas.

Information for Students With Physical Disabilities: See the following Web site for more information: http://www.westga.edu/~sdev.

Application Information:
Send to Graduate Coordinator, Department of Psychology, University of West Georgia, Carrollton, GA 30118. Application available online. URL of online application: http://www.westga.edu/~gradsch/. Students are admitted in the Fall, application deadline February 18; Spring, application deadline September 17; Summer, application deadline April 8. Enrollment for PsyD program in Fall Only. *Fee:* $30.

HAWAII

Hawaii, University of
Department of Educational Psychology
College of Education
1776 University Avenue
Honolulu, HI 96822-2463
Telephone: (808) 956-7775
Fax: (808) 956-6615
E-mail: yamauchi@hawaii.edu
Web: http://www.hawaii.edu/edpsych/

Department Information:
1965. Chairperson: Lois Yamauchi. Number of faculty: total—full-time 8; women—full-time 5; total—minority—full-time 3; women minority—full-time 2.

Programs and Degrees Offered:
Listed in the following order: Program area, degree type (T if terminal Master's), number awarded 7/08–6/09. Educational Psychology MEd (Education) 8, Educational Psychology PhD (Doctor of Philosophy) 5.

Student Applications/Admissions:
Student Applications
Educational Psychology MEd (Education)—Applications 2009–2010, 38. Total applicants accepted 2009–2010, 19. Number full-time enrolled (new admits only) 2009–2010, 7. Number part-time enrolled (new admits only) 2009–2010, 5. Total enrolled 2009–2010 full-time, 16, part-time, 15. The median number of years required for completion of a degree in 2008–2009 were 2. The number of students enrolled full- and part-time who were dismissed or voluntarily withdrew from this program area in 2008–2009 were 2. *Educational Psychology PhD (Doctor of Philosophy)*—Applications 2009–2010, 15. Total applicants accepted 2009–2010, 5. Number full-time enrolled (new admits only) 2009–2010, 2. Number part-time enrolled (new admits only) 2009–2010, 2. Total enrolled 2009–2010 full-time, 5, part-time, 16. The median number of years required for completion of a degree in 2008–2009 were 6. The number of students enrolled full- and part-time who were dismissed or voluntarily withdrew from this program area in 2008–2009 were 0.
Other Criteria: (importance of criteria rated low, medium, or high): GRE scores—high, research experience—medium, work experience—low, extracurricular activity—medium, GPA—high, letters of recommendation—high, statement of goals and objectives—high. The MEd program does not require the GRE or research experience.

Student Characteristics: The following represents characteristics of students in 2009–2010 in all graduate psychology programs in the department: Female—full-time 17, part-time 22; Male—full-time 4, part-time 9; African American/Black—full-time 1, part-time 0; Hispanic/Latino(a)—full-time 0, part-time 0; Asian/Pacific Islander—full-time 12, part-time 18; American Indian/Alaska Native—full-time 0, part-time 0; Caucasian/White—full-time 8, part-time 13; Multi-ethnic—full-time 0, part-time 0; students subject to the Americans With Disabilities Act—full-time 0, part-time 0; Unknown ethnicity—full-time 0, part-time 0; International students who hold an F-1 or J-1 Visa—full-time 3, part-time 0.

Financial Information/Assistance:
Tuition for Full-Time Study: Master's: State residents: per academic year $10,992, $458 per credit hour; Nonstate residents: per academic year $26,784, $1,116 per credit hour. *Doctoral:* State residents: per academic year $10,992, $458 per credit hour; Nonstate residents: per academic year $26,784, $1,116 per credit hour. See the following Web site for updates and changes in tuition costs: http://www.hawaii.edu/admissions/tuition.html.

Financial Assistance:
First-Year Students: Research assistantships available for first year. Average amount paid per academic year: $14,958. Average number of hours worked per week: 20. Fellowships and scholarships available for first year.
Advanced Students: Research assistantships available for advanced students. Average amount paid per academic year: $14,958. Average number of hours worked per week: 20. Fellowships and scholarships available for advanced students.
Additional Information: Of all students currently enrolled full time, 15% benefited from one or more of the listed financial assistance programs. Application and information available online at: http://www.hawaii.edu/fas/.

Internships/Practica: Research and teaching internships are highly recommended for doctoral students; however, financial support continues to be very limited.

Housing and Day Care: On-campus housing is available. See the following Web site for more information: http://www.housing.hawaii.edu/. On-campus day care facilities are available. See the following Web site for more information: http://www.hawaii.edu/childrenscenter/.

Employment of Department Graduates:
Master's Degree Graduates: Of those who graduated in the academic year 2008–2009, the following categories and numbers represent the postgraduate activities and employment of master's degree graduates: Enrolled in a psychology doctoral program (1), enrolled in another graduate/professional program (1), enrolled in a postdoctoral residency/fellowship (n/a), employed in independent practice (n/a), employed in an academic position at a university (1), employed in an academic position at a 2-year/4-year college (0), employed in other positions at a higher education institution (1), employed in a professional position in a school system (4), employed in business or industry (2), employed in government agency (0), employed in a community mental health/counseling center (2), employed in a hospital/medical center (0), still seeking employment (0), not seeking employment (0), other employment position (2), do not know (2), total from the above (master's) (16).

Doctoral Degree Graduates: Of those who graduated in the academic year 2008–2009, the following categories and numbers represent the postgraduate activities and employment of doctoral degree graduates: Enrolled in a psychology doctoral program (n/a), enrolled in another graduate/professional program (0), enrolled in a postdoctoral residency/fellowship (0), employed in independent practice (0), employed in an academic position at a university (1), employed in an academic position at a 2-year/4-year college (1), employed in other positions at a higher education institution (1), employed in a professional position in a school system (2), employed in business or industry (1), employed in government agency (0), employed in a community mental health/counseling center (0), employed in a hospital/medical center (0), still seeking employment (0), not seeking employment (0), other employment position (0), do not know (1), total from the above (doctoral) (7).

Additional Information:
Orientation, Objectives, and Emphasis of Department: The primary objective of graduate training is the development of competent scholars in the discipline of Educational Psychology. Therefore, the faculty seeks students with research interests and abilities, independence of thought, and a willingness to actively participate in both formal and informal teaching and learning experiences. The students' efforts may be directed toward the attainment of the MEd or the PhD degree. Thesis (Plan A) and nonthesis (Plan B) options are available at the MEd level. Members of the faculty share a commitment to a model of graduate education that is humanistic and inquiry oriented. An extensive core of quantitative coursework—measurement, statistics, and research methodology—underlies most programs of study, especially at the doctoral level. In addition, core courses in human learning and development give the student a contextual framework within which inquiry methodologies are applied. The small size of the department ensures a high level of interaction among students and faculty in and out of class. Working closely with the faculty, each student creates a degree plan uniquely suited to his or her academic goals. Interdisciplinary study is particularly encouraged.

Special Facilities or Resources: The college's Curriculum Research and Development Group affords opportunities for involvement in a wide variety of educational research and program evaluation activities, many of which are centered in the K-12 laboratory school on campus.

Information for Students With Physical Disabilities: See the following Web site for more information: http://www.hawaii.edu/kokua/.

Application Information:
Send to Department of Educational Psychology, College of Education, 1776 University Avenue, Honolulu, HI 96822. Application available online. URL of online application: http://www.coe.hawaii.edu/edep/apply. Students are admitted in the Fall, application deadline February 1; Spring, application deadline September 1. PhD program has Fall admission only. Applications from foreign students have deadlines of January 15 and August 1 for Fall and Spring admission, respectively. Fee: $70. Application Fee for non-U.S. Citizens is $70.

Hawaii, University of, Manoa
Department of Psychology
College of Social Sciences
Sakamaki Hall, 2530 Dole Street
Honolulu, HI 96822-2294
Telephone: (808) 956-8414
Fax: (808) 956-4700
E-mail: *gradpsy@hawaii.edu*
Web: *http://www.psychology.hawaii.edu*

Department Information:
1939. Chairperson: Ashley E. Maynard, PhD. Number of faculty: total—full-time 23, part-time 3; women—full-time 8, part-time 1; total—minority—full-time 2.

Programs and Degrees Offered:
Listed in the following order: Program area, degree type (T if terminal Master's), number awarded 7/08–6/09. Social-Personality Psychology PhD (Doctor of Philosophy) 0, Cognition PhD (Doctor of Philosophy) 0, Developmental Psychology PhD (Doctor of Philosophy) 0, Experimental Psychopathology PhD (Doctor of Philosophy) 0, Behavioral Neuroscience PhD (Doctor of Philosophy) 0, Clinical Psychology PhD (Doctor of Philosophy) 7, Community and Cultural Psychology PhD (Doctor of Philosophy) 0.

APA Accreditation: Clinical PhD (Doctor of Philosophy).

Student Applications/Admissions:
Student Applications
Social-Personality Psychology PhD (Doctor of Philosophy)—Applications 2009–2010, 32. Total applicants accepted 2009–2010, 5. Number full-time enrolled (new admits only) 2009–2010, 3. Openings 2010–2011, 5. The number of students enrolled full- and part-time who were dismissed or voluntarily withdrew from this program area in 2008–2009 were 1. *Cognition PhD (Doctor of Philosophy)*—Applications 2009–2010, 6. Total applicants accepted 2009–2010, 2. Number full-time enrolled (new admits only) 2009–2010, 1. Openings 2010–2011, 4. The number of students enrolled full- and part-time who were dismissed or voluntarily withdrew from this program area in 2008–2009 were 0. *Developmental Psychology PhD (Doctor of Philosophy)*—Applications 2009–2010, 6. Total applicants accepted 2009–2010, 2. Number full-time enrolled (new admits only) 2009–2010, 1. Openings 2010–2011, 4. The number of students enrolled full- and part-time who were dismissed or voluntarily withdrew from this program area in 2008–2009 were 0. *Experimental Psychopathology PhD (Doctor of Philosophy)*—Applications 2009–2010, 0. Total applicants accepted 2009–2010, 0. Number full-time enrolled (new admits only) 2009–2010, 0. Openings 2010–2011, 3. The number of students enrolled full- and part-time who were dismissed or voluntarily withdrew from this program area in 2008–2009 were 0. *Behavioral Neuroscience PhD (Doctor of Philosophy)*—Applications 2009–2010, 12. Total applicants accepted 2009–2010, 2. Number full-time enrolled (new admits only) 2009–2010, 2. Openings 2010–2011, 3. The number of students enrolled full- and part-time who were dismissed or voluntarily withdrew from this program area in 2008–2009 were 1. *Clinical Psychology PhD (Doctor of Philosophy)*—Applications 2009–2010, 130. Total applicants accepted 2009–2010, 5. Number full-time

enrolled (new admits only) 2009–2010, 3. Number part-time enrolled (new admits only) 2009–2010, 0. Openings 2010–2011, 10. The median number of years required for completion of a degree in 2008–2009 were 6. The number of students enrolled full- and part-time who were dismissed or voluntarily withdrew from this program area in 2008–2009 were 0. *Community and Cultural Psychology PhD (Doctor of Philosophy)*— Applications 2009–2010, 30. Total applicants accepted 2009–2010, 3. Number full-time enrolled (new admits only) 2009–2010, 2. Openings 2010–2011, 5. The number of students enrolled full- and part-time who were dismissed or voluntarily withdrew from this program area in 2008–2009 were 0.

Other Criteria: (importance of criteria rated low, medium, or high): GRE scores—high, research experience—high, work experience—low, extracurricular activity—low, clinically related public service—low, GPA—high, letters of recommendation—high, statement of goals and objectives—high. For additional information on admission requirements, go to http://www.psychology.hawaii.edu/.

Student Characteristics: The following represents characteristics of students in 2009–2010 in all graduate psychology programs in the department: Female—full-time 64, part-time 0; Male—full-time 24, part-time 0; African American/Black—full-time 0, part-time 0; Hispanic/Latino(a)—full-time 0, part-time 0; Asian/Pacific Islander—full-time 29, part-time 0; American Indian/Alaska Native—full-time 0, part-time 0; Caucasian/White—full-time 0, part-time 0; Multi-ethnic—full-time 0, part-time 0; students subject to the Americans With Disabilities Act—full-time 0, part-time 0; Unknown ethnicity—full-time 0, part-time 0; International students who hold an F-1 or J-1 Visa—full-time 4, part-time 0.

Financial Information/Assistance:

Tuition for Full-Time Study: *Master's:* State residents: per academic year $8,928, $282 per credit hour; Nonstate residents: per academic year $21,552, $372 per credit hour. *Doctoral:* State residents: per academic year $8,928, $282 per credit hour; Nonstate residents: per academic year $21,552, $372 per credit hour. Tuition is subject to change. See the following Web site for updates and changes in tuition costs: http://manoa.hawaii.edu/records/tuition_fees/.

Financial Assistance:

First-Year Students: Teaching assistantships available for first year. Average amount paid per academic year: $13,296. Average number of hours worked per week: 20. Apply by January 1. Research assistantships available for first year. Average amount paid per academic year: $13,296. Average number of hours worked per week: 20. Apply by January 1. Fellowships and scholarships available for first year. Average amount paid per academic year: $6,800. Apply by January 1.

Advanced Students: Teaching assistantships available for advanced students. Average amount paid per academic year: $14,382. Average number of hours worked per week: 20. Apply by January 1. Research assistantships available for advanced students. Average amount paid per academic year: $14,382. Average number of hours worked per week: 20. Apply by January 1. Fellowships and scholarships available for advanced students. Average amount paid per academic year: $6,800. Apply by January 1.

Additional Information: Of all students currently enrolled full time, 31% benefited from one or more of the listed financial assistance programs. Application and information available online at: http://www.hawaii.edu/graduate/.

Internships/Practica: Doctoral Degree (PhD Clinical Psychology): For those doctoral students for whom a professional internship was required in this program prior to graduation, (7) students applied for an internship in 2008–2009, with (7) students obtaining an internship. Of those students who obtained an internship, (7) were paid internships. Of those students who obtained an internship, (7) students placed in APA/CPA accredited internships, (0) students placed in internships not APA/CPA accredited, but listed with the Association of Psychology Postdoctoral and Internship Programs (APPIC), (0) students placed in internships conforming to guidelines of the Council of Directors of School Psychology Programs (CDSPP), (0) students placed in internships that were not APA/CPA accredited, APPIC or CDSPP listed. A minimum of 2 years of practicum experience (18 to 20 hours per week) are required for all 2nd through 4th year graduate students in the Clinical Studies program. A variety of practicum sites are available throughout the state and most include stipend support (average $14,000 per academic year). Sites include the department's Cognitive Behavior Therapy Clinic, community mental health outpatient centers, VA (including PTSD specialty clinics), mental health hospitals, child mental health institutions, UH counseling center, and state supported work with the seriously mentally disabled population.

Housing and Day Care: On-campus housing is available. See the following Web site for more information: http://www.housing.hawaii.edu/. On-campus day care facilities are available. See the following Web site for more information: http://www.hawaii.edu/childrenscenter.

Employment of Department Graduates:

Master's Degree Graduates: Of those who graduated in the academic year 2008–2009, the following categories and numbers represent the postgraduate activities and employment of master's degree graduates: Enrolled in a postdoctoral residency/fellowship (n/a), employed in independent practice (n/a), total from the above (master's) (0).

Doctoral Degree Graduates: Of those who graduated in the academic year 2008–2009, the following categories and numbers represent the postgraduate activities and employment of doctoral degree graduates: Enrolled in a psychology doctoral program (n/a), total from the above (doctoral) (0).

Additional Information:

Orientation, Objectives, and Emphasis of Department: The Department of Psychology's orientation is best characterized as a synthesis of biological, behavioral, social, cognitive and developmental areas, with an overriding emphasis on empiricism (i.e., the study of psychological phenomena based on sound research findings). The graduate concentrations in clinical, developmental, community and cultural, behavioral neuroscience, experimental psychopathology, social-personality, and cognition emphasize the development of research skills and knowledge that are applicable to a wide range of academic and applied settings. The clinical program adheres to the scientist–practitioner model of training, wherein research and clinical skills are equally emphasized. Research opportunities in all graduate concentrations are available. The faculty is particularly interested in admitting students who are interested in pursuing academically related careers.

Special Facilities or Resources: The Psychology Department is mainly housed in Gartley Hall, a historic campus building. Gartley Hall is devoted to facilities for office space, research, and teaching in psychology. Faculty members have specialized laboratories for research, including equipment to support cognitive, social and developmental work. Graduate students are assigned shared office space in Gartley Hall and have access to most departmental facilities. The computing facilities in the department and university are of a high standard, and the campus has good wireless internet coverage. Opportunities for study and research also exist elsewhere at the university and in the community. These include the Pacific Biosciences Research Center, the John A. Burns School of Medicine, the Center for Disability Studies, the Hawaii State Hospital at Kaneohe, Leahi Hospital, the State Departments of Health and Education, and the Osher Lifelong Learning Institute. Beyond the physical facilities available to the department is the unusual opportunity for research provided by the unique social and environmental structure of Hawaii. An important dimension is also provided by the East-West Center for Cultural Interchange, which provides fellowships for Asian and U.S. students and for senior scholars from mainland and foreign universities.

Information for Students With Physical Disabilities: See the following Web site for more information: http://www.hawaii.edu/KOKUA.

Application Information:
Send to Graduate Admissions, Department of Psychology, University of Hawaii at Manoa, Sakamaki Hall, 2530 Dole Street, Honolulu, Hawaii 96822. Application available online. URL of online application: http://apply.hawaii.edu. Students are admitted in the Fall, application deadline January 1.

IDAHO

Idaho State University
Department of Psychology
Arts and Sciences
921 South 8th Avenue, Stop 8112
Pocatello, ID 83209
Telephone: (208) 282-2462
Fax: (208) 282-4832
E-mail: *lyncshan@isu.edu*
Web: *http://www.isu.edu/departments/psych*

Department Information:
1968. Interim Chair: Shannon Lynch. Number of faculty: total—full-time 12, part-time 13; women—full-time 8, part-time 2; total—minority—full-time 1, part-time 1; women minority—full-time 1; faculty subject to the Americans With Disabilities Act 1.

Programs and Degrees Offered:
Listed in the following order: Program area, degree type (T if terminal Master's), number awarded 7/08–6/09. General Experimental Psychology MA/MS (Master of Arts/Science) (T) 1, Clinical Psychology PhD (Doctor of Philosophy) 3.

APA Accreditation: Clinical PhD (Doctor of Philosophy). Student Outcome Data Website: http://www.isu.edu/departments/psych/clinicalprogram.shtml.

Student Applications/Admissions:
Student Applications
General Experimental Psychology MA/MS (*Master of Arts/Science*)—Applications 2009–2010, 8. Total applicants accepted 2009–2010, 4. Number full-time enrolled (new admits only) 2009–2010, 3. Number part-time enrolled (new admits only) 2009–2010, 0. Total enrolled 2009–2010 full-time, 5, part-time, 1. Openings 2010–2011, 5. The median number of years required for completion of a degree in 2008–2009 were 3. The number of students enrolled full- and part-time who were dismissed or voluntarily withdrew from this program area in 2008–2009 were 2. Clinical Psychology PhD (*Doctor of Philosophy*)—Applications 2009–2010, 46. Total applicants accepted 2009–2010, 8. Number full-time enrolled (new admits only) 2009–2010, 6. Number part-time enrolled (new admits only) 2009–2010, 0. Total enrolled 2009–2010 full-time, 29, part-time, 5. Openings 2010–2011, 6. The median number of years required for completion of a degree in 2008–2009 were 6. The number of students enrolled full- and part-time who were dismissed or voluntarily withdrew from this program area in 2008–2009 were 0.
Scores: Entries appear in this order: required test or GPA, minimum score (if required), median score of students entering in 2009–2010. General Experimental Psychology MA/MS (*Master of Arts/Science*): GRE-V no minimum stated, 530, GRE-Q no minimum stated, 630, GRE-Analytical no minimum stated, 4.5, GRE-Subject (Psychology) no minimum stated, 660, last 2 years GPA 3.0, 3.9; Clinical Psychology PhD (*Doctor of Philosophy*): GRE-V no minimum stated, 545, GRE-Q no minimum stated, 615, GRE-Analytical no minimum stated, 4.75, GRE-Subject (Psychology) no minimum stated, 705, last 2 years GPA 3.0, 3.9.
Other Criteria: (importance of criteria rated low, medium, or high): GRE scores—medium, research experience—high, work experience—low, extracurricular activity—low, clinically related public service—medium, GPA—medium, letters of recommendation—medium, interview—medium, statement of goals and objectives—medium, undergraduate major in psychology—medium, specific undergraduate psychology courses taken—low. For the general-experimental MS program, clinically related public service is not relevant. For additional information on admission requirements, go to http://www.isu.edu/psych/apply.shtml.

Student Characteristics: The following represents characteristics of students in 2009–2010 in all graduate psychology programs in the department: Female—full-time 23, part-time 5; Male—full-time 11, part-time 1; African American/Black—full-time 0, part-time 0; Hispanic/Latino(a)—full-time 0, part-time 1; Asian/Pacific Islander—full-time 1, part-time 0; American Indian/Alaska Native—full-time 0, part-time 0; Caucasian/White—full-time 33, part-time 5; Multi-ethnic—full-time 0, part-time 0; students subject to the Americans With Disabilities Act—full-time 1, part-time 0; Unknown ethnicity—full-time 0, part-time 0; International students who hold an F-1 or J-1 Visa—full-time 4, part-time 0.

Financial Information/Assistance:
Tuition for Full-Time Study: Master's: State residents: per academic year $5,848, $297 per credit hour; Nonstate residents: per academic year $15,650, $437 per credit hour. *Doctoral:* State residents: per academic year $5,848, $297 per credit hour; Nonstate residents: per academic year $15,650, $437 per credit hour. Tuition is subject to change. Additional fees are assessed to students beyond the costs of tuition for the following: $647 health insurance premium per semester, unless waived by proof of insurance. See the following Web site for updates and changes in tuition costs: http://www.isu.edu/finserv/costinfo.shtml.

Financial Assistance:
First-Year Students: Teaching assistantships available for first year. Average amount paid per academic year: $11,352. Average number of hours worked per week: 18. Apply by March 1. Traineeships available for first year. Average amount paid per academic year: $6,210. Average number of hours worked per week: 15. Apply by March 1.
Advanced Students: Teaching assistantships available for advanced students. Average amount paid per academic year: $11,352. Average number of hours worked per week: 18. Apply by March 1. Traineeships available for advanced students. Average amount paid per academic year: $10,350. Average number of hours worked per week: 15. Apply by March 1.
Additional Information: Of all students currently enrolled full time, 91% benefited from one or more of the listed financial assistance programs.

Internships/Practica: Doctoral Degree (PhD Clinical Psychology): For those doctoral students for whom a professional internship was required in this program prior to graduation, (9) students applied for an internship in 2008–2009, with (8) students obtaining an internship. Of those students who obtained an internship, (8) were paid internships. Of those students who obtained an internship, (6) students placed in APA/CPA accredited internships, (2) students placed in internships not APA/CPA accredited, but listed with the Association of Psychology Postdoctoral and Internship Programs (APPIC), (0) students placed in internships conforming to guidelines of the Council of Directors of School Psychology Programs (CDSPP), (0) students placed in internships that were not APA/CPA accredited, APPIC or CDSPP listed. Master's Degree (MA/MS General Experimental Psychology): An internship experience, such as a final research project or "capstone" experience is required of graduates. Clinical practica are required for doctoral students admitted into the MS-PhD clinical program. First and second year students complete practica in the ISU Psychology Clinic under the supervision of clinical faculty. Third and fourth year students, however, often participate in community practica and/or clinical externships under the supervision of licensed psychologists employed by local mental health providers/agencies. One semester participation on the ISU Interdisciplinary Evaluation Team is also required. Currently, eight clinical externship sites provide stipends and supervised practice in applied settings for twelve students. The average student entering APPIC internships from ISU during 2009-10 (n = 6) accumulated 1924 hours of supervised professional activities (median = 2,038 hours).

Housing and Day Care: On-campus housing is available. See the following Web site for more information: http://www.isu.edu/housing. On-campus day care facilities are available. See the following Web site for more information: http://www.isu.edu/earlylc.

Employment of Department Graduates:
Master's Degree Graduates: Of those who graduated in the academic year 2008–2009, the following categories and numbers represent the postgraduate activities and employment of master's degree graduates: Enrolled in a postdoctoral residency/fellowship (n/a), employed in independent practice (n/a), employed in an academic position at a 2-year/4-year college (1), total from the above (master's) (1).
Doctoral Degree Graduates: Of those who graduated in the academic year 2008–2009, the following categories and numbers represent the postgraduate activities and employment of doctoral degree graduates: Enrolled in a psychology doctoral program (n/a), enrolled in a postdoctoral residency/fellowship (1), employed in government agency (1), employed in a community mental health/counseling center (1), total from the above (doctoral) (3).

Additional Information:
Orientation, Objectives, and Emphasis of Department: The master of science program in general/experimental psychology provides students with an education in core areas of psychological science, such as personality/social, perception/cognitive, and sensory/physiological. This program of study, culminating in defense of a thesis, is designed to prepare students for doctoral work in psychology or careers in psychology or related fields that require mastery of the principles and methods of general/experimental psychology. The experimental MS in psychology is not intended to prepare students for careers in mental health. The department anticipates offering the doctoral degree in experimental psychology, pending final approval and funding. The mission of the clinical doctoral program is to train competent clinical psychologists who can apply and adapt general conceptual and technical skills in diverse regional and professional settings. An effective clinical psychologist possesses a strong professional identity that includes: (a) a firm grounding in the science of psychology, and (b) knowledge of relevant theories and technical skills that aid in the amelioration of human suffering. Most importantly, a clinical psychologist understands the interactive relationship between science and practice. As such, the educational philosophy of the clinical training program at ISU is based on the traditional scientist-practitioner model of clinical training.

Special Facilities or Resources: The Psychology Department has office and laboratory space for all faculty. The ISU Psychology Clinic, housed in the same building, provides four individual therapy rooms, two child/family rooms, two testing rooms, and a group therapy room, all equipped with observation systems and videotape capabilities. Office space is provided to graduate students. Computer access is available in offices, in the department, the clinic, and a university center located nearby. The university maintains an animal colony at which two Psychology faculty members participate, an Office of Sponsored Programs (grant assistance), and an instructional technical resource center (website assistance).

Information for Students With Physical Disabilities: See the following Web site for more information: http://www.isu.edu/ada4isu/.

Application Information:
Send to Admissions Committee, 921 South 8th Avenue, Stop 8112 Idaho State University, Pocatello, ID 83209. Application available online. URL of online application: http://www.isu.edu/psych/apply.shtml. Students are admitted in the Fall, application deadline January 1; Spring, application deadline November 1. For clinical students the deadline is January 1. Clinical students are only admitted to enter fall semester. For general MS students the fall admission deadline is March 1, and the spring admission deadline is November 1.

Idaho, University of
Department of Psychology and Communication Studies
Letters, Arts, and Social Sciences
University of Idaho
Moscow, ID 83844-3043
Telephone: (208) 885-6324
Fax: (208) 885-7710
E-mail: cberreth@uidaho.edu
Web: http://www.class.uidaho.edu/psychcomm

Department Information:
Chairperson: Kenneth Locke. Number of faculty: total—full-time 15, part-time 2; women—full-time 5, part-time 1; total—minority—full-time 2; women minority—full-time 1.

Programs and Degrees Offered:
Listed in the following order: Program area, degree type (T if terminal Master's), number awarded 7/08–6/09. General Experimental Psychology MA/MS (Master of Arts/Science) (T) 1, Hu-

man Factors MA/MS (Master of Arts/Science) (T) 6, Industrial/Organizational Psychology MA/MS (Master of Arts/Science) (T) 1, Neuroscience PhD (Doctor of Philosophy) 0.

Student Applications/Admissions:
Student Applications
General Experimental Psychology MA/MS (Master of Arts/Science)—Applications 2009–2010, 1. Total applicants accepted 2009–2010, 1. Number full-time enrolled (new admits only) 2009–2010, 1. Number part-time enrolled (new admits only) 2009–2010, 0. Openings 2010–2011, 1. The median number of years required for completion of a degree in 2008–2009 were 2. The number of students enrolled full- and part-time who were dismissed or voluntarily withdrew from this program area in 2008–2009 were 0. *Human Factors MA/MS (Master of Arts/Science)*—Applications 2009–2010, 22. Total applicants accepted 2009–2010, 14. Number full-time enrolled (new admits only) 2009–2010, 12. Number part-time enrolled (new admits only) 2009–2010, 1. Total enrolled 2009–2010 full-time, 20, part-time, 12. Openings 2010–2011, 8. The median number of years required for completion of a degree in 2008–2009 were 2. The number of students enrolled full- and part-time who were dismissed or voluntarily withdrew from this program area in 2008–2009 were 0. *Industrial/Organizational Psychology MA/MS (Master of Arts/Science)*—Applications 2009–2010, 5. Total applicants accepted 2009–2010, 0. Number full-time enrolled (new admits only) 2009–2010, 0. Number part-time enrolled (new admits only) 2009–2010, 0. The median number of years required for completion of a degree in 2008–2009 were 2. The number of students enrolled full- and part-time who were dismissed or voluntarily withdrew from this program area in 2008–2009 were 0. *Neuroscience PhD (Doctor of Philosophy)*—Applications 2009–2010, 0. Total applicants accepted 2009–2010, 0. Number full-time enrolled (new admits only) 2009–2010, 0. Number part-time enrolled (new admits only) 2009–2010, 0. Openings 2010–2011, 1. The median number of years required for completion of a degree in 2008–2009 were 5. The number of students enrolled full- and part-time who were dismissed or voluntarily withdrew from this program area in 2008–2009 were 0.
Scores: Entries appear in this order: required test or GPA, minimum score (if required), median score of students entering in 2009–2010. *General Experimental Psychology MA/MS (Master of Arts/Science)*: GRE-V no minimum stated, GRE-Q no minimum stated, overall undergraduate GPA 3.0; *Human Factors MA/MS (Master of Arts/Science)*: GRE-V no minimum stated, GRE-Q no minimum stated, overall undergraduate GPA 3.0; *Neuroscience PhD (Doctor of Philosophy)*: GRE-V no minimum stated, GRE-Q no minimum stated, GRE-Analytical 4.0, overall undergraduate GPA 3.0.
Other Criteria: (importance of criteria rated low, medium, or high): GRE scores—high, research experience—high, work experience—medium, extracurricular activity—low, GPA—high, letters of recommendation—high, statement of goals and objectives—high, undergraduate major in psychology—low, specific undergraduate psychology courses taken—low. Work experience more important for Human Factors and I/O candidates than General Experimental candidates.

Student Characteristics: The following represents characteristics of students in 2009–2010 in all graduate psychology programs in the department: Female—full-time 5, part-time 8; Male—full-time 14, part-time 5; African American/Black—full-time 0, part-time 0; Hispanic/Latino(a)—full-time 0, part-time 1; Asian/Pacific Islander—full-time 0, part-time 0; American Indian/Alaska Native—full-time 0, part-time 0; Caucasian/White—full-time 16, part-time 9; Multi-ethnic—full-time 0, part-time 0; students subject to the Americans With Disabilities Act—full-time 0, part-time 0; Unknown ethnicity—full-time 3, part-time 3; International students who hold an F-1 or J-1 Visa—full-time 1, part-time 0.

Financial Information/Assistance:
Tuition for Full-Time Study: Master's: State residents: per academic year $4,740, $227 per credit hour; Nonstate residents: per academic year $14,340, $367 per credit hour. Tuition is subject to change. See the following Web site for updates and changes in tuition costs: http://www.uidaho.edu/cogs.aspx.

Financial Assistance:
First-Year Students: Teaching assistantships available for first year. Average amount paid per academic year: $5,000. Average number of hours worked per week: 10. Apply by February 15. Research assistantships available for first year. Average amount paid per academic year: $10,000. Average number of hours worked per week: 20. Apply by February 15.
Advanced Students: Teaching assistantships available for advanced students. Average amount paid per academic year: $10,000. Average number of hours worked per week: 20. Apply by February 15. Research assistantships available for advanced students. Average amount paid per academic year: $10,500. Average number of hours worked per week: 20. Apply by February 15.
Additional Information: Of all students currently enrolled full time, 100% benefited from one or more of the listed financial assistance programs.

Internships/Practica: A few internships are available locally (e.g., human resources, usability testing, web analytics).

Housing and Day Care: On-campus housing is available. See the following Web site for more information: http://www.uidaho.edu/universityhousing.aspx. On-campus day care facilities are available. See the following Web site for more information: http://www.students.uidaho.edu/uikids/.

Employment of Department Graduates:
Master's Degree Graduates: Of those who graduated in the academic year 2008–2009, the following categories and numbers represent the postgraduate activities and employment of master's degree graduates: Enrolled in a psychology doctoral program (2), enrolled in another graduate/professional program (0), enrolled in a postdoctoral residency/fellowship (n/a), employed in independent practice (n/a), employed in an academic position at a university (0), employed in an academic position at a 2-year/4-year college (0), employed in other positions at a higher education institution (0), employed in a professional position in a school system (0), employed in business or industry (2), employed in government agency (2), employed in a community mental health/counseling center (0), employed in a hospital/medical center (0), still seeking employment (0), other employment position (1), total from the above (master's) (7).
Doctoral Degree Graduates: Of those who graduated in the academic year 2008–2009, the following categories and numbers represent the postgraduate activities and employment of doctoral

degree graduates: Enrolled in a psychology doctoral program (n/a), total from the above (doctoral) (0).

Additional Information:
Orientation, Objectives, and Emphasis of Department: In the Land Grant tradition of providing a "practical education," the Department of Psychology at the University of Idaho offers the MS degree in psychology with emphases in either Industrial/Organizational psychology (human resources, personnel, selection, organizational behavior) or Human Factors psychology (human technology interaction, ergonomics, human performance). The Department also provides off-campus and distance educational outreach by offering the MS in Psychology (Human Factors option only) through video and compressed video. The intent of both emphases is to develop knowledge and skills germane to a professional position. However, both programs also provide appropriate preparation for further graduate study. Thus, students are encouraged to develop analytical and problem solving skills that will serve them well in whatever they choose to do after graduation. Student placement figures show that most graduates have been very successful in obtaining positions in technical industries. The department is small, but is able to address the broad needs of its students through working relationships with the College of Business and Economics, the College of Engineering, and the Department of Psychology at nearby (9 miles) Washington State University. The department will consider, and has occasionally admitted, students for the general experimental MS. General experimental students typically use the program to prepare for admission to doctoral programs elsewhere. In 2004, the department began admitting students seeking a PhD degree in Neuroscience. This degree is interdisciplinary, and our primary partner is the Department of Biological Sciences.

Special Facilities or Resources: The department provides over 3000 square feet of research space. Labs are equipped with cutting-edge technology (e.g., driving and flight simulators, immersive virtual reality displays, multiple graphics workstations, eye-and head-tracking technology, six web cameras with a quad multiplexer to allow for simultaneous recording of four camera views simultaneously). Research opportunities are available at remote sites, such as the Motion Analysis Lab at Shriners Hospital in Spokane, WA.

Information for Students With Physical Disabilities: See the following Web site for more information: http://www.access.uidaho.edu/.

Application Information:
Send to Graduate Admissions. Application available online. URL of online application: http://www.uidaho.edu/cogs/admissions.aspx. Students are admitted in the Fall, application deadline February 15. Applications will be considered after the deadline, but availability of funding declines with passage of time. *Fee:* $30.

ILLINOIS

Adler School of Professional Psychology
Professional School
17 North Dearborn Street
Chicago, IL 60603-2301
Telephone: (312) 201-5900
Fax: (312) 201-5917
E-mail: dcastroblanco@adler.edu
Web: http://www.adler.edu

Department Information:
1952. PsyD Program Director: David Castro-Blanco, PhD, ABPP. Number of faculty: total—full-time 38, part-time 4; women—full-time 19; total—minority—full-time 9, part-time 1; women minority—full-time 7.

Programs and Degrees Offered:
Listed in the following order: Program area, degree type (T if terminal Master's), number awarded 7/08–6/09. Rehabilitation Counseling MA/MS (Master of Arts/Science) (T) 0, Art Therapy/Counseling MA/MS (Master of Arts/Science) (T) 27, Marriage and Family Counseling MA/MS (Master of Arts/Science) (T) 16, Clinical Psychology PsyD (Doctor of Psychology) 43, Counseling Psychology MA/MS (Master of Arts/Science) (T) 49, Organizational Psychology MA/MS (Master of Arts/Science) (T) 5, Sport and Health Psychology MA/MS (Master of Arts/Science) (T) 0, Police Psychology MA/MS (Master of Arts/Science) (T) 18, Gerontological Counseling MA/MS (Master of Arts/Science) (T) 0, Forensic Psychology MA/MS (Master of Arts/Science) (T) 0.

APA Accreditation: Clinical PsyD (Doctor of Psychology). Student Outcome Data Website: http://www.adler.edu/about/APAAdditionalInformation.asp.

Student Applications/Admissions:
Student Applications
Rehabilitation Counseling MA/MS (Master of Arts/Science)—Applications 2009–2010, 25. Total applicants accepted 2009–2010, 18. Number full-time enrolled (new admits only) 2009–2010, 9. Number part-time enrolled (new admits only) 2009–2010, 0. Openings 2010–2011, 15. The number of students enrolled full- and part-time who were dismissed or voluntarily withdrew from this program area in 2008–2009 were 0. *Art Therapy/Counseling MA/MS (Master of Arts/Science)*—Applications 2009–2010, 90. Total applicants accepted 2009–2010, 55. Number full-time enrolled (new admits only) 2009–2010, 28. Number part-time enrolled (new admits only) 2009–2010, 0. Total enrolled 2009–2010 full-time, 60, part-time, 4. Openings 2010–2011, 30. The median number of years required for completion of a degree in 2008–2009 were 2. The number of students enrolled full- and part-time who were dismissed or voluntarily withdrew from this program area in 2008–2009 were 3. *Marriage and Family Counseling MA/MS (Master of Arts/Science)*—Applications 2009–2010, 95. Total applicants accepted 2009–2010, 45. Number full-time enrolled (new admits only) 2009–2010, 26. Number part-time enrolled (new admits only) 2009–2010, 0. Total enrolled 2009–2010 full-time, 40, part-time, 1. Openings 2010–2011, 30. The median number of years required for completion of a degree in 2008–2009 were 2. The number of students enrolled full- and part-time who were dismissed or voluntarily withdrew from this program area in 2008–2009 were 0. *Clinical Psychology PsyD (Doctor of Psychology)*—Applications 2009–2010, 480. Total applicants accepted 2009–2010, 202. Number full-time enrolled (new admits only) 2009–2010, 69. Number part-time enrolled (new admits only) 2009–2010, 0. Total enrolled 2009–2010 full-time, 500, part-time, 38. Openings 2010–2011, 80. The median number of years required for completion of a degree in 2008–2009 were 6. The number of students enrolled full- and part-time who were dismissed or voluntarily withdrew from this program area in 2008–2009 were 9. *Counseling Psychology MA/MS (Master of Arts/Science)*—Applications 2009–2010, 200. Total applicants accepted 2009–2010, 90. Number full-time enrolled (new admits only) 2009–2010, 79. Number part-time enrolled (new admits only) 2009–2010, 0. Total enrolled 2009–2010 full-time, 80, part-time, 9. Openings 2010–2011, 40. The median number of years required for completion of a degree in 2008–2009 were 2. The number of students enrolled full- and part-time who were dismissed or voluntarily withdrew from this program area in 2008–2009 were 5. *Organizational Psychology MA/MS (Master of Arts/Science)*—Applications 2009–2010, 40. Total applicants accepted 2009–2010, 25. Number full-time enrolled (new admits only) 2009–2010, 20. Number part-time enrolled (new admits only) 2009–2010, 0. Total enrolled 2009–2010 full-time, 40, part-time, 11. Openings 2010–2011, 15. The median number of years required for completion of a degree in 2008–2009 were 2. The number of students enrolled full- and part-time who were dismissed or voluntarily withdrew from this program area in 2008–2009 were 7. *Sport and Health Psychology MA/MS (Master of Arts/Science)*—Applications 2009–2010, 25. Total applicants accepted 2009–2010, 20. Number full-time enrolled (new admits only) 2009–2010, 0. Number part-time enrolled (new admits only) 2009–2010, 0. Openings 2010–2011, 15. The number of students enrolled full- and part-time who were dismissed or voluntarily withdrew from this program area in 2008–2009 were 0. *Police Psychology MA/MS (Master of Arts/Science)*—Applications 2009–2010, 30. Total applicants accepted 2009–2010, 25. Number full-time enrolled (new admits only) 2009–2010, 13. Number part-time enrolled (new admits only) 2009–2010, 0. Total enrolled 2009–2010 full-time, 57, part-time, 6. Openings 2010–2011, 20. The median number of years required for completion of a degree in 2008–2009 were 2. The number of students enrolled full- and part-time who were dismissed or voluntarily withdrew from this program area in 2008–2009 were 0. *Gerontological Counseling MA/MS (Master of Arts/Science)*—Applications 2009–2010, 20. Total applicants accepted 2009–2010, 15. Number full-time enrolled (new admits only) 2009–2010, 3. Number part-time enrolled (new admits only) 2009–2010, 1. Total enrolled 2009–2010 full-time, 3, part-time, 1. Openings 2010–2011, 12. The number of students enrolled full- and part-time who were dismissed or voluntarily withdrew from this program area in 2008–2009 were 0. *Forensic Psychology MA/MS (Master of Arts/Science)*—Applications 2009–2010, 40. Total applicants accepted 2009–

2010, 25. Number full-time enrolled (new admits only) 2009–2010, 0. Number part-time enrolled (new admits only) 2009–2010, 0. Openings 2010–2011, 15. The number of students enrolled full- and part-time who were dismissed or voluntarily withdrew from this program area in 2008–2009 were 0.

Scores: Entries appear in this order: required test or GPA, minimum score (if required), median score of students entering in 2009–2010. *Rehabilitation Counseling MA/MS (Master of Arts/Science):* overall undergraduate GPA 3.0, 3.21; *Art Therapy/Counseling MA/MS (Master of Arts/Science):* overall undergraduate GPA 3.0, 3.21; *Marriage and Family Counseling MA/MS (Master of Arts/Science):* overall undergraduate GPA 3.0, 3.21; *Clinical Psychology PsyD (Doctor of Psychology):* overall undergraduate GPA 3.25, 3.21, Masters GPA no minimum stated, 3.41; *Counseling Psychology MA/MS (Master of Arts/Science):* overall undergraduate GPA 3.0, 3.21; *Organizational Psychology MA/MS (Master of Arts/Science):* overall undergraduate GPA 3.0, 3.21; *Sport and Health Psychology MA/MS (Master of Arts/Science):* overall undergraduate GPA 3.0, 3.21; *Police Psychology MA/MS (Master of Arts/Science):* overall undergraduate GPA 3.0, 3.21; *Gerontological Counseling MA/MS (Master of Arts/Science):* overall undergraduate GPA 3.0, 3.21; *Forensic Psychology MA/MS (Master of Arts/Science):* overall undergraduate GPA 3.0, 3.21.

Other Criteria: (importance of criteria rated low, medium, or high): research experience—medium, work experience—medium, extracurricular activity—medium, clinically related public service—high, GPA—high, letters of recommendation—high, interview—high, statement of goals and objectives—high, interest in mission—high, undergraduate major in psychology—medium, specific undergraduate psychology courses taken—medium. Masters in Art Therapy must also have 18 studio credits of art and present a portfolio at the time of interview. For additional information on admission requirements, go to http://www.adler.edu.

Student Characteristics: The following represents characteristics of students in 2009–2010 in all graduate psychology programs in the department: Female—full-time 630, part-time 50; Male—full-time 159, part-time 20; African American/Black—full-time 85, part-time 12; Hispanic/Latino(a)—full-time 51, part-time 8; Asian/Pacific Islander—full-time 36, part-time 2; American Indian/Alaska Native—full-time 2, part-time 0; Caucasian/White—full-time 530, part-time 40; Multi-ethnic—full-time 19, part-time 3; students subject to the Americans With Disabilities Act—full-time 18, part-time 7; Unknown ethnicity—full-time 66, part-time 5; International students who hold an F-1 or J-1 Visa—full-time 45, part-time 0.

Financial Information/Assistance:
Tuition for Full-Time Study: Master's: State residents: per academic year $26,400, $880 per credit hour; Nonstate residents: per academic year $26,400, $880 per credit hour. Doctoral: State residents: per academic year $27,600, $920 per credit hour; Nonstate residents: per academic year $27,600, $920 per credit hour. Tuition is subject to change. Additional fees are assessed to students beyond the costs of tuition for the following: Student Services Fee, Lab Fee, Professional Liability Insurances Fee, UPass (for full time students). Tuition costs vary by program. See the following Web site for updates and changes in tuition costs: http://www.adler.edu.

Financial Assistance:
First-Year Students: Teaching assistantships available for first year. Average amount paid per academic year: $5,700. Average number of hours worked per week: 10. Research assistantships available for first year. Average amount paid per academic year: $5,700. Average number of hours worked per week: 10. Fellowships and scholarships available for first year. Average amount paid per academic year: $10,000.

Advanced Students: Teaching assistantships available for advanced students. Average amount paid per academic year: $5,700. Average number of hours worked per week: 10. Research assistantships available for advanced students. Average amount paid per academic year: $5,700. Average number of hours worked per week: 10. Fellowships and scholarships available for advanced students. Average amount paid per academic year: $5,000. Apply by May 15.

Additional Information: Of all students currently enrolled full time, 3% benefited from one or more of the listed financial assistance programs

Internships/Practica: Doctoral Degree (PsyD Clinical Psychology): For those doctoral students for whom a professional internship was required in this program prior to graduation, (53) students applied for an internship in 2008–2009, with (44) students obtaining an internship. Of those students who obtained an internship, (44) were paid internships. Of those students who obtained an internship, (25) students placed in APA/CPA accredited internships, (17) students placed in internships not APA/CPA accredited, but listed with the Association of Psychology Postdoctoral and Internship Programs (APPIC), (0) students placed in internships conforming to guidelines of the Council of Directors of School Psychology Programs (CDSPP), (2) students placed in internships that were not APA/CPA accredited, APPIC or CDSPP listed. Master's Degree (MA/MS Rehabilitation Counseling): An internship experience, such as a final research project or "capstone" experience is required of graduates. Master's Degree (MA/MS Art Therapy/Counseling): An internship experience, such as a final research project or "capstone" experience is required of graduates. Master's Degree (MA/MS Marriage and Family Counseling): An internship experience, such as a final research project or "capstone" experience is required of graduates. Master's Degree (MA/MS Counseling Psychology): An internship experience, such as a final research project or "capstone" experience is required of graduates. Master's Degree (MA/MS Organizational Psychology): An internship experience, such as a final research project or "capstone" experience is required of graduates. Master's Degree (MA/MS Sport and Health Psychology): An internship experience, such as a final research project or "capstone" experience is required of graduates. Master's Degree (MA/MS Police Psychology): An internship experience, such as a final research project or "capstone" experience is required of graduates. Master's Degree (MA/MS Gerontological Counseling): An internship experience, such as a final research project or "capstone" experience is required of graduates. Master's Degree (MA/MS Forensic Psychology): An internship experience, such as a final research project or "capstone" experience is required of graduates. Practicum training is a core component of the educational experience at the Adler School. Students in both the doctoral and masters programs are required to undertake a Community Service Practicum, designed to provide practical application of the principles of socially responsible practice central to the training model. Students in the doctoral program also engage in assessment and intervention practicum experiences, and many engage in advanced practica prior to their internship training. The training department works diligently to match student interests and skills with available training venues, and our affiliation with large, regional social service organizations, such as Heartland Alliance, provide students with a wide array of opportunities to work with diverse and traditionally underserved populations in settings ranging from correctional facilities to family service agencies. The Adler Psychological Services Center, comprised of several mental and general healthcare settings, offers training to practicum students as well as an APA accredited internship site. The Training Department works to prepare students for the internship application process and Adler students have enjoyed considerable success in matching for APPIC affiliated internships. Training is guided by an emphasis on evidence-based practice and the principles of social responsibility and justice.

Housing and Day Care: No on-campus housing is available. No on-campus day care facilities are available.

Employment of Department Graduates:
Master's Degree Graduates: Of those who graduated in the academic year 2008–2009, the following categories and numbers represent the postgraduate activities and employment of master's degree graduates: Enrolled in a postdoctoral residency/fellowship (n/a), employed in independent practice (n/a), total from the above (master's) (0).
Doctoral Degree Graduates: Of those who graduated in the academic year 2008–2009, the following categories and numbers represent the postgraduate activities and employment of doctoral degree graduates: Enrolled in a psychology doctoral program (n/a), total from the above (doctoral) (0).

Additional Information:
Orientation, Objectives, and Emphasis of Department: Established in 1952, the Adler School follows in the tradition of Alfred Adler, founder of community psychology. Adlerian theory, especially its emphasis on social responsibility and justice, forms the theoretical basis for training across programs, and as a platform for exposure to a broad array of theoretical approaches. A core principle common to the doctoral and masters programs at Adler is the incorporation of socially responsible practice in didactic, seminar and applied training experiences. In addition to Adlerian psychotherapy, students in the doctoral program are able to obtain training in a variety of theoretical approaches, including cognitive-behavioral, humanistic, psychodynamic and group therapies. In addition, concentrations in specialty areas, such as integrated healthcare, trauma-related intervention, child and adolescent treatment and clinical hypnosis are available. Graduates of the masters programs are prepared for license-eligible work as counselors in areas as diverse as gerontology, rehabilitation, marriage and family therapy and organizations. Doctoral program graduates often go on to serve their communities as clinicians, advocates, researchers and policy makers. Students learn to think critically, understand and utilize the available evidence in making informed clinical decisions and incorporate what Adler referred to as Social Interest in all their professional endeavors.

Special Facilities or Resources: Our new facility offers state of the art and accessible computer, classroom, lab and common area facilities located in the heart of downtown Chicago. The Adler Institutes for Social Justice (Institute of Social Exclusion and Institute of Public Safety and Social Justice) sponsor national conferences of interest in the areas of social responsibility and public health. In addition, their affiliations with major community organizations provide students at all levels of training with opportunities for practicum and internship training with culturally diverses and traditionally underserved groups. These placements provide a practical application of the principles of social justice and responsibility that form the core of the training experience at the Adler School. The library offers a vast array of electronic journal and print holdings, made more extensive by institutional lending agreements and consortium affiliations. In addition, the library boasts a large collection of the works of both, Alfred Adler and the school's founder, Rudolf Dreikurs. The Institutional Review Board is federally registered and the school possesses a Federal Wide Assurance certificate, facilitating efforts to secure extramural funding for research and educational programming.

Application Information:
Send to Office of Admissions, 65 E Wacker Place Suite 2100, Chicago, IL 60601. Application available online. URL of online application: http://www.adler.edu. Students are admitted in the Fall, application deadline February 15. PsyD priority deadline is February 15. All MA programs are on rolling admissions basis. *Fee:* $50. Fee is waived for McNair Scholars.

Argosy University/Chicago (formerly the Illinois School of Professional Psychology)
Clinical Psychology Programs
225 North Michigan, Suite 1300
Chicago, IL 60601
Telephone: (312) 777-7600
Fax: (312) 777-7750
E-mail: *aslobig@argosy.edu*
Web: *http://www.auconnection.net/chicago/chi_home.asp*

Department Information:
1976. Dean of the Clinical Psychology Programs: Annemarie Slobig. Number of faculty: total—full-time 28, part-time 7; women—full-time 13, part-time 4; total—minority—full-time 7; women minority—full-time 2.

Programs and Degrees Offered:
Listed in the following order: Program area, degree type (T if terminal Master's), number awarded 7/08–6/09. Clinical Psychology PsyD (Doctor of Psychology) 76.

APA Accreditation: Clinical PsyD (Doctor of Psychology).

Student Applications/Admissions:
Student Applications
Clinical Psychology PsyD (Doctor of Psychology)—Applications 2009–2010, 105. Total applicants accepted 2009–2010, 90. Number full-time enrolled (new admits only) 2009–2010, 73. Number part-time enrolled (new admits only) 2009–2010, 4. Total enrolled 2009–2010 full-time, 323, part-time, 103. Openings 2010–2011, 45. The median number of years required for completion of a degree in 2008–2009 were 6. The number of students enrolled full- and part-time who were

dismissed or voluntarily withdrew from this program area in 2008–2009 were 15.

Scores: Entries appear in this order: required test or GPA, minimum score (if required), median score of students entering in 2009–2010. *Clinical Psychology PsyD (Doctor of Psychology):* overall undergraduate GPA 3.25, last 2 years GPA 3.25, Masters GPA 3.25.

Other Criteria: (importance of criteria rated low, medium, or high): GRE scores—low, research experience—medium, work experience—high, extracurricular activity—medium, clinically related public service—high, GPA—high, letters of recommendation—high, interview—high, statement of goals and objectives—high, undergraduate major in psychology—low, specific undergraduate psychology courses taken—low.

Student Characteristics: The following represents characteristics of students in 2009–2010 in all graduate psychology programs in the department: Female—full-time 305, part-time 33; Male—full-time 90, part-time 8; African American/Black—full-time 55, part-time 12; Hispanic/Latino(a)—full-time 18, part-time 3; Asian/Pacific Islander—full-time 27, part-time 3; American Indian/Alaska Native—full-time 0, part-time 0; Caucasian/White—full-time 266, part-time 21; Multi-ethnic—full-time 7, part-time 0; students subject to the Americans With Disabilities Act—full-time 20, part-time 0; Unknown ethnicity—full-time 22, part-time 2; International students who hold an F-1 or J-1 Visa—full-time 3, part-time 0.

Financial Information/Assistance:

Tuition for Full-Time Study: Master's: State residents: per academic year $29,403, $998 per credit hour; Nonstate residents: per academic year $29,403, $998 per credit hour. *Doctoral:* State residents: per academic year $29,403, $998 per credit hour; Nonstate residents: per academic year $29,403, $998 per credit hour. Tuition is subject to change. Additional fees are assessed to students beyond the costs of tuition for the following: testing kit fee, technology fee.

Financial Assistance:

First-Year Students: Teaching assistantships available for first year. Average amount paid per academic year: $750. Average number of hours worked per week: 5. Apply by September 14. Fellowships and scholarships available for first year. Average amount paid per academic year: $25,000. Average number of hours worked per week: 100.

Advanced Students: Teaching assistantships available for advanced students. Average amount paid per academic year: $750. Average number of hours worked per week: 5. Apply by September 14. Fellowships and scholarships available for advanced students. Average amount paid per academic year: $25,000. Average number of hours worked per week: 100. Apply by November 15.

Additional Information: Of all students currently enrolled full time, 7% benefited from one or more of the listed financial assistance programs. Application and information available online at: http://www.auconnection.net/chicago/stfinace.

Internships/Practica: Doctoral Degree (PsyD Clinical Psychology): For those doctoral students for whom a professional internship was required in this program prior to graduation, (74) students applied for an internship in 2008–2009, with (66) students obtaining an internship. Of those students who obtained an internship, (61) were paid internships. Of those students who obtained an internship, (28) students placed in APA/CPA accredited internships, (28) students placed in internships not APA/CPA accredited, but listed with the Association of Psychology Postdoctoral and Internship Programs (APPIC), (0) students placed in internships conforming to guidelines of the Council of Directors of School Psychology Programs (CDSPP), (10) students placed in internships that were not APA/CPA accredited, APPIC or CDSPP listed. The School approves and monitors over 300 practicum sites and assists students in locating and applying for internships across the country and in Canada. Both practicum and internship sites offer a wide range of training populations and approaches to students in the programs.

Housing and Day Care: No on-campus housing is available. No on-campus day care facilities are available.

Employment of Department Graduates:

Master's Degree Graduates: Of those who graduated in the academic year 2008–2009, the following categories and numbers represent the postgraduate activities and employment of master's degree graduates: Enrolled in a postdoctoral residency/fellowship (n/a), employed in independent practice (n/a), total from the above (master's) (0).

Doctoral Degree Graduates: Of those who graduated in the academic year 2008–2009, the following categories and numbers represent the postgraduate activities and employment of doctoral degree graduates: Enrolled in a psychology doctoral program (n/a), enrolled in another graduate/professional program (0), enrolled in a postdoctoral residency/fellowship (28), employed in independent practice (1), employed in an academic position at a university (2), employed in an academic position at a 2-year/4-year college (2), employed in other positions at a higher education institution (2), employed in a professional position in a school system (5), employed in government agency (1), employed in a community mental health/counseling center (8), employed in a hospital/medical center (10), still seeking employment (1), other employment position (4), do not know (14), total from the above (doctoral) (78).

Additional Information:

Orientation, Objectives, and Emphasis of Department: The Argosy University, Chicago programs prepare students for contemporary practice through a clinically focused curriculum, taught by practitioner-scholar faculty, with a strong commitment to quality teaching and supervision. The current curricula have been structured to provide students with the fundamental knowledge and skills in psychological assessment and psychotherapy necessary to work with a wide range of traditional clinical populations. In addition, the required curricula include courses and perspectives designed to prepare students for emerging populations from diverse backgrounds and contemporary practice approaches now addressed by clinical psychology. PsyD students may satisfy basic requirements that address the learning of fundamental knowledge and competencies in intervention, assessment, population diversity, and professional practice areas through elective clusters that also provide choices that may conform to their individualized professional goals. As part of the commitment to providing both general and concentrated education and training for doctoral students, the PsyD program offers nine minors, or optional areas of electives choices for students wishing to focus their predoctoral studies in particular areas.

Special Facilities or Resources: The Argosy, Chicago programs offers predoctoral minors which support students' interests in the following areas: Child/Adolescent Psychology, Health Psychology, Family Psychology, Forensic Psychology, Psychoanalytic Psychology, Client-Centered and Experiential Psychology, Diversity and Multicultural Psychology, Organizational Consulting, and Psychology and Spirituality. The School has over 300 practicum sites available for student training in agencies, schools, clinics, hospitals, and practice organizations. Several faculty at the School have ongoing research projects in the following areas, in which students are invited to participate as they engage in their Clinical Research Projects: Effects of mindfulness meditation techniques on medical residents, intergenerational patterns related to sexual abuse, psychology of women, psychology in the schools, intergenerational cultural patterns in mother-daughter relationships, client-centered therapy with the severely mentally ill, personality disorders.

Application Information:
Send to Admissions Department, Argosy University, Chicago, 225 N. Michigan, Suite 1300, Chicago, IL 60601. Application available online. URL of online application: http://www.argosy.edu. Students are admitted in the Fall, application deadline January 15; Spring, application deadline October 1; *Fee:* $50.

Argosy University/Schaumburg
Clinical Psychology
American School of Professional Psychology
999 North Plaza Drive, Suite 111
Schaumburg, IL 60173
Telephone: (847) 969-4900
Fax: (847) 969-4999
E-mail: *jwasner@argosy.edu*
Web: *http://www.argosy.edu*

Department Information:
1994. Dean, ASPP and Chair, Clinical Psychology: Jim Wasner, PhD. Number of faculty: total—full-time 16, part-time 20; women—full-time 8, part-time 10; total—minority—full-time 4, part-time 2; women minority—full-time 2, part-time 1; faculty subject to the Americans With Disabilities Act 1.

Programs and Degrees Offered:
Listed in the following order: Program area, degree type (T if terminal Master's), number awarded 7/08–6/09. Clinical Psychology MA/MS (Master of Arts/Science) (T) 15, Clinical Psychology PsyD (Doctor of Psychology) 23.

APA Accreditation: Clinical PsyD (Doctor of Psychology).

Student Applications/Admissions:
Student Applications
Clinical Psychology MA/MS (*Master of Arts/Science*)—Applications 2009–2010, 51. Total applicants accepted 2009–2010, 32. Number full-time enrolled (new admits only) 2009–2010, 20. Number part-time enrolled (new admits only) 2009–2010, 0. Total enrolled 2009–2010 full-time, 46, part-time, 4. Openings 2010–2011, 20. The median number of years required for completion of a degree in 2008–2009 were 2. The number of students enrolled full- and part-time who were dismissed or voluntarily withdrew from this program area in 2008–2009 were 6. *Clinical Psychology PsyD (Doctor of Psychology)*—Applications 2009–2010, 147. Total applicants accepted 2009–2010, 65. Number full-time enrolled (new admits only) 2009–2010, 47. Number part-time enrolled (new admits only) 2009–2010, 1. Total enrolled 2009–2010 full-time, 177, part-time, 49. Openings 2010–2011, 47. The median number of years required for completion of a degree in 2008–2009 were 5. The number of students enrolled full- and part-time who were dismissed or voluntarily withdrew from this program area in 2008–2009 were 5.

Other Criteria: (importance of criteria rated low, medium, or high): research experience—low, work experience—medium, extracurricular activity—low, clinically related public service—medium, GPA—high, letters of recommendation—high, interview—high, statement of goals and objectives—high, undergraduate major in psychology—medium, specific undergraduate psychology courses taken—high.

Student Characteristics: The following represents characteristics of students in 2009–2010 in all graduate psychology programs in the department: Female—full-time 192, part-time 41; Male—full-time 31, part-time 12; African American/Black—full-time 9, part-time 2; Hispanic/Latino(a)—full-time 6, part-time 1; Asian/Pacific Islander—full-time 3, part-time 1; American Indian/Alaska Native—full-time 2, part-time 0; Caucasian/White—full-time 197, part-time 47; Multi-ethnic—full-time 6, part-time 2; students subject to the Americans With Disabilities Act—full-time 3, part-time 1; Unknown ethnicity—full-time 0, part-time 0; International students who hold an F-1 or J-1 Visa—full-time 0, part-time 0.

Financial Information/Assistance:
Tuition for Full-Time Study: Master's: State residents: per academic year $24,950, $998 per credit hour; Nonstate residents: per academic year $24,950, $998 per credit hour. *Doctoral:* State residents: per academic year $24,950, $998 per credit hour; Nonstate residents: per academic year $24,950, $998 per credit hour. Tuition is subject to change.

Financial Assistance:
First-Year Students: Teaching assistantships available for first year. Average amount paid per academic year: $2,000. Average number of hours worked per week: 5. Traineeships available for first year. Average amount paid per academic year: $2,000. Average number of hours worked per week: 7. Fellowships and scholarships available for first year. Average amount paid per academic year: $2,000.

Advanced Students: Teaching assistantships available for advanced students. Average amount paid per academic year: $2,000. Average number of hours worked per week: 5. Traineeships available for advanced students. Average amount paid per academic year: $2,000. Average number of hours worked per week: 7. Fellowships and scholarships available for advanced students. Average amount paid per academic year: $2,000.

Additional Information: Of all students currently enrolled full time, 13% benefited from one or more of the listed financial assistance programs.

Internships/Practica: Doctoral Degree (PsyD Clinical Psychology): For those doctoral students for whom a professional internship was required in this program prior to graduation, (44) students applied for an internship in 2008–2009, with (38) students obtaining an internship. Of those students who obtained an internship, (35) were paid internships. Of those students who obtained an internship, (12) students placed in APA/CPA accredited internships, (24) students placed in internships not APA/CPA accredited, but listed with the Association of Psychology Postdoctoral and Internship Programs (APPIC), (0) students placed in internships conforming to guidelines of the Council of Directors of School Psychology Programs (CDSPP), (2) students placed in internships that were not APA/CPA accredited, APPIC or CDSPP listed. Clinical field training is a required component of all programs at the American School of Professional Psychology at Argosy University, Schaumburg and is a direct outgrowth of the practitioner emphasis of professional psychology. The school provides advisement and assistance in placing students in a wide variety of clinical sites, including hospitals, schools, mental health facilities, treatment centers, and social service agencies. The MA in clinical psychology requires a minimum of 750 hours of practicum experience. The PsyD program includes two years of practicum experience, including separate practica for diagnosis and assessment, and psychotherapy, with a minimum of 900 hours per year; plus an additional one-year full-time clinical internship.

Housing and Day Care: No on-campus housing is available. No on-campus day care facilities are available.

Employment of Department Graduates:
Master's Degree Graduates: Of those who graduated in the academic year 2008–2009, the following categories and numbers represent the postgraduate activities and employment of master's degree graduates: Enrolled in a psychology doctoral program (9), enrolled in a postdoctoral residency/fellowship (n/a), employed in independent practice (n/a), employed in a community mental health/counseling center (3), employed in a hospital/medical center (1), other employment position (1), do not know (1), total from the above (master's) (15).
Doctoral Degree Graduates: Of those who graduated in the academic year 2008–2009, the following categories and numbers represent the postgraduate activities and employment of doctoral degree graduates: Enrolled in a psychology doctoral program (n/a), enrolled in another graduate/professional program (0), enrolled in a postdoctoral residency/fellowship (9), employed in independent practice (3), employed in an academic position at a university (2), employed in an academic position at a 2-year/4-year college (1), employed in other positions at a higher education institution (1), employed in a professional position in a school system (3), employed in a community mental health/counseling center (3), employed in a hospital/medical center (1), total from the above (doctoral) (23).

Additional Information:
Orientation, Objectives, and Emphasis of Department: The primary purpose of the Clinical Psychology program of the American School of Professional Psychology at Argosy University, Schaumburg is to educate and train students in the major aspects of clinical practice and prepare students for careers as practitioners. To ensure that students are prepared adequately, the curriculum integrates theory, training, research, and practice in preparing students to work with a wide range of populations in need of psychological services. Faculty are both scholars and practitioners and guide students through coursework and field experiences so that they might learn the work involved in professional psychology and understand how formal knowledge and practice operate to inform and enrich each other. The emphasis of the school is a scholar/practitioner orientation, with faculty skilled in all major theories of assessment and intervention. Working closely with faculty, students are provided with exposure to a variety of diagnostic and therapeutic approaches. Sensitivity to diverse populations, populations with specific needs, and multicultural issues are important components of all programs. The program also has emphasis areas in forensic psychology, neuropsychology, clinical health psychology, child and family psychology, and multicultural psychology. Certificate programs in Forensics, Clinical Health and Neuropsychology are available to both PsyD and postgraduate students.

Special Facilities or Resources: Faculty members actively encourage student involvement in research projects as a means of fostering mentoring relationships. The American School of Professional Psychology at Schaumburg Campus has core faculty with extensive experience, enthusiasm, and expertise in the following areas: clinical research, forensic psychology, clinical health and rehabilitation psychology, brief therapy, cognitive-behavioral therapy, client-centered and experiential therapy, emotion focused therapy, severe psychopathology, substance abuse, addictive disorders, family and couples therapy, child development and therapy, psychodiagnostics, psychology of women, sexual orientation diversity, domestic violence, neuropsychology (adult and pediatric), clinical hypnosis, and psychoanalysis. In addition, the clinical training department has contracts with the Illinois Department of Correction at several correctional facilities to provide training in forensic psychology to practicum students, interns and postdoctoral fellows. These training contracts allow students to blend the knowledge attained in the classroom with professional on-site training in correctional and forensic psychology.

Application Information:
Send to Katie Curran, Director of Admissions, 999 N. Plaza Drive, Suite 111, Schaumburg, Illinois 60173. Application available online. URL of online application: http://www.argosy.edu. Students are admitted in the Fall, application deadline May 15; Spring, application deadline November 15. Deadlines may be extended dependent upon space availability. *Fee:* $50.

Benedictine University
Graduate Department of Clinical Psychology
College of Liberal Arts
5700 College Road
Lisle, IL 60532
Telephone: (630) 829-6230
Fax: (630) 829-6231
E-mail: *jbooth@ben.edu*
Web: *http://www.ben.edu*

Department Information:
1967. Chairperson: James K. Crissman. Number of faculty: total—full-time 5, part-time 7; women—full-time 3, part-time 5.

Programs and Degrees Offered:
Listed in the following order: Program area, degree type (T if terminal Master's), number awarded 7/08–6/09. Clinical Psychology MA/MS (Master of Arts/Science) (T) 20.

Student Applications/Admissions:
Student Applications
Clinical Psychology MA/MS (Master of Arts/Science)—Applications 2009–2010, 30. Total applicants accepted 2009–2010, 16. Number full-time enrolled (new admits only) 2009–2010, 10. Number part-time enrolled (new admits only) 2009–2010, 10. Total enrolled 2009–2010 full-time, 35, part-time, 45. Openings 2010–2011, 25. The median number of years required for completion of a degree in 2008–2009 were 2. The number of students enrolled full- and part-time who were dismissed or voluntarily withdrew from this program area in 2008–2009 were 2.

Other Criteria: (importance of criteria rated low, medium, or high): GRE scores—medium, research experience—low, work experience—medium, extracurricular activity—medium, clinically related public service—high, GPA—medium, letters of recommendation—high, interview—high, statement of goals and objectives—high, undergraduate major in psychology—low, specific undergraduate psychology courses taken—medium. For additional information on admission requirements, go to http://www.ben.edu/admissions/graduate.

Student Characteristics: The following represents characteristics of students in 2009–2010 in all graduate psychology programs in the department: Female—full-time 11, part-time 51; Male—full-time 5, part-time 3; African American/Black—full-time 2, part-time 4; Hispanic/Latino(a)—full-time 4, part-time 1; Asian/Pacific Islander—full-time 2, part-time 0; American Indian/Alaska Native—full-time 0, part-time 0; Caucasian/White—full-time 8, part-time 0; Multi-ethnic—full-time 0, part-time 0; students subject to the Americans With Disabilities Act—full-time 1, part-time 1; Unknown ethnicity—full-time 0, part-time 0; International students who hold an F-1 or J-1 Visa—full-time 0, part-time 0.

Financial Information/Assistance:
Tuition for Full-Time Study: *Master's:* State residents: $490 per credit hour; Nonstate residents: $490 per credit hour. Tuition is subject to change. See the following Web site for updates and changes in tuition costs: http://www.ben.edu/admissions/tuition_fees.asp.

Financial Assistance:
First-Year Students: No information provided.
Advanced Students: No information provided.
Additional Information: Of all students currently enrolled full time, 0% benefited from one or more of the listed financial assistance programs. Application and information available online at: http://www.ben.edu/resources/financialaid/GradProgramTable03.htm.

Internships/Practica: Master's Degree (MA/MS Clinical Psychology): An internship experience, such as, a final research project or "capstone" experience is required of graduates. The program has established relationships with over 100 mental health agencies, in-patient, out-patient, and social service agencies in the Chicago metropolitan area.

Housing and Day Care: On-campus housing is available. See the following Web site for more information: http://www.founderswoods.com. No on-campus day care facilities are available.

Employment of Department Graduates:
Master's Degree Graduates: Of those who graduated in the academic year 2008–2009, the following categories and numbers represent the postgraduate activities and employment of master's degree graduates: Enrolled in a psychology doctoral program (5), enrolled in a postdoctoral residency/fellowship (n/a), employed in independent practice (n/a), total from the above (master's) (5).
Doctoral Degree Graduates: Of those who graduated in the academic year 2008–2009, the following categories and numbers represent the postgraduate activities and employment of doctoral degree graduates: Enrolled in a psychology doctoral program (n/a), total from the above (doctoral) (0).

Additional Information:
Orientation, Objectives, and Emphasis of Department: Our program is a rigorous one, offering two clinical internship experiences that more than meet the number of hours required for state licensure. Our program has a curriculum in place that satisfies all Licensed Clinical Professional Counselor (LCPC) licensure requirements. To date, more than 90% of our alumni have successfully passed the licensure exam. Our program is approved by the Illinois Department of Professional Regulation.

Special Facilities or Resources: The department has lab space provided for role play and audio and video taping. The university opened the state-of-art Kindlon Hall of Learning in fall 2001. The building has a beautiful new library and teaching facilities.

Application Information:
Send to Graduate Admissions, Benedictine University, 5700 College Road, Lisle, IL 60532. Application available online. URL of online application: http://www.ben.edu/admissions/graduate/application.asp. Programs have rolling admissions. *Fee:* $40. Application fee waived for Benedictine University, Illinois Benedictine College, or St. Procopius College alumni.

Chicago, University of (2009 data)
Department of Psychology
5848 South University Avenue
Chicago, IL 60637
Telephone: (773) 702-8861
Fax: (773) 702-0886
E-mail: *marj@uchicago.edu*
Web: *http://psychology.uchicago.edu/*

Department Information:
1893. Chairperson: Howard Nusbaum. Number of faculty: total—full-time 19; women—full-time 9; total—minority—full-time 1.

Programs and Degrees Offered:
Listed in the following order: Program area, degree type (T if terminal Master's), number awarded 7/08–6/09. Social PhD (Doctor of Philosophy) 2, Developmental PhD (Doctor of

GRADUATE STUDY IN PSYCHOLOGY

Philosophy) 2, Integrative Neuroscience PhD (Doctor of Philosophy) 0, Cognition Program PhD (Doctor of Philosophy) 5.

Student Applications/Admissions:

Student Applications

Social PhD (Doctor of Philosophy)—Applications 2009–2010, 93. Total applicants accepted 2009–2010, 0. Number full-time enrolled (new admits only) 2009–2010, 4. Number part-time enrolled (new admits only) 2009–2010, 0. Openings 2010–2011, 2. The median number of years required for completion of a degree in 2008–2009 were 5. The number of students enrolled full- and part-time who were dismissed or voluntarily withdrew from this program area in 2008–2009 were 1. *Developmental PhD (Doctor of Philosophy)*—Applications 2009–2010, 32. Total applicants accepted 2009–2010, 3. Number full-time enrolled (new admits only) 2009–2010, 2. Number part-time enrolled (new admits only) 2009–2010, 0. Openings 2010–2011, 3. The median number of years required for completion of a degree in 2008–2009 were 5. The number of students enrolled full- and part-time who were dismissed or voluntarily withdrew from this program area in 2008–2009 were 1. *Integrative Neuroscience PhD (Doctor of Philosophy)*—Applications 2009–2010, 54. Total applicants accepted 2009–2010, 2. Number full-time enrolled (new admits only) 2009–2010, 2. Number part-time enrolled (new admits only) 2009–2010, 0. Openings 2010–2011, 2. The number of students enrolled full- and part-time who were dismissed or voluntarily withdrew from this program area in 2008–2009 were 0. *Cognition Program PhD (Doctor of Philosophy)*—Applications 2009–2010, 47. Total applicants accepted 2009–2010, 4. Number full-time enrolled (new admits only) 2009–2010, 3. Number part-time enrolled (new admits only) 2009–2010, 0. Openings 2010–2011, 4. The median number of years required for completion of a degree in 2008–2009 were 6. The number of students enrolled full- and part-time who were dismissed or voluntarily withdrew from this program area in 2008–2009 were 0.

Other Criteria: (importance of criteria rated low, medium, or high): GRE scores—high, research experience—high, work experience—low, extracurricular activity—low, GPA—high, letters of recommendation—high, interview—medium, statement of goals and objectives—high, undergraduate major in psychology—medium, specific undergraduate psychology courses taken—medium. Some science background is helpful for the Integrative Neuroscience program. For additional information on admission requirements, go to http://psychology.uchicago.edu.

Student Characteristics: The following represents characteristics of students in 2009–2010 in all graduate psychology programs in the department: Female—full-time 37, part-time 0; Male—full-time 18, part-time 0; African American/Black—full-time 3, part-time 0; Hispanic/Latino(a)—full-time 2, part-time 0; Asian/Pacific Islander—full-time 0, part-time 0; American Indian/Alaska Native—full-time 0, part-time 0; Caucasian/White—full-time 54, part-time 0; Multi-ethnic—full-time 0, part-time 0; students subject to the Americans With Disabilities Act—full-time 0, part-time 0; Unknown ethnicity—full-time 0, part-time 0; International students who hold an F-1 or J-1 Visa—full-time 0, part-time 0.

Financial Information/Assistance:

Tuition for Full-Time Study: *Doctoral*: State residents: per academic year $40,432; Nonstate residents: per academic year $40,432. Tuition is subject to change. Additional fees are assessed to students beyond the costs of tuition for the following: an acitivty fee and a health and wellness fee. See the following Web site for updates and changes in tuition costs: http://bursar.uchicago.edu/tuition.html.

Financial Assistance:

First-Year Students: Research assistantships available for first year. Average number of hours worked per week: 10. Fellowships and scholarships available for first year. Average amount paid per academic year: $19,500. Apply by December 10.

Advanced Students: Teaching assistantships available for advanced students. Average amount paid per academic year: $3,000. Research assistantships available for advanced students. Fellowships and scholarships available for advanced students. Average amount paid per academic year: $19,500.

Additional Information: Of all students currently enrolled full time, 85% benefited from one or more of the listed financial assistance programs.

Housing and Day Care: On-campus housing is available. See the following Web site for more information: http://rs.chicago.edu. No on-campus day care facilities are available.

Employment of Department Graduates:

Master's Degree Graduates: Of those who graduated in the academic year 2008–2009, the following categories and numbers represent the postgraduate activities and employment of master's degree graduates: Enrolled in a postdoctoral residency/fellowship (n/a), employed in independent practice (n/a), total from the above (master's) (0).

Doctoral Degree Graduates: Of those who graduated in the academic year 2008–2009, the following categories and numbers represent the postgraduate activities and employment of doctoral degree graduates: Enrolled in a psychology doctoral program (n/a), enrolled in a postdoctoral residency/fellowship (5), employed in an academic position at a university (1), employed in other positions at a higher education institution (1), still seeking employment (1), other employment position (1), total from the above (doctoral) (9).

Additional Information:

Orientation, Objectives, and Emphasis of Department: The Department of Psychology at the University of Chicago has been for a century a leading center of scholarship, research and teaching in psychology and related fields. Department is organized into specialized programs that reflect the contemporary state of the discipline as well as the wide-ranging interests of its own faculty. The four areas are: the Cognition Program, the Developmental Psychology Program, the Integrative Neuroscience Program, and the Social Psychology Program. The interdisciplinary character of the University is further reflected in the close connections the Department of Psychology maintains with other departments in the University.

Special Facilities or Resources: Facilities include a Laboratory for Conceptual Psychology, an Audio Visual Laboratory, an Early Childhood Initiative, Institute for Mind and Biology, and a Center for Cognitive and Social Neuroscience.

Information for Students With Physical Disabilities: See the following Web site for more information: http://disabilities.uchicago.edu/.

Application Information:
Send to Social Science Division, Office of Admissions, Foster Hall 105, 1130 E. 59th Street, University of Chicago, Chicago, IL 60637. Application available online. URL of online application: https://grad-application.uchicago.edu/. Students are admitted in the Fall, application deadline December 10. *Fee:* $55.

DePaul University
Department of Psychology
2219 North Kenmore - Room 420
Chicago, IL 60614
Telephone: (773) 325-7887
Fax: (773) 325-7888
E-mail: *jmicha12@depaul.edu*
Web: *http://las.depaul.edu/psy/*

Department Information:
1936. Chairperson: Jerry Cleland, PhD. Number of faculty: total—full-time 31, part-time 4; women—full-time 18, part-time 1; total—minority—full-time 5; women minority—full-time 3.

Programs and Degrees Offered:
Listed in the following order: Program area, degree type (T if terminal Master's), number awarded 7/08–6/09. Clinical Psychology PhD (Doctor of Philosophy) 9, Experimental Psychology PhD (Doctor of Philosophy) 3, Industrial/Organizational Psychology PhD (Doctor of Philosophy) 4, Community Psychology PhD (Doctor of Philosophy) 2, General Psychology MA/MS (Master of Arts/Science) (T) 4.

APA Accreditation: Clinical PhD (Doctor of Philosophy).

Student Applications/Admissions:
Student Applications
Clinical Psychology PhD (Doctor of Philosophy)—Applications 2009–2010, 284. Total applicants accepted 2009–2010, 7. Number full-time enrolled (new admits only) 2009–2010, 7. Number part-time enrolled (new admits only) 2009–2010, 0. Openings 2010–2011, 6. The median number of years required for completion of a degree in 2008–2009 were 7. The number of students enrolled full- and part-time who were dismissed or voluntarily withdrew from this program area in 2008–2009 were 1. *Experimental Psychology PhD (Doctor of Philosophy)*—Applications 2009–2010, 43. Total applicants accepted 2009–2010, 3. Number full-time enrolled (new admits only) 2009–2010, 2. Number part-time enrolled (new admits only) 2009–2010, 0. Openings 2010–2011, 3. The median number of years required for completion of a degree in 2008–2009 were 6. The number of students enrolled full- and part-time who were dismissed or voluntarily withdrew from this program area in 2008–2009 were 1. *Industrial/Organizational Psychology PhD (Doctor of Philosophy)*—Applications 2009–2010, 104. Total applicants accepted 2009–2010, 3. Number full-time enrolled (new admits only) 2009–2010, 3. Number part-time enrolled (new admits only) 2009–2010, 0. Openings 2010–2011, 3. The median number of years required for completion of a degree in 2008–2009 were 6. The number of students enrolled full- and part-time who were dismissed or voluntarily withdrew from this program area in 2008–2009 were 0. *Community Psychology PhD (Doctor of Philosophy)*—Applications 2009–2010, 47. Total applicants accepted 2009–2010, 3. Number full-time enrolled (new admits only) 2009–2010, 3. Number part-time enrolled (new admits only) 2009–2010, 0. Openings 2010–2011, 3. The median number of years required for completion of a degree in 2008–2009 were 7. The number of students enrolled full- and part-time who were dismissed or voluntarily withdrew from this program area in 2008–2009 were 0. *General Psychology MA/MS (Master of Arts/Science)*—Applications 2009–2010, 68. Total applicants accepted 2009–2010, 7. Number full-time enrolled (new admits only) 2009–2010, 7. Number part-time enrolled (new admits only) 2009–2010, 0. Openings 2010–2011, 5. The median number of years required for completion of a degree in 2008–2009 were 2. The number of students enrolled full- and part-time who were dismissed or voluntarily withdrew from this program area in 2008–2009 were 1.

Scores: Entries appear in this order: required test or GPA, minimum score (if required), median score of students entering in 2009–2010. *Clinical Psychology PhD (Doctor of Philosophy):* GRE-V no minimum stated, GRE-Q no minimum stated, GRE-Analytical no minimum stated, overall undergraduate GPA no minimum stated, Masters GPA no minimum stated; *Experimental Psychology PhD (Doctor of Philosophy):* GRE-V no minimum stated, GRE-Q no minimum stated, GRE-Analytical no minimum stated, overall undergraduate GPA no minimum stated, Masters GPA no minimum stated; *Industrial/Organizational Psychology PhD (Doctor of Philosophy):* GRE-V no minimum stated, GRE-Q no minimum stated, GRE-Analytical no minimum stated, overall undergraduate GPA no minimum stated, psychology GPA no minimum stated, Masters GPA no minimum stated; *Community Psychology PhD (Doctor of Philosophy):* GRE-V no minimum stated, GRE-Q no minimum stated, GRE-Analytical no minimum stated, overall undergraduate GPA no minimum stated, Masters GPA no minimum stated; *General Psychology MA/MS (Master of Arts/Science):* GRE-V no minimum stated, GRE-Q no minimum stated, GRE-Analytical no minimum stated, overall undergraduate GPA no minimum stated, psychology GPA no minimum stated.

Other Criteria: (importance of criteria rated low, medium, or high): GRE scores—high, research experience—high, work experience—medium, extracurricular activity—medium, clinically related public service—medium, GPA—high, letters of recommendation—high, interview—high, statement of goals and objectives—high. Clinically related public service is not applicable for the Community, Experimental, I/O, or General MS programs. Only the Clinical and Community programs require interviews. For additional information on admission requirements, go to http://www.depaul.edu/admission/types_of_admission/graduate/psychology/index.asp.

Student Characteristics: The following represents characteristics of students in 2009–2010 in all graduate psychology programs in the department: Female—full-time 78, part-time 0; Male—full-time 44, part-time 0; African American/Black—full-time 14, part-time 0; Hispanic/Latino(a)—full-time 10, part-time 0; Asian/Pacific Islander—full-time 5, part-time 0; American Indian/Alaska

Native—full-time 1, part-time 0; Caucasian/White—full-time 86, part-time 0; Multi-ethnic—full-time 2, part-time 0; students subject to the Americans With Disabilities Act—full-time 0, part-time 0; Unknown ethnicity—full-time 0, part-time 0; International students who hold an F-1 or J-1 Visa—full-time 4, part-time 0.

Financial Information/Assistance:
Tuition for Full-Time Study: *Master's:* State residents: per academic year $18,900, $525 per credit hour; Nonstate residents: per academic year $18,900, $525 per credit hour. *Doctoral:* State residents: per academic year $18,900, $525 per credit hour; Nonstate residents: per academic year $18,900, $525 per credit hour. Tuition is subject to change. See the following Web site for updates and changes in tuition costs: http://www.depaul.edu/admission/tuition/index.asp.

Financial Assistance:
First-Year Students: Teaching assistantships available for first year. Average amount paid per academic year: $15,500. Average number of hours worked per week: 20. Research assistantships available for first year. Average amount paid per academic year: $15,500. Average number of hours worked per week: 20.

Advanced Students: Teaching assistantships available for advanced students. Average amount paid per academic year: $15,500. Average number of hours worked per week: 20. Research assistantships available for advanced students. Average amount paid per academic year: $15,500. Average number of hours worked per week: 20. Traineeships available for advanced students. Average amount paid per academic year: $15,500. Average number of hours worked per week: 20.

Additional Information: Of all students currently enrolled full time, 100% benefited from one or more of the listed financial assistance programs. Application and information available online at: http://www.depaul.edu/admissions/types_of_admission/graduate/psychology/index.asp.

Internships/Practica: Doctoral Degree (PhD Clinical Psychology): For those doctoral students for whom a professional internship was required in this program prior to graduation, (8) students applied for an internship in 2008–2009, with (8) students obtaining an internship. Of those students who obtained an internship, (8) were paid internships. Of those students who obtained an internship, (8) students placed in APA/CPA accredited internships, (0) students placed in internships not APA/CPA accredited, but listed with the Association of Psychology Postdoctoral and Internship Programs (APPIC), (0) students placed in internships conforming to guidelines of the Council of Directors of School Psychology Programs (CDSPP), (0) students placed in internships that were not APA/CPA accredited, APPIC or CDSPP listed. All of our clinical students are required to take a practicum course every quarter in their second and third years. Though DePaul does not have an internship program, our students fulfill their internship requirement at top facilities in Chicago and across the nation.

Housing and Day Care: On-campus housing is available. See the following Web site for more information: http://housing.depaul.edu/. No on-campus day care facilities are available.

Employment of Department Graduates:
Master's Degree Graduates: Of those who graduated in the academic year 2008–2009, the following categories and numbers represent the postgraduate activities and employment of master's degree graduates: Enrolled in a postdoctoral residency/fellowship (n/a), employed in independent practice (n/a), total from the above (master's) (0).

Doctoral Degree Graduates: Of those who graduated in the academic year 2008–2009, the following categories and numbers represent the postgraduate activities and employment of doctoral degree graduates: Enrolled in a psychology doctoral program (n/a), do not know (9), total from the above (doctoral) (9).

Additional Information:
Orientation, Objectives, and Emphasis of Department: In addition to several common training experiences, the Clinical program has two areas of emphasis, or tracks: Community and Child. The Community track focuses on prevention, consultation, program development, empowerment, and health promotion, rather than traditional treatment. The Child track emphasizes training in developmental psychopathology, in the development of efficacious treatments for low income African American and Latino families, and the delivery of services for youth living in urban settings, including schools and community mental health centers. Applicants select an area of emphasis and are admitted to one of the two tracks. The two areas of emphasis are complementary to one another. Most of the research and training conducted in the Community track is focused on children, adolescents, and families, and the training received in the Child track is informed by Community principles (e.g., prevention, empowerment, health promotion). The educational philosophy of the Department of Psychology is based upon a recognition of three components of modern psychology. The first of these is academic: the accumulated body of knowledge and theory relevant to the many areas of psychological study. The second is research: the methodologies and skills whereby the science of psychology is advanced. The third is application: the use of psychology for individuals and society. A major function of the graduate curriculum in psychology is to bring to the student an awareness of the real unity of psychological study and practice, despite apparent diversity. The student must come to appreciate the fact that psychology is both a pure science and an applied science, and that these aspects are not mutually exclusive. This educational philosophy underlies all programs within the department. Each seeks to incorporate the three interrelated components of psychology at the graduate and professional levels; hence each program contains an academic, a research, and an applied component. It is the emphasis given to each component that is distinctive for each of our graduate programs. Students are strongly encouraged to work with faculty in research and tutorial settings. Doctoral candidates are given opportunities to gain teaching experience. Many students work in applied or research settings in the metropolitan Chicago area so that they can apply their graduate education to practical settings. Our Experimental program has three tracks: Cognitive, Developmental, and Social Psychology. Students specialize in one of these areas, but are free to change areas during their graduate careers or to work with faculty in multiple areas.

Special Facilities or Resources: Extensive facilities are available to support the graduate programs and research projects. We have state-of-the-art classrooms and computer facilities. The university also has a new library, recreation center, athletic facility, and student center. The Family and Community Services (FCS) Center, which is located in the same building as the psychology department, serves approximately 150,000 people. Our clinical students gain their initial practicum experiences in the Family and Community Services (FCS) Center. In addition, the center serves as a venue for community and applied research. The university has prominent law and business colleges, which are well reputed in the midwestern business community and provide work opportunities for our experimental and industrial/organizational students. The department maintains an active network of our PhD graduates to help in obtaining jobs. There are many educational opportunities in this area, including colloquia, lectures, and regional and national organizations and conferences. We have an active graduate student organization that maintains contact with graduate students from other universities, providing opportunities to share educational experiences and recreational activities.

Information for Students With Physical Disabilities: See the following Web site for more information: http://studentaffairs.depaul.edu/studentswithdisabilities.

Application Information:

Send to Department of Psychology, DePaul University, 2219 North Kenmore, Chicago, IL 60614-3504. Application available online. URL of online application: https://www.depaul.edu/admission/. Students are admitted in the Fall, application deadline Clinical Child and Clinical Community—December 1; Industrial/Organizational—January 5; Community—January 5; Experimental—February 1; General (MS)—May 1. *Fee:* $40. A student in need of financial aid may request a waiver of the application fee by submitting a personal letter requesting this consideration, a letter from the financial aid office of the institution attended outlining need, and official copies of financial aid transcripts.

Eastern Illinois University
Department of Psychology
College of Sciences
Charleston, IL 61920
Telephone: (217) 581-2127
Fax: (217) 581-6764
E-mail: *ahailemariam@eiu.edu; asharma@eiu.edu*
Web: *http://www.eiu.edu/~psych/*

Department Information:

1963. Chairperson: John Mace. Number of faculty: total—full-time 22; women—full-time 10; total—minority—full-time 4; women minority—full-time 3.

Programs and Degrees Offered:

Listed in the following order: Program area, degree type (T if terminal Master's), number awarded 7/08–6/09. Clinical Psychology MA/MS (Master of Arts/Science) (T) 10, School Psychology Other 11.

Student Applications/Admissions:
Student Applications

Clinical Psychology MA/MS (*Master of Arts/Science*)—Applications 2009–2010, 45. Total applicants accepted 2009–2010, 20. Number full-time enrolled (new admits only) 2009–2010, 10. Total enrolled 2009–2010 full-time, 19. Openings 2010–2011, 10. The median number of years required for completion of a degree in 2008–2009 were 2. The number of students enrolled full- and part-time who were dismissed or voluntarily withdrew from this program area in 2008–2009 were 0. *School Psychology Other*—Applications 2009–2010, 55. Total applicants accepted 2009–2010, 25. Number full-time enrolled (new admits only) 2009–2010, 9. Openings 2010–2011, 12. The median number of years required for completion of a degree in 2008–2009 were 3.

Scores: Entries appear in this order: required test or GPA, minimum score (if required), median score of students entering in 2009–2010. *Clinical Psychology MA/MS (Master of Arts/Science):* GRE-V no minimum stated, GRE-Q no minimum stated; *School Psychology Other:* GRE-V no minimum stated, 475, GRE-Q no minimum stated, 625, GRE-Analytical no minimum stated, overall undergraduate GPA no minimum stated, last 2 years GPA no minimum stated, psychology GPA no minimum stated.

Other Criteria: (importance of criteria rated low, medium, or high): GRE scores—high, research experience—medium, work experience—medium, extracurricular activity—medium, clinically related public service—medium, GPA—high, letters of recommendation—high, interview—low, statement of goals and objectives—high, specific undergraduate psychology courses taken—medium.

Student Characteristics: The following represents characteristics of students in 2009–2010 in all graduate psychology programs in the department: Female—full-time 42, part-time 1; Male—full-time 13, part-time 0; African American/Black—full-time 2, part-time 0; Hispanic/Latino(a)—full-time 2, part-time 0; Asian/Pacific Islander—full-time 3, part-time 0; American Indian/Alaska Native—full-time 0, part-time 0; Caucasian/White—full-time 0, part-time 0; Multi-ethnic—full-time 1, part-time 0; students subject to the Americans With Disabilities Act—full-time 0, part-time 0; Unknown ethnicity—full-time 0, part-time 0; International students who hold an F-1 or J-1 Visa—full-time 0, part-time 0.

Financial Information/Assistance:

Tuition for Full-Time Study: Master's: State residents: $239 per credit hour; Nonstate residents: $717 per credit hour. Additional fees are assessed to students beyond the costs of tuition for the following: assessment courses. See the following Web site for updates and changes in tuition costs: http://www.eiu.edu/~graduate/prospective_students/admissions_tuitionfees.php.

Financial Assistance:

First-Year Students: Research assistantships available for first year. Average amount paid per academic year: $7,740. Average number of hours worked per week: 18. Apply by February 15.

Advanced Students: Research assistantships available for advanced students. Average amount paid per academic year: $7,740. Average number of hours worked per week: 18. Apply by February 15.

Additional Information: Of all students currently enrolled full time, 90% benefited from one or more of the listed financial assistance programs. Application and information available online at: http://www.eiu.edu/~finaid/.

Internships/Practica:

A two-semester clinical internship in the second year of graduate study is required for the Master of Arts degree. The 12 semester hour internship includes a weekly seminar emphasizing treatment planning, ethical practice and case management, and requires 600 hours of supervised clinical practice in an approved community agency setting with regular on-campus clinical supervision coordinated with on-site supervision provided by an approved agency supervisor. Some internships carry a stipend and tuition waiver. During the two years of on-campus study required by the school psychology program, students participate in three practica. First-semester students complete a school-based practicum which is designed to orient them to the workings of the public education system. During the first semester of the second year students participate in an assessment practicum centered in the on-campus psychological assessment center. A field-based component of this practicum allows students to also complete assessment activities in a public school setting. During their last semester on campus students participate in a field-based practicum devoted to enhancing counseling and consultation skills.

Housing and Day Care: On-campus housing is available. See the following Web site for more information: http://www.eiu.edu/~housing/. No on-campus day care facilities are available.

Employment of Department Graduates:
Master's Degree Graduates: Of those who graduated in the academic year 2008–2009, the following categories and numbers represent the postgraduate activities and employment of master's degree graduates: Enrolled in a psychology doctoral program (2), enrolled in a postdoctoral residency/fellowship (n/a), employed in independent practice (n/a), employed in a professional position in a school system (12), employed in a community mental health/counseling center (6), total from the above (master's) (20).
Doctoral Degree Graduates: Of those who graduated in the academic year 2008–2009, the following categories and numbers represent the postgraduate activities and employment of doctoral degree graduates: Enrolled in a psychology doctoral program (n/a), total from the above (doctoral) (0).

Additional Information:
Orientation, Objectives, and Emphasis of Department: The Master of Arts degree in Clinical Psychology at Eastern Illinois University is designed to provide graduate training with a solid foundation in the science and practice of clinical psychology. The program is a terminal master's degree training experience, which is approved by the Council of Applied Master's Programs in Psychology. The emphases highlight training and instruction in psychological interventions and therapy, assessment, and research. EIU graduates in Clinical Psychology possess a combination of skills in assessment, data management and analysis that uniquely position them amongst other master's level practitioners when it comes to assisting mental health organizations to meet the increasing demands of accurate evaluation, current, state-of-the-art programming, timely treatment protocols and accountability. The clinical psychology program also provides solid preparation for further graduate study. The purpose of the school psychology program is to prepare students to deliver high quality services to students, parents, and professional personnel in public school settings. The program offers a generalist curriculum designed to allow students to develop the flexibility to practice in varied settings. Particular emphasis is placed on assessment, consultation, behavior management, and counseling. The importance of applied experiences is stressed.

Special Facilities or Resources: The Department of Psychology has a computer/statistics lab, as well as faculty directed research labs, one currently in use as setting for a NIH grant. Training facilities include a three room suite used as a Psychology Assessment Center with one-way-mirror viewing for testing and interviews and video taping facilities. A further Clinical/Observation research suite, with video and one-way mirror equipment is available for clinical training and supervised community services. Both applied programs enjoy viable cooperative agreements with a number of area educational, correctional and mental health agencies which serve as training and practicum sites for graduate clinical experiences in addition to the internship sites.

Information for Students With Physical Disabilities: See the following Web site for more information: http://www.eiu.edu/~disablty/.

Application Information:
Send to Psychology Department, Eastern Illinois University, Charleston, IL 61920. Application available online. URL of online application: http://www.eiu.edu/~psych/clinical/grad_application.php. Students are admitted in the Fall, application deadline February 15. *Fee:* $30.

Illinois Institute of Technology
Institute of Psychology
3105 South Dearborn, LS-252
Chicago, IL 60616
Telephone: (312) 567-3500
Fax: (312) 567-3493
E-mail: *mitchelle@iit.edu*
Web: *http://www.iit.edu/psych/*

Department Information:
1929. Dean: M. Ellen Mitchell. Number of faculty: total—full-time 19, part-time 12; women—full-time 7, part-time 12; total—minority—full-time 2, part-time 1; women minority—full-time 1, part-time 2.

Programs and Degrees Offered:
Listed in the following order: Program area, degree type (T if terminal Master's), number awarded 7/08–6/09. Industrial/Organizational Psychology PhD (Doctor of Philosophy) 2, Personnel and Human Resources Development MA/MS (Master of Arts/Science) (T) 10, Rehabilitation PhD (Doctor of Philosophy) 0, Clinical Psychology PhD (Doctor of Philosophy) 14, Rehabilitation Counseling MA/MS (Master of Arts/Science) (T) 11.

APA Accreditation: Clinical PhD (Doctor of Philosophy).

Student Applications/Admissions:
Student Applications
Industrial/Organizational Psychology PhD (Doctor of Philosophy)—Applications 2009–2010, 58. Total applicants accepted 2009–2010, 27. Number full-time enrolled (new admits only) 2009–2010, 8. Number part-time enrolled (new admits only) 2009–2010, 0. Openings 2010–2011, 8. The median number of years required for completion of a degree in 2008–2009 were 9. The number of students enrolled full- and part-time who were dismissed or voluntarily withdrew from this program area in 2008–2009 were 5. *Personnel and Human Resources Development MA/MS (Master of Arts/Science)*—Applications

2009–2010, 46. Total applicants accepted 2009–2010, 22. Number full-time enrolled (new admits only) 2009–2010, 8. Number part-time enrolled (new admits only) 2009–2010, 0. Openings 2010–2011, 10. The median number of years required for completion of a degree in 2008–2009 were 2. The number of students enrolled full- and part-time who were dismissed or voluntarily withdrew from this program area in 2008–2009 were 0. *Rehabilitation PhD (Doctor of Philosophy)*—Applications 2009–2010, 2. Total applicants accepted 2009–2010, 0. Number full-time enrolled (new admits only) 2009–2010, 0. Number part-time enrolled (new admits only) 2009–2010, 0. Openings 2010–2011, 3. The number of students enrolled full- and part-time who were dismissed or voluntarily withdrew from this program area in 2008–2009 were 0. *Clinical Psychology PhD (Doctor of Philosophy)*—Applications 2009–2010, 133. Total applicants accepted 2009–2010, 27. Number full-time enrolled (new admits only) 2009–2010, 13. Number part-time enrolled (new admits only) 2009–2010, 0. Openings 2010–2011, 13. The median number of years required for completion of a degree in 2008–2009 were 6. The number of students enrolled full- and part-time who were dismissed or voluntarily withdrew from this program area in 2008–2009 were 3. *Rehabilitation Counseling MA/MS (Master of Arts/Science)*—Applications 2009–2010, 32. Total applicants accepted 2009–2010, 18. Number full-time enrolled (new admits only) 2009–2010, 11. Number part-time enrolled (new admits only) 2009–2010, 0. Total enrolled 2009–2010 full-time, 22, part-time, 17. Openings 2010–2011, 15. The median number of years required for completion of a degree in 2008–2009 were 2. The number of students enrolled full- and part-time who were dismissed or voluntarily withdrew from this program area in 2008–2009 were 4.

Other Criteria: (importance of criteria rated low, medium, or high): GRE scores—high, research experience—high, work experience—high, extracurricular activity—low, clinically related public service—medium, GPA—high, letters of recommendation—high, interview—high, statement of goals and objectives—high. GPA and GRE are less important for MS programs; MS in rehabilitation does not require the GRE.

Student Characteristics: The following represents characteristics of students in 2009–2010 in all graduate psychology programs in the department: Female—full-time 138, part-time 13; Male—full-time 54, part-time 4; African American/Black—full-time 5, part-time 3; Hispanic/Latino(a)—full-time 5, part-time 2; Asian/Pacific Islander—full-time 11, part-time 1; American Indian/Alaska Native—full-time 0, part-time 0; Caucasian/White—full-time 110, part-time 10; Multi-ethnic—full-time 0, part-time 0; students subject to the Americans With Disabilities Act—full-time 7, part-time 1; Unknown ethnicity—full-time 61, part-time 1; International students who hold an F-1 or J-1 Visa—full-time 11, part-time 2.

Financial Information/Assistance:
Tuition for Full-Time Study: *Master's:* State residents: $975 per credit hour; Nonstate residents: $975 per credit hour. *Doctoral:* State residents: $975 per credit hour; Nonstate residents: $975 per credit hour. Tuition is subject to change. Tuition costs vary by program. See the following Web site for updates and changes in tuition costs: http://www.iit.edu/psych/admission/graduate/deadlines_and_costs.shtml.

Financial Assistance:
First-Year Students: Teaching assistantships available for first year. Average amount paid per academic year: $5,440. Average number of hours worked per week: 10. Apply by April 1. Fellowships and scholarships available for first year.

Advanced Students: Teaching assistantships available for advanced students. Average amount paid per academic year: $5,440. Average number of hours worked per week: 10. Apply by April 1. Research assistantships available for advanced students. Average amount paid per academic year: $13,300. Average number of hours worked per week: 20. Traineeships available for advanced students. Fellowships and scholarships available for advanced students.

Additional Information: Of all students currently enrolled full time, 68% benefited from one or more of the listed financial assistance programs.

Internships/Practica: Doctoral Degree (PhD Clinical Psychology): For those doctoral students for whom a professional internship was required in this program prior to graduation, (9) students applied for an internship in 2008–2009, with (9) students obtaining an internship. Of those students who obtained an internship, (9) were paid internships. Of those students who obtained an internship, (8) students placed in APA/CPA accredited internships, (0) students placed in internships not APA/CPA accredited, but listed with the Association of Psychology Postdoctoral and Internship Programs (APPIC), (0) students placed in internships conforming to guidelines of the Council of Directors of School Psychology Programs (CDSPP), (1) students placed in internships that were not APA/CPA accredited, APPIC or CDSPP listed. All students are required to complete fieldwork internships and practica. Experiences vary by program. As one of the largest cities in the United States, Chicago provides access to diverse practicum and internship sites.

Housing and Day Care: On-campus housing is available. See the following Web site for more information: http://www.iit.edu/housing. No on-campus day care facilities are available.

Employment of Department Graduates:
Master's Degree Graduates: Of those who graduated in the academic year 2008–2009, the following categories and numbers represent the postgraduate activities and employment of master's degree graduates: Enrolled in a postdoctoral residency/fellowship (n/a), employed in independent practice (n/a), total from the above (master's) (0).

Doctoral Degree Graduates: Of those who graduated in the academic year 2008–2009, the following categories and numbers represent the postgraduate activities and employment of doctoral degree graduates: Enrolled in a psychology doctoral program (n/a), total from the above (doctoral) (0).

Additional Information:
Orientation, Objectives, and Emphasis of Department: The primary emphasis in the Institute is on a scientist–practitioner model of training. Our APA-approved clinical psychology program offers intensive clinical and research training with an emphasis on a cognitive theoretical framework, community involvement, and exposure to underserved populations. The MS in rehabilitation counseling prepares students to function as rehabilitation counselors for disabled persons. The PhD program in rehabilitation psychology prepares students for careers in rehabilitation education,

research, and the practice of rehabilitation psychology. Our industrial/organizational program provides a solid scientific background as well as knowledge and expertise in personnel selection, evaluation, training and development, motivation, and organizational behavior.

Special Facilities or Resources: Facilities include laboratories for human behavior studies, psychophysiological research, infant and maternal attachment, and a testing and interviewing laboratory with attached one-way viewing rooms. Equipment includes programming apparatus for learning studies, specialized computer facilities, and videotaping and other audiovisual equipment. There are graduate student offices, a testing library of assessment equipment, and a student lounge. The Disabilities Resource Center is housed within psychology.

Information for Students With Physical Disabilities: See the following Web site for more information: http://www.iit.edu/cdr/.

Application Information:
Send to Admissions, Institute of Psychology, Illinois Institute of Technology, 3105 S. Dearborn, Suite 252, Chicago, IL 60616. Application available online. URL of online application: http://www.iit.edu/psych/admission/graduate/apply.shtml. Students are admitted in the Fall, application deadline January 15. Clinical deadline is January 15, I/O and PHRD deadline is February 15, Rehabilitation deadline is March 15. *Fee:* $40.

Illinois State University
Department of Psychology
College of Arts and Sciences
Campus Box 4620
Normal, IL 61790-4620
Telephone: (309) 438-8701
Fax: (309) 438-5789
E-mail: *psygrad@ilstu.edu*
Web: *http://psychology.illinoisstate.edu/grad/index.shtml*

Department Information:
1966. Interim Department Chair: J. Scott Jordan. Number of faculty: total—full-time 37, part-time 6; women—full-time 14, part-time 4; total—minority—full-time 2; women minority—full-time 1; faculty subject to the Americans With Disabilities Act 1.

Programs and Degrees Offered:
Listed in the following order: Program area, degree type (T if terminal Master's), number awarded 7/08–6/09. Clinical-Counseling Psychology MA/MS (Master of Arts/Science) (T) 8, Developmental Psychology MA/MS (Master of Arts/Science) (T) 3, Cognitive & Behavioral Sciences MA/MS (Master of Arts/Science) (T) 2, School Psychology PhD (Doctor of Philosophy) 4, Industrial/Organizational-Social Psychology MA/MS (Master of Arts/Science) (T) 3, Quantitative Psychology MA/MS (Master of Arts/Science) (T) 0, School Psychology Other 8.

APA Accreditation: School PhD (Doctor of Philosophy).

Student Applications/Admissions:
Student Applications
Clinical-Counseling Psychology MA/MS (Master of Arts/Science)—Applications 2009–2010, 61. Total applicants accepted 2009–2010, 25. Number full-time enrolled (new admits only) 2009–2010, 13. Number part-time enrolled (new admits only) 2009–2010, 0. Total enrolled 2009–2010 full-time, 24, part-time, 12. Openings 2010–2011, 12. The median number of years required for completion of a degree in 2008–2009 were 3. The number of students enrolled full- and part-time who were dismissed or voluntarily withdrew from this program area in 2008–2009 were 1. *Developmental Psychology MA/MS (Master of Arts/Science)*—Applications 2009–2010, 13. Total applicants accepted 2009–2010, 5. Number full-time enrolled (new admits only) 2009–2010, 2. Number part-time enrolled (new admits only) 2009–2010, 0. Total enrolled 2009–2010 full-time, 6, part-time, 7. Openings 2010–2011, 4. The median number of years required for completion of a degree in 2008–2009 were 2. The number of students enrolled full- and part-time who were dismissed or voluntarily withdrew from this program area in 2008–2009 were 0. *Cognitive & Behavioral Sciences MA/MS (Master of Arts/Science)*—Applications 2009–2010, 18. Total applicants accepted 2009–2010, 9. Number full-time enrolled (new admits only) 2009–2010, 5. Number part-time enrolled (new admits only) 2009–2010, 0. Total enrolled 2009–2010 full-time, 10, part-time, 7. Openings 2010–2011, 5. The median number of years required for completion of a degree in 2008–2009 were 2. The number of students enrolled full- and part-time who were dismissed or voluntarily withdrew from this program area in 2008–2009 were 0. *School Psychology PhD (Doctor of Philosophy)*—Applications 2009–2010, 24. Total applicants accepted 2009–2010, 15. Number full-time enrolled (new admits only) 2009–2010, 8. Number part-time enrolled (new admits only) 2009–2010, 0. Total enrolled 2009–2010 full-time, 28, part-time, 15. Openings 2010–2011, 7. The median number of years required for completion of a degree in 2008–2009 were 8. The number of students enrolled full- and part-time who were dismissed or voluntarily withdrew from this program area in 2008–2009 were 0. *Industrial/Organizational-Social Psychology MA/MS (Master of Arts/Science)*—Applications 2009–2010, 48. Total applicants accepted 2009–2010, 16. Number full-time enrolled (new admits only) 2009–2010, 6. Number part-time enrolled (new admits only) 2009–2010, 0. Total enrolled 2009–2010 full-time, 10, part-time, 20. Openings 2010–2011, 5. The median number of years required for completion of a degree in 2008–2009 were 5. The number of students enrolled full- and part-time who were dismissed or voluntarily withdrew from this program area in 2008–2009 were 1. *Quantitative Psychology MA/MS (Master of Arts/Science)*—Applications 2009–2010, 4. Total applicants accepted 2009–2010, 1. Number full-time enrolled (new admits only) 2009–2010, 0. Number part-time enrolled (new admits only) 2009–2010, 0. Total enrolled 2009–2010 full-time, 1, part-time, 5. Openings 2010–2011, 4. The number of students enrolled full- and part-time who were dismissed or voluntarily withdrew from this program area in 2008–2009 were 0. *School Psychology Other*—Applications 2009–2010, 66. Total applicants accepted 2009–2010, 10. Number full-time enrolled (new admits only) 2009–2010, 6. Number part-time enrolled (new admits only) 2009–2010, 0. Total enrolled 2009–2010 full-time, 18, part-time, 8. Openings 2010–2011, 7. The median number of years required for com-

pletion of a degree in 2008–2009 were 3. The number of students enrolled full- and part-time who were dismissed or voluntarily withdrew from this program area in 2008–2009 were 0.
Scores: Entries appear in this order: required test or GPA, minimum score (if required), median score of students entering in 2009–2010. *Clinical-Counseling Psychology MA/MS (Master of Arts/Science):* GRE-V no minimum stated, GRE-Q no minimum stated, GRE-Analytical no minimum stated, overall undergraduate GPA no minimum stated, last 2 years GPA 3.0, psychology GPA no minimum stated; *Developmental Psychology MA/MS (Master of Arts/Science):* GRE-V no minimum stated, GRE-Q no minimum stated, GRE-Analytical no minimum stated, overall undergraduate GPA no minimum stated, last 2 years GPA 3.0, psychology GPA no minimum stated; *Cognitive & Behavioral Sciences MA/MS (Master of Arts/Science):* GRE-V no minimum stated, GRE-Q no minimum stated, GRE-Analytical no minimum stated, overall undergraduate GPA no minimum stated, last 2 years GPA 3.0, psychology GPA no minimum stated; *School Psychology PhD (Doctor of Philosophy):* GRE-V no minimum stated, GRE-Q no minimum stated, GRE-Analytical no minimum stated, overall undergraduate GPA no minimum stated, last 2 years GPA 3.0, psychology GPA no minimum stated; *Industrial/Organizational-Social Psychology MA/MS (Master of Arts/Science):* GRE-V no minimum stated, GRE-Q no minimum stated, GRE-Analytical no minimum stated, overall undergraduate GPA no minimum stated, last 2 years GPA 3.0, psychology GPA no minimum stated; *Quantitative Psychology MA/MS (Master of Arts/Science):* GRE-V no minimum stated, GRE-Q no minimum stated, GRE-Analytical no minimum stated, overall undergraduate GPA no minimum stated, last 2 years GPA 3.0, psychology GPA no minimum stated; *School Psychology Other:* GRE-V no minimum stated, GRE-Q no minimum stated, GRE-Analytical no minimum stated, overall undergraduate GPA no minimum stated, last 2 years GPA 3.0, psychology GPA no minimum stated.
Other Criteria: (importance of criteria rated low, medium, or high): GRE scores—high, research experience—medium, work experience—medium, extracurricular activity—low, clinically related public service—medium, GPA—high, letters of recommendation—high, interview—high, statement of goals and objectives—medium, undergraduate major in psychology—medium, specific undergraduate psychology courses taken—medium. Interview required only for the PhD degree. Interview (in person, preferably, or by phone) for master's degree. For additional information on admission requirements, go to http://psychology.illinoisstate.edu/grad/application/department.shtml.

Student Characteristics: The following represents characteristics of students in 2009–2010 in all graduate psychology programs in the department: Female—full-time 65, part-time 60; Male—full-time 32, part-time 14; African American/Black—full-time 3, part-time 1; Hispanic/Latino(a)—full-time 1, part-time 0; Asian/Pacific Islander—full-time 5, part-time 3; American Indian/Alaska Native—full-time 0, part-time 0; Caucasian/White—full-time 78, part-time 64; Multi-ethnic—full-time 0, part-time 0; students subject to the Americans With Disabilities Act—full-time 1, part-time 2; Unknown ethnicity—full-time 10, part-time 6; International students who hold an F-1 or J-1 Visa—full-time 6, part-time 3.

Financial Information/Assistance:
Tuition for Full-Time Study: *Master's:* State residents: per academic year $5,280, $220 per credit hour; Nonstate residents: per academic year $10,968, $457 per credit hour. *Doctoral:* State residents: per academic year $5,720, $220 per credit hour; Nonstate residents: per academic year $11,882, $457 per credit hour. Tuition is subject to change. Additional fees are assessed to students beyond the costs of tuition for the following: general fees and student insurance (which may be waived if other coverage is in place). See the following Web site for updates and changes in tuition costs: htthttp://www.comptroller.ilstu.edu/studentaccounts/tuition-rates/.

Financial Assistance:
First-Year Students: Teaching assistantships available for first year. Average amount paid per academic year: $3,994. Average number of hours worked per week: 10. Apply by January 5. Research assistantships available for first year. Average amount paid per academic year: $3,994. Average number of hours worked per week: 10. Apply by January 5. Traineeships available for first year. Average amount paid per academic year: $4,630. Average number of hours worked per week: 10. Apply by January 5. Fellowships and scholarships available for first year. Average amount paid per academic year: $3,366. Average number of hours worked per week: 0.
Advanced Students: Teaching assistantships available for advanced students. Average amount paid per academic year: $4,307. Average number of hours worked per week: 10. Apply by March 15. Research assistantships available for advanced students. Average amount paid per academic year: $4,307. Average number of hours worked per week: 10. Apply by March 15. Traineeships available for advanced students. Average amount paid per academic year: $5,553. Average number of hours worked per week: 10. Apply by March 15. Fellowships and scholarships available for advanced students. Average amount paid per academic year: $3,600. Average number of hours worked per week: 0.
Additional Information: Of all students currently enrolled full time, 88% benefited from one or more of the listed financial assistance programs. Application and information available online at: http://financialaid.illinoisstate.edu/.

Internships/Practica: Doctoral Degree (PhD School Psychology): For those doctoral students for whom a professional internship was required in this program prior to graduation, (3) students applied for an internship in 2008–2009, with (3) students obtaining an internship. Of those students who obtained an internship, (3) were paid internships. Of those students who obtained an internship, (3) students placed in APA/CPA accredited internships, (0) students placed in internships not APA/CPA accredited, but listed with the Association of Psychology Postdoctoral and Internship Programs (APPIC), (0) students placed in internships conforming to guidelines of the Council of Directors of School Psychology Programs (CDSPP), (0) students placed in internships that were not APA/CPA accredited, APPIC or CDSPP listed. Master's Degree (MA/MS Clinical-Counseling Psychology): An internship experience, such as a final research project or "capstone" experience is required of graduates. Master's Degree (MA/MS Developmental Psychology): An internship experience, such as a final research project or "capstone" experience is required of graduates. Master's Degree (MA/MS Cognitive & Behavioral Sciences): An internship experience, such as a final research project or "capstone" experience is required of graduates.

Master's Degree (MA/MS Industrial/Organizational-Social Psychology): An internship experience, such as a final research project or "capstone" experience is required of graduates. Master's Degree (MA/MS Quantitative Psychology): An internship experience, such as a final research project or "capstone" experience is required of graduates. Students in the clinical-counseling master's program are provided with extensive supervised experience in practica in external mental health agencies. Students in the School Psychology specialist (SSP) and doctoral (PhD) programs participate from their first semester in supervised practica in public and private schools, Head Start centers, and the on-campus Psychological Services Center. Full-time internships are required for all school psychology students.

Housing and Day Care: On-campus housing is available. See the following Web site for more information: http://www.housing.ilstu.edu/. On-campus day care facilities are available. See the following Web site for more information: http://childcarecenter.illinoisstate.edu/.

Employment of Department Graduates:
Master's Degree Graduates: Of those who graduated in the academic year 2008–2009, the following categories and numbers represent the postgraduate activities and employment of master's degree graduates: Enrolled in a psychology doctoral program (3), enrolled in a postdoctoral residency/fellowship (n/a), employed in independent practice (n/a), employed in an academic position at a university (1), employed in an academic position at a 2-year/4-year college (1), employed in other positions at a higher education institution (2), employed in a professional position in a school system (8), employed in business or industry (1), employed in government agency (0), employed in a community mental health/counseling center (7), employed in a hospital/medical center (0), still seeking employment (0), not seeking employment (0), other employment position (0), do not know (1), total from the above (master's) (24).
Doctoral Degree Graduates: Of those who graduated in the academic year 2008–2009, the following categories and numbers represent the postgraduate activities and employment of doctoral degree graduates: Enrolled in a psychology doctoral program (n/a), enrolled in another graduate/professional program (0), employed in independent practice (0), employed in an academic position at a 2-year/4-year college (1), employed in other positions at a higher education institution (0), employed in a professional position in a school system (3), employed in business or industry (0), employed in government agency (0), employed in a community mental health/counseling center (0), still seeking employment (0), other employment position (0), do not know (0), total from the above (doctoral) (4).

Additional Information:
Orientation, Objectives, and Emphasis of Department: The department provides training in professional areas supplemented by options in developmental, cognitive and behavioral sciences, and quantitative. Training in the professional areas takes advantage of the professional experience of the faculty in human service settings and industry so that instruction is both practical and theoretical. Programs require a master's thesis, doctoral dissertation, an applied research apprenticeship, or a comprehensive examination project.

Special Facilities or Resources: The department has computer facilities and human and animal laboratories. The department also has a Psychological Services Center for assessment and treatment of children and families. For the clinical-counseling and school psychology programs, a large number of community agencies participate in the one-year practicum (schools, hospitals, mental health centers, and alcohol and drug rehabilitation centers).

Information for Students With Physical Disabilities: See the following Web site for more information: http://www.disabilityconcerns.ilstu.edu/.

Application Information:
Send to Illinois State University, Department of Psychology, Graduate Psychology Programs, Campus Box 4620, Normal, IL 61790-4620. Application available online. URL of online application: http://www.admissions.ilstu.edu/graduate/. Students are admitted in the Fall, application deadline November 15. Fall and Summer application deadline for the PhD program in School Psychology only is November 15. Fall and Summer application deadline for SSP program in School Psychology only is December 1. Fall application deadline for all master's programs is January 5. *Fee:* $40. Fee waiver based on documented financial need, re-enrollment at same level as prior enrollment at ISU, veteran service (active duty for one year or more), McNair, Project 1000, and Fulbright Scholar applicants.

Illinois, University of, Chicago
Department of Psychology (M/C 285)
Liberal Arts and Sciences
1007 West Harrison Street
Chicago, IL 60607-7137
Telephone: (312) 996-2434
Fax: (312) 413-4122
E-mail: *geraney@uic.edu*
Web: *http://www.psch.uic.edu*

Department Information:
1965. Chairperson: Gary E. Raney. Number of faculty: total—full-time 27, part-time 12; women—full-time 8, part-time 9; total—minority—full-time 4; women minority—full-time 4.

Programs and Degrees Offered:
Listed in the following order: Program area, degree type (T if terminal Master's), number awarded 7/08–6/09. Behavioral Neuroscience PhD (Doctor of Philosophy) 0, Clinical Psychology PhD (Doctor of Philosophy) 3, Cognitive Psychology PhD (Doctor of Philosophy) 0, Community and Prevention Research PhD (Doctor of Philosophy) 5, Social and Personality Psychology PhD (Doctor of Philosophy) 4.

APA Accreditation: Clinical PhD (Doctor of Philosophy).

Student Applications/Admissions:
Student Applications
Behavioral Neuroscience PhD (Doctor of Philosophy)—Applications 2009–2010, 28. Total applicants accepted 2009–2010, 2. Number full-time enrolled (new admits only) 2009–2010, 2. Number part-time enrolled (new admits only) 2009–2010, 0. Openings 2010–2011, 2. The median number of years re-

quired for completion of a degree in 2008–2009 were 6. The number of students enrolled full- and part-time who were dismissed or voluntarily withdrew from this program area in 2008–2009 were 0. *Clinical Psychology PhD (Doctor of Philosophy)*—Applications 2009–2010, 363. Total applicants accepted 2009–2010, 10. Number full-time enrolled (new admits only) 2009–2010, 10. Total enrolled 2009–2010 full-time, 47. Openings 2010–2011, 5. The median number of years required for completion of a degree in 2008–2009 were 7. The number of students enrolled full- and part-time who were dismissed or voluntarily withdrew from this program area in 2008–2009 were 0. *Cognitive Psychology PhD (Doctor of Philosophy)*—Applications 2009–2010, 34. Total applicants accepted 2009–2010, 9. Number full-time enrolled (new admits only) 2009–2010, 9. Total enrolled 2009–2010 full-time, 23. Openings 2010–2011, 5. The median number of years required for completion of a degree in 2008–2009 were 6. The number of students enrolled full- and part-time who were dismissed or voluntarily withdrew from this program area in 2008–2009 were 0. *Community and Prevention Research PhD (Doctor of Philosophy)*—Applications 2009–2010, 80. Total applicants accepted 2009–2010, 5. Number full-time enrolled (new admits only) 2009–2010, 5. Total enrolled 2009–2010 full-time, 27. Openings 2010–2011, 5. The median number of years required for completion of a degree in 2008–2009 were 6. The number of students enrolled full- and part-time who were dismissed or voluntarily withdrew from this program area in 2008–2009 were 0. *Social and Personality Psychology PhD (Doctor of Philosophy)*—Applications 2009–2010, 80. Total applicants accepted 2009–2010, 3. Number full-time enrolled (new admits only) 2009–2010, 3. Total enrolled 2009–2010 full-time, 16. Openings 2010–2011, 5. The median number of years required for completion of a degree in 2008–2009 were 6. The number of students enrolled full- and part-time who were dismissed or voluntarily withdrew from this program area in 2008–2009 were 0.

Scores: Entries appear in this order: required test or GPA, minimum score (if required), median score of students entering in 2009–2010. *Behavioral Neuroscience PhD (Doctor of Philosophy)*: GRE-V no minimum stated, 675, GRE-Q no minimum stated, 540, GRE-Analytical no minimum stated, 4.5, last 2 years GPA 3.36; *Clinical Psychology PhD (Doctor of Philosophy)*: GRE-V no minimum stated, 630, GRE-Q no minimum stated, 735, GRE-Analytical no minimum stated, 5.25, last 2 years GPA 3.36; *Cognitive Psychology PhD (Doctor of Philosophy)*: GRE-V no minimum stated, 620, GRE-Q no minimum stated, 760, GRE-Analytical no minimum stated, 5, last 2 years GPA 3.36; *Community and Prevention Research PhD (Doctor of Philosophy)*: GRE-V no minimum stated, 560, GRE-Q no minimum stated, 640, GRE-Analytical no minimum stated, 4.5, last 2 years GPA 3.36; *Social and Personality Psychology PhD (Doctor of Philosophy)*: GRE-V no minimum stated, 570, GRE-Q no minimum stated, 660, GRE-Analytical no minimum stated, 5, last 2 years GPA 3.36.

Other Criteria: (importance of criteria rated low, medium, or high): GRE scores—medium, research experience—high, work experience—medium, extracurricular activity—medium, clinically related public service—low, GPA—high, letters of recommendation—high, interview—high, statement of goals and objectives—high, fit with faculty research—high, undergraduate major in psychology—medium, specific undergraduate psychology courses taken—medium.

Student Characteristics: The following represents characteristics of students in 2009–2010 in all graduate psychology programs in the department: Female—full-time 79, part-time 0; Male—full-time 44, part-time 0; African American/Black—full-time 9, part-time 0; Hispanic/Latino(a)—full-time 5, part-time 0; Asian/Pacific Islander—full-time 10, part-time 0; American Indian/Alaska Native—full-time 0, part-time 0; Caucasian/White—full-time 98, part-time 0; Multi-ethnic—full-time 0, part-time 0; students subject to the Americans With Disabilities Act—part-time 0; Unknown ethnicity—full-time 1, part-time 0; International students who hold an F-1 or J-1 Visa—full-time 3, part-time 0.

Financial Information/Assistance:

Tuition for Full-Time Study: *Doctoral:* State residents: per academic year $8,872; Nonstate residents: per academic year $20,870. Tuition is subject to change. See the following Web site for updates and changes in tuition costs: http://www.uic.edu/depts/oar/grad/tuition_grad.html.

Financial Assistance:

First-Year Students: Teaching assistantships available for first year. Average amount paid per academic year: $14,000. Average number of hours worked per week: 20. Apply by January 1. Research assistantships available for first year. Average amount paid per academic year: $14,000. Average number of hours worked per week: 20. Apply by January 1. Traineeships available for first year. Average amount paid per academic year: $14,000. Average number of hours worked per week: 0. Apply by January 1. Fellowships and scholarships available for first year. Average amount paid per academic year: $20,000. Average number of hours worked per week: 0. Apply by January 1.

Advanced Students: Teaching assistantships available for advanced students. Average amount paid per academic year: $14,000. Average number of hours worked per week: 20. Research assistantships available for advanced students. Average amount paid per academic year: $14,000. Average number of hours worked per week: 20. Traineeships available for advanced students. Average amount paid per academic year: $14,000. Average number of hours worked per week: 0. Fellowships and scholarships available for advanced students. Average amount paid per academic year: $20,000. Average number of hours worked per week: 0.

Additional Information: Of all students currently enrolled full time, 100% benefited from one or more of the listed financial assistance programs.

Internships/Practica: Doctoral Degree (PhD Clinical Psychology): For those doctoral students for whom a professional internship was required in this program prior to graduation, (11) students applied for an internship in 2008–2009, with (11) students obtaining an internship. Of those students who obtained an internship, (11) were paid internships. Of those students who obtained an internship, (10) students placed in APA/CPA accredited internships, (1) students placed in internships not APA/CPA accredited, but listed with the Association of Psychology Postdoctoral and Internship Programs (APPIC), (0) students placed in internships conforming to guidelines of the Council of Directors of School Psychology Programs (CDSPP), (0) students placed in internships that were not APA/CPA accredited, APPIC or CDSPP listed. Access to a wide variety of practicum and research sites is available to advanced students. These include the UIC Counseling Service, Cook County Hospital, Rush-Presbyterian-St. Lukes Medical Center, the Institute for Juvenile Research, the Institute on Disabilities and Human Development, several Veterans Administration hospitals and mental health clinics, schools, and diverse community agencies throughout the Chicago area, in addition to our own Office of Applied Psychology.

Housing and Day Care: On-campus housing is available. See the following Web site for more information: http://www.housing.uic.edu/. On-campus day care facilities are available. See the following Web site for more information: http://www.uic.edu/depts/children/.

Employment of Department Graduates:
Master's Degree Graduates: Of those who graduated in the academic year 2008–2009, the following categories and numbers represent the postgraduate activities and employment of master's degree graduates: Enrolled in a postdoctoral residency/fellowship (n/a), employed in independent practice (n/a), total from the above (master's) (0).
Doctoral Degree Graduates: Of those who graduated in the academic year 2008–2009, the following categories and numbers represent the postgraduate activities and employment of doctoral degree graduates: Enrolled in a psychology doctoral program (n/a), enrolled in a postdoctoral residency/fellowship (1), employed in an academic position at a university (4), employed in a professional position in a school system (1), employed in government agency (2), employed in a hospital/medical center (1), other employment position (1), do not know (3), total from the above (doctoral) (13).

Additional Information:
Orientation, Objectives, and Emphasis of Department: The goal of the psychology department's doctoral program is to educate scholars and researchers who will contribute to the growth of psychological knowledge whether they work in academic, applied, or policy settings. Within the framework of satisfying the requirements of a major division and a minor, the department encourages students in consultation with their advisors to construct programs individually tailored to their research interests. The psychology department has more than 30 faculty and over 100 graduate students. It has 5 major divisions: behavioral neuroscience, clinical, cognitive, community and prevention research, and social and personality. It has a psychology and law minor, a statistics, methods and measurement minor and an interdepartmental specialization in neuroscience. We have close collaborations with the Institute for Juvenile Research, the Institute for Disabilities and Human Development, the School of Public Health, the Center for Urban Educational Research and Development, the Center for the Study of Learning, Instruction and Teacher Development, the Center for Literacy, and the Institute of Government and Public Affairs. These partnerships provide students and faculty having interest in interdisciplinary research an opportunity to work with scholars from diverse fields.

Special Facilities or Resources: The department is located in the Behavioral Sciences Building, a fully equipped facility designed to serve the needs of the behavioral and social sciences. Physical facilities include seminar rooms, animal laboratories, human research labs, clinical observation rooms with one-way observational windows and video-recording and biofeedback equipment, a well-equipped electronics and mechanics shop with an on-staff engineer, a department library, the Office of Applied Psychological Services which coordinates clinical and community interventions, the Office of Social Science Research which provides research support, and faculty-student lounge. The Department maintains its own computer lab, in which personal computer workstations connected to a mainframe and stand alone PCs (MS-DOS based and Macintosh) are offered for student use. The department also offers wireless internet access.

Information for Students With Physical Disabilities: See the following Web site for more information: http://www.uic.edu/index.html/disability.shtml.

Application Information:
Send to Graduate Admissions, University of Illinois at Chicago, Department of Psychology, MC 285, 1007 W. Harrison Street, Chicago, IL 60607-7137. Application available online. URL of online application: http://www.uic.edu/depts/oar/grad/apply_grad.html. Students are admitted in the Fall, application deadline December 15. *Fee:* $50. McNair application fee waivers.

Illinois, University of, Urbana–Champaign
Department of Educational Psychology
College of Education
226 Education Building, 1310 South Sixth Street
Champaign, IL 61820
Telephone: (217) 333-2245
Fax: (217) 244-7620
E-mail: *edpsy@uiuc.edu*
Web: *http://www.education.illinois.edu/edpsy/*

Department Information:
1962. Chairperson: Thomas A. Schwandt. Number of faculty: total—full-time 20; women—full-time 11; total—minority—full-time 3; women minority—full-time 2; faculty subject to the Americans With Disabilities Act 1.

Programs and Degrees Offered:
Listed in the following order: Program area, degree type (T if terminal Master's), number awarded 7/08–6/09. Counseling Psychology PhD (Doctor of Philosophy) 6, Child Development PhD (Doctor of Philosophy) 0, Measurement and Evaluation (Queries) PhD (Doctor of Philosophy) 7, Cognitive Science Of Teaching and Learning PhD (Doctor of Philosophy) 10, Curriculum, Technology and Education Reform MEd (Education) 20.

APA Accreditation: Counseling PhD (Doctor of Philosophy). Student Outcome Data Website: http://education.illinois.edu/edpsy/areasofstudy/counseling/counselingstatistics.html.

Student Applications/Admissions:
Student Applications
Counseling Psychology PhD (Doctor of Philosophy)—Applications 2009–2010, 90. Total applicants accepted 2009–2010, 5. Number full-time enrolled (new admits only) 2009–2010, 4. Number part-time enrolled (new admits only) 2009–2010, 0. Openings 2010–2011, 3. The median number of years required for completion of a degree in 2008–2009 were 6. The number of students enrolled full- and part-time who were dismissed or voluntarily withdrew from this program area in

2008–2009 were 0. *Child Development PhD (Doctor of Philosophy)*—Applications 2009–2010, 9. Total applicants accepted 2009–2010, 3. Number full-time enrolled (new admits only) 2009–2010, 0. Number part-time enrolled (new admits only) 2009–2010, 0. Openings 2010–2011, 7. The number of students enrolled full- and part-time who were dismissed or voluntarily withdrew from this program area in 2008–2009 were 0. *Measurement and Evaluation (Queries) PhD (Doctor of Philosophy)*—Applications 2009–2010, 14. Total applicants accepted 2009–2010, 4. Number full-time enrolled (new admits only) 2009–2010, 4. Number part-time enrolled (new admits only) 2009–2010, 0. Openings 2010–2011, 2. The median number of years required for completion of a degree in 2008–2009 were 5. The number of students enrolled full- and part-time who were dismissed or voluntarily withdrew from this program area in 2008–2009 were 0. *Cognitive Science Of Teaching and Learning PhD (Doctor of Philosophy)*—Applications 2009–2010, 16. Total applicants accepted 2009–2010, 9. Number full-time enrolled (new admits only) 2009–2010, 9. Number part-time enrolled (new admits only) 2009–2010, 0. Openings 2010–2011, 3. The median number of years required for completion of a degree in 2008–2009 were 5. The number of students enrolled full- and part-time who were dismissed or voluntarily withdrew from this program area in 2008–2009 were 0. *Curriculum, Technology and Education Reform MEd (Education)*—Applications 2009–2010, 17. Total applicants accepted 2009–2010, 15. Number full-time enrolled (new admits only) 2009–2010, 0. Number part-time enrolled (new admits only) 2009–2010, 12. Openings 2010–2011, 25. The median number of years required for completion of a degree in 2008–2009 were 2. The number of students enrolled full- and part-time who were dismissed or voluntarily withdrew from this program area in 2008–2009 were 0.

Scores: Entries appear in this order: required test or GPA, minimum score (if required), median score of students entering in 2009–2010. *Counseling Psychology PhD (Doctor of Philosophy):* GRE-V 500, 590, GRE-Q 570, 590, last 2 years GPA 3.2, 3.6, Masters GPA 3.8, 3.85; *Child Development PhD (Doctor of Philosophy):* GRE-V 490, 630, GRE-Q 630, 660, last 2 years GPA 3.82, 3.96, Masters GPA 3.5, 3.5; *Measurement and Evaluation (Queries) PhD (Doctor of Philosophy):* GRE-V 530, 560, GRE-Q 610, 710, last 2 years GPA 3.5, 3.6, Masters GPA 3.9, 3.9; *Cognitive Science of Teaching and Learning (CSTL) PhD (Doctor of Philosophy):* GRE-V 370, 480, GRE-Q 360, 650, last 2 years GPA 3.2, 3.5, Masters GPA 3.5, 3.8; *Curriculum, Technology and Education Reform (CTER) MEd (Education):* last 2 years GPA 2.52, 3.45.

Other Criteria: (importance of criteria rated low, medium, or high): GRE scores—medium, research experience—high, work experience—medium, extracurricular activity—medium, clinically related public service—medium, GPA—medium, letters of recommendation—high, interview—low, statement of goals and objectives—high, research interests—high. For additional information on admission requirements, go to http://education.illinois.edu/edpsy/howtoapply.html.

Student Characteristics: The following represents characteristics of students in 2009–2010 in all graduate psychology programs in the department: Female—full-time 76, part-time 34; Male—full-time 26, part-time 13; African American/Black—full-time 14, part-time 0; Hispanic/Latino(a)—full-time 6, part-time 3; Asian/Pacific Islander—full-time 2, part-time 1; American Indian/Alaska Native—full-time 0, part-time 0; Caucasian/White—full-time 80, part-time 43; Multi-ethnic—full-time 0, part-time 0; students subject to the Americans With Disabilities Act—full-time 0, part-time 0; Unknown ethnicity—full-time 0, part-time 0; International students who hold an F-1 or J-1 Visa—full-time 38, part-time 0.

Financial Information/Assistance:

Tuition for Full-Time Study: *Master's:* State residents: $503 per credit hour; Nonstate residents: $503 per credit hour. *Doctoral:* State residents: per academic year $9,318; Nonstate residents: per academic year $22,584. Tuition is subject to change. See the following Web site for updates and changes in tuition costs: http://www.registrar.illinois.edu/financial/tuition.html.

Financial Assistance:

First-Year Students: Teaching assistantships available for first year. Average amount paid per academic year: $7,000. Average number of hours worked per week: 20. Research assistantships available for first year. Average amount paid per academic year: $7,000. Average number of hours worked per week: 20. Fellowships and scholarships available for first year. Average amount paid per academic year: $10,000.

Advanced Students: Teaching assistantships available for advanced students. Average amount paid per academic year: $14,000. Average number of hours worked per week: 20. Research assistantships available for advanced students. Average amount paid per academic year: $14,000. Average number of hours worked per week: 20. Fellowships and scholarships available for advanced students. Average amount paid per academic year: $10,000.

Additional Information: Of all students currently enrolled full time, 90% benefited from one or more of the listed financial assistance programs. Application and information available online at: http://education.illinois.edu/edpsy/financialaid.html.

Internships/Practica: Doctoral Degree (PhD Counseling Psychology): For those doctoral students for whom a professional internship was required in this program prior to graduation, (4) students applied for an internship in 2008–2009, with (4) students obtaining an internship. Of those students who obtained an internship, (4) were paid internships. Of those students who obtained an internship, (4) students placed in APA/CPA accredited internships, (0) students placed in internships not APA/CPA accredited, but listed with the Association of Psychology Postdoctoral and Internship Programs (APPIC), (0) students placed in internships conforming to guidelines of the Council of Directors of School Psychology Programs (CDSPP), (0) students placed in internships that were not APA/CPA accredited, APPIC or CDSPP listed. The Counseling Psychology Division offers a variety of practica in University and community settings. Within the university, students work in agencies such as the Counseling Center, Career Center, McKinley Health Center, and the Disability Resources and Education Services Center at the University of Illinois and the Counseling Center at Illinois State University. Within the community, students work at the Psychological Services Center, the Champaign County Mental Health Center, Carle Clinic (a multi-specialty medical center), Veterans Administration Medical Center, and Cunningham Children's Home. Supervision is provided by on-site supervisors and by faculty members. Each Counseling Psychology doctoral student is required to complete a year long, full-time predoctoral internship approved by APPIC, or the equivalent. Typical internship sites include university counseling centers, hospitals/VA medical centers, child/adolescent treatment programs, and community mental health agencies.

Housing and Day Care: On-campus housing is available. See the following Web site for more information: http://www.housing.illinois.edu/. On-campus day care facilities are available. See the following Web site for more information: http://cdl.illinois.edu/.

Employment of Department Graduates:

Master's Degree Graduates: Of those who graduated in the academic year 2008–2009, the following categories and numbers represent the postgraduate activities and employment of master's degree graduates: Enrolled in a postdoctoral residency/fellowship (n/a), employed in independent practice (n/a), employed in other positions at a higher education institution (2), employed in a professional position in a school system (14), employed in business or industry (2), do not know (2), total from the above (master's) (20).

Doctoral Degree Graduates: Of those who graduated in the academic year 2008–2009, the following categories and numbers represent the postgraduate activities and employment of doctoral degree graduates: Enrolled in a psychology doctoral program (n/a), enrolled in a postdoctoral residency/fellowship (2), employed in an academic position at a university (7), employed in other positions at a higher education institution (5), employed in a hospital/medical center (1), still seeking employment (1), do not know (7), total from the above (doctoral) (23).

Additional Information:

Orientation, Objectives, and Emphasis of Department: The Department of Educational Psychology has been a leader in placing students as university/college professors, researchers, professional psychologists, and administrators in educational, private and government settings. The Department is composed of four divisions, each with a with distinctive program of doctoral study: (1) Counseling Psychology, offering an APA-accredited program, in which students are trained in the scientist–practitioner model from a multicultural perspective; (2) Child Development, focused on the development of children and adolescents, especially as it is relevant to education and educationally relevant outcomes; (3) Studies in Interpretive, Statistical, Measurement, and Evaluative Methodologies for Education (QUERIES), focused on developing and applying new methodologies in educational measurement, statistics, research design, and evaluation; and (4) the Cognitive Science of Teaching and Learning (CSTL), which is concerned with the study of basic processes in learning, cognition, and language understanding, and the principles through which learning is optimized in diverse contexts across the life span, among individuals who vary with respect to abilities, interests, and goals.

Special Facilities or Resources: The Department of Educational Psychology is under the purview of the College of Education, rated one of the nation's top education colleges, with research and support facilities that include the Graduate Research and Instructional Computing Lab, Children's Research Center, Bureau of Educational Research, Office of Educational Technology, Adult Learning Lab (with eyetracking equipment), Center for the Study of Reading, and classrooms for video demonstration, telecommunications, and computer-based education. Faculty research is funded by the National Science Foundation, National Institutes of Health, Centers for Disease Control, Institute of Educational Sciences, WT Grant Foundation, and the Spencer Foundation. The University of Illinois offers a rich academic environment with top-ranked Departments of Psychology, Computer Science, Engineering, and Speech Communication, as well as the 3rd largest academic library system in the U.S., ranking only behind Harvard and Yale. There are also strong programs in Cognitive Neuroscience (Brain and Cognition Program), Human and Community Development, Gender and Women's Studies, Afro-American Studies and Research Program, and Center for Latin American and Caribbean Studies. Research and support facilities on campus include Beckman Institute for Advanced Science and Technology, Statistical Laboratory for Educational and Psychological Measurement, Language Learning Lab, Survey Research Laboratory, and Illinois Statistical Office (consulting services).

Information for Students With Physical Disabilities: See the following Web site for more information: http://www.disability.uiuc.edu/.

Application Information:
Send to Admissions, Department of Educational Psychology, 226 Education, 1310 S. Sixth Street, Champaign, IL 61820. Application available online. URL of online application: http://www.grad.uiuc.edu/admissions/apply/. Students are admitted in the Fall, application deadline December 1. *Fee:* $60. International applicant fee $75.

Illinois, University of, Urbana–Champaign
Department of Human and Community Development
Agricultural, Consumer and Environmental Sciences
274 Bevier Hall, MC-180
Urbana, IL 61801
Telephone: (217) 333-3790
Fax: (217) 244-7877
E-mail: *roswald@illinois.edu*
Web: *http://www.hcd.uiuc.edu/*

Department Information:
1996. Department Head: Robert Hughes, Jr., PhD. Number of faculty: total—full-time 20; women—full-time 15; total—minority—full-time 4; women minority—full-time 3; faculty subject to the Americans With Disabilities Act 1.

Programs and Degrees Offered:
Listed in the following order: Program area, degree type (T if terminal Master's), number awarded 7/08–6/09. Human Development and Family Studies PhD (Doctor of Philosophy) 1, Marriage and Family Services MA/MS (Master of Arts/Science) (T) 4.

Student Applications/Admissions:
Student Applications
Human Development and Family Studies PhD *(Doctor of Philosophy)*—Applications 2009–2010, 29. Total applicants accepted 2009–2010, 9. Number full-time enrolled (new admits only) 2009–2010, 6. Number part-time enrolled (new admits only) 2009–2010, 0. Openings 2010–2011, 5. The median number of years required for completion of a degree in 2008–2009 were 5. The number of students enrolled full- and part-time who were dismissed or voluntarily withdrew from this program

area in 2008–2009 were 0. *Marriage and Family Services MA/MS (Master of Arts/Science)*—Applications 2009–2010, 13. Total applicants accepted 2009–2010, 3. Number full-time enrolled (new admits only) 2009–2010, 3. Number part-time enrolled (new admits only) 2009–2010, 0. Openings 2010–2011, 3. The median number of years required for completion of a degree in 2008–2009 were 3. The number of students enrolled full- and part-time who were dismissed or voluntarily withdrew from this program area in 2008–2009 were 0.

Scores: Entries appear in this order: required test or GPA, minimum score (if required), median score of students entering in 2009–2010. *Human Development and Family Studies PhD (Doctor of Philosophy)*: GRE-V 550, 570, GRE-Q 550, 620, GRE-Analytical 4.5, 5, last 2 years GPA 3.0, 3.7; *Marriage and Family Services (MS/MSW) MA/MS (Master of Arts/Science)*: GRE-V 500, 630, GRE-Q 500, 660, GRE-Analytical 4.0, 5, overall undergraduate GPA no minimum stated, last 2 years GPA 3.0, 3.7.

Other Criteria: (importance of criteria rated low, medium, or high): GRE scores—medium, research experience—high, GPA—medium, letters of recommendation—high, statement of goals and objectives—high, fit with program—high. For additional information on admission requirements, go to http://www.hcd.uiuc.edu/grad/.

Student Characteristics: The following represents characteristics of students in 2009–2010 in all graduate psychology programs in the department: Female—full-time 29, part-time 0; Male—full-time 5, part-time 0; African American/Black—full-time 5, part-time 0; Hispanic/Latino(a)—full-time 3, part-time 0; Asian/Pacific Islander—full-time 6, part-time 0; American Indian/Alaska Native—full-time 0, part-time 0; Caucasian/White—full-time 18, part-time 0; Multi-ethnic—full-time 1, part-time 0; students subject to the Americans With Disabilities Act—full-time 0, part-time 0; Unknown ethnicity—full-time 1, part-time 0; International students who hold an F-1 or J-1 Visa—full-time 0, part-time 0.

Financial Information/Assistance:
Tuition for Full-Time Study: *Master's:* State residents: per academic year $8,960; Nonstate residents: per academic year $21,714. *Doctoral:* State residents: per academic year $8,960; Nonstate residents: per academic year $21,714. Tuition is subject to change. See the following Web site for updates and changes in tuition costs: http://www.registrar.illinois.edu/financial/tuition.html.

Financial Assistance:
First-Year Students: Teaching assistantships available for first year. Average amount paid per academic year: $13,429. Average number of hours worked per week: 20. Research assistantships available for first year. Average amount paid per academic year: $13,429. Average number of hours worked per week: 20. Fellowships and scholarships available for first year. Average amount paid per academic year: $17,500. Average number of hours worked per week: 0.

Advanced Students: Teaching assistantships available for advanced students. Average amount paid per academic year: $13,961. Average number of hours worked per week: 20. Research assistantships available for advanced students. Average amount paid per academic year: $13,961. Average number of hours worked per week: 20. Fellowships and scholarships available for advanced students. Average amount paid per academic year: $20,000. Average number of hours worked per week: 0.

Additional Information: Of all students currently enrolled full time, 100% benefited from one or more of the listed financial assistance programs. Application and information available online at: http://www.hcd.uiuc.edu/grad/fellow.html.

Internships/Practica: Master's Degree (MA/MS Marriage and Family Services (MS/MSW)): An internship experience, such as a final research project or "capstone" experience is required of graduates. MS/MSW students and doctoral students with the applied option complete at least one semester-long internship, usually within a human services setting.

Housing and Day Care: On-campus housing is available. See the following Web site for more information: http://www.housing.illinois.edu/. On-campus day care facilities are available. See the following Web site for more information: http://cdl.uiuc.edu/; http://www.ccrs.uiuc.edu.

Employment of Department Graduates:
Master's Degree Graduates: Of those who graduated in the academic year 2008–2009, the following categories and numbers represent the postgraduate activities and employment of master's degree graduates: Enrolled in a postdoctoral residency/fellowship (n/a), employed in independent practice (n/a), employed in an academic position at a university (1), employed in a community mental health/counseling center (3), not seeking employment (1), total from the above (master's) (5).

Doctoral Degree Graduates: Of those who graduated in the academic year 2008–2009, the following categories and numbers represent the postgraduate activities and employment of doctoral degree graduates: Enrolled in a psychology doctoral program (n/a), enrolled in a postdoctoral residency/fellowship (3), employed in an academic position at a university (4), employed in other positions at a higher education institution (1), employed in business or industry (1), still seeking employment (0), other employment position (2), total from the above (doctoral) (11).

Additional Information:
Orientation, Objectives, and Emphasis of Department: Our Human Development and Family Studies doctoral program focuses on the positive development and resilience of children, youth, and families within everyday life contexts. Emphases include the social and emotional development of children and youth; parent-child and sibling relationships; and racial, ethnic, and sexual orientation diversity. All topics are studied within specific settings. Faculty have expertise in both qualitative and quantitative research. Students may choose an applied supporting option in program development, evaluation, and outreach.

Special Facilities or Resources: Our department includes two laboratory preschool facilities, a childcare resource and referral service, a lab for community and economic development, and the Family Resiliency Center.

Information for Students With Physical Disabilities: See the following Web site for more information: http://www.disability.uiuc.edu/.

Application Information:
Send to Graduate Secretary, 274 Bevier Hall, 905 South Goodwin, Urbana, IL, 61801. Application available online. URL of online appli-

GRADUATE STUDY IN PSYCHOLOGY

cation: http://www.hcd.uiuc.edu/grad/app-process.html. Students are admitted in the Fall, application deadline January 15. *Fee:* $60. $75.00 for international applicants.

Illinois, University of, Urbana–Champaign
Department of Psychology
Liberal Arts & Sciences
Psychology Building, 603 East Daniel Street
Champaign, IL 61820
Telephone: (217) 333-2169
Fax: (217) 244-5876
E-mail: *garnsey@illinois.edu*
Web: *http://www.psych.illinois.edu*

Department Information:
1904. Head: David E. Irwin. Number of faculty: total—full-time 51, part-time 8; women—full-time 17, part-time 4; total—minority—full-time 9, part-time 2; women minority—full-time 4, part-time 1.

Programs and Degrees Offered:
Listed in the following order: Program area, degree type (T if terminal Master's), number awarded 7/08–6/09. Applied Measurement MA/MS (Master of Arts/Science) (T) 1, Applied Personnel MA/MS (Master of Arts/Science) (T) 0, Biological Psychology PhD (Doctor of Philosophy) 1, Clinical Psychology PhD (Doctor of Philosophy) 7, Cognitive Psychology PhD (Doctor of Philosophy) 3, Developmental Psychology PhD (Doctor of Philosophy) 3, Social-Personality-Organizational PhD (Doctor of Philosophy) 5, Brain and Cognition PhD (Doctor of Philosophy) 2, Quantitative Psychology PhD (Doctor of Philosophy) 2, Visual Cognition & Human Performance PhD (Doctor of Philosophy) 3.

APA Accreditation: Clinical PhD (Doctor of Philosophy). Student Outcome Data Website: http://www.psych.illinois.edu/divisions/clinicalcommunity.php.

Student Applications/Admissions:
Student Applications
Applied Measurement MA/MS (Master of Arts/Science)—Applications 2009–2010, 0. Total applicants accepted 2009–2010, 0. Number full-time enrolled (new admits only) 2009–2010, 1. The median number of years required for completion of a degree in 2008–2009 were 2. The number of students enrolled full- and part-time who were dismissed or voluntarily withdrew from this program area in 2008–2009 were 0. *Applied Personnel MA/MS (Master of Arts/Science)*—Applications 2009–2010, 5. Total applicants accepted 2009–2010, 0. Number full-time enrolled (new admits only) 2009–2010, 0. The number of students enrolled full- and part-time who were dismissed or voluntarily withdrew from this program area in 2008–2009 were 0. *Biological Psychology PhD (Doctor of Philosophy)*—Applications 2009–2010, 15. Total applicants accepted 2009–2010, 2. Number full-time enrolled (new admits only) 2009–2010, 0. The median number of years required for completion of a degree in 2008–2009 were 6. The number of students enrolled full- and part-time who were dismissed or voluntarily withdrew from this program area in 2008–2009 were 1. *Clinical Psychology PhD (Doctor of Philosophy)*—Applications 2009–2010, 241. Total applicants accepted 2009–2010, 10. Number full-time enrolled (new admits only) 2009–2010, 4. The median number of years required for completion of a degree in 2008–2009 were 6. The number of students enrolled full- and part-time who were dismissed or voluntarily withdrew from this program area in 2008–2009 were 1. *Cognitive Psychology PhD (Doctor of Philosophy)*—Applications 2009–2010, 47. Total applicants accepted 2009–2010, 6. Number full-time enrolled (new admits only) 2009–2010, 4. The median number of years required for completion of a degree in 2008–2009 were 6. The number of students enrolled full- and part-time who were dismissed or voluntarily withdrew from this program area in 2008–2009 were 1. *Developmental Psychology PhD (Doctor of Philosophy)*—Applications 2009–2010, 59. Total applicants accepted 2009–2010, 5. Number full-time enrolled (new admits only) 2009–2010, 3. Total enrolled 2009–2010 full-time, 21. The median number of years required for completion of a degree in 2008–2009 were 6. *Social-Personality-Organizational PhD (Doctor of Philosophy)*—Applications 2009–2010, 189. Total applicants accepted 2009–2010, 16. Number full-time enrolled (new admits only) 2009–2010, 10. The median number of years required for completion of a degree in 2008–2009 were 6. *Brain and Cognition PhD (Doctor of Philosophy)*—Applications 2009–2010, 59. Total applicants accepted 2009–2010, 6. Number full-time enrolled (new admits only) 2009–2010, 4. Total enrolled 2009–2010 full-time, 19. The median number of years required for completion of a degree in 2008–2009 were 6. The number of students enrolled full- and part-time who were dismissed or voluntarily withdrew from this program area in 2008–2009 were 1. *Quantitative Psychology PhD (Doctor of Philosophy)*—Applications 2009–2010, 32. Total applicants accepted 2009–2010, 4. Number full-time enrolled (new admits only) 2009–2010, 3. The median number of years required for completion of a degree in 2008–2009 were 6. *Visual Cognition & Human Performance PhD (Doctor of Philosophy)*—Applications 2009–2010, 17. Total applicants accepted 2009–2010, 4. Number full-time enrolled (new admits only) 2009–2010, 1. The median number of years required for completion of a degree in 2008–2009 were 6.

Scores: Entries appear in this order: required test or GPA, minimum score (if required), median score of students entering in 2009–2010. *Applied Measurement MA/MS (Master of Arts/Science):* GRE-V no minimum stated, 555, GRE-Q no minimum stated, 730, last 2 years GPA 3.0, 3.97; *Applied Personnel MA/MS (Master of Arts/Science):* GRE-V no minimum stated, GRE-Q no minimum stated, last 2 years GPA 3.0; *Biological Psychology PhD (Doctor of Philosophy):* GRE-V no minimum stated, 563, GRE-Q no minimum stated, 648, last 2 years GPA 3.0, 3.57; *Clinical Psychology PhD (Doctor of Philosophy):* GRE-V no minimum stated, 610, GRE-Q no minimum stated, 700, last 2 years GPA 3.0, 3.87; *Cognitive Psychology PhD (Doctor of Philosophy):* GRE-V no minimum stated, 666, GRE-Q no minimum stated, 746, last 2 years GPA 3.0, 3.77; *Developmental Psychology PhD (Doctor of Philosophy):* GRE-V no minimum stated, 636, GRE-Q no minimum stated, 653, last 2 years GPA 3.0, 3.95; *Social-Personality-Organizational PhD (Doctor of Philosophy):* GRE-V no minimum stated, 678, GRE-Q no minimum stated, 737, last 2 years GPA 3.0, 3.82; *Brain and Cognition PhD (Doctor of Philosophy):* GRE-V no minimum stated, 585, GRE-Q no minimum stated, 751, last 2 years GPA 3.0, 3.78; *Quantitative Psychology PhD (Doctor of Philosophy):* GRE-V no minimum stated, 526, GRE-Q no minimum stated,

750, last 2 years GPA 3.0, 3.8; *Visual Cognition & Human Performance PhD (Doctor of Philosophy)*: GRE-V no minimum stated, 630, GRE-Q no minimum stated, 640, last 2 years GPA 3.0, 3.8.

Other Criteria: (importance of criteria rated low, medium, or high): GRE scores—high, research experience—high, work experience—medium, clinically related public service—high, GPA—high, letters of recommendation—high, interview—high, statement of goals and objectives—high. For additional information on admission requirements, go to http://www.psych.illinois.edu/graduate/applying.php.

Student Characteristics: The following represents characteristics of students in 2009–2010 in all graduate psychology programs in the department: Female—full-time 106, part-time 0; Male—full-time 63, part-time 0; African American/Black—full-time 7, part-time 0; Hispanic/Latino(a)—full-time 6, part-time 0; Asian/Pacific Islander—full-time 14, part-time 0; American Indian/Alaska Native—full-time 2, part-time 0; Caucasian/White—full-time 93, part-time 0; Multi-ethnic—full-time 1, part-time 0; students subject to the Americans With Disabilities Act—full-time 0, part-time 0; Unknown ethnicity—full-time 1, part-time 0; International students who hold an F-1 or J-1 Visa—full-time 45, part-time 0.

Financial Information/Assistance:

Tuition for Full-Time Study: *Master's:* State residents: per academic year $9,318; Nonstate residents: per academic year $22,582. *Doctoral:* State residents: per academic year $9,318; Nonstate residents: per academic year $22,582. Tuition is subject to change. See the following Web site for updates and changes in tuition costs: http://registrar.illinois.edu/financial/tuition.html.

Financial Assistance:

First-Year Students: Teaching assistantships available for first year. Average amount paid per academic year: $16,182. Average number of hours worked per week: 20. Apply by January 2. Research assistantships available for first year. Average amount paid per academic year: $16,182. Average number of hours worked per week: 20. Apply by January 2. Traineeships available for first year. Average amount paid per academic year: $20,772. Apply by January 2. Fellowships and scholarships available for first year. Average amount paid per academic year: $17,000. Apply by January 2.

Advanced Students: Teaching assistantships available for advanced students. Average amount paid per academic year: $16,182. Average number of hours worked per week: 20. Research assistantships available for advanced students. Average amount paid per academic year: $16,182. Average number of hours worked per week: 20. Traineeships available for advanced students. Average amount paid per academic year: $20,772. Fellowships and scholarships available for advanced students. Average amount paid per academic year: $17,000.

Additional Information: Of all students currently enrolled full time, 100% benefited from one or more of the listed financial assistance programs. Application and information available online at: http://www.osfa.illinois.edu/.

Internships/Practica: Doctoral Degree (PhD Clinical Psychology): For those doctoral students for whom a professional internship was required in this program prior to graduation, (5) students applied for an internship in 2008–2009, with (4) students obtaining an internship. Of those students who obtained an internship, (4) were paid internships. Of those students who obtained an internship, (4) students placed in APA/CPA accredited internships, (0) students placed in internships not APA/CPA accredited, but listed with the Association of Psychology Postdoctoral and Internship Programs (APPIC), (0) students placed in internships conforming to guidelines of the Council of Directors of School Psychology Programs (CDSPP), (0) students placed in internships that were not APA/CPA accredited, APPIC or CDSPP listed. Laboratories in Clinical Psychology—Intensive practice in techniques of clinical assessment and behavior modification with emphasis on recent innovations; small sections of the course formed according to the specialized interests of students and staff.

Housing and Day Care: On-campus housing is available. See the following Web site for more information: http://www.housing.illinois.edu/Future/Graduate.aspx. On-campus day care facilities are available. See the following Web site for more information: http://www.cdl.uiuc.edu.

Employment of Department Graduates:

Master's Degree Graduates: Of those who graduated in the academic year 2008–2009, the following categories and numbers represent the postgraduate activities and employment of master's degree graduates: Enrolled in a postdoctoral residency/fellowship (n/a), employed in independent practice (n/a), total from the above (master's) (0).

Doctoral Degree Graduates: Of those who graduated in the academic year 2008–2009, the following categories and numbers represent the postgraduate activities and employment of doctoral degree graduates: Enrolled in a psychology doctoral program (n/a), employed in an academic position at a university (52), employed in business or industry (8), employed in government agency (2), employed in a community mental health/counseling center (2), other employment position (4), total from the above (doctoral) (68).

Additional Information:

Orientation, Objectives, and Emphasis of Department: The department trains students at the doctoral level for basic research in all areas. Students are admitted in one of the eight divisions: biological, brain and cognition, cognitive, clinical/community, developmental, quantitative, social-personality-organizational, and visual cognition & human performance. Interactions with faculty in other divisions are quite common; interdisciplinary training is encouraged. Applied research training is offered in measurement and personnel psychology. There is a strong emphasis on individualized training programs in an apprenticeship model. Each student's program is tailored to his or her research interests. Wide opportunities exist for students to participate in ongoing research programs. Students are encouraged to develop their own programs.

Special Facilities or Resources: The department has extensive laboratory facilities in all areas, including biological psychology. Excellent departmental and university computer facilities are readily available to graduate students. Most faculty laboratories are computerized. The department maintains a computer system that supports text processing, data management, and communication between laboratories and campus computers. There are very advanced facilities for research in all areas, including psychophysiology, cognitive psychology, neurochemistry, and neuroanatomy. A first-rate animal colony is maintained by the department. There is an excellent machine shop and a fine electronics shop. Programs are coordinated with other campus departments and institutes, including life sciences, communications, labor, education, and child study.

Information for Students With Physical Disabilities: See the following Web site for more information: http://www.disability.uiuc.edu/.

Application Information:
Send to Graduate Student Affairs Office, 314 Psychology Building, 603 East Daniel Street, Champaign, IL 61820. Application available online. URL of online application: http://www.grad.uiuc.edu/admissions/apply/. Students are admitted in the Fall, application deadline January 2. *Fee:* $60. The fee for an international application is $75.

Lewis University
Department of Psychology
One University Parkway
Romeoville, IL 60446
Telephone: (815) 836-5594
Fax: (815) 836-5032
E-mail: Helmka@lewisu.edu
Web: http://www.lewisu.edu

Department Information:
1993. Director of Graduate Programs in Psychology: Katherine Helm. Number of faculty: total—full-time 14, part-time 4; women—full-time 9; total—minority—full-time 4; women minority—full-time 3.

Programs and Degrees Offered:
Listed in the following order: Program area, degree type (T if terminal Master's), number awarded 7/08–6/09. Counseling Psychology MA/MS (Master of Arts/Science) 24, School Counseling MA/MS (Master of Arts/Science) (T) 78.

Student Applications/Admissions:
Student Applications
Counseling Psychology MA/MS (Master of Arts/Science)—Applications 2009–2010, 54. Total applicants accepted 2009–2010, 40. Number full-time enrolled (new admits only) 2009–2010, 7. Number part-time enrolled (new admits only) 2009–2010, 9. Total enrolled 2009–2010 full-time, 17, part-time, 70. Openings 2010–2011, 40. The median number of years required for completion of a degree in 2008–2009 were 3. The number of students enrolled full- and part-time who were dismissed or voluntarily withdrew from this program area in 2008–2009 were 5. School Counseling MA/MS (Master of Arts/Science)—Applications 2009–2010, 78. Total applicants accepted 2009–2010, 68. Number full-time enrolled (new admits only) 2009–2010, 65. Number part-time enrolled (new admits only) 2009–2010, 134. Total enrolled 2009–2010 full-time, 88, part-time, 112. Openings 2010–2011, 55. The median number of years required for completion of a degree in 2008–2009 were 2. The number of students enrolled full- and part-time who were dismissed or voluntarily withdrew from this program area in 2008–2009 were 8.
Other Criteria: (importance of criteria rated low, medium, or high): research experience—low, work experience—high, extracurricular activity—medium, clinically related public service—high, GPA—high, letters of recommendation—high, interview—low, statement of goals and objectives—high, undergraduate major in psychology—medium, specific undergraduate psychology courses taken—medium. The counseling psychology program requires that applicants have taken 15 hours of undergraduate psychology courses prior to being considered for the program.

Student Characteristics: The following represents characteristics of students in 2009–2010 in all graduate psychology programs in the department: Female—full-time 26, part-time 156; Male—full-time 4, part-time 25; African American/Black—full-time 0, part-time 14; Hispanic/Latino(a)—full-time 0, part-time 12; Asian/Pacific Islander—full-time 0, part-time 3; American Indian/Alaska Native—full-time 0, part-time 0; Caucasian/White—full-time 0, part-time 0; Multi-ethnic—full-time 0, part-time 2; students subject to the Americans With Disabilities Act—full-time 0, part-time 2; Unknown ethnicity—full-time 0, part-time 0; International students who hold an F-1 or J-1 Visa—full-time 1, part-time 2.

Financial Information/Assistance:
Tuition for Full-Time Study: Master's: State residents: per academic year $16,640, $720 per credit hour; Nonstate residents: per academic year $16,640, $720 per credit hour. Tuition is subject to change. Tuition costs vary by program.

Financial Assistance:
First-Year Students: Research assistantships available for first year. Average amount paid per academic year: $12,960. Average number of hours worked per week: 15.
Advanced Students: Research assistantships available for advanced students. Average amount paid per academic year: $12,960. Average number of hours worked per week: 15.
Additional Information: Of all students currently enrolled full time, 1% benefited from one or more of the listed financial assistance programs.

Internships/Practica: Numerous practica and internship sites available in the community.

Housing and Day Care: No on-campus housing is available. No on-campus day care facilities are available.

Employment of Department Graduates:
Master's Degree Graduates: Of those who graduated in the academic year 2008–2009, the following categories and numbers represent the postgraduate activities and employment of master's degree graduates: Enrolled in a postdoctoral residency/fellowship (n/a), employed in independent practice (n/a), total from the above (master's) (0).
Doctoral Degree Graduates: Of those who graduated in the academic year 2008–2009, the following categories and numbers represent the postgraduate activities and employment of doctoral degree graduates: Enrolled in a psychology doctoral program (n/a), total from the above (doctoral) (0).

ILLINOIS

Additional Information:
Orientation, Objectives, and Emphasis of Department: The program in counseling psychology is oriented toward individuals who have some experience or great interest in mental health, behavioral, social service or educational interventions or assessment. It is designed primarily as part-time with courses offered primarily in the evenings and on occasional weekends. The Program has two sub-specialty areas: 1. Mental Health counseling; 2. Child and Adolescent Counseling. There is a second program in School Counseling and is designed for those individuals who want to work in the public or private school systems. The School Counseling program has several sites including the main campus and Tinley Park.

Application Information:
Send to Graduate Program Director, Department of Psychology, Lewis University, One University Parkway, Romeoville, IL 60446. Application available online. Programs have rolling admissions. Fee: $40.

Loyola University of Chicago
Counseling Psychology
School of Education
820 North Michigan Avenue
Chicago, IL 60611
Telephone: (312) 915-6836
Fax: (312) 915-6660
E-mail: sbrown@luc.edu
Web: http://www.luc.edu/education/

Department Information:
1969. Graduate Program Director: Steven D. Brown. Number of faculty: total—full-time 5, part-time 10; women—full-time 4, part-time 5; total—minority—full-time 3, part-time 7; women minority—full-time 3, part-time 5.

Programs and Degrees Offered:
Listed in the following order: Program area, degree type (T if terminal Master's), number awarded 7/08–6/09. Counseling Psychology PhD (Doctor of Philosophy) 5, Community Counseling MA/MS (Master of Arts/Science) (T) 11, School Counseling MEd (Education) 18.

APA Accreditation: Counseling PhD (Doctor of Philosophy). Student Outcome Data Website: http://www.luc.edu/education/programs/cpsy-phd_quality_indicators.shtml.

Student Applications/Admissions:
Student Applications
Counseling Psychology PhD (Doctor of Philosophy)—Applications 2009–2010, 55. Total applicants accepted 2009–2010, 4. Number full-time enrolled (new admits only) 2009–2010, 4. Number part-time enrolled (new admits only) 2009–2010, 0. Openings 2010–2011, 4. The median number of years required for completion of a degree in 2008–2009 were 6. The number of students enrolled full- and part-time who were dismissed or voluntarily withdrew from this program area in 2008–2009 were 1. Community Counseling MA/MS (Master of Arts/Science)—Applications 2009–2010, 78. Total applicants accepted 2009–2010, 50. Number full-time enrolled (new admits only) 2009–2010, 10. Number part-time enrolled (new admits only) 2009–2010, 0. Total enrolled 2009–2010 full-time, 28, part-time, 2. Openings 2010–2011, 25. The median number of years required for completion of a degree in 2008–2009 were 2. The number of students enrolled full- and part-time who were dismissed or voluntarily withdrew from this program area in 2008–2009 were 0. School Counseling MEd (Education)—Applications 2009–2010, 62. Total applicants accepted 2009–2010, 50. Number full-time enrolled (new admits only) 2009–2010, 7. Number part-time enrolled (new admits only) 2009–2010, 4. Total enrolled 2009–2010 full-time, 20, part-time, 9. Openings 2010–2011, 25. The median number of years required for completion of a degree in 2008–2009 were 2. The number of students enrolled full- and part-time who were dismissed or voluntarily withdrew from this program area in 2008–2009 were 0.

Scores: Entries appear in this order: required test or GPA, minimum score (if required), median score of students entering in 2009–2010. Counseling Psychology PhD (Doctor of Philosophy): GRE-V 550, 550, GRE-Q 550, 550, GRE-Analytical 4.5, 5.0, GRE-Subject (Psychology) 550, 550, overall undergraduate GPA 3.5, 3.5, last 2 years GPA 3.0, 3.0, Masters GPA 3.5, 3.5; Community Counseling MA/MS (Master of Arts/Science): GRE-V 500, 550, GRE-Q 500, 550, overall undergraduate GPA 3.0, 3.0, last 2 years GPA 3.0, 3.0; School Counseling MEd (Education): GRE-V 500, 550, GRE-Q 500, 550, overall undergraduate GPA 3.0, 3.0, last 2 years GPA 3.0, 3.0.

Other Criteria: (importance of criteria rated low, medium, or high): GRE scores—medium, research experience—high, work experience—medium, clinically related public service—high, GPA—medium, letters of recommendation—high, interview—high, statement of goals and objectives—high, match w/ faculty interest—high, undergraduate major in psychology—medium, specific undergraduate psychology courses taken—low. For additional information on admission requirements, go to http://www.luc.edu/education/admission.shtml.

Student Characteristics: The following represents characteristics of students in 2009–2010 in all graduate psychology programs in the department: Female—full-time 58, part-time 9; Male—full-time 14, part-time 2; African American/Black—full-time 11, part-time 2; Hispanic/Latino(a)—full-time 1, part-time 2; Asian/Pacific Islander—full-time 4, part-time 0; American Indian/Alaska Native—full-time 0, part-time 0; Caucasian/White—full-time 56, part-time 7; Multi-ethnic—full-time 0, part-time 0; students subject to the Americans With Disabilities Act—full-time 0, part-time 0; Unknown ethnicity—full-time 0, part-time 0; International students who hold an F-1 or J-1 Visa—full-time 0, part-time 0.

Financial Information/Assistance:
Tuition for Full-Time Study: Master's: State residents: $830 per credit hour; Nonstate residents: $830 per credit hour. Doctoral: State residents: $830 per credit hour; Nonstate residents: $830 per credit hour. Tuition is subject to change.

Financial Assistance:
First-Year Students: Teaching assistantships available for first year. Average amount paid per academic year: $14,000. Average number of hours worked per week: 20. Apply by December 1. Research assistantships available for first year. Average amount paid per academic year: $14,000. Average number of hours worked

per week: 20. Apply by December 1. Fellowships and scholarships available for first year. Average amount paid per academic year: $14,000. Average number of hours worked per week: 0.

Advanced Students: Teaching assistantships available for advanced students. Average amount paid per academic year: $14,000. Average number of hours worked per week: 20. Apply by December 1. Research assistantships available for advanced students. Average amount paid per academic year: $14,000. Average number of hours worked per week: 20. Apply by December 1. Fellowships and scholarships available for advanced students. Average amount paid per academic year: $14,000. Average number of hours worked per week: 20.

Additional Information: Of all students currently enrolled full time, 50% benefited from one or more of the listed financial assistance programs. Application and information available online at: http://www.luc.edu/education/financialassistance_grad.shtml.

Internships/Practica: Doctoral Degree (PhD Counseling Psychology): For those doctoral students for whom a professional internship was required in this program prior to graduation, (7) students applied for an internship in 2008–2009, with (6) students obtaining an internship. Of those students who obtained an internship, (6) were paid internships. Of those students who obtained an internship, (6) students placed in APA/CPA accredited internships, (0) students placed in internships not APA/CPA accredited, but listed with the Association of Psychology Postdoctoral and Internship Programs (APPIC), (0) students placed in internships conforming to guidelines of the Council of Directors of School Psychology Programs (CDSPP), (0) students placed in internships that were not APA/CPA accredited, APPIC or CDSPP listed. Master's Degree (MA/MS Community Counseling): An internship experience, such as a final research project or "capstone" experience is required of graduates. Internships and practica are available at many excellent training facilities in the greater Chicago-land area, including university counseling centers, hospitals, VA centers, and mental health clinics. There are both therapy-oriented and diagnostic/assessment-oriented practica. Most practicum sites serve a diverse clientele.

Housing and Day Care: On-campus housing is available. Apartment style housing is available for graduate students. No on-campus day care facilities are available.

Employment of Department Graduates:
Master's Degree Graduates: Of those who graduated in the academic year 2008–2009, the following categories and numbers represent the postgraduate activities and employment of master's degree graduates: Enrolled in a psychology doctoral program (5), enrolled in a postdoctoral residency/fellowship (n/a), employed in independent practice (n/a), total from the above (master's) (5).
Doctoral Degree Graduates: Of those who graduated in the academic year 2008–2009, the following categories and numbers represent the postgraduate activities and employment of doctoral degree graduates: Enrolled in a psychology doctoral program (n/a), enrolled in a postdoctoral residency/fellowship (1), employed in an academic position at a university (1), employed in an academic position at a 2-year/4-year college (1), employed in a community mental health/counseling center (1), employed in a hospital/medical center (1), total from the above (doctoral) (5).

Additional Information:
Orientation, Objectives, and Emphasis of Department: The PhD program, accredited by the APA, is based on the scientist–practitioner model of graduate education and emphasizes the interdependence of science and practice. Doctoral students are provided opportunities to collaborate with faculty in terms of research, prevention/intervention, and teaching activities from the first year of enrollment. Faculty research concentrates in three areas: multicultural psychology, preventive psychology, and vocational psychology. Applicant interest in one of these three areas is a major admission criterion since students are expected to apprentice themselves with a faculty member throughout their tenure in the program. Regardless of the field of interest, each student is exposed to the scientist–practitioner model. Graduates are prepared for teaching, research, and professional practice.

Special Facilities or Resources: The school has excellent library and research facilities and computer resources available to students.

Information for Students With Physical Disabilities: See the following Web site for more information: http://www.luc.edu/sswd/index.shtml.

Application Information:
Send to Graduate Enrollment Management, Loyola University Chicago Lewis Towers, 8th Floor, 820 N. Michigan Avenue, Chicago, IL 60611. Application available online. URL of online application: http://www.luc.edu/education/apply1.shtml. Students are admitted in the Fall, application deadline December 1. Master's programs in School and Community Counseling have an application deadline of February 15. *Fee:* $50. Waived if submitted online.

Loyola University of Chicago
Department of Psychology
Arts and Sciences
1032 West Sheridan Road
Chicago, IL 60660
Telephone: (773) 508-3001
Fax: (773) 508-8713
E-mail: *prupert@luc.edu*
Web: *http://www.luc.edu/psychology*

Department Information:
1930. Chairperson: Patricia A. Rupert. Number of faculty: total—full-time 32, part-time 8; women—full-time 16, part-time 3; total—minority—full-time 5, part-time 1; women minority—full-time 3.

Programs and Degrees Offered:
Listed in the following order: Program area, degree type (T if terminal Master's), number awarded 7/08–6/09. Developmental Psychology PhD (Doctor of Philosophy) 1, Social Psychology PhD (Doctor of Philosophy) 3, Clinical Psychology PhD (Doctor of Philosophy) 74, Applied Social Psychology MA/MS (Master of Arts/Science) (T) 4.

APA Accreditation: Clinical PhD (Doctor of Philosophy).

Student Applications/Admissions:
Student Applications
Developmental Psychology PhD (Doctor of Philosophy)—Applications 2009–2010, 12. Total applicants accepted 2009–2010, 3. Number full-time enrolled (new admits only) 2009–2010, 3. Openings 2010–2011, 2. The median number of years required for completion of a degree in 2008–2009 were 6. *Social Psychology PhD (Doctor of Philosophy)*—Applications 2009–2010, 50. Total applicants accepted 2009–2010, 7. Number full-time enrolled (new admits only) 2009–2010, 3. Number part-time enrolled (new admits only) 2009–2010, 0. Openings 2010–2011, 4. The median number of years required for completion of a degree in 2008–2009 were 6. The number of students enrolled full- and part-time who were dismissed or voluntarily withdrew from this program area in 2008–2009 were 0. *Clinical Psychology PhD (Doctor of Philosophy)*—Applications 2009–2010, 327. Total applicants accepted 2009–2010, 10. Number full-time enrolled (new admits only) 2009–2010, 6. Number part-time enrolled (new admits only) 2009–2010, 0. Openings 2010–2011, 6. The median number of years required for completion of a degree in 2008–2009 were 6. The number of students enrolled full- and part-time who were dismissed or voluntarily withdrew from this program area in 2008–2009 were 0. *Applied Social Psychology MA/MS (Master of Arts/Science)*—Applications 2009–2010, 20. Total applicants accepted 2009–2010, 6. Number full-time enrolled (new admits only) 2009–2010, 4. Openings 2010–2011, 4. The median number of years required for completion of a degree in 2008–2009 were 2. The number of students enrolled full- and part-time who were dismissed or voluntarily withdrew from this program area in 2008–2009 were 0.
Other Criteria: (importance of criteria rated low, medium, or high): GRE scores—high, research experience—high, work experience—low, extracurricular activity—low, clinically related public service—medium, GPA—high, letters of recommendation—high, interview—high, statement of goals and objectives—high. Only the Clinical program requires an interview and clinically related public service. For additional information on admission requirements, go to http://www.luc.edu/psychology/.

Student Characteristics: The following represents characteristics of students in 2009–2010 in all graduate psychology programs in the department: Female—full-time 67, part-time 0; Male—full-time 16, part-time 0; African American/Black—full-time 7, part-time 0; Hispanic/Latino(a)—full-time 9, part-time 0; Asian/Pacific Islander—full-time 5, part-time 0; American Indian/Alaska Native—full-time 0, part-time 0; Caucasian/White—full-time 60, part-time 0; Multi-ethnic—full-time 1, part-time 0; students subject to the Americans With Disabilities Act—full-time 0, part-time 0; Unknown ethnicity—full-time 1, part-time 0; International students who hold an F-1 or J-1 Visa—full-time 0, part-time 0.

Financial Information/Assistance:
Tuition for Full-Time Study: *Master's:* State residents: per academic year $17,430, $830 per credit hour. *Doctoral:* State residents: per academic year $17,430, $830 per credit hour. Tuition is subject to change. See the following Web site for updates and changes in tuition costs: http://www.luc.edu/bursar.

Financial Assistance:
First-Year Students: Research assistantships available for first year. Average amount paid per academic year: $15,000. Average number of hours worked per week: 20. Apply by December 1.
Advanced Students: Teaching assistantships available for advanced students. Average amount paid per academic year: $15,000. Average number of hours worked per week: 20. Apply by March 1. Research assistantships available for advanced students. Average amount paid per academic year: $15,000. Average number of hours worked per week: 20. Apply by March 1.
Additional Information: Of all students currently enrolled full time, 80% benefited from one or more of the listed financial assistance programs.

Internships/Practica: Doctoral Degree (PhD Clinical Psychology): For those doctoral students for whom a professional internship was required in this program prior to graduation, (6) students applied for an internship in 2008–2009, with (6) students obtaining an internship. Of those students who obtained an internship, (6) were paid internships. Of those students who obtained an internship, (6) students placed in APA/CPA accredited internships, (0) students placed in internships not APA/CPA accredited, but listed with the Association of Psychology Postdoctoral and Internship Programs (APPIC), (0) students placed in internships conforming to guidelines of the Council of Directors of School Psychology Programs (CDSPP), (0) students placed in internships that were not APA/CPA accredited, APPIC or CDSPP listed. Externship experiences are available for clinical psychology students through our in-house Training Clinic at the Wellness Center. In addition, numerous externship training opportunities are available throughout the Chicago metropolitan area and clinical students apply nationally for APA-accredited internships. Students in the doctoral applied social psychology program serve a 1000-hour planning, research and evaluation internship during their third year, while students in the developmental program complete a 250-hour internship. These positions are usually found in health-related, governmental, and research organizations in the Chicago area.

Housing and Day Care: On-campus housing is available. See the following Web site for more information: http://www.luc.edu/reslife. On-campus day care facilities are available.

Employment of Department Graduates:
Master's Degree Graduates: Of those who graduated in the academic year 2008–2009, the following categories and numbers represent the postgraduate activities and employment of master's degree graduates: Enrolled in a psychology doctoral program (3), enrolled in another graduate/professional program (1), enrolled in a postdoctoral residency/fellowship (n/a), employed in independent practice (n/a), employed in an academic position at a university (0), employed in an academic position at a 2-year/4-year college (0), employed in other positions at a higher education institution (0), employed in a professional position in a school system (0), employed in business or industry (0), employed in

government agency (0), employed in a community mental health/counseling center (0), employed in a hospital/medical center (0), still seeking employment (0), total from the above (master's) (4). **Doctoral Degree Graduates:** Of those who graduated in the academic year 2008–2009, the following categories and numbers represent the postgraduate activities and employment of doctoral degree graduates: Enrolled in a psychology doctoral program (n/a), enrolled in a postdoctoral residency/fellowship (8), employed in independent practice (0), employed in an academic position at a university (1), employed in an academic position at a 2-year/4-year college (1), employed in other positions at a higher education institution (0), employed in a professional position in a school system (0), employed in business or industry (0), employed in government agency (1), employed in a community mental health/counseling center (1), employed in a hospital/medical center (0), still seeking employment (0), other employment position (1), total from the above (doctoral) (13).

Additional Information:

Orientation, Objectives, and Emphasis of Department: Graduate study is organized into three areas: clinical, developmental, and social. All programs offer the PhD; only the social program offers a terminal MA in applied social psychology. The clinical program emphasizes the scientist–practitioner model, with students receiving extensive training in both areas. Students may specialize in work with children or adults. The developmental program provides training for students wishing to pursue the study of human development, particularly among infants, children, and adolescents. Cognition, social, gender role, and personality development are covered. The social psychology program includes training in both basic and applied social psychology. The emphasis in the applied program is on developing social psychologists who are capable of conducting applied research on the planning, evaluating, and modification of social programs in the areas of law and criminal justice, educational systems, health and/or community services, and organizational behavior.

Special Facilities or Resources: Excellent libraries and computer support are available. Departmental facilities include specialized laboratories for audition, vision, and neurophysiology research; a general purpose laboratory for sensory processes; suites of research and observation rooms for clinical research; observation and videotaping rooms and equipment; an extensive psychological test library; a psychophysiology and biofeedback laboratory; and computer facilities.

Information for Students With Physical Disabilities: See the following Web site for more information: http://www.luc.edu/sswd.

Application Information:

Send to Department of Psychology, Loyola University Chicago, 1032 W. Sheridan Road, Chicago, IL 60660. Application available online. URL of online application: http://www.luc.edu/gpem. Students are admitted in the Fall, application deadline December 1. For the Fall semester the deadlines for each program are as follows: Developmental, February 1; Social, January 15; Clinical, December 1. *Fee:* $40. No application fee for online application submissions.

Midwestern University (2009 data)
Department of Behavioral Medicine/Clinical Psychology Program
College of Health Sciences
555 31st Street
Downers Grove, IL 60515
Telephone: (630) 515-7650
Fax: (630) 515-7655
E-mail: *fprero@midwestern.edu*
Web: *http://www.midwestern.edu*

Department Information:
2001. Chairperson: Frank J. Prerost, PhD. Number of faculty: total—full-time 9, part-time 14; women—full-time 6, part-time 8; total—minority—full-time 2, part-time 2; women minority—full-time 1, part-time 1.

Programs and Degrees Offered:
Listed in the following order: Program area, degree type (T if terminal Master's), number awarded 7/08–6/09. Clinical Psychology PsyD (Doctor of Psychology) 8, Clinical Psychology MA/MS (Master of Arts/Science) 18.

Student Applications/Admissions:
Student Applications

Clinical Psychology PsyD (Doctor of Psychology)—Applications 2009–2010, 95. Total applicants accepted 2009–2010, 40. Number full-time enrolled (new admits only) 2009–2010, 26. Number part-time enrolled (new admits only) 2009–2010, 0. Openings 2010–2011, 24. The median number of years required for completion of a degree in 2008–2009 were 4. The number of students enrolled full- and part-time who were dismissed or voluntarily withdrew from this program area in 2008–2009 were 2. Clinical Psychology MA/MS (Master of Arts/Science)—Applications 2009–2010, 0. Total applicants accepted 2009–2010, 0. Number full-time enrolled (new admits only) 2009–2010, 0. Number part-time enrolled (new admits only) 2009–2010, 0. The median number of years required for completion of a degree in 2008–2009 were 2. The number of students enrolled full- and part-time who were dismissed or voluntarily withdrew from this program area in 2008–2009 were 0.

Other Criteria: (importance of criteria rated low, medium, or high): GRE scores—medium, research experience—medium, work experience—medium, extracurricular activity—medium, clinically related public service—high, GPA—high, letters of recommendation—high, interview—high, statement of goals and objectives—medium, health care experience—medium, undergraduate major in psychology—medium, specific undergraduate psychology courses taken—low.

Student Characteristics: The following represents characteristics of students in 2009–2010 in all graduate psychology programs in the department: Female—full-time 5, part-time 0; Male—full-time 3, part-time 0; African American/Black—full-time 1, part-time 0; Hispanic/Latino(a)—full-time 0, part-time 0; Asian/Pacific Islander—full-time 3, part-time 0; American Indian/Alaska Native—full-time 0, part-time 0; Caucasian/White—full-time 4, part-time 0; Multi-ethnic—full-time 0, part-time 0; students subject to the Americans With Disabilities Act—full-time 0, part-time 0; Unknown ethnicity—full-time 0, part-time 0; International students who hold an F-1 or J-1 Visa—full-time 0, part-time 0.

Financial Information/Assistance:
Tuition for Full-Time Study: *Doctoral:* State residents: per academic year $21,462; Nonstate residents: per academic year $21,462. Tuition is subject to change.

Financial Assistance:
First-Year Students: No information provided.
Advanced Students: No information provided.
Additional Information: No information provided.

Internships/Practica: Doctoral Degree (PsyD Clinical Psychology): For those doctoral students for whom a professional internship was required in this program prior to graduation, (18) students applied for an internship in 2008–2009, with (18) students obtaining an internship. Of those students who obtained an internship, (16) were paid internships. Of those students who obtained an internship, (1) students placed in APA/CPA accredited internships, (15) students placed in internships not APA/CPA accredited, but listed with the Association of Psychology Postdoctoral and Internship Programs (APPIC), (0) students placed in internships conforming to guidelines of the Council of Directors of School Psychology Programs (CDSPP), (2) students placed in internships that were not APA/CPA accredited, APPIC or CDSPP listed. Students participate in clerkships during their first year under the supervision of program core faculty. These are clinical experiences at various direct service sites. A diagnostic practicum is completed in the second year and is followed with a therapy practicum. The fourth year of study consists of a full-time internship. Students may opt for an advanced practicum in their third year while postponing internship into the next year. Students are given individualized attention to help secure appropriate clinical training experiences in practica and internship. Midwestern University has numerous affiliation agreements with clinical sites throughout the metropolitan area of Chicago.

Housing and Day Care: On-campus housing is available. No on-campus day care facilities are available.

Employment of Department Graduates:
Master's Degree Graduates: Of those who graduated in the academic year 2008–2009, the following categories and numbers represent the postgraduate activities and employment of master's degree graduates: Enrolled in a postdoctoral residency/fellowship (n/a), employed in independent practice (n/a), total from the above (master's) (0).
Doctoral Degree Graduates: Of those who graduated in the academic year 2008–2009, the following categories and numbers represent the postgraduate activities and employment of doctoral degree graduates: Enrolled in a psychology doctoral program (n/a), employed in a community mental health/counseling center (4), employed in a hospital/medical center (4), total from the above (doctoral) (8).

Additional Information:
Orientation, Objectives, and Emphasis of Department: The program follows a practitioner-scholar model of training entry level mental health professionals with an eclectic focus who can serve a diverse population. The training model adheres to a competency approach in the development of knowledge, skills, and attitudes related to the practice of clinical psychology. Students are systematically evaluated in the development of competency areas including relationship, assessment, intervention, professionalism, diversity, management and supervision, consultation and education, and research/evaluation. The program emphasizes first year supervised clinical experiences to produce a foundation for later clinical training. The program provides an individualized mentoring experience for its students.

Special Facilities or Resources: The clinical psychology program has the full support of the resources available from the Midwestern University Osteopathic Medical School and School of Pharmacy including research scientists and practicing clinicians. The program is housed on a large wooded campus with numerous buildings and research facilities including a state-of-the-art library. The majority of the physical resources have been constructed or remodeled in the past three years.

Application Information:
Send to Office of Admissions, Midwestern University, 555 31st Street, Downers Grove, IL 60515. Application available online. URL of online application: http://www.midwestern.edu. Programs have rolling admissions. *Fee:* $50.

Northern Illinois University
Department of Psychology
College of Liberal Arts and Sciences
DeKalb, IL 60115-2892
Telephone: (815) 753-0372
Fax: (815) 753-8088
E-mail: *mholliday@niu.edu*
Web: *http://www.niu.edu/psyc/*

Department Information:
1959. Chairperson: Greg Waas. Number of faculty: total—full-time 32; women—full-time 18; total—minority—full-time 1.

Programs and Degrees Offered:
Listed in the following order: Program area, degree type (T if terminal Master's), number awarded 7/08–6/09. Clinical Psychology PhD (Doctor of Philosophy) 9, Neuroscience and Behavior PhD (Doctor of Philosophy) 2, Social-Industrial/Organizational Psychology PhD (Doctor of Philosophy) 4, Cognitive Psychology PhD (Doctor of Philosophy) 0, Developmental Psychology PhD (Doctor of Philosophy) 1, School Psychology PhD (Doctor of Philosophy) 4.

APA Accreditation: Clinical PhD (Doctor of Philosophy). Student Outcome Data Website: http://www.niu.edu/psyc/graduate/clinical/admissions.shtml.

Student Applications/Admissions:
Student Applications
Clinical Psychology PhD (Doctor of Philosophy)—Applications 2009–2010, 166. Total applicants accepted 2009–2010, 15. Number full-time enrolled (new admits only) 2009–2010, 8. Number part-time enrolled (new admits only) 2009–2010, 0.

Total enrolled 2009–2010 full-time, 47, part-time, 3. Openings 2010–2011, 8. The median number of years required for completion of a degree in 2008–2009 were 8. The number of students enrolled full- and part-time who were dismissed or voluntarily withdrew from this program area in 2008–2009 were 1. *Neuroscience and Behavior PhD (Doctor of Philosophy)*—Applications 2009–2010, 19. Total applicants accepted 2009–2010, 2. Number full-time enrolled (new admits only) 2009–2010, 1. Openings 2010–2011, 2. The median number of years required for completion of a degree in 2008–2009 were 10. The number of students enrolled full- and part-time who were dismissed or voluntarily withdrew from this program area in 2008–2009 were 0. *Social-Industrial/Organizational Psychology PhD (Doctor of Philosophy)*—Applications 2009–2010, 67. Total applicants accepted 2009–2010, 8. Number full-time enrolled (new admits only) 2009–2010, 4. Total enrolled 2009–2010 full-time, 31, part-time, 5. Openings 2010–2011, 6. The median number of years required for completion of a degree in 2008–2009 were 6. The number of students enrolled full- and part-time who were dismissed or voluntarily withdrew from this program area in 2008–2009 were 0. *Cognitive Psychology PhD (Doctor of Philosophy)*—Applications 2009–2010, 4. Total applicants accepted 2009–2010, 1. Number full-time enrolled (new admits only) 2009–2010, 1. Total enrolled 2009–2010 full-time, 9, part-time, 1. Openings 2010–2011, 2. The number of students enrolled full- and part-time who were dismissed or voluntarily withdrew from this program area in 2008–2009 were 0. *Developmental Psychology PhD (Doctor of Philosophy)*—Applications 2009–2010, 17. Total applicants accepted 2009–2010, 4. Number full-time enrolled (new admits only) 2009–2010, 1. Total enrolled 2009–2010 full-time, 8, part-time, 1. Openings 2010–2011, 2. The median number of years required for completion of a degree in 2008–2009 were 6. The number of students enrolled full- and part-time who were dismissed or voluntarily withdrew from this program area in 2008–2009 were 0. *School Psychology PhD (Doctor of Philosophy)*—Applications 2009–2010, 60. Total applicants accepted 2009–2010, 8. Number full-time enrolled (new admits only) 2009–2010, 7. Total enrolled 2009–2010 full-time, 23, part-time, 3. Openings 2010–2011, 7. The median number of years required for completion of a degree in 2008–2009 were 6. The number of students enrolled full- and part-time who were dismissed or voluntarily withdrew from this program area in 2008–2009 were 0.

Scores: Entries appear in this order: required test or GPA, minimum score (if required), median score of students entering in 2009–2010. *Clinical Psychology PhD (Doctor of Philosophy)*: GRE-V no minimum stated, 520, GRE-Q no minimum stated, 670, overall undergraduate GPA 3.0, 3.78; *Social-Industrial/ Organizational Psychology PhD (Doctor of Philosophy)*: GRE-V no minimum stated, 525, GRE-Q no minimum stated, 616, GRE-Analytical no minimum stated, 5.5, overall undergraduate GPA no minimum stated, 3.55, Masters GPA no minimum stated, 3.79.

Other Criteria: (importance of criteria rated low, medium, or high): GRE scores—high, research experience—high, work experience—low, extracurricular activity—low, clinically related public service—low, GPA—high, letters of recommendation—high, interview—medium, statement of goals and objectives—high. Clinical and School programs interview students; other programs generally do not. For additional information on admission requirements, go to http://www.niu.edu/psyc/graduate/admissions/index.shtml.

Student Characteristics: The following represents characteristics of students in 2009–2010 in all graduate psychology programs in the department: Female—full-time 86, part-time 7; Male—full-time 38, part-time 6; African American/Black—full-time 3, part-time 0; Hispanic/Latino(a)—full-time 6, part-time 6; Asian/Pacific Islander—full-time 8, part-time 1; American Indian/Alaska Native—full-time 4, part-time 0; Caucasian/White—full-time 101, part-time 6; Multi-ethnic—full-time 1, part-time 0; students subject to the Americans With Disabilities Act—full-time 0, part-time 0; Unknown ethnicity—full-time 1, part-time 0; International students who hold an F-1 or J-1 Visa—full-time 4, part-time 1.

Financial Information/Assistance:

Tuition for Full-Time Study: *Master's:* State residents: $274 per credit hour; Nonstate residents: $548 per credit hour. *Doctoral:* State residents: $274 per credit hour; Nonstate residents: $548 per credit hour. Tuition is subject to change. Additional fees are assessed to students beyond the costs of tuition for the following: General university student fees. See the following Web site for updates and changes in tuition costs: http://www.niu.edu/bursar/tuition/graduate.shtml.

Financial Assistance:

First-Year Students: Teaching assistantships available for first year. Average amount paid per academic year: $11,800. Average number of hours worked per week: 20. Research assistantships available for first year. Average amount paid per academic year: $11,800. Average number of hours worked per week: 20. Traineeships available for first year. Average amount paid per academic year: $11,800. Average number of hours worked per week: 20. Fellowships and scholarships available for first year.

Advanced Students: Teaching assistantships available for advanced students. Average amount paid per academic year: $11,800. Average number of hours worked per week: 20. Research assistantships available for advanced students. Average amount paid per academic year: $11,800. Average number of hours worked per week: 20. Traineeships available for advanced students. Average amount paid per academic year: $11,800. Average number of hours worked per week: 20. Fellowships and scholarships available for advanced students.

Additional Information: Of all students currently enrolled full time, 89% benefited from one or more of the listed financial assistance programs. Application and information available online at: http://www.niu.edu/psyc/graduate/admissions/financial.shtml.

Internships/Practica: Doctoral Degree (PhD Clinical Psychology): For those doctoral students for whom a professional internship was required in this program prior to graduation, (12) students applied for an internship in 2008–2009, with (8) students obtaining an internship. Of those students who obtained an internship, (8) were paid internships. Of those students who obtained an internship, (8) students placed in APA/CPA accredited internships, (0) students placed in internships not APA/CPA accredited, but listed with the Association of Psychology Postdoctoral and Internship Programs (APPIC), (0) students placed in internships conforming to guidelines of the Council of Directors of School Psychology Programs (CDSPP), (0) students placed in internships that were not APA/CPA accredited, APPIC or

CDSPP listed. Clinical and school psychology internships are required for students in those areas. Clinical externships (equivalent to in-residence assistantships) are available and recommended.

Housing and Day Care: On-campus housing is available. See the following Web site for more information: http://www.niu.edu/housing/. On-campus day care facilities are available. See the following Web site for more information: http://www.niu.edu/ccc/.

Employment of Department Graduates:
Master's Degree Graduates: Of those who graduated in the academic year 2008–2009, the following categories and numbers represent the postgraduate activities and employment of master's degree graduates: Enrolled in a postdoctoral residency/fellowship (n/a), employed in independent practice (n/a), total from the above (master's) (0).
Doctoral Degree Graduates: Of those who graduated in the academic year 2008–2009, the following categories and numbers represent the postgraduate activities and employment of doctoral degree graduates: Enrolled in a psychology doctoral program (n/a), employed in independent practice (3), employed in an academic position at a university (2), employed in a hospital/medical center (4), total from the above (doctoral) (9).

Additional Information:
Orientation, Objectives, and Emphasis of Department: The PhD program in psychology is designed to prepare graduate students to function in a variety of settings such as academic institutions, which emphasize research and/or teaching, non-academic institutions, which emphasize research on mental health, human factors, or skill acquisition, and various consultative modalities, which emphasize practitioner applications and the delivery of human services. Doctorates in psychology are awarded in four specialty areas: an APA-accredited program in clinical psychology; cognitive/instructional, developmental, and school psychology (NASP approved); neuroscience and behavior; and social and industrial/organizational psychology. Faculty in all areas endorse the value of well-trained researchers and practitioners. Students are equipped to conduct sophisticated, theoretically-based empirical research and to teach at the graduate or undergraduate level. In addition to academic placements, students can also find suitable employment as applied researchers or service practitioners in a variety of mental health (clinical), educational (instructional, developmental, school), physical health (neuroscience), or business (social and industrial/organizational) settings. The overall goal of the graduate program is to produce doctoral graduates who appreciate and are deeply committed to the study of psychological processes and behavior, who are familiar with fundamental knowledge in the field, and who are well-trained in methodology and modern techniques of data analysis.

Special Facilities or Resources: The department has a modern psychology building with offices for faculty, staff, and graduate students; classrooms; shops; a six-story research wing with research equipment, including minicomputers and direct access to the university computer and Internet applications; and a Psychological Services Center for practicum training in clinical, school, industrial/organizational, and other applied psychological areas.

Information for Students With Physical Disabilities: See the following Web site for more information: http://www.niu.edu/caar/.

Application Information:
Send to The Graduate School, Altgeld Hall, Northern Illinois University, DeKalb, IL 60115-2864. Application available online. URL of online application: http://www.grad.niu.edu/grad/apply/index.shtml. Students are admitted in the Fall, application deadline December 1. December 1 deadline for Clinical applicants. December 15 deadline for School. January 15 deadline for Social/Industrial Organizational and Neuroscience and Behavior. February 1 deadline for Cognitive/Instructional or Developmental. *Fee:* $40. Fees waived/deferred if applicant was exempt from GRE fees, is an NIU employee, or is currently enrolled in a graduate program at NIU.

Northwestern University
Department of Psychology
102 Swift Hall, 2029 Sheridan Road
Evanston, IL 60208-2710
Telephone: (847) 491-5190
Fax: (847) 491-7859
E-mail: *f-sales@northwestern.edu*
Web: *http://www.wcas.northwestern.edu/psych/*

Department Information:
1909. Chairperson: Dan P. McAdams. Number of faculty: total—full-time 34, part-time 1; women—full-time 12, part-time 1; total—minority—full-time 3; women minority—full-time 3.

Programs and Degrees Offered:
Listed in the following order: Program area, degree type (T if terminal Master's), number awarded 7/08–6/09. Clinical Psychology PhD (Doctor of Philosophy) 1, Cognitive Psychology PhD (Doctor of Philosophy) 1, Personality Psychology PhD (Doctor of Philosophy) 0, Brain, Behavior, and Cognition PhD (Doctor of Philosophy) 1, Social Psychology PhD (Doctor of Philosophy) 3.

APA Accreditation: Clinical PhD (Doctor of Philosophy). Student Outcome Data Website: http://www.wcas.northwestern.edu/psych/program_areas/clinical/ClinicalStudentOutcomes.htm.

Student Applications/Admissions:
Student Applications
Clinical Psychology PhD (Doctor of Philosophy)—Applications 2009–2010, 80. Total applicants accepted 2009–2010, 3. Number full-time enrolled (new admits only) 2009–2010, 2. Number part-time enrolled (new admits only) 2009–2010, 0. Openings 2010–2011, 3. The median number of years required for completion of a degree in 2008–2009 were 6. The number of students enrolled full- and part-time who were dismissed or voluntarily withdrew from this program area in 2008–2009 were 0. *Cognitive Psychology PhD (Doctor of Philosophy)*—Applications 2009–2010, 60. Total applicants accepted 2009–2010, 12. Number full-time enrolled (new admits only) 2009–2010, 7. Number part-time enrolled (new admits only) 2009–2010, 0. Openings 2010–2011, 5. The median number of years required for completion of a degree in 2008–2009 were 5. The number of students enrolled full- and part-time who were dismissed or voluntarily withdrew from this program area in 2008–2009 were 0. *Personality Psychology PhD (Doctor of Philosophy)*—Applications 2009–2010, 12. Total applicants accepted 2009–2010, 1. Number full-time enrolled (new admits

only) 2009–2010, 1. Number part-time enrolled (new admits only) 2009–2010, 0. The median number of years required for completion of a degree in 2008–2009 were 5. The number of students enrolled full- and part-time who were dismissed or voluntarily withdrew from this program area in 2008–2009 were 0. *Brain, Behavior, and Cognition PhD (Doctor of Philosophy)*—Applications 2009–2010, 47. Total applicants accepted 2009–2010, 6. Number full-time enrolled (new admits only) 2009–2010, 3. Number part-time enrolled (new admits only) 2009–2010, 0. Openings 2010–2011, 4. The median number of years required for completion of a degree in 2008–2009 were 5. The number of students enrolled full- and part-time who were dismissed or voluntarily withdrew from this program area in 2008–2009 were 1. *Social Psychology PhD (Doctor of Philosophy)*—Applications 2009–2010, 121. Total applicants accepted 2009–2010, 6. Number full-time enrolled (new admits only) 2009–2010, 2. Number part-time enrolled (new admits only) 2009–2010, 0. Openings 2010–2011, 4. The median number of years required for completion of a degree in 2008–2009 were 5. The number of students enrolled full- and part-time who were dismissed or voluntarily withdrew from this program area in 2008–2009 were 1.

Other Criteria: (importance of criteria rated low, medium, or high): GRE scores—high, research experience—high, GPA—high, letters of recommendation—medium, interview—medium, statement of goals and objectives—medium. For additional information on admission requirements, go to http://www.wcas.northwestern.edu/psych/graduate_studies/prospective_students/.

Student Characteristics: The following represents characteristics of students in 2009–2010 in all graduate psychology programs in the department: Female—full-time 46, part-time 0; Male—full-time 23, part-time 0; African American/Black—full-time 5, part-time 0; Hispanic/Latino(a)—full-time 2, part-time 0; Asian/Pacific Islander—full-time 9, part-time 0; American Indian/Alaska Native—full-time 0, part-time 0; Caucasian/White—full-time 53, part-time 0; Multi-ethnic—full-time 0, part-time 0; students subject to the Americans With Disabilities Act—full-time 0, part-time 0; Unknown ethnicity—full-time 0, part-time 0; International students who hold an F-1 or J-1 Visa—full-time 7, part-time 0.

Financial Information/Assistance:
Tuition for Full-Time Study: *Doctoral:* State residents: per academic year $38,088; Nonstate residents: per academic year $38,088. Tuition is subject to change. See the following Web site for updates and changes in tuition costs: http://www.northwestern.edu/sfs/tuition/.

Financial Assistance:
First-Year Students: Fellowships and scholarships available for first year. Average amount paid per academic year: $20,520. Apply by December 31.
Advanced Students: Teaching assistantships available for advanced students. Average amount paid per academic year: $21,156. Average number of hours worked per week: 10. Research assistantships available for advanced students. Average amount paid per academic year: $21,156. Fellowships and scholarships available for advanced students. Average amount paid per academic year: $20,520.

Additional Information: Of all students currently enrolled full time, 100% benefited from one or more of the listed financial assistance programs. Application and information available online at: http://www.wcas.northwestern.edu/psych/graduate_studies/fellowship_and_funding/.

Internships/Practica: Doctoral Degree (PhD Clinical Psychology): For those doctoral students for whom a professional internship was required in this program prior to graduation, (1) students applied for an internship in 2008–2009, with (1) students obtaining an internship. Of those students who obtained an internship, (1) were paid internships. Of those students who obtained an internship, (1) students placed in APA/CPA accredited internships, (0) students placed in internships not APA/CPA accredited, but listed with the Association of Psychology Postdoctoral and Internship Programs (APPIC), (0) students placed in internships conforming to guidelines of the Council of Directors of School Psychology Programs (CDSPP), (0) students placed in internships that were not APA/CPA accredited, APPIC or CDSPP listed. A variety of internships in community settings are available.

Housing and Day Care: On-campus housing is available. See the following Web site for more information: http://www.northwestern.edu/gradhousing/. No on-campus day care facilities are available.

Employment of Department Graduates:
Master's Degree Graduates: Of those who graduated in the academic year 2008–2009, the following categories and numbers represent the postgraduate activities and employment of master's degree graduates: Enrolled in a postdoctoral residency/fellowship (n/a), employed in independent practice (n/a), total from the above (master's) (0).
Doctoral Degree Graduates: Of those who graduated in the academic year 2008–2009, the following categories and numbers represent the postgraduate activities and employment of doctoral degree graduates: Enrolled in a psychology doctoral program (n/a), enrolled in a postdoctoral residency/fellowship (1), employed in an academic position at a university (1), total from the above (doctoral) (2).

Additional Information:
Orientation, Objectives, and Emphasis of Department: The faculty in each graduate area has designed programs tailored to the needs of students in that area. Whatever a student's field of interest, the department tries to produce doctoral students with a strong research orientation. Administrative barriers between areas are permeable; most faculty members take an active part in the instruction and research programs of more than one interest area. A significant population of postdoctoral fellows enhances the informal professional education of graduate students. In addition, all graduate students are given opportunities for teaching. Teaching is independent of type of financial aid.

Information for Students With Physical Disabilities: See the following Web site for more information: http://www.northwestern.edu/disability/.

Application Information:
Send to Florence Sales, Graduate Admissions Coordinator, 102 Swift Hall, Dept. of Psychology, Northwestern University, 2029 Sheridan

Road, Evanston, IL 60208-2710. Application available online. URL of online application: https://app.applyyourself.com/?id=nwu-grad. Students are admitted in the Fall, application deadline December 1. *Fee:* $75.

Northwestern University, Feinberg School of Medicine
Department of Psychiatry and Behavioral Sciences, Division of Psychology
Abbott Hall, Suite 1205, 710 North Lake Shore Drive
Chicago, IL 60611
Telephone: (312) 908-8262
Fax: (312) 908-5070
E-mail: *clinpsych@northwestern.edu*
Web: *http://www.clinpsych.northwestern.edu*

Department Information:
1970. Chief: Mark A. Reinecke, PhD. Number of faculty: total—full-time 15, part-time 10; women—full-time 7, part-time 7.

Programs and Degrees Offered:
Listed in the following order: Program area, degree type (T if terminal Master's), number awarded 7/08–6/09. Clinical Psychology PhD (Doctor of Philosophy) 11.

APA Accreditation: Clinical PhD (Doctor of Philosophy).

Student Applications/Admissions:
Student Applications
Clinical Psychology PhD (Doctor of Philosophy)—Applications 2009–2010, 233. Total applicants accepted 2009–2010, 5. Number full-time enrolled (new admits only) 2009–2010, 5. Number part-time enrolled (new admits only) 2009–2010, 0. Openings 2010–2011, 8. The median number of years required for completion of a degree in 2008–2009 were 6. The number of students enrolled full- and part-time who were dismissed or voluntarily withdrew from this program area in 2008–2009 were 1.
Scores: Entries appear in this order: required test or GPA, minimum score (if required), median score of students entering in 2009–2010. Clinical Psychology PhD (Doctor of Philosophy): GRE-V no minimum stated, GRE-Q no minimum stated, GRE-Subject (Psychology) no minimum stated, overall undergraduate GPA no minimum stated.
Other Criteria: (importance of criteria rated low, medium, or high): GRE scores—high, research experience—high, work experience—low, extracurricular activity—low, clinically related public service—medium, GPA—high, letters of recommendation—high, interview—high, statement of goals and objectives—high, undergraduate major in psychology—low. For additional information on admission requirements, go to http://www.clinpsych.northwestern.edu.

Student Characteristics: The following represents characteristics of students in 2009–2010 in all graduate psychology programs in the department: Female—full-time 22, part-time 0; Male—full-time 3, part-time 0; African American/Black—full-time 0, part-time 0; Hispanic/Latino(a)—full-time 1, part-time 0; Asian/Pacific Islander—full-time 2, part-time 0; American Indian/Alaska Native—full-time 0, part-time 0; Caucasian/White—full-time 21, part-time 0; Multi-ethnic—full-time 1, part-time 0; students subject to the Americans With Disabilities Act—full-time 0, part-time 0; Unknown ethnicity—full-time 0, part-time 0; International students who hold an F-1 or J-1 Visa—full-time 0, part-time 0.

Financial Information/Assistance:
Tuition for Full-Time Study: Doctoral: State residents: per academic year $39,940; Nonstate residents: per academic year $39,940. See the following Web site for updates and changes in tuition costs: http://www.tgs.northwestern.edu.

Financial Assistance:
First-Year Students: Research assistantships available for first year. Average number of hours worked per week: 15. Fellowships and scholarships available for first year.
Advanced Students: Research assistantships available for advanced students. Average number of hours worked per week: 15. Fellowships and scholarships available for advanced students.
Additional Information: Of all students currently enrolled full time, 100% benefited from one or more of the listed financial assistance programs. Application and information available online at: http://www.clinpsych.northwestern.edu.

Internships/Practica: Doctoral Degree (PhD Clinical Psychology): For those doctoral students for whom a professional internship was required in this program prior to graduation, (2) students applied for an internship in 2008–2009, with (2) students obtaining an internship. Of those students who obtained an internship, (2) were paid internships. Of those students who obtained an internship, (2) students placed in APA/CPA accredited internships, (0) students placed in internships not APA/CPA accredited, but listed with the Association of Psychology Postdoctoral and Internship Programs (APPIC), (0) students placed in internships conforming to guidelines of the Council of Directors of School Psychology Programs (CDSPP), (0) students placed in internships that were not APA/CPA accredited, APPIC or CDSPP listed. Most practica are located at clinical sites affiliated with the Feinberg School of Medicine, Northwestern Memorial Hospital, or Children's Memorial Hospital. Practicum sites include partial hospitalization programs, outpatient psychiatry clinics, university counseling centers, inpatient and outpatient neuropsychological clinics, and child and adolescent specialty programs.

Housing and Day Care: On-campus housing is available. See the following Web site for more information: http://www.northwestern.edu/gradhousing/. On-campus day care facilities are available. See the following Web site for more information: http://www.northwestern.edu/hr/benefits/childcare/solutions/index.html.

Employment of Department Graduates:
Master's Degree Graduates: Of those who graduated in the academic year 2008–2009, the following categories and numbers represent the postgraduate activities and employment of master's degree graduates: Enrolled in a postdoctoral residency/fellowship (n/a), employed in independent practice (n/a), total from the above (master's) (0).
Doctoral Degree Graduates: Of those who graduated in the academic year 2008–2009, the following categories and numbers represent the postgraduate activities and employment of doctoral

degree graduates: Enrolled in a psychology doctoral program (n/a), enrolled in a postdoctoral residency/fellowship (8), employed in a hospital/medical center (3), total from the above (doctoral) (11).

Additional Information:
Orientation, Objectives, and Emphasis of Department: The goal of our doctoral program is to train academic clinical psychologists using a scientist–practitioner model. The program takes advantage of its placement within the Department of Psychiatry and Behavioral Sciences at the Feinberg School of Medicine by offering a true balance of research and clinical training. This unique setting provides opportunities for translational research and practice that span molecular to social models of disease, and epidemiologic to clinical and neuroimaging methodologies. Our program prepares students to be competitive for careers in academic clinical psychology, particularly in health care settings. Preparation is provided through core and specialty-track curricula, intensive research mentoring and training, and at least two years of clinical practica focused on clinical assessment and treatment. Major milestones include a research qualifying paper, a clinical qualifying exam, an empirical dissertation with original research, and an APA-approved clinical internship. The program is committed to an evidence-based clinical model that provides intensive supervision and training to develop skills in assessment, diagnosis, and treatment. The program offers subspecialties in adult clinical psychology, behavioral medicine, clinical child and adolescent psychology, neuroscience and neuropsychology, and health disparities, public health policy, and mental health policy.

Special Facilities or Resources: The doctoral program has access to research facilities within the Department of Psychiatry and Behavioral Sciences, including psychophysiology methodologies and functional Magnetic Resonance Imaging.

Information for Students With Physical Disabilities: See the following Web site for more information: http://www.northwestern.edu/disability/.

Application Information:
Send to Division of Psychology, Northwestern University Feinberg School of Medicine, Abbott Hall Suite 1205, 710 North Lake Shore Drive, Chicago, IL 60611-3078. Application available online. URL of online application: http://www.tgs.northwestern.edu. Students are admitted in the Fall, application deadline December 15. *Fee:* $50.

Roosevelt University
Department of Psychology
Arts and Sciences
430 South Michigan Avenue
Chicago, IL 60605-1394
Telephone: (312) 341-3760
Fax: (312) 341-6362
E-mail: *jchoca@roosevelt.edu*
Web: *http://www.roosevelt.edu*

Department Information:
1945. Chairperson: Dr. James Choca. Number of faculty: total—full-time 20, part-time 63; women—full-time 11, part-time 39; total—minority—full-time 3, part-time 11; women minority—full-time 2, part-time 6; faculty subject to the Americans With Disabilities Act 1.

Programs and Degrees Offered:
Listed in the following order: Program area, degree type (T if terminal Master's), number awarded 7/08–6/09. Clinical Psychology MA/MS (Master of Arts/Science) (T) 30, Industrial/Organizational Psychology MA/MS (Master of Arts/Science) (T) 23, Clinical Professional Psychology MA/MS (Master of Arts/Science) (T) 62, Counseling Psychology MA/MS (Master of Arts/Science) (T), Clinical Psychology PsyD (Doctor of Psychology) 6.

APA Accreditation: Clinical PsyD (Doctor of Psychology). Student Outcome Data Website: http://legacy.roosevelt.edu/cas/sp/psydapaaccreditation.htm.

Student Applications/Admissions:
Student Applications
Clinical Psychology MA/MS (Master of Arts/Science)—Applications 2009–2010, 82. Total applicants accepted 2009–2010, 37. Number full-time enrolled (new admits only) 2009–2010, 9. Number part-time enrolled (new admits only) 2009–2010, 3. Total enrolled 2009–2010 full-time, 16, part-time, 11. Openings 2010–2011, 40. The median number of years required for completion of a degree in 2008–2009 were 4. The number of students enrolled full- and part-time who were dismissed or voluntarily withdrew from this program area in 2008–2009 were 4. *Industrial/Organizational Psychology MA/MS (Master of Arts/Science)*—Applications 2009–2010, 80. Total applicants accepted 2009–2010, 67. Number full-time enrolled (new admits only) 2009–2010, 21. Number part-time enrolled (new admits only) 2009–2010, 5. Total enrolled 2009–2010 full-time, 46, part-time, 36. Openings 2010–2011, 55. The median number of years required for completion of a degree in 2008–2009 were 3. The number of students enrolled full- and part-time who were dismissed or voluntarily withdrew from this program area in 2008–2009 were 3. *Clinical Professional Psychology MA/MS (Master of Arts/Science)*—Applications 2009–2010, 157. Total applicants accepted 2009–2010, 99. Number full-time enrolled (new admits only) 2009–2010, 39. Number part-time enrolled (new admits only) 2009–2010, 12. Total enrolled 2009–2010 full-time, 102, part-time, 117. Openings 2010–2011, 80. The median number of years required for completion of a degree in 2008–2009 were 3. The number of students enrolled full- and part-time who were dismissed or voluntarily withdrew from this program area in 2008–2009 were 3. *Counseling Psychology MA/MS (Master of Arts/Science)—Clinical Psychology PsyD (Doctor of Psychology)*—Applications 2009–2010, 168. Total applicants accepted 2009–2010, 35. Number full-time enrolled (new admits only) 2009–2010, 20. Number part-time enrolled (new admits only) 2009–2010, 0. Total enrolled 2009–2010 full-time, 72, part-time, 18. Openings 2010–2011, 20. The median number of years required for completion of a degree in 2008–2009 were 6. The number of students enrolled full- and part-time who were dismissed or voluntarily withdrew from this program area in 2008–2009 were 6.

Scores: Entries appear in this order: required test or GPA, minimum score (if required), median score of students entering in 2009–2010. *Clinical Psychology MA/MS (Master of Arts/Science):* overall undergraduate GPA 3.0, last 2 years GPA 3.0, 3.5, psychology GPA 3.0; *Industrial/Organizational Psychology*

MA/MS (*Master of Arts/Science*): overall undergraduate GPA 3.0, last 2 years GPA 3.0, 3.5, psychology GPA 3.0; *Clinical Professional Psychology MA/MS (Master of Arts/Science)*: overall undergraduate GPA 3.0, last 2 years GPA 3.0, 3.50, psychology GPA 3.0; *Clinical Psychology PsyD (Doctor of Psychology)*: GRE-V 500, GRE-Q 500, GRE-Analytical 4.5, overall undergraduate GPA 3.25.

Other Criteria: (importance of criteria rated low, medium, or high): GRE scores—high, research experience—medium, work experience—medium, extracurricular activity—low, clinically related public service—medium, GPA—high, letters of recommendation—medium, interview—high, statement of goals and objectives—medium.

Student Characteristics: The following represents characteristics of students in 2009–2010 in all graduate psychology programs in the department: Female—full-time 185, part-time 148; Male—full-time 51, part-time 34; African American/Black—full-time 33, part-time 34; Hispanic/Latino(a)—full-time 23, part-time 16; Asian/Pacific Islander—full-time 12, part-time 12; American Indian/Alaska Native—full-time 0, part-time 0; Caucasian/White—full-time 147, part-time 108; Multi-ethnic—full-time 8, part-time 3; students subject to the Americans With Disabilities Act—full-time 2, part-time 1; Unknown ethnicity—full-time 13, part-time 9; International students who hold an F-1 or J-1 Visa—full-time 6, part-time 3.

Financial Information/Assistance:

Tuition for Full-Time Study: *Master's:* State residents: $770 per credit hour; Nonstate residents: $770 per credit hour. *Doctoral:* State residents: $1,106 per credit hour; Nonstate residents: $1,106 per credit hour. Tuition is subject to change. See the following Web site for updates and changes in tuition costs: http://www.roosevelt.edu/TuitionAndFees.aspx.

Financial Assistance:

First-Year Students: Research assistantships available for first year. Average amount paid per academic year: $5,200. Average number of hours worked per week: 17. Apply by March 1. Fellowships and scholarships available for first year. Average amount paid per academic year: $3,000. Average number of hours worked per week: 0.

Advanced Students: Research assistantships available for advanced students. Average amount paid per academic year: $5,200. Average number of hours worked per week: 17. Apply by March 1. Fellowships and scholarships available for advanced students. Apply by March 1.

Additional Information: Of all students currently enrolled full time, 17% benefited from one or more of the listed financial assistance programs. Application and information available online at: http://legacy.roosevelt.edu/financialaid/.

Internships/Practica: Doctoral Degree (PsyD Clinical Psychology): For those doctoral students for whom a professional internship was required in this program prior to graduation, (6) students applied for an internship in 2008–2009, with (6) students obtaining an internship. Of those students who obtained an internship, (6) were paid internships. Of those students who obtained an internship, (3) students placed in APA/CPA accredited internships, (2) students placed in internships not APA/CPA accredited, but listed with the Association of Psychology Postdoctoral and Internship Programs (APPIC), (0) students placed in internships conforming to guidelines of the Council of Directors of School Psychology Programs (CDSPP), (1) students placed in internships that were not APA/CPA accredited, APPIC or CDSPP listed. Master's Degree (MA/MS Clinical Psychology): An internship experience, such as a final research project or "capstone" experience is required of graduates. Master's Degree (MA/MS Industrial/Organizational Psychology): An internship experience, such as a final research project or "capstone" experience is required of graduates. Master's Degree (MA/MS Clinical Professional Psychology): An internship experience, such as a final research project or "capstone" experience is required of graduates. Students in our clinical programs have available over 250 sites in the greater Chicago area for practicum experience. We have a full-time Director of Training to assist students with this process. I/O, Clinical MA, and PsyD students have ample opportunities for training; I/O students nearly always obtain paid practicum experience.

Housing and Day Care: On-campus housing is available. See the following Web site for more information: http://www.roosevelt.edu/CampusCommunity/Chicago/ResidenceLife.aspx. On-campus day care facilities are available. See the following Web site for more information: http://www.roosevelt.edu/CampusCommunity/Schaumburg/Childcare.aspx.

Employment of Department Graduates:

Master's Degree Graduates: Of those who graduated in the academic year 2008–2009, the following categories and numbers represent the postgraduate activities and employment of master's degree graduates: Enrolled in a postdoctoral residency/fellowship (n/a), employed in independent practice (n/a), total from the above (master's) (0).

Doctoral Degree Graduates: Of those who graduated in the academic year 2008–2009, the following categories and numbers represent the postgraduate activities and employment of doctoral degree graduates: Enrolled in a psychology doctoral program (n/a), enrolled in a postdoctoral residency/fellowship (1), employed in independent practice (1), employed in an academic position at a university (0), employed in an academic position at a 2-year/4-year college (0), employed in other positions at a higher education institution (2), employed in a professional position in a school system (0), employed in business or industry (0), employed in government agency (1), employed in a community mental health/counseling center (0), employed in a hospital/medical center (1), still seeking employment (0), not seeking employment (0), other employment position (0), do not know (0), total from the above (doctoral) (6).

Additional Information:

Orientation, Objectives, and Emphasis of Department: Roosevelt University was founded over 60 years ago, in 1945, on the principles of social justice and equal educational access for all qualified students. We have a long history of inclusion and multicultural diversity. Our program's orientation reflects the diversity of contemporary psychology practice. A primary goal of the Department of Psychology is to prepare students to work effectively with diverse cultures in metropolitan settings. Master's degree programs in psychology have been offered since 1952, and the PsyD program, the first university-based clinical PsyD program in Illinois, was added in 1996. The PsyD program is designed to provide generalist training in all facets of clinical practice, in preparation for postdoctoral specialization of the student's choice.

Three master's degree programs are offered. Our MA programs offer streamlined and personally tailored predoctoral training designed to help qualified students enter PhD and PsyD programs, including our own, or to prepare for MA-level licensure. Approximately 85% of our graduates who have applied to doctoral programs have been accepted. We prepare students for professional master's-level employment in mental health and I/O careers. Many of our students are several years beyond undergraduate graduation and continue to work full or part-time, while arranging their schedules around evening, daytime, and weekend courses offered at our downtown and suburban campuses.

Special Facilities or Resources: The Department of Psychology has an exceptional faculty who are actively involved in applied research and clinical practice, supplemented by a large and highly trained adjunct faculty who also are involved in clinical, forensic, and experimental work. In addition to the extensive Roosevelt library and other facilities, there is access to clinical, research, computer, and library facilities of major Chicago universities, hospitals, and clinics. Volunteer research assistantships are available to qualified students interested in doing publishable research. A major resource is the urban location with varied employment, educational, and cultural opportunities. The Stress Institute offers basic and advanced certificates in Stress Management, and incorporates a wide range of cognitive-behavioral courses for students and health professionals interested in enhancing their clinical stress management skills. The Children and Family Studies Initiative allows students to train for the clinical treatment of children and families. The Instructor Development Program prepares PsyD students to teach undergraduate courses during the last 2 years of their doctoral training.

Information for Students With Physical Disabilities: See the following Web site for more information: http://legacy.roosevelt.edu/dss/default.htm.

Application Information:
Send to Office of Admission, 1400 North Roosevelt Boulevard, Schaumburg, IL 60173. Application available online. URL of online application: http://www.roosevelt.edu/Admission/HowToApply.aspx. Students are admitted in the Fall, application deadline January 1 PsyD. Clinical MA Program deadlines: Spring - November 1; Fall - May 1 I/O MA Program has rolling admissions. *Fee:* $25.

Rosalind Franklin University of Medicine and Science
Department of Psychology
College of Health Professions
3333 Green Bay Road
North Chicago, IL 60064
Telephone: (847) 578-8747
Fax: (847) 578-8758
E-mail: *john.calamari@rosalindfranklin.edu*
Web: *http://www.rosalindfranklin.edu/dnn/chp/home/chp/psychology.aspx*

Department Information:
1977. Chairperson: John Calamari, PhD. Number of faculty: total—full-time 7, part-time 1; women—full-time 2; total—minority—full-time 1.

Programs and Degrees Offered:
Listed in the following order: Program area, degree type (T if terminal Master's), number awarded 7/08–6/09. Clinical Psychology PhD (Doctor of Philosophy) 9, Clinical Counseling Psychology MA/MS (Master of Arts/Science) (T) 0.

APA Accreditation: Clinical PhD (Doctor of Philosophy). Student Outcome Data Website: http://www.rosalindfranklin.edu/dnn/chp/home/CHP/Psychology/Doctorate/Disclosure/tabid/1704/Default.aspx.

Student Applications/Admissions:
Student Applications

Clinical Psychology PhD (Doctor of Philosophy)—Applications 2009–2010, 52. Total applicants accepted 2009–2010, 14. Number full-time enrolled (new admits only) 2009–2010, 10. Total enrolled 2009–2010 full-time, 48. Openings 2010–2011, 9. The median number of years required for completion of a degree in 2008–2009 were 6. The number of students enrolled full- and part-time who were dismissed or voluntarily withdrew from this program area in 2008–2009 were 0. *Clinical Counseling Psychology MA/MS (Master of Arts/Science)*—Applications 2009–2010, 23. Total applicants accepted 2009–2010, 18. Number full-time enrolled (new admits only) 2009–2010, 11. Number part-time enrolled (new admits only) 2009–2010, 1. Total enrolled 2009–2010 full-time, 22, part-time, 1. Openings 2010–2011, 12. The number of students enrolled full- and part-time who were dismissed or voluntarily withdrew from this program area in 2008–2009 were 0.

Scores: Entries appear in this order: required test or GPA, minimum score (if required), median score of students entering in 2009–2010. *Clinical Psychology PhD (Doctor of Philosophy)*: GRE-V 600, GRE-Q 600, GRE-Analytical 4.5; *Clinical Counseling Psychology MA/MS (Master of Arts/Science)*: overall undergraduate GPA no minimum stated.

Other Criteria: (importance of criteria rated low, medium, or high): GRE scores—medium, research experience—high, work experience—low, extracurricular activity—medium, clinically related public service—medium, GPA—high, letters of recommendation—high, interview—high, statement of goals and objectives—high. For additional information on admission requirements, go to http://www.rosalindfranklin.edu/dnn/chp/home/chp/psychology.aspx.

Student Characteristics: The following represents characteristics of students in 2009–2010 in all graduate psychology programs in the department: Female—full-time 57, part-time 1; Male—full-time 13, part-time 0; African American/Black—full-time 2, part-time 1; Hispanic/Latino(a)—full-time 2, part-time 0; Asian/Pacific Islander—full-time 11, part-time 0; American Indian/Alaska Native—full-time 1, part-time 0; Caucasian/White—full-time 54, part-time 0; Multi-ethnic—full-time 0, part-time 0; students subject to the Americans With Disabilities Act—full-time 0, part-time 0; Unknown ethnicity—full-time 0, part-time 0; International students who hold an F-1 or J-1 Visa—full-time 0, part-time 0.

Financial Information/Assistance:
Tuition for Full-Time Study: *Master's:* State residents: per academic year $22,575; Nonstate residents: per academic year

$22,575. *Doctoral:* State residents: per academic year $22,575; Nonstate residents: per academic year $22,575. Tuition is subject to change.

Financial Assistance:
First-Year Students: Research assistantships available for first year. Average number of hours worked per week: 10. Fellowships and scholarships available for first year.
Advanced Students: Teaching assistantships available for advanced students. Average number of hours worked per week: 10. Research assistantships available for advanced students. Average number of hours worked per week: 10. Traineeships available for advanced students. Average number of hours worked per week: 10. Fellowships and scholarships available for advanced students. Average number of hours worked per week: 10.
Additional Information: Of all students currently enrolled full time, 69% benefited from one or more of the listed financial assistance programs. Application and information available online at: http://www.rosalindfranklin.edu/dnn/administration/FinancialAid/tabid/1942/Default.aspx.

Internships/Practica: Doctoral Degree (PhD Clinical Psychology): For those doctoral students for whom a professional internship was required in this program prior to graduation, (10) students applied for an internship in 2008–2009, with (8) students obtaining an internship. Of those students who obtained an internship, (8) were paid internships. Of those students who obtained an internship, (8) students placed in APA/CPA accredited internships, (0) students placed in internships not APA/CPA accredited, but listed with the Association of Psychology Postdoctoral and Internship Programs (APPIC), (0) students placed in internships conforming to guidelines of the Council of Directors of School Psychology Programs (CDSPP), (0) students placed in internships that were not APA/CPA accredited, APPIC or CDSPP listed. Master's Degree (MA/MS Clinical Counseling Psychology): An internship experience, such as a final research project or "capstone" experience is required of graduates. The Department enjoys formal relationships with many of the major clinical, health and neuropsychology facilities in the catchment area from Chicago to the south and Milwaukee to the north. These include both inpatient and outpatient facilities. Thus, students have the opportunity to obtain experience and clinical training with a diverse range of clinical populations and socio-economic strata.

Housing and Day Care: On-campus housing is available. See the following Web site for more information: http://www.rosalindfranklin.edu/dnn/administration/DOSA/StudentHousing/tabid/565/Default.aspx. No on-campus day care facilities are available.

Employment of Department Graduates:
Master's Degree Graduates: Of those who graduated in the academic year 2008–2009, the following categories and numbers represent the postgraduate activities and employment of master's degree graduates: Enrolled in a postdoctoral residency/fellowship (n/a), employed in independent practice (n/a), total from the above (master's) (0).
Doctoral Degree Graduates: Of those who graduated in the academic year 2008–2009, the following categories and numbers represent the postgraduate activities and employment of doctoral degree graduates: Enrolled in a psychology doctoral program (n/a), enrolled in a postdoctoral residency/fellowship (9), total from the above (doctoral) (9).

Additional Information:
Orientation, Objectives, and Emphasis of Department: The Department of Psychology offers an APA-approved program leading to the PhD degree in clinical psychology, with specialties in Health Psychology, Psychopathology and Clinical Neuropsychology. Within the context of the general clinical training program, students select a specialty emphasis in either clinical neuropsychology, psychopathology or health/behavioral medicine. The program provides students with intensive training in the methods and theories of clinical practice with emphasis in these specialty areas. Research is a vital part of the program and students work closely with professors throughout their training. Research topics include biopsychosocial issues associated with various medical illnesses (e.g., cancer, diabetes, heart disease), aging, psychopathology (e.g., schizophrenia, OCD, psychopathy), and neuropsychological features of various clinical populations (e.g., epilepsy, head injury, multiple sclerosis, AIDS, Alzheimer's disease, dementia, stroke). Subject populations range in age from childhood through adulthood and include those with physical and psychiatric disorders. The Department subscribes to the philosophy that a clinical psychologist is knowledgeable in formulating and solving scientific problems, and skilled in formulating clinical problems and applying empirically supported interventions. To this end, core courses are organized as integrated theory-research-practice units with a problem solving orientation. Our goal is to graduate clinical psychologists who are highly trained, clinically effective, and able to contribute to the continuing development of the profession as practitioners, teachers, and researchers.

Special Facilities or Resources: Research facilities within the Department include an Experimental Neuropsychology Lab, Clinical Health Psychophysiology Lab, Neuroimaging Laboratory, and a Behavioral Therapy Lab. There are ongoing research programs in arthritis, oncology, diabetes, blood pressure regulation, epilepsy, anxiety disorders, schizophrenia, psychopathy, aging and dementia. Collaborative research opportunities are also ongoing with a number of community and academic institutions in the area and include projects using MRI and fMRI to study higher order cognitive processes.

Application Information:
Send to Rosalind Franklin, University of Medicine and Science, CHP Admissions Office, 3333 Green Bay Road, North Chicago, IL 60064. Application available online. URL of online application: http://www.rosalindfranklin.edu/tabid/1862/Default.aspx. Students are admitted in the Fall, application deadline December 1. *Fee:* $50.

Southern Illinois University Carbondale
Department of Psychology
College of Liberal Arts
Life Science Building II, Room 281
Carbondale, IL 62901
Telephone: (618) 453-3564
Fax: (618) 453-3563
E-mail: swanson@siu.edu
Web: http://www.psychology.siu.edu

Department Information:
1948. Chairperson: Jane Swanson. Number of faculty: total—full-time 25, part-time 2; women—full-time 12, part-time 1; total—minority—full-time 3; women minority—full-time 3.

Programs and Degrees Offered:
Listed in the following order: Program area, degree type (T if terminal Master's), number awarded 7/08–6/09. Clinical Psychology PhD (Doctor of Philosophy) 3, Counseling Psychology PhD (Doctor of Philosophy) 5, Applied Psychology PhD (Doctor of Philosophy) 0, Brain and Cognitive Sciences PhD (Doctor of Philosophy) 2.

APA Accreditation: Clinical PhD (Doctor of Philosophy). Counseling PhD (Doctor of Philosophy).

Student Applications/Admissions:
Student Applications
Clinical Psychology PhD (Doctor of Philosophy)—Applications 2009–2010, 130. Total applicants accepted 2009–2010, 10. Number full-time enrolled (new admits only) 2009–2010, 6. Openings 2010–2011, 7. The median number of years required for completion of a degree in 2008–2009 were 6. The number of students enrolled full- and part-time who were dismissed or voluntarily withdrew from this program area in 2008–2009 were 1. Counseling Psychology PhD (Doctor of Philosophy)—Applications 2009–2010, 78. Total applicants accepted 2009–2010, 10. Number full-time enrolled (new admits only) 2009–2010, 5. Total enrolled 2009–2010 full-time, 19. Openings 2010–2011, 5. The median number of years required for completion of a degree in 2008–2009 were 5. The number of students enrolled full- and part-time who were dismissed or voluntarily withdrew from this program area in 2008–2009 were 1. Applied Psychology PhD (Doctor of Philosophy)—Applications 2009–2010, 19. Total applicants accepted 2009–2010, 6. Number full-time enrolled (new admits only) 2009–2010, 4. Number part-time enrolled (new admits only) 2009–2010, 0. Openings 2010–2011, 4. The median number of years required for completion of a degree in 2008–2009 were 6. The number of students enrolled full- and part-time who were dismissed or voluntarily withdrew from this program area in 2008–2009 were 0. Brain and Cognitive Sciences PhD (Doctor of Philosophy)—Applications 2009–2010, 25. Total applicants accepted 2009–2010, 8. Number full-time enrolled (new admits only) 2009–2010, 4. Total enrolled 2009–2010 full-time, 16. Openings 2010–2011, 4. The median number of years required for completion of a degree in 2008–2009 were 5. The number of students enrolled full- and part-time who were dismissed or voluntarily withdrew from this program area in 2008–2009 were 1.

Scores: Entries appear in this order: required test or GPA, minimum score (if required), median score of students entering in 2009–2010. Clinical Psychology PhD (Doctor of Philosophy): GRE-V no minimum stated, GRE-Q no minimum stated, overall undergraduate GPA no minimum stated, last 2 years GPA no minimum stated, psychology GPA no minimum stated; Counseling Psychology PhD (Doctor of Philosophy): GRE-V no minimum stated, GRE-Q no minimum stated, overall undergraduate GPA no minimum stated, last 2 years GPA no minimum stated, psychology GPA no minimum stated; Applied Psychology PhD (Doctor of Philosophy): GRE-V no minimum stated, GRE-Q no minimum stated, overall undergraduate GPA no minimum stated, last 2 years GPA no minimum stated, psychology GPA no minimum stated; Brain and Cognitive Sciences PhD (Doctor of Philosophy): GRE-V no minimum stated, GRE-Q no minimum stated, overall undergraduate GPA no minimum stated, last 2 years GPA no minimum stated, psychology GPA no minimum stated.

Other Criteria: (importance of criteria rated low, medium, or high): GRE scores—medium, research experience—high, work experience—medium, extracurricular activity—medium, clinically related public service—medium, GPA—medium, letters of recommendation—high, interview—low, statement of goals and objectives—high, undergraduate major in psychology—medium, specific undergraduate psychology courses taken—medium. Clinical/work experiences relevant to programs are important. For additional information on admission requirements, go to http://www.psychology.siu.edu.

Student Characteristics: The following represents characteristics of students in 2009–2010 in all graduate psychology programs in the department: Female—full-time 50, part-time 0; Male—full-time 30, part-time 0; African American/Black—full-time 8, part-time 0; Hispanic/Latino(a)—full-time 1, part-time 0; Asian/Pacific Islander—full-time 13, part-time 0; American Indian/Alaska Native—full-time 0, part-time 0; Caucasian/White—full-time 57, part-time 0; Multi-ethnic—full-time 1, part-time 0; students subject to the Americans With Disabilities Act—full-time 1, part-time 0; Unknown ethnicity—full-time 0, part-time 0; International students who hold an F-1 or J-1 Visa—full-time 0, part-time 0.

Financial Information/Assistance:
Tuition for Full-Time Study: *Master's:* State residents: per academic year $7,872, $328 per credit hour; Nonstate residents: per academic year $19,680, $820 per credit hour. *Doctoral:* State residents: per academic year $7,872, $328 per credit hour; Nonstate residents: per academic year $19,680, $820 per credit hour. Tuition is subject to change. Additional fees are assessed to students beyond the costs of tuition for the following: health care and activity fees, approximately $1550 per semester. See the following Web site for updates and changes in tuition costs: http://www.gradschool.siuc.edu.

Financial Assistance:
First-Year Students: Teaching assistantships available for first year. Average amount paid per academic year: $12,060. Average number of hours worked per week: 20. Research assistantships available for first year. Average amount paid per academic year: $12,060. Average number of hours worked per week: 20. Traineeships available for first year. Average amount paid per academic year: $12,060. Average number of hours worked per week: 20.

Fellowships and scholarships available for first year. Average amount paid per academic year: $12,060. Average number of hours worked per week: 20.

Advanced Students: Teaching assistantships available for advanced students. Average amount paid per academic year: $13,518. Average number of hours worked per week: 20. Research assistantships available for advanced students. Average amount paid per academic year: $13,518. Average number of hours worked per week: 20. Traineeships available for advanced students. Average amount paid per academic year: $13,518. Average number of hours worked per week: 20. Fellowships and scholarships available for advanced students. Average amount paid per academic year: $13,518. Average number of hours worked per week: 20.

Additional Information: Of all students currently enrolled full time, 100% benefited from one or more of the listed financial assistance programs.

Internships/Practica: Doctoral Degree (PhD Clinical Psychology): For those doctoral students for whom a professional internship was required in this program prior to graduation, (7) students applied for an internship in 2008–2009, with (6) students obtaining an internship. Of those students who obtained an internship, (6) were paid internships. Of those students who obtained an internship, (6) students placed in APA/CPA accredited internships, (0) students placed in internships not APA/CPA accredited, but listed with the Association of Psychology Postdoctoral and Internship Programs (APPIC), (0) students placed in internships conforming to guidelines of the Council of Directors of School Psychology Programs (CDSPP), (0) students placed in internships that were not APA/CPA accredited, APPIC or CDSPP listed. Doctoral Degree (PhD Counseling Psychology): For those doctoral students for whom a professional internship was required in this program prior to graduation, (5) students applied for an internship in 2008–2009, with (5) students obtaining an internship. Of those students who obtained an internship, (5) were paid internships. Of those students who obtained an internship, (5) students placed in APA/CPA accredited internships, (0) students placed in internships not APA/CPA accredited, but listed with the Association of Psychology Postdoctoral and Internship Programs (APPIC), (0) students placed in internships conforming to guidelines of the Council of Directors of School Psychology Programs (CDSPP), (0) students placed in internships that were not APA/CPA accredited, APPIC or CDSPP listed. A variety of practica and field experiences are available at a department Career Development & Resource Clinic, a university Clinical Center, campus Counseling Center, campus Health Service, Applied Research Consultants, and various local mental health centers, hospitals, and human service agencies.

Housing and Day Care: On-campus housing is available. See the following Web site for more information: http://www.housing.siu.edu/. On-campus day care facilities are available. See the following Web site for more information: http://www.siuc.edu/~rainbowsend/.

Employment of Department Graduates:
Master's Degree Graduates: Of those who graduated in the academic year 2008–2009, the following categories and numbers represent the postgraduate activities and employment of master's degree graduates: Enrolled in a postdoctoral residency/fellowship (n/a), employed in independent practice (n/a), total from the above (master's) (0).

Doctoral Degree Graduates: Of those who graduated in the academic year 2008–2009, the following categories and numbers represent the postgraduate activities and employment of doctoral degree graduates: Enrolled in a psychology doctoral program (n/a), enrolled in a postdoctoral residency/fellowship (1), employed in independent practice (0), employed in an academic position at a university (1), employed in other positions at a higher education institution (1), employed in government agency (1), employed in a community mental health/counseling center (3), employed in a hospital/medical center (3), do not know (1), total from the above (doctoral) (11).

Additional Information:
Orientation, Objectives, and Emphasis of Department: The department maintains a collaborative learning environment that is responsive to student needs, that promotes professional development, and that sustains high academic standards. In all programs the student selects courses from a rich curriculum that promotes mastery of core material while allowing the pursuit of particular interests. A favorable student-faculty ratio permits close supervision of students, whether in student research, clinical/applied practica, or training assignments that provide graduated experience in research, teaching, and service as a complement to formal coursework. Such training serves to expose students to many of the activities in which they will be engaged after receiving their degrees.

Special Facilities or Resources: The department is located in a building with extensive laboratory facilities for human and animal research available to all students. Additional facilities include a clinic and a counseling center for practicum and research experiences.

Information for Students With Physical Disabilities: See the following Web site for more information: http://www.siu.edu/~dss/.

Application Information:
Send to Psychology Graduate Admissions, SIUC, Mailcode 6502, Carbondale, IL 62901-6502. Application available online. URL of online application: http://www.psychology.siu.edu/apply.htm. Students are admitted in the Fall, application deadline Clinical: December 15; Counseling: December 15; Applied Psychology: February 1; Brain and Cognitive Sciences: February 1. *Fee:* $50.

Southern Illinois University Edwardsville
Department of Psychology
Box 1121
Edwardsville, IL 62026-1121
Telephone: (618) 650-2202
Fax: (618) 650-5087
E-mail: *prose@siue.edu*
Web: *http://www.siue.edu/education/psychology/graduate/*

Department Information:
1964. Chairperson: Paul Rose. Number of faculty: total—full-time 17, part-time 3; women—full-time 8, part-time 2; total—minority—full-time 1; women minority—full-time 1.

GRADUATE STUDY IN PSYCHOLOGY

Programs and Degrees Offered:
Listed in the following order: Program area, degree type (T if terminal Master's), number awarded 7/08–6/09. School Psychology EdS (School Psychology) 8, Clinical-Adult Psychology MA/MS (Master of Arts/Science) (T) 11, Industrial/Organizational Psychology MA/MS (Master of Arts/Science) (T) 9, Clinical Child and School Psychology MA/MS (Master of Arts/Science) (T) 15.

Student Applications/Admissions:

Student Applications

School Psychology EdS (School Psychology)—Applications 2009–2010, 12. Total applicants accepted 2009–2010, 6. Number full-time enrolled (new admits only) 2009–2010, 6. Number part-time enrolled (new admits only) 2009–2010, 0. Openings 2010–2011, 10. The median number of years required for completion of a degree in 2008–2009 were 2. The number of students enrolled full- and part-time who were dismissed or voluntarily withdrew from this program area in 2008–2009 were 0. Clinical-Adult Psychology MA/MS (Master of Arts/Science)—Applications 2009–2010, 42. Total applicants accepted 2009–2010, 16. Number full-time enrolled (new admits only) 2009–2010, 10. Number part-time enrolled (new admits only) 2009–2010, 0. Openings 2010–2011, 10. The median number of years required for completion of a degree in 2008–2009 were 2. The number of students enrolled full- and part-time who were dismissed or voluntarily withdrew from this program area in 2008–2009 were 0. Industrial/Organizational Psychology MA/MS (Master of Arts/Science)—Applications 2009–2010, 60. Total applicants accepted 2009–2010, 15. Number full-time enrolled (new admits only) 2009–2010, 9. Number part-time enrolled (new admits only) 2009–2010, 0. Openings 2010–2011, 10. The median number of years required for completion of a degree in 2008–2009 were 2. The number of students enrolled full- and part-time who were dismissed or voluntarily withdrew from this program area in 2008–2009 were 0. Clinical Child and School Psychology MA/MS (Master of Arts/Science)—Applications 2009–2010, 69. Total applicants accepted 2009–2010, 16. Number full-time enrolled (new admits only) 2009–2010, 10. Number part-time enrolled (new admits only) 2009–2010, 0. Openings 2010–2011, 10. The median number of years required for completion of a degree in 2008–2009 were 2. The number of students enrolled full- and part-time who were dismissed or voluntarily withdrew from this program area in 2008–2009 were 2.

Other Criteria: (importance of criteria rated low, medium, or high): GRE scores—medium, research experience—high, work experience—medium, extracurricular activity—medium, clinically related public service—medium, GPA—high, letters of recommendation—high, interview—high, statement of goals and objectives—high, undergraduate major in psychology—medium, specific undergraduate psychology courses taken—high. For additional information on admission requirements, go to http://www.siue.edu/education/psychology/graduate/apinfo.shtml.

Student Characteristics: The following represents characteristics of students in 2009–2010 in all graduate psychology programs in the department: Female—full-time 53, part-time 0; Male—full-time 10, part-time 0; African American/Black—full-time 2, part-time 0; Hispanic/Latino(a)—full-time 2, part-time 0; Asian/Pacific Islander—full-time 1, part-time 0; American Indian/Alaska Native—full-time 0, part-time 0; Caucasian/White—full-time 0, part-time 0; Multi-ethnic—full-time 0, part-time 0; students subject to the Americans With Disabilities Act—full-time 0, part-time 0; Unknown ethnicity—full-time 0, part-time 0; International students who hold an F-1 or J-1 Visa—full-time 0, part-time 0.

Financial Information/Assistance:
Tuition for Full-Time Study: *Master's:* State residents: per academic year $9,305; Nonstate residents: per academic year $20,578. See the following Web site for updates and changes in tuition costs: http://www.siue.edu/apply/tuition/.

Financial Assistance:

First-Year Students: Research assistantships available for first year. Average amount paid per academic year: $3,555. Average number of hours worked per week: 10. Apply by March 1. Fellowships and scholarships available for first year. Average amount paid per academic year: $7,425. Average number of hours worked per week: 0. Apply by January 15.

Advanced Students: Research assistantships available for advanced students. Average amount paid per academic year: $3,825. Average number of hours worked per week: 10. Apply by March 1.

Additional Information: Of all students currently enrolled full time, 75% benefited from one or more of the listed financial assistance programs. Application and information available online at: http://www.siue.edu/education/psychology/graduate/apinfo.shtml.

Internships/Practica: Master's Degree (MA/MS Clinical-Adult Psychology): An internship experience, such as a final research project or "capstone" experience is required of graduates. Master's Degree (MA/MS Industrial/Organizational Psychology): An internship experience, such as a final research project or "capstone" experience is required of graduates. Master's Degree (MA/MS Clinical Child and School Psychology): An internship experience, such as a final research project or "capstone" experience is required of graduates. All graduate programs require at least four credit hours of supervised practicum experience in appropriate professional settings. The Specialist Degree Program also requires a 10-hour paid internship.

Housing and Day Care: On-campus housing is available. See the following Web site for more information: http://www.siue.edu/housing/index.shtml. On-campus day care facilities are available. See the following Web site for more information: http://www.siue.edu/earlychildhood/.

Employment of Department Graduates:

Master's Degree Graduates: Of those who graduated in the academic year 2008–2009, the following categories and numbers represent the postgraduate activities and employment of master's degree graduates: Enrolled in a postdoctoral residency/fellowship (n/a), employed in independent practice (n/a), total from the above (master's) (0).

Doctoral Degree Graduates: Of those who graduated in the academic year 2008–2009, the following categories and numbers represent the postgraduate activities and employment of doctoral degree graduates: Enrolled in a psychology doctoral program (n/a), total from the above (doctoral) (0).

Additional Information:

Orientation, Objectives, and Emphasis of Department: The department, faculty and students have won several awards for teaching excellence, educational outcomes, academic excellence and community contribution. The department is generally eclectic in orientation. Students in each specialization are provided with training that is balanced between scientific and applied orientations.

Special Facilities or Resources: The psychology department facilities house faculty offices, classrooms, and approximately 10,000 square feet of laboratory space. Sophisticated research and instructional equipment is available, including videotaping equipment, computers and a resource center. Special laboratories are available for learning, motivation, information processing, developmental, clinical, and psychometric activities.

Information for Students With Physical Disabilities: See the following Web site for more information: http://www.siue.edu/dss/.

Application Information:

Send to Attention: Graduate Records Secretary, Psychology Department, Box 1121, Edwardsville, IL 62026. Application available online. URL of online application: http://www.siue.edu/education/psychology/graduate/. Students are admitted in the Fall, application deadline February 1. *Fee:* $30.

The Chicago School of Professional Psychology
Professional School
325 North Wells
Chicago, IL 60654
Telephone: (312) 329.6671
Fax: (312) 644.3333
E-mail: ktalley@thechicagoschool.edu
Web: http://www.thechicagoschool.edu

Department Information:

1979. President: Michael Horowitz, PhD. Number of faculty: total—full-time 95, part-time 114; women—full-time 53, part-time 71; total—minority—full-time 22, part-time 26; women minority—full-time 13, part-time 16.

Programs and Degrees Offered:

Listed in the following order: Program area, degree type (T if terminal Master's), number awarded 7/08–6/09. Clinical Psychology PsyD (Doctor of Psychology) 71, Industrial/Organizational Psychology MA/MS (Master of Arts/Science) (T) 63, Forensic Psychology MA/MS (Master of Arts/Science) (T) 39, Clinical Psychology (Counseling) MA/MS (Master of Arts/Science) (T) 64, Clinical Forensic Psychology PsyD (Doctor of Psychology), Business Psychology PsyD (Doctor of Psychology), Clinical Psychology (Applied Behavior Analysis) MA/MS (Master of Arts/Science) (T) 10, Applied Industrial/Organizational Certificate Other 0, Applied Behavior Analysis PsyD (Doctor of Psychology), Board Certified Behavior Analyst Respecialization Respecialization Diploma 0, Applied Forensics Certificate Other 16, Psychology PsyD (Doctor of Psychology), School Psychology EdS (School Psychology) 0, General Psychology MA/MS (Master of Arts/Science) (T), Organizational Leadership PhD (Doctor of Philosophy), International Psychology PhD (Doctor of Philosophy), Clinical Psychology (Marital and Family Therapy) MA/MS (Master of Arts/Science) (T), Marital and Family Therapy PsyD (Doctor of Psychology).

APA Accreditation: Clinical PsyD (Doctor of Psychology). Student Outcome Data Website: http://www.thechicagoschool.edu/resources/content/1/6/8/9/documents/APA-Disclosure-Document-Sept-2009.pdf.

Student Applications/Admissions:

Student Applications

Clinical Psychology PsyD (Doctor of Psychology)—Number full-time enrolled (new admits only) 2009–2010, 106. Total enrolled 2009–2010 full-time, 414, part-time, 10. The median number of years required for completion of a degree in 2008–2009 were 5. *Industrial/Organizational Psychology MA/MS (Master of Arts/Science)*—Number full-time enrolled (new admits only) 2009–2010, 48. Number part-time enrolled (new admits only) 2009–2010, 33. Total enrolled 2009–2010 full-time, 108, part-time, 229. The median number of years required for completion of a degree in 2008–2009 were 2. *Forensic Psychology MA/MS (Master of Arts/Science)*—Number full-time enrolled (new admits only) 2009–2010, 76. Number part-time enrolled (new admits only) 2009–2010, 51. Total enrolled 2009–2010 full-time, 157, part-time, 297. The median number of years required for completion of a degree in 2008–2009 were 2. *Clinical Psychology (Counseling) MA/MS (Master of Arts/Science)*—Number full-time enrolled (new admits only) 2009–2010, 156. Number part-time enrolled (new admits only) 2009–2010, 23. Total enrolled 2009–2010 full-time, 296, part-time, 49. The median number of years required for completion of a degree in 2008–2009 were 2. *Clinical Forensic Psychology PsyD (Doctor of Psychology)*—Number full-time enrolled (new admits only) 2009–2010, 30. Total enrolled 2009–2010 full-time, 30. *Business Psychology PsyD (Doctor of Psychology)*—Number full-time enrolled (new admits only) 2009–2010, 18. Number part-time enrolled (new admits only) 2009–2010, 1. Total enrolled 2009–2010 full-time, 63, part-time, 4. The median number of years required for completion of a degree in 2008–2009 were 7. *Clinical Psychology (Applied Behavior Analysis) MA/MS (Master of Arts/Science)*—Number full-time enrolled (new admits only) 2009–2010, 40. Number part-time enrolled (new admits only) 2009–2010, 2. Total enrolled 2009–2010 full-time, 78, part-time, 23. The median number of years required for completion of a degree in 2008–2009 were 2. *Applied Industrial/Organizational Certificate Other*—Number part-time enrolled (new admits only) 2009–2010, 8. Total enrolled 2009–2010 part-time, 23. *Applied Behavior Analysis PsyD (Doctor of Psychology)*—Number full-time enrolled (new admits only) 2009–2010, 15. Number part-time enrolled (new admits only) 2009–2010, 2. Total enrolled 2009–2010 full-time, 26, part-time, 3. *Board Certified Behavior Analyst Respecialization Respecialization Diploma*—Number full-time enrolled (new admits only) 2009–2010, 0. Number part-time enrolled (new admits only) 2009–2010, 12. *Applied Forensics Certificate Other*—Number part-time enrolled (new admits only) 2009–2010, 19. Total enrolled 2009–2010 part-time, 45. The median number of years required for completion of a degree in 2008–2009 was 1. *Psychology PsyD (Doctor of Psychology)*—*School Psychology EdS (School Psychology)*—Number full-time enrolled

(new admits only) 2009–2010, 39. Number part-time enrolled (new admits only) 2009–2010, 26. Total enrolled 2009–2010 full-time, 125, part-time, 46. The median number of years required for completion of a degree in 2008–2009 were 3. *General Psychology MA/MS (Master of Arts/Science)*—Number part-time enrolled (new admits only) 2009–2010, 64. Total enrolled 2009–2010 part-time, 148. *Organizational Leadership PhD (Doctor of Philosophy)*—Number part-time enrolled (new admits only) 2009–2010, 22. Total enrolled 2009–2010 part-time, 22. *International Psychology PhD (Doctor of Philosophy)*—Number part-time enrolled (new admits only) 2009–2010, 18. Total enrolled 2009–2010 part-time, 18. *Clinical Psychology (Marital and Family Therapy) MA/MS (Master of Arts/Science)—Marital and Family Therapy PsyD (Doctor of Psychology)*
Other Criteria: (importance of criteria rated low, medium, or high): GRE scores—medium, research experience—low, work experience—high, extracurricular activity—low, clinically related public service—high, GPA—high, letters of recommendation—medium, interview—high, statement of goals and objectives—medium. PsyD in Clinical, Business Psychology, Clinical Forensic, and ABA programs - Interviews are required and by invitation. For additional information on admission requirements, go to http://www.thechicagoschool.edu/content.cfm/admission.

Student Characteristics: The following represents characteristics of students in 2009–2010 in all graduate psychology programs in the department: Female—full-time 1032, part-time 774; Male—full-time 265, part-time 174; African American/Black—full-time 122, part-time 151; Hispanic/Latino(a)—full-time 90, part-time 78; Asian/Pacific Islander—full-time 59, part-time 29; American Indian/Alaska Native—full-time 5, part-time 8; Caucasian/White—full-time 826, part-time 453; Multi-ethnic—full-time 25, part-time 7; Unknown ethnicity—full-time 170, part-time 222; International students who hold an F-1 or J-1 Visa—full-time 1, part-time 3.

Financial Information/Assistance:
Financial Assistance:
First-Year Students: Teaching assistantships available for first year. Average amount paid per academic year: $6,000. Average number of hours worked per week: 20. Apply by June 1. Research assistantships available for first year. Average amount paid per academic year: $6,000. Average number of hours worked per week: 20. Apply by June 1. Fellowships and scholarships available for first year. Average amount paid per academic year: $10,000. Average number of hours worked per week: 10. Apply by April 1.
Advanced Students: Teaching assistantships available for advanced students. Average amount paid per academic year: $6,000. Average number of hours worked per week: 20. Research assistantships available for advanced students. Average amount paid per academic year: $6,000. Average number of hours worked per week: 20. Fellowships and scholarships available for advanced students. Average amount paid per academic year: $10,000. Average number of hours worked per week: 10. Apply by April 1.
Additional Information: Of all students currently enrolled full time, 80% benefited from one or more of the listed financial assistance programs. Application and information available online at: http://www.thechicagoschool.edu/content.cfm/financing_your_education.

Internships/Practica: Doctoral Degree (PsyD Clinical Psychology): For those doctoral students for whom a professional internship was required in this program prior to graduation, (66) students applied for an internship in 2008–2009, with (66) students obtaining an internship. Of those students who obtained an internship, (62) were paid internships. Of those students who obtained an internship, (36) students placed in APA/CPA accredited internships, (28) students placed in internships not APA/CPA accredited, but listed with the Association of Psychology Postdoctoral and Internship Programs (APPIC), (0) students placed in internships conforming to guidelines of the Council of Directors of School Psychology Programs (CDSPP), (2) students placed in internships that were not APA/CPA accredited, APPIC or CDSPP listed. Master's Degree (MA/MS Industrial/Organizational Psychology): An internship experience, such as a final research project or "capstone" experience is required of graduates. Master's Degree (MA/MS Forensic Psychology): An internship experience, such as a final research project or "capstone" experience is required of graduates. Master's Degree (MA/MS Clinical Psychology (Counseling)): An internship experience, such as a final research project or "capstone" experience is required of graduates. Master's Degree (MA/MS Clinical Psychology (Applied Behavior Analysis)): An internship experience, such as a final research project or "capstone" experience is required of graduates. Currently there are over 500 assessment and therapy practicum sites in the city and surrounding area at which our students train.

Housing and Day Care: No on-campus housing is available. No on-campus day care facilities are available.

Employment of Department Graduates:
Master's Degree Graduates: Of those who graduated in the academic year 2008–2009, the following categories and numbers represent the postgraduate activities and employment of master's degree graduates: Enrolled in a postdoctoral residency/fellowship (n/a), employed in independent practice (n/a), total from the above (master's) (0).
Doctoral Degree Graduates: Of those who graduated in the academic year 2008–2009, the following categories and numbers represent the postgraduate activities and employment of doctoral degree graduates: Enrolled in a psychology doctoral program (n/a), total from the above (doctoral) (0).

Additional Information:
Orientation, Objectives, and Emphasis of Department: The Chicago School educates students to be competent practitioners by providing curricula that emphasize both a broad knowledge of the scientific and theoretical bases of psychology and the ability to apply that knowledge to specific employment situations. A student-centered environment, with personal advising and supervision provide opportunities for deepening awareness, knowledge, and skills. The programs are designed to integrate the study of cultural and individual differences and their impact in the clinical and work settings. The professional and ethical development of the student is of foremost concern throughout the educational program.

Special Facilities or Resources: The Chicago School offers experiential learning opportunities at the Center for Multicultural and Diversity Studies, the Center for International Studies, the Center for Latino Mental Health, the Forensic Center, and the Platt

Retail Institute. The Naomi Ruth Cohen Institute for Mental Health Education at The Chicago School (TCS) and continues to offer an annual predoctoral fellowship to a TCS student. The mission of the Cohen Institute is to overcome the stigma associated with mental illness through culturally competent community outreach and educational programming.

Information for Students With Physical Disabilities: See the following Web site for more information: http://www.thechicagoschool.edu/content.cfm/disability_accommodations.

Application Information:
Send to Admission Department, Chicago School of Professional Psychology, 325 N Wells, Chicago, IL 60654. Application available online. URL of online application: http://www.thechicagoschool.edu/content.cfm/admission. Students are admitted in the Fall. *Fall Early consideration deadline for PsyD in Clinical Psychology program is December 15. Early consideration deadline for PsyD in Business Psychology, Clinical Forensic Psychology, Applied Behavior Analysis, EdS in School Psychology, all MA programs, and Latino Mental Health Certificate is February 15. General consideration deadline for PsyD in Clinical Psychology program is February 15. General consideration deadline for PsyD in Business Psychology, EdS in School Psychology and all MA programs is April 1. *Space available: Contact the Admission Department after the above deadline for program availability. Fee: $50. McNair Scholars are eligible for an application fee waiver.

Western Illinois University
Department of Psychology
Arts and Sciences
Waggoner Hall
Macomb, IL 61455
Telephone: (309) 298-1919
Fax: (309) 298-2179
E-mail: cj-kreps@wiu.edu
Web: http://www.wiu.edu/psychology

Department Information:
1960. Chairperson: Steven Dworkin. Number of faculty: total—full-time 25, part-time 3; women—full-time 13, part-time 3; total—minority—full-time 1; women minority—full-time 1.

Programs and Degrees Offered:
Listed in the following order: Program area, degree type (T if terminal Master's), number awarded 7/08–6/09. Clinical/Community Mental Health MA/MS (Master of Arts/Science) (T) 5, General Experimental Psychology MA/MS (Master of Arts/Science) (T) 5, School Psychology Other 10.

Student Applications/Admissions:
Student Applications
Clinical/Community Mental Health MA/MS (Master of Arts/Science)—Applications 2009–2010, 39. Total applicants accepted 2009–2010, 8. Number full-time enrolled (new admits only) 2009–2010, 8. Total enrolled 2009–2010 full-time, 18. Openings 2010–2011, 8. The median number of years required for completion of a degree in 2008–2009 were 3. The number of students enrolled full- and part-time who were dismissed or voluntarily withdrew from this program area in 2008–2009 were 0. *General Experimental Psychology MA/MS (Master of Arts/Science)*—Applications 2009–2010, 21. Total applicants accepted 2009–2010, 14. Number full-time enrolled (new admits only) 2009–2010, 9. Number part-time enrolled (new admits only) 2009–2010, 0. Openings 2010–2011, 8. The median number of years required for completion of a degree in 2008–2009 were 2. The number of students enrolled full- and part-time who were dismissed or voluntarily withdrew from this program area in 2008–2009 were 1. *School Psychology Other*—Applications 2009–2010, 20. Total applicants accepted 2009–2010, 18. Number full-time enrolled (new admits only) 2009–2010, 8. Number part-time enrolled (new admits only) 2009–2010, 0. Openings 2010–2011, 12. The median number of years required for completion of a degree in 2008–2009 were 3. The number of students enrolled full- and part-time who were dismissed or voluntarily withdrew from this program area in 2008–2009 were 1.

Scores: Entries appear in this order: required test or GPA, minimum score (if required), median score of students entering in 2009–2010. *Clinical/Community Mental Health MA/MS (Master of Arts/Science)*: GRE-V 500, GRE-Q 500, GRE-Analytical 4.0, last 2 years GPA 3.0, psychology GPA 2.75; *General Experimental Psychology MA/MS (Master of Arts/Science)*: GRE-V 500, GRE-Q 500, GRE-Analytical 4.0, overall undergraduate GPA no minimum stated, last 2 years GPA 3.0, psychology GPA 2.75; *School Psychology Other*: GRE-V 500, GRE-Q 500, GRE-Analytical 4.0, overall undergraduate GPA no minimum stated, last 2 years GPA 3.0, psychology GPA 2.75.

Other Criteria: (importance of criteria rated low, medium, or high): GRE scores—high, research experience—medium, work experience—medium, extracurricular activity—medium, clinically related public service—medium, GPA—high, letters of recommendation—high, interview—low, statement of goals and objectives—high, undergraduate major in psychology—medium, specific undergraduate psychology courses taken—medium.

Student Characteristics: The following represents characteristics of students in 2009–2010 in all graduate psychology programs in the department: Female—full-time 31, part-time 0; Male—full-time 24, part-time 0; African American/Black—part-time 0; Hispanic/Latino(a)—part-time 0; Asian/Pacific Islander—full-time 3, part-time 0; American Indian/Alaska Native—full-time 0, part-time 0; Caucasian/White—full-time 52, part-time 0; Multi-ethnic—full-time 0, part-time 0; students subject to the Americans With Disabilities Act—full-time 0, part-time 0; Unknown ethnicity—full-time 0, part-time 0; International students who hold an F-1 or J-1 Visa—full-time 3, part-time 0.

Financial Information/Assistance:
Tuition for Full-Time Study: *Master's:* State residents: per academic year $6,000, $250 per credit hour; Nonstate residents: per academic year $11,976, $499 per credit hour. Tuition is subject to change. Additional fees are assessed to students beyond the costs of tuition for the following: university fees. See the following Web site for updates and changes in tuition costs: http://www.wiu.edu/grad/resources/fees/php.

Financial Assistance:
First-Year Students: Research assistantships available for first year. Average amount paid per academic year: $5,463. Average number of hours worked per week: 13. Apply by April 15.

GRADUATE STUDY IN PSYCHOLOGY

Advanced Students: Research assistantships available for advanced students. Average amount paid per academic year: $5,463. Average number of hours worked per week: 13. Apply by April 15.

Additional Information: Of all students currently enrolled full time, 90% benefited from one or more of the listed financial assistance programs. Application and information available online at: http://www.wiu.edu/grad/resources/fees/php.

Internships/Practica: Master's Degree (MA/MS Clinical/Community Mental Health): An internship experience, such as a final research project or "capstone" experience is required of graduates. Master's Degree (MA/MS General Experimental Psychology): An internship experience, such as a final research project or "capstone" experience is required of graduates. The Clinical/Community Mental Health program includes a four semester practicum sequence of intensive, supervised work in the department's Psychology Clinic. An internship for which postgraduate credit is given prepares students for jobs in clinical psychology. Practicum work in community schools and the department's psychoeducational clinic under faculty supervision is required throughout both years of the School Psychology program, and a paid internship for which postgraduate credit is given prepares students for certification in Illinois.

Housing and Day Care: On-campus housing is available. On-campus day care facilities are available.

Employment of Department Graduates:
Master's Degree Graduates: Of those who graduated in the academic year 2008–2009, the following categories and numbers represent the postgraduate activities and employment of master's degree graduates: Enrolled in a psychology doctoral program (3), enrolled in another graduate/professional program (3), enrolled in a postdoctoral residency/fellowship (n/a), employed in independent practice (n/a), employed in an academic position at a university (3), employed in an academic position at a 2-year/4-year college (1), employed in other positions at a higher education institution (1), employed in a professional position in a school system (9), employed in business or industry (0), employed in government agency (2), employed in a community mental health/counseling center (2), employed in a hospital/medical center (1), other employment position (4), total from the above (master's) (29).
Doctoral Degree Graduates: Of those who graduated in the academic year 2008–2009, the following categories and numbers represent the postgraduate activities and employment of doctoral degree graduates: Enrolled in a psychology doctoral program (n/a), total from the above (doctoral) (0).

Additional Information:
Orientation, Objectives, and Emphasis of Department: The psychology department offers master's degrees in clinical/community mental health (C/CMH), and general experimental psychology, and a Specialist degree in school psychology. C/CMH-MS and School-Specialist degrees are three year programs with the third year consisting of a paid internship. The emphasis in the Clin/CMH program is to prepare students to assume professional responsibilities in outpatient mental health settings. Central to the program is the practicum experience offered through the University Psychology Clinic. Graduates of the Clin/CMH program have found employment in a variety of mental health agencies, with over 90 percent of all graduates currently employed in mental health positions. Students in the general psychology program engage in one to two years of course work in psychology. The opportunity to specialize in industrial/organizational, social, developmental, or experimental psychology is available within the general psychology program. Many students completing the general program have been admitted to PhD programs in psychology. Students in the school psychology program acquire an academic background in psychology and a practical awareness of public school systems. During the first year of the program, students are placed in elementary schools for practical experience, and during their second year, students work in the university psychoeducational clinic. Graduates of the program have had no difficulty finding employment as school psychologists following their internships. Many have also pursued doctoral training.

Special Facilities or Resources: The Department of Psychology is housed in a large modern structure providing facilities for teaching, clinical training, and human and animal research. The department has 55 rooms, including regular classrooms, seminar rooms, observation rooms, small experimental cubicles, and neuroscience labs. Computers are available throughout the department and campus. The department operates a psychology clinic for community referrals, which aids in clinical training, and a psychoeducational clinic for training in school psychology.

Information for Students With Physical Disabilities: See the following Web site for more information: http://dss.wiu.edu.

Application Information:
Send to School of Graduate Studies, Western Illinois University, #1 University Circle, Macomb, IL 61455. Application available online. URL of online application: http://www.wiu.edu/grad/prospective/index.php. Students are admitted in the Fall, application deadline February 15; Spring, application deadline. Spring and Fall admission pertains to the MS in General Experimental Program. The School Psychology and Clinical/Community Mental Health Programs take Fall semester admission only. Application deadline is February 15 for both C/CMH program and School Psychology Program. *Fee:* $30.

Wheaton College
Department of Psychology
501 College Avenue
Wheaton, IL 60187-5593
Telephone: (630) 752-5762
Fax: (630) 752-7033
E-mail: *ted.kahn@wheaton.edu*
Web: *http://www.wheaton.edu/psychology/*

Department Information:
1979. Chairperson: Robert J. Gregory, PhD. Number of faculty: total—full-time 16, part-time 3; women—full-time 5, part-time 3; total—minority—full-time 1, part-time 1; women minority—part-time 1.

Programs and Degrees Offered:
Listed in the following order: Program area, degree type (T if terminal Master's), number awarded 7/08–6/09. Clinical Psychology MA/MS (Master of Arts/Science) (T) 29, Clinical Psychology

PsyD (Doctor of Psychology) 9, Counseling Ministries MA/MS (Master of Arts/Science) (T) 1.

APA Accreditation: Clinical PsyD (Doctor of Psychology). Student Outcome Data Website: http://www.wheaton.edu/psychology/graduate/costs_outcomes/costs.html.

Student Applications/Admissions:
Student Applications
Clinical Psychology MA/MS (Master of Arts/Science)—Applications 2009–2010, 85. Total applicants accepted 2009–2010, 43. Number full-time enrolled (new admits only) 2009–2010, 31. Total enrolled 2009–2010 full-time, 58, part-time, 2. Openings 2010–2011, 30. The median number of years required for completion of a degree in 2008–2009 were 2. The number of students enrolled full- and part-time who were dismissed or voluntarily withdrew from this program area in 2008–2009 were 0. *Clinical Psychology PsyD (Doctor of Psychology)*—Applications 2009–2010, 67. Total applicants accepted 2009–2010, 30. Number full-time enrolled (new admits only) 2009–2010, 19. Number part-time enrolled (new admits only) 2009–2010, 0. Total enrolled 2009–2010 full-time, 89, part-time, 18. Openings 2010–2011, 20. The median number of years required for completion of a degree in 2008–2009 were 5. The number of students enrolled full- and part-time who were dismissed or voluntarily withdrew from this program area in 2008–2009 were 1. *Counseling Ministries MA/MS (Master of Arts/Science)*—Applications 2009–2010, 7. Total applicants accepted 2009–2010, 3. Number full-time enrolled (new admits only) 2009–2010, 2. Number part-time enrolled (new admits only) 2009–2010, 0. Total enrolled 2009–2010 full-time, 2, part-time, 2. Openings 2010–2011, 5. The median number of years required for completion of a degree in 2008–2009 was 1. The number of students enrolled full- and part-time who were dismissed or voluntarily withdrew from this program area in 2008–2009 were 0.
Scores: Entries appear in this order: required test or GPA, minimum score (if required), median score of students entering in 2009–2010. *Clinical Psychology MA/MS (Master of Arts/Science)*: GRE-V no minimum stated, GRE-Q no minimum stated, GRE-Analytical no minimum stated, overall undergraduate GPA 3.0; *Clinical Psychology PsyD (Doctor of Psychology)*: GRE-V no minimum stated, GRE-Q no minimum stated, GRE-Analytical no minimum stated, overall undergraduate GPA 3.0, Masters GPA no minimum stated; *Counseling Ministries MA/MS (Master of Arts/Science)*: GRE-V no minimum stated, GRE-Q no minimum stated, GRE-Analytical no minimum stated, overall undergraduate GPA 2.75.
Other Criteria: (importance of criteria rated low, medium, or high): GRE scores—medium, research experience—medium, work experience—medium, extracurricular activity—medium, clinically related public service—medium, GPA—medium, letters of recommendation—high, interview—high, statement of goals and objectives—high, undergraduate major in psychology—low, specific undergraduate psychology courses taken—medium, PsyD Program conducts a series of applicant interviews. MA Program works with application packages only. For additional information on admission requirements, go to http://www.wheatongrad.com/Admission_Requirements.

Student Characteristics: The following represents characteristics of students in 2009–2010 in all graduate psychology programs in the department: Female—full-time 107, part-time 14; Male—full-time 42, part-time 8; African American/Black—full-time 9, part-time 1; Hispanic/Latino(a)—full-time 5, part-time 0; Asian/Pacific Islander—full-time 12, part-time 3; American Indian/Alaska Native—full-time 0, part-time 0; Caucasian/White—full-time 123, part-time 18; Multi-ethnic—full-time 0, part-time 0; students subject to the Americans With Disabilities Act—full-time 3, part-time 0; Unknown ethnicity—full-time 0, part-time 0; International students who hold an F-1 or J-1 Visa—full-time 6, part-time 0.

Financial Information/Assistance:
Tuition for Full-Time Study: *Master's:* State residents: per academic year $15,120, $630 per credit hour; Nonstate residents: per academic year $15,120, $630 per credit hour. *Doctoral:* State residents: per academic year $24,900, $830 per credit hour; Nonstate residents: per academic year $24,900, $830 per credit hour. Tuition is subject to change. Tuition costs vary by program. See the following Web site for updates and changes in tuition costs: http://www.wheatongrad.com/Tuition_and_Fees.

Financial Assistance:
First-Year Students: Teaching assistantships available for first year. Average amount paid per academic year: $5,000. Average number of hours worked per week: 10. Research assistantships available for first year. Average amount paid per academic year: $5,000. Average number of hours worked per week: 10. Fellowships and scholarships available for first year. Average amount paid per academic year: $5,400. Average number of hours worked per week: 0.
Advanced Students: Teaching assistantships available for advanced students. Average amount paid per academic year: $5,000. Average number of hours worked per week: 10. Research assistantships available for advanced students. Average amount paid per academic year: $5,000. Average number of hours worked per week: 10. Traineeships available for advanced students. Average amount paid per academic year: $5,000. Average number of hours worked per week: 15. Fellowships and scholarships available for advanced students. Average amount paid per academic year: $6,000. Average number of hours worked per week: 0.
Additional Information: Of all students currently enrolled full time, 80% benefited from one or more of the listed financial assistance programs. Application and information available online at: http://www.wheaton.edu/finaid/grad/index.html.

Internships/Practica: Doctoral Degree (PsyD Clinical Psychology): For those doctoral students for whom a professional internship was required in this program prior to graduation, (17) students applied for an internship in 2008–2009, with (14) students obtaining an internship. Of those students who obtained an internship, (14) were paid internships. Of those students who obtained an internship, (7) students placed in APA/CPA accredited internships, (6) students placed in internships not APA/CPA accredited, but listed with the Association of Psychology Postdoctoral and Internship Programs (APPIC), (0) students placed in internships conforming to guidelines of the Council of Directors of School Psychology Programs (CDSPP), (1) students placed in internships that were not APA/CPA accredited, APPIC or CDSPP listed. Master's Degree (MA/MS Clinical Psychology): An internship experience, such as a final research project or "capstone" experience is required of graduates. Master's Degree (MA/MS Counseling Ministries): An internship experience, such as a final research project or "capstone" experience is required of graduates. The Graduate Psychology Programs have liaisons with over 90 agencies in the Chicago and suburban area with facility types ranging from hospitals, clinics, community agencies, residential, and correctional facilities. The MA Program requires 600 on-site hours and the PsyD requires a minimum of 1200 hours. Faculty are involved through professional development groups while students are placed in field assignments.

Housing and Day Care: On-campus housing is available. See the following Web site for more information: http://www.wheatongrad.com/Housing. No on-campus day care facilities are available.

Employment of Department Graduates:
Master's Degree Graduates: Of those who graduated in the academic year 2008–2009, the following categories and numbers represent the postgraduate activities and employment of master's degree graduates: Enrolled in a postdoctoral residency/fellowship (n/a), employed in independent practice (n/a), total from the above (master's) (0).
Doctoral Degree Graduates: Of those who graduated in the academic year 2008–2009, the following categories and numbers represent the postgraduate activities and employment of doctoral degree graduates: Enrolled in a psychology doctoral program (n/a), total from the above (doctoral) (0).

Additional Information:
Orientation, Objectives, and Emphasis of Department: The doctoral program aims to produce competent scholar-practitioners in clinical psychology who will understand professional practice as service. The primary emphasis of the MA program is the professional preparation of the master's level therapist for employment in clinical settings; a secondary objective is the preparation of selected students for doctoral studies. The departmental orientation is eclectic, with students exposed to the theory, research, and practical clinical skills of the major clinical models in use today. A pre-eminent concern of all faculty is the interface of psychological theory and practice with Christian faith. Thus, students also take coursework in the theory and practice of integrating psychology and Christian faith, and coursework in theology/biblical studies. Students are encouraged to participate in a growth-oriented group therapy experience or an individual therapy experience. The objectives of the department are to produce mature, capable Master's and doctoral-level clinicians who are well grounded in clinical theory and the essentials of professional practice, and who responsibly and capably relate their Christian faith and professional interests.

Personal Behavior Statement: http://www.wheatongrad.com/?p=71.

Special Facilities or Resources: The PsyD Program has its own computer lab/reading room for research and study. The Psychology Department also has a state-of-the-art child development lab equipped with Noldus XT. Many students work with faculty research projects. Opportunities exist for professional conference presentations and involvement in international projects.

Application Information:
Send to Graduate Admissions Office, Wheaton College, 501 College Avenue, Wheaton, IL, 60187. Application available online. URL of online application: http://www.wheatongrad.com/Graduate_Applications. Students are admitted in the Fall, application deadline December 15. December 15 deadline PsyD, March 1 deadline MA in Clinical Psychology, May 1 deadline MA in Counseling Ministries. *Fee:* $50.

INDIANA

Ball State University
Department of Counseling Psychology and Guidance Services
Teachers College, Room 622
Muncie, IN 47306-0585
Telephone: (765) 285-8040
Fax: (765) 285-2067
E-mail: sbowman@bsu.edu
Web: http://www.bsu.edu/counselingpsychology/

Department Information:
1967. Chairperson: Sharon L. Bowman. Number of faculty: total—full-time 11; women—full-time 5; total—minority—full-time 4; women minority—full-time 2; faculty subject to the Americans With Disabilities Act 1.

Programs and Degrees Offered:
Listed in the following order: Program area, degree type (T if terminal Master's), number awarded 7/08–6/09. Social Psychology MA/MS (Master of Arts/Science) (T) 7, Counseling MA/MS (Master of Arts/Science) (T) 41, Counseling Psychology PhD (Doctor of Philosophy) 8.

APA Accreditation: Counseling PhD (Doctor of Philosophy). Student Outcome Data Website: http://www.bsu.edu/counselingpsychology/phdcounpsych/.

Student Applications/Admissions:
Student Applications
Social Psychology MA/MS (Master of Arts/Science)—Applications 2009–2010, 20. Total applicants accepted 2009–2010, 13. Number full-time enrolled (new admits only) 2009–2010, 9. Total enrolled 2009–2010 full-time, 19, part-time, 1. Openings 2010–2011, 10. The median number of years required for completion of a degree in 2008–2009 were 2. The number of students enrolled full- and part-time who were dismissed or voluntarily withdrew from this program area in 2008–2009 were 0. Counseling MA/MS (Master of Arts/Science)—Applications 2009–2010, 90. Total applicants accepted 2009–2010, 65. Number full-time enrolled (new admits only) 2009–2010, 51. Number part-time enrolled (new admits only) 2009–2010, 5. Total enrolled 2009–2010 full-time, 122, part-time, 18. Openings 2010–2011, 43. The median number of years required for completion of a degree in 2008–2009 were 2. The number of students enrolled full- and part-time who were dismissed or voluntarily withdrew from this program area in 2008–2009 were 2. Counseling Psychology PhD (Doctor of Philosophy)—Applications 2009–2010, 116. Total applicants accepted 2009–2010, 15. Number full-time enrolled (new admits only) 2009–2010, 10. Total enrolled 2009–2010 full-time, 36, part-time, 14. Openings 2010–2011, 10. The median number of years required for completion of a degree in 2008–2009 were 5. The number of students enrolled full- and part-time who were dismissed or voluntarily withdrew from this program area in 2008–2009 were 1.

Scores: Entries appear in this order: required test or GPA, minimum score (if required), median score of students entering in 2009–2010. Social Psychology MA/MS (Master of Arts/Science): GRE-V 490, GRE-Q 490, overall undergraduate GPA 3.5; Counseling MA/MS (Master of Arts/Science): GRE-V 480, GRE-Q 500, overall undergraduate GPA no minimum stated, 3.53; Counseling Psychology PhD (Doctor of Philosophy): GRE-V 500, GRE-Q 500, overall undergraduate GPA 3.5.

Other Criteria: (importance of criteria rated low, medium, or high): GRE scores—high, research experience—high, work experience—high, extracurricular activity—medium, clinically related public service—medium, GPA—high, letters of recommendation—high, interview—medium, statement of goals and objectives—high, diversity interest—high. Interview is a requirement for the Doctoral Program, not the Master's programs. For additional information on admission requirements, go to http://www.bsu.edu/counselingpsychology.

Student Characteristics: The following represents characteristics of students in 2009–2010 in all graduate psychology programs in the department: Female—full-time 128, part-time 23; Male—full-time 49, part-time 10; African American/Black—full-time 5, part-time 0; Hispanic/Latino(a)—full-time 0, part-time 0; Asian/Pacific Islander—full-time 5, part-time 0; American Indian/Alaska Native—full-time 0, part-time 0; Caucasian/White—full-time 161, part-time 33; Multi-ethnic—full-time 2, part-time 0; students subject to the Americans With Disabilities Act—full-time 2, part-time 0; Unknown ethnicity—full-time 4, part-time 0; International students who hold an F-1 or J-1 Visa—full-time 11, part-time 0.

Financial Information/Assistance:
Tuition for Full-Time Study: *Master's:* State residents: per academic year $7,428; Nonstate residents: per academic year $19,996. *Doctoral:* State residents: per academic year $7,428; Nonstate residents: per academic year $19,996. Tuition is subject to change. See the following Web site for updates and changes in tuition costs: http://www.bsu.edu/gradschool.

Financial Assistance:
First-Year Students: Teaching assistantships available for first year. Average amount paid per academic year: $9,587. Average number of hours worked per week: 20. Apply by December 15. Research assistantships available for first year. Average amount paid per academic year: $9,587. Average number of hours worked per week: 20. Apply by December 15.

Advanced Students: Teaching assistantships available for advanced students. Average amount paid per academic year: $9,587. Average number of hours worked per week: 20. Apply by March 1. Research assistantships available for advanced students. Average amount paid per academic year: $9,587. Average number of hours worked per week: 20. Apply by March 1. Traineeships available for advanced students. Average amount paid per academic year: $9,587. Average number of hours worked per week: 20. Apply by March 1.

Additional Information: Of all students currently enrolled full time, 80% benefited from one or more of the listed financial assistance programs.

Internships/Practica: Doctoral Degree (PhD Counseling Psychology): For those doctoral students for whom a professional internship was required in this program prior to graduation, (10) students applied for an internship in 2008–2009, with (9) students obtaining an internship. Of those students who obtained an internship, (9) were paid internships. Of those students who obtained an internship, (9) students placed in APA/CPA accredited internships, (0) students placed in internships not APA/CPA accredited, but listed with the Association of Psychology Postdoctoral and Internship Programs (APPIC), (0) students placed in internships conforming to guidelines of the Council of Directors of School Psychology Programs (CDSPP), (0) students placed in internships that were not APA/CPA accredited, APPIC or CDSPP listed. Master's Degree (MA/MS Counseling): An internship experience, such as a final research project or "capstone" experience is required of graduates. The department operates a practicum clinic that serves the surrounding community on a low-cost basis. All counseling master's students and doctoral students are required to complete at least one practicum in this clinic. Other practicum opportunities are available at the university counseling center, a local elementary school, and the nearby medical hospital. Master's students also are required to complete an internship prior to graduation. The Internship Director maintains a listing of available sites and assists students in identifying and securing such a site. Most of these sites are unpaid, although a few are paying sites. Doctoral students typically seek APA-approved predoctoral internship sites. There is one such site on campus, in the university's counseling center. Although that site does not guarantee a slot to students from this program, usually one CPSY student a year is matched there.

Housing and Day Care: On-campus housing is available. See the following Web site for more information: http://www.bsu.edu/housing. On-campus day care facilities are available. See the following Web site for more information: http://www.bsu.edu/fcs/csc.

Employment of Department Graduates:
Master's Degree Graduates: Of those who graduated in the academic year 2008–2009, the following categories and numbers represent the postgraduate activities and employment of master's degree graduates: Enrolled in a psychology doctoral program (10), enrolled in another graduate/professional program (1), enrolled in a postdoctoral residency/fellowship (n/a), employed in independent practice (n/a), employed in an academic position at a university (0), employed in an academic position at a 2-year/4-year college (0), employed in other positions at a higher education institution (2), employed in a professional position in a school system (10), employed in business or industry (0), employed in government agency (4), employed in a community mental health/counseling center (7), employed in a hospital/medical center (1), still seeking employment (1), other employment position (3), total from the above (master's) (39).
Doctoral Degree Graduates: Of those who graduated in the academic year 2008–2009, the following categories and numbers represent the postgraduate activities and employment of doctoral degree graduates: Enrolled in a psychology doctoral program (n/a), enrolled in a postdoctoral residency/fellowship (2), employed in independent practice (0), employed in an academic position at a university (1), employed in an academic position at a 2-year/4-year college (1), employed in other positions at a higher education institution (3), employed in a professional position in a school system (0), employed in business or industry (0), employed in government agency (0), employed in a community mental health/counseling center (2), employed in a hospital/medical center (1), not seeking employment (0), total from the above (doctoral) (10).

Additional Information:
Orientation, Objectives, and Emphasis of Department: The objective of the master's counseling programs is to prepare effective counselors by providing students with a common professional core of courses and experiences. The faculty is committed to keeping abreast of trends, skills, and knowledge and to modifying the program to prepare students for their profession. Students will be able to practice in a variety of settings using therapeutic, preventive, or developmental counseling approaches. The counseling programs also prepare students for doctoral study in counseling psychology. The program goals are to develop an atmosphere conducive to inquiry, creativity, and learning and to the discovery of new knowledge through research, counseling, and interactive involvement between students and faculty. The master's program in social psychology provides a conceptual background for those pursuing careers in education, counseling, criminology, personnel work, etc. and prepares students for entry into doctoral programs in social psychology. The doctoral program is designed to broaden students' knowledge beyond the master's degree. The rigorous program includes a sound theoretical basis, a substantial experiential component, a research component, and a variety of assistantship assignments. A basic core of courses stresses competence in the social, psychological, biological, cognitive, and affective bases of behavior. The counseling psychology PhD program is structured within a scientist-professional model of training.

Special Facilities or Resources: Departmental instructional and research facilities are exceptional. The facilities of the department occupy the sixth floor of the Teachers College building and include ten practicum rooms, an observation corridor, several group observation rooms, and computer access. Most of these facilities are linked to a control room for use of audio and video media. The computer terminals are connected to the university VAX computer cluster. The department operates an outpatient counseling clinic that serves as the training facility for all counseling graduate students. The clinic serves clients from Muncie and surrounding communities as well as Ball State faculty/staff. The university operates a separate state-of-the-art counseling center that serves as a training site for a select number of graduate students from the department.

Information for Students With Physical Disabilities: See the following Web site for more information: http://www.bsu.edu/dsd.

Application Information:
Send to Department of Counseling Psychology and Guidance Services, Teachers College, Ball State University, Muncie, IN 47306. Application available online. URL of online application: http://www.bsu.edu/counselingpsychology. Students are admitted in the Fall, application deadline December 15. Doctoral program - December 15. Master's programs deadlines are February 1 and June 15 for Fall admission. Counseling (Rehabilitation track) has rolling admissions. *Fee:* $50. Graduate School fee: $50; the Department does not charge an application fee. International applicants will pay $40 to apply through the Rinker Center for International Programs.

Ball State University (2009 data)
Department of Educational Psychology
Teachers College
Muncie, IN 47306
Telephone: (765) 285-8500
Fax: (765) 285-3653
E-mail: lhuffman@bsu.edu
Web: http://www.bsu.edu/edpsych

Department Information:
1967. Chairperson: Lisa F. Huffman. Number of faculty: total—full-time 11, part-time 9; women—full-time 11, part-time 8; women minority—full-time 2, part-time 2.

Programs and Degrees Offered:
Listed in the following order: Program area, degree type (T if terminal Master's), number awarded 7/08–6/09. School Psychology PhD (Doctor of Philosophy) 2, Educational Psychology MA/MS (Master of Arts/Science) (T) 11, School Psychology MA/MS (Master of Arts/Science) 8, School Psychology EdS (School Psychology) 5, Educational Psychology PhD (Doctor of Philosophy) 0.

APA Accreditation: School PhD (Doctor of Philosophy).

Student Applications/Admissions:

Student Applications

School Psychology PhD (Doctor of Philosophy)—Applications 2009–2010, 26. Total applicants accepted 2009–2010, 13. Number full-time enrolled (new admits only) 2009–2010, 13. Openings 2010–2011, 10. The median number of years required for completion of a degree in 2008–2009 were 4. The number of students enrolled full- and part-time who were dismissed or voluntarily withdrew from this program area in 2008–2009 were 0. *Educational Psychology MA/MS (Master of Arts/Science)*—Applications 2009–2010, 12. Total applicants accepted 2009–2010, 9. Number full-time enrolled (new admits only) 2009–2010, 9. Openings 2010–2011, 10. The median number of years required for completion of a degree in 2008–2009 were 2. The number of students enrolled full- and part-time who were dismissed or voluntarily withdrew from this program area in 2008–2009 were 0. *School Psychology MA/MS (Master of Arts/Science)*—Applications 2009–2010, 65. Total applicants accepted 2009–2010, 12. Number full-time enrolled (new admits only) 2009–2010, 12. Total enrolled 2009–2010 full-time, 12. Openings 2010–2011, 10. The median number of years required for completion of a degree in 2008–2009 was 1. The number of students enrolled full- and part-time who were dismissed or voluntarily withdrew from this program area in 2008–2009 were 0. *School Psychology EdS (School Psychology)*—Applications 2009–2010, 20. Total applicants accepted 2009–2010, 12. Number full-time enrolled (new admits only) 2009–2010, 12. Total enrolled 2009–2010 full-time, 19. Openings 2010–2011, 5. The median number of years required for completion of a degree in 2008–2009 were 3. The number of students enrolled full- and part-time who were dismissed or voluntarily withdrew from this program area in 2008–2009 were 0. *Educational Psychology PhD (Doctor of Philosophy)*—Applications 2009–2010, 10. Total applicants accepted 2009–2010, 6. Number full-time enrolled (new admits only) 2009–2010, 6. Number part-time enrolled (new admits only) 2009–2010, 0. Openings 2010–2011, 5. The number of students enrolled full- and part-time who were dismissed or voluntarily withdrew from this program area in 2008–2009 were 0.

Other Criteria: (importance of criteria rated low, medium, or high): GRE scores—high, research experience—medium, work experience—medium, extracurricular activity—medium, clinically related public service—high, GPA—medium, letters of recommendation—high, statement of goals and objectives—medium, diversity—high. For additional information on admission requirements, go to http://www.bsu.edu/edpsych/.

Student Characteristics: The following represents characteristics of students in 2009–2010 in all graduate psychology programs in the department: Female—full-time 42, part-time 0; Male—full-time 17, part-time 0; African American/Black—full-time 3, part-time 0; Hispanic/Latino(a)—full-time 1, part-time 0; Asian/Pacific Islander—full-time 0, part-time 0; American Indian/Alaska Native—full-time 0, part-time 0; Caucasian/White—full-time 0, part-time 0; Multi-ethnic—full-time 0, part-time 0; students subject to the Americans With Disabilities Act—full-time 0, part-time 0; Unknown ethnicity—full-time 0, part-time 0; International students who hold an F-1 or J-1 Visa—full-time 0, part-time 0.

Financial Information/Assistance:
Tuition for Full-Time Study: *Master's:* State residents: per academic year $6,030; Nonstate residents: per academic year $15,790. *Doctoral:* State residents: per academic year $6,030; Nonstate residents: per academic year $15,790. Tuition is subject to change.

Financial Assistance:

First-Year Students: Teaching assistantships available for first year. Average amount paid per academic year: $9,967. Average number of hours worked per week: 20. Apply by February 15. Research assistantships available for first year. Average amount paid per academic year: $9,967. Average number of hours worked per week: 20. Apply by February 15. Fellowships and scholarships available for first year. Average amount paid per academic year: $9,967. Average number of hours worked per week: 0. Apply by February 15.

Advanced Students: Teaching assistantships available for advanced students. Average amount paid per academic year: $9,967. Average number of hours worked per week: 20. Apply by February 15. Research assistantships available for advanced students. Average amount paid per academic year: $9,967. Average number of hours worked per week: 20. Apply by February 15. Fellowships and scholarships available for advanced students. Average amount paid per academic year: $9,967. Average number of hours worked per week: 0. Apply by February 15.

Additional Information: Of all students currently enrolled full time, 100% benefited from one or more of the listed financial assistance programs. Application and information available online at: http://www.bsu.edu/edpsych.

Internships/Practica: School psychology students are expected to be involved in practicum experiences from very early in their programs and to continue such experiences until they enroll in internships. (500 clock hours in practicum are expected.) A school-based internship of one academic year is required of School

Psychology MA/EdS students. Internships are not required of graduate students in the Educational Psychology MA or PhD programs.

Housing and Day Care: On-campus housing is available. See the following Web site for more information: http://www.bsu.edu/housing/. On-campus day care facilities are available. See the following Web site for more information: http://www.bsu.edu/fcs/csc/.

Employment of Department Graduates:
Master's Degree Graduates: Of those who graduated in the academic year 2008–2009, the following categories and numbers represent the postgraduate activities and employment of master's degree graduates: Enrolled in a postdoctoral residency/fellowship (n/a), employed in independent practice (n/a), total from the above (master's) (0).
Doctoral Degree Graduates: Of those who graduated in the academic year 2008–2009, the following categories and numbers represent the postgraduate activities and employment of doctoral degree graduates: Enrolled in a psychology doctoral program (n/a), enrolled in a postdoctoral residency/fellowship (6), employed in independent practice (3), employed in an academic position at a university (4), employed in an academic position at a 2-year/4-year college (2), employed in other positions at a higher education institution (3), employed in a professional position in a school system (7), employed in business or industry (0), employed in government agency (0), employed in a community mental health/counseling center (2), employed in a hospital/medical center (4), still seeking employment (0), other employment position (0), total from the above (doctoral) (31).

Additional Information:
Orientation, Objectives, and Emphasis of Department: The mission of the graduate programs is to train research scientists to make significant contributions in specialty areas and to address applied problems in educational settings. Our school psychology track further trains students to render diagnostic and remedial services and educational consultation. Specialty areas include neuropsychology, human development, learning, research methods/statistics, and gifted studies. Doctoral students are encouraged to become involved in on-going research with faculty members. The MA/EdS program is designed to train students for the professional practice of School Psychology, and to meet licensure requirements of Indiana and most states. The MA in Educational Psychology provides specialization options in human development, gifted and talented studies, and educational technology. Other specialization options can be tailored to meet the needs and interests of individual students.

Special Facilities or Resources: The department has an on-campus school psychology clinic, a neuropsychology laboratory, a computer laboratory, videotaping facilities, and adequate research facilities. The department is allied with the Office of Charter School Research and the Center for Gifted Studies and Talent Development.

Information for Students With Physical Disabilities: See the following Web site for more information: http://www.bsu.edu/dsd.

Application Information:
Send to Educational Psychology, TC 524, Ball State University, Muncie, IN 47306. Application available online. URL of online application: http://www.bsu.edu/edpsych/. Students are admitted in the Fall, application deadline February 15. Application for the new PhD in Educational Psychology: March 18. Application for MA/EdS and PhD in School Psychology: February 15. Rolling admissions for the MA in Educational Psychology. *Fee:* $35.

Ball State University
Department of Psychological Science
Sciences and Humanities
Muncie, IN 47306-0520
Telephone: (765) 285-1690
Fax: (765) 285-1702
E-mail: *kpickel@bsu.edu*
Web: *http://www.bsu.edu/psysc/masters/*

Department Information:
1968. Chairperson: Bernie Whitley. Number of faculty: total—full-time 20; women—full-time 8; total—minority—full-time 1; women minority—full-time 1; faculty subject to the Americans With Disabilities Act 2.

Programs and Degrees Offered:
Listed in the following order: Program area, degree type (T if terminal Master's), number awarded 7/08–6/09. Clinical MA/MS (Master of Arts/Science) (T) 12, Cognitive and Social Processes MA/MS (Master of Arts/Science) (T) 8.

Student Applications/Admissions:
Student Applications
Clinical MA/MS (Master of Arts/Science)—Applications 2009–2010, 60. Total applicants accepted 2009–2010, 10. Number full-time enrolled (new admits only) 2009–2010, 10. Number part-time enrolled (new admits only) 2009–2010, 0. Openings 2010–2011, 12. The median number of years required for completion of a degree in 2008–2009 were 2. The number of students enrolled full- and part-time who were dismissed or voluntarily withdrew from this program area in 2008–2009 were 0. Cognitive and Social Processes MA/MS (Master of Arts/Science)—Applications 2009–2010, 23. Total applicants accepted 2009–2010, 7. Number full-time enrolled (new admits only) 2009–2010, 7. Number part-time enrolled (new admits only) 2009–2010, 0. Openings 2010–2011, 8. The median number of years required for completion of a degree in 2008–2009 were 2. The number of students enrolled full- and part-time who were dismissed or voluntarily withdrew from this program area in 2008–2009 were 0.
Scores: Entries appear in this order: required test or GPA, minimum score (if required), median score of students entering in 2009–2010. Clinical MA/MS (Master of Arts/Science): GRE-V no minimum stated, GRE-Q no minimum stated, overall undergraduate GPA 2.75; Cognitive and Social Processes MA/MS (Master of Arts/Science): GRE-V no minimum stated, GRE-Q no minimum stated, overall undergraduate GPA 2.75.

Other Criteria: (importance of criteria rated low, medium, or high): GRE scores—high, research experience—high, work experience—medium, extracurricular activity—low, clinically related public service—medium, GPA—high, letters of recommendation—high, statement of goals and objectives—high, Fit w/ faculty interests—high. Clinical service not important for Cognitive/Social Processes program. For additional information on admission requirements, go to http://www.bsu.edu/psysc/masters/.

Student Characteristics: The following represents characteristics of students in 2009–2010 in all graduate psychology programs in the department: Female—full-time 23, part-time 0; Male—full-time 13, part-time 0; African American/Black—full-time 1, part-time 0; Hispanic/Latino(a)—full-time 1, part-time 0; Asian/Pacific Islander—full-time 0, part-time 0; American Indian/Alaska Native—full-time 1, part-time 0; Caucasian/White—full-time 32, part-time 0; Multi-ethnic—full-time 1, part-time 0; students subject to the Americans With Disabilities Act—full-time 1, part-time 0; Unknown ethnicity—full-time 0, part-time 0; International students who hold an F-1 or J-1 Visa—full-time 1, part-time 0.

Financial Information/Assistance:
Tuition for Full-Time Study: *Master's:* State residents: per academic year $7,508; Nonstate residents: per academic year $20,960. Tuition is subject to change. Additional fees are assessed to students beyond the costs of tuition for the following: technology, recreation, health center, course fees. See the following Web site for updates and changes in tuition costs: http://www.bsu.edu/bursar.

Financial Assistance:
First-Year Students: Teaching assistantships available for first year. Average amount paid per academic year: $8,275. Average number of hours worked per week: 20. Apply by March 1. Research assistantships available for first year. Average amount paid per academic year: $8,275. Average number of hours worked per week: 20. Apply by March 1. Fellowships and scholarships available for first year. Average amount paid per academic year: $8,275. Average number of hours worked per week: 0. Apply by March 1.

Advanced Students: Teaching assistantships available for advanced students. Average amount paid per academic year: $8,275. Average number of hours worked per week: 20. Apply by March 1. Research assistantships available for advanced students. Average amount paid per academic year: $8,275. Average number of hours worked per week: 20. Apply by March 1. Fellowships and scholarships available for advanced students. Average amount paid per academic year: $8,275. Average number of hours worked per week: 0.

Additional Information: Of all students currently enrolled full time, 70% benefited from one or more of the listed financial assistance programs. Application and information available online at: http://www.bsu.edu/psysc/masters/.

Internships/Practica: Master's Degree (MA/MS Clinical): An internship experience, such as a final research project or "capstone" experience is required of graduates. Internships for clinical students are available at the University Counseling Center, Community Mental Health Centers, Youth Opportunity Center, a V.A. hospital, children's hospital, and many other locations.

Housing and Day Care: On-campus housing is available. See the following Web site for more information: http://www.bsu.edu/gradschool/housing/. On-campus day care facilities are available. See the following Web site for more information: http://www.bsu.edu/hrs/worklife/childcare/.

Employment of Department Graduates:
Master's Degree Graduates: Of those who graduated in the academic year 2008–2009, the following categories and numbers represent the postgraduate activities and employment of master's degree graduates: Enrolled in a postdoctoral residency/fellowship (n/a), employed in independent practice (n/a), total from the above (master's) (0).
Doctoral Degree Graduates: Of those who graduated in the academic year 2008–2009, the following categories and numbers represent the postgraduate activities and employment of doctoral degree graduates: Enrolled in a psychology doctoral program (n/a), total from the above (doctoral) (0).

Additional Information:
Orientation, Objectives, and Emphasis of Department: Our Clinical MA program is a two-year, 48-credit hour program based on the scientist practitioner model. Our Cognitive/Social program is a two-year, 43-credit hour program that provides students with intensive training in cognitive and social psychology, research methods, and statistics. We admit a limited number of new students per year, which allows our faculty to work closely with students in terms of providing instruction and research opportunities. Our primary goal is to prepare students for doctoral study; during the past 10 years, 90% of our graduates who applied to a doctoral program and completed a thesis were accepted to a doctoral program. Faculty research interests include stereotyping and prejudice, industrial/organizational psychology, eyewitness memory, juror decision making, gender issues, multicultural issues/diversity, emotion, sexuality, problem solving/critical thinking, sexual behavior, community psychology, identity development, and interpersonal communication.

Special Facilities or Resources: Students have access to university and departmental computers and a wireless network. The department maintains space for faculty and student research. Internal grants are available for student research and travel.

Information for Students With Physical Disabilities: See the following Web site for more information: http://www.bsu.edu/dsd/.

Application Information:
Send to Kerri Pickel, PhD, Director of Graduate Studies, Department of Psychological Science, Ball State University, Muncie, IN 47306-0520. Application available online. URL of online application: http://www.bsu.edu/psysc/masters/. Students are admitted in the Fall, application deadline March 1. For cognitive and social processes program, deadline is 5 weeks prior to either Fall or Spring semester if program is not full. *Fee:* $50. Fee is waived for McNair Scholars.

Indiana State University
Department of Communication Disorders & Counseling, School, & Educational Psychology
Education
Bayh College of Education
Terre Haute, IN 47809
Telephone: (812) 237-2870
Fax: (812) 237-2729
E-mail: Sandie.Edwards@indstate.edu
Web: http://counseling.indstate.edu

Department Information:
1968. Chairperson: Michele C. Boyer. Number of faculty: total—full-time 5, part-time 2; women—full-time 5, part-time 1; total—minority—full-time 1; women minority—full-time 1.

Programs and Degrees Offered:
Listed in the following order: Program area, degree type (T if terminal Master's), number awarded 7/08–6/09. Counseling Psychology PhD (Doctor of Philosophy) 6, Clinical Mental Health Counseling MA/MS (Master of Arts/Science) 10.

APA Accreditation: Counseling PhD (Doctor of Philosophy).

Student Applications/Admissions:
Student Applications
Counseling Psychology PhD (Doctor of Philosophy)—Applications 2009–2010, 1. Total applicants accepted 2009–2010, 1. Number full-time enrolled (new admits only) 2009–2010, 1. Number part-time enrolled (new admits only) 2009–2010, 0. Total enrolled 2009–2010 full-time, 18, part-time, 8. The median number of years required for completion of a degree in 2008–2009 were 5. *Clinical Mental Health Counseling MA/MS (Master of Arts/Science)*—Applications 2009–2010, 27. Total applicants accepted 2009–2010, 18. Number full-time enrolled (new admits only) 2009–2010, 16. Number part-time enrolled (new admits only) 2009–2010, 2. Total enrolled 2009–2010 full-time, 17, part-time, 3. Openings 2010–2011, 25. The median number of years required for completion of a degree in 2008–2009 were 2. The number of students enrolled full- and part-time who were dismissed or voluntarily withdrew from this program area in 2008–2009 were 0.
Scores: Entries appear in this order: required test or GPA, minimum score (if required), median score of students entering in 2009–2010. *Counseling Psychology PhD (Doctor of Philosophy):* GRE-V 500, GRE-Q 500, overall undergraduate GPA 2.5, Masters GPA 3.5; *Clinical Mental Health Counseling MA/MS (Master of Arts/Science):* GRE-V 450, GRE-Q 450, overall undergraduate GPA 2.75.
Other Criteria: (importance of criteria rated low, medium, or high): GRE scores—medium, research experience—medium, work experience—high, extracurricular activity—medium, clinically related public service—high, GPA—medium, letters of recommendation—high, interview—high, statement of goals and objectives—high.

Student Characteristics: The following represents characteristics of students in 2009–2010 in all graduate psychology programs in the department: Female—full-time 25, part-time 8; Male—full-time 10, part-time 3; African American/Black—full-time 3, part-time 1; Hispanic/Latino(a)—full-time 0, part-time 0; Asian/Pacific Islander—full-time 0, part-time 1; American Indian/Alaska Native—full-time 0, part-time 0; Caucasian/White—full-time 0, part-time 0; Multi-ethnic—full-time 0, part-time 0; students subject to the Americans With Disabilities Act—full-time 0, part-time 0; Unknown ethnicity—full-time 0, part-time 0; International students who hold an F-1 or J-1 Visa—full-time 1, part-time 0.

Financial Information/Assistance:
Tuition for Full-Time Study: *Master's:* State residents: per academic year $6,888, $328 per credit hour; Nonstate residents: per academic year $13,545, $645 per credit hour. *Doctoral:* State residents: per academic year $7,872, $328 per credit hour; Nonstate residents: per academic year $15,840, $645 per credit hour. Tuition is subject to change. See the following Web site for updates and changes in tuition costs: http://www.indstate.edu/bursar/academicfees.htm.

Financial Assistance:
First-Year Students: Teaching assistantships available for first year. Average amount paid per academic year: $7,500. Average number of hours worked per week: 15. Apply by March 1. Research assistantships available for first year. Average amount paid per academic year: $7,500. Average number of hours worked per week: 15. Apply by March 1. Fellowships and scholarships available for first year. Average amount paid per academic year: $7,500. Average number of hours worked per week: 15. Apply by March 1.
Advanced Students: Teaching assistantships available for advanced students. Average amount paid per academic year: $7,500. Average number of hours worked per week: 15. Apply by March 1. Research assistantships available for advanced students. Average amount paid per academic year: $7,500. Average number of hours worked per week: 15. Apply by March 1. Fellowships and scholarships available for advanced students. Average amount paid per academic year: $7,500. Average number of hours worked per week: 15. Apply by March 1.
Additional Information: Of all students currently enrolled full time, 50% benefited from one or more of the listed financial assistance programs. Application and information available online at: http://www.indstate.edu/sogs/students.htm.

Internships/Practica: Doctoral Degree (PhD Counseling Psychology): For those doctoral students for whom a professional internship was required in this program prior to graduation, (8) students applied for an internship in 2008–2009, with (8) students obtaining an internship. Of those students who obtained an internship, (8) were paid internships. Of those students who obtained an internship, (8) students placed in APA/CPA accredited internships, (0) students placed in internships not APA/CPA accredited, but listed with the Association of Psychology Postdoctoral and Internship Programs (APPIC), (0) students placed in internships conforming to guidelines of the Council of Directors of School Psychology Programs (CDSPP), (0) students placed in internships that were not APA/CPA accredited, APPIC or CDSPP listed. Master's Degree (MA/MS Clinical Mental Health Counseling): An internship experience, such as a final research project or "capstone" experience is required of graduates. Doctoral practica are available on campus (Student Counseling Center) and in a variety of community settings (CMHC, schools, hospitals, prisons, VAMC, primary care medical settings), residential treatment facilities, and community college counseling centers.

Housing and Day Care: On-campus housing is available. See the following Web site for more information: http://www.indstate.edu/reslife/. On-campus day care facilities are available. See the following Web site for more information: http://www.indstate.edu/childcare/.

Employment of Department Graduates:
Master's Degree Graduates: Of those who graduated in the academic year 2008–2009, the following categories and numbers represent the postgraduate activities and employment of master's degree graduates: Enrolled in a psychology doctoral program (1), enrolled in a postdoctoral residency/fellowship (n/a), employed in independent practice (n/a), employed in government agency (1), do not know (8), total from the above (master's) (10).
Doctoral Degree Graduates: Of those who graduated in the academic year 2008–2009, the following categories and numbers represent the postgraduate activities and employment of doctoral degree graduates: Enrolled in a psychology doctoral program (n/a), employed in independent practice (1), employed in other positions at a higher education institution (1), employed in government agency (1), employed in a hospital/medical center (1), do not know (2), total from the above (doctoral) (6).

Additional Information:
Orientation, Objectives, and Emphasis of Department: The Counseling Psychology program is designed to prepare professional psychologists, through a scientist-professional model of training, for general practice in a variety of practice, service, and educational settings. These setting may include colleges and universities, mental health centers, medical care facilities, government agencies, private practice settings, and in the private corporate sector. The program is seen as an area of applied psychology that helps individuals solve problems by making more effective use of their resources. Toward this end, training and research focus on facilitating the personal, interpersonal, educational, and vocational development of individuals, as well as enhancing the environments in which they live. Attention is focused on individual clients' personal and social assets and strengths as well their sociopsychological liabilities and weaknesses. The program emphasizes human development, personalized assessment, and planned problem-solving, while de emphasizing dichotomies such as sick vs. well and abnormal vs. normal. Our program allows flexibility for students to pursue personal career goals through focused electives, independent study, and specialized training experiences in practica, fieldwork, assistantship assignments, teaching, research, and community and university work experiences. Faculty members represent a broad range of professional and research interests, theoretical perspectives, and treatment modalities.

Special Facilities or Resources: The counseling psychology training area is housed in the Bayh College of Education. This area provides faculty and student offices, and a departmental clinic (individual and group therapy rooms, videotaping equipment with observation rooms, and a career and testing laboratory). Also available in the building are research stations, microcomputer labs, a statistics laboratory, a psychological evaluation library, testing rooms, and an instructional resource center.

Information for Students With Physical Disabilities: See the following Web site for more information: http://www.indstate.edu/sasc/dss/index.htm.

Application Information:
Send to Director of Training, ATTN: S. Edwards, Bayh College of Education 226E, CMHC Program, Indiana State University, Terre Haute, IN 47809. Application available online. URL of online application: http://counseling.indstate.edu/dcp/app.htm. Students are admitted in the Fall, application deadline January 1. MS Program deadline February 1; EdS Program deadline January 15. *Fee:* $35.

Indiana State University
Department of Communication Disorders, Counseling, School, and Educational Psychology
College of Education
Terre Haute, IN 47809
Telephone: (812) 237-2880
Fax: (812) 237-2729
E-mail: *patricia.snyder@indstate.edu*
Web: *http://coe.indstate.edu/cdcsep/edpsych*

Department Information:
1981. Chairperson: Michele Boyer, PhD. Number of faculty: total—full-time 7; women—full-time 5; total—minority—full-time 1; women minority—full-time 1.

Programs and Degrees Offered:
Listed in the following order: Program area, degree type (T if terminal Master's), number awarded 7/08–6/09. School Psychology PhD (Doctor of Philosophy) 3, School Psychology MEd (Education) 5, School Psychology EdS (School Psychology) 1.

APA Accreditation: School PhD (Doctor of Philosophy). Student Outcome Data Website: http://coe.indstate.edu/cdcsep/edpsych/phdstudentinfo.htm.

Student Applications/Admissions:
Student Applications
School Psychology PhD (Doctor of Philosophy)—Applications 2009–2010, 8. Total applicants accepted 2009–2010, 4. Number full-time enrolled (new admits only) 2009–2010, 4. Number part-time enrolled (new admits only) 2009–2010, 0. Total enrolled 2009–2010 full-time, 7, part-time, 6. Openings 2010–2011, 8. The median number of years required for completion of a degree in 2008–2009 were 6. The number of students enrolled full- and part-time who were dismissed or voluntarily withdrew from this program area in 2008–2009 were 0. *School Psychology MEd (Education)*—Applications 2009–2010, 9. Total applicants accepted 2009–2010, 9. Number full-time enrolled (new admits only) 2009–2010, 9. Number part-time enrolled (new admits only) 2009–2010, 0. The median number of years required for completion of a degree in 2008–2009 was 1. The number of students enrolled full- and part-time who were dismissed or voluntarily withdrew from this program area in 2008–2009 were 0. *School Psychology EdS (School Psychology)*—Applications 2009–2010, 13. Total applicants accepted 2009–2010, 8. Number full-time enrolled (new admits only) 2009–2010, 8. Number part-time enrolled (new admits only)

2009–2010, 0. Openings 2010–2011, 10. The median number of years required for completion of a degree in 2008–2009 were 3. The number of students enrolled full- and part-time who were dismissed or voluntarily withdrew from this program area in 2008–2009 were 0.

Other Criteria: (importance of criteria rated low, medium, or high): GRE scores—medium, research experience—medium, work experience—medium, extracurricular activity—high, clinically related public service—high, GPA—high, letters of recommendation—high, interview—high, statement of goals and objectives—high, vita—high, undergraduate major in psychology—medium, specific undergraduate psychology courses taken—medium.

Student Characteristics: The following represents characteristics of students in 2009–2010 in all graduate psychology programs in the department: Female—full-time 25, part-time 4; Male—full-time 5, part-time 2; African American/Black—full-time 1, part-time 0; Hispanic/Latino(a)—full-time 0, part-time 1; Asian/Pacific Islander—full-time 4, part-time 0; American Indian/Alaska Native—full-time 0, part-time 0; Caucasian/White—full-time 21, part-time 9; Multi-ethnic—full-time 1, part-time 0; students subject to the Americans With Disabilities Act—full-time 0, part-time 0; Unknown ethnicity—full-time 0, part-time 0; International students who hold an F-1 or J-1 Visa—full-time 0, part-time 0.

Financial Information/Assistance:
Tuition for Full-Time Study: *Master's:* State residents: per academic year $6,888, $328 per credit hour; Nonstate residents: per academic year $13,545, $645 per credit hour. *Doctoral:* State residents: per academic year $7,872, $328 per credit hour; Nonstate residents: per academic year $15,840, $645 per credit hour. Tuition is subject to change. See the following Web site for updates and changes in tuition costs: http://web.indstate.edu/sogs.

Financial Assistance:
First-Year Students: Teaching assistantships available for first year. Average amount paid per academic year: $5,250. Average number of hours worked per week: 15. Apply by March 1. Research assistantships available for first year. Average amount paid per academic year: $5,250. Average number of hours worked per week: 15. Apply by March 1. Fellowships and scholarships available for first year. Average amount paid per academic year: $5,250. Average number of hours worked per week: 15. Apply by March 1.

Advanced Students: Teaching assistantships available for advanced students. Average amount paid per academic year: $7,500. Average number of hours worked per week: 15. Apply by March 1. Research assistantships available for advanced students. Average amount paid per academic year: $7,500. Average number of hours worked per week: 15. Apply by March 1. Fellowships and scholarships available for advanced students. Average amount paid per academic year: $7,500. Average number of hours worked per week: 15. Apply by March 1.

Additional Information: Of all students currently enrolled full time, 100% benefited from one or more of the listed financial assistance programs. Application and information available online at: http://www.indstate.edu/finaid/.

Internships/Practica: Doctoral Degree (PhD School Psychology): For those doctoral students for whom a professional internship was required in this program prior to graduation, (2) students applied for an internship in 2008–2009, with (2) students obtaining an internship. Of those students who obtained an internship, (2) were paid internships. Of those students who obtained an internship, (2) students placed in APA/CPA accredited internships, (0) students placed in internships not APA/CPA accredited, but listed with the Association of Psychology Postdoctoral and Internship Programs (APPIC), (0) students placed in internships conforming to guidelines of the Council of Directors of School Psychology Programs (CDSPP), (0) students placed in internships that were not APA/CPA accredited, APPIC or CDSPP listed. Students in all programs are required to complete a minimum of 160 direct contact hours each semester they are enrolled in the program. Practicum experiences include observation, consultation, assessment, counseling and intervention with diverse populations ranging from preschool-aged to school-aged students, as well as with college students, parents, teachers, and other professionals. Practicum sites include the local Head Start, public school settings, the Porter School Psychology Clinic, ISU ADHD Clinic, the READ Clinic as well as agencies such as Gibault, Inc. and Riley Children's Hospital. PhD students have the opportunity to complete advanced practicum requirements in school or clinical settings in order to gain additional experiences and to foster increasing autonomy. Final experiences include a 1,200+ hour school-based internship for EdS students and a 1,500+ hour predoctoral internship in clinic and/or school settings for PhD students. Predoctoral internship sites include public school settings, hospitals and mental health agencies.

Housing and Day Care: On-campus housing is available. See the following Web site for more information: http://www.indstate.edu/reslife/. On-campus day care facilities are available. See the following Web site for more information: http://web.indstate.edu/childcare/.

Employment of Department Graduates:
Master's Degree Graduates: Of those who graduated in the academic year 2008–2009, the following categories and numbers represent the postgraduate activities and employment of master's degree graduates: Enrolled in a psychology doctoral program (0), enrolled in another graduate/professional program (0), enrolled in a postdoctoral residency/fellowship (n/a), employed in independent practice (n/a), employed in an academic position at a university (0), employed in an academic position at a 2-year/4-year college (0), employed in other positions at a higher education institution (0), employed in a professional position in a school system (0), employed in business or industry (0), employed in government agency (0), employed in a community mental health/counseling center (0), employed in a hospital/medical center (0), still seeking employment (0), other employment position (0), total from the above (master's) (0).

Doctoral Degree Graduates: Of those who graduated in the academic year 2008–2009, the following categories and numbers represent the postgraduate activities and employment of doctoral degree graduates: Enrolled in a psychology doctoral program (n/a), enrolled in another graduate/professional program (0), enrolled in a postdoctoral residency/fellowship (0), employed in independent practice (0), employed in an academic position at a university (1), employed in an academic position at a 2-year/4-year college (1), employed in other positions at a higher education institution (0), employed in a professional position in a school system (2), employed in business or industry (0), employed in government

agency (0), employed in a community mental health/counseling center (0), employed in a hospital/medical center (0), still seeking employment (0), other employment position (0), total from the above (doctoral) (4).

Additional Information:
Orientation, Objectives, and Emphasis of Department: The PhD program in guidance and psychological services specialization in school psychology follows a scholar-practitioner model which serves as a foundation upon which program goals and objectives are based. The mission of the program is to prepare professional school psychologists as scholar-practitioners with a broad cognitive behavioral orientation through a program that is research-based, theory-driven, school-focused, and experiential in nature.

Special Facilities or Resources: The program has a university-based clinic that provides psychological and educational services to children, youth, and families. The clinic includes programs specifically designed to serve children with autism spectrum disorders, children with reading disorders, and children with behavioral difficulties. The department partners with the Psychology Department to provide services through a university-based ADHD clinic. These clinics provide both clinical and research experiences. Community resources with which the department has established partnerships include a HeadStart facility, public and private schools, a residential facility for children and youth with behavioral disorders, and a local community center.

Information for Students With Physical Disabilities: See the following Web site for more information: http://www.indstate.edu/sasc.

Application Information:
Send to Leah Nellis, Director of School Psychology Training Program, Bayh College of Education, Room 302D, Indiana State University, Terrre Haute, IN 47809. Application available online. URL of online application: http://www.indstate.edu/sogs. Students are admitted in the Fall, application deadline January 15. *Fee:* $35.

Indiana State University (2009 data)
Department of Psychology
Root Hall
Terre Haute, IN 47809
Telephone: (812) 237-4314
Fax: (812) 237-4378
E-mail: *criggs@isugw.indstate.edu*
Web: *http://www.indstate.edu/psychology*

Department Information:
1968. Chairperson: Virgil Sheets. Number of faculty: total—full-time 13; women—full-time 7; total—minority—full-time 1; women minority—full-time 1; faculty subject to the Americans With Disabilities Act 13.

Programs and Degrees Offered:
Listed in the following order: Program area, degree type (T if terminal Master's), number awarded 7/08–6/09. General MA/MS (Master of Arts/Science) (T) 3, Clinical PsyD (Doctor of Psychology) 8.

APA Accreditation: Clinical PsyD (Doctor of Psychology).

Student Applications/Admissions:
Student Applications
General MA/MS *(Master of Arts/Science)*—Applications 2009–2010, 42. Total applicants accepted 2009–2010, 5. Number full-time enrolled (new admits only) 2009–2010, 5. Number part-time enrolled (new admits only) 2009–2010, 0. Openings 2010–2011, 4. The median number of years required for completion of a degree in 2008–2009 were 2. The number of students enrolled full- and part-time who were dismissed or voluntarily withdrew from this program area in 2008–2009 were 0. *Clinical PsyD (Doctor of Psychology)*—Applications 2009–2010, 145. Total applicants accepted 2009–2010, 8. Number full-time enrolled (new admits only) 2009–2010, 8. Total enrolled 2009–2010 full-time, 42. Openings 2010–2011, 8. The median number of years required for completion of a degree in 2008–2009 were 5. The number of students enrolled full- and part-time who were dismissed or voluntarily withdrew from this program area in 2008–2009 were 0.

Other Criteria: (importance of criteria rated low, medium, or high): GRE scores—high, research experience—high, work experience—medium, extracurricular activity—low, clinically related public service—high, GPA—high, letters of recommendation—high, interview—high, statement of goals and objectives—high. Formal interviews are not conducted for the Masters Program. Clinically related public service is low for the Master's Program. For additional information on admission requirements, go to http://web.indstate.edu/psych.

Student Characteristics: The following represents characteristics of students in 2009–2010 in all graduate psychology programs in the department: Female—full-time 30, part-time 0; Male—full-time 12, part-time 0; African American/Black—full-time 1, part-time 0; Hispanic/Latino(a)—full-time 3, part-time 0; Asian/Pacific Islander—full-time 0, part-time 0; American Indian/Alaska Native—full-time 0, part-time 0; Caucasian/White—full-time 0, part-time 0; Multi-ethnic—full-time 0, part-time 0; students subject to the Americans With Disabilities Act—full-time 0, part-time 0; Unknown ethnicity—full-time 0, part-time 0; International students who hold an F-1 or J-1 Visa—full-time 0, part-time 0.

Financial Information/Assistance:
Tuition for Full-Time Study: Master's: State residents: per academic year $7,056, $294 per credit hour; Nonstate residents: per academic year $14,016, $584 per credit hour. *Doctoral:* State residents: per academic year $7,056, $294 per credit hour; Nonstate residents: per academic year $14,016, $584 per credit hour. Tuition is subject to change. Additional fees are assessed to students beyond the costs of tuition for the following: $60 technology fee, $100 recreation fee, $15 Transportation fee. See the following Web site for updates and changes in tuition costs: http://web.indstate.edu/sogs.

Financial Assistance:
First-Year Students: Teaching assistantships available for first year. Average amount paid per academic year: $7,000. Average number of hours worked per week: 20. Apply by March 15.

Research assistantships available for first year. Average amount paid per academic year: $7,000. Average number of hours worked per week: 20. Apply by March 15. Fellowships and scholarships available for first year. Average amount paid per academic year: $7,000. Average number of hours worked per week: 15. Apply by March 15.

Advanced Students: Teaching assistantships available for advanced students. Average amount paid per academic year: $7,000. Average number of hours worked per week: 20. Apply by March 15. Research assistantships available for advanced students. Average amount paid per academic year: $7,000. Average number of hours worked per week: 20. Apply by March 15. Fellowships and scholarships available for advanced students. Average amount paid per academic year: $7,000. Average number of hours worked per week: 15. Apply by March 15.

Additional Information: Of all students currently enrolled full time, 100% benefited from one or more of the listed financial assistance programs.

Internships/Practica: Doctoral Degree (PsyD Clinical): For those doctoral students for whom a professional internship was required in this program prior to graduation, (9) students applied for an internship in 2008–2009, with (9) students obtaining an internship. Of those students who obtained an internship, (9) were paid internships. Of those students who obtained an internship, (9) students placed in APA/CPA accredited internships, (0) students placed in internships not APA/CPA accredited, but listed with the Association of Psychology Postdoctoral and Internship Programs (APPIC), (0) students placed in internships conforming to guidelines of the Council of Directors of School Psychology Programs (CDSPP), (0) students placed in internships that were not APA/CPA accredited, APPIC or CDSPP listed. Master's Degree (MA/MS General): An internship experience, such as a final research project or "capstone" experience is required of graduates. PsyD students are expected to participate in practicum experiences from the beginning of the program, with clinical responsibilities gradually increasing throughout enrollment. Second year and third year PsyD students see clients in the Psychology Clinic and are supervised by clinical faculty. Fourth year students are placed in community mental health facilities under the supervision of a licensed psychologist.

Housing and Day Care: On-campus housing is available. On-campus day care facilities are available.

Employment of Department Graduates:
Master's Degree Graduates: Of those who graduated in the academic year 2008–2009, the following categories and numbers represent the postgraduate activities and employment of master's degree graduates: Enrolled in a psychology doctoral program (1), enrolled in a postdoctoral residency/fellowship (n/a), employed in independent practice (n/a), total from the above (master's) (1).
Doctoral Degree Graduates: Of those who graduated in the academic year 2008–2009, the following categories and numbers represent the postgraduate activities and employment of doctoral degree graduates: Enrolled in a psychology doctoral program (n/a), enrolled in a postdoctoral residency/fellowship (2), employed in independent practice (1), employed in a community mental health/counseling center (10), other employment position (1), total from the above (doctoral) (14).

Additional Information:
Orientation, Objectives, and Emphasis of Department: The Doctor of Psychology program at Indiana State University follows a practitioner-scientist model of training in clinical psychology to guide the preparation and evaluation of its students. The primary goal is the training of skilled clinical psychologists in the assessment and treatment of psychological problems. The program seeks to develop a professional identity which values and pursues: excellence in clinical practice; a spirit of active inquiry and critical thought; a commitment to the development and application of new knowledge in the field; an active sense of social responsibility combined with an appreciation and respect for cultural and individual differences; and an enduring commitment to personal and professional development. The program philosophy is to prepare all students as broad-based general clinicians, with encouragement to specialize through electives, research area, internship selection, and postdoctoral training. The Master's program, with an emphasis on basic psychology and research, is intended to serve as preparatory to entrance into doctoral level study. Students are encouraged to become involved in research beginning with their first term in the program. Although the degree is in general psychology, some concentration is often possible. A main goal of the program is to have students leave with a sense of what it means to be a research psychologist.

Special Facilities or Resources: The department has a psychology clinic, mini- and micro-computers, and good laboratory facilities.

Information for Students With Physical Disabilities: See the following Web site for more information: http://web.indstate.edu/sasc/dss/index.htm.

Application Information:
Send to Department of Psychology, c/o Graduate Admissions, Root Hall, Indiana State University, Terre Haute, IN 47809. Application available online. URL of online application: http:/indstate.edu/sogs. Students are admitted in the Fall, application deadline January 1. Application deadline January 1 (PsyD); March 15 (Master's). Fee: $35.

Indiana University
Department of Counseling and Educational Psychology
School of Education
201 North Rose Avenue
Bloomington, IN 47405-1006
Telephone: (812) 856-8300
Fax: (812) 856-8333
E-mail: *joalexan@indiana.edu*
Web: *http://education.indiana.edu/cep*

Department Information:
1948. Chairperson: Joyce Alexander, PhD. Number of faculty: total—full-time 33, part-time 12; women—full-time 14, part-time 5; total—minority—full-time 4; women minority—full-time 2.

Programs and Degrees Offered:
Listed in the following order: Program area, degree type (T if terminal Master's), number awarded 7/08–6/09. Counseling Psychology PhD (Doctor of Philosophy) 10, Educational Psychology PhD (Doctor of Philosophy) 7, School Psychology PhD (Doctor

of Philosophy) 2, School Psychology EdS (School Psychology) 4, Educational Psychology MA/MS (Master of Arts/Science) 0.

APA Accreditation: Counseling PhD (Doctor of Philosophy). Student Outcome Data Website: http://education.indiana.edu/Doctoral/CounselingPsychologyPhDProgramOverview/tabid/5543/Default.aspx. School PhD (Doctor of Philosophy). Student Outcome Data Website: http://education.indiana.edu/Doctoral/tabid/5586/Default.aspx.

Student Applications/Admissions:
Student Applications
Counseling Psychology PhD (Doctor of Philosophy)—Applications 2009–2010, 103. Total applicants accepted 2009–2010, 6. Number full-time enrolled (new admits only) 2009–2010, 10. Openings 2010–2011, 10. The median number of years required for completion of a degree in 2008–2009 were 6. The number of students enrolled full- and part-time who were dismissed or voluntarily withdrew from this program area in 2008–2009 were 0. *Educational Psychology PhD (Doctor of Philosophy)*—Applications 2009–2010, 40. Total applicants accepted 2009–2010, 14. Number full-time enrolled (new admits only) 2009–2010, 7. Openings 2010–2011, 12. The median number of years required for completion of a degree in 2008–2009 were 5. The number of students enrolled full- and part-time who were dismissed or voluntarily withdrew from this program area in 2008–2009 were 2. *School Psychology PhD (Doctor of Philosophy)*—Applications 2009–2010, 36. Total applicants accepted 2009–2010, 15. Number full-time enrolled (new admits only) 2009–2010, 7. Openings 2010–2011, 8. The median number of years required for completion of a degree in 2008–2009 were 5. The number of students enrolled full- and part-time who were dismissed or voluntarily withdrew from this program area in 2008–2009 were 2. *School Psychology EdS (School Psychology)*—Applications 2009–2010, 32. Total applicants accepted 2009–2010, 18. Number full-time enrolled (new admits only) 2009–2010, 7. Total enrolled 2009–2010 full-time, 25. Openings 2010–2011, 10. The median number of years required for completion of a degree in 2008–2009 were 3. The number of students enrolled full- and part-time who were dismissed or voluntarily withdrew from this program area in 2008–2009 were 1. *Educational Psychology MA/MS (Master of Arts/Science)*—Applications 2009–2010, 20. Total applicants accepted 2009–2010, 10. Number full-time enrolled (new admits only) 2009–2010, 0. Total enrolled 2009–2010 full-time, 9. Openings 2010–2011, 8. The number of students enrolled full- and part-time who were dismissed or voluntarily withdrew from this program area in 2008–2009 were 0.
Scores: Entries appear in this order: required test or GPA, minimum score (if required), median score of students entering in 2009–2010. *Counseling Psychology PhD (Doctor of Philosophy):* GRE-V no minimum stated, 593, GRE-Q no minimum stated, 611, GRE-Analytical no minimum stated, 4.14, overall undergraduate GPA no minimum stated, 3.43, Masters GPA no minimum stated, 3.96; *Educational Psychology PhD (Doctor of Philosophy):* GRE-V no minimum stated, 603, GRE-Q no minimum stated, 667, GRE-Analytical no minimum stated, 4.4, overall undergraduate GPA no minimum stated, 3.53, Masters GPA no minimum stated, 3.89; *School Psychology PhD (Doctor of Philosophy):* GRE-V no minimum stated, 536, GRE-Q no minimum stated, 625, GRE-Analytical no minimum stated, 4.5, overall undergraduate GPA no minimum stated, 3.73; *Educational Psychology MA/MS (Master of Arts/Science):* GRE-V no minimum stated, 589, GRE-Q no minimum stated, 661, GRE-Analytical no minimum stated, 4.2, overall undergraduate GPA no minimum stated, 3.3.
Other Criteria: (importance of criteria rated low, medium, or high): GRE scores—high, research experience—medium, work experience—medium, extracurricular activity—medium, clinically related public service—medium, GPA—high, letters of recommendation—high, interview—high, statement of goals and objectives—high. In the PhD in Counseling Psychology; PhD in School Psychology and Learning Science programs, personal interviews are required. GRE scores are interpreted differently for domestic and international applicants.

Student Characteristics: The following represents characteristics of students in 2009–2010 in all graduate psychology programs in the department: Female—full-time 132, part-time 0; Male—full-time 49, part-time 0; African American/Black—full-time 16, part-time 0; Hispanic/Latino(a)—full-time 12, part-time 0; Asian/Pacific Islander—full-time 25, part-time 0; American Indian/Alaska Native—full-time 0, part-time 0; Caucasian/White—full-time 102, part-time 0; Multi-ethnic—full-time 0, part-time 0; students subject to the Americans With Disabilities Act—full-time 0, part-time 0; Unknown ethnicity—full-time 26, part-time 0; International students who hold an F-1 or J-1 Visa—full-time 37, part-time 0.

Financial Information/Assistance:
Tuition for Full-Time Study: *Master's:* State residents: $330 per credit hour; Nonstate residents: $960 per credit hour. *Doctoral:* State residents: $330 per credit hour; Nonstate residents: $960 per credit hour. Tuition is subject to change. See the following Web site for updates and changes in tuition costs: http://bursar.indiana.edu/fee_schedule.php.

Financial Assistance:
First-Year Students: Teaching assistantships available for first year. Average amount paid per academic year: $14,280. Average number of hours worked per week: 18. Research assistantships available for first year. Average amount paid per academic year: $12,000. Average number of hours worked per week: 18. Fellowships and scholarships available for first year. Average amount paid per academic year: $19,000.
Advanced Students: Teaching assistantships available for advanced students. Average amount paid per academic year: $14,280. Average number of hours worked per week: 18. Research assistantships available for advanced students. Average amount paid per academic year: $12,000. Average number of hours worked per week: 18. Fellowships and scholarships available for advanced students. Average amount paid per academic year: $19,000.
Additional Information: Of all students currently enrolled full time, 50% benefited from one or more of the listed financial assistance programs. Application and information available online at: http://www.indiana.edu/~sfa/.

Internships/Practica: Doctoral Degree (PhD Counseling Psychology): For those doctoral students for whom a professional internship was required in this program prior to graduation, (6) students applied for an internship in 2008–2009, with (6) students obtaining an internship. Of those students who obtained an internship, (6) were paid internships. Of those students who obtained an internship, (6) students placed in APA/CPA accredited internships, (0) students placed in internships not APA/CPA accredited, but listed with the Association of Psychology Postdoctoral and Internship Programs (APPIC), (0) students placed in internships conforming to guidelines of the Council of Directors of School Psychology Programs (CDSPP), (0) students placed in internships that were not APA/CPA accredited, APPIC or CDSPP listed. Doctoral Degree (PhD School Psychology): For those doctoral students for whom a professional internship was required in this program prior to graduation, (8) students applied for an internship in 2008–2009, with (8) students obtaining an internship. Of those students who obtained an internship, (8) were paid internships. Of those students who obtained an internship, (4) students placed in APA/CPA accredited internships, (0) students placed in internships not APA/CPA accredited, but listed with the Association of Psychology Postdoctoral and Internship Programs (APPIC), (0) students placed in internships conforming to guidelines of the Council of Directors of School Psychology Programs (CDSPP), (4) students placed in internships that were not APA/CPA accredited, APPIC or CDSPP listed. All counseling and school psychology students must take both practica and internships.

Housing and Day Care: On-campus housing is available. See the following Web site for more information: http://www.rps.indiana.edu/index.cfml. On-campus day care facilities are available. See the following Web site for more information: http://www.childcare.indiana.edu/.

Employment of Department Graduates:
Master's Degree Graduates: Of those who graduated in the academic year 2008–2009, the following categories and numbers represent the postgraduate activities and employment of master's degree graduates: Enrolled in a postdoctoral residency/fellowship (n/a), employed in independent practice (n/a), total from the above (master's) (0).
Doctoral Degree Graduates: Of those who graduated in the academic year 2008–2009, the following categories and numbers represent the postgraduate activities and employment of doctoral degree graduates: Enrolled in a psychology doctoral program (n/a), enrolled in a postdoctoral residency/fellowship (2), employed in an academic position at a university (7), employed in other positions at a higher education institution (1), employed in business or industry (1), employed in a community mental health/counseling center (2), do not know (3), total from the above (doctoral) (16).

Additional Information:
Orientation, Objectives, and Emphasis of Department: The Department has multiple missions, but at the heart of our enterprise is a community of scholars working to contribute solutions to the problems faced by children, adolescents, and adults in the context of contemporary education. Additionally, the counseling psychology program promotes a broad range of interventions designed to facilitate the maximal adjustment of individuals. Faculty, staff and students share a commitment to open-mindedness and to social justice. We recognize the complex and dynamic nature of the social fabric and welcome qualified students of all ethnic, racial, national, religious, gender, social class, sexual, political, and philosophic orientations. Faculty and students collaboratively investigate numerous facets of child and adolescent development, creativity, learning, metacognition, aging, semiotics, and inquiry methodologies. Our programs require an understanding of both quantitative and qualitative research paradigms. We ascribe to the scientist–practitioner model for preparing professional psychologists. Our graduates work in various research and practice settings; universities, public schools, state departments of education, mental health centers, hospitals, and corporations.

Special Facilities or Resources: Special facilities include the Institute for Child Study, Center for Human Growth, Center for Evaluation and Education Policy, Center for Adolescent & Family Studies, Center for Research on Learning & Technology, and the Indiana Institute on Disability and Community.

Information for Students With Physical Disabilities: See the following Web site for more information: http://www2.dsa.indiana.edu/dss/.

Application Information:
Send to Office of Graduate Studies, Room 4214, W.W. Wright Education Building 201, North Rose Avenue, Bloomington, IN 47405-1006. Application available online. URL of online application: http://education.indiana.edu/cep/ApplicationProcedures/tabid/5624/Default.aspx. Students are admitted in the Fall, application deadline December 1. *Fee:* $55. Application fee of $60 for international students.

Indiana University (2009 data)
Department of Psychological and Brain Sciences
Arts and Sciences
Psychology Building, 1101 East 10th Street
Bloomington, IN 47405
Telephone: (812) 855-2012
Fax: (812) 855-4691
E-mail: *psychgrd@indiana.edu*
Web: *http://www.psych.indiana.edu*

Department Information:
1919. Chairperson: Linda B. Smith. Number of faculty: total—full-time 50; women—full-time 12; total—minority—full-time 1; women minority—full-time 1; faculty subject to the Americans With Disabilities Act 1.

Programs and Degrees Offered:
Listed in the following order: Program area, degree type (T if terminal Master's), number awarded 7/08–6/09. Biology, Behavior, and Neuroscience PhD (Doctor of Philosophy) 3, Clinical Science PhD (Doctor of Philosophy) 3, Cognitive PhD (Doctor of Philosophy) 6, Developmental PhD (Doctor of Philosophy) 1, Social PhD (Doctor of Philosophy) 4, Cognitive Neuroscience PhD (Doctor of Philosophy) 0.

APA Accreditation: Clinical PhD (Doctor of Philosophy).

Student Applications/Admissions:
Student Applications
Biology, Behavior, and Neuroscience PhD (Doctor of Philosophy)—Applications 2009–2010, 25. Total applicants accepted 2009–2010, 1. Number full-time enrolled (new admits only) 2009–2010, 1. Number part-time enrolled (new admits only) 2009–2010, 0. Openings 2010–2011, 4. The median number of years required for completion of a degree in 2008–2009

were 5. The number of students enrolled full- and part-time who were dismissed or voluntarily withdrew from this program area in 2008–2009 were 1. *Clinical Science PhD (Doctor of Philosophy)*—Applications 2009–2010, 80. Total applicants accepted 2009–2010, 5. Number full-time enrolled (new admits only) 2009–2010, 5. Number part-time enrolled (new admits only) 2009–2010, 0. Openings 2010–2011, 7. The median number of years required for completion of a degree in 2008–2009 were 6. The number of students enrolled full- and part-time who were dismissed or voluntarily withdrew from this program area in 2008–2009 were 0. *Cognitive PhD (Doctor of Philosophy)*—Applications 2009–2010, 29. Total applicants accepted 2009–2010, 8. Number full-time enrolled (new admits only) 2009–2010, 5. Number part-time enrolled (new admits only) 2009–2010, 0. Openings 2010–2011, 9. The median number of years required for completion of a degree in 2008–2009 were 6. The number of students enrolled full- and part-time who were dismissed or voluntarily withdrew from this program area in 2008–2009 were 1. *Developmental PhD (Doctor of Philosophy)*—Applications 2009–2010, 10. Total applicants accepted 2009–2010, 4. Number full-time enrolled (new admits only) 2009–2010, 3. Number part-time enrolled (new admits only) 2009–2010, 0. Openings 2010–2011, 1. The median number of years required for completion of a degree in 2008–2009 were 6. The number of students enrolled full- and part-time who were dismissed or voluntarily withdrew from this program area in 2008–2009 were 0. *Social PhD (Doctor of Philosophy)*—Applications 2009–2010, 43. Total applicants accepted 2009–2010, 2. Number full-time enrolled (new admits only) 2009–2010, 2. Number part-time enrolled (new admits only) 2009–2010, 0. Openings 2010–2011, 2. The median number of years required for completion of a degree in 2008–2009 were 6. The number of students enrolled full- and part-time who were dismissed or voluntarily withdrew from this program area in 2008–2009 were 0. *Cognitive Neuroscience PhD (Doctor of Philosophy)*—Applications 2009–2010, 12. Total applicants accepted 2009–2010, 4. Number full-time enrolled (new admits only) 2009–2010, 2. Number part-time enrolled (new admits only) 2009–2010, 0. Openings 2010–2011, 4. The median number of years required for completion of a degree in 2008–2009 were 6. The number of students enrolled full- and part-time who were dismissed or voluntarily withdrew from this program area in 2008–2009 were 0.
Other Criteria: (importance of criteria rated low, medium, or high): GRE scores—high, research experience—high, GPA—high, letters of recommendation—high, interview—high, statement of goals and objectives—medium. For additional information on admission requirements, go to http://www.psych.indiana.edu.

Student Characteristics: The following represents characteristics of students in 2009–2010 in all graduate psychology programs in the department: Female—full-time 46, part-time 0; Male—full-time 41, part-time 0; African American/Black—full-time 3, part-time 0; Hispanic/Latino(a)—full-time 3, part-time 0; Asian/Pacific Islander—full-time 7, part-time 0; American Indian/Alaska Native—full-time 1, part-time 0; Caucasian/White—full-time 73, part-time 0; Multi-ethnic—full-time 0, part-time 0; students subject to the Americans With Disabilities Act—full-time 0, part-time 0; Unknown ethnicity—full-time 0, part-time 0; International students who hold an F-1 or J-1 Visa—full-time 0, part-time 0.

Financial Information/Assistance:
Tuition for Full-Time Study: *Doctoral*: State residents: per academic year $8,760, $292 per credit hour; Nonstate residents: per academic year $25,500, $850 per credit hour. Tuition is subject to change. Additional fees are assessed to students beyond the costs of tuition for the following: activity fee, health fee, technology fee, transportation fee. See the following Web site for updates and changes in tuition costs: http://bursar.indiana.edu/.

Financial Assistance:
First-Year Students: Teaching assistantships available for first year. Average amount paid per academic year: $20,810. Average number of hours worked per week: 20. Research assistantships available for first year. Average amount paid per academic year: $20,810. Average number of hours worked per week: 20. Fellowships and scholarships available for first year. Average amount paid per academic year: $23,000. Average number of hours worked per week: 0.
Advanced Students: Teaching assistantships available for advanced students. Average amount paid per academic year: $20,810. Average number of hours worked per week: 20. Research assistantships available for advanced students. Average amount paid per academic year: $20,810. Average number of hours worked per week: 20. Fellowships and scholarships available for advanced students. Average amount paid per academic year: $23,000. Average number of hours worked per week: 20.
Additional Information: Of all students currently enrolled full time, 100% benefited from one or more of the listed financial assistance programs. Application and information available online at: http://www.gradapp.indiana.edu.

Housing and Day Care: On-campus housing is available. See the following Web site for more information: http://www.rps.indiana.edu/. On-campus day care facilities are available. See the following Web site for more information: http://www.childcare.indiana.edu/.

Employment of Department Graduates:
Master's Degree Graduates: Of those who graduated in the academic year 2008–2009, the following categories and numbers represent the postgraduate activities and employment of master's degree graduates: Enrolled in a postdoctoral residency/fellowship (n/a), employed in independent practice (n/a), total from the above (master's) (0).
Doctoral Degree Graduates: Of those who graduated in the academic year 2008–2009, the following categories and numbers represent the postgraduate activities and employment of doctoral degree graduates: Enrolled in a psychology doctoral program (n/a), total from the above (doctoral) (0).

Additional Information:
Orientation, Objectives, and Emphasis of Department: Students acquire fundamental knowledge and are offered specialized training so that they may develop competence in research, teaching (college and university levels), and service. Close contact between faculty and students is made possible by a low ratio of graduate students to faculty. Extensive laboratory facilities are available for research in the major areas. A psychological clinic is maintained as a specialized unit of the department. The primary emphasis of the clinical training program is on the theoretical and scientific aspects of clinical psychology. However, in view of the diverse and changing nature of the field, the program's goal is to produce

clinical psychologists who are well trained scientifically and clinically and who are capable of achieving excellence in their careers in either a clinical or an academic and research setting.

Special Facilities or Resources: Recently, the Department of Psychological and Brain Sciences became home to the IU Imaging Research Facility. The facility houses a 3T Siemens Magnetom Trio whole body system, used for magnetic resonance imaging (MRI) or functional MRI (fMRI), a noninvasive method for studying patterns of brain activity during mental operations. The facility gives our students the opportunity to be part of research labs doing MRI and fMRI studies and to take classes with the MRI scientists.

Information for Students With Physical Disabilities: See the following Web site for more information: http://www2.dsa.indiana.edu.dss.

Application Information:
Send to Indiana University, Department of Psychological and Brain Scieces, Graduate Admissions, 1101 East 10th Street, Bloomington, IN 47405. Application available online. URL of online application: https://www.gradapp.indiana.edu/. Students are admitted in the Fall, application deadline December 15. December 1 is the application deadline for international graduate student candidates. *Fee:* $50. The application fee is $60 for international students.

Indiana University-Purdue University Indianapolis
Department of Psychology
Science
402 North Blackford Street, LD 124
Indianapolis, IN 46202-3275
Telephone: (317) 274-6945
Fax: (317) 274-6756
E-mail: *gradpsy@iupui.edu*
Web: *http://www.psych.iupui.edu*

Department Information:
1969. Chairperson: Kathy E. Johnson. Number of faculty: total—full-time 33; women—full-time 13; total—minority—full-time 2; women minority—full-time 2.

Programs and Degrees Offered:
Listed in the following order: Program area, degree type (T if terminal Master's), number awarded 7/08–6/09. Industrial/Organizational Psychology MA/MS (Master of Arts/Science) (T) 3, Clinical Psychology PhD (Doctor of Philosophy) 2, Psychobiology PhD (Doctor of Philosophy) 2, Clinical Psychology MA/MS (Master of Arts/Science) (T) 0.

APA Accreditation: Clinical PhD (Doctor of Philosophy).

Student Applications/Admissions:
Student Applications
Industrial/Organizational Psychology MA/MS (Master of Arts/Science)—Applications 2009–2010, 51. Total applicants accepted 2009–2010, 5. Number full-time enrolled (new admits only) 2009–2010, 5. Number part-time enrolled (new admits only) 2009–2010, 0. Openings 2010–2011, 5. The median number of years required for completion of a degree in 2008–2009 were 2. The number of students enrolled full- and part-time who were dismissed or voluntarily withdrew from this program area in 2008–2009 were 0. Clinical Psychology PhD (Doctor of Philosophy)—Applications 2009–2010, 53. Total applicants accepted 2009–2010, 4. Number full-time enrolled (new admits only) 2009–2010, 4. Number part-time enrolled (new admits only) 2009–2010, 0. Openings 2010–2011, 4. The median number of years required for completion of a degree in 2008–2009 were 5. The number of students enrolled full- and part-time who were dismissed or voluntarily withdrew from this program area in 2008–2009 were 0. Psychobiology PhD (Doctor of Philosophy)—Applications 2009–2010, 12. Total applicants accepted 2009–2010, 6. Number full-time enrolled (new admits only) 2009–2010, 6. Openings 2010–2011, 2. The median number of years required for completion of a degree in 2008–2009 were 6. The number of students enrolled full- and part-time who were dismissed or voluntarily withdrew from this program area in 2008–2009 were 0. Clinical Psychology MA/MS (Master of Arts/Science)—Applications 2009–2010, 35. Total applicants accepted 2009–2010, 6. Number full-time enrolled (new admits only) 2009–2010, 6. Total enrolled 2009–2010 full-time, 6. Openings 2010–2011, 2. The number of students enrolled full- and part-time who were dismissed or voluntarily withdrew from this program area in 2008–2009 were 1.

Scores: Entries appear in this order: required test or GPA, minimum score (if required), median score of students entering in 2009–2010. *Industrial/Organizational Psychology MA/MS (Master of Arts/Science):* GRE-V 510, 562, GRE-Q 590, 642, GRE-Analytical 4.5, 4.7, overall undergraduate GPA 3.36, 3.75; *Clinical Psychology PhD (Doctor of Philosophy):* GRE-V 480, 610, GRE-Q 640, 683, GRE-Analytical 4.5, 4.75, GRE-Subject (Psychology) 640, 710, overall undergraduate GPA 3.52, 3.71, Masters GPA no minimum stated; *Psychobiology PhD (Doctor of Philosophy):* GRE-V 470, 538, GRE-Q 570, 643, GRE-Analytical 4, 4, overall undergraduate GPA 2.89, 3.34, Masters GPA no minimum stated; *Clinical Psychology MA/MS (Master of Arts/Science):* GRE-V 430, 497, GRE-Q 550, 635, GRE-Analytical 3, 4.2, overall undergraduate GPA 3.16, 3.56.

Other Criteria: (importance of criteria rated low, medium, or high): GRE scores—high, research experience—high, work experience—low, GPA—high, letters of recommendation—high, interview—medium, statement of goals and objectives—high, undergraduate major in psychology—low, specific undergraduate psychology courses taken—low. For additional information on admission requirements, go to http://psych.iupui.edu.

Student Characteristics: The following represents characteristics of students in 2009–2010 in all graduate psychology programs in the department: Female—full-time 46, part-time 0; Male—full-time 6, part-time 0; African American/Black—full-time 3, part-time 0; Hispanic/Latino(a)—full-time 1, part-time 0; Asian/Pacific Islander—full-time 3, part-time 0; American Indian/Alaska Native—full-time 0, part-time 0; Caucasian/White—full-time 45, part-time 0; Multi-ethnic—full-time 0, part-time 0; students subject to the Americans With Disabilities Act—full-time 0, part-time 0; Unknown ethnicity—full-time 0, part-time 0; Interna-

tional students who hold an F-1 or J-1 Visa—full-time 3, part-time 0.

Financial Information/Assistance:
Tuition for Full-Time Study: *Master's:* State residents: per academic year $2,844, $316 per credit hour; Nonstate residents: per academic year $8,136, $904 per credit hour. *Doctoral:* State residents: per academic year $7,584, $316 per credit hour; Nonstate residents: per academic year $21,696, $904 per credit hour. Tuition is subject to change. Additional fees are assessed to students beyond the costs of tuition for the following: recreational fee, graduate fee and technology fee. Tuition costs vary by program. See the following Web site for updates and changes in tuition costs: http://www.osas.iupui.edu.

Financial Assistance:
First-Year Students: Teaching assistantships available for first year. Average amount paid per academic year: $13,000. Average number of hours worked per week: 20. Research assistantships available for first year. Average amount paid per academic year: $13,000. Average number of hours worked per week: 20. Fellowships and scholarships available for first year. Average amount paid per academic year: $22,000. Average number of hours worked per week: 0.

Advanced Students: Teaching assistantships available for advanced students. Average amount paid per academic year: $13,000. Average number of hours worked per week: 20. Research assistantships available for advanced students. Average amount paid per academic year: $13,000. Average number of hours worked per week: 20. Fellowships and scholarships available for advanced students. Average amount paid per academic year: $13,000. Average number of hours worked per week: 0.

Additional Information: Of all students currently enrolled full time, 72% benefited from one or more of the listed financial assistance programs.

Internships/Practica: Doctoral Degree (PhD Clinical Psychology): For those doctoral students for whom a professional internship was required in this program prior to graduation, (5) students applied for an internship in 2008–2009, with (4) students obtaining an internship. Of those students who obtained an internship, (4) were paid internships. Of those students who obtained an internship, (4) students placed in APA/CPA accredited internships, (0) students placed in internships not APA/CPA accredited, but listed with the Association of Psychology Postdoctoral and Internship Programs (APPIC), (0) students placed in internships conforming to guidelines of the Council of Directors of School Psychology Programs (CDSPP), (0) students placed in internships that were not APA/CPA accredited, APPIC or CDSPP listed. Clinical practicum sites are located at IUPUI and within the Indianapolis area, and involve supervised clinical training individually tailored for each student. A practicum coordinator, the site supervisor, and the student develop specific contracts that emphasize education and the acquisition of clinical skills and knowledge, rather than experience per se. These contractual activities and goals are monitored and evaluated at the end of each placement. Practicum opportunities are varied and numerous and include many different types of clinical settings with different clinical populations. On-site supervisors are psychologists. Many sites in different settings are available. General practicum sites include a university counseling center and several psychiatric clinics. More advanced settings can be categorized as 1) Behavioral Medicine/Health Psychology; 2) Severe Mental Illness/Psychiatric Rehabilitation. The I/O Master's program offers opportunities to achieve applied experience in business settings. Students have the opportunity to sign up for practicum in the spring of their second year. Students are typically placed in an organization for one 8-hour day each week of the semester. Paid summer internships (15-20 hours per week) in the community are also available.

Housing and Day Care: On-campus housing is available. See the following Web site for more information: http://www.housing.iupui.edu/. On-campus day care facilities are available. See the following Web site for more information: http://www.childcare.iupui.edu/.

Employment of Department Graduates:
Master's Degree Graduates: Of those who graduated in the academic year 2008–2009, the following categories and numbers represent the postgraduate activities and employment of master's degree graduates: Enrolled in a postdoctoral residency/fellowship (n/a), employed in independent practice (n/a), employed in business or industry (3), total from the above (master's) (3).

Doctoral Degree Graduates: Of those who graduated in the academic year 2008–2009, the following categories and numbers represent the postgraduate activities and employment of doctoral degree graduates: Enrolled in a psychology doctoral program (n/a), enrolled in a postdoctoral residency/fellowship (1), employed in an academic position at a university (1), employed in other positions at a higher education institution (1), employed in a hospital/medical center (1), total from the above (doctoral) (4).

Additional Information:
Orientation, Objectives, and Emphasis of Department: Graduate education is offered at the PhD level in Clinical Psychology and Psychobiology of Addictions. The APA-accredited Clinical program follows the scientist–practitioner model. A rigorous academic and research education is combined with supervised practical training. The clinical program provides specialization in behavioral medicine/health psychology, and severe mental illness/psychiatric rehabilitation. The PhD program in the psychobiological bases of addictions emphasizes the core content areas of psychology along with specialization in psychobiology and animal models of addiction. Research, scholarship, and close faculty-student mentor relationships are viewed as integral training elements within both programs. Graduate training at the MS level is designed to provide students with theory and practice that will enable them to apply psychological techniques and findings to subsequent jobs. All students are required to take departmental methods courses and then specific area core courses and electives. The MS degree areas are applied in focus and science-based, and this reflects the interests and orientation of the faculty.

Special Facilities or Resources: IUPUI is a unique urban university campus with 27,000 students enrolled in 235 degree programs at the undergraduate and graduate level. The campus includes schools of law, dentistry, and medicine, among others, along with undergraduate programs in the arts, humanities, and science. In addition, there are over 75 research institutes, centers, laboratories and specialized programs. The Department of Psychology at IUPUI occupies teaching and research facilities in a modern science building in the heart of campus. Facilities include a 4,000-square foot space and self-contained area devoted to faculty and graduate student basic animal research in experimental psychology and psychobiology. Many of the research rooms are equipped for online computer recording to one of the faculty offices. Laboratories for human research, research rooms, and teaching laboratories are separately located on the first floor of the building. The Psychology Department maintains ties with the faculty and programs in other schools within IUPUI, including the School of Nursing, and the Departments of Psychiatry, Adolescent Medicine, and Neurology. The clinical program provides an unusually rich array of practicum opportunities in behavioral medicine/health psychology and psychiatric rehabilitation.

Information for Students With Physical Disabilities: See the following Web site for more information: http://www.iupui.edu/~divrsity/aes/.

Application Information:
Send to Kristi S. Combs, Graduate Coordinator, IUPUI, Department of Psychology, LD124, 402 N. Blackford Street, Indianapolis, IN 46202-3275. Application available online. URL of online application: http://psych.iupui.edu. Students are admitted in the Fall, application deadline December 1. Each program has a different application deadline. Clinical PhD is December 1. Psychobiology application deadline is January 1. Industrial/Organizational application deadline is February 1. Clinical MS program application deadline is March 15. *Fee:* $50. International - $60.

Indianapolis, University of
Graduate Psychology Program
School of Psychological Sciences
1400 East Hanna Avenue GH 109
Indianapolis, IN 46227
Telephone: (317) 788-3353
Fax: (317) 788-2120
E-mail: *psychology@uindy.edu*
Web: *http://psych.uindy.edu/*

Department Information:
1994. Dean and Associate Dean: John McIlvried, PhD and Richard Holigrocki, PhD. Number of faculty: total—full-time 15, part-time 1; women—full-time 7, part-time 1; total—minority—full-time 1; faculty subject to the Americans With Disabilities Act 1.

Programs and Degrees Offered:
Listed in the following order: Program area, degree type (T if terminal Master's), number awarded 7/08–6/09. Clinical Psychology MA/MS (Master of Arts/Science) 19, Clinical Psychology PsyD (Doctor of Psychology) 17, Mental Health Counseling MA/MS (Master of Arts/Science) (T) 8.

APA Accreditation: Clinical PsyD (Doctor of Psychology). Student Outcome Data Website: http://psych.uindy.edu/outcomes.php.

Student Applications/Admissions:
Student Applications
Clinical Psychology MA/MS (Master of Arts/Science)—Applications 2009–2010, 60. Total applicants accepted 2009–2010, 3. Number full-time enrolled (new admits only) 2009–2010, 0. Number part-time enrolled (new admits only) 2009–2010, 0. Openings 2010–2011, 3. The median number of years required for completion of a degree in 2008–2009 were 2. The number of students enrolled full- and part-time who were dismissed or voluntarily withdrew from this program area in 2008–2009 were 0. *Clinical Psychology PsyD (Doctor of Psychology)*—Applications 2009–2010, 228. Total applicants accepted 2009–2010, 50. Number full-time enrolled (new admits only) 2009–2010, 22. Number part-time enrolled (new admits only) 2009–2010, 2. Total enrolled 2009–2010 full-time, 123, part-time, 8. Openings 2010–2011, 24. The median number of years required for completion of a degree in 2008–2009 were 6. The number of students enrolled full- and part-time who were dismissed or voluntarily withdrew from this program area in 2008–2009 were 2. *Mental Health Counseling MA/MS (Master of Arts/Science)*—Applications 2009–2010, 108. Total applicants accepted 2009–2010, 37. Number full-time enrolled (new admits only) 2009–2010, 16. Number part-time enrolled (new admits only) 2009–2010, 2. Total enrolled 2009–2010 full-time, 30, part-time, 4. Openings 2010–2011, 17. The median number of years required for completion of a degree in 2008–2009 were 2. The number of students enrolled full- and part-time who were dismissed or voluntarily withdrew from this program area in 2008–2009 were 2.

Scores: Entries appear in this order: required test or GPA, minimum score (if required), median score of students entering in 2009–2010. *Clinical Psychology MA/MS (Master of Arts/Science)*: GRE-V 500, 507, GRE-Q 500, 574, GRE-Analytical 4.0, 4.6, overall undergraduate GPA 3.0, 3.42; *Clinical Psychology PsyD (Doctor of Psychology)*: GRE-V 500, 555, GRE-Q 500, 647, GRE-Analytical 4.0, 4.67, overall undergraduate GPA 3.0, 3.61; *Mental Health Counseling MA/MS (Master of Arts/Science)*: GRE-V 500, 507, GRE-Q 500, 574, GRE-Analytical 4.0, 4.6, overall undergraduate GPA 3.0, 3.42.

Other Criteria: (importance of criteria rated low, medium, or high): GRE scores—high, research experience—medium, work experience—medium, extracurricular activity—low, clinically related public service—medium, GPA—high, letters of recommendation—high, interview—high, statement of goals and objectives—medium, 18 credits in psychology—high. For additional information on admission requirements, go to http://psych.uindy.edu.

Student Characteristics: The following represents characteristics of students in 2009–2010 in all graduate psychology programs in the department: Female—full-time 135, part-time 11; Male—full-time 20, part-time 1; African American/Black—full-time 8, part-time 0; Hispanic/Latino(a)—full-time 1, part-time 0; Asian/Pacific Islander—full-time 5, part-time 0; American Indian/Alaska Native—full-time 0, part-time 0; Caucasian/White—full-time 138, part-time 12; Multi-ethnic—full-time 1, part-time 0; students subject to the Americans With Disabilities Act—full-time 4, part-time 0; Unknown ethnicity—full-time 2, part-time 0; International students who hold an F-1 or J-1 Visa—full-time 6, part-time 0.

Financial Information/Assistance:
Tuition for Full-Time Study: *Master's:* State residents: $675 per credit hour; Nonstate residents: $675 per credit hour. *Doctoral:* State residents: $675 per credit hour; Nonstate residents: $675 per credit hour. Tuition is subject to change. See the following

Web site for updates and changes in tuition costs: http://psych.uindy.edu/tuifinaidpsyd.php.

Financial Assistance:

First-Year Students: Teaching assistantships available for first year. Average amount paid per academic year: $0. Average number of hours worked per week: 11. Apply by January 10. Research assistantships available for first year. Average amount paid per academic year: $0. Average number of hours worked per week: 11. Apply by January 10. Fellowships and scholarships available for first year. Average amount paid per academic year: $0. Average number of hours worked per week: 0. Apply by January 10.

Advanced Students: Teaching assistantships available for advanced students. Average amount paid per academic year: $0. Average number of hours worked per week: 11. Research assistantships available for advanced students. Average amount paid per academic year: $0. Average number of hours worked per week: 11. Fellowships and scholarships available for advanced students. Average amount paid per academic year: $0. Average number of hours worked per week: 0.

Additional Information: Of all students currently enrolled full time, 30% benefited from one or more of the listed financial assistance programs. Application and information available online at: http://finaid.uindy.edu.

Internships/Practica: Doctoral Degree (PsyD Clinical Psychology): For those doctoral students for whom a professional internship was required in this program prior to graduation, (14) students applied for an internship in 2008–2009, with (13) students obtaining an internship. Of those students who obtained an internship, (13) were paid internships. Of those students who obtained an internship, (12) students placed in APA/CPA accredited internships, (1) students placed in internships not APA/CPA accredited, but listed with the Association of Psychology Postdoctoral and Internship Programs (APPIC), (0) students placed in internships conforming to guidelines of the Council of Directors of School Psychology Programs (CDSPP), (0) students placed in internships that were not APA/CPA accredited, APPIC or CDSPP listed. Master's Degree (MA/MS Mental Health Counseling): An internship experience, such as a final research project or "capstone" experience is required of graduates. There are numerous clinical practicum experiences available for both master's (CP and MHC) and doctoral students. Clinical psychology master's students (CP) obtain a minimum of 225 hours of supervised clinical practicum experience, clinical psychology mental health counseling students (MHC) require 1000 hours of supervised clinical practicum experience and doctoral students receive a minimum of 1200 hours of supervised clinical practicum experience. Practica are available at numerous settings, including medical centers, local community hospitals, university counseling centers, forensic settings, private practice placements, schools, social service agencies, and mental health centers. At these placements, students gain supervised experience in clinical assessment and testing, psychotherapy, collaboration and consultation with interdisciplinary teams, program development and evaluation, treatment planning and case management, and participation in development and delivery of services to professional staff. In addition to mainstream psychological services, practicum students have opportunities to obtain specific training in forensics, psychodiagnostic assessment, neuropsychology, health psychology, pain, substance abuse/dependence, eating disorders, developmental disabilities, and HIV/AIDS. All doctoral practica are supervised by licensed, doctoral level psychologists and all master's practica are supervised by licensed, master's level mental health professionals. In conjunction with practica, students enroll in a professional practice seminar that addresses a wide variety of issues that confront mental health professionals and students. This professional practice seminar is taught by full time University faculty. Doctoral students must also complete a 2000-hour internship. The Director of Clinical Training develops training sites, assists students in their placement and ensures the quality of practicum and internship training.

Housing and Day Care: On-campus housing is available. See the following Web site for more information: http://reslife.uindy.edu/. On-campus day care facilities are available. See the following Web site for more information: http://www.universityheightsumc.org/page9.html.

Employment of Department Graduates:

Master's Degree Graduates: Of those who graduated in the academic year 2008–2009, the following categories and numbers represent the postgraduate activities and employment of master's degree graduates: Enrolled in a postdoctoral residency/fellowship (n/a), employed in independent practice (n/a), do not know (8), total from the above (master's) (8).

Doctoral Degree Graduates: Of those who graduated in the academic year 2008–2009, the following categories and numbers represent the postgraduate activities and employment of doctoral degree graduates: Enrolled in a psychology doctoral program (n/a), enrolled in a postdoctoral residency/fellowship (10), employed in independent practice (2), employed in other positions at a higher education institution (1), employed in government agency (3), not seeking employment (1), total from the above (doctoral) (17).

Additional Information:

Orientation, Objectives, and Emphasis of Department: The graduate program in clinical psychology at the University of Indianapolis is based on a practitioner-scholar model of training. As such, the program is committed to developing highly competent and qualified professionals. The focus of the program is on preparing individuals to aid in the prevention and treatment of human problems, as well as the enhancement of human functioning and potential. The program trains students in the general, integrative practice of professional psychology through a broad-based exposure to a variety of psychological approaches and modalities. In addition, the program offers specialized training in three clinical emphasis areas: health psychology/behavioral medicine, childhood and adolescent psychology, adult psychopathology and psychotherapy. The faculty believe that education is most effective when the relationship between students and faculty is characterized by mutual respect, responsibility, and dedication to excellence. The program is founded on a deep and abiding respect for diversity in individuals, the ethical practice of psychology, and a commitment to service to others. These core values are reflected in the selection of students, the coursework and training experiences offered, and the faculty who serve as role models and mentors.

Special Facilities or Resources: Specialized training facilities include several clinical therapy labs designed for supervised assessment, testing, and therapy, and for videotaping of clinical sessions utilized in feedback and instruction. The Large Groups Lab includes interconnected classrooms used for videotaping and monitoring of experiential group or class exercises, psychoeducational programs, and other large group activities. Individualized Study and Research Labs equipped with computers are available for research projects, classroom assignments, and personal study. Computer facilities in the School of Psychological Sciences and throughout the university allow access to the internet, a full range of statistical and office software and library holdings. Wireless internet is available throughout the university. In addition, the capability of conducting direct, online literature searches using a variety of different databases (e.g., PsycBOOKS, PsycINFO [with PsycARTICLES], PsycEXTRA, MedLine, PEP CD) is available. The library subscribes to the major psychology journals and contains the latest publications in the field of clinical psychology. The School has a graduate student lounge in which students meet to confer about class assignments, have group study sessions, practice presentations, or just relax between classes. The School also has an on-site Psychological Services Center, which offers treatment services to community residents on a sliding fee scale. Students receive applied training experience at the Center while conducting intake assessments or providing therapeutic services.

Information for Students With Physical Disabilities: See the following Web site for more information: http://www.uindy.edu/ssd/.

Application Information:
Send to Margie Keaton, PsyD, Director of Student Services, 1400 East Hanna Avenue GH 109, Indianapolis, IN 46227. Application available online. URL of online application: https://www.applyweb.com/apply/uipsych/. Students are admitted in the Fall, application deadline January 10. January 10 PsyD deadline; February 25 MA deadline. *Fee:* $55.

Notre Dame, University of (2009 data)
Department of Psychology
Arts & Letters
118 Haggar Hall
Notre Dame, IN 46556
Telephone: (574) 631-6650
Fax: (574) 631-8883
E-mail: *danlapsley@nd.edu*
Web: *http://psychology.nd.edu*

Department Information:
1965. Chairperson: Daniel K. Lapsley. Number of faculty: total—full-time 36; women—full-time 16; total—minority—full-time 7; women minority—full-time 3.

Programs and Degrees Offered:
Listed in the following order: Program area, degree type (T if terminal Master's), number awarded 7/08–6/09. Cognitive Psychology PhD (Doctor of Philosophy) 0, Counseling Psychology PhD (Doctor of Philosophy) 2, Developmental Psychology PhD (Doctor of Philosophy) 4, Quantitative Psychology PhD (Doctor of Philosophy) 1.

APA Accreditation: Counseling PhD (Doctor of Philosophy).

Student Applications/Admissions:
Student Applications
Cognitive Psychology PhD (Doctor of Philosophy)—Applications 2009–2010, 19. Total applicants accepted 2009–2010, 2. Number full-time enrolled (new admits only) 2009–2010, 4. Total enrolled 2009–2010 full-time, 12. Openings 2010–2011, 5. The median number of years required for completion of a degree in 2008–2009 were 6. The number of students enrolled full- and part-time who were dismissed or voluntarily withdrew from this program area in 2008–2009 were 1. *Counseling Psychology PhD (Doctor of Philosophy)*—Applications 2009–2010, 91. Total applicants accepted 2009–2010, 3. Number full-time enrolled (new admits only) 2009–2010, 4. Total enrolled 2009–2010 full-time, 23. Openings 2010–2011, 4. The median number of years required for completion of a degree in 2008–2009 were 6. The number of students enrolled full- and part-time who were dismissed or voluntarily withdrew from this program area in 2008–2009 were 1. *Developmental Psychology PhD (Doctor of Philosophy)*—Applications 2009–2010, 32. Total applicants accepted 2009–2010, 8. Number full-time enrolled (new admits only) 2009–2010, 8. Total enrolled 2009–2010 full-time, 22. Openings 2010–2011, 4. The median number of years required for completion of a degree in 2008–2009 were 6. The number of students enrolled full- and part-time who were dismissed or voluntarily withdrew from this program area in 2008–2009 were 0. *Quantitative Psychology PhD (Doctor of Philosophy)*—Applications 2009–2010, 21. Total applicants accepted 2009–2010, 3. Number full-time enrolled (new admits only) 2009–2010, 2. Number part-time enrolled (new admits only) 2009–2010, 0. Openings 2010–2011, 4. The median number of years required for completion of a degree in 2008–2009 were 7. The number of students enrolled full- and part-time who were dismissed or voluntarily withdrew from this program area in 2008–2009 were 2.

Other Criteria: (importance of criteria rated low, medium, or high): GRE scores—high, research experience—high, work experience—low, extracurricular activity—low, clinically related public service—low, GPA—high, letters of recommendation—high, interview—medium, statement of goals and objectives—high, undergraduate major in psychology—high, specific undergraduate psychology courses taken—medium.

Student Characteristics: The following represents characteristics of students in 2009–2010 in all graduate psychology programs in the department: Female—full-time 40, part-time 0; Male—full-time 16, part-time 0; African American/Black—full-time 4, part-time 0; Hispanic/Latino(a)—full-time 6, part-time 0; Asian/Pacific Islander—full-time 4, part-time 0; American Indian/Alaska Native—full-time 0, part-time 0; Caucasian/White—full-time 40, part-time 0; Multi-ethnic—full-time 2, part-time 0; students subject to the Americans With Disabilities Act—full-time 0, part-time 0; Unknown ethnicity—full-time 0, part-time 0; International students who hold an F-1 or J-1 Visa—full-time 0, part-time 0.

Financial Information/Assistance:
Tuition for Full-Time Study: *Doctoral:* State residents: per academic year $31,000; Nonstate residents: per academic year $31,000.

Financial Assistance:
First-Year Students: Teaching assistantships available for first year. Average amount paid per academic year: $17,000. Re-

search assistantships available for first year. Average amount paid per academic year: $17,000. Fellowships and scholarships available for first year. Average amount paid per academic year: $20,000.

Advanced Students: Teaching assistantships available for advanced students. Average amount paid per academic year: $16,000. Research assistantships available for advanced students. Average amount paid per academic year: $16,000. Fellowships and scholarships available for advanced students. Average amount paid per academic year: $20.

Additional Information: Of all students currently enrolled full time, 100% benefited from one or more of the listed financial assistance programs. Application and information available online at: http://graduateschool.nd.edu.

Internships/Practica: Doctoral Degree (PhD Counseling Psychology): For those doctoral students for whom a professional internship was required in this program prior to graduation, (4) students applied for an internship in 2008–2009, with (4) students obtaining an internship. Of those students who obtained an internship, (4) were paid internships. Of those students who obtained an internship, (4) students placed in APA/CPA accredited internships, (0) students placed in internships not APA/CPA accredited, but listed with the Association of Psychology Postdoctoral and Internship Programs (APPIC), (0) students placed in internships conforming to guidelines of the Council of Directors of School Psychology Programs (CDSPP), (0) students placed in internships that were not APA/CPA accredited, APPIC or CDSPP listed. All students in the APA-accredited counseling program have an initial practicum 13-17 hours per week at the University Counseling Center. These same students have opportunities for additional practicum placements in agencies in the community. The University Counseling Center also houses an APA-accredited internship. Advanced students in the accredited program are eligible to apply.

Housing and Day Care: On-campus housing is available. See the following Web site for more information: http://orlh.nd.edu. On-campus day care facilities are available.

Employment of Department Graduates:
Master's Degree Graduates: Of those who graduated in the academic year 2008–2009, the following categories and numbers represent the postgraduate activities and employment of master's degree graduates: Enrolled in a postdoctoral residency/fellowship (n/a), employed in independent practice (n/a), total from the above (master's) (0).
Doctoral Degree Graduates: Of those who graduated in the academic year 2008–2009, the following categories and numbers represent the postgraduate activities and employment of doctoral degree graduates: Enrolled in a psychology doctoral program (n/a), enrolled in a postdoctoral residency/fellowship (3), employed in independent practice (3), employed in an academic position at a university (2), employed in other positions at a higher education institution (2), employed in business or industry (3), do not know (1), total from the above (doctoral) (14).

Additional Information:
Orientation, Objectives, and Emphasis of Department: The Department of Psychology at the University of Notre Dame is committed to excellence in psychological science and its applications. To realize this commitment a major focus is upon developing knowledge and expertise in the increasingly sophisticated methodology of the discipline. With this methodological core as its major emphasis and integrating link, the department has emphasized four content areas: cognitive, counseling, developmental and quantitative psychology. In the context of the mores of the academy, the faculty of each content area organize and coordinate work in the three domains of research, graduate education and undergraduate education. Using our methodological understandings as a base, we strive to find intellectual common ground among the content areas within our department and other disciplines throughout the social sciences and the academy.

Special Facilities or Resources: We are involved in the development of innovative science and practice experiences for undergraduate and graduate students in the local community. Currently, many faculty have excellent relationships with community groups (e.g., the local schools, hospitals, Madison Center, Logan center, Center for the Homeless, Head Start). Many faculty conduct research with undergraduate and graduate students in these settings. Over and above these research activities, many students volunteer in these agencies. Finally, counseling psychology graduate students receive supervision to work in Madison Center, Family and Children's Ctr., Michiana EAP, Oaklawn, St. Joseph Medical Ctr., and the Center for the Homeless and, in a new initiative, postdoctoral positions exist in the Multicultural Research Institute.

Information for Students With Physical Disabilities: See the following Web site for more information: http://disabilityservices.nd.edu.

Application Information:
Send to Graduate Admissions, The Graduate School, University of Notre Dame, Notre Dame, IN 46556. Application available online. URL of online application: http://graduateschool.nd.edu/admissions. Students are admitted in the Fall, application deadline January 2. *Fee:* $50. In certain circumstances the Graduate School (at the address above) can approve the waiver of fees. Fee is $35 for applications received before December 1.

Purdue University
Department of Psychological Sciences
College of Health and Human Sciences
701 Third Street
West Lafayette, IN 47906-2004
Telephone: (765) 494-6067
Fax: (765) 496-1264
E-mail: *nobrien@psych.purdue.edu*
Web: *http://www.psych.purdue.edu*

Department Information:
1954. Professor and Head: Christopher R. Agnew. Number of faculty: total—full-time 41, part-time 1; women—full-time 12; total—minority—full-time 3; women minority—full-time 2.

Programs and Degrees Offered:
Listed in the following order: Program area, degree type (T if terminal Master's), number awarded 7/08–6/09. Clinical Psychology PhD (Doctor of Philosophy) 4, Cognitive Psychology PhD (Doctor of Philosophy) 4, Developmental Psychology PhD (Doc-

tor of Philosophy) 1, Industrial/Organizational Psychology PhD (Doctor of Philosophy) 2, Learning and Memory PhD (Doctor of Philosophy) 1, Behavioral Neuroscience PhD (Doctor of Philosophy) 1, Mathematical and Computational Cognitive Science PhD (Doctor of Philosophy) 0, Social Psychology PhD (Doctor of Philosophy) 8.

APA Accreditation: Clinical PhD (Doctor of Philosophy). Student Outcome Data Website: http://www.psych.purdue.edu/index.php?option=com_content&task=view&id=267&Itemid=139.

Student Applications/Admissions:
Student Applications
Clinical Psychology PhD (Doctor of Philosophy)—Applications 2009–2010, 129. Total applicants accepted 2009–2010, 2. Number full-time enrolled (new admits only) 2009–2010, 2. Number part-time enrolled (new admits only) 2009–2010, 0. Openings 2010–2011, 3. The median number of years required for completion of a degree in 2008–2009 were 5. The number of students enrolled full- and part-time who were dismissed or voluntarily withdrew from this program area in 2008–2009 were 1. Cognitive Psychology PhD (Doctor of Philosophy)—Applications 2009–2010, 41. Total applicants accepted 2009–2010, 3. Number full-time enrolled (new admits only) 2009–2010, 2. Number part-time enrolled (new admits only) 2009–2010, 0. Openings 2010–2011, 2. The median number of years required for completion of a degree in 2008–2009 were 6. The number of students enrolled full- and part-time who were dismissed or voluntarily withdrew from this program area in 2008–2009 were 0. Developmental Psychology PhD (Doctor of Philosophy)—Applications 2009–2010, 23. Total applicants accepted 2009–2010, 1. Number full-time enrolled (new admits only) 2009–2010, 0. Number part-time enrolled (new admits only) 2009–2010, 0. Openings 2010–2011, 2. The median number of years required for completion of a degree in 2008–2009 were 3. The number of students enrolled full- and part-time who were dismissed or voluntarily withdrew from this program area in 2008–2009 were 0. Industrial/Organizational Psychology PhD (Doctor of Philosophy)—Applications 2009–2010, 56. Total applicants accepted 2009–2010, 3. Number full-time enrolled (new admits only) 2009–2010, 2. Number part-time enrolled (new admits only) 2009–2010, 0. Openings 2010–2011, 2. The median number of years required for completion of a degree in 2008–2009 were 5. The number of students enrolled full- and part-time who were dismissed or voluntarily withdrew from this program area in 2008–2009 were 0. Learning and Memory PhD (Doctor of Philosophy)—Applications 2009–2010, 0. Total applicants accepted 2009–2010, 0. Number full-time enrolled (new admits only) 2009–2010, 0. Number part-time enrolled (new admits only) 2009–2010, 0. Openings 2010–2011, 2. The median number of years required for completion of a degree in 2008–2009 were 4. The number of students enrolled full- and part-time who were dismissed or voluntarily withdrew from this program area in 2008–2009 were 0. Behavioral Neuroscience PhD (Doctor of Philosophy)—Applications 2009–2010, 15. Total applicants accepted 2009–2010, 2. Number full-time enrolled (new admits only) 2009–2010, 0. Number part-time enrolled (new admits only) 2009–2010, 0. Openings 2010–2011, 2. The median number of years required for completion of a degree in 2008–2009 were 5. The number of students enrolled full- and part-time who were dismissed or voluntarily withdrew from this program area in 2008–2009 were 0. Mathematical and Computational Cognitive Science PhD (Doctor of Philosophy)—Applications 2009–2010, 9. Total applicants accepted 2009–2010, 6. Number full-time enrolled (new admits only) 2009–2010, 2. Number part-time enrolled (new admits only) 2009–2010, 0. Openings 2010–2011, 2. The number of students enrolled full- and part-time who were dismissed or voluntarily withdrew from this program area in 2008–2009 were 0. Social Psychology PhD (Doctor of Philosophy)—Applications 2009–2010, 99. Total applicants accepted 2009–2010, 5. Number full-time enrolled (new admits only) 2009–2010, 3. Number part-time enrolled (new admits only) 2009–2010, 0. Openings 2010–2011, 3. The median number of years required for completion of a degree in 2008–2009 were 5. The number of students enrolled full- and part-time who were dismissed or voluntarily withdrew from this program area in 2008–2009 were 0.

Scores: Entries appear in this order: required test or GPA, minimum score (if required), median score of students entering in 2009–2010. Clinical Psychology PhD (Doctor of Philosophy): GRE-V no minimum stated, 605, GRE-Q no minimum stated, 683, GRE-Analytical no minimum stated, 4.6, overall undergraduate GPA 3.0, 3.69; Cognitive Psychology PhD (Doctor of Philosophy): GRE-V no minimum stated, 597, GRE-Q no minimum stated, 743, GRE-Analytical no minimum stated, 4.7, overall undergraduate GPA 3.0, 3.46; Developmental Psychology PhD (Doctor of Philosophy): GRE-V no minimum stated, 590, GRE-Q no minimum stated, 680, GRE-Analytical no minimum stated, 4.5, overall undergraduate GPA 3.0, 3.95; Industrial/Organizational Psychology PhD (Doctor of Philosophy): GRE-V no minimum stated, 593, GRE-Q no minimum stated, 660, GRE-Analytical no minimum stated, 4.8, overall undergraduate GPA 3.0, 3.58; Learning and Memory PhD (Doctor of Philosophy): GRE-V no minimum stated, GRE-Q no minimum stated, GRE-Analytical no minimum stated, overall undergraduate GPA 3.0; Behavioral Neuroscience PhD (Doctor of Philosophy): GRE-V no minimum stated, 630, GRE-Q no minimum stated, 675, GRE-Analytical no minimum stated, 4.0, overall undergraduate GPA 3.0, 3.79; Mathematical and Computational Cognitive Science PhD (Doctor of Philosophy): GRE-V no minimum stated, 608, GRE-Q no minimum stated, 778, GRE-Analytical no minimum stated, 3.8, overall undergraduate GPA 3.0, 3.66; Social Psychology PhD (Doctor of Philosophy): GRE-V no minimum stated, 618, GRE-Q no minimum stated, 674, GRE-Analytical no minimum stated, 4.9, overall undergraduate GPA 3.0, 3.56.

Other Criteria: (importance of criteria rated low, medium, or high): GRE scores—high, research experience—medium, work experience—low, extracurricular activity—low, clinically related public service—medium, GPA—high, letters of recommendation—high, interview—high, statement of goals and objectives—high, undergraduate major in psychology—medium, specific undergraduate psychology courses taken—low. Not all areas hold formal interviews. Clinically related public service is important if you are applying to the clinical program. For additional information on admission requirements, go to http://www.psych.purdue.edu.

Student Characteristics: The following represents characteristics of students in 2009–2010 in all graduate psychology programs in the department: Female—full-time 66, part-time 0; Male—full-time 21, part-time 0; African American/Black—full-time 6, part-time 0; Hispanic/Latino(a)—full-time 2, part-time 0; Asian/Pa-

cific Islander—full-time 13, part-time 0; American Indian/Alaska Native—full-time 0, part-time 0; Caucasian/White—full-time 66, part-time 0; Multi-ethnic—full-time 0, part-time 0; students subject to the Americans With Disabilities Act—full-time 0, part-time 0; Unknown ethnicity—full-time 0, part-time 0; International students who hold an F-1 or J-1 Visa—full-time 16, part-time 0.

Financial Information/Assistance:
Tuition for Full-Time Study: *Doctoral:* State residents: per academic year $9,070, $325 per credit hour; Nonstate residents: per academic year $26,622, $885 per credit hour. Tuition is subject to change. See the following Web site for updates and changes in tuition costs: http://www.purdue.edu/Bursar/fees.html.

Financial Assistance:
First-Year Students: Teaching assistantships available for first year. Average amount paid per academic year: $15,000. Average number of hours worked per week: 20. Apply by December 3. Research assistantships available for first year. Average amount paid per academic year: $15,000. Average number of hours worked per week: 20. Apply by December 3. Fellowships and scholarships available for first year. Average amount paid per academic year: $16,000. Apply by December 3.

Advanced Students: Teaching assistantships available for advanced students. Average amount paid per academic year: $15,000. Average number of hours worked per week: 20. Research assistantships available for advanced students. Average amount paid per academic year: $15,000. Average number of hours worked per week: 20. Fellowships and scholarships available for advanced students. Average amount paid per academic year: $16,000. Average number of hours worked per week: 20.

Additional Information: Of all students currently enrolled full time, 100% benefited from one or more of the listed financial assistance programs. Application and information available online at: http://www.gradschool.purdue.edu/funding/.

Internships/Practica: Doctoral Degree (PhD Clinical Psychology): For those doctoral students for whom a professional internship was required in this program prior to graduation, (3) students applied for an internship in 2008–2009, with (3) students obtaining an internship. Of those students who obtained an internship, (3) were paid internships. Of those students who obtained an internship, (3) students placed in APA/CPA accredited internships, (0) students placed in internships not APA/CPA accredited, but listed with the Association of Psychology Postdoctoral and Internship Programs (APPIC), (0) students placed in internships conforming to guidelines of the Council of Directors of School Psychology Programs (CDSPP), (0) students placed in internships that were not APA/CPA accredited, APPIC or CDSPP listed. After the first year requirements, clinical psychology students enroll in clinical practica carried out in the Purdue Psychology Treatment and Research Clinics. Practica include providing services for anxiety disorders, depression, personality disorders, Attention Deficit Hyperactivity Disorder, and oppositional disorders. Practicum training emphasizes use of empirically corroborated interventions for particular problems. A year-long clinical internship is required in order to complete training.

Housing and Day Care: On-campus housing is available. See the following Web site for more information: http://www.housing.purdue.edu. On-campus day care facilities are available. See the following Web site for more information: http://www.purdue.edu/hr/Childcare/.

Employment of Department Graduates:
Master's Degree Graduates: Of those who graduated in the academic year 2008–2009, the following categories and numbers represent the postgraduate activities and employment of master's degree graduates: Enrolled in a postdoctoral residency/fellowship (n/a), employed in independent practice (n/a), total from the above (master's) (0).

Doctoral Degree Graduates: Of those who graduated in the academic year 2008–2009, the following categories and numbers represent the postgraduate activities and employment of doctoral degree graduates: Enrolled in a psychology doctoral program (n/a), enrolled in a postdoctoral residency/fellowship (5), employed in an academic position at a university (8), employed in business or industry (3), employed in government agency (2), employed in a hospital/medical center (2), other employment position (1), total from the above (doctoral) (21).

Additional Information:
Orientation, Objectives, and Emphasis of Department: The dominant emphasis of the department is a commitment to research and scholarship as the major core of graduate education. All programs are structured so that students become involved in research activities almost immediately upon beginning their graduate education, and this involvement is expected to continue throughout an individual's entire graduate career.

Special Facilities or Resources: Excellent research facilities are available in many areas, including more than 35 computer-controlled laboratories.

Information for Students With Physical Disabilities: See the following Web site for more information: http://www.purdue.edu/odos/drc/.

Application Information:
Send to Nancy O'Brien, Administrative Assistant, Psychological Sciences, Purdue University, 701 Third Street, West Lafayette, IN 47906-2004. Application available online. URL of online application: http://www.gradschool.purdue.edu/admissions. Students are admitted in the Fall, application deadline December 3. *Fee:* $55.

Saint Francis, University of
Psychology and Counseling
School of Professional Studies
2701 Spring Street
Fort Wayne, IN 46808
Telephone: (260) 399-7700 ext 8422
Fax: (260) 399-8170
E-mail: *mfriedmeyer@sf.edu*
Web: *http://www.sf.edu/psychology*

Department Information:
1971. Chairperson: Mark H. Friedmeyer, MS. Number of faculty: total—full-time 5, part-time 5; women—full-time 1, part-time 5; minority—part-time 1; women minority—part-time 1.

GRADUATE STUDY IN PSYCHOLOGY

Programs and Degrees Offered:
Listed in the following order: Program area, degree type (T if terminal Master's), number awarded 7/08–6/09. Mental Health Counseling MA/MS (Master of Arts/Science) (T) 12, Psychology MA/MS (Master of Arts/Science) (T) 8, School Counseling MEd (Education) 8, Pastoral Counseling MA/MS (Master of Arts/Science) 0, Advanced Certificate in Pastoral Counseling 0.

Student Applications/Admissions:
Student Applications
Mental Health Counseling MA/MS (Master of Arts/Science)—Applications 2009–2010, 18. Total applicants accepted 2009–2010, 16. Number full-time enrolled (new admits only) 2009–2010, 12. Number part-time enrolled (new admits only) 2009–2010, 4. Total enrolled 2009–2010 full-time, 35, part-time, 9. Openings 2010–2011, 10. The median number of years required for completion of a degree in 2008–2009 were 3. The number of students enrolled full- and part-time who were dismissed or voluntarily withdrew from this program area in 2008–2009 were 3. *Psychology MA/MS (Master of Arts/Science)*—Applications 2009–2010, 6. Total applicants accepted 2009–2010, 6. Number full-time enrolled (new admits only) 2009–2010, 4. Number part-time enrolled (new admits only) 2009–2010, 2. Total enrolled 2009–2010 full-time, 13, part-time, 4. Openings 2010–2011, 10. The median number of years required for completion of a degree in 2008–2009 were 2. The number of students enrolled full- and part-time who were dismissed or voluntarily withdrew from this program area in 2008–2009 were 0. *School Counseling MEd (Education)*—Applications 2009–2010, 13. Total applicants accepted 2009–2010, 12. Number full-time enrolled (new admits only) 2009–2010, 10. Number part-time enrolled (new admits only) 2009–2010, 2. Total enrolled 2009–2010 full-time, 21, part-time, 5. Openings 2010–2011, 10. The median number of years required for completion of a degree in 2008–2009 were 2. The number of students enrolled full- and part-time who were dismissed or voluntarily withdrew from this program area in 2008–2009 were 0. *Pastoral Counseling MA/MS (Master of Arts/Science)*—Applications 2009–2010, 0. Total applicants accepted 2009–2010, 0. Number full-time enrolled (new admits only) 2009–2010, 0. Number part-time enrolled (new admits only) 2009–2010, 0. Openings 2010–2011, 8. The median number of years required for completion of a degree in 2008–2009 were 2. The number of students enrolled full- and part-time who were dismissed or voluntarily withdrew from this program area in 2008–2009 were 0. *Advanced Certificate in Pastoral Counseling*—Applications 2009–2010, 0. Total applicants accepted 2009–2010, 0. Number full-time enrolled (new admits only) 2009–2010, 0. Number part-time enrolled (new admits only) 2009–2010, 0. Openings 2010–2011, 10. The median number of years required for completion of a degree in 2008–2009 were 2. The number of students enrolled full- and part-time who were dismissed or voluntarily withdrew from this program area in 2008–2009 were 0.
Scores: Entries appear in this order: required test or GPA, minimum score (if required), median score of students entering in 2009–2010. *Mental Health Counseling MA/MS (Master of Arts/Science)*: overall undergraduate GPA 3.0; *Psychology MA/MS (Master of Arts/Science)*: overall undergraduate GPA 3.0; *School Counseling MEd (Education)*: GRE-V no minimum stated, GRE-Q no minimum stated, overall undergraduate GPA 2.8; *Pastoral Counseling MA/MS (Master of Arts/Science)*: overall undergraduate GPA 3.0.
Other Criteria: (importance of criteria rated low, medium, or high): GRE scores—medium, research experience—medium, work experience—high, extracurricular activity—low, clinically related public service—high, GPA—high, letters of recommendation—high, interview—high, statement of goals and objectives—high, undergraduate major in psychology—high, specific undergraduate psychology courses taken—high. For additional information on admission requirements, go to http://www.sf.edu/sf/graduate-studies/admissions/entrance-requirements.

Student Characteristics: The following represents characteristics of students in 2009–2010 in all graduate psychology programs in the department: Female—full-time 61, part-time 20; Male—full-time 8, part-time 1; African American/Black—full-time 2, part-time 2; Hispanic/Latino(a)—full-time 2, part-time 0; Asian/Pacific Islander—full-time 1, part-time 0; American Indian/Alaska Native—full-time 0, part-time 0; Caucasian/White—full-time 59, part-time 17; Multi-ethnic—full-time 5, part-time 2; students subject to the Americans With Disabilities Act—full-time 3, part-time 0; Unknown ethnicity—full-time 0, part-time 0; International students who hold an F-1 or J-1 Visa—full-time 0, part-time 0.

Financial Information/Assistance:
Tuition for Full-Time Study: *Master's:* State residents: $735 per credit hour; Nonstate residents: $735 per credit hour. Tuition is subject to change. See the following Web site for updates and changes in tuition costs: http://www.sf.edu/sf/graduate-studies/financial-aid/tuition.

Financial Assistance:
First-Year Students: Teaching assistantships available for first year. Average number of hours worked per week: 10. Apply by June 30.
Advanced Students: Teaching assistantships available for advanced students. Average number of hours worked per week: 10. Apply by June 30.
Additional Information: Of all students currently enrolled full time, 30% benefited from one or more of the listed financial assistance programs. Application and information available online at: http://www.sf.edu/sf/graduate-studies/financial-aid.

Internships/Practica: Master's Degree (MA/MS Mental Health Counseling): An internship experience, such as a final research project or "capstone" experience is required of graduates. General Psychology students can elect to do a practicum experience. This experience would be 150 clock hours (10 hours/week) of supervised practical field experience tailored to the individual needs/interests of the students. Students choosing to have a practicum experience have an on-site supervisor who helps define, mentor, and direct the student's activities. Students also have 15 hours of supervision on campus. This experience is designed to give students an opportunity to integrate formal education with work experience. Mental Health Counseling (MS) has required practicum and internship: Practicum: 1 semester-100 hours/60 face-to-face client contact hours. Internship: 1 or 2 semesters - 600 hours/240 face-to-face client contact hours. Advanced Internship: 1 semester-300 hours/120 face-to-face client contact hours. MSEd School Counseling students complete a 105-hour practicum and non-teacher licensed candidates complete a 600-hour, two-semester internship.

Housing and Day Care: No on-campus housing is available. No on-campus day care facilities are available.

Employment of Department Graduates:
Master's Degree Graduates: Of those who graduated in the academic year 2008–2009, the following categories and numbers represent the postgraduate activities and employment of master's degree graduates: Enrolled in a psychology doctoral program (2), enrolled in another graduate/professional program (0), enrolled in a postdoctoral residency/fellowship (n/a), employed in independent practice (n/a), employed in an academic position at a university (0), employed in an academic position at a 2-year/4-year college (0), employed in other positions at a higher education institution (0), employed in a professional position in a school system (8), employed in business or industry (6), employed in government agency (0), employed in a community mental health/counseling center (10), employed in a hospital/medical center (0), still seeking employment (0), not seeking employment (1), other employment position (1), total from the above (master's) (28).
Doctoral Degree Graduates: Of those who graduated in the academic year 2008–2009, the following categories and numbers represent the postgraduate activities and employment of doctoral degree graduates: Enrolled in a psychology doctoral program (n/a), total from the above (doctoral) (0).

Additional Information:
Orientation, Objectives, and Emphasis of Department: The MS in Psychology Program is designed for people who are either interested in preparation for doctoral work, or furthering their professional careers through a greater understanding of basic psychological principles. The primary goal of the program is to give students a solid, graduate-level grounding in psychology. This program emphasizes a mastery of psychological fundamentals, i.e., theories and research methods, areas of specialization (development, social, abnormal behavior, physiological data, personality development and behavior management techniques). The program of study leading to the MS Degree in Mental Health Counseling is designed to prepare persons to function as Licensed Mental Health Counselors (LMHC) in health care residential, private practice, community agency, governmental, business, and industrial settings. To successfully complete the M.S. in Mental Health Counseling, students will: 1. Demonstrate ability to analyze, synthesize, and critique in a scholarly manner academic subject matter, professional journal articles, and other professional resources. Students will demonstrate ability to write coherently and professionally according to the Publication Manual of the American Psychological Association (4th edition) standards. 2. Promote and adhere to the standards/guidelines for ethical and professional conduct in all classroom and field experiences (i.e., American Counseling Association's Ethical Standards for Mental Health Professionals, and the American Psychological Association's Ethical Principles), as well as legal mandates regarding the practice of their profession. 3. Demonstrate an ability to synthesize, evaluate, and articulate broad knowledge of counseling theories and approaches. This will include the ability to apply scientific and measurement principles to the study of psychology. 4. Develop a capacity to communicate respect, empathy, and unconditional positive regard toward others, including demonstration of a tolerant, non-judgmental attitude toward different ethnic/cultural heritage, value orientations, and lifestyles. 5. Recognize and effectively conceptualize the special needs of persons with varying mental, adjustment, developmental and/or chemical dependence disorders. Students will recognize the need for, request, and benefit from consultation and supervision when practicing in areas of insufficient competence. 6. Demonstrate competence to counsel/interview using basic listening and influencing skills in one-to-one, marital, family, and group counseling modalities. 7. Be prepared to seek employment as a Licensed Mental Health Counselor, enter a program of additional education/training, and/or seek other appropriate certifications. The MS in Pastoral Counseling program is designed for active members of the clergy with a minimum of a Bachelor's degree from an accredited college. The program consists of three parts: a core of clinical courses (18 hours) in psychology, a foundation in Pastoral Counseling (27 hours) and elective courses (6 hours). Upon completion of nine additional credits, Master's degree students can qualify to take the examination for licensure as a Licensed Professional Counselor. The Advanced Certificate in Pastoral Counseling is available for licensed mental health professionals, such as licensed clinical social workers, licensed mental health counselors, licensed marriage and family therapists, and licensed psychologists. The certificate program includes six courses (18 hours): Pastoral Theological Methods, History of Pastoral Care and Counseling, Pastoral Diagnosis, Franciscan Intellectual and Spiritual Tradition, Spirituality and Spiritual Formation and Pastoral Care Specialist Training.

Information for Students With Physical Disabilities: See the following Web site for more information: http://www.sf.edu/sf/studentservices/academics/disability.

Application Information:
Send to Office of Admissions, Trinity Hall, Room 110A, University of Saint Francis, 2701 Spring Street, Fort Wayne, IN 46808. Application available online. URL of online application: http://www.sf.edu/sf/graduate-studies/admissions/apply-online. Programs have rolling admissions. *Fee:* $20. Application fee waived if applicant applies online.

IOWA

Iowa State University
Department of Psychology
Liberal Arts & Sciences
Lagomarcino Hall
Ames, IA 50011-3180
Telephone: (515) 294-1743
Fax: (515) 294-6424
E-mail: *madon@iastate.edu*
Web: *http://www.psychology.iastate.edu/*

Department Information:
1924. Chairperson: Carolyn Cutrona. Number of faculty: total—full-time 28, part-time 4; women—full-time 10; total—minority—full-time 5, part-time 1; women minority—full-time 1.

Programs and Degrees Offered:
Listed in the following order: Program area, degree type (T if terminal Master's), number awarded 7/08–6/09. Counseling Psychology PhD (Doctor of Philosophy) 6, Social Psychology PhD (Doctor of Philosophy) 6, Cognitive Psychology PhD (Doctor of Philosophy) 3.

APA Accreditation: Counseling PhD (Doctor of Philosophy). Student Outcome Data Website: http://www.psychology.iastate.edu/index.php?id=187.

Student Applications/Admissions:
Student Applications

Counseling Psychology PhD (Doctor of Philosophy)—Applications 2009–2010, 37. Total applicants accepted 2009–2010, 4. Number full-time enrolled (new admits only) 2009–2010, 4. Number part-time enrolled (new admits only) 2009–2010, 0. Openings 2010–2011, 5. The median number of years required for completion of a degree in 2008–2009 were 6. The number of students enrolled full- and part-time who were dismissed or voluntarily withdrew from this program area in 2008–2009 were 0. *Social Psychology PhD (Doctor of Philosophy)*—Applications 2009–2010, 39. Total applicants accepted 2009–2010, 4. Number full-time enrolled (new admits only) 2009–2010, 4. Number part-time enrolled (new admits only) 2009–2010, 0. Openings 2010–2011, 3. The median number of years required for completion of a degree in 2008–2009 were 5. The number of students enrolled full- and part-time who were dismissed or voluntarily withdrew from this program area in 2008–2009 were 1. *Cognitive Psychology PhD (Doctor of Philosophy)*—Applications 2009–2010, 8. Total applicants accepted 2009–2010, 1. Number full-time enrolled (new admits only) 2009–2010, 1. Number part-time enrolled (new admits only) 2009–2010, 0. Openings 2010–2011, 3. The median number of years required for completion of a degree in 2008–2009 were 5. The number of students enrolled full- and part-time who were dismissed or voluntarily withdrew from this program area in 2008–2009 were 0.

Other Criteria: (importance of criteria rated low, medium, or high): GRE scores—high, research experience—high, work experience—low, extracurricular activity—low, clinically related public service—low, GPA—high, letters of recommendation—high, interview—high, statement of goals and objectives—high, fit with faculty research—high, undergraduate major in psychology—medium, specific undergraduate psychology courses taken—medium. For additional information on admission requirements, go to http://www.psychology.iastate.edu/.

Student Characteristics: The following represents characteristics of students in 2009–2010 in all graduate psychology programs in the department: Female—full-time 37, part-time 0; Male—full-time 19, part-time 0; African American/Black—full-time 4, part-time 0; Hispanic/Latino(a)—full-time 0, part-time 0; Asian/Pacific Islander—full-time 7, part-time 0; American Indian/Alaska Native—full-time 0, part-time 0; Caucasian/White—full-time 39, part-time 0; Multi-ethnic—full-time 0, part-time 0; students subject to the Americans With Disabilities Act—full-time 0, part-time 0; Unknown ethnicity—full-time 6, part-time 0; International students who hold an F-1 or J-1 Visa—full-time 9, part-time 0.

Financial Information/Assistance:
Tuition for Full-Time Study: *Doctoral:* State residents: per academic year $7,120; Nonstate residents: per academic year $18,548. Tuition is subject to change. See the following Web site for updates and changes in tuition costs: http://www.iastate.edu/~registrar/fees/.

Financial Assistance:
First-Year Students: Teaching assistantships available for first year. Average amount paid per academic year: $12,200. Average number of hours worked per week: 20. Apply by January 2. Research assistantships available for first year. Average amount paid per academic year: $12,200. Average number of hours worked per week: 20. Apply by January 2. Fellowships and scholarships available for first year. Average amount paid per academic year: $12,200. Average number of hours worked per week: 20. Apply by January 2.

Advanced Students: Teaching assistantships available for advanced students. Average amount paid per academic year: $12,200. Average number of hours worked per week: 20. Research assistantships available for advanced students. Average amount paid per academic year: $12,200. Average number of hours worked per week: 20.

Additional Information: Of all students currently enrolled full time, 100% benefited from one or more of the listed financial assistance programs. Application and information available online at: http://www.psychology.iastate.edu/index.php?id=28.

Internships/Practica: Doctoral Degree (PhD Counseling Psychology): For those doctoral students for whom a professional internship was required in this program prior to graduation, (4) students applied for an internship in 2008–2009, with (4) students obtaining an internship. Of those students who obtained an internship, (4) were paid internships. Of those students who obtained an internship, (4) students placed in APA/CPA accredited internships, (0) students placed in internships not APA/CPA accredited, but listed with the Association of Psychology Postdoctoral and Internship Programs (APPIC), (0) students placed in internships conforming to guidelines of the Council of Directors of School Psychology Programs (CDSPP), (0) students placed in internships that were not APA/CPA accredited, APPIC or CDSPP listed. Sequential, progressive practica provide students in our professional programs with individually supervised applied training in their specialty area. All supervision is provided by appropriately certified/licensed faculty and adjuncts in a range of settings, including university counseling centers, major hospitals, outpatient clinics, child and adolescent treatment centers, correctional facilities, and the public school system. Based on such practicum experience and their academic training, ISU students compete successfully for select predoctoral internships across the country.

Housing and Day Care: On-campus housing is available. See the following Web site for more information: http://www.housing.iastate.edu/. On-campus day care facilities are available. See the following Web site for more information: http://www.hrs.iastate.edu/childcare/homepage.shtml.

Employment of Department Graduates:
Master's Degree Graduates: Of those who graduated in the academic year 2008–2009, the following categories and numbers represent the postgraduate activities and employment of master's degree graduates: Enrolled in a postdoctoral residency/fellowship (n/a), employed in independent practice (n/a), total from the above (master's) (0).
Doctoral Degree Graduates: Of those who graduated in the academic year 2008–2009, the following categories and numbers represent the postgraduate activities and employment of doctoral degree graduates: Enrolled in a psychology doctoral program (n/a), enrolled in a postdoctoral residency/fellowship (2), employed in independent practice (2), employed in an academic position at a university (7), employed in business or industry (1), employed in a community mental health/counseling center (3), total from the above (doctoral) (15).

Additional Information:
Orientation, Objectives, and Emphasis of Department: Graduate programs emphasize the acquisition of a broad base of knowledge in psychology as well as concentration on the content and methodological skills requisite to performance in teaching, research, and applied activities. A strong research orientation is evident in all areas of the department, with involvement in research being required of all doctoral students throughout their graduate studies. Curriculum requirements for the degrees are based on a core course system, which is designed to enable students to tailor a program best suited to their particular objectives. Subsequent courses, seminars, research, and applied experiences are determined by the student and his or her graduate advisory committee. Additionally, teaching experience is available to all doctoral students, and extensive supervised practicum experience is required of students in the applied programs.

Special Facilities or Resources: The department maintains the full array of physical facilities and equipment required for behavioral research. Observational and videotaping facilities are available for research and applied training. The department maintains a microcomputer lab, and the university maintains a superior computation center.

Information for Students With Physical Disabilities: See the following Web site for more information: http://www.dso.iastate.edu/dr/.

Application Information:
Send to Iowa State University, Graduate Admissions, Department of Psychology, W112 Lagomarcino, Ames, IA 50011. Application available online. URL of online application: http://www.psychology.iastate.edu/index.php?id=29. Students are admitted in the Fall, application deadline January 2. *Fee:* $40. $90 fee for international application. Application fee is waived only for McNair scholars.

Iowa, University of
Department of Psychological and Quantitative Foundations
College of Education
361 Lindquist Center
Iowa City, IA 52242
Telephone: (319) 335-5578
Fax: (319) 335-6145
E-mail: *janet-ervin@uiowa.edu*
Web: *http://www.education.uiowa.edu/pandq/*

Department Information:
Chairperson: Timothy Ansley. Number of faculty: total—full-time 16, part-time 8; women—full-time 9, part-time 1; total—minority—full-time 3; women minority—full-time 2.

Programs and Degrees Offered:
Listed in the following order: Program area, degree type (T if terminal Master's), number awarded 7/08–6/09. Educational PhD (Doctor of Philosophy) 0, Educational Measurement and Statistics MA/MS (Master of Arts/Science) 3, Educational Measurement and Statistics PhD (Doctor of Philosophy) 8, School PhD (Doctor of Philosophy) 5, Counseling PhD (Doctor of Philosophy) 1.

APA Accreditation: School PhD (Doctor of Philosophy). Student Outcome Data Website: http://www.education.uiowa.edu/schpsych/ProgramStatistics.htm. Counseling PhD (Doctor of Philosophy). Student Outcome Data Website: http://www.education.uiowa.edu/counspsy/outcomes/index.htm.

Student Applications/Admissions:
Student Applications
Educational PhD (Doctor of Philosophy)—Applications 2009–2010, 7. Total applicants accepted 2009–2010, 4. Number full-time enrolled (new admits only) 2009–2010, 4. Number part-time enrolled (new admits only) 2009–2010, 0. Openings 2010–2011, 20. The number of students enrolled full- and part-time who were dismissed or voluntarily withdrew from this program area in 2008–2009 were 0. *Educational Measurement and Statistics MA/MS (Master of Arts/Science)*—Applications 2009–2010, 9. Total applicants accepted 2009–2010, 6. Number full-time enrolled (new admits only) 2009–2010, 6. Number part-time enrolled (new admits only) 2009–2010, 0. Openings 2010–2011, 20. The median number of years required for completion of a degree in 2008–2009 were 3. The number of students enrolled full- and part-time who were dismissed or voluntarily withdrew from this program area in 2008–2009 were 0. *Educational Measurement and Statistics PhD*

(Doctor of Philosophy)—Applications 2009–2010, 9. Total applicants accepted 2009–2010, 5. Number full-time enrolled (new admits only) 2009–2010, 5. Number part-time enrolled (new admits only) 2009–2010, 0. Openings 2010–2011, 20. The median number of years required for completion of a degree in 2008–2009 were 4. The number of students enrolled full- and part-time who were dismissed or voluntarily withdrew from this program area in 2008–2009 were 0. *School PhD (Doctor of Philosophy)*—Applications 2009–2010, 35. Total applicants accepted 2009–2010, 20. Number full-time enrolled (new admits only) 2009–2010, 9. Openings 2010–2011, 15. The median number of years required for completion of a degree in 2008–2009 were 5. *Counseling PhD (Doctor of Philosophy)*—Applications 2009–2010, 57. Total applicants accepted 2009–2010, 12. Number full-time enrolled (new admits only) 2009–2010, 10. Number part-time enrolled (new admits only) 2009–2010, 0. Openings 2010–2011, 10. The median number of years required for completion of a degree in 2008–2009 were 5. The number of students enrolled full- and part-time who were dismissed or voluntarily withdrew from this program area in 2008–2009 were 0.

Scores: Entries appear in this order: required test or GPA, minimum score (if required), median score of students entering in 2009–2010. *Educational PhD (Doctor of Philosophy)*: GRE-V no minimum stated, GRE-Q no minimum stated, overall undergraduate GPA 3.0; *Counseling PhD (Doctor of Philosophy)*: GRE-V no minimum stated, GRE-Q no minimum stated, overall undergraduate GPA no minimum stated.

Other Criteria: (importance of criteria rated low, medium, or high): GRE scores—high, research experience—high, work experience—medium, extracurricular activity—low, clinically related public service—high, GPA—high, letters of recommendation—high, interview—medium, statement of goals and objectives—high.

Student Characteristics: The following represents characteristics of students in 2009–2010 in all graduate psychology programs in the department: Female—full-time 136, part-time 0; Male—full-time 56, part-time 0; African American/Black—full-time 15, part-time 0; Hispanic/Latino(a)—full-time 5, part-time 0; Asian/Pacific Islander—full-time 2, part-time 0; American Indian/Alaska Native—full-time 1, part-time 0; Caucasian/White—full-time 119, part-time 0; Multi-ethnic—full-time 0, part-time 0; students subject to the Americans With Disabilities Act—full-time 0, part-time 0; Unknown ethnicity—full-time 0, part-time 0; International students who hold an F-1 or J-1 Visa—full-time 50, part-time 0.

Financial Information/Assistance:

Tuition for Full-Time Study: *Master's:* State residents: per academic year $6,840; Nonstate residents: per academic year $20,444. *Doctoral:* State residents: per academic year $6,840; Nonstate residents: per academic year $20,444. See the following Web site for updates and changes in tuition costs: http://www.uiowa.edu/admissions/graduate/costs/index.html.

Financial Assistance:

First-Year Students: Research assistantships available for first year. Average amount paid per academic year: $16,575. Average number of hours worked per week: 20. Apply by April 1.

Advanced Students: Research assistantships available for advanced students. Average amount paid per academic year: $16,575. Average number of hours worked per week: 20. Apply by April 1. Fellowships and scholarships available for advanced students. Average amount paid per academic year: $16,575. Average number of hours worked per week: 20.

Additional Information: Of all students currently enrolled full time, 5% benefited from one or more of the listed financial assistance programs.

Internships/Practica: Doctoral Degree (PhD Counseling): For those doctoral students for whom a professional internship was required in this program prior to graduation, (9) students applied for an internship in 2008–2009, with (9) students obtaining an internship. Of those students who obtained an internship, (9) were paid internships. Of those students who obtained an internship, (9) students placed in APA/CPA accredited internships, (0) students placed in internships not APA/CPA accredited, but listed with the Association of Psychology Postdoctoral and Internship Programs (APPIC), (0) students placed in internships conforming to guidelines of the Council of Directors of School Psychology Programs (CDSPP), (0) students placed in internships that were not APA/CPA accredited, APPIC or CDSPP listed. There are multiple practicum sites at a variety of agencies, (e.g., university counseling centers, VA medical centers, community mental health centers). In the educational psychology program, formal internship and practicum experiences are not available for MA students, although some students do find paid positions as teaching or research assistants in fields in which they have prior experience. At the PhD level, most students are supported by half-time fellowships or assistantships. In a research-oriented program, these paid positions serve the purpose of an internship or fellowship. In the school psychology program, practica are available in the public schools, The University of Iowa Hospitals and Clinics (Department of Pediatrics, Psychiatry and Neurology), the Berlin-Blank National Center for Gifted, located in the College of Education, The Wendell Johnson Speech and Hearing Clinic at the University of Iowa, and in local mental health agencies.

Housing and Day Care: On-campus housing is available. See the following Web site for more information: http://www.uiowa.edu/admissions/graduate/housing/index.html. On-campus day care facilities are available. See the following Web site for more information: http://www.uiowa.edu/admissions/graduate/community/families.htm.

Employment of Department Graduates:

Master's Degree Graduates: Of those who graduated in the academic year 2008–2009, the following categories and numbers represent the postgraduate activities and employment of master's degree graduates: Enrolled in a psychology doctoral program (1), enrolled in another graduate/professional program (2), enrolled in a postdoctoral residency/fellowship (n/a), employed in independent practice (n/a), employed in other positions at a higher education institution (1), do not know (4), total from the above (master's) (8).

Doctoral Degree Graduates: Of those who graduated in the academic year 2008–2009, the following categories and numbers represent the postgraduate activities and employment of doctoral degree graduates: Enrolled in a psychology doctoral program (n/a), enrolled in another graduate/professional program (1), enrolled in a postdoctoral residency/fellowship (1), employed in independent practice (1), employed in other positions at a higher education institution (3), employed in a professional position in a school system (1), employed in business or industry (2), employed in government agency (1), still seeking employment (1), do not know (10), total from the above (doctoral) (21).

Additional Information:

Orientation, Objectives, and Emphasis of Department: The counseling psychology program endorses a scientist–practitioner model and expects students to be competent researchers and practitioners at the completion of their program. At the PhD level, the educational psychology program at the University of Iowa is designed to provide students with strong grounding in the psychology of learning and instruction. Students are encouraged to become proficient in both quantitative and qualitative research methods with an emphasis on the former. The study of individual differences is one program emphasis. At the MA level, the program provides a broad introduction to educational psychology and flexible accommodation of individual students' interest in diverse areas such as instructional technology, reading acquisition and program evaluation. The doctoral program in school psychology is committed to training professional psychologists who are knowledgeable about providing services to children in school, medical and mental health settings. The students will possess expertise in addressing children's social/emotional needs and learning processes. The program's curriculum has been developed to reflect consideration of multicultural issues within psychological theory, research and professional development. The program strives to produce psychologists who are competent in working in a variety of settings with children/adolescents with a wide array of problems and be able to provide a wide range of psychological services to children and the adults in their lives.

Special Facilities or Resources: The University of Iowa Hospitals and Clinics provide multiple research opportunities. Outstanding computer facilities exist on the campus. Students in the educational psychology program frequently make use of two important resources of the University of Iowa College of Education. The Iowa Testing Programs, creator of the Iowa Tests of Basic Skills and the Iowa Tests of Educational Development, are housed here. Students have access to test databases for research and may work with faculty or research assistantships supported by the Iowa Measurement Research Foundation. The Berlin/Blank International Center for Gifted Education also provides opportunities for research, teaching, and counseling experiences as well as assistantship support. All of the above settings are open to students in the school psychology program for applied research and have existing data available to students as do American College Testing and National Computer Systems, located in Iowa City, IA.

Information for Students With Physical Disabilities: See the following Web site for more information: http://www.uiowa.edu/homepage/diversity/disability.html.

Application Information:
Send to Susan Cline, Student Services Admissions, College of Education, N310 Lindquist Center, Iowa City, IA 52242. Application available online. URL of online application: http://www.education.uiowa.edu/tess/Admissions.htm. Students are admitted in the Fall, application deadline December 1; Spring, application deadline September 1. For students admitted in the Fall, application deadlines are: MA: May 1-Measurement and Statistics, January 1-Educational Psychology; PhD: January 1-Educational Psychology, March 1-Measurement and Statistics, December 1-Counseling Psychology, January 1-School Psychology. For students admitted in the Spring, deadlines are: MA: November 1-Measurement and Statistics; PhD: September 1-Measurement and Statistics. *Fee:* $50.

Iowa, University of
Department of Psychology
Liberal Arts and Sciences
11 Seashore Hall East
Iowa City, IA 52242-1407
Telephone: (319) 335-2406
Fax: (319) 335-0191
E-mail: *alan-christensen@uiowa.edu*
Web: *http://www.psychology.uiowa.edu*

Department Information:
1887. Chairperson: Alan J. Christensen. Number of faculty: total—full-time 31, part-time 5; women—full-time 10, part-time 2; total—minority—full-time 1; women minority—full-time 1.

Programs and Degrees Offered:
Listed in the following order: Program area, degree type (T if terminal Master's), number awarded 7/08–6/09. Behavioral and Cognitive Neuroscience PhD (Doctor of Philosophy) 4, Clinical Psychology PhD (Doctor of Philosophy) 6, Cognition and Perception PhD (Doctor of Philosophy) 4, Developmental Science PhD (Doctor of Philosophy) 2, Personality and Social Psychology PhD (Doctor of Philosophy) 0, Health Psychology PhD (Doctor of Philosophy) 1.

APA Accreditation: Clinical PhD (Doctor of Philosophy).

Student Applications/Admissions:
Student Applications

Behavioral and Cognitive Neuroscience PhD (Doctor of Philosophy)—Applications 2009–2010, 17. Total applicants accepted 2009–2010, 5. Number full-time enrolled (new admits only) 2009–2010, 3. Number part-time enrolled (new admits only) 2009–2010, 0. Openings 2010–2011, 3. The median number of years required for completion of a degree in 2008–2009 were 6. The number of students enrolled full- and part-time who were dismissed or voluntarily withdrew from this program area in 2008–2009 were 0. *Clinical Psychology PhD (Doctor of Philosophy)*—Applications 2009–2010, 121. Total applicants accepted 2009–2010, 8. Number full-time enrolled (new admits only) 2009–2010, 3. Number part-time enrolled (new admits only) 2009–2010, 0. Openings 2010–2011, 5. The median number of years required for completion of a degree in 2008–2009 were 7. The number of students enrolled full- and part-time who were dismissed or voluntarily withdrew from this program area in 2008–2009 were 1. *Cognition and Perception PhD (Doctor of Philosophy)*—Applications 2009–2010, 24. Total applicants accepted 2009–2010, 8. Number full-time enrolled (new admits only) 2009–2010, 3. Number part-time enrolled (new admits only) 2009–2010, 0. Openings 2010–2011, 3. The median number of years required for completion of a degree in 2008–2009 were 5. The number of students enrolled full- and part-time who were dismissed or voluntarily withdrew from this program area in 2008–2009 were 0. *Developmental Science PhD (Doctor of Philosophy)*—Applications

2009–2010, 6. Total applicants accepted 2009–2010, 2. Number full-time enrolled (new admits only) 2009–2010, 2. Number part-time enrolled (new admits only) 2009–2010, 0. Openings 2010–2011, 3. The median number of years required for completion of a degree in 2008–2009 were 6. The number of students enrolled full- and part-time who were dismissed or voluntarily withdrew from this program area in 2008–2009 were 0. *Personality and Social Psychology PhD (Doctor of Philosophy)*—Applications 2009–2010, 45. Total applicants accepted 2009–2010, 1. Number full-time enrolled (new admits only) 2009–2010, 1. Number part-time enrolled (new admits only) 2009–2010, 0. Openings 2010–2011, 3. The number of students enrolled full- and part-time who were dismissed or voluntarily withdrew from this program area in 2008–2009 were 0. *Health Psychology PhD (Doctor of Philosophy)*—Applications 2009–2010, 12. Total applicants accepted 2009–2010, 2. Number full-time enrolled (new admits only) 2009–2010, 1. Number part-time enrolled (new admits only) 2009–2010, 0. Openings 2010–2011, 2. The median number of years required for completion of a degree in 2008–2009 were 6. The number of students enrolled full- and part-time who were dismissed or voluntarily withdrew from this program area in 2008–2009 were 0.

Scores: Entries appear in this order: required test or GPA, minimum score (if required), median score of students entering in 2009–2010. *Behavioral and Cognitive Neuroscience PhD (Doctor of Philosophy)*: GRE-V no minimum stated, GRE-Q no minimum stated, GRE-Analytical no minimum stated, overall undergraduate GPA no minimum stated; *Clinical Psychology PhD (Doctor of Philosophy)*: GRE-V no minimum stated, GRE-Q no minimum stated, GRE-Analytical no minimum stated, overall undergraduate GPA no minimum stated; *Cognition and Perception PhD (Doctor of Philosophy)*: GRE-V no minimum stated, GRE-Q no minimum stated, GRE-Analytical no minimum stated, overall undergraduate GPA no minimum stated; *Developmental Science PhD (Doctor of Philosophy)*: GRE-V no minimum stated, GRE-Q no minimum stated, GRE-Analytical no minimum stated, overall undergraduate GPA no minimum stated; *Personality and Social Psychology PhD (Doctor of Philosophy)*: GRE-V no minimum stated, GRE-Q no minimum stated, GRE-Analytical no minimum stated, overall undergraduate GPA no minimum stated; *Health Psychology PhD (Doctor of Philosophy)*: GRE-V no minimum stated, GRE-Q no minimum stated, GRE-Analytical no minimum stated, overall undergraduate GPA no minimum stated.

Other Criteria: (importance of criteria rated low, medium, or high): GRE scores—high, research experience—high, work experience—low, extracurricular activity—low, clinically related public service—medium, GPA—high, letters of recommendation—high, interview—high, statement of goals and objectives—high, undergraduate major in psychology—low, specific undergraduate psychology courses taken—low. For additional information on admission requirements, go to http://www.psychology.uiowa.edu.

Student Characteristics: The following represents characteristics of students in 2009–2010 in all graduate psychology programs in the department: Female—full-time 53, part-time 0; Male—full-time 30, part-time 0; African American/Black—full-time 3, part-time 0; Hispanic/Latino(a)—full-time 9, part-time 0; Asian/Pacific Islander—full-time 8, part-time 0; American Indian/Alaska Native—full-time 0, part-time 0; Caucasian/White—full-time 63, part-time 0; Multi-ethnic—full-time 0, part-time 0; students subject to the Americans With Disabilities Act—full-time 1, part-time 0; Unknown ethnicity—full-time 0, part-time 0; International students who hold an F-1 or J-1 Visa—full-time 10, part-time 0.

Financial Information/Assistance:
  Tuition for Full-Time Study: Doctoral: State residents: per academic year $7,250; Nonstate residents: per academic year $21,670. Tuition is subject to change. See the following Web site for updates and changes in tuition costs: http://www.registrar.uiowa.edu/.

Financial Assistance:
  First-Year Students: Teaching assistantships available for first year. Average amount paid per academic year: $20,258. Average number of hours worked per week: 20. Research assistantships available for first year. Average amount paid per academic year: $20,258. Average number of hours worked per week: 20. Fellowships and scholarships available for first year. Average amount paid per academic year: $21,500. Average number of hours worked per week: 0.
  Advanced Students: Teaching assistantships available for advanced students. Average amount paid per academic year: $20,381. Average number of hours worked per week: 20. Research assistantships available for advanced students. Average amount paid per academic year: $20,381. Average number of hours worked per week: 20. Fellowships and scholarships available for advanced students. Average amount paid per academic year: $25,000. Average number of hours worked per week: 0.
  Additional Information: Of all students currently enrolled full time, 100% benefited from one or more of the listed financial assistance programs. Application and information available online at: http://www.grad.uiowa.edu/financing-your-education.

Internships/Practica: Doctoral Degree (PhD Clinical Psychology): For those doctoral students for whom a professional internship was required in this program prior to graduation, (6) students applied for an internship in 2008–2009, with (6) students obtaining an internship. Of those students who obtained an internship, (6) were paid internships. Of those students who obtained an internship, (6) students placed in APA/CPA accredited internships, (0) students placed in internships not APA/CPA accredited, but listed with the Association of Psychology Postdoctoral and Internship Programs (APPIC), (0) students placed in internships conforming to guidelines of the Council of Directors of School Psychology Programs (CDSPP), (0) students placed in internships that were not APA/CPA accredited, APPIC or CDSPP listed. Students in our Clinical Psychology program participate in clinical assessment and treatment practica at our department-run clinic (the Carl E. Seashore Psychology Training Clinic) and in clinics run by departments such as Psychiatry and Neurology at the University of Iowa Hospitals and Clinics.

Housing and Day Care: On-campus housing is available. See the following Web site for more information: http://www.uiowa.edu/admissions/graduate/housing/. On-campus day care facilities are available. See the following Web site for more information: http://www.uiowa.edu/hr/famserv/index.html.

Employment of Department Graduates:
  Master's Degree Graduates: Of those who graduated in the academic year 2008–2009, the following categories and numbers

represent the postgraduate activities and employment of master's degree graduates: Enrolled in a postdoctoral residency/fellowship (n/a), employed in independent practice (n/a), total from the above (master's) (0).

Doctoral Degree Graduates: Of those who graduated in the academic year 2008–2009, the following categories and numbers represent the postgraduate activities and employment of doctoral degree graduates: Enrolled in a psychology doctoral program (n/a), enrolled in a postdoctoral residency/fellowship (8), employed in an academic position at a university (6), employed in business or industry (1), employed in government agency (1), employed in a hospital/medical center (1), total from the above (doctoral) (17).

Additional Information:
Orientation, Objectives, and Emphasis of Department: The mission of the PhD program is to produce professional scholars who contribute significantly to the advancement of scientific psychological knowledge and who can effectively teach students about the science of psychology. Some of these scholars are also prepared to deliver psychological services. Our goal is to produce PhDs who have developed world-class programs of research, who have published extensively, and who have both broad and deep knowledge. Graduate training is organized into six broad training areas: Behavioral & Cognitive Neuroscience, Clinical Psychology, Cognition & Perception, Developmental Science, Health Psychology, and Personality & Social Psychology. The training programs are flexible, and there is considerable overlap and interaction among students and faculty in all areas, leading to an exciting intellectual environment. Students in good standing receive full support for at least five years. The student-faculty ratio remains quite low, usually less than 2 to 1. The department has been successful in establishing strong ties with other campus units such as Psychiatry, Neurology, the law school, and the business school. Through these associations, one may study such topics as the law and psychology, aging, consumer behavior, and neuroscience.

Special Facilities or Resources: The Kenneth W. Spence Laboratories of Psychology and adjoining space in Seashore Hall include automated data acquisition and analysis systems, extensive computing facilities, observation suites with remote audiovisual control and recording equipment, multiple animal facilities, several surgeries, a histology laboratory, soundproof chambers, closed-circuit TV systems, electrophysiological recording rooms, conditioning laboratories, the Carl E. Seashore Psychology Training Clinic, and well-equipped electronic, mechanical, woodworking, and computer shops. Well over half of the departmental laboratories have been extensively renovated or created anew within the past 5 years. In addition, many resources are available through collaboration with colleagues at the university hospital, the Iowa Veterans Administration Hospital, community service centers, and the Colleges of Medicine, Nursing, Dentistry, Engineering, Business, Education, and Law.

Information for Students With Physical Disabilities: See the following Web site for more information: http://www.uiowa.edu/~eod/disability/.

Application Information:
Send to Graduate Admissions Office, 11 Seashore Hall E. Application available online. URL of online application: http://www.uiowa.edu/admissions/graduate. Students are admitted in the Fall, application deadline December 15. *Fee:* $60. $100 for international applicants.

Northern Iowa, University of
Department of Psychology
Social and Behavioral Sciences
334 Baker Hall
Cedar Falls, IA 50614-0505
Telephone: (319) 273-2303
Fax: (319) 273-6188
E-mail: *harton@uni.edu*
Web: *http://www.uni.edu/psych/graduate*

Department Information:
1968. Interim Head: Carolyn Hildebrandt. Number of faculty: total—full-time 15, part-time 7; women—full-time 6, part-time 2; minority—part-time 1; women minority—part-time 1.

Programs and Degrees Offered:
Listed in the following order: Program area, degree type (T if terminal Master's), number awarded 7/08–6/09. Social Psychology MA/MS (Master of Arts/Science) (T) 3, Industrial/Organizational Psychology MA/MS (Master of Arts/Science) (T) 8, Clinical Science MA/MS (Master of Arts/Science) (T) 7, Individualized Study MA/MS (Master of Arts/Science) 1.

Student Applications/Admissions:
Student Applications
Social Psychology MA/MS *(Master of Arts/Science)*—Applications 2009–2010, 15. Total applicants accepted 2009–2010, 8. Number full-time enrolled (new admits only) 2009–2010, 3. Number part-time enrolled (new admits only) 2009–2010, 0. Openings 2010–2011, 4. The median number of years required for completion of a degree in 2008–2009 were 2. The number of students enrolled full- and part-time who were dismissed or voluntarily withdrew from this program area in 2008–2009 were 0. *Industrial/Organizational Psychology MA/MS (Master of Arts/Science)*—Applications 2009–2010, 36. Total applicants accepted 2009–2010, 22. Number full-time enrolled (new admits only) 2009–2010, 8. Number part-time enrolled (new admits only) 2009–2010, 0. The median number of years required for completion of a degree in 2008–2009 were 2. The number of students enrolled full- and part-time who were dismissed or voluntarily withdrew from this program area in 2008–2009 were 3. *Clinical Science MA/MS (Master of Arts/Science)*—Applications 2009–2010, 22. Total applicants accepted 2009–2010, 13. Number full-time enrolled (new admits only) 2009–2010, 7. Number part-time enrolled (new admits only) 2009–2010, 0. Openings 2010–2011, 7. The median number of years required for completion of a degree in 2008–2009 were 2. The number of students enrolled full- and part-time who were dismissed or voluntarily withdrew from this program area in 2008–2009 were 1. *Individualized Study MA/MS (Master of Arts/Science)*—Applications 2009–2010, 1. Total applicants accepted 2009–2010, 1. Number full-time enrolled (new admits only) 2009–2010, 1. Number part-time enrolled (new admits only) 2009–2010, 0. Openings 2010–2011, 1. The median number of years required for completion of a degree in 2008–2009 were 2. The number of students enrolled full- and part-time who were dismissed or voluntarily withdrew from this program area in 2008–2009 were 0.

Scores: Entries appear in this order: required test or GPA, minimum score (if required), median score of students entering

in 2009–2010. *Social Psychology MA/MS (Master of Arts/Science)*: GRE-V 450, 520, GRE-Q 450, 630, overall undergraduate GPA 3.2, 3.48; *Industrial/Organizational Psychology MA/MS (Master of Arts/Science)*: GRE-V 450, 450, GRE-Q 450, 610, overall undergraduate GPA 3.2, 3.52; *Clinical Science MA/MS (Master of Arts/Science)*: GRE-V 450, 450, GRE-Q 450, 500, overall undergraduate GPA 3.0; *Individualized Study MA/MS (Master of Arts/Science)*: GRE-V 450, 510, GRE-Q 450, 450, overall undergraduate GPA 3.2, 3.41.

Other Criteria: (importance of criteria rated low, medium, or high): GRE scores—high, research experience—high, work experience—medium, extracurricular activity—low, clinically related public service—medium, GPA—high, letters of recommendation—high, interview—medium, statement of goals and objectives—high, undergraduate major in psychology—high, specific undergraduate psychology courses taken—medium. Clinically related public service is less important for the social and industrial/organizational emphases; work experience is less important for the social emphasis. For additional information on admission requirements, go to http://www.uni.edu/psych/graduate.html.

Student Characteristics: The following represents characteristics of students in 2009–2010 in all graduate psychology programs in the department: Female—full-time 20, part-time 0; Male—full-time 13, part-time 0; African American/Black—full-time 1, part-time 0; Hispanic/Latino(a)—full-time 2, part-time 0; Asian/Pacific Islander—full-time 1, part-time 0; American Indian/Alaska Native—full-time 1, part-time 0; Caucasian/White—full-time 28, part-time 0; Multi-ethnic—full-time 0, part-time 0; students subject to the Americans With Disabilities Act—full-time 0, part-time 0; Unknown ethnicity—full-time 0, part-time 0; International students who hold an F-1 or J-1 Visa—full-time 2, part-time 0.

Financial Information/Assistance:
Tuition for Full-Time Study: *Master's:* State residents: per academic year $6,716; Nonstate residents: per academic year $15,172. Tuition is subject to change. See the following Web site for updates and changes in tuition costs: http://www.uni.edu/tuition/.

Financial Assistance:
First-Year Students: Teaching assistantships available for first year. Average amount paid per academic year: $4,196. Average number of hours worked per week: 10. Apply by February 1. Research assistantships available for first year. Average amount paid per academic year: $4,196. Average number of hours worked per week: 10. Apply by February 1. Traineeships available for first year. Average amount paid per academic year: $4,196. Average number of hours worked per week: 10. Apply by February 1. Fellowships and scholarships available for first year. Average amount paid per academic year: $3,358. Average number of hours worked per week: 0. Apply by February 1.

Advanced Students: Teaching assistantships available for advanced students. Average amount paid per academic year: $4,196. Average number of hours worked per week: 10. Apply by February 1. Research assistantships available for advanced students. Average amount paid per academic year: $4,196. Average number of hours worked per week: 10. Apply by February 1. Traineeships available for advanced students. Average amount paid per academic year: $4,196. Average number of hours worked per week: 10. Apply by February 1. Fellowships and scholarships available for advanced students. Average amount paid per academic year: $3,358. Average number of hours worked per week: 0. Apply by February 1.

Additional Information: Of all students currently enrolled full time, 100% benefited from one or more of the listed financial assistance programs. Application and information available online at: http://www.uni.edu/finaid.

Internships/Practica: Master's Degree (MA/MS Social Psychology): An internship experience, such as a final research project or "capstone" experience is required of graduates. Master's Degree (MA/MS Industrial/Organizational Psychology): An internship experience, such as a final research project or "capstone" experience is required of graduates. Master's Degree (MA/MS Clinical Science): An internship experience, such as a final research project or "capstone" experience is required of graduates. A variety of practicum sites are available for second year students in the clinical science and industrial/organizational emphases. Clinical practicum sites have included the University Counseling Center, the State Psychiatric Hospital, correctional facilities, private hospitals, educational settings, and community-based agencies. I/O practicum sites have included the University's Human Resources Office, John Deere, Waterloo Industries, 3-M, and other local and out-of-state (during summer terms) businesses. Students in the social emphasis conduct independent first-year research projects under faculty supervision and present these research projects at regional and national professional conferences.

Housing and Day Care: On-campus housing is available. See the following Web site for more information: http://www.uni.edu/dor/. No on-campus day care facilities are available.

Employment of Department Graduates:
Master's Degree Graduates: Of those who graduated in the academic year 2008–2009, the following categories and numbers represent the postgraduate activities and employment of master's degree graduates: Enrolled in a psychology doctoral program (8), enrolled in another graduate/professional program (0), enrolled in a postdoctoral residency/fellowship (n/a), employed in independent practice (n/a), employed in an academic position at a university (2), employed in other positions at a higher education institution (1), employed in business or industry (5), employed in government agency (1), not seeking employment (1), do not know (1), total from the above (master's) (19).
Doctoral Degree Graduates: Of those who graduated in the academic year 2008–2009, the following categories and numbers represent the postgraduate activities and employment of doctoral degree graduates: Enrolled in a psychology doctoral program (n/a), total from the above (doctoral) (0).

Additional Information:
Orientation, Objectives, and Emphasis of Department: The MA program in General Psychology provides a strong empirical, research-based approach to the study of human behavior. Students may select one of three emphases: a) clinical science; b) social psychology; or c) industrial-organizational psychology. They may also choose to complete an individualized study program in conjunction with a faculty mentor. The objectives of the program are: a) to develop skills in research methodology; b) to gain knowledge of basic areas of scientific psychology; and c) to obtain competence in research, consulting, and/or clinical skills. The clinical science emphasis is designed for those who wish to either

obtain doctoral degrees in clinical or counseling psychology or become master's-level providers of services operating in clinical settings under appropriate supervision. The social emphasis is designed for students who wish to pursue doctoral degrees in social psychology or master's-level research or teaching positions. The industrial/organizational emphasis is designed for those planning doctoral study in I/O psychology or a position in human resources or consulting.

Special Facilities or Resources: The department provides laboratory space for research with human participants; access to community facilities and populations for applied research; 24/7 access to computers for graduate students; and office space for graduate students. We are affiliated with a laboratory school and a center for social research, and students have access to psychiatric, work, and community populations for research projects.

Information for Students With Physical Disabilities: See the following Web site for more information: http://www.uni.edu/disability/.

Application Information:
Send to Graduate Coordinator, Department of Psychology, University of Northern Iowa, Cedar Falls, IA 50614-0505. Application available online. URL of online application: http://www.uni.edu/psych/graduate.html. Students are admitted in the Fall, application deadline April 30. For full consideration, applications should be received by February 1, although applications will be considered if received by April 30 as space permits. *Fee:* $40. Application fee for international students is $50.

KANSAS

Emporia State University
Department of Psychology, Art Therapy, Rehabilitation, and Mental Health Counseling
The Teachers College
1200 Commercial Street
Emporia, KS 66801-5087
Telephone: (620) 341-5317
Fax: (620) 341-5801
E-mail: *parm@emporia.edu*
Web: *http://www.emporia.edu/parm*

Department Information:
1932. Interim Chair: Brian W. Schrader. Number of faculty: total—full-time 16, part-time 2; women—full-time 8, part-time 1; faculty subject to the Americans With Disabilities Act 2.

Programs and Degrees Offered:
Listed in the following order: Program area, degree type (T if terminal Master's), number awarded 7/08–6/09. General Experimental MA/MS (Master of Arts/Science) (T) 3, School EdS (School Psychology) 6, Clinical Psychology MA/MS (Master of Arts/Science) (T) 9, Industrial/Organizational Psychology MA/MS (Master of Arts/Science) (T) 8.

Student Applications/Admissions:
Student Applications
General Experimental MA/MS (Master of Arts/Science)—Applications 2009–2010, 7. Total applicants accepted 2009–2010, 6. Number full-time enrolled (new admits only) 2009–2010, 4. Number part-time enrolled (new admits only) 2009–2010, 0. Openings 2010–2011, 15. The median number of years required for completion of a degree in 2008–2009 were 2. The number of students enrolled full- and part-time who were dismissed or voluntarily withdrew from this program area in 2008–2009 were 0. School EdS (School Psychology)—Applications 2009–2010, 12. Total applicants accepted 2009–2010, 10. Number full-time enrolled (new admits only) 2009–2010, 8. Number part-time enrolled (new admits only) 2009–2010, 0. Total enrolled 2009–2010 full-time, 15, part-time, 6. Openings 2010–2011, 15. The median number of years required for completion of a degree in 2008–2009 were 3. The number of students enrolled full- and part-time who were dismissed or voluntarily withdrew from this program area in 2008–2009 were 0. Clinical Psychology MA/MS (Master of Arts/Science)—Applications 2009–2010, 14. Total applicants accepted 2009–2010, 10. Number full-time enrolled (new admits only) 2009–2010, 7. Total enrolled 2009–2010 full-time, 18, part-time, 2. Openings 2010–2011, 15. The median number of years required for completion of a degree in 2008–2009 were 2. Industrial/Organizational Psychology MA/MS (Master of Arts/Science)—Applications 2009–2010, 14. Total applicants accepted 2009–2010, 12. Number full-time enrolled (new admits only) 2009–2010, 7. Number part-time enrolled (new admits only) 2009–2010, 0. Total enrolled 2009–2010 full-time, 27, part-time, 5. Openings 2010–2011, 15. The median number of years required for completion of a degree in 2008–2009 were 2. The number of students enrolled full- and part-time who were dismissed or voluntarily withdrew from this program area in 2008–2009 were 0.

Scores: Entries appear in this order: required test or GPA, minimum score (if required), median score of students entering in 2009–2010. *General Experimental MA/MS (Master of Arts/Science)*: GRE-V no minimum stated, GRE-Q no minimum stated, overall undergraduate GPA 3.00, last 2 years GPA 3.25; *School EdS (School Psychology)*: GRE-V no minimum stated, GRE-Q no minimum stated, overall undergraduate GPA 3.00, last 2 years GPA 3.25; *Clinical Psychology MA/MS (Master of Arts/Science)*: GRE-V no minimum stated, GRE-Q no minimum stated, overall undergraduate GPA 3.00, last 2 years GPA 3.25, psychology GPA 3.0; *Industrial/Organizational Psychology MA/MS (Master of Arts/Science)*: GRE-V no minimum stated, GRE-Q no minimum stated, overall undergraduate GPA 3.00, last 2 years GPA 3.25.

Other Criteria: (importance of criteria rated low, medium, or high): GRE scores—low, research experience—medium, work experience—medium, extracurricular activity—low, clinically related public service—low, GPA—high, letters of recommendation—high, statement of goals and objectives—high, undergraduate major in psychology—high, specific undergraduate psychology courses taken—high. For additional information on admission requirements, go to http://www.emporia.edu/parm/.

Student Characteristics: The following represents characteristics of students in 2009–2010 in all graduate psychology programs in the department: Female—full-time 48, part-time 12; Male—full-time 25, part-time 8; African American/Black—full-time 10, part-time 0; Hispanic/Latino(a)—full-time 4, part-time 0; Asian/Pacific Islander—full-time 2, part-time 0; American Indian/Alaska Native—full-time 0, part-time 0; Caucasian/White—full-time 0, part-time 0; Multi-ethnic—full-time 6, part-time 0; students subject to the Americans With Disabilities Act—full-time 1, part-time 0; Unknown ethnicity—full-time 0, part-time 0; International students who hold an F-1 or J-1 Visa—full-time 0, part-time 0.

Financial Information/Assistance:
Tuition for Full-Time Study: *Master's:* State residents: per academic year $5,002, $231 per credit hour; Nonstate residents: per academic year $13,812, $594 per credit hour. Tuition is subject to change. See the following Web site for updates and changes in tuition costs: http://www.emporia.edu/busaff/tuitwaiv.htm.

Financial Assistance:
First-Year Students: Teaching assistantships available for first year. Average amount paid per academic year: $7,009. Average number of hours worked per week: 20. Apply by March 15. Research assistantships available for first year. Average amount paid per academic year: $7,009. Average number of hours worked per week: 20. Apply by March 15. Fellowships and scholarships available for first year. Average amount paid per academic year: $300.

Advanced Students: Teaching assistantships available for advanced students. Average amount paid per academic year:

$7,009. Average number of hours worked per week: 20. Apply by March 15. Research assistantships available for advanced students. Average amount paid per academic year: $7,009. Average number of hours worked per week: 20. Apply by March 15. Fellowships and scholarships available for advanced students. Average amount paid per academic year: $300.

Additional Information: Of all students currently enrolled full time, 70% benefited from one or more of the listed financial assistance programs. Application and information available online at: http://www.emporia.edu/grad/load.htm.

Internships/Practica: Master's Degree (MA/MS Clinical Psychology): An internship experience, such as a final research project or "capstone" experience is required of graduates. Master's Degree (MA/MS Industrial/Organizational Psychology): An internship experience, such as a final research project or "capstone" experience is required of graduates. For Clinical students, internship is 750 clock hours in a mental health setting supervised by a PhD psychologist. For I/O students the internship is 300 clock hours in a business setting performing I/O-related tasks. For Experimental students, the internship is defined as experiences working in a laboratory setting. School Psychology and Special Education students do semester internships/practica in the schools. In addition, there is a one-year, paid, post-EdS internship for School Psychology.

Housing and Day Care: On-campus housing is available. See the following Web site for more information: http://www.emporia.edu/reslife/index.htm. On-campus day care facilities are available. See the following Web site for more information: http://cece.emporia.edu/.

Employment of Department Graduates:
Master's Degree Graduates: Of those who graduated in the academic year 2008–2009, the following categories and numbers represent the postgraduate activities and employment of master's degree graduates: Enrolled in a psychology doctoral program (3), enrolled in another graduate/professional program (1), enrolled in a postdoctoral residency/fellowship (n/a), employed in independent practice (n/a), employed in an academic position at a university (1), employed in an academic position at a 2-year/4-year college (1), employed in a professional position in a school system (6), employed in business or industry (8), employed in government agency (2), employed in a community mental health/counseling center (7), employed in a hospital/medical center (1), still seeking employment (1), do not know (2), total from the above (master's) (33).
Doctoral Degree Graduates: Of those who graduated in the academic year 2008–2009, the following categories and numbers represent the postgraduate activities and employment of doctoral degree graduates: Enrolled in a psychology doctoral program (n/a), total from the above (doctoral) (0).

Additional Information:
Orientation, Objectives, and Emphasis of Department: Emporia State offers the Master of Science degree in general experimental psychology, clinical psychology, and industrial/organizational psychology. Additionally, students may pursue the EdS degree in school psychology.

Special Facilities or Resources: In 1999, all classrooms in the Department of Psychology, Art Therapy, Rehabilitation, and Mental Health Counseling were upgraded with multimedia technology. Facilities include cognitive and animal behavior, and physiological psychology laboratories; a complete animal vivarium; suites of rooms for administration of psychological tests and observation of testing or clinical and counseling sessions; and microprocessors and mainframe computer facilities. The computers and animal lab have been periodically updated every three years.

Information for Students With Physical Disabilities: See the following Web site for more information: http://www.emporia.edu/disability/.

Application Information:
Send to Dean of Graduate Studies and Research, Campus Box 4003, Emporia State University, 1200 Commercial St., Emporia, KS 66801. Application available online. URL of online application: http://www.emporia.edu/parm/. Students are admitted in the Spring, application deadline October 1; Summer, application deadline March 1; Fall, application deadline June 1. Most programs have continuous admission/enrollment but the application deadline dates give the student the optimal opportunity for financial aid, etc. *Fee:* $40.

Fort Hays State University (2009 data)
Department of Psychology
600 Park Street
Hays, KS 67601-4099
Telephone: (785) 628-4405
Fax: (785) 628-5861
E-mail: *hmarrs@fhsu.edu*
Web: *http://www.fhsu.edu/psych/*

Department Information:
1929. Chair: Heath Marrs. Number of faculty: total—full-time 7, part-time 1; women—full-time 4.

Programs and Degrees Offered:
Listed in the following order: Program area, degree type (T if terminal Master's), number awarded 7/08–6/09. Applied Clinical MA/MS (Master of Arts/Science) (T) 6, General MA/MS (Master of Arts/Science) (T) 1, School EdS (School Psychology) 5.

Student Applications/Admissions:
Student Applications
Applied Clinical MA/MS (Master of Arts/Science)—Applications 2009–2010, 6. Total applicants accepted 2009–2010, 4. Number full-time enrolled (new admits only) 2009–2010, 4. Number part-time enrolled (new admits only) 2009–2010, 0. Total enrolled 2009–2010 full-time, 10, part-time, 2. Openings 2010–2011, 7. The median number of years required for completion of a degree in 2008–2009 were 2. The number of students enrolled full- and part-time who were dismissed or voluntarily withdrew from this program area in 2008–2009 were 0. General MA/MS (Master of Arts/Science)—Applications 2009–2010, 3. Total applicants accepted 2009–2010, 3. Number full-time enrolled (new admits only) 2009–2010, 2. Number part-time enrolled (new admits only) 2009–2010, 1. Total enrolled 2009–2010 full-time, 2, part-time, 1. Openings 2010–2011, 5. The median number of years required for com-

pletion of a degree in 2008–2009 were 2. The number of students enrolled full- and part-time who were dismissed or voluntarily withdrew from this program area in 2008–2009 were 0. *School EdS (School Psychology)*—Applications 2009–2010, 6. Total applicants accepted 2009–2010, 6. Number full-time enrolled (new admits only) 2009–2010, 6. Number part-time enrolled (new admits only) 2009–2010, 0. Total enrolled 2009–2010 full-time, 12, part-time, 2. Openings 2010–2011, 7. The median number of years required for completion of a degree in 2008–2009 were 2. The number of students enrolled full- and part-time who were dismissed or voluntarily withdrew from this program area in 2008–2009 were 0.

Other Criteria: (importance of criteria rated low, medium, or high): GRE scores—medium, research experience—medium, work experience—medium, extracurricular activity—medium, clinically related public service—medium, GPA—high, letters of recommendation—high, interview—medium, statement of goals and objectives—medium.

Student Characteristics: The following represents characteristics of students in 2009–2010 in all graduate psychology programs in the department: Female—full-time 22, part-time 3; Male—full-time 9, part-time 3; African American/Black—full-time 0, part-time 0; Hispanic/Latino(a)—full-time 2, part-time 0; Asian/Pacific Islander—full-time 0, part-time 0; American Indian/Alaska Native—full-time 0, part-time 0; Caucasian/White—full-time 0, part-time 0; Multi-ethnic—full-time 0, part-time 1; students subject to the Americans With Disabilities Act—full-time 0, part-time 0; Unknown ethnicity—full-time 0, part-time 0; International students who hold an F-1 or J-1 Visa—full-time 0, part-time 0.

Financial Information/Assistance:
Tuition for Full-Time Study: *Master's:* State residents: $163 per credit hour; Nonstate residents: $431 per credit hour. Tuition is subject to change. See the following Web site for updates and changes in tuition costs: http://www.fhsu.edu/gradschl/.

Financial Assistance:
First-Year Students: Teaching assistantships available for first year. Apply by March 1.
Advanced Students: Teaching assistantships available for advanced students. Apply by March 1. Fellowships and scholarships available for advanced students. Average amount paid per academic year: $600. Apply by March 15.
Additional Information: Of all students currently enrolled full time, 70% benefited from one or more of the listed financial assistance programs. Application and information available online at: http://www.fhsu.edu/gradschl/.

Internships/Practica: Master's Degree (MA/MS Applied Clinical): An internship experience, such as a final research project or "capstone" experience is required of graduates. Master's Degree (MA/MS General): An internship experience, such as a final research project or "capstone" experience is required of graduates. All students in the applied psychology programs (clinical, school) are required to take a practicum in their specialty area. Students in the clinical psychology program receive initial practicum experience in the Kelly Center (an on-campus psychological services center), and then are required to complete an internship off-campus at a regional mental health agency or other approved agency. Students in the school psychology program receive initial practicum experience in a school district. School psychology graduates are also required to complete one year of paid, supervised post-EdS internship before being recommended for full Licensure (certification). Students in the general psychology program have the opportunity to take apprenticeships concentrating on the teaching of psychology.

Housing and Day Care: On-campus housing is available. See the following Web site for more information: http://www.fhsu.edu/reslife/. On-campus day care facilities are available. See the following Web site for more information: http://www.fhsu.edu/tigertots/.

Employment of Department Graduates:
Master's Degree Graduates: Of those who graduated in the academic year 2008–2009, the following categories and numbers represent the postgraduate activities and employment of master's degree graduates: Enrolled in a postdoctoral residency/fellowship (n/a), employed in independent practice (n/a), total from the above (master's) (0).
Doctoral Degree Graduates: Of those who graduated in the academic year 2008–2009, the following categories and numbers represent the postgraduate activities and employment of doctoral degree graduates: Enrolled in a psychology doctoral program (n/a), total from the above (doctoral) (0).

Additional Information:
Orientation, Objectives, and Emphasis of Department: The department emphasizes a research approach to the understanding of behavior. We strive to provide basic empirical and theoretical foundations of psychology to prepare the student for doctoral study, for teaching, or for employment in a service or professional agency. The school program offers broad preparation for students in both psychology and education and includes training as a consultant to work with educators and parents as well as with children. The clinical program emphasizes the preparation of rural mental health workers, although many graduates go on to doctoral programs. The general program is intended to prepare the student for doctoral study.

Special Facilities or Resources: The department of psychology now occupies a newly remodeled building in the center of campus. Some of the new facilities in this building include: a 25-machine computer facility with separate spaces for individualized research and full Internet connections; testing and observation rooms for children, adults, and small groups; separate research and teaching labs for the major areas of psychology; an isolated small animal facility; and several seminar rooms. We are located adjacent to the student psychological services center. There is an active social organization for psychology graduate students. All students at the university have free remote Internet access.

Information for Students With Physical Disabilities: See the following Web site for more information: http://www.fhsu.edu/disability.

Application Information:
Send to Dean of the Graduate School, Fort Hays State University, 600 Park Street, Hays, KS 67601-4099. Application available online. URL of online application: http://www.fhsu.edu/gradschl/forms.shtml. Students are admitted in the Fall; Programs have rolling admissions. Deadline for financial aid is March 1. *Fee:* $35.

Kansas State University
Department of Psychology
College of Arts and Sciences
492 Bluemont Hall - 1100 Mid-Campus Drive
Manhattan, KS 66506-5302
Telephone: (785) 532-6850
Fax: (785) 532-5401
E-mail: psych@ksu.edu
Web: http://www.k-state.edu/psych/index.htm

Department Information:
1951. Head: Jerome Frieman. Number of faculty: total—full-time 17, part-time 7; women—full-time 5, part-time 1.

Programs and Degrees Offered:
Listed in the following order: Program area, degree type (T if terminal Master's), number awarded 7/08–6/09. Animal Learning/Behavioral Neuroscience PhD (Doctor of Philosophy) 2, Cognitive and Human Factors PhD (Doctor of Philosophy) 3, Social/Personality Psychology PhD (Doctor of Philosophy) 3, Industrial/Organizational Psychology PhD (Doctor of Philosophy) 0, Industrial/Organizational (Distance) MA/MS (Master of Arts/Science) (T) 11, Occupational Health Psychology Other 3.

Student Applications/Admissions:
Student Applications
Animal Learning/Behavioral Neuroscience PhD (Doctor of Philosophy)—Applications 2009–2010, 9. Total applicants accepted 2009–2010, 5. Number full-time enrolled (new admits only) 2009–2010, 1. Total enrolled 2009–2010 full-time, 8. The median number of years required for completion of a degree in 2008–2009 were 5. The number of students enrolled full- and part-time who were dismissed or voluntarily withdrew from this program area in 2008–2009 were 0. *Cognitive and Human Factors PhD (Doctor of Philosophy)*—Applications 2009–2010, 18. Total applicants accepted 2009–2010, 4. Number full-time enrolled (new admits only) 2009–2010, 2. Number part-time enrolled (new admits only) 2009–2010, 0. Total enrolled 2009–2010 full-time, 12, part-time, 2. Openings 2010–2011, 3. The median number of years required for completion of a degree in 2008–2009 were 5. The number of students enrolled full- and part-time who were dismissed or voluntarily withdrew from this program area in 2008–2009 were 0. *Social/Personality Psychology PhD (Doctor of Philosophy)*—Applications 2009–2010, 25. Total applicants accepted 2009–2010, 6. Number full-time enrolled (new admits only) 2009–2010, 2. Total enrolled 2009–2010 full-time, 14. Openings 2010–2011, 3. The median number of years required for completion of a degree in 2008–2009 were 5. The number of students enrolled full- and part-time who were dismissed or voluntarily withdrew from this program area in 2008–2009 were 0. *Industrial/Organizational Psychology PhD (Doctor of Philosophy)*—Applications 2009–2010, 27. Total applicants accepted 2009–2010, 6. Number full-time enrolled (new admits only) 2009–2010, 2. Total enrolled 2009–2010 full-time, 16, part-time, 9. Openings 2010–2011, 2. The median number of years required for completion of a degree in 2008–2009 were 5. The number of students enrolled full- and part-time who were dismissed or voluntarily withdrew from this program area in 2008–2009 were 0. *Industrial/Organizational (Distance) MA/MS (Master of Arts/Science)*—Applications 2009–2010, 24. Total applicants accepted 2009–2010, 12. Number part-time enrolled (new admits only) 2009–2010, 12. Total enrolled 2009–2010 part-time, 25. Openings 2010–2011, 15. The median number of years required for completion of a degree in 2008–2009 were 2. The number of students enrolled full- and part-time who were dismissed or voluntarily withdrew from this program area in 2008–2009 were 0. *Occupational Health Psychology Other*—Applications 2009–2010, 5. Total applicants accepted 2009–2010, 4. Number part-time enrolled (new admits only) 2009–2010, 4. Total enrolled 2009–2010 part-time, 6. Openings 2010–2011, 10. The median number of years required for completion of a degree in 2008–2009 were 2. The number of students enrolled full- and part-time who were dismissed or voluntarily withdrew from this program area in 2008–2009 were 1.

Scores: Entries appear in this order: required test or GPA, minimum score (if required), median score of students entering in 2009–2010. *Cognitive and Human Factors PhD (Doctor of Philosophy)*: GRE-V no minimum stated, GRE-Q no minimum stated, overall undergraduate GPA 3.0; *Industrial/Organizational (Distance) MA/MS (Master of Arts/Science)*: overall undergraduate GPA 3.0.

Other Criteria: (importance of criteria rated low, medium, or high): GRE scores—high, research experience—high, work experience—low, extracurricular activity—low, clinically related public service—low, GPA—high, letters of recommendation—high, statement of goals and objectives—high. For additional information on admission requirements, go to http://www.k-state.edu/psych/graduate/graduate_application_procedures.htm.

Student Characteristics: The following represents characteristics of students in 2009–2010 in all graduate psychology programs in the department: Female—full-time 24, part-time 12; Male—full-time 18, part-time 5; African American/Black—full-time 1, part-time 1; Hispanic/Latino(a)—full-time 0, part-time 0; Asian/Pacific Islander—full-time 2, part-time 0; American Indian/Alaska Native—full-time 0, part-time 0; Caucasian/White—full-time 0, part-time 0; Multi-ethnic—full-time 0, part-time 0; students subject to the Americans With Disabilities Act—full-time 0, part-time 0; Unknown ethnicity—full-time 0, part-time 0; International students who hold an F-1 or J-1 Visa—full-time 0, part-time 0.

Financial Information/Assistance:
Tuition for Full-Time Study: *Master's:* State residents: $280 per credit hour; Nonstate residents: $644 per credit hour. *Doctoral:* State residents: $280 per credit hour; Nonstate residents: $644 per credit hour. Tuition is subject to change. See the following Web site for updates and changes in tuition costs: http://www.k-state.edu/controller/cashiers/tuitionfeesinfo.html.

Financial Assistance:
First-Year Students: Teaching assistantships available for first year. Average amount paid per academic year: $10,437. Average number of hours worked per week: 20. Apply by January 15. Research assistantships available for first year. Average amount paid per academic year: $9,627. Average number of hours worked per week: 20. Apply by January 15.

Advanced Students: Teaching assistantships available for advanced students. Average amount paid per academic year:

$10,437. Average number of hours worked per week: 20. Research assistantships available for advanced students. Average amount paid per academic year: $9,627. Average number of hours worked per week: 20.

Additional Information: Of all students currently enrolled full time, 85% benefited from one or more of the listed financial assistance programs. Application and information available online at: http://www.k-state.edu/psych/graduate/graduate_application_procedures.htm.

Internships/Practica: Arrangements for internships in human factors/applied experimental and industrial/organizational psychology vary widely and are made on an individual basis.

Housing and Day Care: On-campus housing is available. See the following Web site for more information: http://www.k-state.edu/grad/gsprospective/orientation/house.htm. On-campus day care facilities are available. See the following Web site for more information: http://www.k-state.edu/ksucdc/.

Employment of Department Graduates:
Master's Degree Graduates: Of those who graduated in the academic year 2008–2009, the following categories and numbers represent the postgraduate activities and employment of master's degree graduates: Enrolled in a psychology doctoral program (4), enrolled in a postdoctoral residency/fellowship (n/a), employed in independent practice (n/a), employed in a professional position in a school system (1), total from the above (master's) (5).
Doctoral Degree Graduates: Of those who graduated in the academic year 2008–2009, the following categories and numbers represent the postgraduate activities and employment of doctoral degree graduates: Enrolled in a psychology doctoral program (n/a), employed in an academic position at a university (1), employed in an academic position at a 2-year/4-year college (3), employed in other positions at a higher education institution (2), employed in business or industry (1), total from the above (doctoral) (7).

Additional Information:
Orientation, Objectives, and Emphasis of Department: Both teaching and research are heavily emphasized. Training prepares students for a variety of positions, including teaching and research positions in colleges and universities. Students have also assumed research and evaluative positions in hospitals, clinics, governmental agencies, and industry.

Special Facilities or Resources: The department has rooms for individual and group research; several computer laboratories and remote terminal access to mainframe computers; a photographic darkroom; one-way observation facilities; an electrically shielded, light-tight, sound-deadened room for auditory and visual research; laboratories for behavioral research with animals; surgical and histological facilities; and colony rooms.

Information for Students With Physical Disabilities: See the following Web site for more information: http://www.k-state.edu/dss/.

Application Information:
Send to Graduate Admissions, Department of Psychology, 492 Bluemont Hall, 1100 Mid-campus Drive, Kansas State University, Manhattan, KS 66506-5302. Application available online. URL of online application: http://www.k-state.edu/grad/gsprospective/apply/index.htm. Students are admitted in the Fall, application deadline January 15. Applicants for the Distance Master's Program in Industrial/Organizational Psychology should apply online at http://www.dce.ksu.edu/industrialpsych/. The deadline for applications is April 30. *Fee:* $40. International applicants must pay a $55 application fee in the form of an international cashier's check or money order.

Kansas, University of (2009 data)
Department of Applied Behavioral Science (formerly Human Development)
College of Liberal Arts and Sciences
1000 Sunnyside Avenue
Lawrence, KS 66045-7555
Telephone: (785) 864-4840
Fax: (785) 864-5202
E-mail: *absc@ku.edu*
Web: *http://www.absc.ku.edu*

Department Information:
1964. Chairperson: Edward K. Morris. Number of faculty: total—full-time 19; women—full-time 7; total—minority—full-time 2; women minority—full-time 2; faculty subject to the Americans With Disabilities Act 1.

Programs and Degrees Offered:
Listed in the following order: Program area, degree type (T if terminal Master's), number awarded 7/08–6/09. Behavioral Psychology PhD (Doctor of Philosophy) 8, Applied Behavioral Science MA/MS (Master of Arts/Science) 8.

Student Applications/Admissions:
Student Applications
Behavioral Psychology PhD (Doctor of Philosophy)—Applications 2009–2010, 30. Total applicants accepted 2009–2010, 10. Number full-time enrolled (new admits only) 2009–2010, 10. Total enrolled 2009–2010 full-time, 56. Openings 2010–2011, 10. The median number of years required for completion of a degree in 2008–2009 were 6. The number of students enrolled full- and part-time who were dismissed or voluntarily withdrew from this program area in 2008–2009 were 0. *Applied Behavioral Science MA/MS (Master of Arts/Science)*—Applications 2009–2010, 12. Total applicants accepted 2009–2010, 0. Number full-time enrolled (new admits only) 2009–2010, 0. Total enrolled 2009–2010 full-time, 3. Openings 2010–2011, 10. The median number of years required for completion of a degree in 2008–2009 were 3. The number of students enrolled full- and part-time who were dismissed or voluntarily withdrew from this program area in 2008–2009 were 0.
Other Criteria: (importance of criteria rated low, medium, or high): GRE scores—medium, research experience—high, work experience—high, extracurricular activity—low, clinically related public service—medium, GPA—high, letters of recommendation—high, interview—high, statement of goals and objectives—high, undergraduate major in psychology—medium, specific undergraduate psychology courses taken—low. For additional information on admission requirements, go to http://www.absc.ku.edu/graduate/.

Student Characteristics: The following represents characteristics of students in 2009–2010 in all graduate psychology programs in the department: Female—full-time 64, part-time 0; Male—full-time 20, part-time 0; African American/Black—full-time 6, part-time 0; Hispanic/Latino(a)—full-time 3, part-time 0; Asian/Pacific Islander—full-time 3, part-time 0; American Indian/Alaska Native—full-time 1, part-time 0; Caucasian/White—full-time 69, part-time 0; Multi-ethnic—full-time 2, part-time 0; students subject to the Americans With Disabilities Act—full-time 5, part-time 0; Unknown ethnicity—full-time 0, part-time 0; International students who hold an F-1 or J-1 Visa—full-time 0, part-time 0.

Financial Information/Assistance:
Financial Assistance:
First-Year Students: Teaching assistantships available for first year. Apply by December 15. Research assistantships available for first year. Apply by December 15. Traineeships available for first year. Apply by December 15. Fellowships and scholarships available for first year. Apply by December 15.
Advanced Students: Teaching assistantships available for advanced students. Research assistantships available for advanced students. Traineeships available for advanced students. Fellowships and scholarships available for advanced students.
Additional Information: Of all students currently enrolled full time, 80% benefited from one or more of the listed financial assistance programs. Application and information available online at: http://www.absc.ku.edu/graduate.

Internships/Practica: A wide variety of research settings and practica sites are available to graduate students. They include: Behavioral Pediatrics; Center for Independent Living; Center for the Study of Mental Retardation and Related Problems; Child and Family Research Center; Community Programs for Adults with Mental Retardation; Edna A. Hill Child Development Center; Experimental Analysis of Behavior Laboratories; Family Enhancement Project; Gerontology Center; Juniper Gardens Project; Research on Children with Retardation; Schiefelbusch Institute for Life Span Studies; Work Group on Health Promotion and Community Development.

Housing and Day Care: On-campus housing is available. See the following Web site for more information: http://www.housing.ku.edu/. On-campus day care facilities are available. See the following Web site for more information: http://www.hilltop.ku.edu/.

Employment of Department Graduates:
Master's Degree Graduates: Of those who graduated in the academic year 2008–2009, the following categories and numbers represent the postgraduate activities and employment of master's degree graduates: Enrolled in a psychology doctoral program (3), enrolled in a postdoctoral residency/fellowship (n/a), employed in independent practice (n/a), other employment position (1), do not know (1), total from the above (master's) (5).
Doctoral Degree Graduates: Of those who graduated in the academic year 2008–2009, the following categories and numbers represent the postgraduate activities and employment of doctoral degree graduates: Enrolled in a psychology doctoral program (n/a), enrolled in a postdoctoral residency/fellowship (1), employed in an academic position at a university (1), total from the above (doctoral) (2).

Additional Information:
Orientation, Objectives, and Emphasis of Department: The primary purpose of the program is to train students in basic and applied research in behavior analysis. It features emphases in applied behavior analysis, early childhood, developmental disabilities, community health and development, the experimental analysis of human and animal behavior, conceptual issues in behavior analysis, independent living, and rehabilitation. Throughout the PhD training sequence, students work closely as junior colleagues with a faculty advisor and a research group. Although students typically work with one faculty advisor, they are free to select a different advisor if their interests change during the course of their training. Students participate in research throughout their graduate careers in an individualized, intensive program. As a result, most students complete more research projects than those required for the degree.

Special Facilities or Resources: A wide range of research settings are available to graduate students. Populations and settings include both typically developing and disabled infants, toddlers, preschool children, elementary school settings, adolescents, adults, and elders. In addition, the department has an animal laboratory facility.

Information for Students With Physical Disabilities: See the following Web site for more information: http://www.ku.edu/~ssdis/.

Application Information:
Send to Graduate Admissions, University of Kansas, Applied Behavioral Science, 1000 Sunnyside Avenue, 4001 Dole, Lawrence, KS 66047. Application available online. URL of online application: http://www.absc.ku.edu/graduate/. Students are admitted in the Fall, application deadline December 15. All admissions are based on selections by individual faculty members willing to serve as a mentor to the student; there is no centralized admission. There is no set number of students admitted in any year. Some admissions occur throughout the year. Fee: $55.

Kansas, University of
Department of Psychology
426 Fraser Hall 1415 Jayhawk Boulevard
Lawrence, KS 66045-7556
Telephone: (785) 864-4131
Fax: (785) 864-5696
E-mail: *ratchley@ku.edu*
Web: *http://www.psych.ku.edu*

Department Information:
1916. Chairperson: Ruth Ann Atchley. Number of faculty: total—full-time 27, part-time 9; women—full-time 8, part-time 4; total—minority—full-time 2, part-time 1; women minority—full-time 1, part-time 1.

Programs and Degrees Offered:
Listed in the following order: Program area, degree type (T if terminal Master's), number awarded 7/08–6/09. Clinical Psychology PhD (Doctor of Philosophy) 4, Cognitive Psychology PhD (Doctor of Philosophy) 2, Quantitative Psychology PhD (Doctor

of Philosophy) 4, Social Psychology PhD (Doctor of Philosophy) 2, Developmental Psychology PhD (Doctor of Philosophy) 0.

APA Accreditation: Clinical PhD (Doctor of Philosophy). Student Outcome Data Website: http://www.psych.ku.edu/clinprog/admissions.shtml.

Student Applications/Admissions:
Student Applications
Clinical Psychology PhD (Doctor of Philosophy)—Applications 2009–2010, 83. Total applicants accepted 2009–2010, 12. Number full-time enrolled (new admits only) 2009–2010, 6. Number part-time enrolled (new admits only) 2009–2010, 0. Openings 2010–2011, 5. The median number of years required for completion of a degree in 2008–2009 were 6. The number of students enrolled full- and part-time who were dismissed or voluntarily withdrew from this program area in 2008–2009 were 1. *Cognitive Psychology PhD (Doctor of Philosophy)*—Applications 2009–2010, 13. Total applicants accepted 2009–2010, 5. Number full-time enrolled (new admits only) 2009–2010, 3. Openings 2010–2011, 3. The median number of years required for completion of a degree in 2008–2009 were 6. The number of students enrolled full- and part-time who were dismissed or voluntarily withdrew from this program area in 2008–2009 were 2. *Quantitative Psychology PhD (Doctor of Philosophy)*—Applications 2009–2010, 15. Total applicants accepted 2009–2010, 6. Number full-time enrolled (new admits only) 2009–2010, 4. Openings 2010–2011, 2. The median number of years required for completion of a degree in 2008–2009 were 5. The number of students enrolled full- and part-time who were dismissed or voluntarily withdrew from this program area in 2008–2009 were 0. *Social Psychology PhD (Doctor of Philosophy)*—Applications 2009–2010, 65. Total applicants accepted 2009–2010, 11. Number full-time enrolled (new admits only) 2009–2010, 4. Openings 2010–2011, 4. The median number of years required for completion of a degree in 2008–2009 were 6. The number of students enrolled full- and part-time who were dismissed or voluntarily withdrew from this program area in 2008–2009 were 0. *Developmental Psychology PhD (Doctor of Philosophy)*—Applications 2009–2010, 10. Total applicants accepted 2009–2010, 0. Number full-time enrolled (new admits only) 2009–2010, 0. Total enrolled 2009–2010 full-time, 4. Openings 2010–2011, 2. The median number of years required for completion of a degree in 2008–2009 were 5. The number of students enrolled full- and part-time who were dismissed or voluntarily withdrew from this program area in 2008–2009 were 1.
Scores: Entries appear in this order: required test or GPA, minimum score (if required), median score of students entering in 2009–2010. *Clinical Psychology PhD (Doctor of Philosophy):* GRE-V no minimum stated, 620, GRE-Q no minimum stated, 705, GRE-Analytical no minimum stated, 4.75, overall undergraduate GPA 3.0, 3.86.
Other Criteria: (importance of criteria rated low, medium, or high): GRE scores—high, research experience—high, work experience—low, extracurricular activity—low, clinically related public service—medium, GPA—high, letters of recommendation—high, interview—high, statement of goals and objectives—high, undergraduate major in psychology—medium, specific undergraduate psychology courses taken—medium. Writing sample for Clinical programs only. For additional information on admission requirements, go to http://www.psych.ku.edu/psych_programs/graduate/graduate_apply.shtml.

Student Characteristics: The following represents characteristics of students in 2009–2010 in all graduate psychology programs in the department: Female—full-time 80, part-time 0; Male—full-time 30, part-time 0; African American/Black—full-time 4, part-time 0; Hispanic/Latino(a)—full-time 2, part-time 0; Asian/Pacific Islander—full-time 13, part-time 0; American Indian/Alaska Native—full-time 1, part-time 0; Caucasian/White—full-time 76, part-time 0; Multi-ethnic—full-time 1, part-time 0; students subject to the Americans With Disabilities Act—full-time 1, part-time 0; Unknown ethnicity—full-time 13, part-time 0; International students who hold an F-1 or J-1 Visa—full-time 7, part-time 0.

Financial Information/Assistance:
Tuition for Full-Time Study: *Master's:* State residents: $270 per credit hour; Nonstate residents: $646 per credit hour. *Doctoral:* State residents: $270 per credit hour; Nonstate residents: $646 per credit hour. Tuition is subject to change. See the following Web site for updates and changes in tuition costs: http://www.tuition.ku.edu/rates.shtml.

Financial Assistance:
First-Year Students: Teaching assistantships available for first year. Average amount paid per academic year: $12,250. Average number of hours worked per week: 20. Apply by December 1. Research assistantships available for first year. Average amount paid per academic year: $12,250. Average number of hours worked per week: 20. Apply by December 1. Fellowships and scholarships available for first year. Apply by December 1.
Advanced Students: Teaching assistantships available for advanced students. Average amount paid per academic year: $13,000. Average number of hours worked per week: 20. Apply by January 15. Research assistantships available for advanced students. Average amount paid per academic year: $13,000. Average number of hours worked per week: 20. Apply by January 15. Fellowships and scholarships available for advanced students. Average number of hours worked per week: 0. Apply by January 15.
Additional Information: Of all students currently enrolled full time, 65% benefited from one or more of the listed financial assistance programs. Application and information available online at: http://www.psych.ku.edu.

Internships/Practica: Doctoral Degree (PhD Clinical Psychology): For those doctoral students for whom a professional internship was required in this program prior to graduation, (6) students applied for an internship in 2008–2009, with (6) students obtaining an internship. Of those students who obtained an internship, (6) were paid internships. Of those students who obtained an internship, (6) students placed in APA/CPA accredited internships, (0) students placed in internships not APA/CPA accredited, but listed with the Association of Psychology Postdoctoral and Internship Programs (APPIC), (0) students placed in internships conforming to guidelines of the Council of Directors of School Psychology Programs (CDSPP), (0) students placed in internships that were not APA/CPA accredited, APPIC or CDSPP listed.

Housing and Day Care: On-campus housing is available. See the following Web site for more information: http://www.housing.ku.

edu/. On-campus day care facilities are available. See the following Web site for more information: http://www.hilltop.ku.edu/.

Employment of Department Graduates:
Master's Degree Graduates: Of those who graduated in the academic year 2008–2009, the following categories and numbers represent the postgraduate activities and employment of master's degree graduates: Enrolled in a postdoctoral residency/fellowship (n/a), employed in independent practice (n/a), total from the above (master's) (0).
Doctoral Degree Graduates: Of those who graduated in the academic year 2008–2009, the following categories and numbers represent the postgraduate activities and employment of doctoral degree graduates: Enrolled in a psychology doctoral program (n/a), enrolled in a postdoctoral residency/fellowship (6), employed in independent practice (4), employed in an academic position at a university (1), employed in an academic position at a 2-year/4-year college (1), employed in other positions at a higher education institution (3), employed in government agency (1), employed in a community mental health/counseling center (1), employed in a hospital/medical center (1), total from the above (doctoral) (18).

Additional Information:
Orientation, Objectives, and Emphasis of Department: With 36 faculty, the department offers a wide range of opportunities for the study and treatment of human psychological and behavioral functioning. Students develop skills in statistics, research methods, and specific content areas with basic and applied emphases, with the flexibility to tailor programs to individual students' needs. Students in all programs (Clinical, Developmental, Quantitative, Cognitive or Social) may also complete coursework toward a minor in quantitative psychology.

Special Facilities or Resources: The department has well-equipped computer labs, and access to university mainframe computers. Clinical and research support facilities include an on-site clinic with a test resource library, individual and group therapy rooms, and play and psychodrama rooms. Specialized research facilities include interview rooms with audio and video capacities, psychophysiological and stress laboratories, ERP facilities, eye-movement monitoring laboratories, and an anechoic chamber. The Kansas University Medical Center houses the Hoglund Brain Imaging Center, a state-of-the-art facility with fMRI and MEG laboratories.

Information for Students With Physical Disabilities: See the following Web site for more information: http://www.disability.ku.edu/.

Application Information:
Send to The University of Kansas Graduate School, 1450 Jayhawk Blvd., Rm 313, Lawrence, KS 66045-7535. Application available online. URL of online application: http://www.psych.ku.edu/psych_programs/graduate/graduate_apply.shtml. Students are admitted in the Fall, application deadline December 1. *Fee:* $45.

Kansas, University of
Psychology and Research in Education
School of Education
Joseph R. Pearson Hall, 1122 West Campus Road, Room 621
Lawrence, KS 66045-3101
Telephone: (785) 864-3931
Fax: (785) 864-3820
E-mail: *kmulton@ku.edu*
Web: *http://www.soe.ku.edu/pre/*

Department Information:
1955. Chairperson: Karen D. Multon, PhD. Number of faculty: total—full-time 14, part-time 2; women—full-time 4, part-time 2; minority—part-time 1; women minority—part-time 1.

Programs and Degrees Offered:
Listed in the following order: Program area, degree type (T if terminal Master's), number awarded 7/08–6/09. Counseling Psychology PhD (Doctor of Philosophy) 5, School Psychology EdS (School Psychology) 1, School Psychology PhD (Doctor of Philosophy) 1, Counseling Psychology MA/MS (Master of Arts/Science) (T) 19, Educational Psychology and Research PhD (Doctor of Philosophy) 0, Educational Psychology and Research MEd (Education) 0.

APA Accreditation: Counseling PhD (Doctor of Philosophy). School PhD (Doctor of Philosophy).

Student Applications/Admissions:
Student Applications
Counseling Psychology PhD (Doctor of Philosophy)—Applications 2009–2010, 63. Total applicants accepted 2009–2010, 5. Number full-time enrolled (new admits only) 2009–2010, 5. Number part-time enrolled (new admits only) 2009–2010, 0. Openings 2010–2011, 7. The median number of years required for completion of a degree in 2008–2009 were 7. The number of students enrolled full- and part-time who were dismissed or voluntarily withdrew from this program area in 2008–2009 were 0. *School Psychology EdS (School Psychology)*—Applications 2009–2010, 22. Total applicants accepted 2009–2010, 8. Number full-time enrolled (new admits only) 2009–2010, 8. Total enrolled 2009–2010 full-time, 20. Openings 2010–2011, 13. The median number of years required for completion of a degree in 2008–2009 were 2. The number of students enrolled full- and part-time who were dismissed or voluntarily withdrew from this program area in 2008–2009 were 0. *School Psychology PhD (Doctor of Philosophy)*—Applications 2009–2010, 20. Total applicants accepted 2009–2010, 3. Number full-time enrolled (new admits only) 2009–2010, 3. Number part-time enrolled (new admits only) 2009–2010, 0. Openings 2010–2011, 6. The median number of years required for completion of a degree in 2008–2009 were 5. The number of students enrolled full- and part-time who were dismissed or voluntarily withdrew from this program area in 2008–2009 were 0. *Counseling Psychology MA/MS (Master of Arts/Science)*—Applications 2009–2010, 55. Total applicants accepted 2009–2010, 15. Number full-time enrolled (new admits only) 2009–2010, 15. Number part-time enrolled (new admits only) 2009–2010, 0. Openings 2010–2011, 15. The median number of years required for completion of a degree

in 2008–2009 were 2. The number of students enrolled full- and part-time who were dismissed or voluntarily withdrew from this program area in 2008–2009 were 0. *Educational Psychology and Research PhD (Doctor of Philosophy)*—Applications 2009–2010, 20. Total applicants accepted 2009–2010, 14. Number full-time enrolled (new admits only) 2009–2010, 14. Number part-time enrolled (new admits only) 2009–2010, 0. Openings 2010–2011, 7. The number of students enrolled full- and part-time who were dismissed or voluntarily withdrew from this program area in 2008–2009 were 0. *Educational Psychology and Research MEd (Education)*—Applications 2009–2010, 8. Total applicants accepted 2009–2010, 4. Number full-time enrolled (new admits only) 2009–2010, 4. Number part-time enrolled (new admits only) 2009–2010, 0. Openings 2010–2011, 6. The number of students enrolled full- and part-time who were dismissed or voluntarily withdrew from this program area in 2008–2009 were 0.

Other Criteria: (importance of criteria rated low, medium, or high): GRE scores—high, research experience—medium, work experience—medium, extracurricular activity—low, clinically related public service—low, GPA—high, letters of recommendation—high, interview—high, statement of goals and objectives—high, The admission criteria above are for applicants to the Counseling Psychology PhD program. The admission criteria for applicants to the School Psychology PhD program are: GRE scores—high; research experience—high; work experience—medium; extracurricular activity—low; clinically related public service—high; UGPA—high; letters of recommendation—high; statement of goals and objectives—high. For additional information on admission requirements, go to http://soe.ku.edu/pre/.

Student Characteristics: The following represents characteristics of students in 2009–2010 in all graduate psychology programs in the department: Female—full-time 106, part-time 0; Male—full-time 46, part-time 0; African American/Black—full-time 7, part-time 0; Hispanic/Latino(a)—full-time 8, part-time 0; Asian/Pacific Islander—full-time 3, part-time 0; American Indian/Alaska Native—full-time 1, part-time 0; Caucasian/White—full-time 94, part-time 0; Multi-ethnic—full-time 0, part-time 0; students subject to the Americans With Disabilities Act—full-time 0, part-time 0; Unknown ethnicity—full-time 39, part-time 0; International students who hold an F-1 or J-1 Visa—full-time 22, part-time 0.

Financial Information/Assistance:
Tuition for Full-Time Study: *Master's:* State residents: $270 per credit hour; Nonstate residents: $646 per credit hour. *Doctoral:* State residents: $270 per credit hour; Nonstate residents: $646 per credit hour. Tuition is subject to change. See the following Web site for updates and changes in tuition costs: http://www.tuition.ku.edu/rates.shtml. Higher tuition cost for this program: The School of Education has a differential tuition fee of $19.30 per credit hour.

Financial Assistance:
First-Year Students: Teaching assistantships available for first year. Average amount paid per academic year: $7,350. Average number of hours worked per week: 10. Apply by February 15. Research assistantships available for first year. Average amount paid per academic year: $6,050. Average number of hours worked per week: 10. Fellowships and scholarships available for first year.

Advanced Students: Teaching assistantships available for advanced students. Average amount paid per academic year: $7,350. Average number of hours worked per week: 10. Apply by February 15. Research assistantships available for advanced students. Average amount paid per academic year: $6,050. Average number of hours worked per week: 10. Fellowships and scholarships available for advanced students.

Additional Information: Of all students currently enrolled full time, 70% benefited from one or more of the listed financial assistance programs. Application and information available online at: http://www.financialaid.ku.edu.

Internships/Practica: Doctoral Degree (PhD Counseling Psychology): For those doctoral students for whom a professional internship was required in this program prior to graduation, (9) students applied for an internship in 2008–2009, with (7) students obtaining an internship. Of those students who obtained an internship, (7) were paid internships. Of those students who obtained an internship, (7) students placed in APA/CPA accredited internships, (0) students placed in internships not APA/CPA accredited, but listed with the Association of Psychology Postdoctoral and Internship Programs (APPIC), (0) students placed in internships conforming to guidelines of the Council of Directors of School Psychology Programs (CDSPP), (0) students placed in internships that were not APA/CPA accredited, APPIC or CDSPP listed. The Counseling Psychology and School Psychology programs require practicum and/or internship courses as part of the degree requirements. Additionally, PRE graduate students enroll in field experience, seminars, and specific PRE courses to obtain additional training with special populations and/or psychological testing procedures. (1) Counseling Psychology doctoral students must participate in three semesters of practicum and one full year of internship. Both master's and doctoral students in the Counseling Psychology programs complete their practica in a variety of local applied settings. Our doctoral students in Counseling Psychology have been successful in obtaining APA accredited internships in university counseling centers, veterans' administration medical centers, community mental health centers, and other human service agencies. (2) Students in the School Psychology EdS program devote a full year to a school psychology internship. These students obtain internships in a variety of elementary, secondary, and special needs school settings throughout the country. Individuals obtaining their doctoral degree in School Psychology are required to participate in a second full year of internship (PRE 992). Course descriptions may be viewed at http://www.catalogs.ku.edu/graduate. Please see the section for the School of Education.

Housing and Day Care: On-campus housing is available. See the following Web site for more information: http://www.housing.ku.edu/.

Employment of Department Graduates:
Master's Degree Graduates: Of those who graduated in the academic year 2008–2009, the following categories and numbers represent the postgraduate activities and employment of master's degree graduates: Enrolled in a psychology doctoral program (7), enrolled in another graduate/professional program (0), enrolled in a postdoctoral residency/fellowship (n/a), employed in independent practice (n/a), employed in an academic position at a university (1), employed in an academic position at a 2-year/4-year college (0), employed in other positions at a higher education

institution (0), employed in a professional position in a school system (0), employed in business or industry (0), employed in government agency (0), employed in a community mental health/counseling center (0), employed in a hospital/medical center (1), still seeking employment (1), not seeking employment (0), other employment position (2), do not know (8), total from the above (master's) (20).

Doctoral Degree Graduates: Of those who graduated in the academic year 2008–2009, the following categories and numbers represent the postgraduate activities and employment of doctoral degree graduates: Enrolled in a psychology doctoral program (n/a), enrolled in another graduate/professional program (0), enrolled in a postdoctoral residency/fellowship (1), employed in independent practice (0), employed in an academic position at a university (0), employed in an academic position at a 2-year/4-year college (0), employed in other positions at a higher education institution (2), employed in a professional position in a school system (1), employed in business or industry (0), employed in government agency (1), employed in a community mental health/counseling center (1), employed in a hospital/medical center (0), still seeking employment (0), not seeking employment (0), other employment position (0), do not know (0), total from the above (doctoral) (6).

Additional Information:

Orientation, Objectives, and Emphasis of Department: Psychology and Research in Education offers graduate degrees in three distinct areas. The doctoral programs in Counseling Psychology and School Psychology are APA accredited. The EdS and PhD degrees in School Psychology are NASP accredited. (1) Counseling Psychology trains professionals to possess the generalist skills to function in a wide array of work settings. This program is strongly committed to the training of scientist–practitioners focused on facilitating the personal, social, educational, and vocational development of individuals. (2) School Psychology endorses the training model of the psychoeducational consultant with multifaceted skills drawn from psychology and education to assist children toward greater realization of their potential. The psychoeducational consultant is vitally concerned with enhancing teacher effectiveness, creating a positive classroom environment for children, and influencing educational thought within the school system. (3) The Educational Psychology and Research program offers instruction in two tracks. The objectives of the program are to prepare students to become faculty members, researchers, and measurement specialists. Students may focus on (a) development and learning, or (b) research, evaluation, measurement, and statistics. Graduate study includes experiences in designing, conducting, and evaluating research and field experiences in a variety of settings.

Special Facilities or Resources: Students have employment and/or research opportunities with diverse populations in a variety of settings, including university-related facilities and public/private schools. (1) KU's Multicultural Resource Center seeks to reshape notions of education, research, and public service to include a multicultural focus. (2) The America Reads Challenge, Institute of Educational Research and Public Service, Center for Educational Testing and Evaluation, Center for Research on Learning, and the Center for Psychoeducational Services are under the umbrella of KU's School of Education. The Center for Psychoeducational Services serves the needs of local schools and community members while offering excellent training opportunities for School Psychology and Counseling Psychology students. Graduate students may work with preschool, school-age children and their families, and college students from the local area. (3) KU's Life Span Institute, has numerous programs such as the Juniper Gardens Children's Project, Beach Center on Disability, Research and Training Center on Independent Living, Gerontology Center, and the Work Group for Community Health and Development. (4) The School of Education provides extensive media and internet technology in its state-of-the-art facility, Joseph R. Pearson Hall. Students have access to mediated classrooms and laboratories, instructional and assessment libraries, audio visual resources, and computer labs.

Information for Students With Physical Disabilities: See the following Web site for more information: http://www.disability.ku.edu/.

Application Information:
Send to KU Psychology and Research in Education, Admissions Committee, 1122 W Campus Rd, Room 621 JRP, Lawrence, KS 66045-3101. Application available online. URL of online application: http://www.soe.ku.edu/pre. Students are admitted in the Fall, application deadline December 15. Counseling Psychology PhD program, School Psychology PhD program, February 15 - Educational Psychology & Research, PhD. Master's Programs: December 15 - School Psychology EdS program, January 15 - Counseling Psychology MS program, February 15 - Educational Psychology & Research, MSEd. *Fee:* $45. Individuals requesting an application fee waiver should send a letter directly to the chair of the Department of Psychology and Research in Education.

Pittsburg State University (2009 data)
Department of Psychology and Counseling
College of Education
207 Whitesitt Hall, 1701 South Broadway
Pittsburg, KS 66762-7551
Telephone: (620) 235-4523
Fax: (620) 235-6102
E-mail: *dhurford@pittstate.edu*
Web: *http://www.pittstate.edu/psych/*

Department Information:
1929. Chairperson: David P. Hurford. Number of faculty: total—full-time 15, part-time 2; women—full-time 7.

Programs and Degrees Offered:
Listed in the following order: Program area, degree type (T if terminal Master's), number awarded 7/08–6/09. Clinical Psychology MA/MS (Master of Arts/Science) (T) 6, General Psychology MA/MS (Master of Arts/Science) (T) 9, School Psychology EdS (School Psychology) 9, School Counseling MA/MS (Master of Arts/Science) (T) 3, Clinical Mental Health Counseling MA/MS (Master of Arts/Science) 9.

Student Applications/Admissions:
Student Applications

Clinical Psychology MA/MS (Master of Arts/Science)—Applications 2009–2010, 31. Total applicants accepted 2009–2010, 12. Number full-time enrolled (new admits only) 2009–2010, 10. Total enrolled 2009–2010 full-time, 12. Openings 2010–2011, 10. *General Psychology MA/MS (Master of Arts/Science)*—

Applications 2009–2010, 16. Total applicants accepted 2009–2010, 14. Number full-time enrolled (new admits only) 2009–2010, 10. Total enrolled 2009–2010 full-time, 11. Openings 2010–2011, 12. *School Psychology EdS (School Psychology)*—Applications 2009–2010, 7. Total applicants accepted 2009–2010, 7. Number full-time enrolled (new admits only) 2009–2010, 7. Total enrolled 2009–2010 full-time, 18, part-time, 4. Openings 2010–2011, 10. *School Counseling MA/MS (Master of Arts/Science)*—Applications 2009–2010, 14. Total applicants accepted 2009–2010, 14. Number full-time enrolled (new admits only) 2009–2010, 5. Number part-time enrolled (new admits only) 2009–2010, 3. Total enrolled 2009–2010 full-time, 14, part-time, 16. Openings 2010–2011, 10. *Clinical Mental Health Counseling MA/MS (Master of Arts/Science)*—Applications 2009–2010, 30. Total applicants accepted 2009–2010, 24. Number full-time enrolled (new admits only) 2009–2010, 12. Number part-time enrolled (new admits only) 2009–2010, 12. The median number of years required for completion of a degree in 2008–2009 were 2.

Other Criteria: (importance of criteria rated low, medium, or high): GRE scores—high, research experience—medium, work experience—high, extracurricular activity—low, clinically related public service—medium, GPA—high, letters of recommendation—high, interview—medium, statement of goals and objectives—high.

Student Characteristics: The following represents characteristics of students in 2009–2010 in all graduate psychology programs in the department: Female—full-time 22, part-time 24; Male—full-time 15, part-time 12; African American/Black—full-time 3, part-time 1; Hispanic/Latino(a)—full-time 2, part-time 0; Asian/Pacific Islander—full-time 6, part-time 0; American Indian/Alaska Native—full-time 2, part-time 1; Caucasian/White—full-time 0, part-time 0; Multi-ethnic—full-time 0, part-time 0; students subject to the Americans With Disabilities Act—full-time 0, part-time 0; Unknown ethnicity—full-time 0, part-time 0; International students who hold an F-1 or J-1 Visa—full-time 0, part-time 0.

Financial Information/Assistance:
Tuition for Full-Time Study: *Master's:* State residents: per academic year $2,441, $206 per credit hour; Nonstate residents: per academic year $5,965, $500 per credit hour. Tuition is subject to change.

Financial Assistance:
First-Year Students: Teaching assistantships available for first year. Average amount paid per academic year: $4,660. Average number of hours worked per week: 20. Apply by March 1.
Advanced Students: Teaching assistantships available for advanced students. Average amount paid per academic year: $4,660. Average number of hours worked per week: 20. Apply by March 1.
Additional Information: Of all students currently enrolled full time, 5% benefited from one or more of the listed financial assistance programs.

Internships/Practica: All MS and EdS practitioner programs include a 3-8 semester hour (150-400 clock hour) practicum sequence and a 4-32 semester hour (600-1200 clock hour) internship at a site appropriate to the specialty, and under the supervision of faculty and site supervisors. The internship in school psychology is post-degree, and is typically a paid internship. Some internships in other programs are also paid. All internships meet guidelines of the professional association or accrediting body of the specialty (i.e., CACREP, MPAC, NASP).

Housing and Day Care: On-campus housing is available. See the following Web site for more information: http://www.pittstate.edu/house/. No on-campus day care facilities are available.

Employment of Department Graduates:
Master's Degree Graduates: Of those who graduated in the academic year 2008–2009, the following categories and numbers represent the postgraduate activities and employment of master's degree graduates: Enrolled in a psychology doctoral program (2), enrolled in another graduate/professional program (3), enrolled in a postdoctoral residency/fellowship (n/a), employed in independent practice (n/a), employed in an academic position at a university (1), employed in an academic position at a 2-year/4-year college (2), employed in other positions at a higher education institution (0), employed in a professional position in a school system (20), employed in business or industry (0), employed in government agency (0), employed in a community mental health/counseling center (16), employed in a hospital/medical center (2), still seeking employment (2), other employment position (3), total from the above (master's) (51).
Doctoral Degree Graduates: Of those who graduated in the academic year 2008–2009, the following categories and numbers represent the postgraduate activities and employment of doctoral degree graduates: Enrolled in a psychology doctoral program (n/a), total from the above (doctoral) (0).

Additional Information:
Orientation, Objectives, and Emphasis of Department: The Department of Psychology and Counseling uses an interdisciplinary model to provide broad-based training, understanding and appreciation of the specialties that we represent. The major objective of the department is to prepare graduates with knowledge in scientific foundations and practical applied skills to function as mental health service providers or to pursue study at the doctoral level. Faculty in the department represent a diverse collection of theoretical backgrounds in scientific and applied psychology. All faculty teach coursework in each program area, providing students with the opportunity to learn multidisciplinary approaches and models. The emphasis in the department is on integrated, cross-disciplinary studies within a close faculty-student colleague model that promotes frequent contact and close supervision, aimed at developing practitioner skills. The department is pleased to have the first accredited master's degree program in clinical psychology in the nation (MPAC accreditation received in May 1997), and enjoys CACREP accreditation of the master's degree program in community counseling. The department also enjoys NCATE accreditation of the M.S. Degree program in school counseling and the EdS Degree program in school psychology.

Special Facilities or Resources: The department has counseling and psychotherapy training facilities equipped with one-way mirrors and audio and video taping equipment. Microcomputer laboratories with network capacity, word processing, and SAS and SPSS software are available in the department. The university library, in addition to a large book collection, currently maintains over 150 periodical subscriptions in psychology. The department operates the Center for Human Services, an on-campus training, research, and service facility, which includes University Testing Services, a family counseling center, an adult assessment center, the Center for Assessment and Remediation of Reading Difficulties, the Attention Deficit/Hyperactivity Disorder Neurofeedback Diagnostic and Treatment Center, and the Welfare to Work Assessment Center. The department has a close working relationship with local hospitals and mental health facilities, and is a constituent member of the regional community service coalition.

Information for Students With Physical Disabilities: See the following Web site for more information: http://www.pittstate.edu/eoaa/.

Application Information:
Send to Chairperson, Department of Psychology and Counseling, Pittsburg State University, 1701 S. Broadway, Pittsburg, KS 66762-7551. Students are admitted in the Fall, application deadline March 1; Spring, application deadline October 1; Summer, application deadline March 1. Applications for the MS in Clinical Psychology are normally accepted for Fall admission. Applications will be considered for Spring admission, but please note that this will extend the student's program of study by one semester. *Fee:* $10. In addition to the application fee, there is also a fee to cover the cost of a required criminal background check.

Washburn University (2009 data)
Department of Psychology
1700 College
Topeka, KS 66621
Telephone: (785) 670-1564
Fax: (785) 670-1239
E-mail: *dave.provorse@washburn.edu*
Web: *http://www.washburn.edu/cas/psychology/*

Department Information:
1940. Chairperson: Dave Provorse. Number of faculty: total—full-time 7, part-time 2; women—full-time 3, part-time 2.

Programs and Degrees Offered:
Listed in the following order: Program area, degree type (T if terminal Master's), number awarded 7/08–6/09. Clinical MA/MS (Master of Arts/Science) (T) 11.

Student Applications/Admissions:
Student Applications
Clinical MA/MS *(Master of Arts/Science)*—Applications 2009–2010, 24. Total applicants accepted 2009–2010, 12. Number full-time enrolled (new admits only) 2009–2010, 12. Openings 2010–2011, 12. The median number of years required for completion of a degree in 2008–2009 were 3. The number of students enrolled full- and part-time who were dismissed or voluntarily withdrew from this program area in 2008–2009 were 1.
Other Criteria: (importance of criteria rated low, medium, or high): GRE scores—low, research experience—medium, work experience—medium, extracurricular activity—low, clinically related public service—medium, GPA—medium, letters of recommendation—high, statement of goals and objectives—medium, undergraduate major in psychology—medium, specific undergraduate psychology courses taken—medium. For additional information on admission requirements, go to http://www.washburn.edu/cas/psychology/ma_program.html.

Student Characteristics: The following represents characteristics of students in 2009–2010 in all graduate psychology programs in the department: Female—full-time 16, part-time 3; Male—full-time 4, part-time 3; African American/Black—full-time 1, part-time 0; Hispanic/Latino(a)—full-time 1, part-time 0; Asian/Pacific Islander—full-time 0, part-time 1; American Indian/Alaska Native—full-time 0, part-time 0; Caucasian/White—full-time 0, part-time 0; Multi-ethnic—full-time 1, part-time 0; students subject to the Americans With Disabilities Act—full-time 0, part-time 0; Unknown ethnicity—full-time 0, part-time 0; International students who hold an F-1 or J-1 Visa—full-time 0, part-time 0.

Financial Information/Assistance:
Tuition for Full-Time Study: Master's: State residents: per academic year $4,896, $272 per credit hour; Nonstate residents: per academic year $9,972, $554 per credit hour. Tuition is subject to change. See the following Web site for updates and changes in tuition costs: http://www.washburn.edu/business-office/.

Financial Assistance:
First-Year Students: Teaching assistantships available for first year. Average amount paid per academic year: $3,500. Average number of hours worked per week: 10. Apply by March 15.
Advanced Students: Teaching assistantships available for advanced students. Average amount paid per academic year: $4,000. Average number of hours worked per week: 10. Apply by May 15. Traineeships available for advanced students. Average amount paid per academic year: $3,000. Average number of hours worked per week: 20. Apply by August 15.
Additional Information: Of all students currently enrolled full time, 50% benefited from one or more of the listed financial assistance programs. Application and information available online at: http://www.washburn.edu/cas/psychology/grad/ma_program.html.

Internships/Practica: Master's Degree (MA/MS Clinical): An internship experience, such as a final research project or "capstone" experience is required of graduates. Psychological services are offered to the community through a clinic staffed by graduate students enrolled in practica. Services offered focus on remediation of anxiety and depression. Student therapists practice skills of diagnostic interviewing, and integrating interview information with personality and intelligence testing into the formulation of a DSM-IV-TR diagnosis. Under the close supervision of a faculty clinical psychologist, they use this information to conceptualize etiologies and develop and deliver therapeutic treatment options. The therapy processes implemented reflect several theoretical orientations, including Interpersonal Process, Cognitive/Behavioral and Brief approaches. Issues of suicide, cross-cultural sensitivity and individual therapist development are also addressed. An internship consisting of 750 supervised hours over an academic year is required of each student prior to graduation. This requirement is met by working twenty hours per week at an assigned site and meeting three hours weekly in a classroom setting. Both on-site and academic supervisors are available to the student throughout the internship. The types of experiences provided student interns include: provision of individual adult and child therapy; cofacilitation of group therapy; psychological testing/assessment; and involvement in multidisciplinary treatment teams.

Housing and Day Care: On-campus housing is available. See the following Web site for more information: http://www.washburn.edu/studentlife/resliving/. No on-campus day care facilities are available.

Employment of Department Graduates:
Master's Degree Graduates: Of those who graduated in the academic year 2008–2009, the following categories and numbers represent the postgraduate activities and employment of master's degree graduates: Enrolled in a psychology doctoral program (2), enrolled in a postdoctoral residency/fellowship (n/a), employed in independent practice (n/a), employed in a community mental health/counseling center (6), employed in a hospital/medical center (1), still seeking employment (1), other employment position (1), total from the above (master's) (11).
Doctoral Degree Graduates: Of those who graduated in the academic year 2008–2009, the following categories and numbers represent the postgraduate activities and employment of doctoral degree graduates: Enrolled in a psychology doctoral program (n/a), total from the above (doctoral) (0).

Additional Information:
Orientation, Objectives, and Emphasis of Department: Training is designed to establish a strong foundation in the content and methods of psychology. Students obtain experience and skills in research, psychological assessment and individual and group therapy. Clinical training reflects an integrative blend of humanistic, cognitive/behavioral, interpersonal process and brief therapies. The MA program is designed to prepare students for the pursuit of a doctoral degree in psychology, or for future employment as providers of psychological services in community mental health centers, hospitals, correctional settings and other social service agencies and clinics that require master's level training. Students with special interests in children, rural psychology or correctional and prison settings have the opportunity to pursue such interests in their thesis research and internship placement.

Special Facilities or Resources: The psychology department, housed with other departments in a modern building, has well-equipped laboratories available for human experimentation. These facilities also include observation areas designed for the direct supervision of psychotherapy and psychological testing. The psychology department provides access to the University Academic Computer Center for computer hardware and software resources. Thesis research can be conducted by accessing participants from the undergraduate subject pool, or a wide array of community-based agencies.

Information for Students With Physical Disabilities: See the following Web site for more information: http://www.washburn.edu/studentlife/stuservices.

Application Information:
Send to Department of Psychology, Washburn University, Topeka, KS 66621. Application available online. URL of online application: http://www.washburn.edu/cas/psychology/ma_application.html. Students are admitted in the Fall, application deadline March 15; Spring, application deadline December 1. *Fee:* $0.

Wichita State University
Department of Psychology
Fairmount College of Liberal Arts and Sciences
1845 Fairmount
Wichita, KS 67260-0034
Telephone: (316) 978-3170
Fax: (316) 978-3086
E-mail: *charles.burdsal@wichita.edu*
Web: *http://psychology.wichita.edu*

Department Information:
1948. Chairperson: Charles A. Burdsal. Number of faculty: total—full-time 15, part-time 1; women—full-time 4, part-time 1; total—minority—full-time 3; women minority—full-time 1.

Programs and Degrees Offered:
Listed in the following order: Program area, degree type (T if terminal Master's), number awarded 7/08–6/09. Clinical Psychology PhD (Doctor of Philosophy) 2, Human Factors PhD (Doctor of Philosophy) 2, Community Psychology PhD (Doctor of Philosophy) 11.

APA Accreditation: Clinical PhD (Doctor of Philosophy). Student Outcome Data Website: http://webs.wichita.edu/?u=psychology&p=/graduate/clinical/clinicalphd/.

Student Applications/Admissions:
Student Applications
Clinical Psychology PhD (Doctor of Philosophy)—Applications 2009–2010, 55. Total applicants accepted 2009–2010, 5. Number full-time enrolled (new admits only) 2009–2010, 5. Openings 2010–2011, 4. The median number of years required for completion of a degree in 2008–2009 were 5. The number of students enrolled full- and part-time who were dismissed or voluntarily withdrew from this program area in 2008–2009 were 2. *Human Factors PhD (Doctor of Philosophy)*—Applications 2009–2010, 13. Total applicants accepted 2009–2010, 3. Number full-time enrolled (new admits only) 2009–2010, 3. Openings 2010–2011, 6. The median number of years required for completion of a degree in 2008–2009 were 8. The number of students enrolled full- and part-time who were dismissed or voluntarily withdrew from this program area in 2008–2009 were 0. *Community Psychology PhD (Doctor of Philosophy)*—Applications 2009–2010, 14. Total applicants accepted 2009–2010, 4. Number full-time enrolled (new admits only) 2009–2010, 4. Openings 2010–2011, 4. The median number of years required for completion of a degree in 2008–2009 were 5. The number of students enrolled full- and part-time who were dismissed or voluntarily withdrew from this program area in 2008–2009 were 0.
Other Criteria: (importance of criteria rated low, medium, or high): GRE scores—medium, research experience—high, work experience—medium, clinically related public service—medium, GPA—high, letters of recommendation—medium, interview—medium, statement of goals and objectives—high, undergraduate major in psychology—low, specific undergraduate psychology courses taken—low. For additional information on admission requirements, go to http://psychology.wichita.edu.

Student Characteristics: The following represents characteristics of students in 2009–2010 in all graduate psychology programs in the department: Female—full-time 45, part-time 0; Male—full-time 24, part-time 0; African American/Black—full-time 4, part-time 0; Hispanic/Latino(a)—full-time 4, part-time 0; Asian/Pacific Islander—full-time 5, part-time 0; American Indian/Alaska Native—full-time 1, part-time 0; Caucasian/White—full-time 54, part-time 0; Multi-ethnic—full-time 1, part-time 0; students subject to the Americans With Disabilities Act—full-time 0, part-time 0; Unknown ethnicity—full-time 0, part-time 0; International students who hold an F-1 or J-1 Visa—full-time 0, part-time 0.

Financial Information/Assistance:
Tuition for Full-Time Study: *Doctoral:* State residents: per academic year $6,157, $256 per credit hour; Nonstate residents: per academic year $15,389, $641 per credit hour. Tuition is subject to change. Additional fees are assessed to students beyond the costs of tuition for the following: Student Fees. See the following Web site for updates and changes in tuition costs: http://www.wichita.edu/tuitionfees.

Financial Assistance:
First-Year Students: Teaching assistantships available for first year. Average amount paid per academic year: $6,864. Average number of hours worked per week: 20. Research assistantships available for first year. Average amount paid per academic year: $10,000. Average number of hours worked per week: 20.
Advanced Students: Teaching assistantships available for advanced students. Average amount paid per academic year: $7,912. Average number of hours worked per week: 20. Research assistantships available for advanced students. Average amount paid per academic year: $10,000. Average number of hours worked per week: 20.
Additional Information: Of all students currently enrolled full time, 70% benefited from one or more of the listed financial assistance programs. Application and information available online at: http://www.wichita.edu/financialaid.

Internships/Practica: Doctoral Degree (PhD Clinical Psychology): For those doctoral students for whom a professional internship was required in this program prior to graduation, (2) students applied for an internship in 2008–2009, with (2) students obtaining an internship. Of those students who obtained an internship, (2) were paid internships. Of those students who obtained an internship, (2) students placed in APA/CPA accredited internships, (0) students placed in internships not APA/CPA accredited, but listed with the Association of Psychology Postdoctoral and Internship Programs (APPIC), (0) students placed in internships conforming to guidelines of the Council of Directors of School Psychology Programs (CDSPP), (0) students placed in internships that were not APA/CPA accredited, APPIC or CDSPP listed. An important aspect of the Human Factors program is its requirement that all students complete an internship. The internship is designed to provide students with practical experience integrating their education in real-world situations. The internships have included positions with the FAA, Google, Bell Laboratories, IBM, Microsoft, and other similar settings. These placements have often led to post-PhD employment opportunities. In the Clinical and Community programs, practicum opportunities, most of them funded, are available in on-campus training facilities and community agencies. Settings include the Psychology Clinic and the Counseling and Testing Center, both at Wichita State University, the Sedgwick County Department of Mental Health, Head Start, and various community-based projects. Students in the Clinical program are required to complete one year of internship experience towards the end of their graduate studies.

Housing and Day Care: On-campus housing is available. See the following Web site for more information: http://www.wichita.edu/thisis/studentlife/campus_housing.asp. On-campus day care facilities are available. See the following Web site for more information: http://www.wichita.edu/childdevelopmentcenter.

Employment of Department Graduates:
Master's Degree Graduates: Of those who graduated in the academic year 2008–2009, the following categories and numbers represent the postgraduate activities and employment of master's degree graduates: Enrolled in a postdoctoral residency/fellowship (n/a), employed in independent practice (n/a), total from the above (master's) (0).
Doctoral Degree Graduates: Of those who graduated in the academic year 2008–2009, the following categories and numbers represent the postgraduate activities and employment of doctoral degree graduates: Enrolled in a psychology doctoral program (n/a), enrolled in a postdoctoral residency/fellowship (1), employed in an academic position at a university (1), employed in an academic position at a 2-year/4-year college (2), employed in other positions at a higher education institution (1), employed in business or industry (2), employed in government agency (1), employed in a community mental health/counseling center (3), employed in a hospital/medical center (1), not seeking employment (1), total from the above (doctoral) (13).

Additional Information:
Orientation, Objectives, and Emphasis of Department: The Psychology Department, open to various theoretical orientations, emphasizes research in its three programs. The Human Factors program is accredited by the Education Committee of the Human Factors and Ergonomics Society. This program provides students with wide exposure to research, training, practice, and literature in the field of Human Factors, as well as to issues in the wider context of basic and applied experimental psychology. Current human factors research involves cognitive functioning, aging, development, human-computer interactions, aerospace issues, perception, attention, vision, and driving related issues, especially with the elderly. The APA-accredited Clinical program seeks to integrate community and clinical psychology. The goal of the program is to educate and license students to be competent clinical psychologists who conceptualize, research, intervene, and treat problems at the individual, group, organizational and societal levels. Special areas of interest and research include parent-child interaction, treatment and prevention of depression, treatment and prevention of delinquency, adolescent health and development, and assessment of personality and psychopathology. The Community program seeks to educate students in Community Psychology with an emphasis on assessing and solving problems at the group, organizational and societal levels. Special areas of research and practice include: adolescent health and development, self-help groups, voluntary and paid helping relationships especially with the elderly, animal welfare, and treatment and prevention of delinquency. All three programs have an applied research focus.

Special Facilities or Resources: The department is located in Jabara Hall and maintains fully equipped laboratories. Currently active research groups include the Software Usability Research Lab, Perception & Attention Lab, Visual Psychophysics Lab, Decision Making Research Lab, Child & Family Research Center, Personality Research Lab, Quantitative Modeling Lab, and the Center for Community Support & Research. Our computer facilities are state-of-the-art and are available to students for coursework and research. The department also has access to the National Institute for Aviation Research, the Social Science Research Laboratory, and the University Computing Center. The Psychology Clinic, which is part of the psychology department, provides outpatient services via individual, group, and family modalities. The clinic has facilities for individual and group research. The statewide Center for Community Support & Research, with a computerized database and an 800 number, also operates out of the psychology department. Faculty maintain working relationships with a number of governmental and community agencies which facilitate student involvement in community practice and research. The agencies include the public school system, the Sedgwick County Department of Mental Health, and COMCARE, among others.

Information for Students With Physical Disabilities: See the following Web site for more information: http://webs.wichita.edu/dss.

Application Information:
Send to Graduate Coordinator, Psychology Department. URL of online application: http://webs.wichita.edu/?u=psychology&p=/application/gradapplication/. Students are admitted in the Fall, application deadline January 15. *Fee:* $50. International Students $65.

KENTUCKY

Eastern Kentucky University
Department of Psychology
Arts and Sciences
Cammack 127
Richmond, KY 40475
Telephone: (859) 622-1105
Fax: (859) 622-5871
E-mail: *robert.brubaker@eku.edu*
Web: *http://www.psychology.eku.edu*

Department Information:
1967. Chairperson: Robert G. Brubaker. Number of faculty: total—full-time 21, part-time 12; women—full-time 11, part-time 8; total—minority—full-time 1, part-time 1; women minority—full-time 1; faculty subject to the Americans With Disabilities Act 1.

Programs and Degrees Offered:
Listed in the following order: Program area, degree type (T if terminal Master's), number awarded 7/08–6/09. Clinical Psychology MA/MS (Master of Arts/Science) (T) 11, Industrial/Organizational Psychology MA/MS (Master of Arts/Science) (T) 7, School Psychology Other 9, General Psychology MA/MS (Master of Arts/Science) (T) 2.

Student Applications/Admissions:
Student Applications
Clinical Psychology MA/MS (Master of Arts/Science)—Applications 2009–2010, 60. Total applicants accepted 2009–2010, 19. Number full-time enrolled (new admits only) 2009–2010, 11. Total enrolled 2009–2010 full-time, 25. Openings 2010–2011, 12. The median number of years required for completion of a degree in 2008–2009 were 2. The number of students enrolled full- and part-time who were dismissed or voluntarily withdrew from this program area in 2008–2009 were 0. *Industrial/Organizational Psychology MA/MS (Master of Arts/Science)*—Applications 2009–2010, 30. Total applicants accepted 2009–2010, 13. Number full-time enrolled (new admits only) 2009–2010, 7. Number part-time enrolled (new admits only) 2009–2010, 2. Total enrolled 2009–2010 full-time, 13, part-time, 2. Openings 2010–2011, 10. The median number of years required for completion of a degree in 2008–2009 were 2. The number of students enrolled full- and part-time who were dismissed or voluntarily withdrew from this program area in 2008–2009 were 0. *School Psychology Other*—Applications 2009–2010, 43. Total applicants accepted 2009–2010, 18. Number full-time enrolled (new admits only) 2009–2010, 8. Number part-time enrolled (new admits only) 2009–2010, 0. Openings 2010–2011, 10. The median number of years required for completion of a degree in 2008–2009 were 3. The number of students enrolled full- and part-time who were dismissed or voluntarily withdrew from this program area in 2008–2009 were 1. *General Psychology MA/MS (Master of Arts/Science)*—Applications 2009–2010, 4. Number full-time enrolled (new admits only) 2009–2010, 2. Total enrolled 2009–2010 full-time, 3. Openings 2010–2011, 4. The median number of years required for completion of a degree in 2008–2009 were 2. The number of students enrolled full- and part-time who were dismissed or voluntarily withdrew from this program area in 2008–2009 were 0.

Scores: Entries appear in this order: required test or GPA, minimum score (if required), median score of students entering in 2009–2010. Clinical Psychology MA/MS (Master of Arts/Science): GRE-V no minimum stated, 550, GRE-Q no minimum stated, 490, overall undergraduate GPA no minimum stated, 3.4, last 2 years GPA no minimum stated, 3.6, psychology GPA no minimum stated, 3.7; *Industrial/Organizational Psychology MA/MS (Master of Arts/Science)*: GRE-V no minimum stated, 470, GRE-Q no minimum stated, 510, overall undergraduate GPA no minimum stated, 3.4, last 2 years GPA no minimum stated, 3.6, psychology GPA no minimum stated, 3.6; *School Psychology Other*: GRE-V no minimum stated, 520, GRE-Q no minimum stated, 480, overall undergraduate GPA no minimum stated, 3.3, last 2 years GPA no minimum stated, 3.5, psychology GPA no minimum stated, 3.7; *General Psychology MA/MS (Master of Arts/Science)*: GRE-V no minimum stated, 500, GRE-Q no minimum stated, 490, overall undergraduate GPA no minimum stated, 3.4, last 2 years GPA no minimum stated, 3.5, psychology GPA no minimum stated, 3.6.

Other Criteria: (importance of criteria rated low, medium, or high): GRE scores—medium, research experience—medium, work experience—medium, extracurricular activity—low, clinically related public service—high, GPA—medium, letters of recommendation—high, statement of goals and objectives—high, undergraduate major in psychology—medium, specific undergraduate psychology courses taken—medium. For additional information on admission requirements, go to http://www.psychology.eku.edu/grad1.php.

Student Characteristics: The following represents characteristics of students in 2009–2010 in all graduate psychology programs in the department: Female—full-time 63, part-time 2; Male—full-time 8, part-time 0; African American/Black—full-time 4, part-time 0; Hispanic/Latino(a)—full-time 0, part-time 0; Asian/Pacific Islander—full-time 1, part-time 0; American Indian/Alaska Native—full-time 0, part-time 0; Caucasian/White—full-time 66, part-time 2; Multi-ethnic—full-time 0, part-time 0; students subject to the Americans With Disabilities Act—full-time 0, part-time 0; Unknown ethnicity—full-time 0, part-time 0; International students who hold an F-1 or J-1 Visa—full-time 0, part-time 0.

Financial Information/Assistance:
Tuition for Full-Time Study: *Master's:* State residents: $383 per credit hour; Nonstate residents: $766 per credit hour. Tuition is subject to change. See the following Web site for updates and changes in tuition costs: http://www.gradschool.eku.edu/tuition.php.

Financial Assistance:
First-Year Students: Research assistantships available for first year. Average amount paid per academic year: $5,280. Average number of hours worked per week: 10. Apply by March 15.

GRADUATE STUDY IN PSYCHOLOGY

Advanced Students: Research assistantships available for advanced students. Average amount paid per academic year: $5,280. Average number of hours worked per week: 10. Apply by May 1.

Additional Information: Of all students currently enrolled full time, 90% benefited from one or more of the listed financial assistance programs. Application and information available online at: http://www.gradschool.eku.edu/awards/default.php.

Internships/Practica: Master's Degree (MA/MS Clinical Psychology): An internship experience, such as, a final research project or "capstone" experience is required of graduates. A variety of field placements are available within easy commuting distance from Richmond. Practicum sites have included private psychiatric and VA hospitals, the University counseling center, a residential treatment facility for children, alcohol and drug abuse treatment programs, and several adult and child outpatient mental health centers. Students also gain experience working in the EKU Psychology Clinic, an outpatient mental health facility operated by the Department. School psychology students can choose from a variety of public and private elementary and secondary schools. Students have completed internships in Kentucky as well as many other states. Students in the I/O program work on practicum projects with various for-profit and non-profit organizations in the region.

Housing and Day Care: On-campus housing is available. See the following Web site for more information: http://www.housing.eku.edu/. No on-campus day care facilities are available.

Employment of Department Graduates:
Master's Degree Graduates: Of those who graduated in the academic year 2008–2009, the following categories and numbers represent the postgraduate activities and employment of master's degree graduates: Enrolled in a psychology doctoral program (3), enrolled in a postdoctoral residency/fellowship (n/a), employed in independent practice (n/a), employed in an academic position at a university (1), employed in a professional position in a school system (9), employed in business or industry (7), employed in a community mental health/counseling center (8), total from the above (master's) (28).
Doctoral Degree Graduates: Of those who graduated in the academic year 2008–2009, the following categories and numbers represent the postgraduate activities and employment of doctoral degree graduates: Enrolled in a psychology doctoral program (n/a), total from the above (doctoral) (0).

Additional Information:
Orientation, Objectives, and Emphasis of Department: The MS program in clinical psychology is designed to train professional psychologists to work in clinics, hospitals, or other agencies, or to continue on to doctoral training. In the clinical program, approximately one-third of the course hours are devoted to theory and research, one-third to clinical skills training, and one-third to practicum and internship placements in the community. The clinical program also offers specialized training and experience serving individuals with autism spectrum disorders leading to an Autism Spectrum Disorder Certificate. The clinical program meets the curriculum standards required for membership in the Council of Applied Master's Programs in Psychology and is accredited nationally by the Master's Program Accreditation Council. The PsyS program in school psychology is designed to train professional psychologists to work in schools and school-related agencies. The program involves 71 graduate hours including internship, is NASP and NCATE-accredited and meets Kentucky certification requirements. The I/O program is designed to meet the education and training guidelines established by the Society for Industrial and Organizational Psychology. The scientist–practitioner I/O program prepares students to work in organizations and/or pursue a doctoral degree. Degree requirements include intensive required courses and electives, and practicum. Research opportunities are available in all programs, and all programs prepare students for doctoral study. The MS in General Psychology program offers a flexible curriculum designed to prepare students for further graduate study in psychology or for a variety of non-applied career options.

Special Facilities or Resources: Laboratories include several multipurpose rooms. The clinical training facility includes a group therapy room, individual therapy rooms, a testing room, and a play therapy room. All rooms have two-way mirror viewing and videotape facilities. The department operates a psychology training clinic providing outpatient services to the community, with its primary mission the training of students.

Information for Students With Physical Disabilities: See the following Web site for more information: http://www.disabled.eku.edu/.

Application Information:
Send to Graduate School, Eastern Kentucky University, 521 Lancaster Avenue, Richmond, KY 40475. Application available online. URL of online application: http://www.gradschool.eku.edu/apply/default.php. Students are admitted in the Fall, application deadline March 15. Applications received after March 15 are considered on a space-available basis. *Fee:* $35.

Kentucky, University of
Department of Educational, School, and Counseling Psychology
Education
Dickey Hall, Room 237
Lexington, KY 40506-0017
Telephone: (859) 257-7881
Fax: (859) 257-5662
E-mail: *fdanner@uky.edu*
Web: *http://education.uky.edu/EDP*

Department Information:
1968. Chairperson: Fred Danner. Number of faculty: total—full-time 14; women—full-time 7; total—minority—full-time 3; women minority—full-time 2.

Programs and Degrees Offered:
Listed in the following order: Program area, degree type (T if terminal Master's), number awarded 7/08–6/09. Counseling Psy-

chology MA/MS (Master of Arts/Science) 9, Educational Psychology MA/MS (Master of Arts/Science) (T) 0, School Psychology MA/MS (Master of Arts/Science) 0, Counseling Psychology PhD (Doctor of Philosophy) 2, Educational Psychology PhD (Doctor of Philosophy) 0, School Psychology PhD (Doctor of Philosophy) 3, School Psychology EdS (School Psychology) 16, Counseling Psychology EdS (School Psychology) 7.

APA Accreditation: Counseling PhD (Doctor of Philosophy). Student Outcome Data Website: http://education.uky.edu/EDP/content/counseling-psych-full-disclosure. School PhD (Doctor of Philosophy). Student Outcome Data Website: http://education.uky.edu/EDP/content/school-psych-full-disclosure.

Student Applications/Admissions:
Student Applications
Counseling Psychology MA/MS (Master of Arts/Science)—Applications 2009–2010, 44. Total applicants accepted 2009–2010, 31. Number full-time enrolled (new admits only) 2009–2010, 10. Number part-time enrolled (new admits only) 2009–2010, 0. Openings 2010–2011, 15. The median number of years required for completion of a degree in 2008–2009 were 2. The number of students enrolled full- and part-time who were dismissed or voluntarily withdrew from this program area in 2008–2009 were 0. *Educational Psychology MA/MS (Master of Arts/Science)*—Applications 2009–2010, 4. Total applicants accepted 2009–2010, 1. Number full-time enrolled (new admits only) 2009–2010, 1. Number part-time enrolled (new admits only) 2009–2010, 0. Openings 2010–2011, 5. The median number of years required for completion of a degree in 2008–2009 were 2. The number of students enrolled full- and part-time who were dismissed or voluntarily withdrew from this program area in 2008–2009 were 1. *School Psychology MA/MS (Master of Arts/Science)*—Applications 2009–2010, 48. Total applicants accepted 2009–2010, 14. Number full-time enrolled (new admits only) 2009–2010, 8. Number part-time enrolled (new admits only) 2009–2010, 0. Openings 2010–2011, 12. The median number of years required for completion of a degree in 2008–2009 were 2. The number of students enrolled full- and part-time who were dismissed or voluntarily withdrew from this program area in 2008–2009 were 0. *Counseling Psychology PhD (Doctor of Philosophy)*—Applications 2009–2010, 48. Total applicants accepted 2009–2010, 9. Number full-time enrolled (new admits only) 2009–2010, 5. Number part-time enrolled (new admits only) 2009–2010, 0. Openings 2010–2011, 9. The median number of years required for completion of a degree in 2008–2009 were 5. The number of students enrolled full- and part-time who were dismissed or voluntarily withdrew from this program area in 2008–2009 were 1. *Educational Psychology PhD (Doctor of Philosophy)*—Applications 2009–2010, 6. Total applicants accepted 2009–2010, 4. Number full-time enrolled (new admits only) 2009–2010, 4. Number part-time enrolled (new admits only) 2009–2010, 0. Openings 2010–2011, 5. The median number of years required for completion of a degree in 2008–2009 were 7. The number of students enrolled full- and part-time who were dismissed or voluntarily withdrew from this program area in 2008–2009 were 0. *School Psychology PhD (Doctor of Philosophy)*—Applications 2009–2010, 20. Total applicants accepted 2009–2010, 5. Number full-time enrolled (new admits only) 2009–2010, 4. Number part-time enrolled (new admits only) 2009–2010, 0. Total enrolled 2009–2010 full-time, 27, part-time, 9. Openings 2010–2011, 7. The median number of years required for completion of a degree in 2008–2009 were 6. The number of students enrolled full- and part-time who were dismissed or voluntarily withdrew from this program area in 2008–2009 were 0. *School Psychology EdS (School Psychology)*—Applications 2009–2010, 6. Total applicants accepted 2009–2010, 6. Number full-time enrolled (new admits only) 2009–2010, 6. Total enrolled 2009–2010 full-time, 8. Openings 2010–2011, 10. The median number of years required for completion of a degree in 2008–2009 were 2. The number of students enrolled full- and part-time who were dismissed or voluntarily withdrew from this program area in 2008–2009 were 0. *Counseling Psychology EdS (School Psychology)*—Applications 2009–2010, 1. Total applicants accepted 2009–2010, 1. Number full-time enrolled (new admits only) 2009–2010, 1. Total enrolled 2009–2010 full-time, 5. Openings 2010–2011, 6. The median number of years required for completion of a degree in 2008–2009 were 2.

Other Criteria: (importance of criteria rated low, medium, or high): GRE scores—medium, research experience—high, work experience—medium, extracurricular activity—medium, clinically related public service—high, GPA—medium, letters of recommendation—high, interview—high, statement of goals and objectives—high. Research experience and statement of goals are the highest priority for Educational Psychology programs. Work experiences, and clinically related service are more important for School and Counseling programs. For additional information on admission requirements, go to http://www.uky.edu/Education/edphead.html.

Student Characteristics: The following represents characteristics of students in 2009–2010 in all graduate psychology programs in the department: Female—full-time 108, part-time 0; Male—full-time 27, part-time 0; African American/Black—full-time 20, part-time 0; Hispanic/Latino(a)—full-time 6, part-time 0; Asian/Pacific Islander—full-time 1, part-time 0; American Indian/Alaska Native—full-time 3, part-time 0; Caucasian/White—full-time 96, part-time 0; Multi-ethnic—full-time 0, part-time 0; students subject to the Americans With Disabilities Act—full-time 0, part-time 0; Unknown ethnicity—full-time 9, part-time 0; International students who hold an F-1 or J-1 Visa—full-time 0, part-time 0.

Financial Information/Assistance:
Tuition for Full-Time Study: *Master's:* State residents: per academic year $8,778, $459 per credit hour; Nonstate residents: per academic year $18,089, $977 per credit hour. *Doctoral:* State residents: per academic year $8,778, $459 per credit hour; Nonstate residents: per academic year $18,089, $977 per credit hour. Tuition is subject to change.

Financial Assistance:
First-Year Students: No information provided.
Advanced Students: No information provided.
Additional Information: Of all students currently enrolled full time, 60% benefited from one or more of the listed financial assistance programs.

Internships/Practica: Doctoral Degree (PhD Counseling Psychology): For those doctoral students for whom a professional internship was required in this program prior to graduation, (2) students applied for an internship in 2008–2009, with (2) students obtaining an internship. Of those students who obtained an internship, (2) were paid internships. Of those students who obtained an internship, (2) students placed in APA/CPA accredited internships, (0) students placed in internships not APA/CPA accredited, but listed with the Association of Psychology Postdoctoral and Internship Programs (APPIC), (0) students placed in internships conforming to guidelines of the Council of Directors of School Psychology Programs (CDSPP), (0) students placed in internships that were not APA/CPA accredited, APPIC or CDSPP listed. Doctoral Degree (PhD School Psychology): For those doctoral students for whom a professional internship was required in this program prior to graduation, (2) students applied for an internship in 2008–2009, with (2) students obtaining an internship. Of those students who obtained an internship, (2) were paid internships. Of those students who obtained an internship, (2) students placed in APA/CPA accredited internships, (0) students placed in internships not APA/CPA accredited, but listed with the Association of Psychology Postdoctoral and Internship Programs (APPIC), (0) students placed in internships conforming to guidelines of the Council of Directors of School Psychology Programs (CDSPP), (0) students placed in internships that were not APA/CPA accredited, APPIC or CDSPP listed. Master's Degree (MA/MS Educational Psychology): An internship experience, such as a final research project or "capstone" experience is required of graduates.

Housing and Day Care: On-campus housing is available. See the following Web site for more information: http://www.uky.edu/Housing. On-campus day care facilities are available.

Employment of Department Graduates:
Master's Degree Graduates: Of those who graduated in the academic year 2008–2009, the following categories and numbers represent the postgraduate activities and employment of master's degree graduates: Enrolled in a psychology doctoral program (6), enrolled in another graduate/professional program (1), enrolled in a postdoctoral residency/fellowship (n/a), employed in independent practice (n/a), employed in an academic position at a university (0), employed in an academic position at a 2-year/4-year college (0), employed in other positions at a higher education institution (0), employed in a professional position in a school system (2), employed in business or industry (1), employed in government agency (0), employed in a community mental health/counseling center (1), employed in a hospital/medical center (0), total from the above (master's) (11).
Doctoral Degree Graduates: Of those who graduated in the academic year 2008–2009, the following categories and numbers represent the postgraduate activities and employment of doctoral degree graduates: Enrolled in a psychology doctoral program (n/a), enrolled in another graduate/professional program (0), enrolled in a postdoctoral residency/fellowship (1), employed in independent practice (1), employed in an academic position at a university (6), employed in an academic position at a 2-year/4-year college (4), employed in other positions at a higher education institution (3), employed in a professional position in a school system (1), employed in business or industry (0), employed in government agency (0), employed in a community mental health/counseling center (2), total from the above (doctoral) (18).

Additional Information:
Orientation, Objectives, and Emphasis of Department: Three programs are housed within the department: counseling psychology, educational psychology, and school psychology. The program faculties in counseling psychology and in school psychology are committed to the scientist–practitioner model for professional training, while educational psychology faculty emphasize the researcher-teacher model. A strong emphasis has been placed upon the psychology core for all professional training. Because we are graduate department with a professional emphasis, a high premium is placed on professional writing skills throughout—from admissions to course papers to final projects (theses and dissertations) in all programs. Counseling faculty research interests focus upon cultural diversity and social justice, counseling issues for sexual minorities, family processes, experiential therapies, and rape awareness. The school psychology faculty research interests focus upon evaluation and assessment, positive mental health outcomes, literacy and social development in young children, and direct interventions. The educational psychology faculty research interests include motivation in educational settings, cardiovascular stress in minority children, culture and socialization in relation to cognition, engagement in risky behaviors, and sleep deprivation. Students in each program are encouraged to establish mentoring relationships with their major professor by the beginning of their second semester. The counseling faculty intends to prepare professionals for diverse settings, e.g., colleges and universities, research facilities, hospitals, regional mental health centers, and private practice. The school psychology faculty aims to prepare scientist–practitioners who will function in school and university settings, in mental health consortia, and in private practice. The educational psychology faculty prepares graduates for research and teaching careers within higher education and applied research settings.

Special Facilities or Resources: The University of Kentucky is located on the western edge of Appalachia, which provides students with the opportunity to interact with a rich and varied American culture. The uniqueness of this potential client and research pool allows our students to examine attributes of the bridge between the old, rural America and the future, more technological America. Microcomputer facilities are available within the department and within the college for student use in word processing, model development, simulation and evaluation, and data analysis. The university provides all the facilities and resources expected of a major research institution (e.g., extensive libraries, computer facilities, research environment, and medical center).

Application Information:
Send to Dr. Rory Remer, Director of Graduate Studies, Department of Educational, School, and Counseling Psychology, College of Education, University of Kentucky, 237 Dickey Hall, Lexington, KY 40506-0017. Application available online. URL of online application: http://education.uky.edu/EDP. Students are admitted in the Fall, application deadline December 15. December 15 deadline for PhD; February 15 deadline for Master's and EdS programs. *Fee:* $50. $65 International.

Kentucky, University of
Department of Psychology
Arts and Sciences
Kastle Hall
Lexington, KY 40506-0044
Telephone: (859) 257-9640
Fax: (859) 323-1979
E-mail: mkkell5@email.uky.edu
Web: http://www.uky.edu/ArtsSciences/Psychology

Department Information:
1917. Chairperson: Robert Lorch, PhD. Number of faculty: total—full-time 30, part-time 6; women—full-time 11, part-time 2; total—minority—full-time 4, part-time 1; women minority—full-time 3, part-time 1.

Programs and Degrees Offered:
Listed in the following order: Program area, degree type (T if terminal Master's), number awarded 7/08–6/09. Clinical Psychology PhD (Doctor of Philosophy) 6, Experimental Psychology PhD (Doctor of Philosophy) 3.

APA Accreditation: Clinical PhD (Doctor of Philosophy).

Student Applications/Admissions:
Student Applications
Clinical Psychology PhD (Doctor of Philosophy)—Applications 2009–2010, 202. Total applicants accepted 2009–2010, 8. Number full-time enrolled (new admits only) 2009–2010, 6. Number part-time enrolled (new admits only) 2009–2010, 0. Openings 2010–2011, 9. The median number of years required for completion of a degree in 2008–2009 were 6. The number of students enrolled full- and part-time who were dismissed or voluntarily withdrew from this program area in 2008–2009 were 1. *Experimental Psychology PhD (Doctor of Philosophy)*—Applications 2009–2010, 77. Total applicants accepted 2009–2010, 12. Number full-time enrolled (new admits only) 2009–2010, 8. Openings 2010–2011, 10. The median number of years required for completion of a degree in 2008–2009 were 5. The number of students enrolled full- and part-time who were dismissed or voluntarily withdrew from this program area in 2008–2009 were 1.
Scores: Entries appear in this order: required test or GPA, minimum score (if required), median score of students entering in 2009–2010. *Clinical Psychology PhD (Doctor of Philosophy):* GRE-V no minimum stated, 562, GRE-Q no minimum stated, 659, GRE-Analytical no minimum stated, 4.67, overall undergraduate GPA no minimum stated, 3.67, psychology GPA no minimum stated, Masters GPA no minimum stated, 3.60; *Experimental Psychology PhD (Doctor of Philosophy):* GRE-V no minimum stated, 517, GRE-Q no minimum stated, 632, GRE-Analytical no minimum stated, 4.17, overall undergraduate GPA no minimum stated, 3.42, psychology GPA no minimum stated, Masters GPA no minimum stated, 3.77.
Other Criteria: (importance of criteria rated low, medium, or high): GRE scores—high, research experience—high, work experience—low, clinically related public service—medium, GPA—high, letters of recommendation—high, interview—high, statement of goals and objectives—high, knowledge of mentor's res—high, undergraduate major in psychology—medium, specific undergraduate psychology courses taken—medium.

Student Characteristics: The following represents characteristics of students in 2009–2010 in all graduate psychology programs in the department: Female—full-time 64, part-time 0; Male—full-time 25, part-time 0; African American/Black—full-time 6, part-time 0; Hispanic/Latino(a)—full-time 1, part-time 0; Asian/Pacific Islander—full-time 2, part-time 0; American Indian/Alaska Native—full-time 0, part-time 0; Caucasian/White—full-time 80, part-time 0; Multi-ethnic—full-time 0, part-time 0; students subject to the Americans With Disabilities Act—full-time 1, part-time 0; Unknown ethnicity—full-time 0, part-time 0; International students who hold an F-1 or J-1 Visa—full-time 1, part-time 0.

Financial Information/Assistance:
Tuition for Full-Time Study: Master's: State residents: per academic year $8,778, $459 per credit hour; Nonstate residents: per academic year $18,089, $977 per credit hour. *Doctoral:* State residents: per academic year $8,778, $459 per credit hour; Nonstate residents: per academic year $18,089, $977 per credit hour. Tuition is subject to change. Additional fees are assessed to students beyond the costs of tuition for the following: health fee/recreation fee: totaling less than $500 per semester. See the following Web site for updates and changes in tuition costs: http://www.uky.edu/Registrar/feesgen.htm.

Financial Assistance:
First-Year Students: Teaching assistantships available for first year. Average amount paid per academic year: $14,000. Average number of hours worked per week: 20. Research assistantships available for first year. Average amount paid per academic year: $14,000. Average number of hours worked per week: 20. Fellowships and scholarships available for first year. Average amount paid per academic year: $14,000. Average number of hours worked per week: 20.
Advanced Students: Teaching assistantships available for advanced students. Average amount paid per academic year: $14,000. Average number of hours worked per week: 20. Research assistantships available for advanced students. Average amount paid per academic year: $14,000. Average number of hours worked per week: 20. Fellowships and scholarships available for advanced students. Average amount paid per academic year: $14,000. Average number of hours worked per week: 20.
Additional Information: Of all students currently enrolled full time, 99% benefited from one or more of the listed financial assistance programs.

Internships/Practica: Doctoral Degree (PhD Clinical Psychology): For those doctoral students for whom a professional internship was required in this program prior to graduation, (8) students applied for an internship in 2008–2009, with (7) students obtaining an internship. Of those students who obtained an internship, (7) were paid internships. Of those students who obtained an internship, (7) students placed in APA/CPA accredited internships, (0) students placed in internships not APA/CPA accredited, but listed with the Association of Psychology Postdoctoral and Internship Programs (APPIC), (0) students placed in internships conforming to guidelines of the Council of Directors of School Psychology Programs (CDSPP), (0) students placed in internships that were not APA/CPA accredited, APPIC or CDSPP listed.

Housing and Day Care: On-campus housing is available. See the following Web site for more information: http://www.uky.edu/Housing/graduate/. On-campus day care facilities are available. See the following Web site for more information: http://www.uky.edu/HR/WorkLife/childcare.html.

Employment of Department Graduates:

Master's Degree Graduates: Of those who graduated in the academic year 2008–2009, the following categories and numbers represent the postgraduate activities and employment of master's degree graduates: Enrolled in a psychology doctoral program (0), enrolled in another graduate/professional program (0), enrolled in a postdoctoral residency/fellowship (n/a), employed in independent practice (n/a), employed in an academic position at a university (0), employed in an academic position at a 2-year/4-year college (0), employed in other positions at a higher education institution (0), employed in a professional position in a school system (0), employed in business or industry (0), employed in government agency (0), employed in a community mental health/counseling center (0), employed in a hospital/medical center (0), still seeking employment (0), not seeking employment (0), other employment position (0), do not know (0), total from the above (master's) (0).

Doctoral Degree Graduates: Of those who graduated in the academic year 2008–2009, the following categories and numbers represent the postgraduate activities and employment of doctoral degree graduates: Enrolled in a psychology doctoral program (n/a), enrolled in another graduate/professional program (0), enrolled in a postdoctoral residency/fellowship (5), employed in independent practice (0), employed in an academic position at a university (3), employed in an academic position at a 2-year/4-year college (0), employed in other positions at a higher education institution (5), employed in a professional position in a school system (0), employed in business or industry (0), employed in government agency (0), employed in a community mental health/counseling center (0), employed in a hospital/medical center (0), still seeking employment (2), not seeking employment (0), other employment position (0), do not know (1), total from the above (doctoral) (16).

Additional Information:

Orientation, Objectives, and Emphasis of Department: The goals of the doctoral program depend partly upon the specific program area in which a student enrolls. The program in Clinical Psychology follows the Boulder scientist–practitioner model. Students in the program receive broad exposure to the major theoretical perspectives influencing clinical psychology. All students are actively engaged in research throughout their graduate training. Beginning in the second year of study, each student also receives extensive clinical experience via placements in mental or behavioral health settings. Graduates of the program are prepared to pursue an academic career or to be a practitioner. Students in the program in Experimental Psychology, Cognitive, Developmental, Social, Animal Learning and Behavioral Neuroscience are trained as research scientists. They are exposed to the important theoretical perspectives and research paradigms of their respective areas. There is considerable latitude for individuals to define their specific programs of study. Graduates are prepared to pursue an academic career or a research position in an applied setting. Graduate study is based on a core curriculum model that would fulfill Graduate School requirements for the PhD degree. All students complete a Master's thesis, written and oral doctoral qualifying examinations, and a dissertation demonstrating accomplishment in independent research.

Special Facilities or Resources: The psychology department occupies its own three-story building located by the computer center and main campus library. Kastle Hall houses faculty and student offices, classrooms, and research space. Research facilities in the building include: animal laboratories for behavioral and physiological research; observation rooms with one-way mirrors; extensive video equipment; and microcomputer equipped rooms for cognitive research. Two additional buildings on campus are available for behavioral research. Current faculty have collaborative arrangements with several facilities on campus, including: the neuropsychology laboratories in the Department of Neurology; the OroFacial Pain Clinic in the College of Dentistry; the Central Animal Research Facility; and the Sanders-Brown Center on Aging. The department maintains a large undergraduate subject pool. Clinical training facilities are excellent and include a departmental clinic housed in a separate building and clinical placement arrangements with a variety of mental and behavioral health facilities in Lexington.

Information for Students With Physical Disabilities: See the following Web site for more information: http://www.uky.edu/StudentAffairs/DisabilityResourceCenter/.

Application Information:
Send to Office of Research and Graduate Studies, Department of Psychology, University of Kentucky, 106B Kastle Hall, Lexington, KY 40506-0044. Application available online. URL of online application: http://www.uky.edu/AS/Psychology/graduate/. Students are admitted in the Fall, application deadline December/January. Clinical Psychology: The application deadline is normally the last Friday of classes before the University's Winter Break. Experimental Psychology: The application deadline is normally the second Friday of the month of January. *Fee:* $50. International Fee: $65.

Louisville, University of
Department of Educational & Counseling Psychology
Education & Human Development
2301 South 3rd Street
Louisville, KY 40292
Telephone: (502) 852-6884
Fax: (502) 852-0629
E-mail: m.leach@louisville.edu
Web: http://www.louisville.edu/education/degrees/phd-cps-counselingpsychology.html

---

Department Information:
Chairperson: Dr. Linda Shapiro. Number of faculty: total—full-time 6; women—full-time 2; total—minority—full-time 1.

Programs and Degrees Offered:
Listed in the following order: Program area, degree type (T if terminal Master's), number awarded 7/08–6/09. Counseling and Personnel Services PhD (Doctor of Philosophy) 4.

APA Accreditation: Counseling PhD (Doctor of Philosophy). Student Outcome Data Website: http://louisville.edu/education/degrees/phd-cps-counselingpsychology.html.

Student Applications/Admissions:

Student Applications

Counseling and Personnel Services PhD (Doctor of Philosophy)—Applications 2009–2010, 72. Total applicants accepted 2009–2010, 6. Number full-time enrolled (new admits only) 2009–2010, 6. Number part-time enrolled (new admits only) 2009–2010, 0. Total enrolled 2009–2010 full-time, 39. Openings 2010–2011, 6. The median number of years required for completion of a degree in 2008–2009 were 4. The number of students enrolled full- and part-time who were dismissed or voluntarily withdrew from this program area in 2008–2009 were 0.

Scores: Entries appear in this order: required test or GPA, minimum score (if required), median score of students entering in 2009–2010. *Counseling and Personnel Services PhD (Doctor of Philosophy)*: GRE-V 500, 590, GRE-Q 500, 690, GRE-Analytical 4.0, 5.0, overall undergraduate GPA 3.0, 3.5.

Other Criteria: (importance of criteria rated low, medium, or high): GRE scores—high, research experience—high, work experience—medium, extracurricular activity—medium, clinically related public service—medium, GPA—high, letters of recommendation—high, interview—high, statement of goals and objectives—high, undergraduate major in psychology—medium, specific undergraduate psychology courses taken—medium.

Student Characteristics: The following represents characteristics of students in 2009–2010 in all graduate psychology programs in the department: Female—full-time 25, part-time 0; Male—full-time 14, part-time 0; African American/Black—full-time 2, part-time 0; Hispanic/Latino(a)—full-time 0, part-time 0; Asian/Pacific Islander—full-time 2, part-time 0; American Indian/Alaska Native—full-time 0, part-time 0; Caucasian/White—full-time 35, part-time 0; Multi-ethnic—full-time 0, part-time 0; students subject to the Americans With Disabilities Act—full-time 0, part-time 0; Unknown ethnicity—full-time 0, part-time 0; International students who hold an F-1 or J-1 Visa—full-time 0, part-time 0.

Financial Information/Assistance:

Tuition for Full-Time Study: *Doctoral:* State residents: per academic year $11,496, $479 per credit hour; Nonstate residents: per academic year $24,672, $1,028 per credit hour. Tuition is subject to change. See the following Web site for updates and changes in tuition costs: http://louisville.edu/finance/bursar/tuition/tuitionrates0910.html.

Financial Assistance:

First-Year Students: Teaching assistantships available for first year. Average amount paid per academic year: $18,000. Average number of hours worked per week: 20. Apply by January 15. Research assistantships available for first year. Average amount paid per academic year: $18,000. Average number of hours worked per week: 20. Apply by January 15. Fellowships and scholarships available for first year. Average amount paid per academic year: $18,000. Average number of hours worked per week: 0. Apply by January 15.

Advanced Students: Teaching assistantships available for advanced students. Average amount paid per academic year: $18,000. Apply by January 15. Research assistantships available for advanced students. Average amount paid per academic year: $18,000. Apply by January 15. Fellowships and scholarships available for advanced students. Average amount paid per academic year: $18,000. Apply by January 15.

Additional Information: Of all students currently enrolled full time, 90% benefited from one or more of the listed financial assistance programs.

Internships/Practica: Doctoral Degree (PhD Counseling and Personnel Services): For those doctoral students for whom a professional internship was required in this program prior to graduation, (3) students applied for an internship in 2008–2009, with (3) students obtaining an internship. Of those students who obtained an internship, (3) were paid internships. Of those students who obtained an internship, (3) students placed in APA/CPA accredited internships, (0) students placed in internships not APA/CPA accredited, but listed with the Association of Psychology Postdoctoral and Internship Programs (APPIC), (0) students placed in internships conforming to guidelines of the Council of Directors of School Psychology Programs (CDSPP), (0) students placed in internships that were not APA/CPA accredited, APPIC or CDSPP listed. Our internship placement rate is over 90%. Due to the wide variety of placement sites in the city and surrounding area prior to internship, students accept internship positions in counseling centers, hospitals, community mental health centers, and VAs. Our community sites include the same, which is a strength of our program.

Housing and Day Care: On-campus housing is available. See the following Web site for more information: http://louisville.edu/student/housing/index/html. On-campus day care facilities are available. See the following Web site for more information: http://louisville.edu/education/elc.

Employment of Department Graduates:

Master's Degree Graduates: Of those who graduated in the academic year 2008–2009, the following categories and numbers represent the postgraduate activities and employment of master's degree graduates: Enrolled in a postdoctoral residency/fellowship (n/a), employed in independent practice (n/a), total from the above (master's) (0).

Doctoral Degree Graduates: Of those who graduated in the academic year 2008–2009, the following categories and numbers represent the postgraduate activities and employment of doctoral degree graduates: Enrolled in a psychology doctoral program (n/a), employed in a community mental health/counseling center (2), employed in a hospital/medical center (1), do not know (1), total from the above (doctoral) (4).

Additional Information:

Orientation, Objectives, and Emphasis of Department: The Counseling Psychology PhD Program adheres to a scientist–practitioner model and we strive to be balanced in each area. Students have a wide variety of applied settings from which to engage in counseling work, many consistent with the mission of an urban university. We tend to focus on applied work with adults, though we do include adolescents. Our faculty emphasize cognitive-behavioral, psychodynamic, and interpersonal models in conjunction with multicultural and feminist approaches. Our research foci include diversity, microaggressions, prevention of depression in adolescents, interpersonal relationships, forgiveness, suicide, religion and spirituality, vocational issues, international counseling, gender issues, and adolescent development. Faculty emphasize student inclusion on research projects.

Special Facilities or Resources: Students have opportunities to collect research data at a variety of sites in the city. General research space is available in the department. A research lab is housed in the college. Ample computers and training opportunities are available in the college and university.

Information for Students With Physical Disabilities: See the following Web site for more information: http://louisville.edu/disability.

Application Information:
Send to Graduate Admissions Office, University of Louisville, Houchens Room 6, Louisville, KY 40292-0001. Application available online. URL of online application: https://graduate.louisville.edu/students/apply/application.html. Students are admitted in the Fall, application deadline December 15. *Fee:* $50.

Louisville, University of
Psychological and Brain Sciences
Arts and Sciences
317 Life Sciences Building
Louisville, KY 40292
Telephone: (502) 852-6775
Fax: (502) 852-8904
E-mail: *smeeks@louisville.edu*
Web: *http://www.louisville.edu/psychology/*

Department Information:
1963. Chairperson: Suzanne Meeks. Number of faculty: total—full-time 27, part-time 3; women—full-time 13, part-time 2; total—minority—full-time 3; women minority—full-time 1; faculty subject to the Americans With Disabilities Act 1.

Programs and Degrees Offered:
Listed in the following order: Program area, degree type (T if terminal Master's), number awarded 7/08–6/09. Experimental Psychology PhD (Doctor of Philosophy) 3, Clinical Psychology PhD (Doctor of Philosophy) 6.

APA Accreditation: Clinical PhD (Doctor of Philosophy). Student Outcome Data Website: http://louisville.edu/psychology/doctorate/clinical-psychology/program-statistics.html.

Student Applications/Admissions:
Student Applications
Experimental Psychology PhD (Doctor of Philosophy)—Applications 2009–2010, 20. Total applicants accepted 2009–2010, 4. Number full-time enrolled (new admits only) 2009–2010, 4. Number part-time enrolled (new admits only) 2009–2010, 0. Openings 2010–2011, 5. The median number of years required for completion of a degree in 2008–2009 were 6. The number of students enrolled full- and part-time who were dismissed or voluntarily withdrew from this program area in 2008–2009 were 0. *Clinical Psychology PhD (Doctor of Philosophy)*—Applications 2009–2010, 136. Total applicants accepted 2009–2010, 5. Number full-time enrolled (new admits only) 2009–2010, 5. Number part-time enrolled (new admits only) 2009–2010, 0. Openings 2010–2011, 5. The median number of years required for completion of a degree in 2008–2009 were 5. The number of students enrolled full- and part-time who were dismissed or voluntarily withdrew from this program area in 2008–2009 were 3.

Scores: Entries appear in this order: required test or GPA, minimum score (if required), median score of students entering in 2009–2010. *Experimental Psychology PhD (Doctor of Philosophy):* GRE-V 550, 550, GRE-Q 550, 660, overall undergraduate GPA 3.0, 3.90; *Clinical Psychology PhD (Doctor of Philosophy):* GRE-V 550, 530, GRE-Q 550, 570, overall undergraduate GPA 3.0, 3.42.

Other Criteria: (importance of criteria rated low, medium, or high): GRE scores—high, research experience—high, work experience—high, extracurricular activity—high, clinically related public service—high, GPA—high, letters of recommendation—high, interview—high, statement of goals and objectives—high, undergraduate major in psychology—medium, specific undergraduate psychology courses taken—medium. Experimental Psychology PhD does not require clinically related public service.

Student Characteristics: The following represents characteristics of students in 2009–2010 in all graduate psychology programs in the department: Female—full-time 47, part-time 0; Male—full-time 19, part-time 0; African American/Black—full-time 3, part-time 0; Hispanic/Latino(a)—full-time 1, part-time 0; Asian/Pacific Islander—full-time 8, part-time 0; American Indian/Alaska Native—full-time 0, part-time 0; Caucasian/White—full-time 53, part-time 0; Multi-ethnic—full-time 1, part-time 0; students subject to the Americans With Disabilities Act—full-time 0, part-time 0; Unknown ethnicity—full-time 0, part-time 0; International students who hold an F-1 or J-1 Visa—full-time 6, part-time 0.

Financial Information/Assistance:
Tuition for Full-Time Study: Doctoral: State residents: per academic year $11,496, $479 per credit hour; Nonstate residents: per academic year $24,672, $1,028 per credit hour. Tuition is subject to change. See the following Web site for updates and changes in tuition costs: http://louisville.edu/finance/bursar/tuition.

Financial Assistance:
First-Year Students: Teaching assistantships available for first year. Average amount paid per academic year: $22,000. Average number of hours worked per week: 20. Apply by December 1. Research assistantships available for first year. Average amount paid per academic year: $22,000. Average number of hours worked per week: 20. Apply by December 1. Fellowships and scholarships available for first year. Average amount paid per academic year: $22,000. Average number of hours worked per week: 0. Apply by December 1.

Advanced Students: Teaching assistantships available for advanced students. Average amount paid per academic year: $22,000. Average number of hours worked per week: 20. Apply by December 1. Research assistantships available for advanced students. Average amount paid per academic year: $22,000. Average number of hours worked per week: 20. Apply by December 1. Traineeships available for advanced students. Average amount paid per academic year: $0. Average number of hours worked per week: 0. Fellowships and scholarships available for advanced students. Average amount paid per academic year: $22,000. Average number of hours worked per week: 0. Apply by December 1.

Additional Information: Of all students currently enrolled full time, 74% benefited from one or more of the listed financial assistance programs.

Internships/Practica: Doctoral Degree (PhD Clinical Psychology): For those doctoral students for whom a professional internship was required in this program prior to graduation, (8) students applied for an internship in 2008–2009, with (8) students obtaining an internship. Of those students who obtained an internship, (8) were paid internships. Of those students who obtained an internship, (8) students placed in APA/CPA accredited internships, (0) students placed in internships not APA/CPA accredited, but listed with the Association of Psychology Postdoctoral and Internship Programs (APPIC), (0) students placed in internships conforming to guidelines of the Council of Directors of School Psychology Programs (CDSPP), (0) students placed in internships that were not APA/CPA accredited, APPIC or CDSPP listed. Most practicum experience takes place in our in-house Psychological Services Center. Paid and unpaid practica are available in community and government agencies. These vary from year to year, but include Central State Hospital, private practices, and the Departments of Psychiatry and Behavioral Sciences, Anesthesiology, and Family Medicine.

Housing and Day Care: On-campus housing is available. See the following Web site for more information: http://louisville.edu/housing/. On-campus day care facilities are available. See the following Web site for more information: http://louisville.edu/education/elc/.

Employment of Department Graduates:
Master's Degree Graduates: Of those who graduated in the academic year 2008–2009, the following categories and numbers represent the postgraduate activities and employment of master's degree graduates: Enrolled in a postdoctoral residency/fellowship (n/a), employed in independent practice (n/a), total from the above (master's) (0).
Doctoral Degree Graduates: Of those who graduated in the academic year 2008–2009, the following categories and numbers represent the postgraduate activities and employment of doctoral degree graduates: Enrolled in a psychology doctoral program (n/a), employed in an academic position at a university (3), employed in government agency (1), employed in a community mental health/counseling center (2), employed in a hospital/medical center (1), other employment position (1), total from the above (doctoral) (8).

Additional Information:
Orientation, Objectives, and Emphasis of Department: The Clinical Psychology PhD Program adheres to a scientist–practitioner model and is designed to provide training in research, psychological assessment, psychological intervention, and legal and professional issues. Faculty research foci are in health psychology, geropsychology and psychopathology. Clinical emphases include interpersonal and cognitive-behavioral approaches. The Experimental Psychology PhD program offers a flexible curriculum tailored to the individual student's interests while providing extensive training in the core processes of psychology, research methodology, and data analysis. Research is an integral component of the Experimental Psychology PhD, thus students begin working in their mentor's laboratory when they arrive on campus. Faculty research interests are varied, but fall into the following areas of strength: cognitive science, developmental science, neuroscience, and vision & hearing sciences. Recent graduates are pursuing careers in academic and non-academic fields in numerous settings, including universities and colleges, industry, government and private consulting organizations.

Special Facilities or Resources: Departmental facilities include modern laboratories and a Psychological Services Center. The University Computing resources are available from departmental stations via a campus-wide network. Additional training opportunities are available through such facilities as the Department of Psychiatry and Behavioral Sciences, the Child Evaluation Center, Central State Hospital, and other community agencies.

Information for Students With Physical Disabilities: See the following Web site for more information: http://louisville.edu/disability/.

Application Information:
Send to Graduate Admissions Office, University of Louisville, Houchens Room 6, Louisville, KY 40292-0001. Application available online. URL of online application: http://graduate.louisville.edu/students/apply/application.html. Students are admitted in the Fall, application deadline December 1. *Fee:* $50.

Morehead State University (Kentucky)
Department of Psychology
Science & Technology
414 Reed Hall
Morehead, KY 40351
Telephone: (606) 783-2981
Fax: (606) 783-5077
E-mail: *l.couch@moreheadstate.edu*
Web: *http://www.moreheadstate.edu/psych*

Department Information:
1968. Interim Chair: Laurie L. Couch, PhD. Number of faculty: total—full-time 10, part-time 3; women—full-time 4, part-time 2; total—minority—full-time 1; women minority—full-time 1.

Programs and Degrees Offered:
Listed in the following order: Program area, degree type (T if terminal Master's), number awarded 7/08–6/09. General Experimental Psychology MA/MS (Master of Arts/Science) (T) 2, Clinical/Counseling Psychology MA/MS (Master of Arts/Science) (T) 9.

Student Applications/Admissions:
Student Applications
General Experimental Psychology MA/MS *(Master of Arts/Science)*—Applications 2009–2010, 12. Number full-time enrolled (new admits only) 2009–2010, 7. Number part-time

enrolled (new admits only) 2009–2010, 0. Total enrolled 2009–2010 full-time, 8, part-time, 1. Openings 2010–2011, 8. The median number of years required for completion of a degree in 2008–2009 were 2. The number of students enrolled full- and part-time who were dismissed or voluntarily withdrew from this program area in 2008–2009 were 0. *Clinical/Counseling Psychology MA/MS (Master of Arts/Science)*—Applications 2009–2010, 30. Total applicants accepted 2009–2010, 14. Number full-time enrolled (new admits only) 2009–2010, 12. Number part-time enrolled (new admits only) 2009–2010, 0. Openings 2010–2011, 14. The median number of years required for completion of a degree in 2008–2009 were 2. The number of students enrolled full- and part-time who were dismissed or voluntarily withdrew from this program area in 2008–2009 were 0.

Scores: Entries appear in this order: required test or GPA, minimum score (if required), median score of students entering in 2009–2010. *General Experimental Psychology MA/MS (Master of Arts/Science)*: GRE-V 420, 460, GRE-Q 470, 540, overall undergraduate GPA 2.5, 3.3; *Clinical/Counseling Psychology MA/MS (Master of Arts/Science)*: GRE-V 410, 460, GRE-Q 410, 510, overall undergraduate GPA 2.8, 3.48.

Other Criteria: (importance of criteria rated low, medium, or high): GRE scores—high, research experience—high, work experience—low, extracurricular activity—low, clinically related public service—low, GPA—high, letters of recommendation—high, interview—high, statement of goals and objectives—medium, undergraduate major in psychology—medium, specific undergraduate psychology courses taken—medium.

Student Characteristics: The following represents characteristics of students in 2009–2010 in all graduate psychology programs in the department: Female—full-time 21, part-time 0; Male—full-time 9, part-time 1; African American/Black—full-time 0, part-time 0; Hispanic/Latino(a)—full-time 0, part-time 0; Asian/Pacific Islander—full-time 0, part-time 0; American Indian/Alaska Native—full-time 0, part-time 0; Caucasian/White—full-time 30, part-time 1; Multi-ethnic—full-time 0, part-time 0; students subject to the Americans With Disabilities Act—full-time 0, part-time 0; Unknown ethnicity—full-time 0, part-time 0; International students who hold an F-1 or J-1 Visa—full-time 1, part-time 0.

Financial Information/Assistance:
Tuition for Full-Time Study: *Master's:* State residents: $351 per credit hour; Nonstate residents: $878 per credit hour. Tuition is subject to change. Additional fees are assessed to students beyond the costs of tuition for the following: laboratory fees for some courses may apply (lab courses and internet courses). See the following Web site for updates and changes in tuition costs: http://www.moreheadstate.edu/bestvalue.

Financial Assistance:
First-Year Students: Teaching assistantships available for first year. Average amount paid per academic year: $10,000. Average number of hours worked per week: 20. Research assistantships available for first year. Average amount paid per academic year: $10,000. Average number of hours worked per week: 20.

Advanced Students: Teaching assistantships available for advanced students. Average amount paid per academic year: $10,000. Average number of hours worked per week: 20. Research assistantships available for advanced students. Average amount paid per academic year: $10,000. Average number of hours worked per week: 20.

Additional Information: Of all students currently enrolled full time, 92% benefited from one or more of the listed financial assistance programs.

Internships/Practica: Master's Degree (MA/MS General Experimental Psychology): An internship experience, such as a final research project or "capstone" experience is required of graduates. Master's Degree (MA/MS Clinical/Counseling Psychology): An internship experience, such as a final research project or "capstone" experience is required of graduates. Internships and practicum placement sites are available in several different states.

Housing and Day Care: On-campus housing is available. See the following Web site for more information: http://www.moreheadstate.edu/housing/. No on-campus day care facilities are available.

Employment of Department Graduates:
Master's Degree Graduates: Of those who graduated in the academic year 2008–2009, the following categories and numbers represent the postgraduate activities and employment of master's degree graduates: Enrolled in a psychology doctoral program (1), enrolled in another graduate/professional program (0), enrolled in a postdoctoral residency/fellowship (n/a), employed in independent practice (n/a), employed in an academic position at a university (0), employed in an academic position at a 2-year/4-year college (2), employed in other positions at a higher education institution (0), employed in a professional position in a school system (0), employed in business or industry (0), employed in government agency (0), employed in a community mental health/counseling center (10), employed in a hospital/medical center (1), still seeking employment (0), other employment position (0), total from the above (master's) (14).

Doctoral Degree Graduates: Of those who graduated in the academic year 2008–2009, the following categories and numbers represent the postgraduate activities and employment of doctoral degree graduates: Enrolled in a psychology doctoral program (n/a), total from the above (doctoral) (0).

Additional Information:
Orientation, Objectives, and Emphasis of Department: The clinical and counseling programs are designed primarily to train Master's level psychologists to practice in a variety of settings, and lead to certification in many states. However, approximately 30% of our students also enter doctoral level programs upon graduation. The scientist–practitioner model is emphasized in the program, with primary emphases on acquisition of applied clinical skills and knowledge of the general field of psychology. Consequently, competencies in critical analysis of theories, experimental design, and quantitative data analysis are expected. Clinical and counseling students are encouraged to participate in or conduct research ongoing in the department. Students interested in pursuing doctoral level training are encouraged to complete a thesis. The purpose of the general/experimental master's program is primarily to prepare students for entry into doctoral programs. Students and faculty are involved in research in several areas including cognitive, perception, animal learning and motivation, psychopharmacology, neurophysiology, developmental, social, and personality.

Special Facilities or Resources: The psychology program provides excellent laboratory facilities for the study of human and animal behavior. Faculty/student research programs often are funded through both intra- and extramural grants. The department maintains several microcomputer laboratories, and offers training in the statistical package SPSS. Most accepted students are supported by graduate assistantships. Financial assistance for paper presentations at professional conferences is normally available.

Application Information:
Send to Graduate Office, Morehead State University, 701 Ginger Hall, Morehead, KY 40351. Application available online. URL of online application: http://acampus21.moreheadstate.edu/prospective/graduate/apply. Students are admitted in the Fall, application deadline March 1; Programs have rolling admissions. Preference will be given to applications received by March 1. Rolling admissions continue through June 15. *Fee:* $30.

Murray State University
Department of Psychology
Humanities and Fine Arts
212 Wells Hall
Murray, KY 42071-3318
Telephone: (270) 809-2851
Fax: (270) 809-2991
E-mail: vickid.anderson@murraystate.edu
Web: http://www.murraystate.edu/chfa/psychology/graduate.htm

Department Information:
1966. Chairperson: Dr. Renae D. Duncan. Number of faculty: total—full-time 9, part-time 1; women—full-time 4, part-time 1.

Programs and Degrees Offered:
Listed in the following order: Program area, degree type (T if terminal Master's), number awarded 7/08–6/09. Clinical Psychology MA/MS (Master of Arts/Science) (T) 6, General Psychology MA/MS (Master of Arts/Science) (T) 1.

Student Applications/Admissions:
Student Applications
Clinical Psychology MA/MS (Master of Arts/Science)—Applications 2009–2010, 32. Total applicants accepted 2009–2010, 14. Number full-time enrolled (new admits only) 2009–2010, 7. Number part-time enrolled (new admits only) 2009–2010, 0. Openings 2010–2011, 11. The median number of years required for completion of a degree in 2008–2009 were 2. The number of students enrolled full- and part-time who were dismissed or voluntarily withdrew from this program area in 2008–2009 were 0. *General Psychology MA/MS (Master of Arts/Science)*—Applications 2009–2010, 4. Total applicants accepted 2009–2010, 2. Number full-time enrolled (new admits only) 2009–2010, 1. Number part-time enrolled (new admits only) 2009–2010, 0. Openings 2010–2011, 5. The median number of years required for completion of a degree in 2008–2009 were 2. The number of students enrolled full- and part-time who were dismissed or voluntarily withdrew from this program area in 2008–2009 were 0.

Scores: Entries appear in this order: required test or GPA, minimum score (if required), median score of students entering in 2009–2010. *Clinical Psychology MA/MS (Master of Arts/Science)*: GRE-V 400, 450, GRE-Q 400, 450, overall undergraduate GPA 3.0, 3.3, psychology GPA 3.0, 3.2.
Other Criteria: (importance of criteria rated low, medium, or high): GRE scores—medium, research experience—medium, work experience—low, extracurricular activity—low, GPA—high, letters of recommendation—high, statement of goals and objectives—medium, undergraduate major in psychology—low, specific undergraduate psychology courses taken—medium.

Student Characteristics: The following represents characteristics of students in 2009–2010 in all graduate psychology programs in the department: Female—full-time 18, part-time 0; Male—full-time 0, part-time 0; African American/Black—full-time 0, part-time 0; Hispanic/Latino(a)—full-time 0, part-time 0; Asian/Pacific Islander—full-time 0, part-time 0; American Indian/Alaska Native—full-time 0, part-time 0; Caucasian/White—full-time 15, part-time 0; Multi-ethnic—full-time 0, part-time 0; students subject to the Americans With Disabilities Act—full-time 0, part-time 0; Unknown ethnicity—full-time 3, part-time 0; International students who hold an F-1 or J-1 Visa—full-time 3, part-time 0.

Financial Information/Assistance:
Tuition for Full-Time Study: *Master's:* State residents: per academic year $3,393, $377 per credit hour; Nonstate residents: per academic year $9,544, $1,060 per credit hour. Tuition is subject to change.

Financial Assistance:
First-Year Students: Research assistantships available for first year. Average amount paid per academic year: $4,575. Average number of hours worked per week: 10. Apply by March 15.
Advanced Students: Research assistantships available for advanced students. Average amount paid per academic year: $4,575. Average number of hours worked per week: 10. Apply by March 15.
Additional Information: Of all students currently enrolled full time, 50% benefited from one or more of the listed financial assistance programs.

Internships/Practica: Master's Degree (MA/MS Clinical Psychology): An internship experience, such as a final research project or "capstone" experience is required of graduates. Master's Degree (MA/MS General Psychology): An internship experience, such as a final research project or "capstone" experience is required of graduates. To gain experience conducting therapy and psychological evaluations, a supervised two-semester, 20 hour per week clinical practicum is required. Clinical psychology students serve their practica at the MSU Psychological Center, an on-campus treatment center, which provides therapy and assessments for children, adults and families from the community as well as for university students and staff. In addition to gaining experience conducting therapy and assessments, our clinical graduate students receive 2½ hours per week of supervision with our PhD level licensed clinical psychologists. This allows for a fine-tuning of clinical skills as well as added assurance that the clinician is providing the best and most ethical services to the Center's clients.

Housing and Day Care: On-campus housing is available. On-campus day care facilities are available.

Employment of Department Graduates:
Master's Degree Graduates: Of those who graduated in the academic year 2008–2009, the following categories and numbers represent the postgraduate activities and employment of master's degree graduates: Enrolled in a psychology doctoral program (2), enrolled in another graduate/professional program (0), enrolled in a postdoctoral residency/fellowship (n/a), employed in independent practice (n/a), employed in an academic position at a university (0), employed in an academic position at a 2-year/4-year college (0), employed in other positions at a higher education institution (0), employed in a professional position in a school system (0), employed in business or industry (0), employed in government agency (0), employed in a community mental health/counseling center (3), employed in a hospital/medical center (1), still seeking employment (0), other employment position (2), total from the above (master's) (8).
Doctoral Degree Graduates: Of those who graduated in the academic year 2008–2009, the following categories and numbers represent the postgraduate activities and employment of doctoral degree graduates: Enrolled in a psychology doctoral program (n/a), total from the above (doctoral) (0).

Additional Information:
Orientation, Objectives, and Emphasis of Department: The clinical program is based on the philosophy that the master's degree is first and foremost a degree in psychology and that students should achieve a broad base of knowledge in the field. Thus, students are required to take 5 psychological foundations courses which prepare the graduate to enter the field of psychology and also provide the general psychology courses required by state licensing boards. Clinical students also receive intensive instruction in psychodiagnostics, which emphasizes the administration, scoring, and interpretation of a variety of intelligence and personality tests. The psychotherapy curriculum is primarily cognitive-behavioral in nature, though a variety of techniques and orientations are presented which teach the student how best to conduct psychotherapy with adults, children, families, and couples. Students are expected to participate in research and a master's thesis is required. The general program emphasizes psychological foundations and research methodology as preparation for doctoral studies, community college teaching, or applied research.

Special Facilities or Resources: The department has research laboratories, an on-site psychological clinic with testing and observation rooms, and complete facilities for practica in diagnostics and therapy. Students also share offices in the department. Each student is assigned a locking desk with personal computer.

Application Information:
Send to Graduate Admissions Committee. Application available online. URL of online application: http://www.murraystate.edu/Admissions/GraduateSchool.aspx. Students are admitted in the Fall, application deadline March 15. Applications will be accepted after the deadline. However, late applications will be considered only if openings remain after review of applications received before the due date. *Fee:* $30.

Northern Kentucky University
Department of Psychological Science
Arts & Sciences
Nunn Drive
Highland Heights, KY 41099
Telephone: (859) 572-5310
Fax: (859) 572-6085
E-mail: *msio@nku.edu*
Web: *http://psychology.nku.edu/programs/graduate.php*

Department Information:
1968. Chairperson: Jeffrey Smith. Number of faculty: total—full-time 18, part-time 18; women—full-time 8, part-time 15; total—minority—full-time 1, part-time 1; women minority—full-time 1, part-time 1.

Programs and Degrees Offered:
Listed in the following order: Program area, degree type (T if terminal Master's), number awarded 7/08–6/09. Industrial/Organizational Psychology MA/MS (Master of Arts/Science) (T) 14.

Student Applications/Admissions:
Student Applications
Industrial/Organizational Psychology MA/MS (Master of Arts/Science)—Applications 2009–2010, 47. Total applicants accepted 2009–2010, 16. Number full-time enrolled (new admits only) 2009–2010, 15. Number part-time enrolled (new admits only) 2009–2010, 1. Total enrolled 2009–2010 full-time, 39, part-time, 5. Openings 2010–2011, 18. The median number of years required for completion of a degree in 2008–2009 were 2. The number of students enrolled full- and part-time who were dismissed or voluntarily withdrew from this program area in 2008–2009 were 1.
Scores: Entries appear in this order: required test or GPA, minimum score (if required), median score of students entering in 2009–2010. Industrial/Organizational Psychology MA/MS (Master of Arts/Science): GRE-V 450, 475, GRE-Q 450, 535, GRE-Analytical 4.0, 4.5, overall undergraduate GPA 3.0, 3.45.
Other Criteria: (importance of criteria rated low, medium, or high): GRE scores—high, research experience—medium, work experience—medium, extracurricular activity—low, GPA—high, letters of recommendation—low, statement of goals and objectives—high, statistics course—high, undergraduate major in psychology—medium, specific undergraduate psychology courses taken—high.

Student Characteristics: The following represents characteristics of students in 2009–2010 in all graduate psychology programs in the department: Female—full-time 33, part-time 4; Male—full-time 6, part-time 1; African American/Black—full-time 1, part-time 1; Hispanic/Latino(a)—full-time 0, part-time 0; Asian/Pacific Islander—full-time 0, part-time 0; American Indian/Alaska Native—full-time 0, part-time 0; Caucasian/White—full-time 38, part-time 4; Multi-ethnic—full-time 0, part-time 0; students subject to the Americans With Disabilities Act—full-time 0, part-time 0; Unknown ethnicity—full-time 0, part-time 0; International students who hold an F-1 or J-1 Visa—full-time 0, part-time 0.

Financial Information/Assistance:
  Tuition for Full-Time Study: Master's: State residents: $384 per credit hour; Nonstate residents: $675 per credit hour. Tuition is subject to change. Additional fees are assessed to students beyond the costs of tuition for the following: Automobile Parking Registration $187 per year. See the following Web site for updates and changes in tuition costs: http://bursar.nku.edu/students/tuitionfees.php. Higher tuition cost for this program: Cincinnati Metropolitan Area Resident Rate $509 per credit hour.

  Financial Assistance:
    First-Year Students: Teaching assistantships available for first year. Average number of hours worked per week: 20. Apply by March 1. Research assistantships available for first year. Average number of hours worked per week: 20. Apply by March 1.
    Advanced Students: Teaching assistantships available for advanced students. Average number of hours worked per week: 20. Apply by March 1. Research assistantships available for advanced students. Average number of hours worked per week: 20. Apply by March 1.
    Additional Information: Of all students currently enrolled full time, 15% benefited from one or more of the listed financial assistance programs. Application and information available online at: http://www.nku.edu/~gradprog/prospectivestudents/financialaid/assistantships.php.

Internships/Practica: Master's Degree (MA/MS Industrial/Organizational Psychology): An internship experience, such as a final research project or "capstone" experience is required of graduates. Applied professional experience is gained through internships, which are competitive in nature and become available depending on sponsor funding, and through community engagement projects that allow graduate students to apply their accumulated professional knowledge, statistical skills, and analytic abilities within a consulting framework to challenges confronting regional non-for-profit organizations.

Housing and Day Care: On-campus housing is available. See the following Web site for more information: http://housing.nku.edu/prospective/residence/index.php. On-campus day care facilities are available. See the following Web site for more information: http://www.nku.edu/~ecc/.

Employment of Department Graduates:
  Master's Degree Graduates: Of those who graduated in the academic year 2008–2009, the following categories and numbers represent the postgraduate activities and employment of master's degree graduates: Enrolled in a psychology doctoral program (1), enrolled in another graduate/professional program (0), enrolled in a postdoctoral residency/fellowship (n/a), employed in independent practice (n/a), employed in an academic position at a university (0), employed in an academic position at a 2-year/4-year college (0), employed in other positions at a higher education institution (0), employed in a professional position in a school system (0), employed in business or industry (11), employed in government agency (0), employed in a community mental health/counseling center (1), employed in a hospital/medical center (1), still seeking employment (0), not seeking employment (0), other employment position (0), do not know (1), total from the above (master's) (15).

  Doctoral Degree Graduates: Of those who graduated in the academic year 2008–2009, the following categories and numbers represent the postgraduate activities and employment of doctoral degree graduates: Enrolled in a psychology doctoral program (n/a), total from the above (doctoral) (0).

Additional Information:
  Orientation, Objectives, and Emphasis of Department: The Department of Psychological Science at Northern Kentucky University embodies a rigorous, comprehensive, and evidence-based approach to the application of empirical science and research in psychology. The graduate program in Industrial and Organizational Psychology reflects this empirical orientation in developing the critical professional competencies identified by the Society for Industrial and Organizational Psychology as essential for practice and research in IO psychology. To ensure that the program reflects contemporary trends, an advisory board comprised of IO psychologists and representatives of major organizations in the greater Cincinnati region provides guidance. Graduate students are encouraged to conduct independent study, practicum, or thesis research with faculty on topics of interest throughout the program. Graduate seminars are presented by four fulltime graduate faculty holding doctoral degrees in IO or applied social psychology, supplemented by adjunct faculty holding advanced degrees accompanied by specialized knowledge or relevant experience.

  Special Facilities or Resources: The Department of Psychological Science employs a digitally equipped instructional computer lab equipped with 24 new Dell personal computers and 6 Apple Macintosh computers for statistics, research methods, and psychometrics seminars. Three additional laboratory spaces are available for graduate student use: a suite of four rooms equipped with 16 Apple Macintosh computers and office space; a computer lab equipped with four Dell desktop computers; and a lab equipped with eight Dell laptop computers. All are hardwired or linked to the campus wireless network. The Steely Library at NKU subscribes to most major databases in addition to PsycArticles (all 61 APA journals), PsycInfo (APA articles, texts, and books), and Psychology and Behavioral Science Collection (575 journals), and participates in a state, regional, and national interlibrary loan system. The Information Systems group at NKU provides lifetime email accounts to graduate students, and operates a contemporary, professional information management system with full access to the internet.

  Information for Students With Physical Disabilities: See the following Web site for more information: http://disability.nku.edu/.

Application Information:
Send to Office of Graduate Programs, Northern Kentucky University, Nunn Drive, Highland Heights, KY 41099. Application available online. URL of online application: http://www.nku.edu/apply/index.php. Students are admitted in the Fall, application deadline July 1; Spring, application deadline December 1; Summer, application deadline April 1. *Fee:* $40.

Spalding University
School of Professional Psychology
College of Social Sciences & Humanities
845 South Third Street
Louisville, KY 40203
Telephone: (502) 585-7127
Fax: (502) 585-7159
E-mail: *esimpson@spalding.edu*
Web: *http://www.spalding.edu/psychology*

Department Information:
1952. Chairperson: Steven Katsikas, PhD. Number of faculty: total—full-time 11, part-time 11; women—full-time 5, part-time 3; total—minority—full-time 2; women minority—full-time 1.

Programs and Degrees Offered:
Listed in the following order: Program area, degree type (T if terminal Master's), number awarded 7/08–6/09. Clinical Psychology PsyD (Doctor of Psychology) 17.

APA Accreditation: Clinical PsyD (Doctor of Psychology). Student Outcome Data Website: http://www.spalding.edu/content.aspx?id=1908&cid=3846.

Student Applications/Admissions:
Student Applications
Clinical Psychology PsyD (Doctor of Psychology)—Applications 2009–2010, 113. Total applicants accepted 2009–2010, 55. Number full-time enrolled (new admits only) 2009–2010, 30. Number part-time enrolled (new admits only) 2009–2010, 0. Openings 2010–2011, 30. The median number of years required for completion of a degree in 2008–2009 were 6. The number of students enrolled full- and part-time who were dismissed or voluntarily withdrew from this program area in 2008–2009 were 2.
Scores: Entries appear in this order: required test or GPA, minimum score (if required), median score of students entering in 2009–2010. Clinical Psychology PsyD (Doctor of Psychology): GRE-V no minimum stated, 510, GRE-Q no minimum stated, 530, GRE-Analytical no minimum stated, 4.5, overall undergraduate GPA no minimum stated, 3.43.
Other Criteria: (importance of criteria rated low, medium, or high): GRE scores—medium, research experience—medium, work experience—medium, extracurricular activity—medium, clinically related public service—medium, GPA—medium, letters of recommendation—medium, interview—medium, statement of goals and objectives—medium, undergraduate major in psychology—low, specific undergraduate psychology courses taken—low.

Student Characteristics: The following represents characteristics of students in 2009–2010 in all graduate psychology programs in the department: Female—full-time 95, part-time 0; Male—full-time 35, part-time 0; African American/Black—full-time 4, part-time 0; Hispanic/Latino(a)—full-time 6, part-time 0; Asian/Pacific Islander—full-time 6, part-time 0; American Indian/Alaska Native—full-time 2, part-time 0; Caucasian/White—full-time 111, part-time 0; Multi-ethnic—full-time 1, part-time 0; students subject to the Americans With Disabilities Act—full-time 1, part-time 0; Unknown ethnicity—full-time 0, part-time 0; International students who hold an F-1 or J-1 Visa—full-time 2, part-time 0.

Financial Information/Assistance:
Tuition for Full-Time Study: *Doctoral:* State residents: $750 per credit hour; Nonstate residents: $750 per credit hour. See the following Web site for updates and changes in tuition costs: http://www.spalding.edu/content.aspx?id=1882&cid=200.

Financial Assistance:
First-Year Students: Research assistantships available for first year. Average amount paid per academic year: $4,260. Average number of hours worked per week: 6. Apply by March 1. Fellowships and scholarships available for first year. Average amount paid per academic year: $4,000. Apply by October 1.
Advanced Students: Teaching assistantships available for advanced students. Average amount paid per academic year: $8,520. Average number of hours worked per week: 14. Apply by March 1. Research assistantships available for advanced students. Average amount paid per academic year: $5,443. Average number of hours worked per week: 6. Apply by March 1. Fellowships and scholarships available for advanced students. Average amount paid per academic year: $4,000. Average number of hours worked per week: 0. Apply by October 1.
Additional Information: Of all students currently enrolled full time, 38% benefited from one or more of the listed financial assistance programs.

Internships/Practica: Doctoral Degree (PsyD Clinical Psychology): For those doctoral students for whom a professional internship was required in this program prior to graduation, (24) students applied for an internship in 2008–2009, with (20) students obtaining an internship. Of those students who obtained an internship, (19) were paid internships. Of those students who obtained an internship, (19) students placed in APA/CPA accredited internships, (0) students placed in internships not APA/CPA accredited, but listed with the Association of Psychology Postdoctoral and Internship Programs (APPIC), (0) students placed in internships conforming to guidelines of the Council of Directors of School Psychology Programs (CDSPP), (1) students placed in internships that were not APA/CPA accredited, APPIC or CDSPP listed. Often referred to as one of the School of Professional Psychology's "gems," our Graduate Practicum Program prides itself on providing incredible opportunity to our students by creating avenues within our communities to take their classroom learning into real-world settings. It is within these venues that our students test their knowledge, gain experience, and contribute to the overall mental and physical health of humankind. Under the professional supervision of committed, licensed psychologists and professional staff, students find voice, presence, silence, and humility when serving those in need of quality mental health care, consultation, assessment, or other professional services best guided by those specifically trained in the science of human behavior. Practicum placements are carefully selected to best meet the training needs of our graduate students. Once partnered with a host site, these placements provide focused challenges and learning opportunities with diverse populations and across a variety of subspecialties, including health/behavioral medicine, forensics/corrections, pediatrics/child/adolescent/family, and adult/geriatrics.

Housing and Day Care: On-campus housing is available. See the following Web site for more information: http://www.spalding.

edu/content.aspx?id=2246&cid=6104. No on-campus day care facilities are available.

Employment of Department Graduates:
Master's Degree Graduates: Of those who graduated in the academic year 2008–2009, the following categories and numbers represent the postgraduate activities and employment of master's degree graduates: Enrolled in a postdoctoral residency/fellowship (n/a), employed in independent practice (n/a), total from the above (master's) (0).
Doctoral Degree Graduates: Of those who graduated in the academic year 2008–2009, the following categories and numbers represent the postgraduate activities and employment of doctoral degree graduates: Enrolled in a psychology doctoral program (n/a), enrolled in a postdoctoral residency/fellowship (5), employed in independent practice (2), employed in government agency (3), employed in a community mental health/counseling center (2), employed in a hospital/medical center (2), do not know (3), total from the above (doctoral) (17).

Additional Information:
Orientation, Objectives, and Emphasis of Department: The Spalding University School of Professional Psychology is dedicated to providing generalist training in clinical psychology based upon scientific principles, grounded in evidence-based practice, and offered in a collaborative and cooperative setting. Furthermore, to train competent professionals to function in a complex and diverse society, the program emphasizes critical thinking, ethical decision-making, and the promotion of social justice. The School of Professional Psychology uses the scholar-practitioner model to train students as local clinical scientists. The curriculum is based on a biopsychosocial approach to understanding human functioning. In addition, doctoral training is organized according to professional competencies set forth by the National Council of Schools of Professional Psychology (NCSPP). Current competencies include: intervention, assessment, research and evaluation, relationship, diversity, and supervision. The faculty share the belief that the most effective approach to training in professional psychology is one of cooperation and mutual support. As such, good relationship skills, compassion and sensitivity to ethical standards are values in our program.

Special Facilities or Resources: The faculty have various areas of expertise and interest and form research and discussion groups around these areas of interest. Current research and interest groups include: a Health Psychology Research Interest Group, a Violence Prevention Research Interest Group, and a Spirituality and Religion Research Interest Group. Because we are a professional training program, research is conducted in applied settings. Students who are active in the Health Psychology Research Interest Group are involved in all phases of research projects. Students and faculty collaborate with other universities, medical centers and specialty medical clinics in conducting clinical research. Students also actively participate in state, regional and national conferences in the presentation of these projects. Students are encouraged to select dissertation and other research projects based on their own desires as well as the interests of the faculty.

Information for Students With Physical Disabilities: See the following Web site for more information: http://www.spalding.edu/content.aspx?id=2246&cid=4996.

Application Information:
Send to Administrative Assistant, School of Professional Psychology, 851 South 4th Street, Louisville, KY 40203. Application available online. URL of online application: http://www.spalding.edu/content.aspx?id=1916&cid=320. Students are admitted in the Fall, application deadline January 15. *Fee:* $30.

LOUISIANA

Louisiana State University Shreveport
Department of Psychology
School of Human Sciences
One University Place
Shreveport, LA 71115
Telephone: (318) 797-5044
Fax: (318) 798-4171
E-mail: *Gary.Jones@lsus.edu*
Web: *http://www.lsus.edu/ehd/psyc/*

Department Information:
1967. Chairperson: Gary E. Jones, PhD Number of faculty: total—full-time 13, part-time 3; women—full-time 6, part-time 2; total—minority—full-time 1.

Programs and Degrees Offered:
Listed in the following order: Program area, degree type (T if terminal Master's), number awarded 7/08–6/09. Counseling Psychology MA/MS (Master of Arts/Science) (T) 15, School Psychology Other 6.

Student Applications/Admissions:
Student Applications
Counseling Psychology MA/MS (Master of Arts/Science)—Applications 2009–2010, 45. Total applicants accepted 2009–2010, 39. Number full-time enrolled (new admits only) 2009–2010, 22. Number part-time enrolled (new admits only) 2009–2010, 0. Total enrolled 2009–2010 full-time, 49, part-time, 8. Openings 2010–2011, 20. The median number of years required for completion of a degree in 2008–2009 were 2. The number of students enrolled full- and part-time who were dismissed or voluntarily withdrew from this program area in 2008–2009 were 3. *School Psychology Other*—Applications 2009–2010, 23. Total applicants accepted 2009–2010, 15. Number full-time enrolled (new admits only) 2009–2010, 12. Number part-time enrolled (new admits only) 2009–2010, 0. Total enrolled 2009–2010 full-time, 20, part-time, 3. Openings 2010–2011, 10. The median number of years required for completion of a degree in 2008–2009 were 3. The number of students enrolled full- and part-time who were dismissed or voluntarily withdrew from this program area in 2008–2009 were 6.
Scores: Entries appear in this order: required test or GPA, minimum score (if required), median score of students entering in 2009–2010. *Counseling Psychology MA/MS (Master of Arts/Science)*: GRE-V 400, 435, GRE-Q 400, 490, overall undergraduate GPA 2.5, 3.03; *School Psychology Other*: GRE-V 400, 503, GRE-Q 400, 483, overall undergraduate GPA 2.5, 3.25.
Other Criteria: (importance of criteria rated low, medium, or high): GRE scores—medium, research experience—low, work experience—low, extracurricular activity—low, clinically related public service—low, GPA—high, letters of recommendation—high, interview—medium, statement of goals and objectives—high, undergraduate major in psychology—medium, specific undergraduate psychology courses taken—low. For additional information on admission requirements, go to http://www.lsus.edu/ehd/psyc/graduate.asp.

Student Characteristics: The following represents characteristics of students in 2009–2010 in all graduate psychology programs in the department: Female—full-time 61, part-time 18; Male—full-time 20, part-time 2; African American/Black—full-time 4, part-time 3; Hispanic/Latino(a)—full-time 1, part-time 2; Asian/Pacific Islander—full-time 0, part-time 1; American Indian/Alaska Native—full-time 0, part-time 0; Caucasian/White—full-time 73, part-time 13; Multi-ethnic—full-time 3, part-time 0; students subject to the Americans With Disabilities Act—full-time 2, part-time 0; Unknown ethnicity—full-time 0, part-time 0; International students who hold an F-1 or J-1 Visa—full-time 0, part-time 0.

Financial Information/Assistance:
Tuition for Full-Time Study: *Master's:* State residents: per academic year $2,552, $212 per credit hour; Nonstate residents: per academic year $5,572, $464 per credit hour. See the following Web site for updates and changes in tuition costs: http://www.lsus.edu/acctserv/fees.asp. Note: We will often waive the out of state tuition charge for students from TX, AR, and MS.

Financial Assistance:
First-Year Students: Research assistantships available for first year. Average amount paid per academic year: $5,000. Average number of hours worked per week: 20. Apply by June 1.
Advanced Students: Teaching assistantships available for advanced students. Average amount paid per academic year: $5,000. Average number of hours worked per week: 20. Apply by June 1.
Additional Information: Of all students currently enrolled full time, 5% benefited from one or more of the listed financial assistance programs. Application and information available online at: http://www.lsus.edu/graduate/finassistance.php.

Internships/Practica: Master's Degree (MA/MS Counseling Psychology): An internship experience, such as a final research project or "capstone" experience is required of graduates. Practica for our Specialist degree students are carried out in surrounding parishes which have cooperative agreements with the university for training purposes. There are two distinct practica experiences for our students. The first involves an observational practicum required during the Introductory to School Psychology course. The second occurs during Psych 754-a formal 200-plus hour practicum that is carried out in cooperating training parishes with supervisory field school psychologists. All students must complete an appropriate internship to qualify for State certification. These internships tend not to be APA-approved, but meet state certification requirements. Students in the MSCP program also are required to serve community-based supervised practicum experiences, in addition to a two semester internship experience supervised by an LPC or other appropriate mental health professional which is acceptable to the program. These internships are not APA-approved, but meet LPC licensure requirements.

Housing and Day Care: On-campus housing is available. See the following Web site for more information: http://www.campushousing.com/lsus/html/index.php. No on-campus day care facilities are available.

Employment of Department Graduates:

Master's Degree Graduates: Of those who graduated in the academic year 2008–2009, the following categories and numbers represent the postgraduate activities and employment of master's degree graduates: Enrolled in a postdoctoral residency/fellowship (n/a), employed in independent practice (n/a), employed in government agency (4), employed in a community mental health/counseling center (7), employed in a hospital/medical center (2), not seeking employment (1), do not know (1), total from the above (master's) (15).

Doctoral Degree Graduates: Of those who graduated in the academic year 2008–2009, the following categories and numbers represent the postgraduate activities and employment of doctoral degree graduates: Enrolled in a psychology doctoral program (n/a), total from the above (doctoral) (0).

Additional Information:

Orientation, Objectives, and Emphasis of Department: The LSUS School Psychology Program curriculum is aligned with the training standards recommended by the National Association of School Psychologists (NASP). The primary focus of training is to develop fluency in data-based problem solving across both academic and behavior domains, and the overarching framework is a tiered model of service delivery based on student response to intervention (RTI). The program features three practicum experiences prior to a culminating 1200-hour internship in a public school setting. In the MSCP program, students are offered a curriculum that will lead to licensure as a professional counselor with a 48 or 60 credit hour program depending on state requirements. Louisiana requires a 48 hour program while many other states require 60 hours. Additionally, the program is designed to prepare students for further graduate study in psychology. The program follows a practitioner-scientist model of training. There are a limited number of competitive graduate assistantships available.

Special Facilities or Resources: The Master's in Counseling Psychology and Specialist in School Psychology have state-of-the-art audio/video equipment for counseling and intervention techniques and skills, all housed in the psychology clinic and Department on campus.

Information for Students With Physical Disabilities: See the following Web site for more information: http://www.lsus.edu/sdcc/services4disabilities/index.asp.

Application Information:
Send to Department Chair Department of Psychology Louisiana State University in Shreveport 1 University Place Shreveport, LA 71115. Application available online. URL of online application: http://www.lsus.edu/ehd/psyc/graduate.asp. Students are admitted in the Fall, application deadline June 30; Spring, application deadline November 30; Summer, application deadline April 30. *Fee:* $10.

Louisiana Tech University
Department of Psychology and Behavioral Sciences
College of Education
Box 10048, T.S.
Ruston, LA 71272
Telephone: (318) 257-4315
Fax: (318) 257-3442
E-mail: *tilman@latech.edu*
Web: *http://www.latech.edu/education/psychology*

Department Information:
1972. Department Head: Tilman Sheets, PhD. Number of faculty: total—full-time 16; women—full-time 8; total—minority—full-time 1; women minority—full-time 2.

Programs and Degrees Offered:
Listed in the following order: Program area, degree type (T if terminal Master's), number awarded 7/08–6/09. Counseling Psychology PhD (Doctor of Philosophy) 6, Industrial/Organizational Psychology MA/MS (Master of Arts/Science) (T) 22, Counseling and Guidance MA/MS (Master of Arts/Science) (T) 30, Industrial/Organizational Psychology PhD (Doctor of Philosophy).

APA Accreditation: Counseling PhD (Doctor of Philosophy). Student Outcome Data Website: http://www.latech.edu/education/psychology/cphd/.

Student Applications/Admissions:

Student Applications

Counseling Psychology PhD (Doctor of Philosophy)—Applications 2009–2010, 40. Total applicants accepted 2009–2010, 6. Number full-time enrolled (new admits only) 2009–2010, 5. Openings 2010–2011, 6. The median number of years required for completion of a degree in 2008–2009 were 6. The number of students enrolled full- and part-time who were dismissed or voluntarily withdrew from this program area in 2008–2009 were 0. *Industrial/Organizational Psychology MA/MS (Master of Arts/Science)*—Applications 2009–2010, 32. Total applicants accepted 2009–2010, 26. Number full-time enrolled (new admits only) 2009–2010, 20. Number part-time enrolled (new admits only) 2009–2010, 6. Total enrolled 2009–2010 full-time, 20, part-time, 11. Openings 2010–2011, 26. The median number of years required for completion of a degree in 2008–2009 was 1. The number of students enrolled full- and part-time who were dismissed or voluntarily withdrew from this program area in 2008–2009 were 4. *Counseling and Guidance MA/MS (Master of Arts/Science)*—Applications 2009–2010, 40. Total applicants accepted 2009–2010, 32. Number full-time enrolled (new admits only) 2009–2010, 20. Number part-time enrolled (new admits only) 2009–2010, 12. Total enrolled 2009–2010 full-time, 36, part-time, 20. Openings 2010–2011, 24. The median number of years required for completion of a degree in 2008–2009 were 2. The number of students enrolled full- and part-time who were dismissed or voluntarily withdrew from this program area in 2008–2009 were 6. *Industrial/Organizational Psychology PhD (Doctor of Philosophy)*—Applications 2009–2010, 26. Total applicants accepted 2009–2010, 6. Number full-time enrolled (new admits only) 2009–2010, 4. Total enrolled 2009–2010 full-time, 4. Openings 2010–2011, 5.

Scores: Entries appear in this order: required test or GPA, minimum score (if required), median score of students entering in 2009–2010. *Counseling Psychology PhD (Doctor of Philosophy):* GRE-V no minimum stated, GRE-Q no minimum stated, GRE-Analytical no minimum stated.

Other Criteria: (importance of criteria rated low, medium, or high): GRE scores—high, research experience—high, work experience—medium, extracurricular activity—low, clinically related public service—medium, GPA—high, letters of recommendation—high, interview—high, statement of goals and objectives—medium, undergraduate major in psychology—medium, These criteria apply to the PhD program.

Student Characteristics: The following represents characteristics of students in 2009–2010 in all graduate psychology programs in the department: Female—full-time 50, part-time 0; Male—full-time 30, part-time 0; African American/Black—full-time 0, part-time 0; Hispanic/Latino(a)—full-time 0, part-time 0; Asian/Pacific Islander—full-time 0, part-time 0; American Indian/Alaska Native—full-time 0, part-time 0; Caucasian/White—full-time 0, part-time 0; Multi-ethnic—full-time 0, part-time 0; students subject to the Americans With Disabilities Act—full-time 0, part-time 0; Unknown ethnicity—full-time 0, part-time 0; International students who hold an F-1 or J-1 Visa—full-time 0, part-time 0.

Financial Information/Assistance:
Financial Assistance:
First-Year Students: Teaching assistantships available for first year. Average amount paid per academic year: $10,000. Average number of hours worked per week: 20. Research assistantships available for first year. Average number of hours worked per week: 20.

Advanced Students: Teaching assistantships available for advanced students. Average amount paid per academic year: $10,000. Average number of hours worked per week: 20. Research assistantships available for advanced students. Average amount paid per academic year: $10,000. Average number of hours worked per week: 20.

Additional Information: Of all students currently enrolled full time, 30% benefited from one or more of the listed financial assistance programs. Application and information available online at: http://www.latech.edu/finaid.

Internships/Practica: Doctoral Degree (PhD Counseling Psychology): For those doctoral students for whom a professional internship was required in this program prior to graduation, (7) students applied for an internship in 2008–2009, with (6) students obtaining an internship. Of those students who obtained an internship, (6) were paid internships. Of those students who obtained an internship, (5) students placed in APA/CPA accredited internships, (1) students placed in internships not APA/CPA accredited, but listed with the Association of Psychology Postdoctoral and Internship Programs (APPIC), (0) students placed in internships conforming to guidelines of the Council of Directors of School Psychology Programs (CDSPP), (0) students placed in internships that were not APA/CPA accredited, APPIC or CDSPP listed. Master's Degree (MA/MS Counseling and Guidance): An internship experience, such as a final research project or "capstone" experience is required of graduates. PhD counseling psychology students must complete a year-long internship. Practica are available throughout the region for PhD and MA students in their respective areas.

Housing and Day Care: On-campus housing is available. On-campus day care facilities are available.

Employment of Department Graduates:
Master's Degree Graduates: Of those who graduated in the academic year 2008–2009, the following categories and numbers represent the postgraduate activities and employment of master's degree graduates: Enrolled in a postdoctoral residency/fellowship (n/a), employed in independent practice (n/a), total from the above (master's) (0).

Doctoral Degree Graduates: Of those who graduated in the academic year 2008–2009, the following categories and numbers represent the postgraduate activities and employment of doctoral degree graduates: Enrolled in a psychology doctoral program (n/a), total from the above (doctoral) (0).

Additional Information:
Orientation, Objectives, and Emphasis of Department: The Department of Psychology and Behavioral Sciences offers master's degree programs in counseling and guidance, educational psychology, and industrial/organizational psychology, in addition to PhD programs in counseling and industrial/organizational psychology. The department strives to provide an eclectic and integrated approach to theory, research, and practice. The scientist–practitioner model provides the framework for most graduate programs. Successful degree candidates develop the knowledge and skills necessary for appropriate level positions in their respective fields in settings such as education, business, mental health, and government. The counseling psychology PhD includes training in assessment, career/vocational, and psychotherapy and is accredited by the American Psychological Association.

Special Facilities or Resources: The Psychological Services Clinic serves as a training center for the Counseling Psychology Doctor of Philosophy (PhD) program in the Louisiana Tech University College of Education.

Information for Students With Physical Disabilities: See the following Web site for more information: http://www.latech.edu/ods/.

Application Information:
Send to Department Chair, Department of Psychology and Behavioral Sciences. Application available online. URL of online application: http://www.latech.edu/graduateschool/. Students are admitted in the Fall, application deadline September 1; Winter, application deadline November 30; Spring, application deadline March 2; Summer, application deadline May 31. PhD: full admissions in the Fall only, Counseling Psychology deadline is December 15 and I/O Psychology deadline is February 15. *Fee:* $35.

Louisiana, University of, Lafayette
Department of Psychology
Liberal Arts
P.O. Box 43131 UL-Lafayette Station
Lafayette, LA 70504-3131
Telephone: (337) 482-6597
Fax: (337) 482-6587
E-mail: *csm5689@louisiana.edu*
Web: *http://psychology.louisiana.edu/*

Department Information:
1970. Department Head: Cheryl S. Lynch. Number of faculty: total—full-time 18; women—full-time 11; total—minority—full-time 3; women minority—full-time 2.

Programs and Degrees Offered:
Listed in the following order: Program area, degree type (T if terminal Master's), number awarded 7/08–6/09. Experimental Psychology MA/MS (Master of Arts/Science) (T) 6, Counselor Education MA/MS (Master of Arts/Science) (T) 20.

Student Applications/Admissions:
Student Applications
Experimental Psychology MA/MS (Master of Arts/Science)—Applications 2009–2010, 36. Total applicants accepted 2009–2010, 23. Number full-time enrolled (new admits only) 2009–2010, 7. Number part-time enrolled (new admits only) 2009–2010, 2. Total enrolled 2009–2010 full-time, 24, part-time, 21. Openings 2010–2011, 18. The median number of years required for completion of a degree in 2008–2009 were 2. The number of students enrolled full- and part-time who were dismissed or voluntarily withdrew from this program area in 2008–2009 were 0. *Counselor Education MA/MS (Master of Arts/Science)*—Applications 2009–2010, 40. Total applicants accepted 2009–2010, 30. Number full-time enrolled (new admits only) 2009–2010, 20. Number part-time enrolled (new admits only) 2009–2010, 10. Total enrolled 2009–2010 full-time, 22, part-time, 30. Openings 2010–2011, 25. The median number of years required for completion of a degree in 2008–2009 were 2. The number of students enrolled full- and part-time who were dismissed or voluntarily withdrew from this program area in 2008–2009 were 1.
Scores: Entries appear in this order: required test or GPA, minimum score (if required), median score of students entering in 2009–2010. *Experimental Psychology MA/MS (Master of Arts/Science):* GRE-V 500, 480, GRE-Q 500, 555, overall undergraduate GPA 3.0, 3.12, last 2 years GPA 3.0, psychology GPA 3.0.
Other Criteria: (importance of criteria rated low, medium, or high): GRE scores—medium, research experience—medium, work experience—medium, extracurricular activity—low, clinically related public service—medium, GPA—medium, letters of recommendation—high, statement of goals and objectives—medium.

Student Characteristics: The following represents characteristics of students in 2009–2010 in all graduate psychology programs in the department: Female—full-time 13, part-time 16; Male—full-time 11, part-time 5; African American/Black—full-time 2, part-time 2; Hispanic/Latino(a)—full-time 0, part-time 0; Asian/Pacific Islander—full-time 1, part-time 1; American Indian/Alaska Native—full-time 0, part-time 0; Caucasian/White—full-time 19, part-time 17; Multi-ethnic—full-time 0, part-time 0; students subject to the Americans With Disabilities Act—full-time 0, part-time 0; Unknown ethnicity—full-time 2, part-time 1; International students who hold an F-1 or J-1 Visa—full-time 0, part-time 0.

Financial Information/Assistance:
Tuition for Full-Time Study: Master's: State residents: per academic year $2,300, $579 per credit hour; Nonstate residents: per academic year $6,585. Tuition is subject to change. See the following Web site for updates and changes in tuition costs: http://bursar.louisiana.edu/.

Financial Assistance:
First-Year Students: Teaching assistantships available for first year. Average amount paid per academic year: $7,500. Average number of hours worked per week: 15. Apply by April 12.
Advanced Students: Teaching assistantships available for advanced students. Average amount paid per academic year: $7,500. Average number of hours worked per week: 15. Apply by April 12.
Additional Information: Of all students currently enrolled full time, 22% benefited from one or more of the listed financial assistance programs. Application and information available online at: http://gradschool.louisiana.edu/moneymatters.shtml.

Internships/Practica: Master's Degree (MA/MS Experimental Psychology): An internship experience, such as a final research project or "capstone" experience is required of graduates. Internships for master's students in the applied option are available at the Community Mental Health Center, local psychiatric and rehabilitation hospitals and facilities, private agencies and practices, and at the University Counseling and Testing Center.

Housing and Day Care: On-campus housing is available. See the following Web site for more information: http://www.louisiana.edu/Student/Housing/. On-campus day care facilities are available. See the following Web site for more information: http://www.louisiana.edu/Student/ChildDev/.

Employment of Department Graduates:
Master's Degree Graduates: Of those who graduated in the academic year 2008–2009, the following categories and numbers represent the postgraduate activities and employment of master's degree graduates: Enrolled in a psychology doctoral program (2), enrolled in a postdoctoral residency/fellowship (n/a), employed in independent practice (n/a), employed in an academic position at a 2-year/4-year college (1), employed in other positions at a higher education institution (2), still seeking employment (1), do not know (0), total from the above (master's) (6).
Doctoral Degree Graduates: Of those who graduated in the academic year 2008–2009, the following categories and numbers represent the postgraduate activities and employment of doctoral degree graduates: Enrolled in a psychology doctoral program (n/a), total from the above (doctoral) (0).

Additional Information:
Orientation, Objectives, and Emphasis of Department: The Department of Psychology at the University of Louisiana at Lafayette strives to promote the study of psychology as a science, as a

profession, and as a means of promoting human welfare. A master's program is offered with options in general experimental or applied psychology. After obtaining their degree, students may pursue the doctorate at other universities. Qualified students also have the option of applying to the university's doctoral program in Cognitive Science. Applied program students who just seek a terminal master's have found employment in the locality working for private and public agencies.

Special Facilities or Resources: The Psychology Department houses a computer laboratory for cognitive and social research. Computer assisted instruction is available for several courses. Major physiological research is conducted at the nearby primate center, The New Iberia Research Center. An additional smaller physiological laboratory is housed in the Psychology Department. The University of Louisiana at Lafayette has excellent computer facilities. Many members of the department are also affiliated with the university's Institute for Cognitive Science, providing additional opportunities for research. There is also the possibility that students may be simultaneously enrolled in the Psychology MS program and the Cognitive Science PhD program.

Information for Students With Physical Disabilities: See the following Web site for more information: http://disability.louisiana.edu/.

Application Information:
Send to Graduate School Director, Martin Hall, University of Louisiana, Lafayette, LA 70504. Application available online. URL of online application: http://gradschool.louisiana.edu/. Students are admitted in the Fall, application deadline 30 days. Fellowships have a deadline of February 15; applicants seeking an assistantship ought to have all materials in by the start of April (for the Fall semester). *Fee:* $25. U.S. students' applications are due 30 days prior to start of semester. For international students, the fee is $30, and the deadline is 90 days prior to the semester.

Louisiana, University of, Monroe
Department of Psychology
University of Louisiana—Monroe
700 University Avenue
Monroe, LA 71209
Telephone: (318) 342-1330
Fax: (318) 342-1352
E-mail: *williamson@ulm.edu*
Web: *http://www.ulm.edu/psychology/*

Department Information:
1965. Head: David Williamson. Number of faculty: total—full-time 9, part-time 3; women—full-time 2, part-time 1; total—minority—full-time 1, part-time 1; women minority—full-time 1, part-time 1.

Programs and Degrees Offered:
Listed in the following order: Program area, degree type (T if terminal Master's), number awarded 7/08–6/09. Experimental Psychology MA/MS (Master of Arts/Science) (T) 2, Psychometrics MA/MS (Master of Arts/Science) 9.

Student Applications/Admissions:
Student Applications
Experimental Psychology MA/MS (Master of Arts/Science)—Applications 2009–2010, 2. Total applicants accepted 2009–2010, 1. Number full-time enrolled (new admits only) 2009–2010, 1. Total enrolled 2009–2010 full-time, 6. Openings 2010–2011, 10. The median number of years required for completion of a degree in 2008–2009 were 2. *Psychometrics MA/MS (Master of Arts/Science)*—Applications 2009–2010, 16. Total applicants accepted 2009–2010, 15. Number full-time enrolled (new admits only) 2009–2010, 15. Total enrolled 2009–2010 full-time, 31. Openings 2010–2011, 10. The median number of years required for completion of a degree in 2008–2009 were 2.

Scores: Entries appear in this order: required test or GPA, minimum score (if required), median score of students entering in 2009–2010. *Experimental Psychology MA/MS (Master of Arts/Science)*: GRE-V 450, GRE-Q 450, overall undergraduate GPA 2.75; *Psychometrics MA/MS (Master of Arts/Science)*: GRE-V 450, GRE-Q 450, overall undergraduate GPA 2.75.

Other Criteria: (importance of criteria rated low, medium, or high): GRE scores—high, research experience—medium, work experience—medium, extracurricular activity—low, clinically related public service—medium, GPA—high, letters of recommendation—high.

Student Characteristics: The following represents characteristics of students in 2009–2010 in all graduate psychology programs in the department: Female—full-time 24, part-time 0; Male—full-time 13, part-time 0; African American/Black—full-time 7, part-time 0; Hispanic/Latino(a)—full-time 0, part-time 0; Asian/Pacific Islander—full-time 1, part-time 0; American Indian/Alaska Native—full-time 0, part-time 0; Caucasian/White—full-time 29, part-time 0; Multi-ethnic—full-time 0, part-time 0; students subject to the Americans With Disabilities Act—full-time 1, part-time 0; Unknown ethnicity—full-time 0, part-time 0; International students who hold an F-1 or J-1 Visa—full-time 0, part-time 0.

Financial Information/Assistance:
Tuition for Full-Time Study: *Master's:* State residents: per academic year $3,511; Nonstate residents: per academic year $9,470. See the following Web site for updates and changes in tuition costs: http://www.ulm.edu/controller/sas/.

Financial Assistance:
First-Year Students: Research assistantships available for first year. Average amount paid per academic year: $5,000. Average number of hours worked per week: 20.

Advanced Students: Research assistantships available for advanced students. Average amount paid per academic year: $5,000.

Additional Information: Of all students currently enrolled full time, 50% benefited from one or more of the listed financial assistance programs.

Internships/Practica: Master's Degree (MA/MS Experimental Psychology): An internship experience, such as a final research project or "capstone" experience is required of graduates. Practica and internships are not required but encouraged for the psychometric concentration of the MS program.

Housing and Day Care: On-campus housing is available. See the following Web site for more information: http://www.ulm.edu/reslife/. On-campus day care facilities are available. See the following Web site for more information: http://www.ulm.edu/cdc/.

Employment of Department Graduates:
Master's Degree Graduates: Of those who graduated in the academic year 2008–2009, the following categories and numbers represent the postgraduate activities and employment of master's degree graduates: Enrolled in a psychology doctoral program (1), enrolled in another graduate/professional program (3), enrolled in a postdoctoral residency/fellowship (n/a), employed in independent practice (n/a), employed in a professional position in a school system (2), employed in government agency (1), total from the above (master's) (7).
Doctoral Degree Graduates: Of those who graduated in the academic year 2008–2009, the following categories and numbers represent the postgraduate activities and employment of doctoral degree graduates: Enrolled in a psychology doctoral program (n/a), total from the above (doctoral) (0).

Additional Information:
Orientation, Objectives, and Emphasis of Department: Two areas of concentration are available in the MS program. The general-experimental option focuses upon the basic science areas of psychology. The psychometric (preclinical) option is structured for those whose primary interest is employment in mental health or related settings. Both programs require a comprehensive examination and a thesis.

Special Facilities or Resources: A psychological services center includes a test library and special rooms. The department also has a computer room with 16 PCs with printer for general student use.

Application Information:
Send to Graduate School, University of Louisiana-Monroe, 700 University Avenue, Monroe, LA 71209. Application available online. URL of online application: http://www.ulm.edu/gradschool/admis.html. Programs have rolling admissions. *Fee:* $20.

New Orleans, University of
Department of Psychology
College of Science
2001 Geology and Psychology Building
New Orleans, LA 70148
Telephone: (504) 280-6291
Fax: (504) 280-6049
E-mail: *lscarame@uno.edu*
Web: *http://psyc.uno.edu/*

Department Information:
1982. Chairperson: Paul Frick. Number of faculty: total—full-time 12; women—full-time 6; faculty subject to the Americans With Disabilities Act 1.

Programs and Degrees Offered:
Listed in the following order: Program area, degree type (T if terminal Master's), number awarded 7/08–6/09. Applied Biopsychology PhD (Doctor of Philosophy) 0, Applied Developmental Psychology PhD (Doctor of Philosophy) 0.

Student Applications/Admissions:
Student Applications
Applied Biopsychology PhD (Doctor of Philosophy)—Applications 2009–2010, 6. Total applicants accepted 2009–2010, 4. Number full-time enrolled (new admits only) 2009–2010, 4. Number part-time enrolled (new admits only) 2009–2010, 0. Openings 2010–2011, 4. The number of students enrolled full- and part-time who were dismissed or voluntarily withdrew from this program area in 2008–2009 were 0. Applied Developmental Psychology PhD (Doctor of Philosophy)—Applications 2009–2010, 28. Total applicants accepted 2009–2010, 6. Number full-time enrolled (new admits only) 2009–2010, 3. Number part-time enrolled (new admits only) 2009–2010, 0. Openings 2010–2011, 5. The number of students enrolled full- and part-time who were dismissed or voluntarily withdrew from this program area in 2008–2009 were 0.
Scores: Entries appear in this order: required test or GPA, minimum score (if required), median score of students entering in 2009–2010. Applied Biopsychology PhD (Doctor of Philosophy): GRE-V no minimum stated, 550, GRE-Q no minimum stated, 635, overall undergraduate GPA no minimum stated; Applied Developmental Psychology PhD (Doctor of Philosophy): GRE-V no minimum stated, 580, GRE-Q no minimum stated, 600, overall undergraduate GPA no minimum stated.
Other Criteria: (importance of criteria rated low, medium, or high): GRE scores—high, research experience—high, work experience—low, extracurricular activity—low, clinically related public service—medium, GPA—high, letters of recommendation—high, statement of goals and objectives—high, undergraduate major in psychology—medium, specific undergraduate psychology courses taken—high. For additional information on admission requirements, go to http://psyc.uno.edu/ApplicationInfo.html.

Student Characteristics: The following represents characteristics of students in 2009–2010 in all graduate psychology programs in the department: Female—full-time 17, part-time 0; Male—full-time 12, part-time 0; African American/Black—full-time 2, part-time 0; Hispanic/Latino(a)—full-time 1, part-time 0; Asian/Pacific Islander—full-time 1, part-time 0; American Indian/Alaska Native—full-time 0, part-time 0; Caucasian/White—full-time 24, part-time 0; Multi-ethnic—full-time 1, part-time 0; students subject to the Americans With Disabilities Act—full-time 0, part-time 0; Unknown ethnicity—full-time 0, part-time 0; International students who hold an F-1 or J-1 Visa—full-time 2, part-time 0.

Financial Information/Assistance:
Tuition for Full-Time Study: *Doctoral:* State residents: per academic year $4,336; Nonstate residents: per academic year $12,474. Tuition is subject to change. See the following Web site for updates and changes in tuition costs: http://bursar.uno.edu/ExplanationFees.cfm.

Financial Assistance:
First-Year Students: Teaching assistantships available for first year. Average amount paid per academic year: $11,278. Average number of hours worked per week: 20. Research assistantships available for first year. Average amount paid per academic year:

$14,514. Average number of hours worked per week: 20. Fellowships and scholarships available for first year. Average amount paid per academic year: $22,000.

Advanced Students: Teaching assistantships available for advanced students. Average amount paid per academic year: $11,303. Average number of hours worked per week: 20. Research assistantships available for advanced students. Average amount paid per academic year: $12,783. Average number of hours worked per week: 20. Fellowships and scholarships available for advanced students. Average amount paid per academic year: $20,000. Average number of hours worked per week: 20.

Additional Information: Of all students currently enrolled full time, 100% benefited from one or more of the listed financial assistance programs. Application and information available online at: http://www.finaid.uno.edu.

Internships/Practica: Students in both applied specialties are required to complete 12 semester hours of practicum for the doctoral degree. There are a wide array of practicum experiences available and student's choice of practicum is based on his or her specific career objectives.

Housing and Day Care: On-campus housing is available. See the following Web site for more information: http://www.housing.uno.edu/. On-campus day care facilities are available.

Employment of Department Graduates:
Master's Degree Graduates: Of those who graduated in the academic year 2008–2009, the following categories and numbers represent the postgraduate activities and employment of master's degree graduates: Enrolled in a postdoctoral residency/fellowship (n/a), employed in independent practice (n/a), total from the above (master's) (0).
Doctoral Degree Graduates: Of those who graduated in the academic year 2008–2009, the following categories and numbers represent the postgraduate activities and employment of doctoral degree graduates: Enrolled in a psychology doctoral program (n/a), enrolled in a postdoctoral residency/fellowship (1), employed in an academic position at a university (1), employed in government agency (2), total from the above (doctoral) (4).

Additional Information:
Orientation, Objectives, and Emphasis of Department: The University of New Orleans, Department of Psychology offers a PhD program with specializations in applied biopsychology and applied developmental psychology. The program was established in 1980 in response to a growing need for persons who are thoroughly trained in the basic content areas of human development or biopsychology, and who are able to translate that knowledge into practical applications. Both specialties emphasize research and service delivery in applied contexts. The applied developmental program has chosen to focus its training in the area of developmental psychopathology. Graduates are trained to work in a variety of settings where they can advance programmatic research focused on understanding psychopathological conditions from a developmental perspective and where they can make practical applications from this research (e.g., design and implement innovative prevention programs, or develop assessments for at-risk children). Similarly, the applied biopsychology program has chosen to focus its training in the area of the biological bases of psychopathology. Graduates are trained to work in a variety of settings where they can advance programmatic research focused on understanding psychopathological conditions from a biological and neuroscience perspective and where they can make practical applications from this research (e.g., test pharmacological treatments for psychological disorders; development of neurological, psychophysiological, or other biological tests for psychological disorders).

Information for Students With Physical Disabilities: See the following Web site for more information: http://www.ods.uno.edu/.

Application Information:
Send to Graduate Coordinator, Department of Psychology, 2001 Geology & Psychology Bldg., New Orleans, LA 70148. Application available online. URL of online application: http://admissions.uno.edu/app.cfm. Students are admitted in the Fall, application deadline February 1. *Fee:* $40.

Southeastern Louisiana University
Department of Psychology
Arts and Sciences
SLU 10831
Hammond, LA 70402
Telephone: (985) 549-2154
Fax: (985) 549-3892
E-mail: pvarnado@selu.edu
Web: http://www.selu.edu/acad_research/depts/psyc/grad_degree/index.html

---

Department Information:
Chairperson: Matt J. Rossano. Number of faculty: total—full-time 11, part-time 4; women—full-time 6, part-time 2; total—minority—full-time 1.

Programs and Degrees Offered:
Listed in the following order: Program area, degree type (T if terminal Master's), number awarded 7/08–6/09. General Psychology MA/MS (Master of Arts/Science) (T) 4, I/O Concentration Other 0.

Student Applications/Admissions:
Student Applications
General Psychology MA/MS (Master of Arts/Science)—Applications 2009–2010, 25. Total applicants accepted 2009–2010, 19. Number full-time enrolled (new admits only) 2009–2010, 8. Number part-time enrolled (new admits only) 2009–2010, 0. Total enrolled 2009–2010 full-time, 16, part-time, 6. Openings 2010–2011, 12. The median number of years required for completion of a degree in 2008–2009 were 2. The number of students enrolled full- and part-time who were dismissed or voluntarily withdrew from this program area in 2008–2009 were 1. *I/O Concentration Other*—Applications 2009–2010, 2. Total applicants accepted 2009–2010, 2. Number full-time enrolled (new admits only) 2009–2010, 2. Number part-time enrolled (new admits only) 2009–2010, 0. Openings 2010–2011, 8. The number of students enrolled full- and part-time who were dismissed or voluntarily withdrew from this program area in 2008–2009 were 1.

Scores: Entries appear in this order: required test or GPA, minimum score (if required), median score of students entering in 2009–2010. *General Psychology MA/MS (Master of Arts/Science):* GRE-V no minimum stated, GRE-Q no minimum stated, overall undergraduate GPA 3.0; *I/O Concentration Other:* GRE-V no minimum stated, GRE-Q no minimum stated, overall undergraduate GPA 3.0.

Other Criteria: (importance of criteria rated low, medium, or high): GRE scores—high, research experience—high, work experience—low, extracurricular activity—low, clinically related public service—low, GPA—high, letters of recommendation—high, statement of goals and objectives—medium.

Student Characteristics: The following represents characteristics of students in 2009–2010 in all graduate psychology programs in the department: Female—full-time 13, part-time 5; Male—full-time 6, part-time 1; African American/Black—full-time 0, part-time 0; Hispanic/Latino(a)—full-time 1, part-time 0; Asian/Pacific Islander—full-time 1, part-time 0; American Indian/Alaska Native—full-time 0, part-time 0; Caucasian/White—full-time 17, part-time 6; Multi-ethnic—full-time 0, part-time 0; students subject to the Americans With Disabilities Act—full-time 1, part-time 0; Unknown ethnicity—full-time 0, part-time 0; International students who hold an F-1 or J-1 Visa—full-time 2, part-time 0.

Financial Information/Assistance:
Tuition for Full-Time Study: *Master's:* State residents: per academic year $3,992; Nonstate residents: per academic year $7,256. Tuition is subject to change.

Financial Assistance:
First-Year Students: Research assistantships available for first year. Average amount paid per academic year: $9,000. Average number of hours worked per week: 20. Apply by March 15. Fellowships and scholarships available for first year. Average amount paid per academic year: $12,500. Average number of hours worked per week: 0. Apply by March 15.

Advanced Students: Research assistantships available for advanced students. Average amount paid per academic year: $9,000. Average number of hours worked per week: 20. Apply by March 15. Fellowships and scholarships available for advanced students. Average amount paid per academic year: $12,500. Average number of hours worked per week: 0. Apply by March 15.

Additional Information: Of all students currently enrolled full time, 40% benefited from one or more of the listed financial assistance programs.

Internships/Practica: Practica are available in clinical, counseling, and business (for I/O concentration) settings.

Housing and Day Care: On-campus housing is available. See the following Web site for more information: http://www.selu.edu/future_students/campus_life/housing/index.html. No on-campus day care facilities are available.

Employment of Department Graduates:
Master's Degree Graduates: Of those who graduated in the academic year 2008–2009, the following categories and numbers represent the postgraduate activities and employment of master's degree graduates: Enrolled in a psychology doctoral program (3), enrolled in another graduate/professional program (0), enrolled in a postdoctoral residency/fellowship (n/a), employed in independent practice (n/a), employed in an academic position at a university (0), employed in an academic position at a 2-year/4-year college (0), employed in other positions at a higher education institution (0), employed in a professional position in a school system (0), employed in business or industry (0), employed in government agency (0), employed in a community mental health/counseling center (0), employed in a hospital/medical center (1), still seeking employment (0), not seeking employment (0), other employment position (0), do not know (0), total from the above (master's) (4).

Doctoral Degree Graduates: Of those who graduated in the academic year 2008–2009, the following categories and numbers represent the postgraduate activities and employment of doctoral degree graduates: Enrolled in a psychology doctoral program (n/a), total from the above (doctoral) (0).

Additional Information:
Orientation, Objectives, and Emphasis of Department: The primary purpose of the MA in general psychology is to prepare the student for doctoral study. This goal is achieved by providing extensive research experience and advanced knowledge in several basic areas within psychology. In recent years, 90% of students who have successfully completed our Master's program in psychology have been placed into doctoral programs.

Special Facilities or Resources: The department has three 5-room laboratory suites for conducting research with humans. There are about 40 microcomputers and 7 printers in the department, about half of which are in a microcomputer laboratory. Statistical packages, such as SPSS, are available on the microcomputers and (via departmental terminal) on the university's mainframe computers.

Application Information:
Application available online. URL of online application: https://www.selu.edu/future_students/apply/g_app.php. Students are admitted in the Fall, application deadline March 15; Spring, application deadline November 15. *Fee:* $20.

Tulane University
Department of Psychology
School of Science and Engineering
2007 Stern Hall
New Orleans, LA 70118
Telephone: (504) 865-5331
Fax: (504) 862-8744
E-mail: *ruscher@tulane.edu*
Web: *http://psych.tulane.edu/*

Department Information:
1911. Chairperson: Janet B. Ruscher. Number of faculty: total—full-time 21; women—full-time 10; total—minority—full-time 4; women minority—full-time 1.

Programs and Degrees Offered:
Listed in the following order: Program area, degree type (T if terminal Master's), number awarded 7/08–6/09. Social Psychology PhD (Doctor of Philosophy) 1, School Psychology PhD (Doctor of Philosophy) 2, Developmental Psychology PhD (Doctor of

Philosophy) 2, Psychobiology/Cognitive Neuroscience PhD (Doctor of Philosophy) 0.

APA Accreditation: School PhD (Doctor of Philosophy). Student Outcome Data Website: http://psych.tulane.edu/graduate/school.php.

Student Applications/Admissions:
Student Applications
Social Psychology PhD (Doctor of Philosophy)—Applications 2009–2010, 10. Total applicants accepted 2009–2010, 1. Number full-time enrolled (new admits only) 2009–2010, 3. Openings 2010–2011, 3. The median number of years required for completion of a degree in 2008–2009 were 5. The number of students enrolled full- and part-time who were dismissed or voluntarily withdrew from this program area in 2008–2009 were 1. *School Psychology PhD (Doctor of Philosophy)*—Applications 2009–2010, 23. Total applicants accepted 2009–2010, 7. Number full-time enrolled (new admits only) 2009–2010, 7. Openings 2010–2011, 5. The median number of years required for completion of a degree in 2008–2009 were 6. The number of students enrolled full- and part-time who were dismissed or voluntarily withdrew from this program area in 2008–2009 were 0. *Developmental Psychology PhD (Doctor of Philosophy)*—Applications 2009–2010, 8. Total applicants accepted 2009–2010, 2. Number full-time enrolled (new admits only) 2009–2010, 0. Openings 2010–2011, 3. The median number of years required for completion of a degree in 2008–2009 were 6. *Psychobiology/Cognitive Neuroscience PhD (Doctor of Philosophy)*—Applications 2009–2010, 12. Total applicants accepted 2009–2010, 3. Number full-time enrolled (new admits only) 2009–2010, 3. Total enrolled 2009–2010 full-time, 10. Openings 2010–2011, 4.

Scores: Entries appear in this order: required test or GPA, minimum score (if required), median score of students entering in 2009–2010. *Social Psychology PhD (Doctor of Philosophy)*: GRE-V no minimum stated, GRE-Q no minimum stated; *School Psychology PhD (Doctor of Philosophy)*: GRE-V no minimum stated, GRE-Q no minimum stated; *Developmental Psychology PhD (Doctor of Philosophy)*: GRE-V no minimum stated, GRE-Q no minimum stated; *Psychobiology/Cognitive Neuroscience PhD (Doctor of Philosophy)*: GRE-V no minimum stated, GRE-Q no minimum stated.

Other Criteria: (importance of criteria rated low, medium, or high): GRE scores—high, research experience—high, work experience—low, extracurricular activity—low, clinically related public service—medium, GPA—high, letters of recommendation—high, interview—high, statement of goals and objectives—medium, undergraduate major in psychology—medium, specific undergraduate psychology courses taken—medium. Clinical experience and interview important for school psychology. Relevant work experience can be looked upon favorably in other programs (e.g., statistical consulting; market research). For additional information on admission requirements, go to http://psych.tulane.edu/graduate/admission.php.

Student Characteristics: The following represents characteristics of students in 2009–2010 in all graduate psychology programs in the department: Female—full-time 29, part-time 0; Male—full-time 11, part-time 0; African American/Black—full-time 5, part-time 0; Hispanic/Latino(a)—full-time 3, part-time 0; Asian/Pacific Islander—full-time 4, part-time 0; American Indian/Alaska Native—full-time 0, part-time 0; Caucasian/White—full-time 28, part-time 0; Multi-ethnic—full-time 0, part-time 0; students subject to the Americans With Disabilities Act—full-time 1, part-time 0; Unknown ethnicity—full-time 0, part-time 0; International students who hold an F-1 or J-1 Visa—full-time 3, part-time 0.

Financial Information/Assistance:
Tuition for Full-Time Study: *Doctoral:* State residents: per academic year $39,000; Nonstate residents: per academic year $39,000. Tuition is subject to change. See the following Web site for updates and changes in tuition costs: http://tulane.edu/sse/academics/graduate/ssegrad_tuition_fees.cfm.

Financial Assistance:
First-Year Students: Teaching assistantships available for first year. Average amount paid per academic year: $17,000. Average number of hours worked per week: 12. Apply by February 1. Research assistantships available for first year. Average amount paid per academic year: $17,000. Average number of hours worked per week: 12. Apply by February 1. Fellowships and scholarships available for first year. Average amount paid per academic year: $18,000. Average number of hours worked per week: 12. Apply by February 1.

Advanced Students: Teaching assistantships available for advanced students. Average amount paid per academic year: $17,000. Average number of hours worked per week: 12. Research assistantships available for advanced students. Average amount paid per academic year: $17,000. Average number of hours worked per week: 12. Fellowships and scholarships available for advanced students. Average amount paid per academic year: $17,000. Average number of hours worked per week: 12.

Additional Information: Of all students currently enrolled full time, 100% benefited from one or more of the listed financial assistance programs. Application and information available online at: http://www.tulane.edu/~finaid/.

Internships/Practica: Doctoral Degree (PhD School Psychology): For those doctoral students for whom a professional internship was required in this program prior to graduation, (2) students applied for an internship in 2008–2009, with (2) students obtaining an internship. Of those students who obtained an internship, (2) were paid internships. Of those students who obtained an internship, (2) students placed in APA/CPA accredited internships, (0) students placed in internships not APA/CPA accredited, but listed with the Association of Psychology Postdoctoral and Internship Programs (APPIC), (0) students placed in internships conforming to guidelines of the Council of Directors of School Psychology Programs (CDSPP), (0) students placed in internships that were not APA/CPA accredited, APPIC or CDSPP listed. Practicum opportunities are available in psychoeducational assessment, school consultation, family-school intervention, and cognitive-behavioral assessment and intervention.

Housing and Day Care: On-campus housing is available. See the following Web site for more information: http://housing.tulane.edu/. On-campus day care facilities are available. See the following Web site for more information: http://newcombkids.tulane.edu/.

Employment of Department Graduates:
Master's Degree Graduates: Of those who graduated in the academic year 2008–2009, the following categories and numbers

represent the postgraduate activities and employment of master's degree graduates: Enrolled in a postdoctoral residency/fellowship (n/a), employed in independent practice (n/a), total from the above (master's) (0).

Doctoral Degree Graduates: Of those who graduated in the academic year 2008–2009, the following categories and numbers represent the postgraduate activities and employment of doctoral degree graduates: Enrolled in a psychology doctoral program (n/a), enrolled in a postdoctoral residency/fellowship (3), total from the above (doctoral) (3).

Additional Information:

Orientation, Objectives, and Emphasis of Department: Tulane's Department of Psychology offers the PhD in social psychology, developmental psychology, and cognitive/behavioral neuroscience, as well as in applied areas of school psychology. The Department does not offer programs in clinical or counseling psychology. All students are expected to articulate an individualized plan of study by the end of the first year of training, a plan developed in consultation with an advisor and a committee of faculty members. Our two broad areas of substantive focus are development (e.g., infant, childhood, adolescence, cognitive aging and neuroscience) and culture & context (e.g., minority youth, stereotyping, ecological systems). Students are required to complete empirical studies for the master's thesis and the dissertation, and are expected to carry out additional research while in training. The program in school psychology, which emphasizes normal developmental processes, will take a minimum of four years to complete, including a year-long internship.

Special Facilities or Resources: The department has research laboratories and computer resources to facilitate research efforts requiring special equipment or space, including physiological, social, sensory, comparative, cognitive, and developmental psychology and human and animal learning. The Newcomb Children's Center, the Hebert facilities at Riverside for natural observation of animals, the laboratories of the Delta Primate Center, and the Audubon Zoological Gardens are available as research sites. There are also opportunities for research in the New Orleans area in organizations and industries, in public and private schools, and in hospitals and other settings serving children.

Information for Students With Physical Disabilities: See the following Web site for more information: http://www.tulane.edu/~erc/disability/index.html.

Application Information:
Send to Dean of the School of Science and Engineering, Tulane University, New Orleans, LA 70118. Application available online. URL of online application: http://psych.tulane.edu/graduate/admission.php. Students are admitted in the Fall, application deadline January 15.

MAINE

Maine, University of (2009 data)
Department of Psychology
Liberal Arts and Sciences
5742 Little Hall
Orono, ME 04469-5742
Telephone: (207) 581-2030
Fax: (207) 581-6128
E-mail: *michael.robbins@umit.maine.edu*
Web: *http://www.umaine.edu/psychology*

Department Information:
1926. Chairperson: Michael A. Robbins. Number of faculty: total—full-time 20, part-time 3; women—full-time 7; total—minority—full-time 1; women minority—full-time 1.

Programs and Degrees Offered:
Listed in the following order: Program area, degree type (T if terminal Master's), number awarded 7/08–6/09. Clinical PhD (Doctor of Philosophy) 2, Development PhD (Doctor of Philosophy) 0, General MA/MS (Master of Arts/Science) 0, Psychological Sciences PhD (Doctor of Philosophy) 0.

APA Accreditation: Clinical PhD (Doctor of Philosophy).

Student Applications/Admissions:
Student Applications
Clinical PhD (Doctor of Philosophy)—Applications 2009–2010, 91. Total applicants accepted 2009–2010, 6. Number full-time enrolled (new admits only) 2009–2010, 4. Number part-time enrolled (new admits only) 2009–2010, 0. Openings 2010–2011, 4. The median number of years required for completion of a degree in 2008–2009 were 6. The number of students enrolled full- and part-time who were dismissed or voluntarily withdrew from this program area in 2008–2009 were 0. *Development PhD (Doctor of Philosophy)*—Applications 2009–2010, 6. Total applicants accepted 2009–2010, 1. Number full-time enrolled (new admits only) 2009–2010, 1. Openings 2010–2011, 1. The number of students enrolled full- and part-time who were dismissed or voluntarily withdrew from this program area in 2008–2009 were 0. *General MA/MS (Master of Arts/Science)*—Applications 2009–2010, 7. Total applicants accepted 2009–2010, 1. Number full-time enrolled (new admits only) 2009–2010, 1. Openings 2010–2011, 1. The median number of years required for completion of a degree in 2008–2009 were 3. The number of students enrolled full- and part-time who were dismissed or voluntarily withdrew from this program area in 2008–2009 were 0. *Psychological Sciences PhD (Doctor of Philosophy)*—Applications 2009–2010, 21. Total applicants accepted 2009–2010, 1. Number full-time enrolled (new admits only) 2009–2010, 1. Total enrolled 2009–2010 full-time, 10. Openings 2010–2011, 2. The number of students enrolled full- and part-time who were dismissed or voluntarily withdrew from this program area in 2008–2009 were 0.
Other Criteria: (importance of criteria rated low, medium, or high): GRE scores—medium, research experience—high, work experience—low, extracurricular activity—low, clinically related public service—medium, GPA—high, letters of recommendation—high, interview—high, statement of goals and objectives—high.

Student Characteristics: The following represents characteristics of students in 2009–2010 in all graduate psychology programs in the department: Female—full-time 24, part-time 0; Male—full-time 8, part-time 0; African American/Black—full-time 0, part-time 0; Hispanic/Latino(a)—full-time 0, part-time 0; Asian/Pacific Islander—full-time 1, part-time 0; American Indian/Alaska Native—full-time 1, part-time 0; Caucasian/White—full-time 30, part-time 0; Multi-ethnic—full-time 1, part-time 0; students subject to the Americans With Disabilities Act—full-time 2, part-time 0; Unknown ethnicity—full-time 0, part-time 0; International students who hold an F-1 or J-1 Visa—full-time 0, part-time 0.

Financial Information/Assistance:
Tuition for Full-Time Study: *Master's*: State residents: $357 per credit hour; Nonstate residents: $1,028 per credit hour. *Doctoral*: State residents: $357 per credit hour; Nonstate residents: $1,028 per credit hour. Tuition is subject to change.

Financial Assistance:
First-Year Students: Teaching assistantships available for first year. Average number of hours worked per week: 12. Research assistantships available for first year. Average number of hours worked per week: 20.
Advanced Students: Teaching assistantships available for advanced students. Average number of hours worked per week: 12. Research assistantships available for advanced students. Average number of hours worked per week: 12. Traineeships available for advanced students. Average number of hours worked per week: 12. Fellowships and scholarships available for advanced students. Average number of hours worked per week: 0.
Additional Information: Of all students currently enrolled full time, 88% benefited from one or more of the listed financial assistance programs.

Internships/Practica: Doctoral Degree (PhD Clinical): For those doctoral students for whom a professional internship was required in this program prior to graduation, (3) students applied for an internship in 2008–2009, with (3) students obtaining an internship. Of those students who obtained an internship, (3) were paid internships. Of those students who obtained an internship, (3) students placed in APA/CPA accredited internships, (0) students placed in internships not APA/CPA accredited, but listed with the Association of Psychology Postdoctoral and Internship Programs (APPIC), (0) students placed in internships conforming to guidelines of the Council of Directors of School Psychology Programs (CDSPP), (0) students placed in internships that were not APA/CPA accredited, APPIC or CDSPP listed. Several settings are used for practicum training: The Psychological Services Center housed within the department, Penobscot Job Corps, Kennebec Valley Mental Health Center, Penqis CAPS Head Start, School Administrative District #4, #68, KidsPeace New England.

Housing and Day Care: On-campus housing is available. See the following Web site for more information: http://www.umaine.edu/

housing/graduate.htm. On-campus day care facilities are available. See the following Web site for more information: http://www.umaine.edu/hr/family/childcare.htm.

Employment of Department Graduates:
Master's Degree Graduates: Of those who graduated in the academic year 2008–2009, the following categories and numbers represent the postgraduate activities and employment of master's degree graduates: Enrolled in a postdoctoral residency/fellowship (n/a), employed in independent practice (n/a), total from the above (master's) (0).
Doctoral Degree Graduates: Of those who graduated in the academic year 2008–2009, the following categories and numbers represent the postgraduate activities and employment of doctoral degree graduates: Enrolled in a psychology doctoral program (n/a), enrolled in a postdoctoral residency/fellowship (2), do not know (0), total from the above (doctoral) (2).

Additional Information:
Orientation, Objectives, and Emphasis of Department: The department believes that the best graduate education involves close working relationships between the faculty and the student. Thus, a high faculty-to-student ratio and small class sizes characterize the department. In addition, incoming students are selected to work with a faculty research mentor. There are also opportunities for individualized study and experience in directed readings, research, and teaching. A faculty committee, selected to represent the student's interests, will assist the student in planning an appropriate graduate program.

Special Facilities or Resources: Psychophysiological, perception, EEG laboratories; animal research laboratory; on-site practicum training center; department-run preschool.

Information for Students With Physical Disabilities: See the following Web site for more information: http://www.ume.maine.edu/disability.

Application Information:
Send to Graduate School, 5782 Winslow Hall, University of Maine, Orono, ME 04469-5782. Students are admitted in the Fall, application deadline December 31. *Fee:* $50.

MARYLAND

Baltimore, University of
Division of Applied Behavioral Sciences
Yale Gordon College of Liberal Arts
1420 North Charles Street
Baltimore, MD 21201-5779
Telephone: (410) 837-5310
Fax: (410) 837-4059
E-mail: *tmitchell@ubalt.edu*
Web: *http://www.ubalt.edu/cla_template.cfm?page=729*

Department Information:
1970. Graduate Program Director: Tom Mitchell, PhD. Number of faculty: total—full-time 8; women—full-time 6; total—minority—full-time 1; women minority—full-time 1.

Programs and Degrees Offered:
Listed in the following order: Program area, degree type (T if terminal Master's), number awarded 7/08–6/09. Psychological Applications MA/MS (Master of Arts/Science) (T) 4, Counseling Psychology MA/MS (Master of Arts/Science) (T) 14, Industrial/Organizational Psychology MA/MS (Master of Arts/Science) (T) 14.

Student Applications/Admissions:
Student Applications
Psychological Applications MA/MS (Master of Arts/Science)—Applications 2009–2010, 18. Total applicants accepted 2009–2010, 12. Number full-time enrolled (new admits only) 2009–2010, 5. Number part-time enrolled (new admits only) 2009–2010, 9. Total enrolled 2009–2010 full-time, 9, part-time, 7. Openings 2010–2011, 10. The median number of years required for completion of a degree in 2008–2009 were 3. The number of students enrolled full- and part-time who were dismissed or voluntarily withdrew from this program area in 2008–2009 were 0. Counseling Psychology MA/MS (Master of Arts/Science)—Applications 2009–2010, 48. Total applicants accepted 2009–2010, 38. Number full-time enrolled (new admits only) 2009–2010, 9. Number part-time enrolled (new admits only) 2009–2010, 22. Total enrolled 2009–2010 full-time, 16, part-time, 38. Openings 2010–2011, 25. The median number of years required for completion of a degree in 2008–2009 were 4. The number of students enrolled full- and part-time who were dismissed or voluntarily withdrew from this program area in 2008–2009 were 2. Industrial/Organizational Psychology MA/MS (Master of Arts/Science)—Applications 2009–2010, 52. Total applicants accepted 2009–2010, 42. Number full-time enrolled (new admits only) 2009–2010, 18. Number part-time enrolled (new admits only) 2009–2010, 8. Total enrolled 2009–2010 full-time, 27, part-time, 21. Openings 2010–2011, 25. The median number of years required for completion of a degree in 2008–2009 were 2. The number of students enrolled full- and part-time who were dismissed or voluntarily withdrew from this program area in 2008–2009 were 3.
Scores: Entries appear in this order: required test or GPA, minimum score (if required), median score of students entering in 2009–2010. *Psychological Applications MA/MS (Master of Arts/Science)*: GRE-V no minimum stated, 440, GRE-Q no minimum stated, 540, GRE-Analytical no minimum stated, 4.0, overall undergraduate GPA 3.0; *Counseling Psychology MA/MS (Master of Arts/Science)*: GRE-V no minimum stated, 440, GRE-Q no minimum stated, 530, GRE-Analytical no minimum stated, 4.0, overall undergraduate GPA 3.0; *Industrial/Organizational Psychology MA/MS (Master of Arts/Science)*: GRE-V no minimum stated, 440, GRE-Q no minimum stated, 535, overall undergraduate GPA 3.0.
Other Criteria: (importance of criteria rated low, medium, or high): GRE scores—medium, GPA—high, letters of recommendation—medium, statement of goals and objectives—medium, specific undergraduate psychology courses taken—low. For additional information on admission requirements, go to http://www.ubalt.edu/cla_template.cfm?page=1348.

Student Characteristics: The following represents characteristics of students in 2009–2010 in all graduate psychology programs in the department: Female—full-time 35, part-time 53; Male—full-time 17, part-time 13; African American/Black—full-time 18, part-time 25; Hispanic/Latino(a)—full-time 2, part-time 2; Asian/Pacific Islander—full-time 2, part-time 1; American Indian/Alaska Native—full-time 0, part-time 0; Caucasian/White—full-time 30, part-time 38; Multi-ethnic—full-time 0, part-time 0; students subject to the Americans With Disabilities Act—full-time 0, part-time 0; Unknown ethnicity—full-time 0, part-time 0; International students who hold an F-1 or J-1 Visa—full-time 3, part-time 0.

Financial Information/Assistance:
Tuition for Full-Time Study: *Master's:* State residents: per academic year $11,196, $622 per credit hour; Nonstate residents: per academic year $15,559, $864 per credit hour. See the following Web site for updates and changes in tuition costs: http://www.ubalt.edu/tuition.

Financial Assistance:
First-Year Students: Research assistantships available for first year. Average amount paid per academic year: $4,260. Average number of hours worked per week: 20. Apply by March 15.
Advanced Students: Research assistantships available for advanced students. Average amount paid per academic year: $4,260. Average number of hours worked per week: 20. Apply by March 15.
Additional Information: Of all students currently enrolled full time, 8% benefited from one or more of the listed financial assistance programs. Application and information available online at: http://www.ubalt.edu/financialaid.

Internships/Practica: The Baltimore/Washington Metropolitan area provides a wide range of settings for paid practicum and internships. The academic and site supervisors work closely with the intern to insure a quality experience.

Housing and Day Care: On-campus housing is available. See the following Web site for more information: http://www.ubalt.edu/

template.cfm?page=94. No on-campus day care facilities are available.

Employment of Department Graduates:
Master's Degree Graduates: Of those who graduated in the academic year 2008–2009, the following categories and numbers represent the postgraduate activities and employment of master's degree graduates: Enrolled in a postdoctoral residency/fellowship (n/a), employed in independent practice (n/a), total from the above (master's) (0).
Doctoral Degree Graduates: Of those who graduated in the academic year 2008–2009, the following categories and numbers represent the postgraduate activities and employment of doctoral degree graduates: Enrolled in a psychology doctoral program (n/a), total from the above (doctoral) (0).

Additional Information:
Orientation, Objectives, and Emphasis of Department: The Division of Applied Behavioral Sciences has a practitioner-oriented faculty of applied psychologists and researchers.

Special Facilities or Resources: Four different university labs and 100% of our classrooms provide Internet access, MS Office, and SPSS for students and faculty members. The Wagman Psychology Lab provides for computer based testing and assessment.

Information for Students With Physical Disabilities: See the following Web site for more information: http://www.ubalt.edu/disability.

Application Information:
Send to Office of Graduate Admissions, University of Baltimore, 1420 N. Charles Street, Baltimore, MD 21201-5779. Application available online. URL of online application: http://www.ubalt.edu/admissions/graduate/dates.html. Students are admitted in the Fall, application deadline July 1; Spring, application deadline December 1. *Fee:* $30.

Frostburg State University
MS in Counseling Psychology Program
College of Liberal Arts and Sciences
Department of Psychology, 101 Braddock Road
Frostburg, MD 21532
Telephone: (301) 687-4446
Fax: (301) 687-7418
E-mail: *mpmurtagh@frostburg.edu*
Web: *http://www.frostburg.edu/dept/psyc/graduate/coupsy.htm*

Department Information:
1977. Michael Murtagh, Graduate Program Coordinator; Kevin Peterson, Chair. Number of faculty: total—full-time 5, part-time 1; women—full-time 2; total—minority—full-time 1; women minority—full-time 1.

Programs and Degrees Offered:
Listed in the following order: Program area, degree type (T if terminal Master's), number awarded 7/08–6/09. Counseling Psychology MA/MS (Master of Arts/Science) (T) 9.

Student Applications/Admissions:
Student Applications
Counseling Psychology MA/MS (Master of Arts/Science)—Applications 2009–2010, 43. Total applicants accepted 2009–2010, 12. Number full-time enrolled (new admits only) 2009–2010, 12. Number part-time enrolled (new admits only) 2009–2010, 0. Total enrolled 2009–2010 full-time, 37, part-time, 2. Openings 2010–2011, 14. The median number of years required for completion of a degree in 2008–2009 were 3. The number of students enrolled full- and part-time who were dismissed or voluntarily withdrew from this program area in 2008–2009 were 3.

Other Criteria: (importance of criteria rated low, medium, or high): GRE scores—low, research experience—low, work experience—high, extracurricular activity—low, clinically related public service—high, GPA—high, letters of recommendation—high, interview—high, statement of goals and objectives—high, internship—high, undergraduate major in psychology—medium, specific undergraduate psychology courses taken—medium. For additional information on admission requirements, go to http://www.frostburg.edu/dept/psyc/graduate/spadmin.htm.

Student Characteristics: The following represents characteristics of students in 2009–2010 in all graduate psychology programs in the department: Female—full-time 35, part-time 2; Male—full-time 2, part-time 0; African American/Black—full-time 2, part-time 0; Hispanic/Latino(a)—full-time 0, part-time 0; Asian/Pacific Islander—full-time 0, part-time 0; American Indian/Alaska Native—full-time 0, part-time 0; Caucasian/White—full-time 34, part-time 2; Multi-ethnic—full-time 1, part-time 0; students subject to the Americans With Disabilities Act—full-time 0, part-time 0; Unknown ethnicity—full-time 0, part-time 0; International students who hold an F-1 or J-1 Visa—full-time 2, part-time 0.

Financial Information/Assistance:
Tuition for Full-Time Study: Master's: State residents: $305 per credit hour; Nonstate residents: $350 per credit hour. Tuition is subject to change. See the following Web site for updates and changes in tuition costs: http://www.frostburg.edu/admin/billing/.

Financial Assistance:
First-Year Students: Research assistantships available for first year. Average amount paid per academic year: $5,000. Average number of hours worked per week: 20. Apply by March 15. Fellowships and scholarships available for first year. Average amount paid per academic year: $6,500. Average number of hours worked per week: 20. Apply by March 15.
Advanced Students: No information provided.
Additional Information: Of all students currently enrolled full time, 57% benefited from one or more of the listed financial assistance programs. Application and information available online at: http://www.frostburg.edu/grad/financ.htm.

Internships/Practica: Master's Degree (MA/MS Counseling Psychology): An internship experience, such as a final research project or "capstone" experience is required of graduates. An extensive, two semester internship experience is required which facilitates students' receptivity to supervisory feedback, enhances self-awareness, and provides a setting in which the transition from student to professional is accomplished. In addition to on-site supervision, students participate in individual and group supervision with FSU faculty. Past graduate internship sites for the M.S. Counseling Psychology program have included: outpatient community mental health (the most frequent internship setting); college counseling; inpatient psychiatric; inpatient and outpatient addictions; family services; K-12 psychological assessment and alternative classroom and after school care programs; community health advocacy and counseling; criminal justice system; nursing homes; hospital-based crisis services; hospice; domestic violence programs. Students construct their internship experiences in order to meet training goals they formulate. Students electing to complete graduate certificate programs in Addictions Counseling Psychology and Child and Family Counseling Psychology must complete at least 150 hours of direct services in settings consistent with the certificate program's focus. Internship experiences, in addition to at least four academic semesters of study, prepare graduates for positions as mental health counselors, marriage and family counselors, crisis counselors, drug and alcohol counselors, community health specialists, and in supervisory positions in a variety of settings.

Housing and Day Care: On-campus housing is available. See the following Web site for more information: http://www.frostburg.edu/clife/reslife. On-campus day care facilities are available. See the following Web site for more information: http://www.frostburg.edu/childrenscenter.

Employment of Department Graduates:
Master's Degree Graduates: Of those who graduated in the academic year 2008–2009, the following categories and numbers represent the postgraduate activities and employment of master's degree graduates: Enrolled in a postdoctoral residency/fellowship (n/a), employed in independent practice (n/a), total from the above (master's) (0).
Doctoral Degree Graduates: Of those who graduated in the academic year 2008–2009, the following categories and numbers represent the postgraduate activities and employment of doctoral degree graduates: Enrolled in a psychology doctoral program (n/a), total from the above (doctoral) (0).

Additional Information:
Orientation, Objectives, and Emphasis of Department: Providing training in professional psychology at the Master's level, FSU's program is designed for those pursuing further study in science-based counseling psychology. Our theoretical perspective is integrative, including cognitive-behavioral, motivational interviewing, family systems, developmental, multicultural, humanistic, and brief therapies. We emphasize training in empirically-supported treatments for children, adolescents, families and adults. Students develop counseling skills through learning about self, client, counselor-client relationships, and the importance of cultural contexts. Considerable attention is given not only to development of professional skills but also to personal development and multicultural awareness. These emphases reflect our belief that an effective counselor is one who is self-aware and receptive to consultation. For continuing study at the doctoral level, experience and knowledge gained in this program provide a firm foundation. Optional research opportunities prepare students for advanced graduate study in psychology. The Center for Children and Families offers unique research, educational and service experiences. Two certificate programs provide specialized training in Addictions Counseling Psychology and Child and Family Counseling Psychology.

These can be completed within the three-year program of study, as well as courses required for licensure. All National Counselor Exam course areas are offered, and FSU offers this exam. The Master's in Psychology Accreditation Council accredits this program.

Special Facilities or Resources: Resources include specially designed counseling practice rooms for individual and group counseling. Two-way mirrors with adjacent observation rooms are available for supervision. Audiotaping and videotaping resources are available for faculty and student use. In addition, students' case conceptualization write-ups and all previous internship papers are available for restricted use by students.

Information for Students With Physical Disabilities: See the following Web site for more information: http://www.frostburg.edu/clife/dss.

Application Information:
Send to Office of Graduate Services, 101 Braddock Road, Frostburg State University, Frostburg, MD 21532. Application available online. URL of online application: http://www.frostburg.edu/grad. Students are admitted in the Fall, application deadline February 1; March 15 for Graduate Assistantship applications. *Fee:* $30.

Johns Hopkins University
Department of Psychological and Brain Sciences
3400 North Charles Street Ames Hall 204
Baltimore, MD 21218
Telephone: (410) 516-6175
Fax: (410) 516-4478
E-mail: *hope.stein@jhu.edu*
Web: *http://pbs.jhu.edu*

Department Information:
1881. Chairperson: Dr. Steven Yantis. Number of faculty: total—full-time 12, part-time 9; women—full-time 4, part-time 1; faculty subject to the Americans With Disabilities Act 1.

Programs and Degrees Offered:
Listed in the following order: Program area, degree type (T if terminal Master's), number awarded 7/08–6/09. Biopsychology PhD (Doctor of Philosophy) 3, Cognitive PhD (Doctor of Philosophy) 1, Cognitive Neuroscience PhD (Doctor of Philosophy) 1, Developmental PhD (Doctor of Philosophy) 1.

Student Applications/Admissions:
Student Applications
Biopsychology PhD (Doctor of Philosophy)—Applications 2009–2010, 45. Total applicants accepted 2009–2010, 4. Number full-time enrolled (new admits only) 2009–2010, 1. Openings 2010–2011, 3. The median number of years required for completion of a degree in 2008–2009 were 5. The number of students enrolled full- and part-time who were dismissed or voluntarily withdrew from this program area in 2008–2009 were 0. *Cognitive PhD (Doctor of Philosophy)*—Applications 2009–2010, 21. Total applicants accepted 2009–2010, 2. Number full-time enrolled (new admits only) 2009–2010, 1. Total

enrolled 2009–2010 full-time, 4. Openings 2010–2011, 2. The median number of years required for completion of a degree in 2008–2009 were 5. The number of students enrolled full- and part-time who were dismissed or voluntarily withdrew from this program area in 2008–2009 were 0. *Cognitive Neuroscience PhD (Doctor of Philosophy)*—Applications 2009–2010, 40. Total applicants accepted 2009–2010, 3. Number full-time enrolled (new admits only) 2009–2010, 3. Openings 2010–2011, 3. The median number of years required for completion of a degree in 2008–2009 were 5. The number of students enrolled full- and part-time who were dismissed or voluntarily withdrew from this program area in 2008–2009 were 0. *Developmental PhD (Doctor of Philosophy)*—Applications 2009–2010, 30. Total applicants accepted 2009–2010, 0. Number full-time enrolled (new admits only) 2009–2010, 0. Openings 2010–2011, 2. The median number of years required for completion of a degree in 2008–2009 were 5. The number of students enrolled full- and part-time who were dismissed or voluntarily withdrew from this program area in 2008–2009 were 1.

Other Criteria: (importance of criteria rated low, medium, or high): GRE scores—high, research experience—high, work experience—medium, extracurricular activity—low, clinically related public service—low, GPA—high, letters of recommendation—high, interview—high, statement of goals and objectives—high, Sample of work—medium, undergraduate major in psychology—medium.

Student Characteristics: The following represents characteristics of students in 2009–2010 in all graduate psychology programs in the department: Female—full-time 13, part-time 0; Male—full-time 15, part-time 0; African American/Black—full-time 1, part-time 0; Hispanic/Latino(a)—full-time 0, part-time 0; Asian/Pacific Islander—full-time 8, part-time 0; American Indian/Alaska Native—full-time 0, part-time 0; Caucasian/White—full-time 15, part-time 0; Multi-ethnic—full-time 1, part-time 0; students subject to the Americans With Disabilities Act—full-time 0, part-time 0; Unknown ethnicity—full-time 0, part-time 0; International students who hold an F-1 or J-1 Visa—full-time 3, part-time 0.

Financial Information/Assistance:
  Tuition for Full-Time Study: *Doctoral:* State residents: per academic year $40,680; Nonstate residents: per academic year $40,680. Tuition is subject to change. See the following Web site for updates and changes in tuition costs: http://www.jhu.edu.

Financial Assistance:
  First-Year Students: Teaching assistantships available for first year. Research assistantships available for first year.
  Advanced Students: Teaching assistantships available for advanced students. Research assistantships available for advanced students.
  Additional Information: Of all students currently enrolled full time, 100% benefited from one or more of the listed financial assistance programs. Application and information available online at: http://pbs.jhu.edu.

Housing and Day Care: No on-campus housing is available. No on-campus day care facilities are available.

Employment of Department Graduates:
  Master's Degree Graduates: Of those who graduated in the academic year 2008–2009, the following categories and numbers represent the postgraduate activities and employment of master's degree graduates: Enrolled in a postdoctoral residency/fellowship (n/a), employed in independent practice (n/a), total from the above (master's) (0).
  Doctoral Degree Graduates: Of those who graduated in the academic year 2008–2009, the following categories and numbers represent the postgraduate activities and employment of doctoral degree graduates: Enrolled in a psychology doctoral program (n/a), enrolled in a postdoctoral residency/fellowship (5), employed in an academic position at a 2-year/4-year college (1), total from the above (doctoral) (6).

Additional Information:
  Orientation, Objectives, and Emphasis of Department: The graduate program in psychology at The Johns Hopkins University emphasizes research training, stressing the application of basic research methodology to theoretical problems in psychology. Students are actively engaged in research projects within the first semester. There is a low student/faculty ratio; students work closely with their advisors. Courses, seminars, and research activities provide training so that students will emerge as independent investigators who can embark on successful research careers in psychology. Courses cover fundamental issues in experimental design and analysis, and provide a broad background in all the major areas of psychology. Advanced seminars deal with topics of current interest in various specific areas. The department has programs in cognitive psychology (including perceptual and cognitive development), cognitive neuroscience, quantitative psychology, and biopsychology. The evaluation of applications to our graduate program is based on many factors. They include both objective indicators, such as required GRE scores and undergraduate GPA, and more subjective information, such as a statement of purpose, a description of applicant's background and experience, and letters of recommendation. To select among the top candidates, we rely on letters of recommendation to provide a personal assessment of applicant's potential for graduate work by faculty mentors and advisors who know the applicant well. Students in good standing can expect to receive both tuition remission and salary.

  Special Facilities or Resources: Each faculty member in the Department of Psychology maintains a laboratory for conducting research. The psychology building was recently renovated, and the research space is both excellent and plentiful. Every lab contains multiple microcomputer systems for experimentation, analysis, and word processing; most machines are connected via a local-area network to one another and to the Internet. In addition, individual laboratories contain special-purpose equipment designed for the research carried out there. Laboratories in cognition, for example, include high-resolution display devices for experiments in visual. Quantitative psychology laboratories include UNIX work stations for computational analysis and simulation studies. Biopsychology laboratories have facilities for animal surgery, histology, electrophysiological recording of single units and evoked potentials, analysis of neurotransmitters through assays and high-pressure liquid chromatography, bioacoustics, and for general behavioral testing.

GRADUATE STUDY IN PSYCHOLOGY

Application Information:
Send to Hope Stein, Academic Program Coordinator, Psychological & Brain Sciences, Johns Hopkins University, 3400 N. Charles St. Ames Hall 204, Baltimore MD 21218 Applications on line at http://pbs.jhu.edu. Application available online. URL of online application: https://app.applyyourself.com/?id=jhu-grad. Students are admitted in the Fall, application deadline December 15. Online applications only. *Fee:* $75.

Loyola University Maryland
Department of Psychology
4501 North Charles Street
Baltimore, MD 21210
Telephone: (410) 617-2696
Fax: (410) 617-5341
E-mail: *tpmartino@loyola.edu*
Web: *http://www.loyola.edu/psychology*

Department Information:
1968. Chairperson: Dr. Beth A. Kotchick. Number of faculty: total—full-time 20, part-time 2; women—full-time 12; total—minority—full-time 4; women minority—full-time 4.

Programs and Degrees Offered:
Listed in the following order: Program area, degree type (T if terminal Master's), number awarded 7/08–6/09. Clinical Psychology MA/MS (Master of Arts/Science) (T) 37, Counseling Psychology MA/MS (Master of Arts/Science) (T) 14, Clinical Psychology PsyD (Doctor of Psychology) 11.

APA Accreditation: Clinical PsyD (Doctor of Psychology). Student Outcome Data Website: http://www.loyola.edu/academics/psychology/doctoral/current/trainingoutcomes.html.

Student Applications/Admissions:
Student Applications
Clinical Psychology MA/MS (Master of Arts/Science)—Applications 2009–2010, 172. Total applicants accepted 2009–2010, 105. Number full-time enrolled (new admits only) 2009–2010, 30. Number part-time enrolled (new admits only) 2009–2010, 8. Total enrolled 2009–2010 full-time, 80, part-time, 13. Openings 2010–2011, 40. The median number of years required for completion of a degree in 2008–2009 were 2. The number of students enrolled full- and part-time who were dismissed or voluntarily withdrew from this program area in 2008–2009 were 4. Counseling Psychology MA/MS (Master of Arts/Science)—Applications 2009–2010, 120. Total applicants accepted 2009–2010, 61. Number full-time enrolled (new admits only) 2009–2010, 19. Number part-time enrolled (new admits only) 2009–2010, 6. Total enrolled 2009–2010 full-time, 45, part-time, 17. Openings 2010–2011, 40. The median number of years required for completion of a degree in 2008–2009 were 2. The number of students enrolled full- and part-time who were dismissed or voluntarily withdrew from this program area in 2008–2009 were 3. Clinical Psychology PsyD (Doctor of Psychology)—Applications 2009–2010, 330. Total applicants accepted 2009–2010, 27. Number full-time enrolled (new admits only) 2009–2010, 19. Total enrolled 2009–2010 full-time, 71. Openings 2010–2011, 15. The median number of years required for completion of a degree in 2008–2009 were 4. The number of students enrolled full- and part-time who were dismissed or voluntarily withdrew from this program area in 2008–2009 were 1.

Scores: Entries appear in this order: required test or GPA, minimum score (if required), median score of students entering in 2009–2010. Clinical Psychology MA/MS (Master of Arts/Science): GRE-V no minimum stated, 530, GRE-Q no minimum stated, 620, GRE-Analytical no minimum stated, 4.5, overall undergraduate GPA 3.0; Counseling Psychology MA/MS (Master of Arts/Science): GRE-V no minimum stated, 510, GRE-Q no minimum stated, 570, GRE-Analytical no minimum stated, 4.5, overall undergraduate GPA 3.0, 3.4; Clinical Psychology PsyD (Doctor of Psychology): GRE-V no minimum stated, 580, GRE-Q no minimum stated, 650, GRE-Analytical no minimum stated, 5.0, overall undergraduate GPA 3.0, 3.55.

Other Criteria: (importance of criteria rated low, medium, or high): GRE scores—high, research experience—high, work experience—high, extracurricular activity—high, clinically related public service—high, GPA—high, letters of recommendation—high, interview—high, statement of goals and objectives—high, undergraduate major in psychology—medium, specific undergraduate psychology courses taken—high, Interviews by invitation only for PsyD program. No interview for Master's programs. For additional information on admission requirements, go to http://www.loyola.edu/graduate/loyola-college/programs/psychology/admission-requirements.aspx.

Student Characteristics: The following represents characteristics of students in 2009–2010 in all graduate psychology programs in the department: Female—full-time 161, part-time 25; Male—full-time 35, part-time 5; African American/Black—full-time 10, part-time 2; Hispanic/Latino(a)—full-time 3, part-time 2; Asian/Pacific Islander—full-time 8, part-time 1; American Indian/Alaska Native—full-time 1, part-time 0; Caucasian/White—full-time 153, part-time 24; Multi-ethnic—full-time 5, part-time 1; Unknown ethnicity—full-time 16, part-time 0; International students who hold an F-1 or J-1 Visa—full-time 3, part-time 0.

Financial Information/Assistance:
Tuition for Full-Time Study: *Master's:* State residents: $645 per credit hour; Nonstate residents: $645 per credit hour. *Doctoral:* State residents: per academic year $26,412; Nonstate residents: per academic year $26,412. Tuition is subject to change. Tuition costs vary by program. See the following Web site for updates and changes in tuition costs: http://www.loyola.edu/Graduate/Loyola-College/financial-aid/costs-per-calendar-year.aspx.

Financial Assistance:
First-Year Students: No information provided.
Advanced Students: Teaching assistantships available for advanced students. Average amount paid per academic year: $1,600. Average number of hours worked per week: 10. Apply by May/November. Research assistantships available for advanced students. Average amount paid per academic year: $1,600. Average number of hours worked per week: 10. Apply by May/November. Fellowships and scholarships available for advanced students.

Additional Information: Of all students currently enrolled full time, 45% benefited from one or more of the listed financial assistance programs. Application and information available online at: http://www.loyola.edu/HR/Student Employment/.

Internships/Practica: Doctoral Degree (PsyD Clinical Psychology): For those doctoral students for whom a professional internship was required in this program prior to graduation, (15) students applied for an internship in 2008–2009, with (15) students obtaining an internship. Of those students who obtained an internship, (14) were paid internships. Of those students who obtained an internship, (11) students placed in APA/CPA accredited internships, (1) students placed in internships not APA/CPA accredited, but listed with the Association of Psychology Postdoctoral and Internship Programs (APPIC), (0) students placed in internships conforming to guidelines of the Council of Directors of School Psychology Programs (CDSPP), (3) students placed in internships that were not APA/CPA accredited, APPIC or CDSPP listed. Master's Degree (MA/MS Clinical Psychology): An internship experience, such as a final research project or "capstone" experience is required of graduates. Master's Degree (MA/MS Counseling Psychology): An internship experience, such as a final research project or "capstone" experience is required of graduates. The MS program, Practitioner Track requires 300 hours of externship experience. The MS program, Thesis Track requires 150 hours of externship experience. Students are able to choose from a wide variety of sites approved by the Department. The PsyD program incorporates field placement training throughout the curriculum; a minimum total of 1,260 hours of field training is required. The final (fifth) year of the PsyD program is a full-time internship.

Housing and Day Care: No on-campus housing is available. No on-campus day care facilities are available.

Employment of Department Graduates:
Master's Degree Graduates: Of those who graduated in the academic year 2008–2009, the following categories and numbers represent the postgraduate activities and employment of master's degree graduates: Enrolled in a psychology doctoral program (11), enrolled in another graduate/professional program (3), enrolled in a postdoctoral residency/fellowship (n/a), employed in independent practice (n/a), employed in a community mental health/counseling center (6), employed in a hospital/medical center (3), do not know (27), total from the above (master's) (50).
Doctoral Degree Graduates: Of those who graduated in the academic year 2008–2009, the following categories and numbers represent the postgraduate activities and employment of doctoral degree graduates: Enrolled in a psychology doctoral program (n/a), enrolled in a postdoctoral residency/fellowship (11), employed in independent practice (0), total from the above (doctoral) (11).

Additional Information:
Orientation, Objectives, and Emphasis of Department: The Master's programs in Clinical and Counseling Psychology at Loyola University Maryland provides training to individuals who wish to promote mental health in individuals, families, organizations, and communities through careers in direct service, leadership, research, and education. We strive to provide a learning environment that facilitates the development of skills in critical thinking, scholarship, assessment and intervention, and that is grounded in an appreciation for both psychological science and human diversity. The goals of the PsyD program in Clinical Psychology are based on the scholar-professional model of training, designed to train autonomous practitioners of professional psychology who will deliver mental health services and lead others in service to the general public in diverse settings.

Special Facilities or Resources: Departmental facilities include the Loyola Clinic, a health psychology/behavioral medicine laboratory, audiovisual recording facilities, assessment and therapy training rooms, and a student lounge. Students have access to a campus-wide computer system, including SPSS and SAS software. All graduate students have telephone voicemail and e-mail addresses. Advanced doctoral students are provided with individual workstations with computers.

Information for Students With Physical Disabilities: See the following Web site for more information: http://www.loyola.edu/campuslife/healthservices/disabilitysupportservices/.

Application Information:
Send to Office of Graduate Admissions, Loyola College in Maryland, 4501 N. Charles Street, Baltimore, MD 21210. Application available online. URL of online application: https://graduate.loyola.edu/graduate/application/. Students are admitted in the Fall, application deadline December 15. Deadline for MS in Clinical or Counseling Psychology is March 15. *Fee:* $50.

Maryland, University of
Department of Counseling and Personnel Services, School and Counseling Psychology Programs
College of Education
3214 Benjamin Building
College Park, MD 20742
Telephone: (301) 405-2858
Fax: (301) 405-9995
E-mail: *caps@umd.edu*
Web: *http://www.education.umd.edu/EDCP/*

Department Information:
1967. Chairperson: Dennis M. Kivlighan, Jr. Number of faculty: total—full-time 16, part-time 3; women—full-time 10, part-time 3; total—minority—full-time 4, part-time 1; women minority—full-time 2, part-time 1.

Programs and Degrees Offered:
Listed in the following order: Program area, degree type (T if terminal Master's), number awarded 7/08–6/09. Counseling Psychology PhD (Doctor of Philosophy) 8, School Psychology PhD (Doctor of Philosophy) 3.

APA Accreditation: Counseling PhD (Doctor of Philosophy). School PhD (Doctor of Philosophy).

Student Applications/Admissions:
Student Applications
Counseling Psychology PhD (Doctor of Philosophy)—Applications 2009–2010, 204. Total applicants accepted 2009–2010, 8. Number full-time enrolled (new admits only) 2009–2010, 4. Number part-time enrolled (new admits only) 2009–2010, 0. Openings 2010–2011, 6. The median number of years required for completion of a degree in 2008–2009 were 6. The number of students enrolled full- and part-time who were dismissed or voluntarily withdrew from this program area in 2008–2009 were 0. School Psychology PhD (Doctor of Philoso-

phy)—Applications 2009–2010, 59. Total applicants accepted 2009–2010, 7. Number full-time enrolled (new admits only) 2009–2010, 2. Number part-time enrolled (new admits only) 2009–2010, 0. Total enrolled 2009–2010 full-time, 24, part-time, 8. Openings 2010–2011, 3. The median number of years required for completion of a degree in 2008–2009 were 6. The number of students enrolled full- and part-time who were dismissed or voluntarily withdrew from this program area in 2008–2009 were 1.

Scores: Entries appear in this order: required test or GPA, minimum score (if required), median score of students entering in 2009–2010. *Counseling Psychology PhD (Doctor of Philosophy)*: GRE-V no minimum stated, GRE-Q no minimum stated, GRE-Analytical no minimum stated, overall undergraduate GPA no minimum stated, last 2 years GPA no minimum stated, psychology GPA no minimum stated, Masters GPA no minimum stated; *School Psychology PhD (Doctor of Philosophy)*: GRE-V 500, 620, GRE-Q 500, 705, GRE-Analytical 4.5, 5.0, overall undergraduate GPA 3.30, 3.72, last 2 years GPA no minimum stated, psychology GPA no minimum stated, Masters GPA no minimum stated.

Other Criteria: (importance of criteria rated low, medium, or high): GRE scores—medium, research experience—high, work experience—medium, extracurricular activity—medium, clinically related public service—low, GPA—high, letters of recommendation—high, interview—medium, statement of goals and objectives—high, undergraduate major in psychology—medium. For additional information on admission requirements, go to http://www.education.umd.edu/edcp.

Student Characteristics: The following represents characteristics of students in 2009–2010 in all graduate psychology programs in the department: Female—full-time 36, part-time 8; Male—full-time 7, part-time 0; African American/Black—full-time 6, part-time 0; Hispanic/Latino(a)—full-time 2, part-time 1; Asian/Pacific Islander—full-time 10, part-time 1; American Indian/Alaska Native—full-time 0, part-time 0; Caucasian/White—full-time 25, part-time 6; Multi-ethnic—full-time 0, part-time 0; students subject to the Americans With Disabilities Act—full-time 1, part-time 0; Unknown ethnicity—full-time 0, part-time 0; International students who hold an F-1 or J-1 Visa—full-time 0, part-time 0.

Financial Information/Assistance:
   Tuition for Full-Time Study: Doctoral: State residents: per academic year $8,880, $444 per credit hour; Nonstate residents: per academic year $19,160, $958 per credit hour. Tuition is subject to change. Additional fees are assessed to students beyond the costs of tuition for the following: various fees total $1140 per year. See the following Web site for updates and changes in tuition costs: http://www.umd.edu/bursar/Tuitionfees.html.

   Financial Assistance:
   First-Year Students: Teaching assistantships available for first year. Average amount paid per academic year: $14,800. Average number of hours worked per week: 20. Apply by December 15. Research assistantships available for first year. Average amount paid per academic year: $14,800. Average number of hours worked per week: 20. Apply by December 15. Fellowships and scholarships available for first year. Average amount paid per academic year: $16,750. Apply by December 15.

   Advanced Students: Teaching assistantships available for advanced students. Average amount paid per academic year: $15,300. Average number of hours worked per week: 20. Apply by April 15. Research assistantships available for advanced students. Average amount paid per academic year: $15,300. Average number of hours worked per week: 20. Apply by April 15.

   Additional Information: Of all students currently enrolled full time, 90% benefited from one or more of the listed financial assistance programs.

Internships/Practica: Doctoral Degree (PhD Counseling Psychology): For those doctoral students for whom a professional internship was required in this program prior to graduation, (6) students applied for an internship in 2008–2009, with (6) students obtaining an internship. Of those students who obtained an internship, (6) were paid internships. Of those students who obtained an internship, (6) students placed in APA/CPA accredited internships, (0) students placed in internships not APA/CPA accredited, but listed with the Association of Psychology Postdoctoral and Internship Programs (APPIC), (0) students placed in internships conforming to guidelines of the Council of Directors of School Psychology Programs (CDSPP), (0) students placed in internships that were not APA/CPA accredited, APPIC or CDSPP listed. Doctoral Degree (PhD School Psychology): For those doctoral students for whom a professional internship was required in this program prior to graduation, (6) students applied for an internship in 2008–2009, with (6) students obtaining an internship. Of those students who obtained an internship, (6) were paid internships. Of those students who obtained an internship, (0) students placed in APA/CPA accredited internships, (0) students placed in internships not APA/CPA accredited, but listed with the Association of Psychology Postdoctoral and Internship Programs (APPIC), (5) students placed in internships conforming to guidelines of the Council of Directors of School Psychology Programs (CDSPP), (1) students placed in internships that were not APA/CPA accredited, APPIC or CDSPP listed. The Washington DC area offers an abundance of training settings which supplement our on-campus training facilities. A number of practica are offered at the University of Maryland Counseling Center. In addition, other practica and externships are offered at schools, community agencies, hospitals, and other counseling centers. Counseling Psychology students all complete APA-approved internships. In order to maximize school-based training, students in the School Psychology program may complete internships that conform to CDSPP guidelines but that are not APA-approved.

Housing and Day Care: No on-campus housing is available. On-campus day care facilities are available. See the following Web site for more information: http://www.union.umd.edu/GH/family/child_care.html.

Employment of Department Graduates:
   Master's Degree Graduates: Of those who graduated in the academic year 2008–2009, the following categories and numbers represent the postgraduate activities and employment of master's degree graduates: Enrolled in a postdoctoral residency/fellowship (n/a), employed in independent practice (n/a), total from the above (master's) (0).
   Doctoral Degree Graduates: Of those who graduated in the academic year 2008–2009, the following categories and numbers represent the postgraduate activities and employment of doctoral

degree graduates: Enrolled in a psychology doctoral program (n/a), employed in an academic position at a university (1), employed in other positions at a higher education institution (2), employed in a professional position in a school system (4), employed in a community mental health/counseling center (1), total from the above (doctoral) (8).

Additional Information:
Orientation, Objectives, and Emphasis of Department: Both the Counseling Psychology and School Psychology programs espouse the scientist practitioner model of training. These programs enable students to become psychologists who are trained in general psychology, competent in providing effective assessment and intervention from a variety of theoretical perspectives, and in conducting research on a wide range of psychological topics. Note: The Counseling Psychology program is administered collaboratively by the departments of Counseling and Personnel Services and Psychology.

Special Facilities or Resources: Observation/training facilities and access to extensive library facilities both on and off campus (e.g., NIH Library of Medicine, Library of Congress).

Information for Students With Physical Disabilities: See the following Web site for more information: http://www.counseling.umd.edu/DSS/.

Application Information:
Send to Graduate Admissions, College of Education, 1210 Benjamin Building, University of Maryland, College Park, MD 20742. Application available online. URL of online application: http://www.gradschool.umd.edu/gss/admission.htm. Students are admitted in the Fall, application deadline December 15. *Fee:* $60.

Maryland, University of
Department of Psychology
College of Behavioral and Social Sciences
Biology and Psychology Building
College Park, MD 20742-4411
Telephone: (301) 405-5865
Fax: (301) 314-9566
E-mail: cgorham@psyc.umd.edu
Web: http://psychology.umd.edu

Department Information:
1937. Chairperson: Thomas Wallsten. Number of faculty: total—full-time 42; women—full-time 16; total—minority—full-time 2.

Programs and Degrees Offered:
Listed in the following order: Program area, degree type (T if terminal Master's), number awarded 7/08–6/09. Clinical Psychology PhD (Doctor of Philosophy) 8, Developmental Psychology PhD (Doctor of Philosophy) 0, Counseling Psychology PhD (Doctor of Philosophy) 2, Cognitive and Neural Systems PhD (Doctor of Philosophy) 2, Social, Decision, and Organizational Sciences PhD (Doctor of Philosophy) 6.

APA Accreditation: Clinical PhD (Doctor of Philosophy). Counseling PhD (Doctor of Philosophy).

Student Applications/Admissions:
Student Applications
Clinical Psychology PhD (Doctor of Philosophy)—Applications 2009–2010, 288. Total applicants accepted 2009–2010, 13. Number full-time enrolled (new admits only) 2009–2010, 4. Openings 2010–2011, 7. The median number of years required for completion of a degree in 2008–2009 were 6. The number of students enrolled full- and part-time who were dismissed or voluntarily withdrew from this program area in 2008–2009 were 0. Developmental Psychology PhD (Doctor of Philosophy)—Applications 2009–2010, 32. Total applicants accepted 2009–2010, 3. Number full-time enrolled (new admits only) 2009–2010, 0. Openings 2010–2011, 3. The number of students enrolled full- and part-time who were dismissed or voluntarily withdrew from this program area in 2008–2009 were 0. Counseling Psychology PhD (Doctor of Philosophy)—Applications 2009–2010, 109. Total applicants accepted 2009–2010, 1. Number full-time enrolled (new admits only) 2009–2010, 1. Total enrolled 2009–2010 full-time, 15. Openings 2010–2011, 3. The median number of years required for completion of a degree in 2008–2009 were 5. The number of students enrolled full- and part-time who were dismissed or voluntarily withdrew from this program area in 2008–2009 were 0. Cognitive and Neural Systems PhD (Doctor of Philosophy)—Applications 2009–2010, 40. Total applicants accepted 2009–2010, 0. Number full-time enrolled (new admits only) 2009–2010, 0. Total enrolled 2009–2010 full-time, 2. The median number of years required for completion of a degree in 2008–2009 were 6. The number of students enrolled full- and part-time who were dismissed or voluntarily withdrew from this program area in 2008–2009 were 0. Social, Decision, and Organizational Sciences PhD (Doctor of Philosophy)—Applications 2009–2010, 155. Total applicants accepted 2009–2010, 5. Number full-time enrolled (new admits only) 2009–2010, 3. Total enrolled 2009–2010 full-time, 25. Openings 2010–2011, 5. The median number of years required for completion of a degree in 2008–2009 were 6. The number of students enrolled full- and part-time who were dismissed or voluntarily withdrew from this program area in 2008–2009 were 0.

Other Criteria: (importance of criteria rated low, medium, or high): GRE scores—high, research experience—high, work experience—low, extracurricular activity—low, clinically related public service—low, GPA—high, letters of recommendation—high, interview—high, statement of goals and objectives—high, specific undergraduate psychology courses taken—medium, The specific criteria vary across our 5 programs. For additional information on admission requirements, go to http://www.psychology.umd.edu.

Student Characteristics: The following represents characteristics of students in 2009–2010 in all graduate psychology programs in the department: Female—full-time 55, part-time 0; Male—full-time 12, part-time 0; African American/Black—full-time 2, part-time 0; Hispanic/Latino(a)—full-time 4, part-time 0; Asian/Pacific Islander—full-time 4, part-time 0; American Indian/Alaska Native—full-time 0, part-time 0; Caucasian/White—full-time 45, part-time 0; Multi-ethnic—full-time 0, part-time 0; students subject to the Americans With Disabilities Act—full-time 0, part-time 0; Unknown ethnicity—full-time 12, part-time 0; International students who hold an F-1 or J-1 Visa—full-time 0, part-time 0.

GRADUATE STUDY IN PSYCHOLOGY

Financial Information/Assistance:
   Tuition for Full-Time Study: Doctoral: State residents: $471 per credit hour; Nonstate residents: $1,016 per credit hour. Tuition is subject to change. Additional fees are assessed to students beyond the costs of tuition for the following: technology, shuttle bus, athletic, recreation, etc. See the following Web site for updates and changes in tuition costs: http://www.umd.edu/bursar/tuition.fees.html.

Financial Assistance:
   First-Year Students: Teaching assistantships available for first year. Average amount paid per academic year: $16,260. Average number of hours worked per week: 20. Research assistantships available for first year. Average amount paid per academic year: $16,260. Average number of hours worked per week: 20. Fellowships and scholarships available for first year. Average amount paid per academic year: $21,260. Average number of hours worked per week: 20.
   Advanced Students: Teaching assistantships available for advanced students. Average amount paid per academic year: $18,271. Average number of hours worked per week: 20. Research assistantships available for advanced students. Average amount paid per academic year: $18,271. Average number of hours worked per week: 20. Fellowships and scholarships available for advanced students.
   Additional Information: Of all students currently enrolled full time, 100% benefited from one or more of the listed financial assistance programs. Application and information available online at: http://www.gradschool.umd.edu/gss.

Internships/Practica: Doctoral Degree (PhD Clinical Psychology): For those doctoral students for whom a professional internship was required in this program prior to graduation, (4) students applied for an internship in 2008–2009, with (4) students obtaining an internship. Of those students who obtained an internship, (4) were paid internships. Of those students who obtained an internship, (4) students placed in APA/CPA accredited internships, (0) students placed in internships not APA/CPA accredited, but listed with the Association of Psychology Postdoctoral and Internship Programs (APPIC), (0) students placed in internships conforming to guidelines of the Council of Directors of School Psychology Programs (CDSPP), (0) students placed in internships that were not APA/CPA accredited, APPIC or CDSPP listed. Doctoral Degree (PhD Counseling Psychology): For those doctoral students for whom a professional internship was required in this program prior to graduation, (2) students applied for an internship in 2008–2009, with (2) students obtaining an internship. Of those students who obtained an internship, (2) were paid internships. Of those students who obtained an internship, (2) students placed in APA/CPA accredited internships, (0) students placed in internships not APA/CPA accredited, but listed with the Association of Psychology Postdoctoral and Internship Programs (APPIC), (0) students placed in internships conforming to guidelines of the Council of Directors of School Psychology Programs (CDSPP), (0) students placed in internships that were not APA/CPA accredited, APPIC or CDSPP listed. The metropolitan area also has many psychologists who can provide students with excellent opportunities for collaboration and/or consultation. The specialty areas have established collaborative relationships with several federal and community agencies and hospitals as well as with businesses and consulting firms, where it is possible for students to arrange for research, practicum and internship placement. These opportunities are available for Clinical and Counseling students at the National Institutes of Health, Veteran's Administration clinics and hospitals in Washington, DC, Baltimore Perry Point, Coatesville, Martinsburg, Kecoughton, and a number of others within a hundred mile radius of the University. Experiences include a wide range of research activities, as well as psychodiagnostic work, psychotherapy, and work within drug and alcohol abuse clinics. Various other hospitals, clinics and research facilities in the Washington, DC and Baltimore metropolitan area are also available. Industrial/Organizational students also have opportunities for practitioner experiences in organizations such as the U.S. Office of Personnel Management, GEICO, Bell Atlantic, and various consulting firms.

Housing and Day Care: No on-campus housing is available. On-campus day care facilities are available.

Employment of Department Graduates:
   Master's Degree Graduates: Of those who graduated in the academic year 2008–2009, the following categories and numbers represent the postgraduate activities and employment of master's degree graduates: Enrolled in a postdoctoral residency/fellowship (n/a), employed in independent practice (n/a), total from the above (master's) (0).
   Doctoral Degree Graduates: Of those who graduated in the academic year 2008–2009, the following categories and numbers represent the postgraduate activities and employment of doctoral degree graduates: Enrolled in a psychology doctoral program (n/a), enrolled in another graduate/professional program (0), enrolled in a postdoctoral residency/fellowship (6), employed in independent practice (0), employed in an academic position at a university (2), employed in an academic position at a 2-year/4-year college (0), employed in other positions at a higher education institution (2), employed in a professional position in a school system (0), employed in business or industry (4), employed in government agency (3), employed in a community mental health/counseling center (0), employed in a hospital/medical center (0), still seeking employment (0), not seeking employment (1), other employment position (0), do not know (0), total from the above (doctoral) (18).

Additional Information:
   Orientation, Objectives, and Emphasis of Department: The department offers a full-time graduate program with an emphasis on intensive individual training made possible by a 3-to-1 student/faculty ratio. All students are expected to participate in a variety of relevant experiences that, in addition to coursework and research training, can include practicum experiences, field training, and teaching. The department offers a variety of programs described in the admissions brochure as well as other emphases that cut across the various specialties. All programs have a strong research emphasis with programs in clinical, counseling, and industrial advocating the scientist–practitioner model.

   Special Facilities or Resources: The Department of Psychology has all of the advantages of a large state university, and also has advantages offered by the many resources available in the metropolitan Washington-Baltimore area. The University is approximately 15 miles from the center of Washington, DC and is in close proximity to a number of libraries and state and federal agencies. Students are able to benefit from the excellent additional library resources of the community, such as the Library of Congress, National Library of Medicine, and the National Archives (which is located on the UMCP campus). The building in which the Department is housed was designed by the faculty to incorporate research and educational facilities for all specialty areas. The building contains special centers for research, with acoustical centers, observational units, video equipment, computer facilities, surgical facilities, and radio frequency shielding. Departmental laboratories are well equipped for research in animal behavior, audition, biopsychology, cognition, coordinated motor control, counseling, industrial/organizational psychology, learning, lifespan development, psycholinguistics, psychotherapy, social psychology, and vision.

Information for Students With Physical Disabilities: See the following Web site for more information: http://www.counseling.umd.edu/DSS/.

Application Information:
Send to University of Maryland College Park, Enrollment Services Operations, Application for Graduate Admission, Rm 0130 Mitchell Building, College Park, MD 20742. Application available online. URL of online application: http://www.gradschool.umd.edu/gss/admission.htm. Students are admitted in the Fall, application deadline December 1. *Fee:* $60.

Maryland, University of
Institute for Child Study/Department of Human Development
College of Education
3304 Benjamin Building
College Park, MD 20742
Telephone: (301) 405-2827
Fax: (301) 405-2891
E-mail: *mkillen@umd.edu*
Web: *http://www.education.umd.edu/EDHD*

Department Information:
1947. Chairperson: Allan Wigfield. Number of faculty: total—full-time 22; women—full-time 16; total—minority—full-time 4; women minority—full-time 4.

Programs and Degrees Offered:
Listed in the following order: Program area, degree type (T if terminal Master's), number awarded 7/08–6/09. Developmental Science PhD (Doctor of Philosophy) 8, Educational Psychology PhD (Doctor of Philosophy) 5.

Student Applications/Admissions:
Student Applications
Developmental Science PhD (Doctor of Philosophy)—Applications 2009–2010, 40. Total applicants accepted 2009–2010, 11. Number full-time enrolled (new admits only) 2009–2010, 5. Total enrolled 2009–2010 full-time, 32. Openings 2010–2011, 10. The median number of years required for completion of a degree in 2008–2009 were 5. The number of students enrolled full- and part-time who were dismissed or voluntarily withdrew from this program area in 2008–2009 were 1. Educational Psychology PhD (Doctor of Philosophy)—Applications 2009–2010, 30. Total applicants accepted 2009–2010, 10. Number full-time enrolled (new admits only) 2009–2010, 6. Number part-time enrolled (new admits only) 2009–2010, 0. Openings 2010–2011, 10. The median number of years required for completion of a degree in 2008–2009 were 5. The number of students enrolled full- and part-time who were dismissed or voluntarily withdrew from this program area in 2008–2009 were 0.

Scores: Entries appear in this order: required test or GPA, minimum score (if required), median score of students entering in 2009–2010. *Developmental Science PhD (Doctor of Philosophy):* GRE-V no minimum stated, GRE-Q no minimum stated, GRE-Analytical no minimum stated, overall undergraduate GPA 3.0, Masters GPA 3.0; *Educational Psychology PhD (Doctor of Philosophy):* GRE-V no minimum stated, GRE-Q no minimum stated, GRE-Analytical no minimum stated, overall undergraduate GPA 3.0, Masters GPA 3.5.

Other Criteria: (importance of criteria rated low, medium, or high): GRE scores—high, research experience—high, work experience—medium, clinically related public service—medium, GPA—medium, letters of recommendation—high, interview—medium, statement of goals and objectives—high, undergraduate major in psychology—high, specific undergraduate psychology courses taken—medium.

Student Characteristics: The following represents characteristics of students in 2009–2010 in all graduate psychology programs in the department: Female—full-time 53, part-time 17; Male—full-time 5, part-time 10; African American/Black—full-time 6, part-time 2; Hispanic/Latino(a)—full-time 5, part-time 1; Asian/Pacific Islander—full-time 11, part-time 2; American Indian/Alaska Native—full-time 0, part-time 0; Caucasian/White—full-time 36, part-time 22; Multi-ethnic—full-time 0, part-time 0; students subject to the Americans With Disabilities Act—full-time 1, part-time 0; Unknown ethnicity—full-time 0, part-time 0; International students who hold an F-1 or J-1 Visa—full-time 10, part-time 0.

Financial Information/Assistance:
Tuition for Full-Time Study: *Master's:* State residents: $471 per credit hour; Nonstate residents: $1,016 per credit hour. *Doctoral:* State residents: $471 per credit hour; Nonstate residents: $1,016 per credit hour. Tuition is subject to change. Additional fees are assessed to students beyond the costs of tuition for the following: campus activities fees. See the following Web site for updates and changes in tuition costs: http://www.umd.edu/bursar/.

Financial Assistance:
First-Year Students: Research assistantships available for first year. Average amount paid per academic year: $15,000. Average number of hours worked per week: 20. Apply by December 15. Fellowships and scholarships available for first year. Average amount paid per academic year: $15,000. Average number of hours worked per week: 20. Apply by December 15.

Advanced Students: Teaching assistantships available for advanced students. Average amount paid per academic year: $15,000. Average number of hours worked per week: 20. Research assistantships available for advanced students. Average amount paid per academic year: $15,000. Average number of hours worked per week: 20. Traineeships available for advanced students. Average amount paid per academic year: $15,000. Average number of hours worked per week: 20. Fellowships and scholarships available for advanced students. Average amount paid per academic year: $15,000. Average number of hours worked per week: 20.

Additional Information: Of all students currently enrolled full time, 85% benefited from one or more of the listed financial assistance programs. Application and information available online at: http://www.gradschool.umd.edu/gss/.

Housing and Day Care: No on-campus housing is available. On-campus day care facilities are available. See the following Web site for more information: http://www.education.umd.edu/EDHD/CYC/.

Employment of Department Graduates:
Master's Degree Graduates: Of those who graduated in the academic year 2008–2009, the following categories and numbers represent the postgraduate activities and employment of master's degree graduates: Enrolled in a psychology doctoral program (0), enrolled in another graduate/professional program (0), enrolled in a postdoctoral residency/fellowship (n/a), employed in independent practice (n/a), total from the above (master's) (0).
Doctoral Degree Graduates: Of those who graduated in the academic year 2008–2009, the following categories and numbers represent the postgraduate activities and employment of doctoral degree graduates: Enrolled in a psychology doctoral program (n/a), enrolled in a postdoctoral residency/fellowship (3), employed in independent practice (1), employed in an academic position at a university (0), employed in an academic position at a 2-year/4-year college (0), employed in other positions at a higher education institution (1), employed in a professional position in a school system (15), employed in business or industry (0), employed in government agency (0), employed in a community mental health/counseling center (0), employed in a hospital/medical center (2), other employment position (1), do not know (3), total from the above (doctoral) (26).

Additional Information:
Orientation, Objectives, and Emphasis of Department: Human development courses are psychological in nature and are intended to increase the student's understanding of human behavior, including development, learning, and adjustment. Areas of concentration that relate to the institute's goals and interests include, but are not limited to, infancy and early childhood, adolescence, adult development and aging, development over the life span, cultural processes, neuropsychology, cognitive processes, personality, and learning. Information is drawn primarily from the major fields of psychology, sociology, and physiology. The graduate specialization in educational psychology is intended to prepare educational psychologists for service in schools and other community agencies dealing with individuals of all ages, to prepare teachers of human development and educational psychology in higher education, and to prepare research-oriented individuals for service in public (state or federal) or private organizations. A graduate specialization in development science is also available. The research thrust of this specialization is primarily concerned with social aspects of development. The developmental science specialization is designed to prepare researchers and teachers in higher education.

Special Facilities or Resources: Special facilities or resources include extensive research and computer facilities. Videotaping studios and observation rooms are located in the building. The Child Development Assessment Laboratory is associated with the department and is heavily used for neuropsychological assessments on children. Testing and observation rooms are available in the Center for Family Relationships and Culture. In addition, the Center for Young Children, a child care center for preschool children, is under the auspices of the unit and is a resource for students studying and researching this age group.

Application Information:
Send to The University of Maryland, Enrollment Services Operations, 0130 Mitchell Building, College Park, MD 20742. Application available online. URL of online application: http://www.gradschool.umd.edu/gss/admission.html. Students are admitted in the Fall, application deadline March 15; Spring, application deadline October 1. For international students the application deadline for Fall admissions is December 15. For international students the application deadline for Spring admissions is June 1. Deadline for financial aid consideration is December 15 for domestic students for Fall admissions. *Fee:* $60.

Maryland, University of, Baltimore County (2009 data)
Department of Psychology
Arts and Sciences
1000 Hilltop Circle
Baltimore, MD 21250
Telephone: (410) 455-2567
Fax: (410) 455-1055
E-mail: *psycdept@umbc.edu*
Web: *http://www.umbc.edu/psyc/index.html*

Department Information:
1966. Chairperson: Linda Baker, PhD. Number of faculty: total—full-time 28, part-time 11; women—full-time 13, part-time 4; total—minority—full-time 3; women minority—full-time 1; faculty subject to the Americans With Disabilities Act 1.

Programs and Degrees Offered:
Listed in the following order: Program area, degree type (T if terminal Master's), number awarded 7/08–6/09. Applied Behavior Analysis MA/MS (Master of Arts/Science) (T) 6, Applied Developmental PhD (Doctor of Philosophy) 1, Human Services PhD (Doctor of Philosophy) 6.

APA Accreditation: Clinical PhD (Doctor of Philosophy).

Student Applications/Admissions:
Student Applications
Applied Behavior Analysis MA/MS (Master of Arts/Science)—Applications 2009–2010, 68. Total applicants accepted 2009–2010, 19. Number full-time enrolled (new admits only) 2009–2010, 13. Number part-time enrolled (new admits only) 2009–2010, 0. Total enrolled 2009–2010 full-time, 27, part-time, 2. Openings 2010–2011, 12. The median number of years required for completion of a degree in 2008–2009 were 2. *Applied Developmental PhD (Doctor of Philosophy)*—Applications 2009–2010, 18. Total applicants accepted 2009–2010, 7. Number full-time enrolled (new admits only) 2009–2010, 6. Number part-time enrolled (new admits only) 2009–2010, 0. Total enrolled 2009–2010 full-time, 29, part-time, 6. Openings 2010–2011, 10. The median number of years required for completion of a degree in 2008–2009 were 9. The number of students enrolled full- and part-time who were dismissed or

voluntarily withdrew from this program area in 2008–2009 were 1. *Human Services PhD (Doctor of Philosophy)*—Applications 2009–2010, 96. Total applicants accepted 2009–2010, 16. Number full-time enrolled (new admits only) 2009–2010, 13. Number part-time enrolled (new admits only) 2009–2010, 0. Total enrolled 2009–2010 full-time, 61, part-time, 6. Openings 2010–2011, 12. The median number of years required for completion of a degree in 2008–2009 were 7. The number of students enrolled full- and part-time who were dismissed or voluntarily withdrew from this program area in 2008–2009 were 2.

Other Criteria: (importance of criteria rated low, medium, or high): GRE scores—high, research experience—high, work experience—medium, extracurricular activity—medium, clinically related public service—medium, GPA—high, letters of recommendation—high, interview—high, statement of goals and objectives—high. ADP puts less weight (low) on clinical service than does HSP. For additional information on admission requirements, go to http://www.umbc.edu/psyc/grad/.

Student Characteristics: The following represents characteristics of students in 2009–2010 in all graduate psychology programs in the department: Female—full-time 57, part-time 29; Male—full-time 14, part-time 5; African American/Black—full-time 13, part-time 5; Hispanic/Latino(a)—full-time 2, part-time 2; Asian/Pacific Islander—full-time 4, part-time 0; American Indian/Alaska Native—full-time 0, part-time 0; Caucasian/White—full-time 58, part-time 0; Multi-ethnic—full-time 6, part-time 2; students subject to the Americans With Disabilities Act—full-time 0, part-time 0; Unknown ethnicity—full-time 0, part-time 0; International students who hold an F-1 or J-1 Visa—full-time 0, part-time 0.

Financial Information/Assistance:
Tuition for Full-Time Study: *Master's:* State residents: $428 per credit hour; Nonstate residents: $708 per credit hour. *Doctoral:* State residents: $428 per credit hour; Nonstate residents: $708 per credit hour. Tuition is subject to change.

Financial Assistance:
First-Year Students: Teaching assistantships available for first year. Average amount paid per academic year: $14,857. Average number of hours worked per week: 20. Research assistantships available for first year. Average amount paid per academic year: $14,857. Average number of hours worked per week: 20.

Advanced Students: Teaching assistantships available for advanced students. Average number of hours worked per week: 20. Research assistantships available for advanced students. Average number of hours worked per week: 20.

Additional Information: Of all students currently enrolled full time, 83% benefited from one or more of the listed financial assistance programs.

Internships/Practica: Doctoral Degree (PhD Human Services): For those doctoral students for whom a professional internship was required in this program prior to graduation, (11) students applied for an internship in 2008–2009, with (9) students obtaining an internship. Of those students who obtained an internship, (9) were paid internships. Of those students who obtained an internship, (9) students placed in APA/CPA accredited internships, (0) students placed in internships not APA/CPA accredited, but listed with the Association of Psychology Postdoctoral and Internship Programs (APPIC), (0) students placed in internships conforming to guidelines of the Council of Directors of School Psychology Programs (CDSPP), (0) students placed in internships that were not APA/CPA accredited, APPIC or CDSPP listed. Course-linked practica provide students with a focused experience in the application of the skills and knowledge presented in the associated course. The course instructor is responsible for arranging these practica. Beyond the course-linked practica, students in the HSP and ADP programs are required to take a minimum of six additional credits of practicum, usually in their second and third years. These practica, in various clinical, research, and human services settings, are intended to give students a broader and more integrative experience in the application of the skills and knowledge that they have acquired in the various courses they have taken.

Housing and Day Care: On-campus housing is available. On-campus day care facilities are available. Child Care Center: (410) 455-6830.

Employment of Department Graduates:
Master's Degree Graduates: Of those who graduated in the academic year 2008–2009, the following categories and numbers represent the postgraduate activities and employment of master's degree graduates: Enrolled in a postdoctoral residency/fellowship (n/a), employed in independent practice (n/a), total from the above (master's) (0).

Doctoral Degree Graduates: Of those who graduated in the academic year 2008–2009, the following categories and numbers represent the postgraduate activities and employment of doctoral degree graduates: Enrolled in a psychology doctoral program (n/a), enrolled in a postdoctoral residency/fellowship (2), total from the above (doctoral) (2).

Additional Information:
Orientation, Objectives, and Emphasis of Department: UMBC Psychology is committed to a scientist–practitioner model and emphasizes science with an applied psychological research focus. The department uses a biopsychosocial interactive framework as the foundation for exploring various problems and issues in psychology. Two doctoral graduate programs are housed in the department: Applied Developmental Psychology (ADP) and Human Services Psychology (HSP). The ADP program has three concentrations: Early Development/Early Intervention, Socioemotional Development of Children, and Educational Contexts of Development; students can affiliate flexibly with one or more concentrations. The ADP program is accredited by the ASPPB/National Register of Health Service Providers in Psychology. The HSP program consists of three subprograms - community/social, behavioral medicine, and an APA approved clinical subprogram. Many HSP students take cross-area training in clinical/behavioral medicine or clinical/community areas. There is also a Master's program in Applied Behavior Analysis; housed at UMBC and in collaboration with the Kennedy Krieger Institute. Faculty represent a broad range of theoretical perspectives and maintain active research programs. The psychology department has many collaborative relationships for research and clinical and practical training opportunities with institutions in the Baltimore-Washington Corridor.

Special Facilities or Resources: The Psychology Department at UMBC has numerous faculty research laboratories on campus in close proximity to faculty offices. Laboratories include equipment for psychological assessments, videotaping and coding, observation as well as an animal laboratory. The department has access to several large computer laboratories on campus and has a small computer laboratory for graduate students. Through collaborative arrangements with the medical school and other University of Maryland System facilities, and Kennedy Krieger Institute, graduate students have access to different patient populations and opportunities for community based projects.

Application Information:
Send to Dean of Graduate School, 1000 Hilltop Circle, Baltimore, MD 21250. Application available online. URL of online application: http://www.umbc.edu/gradschool/. Students are admitted in the Fall, application deadline December 1. Applied Behavior Analysis Masters program deadline is February 1. Doctoral Program in Applied Developmental Psychology is January 9. *Fee:* $50.

Towson University
Department of Psychology
8000 York Road
Towson, MD 21252
Telephone: (410) 704-3080
Fax: (410) 704-3800
E-mail: *cjohnson@towson.edu*
Web: *http://www.towson.edu/psychology/*

Department Information:
1965. Chairperson: Craig T. Johnson, PhD Number of faculty: total—full-time 37, part-time 39; women—full-time 20, part-time 22; total—minority—full-time 4, part-time 1; women minority—full-time 4.

Programs and Degrees Offered:
Listed in the following order: Program area, degree type (T if terminal Master's), number awarded 7/08–6/09. Counseling Psychology MA/MS (Master of Arts/Science) (T) 15, Experimental Psychology MA/MS (Master of Arts/Science) (T) 10, Clinical Psychology MA/MS (Master of Arts/Science) (T) 14, School Psychology MA/MS (Master of Arts/Science) 14, Human Resource Development MA/MS (Master of Arts/Science) 35.

Student Applications/Admissions:
Student Applications
Counseling Psychology MA/MS (Master of Arts/Science)—Applications 2009–2010, 116. Total applicants accepted 2009–2010, 18. Number full-time enrolled (new admits only) 2009–2010, 14. Number part-time enrolled (new admits only) 2009–2010, 1. Total enrolled 2009–2010 full-time, 27, part-time, 4. Openings 2010–2011, 18. The median number of years required for completion of a degree in 2008–2009 were 2. The number of students enrolled full- and part-time who were dismissed or voluntarily withdrew from this program area in 2008–2009 were 2. Experimental Psychology MA/MS (Master of Arts/Science)—Applications 2009–2010, 35. Total applicants accepted 2009–2010, 20. Number full-time enrolled (new admits only) 2009–2010, 10. Number part-time enrolled (new admits only) 2009–2010, 2. Total enrolled 2009–2010 full-time, 24, part-time, 14. Openings 2010–2011, 15. The median number of years required for completion of a degree in 2008–2009 were 3. The number of students enrolled full- and part-time who were dismissed or voluntarily withdrew from this program area in 2008–2009 were 2. Clinical Psychology MA/MS (Master of Arts/Science)—Applications 2009–2010, 92. Total applicants accepted 2009–2010, 14. Number full-time enrolled (new admits only) 2009–2010, 14. Number part-time enrolled (new admits only) 2009–2010, 0. Total enrolled 2009–2010 full-time, 29, part-time, 3. Openings 2010–2011, 16. The median number of years required for completion of a degree in 2008–2009 were 2. The number of students enrolled full- and part-time who were dismissed or voluntarily withdrew from this program area in 2008–2009 were 0. School Psychology MA/MS (Master of Arts/Science)—Applications 2009–2010, 81. Total applicants accepted 2009–2010, 14. Number full-time enrolled (new admits only) 2009–2010, 13. Number part-time enrolled (new admits only) 2009–2010, 0. Openings 2010–2011, 16. The median number of years required for completion of a degree in 2008–2009 were 3. The number of students enrolled full- and part-time who were dismissed or voluntarily withdrew from this program area in 2008–2009 were 2. Human Resource Development MA/MS (Master of Arts/Science)—Applications 2009–2010, 50. Total applicants accepted 2009–2010, 40. Number full-time enrolled (new admits only) 2009–2010, 0. Number part-time enrolled (new admits only) 2009–2010, 25. Openings 2010–2011, 40. The median number of years required for completion of a degree in 2008–2009 were 2. The number of students enrolled full- and part-time who were dismissed or voluntarily withdrew from this program area in 2008–2009 were 5.

Scores: Entries appear in this order: required test or GPA, minimum score (if required), median score of students entering in 2009–2010. Counseling Psychology MA/MS (Master of Arts/Science): GRE-V 400, 460, GRE-Q 400, 514, GRE-Analytical 4, 4, overall undergraduate GPA 3.0, 3.5, last 2 years GPA 3.0, 3.6; Experimental Psychology MA/MS (Master of Arts/Science): overall undergraduate GPA 2.8, 3.5; Clinical Psychology MA/MS (Master of Arts/Science): GRE-V 450, 500, GRE-Q 450, 580, GRE-Analytical 4.0, 4.5, overall undergraduate GPA 3.0, 3.5, last 2 years GPA 3.0, 3.5; School Psychology MA/MS (Master of Arts/Science): GRE-V 400, 500, GRE-Analytical 4.0, 4.5, overall undergraduate GPA 3.2, 3.53; Human Resource Development MA/MS (Master of Arts/Science): overall undergraduate GPA 2.8, 3.2.

Other Criteria: (importance of criteria rated low, medium, or high): GRE scores—medium, research experience—medium, work experience—medium, clinically related public service—medium, GPA—high, letters of recommendation—high, interview—high, statement of goals and objectives—medium, specific undergraduate psychology courses taken—medium, Clinically related public service, letters of recommendation and interview are all used by the clinical, counseling, and school psychology programs only. Research experience is very important for the experimental program and clinical program. Counseling, clinical, experimental, and school psychology also use a letter of intent and consider it very important. For additional information on admission requirements, go to http://www.towson.edu/psychology.

Student Characteristics: The following represents characteristics of students in 2009–2010 in all graduate psychology programs in the department: Female—full-time 99, part-time 135; Male—full-time 22, part-time 36; African American/Black—full-time 6, part-time 15; Hispanic/Latino(a)—full-time 2, part-time 6; Asian/Pacific Islander—full-time 0, part-time 0; American Indian/Alaska Native—full-time 0, part-time 0; Caucasian/White—full-time 93, part-time 125; Multi-ethnic—full-time 0, part-time 0; students subject to the Americans With Disabilities Act—full-time 0, part-time 0; Unknown ethnicity—full-time 20, part-time 25; International students who hold an F-1 or J-1 Visa—full-time 0, part-time 0.

Financial Information/Assistance:
Tuition for Full-Time Study: *Master's:* State residents: $394 per credit hour; Nonstate residents: $734 per credit hour. Tuition is not available at this time. Tuition is subject to change. Additional fees are assessed to students beyond the costs of tuition for the following: Technology fees: $7 per credit with a $75 cap. See the following Web site for updates and changes in tuition costs: http://www.towson.edu/adminfinance/fiscalplanning/bursar/tuitionandfees/.

Financial Assistance:
First-Year Students: Teaching assistantships available for first year. Average amount paid per academic year: $8,000. Average number of hours worked per week: 20. Apply by February 1. Research assistantships available for first year. Average amount paid per academic year: $5,000. Average number of hours worked per week: 20. Apply by February 1.
Advanced Students: Teaching assistantships available for advanced students. Average amount paid per academic year: $8,000. Average number of hours worked per week: 20. Apply by February 1. Research assistantships available for advanced students. Average amount paid per academic year: $5,000. Average number of hours worked per week: 20. Apply by February 1.
Additional Information: Of all students currently enrolled full time, 25% benefited from one or more of the listed financial assistance programs. Application and information available online at: http://grad.towson.edu/finance/index.asp.

Internships/Practica: Master's Degree (MA/MS Counseling Psychology): An internship experience, such as, a final research project or "capstone" experience is required of graduates. Master's Degree (MA/MS Experimental Psychology): An internship experience, such as a final research project or "capstone" experience is required of graduates. Master's Degree (MA/MS Clinical Psychology): An internship experience, such as a final research project or "capstone" experience is required of graduates. School Psychology students are required to complete two 100-hour practica over two consecutive semesters in a local school system. The program culminates in a 1200-hour internship that is to be completed full-time over one year or part-time over two consecutive years. At least 50% of the 1200 hours must be completed in a public school system; however most students complete all hours in public schools. Students in clinical psychology complete a required 500 hour, nine-month internship. Students may elect to complete a clinical or research internship depending upon their personal and professional goals. Students on clinical internships provide supervised psychological services to clients in an off-campus mental health setting. Students on research internships will assist an experienced scientist in conducting clinical trials research. Counseling students are required to complete a 240-hour practicum and a 300-hour internship over two semesters. Students are placed in community mental health centers, college counseling centers, drug and alcohol rehabilitation agencies, domestic violence centers, and other mental health service agencies. A limited number of graduate assistantships are available for students in the experimental psychology program.

Housing and Day Care: No on-campus housing is available. On-campus day care facilities are available. See the following Web site for more information: http://www.towson.edu/daycare/.

Employment of Department Graduates:
Master's Degree Graduates: Of those who graduated in the academic year 2008–2009, the following categories and numbers represent the postgraduate activities and employment of master's degree graduates: Enrolled in a psychology doctoral program (6), enrolled in a postdoctoral residency/fellowship (n/a), employed in independent practice (n/a), employed in an academic position at a 2-year/4-year college (2), employed in a professional position in a school system (15), employed in business or industry (23), employed in government agency (17), employed in a community mental health/counseling center (17), do not know (8), total from the above (master's) (88).
Doctoral Degree Graduates: Of those who graduated in the academic year 2008–2009, the following categories and numbers represent the postgraduate activities and employment of doctoral degree graduates: Enrolled in a psychology doctoral program (n/a), total from the above (doctoral) (0).

Additional Information:
Orientation, Objectives, and Emphasis of Department: The experimental psychology program is designed to prepare students for subsequent enrollment in PhD programs or for research jobs in industrial, government, private consulting, or hospital settings. Students receive comprehensive instruction in research design, statistical methods (both univariate and multivariate), computer applications (for both data collection and analysis), and take a series of courses in specialized areas of psychology (biological, cognitive, and social psychology). Students collaborate on research with faculty mentors and complete an empirical thesis. The Master of Arts in Clinical Psychology is ideally suited to meet the needs of individuals who want to provide clinical services that are informed by science, want to work as masters-level psychometricians or behavioral specialists, want to work as research or clinical staff on applied research studies, or are considering pursuing doctoral training in clinical psychology. The program curriculum provides comprehensive and hands-on training in personality and intellectual assessment, diagnosis, state-of-the-art and empirically-supported treatment, as well as research methods and statistics. Opportunities are also available for students to work on research projects under the direct supervision of a faculty

member. In addition to completing a research thesis, students may also have the opportunity, depending on the faculty member, to assist in developing research conference presentations and manuscripts for publication. The Counseling Psychology program trains students to facilitate personal, educational, and vocational adjustment across the lifespan. The program offers a practitioner track and a research track from which degree candidates choose. Graduates of the program may go on to meet the requirements of the Licensed Clinical Professional Counselor, pursue doctoral degree, and/or find employment in a wide variety of counseling agencies. The Towson University School Psychology program is fully approved by the National Association of School Psychologists (NASP) and trains graduate students to become school psychologists. The program emphasizes consultation and early intervention. It is unique in its close relationship with its surrounding urban and suburban communities, which welcome Towson's school psychology students in both practicum and internship settings. The program offers a single 63-credit degree: the Master of Arts in Psychology with a concentration in School Psychology and the Certificate of Advanced Study (CAS) in School Psychology. The mission of the Towson University HRD Professional Track MS Graduate Degree program is to equip students with the knowledge, skills and abilities needed to assume and perform successfully professional, managerial and administrative positions in various domains of Human Resources practices through the use of well-organized and implemented classroom-based, online and hybrid instructional events by a highly-qualified faculty for students and employers in the greater Baltimore area. It is a 36-credit hour program, and is ideally suited for people looking to enter the human resources profession, for current practitioners seeking to expand their knowledge and expertise, as well as for mid-career professionals wanting to improve their practice and advancement opportunities. Students can specialize in human resource development, human resource management, or organization development and change concentrations.

Special Facilities or Resources: The Psychology Building houses laboratories for histology and computer analysis as well as specialized space for clinical/counseling training as well as the conduct of research in learning/motivation, physiological, comparative, cognitive, social, developmental, and general experimental psychology. Additionally, because of the popularity of the undergraduate Psychology major, there are many students willing to participate in research studies. In Fall 2009, the department began a move to a new building with expanded facilities for training dyadic interactions as well as enhanced laboratory space for research in social and developmental psychology. That move will be completed in 2011 with the opening of additional research space.

Application Information:
Send to Graduate School, Towson University, Towson, MD 21252. Application available online. URL of online application: https://www.applyweb.com/apply/towson/menu.html. Students are admitted in the Fall, application deadline January 15; Spring, application deadline October 15. Clinical, Counseling, Experimental, and School admit for the Fall with an application deadline of January 15. The Experimental program has a deadline of October 15 for Spring admission. Human Resource Development has rolling admission. *Fee:* $50. Fee is $45 for online applications and $50 for paper applications.

Uniformed Services University of the Health Sciences
Medical and Clinical Psychology
F Edward Hebert School of Medicine
4301 Jones Bridge Road
Bethesda, MD 20814
Telephone: (301) 295-9669
Fax: (301) 295-3034
E-mail: *csimmons@usuhs.mil*
Web: *http://www.usuhs.mil/mps/*

Department Information:
1977. Chairperson: David S. Krantz, PhD Number of faculty: total—full-time 9, part-time 1; women—full-time 3, part-time 1.

Programs and Degrees Offered:
Listed in the following order: Program area, degree type (T if terminal Master's), number awarded 7/08–6/09. Medical Psychology PhD (Doctor of Philosophy) 0, Clinical Psychology PhD (Doctor of Philosophy) 4, Medical Psychology (Clinical Track) PhD (Doctor of Philosophy) 1.

APA Accreditation: Clinical PhD (Doctor of Philosophy).

Student Applications/Admissions:
Student Applications
Medical Psychology PhD (Doctor of Philosophy)—Applications 2009–2010, 9. Total applicants accepted 2009–2010, 1. Number full-time enrolled (new admits only) 2009–2010, 1. Number part-time enrolled (new admits only) 2009–2010, 0. Openings 2010–2011, 3. The median number of years required for completion of a degree in 2008–2009 were 5. The number of students enrolled full- and part-time who were dismissed or voluntarily withdrew from this program area in 2008–2009 were 0. Clinical Psychology PhD (Doctor of Philosophy)—Applications 2009–2010, 28. Total applicants accepted 2009–2010, 4. Number full-time enrolled (new admits only) 2009–2010, 4. Number part-time enrolled (new admits only) 2009–2010, 0. Openings 2010–2011, 7. The median number of years required for completion of a degree in 2008–2009 were 5. The number of students enrolled full- and part-time who were dismissed or voluntarily withdrew from this program area in 2008–2009 were 0. Medical Psychology (Clinical Track) PhD (Doctor of Philosophy)—Applications 2009–2010, 34. Total applicants accepted 2009–2010, 2. Number full-time enrolled (new admits only) 2009–2010, 2. Number part-time enrolled (new admits only) 2009–2010, 0. Openings 2010–2011, 4. The median number of years required for completion of a degree in 2008–2009 were 6. The number of students enrolled full- and part-time who were dismissed or voluntarily withdrew from this program area in 2008–2009 were 0.
Scores: Entries appear in this order: required test or GPA, minimum score (if required), median score of students entering in 2009–2010. *Medical Psychology PhD (Doctor of Philosophy):* GRE-V 550, 600, GRE-Q 550, 600, GRE-Analytical 4.5, 5, overall undergraduate GPA 3.2, 3.5; *Clinical Psychology PhD (Doctor of Philosophy):* GRE-V 550, 600, GRE-Q 550, 600, GRE-Analytical 4.5, 5, overall undergraduate GPA 3.2, 3.5; *Medical Psychology (Clinical Track) PhD (Doctor of Philosophy):* GRE-V 550, 600, GRE-Q 550, 600, GRE-Analytical 4.5, 5,

overall undergraduate GPA 3.2, 3.5, Masters GPA no minimum stated.

Other Criteria: (importance of criteria rated low, medium, or high): GRE scores—high, research experience—high, work experience—low, extracurricular activity—low, clinically related public service—medium, GPA—high, letters of recommendation—high, interview—high, statement of goals and objectives—high, undergraduate major in psychology—medium, specific undergraduate psychology courses taken—medium. For additional information on admission requirements, go to http://www.usuhs.mil/mps/.

Student Characteristics: The following represents characteristics of students in 2009–2010 in all graduate psychology programs in the department: Female—full-time 28, part-time 0; Male—full-time 10, part-time 0; African American/Black—full-time 1, part-time 0; Hispanic/Latino(a)—full-time 1, part-time 0; Asian/Pacific Islander—full-time 2, part-time 0; American Indian/Alaska Native—full-time 0, part-time 0; Caucasian/White—full-time 34, part-time 0; Multi-ethnic—full-time 0, part-time 0; students subject to the Americans With Disabilities Act—full-time 0, part-time 0; Unknown ethnicity—full-time 0, part-time 0; International students who hold an F-1 or J-1 Visa—full-time 1, part-time 0.

Financial Information/Assistance:
Tuition for Full-Time Study: *Master's:* State residents: per academic year $0; Nonstate residents: per academic year $0. *Doctoral:* State residents: per academic year $0; Nonstate residents: per academic year $0.

Financial Assistance:
First-Year Students: Traineeships available for first year. Average amount paid per academic year: $26,000. Average number of hours worked per week: 20. Fellowships and scholarships available for first year. Average amount paid per academic year: $26,000. Average number of hours worked per week: 20.

Advanced Students: Teaching assistantships available for advanced students. Average amount paid per academic year: $26,000. Average number of hours worked per week: 20. Research assistantships available for advanced students. Average amount paid per academic year: $26,000. Average number of hours worked per week: 20. Traineeships available for advanced students. Average amount paid per academic year: $26,000. Average number of hours worked per week: 20. Fellowships and scholarships available for advanced students. Average amount paid per academic year: $26,000. Average number of hours worked per week: 20.

Additional Information: Of all students currently enrolled full time, 90% benefited from one or more of the listed financial assistance programs. Application and information available online at: http://www.usuhs.mil/mps/.

Internships/Practica: Doctoral Degree (PhD Clinical Psychology): For those doctoral students for whom a professional internship was required in this program prior to graduation, (3) students applied for an internship in 2008–2009, with (3) students obtaining an internship. Of those students who obtained an internship, (3) were paid internships. Of those students who obtained an internship, (3) students placed in APA/CPA accredited internships, (0) students placed in internships not APA/CPA accredited, but listed with the Association of Psychology Postdoctoral and Internship Programs (APPIC), (0) students placed in internships conforming to guidelines of the Council of Directors of School Psychology Programs (CDSPP), (0) students placed in internships that were not APA/CPA accredited, APPIC or CDSPP listed. Doctoral Degree (PhD Medical Psychology (Clinical Track)): For those doctoral students for whom a professional internship was required in this program prior to graduation, (1) students applied for an internship in 2008–2009, with (1) students obtaining an internship. Of those students who obtained an internship, (1) were paid internships. Of those students who obtained an internship, (1) students placed in APA/CPA accredited internships, (0) students placed in internships not APA/CPA accredited, but listed with the Association of Psychology Postdoctoral and Internship Programs (APPIC), (0) students placed in internships conforming to guidelines of the Council of Directors of School Psychology Programs (CDSPP), (0) students placed in internships that were not APA/CPA accredited, APPIC or CDSPP listed. Military Clinical Psychology and Clinical/Medical Psychology students complete the 12-month internship during the fifth and final year of the program within an APA-approved military or civilian clinical psychology training program. Practicum training occurs during the Fall, Winter, and Spring quarters of the second, third and fourth years. Students work at practicum sites at local facilities for 6 to 10 hours per week.

Housing and Day Care: No on-campus housing is available. No on-campus day care facilities are available.

Employment of Department Graduates:
Master's Degree Graduates: Of those who graduated in the academic year 2008–2009, the following categories and numbers represent the postgraduate activities and employment of master's degree graduates: Enrolled in a postdoctoral residency/fellowship (n/a), employed in independent practice (n/a), total from the above (master's) (0).

Doctoral Degree Graduates: Of those who graduated in the academic year 2008–2009, the following categories and numbers represent the postgraduate activities and employment of doctoral degree graduates: Enrolled in a psychology doctoral program (n/a), enrolled in a postdoctoral residency/fellowship (1), employed in a hospital/medical center (4), total from the above (doctoral) (5).

Additional Information:
Orientation, Objectives, and Emphasis of Department: The Department's educational programs provide a background in general psychological principles. Two content areas are emphasized: Health Psychology and Clinical Psychology. Educational and research activities focus on the application of principles and methods of scientific psychology relevant to physical and mental health. The Department is set in a School of Medicine and has an interdisciplinary focus. A Clinical Psychology program for uniformed military personnel and a Medical Psychology clinical track for civilians are APA-accredited and follow the scientist'-practitioner model. A research/academic program in Medical Psychology encompasses the fields of Health Psychology and Behavioral Medicine. The Department provides many research opportunities for students in the graduate programs and opportunities for mentorship because of the active and varied research programs conducted by the full-time faculty. Research opportunities available for students all involve the study of behavioral, psychological and biobehavioral factors in physical and mental health. In addition, several faculty in the Department participate

in an NIH-funded predoctoral and postdoctoral training programs in cardiovascular behavioral medicine.

Special Facilities or Resources: The Department has office space, laboratory space for human and animal experimentation, multiple psychophysiology laboratories, and a biochemistry laboratory. There is access to classrooms, conference rooms, an excellent library, a computer center, audiovisual support, teaching hospitals, and a laboratory animal facility that is accredited by the Association for the Assessment and Accreditation of Laboratory Animal Care (AAALAC). The Bethesda campus of the National Institutes of Health, including the National Library of Medicine, is within walking distance from USUHS. The NIH is a resource for lecture series, specialized courses, funding information, and research collaborations. The major military training hospitals also are nearby, as are all the social and cultural offerings of Washington, D.C.

Application Information:
Send to Eleanor Metcalf, PhD Associate Dean for Graduate Education USUHS 4301 Jones Bridge Road Bethesda, MD 20814-4799. Application available online. URL of online application: http://www.usuhs.mil/graded/application.html. Students are admitted in the Fall, application deadline January 15. *Fee:* $0.

Washington College (2009 data)
Department of Psychology
Washington Avenue
Chestertown, MD 21620-1197
Telephone: (410) 778-2800
Fax: (410) 778-7275
E-mail: *llittlefield2@washcoll.edu*
Web: *http://psychology.washcoll.edu*

Department Information:
1953. Chairperson: Lauren M. Littlefield, PhD. Number of faculty: total—full-time 6, part-time 7; women—full-time 2, part-time 2.

Programs and Degrees Offered:
Listed in the following order: Program area, degree type (T if terminal Master's), number awarded 7/08–6/09. General Experimental MA/MS (Master of Arts/Science) (T) 8.

Student Applications/Admissions:
Student Applications
General Experimental MA/MS (Master of Arts/Science)—Applications 2009–2010, 14. Total applicants accepted 2009–2010, 8. Number full-time enrolled (new admits only) 2009–2010, 1. Number part-time enrolled (new admits only) 2009–2010, 7. Total enrolled 2009–2010 full-time, 4, part-time, 13. Openings 2010–2011, 15. The median number of years required for completion of a degree in 2008–2009 were 2. The number of students enrolled full- and part-time who were dismissed or voluntarily withdrew from this program area in 2008–2009 were 0.

Other Criteria: (importance of criteria rated low, medium, or high): GRE scores—medium, research experience—medium, work experience—medium, extracurricular activity—low, clinically related public service—medium, GPA—high, letters of recommendation—high, statement of goals and objectives—medium, undergraduate major in psychology—medium, specific undergraduate psychology courses taken—medium. Applicants who do not have an undergraduate degree in Psychology who earn a score at or above the 50th percentile on the Psychology GRE achievement test are given positive consideration. In unusual circumstances, individuals with degrees in areas other than Psychology may receive provisional admission but need to earn a B or higher score in Statistics before full admission is granted. For additional information on admission requirements, go to http://grad.washcoll.edu/.

Student Characteristics: The following represents characteristics of students in 2009–2010 in all graduate psychology programs in the department: Female—full-time 2, part-time 18; Male—full-time 1, part-time 5; African American/Black—full-time 0, part-time 1; Hispanic/Latino(a)—full-time 0, part-time 0; Asian/Pacific Islander—full-time 0, part-time 0; American Indian/Alaska Native—full-time 0, part-time 0; Caucasian/White—full-time 3, part-time 15; Multi-ethnic—full-time 0, part-time 7; students subject to the Americans With Disabilities Act—full-time 0, part-time 0; Unknown ethnicity—full-time 0, part-time 0; International students who hold an F-1 or J-1 Visa—full-time 0, part-time 0.

Financial Information/Assistance:
Tuition for Full-Time Study: *Master's:* State residents: $292 per credit hour; Nonstate residents: $292 per credit hour. Tuition is subject to change. Additional fees are assessed to students beyond the costs of tuition for the following: $75 registration fee per course.

Financial Assistance:
First-Year Students: No information provided.
Advanced Students: No information provided.
Additional Information: No information provided.

Internships/Practica: The department enjoys excellent ties to local agencies such as the Upper Shore Community Mental Health Center (the regional residential facility located in Chestertown), Upper Shore Aging, both Kent and Queen Anne's counties school systems, residential facilities for developmentally disadvantaged individuals, troubled adolescents, etc. A variety of internships are available through the cooperation of these agencies.

Housing and Day Care: No on-campus housing is available. No on-campus day care facilities are available.

Employment of Department Graduates:
Master's Degree Graduates: Of those who graduated in the academic year 2008–2009, the following categories and numbers represent the postgraduate activities and employment of master's degree graduates: Enrolled in a postdoctoral residency/fellowship (n/a), employed in independent practice (n/a), total from the above (master's) (0).
Doctoral Degree Graduates: Of those who graduated in the academic year 2008–2009, the following categories and numbers represent the postgraduate activities and employment of doctoral degree graduates: Enrolled in a psychology doctoral program (n/a), total from the above (doctoral) (0).

Additional Information:

Orientation, Objectives, and Emphasis of Department: The goal of this program is to prepare graduate students for entry into a doctoral program of their choice and to generate master's level professionals. The emphasis of the curriculum is on psychology as a scientific endeavor and the applications of that scientific discipline to real-world problems.

Special Facilities or Resources: The department has just moved into a newly renovated science center and has more than tripled its available classroom and laboratory space. Newly expanded resources include a computerized learning lab, preclinical behavioral pharmacology laboratory, digital video and audio taping facilities for clinical and social research, a biofeedback-based health psychology laboratory, a 64 channel EEG/ERP and a Transcranial Doppler facility, an eye movement lab, a small mammal surgery suite, and a computerized cognitive laboratory utilizing E-prime.

Application Information:
Send to Director of The Graduate Programs, 300 Washington Avenue, Chestertown, MD 21620-1197. Application available online. URL of online application: http://grad.washcoll.edu/. Students are admitted in the Fall, application deadline August 1; Spring, application deadline December 1; Summer, application deadline April 15. *Fee:* $55.

MASSACHUSETTS

American International College
Department of Graduate Psychology
1000 State Street
Springfield, MA 01109
Telephone: (800) 242-3142
Fax: (413) 737-2803
E-mail: john.defrancesco@aic.edu
Web: http://www.aic.edu/academics/aes/

Department Information:
1979. Chairperson: John J. DeFrancesco, PhD Number of faculty: total—full-time 5, part-time 8; women—full-time 1, part-time 4; faculty subject to the Americans With Disabilities Act 1.

Programs and Degrees Offered:
Listed in the following order: Program area, degree type (T if terminal Master's), number awarded 7/08–6/09. Clinical MA/MS (Master of Arts/Science) (T) 111, Educational MA/MS (Master of Arts/Science) 1, Educational Psychology EdD (Doctor of Education) 9, Forensic Psychology MA/MS (Master of Arts/Science) (T) 20.

Student Applications/Admissions:
Student Applications
Clinical MA/MS (Master of Arts/Science)—Applications 2009–2010, 30. Total applicants accepted 2009–2010, 17. Number full-time enrolled (new admits only) 2009–2010, 10. Number part-time enrolled (new admits only) 2009–2010, 7. Total enrolled 2009–2010 full-time, 27, part-time, 16. Openings 2010–2011, 15. The median number of years required for completion of a degree in 2008–2009 were 3. The number of students enrolled full- and part-time who were dismissed or voluntarily withdrew from this program area in 2008–2009 were 4. Educational MA/MS (Master of Arts/Science)—Applications 2009–2010, 4. Total applicants accepted 2009–2010, 2. Number full-time enrolled (new admits only) 2009–2010, 2. Number part-time enrolled (new admits only) 2009–2010, 0. Openings 2010–2011, 10. The median number of years required for completion of a degree in 2008–2009 were 2. Educational Psychology EdD (Doctor of Education)—Applications 2009–2010, 31. Total applicants accepted 2009–2010, 11. Number full-time enrolled (new admits only) 2009–2010, 8. Number part-time enrolled (new admits only) 2009–2010, 3. Total enrolled 2009–2010 full-time, 26, part-time, 20. Openings 2010–2011, 10. The median number of years required for completion of a degree in 2008–2009 were 5. The number of students enrolled full- and part-time who were dismissed or voluntarily withdrew from this program area in 2008–2009 were 2. Forensic Psychology MA/MS (Master of Arts/Science)—Applications 2009–2010, 35. Total applicants accepted 2009–2010, 15. Number full-time enrolled (new admits only) 2009–2010, 10. Number part-time enrolled (new admits only) 2009–2010, 5. Total enrolled 2009–2010 full-time, 40, part-time, 6. Openings 2010–2011, 15. The median number of years required for completion of a degree in 2008–2009 were 2. The number of students enrolled full- and part-time who were dismissed or voluntarily withdrew from this program area in 2008–2009 were 4.

Scores: Entries appear in this order: required test or GPA, minimum score (if required), median score of students entering in 2009–2010. Clinical MA/MS (Master of Arts/Science): overall undergraduate GPA 2.50, 3.25; Educational MA/MS (Master of Arts/Science): overall undergraduate GPA 2.50, 3.25; Educational Psychology EdD (Doctor of Education): GRE-V no minimum stated, GRE-Q no minimum stated, overall undergraduate GPA 3.00, 3.25, Masters GPA 3.00, 3.25; Forensic Psychology MA/MS (Master of Arts/Science): overall undergraduate GPA 2.50, 3.00.

Other Criteria: (importance of criteria rated low, medium, or high): GRE scores—medium, research experience—high, work experience—high, extracurricular activity—medium, clinically related public service—high, GPA—high, letters of recommendation—high, interview—high, statement of goals and objectives—high, undergraduate major in psychology—medium, specific undergraduate psychology courses taken—medium, GRE only for Doctoral Program.

Student Characteristics: The following represents characteristics of students in 2009–2010 in all graduate psychology programs in the department: Female—full-time 30, part-time 25; Male—full-time 19, part-time 20; African American/Black—full-time 12, part-time 4; Hispanic/Latino(a)—full-time 6, part-time 4; Asian/Pacific Islander—full-time 2, part-time 0; American Indian/Alaska Native—full-time 0, part-time 0; Caucasian/White—full-time 0, part-time 0; Multi-ethnic—full-time 0, part-time 0; students subject to the Americans With Disabilities Act—full-time 0, part-time 0; Unknown ethnicity—full-time 0, part-time 0; International students who hold an F-1 or J-1 Visa—full-time 0, part-time 0.

Financial Information/Assistance:
Tuition for Full-Time Study: *Master's:* State residents: per academic year $15,000, $625 per credit hour; Nonstate residents: per academic year $15,000, $625 per credit hour. *Doctoral:* State residents: per academic year $15,000, $625 per credit hour; Nonstate residents: per academic year $15,000, $625 per credit hour. Tuition is subject to change. See the following Web site for updates and changes in tuition costs: http://www.aic.edu/admissions/graduate/costs.

Financial Assistance:
First-Year Students: Research assistantships available for first year. Average number of hours worked per week: 15. Apply by Apr 15. Fellowships and scholarships available for first year. Average number of hours worked per week: 15. Apply by Apr 15.

Advanced Students: Teaching assistantships available for advanced students. Average number of hours worked per week: 15. Apply by Apr 15. Research assistantships available for advanced students. Average number of hours worked per week: 15. Apply by Apr 15. Fellowships and scholarships available for advanced students. Average number of hours worked per week: 15. Apply by Apr 15.

Additional Information: Of all students currently enrolled full time, 25% benefited from one or more of the listed financial

assistance programs. Application and information available online at: http://www.aic.edu/admissions/graduate/ga.

Internships/Practica: Doctoral Degree (EdD Educational Psychology): For those doctoral students for whom a professional internship was required in this program prior to graduation, (5) students applied for an internship in 2008–2009, with (5) students obtaining an internship. Of those students who obtained an internship, (0) were paid internships. Of those students who obtained an internship, (0) students placed in APA/CPA accredited internships, (1) students placed in internships not APA/CPA accredited, but listed with the Association of Psychology Postdoctoral and Internship Programs (APPIC), (0) students placed in internships conforming to guidelines of the Council of Directors of School Psychology Programs (CDSPP), (4) students placed in internships that were not APA/CPA accredited, APPIC or CDSPP listed. Master's Degree (MA/MS Clinical): An internship experience, such as a final research project or "capstone" experience is required of graduates. Master's Degree (MA/MS Forensic Psychology): An internship experience, such as a final research project or "capstone" experience is required of graduates. Internships and practica are secured at various institutions and facilities throughout the area.

Housing and Day Care: On-campus housing is available. Dean Blaine Stevens, American International College, 1000 State Street, Springfield, MA 01109. No on-campus day care facilities are available.

Employment of Department Graduates:
Master's Degree Graduates: Of those who graduated in the academic year 2008–2009, the following categories and numbers represent the postgraduate activities and employment of master's degree graduates: Enrolled in a postdoctoral residency/fellowship (n/a), employed in independent practice (n/a), total from the above (master's) (0).
Doctoral Degree Graduates: Of those who graduated in the academic year 2008–2009, the following categories and numbers represent the postgraduate activities and employment of doctoral degree graduates: Enrolled in a psychology doctoral program (n/a), total from the above (doctoral) (0).

Additional Information:
Orientation, Objectives, and Emphasis of Department: All graduate programs are based on a balanced scientific/practitioner model that emphasizes the interrelatedness of theory, research, and practice. Our focus is to develop competent, ethical, and self-aware professionals who can function effectively in a diverse, global, and increasingly interdependent world. Graduates of the MA Program in Clinical Psychology are eligible for master's level licensure. Graduates of the Ed.D. Program in Educational Psychology who are interested in seeking certification or licensure will generally meet academic, experiential, and other requirements depending upon the type of certification/license sought, however, each state or jurisdiction may have additional requirements. For specific information, the state or provisional certification/licensing board should be contacted.

Special Facilities or Resources: Curtis Blake Child Development Center.

Application Information:
Send to Graduate Admissions Office. Application available online. URL of online application: http://www.aic.edu/admissions/graduate. Students are admitted in the Fall, application deadline April 1; *Fee:* $50.

Assumption College
Division of Counseling Psychology
500 Salisbury Street
Worcester, MA 01609-1296
Telephone: (508) 767-7390
Fax: (508) 767-7263
E-mail: *doerfler@assumption.edu*
Web: *http://www.assumption.edu/gradce/grad/counspsych/*

Department Information:
1962. Program Director: Leonard A. Doerfler. Number of faculty: total—full-time 4, part-time 7; women—full-time 1, part-time 4; minority—part-time 2; women minority—part-time 2.

Programs and Degrees Offered:
Listed in the following order: Program area, degree type (T if terminal Master's), number awarded 7/08–6/09. Counseling Psychology MA/MS (Master of Arts/Science) (T) 32.

Student Applications/Admissions:
Student Applications
Counseling Psychology MA/MS (Master of Arts/Science)—Applications 2009–2010, 110. Total applicants accepted 2009–2010, 75. Number full-time enrolled (new admits only) 2009–2010, 25. Number part-time enrolled (new admits only) 2009–2010, 25. Total enrolled 2009–2010 full-time, 60, part-time, 49. Openings 2010–2011, 35. The median number of years required for completion of a degree in 2008–2009 were 3. The number of students enrolled full- and part-time who were dismissed or voluntarily withdrew from this program area in 2008–2009 were 5.
Scores: Entries appear in this order: required test or GPA, minimum score (if required), median score of students entering in 2009–2010. Counseling Psychology MA/MS (Master of Arts/Science): overall undergraduate GPA 3.0, 3.4, last 2 years GPA 3.0, 3.4, psychology GPA 3.0, 3.5.
Other Criteria: (importance of criteria rated low, medium, or high): research experience—low, work experience—medium, extracurricular activity—low, clinically related public service—low, GPA—high, letters of recommendation—high, statement of goals and objectives—medium. For additional information on admission requirements, go to http://www.assumption.edu/gradce/grad/counspsych/CP_AdmissionDegreeRequirements.html.

Student Characteristics: The following represents characteristics of students in 2009–2010 in all graduate psychology programs in the department: Female—full-time 45, part-time 45; Male—full-time 10, part-time 10; African American/Black—full-time 0, part-time 2; Hispanic/Latino(a)—full-time 3, part-time 2; Asian/Pacific Islander—full-time 2, part-time 1; American Indian/Alaska Native—full-time 0, part-time 0; Caucasian/White—full-time 50, part-time 50; Multi-ethnic—full-time 0, part-time 0; students subject to the Americans With Disabilities Act—full-time 0, part-time 1; Unknown ethnicity—full-time 0, part-time 0; International students who hold an F-1 or J-1 Visa—full-time 0, part-time 0.

Financial Information/Assistance:
Tuition for Full-Time Study: *Master's:* State residents: $503 per credit hour; Nonstate residents: $503 per credit hour. See the following Web site for updates and changes in tuition costs: http://www1.assumption.edu/gradce/grad/TuitionAid.html.

Financial Assistance:
First-Year Students: Fellowships and scholarships available for first year. Apply by March 1.
Advanced Students: Fellowships and scholarships available for advanced students. Apply by March 1.
Additional Information: Of all students currently enrolled full time, 10% benefited from one or more of the listed financial assistance programs. Application and information available online at: http://www.assumption.edu/gradce/grad/FinancialAidPrograms.html.

Internships/Practica: Practicum and internship placements are available in a wide range of community settings. Students can elect to work in outpatient/community, college counseling centers, substance abuse, inpatient, residential, and correctional settings. Opportunities to work with children, adolescents, adults, and families are available. The department maintains a close working relationship with the University of Massachusetts Medical Center, McLean Hospital/Harvard Medical School, and other mental health training agencies; students attend clinical case conferences, workshops, and lectures at these agencies. Students often receive training in innovative treatment models like home-based, brief problem-focused, or cognitive-behavioral treatments.

Housing and Day Care: On-campus housing is available. See the following Web site for more information: http://www.assumption.edu/living/. No on-campus day care facilities are available.

Employment of Department Graduates:
Master's Degree Graduates: Of those who graduated in the academic year 2008–2009, the following categories and numbers represent the postgraduate activities and employment of master's degree graduates: Enrolled in a psychology doctoral program (2), enrolled in a postdoctoral residency/fellowship (n/a), employed in independent practice (n/a), total from the above (master's) (2).
Doctoral Degree Graduates: Of those who graduated in the academic year 2008–2009, the following categories and numbers represent the postgraduate activities and employment of doctoral degree graduates: Enrolled in a psychology doctoral program (n/a), total from the above (doctoral) (0).

Additional Information:
Orientation, Objectives, and Emphasis of Department: The program is organized to prepare students for entrance into doctoral programs in clinical and counseling psychology and for master's degree entry-level positions in a variety of mental health and related social service settings. Students are given conceptual preparation in a variety of theoretical positions in clinical and counseling psychology. A number of skill courses in counseling, testing, and research are an integral part of the program at both the entry and advanced levels. The goal of the program is to produce master's level psychologists who show conceptual versatility in theory and practice and depth of preparation in one of several special areas of counseling work. The student takes classes in areas such as personality theory, abnormal psychology, child development, counseling, advanced therapeutic procedure, measurement and research. Outside of class the student gains applied experience in clinical practice in the one-semester practicum and two-semester internship.

Special Facilities or Resources: Special facilities on campus include a well-equipped media center and an observation laboratory. Students also have access to in-service training at a local medical school, agencies, and hospitals. The college is located within commuting distance of Boston training facilities. College libraries in Worcester operate on a consortium basis. Programs of study are available on campus in the summer.

Information for Students With Physical Disabilities: See the following Web site for more information: http://www.assumption.edu/ds/default.html.

Application Information:
Send to Dean of Graduate Studies, Graduate Office, Assumption College, 500 Salisbury Street, Worcester, MA 01609-1296. Application available online. URL of online application: http://www.assumption.edu/gradce/grad/Admissions. Programs have rolling admissions. *Fee:* $30. Application fee waived for Assumption College alumni.

Boston College
Department of Counseling, Developmental, and Educational Psychology
309 Campion Hall, School of Education
Chestnut Hill, MA 02467
Telephone: (617) 552-4710
Fax: (617) 552-1981
E-mail: *lykes@bc.edu*
Web: *http://www.bc.edu/schools/lsoe/academics/departments/cdep.html*

Department Information:
1950. Chairperson: M. Brinton Lykes, PhD Number of faculty: total—full-time 18, part-time 2; women—full-time 13, part-time 2; total—minority—full-time 4; women minority—full-time 3.

Programs and Degrees Offered:
Listed in the following order: Program area, degree type (T if terminal Master's), number awarded 7/08–6/09. School Counseling MA/MS (Master of Arts/Science) (T) 16, Counseling Psychology PhD (Doctor of Philosophy) 7, Mental Health Counseling MA/MS (Master of Arts/Science) (T) 49, Developmental and Educational Psychology MA/MS (Master of Arts/Science) (T) 14, Developmental and Educational Psychology PhD (Doctor of Philosophy) 4.

APA Accreditation: Counseling PhD (Doctor of Philosophy). Student Outcome Data Website: http://www.bc.edu/schools/lsoe/academics/graduate/phd/counsel.html.

Student Applications/Admissions:

Student Applications

School Counseling MA/MS (Master of Arts/Science)—Applications 2009–2010, 62. Total applicants accepted 2009–2010, 47. Number full-time enrolled (new admits only) 2009–2010, 18. Number part-time enrolled (new admits only) 2009–2010, 0. Total enrolled 2009–2010 full-time, 39, part-time, 2. Openings 2010–2011, 25. The median number of years required for completion of a degree in 2008–2009 were 2. The number of students enrolled full- and part-time who were dismissed or voluntarily withdrew from this program area in 2008–2009 were 0. *Counseling Psychology PhD (Doctor of Philosophy)*—Applications 2009–2010, 253. Total applicants accepted 2009–2010, 9. Number full-time enrolled (new admits only) 2009–2010, 7. Number part-time enrolled (new admits only) 2009–2010, 0. Openings 2010–2011, 7. The median number of years required for completion of a degree in 2008–2009 were 5. The number of students enrolled full- and part-time who were dismissed or voluntarily withdrew from this program area in 2008–2009 were 0. *Mental Health Counseling MA/MS (Master of Arts/Science)*—Applications 2009–2010, 251. Total applicants accepted 2009–2010, 214. Number full-time enrolled (new admits only) 2009–2010, 61. Number part-time enrolled (new admits only) 2009–2010, 1. Total enrolled 2009–2010 full-time, 123, part-time, 3. Openings 2010–2011, 65. The median number of years required for completion of a degree in 2008–2009 were 2. The number of students enrolled full- and part-time who were dismissed or voluntarily withdrew from this program area in 2008–2009 were 0. *Developmental and Educational Psychology MA/MS (Master of Arts/Science)*—Applications 2009–2010, 85. Total applicants accepted 2009–2010, 59. Number full-time enrolled (new admits only) 2009–2010, 16. Number part-time enrolled (new admits only) 2009–2010, 4. Total enrolled 2009–2010 full-time, 30, part-time, 8. Openings 2010–2011, 25. The median number of years required for completion of a degree in 2008–2009 were 2. The number of students enrolled full- and part-time who were dismissed or voluntarily withdrew from this program area in 2008–2009 were 0. *Developmental and Educational Psychology PhD (Doctor of Philosophy)*—Applications 2009–2010, 46. Total applicants accepted 2009–2010, 5. Number full-time enrolled (new admits only) 2009–2010, 4. Number part-time enrolled (new admits only) 2009–2010, 0. Openings 2010–2011, 5. The median number of years required for completion of a degree in 2008–2009 were 5. The number of students enrolled full- and part-time who were dismissed or voluntarily withdrew from this program area in 2008–2009 were 0.

Other Criteria: (importance of criteria rated low, medium, or high): GRE scores—medium, research experience—high, work experience—medium, extracurricular activity—low, clinically related public service—high, GPA—high, letters of recommendation—high, interview—high, statement of goals and objectives—high, social justice commitment—high. For developmental programs, clinically related public service is low. For counsleing programs, social justice commitment is high.

Student Characteristics: The following represents characteristics of students in 2009–2010 in all graduate psychology programs in the department: Female—full-time 192, part-time 12; Male—full-time 47, part-time 2; African American/Black—full-time 13, part-time 1; Hispanic/Latino(a)—full-time 13, part-time 0; Asian/Pacific Islander—full-time 16, part-time 0; American Indian/Alaska Native—full-time 1, part-time 0; Caucasian/White—full-time 147, part-time 11; Multi-ethnic—full-time 3, part-time 0; students subject to the Americans With Disabilities Act—full-time 0, part-time 0; Unknown ethnicity—full-time 14, part-time 0; International students who hold an F-1 or J-1 Visa—full-time 0, part-time 0.

Financial Information/Assistance:

Tuition for Full-Time Study: *Master's:* State residents: $1,020 per credit hour; Nonstate residents: $1,020 per credit hour. *Doctoral:* State residents: $1,020 per credit hour; Nonstate residents: $1,020 per credit hour. Tuition is subject to change.

Financial Assistance:

First-Year Students: Research assistantships available for first year. Average amount paid per academic year: $17,000. Average number of hours worked per week: 20.

Advanced Students: Teaching assistantships available for advanced students. Average amount paid per academic year: $17,000. Average number of hours worked per week: 20. Research assistantships available for advanced students. Average amount paid per academic year: $17,000. Average number of hours worked per week: 20.

Additional Information: Of all students currently enrolled full time, 50% benefited from one or more of the listed financial assistance programs. Application and information available online at: http://www.bc.edu/schools/lsoe/gradadmission/funding.html.

Internships/Practica: Doctoral Degree (PhD Counseling Psychology): For those doctoral students for whom a professional internship was required in this program prior to graduation, (6) students applied for an internship in 2008–2009, with (5) students obtaining an internship. Of those students who obtained an internship, (5) were paid internships. Of those students who obtained an internship, (5) students placed in APA/CPA accredited internships, (0) students placed in internships not APA/CPA accredited, but listed with the Association of Psychology Postdoctoral and Internship Programs (APPIC), (0) students placed in internships conforming to guidelines of the Council of Directors of School Psychology Programs (CDSPP), (0) students placed in internships that were not APA/CPA accredited, APPIC or CDSPP listed. Doctoral students in Counseling Psychology complete an Advanced Practicum in community mental health agencies, schools, clinics, hospitals, and college counseling centers. They also complete a one year predoctoral internship. Master's students in mental health and school counseling work with the Masters Program Coordinator to identify internships that meet requirements for mental health licensure or school counselor certification. Masters and Doctoral students in the Applied Developmental and Educational Psychology program can complete a non-required internship.

Housing and Day Care: On-campus housing is available. See the following Web site for more information: http://www.bc.edu/offices/reslife/. On-campus day care facilities are available. See the following Web site for more information: http://www.bc.edu/offices/hr/resources/docs/ccquickreference.html.

Employment of Department Graduates:

Master's Degree Graduates: Of those who graduated in the academic year 2008–2009, the following categories and numbers

represent the postgraduate activities and employment of master's degree graduates: Enrolled in a postdoctoral residency/fellowship (n/a), employed in independent practice (n/a), total from the above (master's) (0).

Doctoral Degree Graduates: Of those who graduated in the academic year 2008–2009, the following categories and numbers represent the postgraduate activities and employment of doctoral degree graduates: Enrolled in a psychology doctoral program (n/a), enrolled in a postdoctoral residency/fellowship (1), employed in independent practice (1), employed in a professional position in a school system (1), employed in government agency (1), employed in a community mental health/counseling center (1), do not know (3), total from the above (doctoral) (8).

Additional Information:
Orientation, Objectives, and Emphasis of Department: The Programs in Counseling, Developmental and Educational Psychology emphasize a foundation in developmental theory, research skills, and a commitment to preparing professionals to work in public practice, public service, academic or research institutions. The counseling psychology doctoral program espouses a scientist–practitioner model and provides broad-based training with special attention to group and individual counseling processes, theory and skill in research and assessment, and understanding individual development within a social context. Master's counseling students specialize in mental health counseling or school counseling. The program in Applied Developmental and Educational Psychology focuses on application and draws on psychology, educational and community programs, and engages public policies to enhance the development of individuals and their key institutional contexts- schools, families, and work settings- across the life span. Faculty research interests include psychotherapy, process and outcome, career and moral development, individual differences in cognitive and affective development including developmental disabilities, influence of gender role strain on the well-being of men, Asian-American and Latino mental health, racial identity, marital and community violence, marital satisfaction, and prevention and intervention for promoting positive development among youth.

Special Facilities or Resources: Boston College offers ample student access to computing facilities (Alpha mainframe, Macintosh and PCs) at no charge to students. The Educational Resource Center houses current psychological assessment kits and computerized instructional software. The Thomas P. O'Neill Library is fully automated with all major computerized databases. Through the consortium, students may cross-register in courses in other greater Boston universities (Boston University, Brandeis, and Tufts). The career center provides comprehensive resources and information regarding career planning and placement. The Institute for the Study and Promotion of Race and Culture (ISPRC), under the direction of Dr. Janet E. Helms, promotes the assets and address of the societal conflicts associated with race or culture in theory, and research, mental health practice, education, business, and society at large. The Center for Human Rights and International Justice at Boston College addresses the increasingly interdisciplinary needs of human rights work. Through multidisciplinary training programs, applied research, and the interaction of scholars with practitioners, the Center aims to nurture a new generation of scholars and practitioners in the United States and abroad who draw upon the strengths of many disciplines, and the wisdom of rigorous ethical training in the attainment of human rights and international justice.

Application Information:
Send to Boston College LSOE Data Processing Center P.O. Box 226 Randolph, MA 02368-9998. Application available online. URL of online application: http://www.bc.edu/schools/lsoe/gradadmission. Students are admitted in the Fall, application deadline December 1; Summer, application deadline June 15. Counseling MA programs January 1; Counseling PhD December 1. Developmental PhD January 1. Developmental MA June 15 and January 1. *Fee:* $60.

Boston College
Department of Psychology
College of Arts and Sciences
140 Commonwealth Avenue, McGuinn 300
Chestnut Hill, MA 02467
Telephone: (617) 552-4100
Fax: (617) 552-0523
E-mail: *psychoffice@bc.edu*
Web: *http://www.bc.edu/schools/cas/psych/*

Department Information:
1950. Chairperson: Ellen Winner. Number of faculty: total—full-time 20, part-time 6; women—full-time 10, part-time 5; total—minority—full-time 2; women minority—full-time 1.

Programs and Degrees Offered:
Listed in the following order: Program area, degree type (T if terminal Master's), number awarded 7/08–6/09. Cognitive & Cognitive Neuroscience PhD (Doctor of Philosophy) 2, Social-Personality Psychology PhD (Doctor of Philosophy), Developmental Psychology PhD (Doctor of Philosophy) 1, Behavioral Neuroscience PhD (Doctor of Philosophy), Quantitative Psychology PhD (Doctor of Philosophy).

Student Applications/Admissions:
Student Applications
Cognitive & Cognitive Neuroscience PhD (Doctor of Philosophy)—Applications 2009–2010, 79. Total applicants accepted 2009–2010, 2. Number full-time enrolled (new admits only) 2009–2010, 0. Total enrolled 2009–2010 full-time, 6. The median number of years required for completion of a degree in 2008–2009 were 5. *Social-Personality Psychology PhD (Doctor of Philosophy)*—Applications 2009–2010, 80. Total applicants accepted 2009–2010, 0. Number full-time enrolled (new admits only) 2009–2010, 4. Total enrolled 2009–2010 full-time, 6. *Developmental Psychology PhD (Doctor of Philosophy)*—Applications 2009–2010, 62. Total applicants accepted 2009–2010, 3. Total enrolled 2009–2010 full-time, 7. The median number of years required for completion of a degree in 2008–2009 were 5. *Behavioral Neuroscience PhD (Doctor of Philosophy)*—Applications 2009–2010, 20. Total applicants accepted 2009–2010, 3. Total enrolled 2009–2010 full-time, 3. *Quantitative Psychology PhD (Doctor of Philosophy)*—Applications 2009–2010, 5. Total applicants accepted 2009–2010, 0.

Scores: Entries appear in this order: required test or GPA, minimum score (if required), median score of students entering in 2009–2010. *Behavioral Neuroscience PhD (Doctor of Philosophy):* GRE-V no minimum stated, GRE-Q no minimum stated.
Other Criteria: (importance of criteria rated low, medium, or high): GRE scores—high, research experience—high, work experience—low, extracurricular activity—low, clinically related public service—low, GPA—high, letters of recommendation—high, interview—high, statement of goals and objectives—high. For additional information on admission requirements, go to http://www.bc.edu/schools/cas/psych/graduate.html.

Student Characteristics: The following represents characteristics of students in 2009–2010 in all graduate psychology programs in the department: Female—full-time 17, part-time 0; Male—full-time 4, part-time 0; African American/Black—full-time 0, part-time 0; Hispanic/Latino(a)—full-time 0, part-time 0; Asian/Pacific Islander—full-time 1, part-time 0; American Indian/Alaska Native—full-time 0, part-time 0; Caucasian/White—full-time 19, part-time 0; Multi-ethnic—full-time 0, part-time 0; students subject to the Americans With Disabilities Act—full-time 0, part-time 0; Unknown ethnicity—full-time 1, part-time 0; International students who hold an F-1 or J-1 Visa—full-time 2, part-time 0.

Financial Information/Assistance:
Tuition for Full-Time Study: *Doctoral:* State residents: $1,206 per credit hour; Nonstate residents: $1,206 per credit hour. Tuition is subject to change. See the following Web site for updates and changes in tuition costs: http://www.bc.edu/schools/gsas/admissions/faq.html.

Financial Assistance:
First-Year Students: Teaching assistantships available for first year. Average amount paid per academic year: $19,500. Average number of hours worked per week: 20. Apply by January 2. Fellowships and scholarships available for first year.
Advanced Students: Teaching assistantships available for advanced students. Average amount paid per academic year: $19,500. Average number of hours worked per week: 20. Apply by January 2. Fellowships and scholarships available for advanced students.
Additional Information: Of all students currently enrolled full time, 100% benefited from one or more of the listed financial assistance programs. Application and information available online at: http://www.bc.edu/schools/gsas/admissions/financial-aid.html.

Housing and Day Care: No on-campus housing is available. On-campus day care facilities are available. Contact the Children's Center at (617) 552-3089.

Employment of Department Graduates:
Master's Degree Graduates: Of those who graduated in the academic year 2008–2009, the following categories and numbers represent the postgraduate activities and employment of master's degree graduates: Enrolled in a postdoctoral residency/fellowship (n/a), employed in independent practice (n/a), total from the above (master's) (0).

Doctoral Degree Graduates: Of those who graduated in the academic year 2008–2009, the following categories and numbers represent the postgraduate activities and employment of doctoral degree graduates: Enrolled in a psychology doctoral program (n/a), total from the above (doctoral) (0).

Additional Information:
Orientation, Objectives, and Emphasis of Department: We emphasize rigorous research and a close working relationship between student and professor.

Special Facilities or Resources: Individual faculty maintain separate research laboratories. There is a shared psychophysiology lab. An animal lab facility contains two components: an animal facility and research laboratory space. The animal facility includes small animal housing and behavioral testing rooms, a surgery suite, and special procedure rooms equipped with hoods. The animal research space includes a (1) microscopy suite, (2) dark room, (3) data analysis room, (4) 3 research labs/wet labs equipped with hoods, sinks, and workspace.

Information for Students With Physical Disabilities: See the following Web site for more information: http://www.bc.edu/disability.

Application Information:
Send to Boston College, Graduate School of Arts and Sciences 140 Commonwealth Avenue McGuinn 221 Chestnut Hill, MA 02467. Application available online. URL of online application: http://www.bc.edu/schools/gsas/admissions/applynow.html. Students are admitted in the Fall, application deadline January 2nd. *Fee:* $70.

Boston University
Department of Psychology
64 Cummington Street
Boston, MA 02215
Telephone: (617) 353-2580
Fax: (617) 353-6933
E-mail: *mlyons@bu.edu*
Web: *http://www.bu.edu/psych*

Department Information:
1935. Chairperson: Michael Lyons. Number of faculty: total—full-time 28, part-time 2; women—full-time 15, part-time 1; minority—part-time 1.

Programs and Degrees Offered:
Listed in the following order: Program area, degree type (T if terminal Master's), number awarded 7/08–6/09. Clinical Psychology PhD (Doctor of Philosophy) 7, General Psychology MA/MS (Master of Arts/Science) (T) 31, Developmental Science PhD (Doctor of Philosophy) 2, Brain, Behavior, and Cognition PhD (Doctor of Philosophy) 3.

APA Accreditation: Clinical PhD (Doctor of Philosophy).

Student Applications/Admissions:
Student Applications
Clinical Psychology PhD (Doctor of Philosophy)—Applications 2009–2010, 614. Total applicants accepted 2009–2010, 14.

Number full-time enrolled (new admits only) 2009–2010, 8. Number part-time enrolled (new admits only) 2009–2010, 0. Total enrolled 2009–2010 full-time, 58, part-time, 4. Openings 2010–2011, 10. The median number of years required for completion of a degree in 2008–2009 were 6. The number of students enrolled full- and part-time who were dismissed or voluntarily withdrew from this program area in 2008–2009 were 0. *General Psychology MA/MS (Master of Arts/Science)*—Applications 2009–2010, 212. Total applicants accepted 2009–2010, 147. Number full-time enrolled (new admits only) 2009–2010, 38. Number part-time enrolled (new admits only) 2009–2010, 3. Total enrolled 2009–2010 full-time, 46, part-time, 6. Openings 2010–2011, 40. The median number of years required for completion of a degree in 2008–2009 was 1. The number of students enrolled full- and part-time who were dismissed or voluntarily withdrew from this program area in 2008–2009 were 1. *Developmental Science PhD (Doctor of Philosophy)*—Applications 2009–2010, 31. Total applicants accepted 2009–2010, 7. Number full-time enrolled (new admits only) 2009–2010, 5. Number part-time enrolled (new admits only) 2009–2010, 0. Total enrolled 2009–2010 full-time, 13, part-time, 1. Openings 2010–2011, 4. The median number of years required for completion of a degree in 2008–2009 were 5. The number of students enrolled full- and part-time who were dismissed or voluntarily withdrew from this program area in 2008–2009 were 1. *Brain, Behavior, and Cognition PhD (Doctor of Philosophy)*—Applications 2009–2010, 72. Total applicants accepted 2009–2010, 4. Number full-time enrolled (new admits only) 2009–2010, 3. Number part-time enrolled (new admits only) 2009–2010, 0. Openings 2010–2011, 4. The median number of years required for completion of a degree in 2008–2009 were 5. The number of students enrolled full- and part-time who were dismissed or voluntarily withdrew from this program area in 2008–2009 were 0.

Scores: Entries appear in this order: required test or GPA, minimum score (if required), median score of students entering in 2009–2010. *Clinical Psychology PhD (Doctor of Philosophy)*: GRE-V no minimum stated, GRE-Q no minimum stated, GRE-Analytical no minimum stated, overall undergraduate GPA no minimum stated, last 2 years GPA no minimum stated, psychology GPA no minimum stated, Masters GPA no minimum stated; *General Psychology MA/MS (Master of Arts/Science)*: GRE-V no minimum stated, GRE-Q no minimum stated, GRE-Analytical no minimum stated, overall undergraduate GPA no minimum stated, last 2 years GPA no minimum stated, psychology GPA no minimum stated; *Developmental Science PhD (Doctor of Philosophy)*: GRE-V no minimum stated, GRE-Q no minimum stated, GRE-Analytical no minimum stated, overall undergraduate GPA no minimum stated, last 2 years GPA no minimum stated, psychology GPA no minimum stated, Masters GPA no minimum stated; *Brain, Behavior, and Cognition PhD (Doctor of Philosophy)*: GRE-V no minimum stated, GRE-Q no minimum stated, GRE-Analytical no minimum stated, overall undergraduate GPA no minimum stated, last 2 years GPA no minimum stated, psychology GPA no minimum stated, Masters GPA no minimum stated.

Other Criteria: (importance of criteria rated low, medium, or high): GRE scores—high, research experience—high, work experience—low, extracurricular activity—low, clinically related public service—high, GPA—high, letters of recommendation—high, interview—high, statement of goals and objectives—high. For additional information on admission requirements, go to http://www.bu.edu/psych.

Student Characteristics: The following represents characteristics of students in 2009–2010 in all graduate psychology programs in the department: Female—full-time 103, part-time 9; Male—full-time 26, part-time 2; African American/Black—full-time 6, part-time 1; Hispanic/Latino(a)—full-time 4, part-time 0; Asian/Pacific Islander—full-time 15, part-time 0; American Indian/Alaska Native—full-time 1, part-time 0; Caucasian/White—full-time 78, part-time 5; Multi-ethnic—full-time 0, part-time 0; students subject to the Americans With Disabilities Act—full-time 0, part-time 0; Unknown ethnicity—full-time 25, part-time 5; International students who hold an F-1 or J-1 Visa—full-time 22, part-time 1.

Financial Information/Assistance:
Tuition for Full-Time Study: *Master's:* State residents: per academic year $38,280, $1,184 per credit hour; Nonstate residents: per academic year $38,280, $1,184 per credit hour. *Doctoral:* State residents: per academic year $38,280, $1,184 per credit hour; Nonstate residents: per academic year $38,280, $1,184 per credit hour.

Financial Assistance:
First-Year Students: Teaching assistantships available for first year. Average amount paid per academic year: $18,400. Average number of hours worked per week: 20. Research assistantships available for first year. Average amount paid per academic year: $27,600. Average number of hours worked per week: 20. Fellowships and scholarships available for first year. Average amount paid per academic year: $18,400. Average number of hours worked per week: 0.

Advanced Students: Teaching assistantships available for advanced students. Average amount paid per academic year: $18,400. Average number of hours worked per week: 20. Research assistantships available for advanced students. Average amount paid per academic year: $27,600. Average number of hours worked per week: 20. Traineeships available for advanced students. Average amount paid per academic year: $18,400. Average number of hours worked per week: 20.

Additional Information: Of all students currently enrolled full time, 81% benefited from one or more of the listed financial assistance programs. Application and information available online at: www.bu.edu/cas/admissions/graduate/aid.

Internships/Practica: Doctoral Degree (PhD Clinical Psychology): For those doctoral students for whom a professional internship was required in this program prior to graduation, (10) students applied for an internship in 2008–2009, with (9) students obtaining an internship. Of those students who obtained an internship, (9) were paid internships. Of those students who obtained an internship, (9) students placed in APA/CPA accredited internships, (0) students placed in internships not APA/CPA accredited, but listed with the Association of Psychology Postdoctoral and Internship Programs (APPIC), (0) students placed in internships conforming to guidelines of the Council of Directors of School Psychology Programs (CDSPP), (0) students placed in internships that were not APA/CPA accredited, APPIC or

CDSPP listed. Students in the clinical doctoral program are involved in internships and practica as part of their degree requirements.

Housing and Day Care: No on-campus housing is available. No on-campus day care facilities are available.

Employment of Department Graduates:
Master's Degree Graduates: Of those who graduated in the academic year 2008–2009, the following categories and numbers represent the postgraduate activities and employment of master's degree graduates: Enrolled in a postdoctoral residency/fellowship (n/a), employed in independent practice (n/a), total from the above (master's) (0).
Doctoral Degree Graduates: Of those who graduated in the academic year 2008–2009, the following categories and numbers represent the postgraduate activities and employment of doctoral degree graduates: Enrolled in a psychology doctoral program (n/a), total from the above (doctoral) (0).

Additional Information:
Orientation, Objectives, and Emphasis of Department: The department offers specialized training leading to the PhD degree in three areas of concentration: clinical; brain, behavior, and cognition; and development science. The PhD degree in psychology is awarded to students of scholarly competence as reflected by course achievement and by performance on written and oral examinations and of research competence as reflected by student's skillful application and communication of knowledge in the area of specialization. Breadth is encouraged within psychology and in related social, behavioral, and biological sciences, but it is also expected that the student will engage in intensive and penetrating study of a specialized area of the field.

Special Facilities or Resources: Laboratories for research pursuits in animal behavior, behavior disorders, child development, cognition, neurophysiology, molecular biology and psychopharmacology add to the department's facilities. The Center for Anxiety and Related Disorders (CARD), a nationally recognized clinical research and treatment center, is a recent addition to the department and allows students to engage in a variety of ongoing research projects and receive training in focused clinical interventions. In addition, the Boston area is fortunate to have a number of nationally known hospitals, counseling centers, and community mental health centers directly affiliated with our clinical program where students have opportunities to gain experience in a variety of clinical settings with different client populations. The New England Regional Primate Center, which is supported by the National Institutes of Health, is also available to Boston University faculty and students.

Application Information:
Application available online. URL of online application: http://www.bu.edu/cas/admissions. Students are admitted in the Fall, application deadline December 1. *The deadline for applications to the Clinical PhD program, the Brain, Behavior & Cognition PhD Program and the Development Science PhD Program is December 1. The application deadline for the MA-only program is May 15. Applications will be reviewed beginning March 1.

Boston University
Divison of Graduate Medical Sciences, Program in Mental Health Counseling and Behavioral Medicine
School of Medicine
715 Albany Street, Robinson Building, Suite B-2903
Boston, MA 02118
Telephone: (617) 414-2320
Fax: (617) 414-2323
E-mail: *nicey@bu.edu*
Web: *http://www.bumc.bu.edu/mhbm*

Department Information:
2001. Chairperson: Stephen Brady, PhD. Number of faculty: total—full-time 5, part-time 3; women—full-time 4, part-time 2.

Programs and Degrees Offered:
Listed in the following order: Program area, degree type (T if terminal Master's), number awarded 7/08–6/09. Mental Health Counseling and Behavioral Medicine MA/MS (Master of Arts/Science) (T) 19.

Student Applications/Admissions:
Student Applications
Mental Health Counseling and Behavioral Medicine MA/MS (Master of Arts/Science)—Applications 2009–2010, 68. Total applicants accepted 2009–2010, 38. Number full-time enrolled (new admits only) 2009–2010, 31. Number part-time enrolled (new admits only) 2009–2010, 2. Total enrolled 2009–2010 full-time, 41, part-time, 2. Openings 2010–2011, 30. The median number of years required for completion of a degree in 2008–2009 were 2. The number of students enrolled full- and part-time who were dismissed or voluntarily withdrew from this program area in 2008–2009 were 1.
Other Criteria: (importance of criteria rated low, medium, or high): GRE scores—medium, research experience—medium, work experience—medium, extracurricular activity—medium, clinically related public service—medium, GPA—medium, letters of recommendation—high, interview—high, statement of goals and objectives—high. For additional information on admission requirements, go to http://www.bumc.bu.edu/mhbm/program.

Student Characteristics: The following represents characteristics of students in 2009–2010 in all graduate psychology programs in the department: Female—full-time 0, part-time 0; Male—full-time 0, part-time 0; African American/Black—full-time 0, part-time 0; Hispanic/Latino(a)—full-time 0, part-time 0; Asian/Pacific Islander—full-time 0, part-time 0; American Indian/Alaska Native—full-time 0, part-time 0; Caucasian/White—full-time 0, part-time 0; Multi-ethnic—full-time 0, part-time 0; students subject to the Americans With Disabilities Act—full-time 0, part-time 0; Unknown ethnicity—full-time 0, part-time 0; International students who hold an F-1 or J-1 Visa—full-time 0, part-time 0.

Financial Information/Assistance:
Tuition for Full-Time Study: *Master's:* State residents: per academic year $39,314, $1,228 per credit hour; Nonstate residents: per academic year $39,314, $1,228 per credit hour.

Financial Assistance:
  First-Year Students: No information provided.
  Advanced Students: No information provided.
  Additional Information: No information provided.

Internships/Practica: Completion of the Masters in Mental Health Counseling and Behavioral Medicine program prepares students for independent licensure as a Mental Health Counselor (LMHC). Our students are primarily trained to conduct clinical practice with urban multicultural underserved populations. Our clinical training program includes curricula in mental health, behavioral medicine, and neuroscience offered in an urban hospital and medical school environment. The coursework is intended to prepare students to provide clinical services to a range of individuals in diversified settings. More specifically, students are trained to perform brief forms of assessment and psychotherapeutic interventions in medical and behavioral health care settings. We offer clinical training opportunities in diverse settings such as psychiatric emergency department services, child, adolescent, and adult outpatient psychiatric clinics, medical and psychiatric inpatient services, adolescent substance abuse treatment centers, college counseling centers, and community mental health clinics. Our practicum program is a 16 hour a week commitment over the course of one semester and our internship training is a 24 hour a week commitment over the course of an academic year. At the completion of the Program students will have accumulated approximately 1,000 hours of clinical training.

Housing and Day Care: On-campus housing is available. No on-campus day care facilities are available.

Employment of Department Graduates:
  Master's Degree Graduates: Of those who graduated in the academic year 2008–2009, the following categories and numbers represent the postgraduate activities and employment of master's degree graduates: Enrolled in a psychology doctoral program (5), enrolled in another graduate/professional program (2), enrolled in a postdoctoral residency/fellowship (n/a), employed in independent practice (n/a), employed in a professional position in a school system (3), employed in government agency (4), employed in a community mental health/counseling center (4), employed in a hospital/medical center (1), other employment position (1), do not know (3), total from the above (master's) (23).
  Doctoral Degree Graduates: Of those who graduated in the academic year 2008–2009, the following categories and numbers represent the postgraduate activities and employment of doctoral degree graduates: Enrolled in a psychology doctoral program (n/a), total from the above (doctoral) (0).

Additional Information:
  Orientation, Objectives, and Emphasis of Department: The Mental Health Counseling and Behavioral Medicine Program is the first of its kind in the United States, as it is located within a School of Medicine. Our program curriculum blends scholarship, practical experience and an appreciation of the scientific bases of assessment and treatments for behavioral and neurological disorders. Our objective is to provide Master's level counselors with a strong foundation in psychopathology and psychotherapeutic intervention, as well as a background in behavioral medicine and neuroscience. Our primary focus is the development of professional counselors with the skills to develop as scholars, teachers, researchers and clinicians. Our program fills a major gap in the delivery of mental health services in health care settings and to patients with healthcare concerns. Students have a unique opportunity to work with outstanding mentors in psychology, psychiatry, neuroscience and medicine. Graduates of the program assume positions in a variety of settings, including community mental health centers, college/university settings, clinical research settings, and government facilities. Approximately one-half of our students pursue doctoral level training either immediately upon graduation or soon thereafter.

Special Facilities or Resources: Because the program is housed within the Boston University School of Medicine and is part of Boston University, our students and faculty have access to a wide variety of academic and medical resources. Although not a required part of students' experiences in the program, many of our students collaborate in clinical research activities, which are always a part of our campus. Books, journals, and access to computerized literature searches currently are available in the Alumni Medical Library at BUSM. This full service medical library contains most relevant publications for students in a mental health related program. On the Charles River Campus, the Charles Mugar Library is available for any students who wish further supplementary readings in the behavioral and social sciences. As a member of the Boston Library Consortium, Boston University students have access to additional library collections through inter-library loans. Overall, the library resources available to these students are excellent and do not require additional acquisitions. The current Mental Health Counseling and Behavioral Medicine program occupies a newly renovated space with approximately 1,200 square feet for its administrative and core faculty office space.

Application Information:
Application available online. URL of online application: http://www.bumc.bu.edu/mhbm. Students are admitted in the Fall. Programs have rolling admissions. *Fee:* $50. All online applications are $60.

Brandeis University (2009 data)
Department of Psychology
415 South Street, Mail Stop 62
Waltham, MA 02454-9110
Telephone: (781) 736-3300
Fax: (781) 736-3291
E-mail: *gnat@brandeis.edu*
Web: *http://www.brandeis.edu/departments/psych*

Department Information:
  1948. Chairperson: Malcolm W. Watson, PhD. Number of faculty: total—full-time 17, part-time 3; women—full-time 4, part-time 1.

Programs and Degrees Offered:
  Listed in the following order: Program area, degree type (T if terminal Master's), number awarded 7/08–6/09. Cognitive Neuroscience PhD (Doctor of Philosophy) 0, General Psychology MA/MS (Master of Arts/Science) (T) 5, Social/ Developmental PhD (Doctor of Philosophy) 3, Brain, Body, Behavior PhD (Doctor of Philosophy) 0.

Student Applications/Admissions:
Student Applications
Cognitive Neuroscience PhD (Doctor of Philosophy)—Applications 2009–2010, 15. Total applicants accepted 2009–2010, 3. Number full-time enrolled (new admits only) 2009–2010, 1. Number part-time enrolled (new admits only) 2009–2010, 0. Openings 2010–2011, 2. The number of students enrolled full- and part-time who were dismissed or voluntarily withdrew from this program area in 2008–2009 were 0. *General Psychology MA/MS (Master of Arts/Science)*—Applications 2009–2010, 43. Total applicants accepted 2009–2010, 10. Number full-time enrolled (new admits only) 2009–2010, 5. Number part-time enrolled (new admits only) 2009–2010, 1. Total enrolled 2009–2010 full-time, 7, part-time, 2. Openings 2010–2011, 10. The median number of years required for completion of a degree in 2008–2009 was 1. The number of students enrolled full- and part-time who were dismissed or voluntarily withdrew from this program area in 2008–2009 were 0. *Social/Developmental PhD (Doctor of Philosophy)*—Applications 2009–2010, 49. Total applicants accepted 2009–2010, 7. Number full-time enrolled (new admits only) 2009–2010, 4. Number part-time enrolled (new admits only) 2009–2010, 0. Openings 2010–2011, 3. The median number of years required for completion of a degree in 2008–2009 were 6. The number of students enrolled full- and part-time who were dismissed or voluntarily withdrew from this program area in 2008–2009 were 0. *Brain, Body, Behavior PhD (Doctor of Philosophy)*—Applications 2009–2010, 0. Total applicants accepted 2009–2010, 0. Number full-time enrolled (new admits only) 2009–2010, 0. Number part-time enrolled (new admits only) 2009–2010, 0. Openings 2010–2011, 2. The number of students enrolled full- and part-time who were dismissed or voluntarily withdrew from this program area in 2008–2009 were 0.
Other Criteria: (importance of criteria rated low, medium, or high): GRE scores—high, research experience—high, work experience—medium, extracurricular activity—low, clinically related public service—low, GPA—high, letters of recommendation—high, interview—high, statement of goals and objectives—high.

Student Characteristics: The following represents characteristics of students in 2009–2010 in all graduate psychology programs in the department: Female—full-time 22, part-time 1; Male—full-time 4, part-time 0; African American/Black—full-time 0, part-time 0; Hispanic/Latino(a)—full-time 2, part-time 0; Asian/Pacific Islander—full-time 7, part-time 0; American Indian/Alaska Native—full-time 0, part-time 0; Caucasian/White—full-time 16, part-time 1; Multi-ethnic—full-time 0, part-time 0; students subject to the Americans With Disabilities Act—full-time 0, part-time 1; Unknown ethnicity—full-time 0, part-time 0; International students who hold an F-1 or J-1 Visa—full-time 0, part-time 0.

Financial Information/Assistance:
Tuition for Full-Time Study: *Master's:* State residents: per academic year $37,566; Nonstate residents: per academic year $37,566. *Doctoral:* State residents: per academic year $37,566; Nonstate residents: per academic year $37,566. Additional fees are assessed to students beyond the costs of tuition for the following: health insurance. See the following Web site for updates and changes in tuition costs: http://www.brandeis.edu/gsas/.

Financial Assistance:
First-Year Students: Fellowships and scholarships available for first year. Average amount paid per academic year: $20,000. Apply by January 15.

Advanced Students: Teaching assistantships available for advanced students. Fellowships and scholarships available for advanced students. Average amount paid per academic year: $18,500.

Additional Information: Of all students currently enrolled full time, 80% benefited from one or more of the listed financial assistance programs. Application and information available online at: http://www.brandeis.edu/gsas/prospectives/financial-assistance.html; http://www.brandeis.edu/gsas/financing.

Internships/Practica: Master's Degree (MA/MS General Psychology): An internship experience, such as a final research project or "capstone" experience is required of graduates.

Housing and Day Care: No on-campus housing is available. On-campus day care facilities are available. See the following Web site for more information: http://www.brandeis.edu/lemberg/.

Employment of Department Graduates:
Master's Degree Graduates: Of those who graduated in the academic year 2008–2009, the following categories and numbers represent the postgraduate activities and employment of master's degree graduates: Enrolled in a psychology doctoral program (0), enrolled in another graduate/professional program (0), enrolled in a postdoctoral residency/fellowship (n/a), employed in independent practice (n/a), employed in an academic position at a university (0), employed in an academic position at a 2-year/4-year college (0), employed in other positions at a higher education institution (0), employed in a professional position in a school system (1), employed in business or industry (0), employed in government agency (0), employed in a community mental health/counseling center (0), employed in a hospital/medical center (1), still seeking employment (0), other employment position (1), do not know (2), total from the above (master's) (5).
Doctoral Degree Graduates: Of those who graduated in the academic year 2008–2009, the following categories and numbers represent the postgraduate activities and employment of doctoral degree graduates: Enrolled in a psychology doctoral program (n/a), enrolled in another graduate/professional program (0), enrolled in a postdoctoral residency/fellowship (1), employed in independent practice (0), employed in an academic position at a university (1), employed in an academic position at a 2-year/4-year college (0), employed in other positions at a higher education institution (0), employed in a professional position in a school system (0), employed in business or industry (0), employed in government agency (0), employed in a community mental health/counseling center (0), employed in a hospital/medical center (0), still seeking employment (0), other employment position (0), do not know (1), total from the above (doctoral) (3).

Additional Information:
Orientation, Objectives, and Emphasis of Department: The goal of the PhD program is to develop excellent researchers and teachers who will become leaders in psychological science. From the start of graduate study, research activity is emphasized. The program helps students develop an area of research specialization, and gives them opportunities to work in one of two general areas: social/developmental psychology or cognitive neuroscience. In

both areas, dissertation supervisors are leaders in the following areas: motor control, visual perception, taste physiology and psychophysics, memory, learning, aggression, emotion, personality and cognition in adulthood and old age, social relations and health, stereotypes, and nonverbal communication.

Special Facilities or Resources: Laboratories in the Psychology Department are well-equipped for research on memory, speech recognition, psycholinguistics, visual psychophysics, visual perception, motor control, and spatial orientation, including a NASA-sponsored laboratory for research on human spatial orientation in unusual gravitational environments. Social and developmental psychology laboratories include one-way observation rooms, videorecording and eye-tracking apparatus. There are also opportunities for social neuroscience research through a collaborative grant with the MGH-NMR center. Child development research is facilitated by cooperative relations with the Lemberg Children's Center on the Brandeis campus; applied social research is facilitated by cooperative relations with the Brandeis University Florence Heller Graduate School for Advanced Studies in Social Welfare and the Graduate School of International Economics and Finance. Research on cognitive aging is supported by a training grant from the National Institute on Aging. A special feature of the aging program is an interest in the interaction of cognitive, social and personality factors in healthy aging. The psychology department also participates in an interdisciplinary neuroscience program at the Volen National Center for Complex Systems located on the Brandeis campus.

Information for Students With Physical Disabilities: See the following Web site for more information: http://www.brandeis.edu/as/dis/disabilities.html.

Application Information:
Send to Graduate School of Arts & Sciences, Brandeis University, 415 South Street, MS-031, Waltham, MA 02454-9110. Application available online. URL of online application: http://www.brandeis.edu/gsas/apply/index.html. Students are admitted in the Fall, application deadline January 15. PhD Fall Deadline is January 15. MA applications are accepted on a continuous basis with rolling admission. Review of applications will begin January 15 and continue until the incoming class is filled. *Fee:* $55.

Clark University (2009 data)
Frances L. Hiatt School of Psychology
950 Main Street
Worcester, MA 01610
Telephone: (508) 793-7274
Fax: (508) 793-7265
E-mail: *wgrolnick@clarku.edu*
Web: *http://www.clarku.edu/departments/psychology/*

Department Information:
1889. Chairperson: Wendy Grolnick, PhD. Number of faculty: total—full-time 17, part-time 4; women—full-time 10, part-time 1; total—minority—full-time 3, part-time 1; women minority—full-time 1.

Programs and Degrees Offered:
Listed in the following order: Program area, degree type (T if terminal Master's), number awarded 7/08–6/09. Clinical PhD (Doctor of Philosophy) 3, Developmental PhD (Doctor of Philosophy) 2, Social PhD (Doctor of Philosophy) 1.

APA Accreditation: Clinical PhD (Doctor of Philosophy).

Student Applications/Admissions:
Student Applications
Clinical PhD (Doctor of Philosophy)—Applications 2009–2010, 115. Total applicants accepted 2009–2010, 13. Number full-time enrolled (new admits only) 2009–2010, 5. Total enrolled 2009–2010 full-time, 30. Openings 2010–2011, 4. The median number of years required for completion of a degree in 2008–2009 were 7. The number of students enrolled full- and part-time who were dismissed or voluntarily withdrew from this program area in 2008–2009 were 0. *Developmental PhD (Doctor of Philosophy)*—Applications 2009–2010, 13. Total applicants accepted 2009–2010, 6. Number full-time enrolled (new admits only) 2009–2010, 4. Total enrolled 2009–2010 full-time, 14. Openings 2010–2011, 2. The median number of years required for completion of a degree in 2008–2009 were 6. The number of students enrolled full- and part-time who were dismissed or voluntarily withdrew from this program area in 2008–2009 were 0. *Social PhD (Doctor of Philosophy)*—Applications 2009–2010, 29. Total applicants accepted 2009–2010, 3. Number full-time enrolled (new admits only) 2009–2010, 2. Total enrolled 2009–2010 full-time, 9. Openings 2010–2011, 2. The median number of years required for completion of a degree in 2008–2009 were 4. The number of students enrolled full- and part-time who were dismissed or voluntarily withdrew from this program area in 2008–2009 were 0.
Other Criteria: (importance of criteria rated low, medium, or high): GRE scores—medium, research experience—high, work experience—medium, extracurricular activity—medium, clinically related public service—medium, GPA—high, letters of recommendation—high, interview—medium, statement of goals and objectives—high, specific undergraduate psychology courses taken—medium. Interview by phone or in person is required for prospective clinical students.

Student Characteristics: The following represents characteristics of students in 2009–2010 in all graduate psychology programs in the department: Female—full-time 52, part-time 0; Male—full-time 9, part-time 0; African American/Black—full-time 0, part-time 0; Hispanic/Latino(a)—full-time 5, part-time 0; Asian/Pacific Islander—full-time 5, part-time 0; American Indian/Alaska Native—full-time 0, part-time 0; Caucasian/White—full-time 50, part-time 0; Multi-ethnic—full-time 1, part-time 0; students subject to the Americans With Disabilities Act—full-time 0, part-time 0; Unknown ethnicity—full-time 0, part-time 0; International students who hold an F-1 or J-1 Visa—full-time 0, part-time 0.

Financial Information/Assistance:
Tuition for Full-Time Study: *Doctoral:* State residents: per academic year $34,900; Nonstate residents: per academic year $34,900. Tuition is subject to change.

Financial Assistance:

First-Year Students: Teaching assistantships available for first year. Average amount paid per academic year: $16,700. Average number of hours worked per week: 17. Research assistantships available for first year. Average amount paid per academic year: $16,700. Average number of hours worked per week: 17.

Advanced Students: Teaching assistantships available for advanced students. Average amount paid per academic year: $16,700. Average number of hours worked per week: 17. Research assistantships available for advanced students. Average amount paid per academic year: $16,700. Average number of hours worked per week: 17.

Additional Information: Of all students currently enrolled full time, 100% benefited from one or more of the listed financial assistance programs.

Internships/Practica: Doctoral Degree (PhD Clinical): For those doctoral students for whom a professional internship was required in this program prior to graduation, (4) students applied for an internship in 2008–2009, with (4) students obtaining an internship. Of those students who obtained an internship, (4) were paid internships. Of those students who obtained an internship, (4) students placed in APA/CPA accredited internships, (0) students placed in internships not APA/CPA accredited, but listed with the Association of Psychology Postdoctoral and Internship Programs (APPIC), (0) students placed in internships conforming to guidelines of the Council of Directors of School Psychology Programs (CDSPP), (0) students placed in internships that were not APA/CPA accredited, APPIC or CDSPP listed. Doctoral students in clinical psychology enroll in a supervised practicum each year. These practica involve college students, children, couples and families. In the 3rd year, practicum sites are individually arranged to provide experience in the student's special area of interest. These sites have included state mental institutions, VA neuropsychological units, residential child treatment facilities, etc. Doctoral clinical students also take one full-time year of internship training in APA accredited agencies around the country.

Housing and Day Care: On-campus housing is available. See the following Web site for more information: http://www.clarku.edu/offices/housing/index.cfm. No on-campus day care facilities are available.

Employment of Department Graduates:

Master's Degree Graduates: Of those who graduated in the academic year 2008–2009, the following categories and numbers represent the postgraduate activities and employment of master's degree graduates: Enrolled in a postdoctoral residency/fellowship (n/a), employed in independent practice (n/a), total from the above (master's) (0).

Doctoral Degree Graduates: Of those who graduated in the academic year 2008–2009, the following categories and numbers represent the postgraduate activities and employment of doctoral degree graduates: Enrolled in a psychology doctoral program (n/a), enrolled in a postdoctoral residency/fellowship (2), employed in an academic position at a university (2), employed in a hospital/medical center (1), do not know (1), total from the above (doctoral) (6).

Additional Information:

Orientation, Objectives, and Emphasis of Department: The Department's philosophy affirms the unity of psychology as a subject matter and discourages rigid distinctions among kinds of psychologists and kinds of department programs. Nonetheless, the Department provides in-depth training in the student's area of specialization with a primary concern for theory development, conceptual analysis and empirical investigation. A diversity of theoretical viewpoints is represented, including various developmental viewpoints. Students become acquainted with a variety of methods of investigation, not only with traditional experimental and naturalistic methods, but also with phenomenological, structural, hermeneutic, and other qualitative methodologies. Each student's program is individualized to some degree, and education takes place through small seminars, one-to-one research and practicum training, individualized papers, and MA thesis and PhD dissertation work. Research and other scholarly work are strongly encouraged throughout the graduate experience.

Special Facilities or Resources: The Psychology Department possesses ample space, two entire floors and substantial parts of two others, most of it recently renovated, for offices, classes, laboratories, and clinical training. These include a child study area, facilities for studying family interactions, a human physiology laboratory, a personality-social research area, and dyadic and group clinical training facilities, all with one-way vision and recording facilities. Additional opportunities for research exist in connection with the University of Massachusetts Medical School, the Worcester Foundation for Experimental Biology, schools, and other community settings. Clinical practicum settings include various area agencies.

Application Information:
Send to Graduate Admissions, Frances L. Hiatt School of Psychology, Clark University, 950 Main Street, Worcester, MA 01610. Application available online. URL of online application: http://www.clarku.edu/departments/psychology/grad/app.cfm. Students are admitted in the Fall, application deadline December 28. *Fee:* $50. Fees waived in cases of financial need.

Harvard University
Department of Psychology
33 Kirkland Street
Cambridge, MA 02138
Telephone: (617) 495-3800
E-mail: cir@wjh.harvard.edu
Web: http://wjh.harvard.edu/psych/grad_main.html

Department Information:
1936. Chairperson: Susan Carey. Number of faculty: total—full-time 24, part-time 6; women—full-time 9, part-time 3; total—minority—full-time 4; women minority—full-time 1.

Programs and Degrees Offered:
Listed in the following order: Program area, degree type (T if terminal Master's), number awarded 7/08–6/09. Developmental Psychology PhD (Doctor of Philosophy) 5, Organizational Behavior PhD (Doctor of Philosophy) 1, Social Psychology PhD (Doctor of Philosophy) 1, Clinical Psychology PhD (Doctor of Philosophy) 0, Cognition, Brain, and Behavior PhD (Doctor of Philosophy) 4, Common Curriculum PhD (Doctor of Philosophy) 0.

APA Accreditation: Clinical PhD (Doctor of Philosophy).

GRADUATE STUDY IN PSYCHOLOGY

Student Applications/Admissions:
Student Applications
Developmental Psychology PhD (Doctor of Philosophy)—Applications 2009–2010, 0. Total applicants accepted 2009–2010, 0. Number full-time enrolled (new admits only) 2009–2010, 0. Number part-time enrolled (new admits only) 2009–2010, 0. The median number of years required for completion of a degree in 2008–2009 were 5. The number of students enrolled full- and part-time who were dismissed or voluntarily withdrew from this program area in 2008–2009 were 0. *Organizational Behavior PhD (Doctor of Philosophy)*—Number full-time enrolled (new admits only) 2009–2010, 0. Openings 2010–2011, 2. The median number of years required for completion of a degree in 2008–2009 were 5. The number of students enrolled full- and part-time who were dismissed or voluntarily withdrew from this program area in 2008–2009 were 0. *Social Psychology PhD (Doctor of Philosophy)*—Applications 2009–2010, 0. Total applicants accepted 2009–2010, 0. Number full-time enrolled (new admits only) 2009–2010, 0. Number part-time enrolled (new admits only) 2009–2010, 0. The median number of years required for completion of a degree in 2008–2009 were 6. The number of students enrolled full- and part-time who were dismissed or voluntarily withdrew from this program area in 2008–2009 were 0. *Clinical Psychology PhD (Doctor of Philosophy)*—Applications 2009–2010, 178. Total applicants accepted 2009–2010, 4. Number full-time enrolled (new admits only) 2009–2010, 4. Number part-time enrolled (new admits only) 2009–2010, 0. Openings 2010–2011, 5. The number of students enrolled full- and part-time who were dismissed or voluntarily withdrew from this program area in 2008–2009 were 0. *Cognition, Brain, and Behavior PhD (Doctor of Philosophy)*—Total applicants accepted 2009–2010, 0. Number full-time enrolled (new admits only) 2009–2010, 0. Number part-time enrolled (new admits only) 2009–2010, 0. The median number of years required for completion of a degree in 2008–2009 were 4. The number of students enrolled full- and part-time who were dismissed or voluntarily withdrew from this program area in 2008–2009 were 0. *Common Curriculum PhD (Doctor of Philosophy)*—Applications 2009–2010, 333. Total applicants accepted 2009–2010, 15. Number full-time enrolled (new admits only) 2009–2010, 12. Total enrolled 2009–2010 full-time, 24. Openings 2010–2011, 9. The number of students enrolled full- and part-time who were dismissed or voluntarily withdrew from this program area in 2008–2009 were 0.
Other Criteria: (importance of criteria rated low, medium, or high): GRE scores—high, research experience—high, work experience—high, extracurricular activity—low, clinically related public service—medium, GPA—high, letters of recommendation—high, interview—high, statement of goals and objectives—high, undergraduate major in psychology—medium, specific undergraduate psychology courses taken—medium.

Student Characteristics: The following represents characteristics of students in 2009–2010 in all graduate psychology programs in the department: Female—full-time 45, part-time 0; Male—full-time 38, part-time 0; African American/Black—part-time 0; Hispanic/Latino(a)—part-time 0; Asian/Pacific Islander—full-time 14, part-time 0; American Indian/Alaska Native—part-time 0; Caucasian/White—full-time 69, part-time 0; Multi-ethnic—full-time 0, part-time 0; students subject to the Americans With Disabilities Act—full-time 1, part-time 0; Unknown ethnicity—full-time 0, part-time 0; International students who hold an F-1 or J-1 Visa—full-time 13, part-time 0.

Financial Information/Assistance:
Tuition for Full-Time Study: *Doctoral:* State residents: per academic year $37,830; Nonstate residents: per academic year $37,830. Tuition is subject to change. See the following Web site for updates and changes in tuition costs: http://www.gsas.harvard.edu/prospective_students/financial_aid.php. Higher tuition cost for this program: Tuition is highest in first two years.

Financial Assistance:
First-Year Students: Research assistantships available for first year. Fellowships and scholarships available for first year. Apply by December 15.
Advanced Students: Teaching assistantships available for advanced students. Average amount paid per academic year: $23,000. Average number of hours worked per week: 20. Apply by May 1. Research assistantships available for advanced students. Average amount paid per academic year: $23,000. Average number of hours worked per week: 20. Fellowships and scholarships available for advanced students.
Additional Information: Of all students currently enrolled full time, 95% benefited from one or more of the listed financial assistance programs. Application and information available online at: http://www.gsas.harvard.edu/prospective_students/financial_aid.php.

Internships/Practica: Doctoral Degree (PhD Clinical Psychology): For those doctoral students for whom a professional internship was required in this program prior to graduation, (3) students applied for an internship in 2008–2009, with (3) students obtaining an internship. Of those students who obtained an internship, (3) were paid internships. Of those students who obtained an internship, (3) students placed in APA/CPA accredited internships, (0) students placed in internships not APA/CPA accredited, but listed with the Association of Psychology Postdoctoral and Internship Programs (APPIC), (0) students placed in internships conforming to guidelines of the Council of Directors of School Psychology Programs (CDSPP), (0) students placed in internships that were not APA/CPA accredited, APPIC or CDSPP listed. Students in the clinical program will have predoctoral practicum placements in a local Harvard-affiliated hospital. Students are required to have defended their thesis prospectus, and are strongly encouraged to collect most of the data prior to departing for internship, but the thesis project need not be completed before beginning the internship. Clinical internship applicants use the APPIC system.

Housing and Day Care: On-campus housing is available. See the following Web site for more information: http://www.gsas.harvard.edu/current_students/housing.php. On-campus day care facilities are available. See the following Web site for more information: http://www.childcare.harvard.edu/.

Employment of Department Graduates:
Master's Degree Graduates: Of those who graduated in the academic year 2008–2009, the following categories and numbers represent the postgraduate activities and employment of master's

degree graduates: Enrolled in a postdoctoral residency/fellowship (n/a), employed in independent practice (n/a), total from the above (master's) (0).

Doctoral Degree Graduates: Of those who graduated in the academic year 2008–2009, the following categories and numbers represent the postgraduate activities and employment of doctoral degree graduates: Enrolled in a psychology doctoral program (n/a), enrolled in another graduate/professional program (0), enrolled in a postdoctoral residency/fellowship (9), employed in an academic position at a university (1), employed in business or industry (1), employed in a hospital/medical center (1), do not know (1), total from the above (doctoral) (13).

Additional Information:
Orientation, Objectives, and Emphasis of Department: The psychology department offers PhDs in psychology and social psychology. In conjunction with the Harvard Business School, there is also a PhD program in organizational behavior. The psychology department is divided into two main curricula: an APA-accredited clinical science program, and a common curriculum covering all other areas. The aim of the program is to train students for careers in psychological research and teaching. These careers are mainly in academia. The emphasis of the program is heavily on research training; in addition to a small number of required courses, students do a first-year research project, a second-year research project, and the doctoral dissertation. Students take a major examination or intense seminar(s) in their major specialty fields. Since most students prepare for academic careers, there is ample opportunity to serve as teaching fellows.

Special Facilities or Resources: The department is well equipped with facilities for conducting research. Faculty are the recipients of many grants in various areas of psychology, and graduate students play an essential role in the conduct of most of this research. William James Hall houses a well-staffed computer lab to serve faculty and students. The building also houses a psychology research library. Students are given offices, the use of laboratory space, and a sum of money for research support. The department encourages interdisciplinary study, and students have the benefit of taking courses and working with the faculty at other Harvard graduate schools (Education, Medical School, Public Health, etc.), and at MIT. The Cambridge and Boston areas are well endowed with research facilities and hospitals that offer resources, such as MRI equipment, to students.

Information for Students With Physical Disabilities: See the following Web site for more information: http://www.fas.harvard.edu/~aeo/.

Application Information:
Send to Harvard University, Office of Admissions, The Graduate School of Arts and Sciences, P.O. Box 9129, Cambridge, MA 02238-9129. Application available online. URL of online application: http://apply.embark.com/grad/harvard/gsas/. Students are admitted in the Fall, application deadline December 15. *Fee:* $105. Requests for waivers should be submitted in writing to the Graduate School of Arts and Sciences Admissions Office.

Massachusetts School of Professional Psychology
Professional School
221 Rivermoor Street
Boston, MA 02132
Telephone: (617) 327-6777
Fax: (617) 327-4447
E-mail: *katie_ohare@mspp.edu*
Web: *http://www.mspp.edu*

Department Information:
1974. President: Nicholas A. Covino, PsyD Number of faculty: total—full-time 15, part-time 53; women—full-time 8, part-time 26; total—minority—full-time 6, part-time 2; women minority—full-time 4, part-time 1.

Programs and Degrees Offered:
Listed in the following order: Program area, degree type (T if terminal Master's), number awarded 7/08–6/09. Clinical Psychology PsyD (Doctor of Psychology) 50, Respecialization in Clinical Psychology Respecialization Diploma 2, School Psychology PsyD (Doctor of Psychology) 0, Organizational Psychology MA/MS (Master of Arts/Science) (T) 11, Graduate Certificate in Executive Coaching Other, Forensic Psychology MA/MS (Master of Arts/Science) (T) 0, Counseling Psychology MA/MS (Master of Arts/Science) (T) 30, School Psychology MA/MS (Master of Arts/Science) (T) 0.

APA Accreditation: Clinical PsyD (Doctor of Psychology). Student Outcome Data Website: http://www.mspp.edu/academics/degree-programs/psyd/default.asp.

Student Applications/Admissions:
Student Applications
Clinical Psychology PsyD (Doctor of Psychology)—Applications 2009–2010, 405. Total applicants accepted 2009–2010, 171. Number full-time enrolled (new admits only) 2009–2010, 70. Number part-time enrolled (new admits only) 2009–2010, 11. Total enrolled 2009–2010 full-time, 200, part-time, 61. Openings 2010–2011, 60. The median number of years required for completion of a degree in 2008–2009 were 4. *Respecialization in Clinical Psychology Respecialization Diploma*—Applications 2009–2010, 1. Total applicants accepted 2009–2010, 1. Number full-time enrolled (new admits only) 2009–2010, 1. Number part-time enrolled (new admits only) 2009–2010, 0. Openings 2010–2011, 4. The median number of years required for completion of a degree in 2008–2009 were 3. The number of students enrolled full- and part-time who were dismissed or voluntarily withdrew from this program area in 2008–2009 were 0. *School Psychology PsyD (Doctor of Psychology)*—Applications 2009–2010, 0. Total applicants accepted 2009–2010, 0. Number full-time enrolled (new admits only) 2009–2010, 0. The median number of years required for completion of a degree in 2008–2009 were 4. The number of students enrolled full- and part-time who were dismissed or voluntarily withdrew from this program area in 2008–2009 were 0. *Organizational Psychology MA/MS (Master of Arts/Science)*—Applications 2009–2010, 35. Total applicants accepted 2009–2010, 21. Number full-time enrolled (new admits only) 2009–2010, 19. Total enrolled 2009–2010 full-time, 19. Openings 2010–2011, 15. The median number of years required for

completion of a degree in 2008–2009 was 1. The number of students enrolled full- and part-time who were dismissed or voluntarily withdrew from this program area in 2008–2009 were 0. *Graduate Certificate in Executive Coaching Other—Forensic Psychology MA/MS (Master of Arts/Science)*—Applications 2009–2010, 76. Total applicants accepted 2009–2010, 34. Number full-time enrolled (new admits only) 2009–2010, 22. Number part-time enrolled (new admits only) 2009–2010, 0. Openings 2010–2011, 15. The median number of years required for completion of a degree in 2008–2009 were 2. The number of students enrolled full- and part-time who were dismissed or voluntarily withdrew from this program area in 2008–2009 were 0. *Counseling Psychology MA/MS (Master of Arts/Science)*—Applications 2009–2010, 143. Total applicants accepted 2009–2010, 69. Number full-time enrolled (new admits only) 2009–2010, 35. Total enrolled 2009–2010 full-time, 35. Openings 2010–2011, 40. The median number of years required for completion of a degree in 2008–2009 were 2. The number of students enrolled full- and part-time who were dismissed or voluntarily withdrew from this program area in 2008–2009 were 0. *School Psychology MA/MS (Master of Arts/Science)*—Applications 2009–2010, 44. Total applicants accepted 2009–2010, 25. Number full-time enrolled (new admits only) 2009–2010, 16. Total enrolled 2009–2010 full-time, 26. Openings 2010–2011, 20. The median number of years required for completion of a degree in 2008–2009 were 3. The number of students enrolled full- and part-time who were dismissed or voluntarily withdrew from this program area in 2008–2009 were 0.

Scores: Entries appear in this order: required test or GPA, minimum score (if required), median score of students entering in 2009–2010. *School Psychology PsyD (Doctor of Psychology):* GRE-V no minimum stated, GRE-Q no minimum stated, overall undergraduate GPA 3.0.

Other Criteria: (importance of criteria rated low, medium, or high): GRE scores—medium, research experience—low, work experience—medium, extracurricular activity—high, clinically related public service—high, GPA—high, letters of recommendation—high, interview—high, statement of goals and objectives—high. For additional information on admission requirements, go to http://www.mspp.edu/admissions/apply/default.asp.

Student Characteristics: The following represents characteristics of students in 2009–2010 in all graduate psychology programs in the department: Female—full-time 269, part-time 271; Male—full-time 77, part-time 64; African American/Black—full-time 4, part-time 8; Hispanic/Latino(a)—full-time 19, part-time 17; Asian/Pacific Islander—full-time 10, part-time 6; American Indian/Alaska Native—full-time 0, part-time 0; Caucasian/White—full-time 192, part-time 173; Multi-ethnic—full-time 0, part-time 0; students subject to the Americans With Disabilities Act—full-time 0, part-time 0; Unknown ethnicity—full-time 121, part-time 133; International students who hold an F-1 or J-1 Visa—full-time 2, part-time 6.

Financial Information/Assistance:
Tuition for Full-Time Study: Master's: State residents: per academic year $30,592, $956 per credit hour; Nonstate residents: per academic year $30,592, $956 per credit hour. *Doctoral:* State residents: per academic year $30,592, $956 per credit hour; Nonstate residents: per academic year $30,592, $956 per credit hour. Tuition is subject to change. See the following Web site for updates and changes in tuition costs: http://www.mspp.edu/admissions/tuition.asp.

Financial Assistance:
First-Year Students: Fellowships and scholarships available for first year. Average amount paid per academic year: $2,000. Apply by February 14.

Advanced Students: Teaching assistantships available for advanced students. Research assistantships available for advanced students. Fellowships and scholarships available for advanced students. Average amount paid per academic year: $2,000. Apply by April 16.

Additional Information: Of all students currently enrolled full time, 43% benefited from one or more of the listed financial assistance programs. Application and information available online at: http://www.mspp.edu/admissions/financial-aid/default.asp.

Internships/Practica: Doctoral Degree (PsyD Clinical Psychology): For those doctoral students for whom a professional internship was required in this program prior to graduation, (109) students applied for an internship in 2008–2009, with (108) students obtaining an internship. Of those students who obtained an internship, (46) were paid internships. Of those students who obtained an internship, (8) students placed in APA/CPA accredited internships, (0) students placed in internships not APA/CPA accredited, but listed with the Association of Psychology Postdoctoral and Internship Programs (APPIC), (0) students placed in internships conforming to guidelines of the Council of Directors of School Psychology Programs (CDSPP), (100) students placed in internships that were not APA/CPA accredited, APPIC or CDSPP listed. Master's Degree (MA/MS Organizational Psychology): An internship experience, such as, a final research project or "capstone" experience is required of graduates. Master's Degree (MA/MS Forensic Psychology): An internship experience, such as a final research project or "capstone" experience is required of graduates. Master's Degree (MA/MS Counseling Psychology): An internship experience, such as a final research project or "capstone" experience is required of graduates. Master's Degree (MA/MS School Psychology): An internship experience, such as a final research project or "capstone" experience is required of graduates. Field placements are an integral part of the program throughout the duration of the program. The practicum and internship experiences are integrated with the curriculum and individual's educational needs at each level of the program. Over 200 training sites are available in the greater Boston area including hospitals, mental health centers, court clinics, and other agencies offering mental health services. They provide students the opportunity to work with varied populations, life span issues, theoretical orientations, and treatment modalities in the context of supervised training. The large number of qualified agencies included in our training network enable students the option of applying for full or half-time APA-approved internships or securing suitable, high quality, local internships.

Housing and Day Care: No on-campus housing is available. No on-campus day care facilities are available.

Employment of Department Graduates:
Master's Degree Graduates: Of those who graduated in the academic year 2008–2009, the following categories and numbers represent the postgraduate activities and employment of master's

degree graduates: Enrolled in a postdoctoral residency/fellowship (n/a), employed in independent practice (n/a), total from the above (master's) (0).

Doctoral Degree Graduates: Of those who graduated in the academic year 2008–2009, the following categories and numbers represent the postgraduate activities and employment of doctoral degree graduates: Enrolled in a psychology doctoral program (n/a), total from the above (doctoral) (0).

Additional Information:
Orientation, Objectives, and Emphasis of Department: MSPP strives to be a preeminent school of psychology that integrates rigorous academic instruction with extensive field education and close attention to professional development. We assume an ongoing social responsibility to create programs to educate specialists of many disciplines to meet the evolving mental health needs of society.

Application Information:
Send to Admissions Office MSPP 221 Rivermoor Street Boston, MA 02132. Application available online. URL of online application: http://www.mspp.edu/admissions/apply/default.asp. Students are admitted in the Fall, application deadline January 13; Programs have rolling admissions. Applications received after the deadline will be considered on a space-available basis. Respecialization diploma has rolling admissions. *Fee:* $50.

Massachusetts, University of
Department of Psychology
Tobin Hall
Amherst, MA 01003
Telephone: (413) 545-2383
Fax: (413) 545-0996
E-mail: *lisbell@psych.umass.edu*
Web: *http://www.psych.umass.edu/*

Department Information:
1947. Chairperson: Melinda Novak. Number of faculty: total—full-time 43; women—full-time 22; total—minority—full-time 3, part-time 2; women minority—full-time 2, part-time 1.

Programs and Degrees Offered:
Listed in the following order: Program area, degree type (T if terminal Master's), number awarded 7/08–6/09. Developmental Psychology PhD (Doctor of Philosophy) 1, Clinical Psychology PhD (Doctor of Philosophy) 4, Cognitive Psychology PhD (Doctor of Philosophy) 1, Neuroscience and Behavior PhD (Doctor of Philosophy), Social Psychology PhD (Doctor of Philosophy) 1, Psychology Of Peace and The Prevention Of Violence PhD (Doctor of Philosophy) 2.

APA Accreditation: Clinical PhD (Doctor of Philosophy).

Student Applications/Admissions:
Student Applications
Developmental Psychology PhD (Doctor of Philosophy)—Applications 2009–2010, 30. Total applicants accepted 2009–2010, 2. Number full-time enrolled (new admits only) 2009–2010, 0. Openings 2010–2011, 2. The median number of years required for completion of a degree in 2008–2009 were 5. The number of students enrolled full- and part-time who were dismissed or voluntarily withdrew from this program area in 2008–2009 were 0. *Clinical Psychology PhD (Doctor of Philosophy)*—Applications 2009–2010, 236. Total applicants accepted 2009–2010, 8. Number full-time enrolled (new admits only) 2009–2010, 5. Openings 2010–2011, 4. The median number of years required for completion of a degree in 2008–2009 were 5. The number of students enrolled full- and part-time who were dismissed or voluntarily withdrew from this program area in 2008–2009 were 0. *Cognitive Psychology PhD (Doctor of Philosophy)*—Applications 2009–2010, 42. Total applicants accepted 2009–2010, 2. Number full-time enrolled (new admits only) 2009–2010, 2. Openings 2010–2011, 2. The median number of years required for completion of a degree in 2008–2009 were 5. The number of students enrolled full- and part-time who were dismissed or voluntarily withdrew from this program area in 2008–2009 were 0. *Neuroscience and Behavior PhD (Doctor of Philosophy)*—*Social Psychology PhD (Doctor of Philosophy)*—Applications 2009–2010, 87. Total applicants accepted 2009–2010, 3. Number full-time enrolled (new admits only) 2009–2010, 1. Openings 2010–2011, 2. The median number of years required for completion of a degree in 2008–2009 were 5. The number of students enrolled full- and part-time who were dismissed or voluntarily withdrew from this program area in 2008–2009 were 1. *Psychology Of Peace and The Prevention Of Violence PhD (Doctor of Philosophy)*—Applications 2009–2010, 27. Total applicants accepted 2009–2010, 1. Number full-time enrolled (new admits only) 2009–2010, 2. Total enrolled 2009–2010 full-time, 6. Openings 2010–2011, 1. The median number of years required for completion of a degree in 2008–2009 were 5.

Other Criteria: (importance of criteria rated low, medium, or high): GRE scores—high, research experience—high, work experience—low, clinically related public service—low, GPA—high, letters of recommendation—high, interview—medium, statement of goals and objectives—medium, undergraduate major in psychology—medium, specific undergraduate psychology courses taken—medium. Only clinical requires an interview. Clinically related public service also is a criteria (low) in admission to clinical. Undergraduate major in psychology and specific undergraduate courses will be weighed differently depending on division.

Student Characteristics: The following represents characteristics of students in 2009–2010 in all graduate psychology programs in the department: Female—full-time 60, part-time 0; Male—full-time 15, part-time 0; African American/Black—full-time 4, part-time 0; Hispanic/Latino(a)—full-time 1, part-time 0; Asian/Pacific Islander—full-time 7, part-time 0; American Indian/Alaska Native—full-time 0, part-time 0; Caucasian/White—full-time 50, part-time 0; Multi-ethnic—full-time 3, part-time 0; students subject to the Americans With Disabilities Act—full-time 0, part-time 0; Unknown ethnicity—full-time 10, part-time 0; International students who hold an F-1 or J-1 Visa—full-time 6, part-time 0.

Financial Information/Assistance:
Tuition for Full-Time Study: *Doctoral:* State residents: $110 per credit hour; Nonstate residents: $414 per credit hour. Tuition is

subject to change. See the following Web site for updates and changes in tuition costs: http://www.umass.edu/bursar.

Financial Assistance:
First-Year Students: Teaching assistantships available for first year. Average amount paid per academic year: $14,516. Average number of hours worked per week: 20. Research assistantships available for first year. Average amount paid per academic year: $14,516. Average number of hours worked per week: 20. Traineeships available for first year. Average amount paid per academic year: $14,516. Average number of hours worked per week: 20. Fellowships and scholarships available for first year. Average amount paid per academic year: $16,000. Average number of hours worked per week: 0.

Advanced Students: Teaching assistantships available for advanced students. Average amount paid per academic year: $14,516. Average number of hours worked per week: 20. Research assistantships available for advanced students. Average amount paid per academic year: $14,516. Average number of hours worked per week: 20. Traineeships available for advanced students. Average amount paid per academic year: $14,516. Average number of hours worked per week: 20. Fellowships and scholarships available for advanced students. Average amount paid per academic year: $16,000. Average number of hours worked per week: 0.

Additional Information: Of all students currently enrolled full time, 100% benefited from one or more of the listed financial assistance programs. Application and information available online at: http://www.umass.edu/umfa.

Internships/Practica: Doctoral Degree (PhD Clinical Psychology): For those doctoral students for whom a professional internship was required in this program prior to graduation, (8) students applied for an internship in 2008–2009, with (8) students obtaining an internship. Of those students who obtained an internship, (8) were paid internships. Of those students who obtained an internship, (8) students placed in APA/CPA accredited internships, (0) students placed in internships not APA/CPA accredited, but listed with the Association of Psychology Postdoctoral and Internship Programs (APPIC), (0) students placed in internships conforming to guidelines of the Council of Directors of School Psychology Programs (CDSPP), (0) students placed in internships that were not APA/CPA accredited, APPIC or CDSPP listed. Clinical students must complete an APA-approved clinical internship. None of these required internships are offered by our program.

Housing and Day Care: On-campus housing is available. See the following Web site for more information: http://www.housing.umass.edu. On-campus day care facilities are available.

Employment of Department Graduates:
Master's Degree Graduates: Of those who graduated in the academic year 2008–2009, the following categories and numbers represent the postgraduate activities and employment of master's degree graduates: Enrolled in a postdoctoral residency/fellowship (n/a), employed in independent practice (n/a), total from the above (master's) (0).
Doctoral Degree Graduates: Of those who graduated in the academic year 2008–2009, the following categories and numbers represent the postgraduate activities and employment of doctoral degree graduates: Enrolled in a psychology doctoral program (n/a), total from the above (doctoral) (0).

Additional Information:
Orientation, Objectives, and Emphasis of Department: The psychology program is designed to develop research scholars, college teachers, and scientific/professional psychologists in the six areas listed. Individual student programs combine basic courses and seminars in a variety of specialized areas, research experience, and practica in both on- and off-campus settings. Students may elect to minor in certain areas as well, including social, quantitative methods, and applied social research. In addition, the social area has begun a new specialization in the Psychology of Peace and Prevention of Violence. Students with applied interests, such as clinical and developmental, have ample opportunity for in-depth practical experience.

Special Facilities or Resources: The Department has specialized laboratory facilities, including biochemistry, eyetracking, video data analysis, and other laboratories. It maintains its own clinic for research, clinical training, and service to the community. It provides students with access to microcomputers and to the VAX mainframes at University Computing Services. Departmental facilities and faculty are supplemented by the University's participation in Five-College programs (with Amherst, Hampshire, Mount Holyoke, and Smith Colleges) and by cooperation with other University departments including Computer and Information Science, Industrial Engineering, Education, Linguistics, Sociology, and Biology. The University of Massachusetts also offers a separate PhD degree-granting program in neuroscience and behavior. Many of the students in this program receive the bulk of their training in the Psychology Department and work primarily with Psychology faculty. Students interested in training in neuroscience and behavior should apply for admission directly to that program.

Information for Students With Physical Disabilities: See the following Web site for more information: http://www.umass.edu/disability/.

Application Information:
Send to Graduate Admissions Office, Goodell Building; University of Massachusetts, Amherst, MA 01003. Application available online. URL of online application: http://www.umass.edu/gradschool. Students are admitted in the Fall, application deadline see below. December 1 for Clinical; January 2 for all other programs. *Fee:* $50. Application fee can be waived if GRE fees were waived.

Massachusetts, University of, Boston
Counseling and School Psychology
Graduate College of Education
100 Morrissey Boulevard
Boston, MA 02125-3393
Telephone: (617) 287-7631
Fax: (617) 287-7667
E-mail: *sharon.lamb@umb.edu*
Web: *http://www.umb.edu/academics/departments/gce/programs/counseling/*

Department Information:
1982. Chairperson: Sharon Lamb. Number of faculty: total—full-time 16, part-time 43; women—full-time 12, part-time 30; total—

minority—full-time 3, part-time 2; women minority—full-time 1, part-time 1.

Programs and Degrees Offered:
Listed in the following order: Program area, degree type (T if terminal Master's), number awarded 7/08–6/09. School Psychology EdS (School Psychology) 25, Mental Health Counseling MA/MS (Master of Arts/Science) (T) 45, Rehabilitation Counseling MA/MS (Master of Arts/Science) (T) 7, School Counseling MA/MS (Master of Arts/Science) (T) 16, Family Therapy MA/MS (Master of Arts/Science) (T) 6.

Student Applications/Admissions:
Student Applications
School Psychology EdS (School Psychology)—Applications 2009–2010, 165. Total applicants accepted 2009–2010, 52. Number full-time enrolled (new admits only) 2009–2010, 17. Number part-time enrolled (new admits only) 2009–2010, 8. Total enrolled 2009–2010 full-time, 60, part-time, 34. Openings 2010–2011, 30. The median number of years required for completion of a degree in 2008–2009 were 3. *Mental Health Counseling MA/MS (Master of Arts/Science)*—Applications 2009–2010, 91. Total applicants accepted 2009–2010, 45. Number full-time enrolled (new admits only) 2009–2010, 13. Number part-time enrolled (new admits only) 2009–2010, 14. Total enrolled 2009–2010 full-time, 42, part-time, 42. Openings 2010–2011, 30. *Rehabilitation Counseling MA/MS (Master of Arts/Science)*—Applications 2009–2010, 12. Total applicants accepted 2009–2010, 10. Number full-time enrolled (new admits only) 2009–2010, 4. Number part-time enrolled (new admits only) 2009–2010, 3. Total enrolled 2009–2010 full-time, 12, part-time, 12. Openings 2010–2011, 15. The median number of years required for completion of a degree in 2008–2009 were 2. *School Counseling MA/MS (Master of Arts/Science)*—Applications 2009–2010, 90. Total applicants accepted 2009–2010, 50. Number full-time enrolled (new admits only) 2009–2010, 10. Number part-time enrolled (new admits only) 2009–2010, 10. Total enrolled 2009–2010 full-time, 42, part-time, 42. Openings 2010–2011, 20. The median number of years required for completion of a degree in 2008–2009 were 2. *Family Therapy MA/MS (Master of Arts/Science)*—Applications 2009–2010, 52. Total applicants accepted 2009–2010, 19. Number full-time enrolled (new admits only) 2009–2010, 4. Number part-time enrolled (new admits only) 2009–2010, 4. Total enrolled 2009–2010 full-time, 12, part-time, 13. Openings 2010–2011, 15.

Scores: Entries appear in this order: required test or GPA, minimum score (if required), median score of students entering in 2009–2010. *School Psychology EdS (School Psychology):* GRE-V no minimum stated, GRE-Q no minimum stated, overall undergraduate GPA 3.0; *Mental Health Counseling MA/MS (Master of Arts/Science):* GRE-V no minimum stated, GRE-Q no minimum stated, overall undergraduate GPA 3.0; *Rehabilitation Counseling MA/MS (Master of Arts/Science):* GRE-V no minimum stated, GRE-Q no minimum stated, overall undergraduate GPA 3.0; *School Counseling MA/MS (Master of Arts/Science):* GRE-V no minimum stated, GRE-Q no minimum stated, overall undergraduate GPA 3.0; *Family Therapy MA/MS (Master of Arts/Science):* GRE-V no minimum stated, GRE-Q no minimum stated, overall undergraduate GPA 3.0.

Other Criteria: (importance of criteria rated low, medium, or high): GRE scores—medium, research experience—low, work experience—high, extracurricular activity—medium, clinically related public service—medium, GPA—medium, letters of recommendation—high, interview—high, statement of goals and objectives—high, undergraduate major in psychology—low, specific undergraduate psychology courses taken—medium. For additional information on admission requirements, go to http://www.umb.edu/academics/departments/gce/programs/counseling/.

Student Characteristics: The following represents characteristics of students in 2009–2010 in all graduate psychology programs in the department: Female—full-time 35, part-time 203; Male—full-time 5, part-time 50; African American/Black—full-time 0, part-time 21; Hispanic/Latino(a)—full-time 0, part-time 12; Asian/Pacific Islander—full-time 0, part-time 10; American Indian/Alaska Native—full-time 0, part-time 1; Caucasian/White—full-time 0, part-time 253; Multi-ethnic—full-time 0, part-time 18; students subject to the Americans With Disabilities Act—full-time 0, part-time 0; Unknown ethnicity—full-time 0, part-time 0; International students who hold an F-1 or J-1 Visa—full-time 0, part-time 0.

Financial Information/Assistance:
Tuition for Full-Time Study: *Master's:* State residents: per academic year $11,991; Nonstate residents: per academic year $22,823. Tuition is subject to change. See the following Web site for updates and changes in tuition costs: http://umb.edu/administration_finance/bursar/tuition_fees.html.

Financial Assistance:
First-Year Students: Teaching assistantships available for first year. Average amount paid per academic year: $3,500. Average number of hours worked per week: 5. Research assistantships available for first year. Average amount paid per academic year: $3,500. Average number of hours worked per week: 5.

Advanced Students: Teaching assistantships available for advanced students. Average amount paid per academic year: $3,500. Average number of hours worked per week: 5. Research assistantships available for advanced students. Average amount paid per academic year: $3,500. Average number of hours worked per week: 5.

Additional Information: Of all students currently enrolled full time, 10% benefited from one or more of the listed financial assistance programs. Application and information available online at: http://www.umb.edu/students/financial_aid/.

Internships/Practica: The department maintains collaborative partnerships with a number of Greater Boston area schools, mental health clinics, rehabilitation centers, and other facilities which provide practicum and internship sites for students.

Housing and Day Care: No on-campus housing is available. On-campus day care facilities are available. See the following Web site for more information: http://www.umb.edu/student_affairs/elc/.

GRADUATE STUDY IN PSYCHOLOGY

Employment of Department Graduates:
Master's Degree Graduates: Of those who graduated in the academic year 2008–2009, the following categories and numbers represent the postgraduate activities and employment of master's degree graduates: Enrolled in a postdoctoral residency/fellowship (n/a), employed in independent practice (n/a), total from the above (master's) (0).

Doctoral Degree Graduates: Of those who graduated in the academic year 2008–2009, the following categories and numbers represent the postgraduate activities and employment of doctoral degree graduates: Enrolled in a psychology doctoral program (n/a), total from the above (doctoral) (0).

Additional Information:
Orientation, Objectives, and Emphasis of Department: The Department and our programs are committed to the preparation of highly qualified professionals who will seek to promote maximum growth and development of individuals (children, adolescents, and adults) with whom they work. This is accomplished through a carefully planned curriculum which includes the following: interdisciplinary and multidisciplinary approaches; theory linked to practice; a practitioner-scientist approach; self awareness and self-exploration activities; opportunities to learn and demonstrate respect for others; and socialization into the role of the profession. We value respect for the social foundations and cultural diversity of others and promote opportunities for students to learn how others construct their world. We emphasize to our students to focus on the assets and coping abilities of the people with whom they work rather than focusing on deficits. Additionally, we encourage the promotion of preventative services, which maximize individual functioning. Our programs are grounded in a systematic eclectic philosophical orientation, which includes: systemic theory; social constructionism; cognitive behavioral; psychodynamic; and person-centered approaches.

Special Facilities or Resources: We work in collaboration and have partnerships with the Mass Rehabilitation Commission, the Institute of Community Inclusion, the International Institute of Boston, and several school districts. Our students often find Graduate Assistantships outside of our department which come with partial tuition remission.

Information for Students With Physical Disabilities: See the following Web site for more information: http://www.rosscenter.umb.edu/.

Application Information:
Send to Graduate Admissions, Quinn Adminstration Building, University of Massachusetts Boston, 100 Morrissey Blvd., Boston, MA 02125. Application available online. URL of online application: http://www.umb.edu/admissions/graduate/apply/index.html. Students are admitted in the Fall, application deadline January 2. Application deadline for School Psychology program is January 2. Deadline is February 1 for School Counseling, Mental Health Counseling, and Family Therapy. Deadline for Rehabilitation Counseling is June 1. *Fee:* $40. $40 application fee for Massachusetts residents, $60 for non-residents.

Massachusetts, University of, Dartmouth
Psychology Department
College of Arts & Sciences
285 Old Westport Road
North Dartmouth, MA 02747-2300
Telephone: (508) 999-8380
Fax: (508) 999-9169
E-mail: bhaimson@umassd.edu
Web: http://www.umassd.edu/cas/psychology/welcome.cfm

Department Information:
1962. Chairperson: Barry Haimson. Number of faculty: total—full-time 18, part-time 8; women—full-time 9, part-time 4.

Programs and Degrees Offered:
Listed in the following order: Program area, degree type (T if terminal Master's), number awarded 7/08–6/09. Clinical Psychology MA/MS (Master of Arts/Science) (T) 6, Research MA/MS (Master of Arts/Science) (T) 1, Applied Behavior Analysis MA/MS (Master of Arts/Science) (T), Applied Behavior Analysis Certificate 0.

Student Applications/Admissions:
Student Applications

Clinical Psychology MA/MS (Master of Arts/Science)—Applications 2009–2010, 57. Total applicants accepted 2009–2010, 24. Number full-time enrolled (new admits only) 2009–2010, 13. Total enrolled 2009–2010 full-time, 39. Openings 2010–2011, 15. The median number of years required for completion of a degree in 2008–2009 were 3. The number of students enrolled full- and part-time who were dismissed or voluntarily withdrew from this program area in 2008–2009 were 1. *Research MA/MS (Master of Arts/Science)*—Applications 2009–2010, 16. Total applicants accepted 2009–2010, 10. Number full-time enrolled (new admits only) 2009–2010, 6. Number part-time enrolled (new admits only) 2009–2010, 0. Openings 2010–2011, 8. The median number of years required for completion of a degree in 2008–2009 were 2. The number of students enrolled full- and part-time who were dismissed or voluntarily withdrew from this program area in 2008–2009 were 0. *Applied Behavior Analysis MA/MS (Master of Arts/Science)*—Applications 2009–2010, 13. Total applicants accepted 2009–2010, 8. Number full-time enrolled (new admits only) 2009–2010, 8. Total enrolled 2009–2010 full-time, 8. Openings 2010–2011, 18. The number of students enrolled full- and part-time who were dismissed or voluntarily withdrew from this program area in 2008–2009 were 0. *Applied Behavior Analysis Certificate*—Applications 2009–2010, 5. Total applicants accepted 2009–2010, 4. Number full-time enrolled (new admits only) 2009–2010, 0. Number part-time enrolled (new admits only) 2009–2010, 3. Openings 2010–2011, 10. The number of students enrolled full- and part-time who were dismissed or voluntarily withdrew from this program area in 2008–2009 were 0.

Scores: Entries appear in this order: required test or GPA, minimum score (if required), median score of students entering in 2009–2010. *Research MA/MS (Master of Arts/Science):* GRE-V 440, 600, GRE-Q 670, 710, GRE-Analytical 4, 4.5; *Applied Behavior Analysis MA/MS (Master of Arts/Science):* GRE-V 230, 415, GRE-Q 240, 455.

Other Criteria: (importance of criteria rated low, medium, or high): GRE scores—medium, research experience—high, work experience—high, clinically related public service—high, GPA—medium, letters of recommendation—high, interview—high, statement of goals and objectives—high, These criteria vary across options. The Research track does not require work experience or clinical services. The clinical and ABA tracks do not require research experience. Interview is important for clinical track.

Student Characteristics: The following represents characteristics of students in 2009–2010 in all graduate psychology programs in the department: Female—full-time 30, part-time 0; Male—full-time 5, part-time 0; African American/Black—full-time 0, part-time 0; Hispanic/Latino(a)—full-time 3, part-time 0; Asian/Pacific Islander—full-time 0, part-time 0; American Indian/Alaska Native—full-time 0, part-time 0; Caucasian/White—full-time 30, part-time 0; Multi-ethnic—full-time 2, part-time 0; students subject to the Americans With Disabilities Act—full-time 0, part-time 0; Unknown ethnicity—full-time 0, part-time 0; International students who hold an F-1 or J-1 Visa—full-time 0, part-time 0.

Financial Information/Assistance:
Tuition for Full-Time Study: *Master's:* State residents: per academic year $2,071; Nonstate residents: per academic year $8,099. Additional fees are assessed to students beyond the costs of tuition for the following: curriculum support, athletic fee, student fee, campus center, & health. See the following Web site for updates and changes in tuition costs: http://www.umassd.edu/graduate/tuition/.

Financial Assistance:
First-Year Students: Teaching assistantships available for first year. Average amount paid per academic year: $3,500. Average number of hours worked per week: 10. Research assistantships available for first year. Average amount paid per academic year: $10,000. Average number of hours worked per week: 20.
Advanced Students: Teaching assistantships available for advanced students. Average amount paid per academic year: $3,500. Average number of hours worked per week: 10. Research assistantships available for advanced students. Average amount paid per academic year: $10,000. Average number of hours worked per week: 20.
Additional Information: Of all students currently enrolled full time, 21% benefited from one or more of the listed financial assistance programs.

Internships/Practica: Master's Degree (MA/MS Clinical Psychology): An internship experience, such as a final research project or "capstone" experience is required of graduates. Master's Degree (MA/MS Applied Behavior Analysis): An internship experience, such as a final research project or "capstone" experience is required of graduates. We have a wide variety of internship and practicum experiences available for clinical students. Field experiences are tailored to specific student needs. In addition, we have a number of paid internships and scholarships for students matriculated in the ABA track.

Housing and Day Care: No on-campus housing is available. No on-campus day care facilities are available.

Employment of Department Graduates:
Master's Degree Graduates: Of those who graduated in the academic year 2008–2009, the following categories and numbers represent the postgraduate activities and employment of master's degree graduates: Enrolled in a psychology doctoral program (2), enrolled in another graduate/professional program (8), enrolled in a postdoctoral residency/fellowship (n/a), employed in independent practice (n/a), employed in a community mental health/counseling center (9), total from the above (master's) (19).
Doctoral Degree Graduates: Of those who graduated in the academic year 2008–2009, the following categories and numbers represent the postgraduate activities and employment of doctoral degree graduates: Enrolled in a psychology doctoral program (n/a), total from the above (doctoral) (0).

Additional Information:
Orientation, Objectives, and Emphasis of Department: The research track of the MA program in psychology is designed to prepare students for doctoral work in psychology and related fields, including cognitive science. The program combines coursework in basic areas of psychology with the opportunity to do collaborative research with faculty members. Students have considerable flexibility to tailor their programs to their individual needs. The outstanding feature of this program is the opportunity for close interaction between faculty and students, both in the classroom and in the laboratory, because of the low student/faculty ratio. The objectives of the Clinical track are: to train competent MA-level clinicians; to provide students with applied research and problem-solving skills; to provide students with a broad exposure to a variety of therapy modalities; to provide students with extensive experiential learning opportunities, practica, internships and intensive supervision; and to prepare students to be Licensed Mental Health Counselors. The ABA MA track is designed to prepare students to sit for the BCBA (Board Certified Behavior Analyst) exam administered by the Behavior Analyst Certification Board (BACB). The ABA certificate program is designed to prepare individuals with Master's degrees in other areas and appropriate internship experience to sit for the BCBA exam. All ABA specific courses have been approved by the BACB.

Special Facilities or Resources: Our ABA MA track and certificate programs are offered in collaboration with Evergreen Center and Beacon Services. The Evergreen Center is a residential school serving children with severe developmental disabilities. Beacon Services provides ABA consulting services to schools and families with children requiring behavioral support. Students may also receive field work experience at other ABA sites in the area.

Application Information:
Send to Office of Graduate Studies. Application available online. URL of online application: http://www.umassd.edu/graduate/prospects/waystoapply.cfm. Students are admitted in the Fall, Programs have rolling admissions. March 31 for Clinical Option; rolling admissions for Research and ABA. *Fee:* $60. $40 if resident of Massachusetts.

Massachusetts, University of, Lowell
Community Social Psychology Master's Program
Arts and Sciences
870 Broadway Street, Suite 1
Lowell, MA 01854-3043
Telephone: (978) 934-3950
Fax: (978) 934-3074
E-mail: *csp@uml.edu*
Web: *http://www.uml.edu/csp*

Department Information:
1980. Chairperson: Richard Siegel. Number of faculty: total—full-time 17, part-time 3; women—full-time 12, part-time 2; total—minority—full-time 3; women minority—full-time 2.

Programs and Degrees Offered:
Listed in the following order: Program area, degree type (T if terminal Master's), number awarded 7/08–6/09. Community Social Psychology MA/MS (Master of Arts/Science) (T) 20.

Student Applications/Admissions:
Student Applications
Community Social Psychology MA/MS (Master of Arts/Science)—Applications 2009–2010, 35. Total applicants accepted 2009–2010, 28. Number full-time enrolled (new admits only) 2009–2010, 12. Number part-time enrolled (new admits only) 2009–2010, 6. Total enrolled 2009–2010 full-time, 30, part-time, 20. Openings 2010–2011, 25. The median number of years required for completion of a degree in 2008–2009 were 2. The number of students enrolled full- and part-time who were dismissed or voluntarily withdrew from this program area in 2008–2009 were 0.
Other Criteria: (importance of criteria rated low, medium, or high): GRE scores—medium, research experience—medium, work experience—high, extracurricular activity—low, clinically related public service—medium, GPA—high, letters of recommendation—high, statement of goals and objectives—high, undergraduate major in psychology—medium, specific undergraduate psychology courses taken—low. For additional information on admission requirements, go to http://www.uml.edu/grad/Overview.html.

Student Characteristics: The following represents characteristics of students in 2009–2010 in all graduate psychology programs in the department: Female—full-time 32, part-time 11; Male—full-time 7, part-time 0; African American/Black—full-time 0, part-time 2; Hispanic/Latino(a)—full-time 3, part-time 0; Asian/Pacific Islander—full-time 6, part-time 2; American Indian/Alaska Native—full-time 0, part-time 0; Caucasian/White—full-time 30, part-time 7; Multi-ethnic—full-time 0, part-time 0; students subject to the Americans With Disabilities Act—full-time 0, part-time 0; Unknown ethnicity—full-time 0, part-time 0; International students who hold an F-1 or J-1 Visa—full-time 6, part-time 0.

Financial Information/Assistance:
Tuition for Full-Time Study: *Master's:* State residents: per academic year $10,000, $570 per credit hour; Nonstate residents: per academic year $18,730, $1,055 per credit hour. See the following Web site for updates and changes in tuition costs: http://www.uml.edu/grad/Financial_Information.html. Higher tuition cost for this program: online graduate courses are $1,320 for all students, regardless of residence.

Financial Assistance:
First-Year Students: Teaching assistantships available for first year. Average amount paid per academic year: $6,504. Average number of hours worked per week: 9. Apply by May 1.
Advanced Students: Teaching assistantships available for advanced students. Average amount paid per academic year: $6,504. Average number of hours worked per week: 9. Apply by May 1.
Additional Information: Of all students currently enrolled full time, 20% benefited from one or more of the listed financial assistance programs. Application and information available online at: http://www.uml.edu/college/arts_sciences/psychology/Graduate/Forms_Manuals.html.

Internships/Practica: Master's Degree (MA/MS Community Social Psychology): An internship experience, such as, a final research project or "capstone" experience is required of graduates. There is a one-year practicum requirement of 10 to 12 hours a week. Settings vary but much of the fieldwork takes place directly in Lowell, MA, perhaps the most culturally diverse mid-size city in the United States, located just 25 miles from Boston.

Housing and Day Care: On-campus housing is available. See the following Web site for more information: http://www.uml.edu/student-services/. On-campus day care facilities are available.

Employment of Department Graduates:
Master's Degree Graduates: Of those who graduated in the academic year 2008–2009, the following categories and numbers represent the postgraduate activities and employment of master's degree graduates: Enrolled in a psychology doctoral program (2), enrolled in another graduate/professional program (1), enrolled in a postdoctoral residency/fellowship (n/a), employed in independent practice (n/a), employed in an academic position at a university (2), employed in an academic position at a 2-year/4-year college (3), employed in other positions at a higher education institution (0), employed in a professional position in a school system (1), employed in business or industry (4), employed in government agency (2), employed in a community mental health/counseling center (0), employed in a hospital/medical center (0), still seeking employment (2), other employment position (3), do not know (1), total from the above (master's) (21).
Doctoral Degree Graduates: Of those who graduated in the academic year 2008–2009, the following categories and numbers represent the postgraduate activities and employment of doctoral degree graduates: Enrolled in a psychology doctoral program (n/a), total from the above (doctoral) (0).

Additional Information:
Orientation, Objectives, and Emphasis of Department: The Community Social Psychology faculty and students share a commitment to social justice and the empowerment of all citizens. To those ends, our program is designed to help students understand the complex relationships between individual, family, and community well-being and the broader environment in which we live and work. Our mission is to provide students with the analytic, creative, organizational and evaluative skills needed to design, implement, and assess programs that will facilitate positive

changes within and across communities ' changes that will empower all people to reach their full potential and empower social organizations, public and private, to be more responsive to human needs. CSP is a 36-credit master's degree program, providing opportunities for in-class learning experiences, field study, independent study, and interdisciplinary collaboration. Students admitted to our program will work with recognized faculty and talented students from diverse backgrounds. Our graduates are prepared for leadership positions in government, health and human services, and community and educational organizations in a variety of professional roles and capacities. Many also proceed on toward doctoral degrees.

Special Facilities or Resources: Special facilities and resources consist of a graduate student lounge/computer lab, grant-related technical services from the Office of Research Administration, numerous research centers such as the Center for Family, Work and Community and the Center for Women and Work, and a unique multi-ethnic urban setting in a mid-sized city accessible to Boston.

Information for Students With Physical Disabilities: See the following Web site for more information: http://www.uml.edu/student-services/disability/default.html.

Application Information:
Send to Office of Graduate School Admissions, 883 Broadway Street, Suite 110, Lowell, MA 01854-5130. Application available online. URL of online application: http://www.uml.edu/grad/Overview.html. Programs have rolling admissions. We accept and act on applications year-round. Most of our students start our program in the Fall semester. For students planning full-time study who wish to apply for graduate assistant support, that deadline is May 1 for Fall enrollment. We accept GA applications only once each year. *Fee:* $50.

Northeastern University
Department of Counseling & Applied Educational Psychology
Bouve College of Health Sciences
360 Huntington Avenue, 404 INV
Boston, MA 02115
Telephone: (617) 373-2485
Fax: (617) 373-8892
E-mail: *y.chung@neu.edu*
Web: *http://www.northeastern.edu/bouve/healthprofessions/dept/caep.html*

Department Information:
1983. Chair: Y. Barry Chung, PhD. Number of faculty: total—full-time 20, part-time 27; women—full-time 12, part-time 17; total—minority—full-time 7, part-time 4; women minority—full-time 4, part-time 3; faculty subject to the Americans With Disabilities Act 1.

Programs and Degrees Offered:
Listed in the following order: Program area, degree type (T if terminal Master's), number awarded 7/08–6/09. Combined Counseling/School Psychology PhD (Doctor of Philosophy) 5, College Student Development MA/MS (Master of Arts/Science) (T) 26, Counseling Psychology MA/MS (Master of Arts/Science) (T) 28, Applied Behavioral Analysis MA/MS (Master of Arts/Science) (T) 13, School Counseling MA/MS (Master of Arts/Science) (T) 12, Counseling Psychology PhD (Doctor of Philosophy), School Psychology MA/MS (Master of Arts/Science) (T), Early Intervention Other 4, School Psychology PhD (Doctor of Philosophy).

APA Accreditation: Combination PhD (Doctor of Philosophy). Student Outcome Data Website: http://www.northeastern.edu/bouve/pdfs/Admin/Program_Information_.pdf.

Student Applications/Admissions:
Student Applications

Combined Counseling/School Psychology PhD (Doctor of Philosophy)—Applications 2009–2010, 93. Total applicants accepted 2009–2010, 10. Number full-time enrolled (new admits only) 2009–2010, 5. Number part-time enrolled (new admits only) 2009–2010, 0. Openings 2010–2011, 6. The median number of years required for completion of a degree in 2008–2009 were 6. The number of students enrolled full- and part-time who were dismissed or voluntarily withdrew from this program area in 2008–2009 were 2. *College Student Development MA/MS (Master of Arts/Science)*—Applications 2009–2010, 60. Total applicants accepted 2009–2010, 28. Number full-time enrolled (new admits only) 2009–2010, 16. Number part-time enrolled (new admits only) 2009–2010, 5. Total enrolled 2009–2010 full-time, 34, part-time, 10. Openings 2010–2011, 16. The median number of years required for completion of a degree in 2008–2009 were 2. The number of students enrolled full- and part-time who were dismissed or voluntarily withdrew from this program area in 2008–2009 were 0. *Counseling Psychology MA/MS (Master of Arts/Science)*—Applications 2009–2010, 80. Total applicants accepted 2009–2010, 28. Number full-time enrolled (new admits only) 2009–2010, 20. Number part-time enrolled (new admits only) 2009–2010, 1. Total enrolled 2009–2010 full-time, 38, part-time, 4. Openings 2010–2011, 25. The median number of years required for completion of a degree in 2008–2009 were 2. The number of students enrolled full- and part-time who were dismissed or voluntarily withdrew from this program area in 2008–2009 were 1. *Applied Behavioral Analysis MA/MS (Master of Arts/Science)*—Applications 2009–2010, 56. Total applicants accepted 2009–2010, 22. Number full-time enrolled (new admits only) 2009–2010, 0. Number part-time enrolled (new admits only) 2009–2010, 26. Total enrolled 2009–2010 full-time, 16, part-time, 44. Openings 2010–2011, 12. The median number of years required for completion of a degree in 2008–2009 were 2. The number of students enrolled full- and part-time who were dismissed or voluntarily withdrew from this program area in 2008–2009 were 0. *School Counseling MA/MS (Master of Arts/Science)*—Applications 2009–2010, 45. Total applicants accepted 2009–2010, 20. Number full-time enrolled (new admits only) 2009–2010, 14. Number part-time enrolled (new admits only) 2009–2010, 2. Total enrolled 2009–2010 full-time, 28, part-time, 6. Openings 2010–2011, 16. The median number of years required for completion of a degree in 2008–2009 were 2. The number of students enrolled full- and part-time who were dismissed or voluntarily withdrew from this program area in 2008–2009 were 0. *Counseling Psychology PhD (Doctor of Philosophy)—School Psychology MA/MS (Master of Arts/Science)—Early Intervention Other*—Applications 2009–2010, 20. Total applicants accepted 2009–2010, 10. Number full-time enrolled (new admits only) 2009–2010, 6. Number part-time enrolled (new admits only) 2009–2010, 2. Total enrolled 2009–2010 full-time, 7, part-time, 4. Openings 2010–2011, 6. The median number of years required for completion of a degree in 2008–2009 were 2. The number of students enrolled full- and part-time who were dismissed or voluntarily withdrew from this program area in 2008–2009 were 0. *School Psychology PhD (Doctor of Philosophy)*—

Scores: Entries appear in this order: required test or GPA, minimum score (if required), median score of students entering in 2009–2010. *College Student Development MA/MS (Master of Arts/Science)*: GRE-V no minimum stated, GRE-Q no minimum stated; *Counseling Psychology MA/MS (Master of Arts/Science)*: GRE-V no minimum stated, 550, GRE-Q no minimum stated, 600, overall undergraduate GPA no minimum stated, 3.5; *Counseling Psychology PhD (Doctor of Philosophy)*: GRE-V no minimum stated, GRE-Q no minimum stated; *Early Intervention Other:* overall undergraduate GPA 3.0; *School Psychology PhD (Doctor of Philosophy)*: GRE-V 600, GRE-Q 600, overall undergraduate GPA 3.0.

Other Criteria: (importance of criteria rated low, medium, or high): GRE scores—medium, research experience—medium, work experience—high, extracurricular activity—medium, clinically related public service—high, GPA—medium, letters of recommendation—high, interview—high, statement of goals and objectives—high.

Student Characteristics: The following represents characteristics of students in 2009–2010 in all graduate psychology programs in the department: Female—full-time 113, part-time 59; Male—full-time 250, part-time 64; African American/Black—full-time 11, part-time 3; Hispanic/Latino(a)—full-time 9, part-time 5; Asian/Pacific Islander—full-time 6, part-time 2; American Indian/Alaska Native—full-time 0, part-time 0; Caucasian/White—full-time 0, part-time 0; Multi-ethnic—full-time 0, part-time 2; students subject to the Americans With Disabilities Act—full-time 0, part-time 0; Unknown ethnicity—full-time 0, part-time 0; International students who hold an F-1 or J-1 Visa—full-time 0, part-time 0.

Financial Information/Assistance:
Tuition for Full-Time Study: *Master's:* State residents: $1,035 per credit hour; Nonstate residents: $1,035 per credit hour. *Doctoral:* State residents: $1,035 per credit hour; Nonstate residents: $1,035 per credit hour. Tuition is subject to change.

Financial Assistance:
First-Year Students: No information provided.
Advanced Students: Teaching assistantships available for advanced students. Average amount paid per academic year: $14,125. Average number of hours worked per week: 20. Fellowships and scholarships available for advanced students. Average number of hours worked per week: 0.
Additional Information: Of all students currently enrolled full time, 10% benefited from one or more of the listed financial assistance programs.

Internships/Practica: Doctoral Degree (PhD Combined Counseling/School Psychology): For those doctoral students for whom a professional internship was required in this program prior to graduation, (6) students applied for an internship in 2008–2009, with (5) students obtaining an internship. Of those students who obtained an internship, (5) were paid internships. Of those students who obtained an internship, (5) students placed in APA/CPA accredited internships, (0) students placed in internships not APA/CPA accredited, but listed with the Association of Psychology Postdoctoral and Internship Programs (APPIC), (0) students placed in internships conforming to guidelines of the Council of Directors of School Psychology Programs (CDSPP), (0) students placed in internships that were not APA/CPA accredited, APPIC or CDSPP listed. Master's Degree (MA/MS Counseling Psychology): An internship experience, such as a final research project or "capstone" experience is required of graduates. Master's Degree (MA/MS School Counseling): An internship experience, such as a final research project or "capstone" experience is required of graduates. Master's Degree (MA/MS School Psychology): An internship experience, such as a final research project or "capstone" experience is required of graduates. Internship and field placement sites are varied depending on the program and specialization. Sites are in the Boston metropolitan area and include some of the most desirable and prestigious settings in the field.

Housing and Day Care: No on-campus housing is available. On-campus day care facilities are available.

Employment of Department Graduates:
Master's Degree Graduates: Of those who graduated in the academic year 2008–2009, the following categories and numbers represent the postgraduate activities and employment of master's degree graduates: Enrolled in a postdoctoral residency/fellowship (n/a), employed in independent practice (n/a), total from the above (master's) (0).
Doctoral Degree Graduates: Of those who graduated in the academic year 2008–2009, the following categories and numbers represent the postgraduate activities and employment of doctoral degree graduates: Enrolled in a psychology doctoral program (n/a), total from the above (doctoral) (0).

Additional Information:
Orientation, Objectives, and Emphasis of Department: Philosophically, the school and counseling psychology programs are based on an ecological model. This model focuses on the contexts in which people and their environments intersect, including individuals' families, groups, cultures, and social, political, and economic institutions. Thus, the ecological model includes individual and interpersonal relationships along with their interactive physical and sociocultural environments. It employs a general systems perspective to understand the mutually reciprocal interactions of all of these elements. Central to this theoretical stance are assumptions of interdependence, circular and multilevel influence and causality, and interactive identities. Issues of gender, status, and culture are given special emphasis as well as the developmental stages of the individual, family, or group. The ecological model is large enough and sufficiently comprehensive to allow for teaching and using other models such as psychodynamic, behaviorist, and humanistic, as they help to explain behavior and phenomena in individuals, families, and groups. This allows faculty and students to teach, understand, and use many explanations of human activities. This ecological orientation provides the lenses through which students study psychological and counseling theory and research. In their varied fieldwork settings, students have the opportunity to translate this orientation into practice.

Special Facilities or Resources: Northeastern University, one of the largest private universities in the country, is located in Boston, a center of academic excellence and psychological research. There are numerous opportunities for diverse experiences, such as placements specializing in neuropsychology, early intervention, and sexual abuse. The campus is in the Back Bay, an area with a large student population and rich cultural opportunities. The Snell Library, one of the most advanced college libraries in the Boston area, provides access for students not only to its large psychology and education collections, but also to media and microcomputer centers and an extensive global academic computer networking system. Northeastern students also have privileges at the other Boston area research libraries.

Information for Students With Physical Disabilities: See the following Web site for more information: http://www.drc.neu.edu/.

Application Information:
Send to Graduate Dean, Bouve College of Health Sciences, 123 Beharakis Health Science Building, Boston, MA 02115. Application available online. URL of online application: http://www.northeastern.edu/graduate/apply_now/. Students are admitted in the Fall, application deadline. Deadlines: combined School and Counseling Psychology PhD- December 15 for admission following fall; MS Counseling Psychology - December 1 for admission following fall; MS/CAGS School Psychology - Suggested January 15 for admission following fall. All other program have a suggested May 1 deadline. *Fee:* $50.

Northeastern University
Department of Psychology
College of Science
125 Nightingale Hall
Boston, MA 02115
Telephone: (617) 373-3076
Fax: (617) 373-8714
E-mail: *j.miller@neu.edu*
Web: *http://www.psych.neu.edu*

Department Information:
1966. Chairperson: Joanne L. Miller. Number of faculty: total—full-time 20; women—full-time 5; total—minority—full-time 4; women minority—full-time 2.

Programs and Degrees Offered:
Listed in the following order: Program area, degree type (T if terminal Master's), number awarded 7/08–6/09. Language & Cognition PhD (Doctor of Philosophy) 1, Behavioral Neuroscience PhD (Doctor of Philosophy) 2, Social/Personality Psychology PhD (Doctor of Philosophy) 4, Perception PhD (Doctor of Philosophy) 3.

Student Applications/Admissions:
Student Applications
 Language & Cognition PhD (Doctor of Philosophy)—Applications 2009–2010, 29. Total applicants accepted 2009–2010, 5. Number full-time enrolled (new admits only) 2009–2010, 1. Number part-time enrolled (new admits only) 2009–2010, 0. Openings 2010–2011, 2. The median number of years required for completion of a degree in 2008–2009 were 5. The number of students enrolled full- and part-time who were dismissed or voluntarily withdrew from this program area in 2008–2009 were 1. *Behavioral Neuroscience PhD (Doctor of Philosophy)*—Applications 2009–2010, 25. Total applicants accepted 2009–2010, 0. Number full-time enrolled (new admits only) 2009–2010, 1. Number part-time enrolled (new admits only) 2009–2010, 0. Openings 2010–2011, 2. The median number of years required for completion of a degree in 2008–2009 were 5. The number of students enrolled full- and part-time who were dismissed or voluntarily withdrew from this program area in 2008–2009 were 0. *Social/Personality Psychology PhD (Doctor of Philosophy)*—Applications 2009–2010, 50. Total applicants accepted 2009–2010, 2. Number full-time enrolled (new admits only) 2009–2010, 3. Number part-time enrolled (new admits only) 2009–2010, 0. Openings 2010–2011, 2. The median number of years required for completion of a degree in 2008–2009 were 5. The number of students enrolled full- and part-time who were dismissed or voluntarily withdrew from this program area in 2008–2009 were 0. *Perception PhD (Doctor of Philosophy)*—Applications 2009–2010, 11. Total applicants accepted 2009–2010, 1. Number full-time enrolled (new admits only) 2009–2010, 1. Number part-time enrolled (new admits only) 2009–2010, 0. Openings 2010–2011, 2. The median number of years required for completion of a degree in 2008–2009 were 5. The number of students enrolled full- and part-time who were dismissed or voluntarily withdrew from this program area in 2008–2009 were 0.
Other Criteria: (importance of criteria rated low, medium, or high): GRE scores—high, research experience—high, work experience—low, GPA—high, letters of recommendation—high, interview—high, statement of goals and objectives—high, undergraduate major in psychology—low, specific undergraduate psychology courses taken—low.

Student Characteristics: The following represents characteristics of students in 2009–2010 in all graduate psychology programs in the department: Female—full-time 19, part-time 0; Male—full-time 6, part-time 0; African American/Black—full-time 0, part-time 0; Hispanic/Latino(a)—full-time 2, part-time 0; Asian/Pacific Islander—full-time 3, part-time 0; American Indian/Alaska Native—full-time 0, part-time 0; Caucasian/White—full-time 20, part-time 0; Multi-ethnic—full-time 0, part-time 0; students subject to the Americans With Disabilities Act—full-time 0, part-time 0; Unknown ethnicity—full-time 0, part-time 0; International students who hold an F-1 or J-1 Visa—full-time 4, part-time 0.

Financial Information/Assistance:
 Tuition for Full-Time Study: *Doctoral:* State residents: $1,065 per credit hour; Nonstate residents: $1,065 per credit hour.

Financial Assistance:
 First-Year Students: Teaching assistantships available for first year. Average amount paid per academic year: $24,060. Average number of hours worked per week: 20. Apply by January 1. Research assistantships available for first year. Average amount paid per academic year: $24,060. Average number of hours worked per week: 20. Apply by January 1.
 Advanced Students: Teaching assistantships available for advanced students. Average amount paid per academic year: $24,060. Average number of hours worked per week: 20. Apply by January 1. Research assistantships available for advanced students.

Average amount paid per academic year: $24,060. Average number of hours worked per week: 20. Apply by January 1.

Additional Information: Of all students currently enrolled full time, 100% benefited from one or more of the listed financial assistance programs. Application and information available online at: www.northeastern.edu/cas/graduate/financial_aid.

Housing and Day Care: No on-campus housing is available. On-campus day care facilities are available. See the following Web site for more information: http://www.northeastern.edu/hrm/benefits/child.html.

Employment of Department Graduates:
Master's Degree Graduates: Of those who graduated in the academic year 2008–2009, the following categories and numbers represent the postgraduate activities and employment of master's degree graduates: Enrolled in a postdoctoral residency/fellowship (n/a), employed in independent practice (n/a), total from the above (master's) (0).

Doctoral Degree Graduates: Of those who graduated in the academic year 2008–2009, the following categories and numbers represent the postgraduate activities and employment of doctoral degree graduates: Enrolled in a psychology doctoral program (n/a), enrolled in a postdoctoral residency/fellowship (7), employed in independent practice (0), employed in an academic position at a university (2), employed in an academic position at a 2-year/4-year college (1), employed in other positions at a higher education institution (0), employed in a professional position in a school system (0), employed in business or industry (0), employed in government agency (0), employed in a community mental health/counseling center (0), employed in a hospital/medical center (0), still seeking employment (0), not seeking employment (0), other employment position (0), do not know (0), total from the above (doctoral) (10).

Additional Information:
Orientation, Objectives, and Emphasis of Department: The PhD program aims to train students to undertake basic research in the following areas: behavioral neuroscience; perception; language & cognition; and experimental social/personality. Students may expect to collaborate with faculty in conducting research in state-of-the-art laboratories. The doctoral program also provides opportunities to gain teaching experience. The program does not provide training in clinical/counseling psychology.

Special Facilities or Resources: The department has a wide range of research laboratories containing state-of-the-art facilities in the following areas: behavioral neuroscience; perception; language & cognition; and experimental social/personality. These facilities include an array of computer systems used for subject testing, data acquisition and analysis, graphics, and word processing, as well as numerous special-purpose systems, such as eye-trackers, histology facilities, multiple electrode EEG, small animal fMRI, and speech processing systems. In addition, laboratory resources outside the department are available to students through the collaborative network the department maintains with other institutions in the Boston/Cambridge area.

Application Information:
Send to Applications should be submitted online. Application available online. URL of online application: http://www.northeastern.edu/cas/graduate/admissions.html. Students are admitted in the Fall, application deadline January 1. *Fee:* $50.

Springfield College (2009 data)
Department of Psychology
School of Arts and Sciences and Professional Studies
263 Alden Street
Springfield, MA 01109
Telephone: (413) 748-3322
Fax: (413) 748-3854
E-mail: *Glenn_Lowery@spfldcol.edu*
Web: *http://www.spfldcol.edu/psychology*

Department Information:
1946. Chairperson: Glenn Lowery. Number of faculty: total—full-time 15, part-time 1; women—full-time 8; minority—part-time 1.

Programs and Degrees Offered:
Listed in the following order: Program area, degree type (T if terminal Master's), number awarded 7/08–6/09. Athletic Counseling MA/MS (Master of Arts/Science) (T) 12, Industrial/Organizational MA/MS (Master of Arts/Science) (T) 18, Marriage and Family Therapy MA/MS (Master of Arts/Science) (T) 11, Mental Health Counseling MA/MS (Master of Arts/Science) (T) 11, School Guidance Counseling EdS (School Psychology) 18, Student Personnel Administration MA/MS (Master of Arts/Science) (T) 17.

Student Applications/Admissions:
Student Applications

Athletic Counseling MA/MS (Master of Arts/Science)—Applications 2009–2010, 50. Total applicants accepted 2009–2010, 20. Number full-time enrolled (new admits only) 2009–2010, 12. Total enrolled 2009–2010 full-time, 25. Openings 2010–2011, 12. The median number of years required for completion of a degree in 2008–2009 were 2. The number of students enrolled full- and part-time who were dismissed or voluntarily withdrew from this program area in 2008–2009 were 1. *Industrial/Organizational MA/MS (Master of Arts/Science)*—Applications 2009–2010, 40. Total applicants accepted 2009–2010, 28. Number full-time enrolled (new admits only) 2009–2010, 16. Number part-time enrolled (new admits only) 2009–2010, 5. Total enrolled 2009–2010 full-time, 35, part-time, 5. Openings 2010–2011, 17. The median number of years required for completion of a degree in 2008–2009 were 2. The number of students enrolled full- and part-time who were dismissed or voluntarily withdrew from this program area in 2008–2009 were 1. *Marriage and Family Therapy MA/MS (Master of Arts/Science)*—Applications 2009–2010, 30. Total applicants accepted 2009–2010, 26. Number full-time enrolled (new admits only) 2009–2010, 14. Number part-time enrolled (new admits only) 2009–2010, 2. Total enrolled 2009–2010 full-time, 30, part-time, 2. Openings 2010–2011, 15. The median number of years required for completion of a degree in 2008–2009 were 2. The number of students enrolled full- and part-time who were dismissed or voluntarily withdrew from this program area in 2008–2009 were 1. *Mental Health Counseling MA/MS (Master of Arts/Science)*—Applications 2009–2010, 88. Total applicants accepted 2009–2010, 32. Number full-time enrolled (new admits only) 2009–2010, 32. Number part-time enrolled (new admits only) 2009–2010, 3. Total enrolled 2009–2010 full-time, 73, part-time, 2. Openings 2010–2011, 15. The median number of years required for completion of a degree in 2008–2009 were 2. The number of students enrolled full- and part-time who were dismissed or voluntarily withdrew from this program area in 2008–2009 were 0. *School Guidance Counseling EdS (School Psychology)*—Applications 2009–2010, 40. Total applicants accepted 2009–2010, 20. Number full-time enrolled (new admits only) 2009–2010, 8. Number part-time enrolled (new admits only) 2009–2010, 2. Total enrolled 2009–2010 full-time, 20, part-time, 16. Openings 2010–2011, 11. The median number of years required for completion of a degree in 2008–2009 were 2. The number of students enrolled full- and part-time who were dismissed or voluntarily withdrew from this program area in 2008–2009 were 0. *Student Personnel Administration MA/MS (Master of Arts/Science)*—Applications 2009–2010, 47. Total applicants accepted 2009–2010, 40. Number full-time enrolled (new admits only) 2009–2010, 19. Number part-time enrolled (new admits only) 2009–2010, 4. Total enrolled 2009–2010 full-time, 34, part-time, 10. Openings 2010–2011, 12. The median number of years required for completion of a degree in 2008–2009 were 2. The number of students enrolled full- and part-time who were dismissed or voluntarily withdrew from this program area in 2008–2009 were 0.

Other Criteria: (importance of criteria rated low, medium, or high): research experience—low, work experience—medium, extracurricular activity—medium, clinically related public service—high, GPA—medium, letters of recommendation—high, interview—medium, statement of goals and objectives—high, undergraduate major in psychology—medium, specific undergraduate psychology courses taken—medium.

Student Characteristics: The following represents characteristics of students in 2009–2010 in all graduate psychology programs in the department: Female—full-time 91, part-time 12; Male—full-time 55, part-time 17; African American/Black—full-time 8, part-time 0; Hispanic/Latino(a)—full-time 5, part-time 0; Asian/Pacific Islander—full-time 1, part-time 0; American Indian/Alaska Native—full-time 0, part-time 0; Caucasian/White—full-time 0, part-time 0; Multi-ethnic—full-time 0, part-time 0; students subject to the Americans With Disabilities Act—full-time 1, part-time 0; Unknown ethnicity—full-time 0, part-time 0; International students who hold an F-1 or J-1 Visa—full-time 0, part-time 0.

Financial Information/Assistance:
Tuition for Full-Time Study: *Master's:* State residents: $812 per credit hour; Nonstate residents: $812 per credit hour.

Financial Assistance:
First-Year Students: Teaching assistantships available for first year. Research assistantships available for first year. Fellowships and scholarships available for first year. Average amount paid per academic year: $2,000. Apply by March 1.
Advanced Students: Teaching assistantships available for advanced students. Research assistantships available for advanced students. Fellowships and scholarships available for advanced students. Average amount paid per academic year: $2,000. Apply by March 1.

Additional Information: Of all students currently enrolled full time, 30% benefited from one or more of the listed financial assistance programs.

Internships/Practica: Master's Degree (MA/MS Athletic Counseling): An internship experience, such as a final research project or "capstone" experience is required of graduates. Master's Degree (MA/MS Marriage and Family Therapy): An internship experience, such as a final research project or "capstone" experience is required of graduates. Master's Degree (MA/MS Mental Health Counseling): An internship experience, such as a final research project or "capstone" experience is required of graduates. Master's Degree (MA/MS Student Personnel Administration): An internship experience, such as a final research project or "capstone" experience is required of graduates. Numerous internships, paid and unpaid, exist for students in their field of study. Established affiliation agreements are in place with regional corporate, clinical and counseling settings. A Cooperative Education Program provides students with opportunities for credited, paid internships.

Housing and Day Care: On-campus housing is available. On-campus day care facilities are available.

Employment of Department Graduates:
Master's Degree Graduates: Of those who graduated in the academic year 2008–2009, the following categories and numbers represent the postgraduate activities and employment of master's degree graduates: Enrolled in another graduate/professional program (33), enrolled in a postdoctoral residency/fellowship (n/a), employed in independent practice (n/a), employed in other positions at a higher education institution (12), employed in a professional position in a school system (10), employed in business or industry (11), employed in a community mental health/counseling center (27), employed in a hospital/medical center (3), total from the above (master's) (96).
Doctoral Degree Graduates: Of those who graduated in the academic year 2008–2009, the following categories and numbers represent the postgraduate activities and employment of doctoral degree graduates: Enrolled in a psychology doctoral program (n/a), total from the above (doctoral) (0).

Additional Information:
Orientation, Objectives, and Emphasis of Department: Understanding of personal values, attitudes, and needs is a primary characteristic of effective facilitators. The psychology and counseling programs, therefore, design many of the experiences to help students increase their awareness of self and the ways in which personal behavior affects others. While mastery of content areas is expected, continual reference to personal relevance of that content is encouraged. Frequent opportunities are afforded for students to understand themselves better through participation in group and individual experiences. As a reflection of the value placed upon individual program development, the comprehensive examination requirement is not the traditional written and oral exercise. Some of the Psychology and Counseling programs use the portfolio system, which is an ongoing, active evaluation process. A more traditional thesis or research project is also offered and supported when chosen, and individual attention is readily available for both options.

Special Facilities or Resources: The department offers fully equipped counseling and research laboratories and audiovisual facilities. Access to computers and excellent physiological and fitness laboratories are available. The Department also sponsors the Center for Performance Enhancement and Applied Research (CPEAR), which serves as a clearinghouse for information about grants and research opportunities.

Application Information:
Send to Graduate Admissions, 263 Alden Street, Springfield, MA 01109. Application available online. URL of online application: http://www.spfldcol.edu. Summer, application deadline rolling. *Fee:* $50.

Suffolk University
Department of Psychology
College of Arts and Sciences
41 Temple Street
Boston, MA 02114
Telephone: (617) 573-8293
Fax: (617) 367-2924
E-mail: *sorsillo@suffolk.edu*
Web: *http://www.suffolk.edu/psychology*

Department Information:
1968. Director of Clinical Training: Sue Orsillo. Number of faculty: total—full-time 13, part-time 5; women—full-time 8, part-time 2; total—minority—full-time 3; women minority—full-time 3.

Programs and Degrees Offered:
Listed in the following order: Program area, degree type (T if terminal Master's), number awarded 7/08–6/09. Clinical Psychology PhD (Doctor of Philosophy) 14, Clinical Psychology Respecialization Respecialization Diploma 0.

APA Accreditation: Clinical PhD (Doctor of Philosophy). Student Outcome Data Website: http://www.suffolk.edu/college/23107.html.

Student Applications/Admissions:
Student Applications
Clinical Psychology PhD (Doctor of Philosophy)—Applications 2009–2010, 268. Total applicants accepted 2009–2010, 12. Number full-time enrolled (new admits only) 2009–2010, 12. Number part-time enrolled (new admits only) 2009–2010, 0. Openings 2010–2011, 12. The median number of years required for completion of a degree in 2008–2009 were 6. The number of students enrolled full- and part-time who were dismissed or voluntarily withdrew from this program area in 2008–2009 were 1. *Clinical Psychology Respecialization Respecialization Diploma*—Applications 2009–2010, 4. Total applicants accepted 2009–2010, 3. Number full-time enrolled (new admits only) 2009–2010, 1. Number part-time enrolled (new admits only) 2009–2010, 0. Openings 2010–2011, 2. The number of students enrolled full- and part-time who were dismissed or voluntarily withdrew from this program area in 2008–2009 were 0.

Scores: Entries appear in this order: required test or GPA, minimum score (if required), median score of students entering in 2009–2010. *Clinical Psychology PhD (Doctor of Philosophy):* GRE-V no minimum stated, 615, GRE-Q no minimum stated, 640, GRE-Analytical no minimum stated, 5.0, overall undergraduate GPA no minimum stated, 3.58.

Other Criteria: (importance of criteria rated low, medium, or high): GRE scores—medium, research experience—high, work experience—medium, extracurricular activity—low, clinically related public service—medium, GPA—high, letters of recommendation—high, interview—high, statement of goals and objectives—high, research mentor match—high, undergraduate major in psychology—high, specific undergraduate psychology courses taken—medium. For additional information on admission requirements, go to http://www.suffolk.edu/college/12093.html.

Student Characteristics: The following represents characteristics of students in 2009–2010 in all graduate psychology programs in the department: Female—full-time 74, part-time 0; Male—full-time 14, part-time 0; African American/Black—full-time 3, part-time 0; Hispanic/Latino(a)—full-time 5, part-time 0; Asian/Pacific Islander—full-time 5, part-time 0; American Indian/Alaska Native—full-time 0, part-time 0; Caucasian/White—full-time 75, part-time 0; Multi-ethnic—full-time 0, part-time 0; students subject to the Americans With Disabilities Act—full-time 0, part-time 0; Unknown ethnicity—full-time 0, part-time 0; International students who hold an F-1 or J-1 Visa—full-time 3, part-time 0.

Financial Information/Assistance:
Tuition for Full-Time Study: *Doctoral:* State residents: per academic year $31,078, $1,294 per credit hour; Nonstate residents: per academic year $31,078, $1,294 per credit hour. Tuition is subject to change. See the following Web site for updates and changes in tuition costs: http://www.suffolk.edu/admission/27864.html.

Financial Assistance:
First-Year Students: Research assistantships available for first year. Average amount paid per academic year: $4,800. Average number of hours worked per week: 10. Apply by April 1. Fellowships and scholarships available for first year. Average amount paid per academic year: $5,550. Average number of hours worked per week: 15. Apply by April 1.

Advanced Students: Research assistantships available for advanced students. Average amount paid per academic year: $4,800. Average number of hours worked per week: 10. Apply by April 1. Fellowships and scholarships available for advanced students. Average amount paid per academic year: $5,550. Average number of hours worked per week: 15. Apply by April 1.

Additional Information: Of all students currently enrolled full time, 75% benefited from one or more of the listed financial assistance programs. Application and information available online at: http://www.suffolk.edu/college/24767.html.

Internships/Practica: Doctoral Degree (PhD Clinical Psychology): For those doctoral students for whom a professional internship was required in this program prior to graduation, (13) students applied for an internship in 2008–2009, with (12) students obtaining an internship. Of those students who obtained an internship, (11) were paid internships. Of those students who obtained

an internship, (11) students placed in APA/CPA accredited internships, (0) students placed in internships not APA/CPA accredited, but listed with the Association of Psychology Postdoctoral and Internship Programs (APPIC), (0) students placed in internships conforming to guidelines of the Council of Directors of School Psychology Programs (CDSPP), (1) students placed in internships that were not APA/CPA accredited, APPIC or CDSPP listed. Students in the doctoral program begin their official practicum training in the fall of their second year. All students are required to complete at least two years of practicum training, though many elect to do an optional summer or third year prior to applying for predoctoral internship. A limited number of pre-practicum training experiences are also available to students during their first year in the program. Students are placed with partner sites (medical centers, community mental health clinics and schools) in the greater Boston area that are committed to providing quality supervision and that provide training that is consistent with our program philosophy. While placed at these sites, students take two year-long practicum classes which serve to: 1) integrate the external practicum training experience with other elements of our program, and 2) provide knowledge regarding professional standards and ethics, diversity, treatment and assessment process and outcomes, consultation and supervision. Students who opt to pursue an additional year of clinical training are supported in their efforts to obtain a training experience that is consistent with their emerging areas of specific interest. Two years of practicum experience are required of our doctoral students beginning in their second academic year. A third year is optional, but strongly recommended. Students receive weekly supervision by professionals at their practicum sites and attend a weekly practicum seminar at Suffolk University where they are able to integrate their practical experiences and educational training within the program. Students receive a total of four hours a week, on average, of individual and group supervision during each of their three years of practicum training.

Housing and Day Care: No on-campus housing is available. No on-campus day care facilities are available.

Employment of Department Graduates:
Master's Degree Graduates: Of those who graduated in the academic year 2008–2009, the following categories and numbers represent the postgraduate activities and employment of master's degree graduates: Enrolled in a postdoctoral residency/fellowship (n/a), employed in independent practice (n/a), total from the above (master's) (0).
Doctoral Degree Graduates: Of those who graduated in the academic year 2008–2009, the following categories and numbers represent the postgraduate activities and employment of doctoral degree graduates: Enrolled in a psychology doctoral program (n/a), enrolled in a postdoctoral residency/fellowship (12), employed in a community mental health/counseling center (1), employed in a hospital/medical center (1), total from the above (doctoral) (14).

Additional Information:
Orientation, Objectives, and Emphasis of Department: Suffolk University's PhD program in clinical psychology is based on the philosophy that clinical practice should be grounded in scientific knowledge and that scientific research should be informed by and be relevant to clinical practice. The program's orientation is that of understanding the processes underlying adaptation and maladaptation within a cultural frame. Our faculty approach clinical work from a variety of perspectives including developmental, psychodynamic, systemic, behavioral, cognitive-behavioral, humanistic and integrative/eclectic. Our intent is to enable students to take a creative, empirical, and ethical approach to clinical problems among diverse populations; to critically evaluate and contribute to the evolving body of scholarly literature in the science and practice of psychology; and to integrate the clinical, theoretical, and scientific foundations of psychology. Our program adheres to a generalist model of clinical training, although we also offer concentrated experiences in neuropsychology and child clinical psychology. Across all aspects of our training program we strive to train our students to be knowledgeable about and conduct culturally competent clinical practice and research. Implications of this framework include the recognition that: (a) knowledge of a breadth of psychological subdisciplines such as neuropsychology, developmental psychology, cultural psychology, is required to effectively work within the clinical developmental model; (b) professional psychologists can complement the roles of natural contexts such as families, relationships, schools, and workplaces in fostering development; and (c) psychological pain and conflict can be understood as indicative of a continuum of ongoing life span transformational processes, which include what is typically labeled normal development as well as the development or manifestation of psychopathology. Thus, the program emphasizes that clinical problems are best understood in the context of knowledge about normal and optimal development over the lifespan. The program strives to develop student competencies necessary for successfully working in a range of clinical, educational, research, organizational, and public policy settings. Throughout content and applied areas of training, the program encourages awareness of and respect for diversity of culture, language, national origin, race, gender, age, disability, religious beliefs, sexual orientation, lifestyle, and other individual differences. The program combines a strong theoretical and research background (in both quantitative and qualitative methodologies) with preparation to deliver high-quality psychological services to children, adolescents, and adults.

Special Facilities or Resources: The department has a variety of laboratory spaces available for general use by faculty and doctoral students. Special equipment includes one-way mirrors and video cameras. A great deal of research occurs off-site in the clinical, medical, and scholastic institutions of the Boston area. There are two computer labs for graduate student use within the department in addition to larger computer labs throughout the university; all provide access to SPSS, the Internet, and electronic databases. Graduate students receive inter-library loan and online document delivery privileges and have access to most of the academic libraries in the Boston area.

Information for Students With Physical Disabilities: See the following Web site for more information: http://www.suffolk.edu/campuslife/disabilityservices.html.

Application Information:
Send to Office of Graduate Admissions, 8 Ashburton Place, Boston, MA 02108. Application available online. URL of online application: https://www.applyweb.com/apply/suffcas. Students are admitted in the Fall, application deadline December 1. *Fee:* $50.

Tufts University
Department of Education; School Psychology Program
Graduate School of Arts and Sciences
Paige Hall
Medford, MA 02155
Telephone: (617) 627-2390
Fax: (617) 627-3901
E-mail: steven.luz-alterman@tufts.edu
Web: http://ase.tufts.edu/education/programs/schoolPsych/

Department Information:
1910. Co-Director, School Psychology Program: Steven Luz-Alterman. Number of faculty: total—full-time 15, part-time 13; women—full-time 11, part-time 9; total—minority—full-time 6, part-time 1; women minority—full-time 5, part-time 1.

Programs and Degrees Offered:
Listed in the following order: Program area, degree type (T if terminal Master's), number awarded 7/08–6/09. School Psychology EdS (School Psychology) 15.

Student Applications/Admissions:
Student Applications
School Psychology EdS (School Psychology)—Applications 2009–2010, 93. Total applicants accepted 2009–2010, 32. Number full-time enrolled (new admits only) 2009–2010, 17. Number part-time enrolled (new admits only) 2009–2010, 0. Openings 2010–2011, 16. The median number of years required for completion of a degree in 2008–2009 were 3. The number of students enrolled full- and part-time who were dismissed or voluntarily withdrew from this program area in 2008–2009 were 1.
Scores: Entries appear in this order: required test or GPA, minimum score (if required), median score of students entering in 2009–2010. School Psychology EdS (School Psychology): GRE-V 500, 551, GRE-Q 500, 648, GRE-Analytical 4.5, 5.0, overall undergraduate GPA no minimum stated.
Other Criteria: (importance of criteria rated low, medium, or high): GRE scores—medium, research experience—medium, work experience—high, extracurricular activity—medium, clinically related public service—high, GPA—high, letters of recommendation—high, interview—high, statement of goals and objectives—high, multicultural interest—high, undergraduate major in psychology—low, specific undergraduate psychology courses taken—medium. For additional information on admission requirements, go to http://gradstudy.tufts.edu/admissions/index.htm.

Student Characteristics: The following represents characteristics of students in 2009–2010 in all graduate psychology programs in the department: Female—full-time 37, part-time 0; Male—full-time 9, part-time 0; African American/Black—full-time 1, part-time 0; Hispanic/Latino(a)—full-time 3, part-time 0; Asian/Pacific Islander—full-time 3, part-time 0; American Indian/Alaska Native—full-time 0, part-time 0; Caucasian/White—full-time 36, part-time 1; Multi-ethnic—full-time 3, part-time 0; students subject to the Americans With Disabilities Act—full-time 1, part-time 0; Unknown ethnicity—full-time 0, part-time 0; International students who hold an F-1 or J-1 Visa—full-time 0, part-time 0.

Financial Information/Assistance:
Tuition for Full-Time Study: Master's: State residents: per academic year $34,670; Nonstate residents: per academic year $34,670. See the following Web site for updates and changes in tuition costs: http://gradstudy.tufts.edu/admissions/expensesfinaid/index.htm.

Financial Assistance:
First-Year Students: Teaching assistantships available for first year. Average amount paid per academic year: $1,500. Average number of hours worked per week: 4. Apply by September 1. Research assistantships available for first year. Average amount paid per academic year: $1,500. Average number of hours worked per week: 4. Apply by September 1. Fellowships and scholarships available for first year. Average amount paid per academic year: $14,000. Apply by February 1.
Advanced Students: Teaching assistantships available for advanced students. Average amount paid per academic year: $1,500. Average number of hours worked per week: 4. Apply by September 1. Research assistantships available for advanced students. Average amount paid per academic year: $1,500. Average number of hours worked per week: 4. Apply by September 1. Fellowships and scholarships available for advanced students. Average amount paid per academic year: $14,000. Apply by February 1.
Additional Information: Of all students currently enrolled full time, 90% benefited from one or more of the listed financial assistance programs. Application and information available online at: http://ase.tufts.edu/education/admissions/.

Internships/Practica: Students complete a school-based pre-practicum experience of 150 hours during their first year and a school-based practicum of 600 hours during their second year. Students complete a 1200-hour internship during their third year. This may be completed through 600 hours in a school setting and 600 hours in a clinical setting, or all 1200 hours in a school setting. Internship sites must be approved by the program faculty and may be pursued anywhere in the United States.

Housing and Day Care: On-campus housing is available. See the following Web site for more information: http://ase.tufts.edu/reslife/housing/graduate.asp. On-campus day care facilities are available. See the following Web site for more information: http://ase.tufts.edu/tedcc/.

Employment of Department Graduates:
Master's Degree Graduates: Of those who graduated in the academic year 2008–2009, the following categories and numbers represent the postgraduate activities and employment of master's degree graduates: Enrolled in a postdoctoral residency/fellowship (n/a), employed in independent practice (n/a), employed in a professional position in a school system (15), total from the above (master's) (15).
Doctoral Degree Graduates: Of those who graduated in the academic year 2008–2009, the following categories and numbers represent the postgraduate activities and employment of doctoral degree graduates: Enrolled in a psychology doctoral program (n/a), total from the above (doctoral) (0).

Additional Information:
Orientation, Objectives, and Emphasis of Department: Our mission is to prepare highly effective, culturally competent problem

solvers ready to serve all children in general public education and children with disabilities. We are committed to preparing professional school psychologists who will work effectively with children from racially, ethnically, and linguistically diverse backgrounds in a variety of settings. These include urban, urban-rim, suburban, and rural communities. Providing high quality services in urban and urban-rim schools is a program priority. We seek a diverse cohort of students who think critically and are prepared to engage issues of social justice and cultural and linguistic diversity as they are reproduced in our schools.

Special Facilities or Resources: Tufts offers the resources of a major research university with the campus atmosphere of a small liberal arts college. Several courses of interest are offered through the Eliot-Pearson Department of Child Development. Tufts students may also cross-register for courses at several other Boston universities at no additional charge through a consortium arrangement. We have a variety of urban, urban rim, and suburban field sites, including partnerships with Children's Hospital and Wediko Children's Services in Boston.

Information for Students With Physical Disabilities: See the following Web site for more information: http://uss.tufts.edu/arc/disability/.

Application Information:
Send to Office of Graduate and Professional Studies, Tufts University Ballou Hall, Medford, MA 02155. Application available online. URL of online application: http://gradstudy.tufts.edu/admissions/howtoapply.htm. Students are admitted in the Fall, application deadline February 1. *Fee:* $75.

Tufts University
Department of Psychology
Psychology Building, 490 Boston Avenue
Medford, MA 02155
Telephone: (617) 627-3523
Fax: (617) 627-3181
E-mail: cynthia.goddard@tufts.edu
Web: http://ase.tufts.edu/psychology/

Department Information:
Chairperson: Robert Cook. Number of faculty: total—full-time 20; women—full-time 9; total—minority—full-time 4; women minority—full-time 2.

Programs and Degrees Offered:
Listed in the following order: Program area, degree type (T if terminal Master's), number awarded 7/08–6/09. General Experimental Psychology PhD (Doctor of Philosophy) 8.

Student Applications/Admissions:
Student Applications
General Experimental Psychology PhD (Doctor of Philosophy)—Applications 2009–2010, 163. Total applicants accepted 2009–2010, 8. Number full-time enrolled (new admits only) 2009–2010, 8. Total enrolled 2009–2010 full-time, 40. Openings 2010–2011, 8. The median number of years required for completion of a degree in 2008–2009 were 6. The number of students enrolled full- and part-time who were dismissed or voluntarily withdrew from this program area in 2008–2009 were 0.

Other Criteria: (importance of criteria rated low, medium, or high): GRE scores—medium, research experience—high, work experience—medium, extracurricular activity—low, GPA—medium, letters of recommendation—high, interview—medium, statement of goals and objectives—high, research fit—high, undergraduate major in psychology—medium, specific undergraduate psychology courses taken—medium.

Student Characteristics: The following represents characteristics of students in 2009–2010 in all graduate psychology programs in the department: Female—full-time 24, part-time 0; Male—full-time 16, part-time 0; African American/Black—full-time 1, part-time 0; Hispanic/Latino(a)—full-time 2, part-time 0; Asian/Pacific Islander—full-time 4, part-time 0; American Indian/Alaska Native—full-time 0, part-time 0; Caucasian/White—full-time 32, part-time 0; Multi-ethnic—full-time 1, part-time 0; students subject to the Americans With Disabilities Act—full-time 1, part-time 0; Unknown ethnicity—full-time 0, part-time 0; International students who hold an F-1 or J-1 Visa—full-time 6, part-time 0.

Financial Information/Assistance:
Tuition for Full-Time Study: Doctoral: State residents: per academic year $38,840; Nonstate residents: per academic year $38,840. See the following Web site for updates and changes in tuition costs: http://ase.tufts.edu/admissions/expensesfinaid.

Financial Assistance:
First-Year Students: Teaching assistantships available for first year. Average amount paid per academic year: $20,052. Average number of hours worked per week: 20. Research assistantships available for first year. Average amount paid per academic year: $20,052. Average number of hours worked per week: 20.

Advanced Students: Teaching assistantships available for advanced students. Average amount paid per academic year: $20,452. Average number of hours worked per week: 20. Research assistantships available for advanced students. Average amount paid per academic year: $20,452. Average number of hours worked per week: 20.

Additional Information: Of all students currently enrolled full time, 100% benefited from one or more of the listed financial assistance programs.

Housing and Day Care: No on-campus housing is available. On-campus day care facilities are available. See the following Web site for more information: http://ase.tufts.edu/tedcc/.

Employment of Department Graduates:
Master's Degree Graduates: Of those who graduated in the academic year 2008–2009, the following categories and numbers represent the postgraduate activities and employment of master's degree graduates: Enrolled in a postdoctoral residency/fellowship (n/a), employed in independent practice (n/a), total from the above (master's) (0).

Doctoral Degree Graduates: Of those who graduated in the academic year 2008–2009, the following categories and numbers represent the postgraduate activities and employment of doctoral

degree graduates: Enrolled in a psychology doctoral program (n/a), enrolled in a postdoctoral residency/fellowship (4), employed in an academic position at a 2-year/4-year college (1), employed in business or industry (1), not seeking employment (1), total from the above (doctoral) (7).

Additional Information:
Orientation, Objectives, and Emphasis of Department: The Department of Psychology offers a graduate program in experimental psychology, with specializations in cognition, neuroscience, psychopathology, developmental, and social psychology. The program is designed to produce broadly trained graduates who are prepared for careers in teaching, research, or applied psychology. The department does not offer clinical training. Accepted applicants generally possess a substantial college background in psychology, including familiarity with fundamental statistical concepts and research design. The university is a PhD track program although completion of an MS is required as an integral part of the program. Students who already possess a master's degree may be admitted to the PhD program if a sufficient number of credits are acceptable for transfer and a thesis has been done. Areas of faculty research include infant perception, memory processes, animal cognition and learning, neural and hormonal control of animal sexual behavior, psychopharmacology, event-related brain potentials, neuropsychology of language processes, nutrition and behavior, experimental psychopathology, emotion, human factors, decision making, spatial cognition, psychology and law, and the social psychology of prejudicial attitudes. All graduate students participate in supervised research and/or teaching activities each semester. The department provides laboratory space and equipment for many kinds of research, and facilities are available for the behavioral and physiological study of humans and experimental animals.

Special Facilities or Resources: Department has relatively new research facilities for both human and animal research in areas of cognition, biopsychology, neuroscience, developmental and social psychology.

Application Information:
Send to Graduate School, Tufts University, Ballou Hall, Medford, MA 02155. Application available online. URL of online application: http://ase.tufts.edu/gradstudy/admissions.htm. Students are admitted in the Fall, application deadline December 15. *Fee:* $50.

Tufts University
Eliot-Pearson Department of Child Development
105 College Avenue
Medford, MA 02155
Telephone: (617) 627-3355
Fax: (617) 627-3503
E-mail: *jayanthi.mistry@tufts.edu*
Web: *http://ase.tufts.edu/epcd/*

Department Information:
1964. Chairperson: Jayanthi Mistry. Number of faculty: total—full-time 16, part-time 11; women—full-time 10, part-time 9; total—minority—full-time 4, part-time 1; women minority—full-time 3, part-time 1.

Programs and Degrees Offered:
Listed in the following order: Program area, degree type (T if terminal Master's), number awarded 7/08–6/09. Child Development (Thesis) MA/MS (Master of Arts/Science) (T) 0, Child Development MA/MS (Master of Arts/Science) (T) 25, Applied Child Development MA/MS (Master of Arts/Science) 0, Applied Child Development PhD (Doctor of Philosophy) 6, Applied Child Development Certificate 0.

Student Applications/Admissions:
Student Applications
Child Development (Thesis) MA/MS (Master of Arts/Science)—Applications 2009–2010, 2. Total applicants accepted 2009–2010, 2. Number full-time enrolled (new admits only) 2009–2010, 2. Total enrolled 2009–2010 full-time, 10, part-time, 2. Openings 2010–2011, 2. The number of students enrolled full- and part-time who were dismissed or voluntarily withdrew from this program area in 2008–2009 were 0. *Child Development MA/MS (Master of Arts/Science)*—Applications 2009–2010, 82. Total applicants accepted 2009–2010, 55. Number full-time enrolled (new admits only) 2009–2010, 29. Total enrolled 2009–2010 full-time, 36, part-time, 3. Openings 2010–2011, 55. The median number of years required for completion of a degree in 2008–2009 were 2. The number of students enrolled full- and part-time who were dismissed or voluntarily withdrew from this program area in 2008–2009 were 0. *Applied Child Development MA/MS (Master of Arts/Science)*—Applications 2009–2010, 9. Total applicants accepted 2009–2010, 4. Number full-time enrolled (new admits only) 2009–2010, 1. Number part-time enrolled (new admits only) 2009–2010, 0. Openings 2010–2011, 2. The number of students enrolled full- and part-time who were dismissed or voluntarily withdrew from this program area in 2008–2009 were 0. *Applied Child Development PhD (Doctor of Philosophy)*—Applications 2009–2010, 102. Total applicants accepted 2009–2010, 6. Number full-time enrolled (new admits only) 2009–2010, 2. Total enrolled 2009–2010 full-time, 34. Openings 2010–2011, 4. The median number of years required for completion of a degree in 2008–2009 were 5. The number of students enrolled full- and part-time who were dismissed or voluntarily withdrew from this program area in 2008–2009 were 0. *Applied Child Development Certificate Other*—Applications 2009–2010, 0. Total applicants accepted 2009–2010, 0. Number full-time enrolled (new admits only) 2009–2010, 0. Number part-time enrolled (new admits only) 2009–2010, 0. The number of students enrolled full- and part-time who were dismissed or voluntarily withdrew from this program area in 2008–2009 were 0.

Scores: Entries appear in this order: required test or GPA, minimum score (if required), median score of students entering in 2009–2010. *Child Development (Thesis) MA/MS (Master of Arts/Science):* GRE-V no minimum stated, GRE-Q no minimum stated, overall undergraduate GPA no minimum stated, last 2 years GPA no minimum stated; *Child Development MA/MS (Master of Arts/Science):* GRE-V no minimum stated, GRE-Q no minimum stated, overall undergraduate GPA no minimum stated, last 2 years GPA no minimum stated; *Applied Child Development MA/MS (Master of Arts/Science):* GRE-V no minimum stated, GRE-Q no minimum stated, overall undergraduate GPA no minimum stated, last 2 years GPA no minimum stated; *Applied Child Development PhD (Doctor of Philosophy):* GRE-V no minimum stated, GRE-Q no minimum stated, overall undergraduate GPA no minimum stated, last

2 years GPA no minimum stated, Masters GPA no minimum stated; *Applied Child Development Certificate:* GRE-V no minimum stated, GRE-Q no minimum stated, overall undergraduate GPA no minimum stated, last 2 years GPA no minimum stated.

Other Criteria: (importance of criteria rated low, medium, or high): GRE scores—medium, research experience—low, work experience—high, extracurricular activity—low, clinically related public service—low, GPA—high, letters of recommendation—high, statement of goals and objectives—medium, undergraduate major in psychology—low, specific undergraduate psychology courses taken—low. The criteria filled in above is for consideration to our MA programs. The criteria for application to our PhD program is as follows: GRE: high, Research Exp: high, Work Exp: high, Extracurricular: low, Clinically Related Public Serv: low, GPA: high, Letters of Rec: high, Interview: low, Statement of Goals/Obj: high, UG major psych: medium, Spec UG courses: medium.

Student Characteristics: The following represents characteristics of students in 2009–2010 in all graduate psychology programs in the department: Female—full-time 32, part-time 7; Male—full-time 0, part-time 2; African American/Black—full-time 0, part-time 1; Hispanic/Latino(a)—full-time 3, part-time 1; Asian/Pacific Islander—full-time 1, part-time 0; American Indian/Alaska Native—full-time 0, part-time 0; Caucasian/White—full-time 19, part-time 6; Multi-ethnic—full-time 0, part-time 0; students subject to the Americans With Disabilities Act—full-time 0, part-time 0; Unknown ethnicity—full-time 7, part-time 1; International students who hold an F-1 or J-1 Visa—full-time 2, part-time 0.

Financial Information/Assistance:

Tuition for Full-Time Study: Master's: State residents: per academic year $39,624; Nonstate residents: per academic year $39,624. *Doctoral:* State residents: per academic year $23,774; Nonstate residents: per academic year $23,774. Tuition is subject to change. Tuition costs vary by program. See the following Web site for updates and changes in tuition costs: http://gradstudy.tufts.edu/admissions/expensesfinaid/tuitionartssciences.htm.

Financial Assistance:

First-Year Students: Teaching assistantships available for first year. Research assistantships available for first year. Fellowships and scholarships available for first year.

Advanced Students: Teaching assistantships available for advanced students. Research assistantships available for advanced students. Fellowships and scholarships available for advanced students.

Additional Information: Of all students currently enrolled full time, 70% benefited from one or more of the listed financial assistance programs. Application and information available online at: http://ase.tufts.edu/epcd/programsGradFinAid.asp.

Internships/Practica: Master's Degree (MA/MS Child Development (Thesis)): An internship experience, such as a final research project or "capstone" experience is required of graduates. Master's Degree (MA/MS Child Development): An internship experience, such as a final research project or "capstone" experience is required of graduates. MA students engage in semester-long internship in applied settings such as hospitals, after-school centers, arts programs, policy centers, museums. PhD students engage in full-time 1-semester or half time full-year applied and research internships in varied settings.

Housing and Day Care: On-campus housing is available. On-campus day care facilities are available.

Employment of Department Graduates:

Master's Degree Graduates: Of those who graduated in the academic year 2008–2009, the following categories and numbers represent the postgraduate activities and employment of master's degree graduates: Enrolled in a psychology doctoral program (15), enrolled in another graduate/professional program (5), enrolled in a postdoctoral residency/fellowship (n/a), employed in independent practice (n/a), employed in an academic position at a university (0), employed in an academic position at a 2-year/4-year college (10), employed in other positions at a higher education institution (0), employed in a professional position in a school system (20), employed in business or industry (5), employed in government agency (10), employed in a community mental health/counseling center (15), employed in a hospital/medical center (10), still seeking employment (10), not seeking employment (0), other employment position (0), do not know (0), total from the above (master's) (100).

Doctoral Degree Graduates: Of those who graduated in the academic year 2008–2009, the following categories and numbers represent the postgraduate activities and employment of doctoral degree graduates: Enrolled in a psychology doctoral program (n/a), enrolled in a postdoctoral residency/fellowship (10), employed in independent practice (10), employed in an academic position at a university (25), employed in an academic position at a 2-year/4-year college (10), employed in other positions at a higher education institution (10), employed in a professional position in a school system (10), employed in business or industry (0), employed in government agency (10), employed in a community mental health/counseling center (0), employed in a hospital/medical center (5), still seeking employment (0), not seeking employment (0), other employment position (10), do not know (0), total from the above (doctoral) (100).

Additional Information:

Orientation, Objectives, and Emphasis of Department: The department prepares students for a variety of careers that have, as their common prerequisite, a comprehensive understanding of children and their development. Students receive a foundation in psychological theory and research concerning the social, emotional, intellectual, linguistic, and physiological growth of children. Course material is complemented with progressively more involved practica encompassing observations and work with children in a wide variety of applied and research settings. The major aim of the program is to train people who can translate their knowledge about development into effective strategies for working with and on behalf of children. We believe that a background in child development is the best possible preparation for teaching and administrative careers in schools, children's advocacy and mental health agencies, hospitals, after-school programs, daycare centers, arts programs, museums, the media, government agencies concerned with the rights and welfare of children, and related fields. There is considerable room for flexibility in the program. Also, students may chose from a rich variety of elective courses that touch upon such diverse topics as child advocacy, the arts and children's development, children and technology, arts and social activism, and children's literature.

Special Facilities or Resources: The department is housed in a complex of buildings on the Medford campus. The main building contains faculty and staff offices, class meeting rooms, and a library. Another building houses the Eliot-Pearson Children's School, which serves normal and special-needs children aged 2 to 6. The school has observation booths for student use. The department is also associated with the Tufts Educational Day Care Center. Students may work, as well as observe, in all of these settings. Both facilities are integrated into faculty research and research training for graduate students.

Application Information:
Send to Office of Graduate Studies, Tufts University, Ballou Hall, Medford, MA 02155. Application available online. URL of online application: https://apply.embark.com/Grad/Tufts/grad/16/. Students are admitted in the Fall, application deadline January 15. *Fee:* $75. The application fee is waived only for current Tufts undergraduates and graduate students, students in Tufts certificate programs, Project 1000 applicants, and IRT and McNair Scholars. No other fee waivers are considered.

MICHIGAN

Central Michigan University
Department of Psychology
Humanities and Social and Behavioral Sciences
Sloan Hall
Mount Pleasant, MI 48859
Telephone: (989) 774-3001
Fax: (989) 774-2553
E-mail: *hough1ba@cmich.edu*
Web: *http://www.chsbs.cmich.edu/psychology*

Department Information:
1965. Chairperson: Hajime Otani. Number of faculty: total—full-time 31, part-time 7; women—full-time 10, part-time 3; total—minority—full-time 4; women minority—full-time 1.

Programs and Degrees Offered:
Listed in the following order: Program area, degree type (T if terminal Master's), number awarded 7/08–6/09. Experimental Psychology PhD (Doctor of Philosophy) 2, Clinical Psychology PhD (Doctor of Philosophy) 7, General Psychology MA/MS (Master of Arts/Science) (T) 5, School Psychology PhD (Doctor of Philosophy) 1, Specialist in School Psychology 5, Industrial/Organizational Psychology MA/MS (Master of Arts/Science) (T) 1, Industrial/Organizational Psychology PhD (Doctor of Philosophy) 1.

APA Accreditation: Clinical PhD (Doctor of Philosophy). Student Outcome Data Website: http://www.cmich.edu/chsbs/x20746.xml. School PhD (Doctor of Philosophy). Student Outcome Data Website: http://www.cmich.edu/chsbs/x20694.xml.

Student Applications/Admissions:
Student Applications
Experimental Psychology PhD (Doctor of Philosophy)—Applications 2009–2010, 21. Total applicants accepted 2009–2010, 4. Number full-time enrolled (new admits only) 2009–2010, 4. Openings 2010–2011, 3. The median number of years required for completion of a degree in 2008–2009 were 6. Clinical Psychology PhD (Doctor of Philosophy)—Applications 2009–2010, 157. Total applicants accepted 2009–2010, 4. Number full-time enrolled (new admits only) 2009–2010, 4. Openings 2010–2011, 5. The median number of years required for completion of a degree in 2008–2009 were 6. The number of students enrolled full- and part-time who were dismissed or voluntarily withdrew from this program area in 2008–2009 were 2. General Psychology MA/MS (Master of Arts/Science)—Applications 2009–2010, 15. Total applicants accepted 2009–2010, 4. Number full-time enrolled (new admits only) 2009–2010, 4. Openings 2010–2011, 2. The median number of years required for completion of a degree in 2008–2009 were 4. The number of students enrolled full- and part-time who were dismissed or voluntarily withdrew from this program area in 2008–2009 were 1. School Psychology PhD (Doctor of Philosophy)—Applications 2009–2010, 29. Total applicants accepted 2009–2010, 10. Number full-time enrolled (new admits only) 2009–2010, 10. Total enrolled 2009–2010 full-time, 24. Openings 2010–2011, 3. The median number of years required for completion of a degree in 2008–2009 were 5. Specialist in School Psychology—Applications 2009–2010, 35. Total applicants accepted 2009–2010, 4. Number full-time enrolled (new admits only) 2009–2010, 4. Total enrolled 2009–2010 full-time, 22. The median number of years required for completion of a degree in 2008–2009 were 4. The number of students enrolled full- and part-time who were dismissed or voluntarily withdrew from this program area in 2008–2009 were 0. Industrial/Organizational Psychology MA/MS (Master of Arts/Science)—Applications 2009–2010, 21. Total applicants accepted 2009–2010, 2. Number full-time enrolled (new admits only) 2009–2010, 2. Total enrolled 2009–2010 full-time, 5. Openings 2010–2011, 1. The median number of years required for completion of a degree in 2008–2009 were 2. The number of students enrolled full- and part-time who were dismissed or voluntarily withdrew from this program area in 2008–2009 were 0. Industrial/Organizational Psychology PhD (Doctor of Philosophy)—Applications 2009–2010, 58. Total applicants accepted 2009–2010, 8. Number full-time enrolled (new admits only) 2009–2010, 8. Total enrolled 2009–2010 full-time, 35. Openings 2010–2011, 3. The median number of years required for completion of a degree in 2008–2009 were 6. The number of students enrolled full- and part-time who were dismissed or voluntarily withdrew from this program area in 2008–2009 were 1.

Scores: Entries appear in this order: required test or GPA, minimum score (if required), median score of students entering in 2009–2010. Experimental Psychology PhD (Doctor of Philosophy): overall undergraduate GPA 3.0; Clinical Psychology PhD (Doctor of Philosophy): GRE-V no minimum stated, 650, GRE-Q no minimum stated, 670, GRE-Analytical no minimum stated, 5.0, GRE-Subject (Psychology) no minimum stated, 680, overall undergraduate GPA no minimum stated, 3.91; School Psychology PhD (Doctor of Philosophy): GRE-V no minimum stated, 485, GRE-Q no minimum stated, 595, GRE-Analytical no minimum stated, 4.5, overall undergraduate GPA no minimum stated, 3.63; Specialist in School Psychology: GRE-V no minimum stated, 420, GRE-Q no minimum stated, 565, GRE-Analytical no minimum stated, 4.25, overall undergraduate GPA no minimum stated, 3.71; Industrial/Organizational Psychology MA/MS (Master of Arts/Science): GRE-V no minimum stated, 536, GRE-Q no minimum stated, 596, overall undergraduate GPA no minimum stated, 3.63.

Other Criteria: (importance of criteria rated low, medium, or high): GRE scores—medium, research experience—high, work experience—medium, extracurricular activity—low, clinically related public service—medium, GPA—high, letters of recommendation—high, statement of goals and objectives—high. For additional information on admission requirements, go to http://www.cmich.edu/chsbs/x18841.xml.

Student Characteristics: The following represents characteristics of students in 2009–2010 in all graduate psychology programs in the department: Female—full-time 93, part-time 0; Male—full-time 56, part-time 0; African American/Black—full-time 1, part-time 0; Hispanic/Latino(a)—full-time 1, part-time 0; Asian/Pacific Islander—full-time 5, part-time 0; American Indian/Alaska Native—full-time 2, part-time 0; Caucasian/White—full-time

131, part-time 0; Multi-ethnic—part-time 0; students subject to the Americans With Disabilities Act—full-time 0, part-time 0; Unknown ethnicity—full-time 9, part-time 0; International students who hold an F-1 or J-1 Visa—full-time 0, part-time 0.

Financial Information/Assistance:
Tuition for Full-Time Study: *Master's:* State residents: $434 per credit hour; Nonstate residents: $766 per credit hour. *Doctoral:* State residents: $508 per credit hour; Nonstate residents: $850 per credit hour. Tuition is subject to change. See the following Web site for updates and changes in tuition costs: http://cmich.edu/Office_of_the_Registrar/Registration_/Tuition_and_Fee_Schedule.htm.

Financial Assistance:
First-Year Students: Research assistantships available for first year. Average amount paid per academic year: $10,300. Average number of hours worked per week: 20. Apply by February 6. Fellowships and scholarships available for first year. Average amount paid per academic year: $10,300. Average number of hours worked per week: 24. Apply by February 6.
Advanced Students: Teaching assistantships available for advanced students. Average amount paid per academic year: $13,600. Average number of hours worked per week: 20. Apply by February 6. Research assistantships available for advanced students. Average amount paid per academic year: $12,600. Average number of hours worked per week: 20. Apply by February 6. Fellowships and scholarships available for advanced students. Average amount paid per academic year: $12,600. Average number of hours worked per week: 24. Apply by February 6.
Additional Information: Of all students currently enrolled full time, 68% benefited from one or more of the listed financial assistance programs. Application and information available online at: http://www.cmich.edu/chsbs/x3837.xml.

Internships/Practica: Doctoral Degree (PhD Clinical Psychology): For those doctoral students for whom a professional internship was required in this program prior to graduation, (4) students applied for an internship in 2008–2009, with (4) students obtaining an internship. Of those students who obtained an internship, (4) were paid internships. Of those students who obtained an internship, (4) students placed in APA/CPA accredited internships, (0) students placed in internships not APA/CPA accredited, but listed with the Association of Psychology Postdoctoral and Internship Programs (APPIC), (0) students placed in internships conforming to guidelines of the Council of Directors of School Psychology Programs (CDSPP), (0) students placed in internships that were not APA/CPA accredited, APPIC or CDSPP listed. Doctoral Degree (PhD School Psychology): For those doctoral students for whom a professional internship was required in this program prior to graduation, (3) students applied for an internship in 2008–2009, with (3) students obtaining an internship. Of those students who obtained an internship, (3) were paid internships. Of those students who obtained an internship, (3) students placed in APA/CPA accredited internships, (0) students placed in internships not APA/CPA accredited, but listed with the Association of Psychology Postdoctoral and Internship Programs (APPIC), (0) students placed in internships conforming to guidelines of the Council of Directors of School Psychology Programs (CDSPP), (0) students placed in internships that were not APA/CPA accredited, APPIC or CDSPP listed. Master's Degree (MA/MS General Psychology): An internship experience, such as a final research project or "capstone" experience is required of graduates. Master's Degree (MA/MS Industrial/Organizational Psychology): An internship experience, such as a final research project or "capstone" experience is required of graduates. Most practica and internships are arranged through agencies and schools outside the University. However, practicum experiences are available through the Department's Psychological Training and Consultation Center. Second-year clinical students routinely have their first practicum at the Center.

Housing and Day Care: On-campus housing is available. See the following Web site for more information: http://www.reslife.cmich.edu/. No on-campus day care facilities are available.

Employment of Department Graduates:
Master's Degree Graduates: Of those who graduated in the academic year 2008–2009, the following categories and numbers represent the postgraduate activities and employment of master's degree graduates: Enrolled in a postdoctoral residency/fellowship (n/a), employed in independent practice (n/a), total from the above (master's) (0).
Doctoral Degree Graduates: Of those who graduated in the academic year 2008–2009, the following categories and numbers represent the postgraduate activities and employment of doctoral degree graduates: Enrolled in a psychology doctoral program (n/a), total from the above (doctoral) (0).

Additional Information:
Orientation, Objectives, and Emphasis of Department: Specialization is possible in the areas of clinical, applied experimental, industrial/organizational, and school psychology. There is also a general/experimental MS program with emphasis on foundations, statistics, methodology, and research, which is designed to prepare students for doctoral training or research positions in the public or private sectors. The clinical program follows a practitioner-scientist model, focusing on training for applied settings. The industrial/organizational program is oriented toward training students for careers in research, university, or business settings. The school program prepares school psychologists to provide consultation, intervention, and diagnostic services to schools and school children. The program meets Michigan requirements for certification.

Special Facilities or Resources: Space is reserved for student research with human subjects. Special equipment permits studies in learning, cognition, human factors, psychophysiology, neuropsychology, and perception. Computer laboratories are available, one specifically designated for clinical and school students. All computer labs have direct email and Internet access, as well as statistical and research software. The Psychology Training and Consultation Center provides training, research, and service functions. In a separate building, space is devoted to animal research and teaching of behavioral neuroscience and experimental behavior analysis. The behavioral neuroscience laboratory contains a fully equipped surgical/histological suite, behavioral testing area and equipment, and a data analysis room including microscopes and an image analysis system. The experimental analysis laboratory is equipped with automated operant chambers for both birds and rodents. A Life-Span Development Research Center has been established in the Department.

Information for Students With Physical Disabilities: See the following Web site for more information: http://www.cmich.edu/student-disability/.

Application Information:
Send to Psychology Department, Sloan Hall, Central Michigan University, Mt. Pleasant, MI 48859. Application available online. URL of online application: https://apply.cmich.edu/. Students are admitted in the Fall, application deadline January 1. Industrial/Organizational deadline is January 1, Clinical and School deadlines are January 15, and Experimental program deadline is February 1. *Fee:* $35.

Eastern Michigan University
Department of Psychology
College of Arts and Sciences
537 Mark Jefferson Hall
Ypsilanti, MI 48197
Telephone: (734) 487-1155
Fax: (734) 487-6553
E-mail: *cfreedman@emich.edu*
Web: *http://www.emich.edu/psychology*

Department Information:
1962. Interim Department Head: Carol Freedman-Doan. Number of faculty: total—full-time 23; women—full-time 12; total—minority—full-time 1; women minority—full-time 1.

Programs and Degrees Offered:
Listed in the following order: Program area, degree type (T if terminal Master's), number awarded 7/08–6/09. Clinical Psychology PhD (Doctor of Philosophy) 8, General Clinical Psychology MA/MS (Master of Arts/Science) (T) 5, Clinical Behavioral Psychology MA/MS (Master of Arts/Science) (T) 7, General Experimental Psychology MA/MS (Master of Arts/Science) (T) 0.

APA Accreditation: Clinical PhD (Doctor of Philosophy). Student Outcome Data Website: http://www.emich.edu/psychology/programs-grad.html.

Student Applications/Admissions:
Student Applications
Clinical Psychology PhD (Doctor of Philosophy)—Applications 2009–2010, 139. Total applicants accepted 2009–2010, 10. Number full-time enrolled (new admits only) 2009–2010, 8. Number part-time enrolled (new admits only) 2009–2010, 0. Openings 2010–2011, 8. The median number of years required for completion of a degree in 2008–2009 were 6. The number of students enrolled full- and part-time who were dismissed or voluntarily withdrew from this program area in 2008–2009 were 2. *General Clinical Psychology MA/MS (Master of Arts/Science)*—Applications 2009–2010, 63. Total applicants accepted 2009–2010, 12. Number full-time enrolled (new admits only) 2009–2010, 10. Number part-time enrolled (new admits only) 2009–2010, 0. Total enrolled 2009–2010 full-time, 18, part-time, 4. Openings 2010–2011, 10. The median number of years required for completion of a degree in 2008–2009 were 2. The number of students enrolled full- and part-time who were dismissed or voluntarily withdrew from this program area in 2008–2009 were 1. *Clinical Behavioral Psychology MA/MS (Master of Arts/Science)*—Applications 2009–2010, 20. Total applicants accepted 2009–2010, 9. Number full-time enrolled (new admits only) 2009–2010, 8. Number part-time enrolled (new admits only) 2009–2010, 1. Total enrolled 2009–2010 full-time, 16, part-time, 4. Openings 2010–2011, 12. The median number of years required for completion of a degree in 2008–2009 were 3. The number of students enrolled full- and part-time who were dismissed or voluntarily withdrew from this program area in 2008–2009 were 2. *General Experimental Psychology MA/MS (Master of Arts/Science)*—Applications 2009–2010, 4. Total applicants accepted 2009–2010, 1. Number full-time enrolled (new admits only) 2009–2010, 0. Number part-time enrolled (new admits only) 2009–2010, 1. Openings 2010–2011, 3. The number of students enrolled full- and part-time who were dismissed or voluntarily withdrew from this program area in 2008–2009 were 0.

Scores: Entries appear in this order: required test or GPA, minimum score (if required), median score of students entering in 2009–2010. Clinical Psychology PhD (Doctor of Philosophy): GRE-V 500, 555, GRE-Q 500, 720, GRE-Analytical 4.0, 4.5, overall undergraduate GPA 3.0, 3.43, last 2 years GPA 3.0, psychology GPA 3.0; *General Clinical Psychology MA/MS (Master of Arts/Science)*: GRE-V 500, GRE-Q 500, GRE-Analytical 4.0, overall undergraduate GPA 3.0; *Clinical Behavioral Psychology MA/MS (Master of Arts/Science)*: GRE-V 500, GRE-Q 500, GRE-Analytical 4.0, overall undergraduate GPA 3.0, last 2 years GPA 3.0, psychology GPA 3.0; *General Experimental Psychology MA/MS (Master of Arts/Science)*: GRE-V no minimum stated, GRE-Q no minimum stated, GRE-Analytical no minimum stated, overall undergraduate GPA no minimum stated.

Other Criteria: (importance of criteria rated low, medium, or high): GRE scores—high, research experience—medium, work experience—low, extracurricular activity—low, clinically related public service—medium, GPA—high, letters of recommendation—medium, interview—high, statement of goals and objectives—medium, fit with faculty research—high, undergraduate major in psychology—medium, specific undergraduate psychology courses taken—medium. Weight given to criteria vary among each of the programs, but all programs require 20 undergraduate Psychology credit hours and a course in statistics and experimental psychology.

Student Characteristics: The following represents characteristics of students in 2009–2010 in all graduate psychology programs in the department: Female—full-time 42, part-time 6; Male—full-time 13, part-time 2; African American/Black—full-time 2, part-time 0; Hispanic/Latino(a)—full-time 1, part-time 1; Asian/Pacific Islander—full-time 4, part-time 0; American Indian/Alaska Native—full-time 0, part-time 0; Caucasian/White—full-time 53, part-time 7; Multi-ethnic—full-time 0, part-time 0; students subject to the Americans With Disabilities Act—full-time 0, part-time 0; Unknown ethnicity—full-time 0, part-time 0; International students who hold an F-1 or J-1 Visa—full-time 0, part-time 0.

Financial Information/Assistance:
Tuition for Full-Time Study: *Master's:* State residents: $432 per credit hour; Nonstate residents: $831 per credit hour. *Doctoral:* State residents: $462 per credit hour; Nonstate residents: $892 per credit hour. Tuition is subject to change. Additional fees are assessed to students beyond the costs of tuition for the following:

student and program fees are assessed by the university. Tuition costs vary by program. See the following Web site for updates and changes in tuition costs: http://www.emich.edu/sbs/tuitionfeesoutline.html.

Financial Assistance:
First-Year Students: Teaching assistantships available for first year. Average amount paid per academic year: $8,400. Average number of hours worked per week: 20. Apply by February 15. Fellowships and scholarships available for first year. Average amount paid per academic year: $15,000. Average number of hours worked per week: 20. Apply by December 15.

Advanced Students: Research assistantships available for advanced students. Average amount paid per academic year: $8,400. Average number of hours worked per week: 20. Apply by February 15. Fellowships and scholarships available for advanced students. Average amount paid per academic year: $15,000. Average number of hours worked per week: 20. Apply by December 15.

Additional Information: Of all students currently enrolled full time, 70% benefited from one or more of the listed financial assistance programs. Application and information available online at: http://www.gradschool.emich.edu/student/student_subdir/finasst_gradassist/finasst.html.

Internships/Practica: Doctoral Degree (PhD Clinical Psychology): For those doctoral students for whom a professional internship was required in this program prior to graduation, (9) students applied for an internship in 2008–2009, with (7) students obtaining an internship. Of those students who obtained an internship, (7) were paid internships. Of those students who obtained an internship, (7) students placed in APA/CPA accredited internships, (0) students placed in internships not APA/CPA accredited, but listed with the Association of Psychology Postdoctoral and Internship Programs (APPIC), (0) students placed in internships conforming to guidelines of the Council of Directors of School Psychology Programs (CDSPP), (0) students placed in internships that were not APA/CPA accredited, APPIC or CDSPP listed. Master's Degree (MA/MS General Experimental Psychology): An internship experience, such as a final research project or "capstone" experience is required of graduates. Practicum settings (unpaid) are available in the surrounding community for clinical and clinical behavioral students. In addition, the university offers mental health services involving practicum experiences at both the campus Snow Health Center and the EMU Psychology Clinic. Both terminal MS and PhD programs require sufficient practicum hours to meet the State of Michigan requirements for the Limited License in Psychology (LLP).

Housing and Day Care: On-campus housing is available. See the following Web site for more information: https://www.emich.edu/housing/. On-campus day care facilities are available. See the following Web site for more information: http://www.emich.edu/uhs/childcare.html.

Employment of Department Graduates:
Master's Degree Graduates: Of those who graduated in the academic year 2008–2009, the following categories and numbers represent the postgraduate activities and employment of master's degree graduates: Enrolled in a psychology doctoral program (2), enrolled in a postdoctoral residency/fellowship (n/a), employed in independent practice (n/a), total from the above (master's) (2).

Doctoral Degree Graduates: Of those who graduated in the academic year 2008–2009, the following categories and numbers represent the postgraduate activities and employment of doctoral degree graduates: Enrolled in a psychology doctoral program (n/a), enrolled in a postdoctoral residency/fellowship (3), employed in independent practice (3), employed in an academic position at a university (1), employed in an academic position at a 2-year/4-year college (2), employed in other positions at a higher education institution (5), employed in a hospital/medical center (4), total from the above (doctoral) (18).

Additional Information:
Orientation, Objectives, and Emphasis of Department: The Psychology Department offers three terminal Master's Degree programs and courses in several orientations, including behavioral, social, insight, developmental, and physiological. Within the two Master's clinical programs, the major emphases are on psychological assessment (Clinical program) and behavioral treatment (Clinical Behavioral program). Within each program there are a wide variety of theoretical, applied, and research interests. The goal of the Clinical and Clinical Behavioral programs is on giving students the background to immediately begin work in clinical treatment settings or to prepare them for entry into doctoral programs, as matches the student's educational objectives. The emphasis of the Master's in General Experimental Psychology is to prepare students for entry into higher level study in psychology or as researchers in applied/research settings. Because Psychology is considered a natural science at Eastern Michigan University, there is also an emphasis on basing clinical practice on research findings. Theses, although optional in the clinical master's programs, are expected to be research based. The PhD program in Clinical Psychology is designed to give advanced training in the supervision of mental health professionals in mental health care settings. The entry requirements for this program are more stringent than those of our Master's program with a more competitive applicant pool. The PhD offers specializations in either general clinical or behavioral psychology, a terminal Master's Degree en route, a full four-year doctoral fellowship which covers tuition and fees plus an annual stipend.

Special Facilities or Resources: The faculty, which consists of approximately 25 full-time members with PhDs and varying numbers of part-time lecturers, is eclectic in orientation with a wide variety of interests and professional backgrounds. Research interests and publication records of the faculty include psychological test construction and validation, basic behavioral research with humans and non-humans, the history of psychology, applied behavior analysis, physiological psychology, forensic psychology, personality, social psychology, and many more. Student enrollment is intentionally kept low in order to provide the students with ample opportunities to develop close working relationships with the faculty. Students regularly present at regional, national, and international conventions, as well as co-author published papers with faculty. The facilities of the Psychology Department are located in the Mark Jefferson Science building and in the newly renovated Psychology Clinic at 611 West Cross. The department features a state-of-the-art computer laboratory, IEEE 802.11 (AirPort) wireless networking capabilities, human and animal research facilities, seminar rooms, a clinic with one-way observation capabilities, a new university library less than three minutes away on foot, and other equipment and supplies needed for advanced study.

Information for Students With Physical Disabilities: See the following Web site for more information: http://www.emich.edu/access_services/.

Application Information:
Send to Department of Psychology, Graduate Admissions Committee, 537 Mark Jefferson, Eastern Michigan University, Ypsilanti, MI 48197. Application available online. URL of online application: http://www.emich.edu/admissions/apply.php. Students are admitted in the Fall, application deadline for PhD applications is December 15. The application deadline for the MS programs is February 15. *Fee:* $35. Graduate Admission has a separate application. Applications that are submitted electronically via http://www.emich.edu/admissions/apply/index.html#gradm involve a fee of $25. If the applicant mails in a paper Graduate Admission application, the fee is $35. No applicant will be considered without a Graduate Admissions application.

Michigan School of Professional Psychology (2009 data)
26811 Orchard Lake Road
Farmington Hills, MI 48334-4512
Telephone: (248) 476-1122
Fax: (248) 476-1125
E-mail: *lpgallant@mispp.edu*
Web: *http://www.mispp.edu*

Department Information:
1980. President: Kerry Moustakas, PhD Number of faculty: total—full-time 4, part-time 19; women—full-time 2, part-time 10; minority—part-time 1; women minority—part-time 1.

Programs and Degrees Offered:
Listed in the following order: Program area, degree type (T if terminal Master's), number awarded 7/08–6/09. Clinical Psychology PsyD (Doctor of Psychology) 11, Counseling Psychology MA/MS (Master of Arts/Science) (T) 34.

Student Applications/Admissions:
Student Applications

Clinical Psychology PsyD (Doctor of Psychology)—Applications 2009–2010, 39. Total applicants accepted 2009–2010, 26. Number full-time enrolled (new admits only) 2009–2010, 24. Number part-time enrolled (new admits only) 2009–2010, 0. Total enrolled 2009–2010 full-time, 64, part-time, 9. Openings 2010–2011, 24. The median number of years required for completion of a degree in 2008–2009 were 4. The number of students enrolled full- and part-time who were dismissed or voluntarily withdrew from this program area in 2008–2009 were 3. *Counseling Psychology MA/MS (Master of Arts/Science)*—Applications 2009–2010, 78. Total applicants accepted 2009–2010, 44. Number full-time enrolled (new admits only) 2009–2010, 41. Number part-time enrolled (new admits only) 2009–2010, 0. Total enrolled 2009–2010 full-time, 41, part-time, 3. Openings 2010–2011, 44. The number of students enrolled full- and part-time who were dismissed or voluntarily withdrew from this program area in 2008–2009 were 3.

Other Criteria: (importance of criteria rated low, medium, or high): research experience—medium, work experience—high, extracurricular activity—medium, clinically related public service—high, GPA—medium, letters of recommendation—high, interview—high, statement of goals and objectives—high, scholarly writing sample—medium, undergraduate major in psychology—high, specific undergraduate psychology courses taken—medium. Writing sample is needed for PsyD program only.

Student Characteristics: The following represents characteristics of students in 2009–2010 in all graduate psychology programs in the department: Female—full-time 61, part-time 1; Male—full-time 17, part-time 0; African American/Black—full-time 9, part-time 0; Hispanic/Latino(a)—full-time 0, part-time 0; Asian/Pacific Islander—full-time 1, part-time 0; American Indian/Alaska Native—full-time 1, part-time 0; Caucasian/White—full-time 0, part-time 0; Multi-ethnic—full-time 0, part-time 0; students subject to the Americans With Disabilities Act—full-time 0, part-time 0; Unknown ethnicity—full-time 0, part-time 0; International students who hold an F-1 or J-1 Visa—full-time 0, part-time 0.

Financial Information/Assistance:
Tuition for Full-Time Study: *Master's:* State residents: per academic year $21,255, $490 per credit hour; Nonstate residents: per academic year $21,255, $490 per credit hour. *Doctoral:* State residents: per academic year $18,930, $610 per credit hour; Nonstate residents: per academic year $18,930, $610 per credit hour. Tuition is subject to change. Additional fees are assessed to students beyond the costs of tuition for the following: technology fee, electronic resources, testing/assessment per class, thesis, supervision.

Financial Assistance:
First-Year Students: No information provided.
Advanced Students: No information provided.
Additional Information: Of all students currently enrolled full time, 80% benefited from one or more of the listed financial assistance programs.

Internships/Practica:
Doctoral Degree (PsyD Clinical Psychology): For those doctoral students for whom a professional internship was required in this program prior to graduation, (24) students applied for an internship in 2008–2009, with (24) students obtaining an internship. Of those students who obtained an internship, (2) were paid internships. Of those students who obtained an internship, (2) students placed in APA/CPA accredited internships, (0) students placed in internships not APA/CPA accredited, but listed with the Association of Psychology Postdoctoral and Internship Programs (APPIC), (0) students placed in internships conforming to guidelines of the Council of Directors of School Psychology Programs (CDSPP), (22) students placed in internships that were not APA/CPA accredited, APPIC or CDSPP listed. Master's Degree (MA/MS Counseling Psychology):

GRADUATE STUDY IN PSYCHOLOGY

An internship experience, such as a final research project or "capstone" experience is required of graduates. There is a mandatory 500 hour practicum for master's students. A 500 hour practicum is required for doctoral students with a two-thousand hour internship in order to receive their PsyD degree and satisfy the state licensing board's requirements.

Housing and Day Care: No on-campus housing is available. No on-campus day care facilities are available.

Employment of Department Graduates:
Master's Degree Graduates: Of those who graduated in the academic year 2008–2009, the following categories and numbers represent the postgraduate activities and employment of master's degree graduates: Enrolled in a psychology doctoral program (9), enrolled in another graduate/professional program (1), enrolled in a postdoctoral residency/fellowship (n/a), employed in independent practice (n/a), employed in an academic position at a university (0), employed in an academic position at a 2-year/4-year college (4), employed in a professional position in a school system (0), employed in business or industry (0), employed in government agency (1), employed in a community mental health/counseling center (9), employed in a hospital/medical center (3), still seeking employment (2), not seeking employment (0), do not know (2), total from the above (master's) (31).
Doctoral Degree Graduates: Of those who graduated in the academic year 2008–2009, the following categories and numbers represent the postgraduate activities and employment of doctoral degree graduates: Enrolled in a psychology doctoral program (n/a), enrolled in another graduate/professional program (0), enrolled in a postdoctoral residency/fellowship (0), employed in independent practice (5), employed in an academic position at a university (1), employed in an academic position at a 2-year/4-year college (1), employed in a professional position in a school system (0), employed in business or industry (1), employed in government agency (0), employed in a community mental health/counseling center (0), employed in a hospital/medical center (1), still seeking employment (0), do not know (2), total from the above (doctoral) (11).

Additional Information:
Orientation, Objectives, and Emphasis of Department: The mission of the Michigan School of Professional Psychology is to educate and train individuals to become reflective scholar-practitioners with the competencies necessary to serve diverse populations as professional humanistic psychologists and psychotherapists.

Application Information:
Send to Linda Potter-Gallant, MA Admissions Advisor Michigan School of Professional Psychology, 26811 Orchard Lake Road, Farmington Hills, MI 48334-4512. Students are admitted in the Fall. We accept applications all year round on a rolling basis. Our early admission deadline is January 15 and general admission deadline is May 1. We will continue to accept applications if there are spaces available. Enrollment is one time per year in September. *Fee:* $75.

Michigan State University (2009 data)
Department of Psychology
Social Science
262A Psychology Building
East Lansing, MI 48824-1116
Telephone: (517) 353-5258
Fax: (517) 432-2476
E-mail: *detwiler@msu.edu*
Web: *http://www.psychology.msu.edu*

Department Information:
1946. Chairperson: Neal Schmitt. Number of faculty: total—full-time 52; women—full-time 22; total—minority—full-time 7; women minority—full-time 1.

Programs and Degrees Offered:
Listed in the following order: Program area, degree type (T if terminal Master's), number awarded 7/08–6/09. Behavioral Neuroscience PhD (Doctor of Philosophy) 1, Clinical PhD (Doctor of Philosophy) 7, Ecological/Community PhD (Doctor of Philosophy), Industrial/Organizational PhD (Doctor of Philosophy) 6, Social/Personality PhD (Doctor of Philosophy), Cognitive PhD (Doctor of Philosophy).

APA Accreditation: Clinical PhD (Doctor of Philosophy).

Student Applications/Admissions:
Student Applications
Behavioral Neuroscience PhD (Doctor of Philosophy)—Applications 2009–2010, 9. Total applicants accepted 2009–2010, 2. Openings 2010–2011, 2. The median number of years required for completion of a degree in 2008–2009 were 6. The number of students enrolled full- and part-time who were dismissed or voluntarily withdrew from this program area in 2008–2009 were 0. Clinical PhD (Doctor of Philosophy)—Applications 2009–2010, 218. Total applicants accepted 2009–2010, 5. Openings 2010–2011, 5. The median number of years required for completion of a degree in 2008–2009 were 6. The number of students enrolled full- and part-time who were dismissed or voluntarily withdrew from this program area in 2008–2009 were 4. Ecological/Community PhD (Doctor of Philosophy)—Applications 2009–2010, 21. Total applicants accepted 2009–2010, 5. Openings 2010–2011, 5. The median number of years required for completion of a degree in 2008–2009 were 6. Industrial/Organizational PhD (Doctor of Philosophy)—Applications 2009–2010, 70. Total applicants accepted 2009–2010, 5. Openings 2010–2011, 5. The median number of years required for completion of a degree in 2008–2009 were 5. The number of students enrolled full- and part-time who were dismissed or voluntarily withdrew from this program area in 2008–2009 were 0. Social/Personality PhD (Doctor of Philosophy)—Applications 2009–2010, 42. Total applicants accepted 2009–2010, 5. Openings 2010–2011, 5. The median number of years required for completion of a degree in 2008–2009 were 6. The number of students enrolled full- and part-time who were dismissed or voluntarily withdrew from this program

area in 2008–2009 were 0. *Cognitive PhD (Doctor of Philosophy)*—Applications 2009–2010, 29. Total applicants accepted 2009–2010, 5. Openings 2010–2011, 5. The median number of years required for completion of a degree in 2008–2009 were 6. The number of students enrolled full- and part-time who were dismissed or voluntarily withdrew from this program area in 2008–2009 were 0.

Other Criteria: (importance of criteria rated low, medium, or high): GRE scores—high, research experience—high, work experience—medium, extracurricular activity—medium, GPA—high, letters of recommendation—high, interview—high, statement of goals and objectives—high, undergraduate major in psychology—medium, specific undergraduate psychology courses taken—medium, Extra curricular, public service and clinical activities are important for applicants to the clinical and ecological/community programs. For additional information on admission requirements, go to http://psychology.msu.edu.

Student Characteristics: The following represents characteristics of students in 2009–2010 in all graduate psychology programs in the department: Female—full-time 73, part-time 23; Male—full-time 30, part-time 12; African American/Black—full-time 5, part-time 0; Hispanic/Latino(a)—full-time 2, part-time 0; Asian/Pacific Islander—full-time 3, part-time 0; American Indian/Alaska Native—full-time 0, part-time 0; Caucasian/White—full-time 0, part-time 0; Multi-ethnic—full-time 0, part-time 0; students subject to the Americans With Disabilities Act—full-time 0, part-time 0; Unknown ethnicity—full-time 0, part-time 0; International students who hold an F-1 or J-1 Visa—full-time 0, part-time 0.

Financial Information/Assistance:
Financial Assistance:
First-Year Students: Teaching assistantships available for first year. Average amount paid per academic year: $18,960. Average number of hours worked per week: 20. Apply by December 15. Research assistantships available for first year. Average amount paid per academic year: $18,960. Average number of hours worked per week: 20. Apply by December 15. Fellowships and scholarships available for first year. Average amount paid per academic year: $24,000. Average number of hours worked per week: 0. Apply by December 15.

Advanced Students: Teaching assistantships available for advanced students. Average amount paid per academic year: $18,960. Average number of hours worked per week: 20. Research assistantships available for advanced students. Average amount paid per academic year: $18,960. Average number of hours worked per week: 20. Fellowships and scholarships available for advanced students. Average amount paid per academic year: $24,000.

Additional Information: Of all students currently enrolled full time, 95% benefited from one or more of the listed financial assistance programs.

Internships/Practica: Doctoral Degree (PhD Clinical): For those doctoral students for whom a professional internship was required in this program prior to graduation, (4) students applied for an internship in 2008–2009, with (4) students obtaining an internship. Of those students who obtained an internship, (4) were paid internships. Of those students who obtained an internship, (4) students placed in APA/CPA accredited internships, (0) students placed in internships not APA/CPA accredited, but listed with the Association of Psychology Postdoctoral and Internship Programs (APPIC), (0) students placed in internships conforming to guidelines of the Council of Directors of School Psychology Programs (CDSPP), (0) students placed in internships that were not APA/CPA accredited, APPIC or CDSPP listed. Clinical practica are provided by the clinical program at the department's Psychological Clinic.

Housing and Day Care: On-campus housing is available. See the following Web site for more information: http://www.liveon.msu.edu/. On-campus day care facilities are available. See the following Web site for more information: http://www.frc.msu.edu.

Employment of Department Graduates:
Master's Degree Graduates: Of those who graduated in the academic year 2008–2009, the following categories and numbers represent the postgraduate activities and employment of master's degree graduates: Enrolled in a postdoctoral residency/fellowship (n/a), employed in independent practice (n/a), total from the above (master's) (0).
Doctoral Degree Graduates: Of those who graduated in the academic year 2008–2009, the following categories and numbers represent the postgraduate activities and employment of doctoral degree graduates: Enrolled in a psychology doctoral program (n/a), total from the above (doctoral) (0).

Additional Information:
Orientation, Objectives, and Emphasis of Department: The main objective of our programs is to train researchers who will engage in the generation and application of knowledge in a wide range of areas in psychology.

Special Facilities or Resources: Facilities include the Psychological Clinic for the clinical program, which includes playrooms equipped for audio and video recording, testing equipment, computer-based record keeping system, and neuropsychological assessment lab. The Neuroscience-Biological Psychology Laboratories include research animal facilities, computers, light and electron-microscopy, histology and endocrinology labs. The Vision Research Laboratory, Cognitive Processes Laboratories, Eye-Movement Lab, and Speech Processing Lab provide automated facilities for conducting research in cognitive science. Additional observational labs equipped with video remote control equipment, one-way windows, and automated data recording equipment are available. Computer labs are available within the department and across campus.

Information for Students With Physical Disabilities: See the following Web site for more information: http://www.rcpd.msu.edu/.

Application Information:
Application available online. URL of online application: http://grad.msu.edu/apply. Students are admitted in the Fall, application deadline December 15. *Fee:* $50.

GRADUATE STUDY IN PSYCHOLOGY

Michigan, University of
Combined Program in Education and Psychology
1406 School of Education, 610 East University Avenue
Ann Arbor, MI 48109-1259
Telephone: (734) 647-0626
Fax: (734) 615-2164
E-mail: *cpep@umich.edu*
Web: *http://www.soe.umich.edu/edpsych/index.html*

Department Information:
1956. Chairperson: Tabbye Chavous. Number of faculty: total—part-time 20; women—part-time 9; minority—part-time 4; women minority—part-time 3.

Programs and Degrees Offered:
Listed in the following order: Program area, degree type (T if terminal Master's), number awarded 7/08–6/09. Education and Psychology PhD (Doctor of Philosophy) 3.

Student Applications/Admissions:
Student Applications
Education and Psychology PhD (Doctor of Philosophy)—Applications 2009–2010, 47. Total applicants accepted 2009–2010, 9. Number full-time enrolled (new admits only) 2009–2010, 7. Number part-time enrolled (new admits only) 2009–2010, 0. Openings 2010–2011, 5. The median number of years required for completion of a degree in 2008–2009 were 5. The number of students enrolled full- and part-time who were dismissed or voluntarily withdrew from this program area in 2008–2009 were 1.
Scores: Entries appear in this order: required test or GPA, minimum score (if required), median score of students entering in 2009–2010. *Education and Psychology PhD (Doctor of Philosophy)*: GRE-V no minimum stated, 590, GRE-Q no minimum stated, 677, GRE-Analytical no minimum stated, 4.7, overall undergraduate GPA no minimum stated, 3.72.
Other Criteria: (importance of criteria rated low, medium, or high): GRE scores—medium, research experience—high, work experience—medium, extracurricular activity—medium, clinically related public service—low, GPA—medium, letters of recommendation—high, interview—high, statement of goals and objectives—high, teaching/education—high, undergraduate major in psychology—low, specific undergraduate psychology courses taken—low. For additional information on admission requirements, go to http://www.soe.umich.edu/edpsych/admissions/index.html.

Student Characteristics: The following represents characteristics of students in 2009–2010 in all graduate psychology programs in the department: Female—full-time 21, part-time 0; Male—full-time 9, part-time 0; African American/Black—full-time 8, part-time 0; Hispanic/Latino(a)—full-time 4, part-time 0; Asian/Pacific Islander—full-time 2, part-time 0; American Indian/Alaska Native—full-time 0, part-time 0; Caucasian/White—full-time 11, part-time 0; Multi-ethnic—full-time 0, part-time 0; students subject to the Americans With Disabilities Act—full-time 1, part-time 0; Unknown ethnicity—full-time 5, part-time 0; International students who hold an F-1 or J-1 Visa—full-time 5, part-time 0.

Financial Information/Assistance:
Tuition for Full-Time Study: *Doctoral:* State residents: per academic year $17,286, $1,277 per credit hour; Nonstate residents: per academic year $34,944, $2,258 per credit hour. See the following Web site for updates and changes in tuition costs: http://ro.umich.edu/tuition/.

Financial Assistance:
First-Year Students: Research assistantships available for first year. Average amount paid per academic year: $24,942. Average number of hours worked per week: 20. Apply by December 5. Fellowships and scholarships available for first year. Average amount paid per academic year: $22,800. Average number of hours worked per week: 20. Apply by December 5.
Advanced Students: Teaching assistantships available for advanced students. Average amount paid per academic year: $25,041. Average number of hours worked per week: 20. Apply by varies. Research assistantships available for advanced students. Average amount paid per academic year: $24,942. Average number of hours worked per week: 20. Apply by varies. Fellowships and scholarships available for advanced students. Average amount paid per academic year: $22,800. Average number of hours worked per week: 20. Apply by varies.
Additional Information: Of all students currently enrolled full time, 96% benefited from one or more of the listed financial assistance programs. Application and information available online at: http://www.rackham.umich.edu/funding_resources/.

Housing and Day Care: On-campus housing is available. See the following Web site for more information: http://www.housing.umich.edu. On-campus day care facilities are available. See the following Web site for more information: http://hr.umich.edu/childcare/.

Employment of Department Graduates:
Master's Degree Graduates: Of those who graduated in the academic year 2008–2009, the following categories and numbers represent the postgraduate activities and employment of master's degree graduates: Enrolled in a postdoctoral residency/fellowship (n/a), employed in independent practice (n/a), total from the above (master's) (0).
Doctoral Degree Graduates: Of those who graduated in the academic year 2008–2009, the following categories and numbers represent the postgraduate activities and employment of doctoral degree graduates: Enrolled in a psychology doctoral program (n/a), enrolled in a postdoctoral residency/fellowship (1), employed in an academic position at a university (1), employed in other positions at a higher education institution (1), total from the above (doctoral) (3).

Additional Information:
Orientation, Objectives, and Emphasis of Department: The Combined Program in Education and Psychology focuses on re-

search training in instructional psychology, broadly defined. Students are trained to study educational issues and do research in educational settings, on significant educational problems related to learning. There are currently four main research foci: 1) human development in context of schools, families, and communities; 2) cognitive and learning sciences; 3) motivation and self-regulated learning; 4) resilience and development. Faculty affiliated with the program have ongoing research programs on various important issues. These include projects on children's cognitive development and reading skills, children's achievement motivation, socialization in the schools, how computers are changing the ways in which children learn, and learning and achievement of ethnically diverse students. Students in the program work with faculty on these projects and learn to design projects in their own areas of interest. They take courses taught by faculty members in the program, and also courses taught by faculty in the Psychology Department and the School of Education. Because the department is an independent interdepartmental unit, students have the unique opportunity to work with faculty in both the Psychology Department and the School of Education, in addition to the faculty directly affiliated with the program. Graduates are well prepared for teaching and research careers in academic and non-academic settings. We are not a School Psychology or a Counseling Psychology program.

Special Facilities or Resources: The University of Michigan is blessed with an extensive scientific-scholarly community of psychologists that is virtually unique in breadth, diversity, and quality. Because of the close collaborative relationships that have evolved over the years, graduate and postgraduate students have the opportunity to learn and work in a wide variety of well-developed specialty centers. These include: the Center for Human Growth and Development, the Center for Research on Learning and Teaching, the Center for Research on Women and Gender, the Human Performance Center, the Institute of Gerontology, the Institute for Social Research (i.e., Survey Research Center, Research Center for Group Dynamics, Center for Political Studies), the NASA Center of Excellence in Man-Systems Research, the Cognitive Science and Machine Intelligence Laboratory, the Human Factors Division of the University of Michigan Transportation Research Institute, the Kresge Hearing Research Institute, the Neuroscience Laboratory, the Evolution and Human Behavior Program, the Children's Center, the Vision Research Laboratory, and the Women's Studies Program. In addition to these resources, the Michigan campus also offers an unusually diverse series of stimulating colloquium and seminar presentations, involving both local and visiting speakers, that contributes significantly to the available opportunities for professional growth and development.

Information for Students With Physical Disabilities: See the following Web site for more information: http://www.umich.edu/~sswd/.

Application Information:
Send to Department Chair. Application available online. URL of online application: http://www.rackham.umich.edu/admissions/index.html/. Students are admitted in the Fall, application deadline December 5. *Fee:* $60. $75 for non-U.S. citizens.

Michigan, University of
Department of Psychology
Literature, Science & Arts
530 Church Street, 1343 East Hall
Ann Arbor, MI 48109-1043
Telephone: (734) 764-2580
Fax: (734) 615-7584
E-mail: *psych.saa@umich.edu*
Web: *http://www.lsa.umich.edu/psych/grad/*

Department Information:
1929. Chairperson: Theresa Lee. Number of faculty: total—full-time 51, part-time 30; women—full-time 22, part-time 18; total—minority—full-time 14, part-time 7; women minority—full-time 6, part-time 4.

Programs and Degrees Offered:
Listed in the following order: Program area, degree type (T if terminal Master's), number awarded 7/08–6/09. Personality and Social Contexts PhD (Doctor of Philosophy) 3, Biopsychology PhD (Doctor of Philosophy) 9, Cognition and Cognitive Neuroscience PhD (Doctor of Philosophy) 2, Developmental Psychology PhD (Doctor of Philosophy) 5, Social Psychology PhD (Doctor of Philosophy) 8, Clinical Psychology PhD (Doctor of Philosophy) 2.

APA Accreditation: Clinical PhD (Doctor of Philosophy).

Student Applications/Admissions:
Student Applications
Personality and Social Contexts PhD (Doctor of Philosophy)—Applications 2009–2010, 45. Total applicants accepted 2009–2010, 7. Number full-time enrolled (new admits only) 2009–2010, 5. Number part-time enrolled (new admits only) 2009–2010, 0. The median number of years required for completion of a degree in 2008–2009 were 5. The number of students enrolled full- and part-time who were dismissed or voluntarily withdrew from this program area in 2008–2009 were 0. *Biopsychology PhD (Doctor of Philosophy)*—Applications 2009–2010, 51. Total applicants accepted 2009–2010, 5. Number full-time enrolled (new admits only) 2009–2010, 2. Total enrolled 2009–2010 full-time, 16. The median number of years required for completion of a degree in 2008–2009 were 5. The number of students enrolled full- and part-time who were dismissed or voluntarily withdrew from this program area in 2008–2009 were 1. *Cognition and Cognitive Neuroscience PhD (Doctor of Philosophy)*—Applications 2009–2010, 69. Total applicants accepted 2009–2010, 1. Number full-time enrolled (new admits only) 2009–2010, 8. Total enrolled 2009–2010 full-time, 24. The median number of years required for completion of a degree in 2008–2009 were 5. The number of students enrolled full- and part-time who were dismissed or voluntarily withdrew from this program area in 2008–2009 were 0. *Developmental Psychology PhD (Doctor of Philosophy)*—Applications 2009–2010, 83. Total applicants accepted 2009–2010, 7. Number full-time enrolled (new admits only) 2009–2010, 6. Total enrolled 2009–2010 full-time, 33. The median number of years

required for completion of a degree in 2008–2009 were 5. The number of students enrolled full- and part-time who were dismissed or voluntarily withdrew from this program area in 2008–2009 were 0. *Social Psychology PhD (Doctor of Philosophy)*—Applications 2009–2010, 144. Total applicants accepted 2009–2010, 4. Number full-time enrolled (new admits only) 2009–2010, 2. Total enrolled 2009–2010 full-time, 31. The median number of years required for completion of a degree in 2008–2009 were 5. The number of students enrolled full- and part-time who were dismissed or voluntarily withdrew from this program area in 2008–2009 were 0. *Clinical Psychology PhD (Doctor of Philosophy)*—Applications 2009–2010, 218. Total applicants accepted 2009–2010, 6. Number full-time enrolled (new admits only) 2009–2010, 6. Total enrolled 2009–2010 full-time, 41. The median number of years required for completion of a degree in 2008–2009 were 6. The number of students enrolled full- and part-time who were dismissed or voluntarily withdrew from this program area in 2008–2009 were 0.
Scores: Entries appear in this order: required test or GPA, minimum score (if required), median score of students entering in 2009–2010. *Personality and Social Contexts PhD (Doctor of Philosophy)*: GRE-V no minimum stated, 570, GRE-Q no minimum stated, 690, GRE-Analytical no minimum stated, 4.0, overall undergraduate GPA no minimum stated; *Biopsychology PhD (Doctor of Philosophy)*: GRE-V no minimum stated, 655, GRE-Q no minimum stated, 770, GRE-Analytical no minimum stated, 4.5, overall undergraduate GPA no minimum stated; *Cognition and Cognitive Neuroscience PhD (Doctor of Philosophy)*: GRE-V no minimum stated, 665, GRE-Q no minimum stated, 750, GRE-Analytical no minimum stated, 4.8, overall undergraduate GPA no minimum stated; *Developmental Psychology PhD (Doctor of Philosophy)*: GRE-V no minimum stated, 655, GRE-Q no minimum stated, 760, GRE-Analytical no minimum stated, 5.0, overall undergraduate GPA no minimum stated; *Social Psychology PhD (Doctor of Philosophy)*: GRE-V no minimum stated, 680, GRE-Q no minimum stated, 770, GRE-Analytical no minimum stated, 5.5, overall undergraduate GPA no minimum stated; *Clinical Psychology PhD (Doctor of Philosophy)*: GRE-V no minimum stated, 595, GRE-Q no minimum stated, 655, GRE-Analytical no minimum stated, 5.0, overall undergraduate GPA no minimum stated.
Other Criteria: (importance of criteria rated low, medium, or high): GRE scores—medium, research experience—high, work experience—high, extracurricular activity—low, clinically related public service—low, GPA—medium, letters of recommendation—high, interview—high, statement of goals and objectives—high. For additional information on admission requirements, go to http://www.lsa.umich.edu/psych/grad/prospective/.

Student Characteristics: The following represents characteristics of students in 2009–2010 in all graduate psychology programs in the department: Female—full-time 129, part-time 0; Male—full-time 48, part-time 0; African American/Black—full-time 18, part-time 0; Hispanic/Latino(a)—full-time 12, part-time 0; Asian/Pacific Islander—full-time 41, part-time 0; American Indian/Alaska Native—full-time 2, part-time 0; Caucasian/White—full-time 103, part-time 0; Multi-ethnic—full-time 0, part-time 0; students subject to the Americans With Disabilities Act—full-time 0, part-time 0; Unknown ethnicity—full-time 1, part-time 0; International students who hold an F-1 or J-1 Visa—full-time 26, part-time 0.

Financial Information/Assistance:
  Tuition for Full-Time Study: *Doctoral:* State residents: per academic year $17,475; Nonstate residents: per academic year $35,133. Tuition is subject to change. See the following Web site for updates and changes in tuition costs: http://ro.umich.edu/tuition/.

Financial Assistance:
  First-Year Students: Fellowships and scholarships available for first year. Average amount paid per academic year: $20,900. Average number of hours worked per week: 20. Apply by December 1.
  Advanced Students: Teaching assistantships available for advanced students. Average amount paid per academic year: $25,041. Average number of hours worked per week: 20. Apply by December 1. Research assistantships available for advanced students. Average amount paid per academic year: $25,041. Average number of hours worked per week: 20. Apply by December 1. Fellowships and scholarships available for advanced students. Average amount paid per academic year: $20,900. Average number of hours worked per week: 20. Apply by December 1.
  Additional Information: Of all students currently enrolled full time, 100% benefited from one or more of the listed financial assistance programs. Application and information available online at: http://www.lsa.umich.edu/psych/grad/prospective/financial-aid/.

Internships/Practica: Doctoral Degree (PhD Clinical Psychology): For those doctoral students for whom a professional internship was required in this program prior to graduation, (14) students applied for an internship in 2008–2009, with (14) students obtaining an internship. Of those students who obtained an internship, (14) were paid internships. Of those students who obtained an internship, (14) students placed in APA/CPA accredited internships, (0) students placed in internships not APA/CPA accredited, but listed with the Association of Psychology Postdoctoral and Internship Programs (APPIC), (0) students placed in internships conforming to guidelines of the Council of Directors of School Psychology Programs (CDSPP), (0) students placed in internships that were not APA/CPA accredited, APPIC or CDSPP listed. Students in the clinical area begin practica [e.g., psychological testing] during their first year and continue the practicum experience in the second year [usually in local agencies] on a 6-8 hour a week basis. During the same two year period students are engaged in their Master's level research project. Students begin half-time clinical work [internships] during their third year of training [again, most likely in one of the local training agencies] and at the same time continue to make progress toward their degree.

Housing and Day Care: On-campus housing is available. See the following Web site for more information: http://www.housing.umich.edu. On-campus day care facilities are available. See the following Web site for more information: http://www.studentswithchildren.umich.edu/.

Employment of Department Graduates:
  Master's Degree Graduates: Of those who graduated in the academic year 2008–2009, the following categories and numbers

represent the postgraduate activities and employment of master's degree graduates: Enrolled in a postdoctoral residency/fellowship (n/a), employed in independent practice (n/a), total from the above (master's) (0).

Doctoral Degree Graduates: Of those who graduated in the academic year 2008–2009, the following categories and numbers represent the postgraduate activities and employment of doctoral degree graduates: Enrolled in a psychology doctoral program (n/a), enrolled in a postdoctoral residency/fellowship (16), employed in an academic position at a university (5), employed in government agency (3), still seeking employment (1), do not know (5), total from the above (doctoral) (30).

Additional Information:
Orientation, Objectives, and Emphasis of Department: The Department of Psychology is committed to a broad mission of excellence in research, teaching, and apprenticeship: to create new scientific knowledge about psychological processes through first-rate scholarship; -to teach innovative courses and engage students in our research and service activities; and to maintain our record of outstanding graduate training that produces tomorrow's leading researchers. We strive to accomplish these goals as a large, diverse and interdisciplinary community of scholars.

Special Facilities or Resources: The University of Michigan provides a rich environment for graduate studies. The faculty in both education and psychology are internationally known for their scholarly productivity, and so students receive excellent training in how to conduct educational research. Faculty in the Psychology Department have ties to school officials in Ann Arbor and the greater Detroit area, which means students receive ample opportunities to work on many different kinds of educational projects. Students can take advantage of the university's excellent library and computer facilities, both of which are among the best in the country. A distinct advantage of the program is that it is interdepartmental in the graduate school with full resources and faculty available from the Psychology Department, the School of Education, the School of Social Work, and the Women's Studies Department. The department has close collaborative relationships with the Center for Human Growth and Development, the Center for Research on Learning and Teaching, the Center for Research on Women and Gender, the Human Performance Center, the Institute of Gerontology, the Institute for Social Research, the Cognitive Science and Machine Intelligence Laboratory, the Evolution and Human Behavior Program, and the Children's Center.

Information for Students With Physical Disabilities: See the following Web site for more information: http://www.umich.edu/~sswd.

Application Information:
Send to Graduate Admissions, Rackham Graduate School, 915 East Washington, Ann Arbor, MI 48109-1070. Application available online. URL of online application: http://www.lsa.umich.edu/psych/grad/prospective/. Students are admitted in the Fall, application deadline December 1. *Fee:* $60. $75 for International Applications.

Northern Michigan University (2009 data)
Department of Psychology
Arts and Sciences
1401 Presque Isle Avenue
Marquette, MI 49855
Telephone: (906) 227-2935
Fax: (906) 227-2954
E-mail: *pandroni@nmu.edu or sburns@nmu.edu*
Web: *http://www.nmu.edu/psychology*

Department Information:
1950. Head and Professor: Sheila Burns. Number of faculty: total—full-time 12, part-time 2; women—full-time 5, part-time 1; minority—part-time 1.

Programs and Degrees Offered:
Listed in the following order: Program area, degree type (T if terminal Master's), number awarded 7/08–6/09. Experimental Psychology MA/MS (Master of Arts/Science) 0, Training, Development, and Performance Improvement MA/MS (Master of Arts/Science) (T) 12.

Student Applications/Admissions:
Student Applications
Experimental Psychology MA/MS (Master of Arts/Science)—Applications 2009–2010, 15. Total applicants accepted 2009–2010, 14. Number full-time enrolled (new admits only) 2009–2010, 10. Number part-time enrolled (new admits only) 2009–2010, 0. Openings 2010–2011, 15. The median number of years required for completion of a degree in 2008–2009 were 3. The number of students enrolled full- and part-time who were dismissed or voluntarily withdrew from this program area in 2008–2009 were 0. *Training, Development, and Performance Improvement MA/MS (Master of Arts/Science)*—Applications 2009–2010, 20. Total applicants accepted 2009–2010, 17. Openings 2010–2011, 25. The median number of years required for completion of a degree in 2008–2009 were 3.
Other Criteria: (importance of criteria rated low, medium, or high): GRE scores—medium, research experience—medium, work experience—medium, extracurricular activity—medium, clinically related public service—low, GPA—high, letters of recommendation—high, statement of goals and objectives—high, undergraduate major in psychology—low. Experimental Psychology program looks for a variety of psychology courses and expects students to have completed undergraduate statistics.

Student Characteristics: The following represents characteristics of students in 2009–2010 in all graduate psychology programs in the department: Female—full-time 5, part-time 1; Male—full-time 5, part-time 1; African American/Black—full-time 0, part-time 0; Hispanic/Latino(a)—full-time 0, part-time 0; Asian/Pacific Islander—full-time 1, part-time 0; American Indian/Alaska Native—full-time 0, part-time 0; Caucasian/White—full-time 0, part-time 0; Multi-ethnic—full-time 0, part-time 0; students subject to the Americans With Disabilities Act—full-time 1, part-time 0; Unknown ethnicity—full-time 0, part-time 0; International students who hold an F-1 or J-1 Visa—full-time 0, part-time 0.

Financial Information/Assistance:
Tuition for Full-Time Study: Master's: State residents: $325 per credit hour; Nonstate residents: $479 per credit hour. Tuition is subject to change. See the following Web site for updates and changes in tuition costs: http://www.nmu.edu/facts/tuifees.htm.

Financial Assistance:
First-Year Students: Teaching assistantships available for first year. Average amount paid per academic year: $7,500. Average number of hours worked per week: 20. Apply by May 1. Fellowships and scholarships available for first year. Average amount paid per academic year: $5,000. Average number of hours worked per week: 0. Apply by May 1.
Advanced Students: No information provided.
Additional Information: Of all students currently enrolled full time, 10% benefited from one or more of the listed financial assistance programs. Application and information available online at: http://www.nmu.edu/graduate_studies/.

Internships/Practica: Training, Development, and Performance Improvement program may provide workplace placement in practica or internships for its students.

Housing and Day Care: On-campus housing is available. See the following Web site for more information: http://www.nmu.edu/housing. No on-campus day care facilities are available.

Employment of Department Graduates:
Master's Degree Graduates: Of those who graduated in the academic year 2008–2009, the following categories and numbers represent the postgraduate activities and employment of master's degree graduates: Enrolled in a psychology doctoral program (4), enrolled in another graduate/professional program (0), enrolled in a postdoctoral residency/fellowship (n/a), employed in independent practice (n/a), employed in an academic position at a university (0), employed in an academic position at a 2-year/4-year college (0), employed in other positions at a higher education institution (0), employed in a professional position in a school system (0), employed in business or industry (0), employed in government agency (0), employed in a community mental health/counseling center (0), employed in a hospital/medical center (0), still seeking employment (0), other employment position (0), total from the above (master's) (4).
Doctoral Degree Graduates: Of those who graduated in the academic year 2008–2009, the following categories and numbers represent the postgraduate activities and employment of doctoral degree graduates: Enrolled in a psychology doctoral program (n/a), enrolled in a postdoctoral residency/fellowship (0), employed in independent practice (0), employed in an academic position at a university (0), employed in an academic position at a 2-year/4-year college (0), employed in other positions at a higher education institution (0), employed in a professional position in a school system (0), employed in business or industry (0), employed in government agency (0), employed in a community mental health/counseling center (0), employed in a hospital/medical center (0), still seeking employment (0), other employment position (0), total from the above (doctoral) (0).

Additional Information:
Orientation, Objectives, and Emphasis of Department: The Experimental Psychology MS program is designed to prepare students for PhD programs and specialty jobs in the workplace. The Training, Performance and Performance Improvement MS program is designed for students who will be seeking related jobs upon graduation.

Special Facilities or Resources: Active research labs in the department: learning, perception, developmental, social, physiological (2), behavioral and historical. There is an up-to-date statistics lab. Grad students are provided office and research space.

Information for Students With Physical Disabilities: See the following Web site for more information: http://www.nmu.edu/disserve.

Application Information:
Send to Department Head Director of Graduate Studies, Department of Psychology, Northern Michigan University, Marquette, MI 49855. Application available online. URL of online application: http://www.nmu.edu/graduate_studies/. Students are admitted in the Fall, application deadline May 1; Spring, application deadline November 1; Programs have rolling admissions. Graduate study applications are open until the semester begins. However, most decisions about graduate assistantships are made in May and if necessary, November. Fee: $50.

Wayne State University
Department of Psychology
Science
5057 Woodward Avenue, 7th Floor
Detroit, MI 48202
Telephone: (313) 577-2800
Fax: (313) 577-7636
E-mail: *aallen@wayne.edu*
Web: *http://www.psych.wayne.edu*

Department Information:
1923. Chairperson: R. Douglas Whitman. Number of faculty: total—full-time 42, part-time 12; women—full-time 19, part-time 7; total—minority—full-time 1; women minority—full-time 1; faculty subject to the Americans With Disabilities Act 1.

Programs and Degrees Offered:
Listed in the following order: Program area, degree type (T if terminal Master's), number awarded 7/08–6/09. Cognitive, Developmental & Social Psychology PhD (Doctor of Philosophy) 1, Industrial/Organizational Psychology MA/MS (Master of Arts/Science) (T) 0, Clinical Psychology PhD (Doctor of Philosophy) 14, Behavioral and Cognitive Neuroscience PhD (Doctor of Philosophy) 0, Industrial/Organizational Psychology PhD (Doctor of Philosophy) 4.

APA Accreditation: Clinical PhD (Doctor of Philosophy). Student Outcome Data Website: http://www.clas.wayne.edu/unit-inner.asp?UnitID=20&WebPageID=307&site=candle.

Student Applications/Admissions:
Student Applications
Cognitive, Developmental & Social Psychology PhD (Doctor of Philosophy)—Applications 2009–2010, 43. Total applicants accepted 2009–2010, 9. Number full-time enrolled (new admits

only) 2009–2010, 4. Total enrolled 2009–2010 full-time, 31. Openings 2010–2011, 5. The median number of years required for completion of a degree in 2008–2009 were 5. The number of students enrolled full- and part-time who were dismissed or voluntarily withdrew from this program area in 2008–2009 were 1. *Industrial/Organizational Psychology MA/MS (Master of Arts/Science)*—Applications 2009–2010, 22. Total applicants accepted 2009–2010, 10. Number full-time enrolled (new admits only) 2009–2010, 0. Number part-time enrolled (new admits only) 2009–2010, 4. Openings 2010–2011, 15. The median number of years required for completion of a degree in 2008–2009 were 2. The number of students enrolled full- and part-time who were dismissed or voluntarily withdrew from this program area in 2008–2009 were 0. *Clinical Psychology PhD (Doctor of Philosophy)*—Applications 2009–2010, 157. Total applicants accepted 2009–2010, 14. Number full-time enrolled (new admits only) 2009–2010, 8. Total enrolled 2009–2010 full-time, 64. Openings 2010–2011, 9. The median number of years required for completion of a degree in 2008–2009 were 7. The number of students enrolled full- and part-time who were dismissed or voluntarily withdrew from this program area in 2008–2009 were 1. *Behavioral and Cognitive Neuroscience PhD (Doctor of Philosophy)*—Applications 2009–2010, 19. Total applicants accepted 2009–2010, 3. Number full-time enrolled (new admits only) 2009–2010, 2. Total enrolled 2009–2010 full-time, 18. Openings 2010–2011, 5. The number of students enrolled full- and part-time who were dismissed or voluntarily withdrew from this program area in 2008–2009 were 2. *Industrial/Organizational Psychology PhD (Doctor of Philosophy)*—Applications 2009–2010, 32. Total applicants accepted 2009–2010, 0. Number full-time enrolled (new admits only) 2009–2010, 4. Total enrolled 2009–2010 full-time, 24. The median number of years required for completion of a degree in 2008–2009 were 6. The number of students enrolled full- and part-time who were dismissed or voluntarily withdrew from this program area in 2008–2009 were 0.

Scores: Entries appear in this order: required test or GPA, minimum score (if required), median score of students entering in 2009–2010. *Cognitive, Developmental & Social Psychology PhD (Doctor of Philosophy)*: GRE-V no minimum stated, GRE-Q no minimum stated, GRE-Analytical no minimum stated, overall undergraduate GPA 3.0; *Industrial/Organizational Psychology MA/MS (Master of Arts/Science)*: GRE-V no minimum stated, GRE-Q no minimum stated, GRE-Analytical no minimum stated, overall undergraduate GPA 3.0; *Clinical Psychology PhD (Doctor of Philosophy)*: GRE-V no minimum stated, GRE-Q no minimum stated, GRE-Analytical no minimum stated, overall undergraduate GPA 3.0; *Behavioral and Cognitive Neuroscience PhD (Doctor of Philosophy)*: GRE-V no minimum stated, GRE-Q no minimum stated, GRE-Analytical no minimum stated, overall undergraduate GPA 3.0; *Industrial/Organizational Psychology PhD (Doctor of Philosophy)*: GRE-V no minimum stated, GRE-Q no minimum stated, overall undergraduate GPA 3.0.

Other Criteria: (importance of criteria rated low, medium, or high): GRE scores—high, research experience—high, work experience—low, extracurricular activity—low, clinically related public service—low, GPA—high, letters of recommendation—high, interview—high, statement of goals and objectives—high, undergraduate major in psychology—medium, specific undergraduate psychology courses taken—high. For additional information on admission requirements, go to http://www.clas.wayne.edu/psychology/.

Student Characteristics: The following represents characteristics of students in 2009–2010 in all graduate psychology programs in the department: Female—full-time 99, part-time 14; Male—full-time 38, part-time 9; African American/Black—full-time 15, part-time 0; Hispanic/Latino(a)—full-time 5, part-time 0; Asian/Pacific Islander—full-time 14, part-time 0; American Indian/Alaska Native—full-time 0, part-time 0; Caucasian/White—full-time 106, part-time 0; Multi-ethnic—full-time 3, part-time 0; students subject to the Americans With Disabilities Act—full-time 0, part-time 0; Unknown ethnicity—full-time 0, part-time 0; International students who hold an F-1 or J-1 Visa—full-time 0, part-time 0.

Financial Information/Assistance:

Tuition for Full-Time Study: *Master's:* State residents: $456 per credit hour; Nonstate residents: $1,008 per credit hour. *Doctoral:* State residents: $456 per credit hour; Nonstate residents: $1,008 per credit hour. Tuition is subject to change. Additional fees are assessed to students beyond the costs of tuition for the following: omnibus credits hour fee: $34.05, registration fee: $155.45, Fitness Center Fee: $25.00. See the following Web site for updates and changes in tuition costs: http://reg.wayne.edu/students/tuition.php.

Financial Assistance:

First-Year Students: Teaching assistantships available for first year. Average amount paid per academic year: $15,181. Average number of hours worked per week: 20. Research assistantships available for first year. Average amount paid per academic year: $15,181. Average number of hours worked per week: 20. Traineeships available for first year. Average amount paid per academic year: $15,181. Average number of hours worked per week: 20. Fellowships and scholarships available for first year. Average amount paid per academic year: $15,181. Average number of hours worked per week: 20.

Advanced Students: Teaching assistantships available for advanced students. Average amount paid per academic year: $15,181. Average number of hours worked per week: 20. Research assistantships available for advanced students. Average amount paid per academic year: $15,181. Average number of hours worked per week: 20. Traineeships available for advanced students. Average amount paid per academic year: $15,181. Average number of hours worked per week: 20. Fellowships and scholarships available for advanced students. Average amount paid per academic year: $15,181. Average number of hours worked per week: 20.

Additional Information: Of all students currently enrolled full time, 80% benefited from one or more of the listed financial assistance programs. Application and information available online at: http://www.gradschool.wayne.edu/Funding.html.

Internships/Practica: Doctoral Degree (PhD Clinical Psychology): For those doctoral students for whom a professional internship was required in this program prior to graduation, (10) students applied for an internship in 2008–2009, with (9) students obtaining an internship. Of those students who obtained an internship, (9) were paid internships. Of those students who obtained an internship, (9) students placed in APA/CPA accredited internships, (0) students placed in internships not APA/CPA accredited, but listed with the Association of Psychology Postdoctoral and Internship Programs (APPIC), (0) students placed in internships conforming to guidelines of the Council of Directors of School Psychology Programs (CDSPP), (0) students placed in internships that were not APA/CPA accredited, APPIC or CDSPP listed.

Housing and Day Care: On-campus housing is available. See the following Web site for more information: http://www.housing.wayne.edu. On-campus day care facilities are available. See the following Web site for more information: http://mpsi.wayne.edu/.

Employment of Department Graduates:
Master's Degree Graduates: Of those who graduated in the academic year 2008–2009, the following categories and numbers represent the postgraduate activities and employment of master's degree graduates: Enrolled in a postdoctoral residency/fellowship (n/a), employed in independent practice (n/a), total from the above (master's) (0).
Doctoral Degree Graduates: Of those who graduated in the academic year 2008–2009, the following categories and numbers represent the postgraduate activities and employment of doctoral degree graduates: Enrolled in a psychology doctoral program (n/a), total from the above (doctoral) (0).

Additional Information:
Orientation, Objectives, and Emphasis of Department: This department strives to select graduate students with a strong educational background and outstanding potential and to train them to be knowledgeable, ethical practitioners and research scholars in their chosen areas. Program admission is limited to persons planning to obtain the doctoral degree. Initial broad training is followed by specialized training.

Special Facilities or Resources: The behavioral and cognitive neuroscience area participates in the university neuroscience program. Excellent laboratory facilities are available in neurobiology, neuropharmacology, psychopharmacology, neuropsychology, and ethology. Several faculty in behavioral and cognitive neuroscience and other areas in the department work in the area of substance abuse. The clinical program emphasizes psychotherapy, community mental health, diagnostics, alcohol abuse issues, neuropsychology, and child and geropsychology. Clinical practice and research experience are obtained in a variety of clinical placements and in our own clinic. The cognitive program emphasizes cognition theory and its application to applied problems. The developmental area emphasizes life-span studies and is affiliated with the Institute of Gerontology. The social psychology program has both basic and applied research emphases. Well-equipped laboratories in the department and at the Merrill-Palmer Institute, which is affiliated with the department, are available for cognitive, social, and developmental research. In addition, social psychology uses its urban setting to carry out field studies. The industrial/organizational area emphasizes organizational psychology, personnel research, and field placements. Excellent computer facilities and libraries support research in all areas.

Application Information:
Send to Graduate Office, Psychology Department, WSU, 5057 Woodward Avenue, 7th Floor, Detroit, MI 48202. Application available online. URL of online application: http://www.gradadmissions.wayne.edu/apply.php. Students are admitted in the Fall, application deadline December 15. I/O Master's Program: Fall application deadline- June 15; Spring application deadline-October 15; Summer application deadline-March 15. *Fee:* $50.

Wayne State University
Division of Theoretical and Behavioral Foundations-Educational Psychology
College of Education
Detroit, MI 48202
Telephone: (313) 557-1614
Fax: (313) 577-5235
E-mail: *s.b.hillman@wayne.edu*
Web: *http://tbf.coe.wayne.edu.edp*

Department Information:
1957. Chairperson: Stephen B. Hillman. Number of faculty: total—full-time 6, part-time 12; women—full-time 3, part-time 8; total—minority—full-time 1, part-time 1; women minority—full-time 1.

Programs and Degrees Offered:
Listed in the following order: Program area, degree type (T if terminal Master's), number awarded 7/08–6/09. Educational Psychology PhD (Doctor of Philosophy) 7, School Psychology MA/MS (Master of Arts/Science) 14, Marriage and Family Psychology MA/MS (Master of Arts/Science) 10.

Student Applications/Admissions:
Student Applications
Educational Psychology PhD (Doctor of Philosophy)—Applications 2009–2010, 15. Total applicants accepted 2009–2010, 9. Number full-time enrolled (new admits only) 2009–2010, 9. Number part-time enrolled (new admits only) 2009–2010, 0. Total enrolled 2009–2010 full-time, 9, part-time, 24. Openings 2010–2011, 10. The median number of years required for completion of a degree in 2008–2009 were 7. The number of students enrolled full- and part-time who were dismissed or voluntarily withdrew from this program area in 2008–2009 were 0. *School Psychology MA/MS (Master of Arts/Science)*—Applications 2009–2010, 38. Total applicants accepted 2009–2010, 13. Number full-time enrolled (new admits only) 2009–2010, 13. Total enrolled 2009–2010 full-time, 26, part-time, 12. Openings 2010–2011, 14. The median number of years required for completion of a degree in 2008–2009 were 2. The number of students enrolled full- and part-time who were dismissed or voluntarily withdrew from this program area in 2008–2009 were 2. *Marriage and Family Psychology MA/MS (Master of Arts/Science)*—Applications 2009–2010, 28. Total applicants accepted 2009–2010, 14. Number full-time enrolled (new admits only) 2009–2010, 14. Total enrolled 2009–2010 full-time, 28. Openings 2010–2011, 14. The median number of years required for completion of a degree in 2008–2009 were 2. The number of students enrolled full- and part-time who were dismissed or voluntarily withdrew from this program area in 2008–2009 were 2.
Other Criteria: (importance of criteria rated low, medium, or high): GRE scores—medium, research experience—medium, work experience—medium, extracurricular activity—medium, clinically related public service—medium, GPA—high, letters of recommendation—high, interview—high, statement of

goals and objectives—high. For additional information on admission requirements, go to wayne.edu.

Student Characteristics: The following represents characteristics of students in 2009–2010 in all graduate psychology programs in the department: Female—full-time 31, part-time 43; Male—full-time 5, part-time 12; African American/Black—full-time 0, part-time 7; Hispanic/Latino(a)—full-time 0, part-time 0; Asian/Pacific Islander—full-time 0, part-time 1; American Indian/Alaska Native—full-time 0, part-time 0; Caucasian/White—full-time 0, part-time 54; Multi-ethnic—full-time 0, part-time 0; students subject to the Americans With Disabilities Act—full-time 0, part-time 0; Unknown ethnicity—full-time 0, part-time 0; International students who hold an F-1 or J-1 Visa—full-time 0, part-time 0.

Financial Information/Assistance:
Tuition for Full-Time Study: *Master's:* State residents: $403 per credit hour; Nonstate residents: $890 per credit hour. *Doctoral:* State residents: $403 per credit hour; Nonstate residents: $890 per credit hour. Tuition is subject to change. Additional fees are assessed to students beyond the costs of tuition for the following: testing materials. Tuition costs vary by program. See the following Web site for updates and changes in tuition costs: http://reg.wayne.edu/students/tuition.php.

Financial Assistance:
First-Year Students: Fellowships and scholarships available for first year. Apply by March 1.
Advanced Students: Fellowships and scholarships available for advanced students. Apply by March 1.
Additional Information: Of all students currently enrolled full time, 15% benefited from one or more of the listed financial assistance programs.

Housing and Day Care: On-campus housing is available. On-campus day care facilities are available.

Employment of Department Graduates:
Master's Degree Graduates: Of those who graduated in the academic year 2008–2009, the following categories and numbers represent the postgraduate activities and employment of master's degree graduates: Enrolled in a psychology doctoral program (5), enrolled in another graduate/professional program (0), enrolled in a postdoctoral residency/fellowship (n/a), employed in independent practice (n/a), employed in a professional position in a school system (12), employed in a community mental health/counseling center (3), total from the above (master's) (20).
Doctoral Degree Graduates: Of those who graduated in the academic year 2008–2009, the following categories and numbers represent the postgraduate activities and employment of doctoral degree graduates: Enrolled in a psychology doctoral program (n/a), enrolled in another graduate/professional program (0), enrolled in a postdoctoral residency/fellowship (0), employed in independent practice (3), employed in an academic position at a university (0), employed in a professional position in a school system (6), do not know (2), total from the above (doctoral) (11).

Additional Information:
Orientation, Objectives, and Emphasis of Department: The department offers MA programs in school and community psychology, marriage and family psychology, and MEd and PhD programs in educational psychology. The program orientations are eclectic, using the scientist-practitioner model, with emphasis on application of theory at the master's degree level and on theoretical issues at the PhD level.

Information for Students With Physical Disabilities: http://studentdisability.wayne.edu.

Application Information:
Send to Department Chair. Students are admitted in the Fall, application deadline February 15. MEd Program rolling admissions throughout the year. *Fee:* $50.

Western Michigan University
Counselor Education & Counseling Psychology
College of Education
3102 Sangren Hall, WMU, 1903 West Michigan Avenue
Kalamazoo, MI 49008-5226
Telephone: (269) 387-5100
Fax: (269) 387-5090
E-mail: *patrick.munley@wmich.edu*
Web: *http://www.wmich.edu/coe/cecp*

Department Information:
1970. Chairperson: Patrick H. Munley. Number of faculty: total—full-time 17, part-time 12; women—full-time 6, part-time 3; total—minority—full-time 4, part-time 3; women minority—full-time 1, part-time 3; faculty subject to the Americans With Disabilities Act 1.

Programs and Degrees Offered:
Listed in the following order: Program area, degree type (T if terminal Master's), number awarded 7/08–6/09. Counseling Psychology MA/MS (Master of Arts/Science) (T) 45, Counseling Psychology PhD (Doctor of Philosophy) 5.

APA Accreditation: Counseling PhD (Doctor of Philosophy).

Student Applications/Admissions:
Student Applications
Counseling Psychology MA/MS (Master of Arts/Science)—Applications 2009–2010, 101. Total applicants accepted 2009–2010, 85. Number full-time enrolled (new admits only) 2009–2010, 68. Number part-time enrolled (new admits only) 2009–2010, 17. Total enrolled 2009–2010 full-time, 106, part-time, 76. Openings 2010–2011, 55. The median number of years required for completion of a degree in 2008–2009 were 3. The number of students enrolled full- and part-time who were dismissed or voluntarily withdrew from this program area in 2008–2009 were 12. *Counseling Psychology PhD (Doctor of Philosophy)*—Applications 2009–2010, 70. Total applicants accepted 2009–2010, 8. Number full-time enrolled (new admits only) 2009–2010, 8. Number part-time enrolled (new admits only) 2009–2010, 0. Openings 2010–2011, 8. The median number of years required for completion of a degree in 2008–2009 were 6. The number of students enrolled full- and part-time who were dismissed or voluntarily withdrew from this program area in 2008–2009 were 0.

Other Criteria: (importance of criteria rated low, medium, or high): GRE scores—high, research experience—high, work experience—medium, extracurricular activity—low, clinically related public service—low, GPA—high, letters of recommendation—high, interview—high, statement of goals and objectives—high, multicultural awareness—high, undergraduate major in psychology—low, specific undergraduate psychology courses taken—medium. For additional information on admission requirements, go to http://www.wmich.edu/coe/cecp/.

Student Characteristics: The following represents characteristics of students in 2009–2010 in all graduate psychology programs in the department: Female—full-time 164, part-time 49; Male—full-time 48, part-time 12; African American/Black—full-time 35, part-time 5; Hispanic/Latino(a)—full-time 4, part-time 1; Asian/Pacific Islander—full-time 9, part-time 2; American Indian/Alaska Native—full-time 2, part-time 0; Caucasian/White—full-time 159, part-time 51; Multi-ethnic—full-time 0, part-time 0; students subject to the Americans With Disabilities Act—full-time 0, part-time 0; Unknown ethnicity—full-time 0, part-time 0; International students who hold an F-1 or J-1 Visa—full-time 0, part-time 0.

Financial Information/Assistance:
Tuition for Full-Time Study: *Master's:* State residents: $401 per credit hour; Nonstate residents: $850 per credit hour. *Doctoral:* State residents: $401 per credit hour; Nonstate residents: $850 per credit hour. See the following Web site for updates and changes in tuition costs: http://www.wmich.edu/registrar/tuition.

Financial Assistance:
First-Year Students: Teaching assistantships available for first year. Average amount paid per academic year: $16,620. Average number of hours worked per week: 20. Apply by February 15. Research assistantships available for first year. Average amount paid per academic year: $16,620. Average number of hours worked per week: 20. Apply by February 15. Fellowships and scholarships available for first year. Average amount paid per academic year: $10,400. Average number of hours worked per week: 10. Apply by February 15.

Advanced Students: Teaching assistantships available for advanced students. Average amount paid per academic year: $16,620. Average number of hours worked per week: 20. Apply by February 15. Research assistantships available for advanced students. Average amount paid per academic year: $16,620. Average number of hours worked per week: 20. Apply by February 15. Fellowships and scholarships available for advanced students.

Additional Information: Of all students currently enrolled full time, 95% benefited from one or more of the listed financial assistance programs. Application and information available online at: http://www.wmich.edu/grad/funding/.

Internships/Practica: Doctoral Degree (PhD Counseling Psychology): For those doctoral students for whom a professional internship was required in this program prior to graduation, (14) students applied for an internship in 2008–2009, with (11) students obtaining an internship. Of those students who obtained an internship, (11) were paid internships. Of those students who obtained an internship, (11) students placed in APA/CPA accredited internships, (0) students placed in internships not APA/CPA accredited, but listed with the Association of Psychology Postdoctoral and Internship Programs (APPIC), (0) students placed in internships conforming to guidelines of the Council of Directors of School Psychology Programs (CDSPP), (0) students placed in internships that were not APA/CPA accredited, APPIC or CDSPP listed. Master's Degree (MA/MS Counseling Psychology): An internship experience, such as a final research project or "capstone" experience is required of graduates. Master's level practica are available in a wide range of settings. Doctoral practica are also available in hospitals, clinics, university counseling centers, etc.

Housing and Day Care: On-campus housing is available. See the following Web site for more information: http://www.wmich.edu/housing/. On-campus day care facilities are available. See the following Web site for more information: http://www.wmich.edu/childrensplace/index.html.

Employment of Department Graduates:
Master's Degree Graduates: Of those who graduated in the academic year 2008–2009, the following categories and numbers represent the postgraduate activities and employment of master's degree graduates: Enrolled in a postdoctoral residency/fellowship (n/a), employed in independent practice (n/a), total from the above (master's) (0).
Doctoral Degree Graduates: Of those who graduated in the academic year 2008–2009, the following categories and numbers represent the postgraduate activities and employment of doctoral degree graduates: Enrolled in a psychology doctoral program (n/a), employed in government agency (2), employed in a community mental health/counseling center (1), employed in a hospital/medical center (1), do not know (1), total from the above (doctoral) (5).

Additional Information:
Orientation, Objectives, and Emphasis of Department: The department prepares professional counseling psychologists at the master's and doctoral levels. The counseling psychology doctoral program's philosophy holds that theory, research, and practice are interdependent and complementary. The curriculum and practical experiences are designed to ensure professional competency in all three dimensions and facilitate their integration. Program graduates are typically employed in a variety of settings including academic departments, university counseling centers, community mental health agencies, hospitals, and independent practices. The curriculum was developed by the Counseling Psychology faculty and is based on guidelines and principles of the American Psychological Association (APA) for accreditation of professional psychology programs. Requirements include course work in the basic scientific core of psychology including research design and statistics, the biological bases of behavior, cognitive-affective bases of behavior, social bases of behavior, individual behavior and human development, and the history and systems of psychology. Requirements also involve course work in the specialization of Counseling Psychology including professional issues and ethics in counseling psychology, counseling theory and practice, consultation, supervision, vocational psychology, intellectual and personality assessment, supervised practica, and an emphasis in multicultural counseling psychology. Students are able to pursue specialty interests in Counseling Psychology through elective courses and other adjunctive experiences (e.g. involvement in faculty research, individual or group clinical supervision, etc). In addition to course work and practica, students are required to successfully complete

comprehensive examinations, a supervised APA approved predoctoral internship, and a dissertation that is psychologically focused. The student's doctoral chair and committee, along with the Counseling Psychology Training Committee, are responsible for helping the student develop a program of study and for monitoring the student's progress through the program.

Special Facilities or Resources: The department's primary training facility is the Center for Counseling and Psychological Services, which includes interview rooms, two group/family therapy rooms, and a seminar room; it is equipped with audio and video recording systems and provides for observation and telephone supervision. The department also maintains a comparable training clinic at the Graduate Center in Grand Rapids, Michigan. A wide variety of regional resources, including community clinics, schools, hospitals, and private clinics, are available to students.

Information for Students With Physical Disabilities: See the following Web site for more information: http://www.dsrs.wmich.edu.

Application Information:
Send to Department of Counselor Education & Counseling Psychology, 1903 West Michigan Ave, WMU, Kalamazoo, MI 49008-5226. Application available online. URL of online application: http://www.wmich.edu/coe/cecp/admission/. Students are admitted in the Fall, application deadline January 10. The application deadline for PhD admissions is January 10. Application deadlines for MA admission are January 15, May 15 and September 15. *Fee:* $40.

MINNESOTA

Metropolitan State University
Psychology/MA in Psychology Program
College of Professional Studies
1450 Energy Park Drive
St. Paul, MN 55108-5218
Telephone: (651) 999-5820
Fax: (651) 999-5803
E-mail: mark.stasson@metrostate.edu
Web: http://www.metrostate.edu/msweb/explore/gradstudies/masters/psych

Department Information:
1990. Chairperson: Gary Starr. Number of faculty: total—full-time 9, part-time 38; women—full-time 4, part-time 33; total—minority—full-time 2, part-time 7; women minority—full-time 1, part-time 6.

Programs and Degrees Offered:
Listed in the following order: Program area, degree type (T if terminal Master's), number awarded 7/08–6/09. Psychology MA/MS (Master of Arts/Science) (T) 1.

Student Applications/Admissions:
Student Applications
Psychology MA/MS (*Master of Arts/Science*)—Applications 2009–2010, 24. Total applicants accepted 2009–2010, 11. Number full-time enrolled (new admits only) 2009–2010, 2. Number part-time enrolled (new admits only) 2009–2010, 5. Total enrolled 2009–2010 full-time, 8, part-time, 16. Openings 2010–2011, 15. The median number of years required for completion of a degree in 2008–2009 were 3. The number of students enrolled full- and part-time who were dismissed or voluntarily withdrew from this program area in 2008–2009 were 1.
Scores: Entries appear in this order: required test or GPA, minimum score (if required), median score of students entering in 2009–2010. Psychology MA/MS (*Master of Arts/Science*): overall undergraduate GPA 3.00.
Other Criteria: (importance of criteria rated low, medium, or high): research experience—medium, work experience—high, extracurricular activity—medium, clinically related public service—low, GPA—high, letters of recommendation—medium, interview—high, statement of goals and objectives—high, community-based work—high.

Student Characteristics: The following represents characteristics of students in 2009–2010 in all graduate psychology programs in the department: Female—full-time 12, part-time 10; Male—full-time 2, part-time 3; African American/Black—full-time 4, part-time 2; Hispanic/Latino(a)—full-time 0, part-time 0; Asian/Pacific Islander—full-time 1, part-time 0; American Indian/Alaska Native—full-time 0, part-time 1; Caucasian/White—full-time 0, part-time 0; Multi-ethnic—full-time 0, part-time 0; students subject to the Americans With Disabilities Act—full-time 0, part-time 0; Unknown ethnicity—full-time 0, part-time 0; International students who hold an F-1 or J-1 Visa—full-time 0, part-time 0.

Financial Information/Assistance:
Tuition for Full-Time Study: Master's: State residents: $252 per credit hour; Nonstate residents: $496 per credit hour. Tuition is subject to change. See the following Web site for updates and changes in tuition costs: http://www.metrostate.edu/tuition/.

Financial Assistance:
First-Year Students: No information provided.
Advanced Students: No information provided.
Additional Information: Of all students currently enrolled full time, 0% benefited from one or more of the listed financial assistance programs. Application and information available online at: http://www.metrostate.edu/aid/.

Internships/Practica: Master's Degree (MA/MS Psychology): An internship experience, such as a final research project or "capstone" experience is required of graduates. Community-based practica are arranged in consultation between the student and their faculty advisor. Practica are developed and implemented in cooperation with Metropolitan State University's Center for Community Based Learning.

Housing and Day Care: No on-campus housing is available. No on-campus day care facilities are available.

Employment of Department Graduates:
Master's Degree Graduates: Of those who graduated in the academic year 2008–2009, the following categories and numbers represent the postgraduate activities and employment of master's degree graduates: Enrolled in another graduate/professional program (2), enrolled in a postdoctoral residency/fellowship (n/a), employed in independent practice (n/a), employed in other positions at a higher education institution (1), not seeking employment (1), other employment position (4), total from the above (master's) (10).
Doctoral Degree Graduates: Of those who graduated in the academic year 2008–2009, the following categories and numbers represent the postgraduate activities and employment of doctoral degree graduates: Enrolled in a psychology doctoral program (n/a), total from the above (doctoral) (0).

Additional Information:
Orientation, Objectives, and Emphasis of Department: The Master of Arts in Psychology program emphasizes the application of psychology in the form of community-based interventions that are rooted in the wisdom and work of members of each community. It is an innovative program, rooted in a community psychology model, in which students learn to combine theory, research, and practice to achieve positive social and community change. Prevention (rather than treatment) is a primary focus along with empowerment, health promotion, community organizing and community development.

Application Information:
Send to MA Psychology Program Coordinator 1450 Energy Park Drive St. Paul, MN 55108-5218. Students are admitted in the Fall, applica-

tion deadline March 1. If openings remain, applications might be considered in the order received until as late as June 1. *Fee:* $20. Metropolitan State University graduates are exempt from this fee.

Minnesota State University—Mankato
Department of Psychology
AH 23
Mankato, MN 56001
Telephone: (507) 389-2724
Fax: (507) 389-5831
E-mail: *carol.seifert@mnsu.edu*
Web: *http://www.mnsu.edu/psych/psych.html*

Department Information:
1964. Chairperson: Barry Ries. Number of faculty: total—full-time 16; women—full-time 7; total—minority—full-time 3; women minority—full-time 1; faculty subject to the Americans With Disabilities Act 1.

Programs and Degrees Offered:
Listed in the following order: Program area, degree type (T if terminal Master's), number awarded 7/08–6/09. Industrial/Organizational Psychology MA/MS (Master of Arts/Science) (T) 10, Clinical Psychology MA/MS (Master of Arts/Science) 10, School Psychology PsyD (Doctor of Psychology) 0.

Student Applications/Admissions:
Student Applications
Industrial/Organizational Psychology MA/MS (Master of Arts/Science)—Applications 2009–2010, 57. Total applicants accepted 2009–2010, 18. Number full-time enrolled (new admits only) 2009–2010, 11. Number part-time enrolled (new admits only) 2009–2010, 0. Openings 2010–2011, 10. The median number of years required for completion of a degree in 2008–2009 were 2. The number of students enrolled full- and part-time who were dismissed or voluntarily withdrew from this program area in 2008–2009 were 0. *Clinical Psychology MA/MS (Master of Arts/Science)*—Applications 2009–2010, 42. Total applicants accepted 2009–2010, 20. Number full-time enrolled (new admits only) 2009–2010, 8. Number part-time enrolled (new admits only) 2009–2010, 0. Openings 2010–2011, 8. The median number of years required for completion of a degree in 2008–2009 were 2. The number of students enrolled full- and part-time who were dismissed or voluntarily withdrew from this program area in 2008–2009 were 0. *School Psychology PsyD (Doctor of Psychology)*—Applications 2009–2010, 11. Total applicants accepted 2009–2010, 6. Number full-time enrolled (new admits only) 2009–2010, 3. Number part-time enrolled (new admits only) 2009–2010, 1. Total enrolled 2009–2010 full-time, 12, part-time, 1. Openings 2010–2011, 6. The number of students enrolled full- and part-time who were dismissed or voluntarily withdrew from this program area in 2008–2009 were 0.
Other Criteria: (importance of criteria rated low, medium, or high): GRE scores—high, research experience—medium, work experience—low, extracurricular activity—low, clinically related public service—medium, GPA—medium, letters of recommendation—high, interview—medium, statement of goals and objectives—medium, undergraduate major in psychology—high, specific undergraduate psychology courses taken—medium.

Student Characteristics: The following represents characteristics of students in 2009–2010 in all graduate psychology programs in the department: Female—full-time 33, part-time 1; Male—full-time 17, part-time 0; African American/Black—full-time 1, part-time 0; Hispanic/Latino(a)—full-time 0, part-time 0; Asian/Pacific Islander—full-time 6, part-time 0; American Indian/Alaska Native—full-time 0, part-time 0; Caucasian/White—full-time 41, part-time 1; Multi-ethnic—full-time 2, part-time 0; students subject to the Americans With Disabilities Act—full-time 0, part-time 0; Unknown ethnicity—full-time 0, part-time 0; International students who hold an F-1 or J-1 Visa—full-time 0, part-time 0.

Financial Information/Assistance:
Tuition for Full-Time Study: *Master's:* State residents: $283 per credit hour; Nonstate residents: $467 per credit hour. *Doctoral:* State residents: $412 per credit hour; Nonstate residents: $412 per credit hour. Tuition is subject to change. See the following Web site for updates and changes in tuition costs: http://www.mnsu.edu/campushub/tuition_fees/.

Financial Assistance:
First-Year Students: Teaching assistantships available for first year. Average amount paid per academic year: $4,500. Average number of hours worked per week: 10. Apply by March 15.
Advanced Students: Teaching assistantships available for advanced students. Average amount paid per academic year: $4,500. Average number of hours worked per week: 10. Apply by March 15.
Additional Information: Of all students currently enrolled full time, 50% benefited from one or more of the listed financial assistance programs.

Internships/Practica: Master's Degree (MA/MS Industrial/Organizational Psychology): An internship experience, such as a final research project or "capstone" experience is required of graduates. A variety of clinical practica are available to our clinical students. Sites have included the Mayo Clinic, the Munroe-Meyer Institute, Minneapolis VA Hospital and local Riverview Clinic. I/O internship sites include Chiquita, ePredix, Minnesota Twins, Thrivent, 3-M and Army research labs.

Housing and Day Care: On-campus housing is available. See the following Web site for more information: http://www.mnsu.edu/reslife/. On-campus day care facilities are available. See the following Web site for more information: http://ed.mnsu.edu/tch/.

Employment of Department Graduates:
Master's Degree Graduates: Of those who graduated in the academic year 2008–2009, the following categories and numbers represent the postgraduate activities and employment of master's degree graduates: Enrolled in a psychology doctoral program (7), enrolled in another graduate/professional program (1), enrolled in a postdoctoral residency/fellowship (n/a), employed in independent practice (n/a), total from the above (master's) (8).
Doctoral Degree Graduates: Of those who graduated in the academic year 2008–2009, the following categories and numbers represent the postgraduate activities and employment of doctoral

degree graduates: Enrolled in a psychology doctoral program (n/a), total from the above (doctoral) (0).

Additional Information:
Orientation, Objectives, and Emphasis of Department: The school psychology doctoral program emphasizes data-based decision-making, multiculturalism, mental health, and prevention. Graduates will be prepared to pursue certification and licensure at state and national levels. The clinical program is a research-based, predoctoral program with a strong behavioral emphasis. The goal of the I/O program is to provide broad theoretical and technical training for individuals who will function as human resource professionals or who will go on to doctoral programs in I/O psychology.

Special Facilities or Resources: I/O faculty have ongoing research partnerships with major organizations such as U.S. Airforce Department of Special Investigations, United Health group, 3-M Corporation, Scholarship America, and the national Pork Board. Clinical faculty maintain professional relationships with Immanuel-St. Joseph Hospital, Mayo Health System and with area schools.

Information for Students With Physical Disabilities: See the following Web site for more information: http://www.mnsu.edu/dso/.

Application Information:
Send to Department of Psychology, AH 23, Minnesota State University, Mankato, Mankato, MN 56001. Students are admitted in the Fall, application deadline for School Psychology PsyD program: January 15, Deadline for Clinical Psychology Program: February 15, Deadline for I/O Psychology Program: March 1. *Fee:* $40.

Minnesota State University—Moorhead
School Psychology Program
Social and Natural Sciences
1104 7th Avenue South
Moorhead, MN 56563
Telephone: (218) 477-2802
Fax: (218) 477-2602
E-mail: *schpsych@mnstate.edu*
Web: *http://www.mnstate.edu/gradpsyc*

Department Information:
1970. Program Director: Olivia Melroe. Number of faculty: total—full-time 11; women—full-time 7; total—minority—full-time 1.

Programs and Degrees Offered:
Listed in the following order: Program area, degree type (T if terminal Master's), number awarded 7/08–6/09. School Psychology EdS (School Psychology) 11.

Student Applications/Admissions:
Student Applications
School Psychology EdS (School Psychology)—Applications 2009–2010, 27. Total applicants accepted 2009–2010, 17. Number full-time enrolled (new admits only) 2009–2010, 12. Number part-time enrolled (new admits only) 2009–2010, 0. Total enrolled 2009–2010 full-time, 19, part-time, 2. Openings 2010–2011, 10. The median number of years required for completion of a degree in 2008–2009 were 3.

Scores: Entries appear in this order: required test or GPA, minimum score (if required), median score of students entering in 2009–2010. *School Psychology EdS (School Psychology):* GRE-V 400, 470, GRE-Q 440, 560, overall undergraduate GPA 3.19, 3.45.

Other Criteria: (importance of criteria rated low, medium, or high): GRE scores—high, research experience—medium, work experience—medium, extracurricular activity—medium, clinically related public service—low, GPA—high, letters of recommendation—high, interview—low, statement of goals and objectives—high, undergraduate major in psychology—medium, specific undergraduate psychology courses taken—medium.

Student Characteristics: The following represents characteristics of students in 2009–2010 in all graduate psychology programs in the department: Female—full-time 14, part-time 2; Male—full-time 5, part-time 0; African American/Black—full-time 0, part-time 0; Hispanic/Latino(a)—full-time 0, part-time 0; Asian/Pacific Islander—full-time 0, part-time 0; American Indian/Alaska Native—full-time 0, part-time 0; Caucasian/White—full-time 0, part-time 0; Multi-ethnic—full-time 1, part-time 0; students subject to the Americans With Disabilities Act—full-time 0, part-time 0; Unknown ethnicity—full-time 0, part-time 0; International students who hold an F-1 or J-1 Visa—full-time 0, part-time 0.

Financial Information/Assistance:
Tuition for Full-Time Study: *Master's:* State residents: per academic year $6,774, $282 per credit hour; Nonstate residents: per academic year $6,774, $282 per credit hour. Tuition is subject to change. Additional fees are assessed to students beyond the costs of tuition for the following: basic university activity, health, etc. fees. See the following Web site for updates and changes in tuition costs: http://www.mnstate.edu/busoff/tuitionfees.

Financial Assistance:
First-Year Students: Research assistantships available for first year. Average amount paid per academic year: $1,700. Average number of hours worked per week: 5. Apply by May 15.

Advanced Students: Research assistantships available for advanced students. Average amount paid per academic year: $2,000. Average number of hours worked per week: 6. Apply by May 15.

Additional Information: Of all students currently enrolled full time, 90% benefited from one or more of the listed financial assistance programs.

Internships/Practica: Field-based practica in both first and second years of study provide hands-on experience to students. Practica are supervised by local educators and school psychologists and are coordinated with on-campus course work so students can apply concepts and techniques learned in class. A 1200-hour internship during the third year of study serves as a capstone experience for student's training. Internships are usually positions within school districts or special education cooperatives in the tri-state area, however students have completed internships in sites across the country.

Housing and Day Care: On-campus housing is available. See the following Web site for more information: http://www.mnstate.edu/housing. On-campus day care facilities are available. See the following Web site for more information: http://www.mnstate.edu/childcare.

Employment of Department Graduates:
Master's Degree Graduates: Of those who graduated in the academic year 2008–2009, the following categories and numbers represent the postgraduate activities and employment of master's degree graduates: Enrolled in a postdoctoral residency/fellowship (n/a), employed in independent practice (n/a), employed in a professional position in a school system (5), total from the above (master's) (5).
Doctoral Degree Graduates: Of those who graduated in the academic year 2008–2009, the following categories and numbers represent the postgraduate activities and employment of doctoral degree graduates: Enrolled in a psychology doctoral program (n/a), total from the above (doctoral) (0).

Additional Information:
Orientation, Objectives, and Emphasis of Department: Our goal is to provide the training necessary for our graduates to be skilled problem solvers in dealing with the needs of children, families, and others involved in the learning enterprise. Within a scientist–practitioner model and integrative perspective, the program's primary focus is on educating specialist-level professionals capable of working effectively in educational agencies and in collaboration with other human services providers. Our graduates are highly regarded by the schools and agencies within which they work because of their knowledge of current best practices in the field and because of their skills as team members.

Information for Students With Physical Disabilities: See the following Web site for more information: http://www.mnstate.edu/disability.

Application Information:
Send to Graduate Studies Office, Minnesota State University Moorhead, 1104 7th Avenue S., Moorhead, Minnesota 56563. Application available online. URL of online application: http://www.mnstate.edu/graduate. Students are admitted in the Fall, application deadline February 15. Applications will be accepted after February 15 if space is available. *Fee:* $20.

Minnesota, University of
Department of Educational Psychology: Counseling and Student Personnel; School Psychology
Education and Human Development
178 Pillsbury Drive South East, 206 Burton Hall
Minneapolis, MN 55455
Telephone: (612) 624-1698
Fax: (612) 624-8241
E-mail: *shupp@umn.edu*
Web: *http://education.umn.edu/EdPsych*

Department Information:
1947. Chairperson: Susan Hupp. Number of faculty: total—full-time 35; women—full-time 12; total—minority—full-time 7; women minority—full-time 3; faculty subject to the Americans With Disabilities Act 1.

Programs and Degrees Offered:
Listed in the following order: Program area, degree type (T if terminal Master's), number awarded 7/08–6/09. Counseling and Student Personnel MA/MS (Master of Arts/Science) (T) 33, School Psychology PhD (Doctor of Philosophy) 7, Counseling and Student Personnel PhD (Doctor of Philosophy) 4, School Psychology EdS (School Psychology) 1.

APA Accreditation: School PhD (Doctor of Philosophy). Student Outcome Data Website: http://www.cehd.umn.edu/EdPsych/SchoolPsych/doctor.html. Counseling PhD (Doctor of Philosophy). Student Outcome Data Website: http://www.cehd.umn.edu/EdPsych/CSPP/outcomes.html.

Student Applications/Admissions:
Student Applications
Counseling and Student Personnel MA/MS (Master of Arts/Science)—Applications 2009–2010, 94. Total applicants accepted 2009–2010, 52. Number full-time enrolled (new admits only) 2009–2010, 33. Total enrolled 2009–2010 full-time, 77. Openings 2010–2011, 30. The median number of years required for completion of a degree in 2008–2009 were 2. The number of students enrolled full- and part-time who were dismissed or voluntarily withdrew from this program area in 2008–2009 were 1. *School Psychology PhD (Doctor of Philosophy)*—Applications 2009–2010, 32. Total applicants accepted 2009–2010, 18. Number full-time enrolled (new admits only) 2009–2010, 9. Total enrolled 2009–2010 full-time, 47. Openings 2010–2011, 9. The median number of years required for completion of a degree in 2008–2009 were 7. The number of students enrolled full- and part-time who were dismissed or voluntarily withdrew from this program area in 2008–2009 were 0. *Counseling and Student Personnel PhD (Doctor of Philosophy)*—Applications 2009–2010, 74. Total applicants accepted 2009–2010, 11. Number full-time enrolled (new admits only) 2009–2010, 6. Total enrolled 2009–2010 full-time, 42. Openings 2010–2011, 6. The median number of years required for completion of a degree in 2008–2009 were 8. The number of students enrolled full- and part-time who were dismissed or voluntarily withdrew from this program area in 2008–2009 were 0. *School Psychology EdS (School Psychology)*—Applications 2009–2010, 37. Total applicants accepted 2009–2010, 14. Number full-time enrolled (new admits only) 2009–2010, 6. Total enrolled 2009–2010 full-time, 26. Openings 2010–2011, 6. The median number of years required for completion of a degree in 2008–2009 were 3. The number of students enrolled full- and part-time who were dismissed or voluntarily withdrew from this program area in 2008–2009 were 0.

Scores: Entries appear in this order: required test or GPA, minimum score (if required), median score of students entering in 2009–2010. *Counseling and Student Personnel MA/MS (Master of Arts/Science):* GRE-V no minimum stated, 546, GRE-Q no minimum stated, 637, GRE-Analytical no minimum stated, 4.6, overall undergraduate GPA 3.0, 3.62; *School Psychology PhD (Doctor of Philosophy):* GRE-V no minimum stated, 591, GRE-Q no minimum stated, 695, overall undergraduate GPA no minimum stated, 3.68; *Counseling and Student Personnel PhD (Doctor of Philosophy):* GRE-V no minimum stated, 599, GRE-Q no minimum stated, 686, GRE-Analytical no minimum stated, 4.9, overall undergraduate GPA 3.0, 3.67; *School Psychology EdS (School Psychology)*: GRE-V no minimum stated, 554, GRE-Q no minimum stated, 672, overall undergraduate GPA no minimum stated, 3.53.

Other Criteria: (importance of criteria rated low, medium, or high): GRE scores—high, research experience—medium, work experience—medium, extracurricular activity—medium, clinically related public service—low, GPA—medium, letters of recommendation—high, interview—high, statement of goals and objectives—high. CSPP/PhD: research: high; work: high; extracurricular: high; public service: high; letters of rec: high; statement of goals: high; interview: none. For additional information on admission requirements, go to http://www.cehd.umn.edu/EdPsych/.

Student Characteristics: The following represents characteristics of students in 2009–2010 in all graduate psychology programs in the department: Female—full-time 165, part-time 57; Male—full-time 59, part-time 17; African American/Black—full-time 9, part-time 2; Hispanic/Latino(a)—full-time 5, part-time 1; Asian/Pacific Islander—full-time 13, part-time 3; American Indian/Alaska Native—full-time 1, part-time 1; Caucasian/White—full-time 148, part-time 56; Multi-ethnic—full-time 0, part-time 0; students subject to the Americans With Disabilities Act—full-time 0, part-time 0; Unknown ethnicity—full-time 5, part-time 4; International students who hold an F-1 or J-1 Visa—full-time 43, part-time 7.

Financial Information/Assistance:
Tuition for Full-Time Study: *Master's:* State residents: per academic year $11,212, $934 per credit hour; Nonstate residents: per academic year $18,310, $1,526 per credit hour. *Doctoral:* State residents: per academic year $11,212, $934 per credit hour; Nonstate residents: per academic year $18,310, $1,526 per credit hour. Tuition is subject to change. See the following Web site for updates and changes in tuition costs: http://onestop.umn.edu/finances/costs_and_tuition/index.html.

Financial Assistance:
First-Year Students: Teaching assistantships available for first year. Average amount paid per academic year: $6,533. Average number of hours worked per week: 10. Apply by December 1. Research assistantships available for first year. Average amount paid per academic year: $6,533. Average number of hours worked per week: 10. Apply by December 1. Fellowships and scholarships available for first year. Average amount paid per academic year: $22,500. Average number of hours worked per week: 0. Apply by December 1.

Advanced Students: Teaching assistantships available for advanced students. Average amount paid per academic year: $6,533. Average number of hours worked per week: 10. Apply by December 1. Research assistantships available for advanced students. Average amount paid per academic year: $6,533. Average number of hours worked per week: 10. Apply by December 1. Fellowships and scholarships available for advanced students. Average amount paid per academic year: $22,500. Average number of hours worked per week: 0. Apply by December 1.

Additional Information: Of all students currently enrolled full time, 75% benefited from one or more of the listed financial assistance programs. Application and information available online at: http://onestop.umn.edu/finances/financial_aid/index.html.

Internships/Practica: Doctoral Degree (PhD School Psychology): For those doctoral students for whom a professional internship was required in this program prior to graduation, (3) students applied for an internship in 2008–2009, with (3) students obtaining an internship. Of those students who obtained an internship, (3) were paid internships. Of those students who obtained an internship, (0) students placed in APA/CPA accredited internships, (0) students placed in internships not APA/CPA accredited, but listed with the Association of Psychology Postdoctoral and Internship Programs (APPIC), (1) students placed in internships conforming to guidelines of the Council of Directors of School Psychology Programs (CDSPP), (2) students placed in internships that were not APA/CPA accredited, APPIC or CDSPP listed. Doctoral Degree (PhD Counseling and Student Personnel): For those doctoral students for whom a professional internship was required in this program prior to graduation, (7) students applied for an internship in 2008–2009, with (7) students obtaining an internship. Of those students who obtained an internship, (7) were paid internships. Of those students who obtained an internship, (7) students placed in APA/CPA accredited internships, (0) students placed in internships not APA/CPA accredited, but listed with the Association of Psychology Postdoctoral and Internship Programs (APPIC), (0) students placed in internships conforming to guidelines of the Council of Directors of School Psychology Programs (CDSPP), (0) students placed in internships that were not APA/CPA accredited, APPIC or CDSPP listed. Counseling and Student Personnel Psychology MA students complete an academic year practicum in the second year with a focus on community counseling, school counseling or college student development. The practicum consists of direct work with clients/students, individual supervision on-site and an academic seminar at the university. PhD students complete one or more practica and then a year-long internship. Some students stay in the Twin Cities for the internship; others go nationally. School Psychology Doctoral students have three tiers of applied training. Tier 1 - Year-long practicum tied to assessment coursework followed by a second year of practicum tied to intervention coursework. Most of these experiences occur in metro area schools. Tier 2 - Formal school practicum under the supervision of a school psychologist in Twin Cities area schools. In addition, doctoral students complete a community/clinical practicum. These practica occur in a wide variety of settings including mental health and community agencies such as Indian Health Board, Washburn Child Guidance Center, Community University Health Care Center, Fraser Family and Children services. Tier 3 - Internship. The majority of students complete their year-long internships in public schools settings, although some have found internships in settings that are a collaboration of community and educational settings. In one setting, interns work as part of a mental health and educational team providing school-based services to identified students with emotional and behavioral disorders.

Housing and Day Care: On-campus housing is available. See the following Web site for more information: http://www.housing.umn.edu/graduate. On-campus day care facilities are available. See the following Web site for more information: http://www.sphc.umn.edu/childcare.html.

Employment of Department Graduates:
Master's Degree Graduates: Of those who graduated in the academic year 2008–2009, the following categories and numbers

represent the postgraduate activities and employment of master's degree graduates: Enrolled in a psychology doctoral program (3), enrolled in a postdoctoral residency/fellowship (n/a), employed in independent practice (n/a), employed in an academic position at a university (2), employed in an academic position at a 2-year/4-year college (2), employed in a professional position in a school system (13), employed in business or industry (1), employed in government agency (3), employed in a community mental health/counseling center (3), employed in a hospital/medical center (1), still seeking employment (1), do not know (13), total from the above (master's) (42).

Doctoral Degree Graduates: Of those who graduated in the academic year 2008–2009, the following categories and numbers represent the postgraduate activities and employment of doctoral degree graduates: Enrolled in a psychology doctoral program (n/a), employed in independent practice (1), employed in an academic position at a university (2), employed in other positions at a higher education institution (1), employed in a professional position in a school system (3), employed in business or industry (1), employed in a hospital/medical center (1), total from the above (doctoral) (9).

Additional Information:
Orientation, Objectives, and Emphasis of Department: Counseling and Student Personnel Psychology is intended to provide a fundamental body of knowledge and skills to prepare counselors and counseling psychologists for work in a variety of settings—counseling and human development, career development, staff development, and student personnel work. While the focus is primarily on facilitating human development in educational settings, it is possible for individuals to prepare for community and agency settings as well. The faculty is committed to addressing current social issues such as diversity concerns and adolescent well-being. The CSPP program is designed for a select group of individuals with a demonstrated capacity for leadership and a commitment in the human services. School Psychology: The range of the school psychologist's impact includes, but is not limited to, the application of theory and research in the psychosocial development and learning of children and youth, social interaction processes, prevention and competence enhancement strategies, instructional intervention and program development, and delivery of mental health services. Our major training goal is to prepare school psychologists for roles within higher education and school systems. Competencies needed include knowledge in developmental psychology, personality and learning theory, and social psychology; assessing individual and systems needs; generating and implementing prevention programs and intervention strategies; collaborative consultation; diversity; and evaluating and redesigning programs. Training modalities include a variety of seminars and independent study projects. A wide range of community resources are available to facilitate goals of the program.

Special Facilities or Resources: Our graduate program is located within a major research university where many research projects are ongoing. The program is also located within a state—Minnesota—and major metropolitan area—the Twin Cities—that are known for innovations in human services. The result is that both the research climate and the practice climate are good ones for students. CSPP: The department has some flexibility in the design of student programs. Excellent facilities for research opportunities exist throughout the university. There is a time-shared instructional computing laboratory with batch and online computer facilities available for student use; and free access to the central university computer. Students may borrow laptops, video cameras, LCD projectors, audiorecorders, overheads, and VCRs. Students record counseling role-play sessions in a state-of-the-art digital counseling laboratory. School Psychology: Two job files (academic and professional service positions) exist. School Psychology Resources houses journals, books, and intervention and assessment materials. This collection supplements the Psychology Department Journal Seminar Room (for psychology majors) and the Florence Goodenough Reading Room (for child psychology majors), the University Psychology and Educational Library with its specialized computer search facilities, and the extensive University libraries system with holdings numbering approximately 3.5 million volumes. School psychology also maintains a collection of standardized, individual, and group psychometric tests, measures, and protocols which can be borrowed for coursework use.

Information for Students With Physical Disabilities: See the following Web site for more information: http://ds.umn.edu.

Application Information:
Send to Department of Educational Psychology University of Minnesota 250 Education Sciences Building 56 East River Road Minneapolis, MN 55455. Application available online. URL of online application: http://www.grad.umn.edu/prospective_students/apply_online.html. Students are admitted in the Fall, application deadline December 1. *Fee:* $75.

Minnesota, University of
Department of Psychology
N218 Elliott Hall, 75 East River Road
Minneapolis, MN 55455
Telephone: (612) 625-4042
Fax: (612) 626-2079
E-mail: *psyapply@umn.edu*
Web: *http://www.psych.umn.edu*

Department Information:
1919. Chairperson: Gordon Legge. Number of faculty: total—full-time 44, part-time 36; women—full-time 10, part-time 16; total—minority—full-time 5, part-time 2; women minority—full-time 2, part-time 2; faculty subject to the Americans With Disabilities Act 1.

Programs and Degrees Offered:
Listed in the following order: Program area, degree type (T if terminal Master's), number awarded 7/08–6/09. Biological Psychopathology PhD (Doctor of Philosophy) 2, Clinical Psychology PhD (Doctor of Philosophy) 6, Cognitive and Biological Psychology PhD (Doctor of Philosophy) 5, Counseling Psychology PhD (Doctor of Philosophy) 2, Personality, Individual Diff. & Behav. Genetics PhD (Doctor of Philosophy) 2, Industrial/Organizational Psychology PhD (Doctor of Philosophy) 5, Quantitative/Psychometric Methods PhD (Doctor of Philosophy) 1, School Psychology PhD (Doctor of Philosophy) 1, Social Psychology PhD (Doctor of Philosophy) 3.

GRADUATE STUDY IN PSYCHOLOGY

APA Accreditation: Clinical PhD (Doctor of Philosophy). Student Outcome Data Website: http://www.psych.umn.edu/areas/clinical/index.htm. Counseling PhD (Doctor of Philosophy). Student Outcome Data Website: http://www.psych.umn.edu/areas/counseling/index.htm.

Student Applications/Admissions:
   Student Applications
   Biological Psychopathology PhD (Doctor of Philosophy)—Applications 2009–2010, 6. Total applicants accepted 2009–2010, 1. Number full-time enrolled (new admits only) 2009–2010, 1. Number part-time enrolled (new admits only) 2009–2010, 0. Openings 2010–2011, 1. The median number of years required for completion of a degree in 2008–2009 were 6. The number of students enrolled full- and part-time who were dismissed or voluntarily withdrew from this program area in 2008–2009 were 0. *Clinical Psychology PhD (Doctor of Philosophy)*—Applications 2009–2010, 105. Total applicants accepted 2009–2010, 7. Number full-time enrolled (new admits only) 2009–2010, 3. Number part-time enrolled (new admits only) 2009–2010, 0. Openings 2010–2011, 5. The median number of years required for completion of a degree in 2008–2009 were 6. The number of students enrolled full- and part-time who were dismissed or voluntarily withdrew from this program area in 2008–2009 were 1. *Cognitive and Biological Psychology PhD (Doctor of Philosophy)*—Applications 2009–2010, 43. Total applicants accepted 2009–2010, 7. Number full-time enrolled (new admits only) 2009–2010, 3. Number part-time enrolled (new admits only) 2009–2010, 0. Openings 2010–2011, 5. The median number of years required for completion of a degree in 2008–2009 were 6. The number of students enrolled full- and part-time who were dismissed or voluntarily withdrew from this program area in 2008–2009 were 0. *Counseling Psychology PhD (Doctor of Philosophy)*—Applications 2009–2010, 68. Total applicants accepted 2009–2010, 5. Number full-time enrolled (new admits only) 2009–2010, 3. Number part-time enrolled (new admits only) 2009–2010, 0. Openings 2010–2011, 4. The median number of years required for completion of a degree in 2008–2009 were 6. The number of students enrolled full- and part-time who were dismissed or voluntarily withdrew from this program area in 2008–2009 were 0. *Personality, Individual Diff. & Behav. Genetics PhD (Doctor of Philosophy)*—Applications 2009–2010, 14. Total applicants accepted 2009–2010, 3. Number full-time enrolled (new admits only) 2009–2010, 1. Number part-time enrolled (new admits only) 2009–2010, 0. Openings 2010–2011, 2. The median number of years required for completion of a degree in 2008–2009 were 8. The number of students enrolled full- and part-time who were dismissed or voluntarily withdrew from this program area in 2008–2009 were 0. *Industrial/Organizational Psychology PhD (Doctor of Philosophy)*—Applications 2009–2010, 36. Total applicants accepted 2009–2010, 5. Number full-time enrolled (new admits only) 2009–2010, 3. Number part-time enrolled (new admits only) 2009–2010, 0. Openings 2010–2011, 3. The median number of years required for completion of a degree in 2008–2009 were 5. The number of students enrolled full- and part-time who were dismissed or voluntarily withdrew from this program area in 2008–2009 were 0. *Quantitative/Psychometric Methods PhD (Doctor of Philosophy)*—Applications 2009–2010, 11. Total applicants accepted 2009–2010, 3. Number full-time enrolled (new admits only) 2009–2010, 1. Number part-time enrolled (new admits only) 2009–2010, 0. Openings 2010–2011, 1. The median number of years required for completion of a degree in 2008–2009 were 8. The number of students enrolled full- and part-time who were dismissed or voluntarily withdrew from this program area in 2008–2009 were 0. *School Psychology PhD (Doctor of Philosophy)*—Applications 2009–2010, 0. Total applicants accepted 2009–2010, 0. Number full-time enrolled (new admits only) 2009–2010, 0. Number part-time enrolled (new admits only) 2009–2010, 0. Openings 2010–2011, 1. The median number of years required for completion of a degree in 2008–2009 were 8. The number of students enrolled full- and part-time who were dismissed or voluntarily withdrew from this program area in 2008–2009 were 0. *Social Psychology PhD (Doctor of Philosophy)*—Applications 2009–2010, 75. Total applicants accepted 2009–2010, 8. Number full-time enrolled (new admits only) 2009–2010, 7. Number part-time enrolled (new admits only) 2009–2010, 0. Openings 2010–2011, 4. The median number of years required for completion of a degree in 2008–2009 were 6. The number of students enrolled full- and part-time who were dismissed or voluntarily withdrew from this program area in 2008–2009 were 0.

Other Criteria: (importance of criteria rated low, medium, or high): GRE scores—high, research experience—high, work experience—medium, extracurricular activity—medium, clinically related public service—medium, GPA—high, letters of recommendation—high, interview—high, statement of goals and objectives—high. Please note that applicants to the Clinical Psychology program are the only applicants interviewed. For additional information on admission requirements, go to http://www.psych.umn.edu/graduate.

Student Characteristics: The following represents characteristics of students in 2009–2010 in all graduate psychology programs in the department: Female—full-time 82, part-time 0; Male—full-time 57, part-time 0; African American/Black—full-time 0, part-time 0; Hispanic/Latino(a)—full-time 3, part-time 0; Asian/Pacific Islander—full-time 17, part-time 0; American Indian/Alaska Native—full-time 2, part-time 0; Caucasian/White—full-time 117, part-time 0; Multi-ethnic—full-time 0, part-time 0; students subject to the Americans With Disabilities Act—full-time 1, part-time 0; Unknown ethnicity—full-time 0, part-time 0; International students who hold an F-1 or J-1 Visa—full-time 17, part-time 0.

Financial Information/Assistance:
   Tuition for Full-Time Study: *Doctoral:* State residents: per academic year $11,212, $934 per credit hour; Nonstate residents: per academic year $18,310, $1,525 per credit hour. Tuition is subject to change. Additional fees are assessed to students beyond the costs of tuition for the following: student services fee of $348/semester; CLA fee of $105/semester; university fee of $600/semster. See the following Web site for updates and changes in tuition costs: http://www.grad.umn.edu/prospective_students/.

   Financial Assistance:
   First-Year Students: Teaching assistantships available for first year. Average amount paid per academic year: $13,845. Average number of hours worked per week: 20. Apply by December 1. Research assistantships available for first year. Average amount paid per academic year: $13,845. Average number of hours worked per week: 20. Apply by December 1. Traineeships available for first year. Average amount paid per academic year: $0. Average number of hours worked per week: 0. Apply by December 1.

Fellowships and scholarships available for first year. Average amount paid per academic year: $22,500. Average number of hours worked per week: 0. Apply by December 1.

Advanced Students: Teaching assistantships available for advanced students. Average amount paid per academic year: $13,845. Average number of hours worked per week: 20. Research assistantships available for advanced students. Average amount paid per academic year: $13,845. Average number of hours worked per week: 20. Traineeships available for advanced students. Average amount paid per academic year: $20,976. Average number of hours worked per week: 0. Fellowships and scholarships available for advanced students. Average amount paid per academic year: $23,187. Average number of hours worked per week: 0.

Additional Information: Of all students currently enrolled full time, 84% benefited from one or more of the listed financial assistance programs. Application and information available online at: http://www.psych.umn.edu/graduate/finsup.htm.

Internships/Practica: Doctoral Degree (PhD Clinical Psychology): For those doctoral students for whom a professional internship was required in this program prior to graduation, (8) students applied for an internship in 2008–2009, with (8) students obtaining an internship. Of those students who obtained an internship, (8) were paid internships. Of those students who obtained an internship, (8) students placed in APA/CPA accredited internships, (0) students placed in internships not APA/CPA accredited, but listed with the Association of Psychology Postdoctoral and Internship Programs (APPIC), (0) students placed in internships conforming to guidelines of the Council of Directors of School Psychology Programs (CDSPP), (0) students placed in internships that were not APA/CPA accredited, APPIC or CDSPP listed. Doctoral Degree (PhD Counseling Psychology): For those doctoral students for whom a professional internship was required in this program prior to graduation, (5) students applied for an internship in 2008–2009, with (5) students obtaining an internship. Of those students who obtained an internship, (5) were paid internships. Of those students who obtained an internship, (5) students placed in APA/CPA accredited internships, (0) students placed in internships not APA/CPA accredited, but listed with the Association of Psychology Postdoctoral and Internship Programs (APPIC), (0) students placed in internships conforming to guidelines of the Council of Directors of School Psychology Programs (CDSPP), (0) students placed in internships that were not APA/CPA accredited, APPIC or CDSPP listed. Internships are available at the university hospitals, the department's Vocational Assessment Clinic, the University Counseling and Consulting Services, the Veterans Administration, and several other governmental and private agencies throughout the area.

Housing and Day Care: On-campus housing is available. See the following Web site for more information: http://www.housing.umn.edu. On-campus day care facilities are available. See the following Web site for more information: http://cehd.umn.edu/ChildCareCenter/.

Employment of Department Graduates:

Master's Degree Graduates: Of those who graduated in the academic year 2008–2009, the following categories and numbers represent the postgraduate activities and employment of master's degree graduates: Enrolled in a psychology doctoral program (7), enrolled in another graduate/professional program (1), enrolled in a postdoctoral residency/fellowship (n/a), employed in independent practice (n/a), employed in an academic position at a university (0), employed in an academic position at a 2-year/4-year college (0), employed in other positions at a higher education institution (0), employed in a professional position in a school system (0), employed in business or industry (0), employed in government agency (1), employed in a community mental health/counseling center (0), employed in a hospital/medical center (0), still seeking employment (0), not seeking employment (0), other employment position (0), do not know (1), total from the above (master's) (10).

Doctoral Degree Graduates: Of those who graduated in the academic year 2008–2009, the following categories and numbers represent the postgraduate activities and employment of doctoral degree graduates: Enrolled in a psychology doctoral program (n/a), enrolled in another graduate/professional program (0), enrolled in a postdoctoral residency/fellowship (9), employed in independent practice (0), employed in an academic position at a university (8), employed in an academic position at a 2-year/4-year college (0), employed in other positions at a higher education institution (4), employed in a professional position in a school system (0), employed in business or industry (2), employed in government agency (0), employed in a community mental health/counseling center (1), employed in a hospital/medical center (1), still seeking employment (0), not seeking employment (0), other employment position (1), do not know (1), total from the above (doctoral) (27).

Additional Information:

Orientation, Objectives, and Emphasis of Department: Minnesota has a broad range of areas of specialization in the department. The overall goal is to train the people who will become leaders in their chosen area of specialization. Consequently, the graduate training programs in the department are oriented first to the training of skilled researchers and teachers in psychology, and then to the training of specialists and practitioners. The PhD programs in Clinical, Counseling, and School Psychology are accredited by APA. Department faculty also participate in independent degree programs in neuroscience and cognitive science. The Department of Psychology and the Institute of Child Development offer a training program in child clinical psychology focused on the study of psychopathology in the context of development. The Developmental Psychopathology and Clinical Science (DPCS) training program is APA-accredited as part of the Clinical Psychology Program. Admission to the DPCS program is coordinated by the Institute of Child Development, 51 East River Road, University of Minnesota, Minneapolis, MN 55455. The school psychology PhD is offered jointly with the School Psychology program.

Special Facilities or Resources: The department offers extensive laboratory and computer facilities, a wide variety of resources and collaborative relationships both on and off campus, and several federally funded research projects. For example, three research centers are headquartered in the Department: Center for Cognitive Sciences, Center for the Study of Political Psychology, and the Center for the Study of the Individual and Society. Other research centers with which the faculty are involved are located in Neuroscience, Radiology, Epidemiology, and Public Health. We have adjunct faculty at the University of Minnesota Counseling and Consulting Services, Carlson School of Management, Institute of Child Development, and Department of Educational

GRADUATE STUDY IN PSYCHOLOGY

Psychology; and in the VA Medical Center, Hennepin County Medical Center (Minneapolis), Ramsey County Medical Center (St. Paul), and Personnel Decisions International (Minneapolis).

Information for Students With Physical Disabilities: See the following Web site for more information: http://ds.umn.edu.

Application Information:
Send to Coordinator of Graduate Admissions, University of Minnesota, Department of Psychology, S253 Elliott Hall, 75 East River Road, Minneapolis, MN 55455. Students are admitted in the Fall, application deadline December 1. *Fee:* $75. $95 for international applicants.

Minnesota, University of
Institute of Child Development
College of Education and Human Development
51 East River Road
Minneapolis, MN 55455
Telephone: (612) 624-0526
Fax: (612) 624-6373
E-mail: *icd@umn.edu*
Web: *http://www.cehd.umn.edu/icd/*

Department Information:
1925. Director: Nicki Crick. Number of faculty: total—full-time 19; women—full-time 9; total—minority—full-time 1; women minority—full-time 1.

Programs and Degrees Offered:
Listed in the following order: Program area, degree type (T if terminal Master's), number awarded 7/08–6/09. Child Psychology PhD (Doctor of Philosophy) 5, Child/Clinical Psychology PhD (Doctor of Philosophy) 2, Child/School Psychology PhD (Doctor of Philosophy) 0.

Student Applications/Admissions:
Student Applications
Child Psychology PhD (Doctor of Philosophy)—Applications 2009–2010, 35. Total applicants accepted 2009–2010, 10. Number full-time enrolled (new admits only) 2009–2010, 5. Total enrolled 2009–2010 full-time, 34, part-time, 3. Openings 2010–2011, 6. The median number of years required for completion of a degree in 2008–2009 were 6. The number of students enrolled full- and part-time who were dismissed or voluntarily withdrew from this program area in 2008–2009 were 1. *Child/Clinical Psychology PhD (Doctor of Philosophy)*—Applications 2009–2010, 60. Total applicants accepted 2009–2010, 4. Number full-time enrolled (new admits only) 2009–2010, 4. Total enrolled 2009–2010 full-time, 20, part-time, 2. Openings 2010–2011, 4. The median number of years required for completion of a degree in 2008–2009 were 6. The number of students enrolled full- and part-time who were dismissed or voluntarily withdrew from this program area in 2008–2009 were 0. *Child/School Psychology PhD (Doctor of Philosophy)*—Applications 2009–2010, 3. Total applicants accepted 2009–2010, 0. Number full-time enrolled (new admits only) 2009–2010, 0. The number of students enrolled full- and part-time who were dismissed or voluntarily withdrew from this program area in 2008–2009 were 0.

Scores: Entries appear in this order: required test or GPA, minimum score (if required), median score of students entering in 2009–2010. *Child Psychology PhD (Doctor of Philosophy):* GRE-V no minimum stated, 650, GRE-Q no minimum stated, 750, GRE-Analytical no minimum stated, 5.0, overall undergraduate GPA no minimum stated, 3.89.

Other Criteria: (importance of criteria rated low, medium, or high): GRE scores—medium, research experience—high, work experience—low, extracurricular activity—low, clinically related public service—low, GPA—high, letters of recommendation—high, statement of goals and objectives—high. Clinically related public service rated low for joint child/clinical program. For additional information on admission requirements, go to http://www.cehd.umn.edu/icd/GradInfo/future.html.

Student Characteristics: The following represents characteristics of students in 2009–2010 in all graduate psychology programs in the department: Female—full-time 46, part-time 3; Male—full-time 8, part-time 2; African American/Black—full-time 1, part-time 0; Hispanic/Latino(a)—full-time 4, part-time 0; Asian/Pacific Islander—full-time 7, part-time 1; American Indian/Alaska Native—full-time 0, part-time 0; Caucasian/White—full-time 41, part-time 4; Multi-ethnic—full-time 1, part-time 0; students subject to the Americans With Disabilities Act—full-time 0, part-time 1; Unknown ethnicity—full-time 0, part-time 0; International students who hold an F-1 or J-1 Visa—full-time 9, part-time 0.

Financial Information/Assistance:
Tuition for Full-Time Study: *Doctoral:* State residents: per academic year $11,212, $934 per credit hour; Nonstate residents: per academic year $18,310, $1,526 per credit hour. Tuition is subject to change. See the following Web site for updates and changes in tuition costs: http://www.grad.umn.edu/Prospective_Students/Financing/index.html.

Financial Assistance:
First-Year Students: Teaching assistantships available for first year. Average amount paid per academic year: $13,065. Average number of hours worked per week: 20. Research assistantships available for first year. Average amount paid per academic year: $13,065. Average number of hours worked per week: 20. Fellowships and scholarships available for first year. Average amount paid per academic year: $22,500.

Advanced Students: Teaching assistantships available for advanced students. Average amount paid per academic year: $13,065. Average number of hours worked per week: 20. Research assistantships available for advanced students. Average amount paid per academic year: $13,065. Average number of hours worked per week: 20. Traineeships available for advanced students. Average amount paid per academic year: $20,772. Fellowships and scholarships available for advanced students. Average amount paid per academic year: $22,500.

Additional Information: Of all students currently enrolled full time, 100% benefited from one or more of the listed financial assistance programs. Application and information available online at: http://www.grad.umn.edu/prospective_students/Financing/index.html.

Internships/Practica: Clinical and school psychology practica and internships are available within the local community to joint program students and are offered through our departmental affiliates. Field experiences are also offered to students in our Applied Developmental Psychology Certificate program.

Housing and Day Care: On-campus housing is available. See the following Web site for more information: http://www.housing.umn.edu/graduate/. On-campus day care facilities are available. See the following Web site for more information: http://www.cehd.umn.edu/ChildCareCenter/.

Employment of Department Graduates:
Master's Degree Graduates: Of those who graduated in the academic year 2008–2009, the following categories and numbers represent the postgraduate activities and employment of master's degree graduates: Enrolled in a postdoctoral residency/fellowship (n/a), employed in independent practice (n/a), total from the above (master's) (0).
Doctoral Degree Graduates: Of those who graduated in the academic year 2008–2009, the following categories and numbers represent the postgraduate activities and employment of doctoral degree graduates: Enrolled in a psychology doctoral program (n/a), employed in an academic position at a university (5), employed in other positions at a higher education institution (2), total from the above (doctoral) (7).

Additional Information:
Orientation, Objectives, and Emphasis of Department: The Institute program emphasizes training for research and academic careers and provides supplementary opportunities in areas of applied developmental psychology. The program offers a diversity of substantive and methodological approaches. In the core program, special strengths are in infancy, personality and social development, perception, cognitive processes, language development, biological bases of development, and developmental neuroscience. Formal applied training is available through the Developmental Psychopathology and Clinical Science (DPCS) and School Psychology joint programs. Formal minor programs are offered in Neuroscience, Cognitive Science, Prevention Science and Interpersonal Relationships Research. Students can complete an Applied Developmental Psychology Certificate program, focusing on such areas as educational programs and research, public policy, and policy-relevant research. Special training is also available through affiliations with the Center for Cognitive Sciences, the Center for Neurobehavioral Development, the Center for Early Education and Development and the Consortium on Children, Youth, and Families.

Special Facilities or Resources: Physical and research facilities include an office for every student each equipped with an Ethernet connected computer plus exclusive use of a laptop computer during the program, a reference room with more than 4,500 volumes and 4 computers, twenty-five experiment rooms, and a laboratory nursery school. In addition, state-of-the-art research facilities and interdisciplinary collaborations facilitate cutting-edge neuroscience research in the areas of cognitive, behavioral, and social/emotional development. Onsite facilities include both high density (128 channels) and low density (32 channels) electrophysiological recording equipment and eyetracking equipment. Facilities at the Center for Neurobehavioral Development (opened in 2001) include autonomic and electrophysiological laboratories equipped with functional magnetic resonance imaging (fMRI) and event-related potential (ERP) equipment; audiovisual systems for online data collection, videotaping, presentations, and training; research suites, computer workroom, library/conference room; and subject exam rooms and family waiting/play rooms. At the Center for Magnetic Resonance Research, structural and functional MRI equipment is available.

Information for Students With Physical Disabilities: See the following Web site for more information: http://ds.umn.edu/.

Application Information:
Send to Chair of Admissions, Institute of Child Development, University of Minnesota, 51 E River Road, Minneapolis, MN 55455-0345. Application available online. URL of online application: http://www.cehd.umn.edu/icd/GradInfo/apply.html. Students are admitted in the Fall, application deadline December 1. *Fee:* $75. $95 for international applicants.

Saint Mary's University of Minnesota
Counseling and Psychological Services
School of Graduate Studies
2500 Park Avenue
Minneapolis, MN 55404
Telephone: (612) 728-5113
Fax: (612) 728-5121
E-mail: *chuck@smumn.edu*
Web: *http://www.smumn.edu/GraduateAreasOfStudy.aspx*

Department Information:
1982. Program Director: Christina Huck, PhD, L.P. Number of faculty: total—full-time 2, part-time 77; women—full-time 2, part-time 35; minority—part-time 7; women minority—part-time 4.

Programs and Degrees Offered:
Listed in the following order: Program area, degree type (T if terminal Master's), number awarded 7/08–6/09. Counseling and Psychological Services MA/MS (Master of Arts/Science) (T) 60, Marriage and Family Therapy MA/MS (Master of Arts/Science) (T) 60, Graduate Certificate Marriage and Family Therapy 17.

Student Applications/Admissions:
Student Applications
Counseling and Psychological Services MA/MS (Master of Arts/Science)—Applications 2009–2010, 93. Total applicants accepted 2009–2010, 91. Number full-time enrolled (new admits only) 2009–2010, 26. Number part-time enrolled (new admits only) 2009–2010, 46. Total enrolled 2009–2010 full-time, 68, part-time, 224. *Marriage and Family Therapy MA/MS (Master of Arts/Science)*—Applications 2009–2010, 79. Total applicants accepted 2009–2010, 77. Number full-time enrolled (new admits only) 2009–2010, 16. Number part-time enrolled (new admits only) 2009–2010, 48. Total enrolled 2009–2010 full-time, 71, part-time, 165. *Graduate Certificate Marriage and Family Therapy*—Applications 2009–2010, 27. Total applicants accepted 2009–2010, 27. Number full-time enrolled (new admits only) 2009–2010, 0. Number part-time enrolled (new admits only) 2009–2010, 14. Total enrolled 2009–2010 full-time, 2, part-time, 43.

Scores: Entries appear in this order: required test or GPA, minimum score (if required), median score of students entering in 2009–2010. Counseling and Psychological Services MA/MS (Master of Arts/Science): overall undergraduate GPA 2.75; Marriage and Family Therapy MA/MS (Master of Arts/Science): overall undergraduate GPA 2.75.

Other Criteria: (importance of criteria rated low, medium, or high): research experience—medium, work experience—high, extracurricular activity—medium, clinically related public service—high, GPA—high, letters of recommendation—high, interview—high, statement of goals and objectives—high, undergraduate major in psychology—medium. For additional information on admission requirements, go to http://www.smumn.edu/AdvancedDegreeAdmission.aspx.

Student Characteristics: The following represents characteristics of students in 2009–2010 in all graduate psychology programs in the department: Female—full-time 113, part-time 367; Male—full-time 28, part-time 65; African American/Black—full-time 2, part-time 32; Hispanic/Latino(a)—full-time 2, part-time 10; Asian/Pacific Islander—full-time 3, part-time 14; American Indian/Alaska Native—full-time 1, part-time 3; Caucasian/White—full-time 82, part-time 287; Multi-ethnic—full-time 0, part-time 0; students subject to the Americans With Disabilities Act—full-time 0, part-time 1; Unknown ethnicity—full-time 51, part-time 86; International students who hold an F-1 or J-1 Visa—full-time 2, part-time 1.

Financial Information/Assistance:
Tuition for Full-Time Study: *Master's:* State residents: $350 per credit hour; Nonstate residents: $350 per credit hour. See the following Web site for updates and changes in tuition costs: http://www.smumn.edu/AdvancedDegreeTuitionFees.aspx.

Financial Assistance:
First-Year Students: Fellowships and scholarships available for first year.
Advanced Students: Fellowships and scholarships available for advanced students.
Additional Information: Of all students currently enrolled full time, 1% benefited from one or more of the listed financial assistance programs. Application and information available online at: http://www.smumn.edu/AdvancedDegreeFinancialAidPolicies.aspx.

Internships/Practica: Master's Degree (MA/MS Counseling and Psychological Services): An internship experience, such as a final research project or "capstone" experience is required of graduates. Master's Degree (MA/MS Marriage and Family Therapy): An internship experience, such as a final research project or "capstone" experience is required of graduates. A wide variety of practicum sites are available for students.

Housing and Day Care: No on-campus housing is available. No on-campus day care facilities are available.

Employment of Department Graduates:
Master's Degree Graduates: Of those who graduated in the academic year 2008–2009, the following categories and numbers represent the postgraduate activities and employment of master's degree graduates: Enrolled in a postdoctoral residency/fellowship (n/a), employed in independent practice (n/a), total from the above (master's) (0).
Doctoral Degree Graduates: Of those who graduated in the academic year 2008–2009, the following categories and numbers represent the postgraduate activities and employment of doctoral degree graduates: Enrolled in a psychology doctoral program (n/a), total from the above (doctoral) (0).

Additional Information:
Orientation, Objectives, and Emphasis of Department: The Master of Arts Program in Counseling and Psychological Services prepares graduates for professional work in counseling, psychotherapy, and other psychological services. It is designed to enhance the student's understanding of the complex nature of human behavior and social interaction, and to develop tools for assessing human problems and assisting individuals in developing greater understanding and acceptance of themselves and their relationships with others. The program is designed to meet the educational requirements for Minnesota licensure for Licensed Professional Counselors. Additional coursework is available for those seeking Minnesota licensure for Licensed Professional Clinical Counselors. The Counseling and Psychological Services program is offered in Rochester, MN, as well as in Minneapolis.

Special Facilities or Resources: The majority of our faculty are adjunct (part-time) instructors who are practicing in the field. They bring a wealth of real-world experience to their teaching and possess strong academic credentials. Since our emphasis is on applied psychological competence, we consider the backgrounds of these practitioner-scholars to be a major strength of the program.

Information for Students With Physical Disabilities: See the following Web site for more information: http://www.smumn.edu/AdvancedDegreeDisabilityServices.aspx.

Application Information:
Send to Admissions, Saint Mary's University of MN, 2500 Park Avenue, Minneapolis, MN 55404. Application available online. URL of online application: http://www.smumn.edu. Students are admitted in the Fall, application deadline; Spring, application deadline; Summer, application deadline. Deadlines are somewhat flexible. Recommend applying 3 months before the start of the semester. *Fee:* $25.

St. Cloud State University
Department of Psychology
Social Sciences
720 4th Avenue South
Saint Cloud, MN 56301
Telephone: (320) 308-4157
Fax: (320) 308-3098
E-mail: *dsprotolipac@stcloudstate.edu*
Web: *http://www.stcloudstate.edu/psychology/io/*

Department Information:
1963. Chairperson: Dr. Leslie Valdes. Number of faculty: total—full-time 12, part-time 9; women—full-time 7, part-time 5; total—minority—full-time 1; women minority—full-time 1.

Programs and Degrees Offered:
Listed in the following order: Program area, degree type (T if terminal Master's), number awarded 7/08–6/09. Industrial/Organizational Psychology MA/MS (Master of Arts/Science) (T) 8.

Student Applications/Admissions:
Student Applications
Industrial/Organizational Psychology MA/MS (Master of Arts/Science)—Applications 2009–2010, 35. Total applicants accepted 2009–2010, 15. Number full-time enrolled (new admits only) 2009–2010, 9. Openings 2010–2011, 10. The median number of years required for completion of a degree in 2008–2009 were 2. The number of students enrolled full- and part-time who were dismissed or voluntarily withdrew from this program area in 2008–2009 were 0.

Scores: Entries appear in this order: required test or GPA, minimum score (if required), median score of students entering in 2009–2010. Industrial/Organizational Psychology MA/MS (Master of Arts/Science): GRE-V 450, GRE-Q 550, overall undergraduate GPA 2.75, last 2 years GPA 2.75.

Other Criteria: (importance of criteria rated low, medium, or high): GRE scores—high, research experience—medium, work experience—medium, extracurricular activity—low, GPA—high, letters of recommendation—medium, statement of goals and objectives—medium.

Student Characteristics: The following represents characteristics of students in 2009–2010 in all graduate psychology programs in the department: Female—full-time 13, part-time 0; Male—full-time 3, part-time 1; African American/Black—full-time 1, part-time 0; Hispanic/Latino(a)—full-time 0, part-time 0; Asian/Pacific Islander—full-time 2, part-time 0; American Indian/Alaska Native—full-time 0, part-time 0; Caucasian/White—full-time 13, part-time 1; Multi-ethnic—full-time 0, part-time 0; students subject to the Americans With Disabilities Act—full-time 0, part-time 0; Unknown ethnicity—full-time 0, part-time 0; International students who hold an F-1 or J-1 Visa—full-time 2, part-time 0.

Financial Information/Assistance:
Tuition for Full-Time Study: *Master's:* State residents: $289 per credit hour; Nonstate residents: $451 per credit hour. Tuition is subject to change. See the following Web site for updates and changes in tuition costs: http://www.stcloudstate.edu/billing/tuition.

Financial Assistance:
First-Year Students: Teaching assistantships available for first year. Average amount paid per academic year: $5,150. Average number of hours worked per week: 10. Research assistantships available for first year. Average amount paid per academic year: $5,150. Average number of hours worked per week: 10. Fellowships and scholarships available for first year.

Advanced Students: Teaching assistantships available for advanced students. Average amount paid per academic year: $5,150. Average number of hours worked per week: 10. Research assistantships available for advanced students. Average amount paid per academic year: $5,150. Average number of hours worked per week: 10. Fellowships and scholarships available for advanced students.

Additional Information: Of all students currently enrolled full time, 75% benefited from one or more of the listed financial assistance programs. Application and information available online at: http://www.stcloudstate.edu/financialaid.

Internships/Practica: Students pursuing the Master's Degree in Industrial-Organizational Psychology have the option of completing either a practicum/internship or a thesis. The practicum/internship option is designed for students planning to seek employment upon completion of their degree. The thesis option is designed for students planning to seek a doctoral degree in Industrial-Organizational Psychology.

Housing and Day Care: On-campus housing is available. See the following Web site for more information: http://www.stcloudstate.edu/reslife/. On-campus day care facilities are available. See the following Web site for more information: http://www.stcloudstate.edu/childcare/.

Employment of Department Graduates:
Master's Degree Graduates: Of those who graduated in the academic year 2008–2009, the following categories and numbers represent the postgraduate activities and employment of master's degree graduates: Enrolled in a psychology doctoral program (1), enrolled in a postdoctoral residency/fellowship (n/a), employed in independent practice (n/a), employed in business or industry (5), still seeking employment (2), total from the above (master's) (8).

Doctoral Degree Graduates: Of those who graduated in the academic year 2008–2009, the following categories and numbers represent the postgraduate activities and employment of doctoral degree graduates: Enrolled in a psychology doctoral program (n/a), total from the above (doctoral) (0).

Additional Information:
Orientation, Objectives, and Emphasis of Department: The St. Cloud State University Department of Psychology is dedicated to providing students with a quality graduate education. The Industrial-Organizational Psychology Master's Degree Program is designed to provide graduate students with the knowledge and skills that will prepare them for jobs in consulting, business, and government, or to continue their education. The curriculum reflects a commitment to the scientist–practitioner model of graduate education in psychology by including training in the theoretical and empirical bases of industrial-organizational psychology and in the application of these perspectives to work settings. Following the recommendations of the Society for Industrial-Organizational Psychology for master's level education, students' graduate experience will include: (a) training in the core areas of industrial-organizational psychology, including personnel selection, training and organizational development, criterion development, and organizational theory, (b) a firm foundation in psychological theory, research methods, statistics, and psychometrics, and (c) the opportunity to obtain both research experience and applied experience while completing their education.

Special Facilities or Resources: The St. Cloud State University Psychology Department has a dedicated psychology laboratory facility (new space established in 1999). It has 10 rooms for individual and group testing. The lab has networked computers and a laser printer. Activities that take place in this lab include: faculty and student research, meetings of student organizations, research seminars, and classroom demonstrations.

Information for Students With Physical Disabilities: See the following Web site for more information: http://www.stcloudstate.edu/sds/.

Application Information:
Send to School of Graduate Studies, 121 Administrative Services, St. Cloud State University, 720-4th Avenue South, St. Cloud, MN 56301. Application available online. URL of online application: http://www.stcloudstate.edu/graduatestudies/. Students are admitted in the Fall, application deadline March 1. *Fee:* $35.

St. Thomas, University of (2009 data)
Graduate School of Professional Psychology
College of Applied Professional Studies
1000 La Salle Avenue, TMH 451
Minneapolis, MN 55403-2005
Telephone: (651) 962-4650
Fax: (651) 962-4651
E-mail: *gradpsych@stthomas.edu*
Web: *http://www.stthomas.edu/gradpsych*

Department Information:
1960. Associate Dean: Skip Nolan. Number of faculty: total—full-time 10, part-time 10; women—full-time 4, part-time 4; total—minority—full-time 2; women minority—full-time 1.

Programs and Degrees Offered:
Listed in the following order: Program area, degree type (T if terminal Master's), number awarded 7/08–6/09. Counseling MA/MS (Master of Arts/Science) (T) 11, Counseling Psychology PsyD (Doctor of Psychology) 9.

APA Accreditation: Counseling PsyD (Doctor of Psychology).

Student Applications/Admissions:
Student Applications
Counseling MA/MS (Master of Arts/Science)—Applications 2009–2010, 154. Total applicants accepted 2009–2010, 65. Number full-time enrolled (new admits only) 2009–2010, 46. Number part-time enrolled (new admits only) 2009–2010, 10. Total enrolled 2009–2010 full-time, 125, part-time, 35. Openings 2010–2011, 80. The median number of years required for completion of a degree in 2008–2009 were 3. The number of students enrolled full- and part-time who were dismissed or voluntarily withdrew from this program area in 2008–2009 were 1. *Counseling Psychology PsyD (Doctor of Psychology)*—Applications 2009–2010, 57. Total applicants accepted 2009–2010, 15. Number full-time enrolled (new admits only) 2009–2010, 15. Number part-time enrolled (new admits only) 2009–2010, 0. Total enrolled 2009–2010 full-time, 66, part-time, 4. Openings 2010–2011, 12. The median number of years required for completion of a degree in 2008–2009 were 4. The number of students enrolled full- and part-time who were dismissed or voluntarily withdrew from this program area in 2008–2009 were 0.
Other Criteria: (importance of criteria rated low, medium, or high): GRE scores—medium, research experience—low, work experience—high, extracurricular activity—low, clinically related public service—high, GPA—high, letters of recommendation—high, interview—high, statement of goals and objectives—high, Writing Sample—medium, undergraduate major in psychology—medium, specific undergraduate psychology courses taken—medium. For additional information on admission requirements, go to http://www.stthomas.edu/gradpsych/admissions/default.html.

Student Characteristics: The following represents characteristics of students in 2009–2010 in all graduate psychology programs in the department: Female—full-time 39, part-time 95; Male—full-time 20, part-time 35; African American/Black—full-time 1, part-time 3; Hispanic/Latino(a)—full-time 0, part-time 3; Asian/Pacific Islander—full-time 1, part-time 3; American Indian/Alaska Native—full-time 0, part-time 0; Caucasian/White—full-time 45, part-time 143; Multi-ethnic—full-time 0, part-time 0; students subject to the Americans With Disabilities Act—full-time 0, part-time 0; Unknown ethnicity—full-time 0, part-time 0; International students who hold an F-1 or J-1 Visa—full-time 0, part-time 0.

Financial Information/Assistance:
Tuition for Full-Time Study: Master's: State residents: $616 per credit hour; Nonstate residents: $616 per credit hour. *Doctoral:* State residents: $823 per credit hour; Nonstate residents: $823 per credit hour. See the following Web site for updates and changes in tuition costs: http://www.stthomas.edu/businessoffice.

Financial Assistance:
First-Year Students: Traineeships available for first year. Average amount paid per academic year: $12. Apply by August 1. Fellowships and scholarships available for first year. Average amount paid per academic year: $2,500. Average number of hours worked per week: 0. Apply by August 1.
Advanced Students: Research assistantships available for advanced students. Average amount paid per academic year: $2,500. Average number of hours worked per week: 5. Apply by August 1.
Additional Information: Of all students currently enrolled full time, 1% benefited from one or more of the listed financial assistance programs. Application and information available online at: http://www.stthomas.edu/financialservices.

Internships/Practica: Doctoral Degree (PsyD Counseling Psychology): For those doctoral students for whom a professional internship was required in this program prior to graduation, (13) students applied for an internship in 2008–2009, with (13) students obtaining an internship. Of those students who obtained an internship, (12) were paid internships. Of those students who obtained an internship, (4) students placed in APA/CPA accredited internships, (8) students placed in internships not APA/CPA accredited, but listed with the Association of Psychology Postdoctoral and Internship Programs (APPIC), (0) students placed in internships conforming to guidelines of the Council of Directors of School Psychology Programs (CDSPP), (1) students placed in internships that were not APA/CPA accredited, APPIC or CDSPP listed. Master's and doctoral students have available a wide variety of practica and internships in the surrounding community in the Twin Cities area. Application is competitive and supported by the practicum coordinator at UST. Students also participate in APPIC internships locally and across the country. Recent sites have included community mental health centers, regional hospitals, VA medical centers, residential chemical dependency centers, career and vocational services, college/university counseling and career centers, vocational rehabilitation programs, employee assistance counseling programs, health maintenance organizations, MN state hospitals, and the MN state prison system.

Housing and Day Care: No on-campus housing is available. On-campus day care facilities are available. See the following Web site for more information: http://www.stthomas.edu/childdevelopment/.

Employment of Department Graduates:
Master's Degree Graduates: Of those who graduated in the academic year 2008–2009, the following categories and numbers represent the postgraduate activities and employment of master's degree graduates: Enrolled in a psychology doctoral program (3), enrolled in a postdoctoral residency/fellowship (n/a), employed in independent practice (n/a), employed in other positions at a higher education institution (2), employed in a community mental health/counseling center (6), total from the above (master's) (11).
Doctoral Degree Graduates: Of those who graduated in the academic year 2008–2009, the following categories and numbers represent the postgraduate activities and employment of doctoral degree graduates: Enrolled in a psychology doctoral program (n/a), employed in an academic position at a university (1), employed in a community mental health/counseling center (4), other employment position (2), do not know (2), total from the above (doctoral) (9).

Additional Information:
Orientation, Objectives, and Emphasis of Department: The Graduate School of Professional Psychology is dedicated to the development of general practitioners who will make ethical, professional, creative contributions to their communities and their profession. The programs strive toward leadership in emphasizing a practitioner focus with adult learners. Teaching, scholarship, and service are responsive to diverse perspectives, a blend of practical and reflective inquiry, and social needs. The PsyD is accredited by the APA.

Special Facilities or Resources: UST has developed the Center for Counseling Legal Services (IPC) which is an inter-professional clinic involving counseling psychology, social work and law. This unique center provides free counseling and legal services to underserved populations in the Minneapolis/St. Paul vicinity.

Information for Students With Physical Disabilities: See the following Web site for more information: http://www.stthomas.edu/enhancementprog.

Application Information:
Send to Admissions, Graduate School of Professional Psychology, University of St. Thomas, 1000 La Salle Avenue, TMH451, Minneapolis, MN 55403. Application available online. URL of online application: http://www.stthomas.edu/gradpsych/admissions/applications/default.html. Students are admitted in the Fall, application deadline February 1. Application deadlines for the Fall - March 1 and October 15 for MA; February 1 for PsyD. *Fee:* $50.

Walden University (2009 data)
Psychology
School of Psychology
155 Fifth Avenue South
Minneapolis, MN 55401
Telephone: (800) 925-3368 X2431
Fax: (612) 338-5092
E-mail: *nina.nabors@waldenu.edu*
Web: *http://www.waldenu.edu*

Department Information:
1996. Associate Dean: Nina A. Nabors. Number of faculty: total—full-time 21, part-time 193; women—full-time 12, part-time 106; total—minority—full-time 5, part-time 26; women minority—full-time 4, part-time 17; faculty subject to the Americans With Disabilities Act 4.

Programs and Degrees Offered:
Listed in the following order: Program area, degree type (T if terminal Master's), number awarded 7/08–6/09. Counseling Psychology PhD (Doctor of Philosophy) 2, Organizational Psychology PhD (Doctor of Philosophy) 5, Health Psychology PhD (Doctor of Philosophy) 6, School Psychology PhD (Doctor of Philosophy) 0, General Psychology MA/MS (Master of Arts/Science) (T) 170, Clinical Psychology PhD (Doctor of Philosophy) 8, Organizational Psychology and Development MA/MS (Master of Arts/Science) (T) 0, General Psychology PhD (Doctor of Philosophy) 1.

Student Applications/Admissions:
Student Applications

Counseling Psychology PhD (Doctor of Philosophy)—Applications 2009–2010, 182. Total applicants accepted 2009–2010, 260. Number full-time enrolled (new admits only) 2009–2010, 182. Total enrolled 2009–2010 full-time, 260. The median number of years required for completion of a degree in 2008–2009 were 6. The number of students enrolled full- and part-time who were dismissed or voluntarily withdrew from this program area in 2008–2009 were 130. *Organizational Psychology PhD (Doctor of Philosophy)*—Total applicants accepted 2009–2010, 163. Number full-time enrolled (new admits only) 2009–2010, 163. Total enrolled 2009–2010 full-time, 339. The median number of years required for completion of a degree in 2008–2009 were 5. The number of students enrolled full- and part-time who were dismissed or voluntarily withdrew from this program area in 2008–2009 were 88. *Health Psychology PhD (Doctor of Philosophy)*—Total applicants accepted 2009–2010, 133. Number full-time enrolled (new admits only) 2009–2010, 133. Total enrolled 2009–2010 full-time, 262. The median number of years required for completion of a degree in 2008–2009 were 5. The number of students enrolled full- and part-time who were dismissed or voluntarily withdrew from this program area in 2008–2009 were 92. *School Psychology PhD (Doctor of Philosophy)*—Total applicants accepted 2009–2010, 34. Number full-time enrolled (new admits only) 2009–2010, 34. Total enrolled 2009–2010 full-time, 82. The median number of years required for completion of a degree in 2008–2009 were 9. The number of students enrolled full- and part-time who were dismissed or voluntarily withdrew from this program area in 2008–2009 were 31. *General Psychology MA/*

MS *(Master of Arts/Science)*—Total applicants accepted 2009–2010, 664. Number full-time enrolled (new admits only) 2009–2010, 664. Total enrolled 2009–2010 full-time, 893. The median number of years required for completion of a degree in 2008–2009 were 3. The number of students enrolled full- and part-time who were dismissed or voluntarily withdrew from this program area in 2008–2009 were 338. *Clinical Psychology PhD (Doctor of Philosophy)*—Total applicants accepted 2009–2010, 309. Number full-time enrolled (new admits only) 2009–2010, 309. Total enrolled 2009–2010 full-time, 631. The median number of years required for completion of a degree in 2008–2009 were 6. The number of students enrolled full- and part-time who were dismissed or voluntarily withdrew from this program area in 2008–2009 were 218. *Organizational Psychology and Development MA/MS (Master of Arts/Science)*—Total applicants accepted 2009–2010, 104. Number full-time enrolled (new admits only) 2009–2010, 104. Total enrolled 2009–2010 full-time, 225. The median number of years required for completion of a degree in 2008–2009 were 2. The number of students enrolled full- and part-time who were dismissed or voluntarily withdrew from this program area in 2008–2009 were 77. *General Psychology PhD (Doctor of Philosophy)*—Total applicants accepted 2009–2010, 215. Number full-time enrolled (new admits only) 2009–2010, 215. Total enrolled 2009–2010 full-time, 470. The median number of years required for completion of a degree in 2008–2009 were 4. The number of students enrolled full- and part-time who were dismissed or voluntarily withdrew from this program area in 2008–2009 were 117.

Other Criteria: (importance of criteria rated low, medium, or high): research experience—low, extracurricular activity—low, clinically related public service—high, GPA—high, letters of recommendation—low, statement of goals and objectives—high, undergraduate major in psychology—low, specific undergraduate psychology courses taken—medium.

Student Characteristics: The following represents characteristics of students in 2009–2010 in all graduate psychology programs in the department: Female—full-time 0, part-time 0; Male—full-time 0, part-time 0; African American/Black—full-time 122, part-time 0; Hispanic/Latino(a)—full-time 26, part-time 0; Asian/Pacific Islander—full-time 10, part-time 0; American Indian/Alaska Native—full-time 9, part-time 0; Caucasian/White—full-time 0, part-time 0; Multi-ethnic—full-time 13, part-time 0; students subject to the Americans With Disabilities Act—full-time 9, part-time 0; Unknown ethnicity—full-time 0, part-time 0; International students who hold an F-1 or J-1 Visa—full-time 0, part-time 0.

Financial Information/Assistance:

Tuition for Full-Time Study: *Master's:* State residents: $360 per credit hour; Nonstate residents: $360 per credit hour. *Doctoral:* State residents: $435 per credit hour; Nonstate residents: $435 per credit hour. Tuition is subject to change. Tuition costs vary by program.

Financial Assistance:
First-Year Students: No information provided.
Advanced Students: Research assistantships available for advanced students. Average amount paid per academic year: $6,000. Average number of hours worked per week: 10. Fellowships and scholarships available for advanced students.

Additional Information: Of all students currently enrolled full time, 1% benefited from one or more of the listed financial assistance programs.

Internships/Practica: Doctoral Degree (PhD Counseling Psychology): For those doctoral students for whom a professional internship was required in this program prior to graduation, (13) students applied for an internship in 2008–2009, with (13) students obtaining an internship. Of those students who obtained an internship, (1) were paid internships. Of those students who obtained an internship, (0) students placed in APA/CPA accredited internships, (1) students placed in internships not APA/CPA accredited, but listed with the Association of Psychology Postdoctoral and Internship Programs (APPIC), (0) students placed in internships conforming to guidelines of the Council of Directors of School Psychology Programs (CDSPP), (12) students placed in internships that were not APA/CPA accredited, APPIC or CDSPP listed. Doctoral Degree (PhD School Psychology): For those doctoral students for whom a professional internship was required in this program prior to graduation, (2) students applied for an internship in 2008–2009, with (2) students obtaining an internship. Of those students who obtained an internship, (1) were paid internships. Of those students who obtained an internship, (0) students placed in APA/CPA accredited internships, (0) students placed in internships not APA/CPA accredited, but listed with the Association of Psychology Postdoctoral and Internship Programs (APPIC), (0) students placed in internships conforming to guidelines of the Council of Directors of School Psychology Programs (CDSPP), (2) students placed in internships that were not APA/CPA accredited, APPIC or CDSPP listed. Doctoral Degree (PhD Clinical Psychology): For those doctoral students for whom a professional internship was required in this program prior to graduation, (31) students applied for an internship in 2008–2009, with (29) students obtaining an internship. Of those students who obtained an internship, (3) were paid internships. Of those students who obtained an internship, (2) students placed in APA/CPA accredited internships, (4) students placed in internships not APA/CPA accredited, but listed with the Association of Psychology Postdoctoral and Internship Programs (APPIC), (0) students placed in internships conforming to guidelines of the Council of Directors of School Psychology Programs (CDSPP), (23) students placed in internships that were not APA/CPA accredited, APPIC or CDSPP listed. Master's Degree (MA/MS General Psychology): An internship experience, such as a final research project or "capstone" experience is required of graduates. Our field placement coordinators work with students to arrange for practicum and internship sites. We do not at this time have available internship or practicum sites.

Housing and Day Care: No on-campus housing is available. No on-campus day care facilities are available.

Employment of Department Graduates:

Master's Degree Graduates: Of those who graduated in the academic year 2008–2009, the following categories and numbers represent the postgraduate activities and employment of master's degree graduates: Enrolled in a psychology doctoral program (49), enrolled in a postdoctoral residency/fellowship (n/a), employed in independent practice (n/a), do not know (75), total from the above (master's) (124).

Doctoral Degree Graduates: Of those who graduated in the academic year 2008–2009, the following categories and numbers

represent the postgraduate activities and employment of doctoral degree graduates: Enrolled in a psychology doctoral program (n/a), employed in independent practice (3), employed in an academic position at a university (3), employed in a professional position in a school system (5), employed in a community mental health/counseling center (5), other employment position (4), do not know (11), total from the above (doctoral) (31).

Additional Information:
Orientation, Objectives, and Emphasis of Department: The program is based on a scholar-practitioner model and reflects the university mission of social change. Students have the opportunity to work with faculty with a diverse array of theoretical orientations.

Application Information:
Send to Office of Student Enrollment, Walden University, 650 S. Exeter Street, Baltimore, MD 21202 USA. Students are admitted in the Fall, application deadline August 15; Winter, application deadline November 15; Spring, application deadline February 15; Summer, application deadline May 15; Programs have rolling admissions. *Fee:* $50.

MISSISSIPPI

Mississippi State University
Department of Counseling and Educational Psychology
College of Education
P.O. Box 9727
Mississippi State, MS 39762-5670
Telephone: (662) 325-3426
Fax: (662) 325-3263
E-mail: *tdoggett@colled.msstate.edu*
Web: *http://www.cep.msstate.edu/*

Department Information:
1954. Department Head: Dr. Daniel Wong. Number of faculty: total—full-time 17, part-time 4; women—full-time 13; total—minority—full-time 4, part-time 1; women minority—full-time 3.

Programs and Degrees Offered:
Listed in the following order: Program area, degree type (T if terminal Master's), number awarded 7/08–6/09. School Psychology PhD (Doctor of Philosophy) 6, Educational PhD (Doctor of Philosophy) 2.

APA Accreditation: School PhD (Doctor of Philosophy). Student Outcome Data Website: http://www.msstate.edu/dept/SchoolPsych/SchoolPsych/Home_Page.html.

Student Applications/Admissions:
Student Applications
School Psychology PhD (Doctor of Philosophy)—Applications 2009–2010, 16. Total applicants accepted 2009–2010, 8. Number full-time enrolled (new admits only) 2009–2010, 4. Number part-time enrolled (new admits only) 2009–2010, 0. Total enrolled 2009–2010 full-time, 13, part-time, 10. Openings 2010–2011, 6. The median number of years required for completion of a degree in 2008–2009 were 5. The number of students enrolled full- and part-time who were dismissed or voluntarily withdrew from this program area in 2008–2009 were 2. *Educational PhD (Doctor of Philosophy)*—Applications 2009–2010, 5. Total applicants accepted 2009–2010, 5. Number full-time enrolled (new admits only) 2009–2010, 4. Number part-time enrolled (new admits only) 2009–2010, 1. Total enrolled 2009–2010 full-time, 7, part-time, 1. Openings 2010–2011, 5. The median number of years required for completion of a degree in 2008–2009 were 6. The number of students enrolled full- and part-time who were dismissed or voluntarily withdrew from this program area in 2008–2009 were 0.
Other Criteria: (importance of criteria rated low, medium, or high): GRE scores—high, research experience—high, work experience—high, extracurricular activity—low, clinically related public service—low, GPA—high, letters of recommendation—high, interview—high, statement of goals and objectives—high.

Student Characteristics: The following represents characteristics of students in 2009–2010 in all graduate psychology programs in the department: Female—full-time 18, part-time 11; Male—full-time 3, part-time 1; African American/Black—full-time 3, part-time 3; Hispanic/Latino(a)—full-time 0, part-time 0; Asian/Pacific Islander—full-time 2, part-time 1; American Indian/Alaska Native—full-time 0, part-time 0; Caucasian/White—full-time 16, part-time 8; Multi-ethnic—full-time 0, part-time 0; students subject to the Americans With Disabilities Act—full-time 0, part-time 0; Unknown ethnicity—full-time 0, part-time 0; International students who hold an F-1 or J-1 Visa—full-time 3, part-time 0.

Financial Information/Assistance:
Tuition for Full-Time Study: *Master's:* State residents: per academic year $5,151, $286 per credit hour; Nonstate residents: per academic year $13,020, $723 per credit hour. *Doctoral:* State residents: per academic year $5,151, $286 per credit hour; Nonstate residents: per academic year $13,020, $723 per credit hour. Tuition is subject to change. See the following Web site for updates and changes in tuition costs: http://www.grad.msstate.edu/prospective/tuition/.

Financial Assistance:
First-Year Students: Teaching assistantships available for first year. Average amount paid per academic year: $14,151. Average number of hours worked per week: 20. Research assistantships available for first year. Average amount paid per academic year: $14,151. Average number of hours worked per week: 20.

Advanced Students: Teaching assistantships available for advanced students. Average amount paid per academic year: $14,151. Average number of hours worked per week: 20. Research assistantships available for advanced students. Average amount paid per academic year: $14,151. Average number of hours worked per week: 20.

Additional Information: Of all students currently enrolled full time, 75% benefited from one or more of the listed financial assistance programs. Application and information available online at: http://www.grad.msstate.edu/financial/assist/.

Internships/Practica: Doctoral Degree (PhD School Psychology): For those doctoral students for whom a professional internship was required in this program prior to graduation, (6) students applied for an internship in 2008–2009, with (5) students obtaining an internship. Of those students who obtained an internship, (5) were paid internships. Of those students who obtained an internship, (4) students placed in APA/CPA accredited internships, (0) students placed in internships not APA/CPA accredited, but listed with the Association of Psychology Postdoctoral and Internship Programs (APPIC), (1) students placed in internships conforming to guidelines of the Council of Directors of School Psychology Programs (CDSPP), (0) students placed in internships that were not APA/CPA accredited, APPIC or CDSPP listed. The school psychology program offers students numerous practica and internship opportunities. Most practica are coordinated with local school districts. Some externships have also been coordinated with medical centers/hospitals and/or mental health or community counseling centers both within and outside of the state. Doctoral students are strongly encouraged to seek APA-accredited predoctoral internships.

Housing and Day Care: On-campus housing is available. See the following Web site for more information: http://www.housing.

msstate.edu/. On-campus day care facilities are available. See the following Web site for more information: http://www.msstate.edu/school/humansciences/cdfsc.html; http://earlychildhood.msstate.edu/initiatives/aiken.htm.

Employment of Department Graduates:
Master's Degree Graduates: Of those who graduated in the academic year 2008–2009, the following categories and numbers represent the postgraduate activities and employment of master's degree graduates: Enrolled in a psychology doctoral program (0), enrolled in another graduate/professional program (0), enrolled in a postdoctoral residency/fellowship (n/a), employed in independent practice (n/a), employed in an academic position at a university (0), employed in an academic position at a 2-year/4-year college (0), employed in other positions at a higher education institution (0), employed in a professional position in a school system (0), employed in business or industry (0), employed in government agency (0), employed in a community mental health/counseling center (0), employed in a hospital/medical center (0), still seeking employment (0), not seeking employment (0), other employment position (0), do not know (0), total from the above (master's) (0).

Doctoral Degree Graduates: Of those who graduated in the academic year 2008–2009, the following categories and numbers represent the postgraduate activities and employment of doctoral degree graduates: Enrolled in a psychology doctoral program (n/a), enrolled in another graduate/professional program (0), enrolled in a postdoctoral residency/fellowship (0), employed in independent practice (0), employed in an academic position at a university (2), employed in an academic position at a 2-year/4-year college (0), employed in other positions at a higher education institution (1), employed in a professional position in a school system (2), employed in business or industry (0), employed in government agency (1), employed in a community mental health/counseling center (0), employed in a hospital/medical center (1), still seeking employment (0), not seeking employment (0), other employment position (1), do not know (0), total from the above (doctoral) (8).

Additional Information:
Orientation, Objectives, and Emphasis of Department: Our psychology graduate programs are designed primarily to help develop and train competent and ethical psychologists in the areas of school psychology and educational psychology. The school psychology program is based on a scientist–practitioner model and trains students to implement empirically-based assessment, consultation, and intervention techniques. The flexibility of these offerings gives the student the option of functioning as an educational or school psychologist in a variety of settings, thereby enhancing employment opportunities.

Special Facilities or Resources: The Educational and School Psychology faculty maintain close working relationships with faculty in other programs and departments such as Counseling, Psychology and Special Education. Such relationships afford students the opportunity to work closely with diverse faculty members with various human services backgrounds. Moreover, students are encouraged to work closely with their faculty on various creative projects and research. Additional opportunities exist at the Rehabilitation Research and Training Center on Blindness and Low Vision, the Bureau of Educational Research and Evaluation, and the Research and Curriculum Unit for Vocational-Technical Education, Social Science Research Center, Child Development Center, and T.K. Martin Center, all of which are connected with Mississippi State University.

Information for Students With Physical Disabilities: See the following Web site for more information: http://www.sss.msstate.edu/.

Application Information:
Send to Mississippi State University, Office of the Graduate School, P. O. Box G, Mississippi State, MS 39762-5507. Application available online. URL of online application: http://www.grad.msstate.edu/prospective/. Students are admitted in the Fall, application deadline January 15; The Doctoral (PhD) program in School Psychology and the Educational Specialist (EdS) program in School Psychology applications are due January 15 each year. The Masters (MS) and Doctoral (PhD) programs in Educational Psychology have a rolling admissions for programs spring, summer, and fall admissions. *Fee:* $40.

Mississippi State University
Department of Psychology
Arts and Sciences
P.O. Drawer 6161
Mississippi State, MS 39762
Telephone: (662) 325-3202
Fax: (662) 325-7212
E-mail: *kja3@psychology.msstate.edu*
Web: *http://psychology.msstate.edu*

Department Information:
1966. Department Head: Stephen B. Klein. Number of faculty: total—full-time 15, part-time 4; women—full-time 6, part-time 1.

Programs and Degrees Offered:
Listed in the following order: Program area, degree type (T if terminal Master's), number awarded 7/08–6/09. Clinical Psychology MA/MS (Master of Arts/Science) (T) 16, Experimental Psychology MA/MS (Master of Arts/Science) (T) 2, Cognitive Science PhD (Doctor of Philosophy) 2.

Student Applications/Admissions:
Student Applications

Clinical Psychology MA/MS (Master of Arts/Science)—Applications 2009–2010, 30. Total applicants accepted 2009–2010, 15. Number full-time enrolled (new admits only) 2009–2010, 7. Number part-time enrolled (new admits only) 2009–2010, 0. Total enrolled 2009–2010 full-time, 14, part-time, 1. Openings 2010–2011, 10. The median number of years required for completion of a degree in 2008–2009 were 2. The number of students enrolled full- and part-time who were dismissed or voluntarily withdrew from this program area in 2008–2009 were 1. *Experimental Psychology MA/MS (Master of Arts/Science)*—Applications 2009–2010, 14. Total applicants accepted 2009–2010, 9. Number full-time enrolled (new admits only) 2009–2010, 9. Number part-time enrolled (new admits only) 2009–2010, 0. Total enrolled 2009–2010 full-time, 13, part-time, 4. Openings 2010–2011, 4. The median number of years required for completion of a degree in 2008–2009 were 3. The number of students enrolled full- and part-time who were dismissed or voluntarily withdrew from this program area in

2008–2009 were 1. *Cognitive Science PhD (Doctor of Philosophy)*—Applications 2009–2010, 17. Total applicants accepted 2009–2010, 7. Number full-time enrolled (new admits only) 2009–2010, 4. Number part-time enrolled (new admits only) 2009–2010, 0. Total enrolled 2009–2010 full-time, 10, part-time, 1. Openings 2010–2011, 3. The median number of years required for completion of a degree in 2008–2009 were 8. The number of students enrolled full- and part-time who were dismissed or voluntarily withdrew from this program area in 2008–2009 were 0.

Scores: Entries appear in this order: required test or GPA, minimum score (if required), median score of students entering in 2009–2010. *Clinical Psychology MA/MS (Master of Arts/Science):* GRE-V no minimum stated, 480, GRE-Q no minimum stated, 560, GRE-Analytical no minimum stated, 4.0, overall undergraduate GPA no minimum stated, last 2 years GPA no minimum stated, 3.6, psychology GPA no minimum stated; *Experimental Psychology MA/MS (Master of Arts/Science):* GRE-V no minimum stated, 440, GRE-Q no minimum stated, 560, GRE-Analytical no minimum stated, 4.0, overall undergraduate GPA no minimum stated, last 2 years GPA no minimum stated, 3.5, psychology GPA no minimum stated; *Cognitive Science PhD (Doctor of Philosophy):* GRE-V no minimum stated, 550, GRE-Q no minimum stated, 640, GRE-Analytical no minimum stated, 4.0, overall undergraduate GPA no minimum stated, last 2 years GPA no minimum stated, 3.6, psychology GPA no minimum stated, Masters GPA no minimum stated.

Other Criteria: (importance of criteria rated low, medium, or high): GRE scores—medium, research experience—high, work experience—medium, extracurricular activity—low, clinically related public service—medium, GPA—high, letters of recommendation—high, interview—low, statement of goals and objectives—high, undergraduate major in psychology—medium, specific undergraduate psychology courses taken—medium. The clinically related public service would be relevant for applicants to the master's program (clinical concentration). Computer-related experience is relevant to the Cognitive PhD program. For additional information on admission requirements, go to http://www.psychology.msstate.edu.

Student Characteristics: The following represents characteristics of students in 2009–2010 in all graduate psychology programs in the department: Female—full-time 25, part-time 3; Male—full-time 12, part-time 3; African American/Black—full-time 1, part-time 0; Hispanic/Latino(a)—full-time 0, part-time 0; Asian/Pacific Islander—full-time 2, part-time 1; American Indian/Alaska Native—full-time 0, part-time 0; Caucasian/White—full-time 34, part-time 5; Multi-ethnic—full-time 0, part-time 0; students subject to the Americans With Disabilities Act—full-time 0, part-time 0; Unknown ethnicity—full-time 0, part-time 0; International students who hold an F-1 or J-1 Visa—full-time 4, part-time 0.

Financial Information/Assistance:

Tuition for Full-Time Study: *Master's:* State residents: per academic year $5,151, $286 per credit hour; Nonstate residents: per academic year $13,020, $723 per credit hour. *Doctoral:* State residents: per academic year $5,151, $286 per credit hour; Nonstate residents: per academic year $13,020, $723 per credit hour. Tuition is subject to change. See the following Web site for updates and changes in tuition costs: http://www.grad.msstate.edu/prospective/tuition/.

Financial Assistance:
   First-Year Students: Teaching assistantships available for first year. Average number of hours worked per week: 20.
   Advanced Students: Teaching assistantships available for advanced students. Average amount paid per academic year: $11,950. Average number of hours worked per week: 20. Research assistantships available for advanced students. Average amount paid per academic year: $11,950. Average number of hours worked per week: 20. Traineeships available for advanced students. Average number of hours worked per week: 20.
   Additional Information: Of all students currently enrolled full time, 84% benefited from one or more of the listed financial assistance programs. Application and information available online at: No separate app for TA is required. Some RAs available, esp for advanced students.

Internships/Practica: Master's Degree (MA/MS Clinical Psychology): An internship experience, such as a final research project or "capstone" experience is required of graduates. Master's Degree (MA/MS Experimental Psychology): An internship experience, such as a final research project or "capstone" experience is required of graduates. Students in the clinical-emphasis program complete two 300 clock-hour practicum courses. These practica occur in a variety of settings (including public and private psychiatric hospitals and mental retardation facilities, community mental health centers) and can be completed in other states with prior approval from the program faculty. Students are exposed to diverse client populations (e.g., in- and outpatient, children and adults with varied diagnoses and ethnic backgrounds).

Housing and Day Care: On-campus housing is available. See the following Web site for more information: http://www.housing.msstate.edu/. On-campus day care facilities are available. See the following Web site for more information: http://earlychildhood.msstate.edu/initiatives/aiken.htm and http://www.msstate.edu/school/humansciences/cdfsc.html.

Employment of Department Graduates:
   Master's Degree Graduates: Of those who graduated in the academic year 2008–2009, the following categories and numbers represent the postgraduate activities and employment of master's degree graduates: Enrolled in a psychology doctoral program (3), enrolled in another graduate/professional program (0), enrolled in a postdoctoral residency/fellowship (n/a), employed in independent practice (n/a), employed in an academic position at a university (1), employed in government agency (1), employed in a community mental health/counseling center (2), total from the above (master's) (7).
   Doctoral Degree Graduates: Of those who graduated in the academic year 2008–2009, the following categories and numbers represent the postgraduate activities and employment of doctoral degree graduates: Enrolled in a psychology doctoral program (n/a), employed in other positions at a higher education institution (0), employed in government agency (1), total from the above (doctoral) (1).

Additional Information:
   Orientation, Objectives, and Emphasis of Department: Currently we offer both an MS and a PhD degree through different

programs. Our master's degree programs offer concentrations in either experimental or clinical psychology. The clinical Master's program is accredited by the Master's in Psychology Accreditation Council (MPAC). Our PhD program awards a degree in Applied Cognitive Science through an interdisciplinary program housed in the Psychology Department but operated in cooperation with the Computer Science Department, the Industrial Engineering Department, and other units on campus.

Special Facilities or Resources: The department houses a state-of-the-art computer lab for human subject data collection. Faculty laboratories include extensive computer labs for data collection, eye trackers, high-speed servers, and fast network access. Other research facilities, including an f-MRI, are available through connections to other research facilities, both on-campus and off. Clinical students have research/training opportunities in the on-site Psychology Training Clinic and in several off-campus practicum placements.

Application Information:
Send to Please submit application via electronic system. Go to http://www.grad.msstate.edu/prospective/admissions/domestic to begin the process. Application available online. URL of online application: http://www.grad.msstate.edu/prospective/admissions/domestic. Students are admitted in the Fall, application deadline February 1; Spring, application deadline November 1. The application deadline for the Cognitive Science PhD program is February 1. Although the deadline for full financial consideration is February 1, we will continue to review applications until May 1. Applications to the Master's Degree concentrations in Clinical and Experimental Psychology are reviewed continuously beginning February 1. The masters programs do "rolling" admissions and encourage well qualified applicants to apply up until May 1 presuming slots are still available. *Fee:* $40.

Mississippi, University of (2009 data)
Department of Psychology
Liberal Arts
205 Peabody Hall
University, MS 38677
Telephone: (662) 915-7383
Fax: (662) 915-5398
E-mail: *psych@olemiss.edu*
Web: *http://www.olemiss.edu/depts/psychology*

Department Information:
1932. Chairperson: Michael T. Allen. Number of faculty: total—full-time 16, part-time 4; women—full-time 8, part-time 2.

Programs and Degrees Offered:
Listed in the following order: Program area, degree type (T if terminal Master's), number awarded 7/08–6/09. Clinical PhD (Doctor of Philosophy) 8, Experimental PhD (Doctor of Philosophy) 0.

APA Accreditation: Clinical PhD (Doctor of Philosophy).

Student Applications/Admissions:
Student Applications
Clinical PhD (Doctor of Philosophy)—Applications 2009–2010, 90. Total applicants accepted 2009–2010, 8. Number full-time enrolled (new admits only) 2009–2010, 8. Openings 2010–2011, 8. The median number of years required for completion of a degree in 2008–2009 were 6. The number of students enrolled full- and part-time who were dismissed or voluntarily withdrew from this program area in 2008–2009 were 1. *Experimental PhD (Doctor of Philosophy)*—Applications 2009–2010, 20. Total applicants accepted 2009–2010, 3. Number full-time enrolled (new admits only) 2009–2010, 3. Number part-time enrolled (new admits only) 2009–2010, 0. Openings 2010–2011, 4. The median number of years required for completion of a degree in 2008–2009 were 5. The number of students enrolled full- and part-time who were dismissed or voluntarily withdrew from this program area in 2008–2009 were 0.

Other Criteria: (importance of criteria rated low, medium, or high): GRE scores—medium, research experience—high, work experience—medium, extracurricular activity—medium, clinically related public service—medium, GPA—medium, letters of recommendation—high, interview—high, statement of goals and objectives—high.

Student Characteristics: The following represents characteristics of students in 2009–2010 in all graduate psychology programs in the department: Female—full-time 41, part-time 0; Male—full-time 27, part-time 0; African American/Black—full-time 5, part-time 0; Hispanic/Latino(a)—full-time 1, part-time 0; Asian/Pacific Islander—full-time 3, part-time 0; American Indian/Alaska Native—full-time 0, part-time 0; Caucasian/White—full-time 59, part-time 0; Multi-ethnic—full-time 0, part-time 0; students subject to the Americans With Disabilities Act—full-time 0, part-time 0; Unknown ethnicity—full-time 0, part-time 0; International students who hold an F-1 or J-1 Visa—full-time 0, part-time 0.

Financial Information/Assistance:
Tuition for Full-Time Study: *Master's:* State residents: per academic year $5,103, $284 per credit hour; Nonstate residents: per academic year $12,465, $693 per credit hour. *Doctoral:* State residents: per academic year $5,103, $284 per credit hour; Nonstate residents: per academic year $12,465, $693 per credit hour. Tuition is subject to change.

Financial Assistance:
First-Year Students: Teaching assistantships available for first year. Average amount paid per academic year: $4,250. Average number of hours worked per week: 10. Apply by January 15. Research assistantships available for first year. Average amount paid per academic year: $4,250. Average number of hours worked per week: 10. Apply by January 15.
Advanced Students: Teaching assistantships available for advanced students. Average amount paid per academic year: $5,000. Average number of hours worked per week: 10. Apply by January 15. Research assistantships available for advanced students. Average amount paid per academic year: $4,250. Average number of hours worked per week: 10. Apply by January 15. Traineeships available for advanced students. Average amount paid per academic year: $8,000. Average number of hours worked per week: 20. Apply by January 15. Fellowships and scholarships available for advanced students. Average amount paid per academic year: $3,000. Apply by January 15.
Additional Information: Of all students currently enrolled full time, 95% benefited from one or more of the listed financial

assistance programs. Application and information available online at: http://www.olemiss.edu/gradschool/finaid.php.

Internships/Practica: Doctoral Degree (PhD Clinical): For those doctoral students for whom a professional internship was required in this program prior to graduation, (7) students applied for an internship in 2008–2009, with (7) students obtaining an internship. Of those students who obtained an internship, (7) were paid internships. Of those students who obtained an internship, (7) students placed in APA/CPA accredited internships, (0) students placed in internships not APA/CPA accredited, but listed with the Association of Psychology Postdoctoral and Internship Programs (APPIC), (0) students placed in internships conforming to guidelines of the Council of Directors of School Psychology Programs (CDSPP), (0) students placed in internships that were not APA/CPA accredited, APPIC or CDSPP listed. Practica and field placements are available for clinical students beginning in the second year of the program. Students serve as therapists on practicum teams in our in house clinic for a minimum of three years under the direct supervision of the members of our clinical faculty, all of whom are licensed psychologists. After students have demonstrated a minimum level of competence in the clinic, they are allowed to apply for practicum positions at field placement agencies in the community where they are supervised by licensed practitioners who are employed by the field placement agency. In recent years, students have completed field placements at Community Mental Health Centers in Oxford and Tupelo; North Mississippi Regional Center in Oxford; North Mississippi Medical Center in Tupelo; St. Jude Children's Research Hospital in Memphis, and the DeSoto County (MS) School District. Students are assisted and advised by faculty in choosing field placements most appropriate to their individual career goals.

Housing and Day Care: On-campus housing is available. On-campus day care facilities are available. See the following Web site for more information: http://www.outreach.olemiss.edu/willieprice/.

Employment of Department Graduates:
Master's Degree Graduates: Of those who graduated in the academic year 2008–2009, the following categories and numbers represent the postgraduate activities and employment of master's degree graduates: Enrolled in a postdoctoral residency/fellowship (n/a), employed in independent practice (n/a), total from the above (master's) (0).
Doctoral Degree Graduates: Of those who graduated in the academic year 2008–2009, the following categories and numbers represent the postgraduate activities and employment of doctoral degree graduates: Enrolled in a psychology doctoral program (n/a), enrolled in another graduate/professional program (0), enrolled in a postdoctoral residency/fellowship (7), employed in independent practice (0), employed in an academic position at a university (0), employed in an academic position at a 2-year/4-year college (0), employed in a community mental health/counseling center (1), total from the above (doctoral) (8).

Additional Information:
Orientation, Objectives, and Emphasis of Department: The Department of Psychology offers programs of study in clinical and experimental psychology leading to the Doctor of Philosophy degree. The clinical program, which is fully accredited by the American Psychological Association, ordinarily requires five years beyond the bachelor's level to complete. Four of the five years are devoted to coursework and research, and the remaining year entails a clinical internship at an APA-approved training site. Requirements for the master's degree are also fulfilled during this period; however, the MA is considered to be a step in the doctoral training. The clinical program adheres to the scientist–practitioner model and emphasizes an empirical approach to clinical practice. A social learning or behavioral approach characterizes the clinical training offered. The experimental program is designed to prepare psychologists for careers in teaching and research. Specific programs include Behavioral Neuroscience, Cognitive Psychology, and Social Psychology. Students entering the experimental program are assigned a faculty mentor (major professor) whose research interests match their training goals. All students are required to engage in significant research projects.

Special Facilities or Resources: Most of the department's offices and laboratories are housed in the George Peabody Building. State-of-the-art facilities for animal research are available in a new centralized animal facility on campus. The psychology clinic has recently moved to a new location on campus which provides for a more professional office environment and better client accessibility. The psychology clinic includes multipurpose rooms for evaluation, consultation, and therapy and observation rooms equipped with one-way mirrors and videotape equipment. The department offers computer-based laboratories for psychopharmacology, psychophysiology, operant conditioning, and behavioral toxicology. The department has close ties with the pharmacy and law schools (located on the Oxford campus) and with the medical school in Jackson.

Application Information:
Application available online. URL of online application: http://www.olemiss.edu/gradschool/applyonline.php. Students are admitted in the Fall, application deadline January 15. *Fee:* $25. The application fee is $25 for Mississippi residents; $40 for out of state applicants. If an application is transmitted via an online application service, an additional charge may be required by the service.

MISSOURI

Missouri State University
Psychology Department
Health and Human Services
901 South National Avenue
Springfield, MO 65897
Telephone: (417) 836-5797
Fax: (417) 836-8330
E-mail: *hollyrobison@missouristate.edu*
Web: *http://psychology.missouristate.edu*

Department Information:
1967. Head: Robert G. Jones. Number of faculty: total—full-time 32, part-time 21; women—full-time 16, part-time 11; total—minority—full-time 2, part-time 2; women minority—full-time 1, part-time 2.

Programs and Degrees Offered:
Listed in the following order: Program area, degree type (T if terminal Master's), number awarded 7/08–6/09. Clinical Psychology MA/MS (Master of Arts/Science) (T) 9, Experimental Psychology MA/MS (Master of Arts/Science) (T) 1, Industrial/Organizational Psychology MA/MS (Master of Arts/Science) (T) 12.

Student Applications/Admissions:
Student Applications
Clinical Psychology MA/MS (Master of Arts/Science)—Applications 2009–2010, 27. Total applicants accepted 2009–2010, 9. Number full-time enrolled (new admits only) 2009–2010, 9. Number part-time enrolled (new admits only) 2009–2010, 0. Openings 2010–2011, 8. The median number of years required for completion of a degree in 2008–2009 were 2. The number of students enrolled full- and part-time who were dismissed or voluntarily withdrew from this program area in 2008–2009 were 0. *Experimental Psychology MA/MS (Master of Arts/Science)*—Applications 2009–2010, 4. Total applicants accepted 2009–2010, 2. Number full-time enrolled (new admits only) 2009–2010, 2. Number part-time enrolled (new admits only) 2009–2010, 0. Total enrolled 2009–2010 full-time, 6, part-time, 1. Openings 2010–2011, 3. The median number of years required for completion of a degree in 2008–2009 were 2. The number of students enrolled full- and part-time who were dismissed or voluntarily withdrew from this program area in 2008–2009 were 0. *Industrial/Organizational Psychology MA/MS (Master of Arts/Science)*—Applications 2009–2010, 24. Total applicants accepted 2009–2010, 12. Number full-time enrolled (new admits only) 2009–2010, 12. Number part-time enrolled (new admits only) 2009–2010, 0. Openings 2010–2011, 12. The median number of years required for completion of a degree in 2008–2009 were 2. The number of students enrolled full- and part-time who were dismissed or voluntarily withdrew from this program area in 2008–2009 were 2.
Scores: Entries appear in this order: required test or GPA, minimum score (if required), median score of students entering in 2009–2010. *Experimental Psychology MA/MS (Master of Arts/Science):* GRE-V 350, 500, GRE-Q 380, 600, overall undergraduate GPA 3.0, 3.48, psychology GPA 3.4, 3.6.
Other Criteria: (importance of criteria rated low, medium, or high): GRE scores—medium, research experience—high, work experience—medium, extracurricular activity—medium, clinically related public service—high, GPA—high, letters of recommendation—high, statement of goals and objectives—high, undergraduate major in psychology—high, specific undergraduate psychology courses taken—high. For additional information on admission requirements, go to http://psychology.missouristate.edu/io/apply.htm.

Student Characteristics: The following represents characteristics of students in 2009–2010 in all graduate psychology programs in the department: Female—full-time 31, part-time 1; Male—full-time 12, part-time 0; African American/Black—full-time 2, part-time 0; Hispanic/Latino(a)—full-time 2, part-time 0; Asian/Pacific Islander—full-time 0, part-time 0; American Indian/Alaska Native—full-time 1, part-time 0; Caucasian/White—full-time 29, part-time 1; Multi-ethnic—full-time 1, part-time 0; students subject to the Americans With Disabilities Act—full-time 0, part-time 0; Unknown ethnicity—full-time 8, part-time 0; International students who hold an F-1 or J-1 Visa—full-time 0, part-time 0.

Financial Information/Assistance:
Tuition for Full-Time Study: *Master's:* State residents: per academic year $3,852, $214 per credit hour; Nonstate residents: per academic year $7,524, $418 per credit hour. Tuition is subject to change. Additional fees are assessed to students beyond the costs of tuition for the following: student services Fees $676, parking $96, estimated supplemental course fees $800. See the following Web site for updates and changes in tuition costs: http://graduate.missouristate.edu/Graduate%20Education%20Costs.htm.

Financial Assistance:
First-Year Students: Research assistantships available for first year. Average amount paid per academic year: $7,340. Average number of hours worked per week: 20. Apply by July.
Advanced Students: Teaching assistantships available for advanced students. Average amount paid per academic year: $9,730. Average number of hours worked per week: 20. Apply by March. Research assistantships available for advanced students. Average amount paid per academic year: $7,340. Average number of hours worked per week: 20. Apply by July.
Additional Information: Of all students currently enrolled full time, 90% benefited from one or more of the listed financial assistance programs. Application and information available online at: http://graduate.missouristate.edu/assistantship.htm.

Internships/Practica: Clinical—students must complete two 175 contact hour practica. Placements are in a variety of mental health settings. Students who choose a nonthesis option must complete an additional 175 contact hour internship. Experimental—practicum experience is acquired through basic laboratory research work tailored specifically to the graduate student's research area of interest. The goal of the practicum is for the student to develop or acquire competence in various research methods and behavioral/

cognitive measurement skills that will prepare the student for later doctoral work.

Housing and Day Care: On-campus housing is available. See the following website for more information: http://reslife.missouristate.edu/. On-campus day care facilities are available. See the following website for more information: http://education.missouristate.edu/cdc/.

Employment of Department Graduates:
Master's Degree Graduates: Of those who graduated in the academic year 2008–2009, the following categories and numbers represent the postgraduate activities and employment of master's degree graduates: Enrolled in a psychology doctoral program (7), enrolled in a postdoctoral residency/fellowship (n/a), employed in independent practice (n/a), employed in an academic position at a university (2), employed in an academic position at a 2-year/4-year college (3), employed in other positions at a higher education institution (2), employed in business or industry (2), employed in government agency (13), employed in a community mental health/counseling center (8), employed in a hospital/medical center (1), still seeking employment (2), not seeking employment (1), total from the above (master's) (41).
Doctoral Degree Graduates: Of those who graduated in the academic year 2008–2009, the following categories and numbers represent the postgraduate activities and employment of doctoral degree graduates: Enrolled in a psychology doctoral program (n/a), total from the above (doctoral) (0).

Additional Information:
Orientation, Objectives, and Emphasis of Department: We are an eclectic department of 32 full-time faculty serving over 500 undergraduate majors. The faculty have diverse research interests including clinical, I/O, stress management, sport psychology, human learning, perception, motivation, animal learning, human skills, and memory. The department operates the Learning Diagnostic Clinic for diagnosis and remediation of special populations, as well as limited therapy for other psychological disorders.

Special Facilities or Resources: The department has 14 separate labs that serve the Experimental, Clinical, and Industrial-Organizational tracks. The experimental track has three research labs that provide the means and opportunity for graduate students to conduct basic research. These include: 1) the Infant Perception Laboratory housing computer hardware and software to accommodate basic research in visual scanning and psychophysiological testing; 2) the Implicit and Explicit Motivation Research Lab, which is designed to conduct research in automatic processing and to conduct Structural Equation Modeling and HLM analyses; 3) the Cognitive Strategies Research Lab provides a facility to test and design stimulus materials to conduct applied memory research. Other laboratories support research focusing on cognition, gender issues, life-span development, motivation, body image, music, sport psychology, and animal behavior are available to all students regardless of their track. The department also has excellent computer support facilities in all labs. The department oversees the Learning Diagnostic Clinic that supports student learning and University ADA compliance. The clinic provides an excellent training facility for our clinical graduate students. Faculty in the department provide direct service to faculty and students throughout the College through the RStat Institute, which employs graduate student assistants in research and analysis consultation.

Information for Students With Physical Disabilities: See the following website for more information: http://www.missouristate.edu/disability/.

Application Information:
Send to Academic Administrative Assistant. Application available online. URL of online application: http://psychology.missouristate.edu/io/apply.htm. Students are admitted in the Fall, application deadline March 1. We will accept applications up to June 1 if all openings in each track aren't filled. *Fee:* $35.

Missouri, University of
Department of Psychological Sciences
College of Arts and Science
210 McAlester Hall
Columbia, MO 65211
Telephone: (573) 882-0838
Fax: (573) 882-7710
E-mail: *gradpsych@missouri.edu*
Web: *http://psychology.missouri.edu/*

Department Information:
1900. Chairperson: Ann Bettencourt. Number of faculty: total—full-time 33, part-time 11; women—full-time 10, part-time 6; total—minority—full-time 1; women minority—full-time 1.

Programs and Degrees Offered:
Listed in the following order: Program area, degree type (T if terminal Master's), number awarded 7/08–6/09. Quantitative Psychology PhD (Doctor of Philosophy) 1, Clinical Psychology PhD (Doctor of Philosophy) 2, Cognition and Neuroscience PhD (Doctor of Philosophy) 2, Social/Personality Psychology PhD (Doctor of Philosophy) 5, Developmental Psychology PhD (Doctor of Philosophy) 0, Joint Child Clinical/Developmental PhD (Doctor of Philosophy) 1.

APA Accreditation: Clinical PhD (Doctor of Philosophy). Student Outcome Data Website: http://psychology.missouri.edu/clinical.

Student Applications/Admissions:
Student Applications
Quantitative Psychology PhD (Doctor of Philosophy)—Applications 2009–2010, 10. Total applicants accepted 2009–2010, 3. Number full-time enrolled (new admits only) 2009–2010, 0. Number part-time enrolled (new admits only) 2009–2010, 0. Openings 2010–2011, 2. The number of students enrolled full- and part-time who were dismissed or voluntarily withdrew

from this program area in 2008–2009 were 0. *Clinical Psychology PhD (Doctor of Philosophy)*—Applications 2009–2010, 118. Total applicants accepted 2009–2010, 8. Number full-time enrolled (new admits only) 2009–2010, 4. Number part-time enrolled (new admits only) 2009–2010, 0. Openings 2010–2011, 5. The median number of years required for completion of a degree in 2008–2009 were 8. The number of students enrolled full- and part-time who were dismissed or voluntarily withdrew from this program area in 2008–2009 were 1. *Cognition and Neuroscience PhD (Doctor of Philosophy)*—Applications 2009–2010, 21. Total applicants accepted 2009–2010, 3. Number full-time enrolled (new admits only) 2009–2010, 2. Openings 2010–2011, 2. The median number of years required for completion of a degree in 2008–2009 were 7. The number of students enrolled full- and part-time who were dismissed or voluntarily withdrew from this program area in 2008–2009 were 0. *Social/Personality Psychology PhD (Doctor of Philosophy)*—Applications 2009–2010, 57. Total applicants accepted 2009–2010, 3. Number full-time enrolled (new admits only) 2009–2010, 2. Number part-time enrolled (new admits only) 2009–2010, 0. Openings 2010–2011, 3. The median number of years required for completion of a degree in 2008–2009 were 6. The number of students enrolled full- and part-time who were dismissed or voluntarily withdrew from this program area in 2008–2009 were 0. *Developmental Psychology PhD (Doctor of Philosophy)*—Applications 2009–2010, 14. Total applicants accepted 2009–2010, 4. Number full-time enrolled (new admits only) 2009–2010, 2. Total enrolled 2009–2010 full-time, 9. Openings 2010–2011, 3. The number of students enrolled full- and part-time who were dismissed or voluntarily withdrew from this program area in 2008–2009 were 0. *Joint Child Clinical/Developmental PhD (Doctor of Philosophy)*—Applications 2009–2010, 26. Total applicants accepted 2009–2010, 3. Number full-time enrolled (new admits only) 2009–2010, 2. Total enrolled 2009–2010 full-time, 6. Openings 2010–2011, 1. The number of students enrolled full- and part-time who were dismissed or voluntarily withdrew from this program area in 2008–2009 were 0.

Other Criteria: (importance of criteria rated low, medium, or high): GRE scores—high, research experience—high, work experience—low, extracurricular activity—low, clinically related public service—low, GPA—medium, letters of recommendation—medium, interview—high, statement of goals and objectives—high, undergraduate major in psychology—medium, specific undergraduate psychology courses taken—low. For additional information on admission requirements, go to http://psychology.missouri.edu/grad-chances.

Student Characteristics: The following represents characteristics of students in 2009–2010 in all graduate psychology programs in the department: Female—full-time 51, part-time 0; Male—full-time 31, part-time 0; African American/Black—full-time 3, part-time 0; Hispanic/Latino(a)—full-time 7, part-time 0; Asian/Pacific Islander—full-time 11, part-time 0; American Indian/Alaska Native—full-time 0, part-time 0; Caucasian/White—full-time 59, part-time 0; Multi-ethnic—full-time 0, part-time 0; students subject to the Americans With Disabilities Act—full-time 0, part-time 0; Unknown ethnicity—full-time 2, part-time 0; International students who hold an F-1 or J-1 Visa—full-time 10, part-time 0.

Financial Information/Assistance:
Tuition for Full-Time Study: *Doctoral:* State residents: $298 per credit hour; Nonstate residents: $771 per credit hour. Tuition is subject to change. Additional fees are assessed to students beyond the costs of tuition for the following: Information technology, student activity, recreation facility, health. See the following Web site for updates and changes in tuition costs: http://cashiers.missouri.edu/cost.htm.

Financial Assistance:
 First-Year Students: Teaching assistantships available for first year. Average amount paid per academic year: $13,123. Average number of hours worked per week: 20. Research assistantships available for first year. Average amount paid per academic year: $13,123. Average number of hours worked per week: 20. Fellowships and scholarships available for first year. Average amount paid per academic year: $13,500. Average number of hours worked per week: 20.
 Advanced Students: Teaching assistantships available for advanced students. Average amount paid per academic year: $13,897. Average number of hours worked per week: 20. Research assistantships available for advanced students. Average amount paid per academic year: $13,897. Average number of hours worked per week: 20. Traineeships available for advanced students. Average amount paid per academic year: $20,772. Average number of hours worked per week: 20. Fellowships and scholarships available for advanced students. Average amount paid per academic year: $13,500. Average number of hours worked per week: 20.
 Additional Information: Of all students currently enrolled full time, 91% benefited from one or more of the listed financial assistance programs. Application and information available online at: http://psychology.missouri.edu/grad-financial.

Internships/Practica: Doctoral Degree (PhD Clinical Psychology): For those doctoral students for whom a professional internship was required in this program prior to graduation, (4) students applied for an internship in 2008–2009, with (4) students obtaining an internship. Of those students who obtained an internship, (4) were paid internships. Of those students who obtained an internship, (4) students placed in APA/CPA accredited internships, (0) students placed in internships not APA/CPA accredited, but listed with the Association of Psychology Postdoctoral and Internship Programs (APPIC), (0) students placed in internships conforming to guidelines of the Council of Directors of School Psychology Programs (CDSPP), (0) students placed in internships that were not APA/CPA accredited, APPIC or CDSPP listed. Doctoral Degree (PhD Joint Child Clinical/Developmental): For those doctoral students for whom a professional internship was required in this program prior to graduation, (1) students applied for an internship in 2008–2009, with (1) students obtaining an internship. Of those students who obtained an internship, (1) were paid internships. Of those students who obtained an internship, (1) students placed in APA/CPA accredited internships, (0) students placed in internships not APA/CPA accredited, but listed with the Association of Psychology Postdoctoral and Internship Programs (APPIC), (0) students placed in internships conforming to guidelines of the Council of Directors of School Psychology Programs (CDSPP), (0) students placed in internships that were not APA/CPA accredited, APPIC or CDSPP listed.

Housing and Day Care: On-campus housing is available. See the following Web site for more information: http://reslife.missouri.edu/. On-campus day care facilities are available. See the following Web site for more information: http://www.studentparentcenter.missouri.edu/.

Employment of Department Graduates:
Master's Degree Graduates: Of those who graduated in the academic year 2008–2009, the following categories and numbers represent the postgraduate activities and employment of master's degree graduates: Enrolled in a postdoctoral residency/fellowship (n/a), employed in independent practice (n/a), total from the above (master's) (0).
Doctoral Degree Graduates: Of those who graduated in the academic year 2008–2009, the following categories and numbers represent the postgraduate activities and employment of doctoral degree graduates: Enrolled in a psychology doctoral program (n/a), enrolled in a postdoctoral residency/fellowship (1), employed in an academic position at a university (6), employed in an academic position at a 2-year/4-year college (1), employed in other positions at a higher education institution (1), employed in government agency (1), do not know (2), total from the above (doctoral) (12).

Additional Information:
Orientation, Objectives, and Emphasis of Department: The Department's mission is defined through research, graduate and undergraduate education, and service. The Department contributes to the theoretical and empirical body of knowledge in the discipline of psychology through research and other scholarly activities, trains graduate students to become contributors to psychology as scientists, disseminates the most current knowledge to students through high quality teaching at both the undergraduate and graduate level, and contributes through community, state, and professional service activities. The clinical program is fully accredited by the American Psychological Association and is a charter member of the Academy of Psychological Clinical Science.

Special Facilities or Resources: The department has the following special facilities or resources: a psychology research facility, a psychological clinic, a medical school, a VA hospital, Mid-Missouri Mental Health Center, a counseling center, human experimental laboratories, and a university central computer system and departmental computers.

Information for Students With Physical Disabilities: See the following Web site for more information: http://disabilityservices.missouri.edu.

Application Information:
Send to Graduate Admissions, Graduate Student Services, 210 McAlester Hall, Department of Psychological Sciences, University of Missouri, Columbia, MO 65211. Application available online. URL of online application: http://psychology.missouri.edu/apply-gen. Students are admitted in the Fall, application deadline December 1. The Graduate School would like to receive official transcripts by November 20. *Fee:* $45. The graduate school application fee for non-resident international students is $60.

Missouri, University of, Kansas City
Department of Psychology
4825 Troost Avenue, Suite 124
Kansas City, MO 64110
Telephone: (816) 235-1318
Fax: (816) 235-1062
E-mail: *psychology@umkc.edu*
Web: *http://www.cas.umkc.edu/psyc*

Department Information:
1940. Chairperson: Tamera Murdock, PhD. Number of faculty: total—full-time 14; women—full-time 11; total—minority—full-time 1; women minority—full-time 1.

Programs and Degrees Offered:
Listed in the following order: Program area, degree type (T if terminal Master's), number awarded 7/08–6/09. Clinical Psychology PhD (Doctor of Philosophy) 4.

APA Accreditation: Clinical PhD (Doctor of Philosophy). Student Outcome Data Website: http://cas.umkc.edu/psyc/grad/full-disclosure.asp.

Student Applications/Admissions:
Student Applications
Clinical Psychology PhD (Doctor of Philosophy)—Applications 2009–2010, 98. Total applicants accepted 2009–2010, 4. Number full-time enrolled (new admits only) 2009–2010, 4. Number part-time enrolled (new admits only) 2009–2010, 0. Total enrolled 2009–2010 full-time, 21, part-time, 4. Openings 2010–2011, 4. The median number of years required for completion of a degree in 2008–2009 were 6. The number of students enrolled full- and part-time who were dismissed or voluntarily withdrew from this program area in 2008–2009 were 0.
Scores: Entries appear in this order: required test or GPA, minimum score (if required), median score of students entering in 2009–2010. Clinical Psychology PhD (Doctor of Philosophy): GRE-V no minimum stated, 530, GRE-Q no minimum stated, 710, GRE-Analytical no minimum stated, 5.0, overall undergraduate GPA no minimum stated, 3.74.
Other Criteria: (importance of criteria rated low, medium, or high): GRE scores—high, research experience—high, work experience—medium, extracurricular activity—low, clinically related public service—medium, GPA—high, letters of recommendation—high, interview—high, statement of goals and objectives—high. For additional information on admission requirements, go to http://cas.umkc.edu/psyc/GCPhD.asp.

Student Characteristics: The following represents characteristics of students in 2009–2010 in all graduate psychology programs in the department: Female—full-time 17, part-time 2; Male—full-time 4, part-time 2; African American/Black—full-time 1, part-time 0; Hispanic/Latino(a)—full-time 1, part-time 0; Asian/Pacific Islander—full-time 0, part-time 0; American Indian/Alaska Native—full-time 0, part-time 0; Caucasian/White—full-time 19, part-time 2; Multi-ethnic—full-time 0, part-time 0; students subject to the Americans With Disabilities Act—full-time 0, part-time 0; Unknown ethnicity—full-time 0, part-time 2; Interna-

tional students who hold an F-1 or J-1 Visa—full-time 0, part-time 0.

Financial Information/Assistance:
Tuition for Full-Time Study: *Doctoral:* State residents: $363 per credit hour; Nonstate residents: $835 per credit hour. Tuition is subject to change. See the following Web site for updates and changes in tuition costs: http://www.umkc.edu/adminfinance/finance/cashiers/.

Financial Assistance:
First-Year Students: Teaching assistantships available for first year. Average amount paid per academic year: $9,000. Average number of hours worked per week: 20. Research assistantships available for first year. Average amount paid per academic year: $9,000. Average number of hours worked per week: 20. Fellowships and scholarships available for first year.
Advanced Students: Teaching assistantships available for advanced students. Average amount paid per academic year: $9,000. Average number of hours worked per week: 20. Research assistantships available for advanced students. Average amount paid per academic year: $9,000. Average number of hours worked per week: 20. Fellowships and scholarships available for advanced students.
Additional Information: Of all students currently enrolled full time, 100% benefited from one or more of the listed financial assistance programs. Application and information available online at: http://www.sfa.umkc.edu/.

Internships/Practica: Doctoral Degree (PhD Clinical Psychology): For those doctoral students for whom a professional internship was required in this program prior to graduation, (3) students applied for an internship in 2008–2009, with (3) students obtaining an internship. Of those students who obtained an internship, (3) were paid internships. Of those students who obtained an internship, (1) students placed in APA/CPA accredited internships, (1) students placed in internships not APA/CPA accredited, but listed with the Association of Psychology Postdoctoral and Internship Programs (APPIC), (0) students placed in internships conforming to guidelines of the Council of Directors of School Psychology Programs (CDSPP), (1) students placed in internships that were not APA/CPA accredited, APPIC or CDSPP listed. With a population of over 1.5 million, Kansas City offers numerous opportunities for practicum and research opportunities. A wide range of formal community practicum opportunities are offered to Clinical Psychology PhD students including placements at community agencies, medical centers, and other applied settings. Clinical psychology students are required to enroll in six semesters of practicum during which they are involved in many different types of clinical experiences, ranging from supervised work in specialized health care programs to more general outpatient settings for psychotherapy and psychological assessment. Basic clinical practica include training in general mental health assessment and treatment areas such as crisis intervention, depression screening, personnel and disability evaluations, and treatment of adjustment problems, depression, and anxiety disorders. Advanced training opportunities are available in the assessment and treatment of obesity and eating disorders, smoking and other substance abuse, and chronic pain. In the fifth year of study, students are required to complete a one year clinical internship.

Housing and Day Care: On-campus housing is available. See the following Web site for more information: http://www.umkc.edu/housing/. On-campus day care facilities are available. See the following Web site for more information: http://education.umkc.edu/berkley/.

Employment of Department Graduates:
Master's Degree Graduates: Of those who graduated in the academic year 2008–2009, the following categories and numbers represent the postgraduate activities and employment of master's degree graduates: Enrolled in a postdoctoral residency/fellowship (n/a), employed in independent practice (n/a), total from the above (master's) (0).
Doctoral Degree Graduates: Of those who graduated in the academic year 2008–2009, the following categories and numbers represent the postgraduate activities and employment of doctoral degree graduates: Enrolled in a psychology doctoral program (n/a), employed in an academic position at a university (1), employed in government agency (1), employed in a hospital/medical center (2), total from the above (doctoral) (4).

Additional Information:
Orientation, Objectives, and Emphasis of Department: The psychology program integrates clinical and epidemiological research with the health and life sciences. The department seeks to enhance the public health, broadly defined, through rigorous training of students (education mission); provide an accessible resource for the integration of behavioral sciences and health research and healthcare (service mission); develop knowledge and enhance health outcomes through empirical research (research and evaluation mission); and incorporate integrity and respect for human and intellectual diversity in all our activities (human mission).

Information for Students With Physical Disabilities: See the following Web site for more information: http://www.umkc.edu/disability/.

Application Information:
Send to UMKC Department of Psychology, Clinical PhD Program Admissions, 4825 Troost #124, Kansas City, MO 64110. Application available online. URL of online application: http://www.umkc.edu/admissions/umkc-graduate.asp. Students are admitted in the Fall, application deadline January 15. *Fee:* $35.

Missouri, University of, Kansas City
Division of Counseling and Educational Psychology
School of Education
5100 Rockhill Road, 215
Kansas City, MO 64110
Telephone: (816) 235-2722
Fax: (816) 235-5270
E-mail: *umkccep@umkc.edu*
Web: *http://education.umkc.edu/programs/view/18*

Department Information:
Chairperson: Nancy L. Murdock, PhD. Number of faculty: total—full-time 10, part-time 1; women—full-time 8; total—minority—full-time 4; women minority—full-time 3.

GRADUATE STUDY IN PSYCHOLOGY

Programs and Degrees Offered:
Listed in the following order: Program area, degree type (T if terminal Master's), number awarded 7/08–6/09. Counseling Psychology PhD (Doctor of Philosophy) 6, Counseling and Guidance EdS (School Psychology), Counseling and Guidance MA/MS (Master of Arts/Science) (T) 49.

APA Accreditation: Counseling PhD (Doctor of Philosophy). Student Outcome Data Website: http://education.umkc.edu/cep/PhD/PhDdata.html.

Student Applications/Admissions:
Student Applications
Counseling Psychology PhD (Doctor of Philosophy)—Applications 2009–2010, 73. Total applicants accepted 2009–2010, 7. Number full-time enrolled (new admits only) 2009–2010, 7. Openings 2010–2011, 7. The median number of years required for completion of a degree in 2008–2009 were 6. The number of students enrolled full- and part-time who were dismissed or voluntarily withdrew from this program area in 2008–2009 were 0. *Counseling and Guidance EdS (School Psychology)*—Total enrolled 2009–2010 part-time, 24. *Counseling and Guidance MA/MS (Master of Arts/Science)*—Applications 2009–2010, 127. Total applicants accepted 2009–2010, 66. Total enrolled 2009–2010 part-time, 118. Openings 2010–2011, 50. The median number of years required for completion of a degree in 2008–2009 were 3. The number of students enrolled full- and part-time who were dismissed or voluntarily withdrew from this program area in 2008–2009 were 0.
Other Criteria: (importance of criteria rated low, medium, or high): GRE scores—medium, research experience—high, work experience—medium, extracurricular activity—medium, clinically related public service—medium, GPA—high, letters of recommendation—high, interview—high, statement of goals and objectives—high, research interests—high, undergraduate major in psychology—medium. For additional information on admission requirements, go to http://education.umkc.edu/programs/view/18.

Student Characteristics: The following represents characteristics of students in 2009–2010 in all graduate psychology programs in the department: Female—full-time 24, part-time 0; Male—full-time 10, part-time 0; African American/Black—full-time 3, part-time 0; Hispanic/Latino(a)—full-time 3, part-time 0; Asian/Pacific Islander—full-time 5, part-time 0; American Indian/Alaska Native—full-time 0, part-time 0; Caucasian/White—full-time 23, part-time 0; Multi-ethnic—full-time 0, part-time 0; students subject to the Americans With Disabilities Act—full-time 2, part-time 0; Unknown ethnicity—full-time 0, part-time 0; International students who hold an F-1 or J-1 Visa—full-time 2, part-time 0.

Financial Information/Assistance:
Tuition for Full-Time Study: *Doctoral:* State residents: per academic year $5,865, $363 per credit hour; Nonstate residents: per academic year $5,865, $363 per credit hour. Tuition is subject to change. See the following Web site for updates and changes in tuition costs: http://www.umkc.edu/Adminfinance/finance/cashiers/.

Financial Assistance:
First-Year Students: Teaching assistantships available for first year. Average amount paid per academic year: $12,000. Average number of hours worked per week: 20. Apply by varies. Research assistantships available for first year. Average amount paid per academic year: $12,000. Average number of hours worked per week: 20. Apply by varies. Fellowships and scholarships available for first year. Apply by February 1.
Advanced Students: No information provided.
Additional Information: Of all students currently enrolled full time, 80% benefited from one or more of the listed financial assistance programs. Application and information available online at: http://www.sfa.umkc.edu.

Internships/Practica: Doctoral Degree (PhD Counseling Psychology): For those doctoral students for whom a professional internship was required in this program prior to graduation, (2) students applied for an internship in 2008–2009, with (2) students obtaining an internship. Of those students who obtained an internship, (2) were paid internships. Of those students who obtained an internship, (2) students placed in APA/CPA accredited internships, (0) students placed in internships not APA/CPA accredited, but listed with the Association of Psychology Postdoctoral and Internship Programs (APPIC), (0) students placed in internships conforming to guidelines of the Council of Directors of School Psychology Programs (CDSPP), (0) students placed in internships that were not APA/CPA accredited, APPIC or CDSPP listed. Master's Degree (MA/MS Counseling and Guidance): An internship experience, such as a final research project or "capstone" experience is required of graduates. All programs offer a wide range of practicum and internship placements. The Division of Counseling and Educational Psychology operates the Community Counseling and Assessment Services, an in-house training facility serving individuals, couples, and families in the surrounding community. Advanced practica are also available in a variety of agencies including local community mental health centers, Veterans Affairs Hospitals, and other local service provision agencies.

Housing and Day Care: On-campus housing is available. See the following Web site for more information: http://www.umkc.edu/housing. No on-campus day care facilities are available.

Employment of Department Graduates:
Master's Degree Graduates: Of those who graduated in the academic year 2008–2009, the following categories and numbers represent the postgraduate activities and employment of master's degree graduates: Enrolled in a psychology doctoral program (0), enrolled in another graduate/professional program (0), enrolled in a postdoctoral residency/fellowship (n/a), employed in independent practice (n/a), employed in an academic position at a university (0), employed in an academic position at a 2-year/4-year college (0), employed in other positions at a higher education institution (0), employed in a professional position in a school system (0), employed in business or industry (0), employed in government agency (0), employed in a community

mental health/counseling center (0), employed in a hospital/medical center (0), still seeking employment (0), not seeking employment (0), other employment position (0), do not know (0), total from the above (master's) (0).

Doctoral Degree Graduates: Of those who graduated in the academic year 2008–2009, the following categories and numbers represent the postgraduate activities and employment of doctoral degree graduates: Enrolled in a psychology doctoral program (n/a), enrolled in a postdoctoral residency/fellowship (2), employed in an academic position at a 2-year/4-year college (1), employed in other positions at a higher education institution (2), employed in a hospital/medical center (1), total from the above (doctoral) (6).

Additional Information:
Orientation, Objectives, and Emphasis of Department: Our Counseling Psychology program emphasizes the study of multicultural and individual diversity within a scientist–practitioner model. Consistent with the University of Missouri-Kansas City urban/metropolitan mission, the faculty is committed to educating future Counseling Psychologists to improve the welfare of individuals and communities through scholarship and applied interventions. 1. The program faculty encourages students to develop primary identification with the core values of counseling psychology. These values emphasize: a) assets, strengths, and positive mental health; b) respect for cultural and individual diversity; c) scientific foundation for all activities; d) developmental models of human growth; e) relatively brief counseling interventions; f) person-environment interaction; g) education and prevention; h) career/vocational development. 2. Our commitment to cultural and individual diversity is reflected in: a) faculty composition; b) student recruitment; c) scholarship ; d) course content and offerings; e) practicum opportunities; f) community service and consultation. 3. Education in counseling psychology follows a developmental model in which science-practice integration is emphasized throughout the program. Early and progressive training is provided in research, culminating in professionals who can design, conduct, and evaluate research relevant for counseling psychologists. Similarly, early and progressive training in practice activity is emphasized. 4. Program graduates will apply the values of counseling psychology to their work in a variety of employment settings, and as scientist–practitioners, their practice is informed by research and approached with a scientific attitude. 5. Counseling psychologists abide by the American Psychological Association code of conduct. Students will understand the ethical, legal, and professional issues related to the science and practice of counseling psychology.

Information for Students With Physical Disabilities: See the following Web site for more information: http://www.umkc.edu/disability.

Application Information:
Send to Counseling Psychology Program, University of Missouri-Kansas City, ED 215, 5100 Rockhill Road, Kansas City, Missouri 64110. Students are admitted in the Fall, application deadline January 1. *Fee:* $35. Online application fee $35; in-person (paper) application fee is $45.

Missouri, University of, St. Louis
Department of Psychology
One University Boulevard
St. Louis, MO 63121
Telephone: (314) 516-5391
Fax: (314) 516-5392
E-mail: *geot@UMSL.EDU*
Web: *http://www.umsl.edu/divisions/artscience/psychology*

Department Information:
1967. Chairperson: George T. Taylor. Number of faculty: total—full-time 23, part-time 1; women—full-time 12; total—minority—full-time 2; women minority—full-time 1.

Programs and Degrees Offered:
Listed in the following order: Program area, degree type (T if terminal Master's), number awarded 7/08–6/09. Clinical Psychology PhD (Doctor of Philosophy) 8, Industrial/Organizational Psychology PhD (Doctor of Philosophy) 3, Behavioral Neuroscience PhD (Doctor of Philosophy) 2.

APA Accreditation: Clinical PhD (Doctor of Philosophy).

Student Applications/Admissions:
Student Applications

Clinical Psychology PhD (Doctor of Philosophy)—Applications 2009–2010, 125. Total applicants accepted 2009–2010, 6. Number full-time enrolled (new admits only) 2009–2010, 6. Number part-time enrolled (new admits only) 2009–2010, 0. Openings 2010–2011, 6. The median number of years required for completion of a degree in 2008–2009 were 6. The number of students enrolled full- and part-time who were dismissed or voluntarily withdrew from this program area in 2008–2009 were 1. *Industrial/Organizational Psychology PhD (Doctor of Philosophy)*—Applications 2009–2010, 80. Total applicants accepted 2009–2010, 8. Number full-time enrolled (new admits only) 2009–2010, 4. Number part-time enrolled (new admits only) 2009–2010, 0. Openings 2010–2011, 5. The median number of years required for completion of a degree in 2008–2009 were 7. The number of students enrolled full- and part-time who were dismissed or voluntarily withdrew from this program area in 2008–2009 were 1. *Behavioral Neuroscience PhD (Doctor of Philosophy)*—Applications 2009–2010, 18. Total applicants accepted 2009–2010, 4. Number full-time enrolled (new admits only) 2009–2010, 2. Number part-time enrolled (new admits only) 2009–2010, 0. Openings 2010–2011, 4. The median number of years required for completion of a degree in 2008–2009 were 5. The number of students enrolled full- and part-time who were dismissed or voluntarily withdrew from this program area in 2008–2009 were 0.

Other Criteria: (importance of criteria rated low, medium, or high): GRE scores—high, research experience—high, work experience—medium, extracurricular activity—low, clinically related public service—medium, GPA—high, letters of recommendation—high, interview—medium, statement of goals and objectives—high, undergraduate major in psychology—medium. Only the clinical and behavioral neuroscience programs have a formal interview procedure.

Student Characteristics: The following represents characteristics of students in 2009–2010 in all graduate psychology programs in the department: Female—full-time 53, part-time 0; Male—full-time 19, part-time 0; African American/Black—full-time 1, part-time 0; Hispanic/Latino(a)—full-time 0, part-time 0; Asian/Pacific Islander—full-time 4, part-time 0; American Indian/Alaska Native—full-time 0, part-time 0; Caucasian/White—full-time 63, part-time 0; Multi-ethnic—full-time 4, part-time 0; students subject to the Americans With Disabilities Act—full-time 0, part-time 0; Unknown ethnicity—full-time 0, part-time 0; International students who hold an F-1 or J-1 Visa—full-time 0, part-time 0.

Financial Information/Assistance:
Tuition for Full-Time Study: *Master's:* State residents: $298 per credit hour; Nonstate residents: $771 per credit hour. *Doctoral:* State residents: $298 per credit hour; Nonstate residents: $771 per credit hour. Tuition is subject to change. Additional fees are assessed to students beyond the costs of tuition for the following: computer, parking, activities.

Financial Assistance:
First-Year Students: Teaching assistantships available for first year. Average amount paid per academic year: $10,500. Average number of hours worked per week: 20. Apply by January 15. Research assistantships available for first year. Average amount paid per academic year: $12,500. Average number of hours worked per week: 20. Apply by January 15. Fellowships and scholarships available for first year. Average amount paid per academic year: $4,000. Average number of hours worked per week: 0

Advanced Students: Teaching assistantships available for advanced students. Average amount paid per academic year: $11,500. Average number of hours worked per week: 20. Apply by January 15. Research assistantships available for advanced students. Average amount paid per academic year: $13,500. Average number of hours worked per week: 20. Apply by January 15. Fellowships and scholarships available for advanced students. Average amount paid per academic year: $4,000. Average number of hours worked per week: 0.

Additional Information: Of all students currently enrolled full time, 80% benefited from one or more of the listed financial assistance programs.

Internships/Practica: Doctoral Degree (PhD Clinical Psychology): For those doctoral students for whom a professional internship was required in this program prior to graduation, (1) students applied for an internship in 2008–2009, with (1) students obtaining an internship. Of those students who obtained an internship, (1) were paid internships. Of those students who obtained an internship, (1) students placed in APA/CPA accredited internships, (0) students placed in internships not APA/CPA accredited, but listed with the Association of Psychology Postdoctoral and Internship Programs (APPIC), (0) students placed in internships conforming to guidelines of the Council of Directors of School Psychology Programs (CDSPP), (0) students placed in internships that were not APA/CPA accredited, APPIC or CDSPP listed. Students (clinical) participate in practica in our Community Psychological Service (the psychology clinic), and a paid clinical clerkship, which may be in a community or university-based program. Advanced students in behavioral neuroscience have internship opportunities with research labs at local medical schools, Washington University and St. Louis University.

Housing and Day Care: On-campus housing is available. On-campus day care facilities are available. Child Development Center: (314) 516-5658.

Employment of Department Graduates:
Master's Degree Graduates: Of those who graduated in the academic year 2008–2009, the following categories and numbers represent the postgraduate activities and employment of master's degree graduates: Enrolled in a psychology doctoral program (0), enrolled in another graduate/professional program (1), enrolled in a postdoctoral residency/fellowship (n/a), employed in independent practice (n/a), employed in an academic position at a university (0), employed in an academic position at a 2-year/4-year college (0), employed in other positions at a higher education institution (0), employed in a professional position in a school system (0), employed in business or industry (0), employed in government agency (0), employed in a community mental health/counseling center (0), employed in a hospital/medical center (3), still seeking employment (0), not seeking employment (0), other employment position (0), do not know (0), total from the above (master's) (4).

Doctoral Degree Graduates: Of those who graduated in the academic year 2008–2009, the following categories and numbers represent the postgraduate activities and employment of doctoral degree graduates: Enrolled in a psychology doctoral program (n/a), enrolled in a postdoctoral residency/fellowship (5), employed in independent practice (0), employed in an academic position at a university (0), employed in an academic position at a 2-year/4-year college (0), employed in other positions at a higher education institution (0), employed in a professional position in a school system (0), employed in business or industry (3), employed in government agency (0), employed in a community mental health/counseling center (0), employed in a hospital/medical center (0), still seeking employment (0), not seeking employment (0), other employment position (0), do not know (0), total from the above (doctoral) (8).

Additional Information:
Orientation, Objectives, and Emphasis of Department: The orientation of the department emphasizes psychology as science yet also recognizes the important social responsibilities of psychology, especially in the clinical and applied areas. Emphasis of behavioral neuroscience is in neuropsychology, cognitive behaviors, psychophysiology and animal models of psychopathology, and behavioral neuropharmacology/endocrinology. The department offers a broad spectrum of high-quality programs at the undergraduate and graduate levels.

Special Facilities or Resources: The Department of Psychology is housed in Stadler Hall, and research laboratories and computers are conveniently located in the building. The psychological clinic (Community Psychological Service) is also contained within Stadler Hall. The Center for Trauma Recovery and Child Advocacy Center each have community clinics, which are housed on campus. Physical facilities include workshops and animal, social, and human experimental laboratories. A wide range of research equipment is available, including videotaping facilities, computer terminals, and personal computers.

Information for Students With Physical Disabilities: See the following Web site for more information: http://www.umsl.edu/services/disabled/.

Application Information:
Send to Graduate Admissions, University of Missouri-St. Louis, 358 Millennium Student Center, One University Boulevard, St. Louis, MO 63121. Application available online. URL of online application: http://www.umsl.edu/divisions/graduate. Students are admitted in the Fall. Clinical program deadline: December 15. Behavioral Neuroscience deadline: January 15. Industrial/Organizational deadline: January 15. *Fee:* $35.

The School of Professional Psychology at Forest Institute (2009 data)
Clinical Psychology
2885 West Battlefield Road
Springfield, MO 65807
Telephone: (417) 823-3477
Fax: (417) 823-3442
E-mail: *info@forest.edu*
Web: *http://www.forest.edu*

Department Information:
1979. President: Mark E. Skrade, PsyD. Number of faculty: total—full-time 17, part-time 34; women—full-time 9, part-time 19; total—minority—full-time 2, part-time 1; women minority—full-time 2, part-time 1; faculty subject to the Americans With Disabilities Act 1.

Programs and Degrees Offered:
Listed in the following order: Program area, degree type (T if terminal Master's), number awarded 7/08–6/09. Psychology MA/MS (Master of Arts/Science) (T) 36, Clinical Psychology PsyD (Doctor of Psychology) 36.

APA Accreditation: Clinical PsyD (Doctor of Psychology).

Student Applications/Admissions:
Student Applications
Psychology MA/MS (Master of Arts/Science)—Applications 2009–2010, 13. Total applicants accepted 2009–2010, 7. Number full-time enrolled (new admits only) 2009–2010, 13. Number part-time enrolled (new admits only) 2009–2010, 0. Total enrolled 2009–2010 full-time, 17, part-time, 13. Openings 2010–2011, 30. The median number of years required for completion of a degree in 2008–2009 were 2. The number of students enrolled full- and part-time who were dismissed or voluntarily withdrew from this program area in 2008–2009 were 0. *Clinical Psychology PsyD (Doctor of Psychology)*—Applications 2009–2010, 159. Total applicants accepted 2009–2010, 64. Number full-time enrolled (new admits only) 2009–2010, 42. Number part-time enrolled (new admits only) 2009–2010, 0. Total enrolled 2009–2010 full-time, 191, part-time, 21. Openings 2010–2011, 70. The median number of years required for completion of a degree in 2008–2009 were 4. The number of students enrolled full- and part-time who were dismissed or voluntarily withdrew from this program area in 2008–2009 were 8.
Other Criteria: (importance of criteria rated low, medium, or high): GRE scores—medium, research experience—medium, work experience—medium, extracurricular activity—low, clinically related public service—medium, GPA—high, letters of recommendation—high, interview—high, statement of goals and objectives—high, undergraduate major in psychology—low, specific undergraduate psychology courses taken—medium. For additional information on admission requirements, go to http://www.forest.edu/admissions.

Student Characteristics: The following represents characteristics of students in 2009–2010 in all graduate psychology programs in the department: Female—full-time 136, part-time 9; Male—full-time 75, part-time 7; African American/Black—full-time 16, part-time 0; Hispanic/Latino(a)—full-time 3, part-time 0; Asian/Pacific Islander—full-time 8, part-time 0; American Indian/Alaska Native—full-time 3, part-time 0; Caucasian/White—full-time 0, part-time 0; Multi-ethnic—full-time 4, part-time 0; students subject to the Americans With Disabilities Act—full-time 12, part-time 0; Unknown ethnicity—full-time 0, part-time 0; International students who hold an F-1 or J-1 Visa—full-time 0, part-time 0.

Financial Information/Assistance:
Tuition for Full-Time Study: Master's: State residents: $425 per credit hour; Nonstate residents: $425 per credit hour. *Doctoral:* State residents: $627 per credit hour; Nonstate residents: $627 per credit hour. Tuition is subject to change. See the following Web site for updates and changes in tuition costs: http://www.forest.edu/ad-financial-aid-through-forest.aspx.

Financial Assistance:
First-Year Students: Fellowships and scholarships available for first year. Apply by January 15.
Advanced Students: Fellowships and scholarships available for advanced students. Apply by June 1.
Additional Information: No information provided.

Internships/Practica: Doctoral Degree (PsyD Clinical Psychology): For those doctoral students for whom a professional internship was required in this program prior to graduation, (42) students applied for an internship in 2008–2009, with (38) students obtaining an internship. Of those students who obtained an internship, (36) were paid internships. Of those students who obtained an internship, (8) students placed in APA/CPA accredited internships, (30) students placed in internships not APA/CPA accredited, but listed with the Association of Psychology Postdoctoral and Internship Programs (APPIC), (0) students placed in internships conforming to guidelines of the Council of Directors of School Psychology Programs (CDSPP), (0) students placed in internships that were not APA/CPA accredited, APPIC or CDSPP listed. Master's Degree (MA/MS Psychology): An internship experience, such as a final research project or "capstone" experience is required of graduates. The School of Professional Psychology at Forest Institute enjoys a close relationship with the major state and city mental health facilities in the metropolitan and rural areas. Currently, there are 60 practica available to students. These opportunities provide a vast array of clinical experiences for a total of 1,200 practicum hours accumulated by the end of your required course work. During the fourth year of study, all students are required to complete a 2000 hour internship. Forest Institute has several on-site APA internship opportunities with clinical experiences.

Housing and Day Care: On-campus housing is available. No on-campus day care facilities are available.

GRADUATE STUDY IN PSYCHOLOGY

Employment of Department Graduates:
Master's Degree Graduates: Of those who graduated in the academic year 2008–2009, the following categories and numbers represent the postgraduate activities and employment of master's degree graduates: Enrolled in a postdoctoral residency/fellowship (n/a), employed in independent practice (n/a), total from the above (master's) (0).
Doctoral Degree Graduates: Of those who graduated in the academic year 2008–2009, the following categories and numbers represent the postgraduate activities and employment of doctoral degree graduates: Enrolled in a psychology doctoral program (n/a), enrolled in a postdoctoral residency/fellowship (26), do not know (11), total from the above (doctoral) (37).

Additional Information:
Orientation, Objectives, and Emphasis of Department: The design of the clinical psychology PsyD program is based on the belief that a thorough understanding of the comprehensive body of psychological knowledge, skills, and attitudes is essential for professional practitioners. The acquisition of this broad-based understanding and these abilities requires that the curriculum cover a combination of didactic knowledge, skill training, and supervised clinical experience with faculty and supervisors who provide appropriate role models. The PsyD degree is designed for individuals seeking an educational and training program geared toward professional application. Students are prepared to offer professional services in diagnostic, therapeutic, consultative, and administrative settings. Research and investigation skills are complemented by an increased focus on the use of research findings and theoretical formulations. The field practicum and internship are supervised clinical experiences that are integrated with the academic coursework. The faculty represents a variety of theoretical orientations and is committed to the rigorous preparation of students to become competent providers of service as well as ethical contributing members of the professional community. The MA in psychology program is intended to provide comprehensive exposure to the scientific foundations of psychology, including theories, concepts, and empirical knowledge of human development and behavior. The master's program is valuable to those who wish to increase their understanding of human behavior. These would include teachers, clergy, and training and personnel officers. The program also provides a solid foundation for eventual pursuit of a doctoral degree. The MA program provides the necessary course work to obtain counseling licensure at the master's level in most, if not all states.

Special Facilities or Resources: Forest Institute is located in the heart of the Ozarks. The academic/administrative center sits on 58 acres of land and provides students with a modern facility and state of the art equipment. Forest operates an on-site outpatient community mental health clinic, as well as providing students with access to local, state, and federal facilities. Practicum involves a high degree of community services and resources. Students provide services in the rural Ozarks, are actively involved with the homeless organizations of the Ozarks, correctional facilities, schools, and many other community based counseling opportunities.

Application Information:
Send to The School of Professional Psychology at Forest Institute, Office of Admissions, 2885 W Battlefield Road, Springfield, MO 65807. Application available online. URL of online application: http://www.forest.edu. Students are admitted in the Fall, application deadline January 15; Winter, application deadline September 15; Summer, application deadline November 15; *Fee:* $50.

Washington University in St. Louis
Department of Psychology
One Brookings Drive, Box 1125
St. Louis, MO 63130
Telephone: (314) 935-6520
Fax: (314) 935-7588
E-mail: *mcclelland@wustl.edu*
Web: *http://www.psych.wustl.edu*

Department Information:
1924. Chairperson: Randy J. Larsen. Number of faculty: total—full-time 34, part-time 1; women—full-time 12; total—minority—full-time 3; women minority—full-time 1.

Programs and Degrees Offered:
Listed in the following order: Program area, degree type (T if terminal Master's), number awarded 7/08–6/09. Clinical Psychology PhD (Doctor of Philosophy) 6, Aging and Development PhD (Doctor of Philosophy) 0, Behavior/Brain/Cognition PhD (Doctor of Philosophy) 7, Social/Personality Psychology PhD (Doctor of Philosophy) 1.

APA Accreditation: Clinical PhD (Doctor of Philosophy).

Student Applications/Admissions:
Student Applications
Clinical Psychology PhD (Doctor of Philosophy)—Applications 2009–2010, 214. Total applicants accepted 2009–2010, 9. Number full-time enrolled (new admits only) 2009–2010, 7. Number part-time enrolled (new admits only) 2009–2010, 0. Openings 2010–2011, 4. The median number of years required for completion of a degree in 2008–2009 were 6. The number of students enrolled full- and part-time who were dismissed or voluntarily withdrew from this program area in 2008–2009 were 0. *Aging and Development PhD (Doctor of Philosophy)*—Applications 2009–2010, 14. Total applicants accepted 2009–2010, 4. Number full-time enrolled (new admits only) 2009–2010, 5. Number part-time enrolled (new admits only) 2009–2010, 0. Openings 2010–2011, 2. The number of students enrolled full- and part-time who were dismissed or voluntarily withdrew from this program area in 2008–2009 were 0. *Behavior/Brain/Cognition PhD (Doctor of Philosophy)*—Applications 2009–2010, 77. Total applicants accepted 2009–2010, 10. Number full-time enrolled (new admits only) 2009–2010, 5. Number part-time enrolled (new admits only) 2009–2010, 0. Openings 2010–2011, 5. The median number of years required for completion of a degree in 2008–2009 were 6. The number of students enrolled full- and part-time who were dismissed or voluntarily withdrew from this program area in 2008–2009 were 0. *Social/Personality Psychology PhD (Doctor of Philosophy)*—Applications 2009–2010, 20. Total applicants accepted 2009–2010, 6. Number full-time enrolled (new admits only) 2009–2010, 0. Number part-time enrolled (new admits only) 2009–2010, 0. Openings 2010–2011, 3. The median number of years required for completion of a degree in 2008–2009

were 8. The number of students enrolled full- and part-time who were dismissed or voluntarily withdrew from this program area in 2008–2009 were 0.

Scores: Entries appear in this order: required test or GPA, minimum score (if required), median score of students entering in 2009–2010. *Clinical Psychology PhD (Doctor of Philosophy):* GRE-V no minimum stated, GRE-Q no minimum stated, GRE-Analytical no minimum stated, overall undergraduate GPA no minimum stated; *Aging and Development PhD (Doctor of Philosophy):* GRE-V no minimum stated, GRE-Q no minimum stated, GRE-Analytical no minimum stated, overall undergraduate GPA no minimum stated; *Behavior/Brain/Cognition PhD (Doctor of Philosophy):* GRE-V no minimum stated, GRE-Q no minimum stated, GRE-Analytical no minimum stated, overall undergraduate GPA no minimum stated; *Social/Personality Psychology PhD (Doctor of Philosophy):* GRE-V no minimum stated, GRE-Q no minimum stated, GRE-Analytical no minimum stated, overall undergraduate GPA no minimum stated.

Other Criteria: (importance of criteria rated low, medium, or high): GRE scores—high, research experience—high, work experience—low, clinically related public service—low, GPA—medium, letters of recommendation—high, interview—high, statement of goals and objectives—high, undergraduate major in psychology—medium, specific undergraduate psychology courses taken—medium. Interview is required for applicants prior to acceptance.

Student Characteristics: The following represents characteristics of students in 2009–2010 in all graduate psychology programs in the department: Female—full-time 52, part-time 0; Male—full-time 30, part-time 0; African American/Black—full-time 5, part-time 0; Hispanic/Latino(a)—full-time 4, part-time 0; Asian/Pacific Islander—full-time 15, part-time 0; American Indian/Alaska Native—full-time 0, part-time 0; Caucasian/White—full-time 54, part-time 0; Multi-ethnic—full-time 0, part-time 0; students subject to the Americans With Disabilities Act—full-time 1, part-time 0; Unknown ethnicity—full-time 4, part-time 0; International students who hold an F-1 or J-1 Visa—full-time 10, part-time 0.

Financial Information/Assistance:
Tuition for Full-Time Study: *Doctoral:* State residents: per academic year $37,800; Nonstate residents: per academic year $37,800.

Financial Assistance:
First-Year Students: Research assistantships available for first year. Average amount paid per academic year: $19,110. Average number of hours worked per week: 10. Traineeships available for first year. Average number of hours worked per week: 0. Fellowships and scholarships available for first year. Average amount paid per academic year: $20,000. Average number of hours worked per week: 0. Apply by January 25.

Advanced Students: Teaching assistantships available for advanced students. Average amount paid per academic year: $19,110. Average number of hours worked per week: 10. Research assistantships available for advanced students. Average amount paid per academic year: $19,110. Average number of hours worked per week: 15. Traineeships available for advanced students. Average amount paid per academic year: $19,110. Average number of hours worked per week: 0. Fellowships and scholarships available for advanced students. Average amount paid per academic year: $19,110. Average number of hours worked per week: 0.

Additional Information: Of all students currently enrolled full time, 100% benefited from one or more of the listed financial assistance programs.

Internships/Practica: Doctoral Degree (PhD Clinical Psychology): For those doctoral students for whom a professional internship was required in this program prior to graduation, (5) students applied for an internship in 2008–2009, with (5) students obtaining an internship. Of those students who obtained an internship, (5) were paid internships. Of those students who obtained an internship, (5) students placed in APA/CPA accredited internships, (0) students placed in internships not APA/CPA accredited, but listed with the Association of Psychology Postdoctoral and Internship Programs (APPIC), (0) students placed in internships conforming to guidelines of the Council of Directors of School Psychology Programs (CDSPP), (0) students placed in internships that were not APA/CPA accredited, APPIC or CDSPP listed.

Housing and Day Care: No on-campus housing is available. On-campus day care facilities are available. See the following Web site for more information: http://nurseryschool.wustl.edu/.

Employment of Department Graduates:
Master's Degree Graduates: Of those who graduated in the academic year 2008–2009, the following categories and numbers represent the postgraduate activities and employment of master's degree graduates: Enrolled in a postdoctoral residency/fellowship (n/a), employed in independent practice (n/a), total from the above (master's) (0).

Doctoral Degree Graduates: Of those who graduated in the academic year 2008–2009, the following categories and numbers represent the postgraduate activities and employment of doctoral degree graduates: Enrolled in a psychology doctoral program (n/a), enrolled in another graduate/professional program (0), enrolled in a postdoctoral residency/fellowship (3), employed in independent practice (0), employed in an academic position at a university (4), employed in an academic position at a 2-year/4-year college (1), employed in other positions at a higher education institution (1), employed in a professional position in a school system (0), employed in business or industry (2), employed in government agency (2), employed in a community mental health/counseling center (0), employed in a hospital/medical center (1), still seeking employment (0), not seeking employment (1), other employment position (0), do not know (0), total from the above (doctoral) (15).

Additional Information:
Orientation, Objectives, and Emphasis of Department: The emphasis within the clinical program is on training clinical scientists and promoting an integration of science and practice. Its goal is to train students who will lead the search for knowledge regarding the assessment, understanding, and treatment of psychological

disorders. In the experimental programs, the development of generalists with one or more areas of specialization is the department's orientation.

Special Facilities or Resources: The department's extensive facilities include animal, human psychophysiological, psychoacoustic, and clinical training laboratories; computer labs; closed circuit TV; and Neuroimaging (fMRI) and Image Analysis Laboratory.

Application Information:
Send to Meg McClelland, Graduate Program Coordinator, Washington University, Department of Psychology, Campus Box 1125, St. Louis, MO 63130-4899. Application available online. URL of online application: https://apply.embark.com/grad/washu/gsas/. Students are admitted in the Fall, application deadline December 15. *Fee:* $45.

MONTANA

Montana State University (2009 data)
Department of Psychology
Letters and Science
304 Traphagen Hall, P.O. Box 173440
Bozeman, MT 59717-3440
Telephone: (406) 994-3801
Fax: (406) 994-3804
E-mail: brenda.lewis1@montana.edu
Web: http://www.montana.edu/wwwpy

Department Information:
1950. Chairperson: Ruth Striegel-Moore, PhD. Number of faculty: total—full-time 9, part-time 3; women—full-time 3, part-time 2.

Programs and Degrees Offered:
Listed in the following order: Program area, degree type (T if terminal Master's), number awarded 7/08–6/09. Psychological Science MA/MS (Master of Arts/Science) 6.

Student Applications/Admissions:
Student Applications
Psychological Science MA/MS (Master of Arts/Science)—Applications 2009–2010, 15. Total applicants accepted 2009–2010, 6. Number full-time enrolled (new admits only) 2009–2010, 5. Total enrolled 2009–2010 full-time, 11. Openings 2010–2011, 6. The median number of years required for completion of a degree in 2008–2009 were 2. The number of students enrolled full- and part-time who were dismissed or voluntarily withdrew from this program area in 2008–2009 were 1.
Other Criteria: (importance of criteria rated low, medium, or high): GRE scores—medium, research experience—high, work experience—low, extracurricular activity—low, GPA—high, letters of recommendation—high, interview—medium, statement of goals and objectives—high, undergraduate major in psychology—medium, specific undergraduate psychology courses taken—medium. For additional information on admission requirements, go to http://www.montana.edu/wwwpy.

Student Characteristics: The following represents characteristics of students in 2009–2010 in all graduate psychology programs in the department: Female—full-time 4, part-time 0; Male—full-time 6, part-time 0; African American/Black—full-time 0, part-time 0; Hispanic/Latino(a)—full-time 0, part-time 0; Asian/Pacific Islander—full-time 0, part-time 0; American Indian/Alaska Native—full-time 0, part-time 0; Caucasian/White—full-time 10, part-time 0; Multi-ethnic—full-time 0, part-time 0; students subject to the Americans With Disabilities Act—full-time 0, part-time 0; Unknown ethnicity—full-time 0, part-time 0; International students who hold an F-1 or J-1 Visa—full-time 0, part-time 0.

Financial Information/Assistance:
Tuition for Full-Time Study: *Master's:* State residents: $320 per credit hour; Nonstate residents: $731 per credit hour. Tuition is subject to change. See the following Web site for updates and changes in tuition costs: http://www.montana.edu/wwwcat/expenses/FeeGrad.html.

Financial Assistance:
First-Year Students: Teaching assistantships available for first year. Average amount paid per academic year: $10,011. Average number of hours worked per week: 20. Apply by February 1. Fellowships and scholarships available for first year. Average amount paid per academic year: $1,000. Apply by February 1.

Advanced Students: Teaching assistantships available for advanced students. Average amount paid per academic year: $10,011. Average number of hours worked per week: 20. Apply by February 1.

Additional Information: Of all students currently enrolled full time, 100% benefited from one or more of the listed financial assistance programs. Application and information available online at: http://www.montana.edu/wwwpy/msprogram.htm.

Housing and Day Care: On-campus housing is available. See the following Web site for more information: http://www.montana.edu/fgh. On-campus day care facilities are available. See the following Web site for more information: http://www.montana.edu/wwwecp.

Employment of Department Graduates:
Master's Degree Graduates: Of those who graduated in the academic year 2008–2009, the following categories and numbers represent the postgraduate activities and employment of master's degree graduates: Enrolled in a psychology doctoral program (2), enrolled in another graduate/professional program (0), enrolled in a postdoctoral residency/fellowship (n/a), employed in independent practice (n/a), employed in an academic position at a university (0), employed in an academic position at a 2-year/4-year college (1), employed in other positions at a higher education institution (0), employed in a professional position in a school system (0), employed in business or industry (3), employed in government agency (0), employed in a community mental health/counseling center (0), employed in a hospital/medical center (0), still seeking employment (0), not seeking employment (0), other employment position (0), do not know (0), total from the above (master's) (6).
Doctoral Degree Graduates: Of those who graduated in the academic year 2008–2009, the following categories and numbers represent the postgraduate activities and employment of doctoral degree graduates: Enrolled in a psychology doctoral program (n/a), total from the above (doctoral) (0).

Additional Information:
Orientation, Objectives, and Emphasis of Department: Our two-year, research-oriented MS program in psychological science is designed for students interested mainly in obtaining a PhD degree. Areas of faculty interest include cognitive psychology, social psychology, physiological psychology, and health psychology.

Special Facilities or Resources: Office space provided for graduate students, all of whom are graduate teaching assistants. Laboratory space for human and animal research is available.

GRADUATE STUDY IN PSYCHOLOGY

Information for Students With Physical Disabilities: See the following Web site for more information: http://www.montana.edu/wwwres/disability/index.shtml.

Application Information:
Send to Graduate Admissions, Department of Psychology, 304 Traphagen Hall, Montana State University, P O Box 173440, Bozeman, MT 59717-3440. Application available online. URL of online application: http://www.montana.edu/gradstudies/apply.shtml. Students are admitted in the Fall, application deadline February 1. *Fee:* $50.

Montana State University Billings
Department of Psychology
College of Arts and Sciences
1500 North University Drive
Billings, MT 59101
Telephone: (406) 657-2242
Fax: (406) 657-2187
E-mail: bhengelfelt@msubillings.edu
Web: http://www.msubillings.edu

Department Information:
1967. Chairperson: Dr. Michael Havens. Number of faculty: total—full-time 4, part-time 1; women—full-time 1.

Programs and Degrees Offered:
Listed in the following order: Program area, degree type (T if terminal Master's), number awarded 7/08–6/09. Psychology MA/MS (Master of Arts/Science) (T) 12.

Student Applications/Admissions:
Student Applications
Psychology MA/MS (*Master of Arts/Science*)—Applications 2009–2010, 4. Total applicants accepted 2009–2010, 3. Number full-time enrolled (new admits only) 2009–2010, 3. Number part-time enrolled (new admits only) 2009–2010, 0. Openings 2010–2011, 10. The median number of years required for completion of a degree in 2008–2009 were 2. The number of students enrolled full- and part-time who were dismissed or voluntarily withdrew from this program area in 2008–2009 were 1.
Scores: Entries appear in this order: required test or GPA, minimum score (if required), median score of students entering in 2009–2010. Psychology MA/MS (*Master of Arts/Science*): GRE-V no minimum stated, 442, GRE-Q no minimum stated, 440, GRE-Analytical no minimum stated, 4, overall undergraduate GPA no minimum stated, 3.29.
Other Criteria: (importance of criteria rated low, medium, or high): GRE scores—medium, research experience—medium, work experience—low, extracurricular activity—low, clinically related public service—low, GPA—high, letters of recommendation—high, statement of goals and objectives—high, undergraduate major in psychology—medium, specific undergraduate psychology courses taken—medium.

Student Characteristics: The following represents characteristics of students in 2009–2010 in all graduate psychology programs in the department: Female—full-time 7, part-time 0; Male—full-time 3, part-time 0; African American/Black—full-time 0, part-time 0; Hispanic/Latino(a)—full-time 0, part-time 0; Asian/Pacific Islander—full-time 0, part-time 0; American Indian/Alaska Native—full-time 0, part-time 0; Caucasian/White—full-time 10, part-time 0; Multi-ethnic—full-time 0, part-time 0; students subject to the Americans With Disabilities Act—full-time 0, part-time 0; Unknown ethnicity—full-time 0, part-time 0; International students who hold an F-1 or J-1 Visa—full-time 0, part-time 0.

Financial Information/Assistance:
Tuition for Full-Time Study: Master's: State residents: per academic year $4,737, $263 per credit hour; Nonstate residents: per academic year $11,819, $656 per credit hour. Tuition is subject to change. See the following Web site for updates and changes in tuition costs: http://www.msubillings.edu/cost-GradStudies.htm.

Financial Assistance:
First-Year Students: Research assistantships available for first year.
Advanced Students: Teaching assistantships available for advanced students. Research assistantships available for advanced students.
Additional Information: Of all students currently enrolled full time, 25% benefited from one or more of the listed financial assistance programs. Application and information available online at: http://www.msubillings.edu/finaid/.

Internships/Practica: Our students do internships at several clinics around Billings, including two residential treatment facilities for children and adolescents and a prison prerelease center. Clinical psychologists in private practice also frequently take on our students as testing technicians. Students interested in a teaching career are offered the opportunity to teach undergraduate courses in our department.

Housing and Day Care: On-campus housing is available. See the following Web site for more information: http://www.msubillings.edu/reslife/. On-campus day care facilities are available. See the following Web site for more information: http://www.msubillings.edu/childcare/.

Employment of Department Graduates:
Master's Degree Graduates: Of those who graduated in the academic year 2008–2009, the following categories and numbers represent the postgraduate activities and employment of master's degree graduates: Enrolled in a psychology doctoral program (2), enrolled in another graduate/professional program (1), enrolled in a postdoctoral residency/fellowship (n/a), employed in independent practice (n/a), employed in an academic position at a university (0), employed in an academic position at a 2-year/4-year college (0), do not know (4), total from the above (master's) (7).
Doctoral Degree Graduates: Of those who graduated in the academic year 2008–2009, the following categories and numbers represent the postgraduate activities and employment of doctoral degree graduates: Enrolled in a psychology doctoral program (n/a), total from the above (doctoral) (0).

Additional Information:
Orientation, Objectives, and Emphasis of Department: Ours is a fairly small department with faculty members representing clinical, social, developmental, and physiological psychology. We have

been successful in preparing students for doctoral training, mostly in clinical psychology programs. Some of our students have gone on to successful careers as master's-level clinicians.

Special Facilities or Resources: One faculty member has a laboratory set up to study neural regeneration in planarians. Another is currently collaborating with researchers at a local hospital in a study assessing treatments for methamphetamine addiction. Graduate students have participated in both of these.

Information for Students With Physical Disabilities: See the following Web site for more information: http://www.msubillings.edu/dss/.

Application Information:
Application available online. URL of online application: http://www.msubillings.edu/grad. Students are admitted in the Fall, application deadline April 15; Spring, application deadline October 15. Applications received by dates specified will be given priority, but late applications will be considered until classes are full. *Fee:* $40.

Montana, The University of
Department of Psychology
Arts and Sciences
143 Skaggs Building
Missoula, MT 59812-1584
Telephone: (406) 243-4521
Fax: (406) 243-6366
E-mail: *allen.szalda-petree@umontana.edu*
Web: *http://www.umt.edu/psych/*

Department Information:
1920. Chairperson: Allen Szalda-Petree. Number of faculty: total—full-time 21, part-time 1; women—full-time 10, part-time 1; total—minority—full-time 1; women minority—full-time 1.

Programs and Degrees Offered:
Listed in the following order: Program area, degree type (T if terminal Master's), number awarded 7/08–6/09. Clinical Psychology PhD (Doctor of Philosophy) 6, Developmental Psychology PhD (Doctor of Philosophy) 4, School Psychology MA/MS (Master of Arts/Science) 7, Animal Behavior-Cognition PhD (Doctor of Philosophy) 0, School Psychology PhD (Doctor of Philosophy) 0.

APA Accreditation: Clinical PhD (Doctor of Philosophy). Student Outcome Data Website: http://psychweb.psy.umt.edu/www/graduate_clinical_applicant.asp.

Student Applications/Admissions:
Student Applications
Clinical Psychology PhD (Doctor of Philosophy)—Applications 2009–2010, 108. Total applicants accepted 2009–2010, 12. Number full-time enrolled (new admits only) 2009–2010, 7. Number part-time enrolled (new admits only) 2009–2010, 0. Total enrolled 2009–2010 full-time, 21, part-time, 14. Openings 2010–2011, 6. The median number of years required for completion of a degree in 2008–2009 were 7. The number of students enrolled full- and part-time who were dismissed or voluntarily withdrew from this program area in 2008–2009 were 3. *Developmental Psychology PhD (Doctor of Philosophy)*— Applications 2009–2010, 4. Total applicants accepted 2009–2010, 2. Number full-time enrolled (new admits only) 2009–2010, 1. Number part-time enrolled (new admits only) 2009–2010, 0. Total enrolled 2009–2010 full-time, 3, part-time, 1. Openings 2010–2011, 2. The median number of years required for completion of a degree in 2008–2009 were 6. The number of students enrolled full- and part-time who were dismissed or voluntarily withdrew from this program area in 2008–2009 were 0. *School Psychology MA/MS (Master of Arts/Science)*— Applications 2009–2010, 13. Total applicants accepted 2009–2010, 7. Number full-time enrolled (new admits only) 2009–2010, 2. Number part-time enrolled (new admits only) 2009–2010, 0. Total enrolled 2009–2010 full-time, 4, part-time, 7. Openings 2010–2011, 4. The median number of years required for completion of a degree in 2008–2009 were 2. The number of students enrolled full- and part-time who were dismissed or voluntarily withdrew from this program area in 2008–2009 were 0. *Animal Behavior-Cognition PhD (Doctor of Philosophy)*— Applications 2009–2010, 3. Total applicants accepted 2009–2010, 1. Number full-time enrolled (new admits only) 2009–2010, 1. Number part-time enrolled (new admits only) 2009–2010, 0. Total enrolled 2009–2010 full-time, 1, part-time, 2. Openings 2010–2011, 1. The number of students enrolled full- and part-time who were dismissed or voluntarily withdrew from this program area in 2008–2009 were 0. *School Psychology PhD (Doctor of Philosophy)*—Applications 2009–2010, 12. Total applicants accepted 2009–2010, 4. Number full-time enrolled (new admits only) 2009–2010, 4. Number part-time enrolled (new admits only) 2009–2010, 0. Openings 2010–2011, 3. The number of students enrolled full- and part-time who were dismissed or voluntarily withdrew from this program area in 2008–2009 were 1.

Scores: Entries appear in this order: required test or GPA, minimum score (if required), median score of students entering in 2009–2010. Clinical Psychology PhD (Doctor of Philosophy): GRE-V no minimum stated, 540, GRE-Q no minimum stated, 630, GRE-Analytical no minimum stated, GRE-Subject (Psychology) no minimum stated, 660; *Developmental Psychology PhD (Doctor of Philosophy)*: GRE-V no minimum stated, GRE-Q no minimum stated, GRE-Analytical no minimum stated, GRE-Subject (Psychology) no minimum stated; *School Psychology MA/MS (Master of Arts/Science)*: GRE-V no minimum stated, GRE-Q no minimum stated, GRE-Analytical no minimum stated; *Animal Behavior-Cognition PhD (Doctor of Philosophy)*: GRE-V no minimum stated, GRE-Q no minimum stated, GRE-Analytical no minimum stated, GRE-Subject (Psychology) no minimum stated, overall undergraduate GPA no minimum stated; *School Psychology PhD (Doctor of Philosophy)*: GRE-V no minimum stated, GRE-Q no minimum stated, GRE-Analytical no minimum stated, overall undergraduate GPA no minimum stated.

Other Criteria: (importance of criteria rated low, medium, or high): GRE scores—high, research experience—medium, work experience—medium, extracurricular activity—low, clinically related public service—medium, GPA—high, letters of recommendation—high, interview—medium, statement of goals and objectives—medium. Clinical service is a criterion for clinical program only. For additional information on admission requirements, go to http://psychweb.psy.umt.edu/www/graduate.asp.

Student Characteristics: The following represents characteristics of students in 2009–2010 in all graduate psychology programs in the department: Female—full-time 25, part-time 20; Male—full-time 11, part-time 4; African American/Black—full-time 0, part-time 2; Hispanic/Latino(a)—full-time 1, part-time 0; Asian/Pacific Islander—full-time 2, part-time 1; American Indian/Alaska Native—full-time 3, part-time 3; Caucasian/White—full-time 27, part-time 17; Multi-ethnic—full-time 0, part-time 0; students subject to the Americans With Disabilities Act—full-time 0, part-time 1; Unknown ethnicity—full-time 3, part-time 1; International students who hold an F-1 or J-1 Visa—full-time 0, part-time 0.

Financial Information/Assistance:

Tuition for Full-Time Study: *Master's:* State residents: per academic year $4,558, $296 per credit hour; Nonstate residents: per academic year $13,642, $868 per credit hour. *Doctoral:* State residents: per academic year $5,150, $321 per credit hour; Nonstate residents: per academic year $13,772, $898 per credit hour. Tuition is subject to change. Additional fees are assessed to students beyond the costs of tuition for the following: registration, facilities, equip, tech, ASUM, campus rec, transportation, UCenter, hlth svcs. See the following Web site for updates and changes in tuition costs: http://life.umt.edu/grad/name/tuitionandfees.

Financial Assistance:

First-Year Students: Teaching assistantships available for first year. Average amount paid per academic year: $14,800. Average number of hours worked per week: 15. Apply by January 1. Research assistantships available for first year. Average amount paid per academic year: $12,000. Average number of hours worked per week: 15.

Advanced Students: Teaching assistantships available for advanced students. Average amount paid per academic year: $14,800. Average number of hours worked per week: 15. Apply by January 15. Research assistantships available for advanced students. Average amount paid per academic year: $12,000. Average number of hours worked per week: 15.

Additional Information: Of all students currently enrolled full time, 70% benefited from one or more of the listed financial assistance programs. Application and information available online at: http://life.umt.edu/grad/folder/finassist.

Internships/Practica: Doctoral Degree (PhD Clinical Psychology): For those doctoral students for whom a professional internship was required in this program prior to graduation, (4) students applied for an internship in 2008–2009, with (3) students obtaining an internship. Of those students who obtained an internship, (3) were paid internships. Of those students who obtained an internship, (3) students placed in APA/CPA accredited internships, (0) students placed in internships not APA/CPA accredited, but listed with the Association of Psychology Postdoctoral and Internship Programs (APPIC), (0) students placed in internships conforming to guidelines of the Council of Directors of School Psychology Programs (CDSPP), (0) students placed in internships that were not APA/CPA accredited, APPIC or CDSPP listed. Doctoral Degree (PhD School Psychology): For those doctoral students for whom a professional internship was required in this program prior to graduation, (0) students applied for an internship in 2008–2009, with (0) students obtaining an internship. Of those students who obtained an internship, (0) were paid internships. Of those students who obtained an internship, (0) students placed in APA/CPA accredited internships, (0) students placed in internships not APA/CPA accredited, but listed with the Association of Psychology Postdoctoral and Internship Programs (APPIC), (0) students placed in internships conforming to guidelines of the Council of Directors of School Psychology Programs (CDSPP), (0) students placed in internships that were not APA/CPA accredited, APPIC or CDSPP listed.

Housing and Day Care: On-campus housing is available. See the following Web site for more information: http://www.umt.edu/reslife/. On-campus day care facilities are available. See the following Web site for more information: http://www.umt.edu/childcare.

Employment of Department Graduates:

Master's Degree Graduates: Of those who graduated in the academic year 2008–2009, the following categories and numbers represent the postgraduate activities and employment of master's degree graduates: Enrolled in a postdoctoral residency/fellowship (n/a), employed in independent practice (n/a), employed in a professional position in a school system (7), total from the above (master's) (7).

Doctoral Degree Graduates: Of those who graduated in the academic year 2008–2009, the following categories and numbers represent the postgraduate activities and employment of doctoral degree graduates: Enrolled in a psychology doctoral program (n/a), enrolled in a postdoctoral residency/fellowship (4), employed in independent practice (1), employed in an academic position at a university (1), employed in an academic position at a 2-year/4-year college (1), employed in a community mental health/counseling center (1), employed in a hospital/medical center (1), other employment position (1), total from the above (doctoral) (10).

Additional Information:

Orientation, Objectives, and Emphasis of Department: The clinical psychology PhD program trains students in basic psychological science and clinical skills including assessment, diagnosis, and therapeutic interventions. The program is based on the scientist–practitioner model and a variety of theoretical orientations are represented and taught. The training is a balanced combination of coursework, practicum and research. Upon completion of the program, graduates are well prepared for professional careers as clinical psychologists in institutional, academic, and private settings. In addition to generalist training, two specialty emphases are also offered: child and family and neuropsychology. The experimental psychology PhD program offers major emphases in the fields of animal behavior-cognition and lifespan developmental psychology. Minor areas are offered in quantitative, program evaluation, and special areas of psychology, e.g., cognitive and social, as well as those fields in which majors are offered. Graduates have found placement in academic, research, and applied settings. The School Psychology Program offers both doctoral (PhD) and specialist (EdS) level training based on the scientist-scholar-practitioner model and is aimed at professional preparation of school psychologists who are grounded thoroughly in the principles of human development, behavior and educational psychology. Doctoral candidates are trained to assume leadership roles in academia, research and clinical/school practice. Specialist level candidates are trained to provide psychoeducational services on a systems and individual basis.

Special Facilities or Resources: The Department of Psychology is housed in a modern building. It has classrooms; offices; research laboratories for social, developmental, and learning experimentation; and colony rooms for small animals. A clinical psychology center opened in the fall of 1983 and serves as a meeting place for clinical classes, seminars, research groups, and clinical services.

Information for Students With Physical Disabilities: See the following Web site for more information: http://www.umt.edu/dss/.

Application Information:
Send to Graduate Admissions, Department of Psychology, The University of Montana, Skaggs Building 143, Missoula, MT 59812-1584. Application available online. URL of online application: http://www.applyweb.com/apply/uomont/menu.html. Students are admitted in the Fall, application deadline January 1. The January 1 deadline is a firm date for the Clinical program. For Developmental and Animal Behavior/Cognition, October 15 is also acceptable. Late applications may be reviewed for the School Psychology programs. *Fee:* $45.

NEBRASKA

Nebraska, University of, Lincoln
Department of Educational Psychology
Teachers College
114 Teachers College Hall
Lincoln, NE 68588-0345
Telephone: (402) 472-2223
Fax: (402) 472-8319
E-mail: *rdeayala@unlserve.unl.edu*
Web: *http://cehs.unl.edu/edpsych/*

Department Information:
1908. Chairperson: R.J. De Ayala. Number of faculty: total—full-time 23; women—full-time 9; total—minority—full-time 2; women minority—full-time 1.

Programs and Degrees Offered:
Listed in the following order: Program area, degree type (T if terminal Master's), number awarded 7/08–6/09. Cognition, Learning, and Development PhD (Doctor of Philosophy) 9, Counseling Psychology PhD (Doctor of Philosophy) 4, Quantitative, Qualitative, & Psychometric Methods PhD (Doctor of Philosophy) 4, School Psychology PhD (Doctor of Philosophy) 6.

APA Accreditation: Counseling PhD (Doctor of Philosophy). Student Outcome Data Website: http://cehs.unl.edu/edpsych/graduate/copsych.shtml. School PhD (Doctor of Philosophy). Student Outcome Data Website: http://cehs.unl.edu/edpsych/graduate/schpsych.shtml.

Student Applications/Admissions:
Student Applications
Cognition, Learning, and Development PhD (Doctor of Philosophy)—Applications 2009–2010, 11. Total applicants accepted 2009–2010, 3. Total enrolled 2009–2010 full-time, 23, part-time, 6. Openings 2010–2011, 5. *Counseling Psychology PhD (Doctor of Philosophy)*—Applications 2009–2010, 75. Total applicants accepted 2009–2010, 17. Number full-time enrolled (new admits only) 2009–2010, 15. Total enrolled 2009–2010 full-time, 50, part-time, 1. Openings 2010–2011, 6. *Quantitative, Qualitative, & Psychometric Methods PhD (Doctor of Philosophy)*—Applications 2009–2010, 11. Total applicants accepted 2009–2010, 6. Number full-time enrolled (new admits only) 2009–2010, 5. Total enrolled 2009–2010 full-time, 15, part-time, 11. Openings 2010–2011, 5. *School Psychology PhD (Doctor of Philosophy)*—Applications 2009–2010, 54. Total applicants accepted 2009–2010, 12. Number full-time enrolled (new admits only) 2009–2010, 4. Openings 2010–2011, 8.
Other Criteria: (importance of criteria rated low, medium, or high): GRE scores—high, research experience—high, work experience—high, extracurricular activity—medium, clinically related public service—high, GPA—high, letters of recommendation—high, interview—high, statement of goals and objectives—high. For additional information on admission requirements, go to http://cehs.unl.edu/edpsych/graduate/Programs.shtml.

Student Characteristics: The following represents characteristics of students in 2009–2010 in all graduate psychology programs in the department: Female—full-time 86, part-time 10; Male—full-time 35, part-time 8; African American/Black—full-time 5, part-time 0; Hispanic/Latino(a)—full-time 4, part-time 0; Asian/Pacific Islander—full-time 5, part-time 3; American Indian/Alaska Native—full-time 1, part-time 0; Caucasian/White—full-time 106, part-time 15; Multi-ethnic—full-time 0, part-time 0; students subject to the Americans With Disabilities Act—full-time 1, part-time 0; Unknown ethnicity—full-time 0, part-time 0; International students who hold an F-1 or J-1 Visa—full-time 18, part-time 0.

Financial Information/Assistance:
Tuition for Full-Time Study: *Master's:* State residents: $247 per credit hour; Nonstate residents: $665 per credit hour. *Doctoral:* State residents: $247 per credit hour; Nonstate residents: $665 per credit hour. Tuition is subject to change. See the following Web site for updates and changes in tuition costs: http://www.unl.edu/gradstudies/prospective/money.shtml.

Financial Assistance:
First-Year Students: Teaching assistantships available for first year. Average amount paid per academic year: $14,269. Average number of hours worked per week: 20. Research assistantships available for first year. Average amount paid per academic year: $14,269. Average number of hours worked per week: 20. Fellowships and scholarships available for first year. Average amount paid per academic year: $9,275. Average number of hours worked per week: 13.
Advanced Students: Teaching assistantships available for advanced students. Average number of hours worked per week: 20. Research assistantships available for advanced students. Average number of hours worked per week: 20. Fellowships and scholarships available for advanced students.
Additional Information: Of all students currently enrolled full time, 52% benefited from one or more of the listed financial assistance programs. Application and information available online at: http://cehs.unl.edu/edpsych/graduate/finaid.shtml.

Internships/Practica: Doctoral Degree (PhD Counseling Psychology): For those doctoral students for whom a professional internship was required in this program prior to graduation, (3) students applied for an internship in 2008–2009, with (3) students obtaining an internship. Of those students who obtained an internship, (3) were paid internships. Of those students who obtained an internship, (3) students placed in APA/CPA accredited internships, (0) students placed in internships not APA/CPA accredited, but listed with the Association of Psychology Postdoctoral and Internship Programs (APPIC), (0) students placed in internships conforming to guidelines of the Council of Directors of

School Psychology Programs (CDSPP), (0) students placed in internships that were not APA/CPA accredited, APPIC or CDSPP listed. Doctoral Degree (PhD School Psychology): For those doctoral students for whom a professional internship was required in this program prior to graduation, (7) students applied for an internship in 2008–2009, with (7) students obtaining an internship. Of those students who obtained an internship, (7) were paid internships. Of those students who obtained an internship, (7) students placed in APA/CPA accredited internships, (0) students placed in internships not APA/CPA accredited, but listed with the Association of Psychology Postdoctoral and Internship Programs (APPIC), (0) students placed in internships conforming to guidelines of the Council of Directors of School Psychology Programs (CDSPP), (0) students placed in internships that were not APA/CPA accredited, APPIC or CDSPP listed. The Counseling Psychology and School Psychology programs both have sets of practicum courses wherein students provide direct and consultation services to students, staff and families in urban school settings. The Nebraska Internship Consortium in Professional Psychology is affiliated with the School Psychology program. Doctoral students in the QQPM program are encouraged to obtain internships.

Housing and Day Care: On-campus housing is available. See the following Web site for more information: http://housing.unl.edu/. On-campus day care facilities are available. See the following Web site for more information: http://childcare.unl.edu/.

Employment of Department Graduates:
Master's Degree Graduates: Of those who graduated in the academic year 2008–2009, the following categories and numbers represent the postgraduate activities and employment of master's degree graduates: Enrolled in a postdoctoral residency/fellowship (n/a), employed in independent practice (n/a), total from the above (master's) (0).
Doctoral Degree Graduates: Of those who graduated in the academic year 2008–2009, the following categories and numbers represent the postgraduate activities and employment of doctoral degree graduates: Enrolled in a psychology doctoral program (n/a), total from the above (doctoral) (0).

Additional Information:
Orientation, Objectives, and Emphasis of Department: The objective of the program is to develop applied behavioral scientists able to function in a variety of settings and roles ranging from educational settings to private practice. The broad base of the department offers a diversity of orientations and role models for students.

Special Facilities or Resources: The department operates the Counseling and School Psychology Clinic serves as a practicum site for School Psychology and Counseling Psychology programs. In addition, the department maintains excellent contact with the community, which promotes access to practical experiences and research subject pools. The department contains the Buros Center for Testing and its comprehensive reference library of assessment devices. The department also is home to the Center for Instructional Innovation, which conducts research on teaching and learning as well as the Nebraska Research Center on Children, Youth, Families and Schools.

Information for Students With Physical Disabilities: See the following Web site for more information: http://www.unl.edu/equity/.

Application Information:
Send to Attention: Emily Burgess, Admissions Coordinator, Department of Educational Psychology, 114 Teachers College Hall, University of Nebraska-Lincoln, Lincoln, NE 68405. Application available online. URL of online application: http://cehs.unl.edu/edpsych/graduate/apply.shtml. Students are admitted in the Fall, application deadline December 1; Spring, application deadline October 1. School Psychology program deadline is December 1; Counseling Psychology program is December 5. Cognition, Learning, & Developmental, consider applications for admissions at October 1, January 15, & May 15 deadlines. Quantitative, Qualitative, & Psychometric Methods (QQPM) considers applications for admissions at October 1 and January 15 deadline. *Fee:* $45. Written request for waiver of fee indicating need/justification for waiver or deferral of application fee.

Nebraska, University of, Lincoln
Department of Psychology
Arts & Sciences
238 Burnett Hall
Lincoln, NE 68588-0308
Telephone: (402) 472-3721
Fax: (402) 472-4637
E-mail: jlongwell1@unl.edu
Web: http://www.unl.edu/psypage

Department Information:
1889. Chairperson: David J. Hansen. Number of faculty: total—full-time 25, part-time 4; women—full-time 8, part-time 1; total—minority—full-time 4; women minority—full-time 1.

Programs and Degrees Offered:
Listed in the following order: Program area, degree type (T if terminal Master's), number awarded 7/08–6/09. Developmental Psychology PhD (Doctor of Philosophy) 1, Clinical Psychology PhD (Doctor of Philosophy) 11, Cognitive Psychology PhD (Doctor of Philosophy) 0, Biopsychology PhD (Doctor of Philosophy) 2, Law and Psychology PhD (Doctor of Philosophy) 2, Social/Personality Psychology PhD (Doctor of Philosophy) 1.

APA Accreditation: Clinical PhD (Doctor of Philosophy). Student Outcome Data Website: http://www.unl.edu/psypage/grad/clinical.shtml.

Student Applications/Admissions:
Student Applications
Developmental Psychology PhD (Doctor of Philosophy)—Applications 2009–2010, 20. Total applicants accepted 2009–2010, 1. Number full-time enrolled (new admits only) 2009–2010, 1. Number part-time enrolled (new admits only) 2009–2010, 0. Openings 2010–2011, 3. The median number of years required for completion of a degree in 2008–2009 were 5. The number of students enrolled full- and part-time who were dismissed or voluntarily withdrew from this program area in 2008–2009 were 0. *Clinical Psychology PhD (Doctor of Philosophy)*—Applications 2009–2010, 219. Total applicants ac-

cepted 2009–2010, 7. Number full-time enrolled (new admits only) 2009–2010, 7. Total enrolled 2009–2010 full-time, 63. Openings 2010–2011, 10. The median number of years required for completion of a degree in 2008–2009 were 6. The number of students enrolled full- and part-time who were dismissed or voluntarily withdrew from this program area in 2008–2009 were 0. *Cognitive Psychology PhD (Doctor of Philosophy)*—Applications 2009–2010, 18. Total applicants accepted 2009–2010, 1. Number full-time enrolled (new admits only) 2009–2010, 1. Number part-time enrolled (new admits only) 2009–2010, 0. Openings 2010–2011, 3. The number of students enrolled full- and part-time who were dismissed or voluntarily withdrew from this program area in 2008–2009 were 0. *Biopsychology PhD (Doctor of Philosophy)*—Applications 2009–2010, 24. Total applicants accepted 2009–2010, 3. Number full-time enrolled (new admits only) 2009–2010, 3. Openings 2010–2011, 2. The median number of years required for completion of a degree in 2008–2009 were 5. The number of students enrolled full- and part-time who were dismissed or voluntarily withdrew from this program area in 2008–2009 were 0. *Law and Psychology PhD (Doctor of Philosophy)*—Applications 2009–2010, 12. Total applicants accepted 2009–2010, 1. Number full-time enrolled (new admits only) 2009–2010, 1. Number part-time enrolled (new admits only) 2009–2010, 0. Openings 2010–2011, 4. The median number of years required for completion of a degree in 2008–2009 were 5. The number of students enrolled full- and part-time who were dismissed or voluntarily withdrew from this program area in 2008–2009 were 0. *Social/Personality Psychology PhD (Doctor of Philosophy)*—Applications 2009–2010, 28. Total applicants accepted 2009–2010, 1. Number full-time enrolled (new admits only) 2009–2010, 1. Number part-time enrolled (new admits only) 2009–2010, 0. Openings 2010–2011, 2. The median number of years required for completion of a degree in 2008–2009 were 5. The number of students enrolled full- and part-time who were dismissed or voluntarily withdrew from this program area in 2008–2009 were 0.
Scores: Entries appear in this order: required test or GPA, minimum score (if required), median score of students entering in 2009–2010. *Developmental Psychology PhD (Doctor of Philosophy)*: GRE-V no minimum stated, GRE-Q no minimum stated, GRE-Analytical no minimum stated, overall undergraduate GPA no minimum stated, psychology GPA no minimum stated, Masters GPA no minimum stated; *Clinical Psychology PhD (Doctor of Philosophy)*: GRE-V no minimum stated, GRE-Q no minimum stated, GRE-Analytical no minimum stated, overall undergraduate GPA no minimum stated, psychology GPA no minimum stated, Masters GPA no minimum stated; *Cognitive Psychology PhD (Doctor of Philosophy)*: GRE-V no minimum stated, GRE-Q no minimum stated, GRE-Analytical no minimum stated, overall undergraduate GPA no minimum stated, psychology GPA no minimum stated, Masters GPA no minimum stated; *Biopsychology PhD (Doctor of Philosophy)*: GRE-V no minimum stated, GRE-Q no minimum stated, GRE-Analytical no minimum stated, overall undergraduate GPA no minimum stated, psychology GPA no minimum stated, Masters GPA no minimum stated; *Law and Psychology PhD (Doctor of Philosophy)*: GRE-V no minimum stated, GRE-Q no minimum stated, GRE-Analytical no minimum stated, overall undergraduate GPA no minimum stated, psychology GPA no minimum stated, Masters GPA no minimum stated; *Social/Personality Psychology PhD (Doctor of Philosophy)*: GRE-V no minimum stated, GRE-Q no minimum stated, GRE-Analytical no minimum stated, overall undergraduate GPA no minimum stated, psychology GPA no minimum stated, Masters GPA no minimum stated.

Other Criteria: (importance of criteria rated low, medium, or high): GRE scores—medium, research experience—medium, work experience—medium, extracurricular activity—low, clinically related public service—medium, GPA—medium, letters of recommendation—high, interview—medium, statement of goals and objectives—medium, undergraduate major in psychology—low, specific undergraduate psychology courses taken—low. For additional information on admission requirements, go to http://www.unl.edu/psypage/grad/admission_requirements.shtml.

Student Characteristics: The following represents characteristics of students in 2009–2010 in all graduate psychology programs in the department: Female—full-time 81, part-time 0; Male—full-time 30, part-time 0; African American/Black—full-time 1, part-time 0; Hispanic/Latino(a)—full-time 12, part-time 0; Asian/Pacific Islander—full-time 5, part-time 0; American Indian/Alaska Native—full-time 1, part-time 0; Caucasian/White—full-time 90, part-time 0; Multi-ethnic—full-time 2, part-time 0; students subject to the Americans With Disabilities Act—full-time 0, part-time 0; Unknown ethnicity—full-time 0, part-time 0; International students who hold an F-1 or J-1 Visa—full-time 0, part-time 0.

Financial Information/Assistance:
Tuition for Full-Time Study: *Doctoral:* State residents: $247 per credit hour; Nonstate residents: $665 per credit hour. Tuition is subject to change. See the following Web site for updates and changes in tuition costs: http://stuaccts.unl.edu/tuitionfee/.

Financial Assistance:
First-Year Students: Teaching assistantships available for first year. Average number of hours worked per week: 19. Research assistantships available for first year. Average number of hours worked per week: 19. Fellowships and scholarships available for first year. Average number of hours worked per week: 19.
Advanced Students: Teaching assistantships available for advanced students. Average number of hours worked per week: 19. Research assistantships available for advanced students. Average number of hours worked per week: 19. Fellowships and scholarships available for advanced students.
Additional Information: Of all students currently enrolled full time, 100% benefited from one or more of the listed financial assistance programs. Application and information available online at: http://www.unl.edu/gradstudies/prospective/money.shtml.

Internships/Practica: Doctoral Degree (PhD Clinical Psychology): For those doctoral students for whom a professional internship was required in this program prior to graduation, (11) students applied for an internship in 2008–2009, with (11) students obtaining an internship. Of those students who obtained an internship, (11) were paid internships. Of those students who obtained an internship, (11) students placed in APA/CPA accredited internships, (0) students placed in internships not APA/CPA accredited, but listed with the Association of Psychology Postdoctoral and Internship Programs (APPIC), (0) students placed in internships conforming to guidelines of the Council of Directors of School Psychology Programs (CDSPP), (0) students placed in internships that were not APA/CPA accredited, APPIC or CDSPP listed. The clinical program offers numerous internship opportunities for students. We have an excellent record of placements for our students at high-quality internship sites throughout North America and participate in the APPIC internship match process.

Housing and Day Care: On-campus housing is available. See the following Web site for more information: http://housing.unl.edu/. On-campus day care facilities are available. See the following Web site for more information: http://childcare.unl.edu/.

Employment of Department Graduates:
Master's Degree Graduates: Of those who graduated in the academic year 2008–2009, the following categories and numbers represent the postgraduate activities and employment of master's degree graduates: Enrolled in a postdoctoral residency/fellowship (n/a), employed in independent practice (n/a), total from the above (master's) (0).
Doctoral Degree Graduates: Of those who graduated in the academic year 2008–2009, the following categories and numbers represent the postgraduate activities and employment of doctoral degree graduates: Enrolled in a psychology doctoral program (n/a), total from the above (doctoral) (0).

Additional Information:
Orientation, Objectives, and Emphasis of Department: The Department of Psychology at the University of Nebraska-Lincoln offers PhD programs that emphasize the development of research and teaching excellence, collegial partnerships between students and faculty, and the cross-fertilization of ideas between specializations in the context of a rigorous, but flexible, training program. The goal of the clinical program is to produce broadly trained, scientifically-oriented psychologists who have skills in both research and professional activities. The cognitive, biopsychology, developmental, and social-personality programs all emphasize research training but also place equal importance upon training for college or university teaching and policy/applied careers. Students in the PhD/JD program take their first year in the Law College, and then concentrate on psychology plus law to graduate with a double doctorate.

Special Facilities or Resources: The department has a number of resources including the Ruth Staples Child Development Laboratory, the Center for Children, Families and the Law, the BUROS Mental Measurement Institute, the NEAR Center, the UNL Public Policy Center, and the Lincoln Regional Mental Health Center.

Information for Students With Physical Disabilities: See the following Web site for more information: http://www.unl.edu/ssd/.

Application Information:
Send to Admissions Coordinator, Dept. of Psychology, UNL, 238 Burnett, Lincoln, NE 68588-0308. Application available online. URL of online application: http://www.unl.edu/gradstudies/. Students are admitted in the Fall, application deadline January 1. The deadlines are January 1 for clinical, January 15 for all others. *Fee:* $45.

Nebraska, University of, Omaha
Department of Psychology
Arts and Sciences
6001 Dodge Street
Omaha, NE 68182-0274
Telephone: (402) 554-2592; 2313 Joseph Brown
Fax: (402) 554-2556
E-mail: *josephbrown@unomaha.edu*
Web: *http://www.unomaha.edu/psych/*

Department Information:
Chairperson: Brigette Ryalls. Number of faculty: total—full-time 18; women—full-time 8; total—minority—full-time 3; women minority—full-time 2.

Programs and Degrees Offered:
Listed in the following order: Program area, degree type (T if terminal Master's), number awarded 7/08–6/09. Experimental Psychology MA/MS (Master of Arts/Science) 1, School Psychology MA/MS (Master of Arts/Science) 10, Psychobiology PhD (Doctor of Philosophy) 0, Developmental Psychology MA/MS (Master of Arts/Science) 1, School Psychology EdS (School Psychology) 7, Developmental Psychology PhD (Doctor of Philosophy) 0, Industrial/Organizational Psychology PhD (Doctor of Philosophy) 0, Industrial/Organizational Psychology MA/MS (Master of Arts/Science) 8, Industrial/Organizational Psychology MA/MS (Master of Arts/Science) (T) 4, Psychobiology MA/MS (Master of Arts/Science) 1, Developmental Psychology MA/MS (Master of Arts/Science) (T) 0.

Student Applications/Admissions:
Student Applications
Experimental Psychology MA/MS (Master of Arts/Science)—Applications 2009–2010, 17. Total applicants accepted 2009–2010, 3. Number full-time enrolled (new admits only) 2009–2010, 3. Number part-time enrolled (new admits only) 2009–2010, 0. Openings 2010–2011, 2. The median number of years required for completion of a degree in 2008–2009 were 3. The number of students enrolled full- and part-time who were dismissed or voluntarily withdrew from this program area in 2008–2009 were 0. *School Psychology MA/MS (Master of Arts/Science)*—Applications 2009–2010, 30. Total applicants accepted 2009–2010, 11. Number full-time enrolled (new admits only) 2009–2010, 9. Openings 2010–2011, 12. The median number of years required for completion of a degree in 2008–2009 were 2. The number of students enrolled full- and part-time who were dismissed or voluntarily withdrew from this program area in 2008–2009 were 0. *Psychobiology PhD (Doctor of Philosophy)*—Applications 2009–2010, 5. Total applicants accepted 2009–2010, 4. Number full-time enrolled (new admits only) 2009–2010, 3. Number part-time enrolled (new admits only) 2009–2010, 0. Openings 2010–2011, 1. The number of students enrolled full- and part-time who were dismissed or voluntarily withdrew from this program area in 2008–2009 were 0. *Developmental Psychology MA/MS (Master of Arts/Science)*—Applications 2009–2010, 3. Total applicants accepted 2009–2010, 1. Number full-time enrolled (new admits only) 2009–2010, 1. Openings 2010–2011, 3. The median number of years required for completion of a degree in 2008–2009 were 3. The number of students enrolled full- and part-time

who were dismissed or voluntarily withdrew from this program area in 2008–2009 were 0. *School Psychology EdS (School Psychology)*—Applications 2009–2010, 8. Total applicants accepted 2009–2010, 8. Number full-time enrolled (new admits only) 2009–2010, 8. Number part-time enrolled (new admits only) 2009–2010, 0. Openings 2010–2011, 5. The median number of years required for completion of a degree in 2008–2009 were 4. The number of students enrolled full- and part-time who were dismissed or voluntarily withdrew from this program area in 2008–2009 were 0. *Developmental Psychology PhD (Doctor of Philosophy)*—Applications 2009–2010, 2. Total applicants accepted 2009–2010, 0. Number full-time enrolled (new admits only) 2009–2010, 0. Number part-time enrolled (new admits only) 2009–2010, 0. Openings 2010–2011, 2. The number of students enrolled full- and part-time who were dismissed or voluntarily withdrew from this program area in 2008–2009 were 0. *Industrial/Organizational Psychology PhD (Doctor of Philosophy)*—Applications 2009–2010, 16. Total applicants accepted 2009–2010, 9. Number full-time enrolled (new admits only) 2009–2010, 5. Total enrolled 2009–2010 full-time, 25. Openings 2010–2011, 10. The number of students enrolled full- and part-time who were dismissed or voluntarily withdrew from this program area in 2008–2009 were 0. *Industrial/Organizational Psychology MA/MS (Master of Arts/Science)*—Applications 2009–2010, 5. Total applicants accepted 2009–2010, 2. Number full-time enrolled (new admits only) 2009–2010, 1. Number part-time enrolled (new admits only) 2009–2010, 0. Openings 2010–2011, 5. The median number of years required for completion of a degree in 2008–2009 were 3. The number of students enrolled full- and part-time who were dismissed or voluntarily withdrew from this program area in 2008–2009 were 0. *Industrial/Organizational Psychology MA/MS (Master of Arts/Science)*—Applications 2009–2010, 12. Total applicants accepted 2009–2010, 3. Number full-time enrolled (new admits only) 2009–2010, 1. Number part-time enrolled (new admits only) 2009–2010, 0. Openings 2010–2011, 3. The median number of years required for completion of a degree in 2008–2009 were 2. The number of students enrolled full- and part-time who were dismissed or voluntarily withdrew from this program area in 2008–2009 were 0. *Psychobiology MA/MS (Master of Arts/Science)*—Applications 2009–2010, 3. Total applicants accepted 2009–2010, 2. Number full-time enrolled (new admits only) 2009–2010, 2. Total enrolled 2009–2010 full-time, 3. Openings 2010–2011, 2. The median number of years required for completion of a degree in 2008–2009 were 3. The number of students enrolled full- and part-time who were dismissed or voluntarily withdrew from this program area in 2008–2009 were 0. *Developmental Psychology MA/MS (Master of Arts/Science)*—Applications 2009–2010, 4. Total applicants accepted 2009–2010, 1. Number full-time enrolled (new admits only) 2009–2010, 1. Total enrolled 2009–2010 full-time, 3. Openings 2010–2011, 2. The number of students enrolled full- and part-time who were dismissed or voluntarily withdrew from this program area in 2008–2009 were 0.

Other Criteria: (importance of criteria rated low, medium, or high): GRE scores—high, research experience—high, work experience—medium, extracurricular activity—medium, clinically related public service—low, GPA—high, letters of recommendation—high, interview—medium, statement of goals and objectives—high. For additional information on admission requirements, go to http://www.unomaha.edu/psych/graduate.php.

Student Characteristics: The following represents characteristics of students in 2009–2010 in all graduate psychology programs in the department: Female—full-time 77, part-time 0; Male—full-time 25, part-time 0; African American/Black—full-time 2, part-time 0; Hispanic/Latino(a)—full-time 1, part-time 0; Asian/Pacific Islander—full-time 1, part-time 0; American Indian/Alaska Native—full-time 0, part-time 0; Caucasian/White—full-time 98, part-time 0; Multi-ethnic—full-time 0, part-time 0; students subject to the Americans With Disabilities Act—full-time 0, part-time 0; Unknown ethnicity—full-time 0, part-time 0; International students who hold an F-1 or J-1 Visa—full-time 2, part-time 0.

Financial Information/Assistance:
Tuition for Full-Time Study: *Master's:* State residents: $212 per credit hour; Nonstate residents: $559 per credit hour. *Doctoral:* State residents: $212 per credit hour; Nonstate residents: $559 per credit hour. Tuition is subject to change. See the following Web site for updates and changes in tuition costs: http://cashiering.unomaha.edu/tuition.php.

Financial Assistance:
First-Year Students: Teaching assistantships available for first year. Average amount paid per academic year: $11,921. Average number of hours worked per week: 20. Apply by January 5. Research assistantships available for first year. Average amount paid per academic year: $11,921. Average number of hours worked per week: 20. Apply by January 5. Fellowships and scholarships available for first year. Average amount paid per academic year: $11,921. Average number of hours worked per week: 20. Apply by January 5.

Advanced Students: Teaching assistantships available for advanced students. Average amount paid per academic year: $11,921. Average number of hours worked per week: 20. Apply by January 5. Research assistantships available for advanced students. Average amount paid per academic year: $11,921. Average number of hours worked per week: 20. Apply by January 5. Traineeships available for advanced students. Average number of hours worked per week: 20. Fellowships and scholarships available for advanced students. Average amount paid per academic year: $11,921. Average number of hours worked per week: 20. Apply by January 5.

Additional Information: Of all students currently enrolled full time, 50% benefited from one or more of the listed financial assistance programs. Application and information available online at: http://www.unomaha.edu/psych/graduate.php.

Internships/Practica: An internship in school psychology is available and required within the EdS program leading to certification in the field of school psychology. Practica are also available (and for some degrees required) in industrial/organizational psychology and developmental psychology.

Housing and Day Care: On-campus housing is available. See the following Web site for more information: http://housing.unomaha.edu/index.php. On-campus day care facilities are available. See the following Web site for more information: http://mbsc.unomaha.edu/child.php.

Employment of Department Graduates:

Master's Degree Graduates: Of those who graduated in the academic year 2008–2009, the following categories and numbers represent the postgraduate activities and employment of master's degree graduates: Enrolled in a postdoctoral residency/fellowship (n/a), employed in independent practice (n/a), total from the above (master's) (0).

Doctoral Degree Graduates: Of those who graduated in the academic year 2008–2009, the following categories and numbers represent the postgraduate activities and employment of doctoral degree graduates: Enrolled in a psychology doctoral program (n/a), total from the above (doctoral) (0).

Additional Information:

Orientation, Objectives, and Emphasis of Department: The department is broadly eclectic, placing emphasis on theory, research, and application. The MA program is primarily for students who anticipate continuing their education at the PhD level. The MA degree may be completed in eight areas of psychology. The MS program is primarily for students who view the master's degree as terminal and who wish to emphasize application in the fields of educational-school or industrial/organizational psychology. These two areas may be emphasized within the MA program as well.

Special Facilities or Resources: The department maintains extensive laboratory facilities in a variety of experimental areas, both human and animal. The animal colony consists of rats, gerbils, mice, and golden-lion tamarins. Up-to-date interactive computer facilities are readily available. The Center for Applied Psychological Services is a departmentally controlled, faculty-student consulting service that provides an opportunity to gain practical experience in industrial psychology and school psychology. The department maintains working relationships with the Children's Rehabilitation Institute, the Department of Pediatrics, the Department of Physiology, and the University of Nebraska Medical Center. In addition, contact exists with the Boys Town Institute, Boys Town Home, Henry Doorly Zoo, Union Pacific Railroad, and Mutual of Omaha.

Information for Students With Physical Disabilities: See the following Web site for more information: http://www.unomaha.edu/disability/.

Application Information:
Send to Graduate Programs Chair, 6001 Dodge St., ASH 347, Omaha, NE 68182-0274. Application available online. URL of online application: https://admit.nebraska.edu/applyUNO/login.action. Students are admitted in the Fall, application deadline January 5. *Fee:* $45.

NEVADA

Nevada, University of, Las Vegas
Department of Psychology
Liberal Arts
4505 South Maryland Parkway, Box 455030
Las Vegas, NV 89154-5030
Telephone: (702) 895-3305
Fax: (702) 895-0195
E-mail: *mark.ashcraft@unlv.edu*
Web: *http://psychology.unlv.edu*

Department Information:
1960. Chairperson: Mark H. Ashcraft. Number of faculty: total—full-time 21, part-time 12; women—full-time 9, part-time 6; total—minority—full-time 1, part-time 2; women minority—full-time 1, part-time 2.

Programs and Degrees Offered:
Listed in the following order: Program area, degree type (T if terminal Master's), number awarded 7/08–6/09. Clinical Psychology PhD (Doctor of Philosophy) 7, Experimental Psychology PhD (Doctor of Philosophy) 2.

APA Accreditation: Clinical PhD (Doctor of Philosophy).

Student Applications/Admissions:
Student Applications
Clinical Psychology PhD (Doctor of Philosophy)—Applications 2009–2010, 179. Total applicants accepted 2009–2010, 6. Number full-time enrolled (new admits only) 2009–2010, 6. Number part-time enrolled (new admits only) 2009–2010, 0. Openings 2010–2011, 8. The median number of years required for completion of a degree in 2008–2009 were 6. The number of students enrolled full- and part-time who were dismissed or voluntarily withdrew from this program area in 2008–2009 were 1. Experimental Psychology PhD (Doctor of Philosophy)—Applications 2009–2010, 42. Total applicants accepted 2009–2010, 5. Number full-time enrolled (new admits only) 2009–2010, 5. Number part-time enrolled (new admits only) 2009–2010, 0. Openings 2010–2011, 8. The median number of years required for completion of a degree in 2008–2009 were 7. The number of students enrolled full- and part-time who were dismissed or voluntarily withdrew from this program area in 2008–2009 were 2.
Scores: Entries appear in this order: required test or GPA, minimum score (if required), median score of students entering in 2009–2010. Clinical Psychology PhD (Doctor of Philosophy): GRE-V 550, 597, GRE-Q 550, 723, overall undergraduate GPA 3.5, 3.62, psychology GPA 3.5, 3.8; Experimental Psychology PhD (Doctor of Philosophy): GRE-V 550, 655, GRE-Q 550, 725, overall undergraduate GPA 3.5, 3.72, psychology GPA 3.5, 3.78.
Other Criteria: (importance of criteria rated low, medium, or high): GRE scores—high, research experience—high, work experience—medium, extracurricular activity—low, clinically related public service—medium, GPA—high, letters of recommendation—high, interview—high, statement of goals and objectives—high, undergraduate major in psychology—high, specific undergraduate psychology courses taken—low. Our experimental program ranks clinical related public services as low. For additional information on admission requirements, go to http://psychology.unlv.edu/html/graduate_programs.html.

Student Characteristics: The following represents characteristics of students in 2009–2010 in all graduate psychology programs in the department: Female—full-time 49, part-time 0; Male—full-time 24, part-time 0; African American/Black—full-time 2, part-time 0; Hispanic/Latino(a)—full-time 4, part-time 0; Asian/Pacific Islander—full-time 5, part-time 0; American Indian/Alaska Native—full-time 1, part-time 0; Caucasian/White—full-time 55, part-time 0; Multi-ethnic—full-time 3, part-time 0; students subject to the Americans With Disabilities Act—full-time 0, part-time 0; Unknown ethnicity—full-time 3, part-time 0; International students who hold an F-1 or J-1 Visa—full-time 3, part-time 0.

Financial Information/Assistance:
Tuition for Full-Time Study: *Doctoral:* State residents: $222 per credit hour; Nonstate residents: $460 per credit hour. Tuition is subject to change. Additional fees are assessed to students beyond the costs of tuition for the following: lab assessment materials for some courses. See the following Web site for updates and changes in tuition costs: http://www.unlv.edu/Controller/bursar/tuition.html.

Financial Assistance:
First-Year Students: Teaching assistantships available for first year. Average amount paid per academic year: $15,000. Average number of hours worked per week: 20. Apply by January 15. Research assistantships available for first year. Average amount paid per academic year: $15,000. Average number of hours worked per week: 20. Apply by January 15.
Advanced Students: Teaching assistantships available for advanced students. Average amount paid per academic year: $12,000. Average number of hours worked per week: 20. Apply by March 1. Research assistantships available for advanced students. Average amount paid per academic year: $12,000. Average number of hours worked per week: 20. Apply by March 1. Fellowships and scholarships available for advanced students. Average amount paid per academic year: $15,000. Average number of hours worked per week: 20. Apply by March 1.
Additional Information: Of all students currently enrolled full time, 94% benefited from one or more of the listed financial assistance programs. Application and information available online at: http://graduatecollege.unlv.edu/financing/.

Internships/Practica: Doctoral Degree (PhD Clinical Psychology): For those doctoral students for whom a professional internship was required in this program prior to graduation, (9) students applied for an internship in 2008–2009, with (8) students obtaining an internship. Of those students who obtained an internship, (8) were paid internships. Of those students who obtained an internship, (8) students placed in APA/CPA accredited internships, (0) students placed in internships not APA/CPA accredited, but listed with the Association of Psychology Postdoctoral and Internship Programs (APPIC), (0) students placed in internships conforming to guidelines of the Council of Directors of School Psychology Programs (CDSPP), (0) students placed in internships that were not APA/CPA accredited, APPIC or CDSPP listed. Students work in various community practicum settings as part of their training experience.

Housing and Day Care: No on-campus housing is available. On-campus day care facilities are available. See the following Web site for more information: http://preschool.unlv.edu/.

Employment of Department Graduates:

Master's Degree Graduates: Of those who graduated in the academic year 2008–2009, the following categories and numbers represent the postgraduate activities and employment of master's degree graduates: Enrolled in a postdoctoral residency/fellowship (n/a), employed in independent practice (n/a), total from the above (master's) (0).

Doctoral Degree Graduates: Of those who graduated in the academic year 2008–2009, the following categories and numbers represent the postgraduate activities and employment of doctoral degree graduates: Enrolled in a psychology doctoral program (n/a), employed in independent practice (2), employed in a professional position in a school system (1), employed in a community mental health/counseling center (1), employed in a hospital/medical center (4), total from the above (doctoral) (8).

Additional Information:

Orientation, Objectives, and Emphasis of Department: Our programs combine a strong focus on major content areas of experimental psychology (emphasis in cognitive, neuroscience and developmental studies) and methodology/statistics, while also providing opportunities to learn skills and conduct research that can be applied to real-world problems. In short, graduate training will produce experimental psychologists who can be employed in both academic and non-academic settings. The department has the following goals: Generating new psychological knowledge through original scholarly research. Disseminating psychological knowledge through scholarly articles, books, and other relevant media, and the development of professional conduct through mentorship and supervision of graduate and undergraduate students, and through effective teaching at the graduate and undergraduate levels. Promoting self-exploration and self-awareness among students to develop an appreciation of diversity. Creating a just, diverse, and humane working and learning environment. Enhancing organizational climate, research, teaching/mentoring, and services related to multiculturalism and diversity. Creating an effective and responsive administrative infrastructure to serve all stakeholders, including faculty, graduate and undergraduate students, other administrative units within the College and University, and the larger public. Serving the community by bringing faculty and student expertise to bear on important local and regional issues. The UNLV Experimental Psychology doctoral program is designed to prepare experimental psychologists for the rich opportunities that are presented by a changing employment picture. This program addresses the training needs of new psychologists in ways that traditional programs do not.

Special Facilities or Resources: The strongest resource of the UNLV Psychology Department is the many talents of its diverse faculty. Our graduate program is small enough to provide close personal interaction experiences for training, and yet we encourage students to demonstrate initiative and to undertake the major responsibility for their graduate learning experiences. Student research is encouraged within the department and throughout the university.

Information for Students With Physical Disabilities: See the following Web site for more information: http://www.unlv.edu/studentlife/disability/index.html.

Application Information:

Send to UNLV - Department of Psychology, Doctoral Program Admissions Committee, 4505 Maryland Parkway Box 455030, Las Vegas, NV 89154-5030. Students are admitted in the Fall, application deadline December 15. The application deadline for our Experimental Psychology Graduate Program is January 1. *Fee:* $75. Waivers are obtained through the Graduate College office.

Nevada, University of, Reno
Department of Psychology/296
Liberal Arts
1664 North Virginia
Reno, NV 89557
Telephone: (775) 784-6828
Fax: (775) 784-1126
E-mail: vmf@unr.edu
Web: http://www.unr.edu/psych/

Department Information:
1920. Chairperson: Victoria M. Follette. Number of faculty: total—full-time 21; women—full-time 7; total—minority—full-time 2; women minority—full-time 2.

Programs and Degrees Offered:
Listed in the following order: Program area, degree type (T if terminal Master's), number awarded 7/08–6/09. Behavior Analysis PhD (Doctor of Philosophy) 9, Clinical Psychology PhD (Doctor of Philosophy) 5, Cognitive and Brain Sciences PhD (Doctor of Philosophy) 4.

APA Accreditation: Clinical PhD (Doctor of Philosophy). Student Outcome Data Website: http://www.unr.edu/psych/clinical/student_disclosure_data.html.

Student Applications/Admissions:
Student Applications

Behavior Analysis PhD (Doctor of Philosophy)—Applications 2009–2010, 34. Total applicants accepted 2009–2010, 6. Number full-time enrolled (new admits only) 2009–2010, 6. Number part-time enrolled (new admits only) 2009–2010, 0. Total enrolled 2009–2010 full-time, 26, part-time, 14. Openings 2010–2011, 6. The median number of years required for completion of a degree in 2008–2009 were 6. The number of students enrolled full- and part-time who were dismissed or voluntarily withdrew from this program area in 2008–2009 were 0. *Clinical Psychology PhD (Doctor of Philosophy)*—Applications 2009–2010, 110. Total applicants accepted 2009–2010, 3. Number full-time enrolled (new admits only) 2009–

2010, 3. Number part-time enrolled (new admits only) 2009–2010, 0. Total enrolled 2009–2010 full-time, 35, part-time, 10. Openings 2010–2011, 6. The median number of years required for completion of a degree in 2008–2009 were 7. The number of students enrolled full- and part-time who were dismissed or voluntarily withdrew from this program area in 2008–2009 were 0. *Cognitive and Brain Sciences PhD (Doctor of Philosophy)*—Applications 2009–2010, 11. Total applicants accepted 2009–2010, 4. Number full-time enrolled (new admits only) 2009–2010, 4. Number part-time enrolled (new admits only) 2009–2010, 0. Total enrolled 2009–2010 full-time, 13, part-time, 8. Openings 2010–2011, 4. The median number of years required for completion of a degree in 2008–2009 were 6. The number of students enrolled full- and part-time who were dismissed or voluntarily withdrew from this program area in 2008–2009 were 0.

Other Criteria: (importance of criteria rated low, medium, or high): GRE scores—high, research experience—high, work experience—high, extracurricular activity—medium, clinically related public service—medium, GPA—high, letters of recommendation—high, interview—high, statement of goals and objectives—high. Interview for admission in behavior analysis and clinical psychology is required. For additional information on admission requirements, go to http://www.unr.edu/psych/grad.html.

Student Characteristics: The following represents characteristics of students in 2009–2010 in all graduate psychology programs in the department: Female—full-time 46, part-time 33; Male—full-time 28, part-time 11; African American/Black—full-time 0, part-time 1; Hispanic/Latino(a)—full-time 0, part-time 3; Asian/Pacific Islander—full-time 3, part-time 10; American Indian/Alaska Native—full-time 0, part-time 0; Caucasian/White—full-time 62, part-time 23; Multi-ethnic—full-time 0, part-time 0; students subject to the Americans With Disabilities Act—full-time 0, part-time 0; Unknown ethnicity—full-time 3, part-time 5; International students who hold an F-1 or J-1 Visa—full-time 6, part-time 2.

Financial Information/Assistance:

Tuition for Full-Time Study: Doctoral: State residents: per academic year $4,050, $225 per credit hour; Nonstate residents: per academic year $16,331, $240 per credit hour. Tuition is subject to change. Additional fees are assessed to students beyond the costs of tuition for the following: Health Center (enrolled in six credits or more) $79. See the following Web site for updates and changes in tuition costs: http://www.unr.edu/vpaf/controller/cashiers-office/student-fees.html.

Financial Assistance:

First-Year Students: Teaching assistantships available for first year. Average amount paid per academic year: $14,000. Average number of hours worked per week: 20. Research assistantships available for first year. Average amount paid per academic year: $14,000. Average number of hours worked per week: 20.

Advanced Students: Teaching assistantships available for advanced students. Average amount paid per academic year: $14,000. Average number of hours worked per week: 20. Research assistantships available for advanced students. Average amount paid per academic year: $14,000. Average number of hours worked per week: 20.

Additional Information: Of all students currently enrolled full time, 90% benefited from one or more of the listed financial assistance programs. Application and information available online at: http://www.finaid.unr.edu/.

Internships/Practica: Doctoral Degree (PhD Clinical Psychology): For those doctoral students for whom a professional internship was required in this program prior to graduation, (11) students applied for an internship in 2008–2009, with (9) students obtaining an internship. Of those students who obtained an internship, (9) were paid internships. Of those students who obtained an internship, (9) students placed in APA/CPA accredited internships, (0) students placed in internships not APA/CPA accredited, but listed with the Association of Psychology Postdoctoral and Internship Programs (APPIC), (0) students placed in internships conforming to guidelines of the Council of Directors of School Psychology Programs (CDSPP), (0) students placed in internships that were not APA/CPA accredited, APPIC or CDSPP listed. The department offers several teaching/research assistantships. Experimental—Some students receive support as research assistants through individual faculty grants. Behavior Analysis—All doctoral students and most master's students receive full support from assistantships or consultation services. Clinical—Participation in clinical practica is required for students. From the last half of the first year through the third year, students see clients at the Psychological Service Center, an in-house clinic. During the fourth year, students are required to complete a 1000-hour practicum (externship) on campus or at agencies in the area. Finally, students are required to complete a 2,000 hour, APA-approved internship during their final year.

Housing and Day Care: On-campus housing is available. See the following Web site for more information: http://www.reslife.unr.edu/. On-campus day care facilities are available. See the following Web site for more information: http://www.unr.edu/educ/cfrc/.

Employment of Department Graduates:

Master's Degree Graduates: Of those who graduated in the academic year 2008–2009, the following categories and numbers represent the postgraduate activities and employment of master's degree graduates: Enrolled in a postdoctoral residency/fellowship (n/a), employed in independent practice (n/a), total from the above (master's) (0).

Doctoral Degree Graduates: Of those who graduated in the academic year 2008–2009, the following categories and numbers represent the postgraduate activities and employment of doctoral degree graduates: Enrolled in a psychology doctoral program (n/a), total from the above (doctoral) (0).

Additional Information:

Orientation, Objectives, and Emphasis of Department: The Cognitive and Brain Science (previously Experimental) program in psychology is research-oriented. The division offers specialized work in human cognition and cognitive neuroscience; learning, perception and psychophysics; and animal communication. The clinical program has a scientist–practitioner emphasis and offers skills in psychotherapy, assessment, evaluation, and community psychology. The behavior analysis program emphasizes applied behavior analysis, especially in institutional settings, and examines both the theoretical and applied ramifications of the behavioral programs.

Special Facilities or Resources: Cognitive and Brain Science—the program has active labs with facilities for research in visual perception, memory, cognition, and animal behavior and communication (including opportunities for research at the primate center at Central Washington University). Behavior Analysis—the program has a lab where students work with autistic children and developmentally disabled clients. Clinical—the primary academic/research facility of the program is the Psychological Service Center, an in-house training clinic that serves the community by offering services on a sliding fee basis.

Information for Students With Physical Disabilities: See the following Web site for more information: http://www.unr.edu/stsv/slservices/drc/.

Application Information:
Send to Admissions, Psychology Department/296, University of Nevada, Reno, NV 89557. Application available online. URL of online application: http://www.unr.edu/psych/gradappl.html. Students are admitted in the Fall, application deadline January 1; Spring, application deadline November 1. For the Fall semester, the deadline for Clinical Psychology and Behavior Analysis is January 1, and March 1 for Cognitive and Brain Sciences. For the Spring semester, the deadline is November 1 for Cognitive and Brain Sciences only. *Fee:* $60. $40 if previously enrolled in UNR. International applicants pay non refundable application fee of $95. If applying to more than one graduate program, a fee for each additional application is $40 for all applicants.

NEW HAMPSHIRE

Antioch University New England (2009 data)
Clinical Psychology
40 Avon Street
Keene, NH 03431-3552
Telephone: (603) 283-2183
Fax: (603) 357-1679
E-mail: cpeterson@antioch.edu
Web: http://www.antiochne.edu/cp

Department Information:
1982. Professor & Chair: Kathi A. Borden, PhD. Number of faculty: total—full-time 11, part-time 18; women—full-time 5, part-time 8; total—minority—full-time 1; women minority—full-time 1.

Programs and Degrees Offered:
Listed in the following order: Program area, degree type (T if terminal Master's), number awarded 7/08–6/09. Clinical Psychology PsyD (Doctor of Psychology) 25.

APA Accreditation: Clinical PsyD (Doctor of Psychology).

Student Applications/Admissions:
Student Applications
Clinical Psychology PsyD (Doctor of Psychology)—Applications 2009–2010, 83. Total applicants accepted 2009–2010, 48. Number full-time enrolled (new admits only) 2009–2010, 24. Number part-time enrolled (new admits only) 2009–2010, 0. Openings 2010–2011, 27. The median number of years required for completion of a degree in 2008–2009 were 6. The number of students enrolled full- and part-time who were dismissed or voluntarily withdrew from this program area in 2008–2009 were 4.
Other Criteria: (importance of criteria rated low, medium, or high): GRE scores—high, research experience—medium, work experience—medium, extracurricular activity—low, clinically related public service—medium, GPA—high, letters of recommendation—high, interview—high, statement of goals and objectives—high, undergraduate major in psychology—medium, specific undergraduate psychology courses taken—medium. For additional information on admission requirements, go to http://www.antiochne.edu/CP/.

Student Characteristics: The following represents characteristics of students in 2009–2010 in all graduate psychology programs in the department: Female—full-time 95, part-time 0; Male—full-time 25, part-time 0; African American/Black—full-time 2, part-time 0; Hispanic/Latino(a)—full-time 2, part-time 0; Asian/Pacific Islander—full-time 1, part-time 0; American Indian/Alaska Native—full-time 0, part-time 0; Caucasian/White—full-time 115, part-time 0; Multi-ethnic—full-time 0, part-time 0; students subject to the Americans With Disabilities Act—full-time 4, part-time 0; Unknown ethnicity—full-time 0, part-time 0; International students who hold an F-1 or J-1 Visa—full-time 0, part-time 0.

Financial Information/Assistance:
Tuition for Full-Time Study: Doctoral: State residents: per academic year $28,200; Nonstate residents: per academic year $28,200. Tuition is subject to change.

Financial Assistance:
First-Year Students: Teaching assistantships available for first year. Average amount paid per academic year: $1,764. Average number of hours worked per week: 9. Research assistantships available for first year. Average amount paid per academic year: $2,338. Average number of hours worked per week: 6.
Advanced Students: Teaching assistantships available for advanced students. Average amount paid per academic year: $1,764. Average number of hours worked per week: 9. Research assistantships available for advanced students. Average amount paid per academic year: $2,338. Average number of hours worked per week: 6. Fellowships and scholarships available for advanced students. Average amount paid per academic year: $1,900. Apply by March 1.
Additional Information: Of all students currently enrolled full time, 18% benefited from one or more of the listed financial assistance programs. Application and information available online at: http://www.antiochne.edu/cp/.

Internships/Practica: Doctoral Degree (PsyD Clinical Psychology): For those doctoral students for whom a professional internship was required in this program prior to graduation, (22) students applied for an internship in 2008–2009, with (21) students obtaining an internship. Of those students who obtained an internship, (20) were paid internships. Of those students who obtained an internship, (13) students placed in APA/CPA accredited internships, (4) students placed in internships not APA/CPA accredited, but listed with the Association of Psychology Postdoctoral and Internship Programs (APPIC), (0) students placed in internships conforming to guidelines of the Council of Directors of School Psychology Programs (CDSPP), (4) students placed in internships that were not APA/CPA accredited, APPIC or CDSPP listed. Students complete practica at agencies around New England. About 11 students per year do practicum training at the Antioch Family Therapy and Psychological Services Center (PSC), within the Department of Clinical Psychology. It functions as a mental health clinic providing a range of psychological services to residents from Keene and surrounding communities, and to Antioch New England students in departments other than Clinical Psychology. These services include individual psychotherapy, couple and family therapy, individual and family assessment, and various problem-specific psychoeducational groups and seminars. In addition, the PSC is actively involved in community outreach services; clinicians are encouraged to develop public psychoeducation and consultation activities, and to work in collaboration with other social service agencies for the purpose of ongoing community needs assessment and program development. A practicum at the PSC offers the student a unique opportunity for more concentrated interaction with core faculty—through supervision, training, and involvement in applied clinical and research projects of mutual interest. Specialized training opportunities exist for students interested in health psychology, family therapy, and assessment. Students seek internships through APPIC match.

Housing and Day Care: No on-campus housing is available. No on-campus day care facilities are available.

Employment of Department Graduates:
Master's Degree Graduates: Of those who graduated in the academic year 2008–2009, the following categories and numbers represent the postgraduate activities and employment of master's degree graduates: Enrolled in a postdoctoral residency/fellowship (n/a), employed in independent practice (n/a), total from the above (master's) (0).
Doctoral Degree Graduates: Of those who graduated in the academic year 2008–2009, the following categories and numbers represent the postgraduate activities and employment of doctoral degree graduates: Enrolled in a psychology doctoral program (n/a), enrolled in a postdoctoral residency/fellowship (7), employed in a community mental health/counseling center (4), employed in a hospital/medical center (3), other employment position (2), do not know (4), total from the above (doctoral) (20).

Additional Information:
Orientation, Objectives, and Emphasis of Department: Our practitioner-scholar program prepares professional psychologists for multiple roles for the expanded world of 21st century clinical psychology, including not only intervention, assessment, and research but also supervision, management, administration, consultation, and public policy. With a commitment to social responsibility, social justice, and diversity, we emphasize a social vision of clinical psychology, responsive to the needs of the larger society. The program includes broad training with a range of theoretical perspectives, a sound psychological knowledge base, and supervised practice. It follows the educational model developed by the National Council of Schools and Programs of Professional Psychology (NCSPP). This model specifies seven core professional competency areas: relationship, assessment, intervention, research and evaluation, consultation and education, management and supervision, and diversity (we have required courses in each) and, of course, includes basic psychological science. Research for clinical psychology is rooted in solving professional and social problems, where science and practice are integrated and complementary in the required dissertation. Preparation as "local clinical scientists" includes opportunities for training in program evaluation, as well as a range of other psychological topics and methodologies. Our pedagogy brings together theory, practice, and research through integrative, reflective learning experiences which help students develop their professional voice.

Special Facilities or Resources: The Center for Research on Psychological Practice (CROPP) in the Department of Clinical Psychology serves both the department and the community. This center is designed to address particular emerging educational aspects of doctoral training in clinical psychology that are not regularly included within the usual professional psychology curriculum—those relevant to applied clinical research skills and the associated administrative, consultative, and policy-creation roles of doctoral level psychologists. Several specific areas of research are priorities for CROPP. These include program evaluation and quality assurance issues, such as needs assessment, outcome and satisfaction research, cost-benefit analysis, policy analysis, and other topics relevant to mental health service management: public welfare issues such as treatment access, utilization, and outcome for underserved, rural, low socioeconomic, and minority populations; development of novel treatment and delivery systems; and methodological issues including the assessment and development of methods and measures appropriate for practice research. The research is done primarily in community service settings and entails collaboration with agencies and caregivers throughout the region. The development of this kind of research center, particularly within the context of a doctoral program in clinical psychology, has not, to our knowledge, been done elsewhere in the country. The Antioch University New England Multicultural Center for Research and Practice addresses the diverse array of emerging multicultural information which represents an enormous and unique opportunity to revolutionize and improve education, training, research, and human services, while addressing concerns of social justice. The Center has a particular focus on racial and ethnic minority and immigrant youth, adults, and families. It provides an excellent model of how the combination of research and practice can have a positive impact on communities across New England and beyond. The services of the Multicultural Center include social support for racial and ethnic minority people; individual and group multicultural interactions; workshops on multicultural awareness and acceptance; workshops on racism and stereotypes; consultation with professionals, educators, and businesses on multicultural applications and services; and coalition-building among disenfranchised groups. Its Web-based services include access to multicultural tests housed in the Center, resources of multicultural test titles and reviews, multicultural lecture notes, awareness exercises, documentation of process and outcome of multicultural service delivery, and a national multicultural course syllabus archive.

Application Information:
Send to Office of Doctoral Admissions, Antioch University New England, 40 Avon Street, Keene, NH 03431-3552. Application available online. URL of online application: http://www.antiochne.edu/admissions/. Students are admitted in the Fall, application deadline January 7. *Fee:* $75.

New Hampshire, University of
Department of Psychology
College of Liberal Arts
Conant Hall
Durham, NH 03824
Telephone: (603) 862-2360
Fax: (603) 862-4986
E-mail: *janicec@unh.edu*
Web: *http://www.unh.edu/psychology/*

Department Information:
1923. Chairperson: Robert G. Mair. Number of faculty: total—full-time 20; women—full-time 6; total—minority—full-time 1.

Programs and Degrees Offered:
Listed in the following order: Program area, degree type (T if terminal Master's), number awarded 7/08–6/09. Brain, Behavior and Cognition PhD (Doctor of Philosophy), Social/Personality Psychology PhD (Doctor of Philosophy), Developmental Psychology PhD (Doctor of Philosophy).

GRADUATE STUDY IN PSYCHOLOGY

Student Applications/Admissions:
Student Applications
Brain, Behavior and Cognition PhD (Doctor of Philosophy)—Social/Personality Psychology PhD (Doctor of Philosophy)—Developmental Psychology PhD (Doctor of Philosophy)—
Scores: Entries appear in this order: required test or GPA, minimum score (if required), median score of students entering in 2009–2010. Social/Personality Psychology PhD (Doctor of Philosophy): GRE-V no minimum stated, GRE-Q no minimum stated.
Other Criteria: (importance of criteria rated low, medium, or high): GRE scores—high, research experience—high, work experience—low, extracurricular activity—low, GPA—high, letters of recommendation—high, interview—low, statement of goals and objectives—high, Interests match program—high, undergraduate major in psychology—medium, specific undergraduate psychology courses taken—medium. For additional information on admission requirements, go to http://www.unh.edu/psychology/.

Student Characteristics: The following represents characteristics of students in 2009–2010 in all graduate psychology programs in the department: Female—full-time 21, part-time 0; Male—full-time 9, part-time 0; African American/Black—full-time 0, part-time 0; Hispanic/Latino(a)—full-time 0, part-time 0; Asian/Pacific Islander—full-time 0, part-time 0; American Indian/Alaska Native—full-time 0, part-time 0; Caucasian/White—full-time 29, part-time 0; Multi-ethnic—full-time 1, part-time 0; students subject to the Americans With Disabilities Act—full-time 0, part-time 0; Unknown ethnicity—full-time 0, part-time 0; International students who hold an F-1 or J-1 Visa—full-time 0, part-time 0.

Financial Information/Assistance:
Tuition for Full-Time Study: *Doctoral:* State residents: per academic year $10,380, $577 per credit hour; Nonstate residents: per academic year $24,350, $1,002 per credit hour. Tuition is subject to change. See the following Web site for updates and changes in tuition costs: http://www.unh.edu/business-services/tuitfees.html.

Financial Assistance:
First-Year Students: Teaching assistantships available for first year. Average amount paid per academic year: $14,500. Average number of hours worked per week: 20.
Advanced Students: Teaching assistantships available for advanced students. Average amount paid per academic year: $15,500. Average number of hours worked per week: 20. Fellowships and scholarships available for advanced students. Average amount paid per academic year: $16,500.
Additional Information: Of all students currently enrolled full time, 100% benefited from one or more of the listed financial assistance programs. Application and information available online at: http://financialaid.unh.edu/.

Housing and Day Care: On-campus housing is available. See the following Web site for more information: http://www.unh.edu/housing/gradhousing/. On-campus day care facilities are available. See the following Web site for more information: http://csdc.unh.edu/.

Employment of Department Graduates:
Master's Degree Graduates: Of those who graduated in the academic year 2008–2009, the following categories and numbers represent the postgraduate activities and employment of master's degree graduates: Enrolled in a postdoctoral residency/fellowship (n/a), employed in independent practice (n/a), total from the above (master's) (0).
Doctoral Degree Graduates: Of those who graduated in the academic year 2008–2009, the following categories and numbers represent the postgraduate activities and employment of doctoral degree graduates: Enrolled in a psychology doctoral program (n/a), employed in an academic position at a university (4), employed in other positions at a higher education institution (2), not seeking employment (1), total from the above (doctoral) (7).

Additional Information:
Orientation, Objectives, and Emphasis of Department: The program's basic goal is the preparation of doctoral students for academic careers. We focus on the development of psychologists who have a broad knowledge of psychology, who can teach and communicate effectively, and who can carry out sound research. Specialties are offered in the following areas: Brain, Behavior and Cognition (behavioral and cognitive neuroscience, cognition, vision); Developmental Psychology; and Social/Personality Psychology. Besides completing academic courses, our program places a distinctive emphasis on preparing graduate students for future roles as faculty members in college or university settings. Students complete a year-long seminar and practicum in the teaching of psychology, which introduces them to the theory and practice of teaching, while they concurrently teach under the supervision of master-teachers. Students also gain experience in other faculty roles such as sponsoring undergraduate students' research and serving on committees. Students are involved in research activities throughout the program. After graduation, most students secure academic positions. All students receive tuition waivers and stipends for at least 4 years, in exchange for serving as teaching or research assistants in their early years and as teachers in their later years. Students can apply for research and summer funding.

Special Facilities or Resources: The department occupies several buildings and offers research facilities, equipment, and resources in all of its areas of specialization. In addition, the department has up-to-date computing and related resources.

Information for Students With Physical Disabilities: See the following Web site for more information: http://www.unh.edu/disabilityservices/.

Application Information:
Send to Dean of the Graduate School, University of New Hampshire, Thompson Hall, Durham, NH 03824. Application available online. URL of online application: http://www.gradschool.unh.edu/apply.html. Students are admitted in the Fall, application deadline January 15. Review of applications begins January 15 and continues until the incoming class is filled. *Fee:* $65.

NEW JERSEY

Fairleigh Dickinson University, Metropolitan Campus
School of Psychology
University College: Arts–Sciences–Professional Studies
1000 River Road
Teaneck, NJ 07666
Telephone: (201) 692-2300
Fax: (201) 692-2304
E-mail: dumont@fdu.edu
Web: http://view.fdu.edu/default.aspx?id=169

Department Information:
1960. Director: Ron Dumont EdD, NCSP. Number of faculty: total—full-time 19, part-time 19; women—full-time 9, part-time 12.

Programs and Degrees Offered:
Listed in the following order: Program area, degree type (T if terminal Master's), number awarded 7/08–6/09. General/Theoretical Psychology MA/MS (Master of Arts/Science) (T) 12, Clinical Psychology PhD (Doctor of Philosophy) 13, School Psychology PsyD (Doctor of Psychology) 7, Psychopharmacology MA/MS (Master of Arts/Science) (T) 13, School Psychology MA/MS (Master of Arts/Science) (T) 8, Forensic Psychology MA/MS (Master of Arts/Science) (T) 0.

APA Accreditation: Clinical PhD (Doctor of Philosophy). Student Outcome Data Website: http://view.fdu.edu/default.aspx?id=6281.

Student Applications/Admissions:
Student Applications
General/Theoretical Psychology MA/MS (Master of Arts/Science)—Applications 2009–2010, 34. Total applicants accepted 2009–2010, 14. Number full-time enrolled (new admits only) 2009–2010, 5. Number part-time enrolled (new admits only) 2009–2010, 9. Total enrolled 2009–2010 full-time, 9, part-time, 25. Openings 2010–2011, 14. The median number of years required for completion of a degree in 2008–2009 were 2. The number of students enrolled full- and part-time who were dismissed or voluntarily withdrew from this program area in 2008–2009 were 2. Clinical Psychology PhD (Doctor of Philosophy)—Applications 2009–2010, 202. Total applicants accepted 2009–2010, 24. Number full-time enrolled (new admits only) 2009–2010, 17. Number part-time enrolled (new admits only) 2009–2010, 0. Openings 2010–2011, 14. The median number of years required for completion of a degree in 2008–2009 were 5. The number of students enrolled full- and part-time who were dismissed or voluntarily withdrew from this program area in 2008–2009 were 3. School Psychology PsyD (Doctor of Psychology)—Applications 2009–2010, 45. Total applicants accepted 2009–2010, 16. Number full-time enrolled (new admits only) 2009–2010, 15. Total enrolled 2009–2010 full-time, 59. Openings 2010–2011, 15. The median number of years required for completion of a degree in 2008–2009 were 3. The number of students enrolled full- and part-time who were dismissed or voluntarily withdrew from this program area in 2008–2009 were 1. Psychopharmacology MA/MS (Master of Arts/Science)—Applications 2009–2010, 25. Total applicants accepted 2009–2010, 25. Number part-time enrolled (new admits only) 2009–2010, 20. Total enrolled 2009–2010 part-time, 45. Openings 2010–2011, 20. The median number of years required for completion of a degree in 2008–2009 were 2. The number of students enrolled full- and part-time who were dismissed or voluntarily withdrew from this program area in 2008–2009 were 3. School Psychology MA/MS (Master of Arts/Science)—Applications 2009–2010, 52. Total applicants accepted 2009–2010, 18. Number full-time enrolled (new admits only) 2009–2010, 13. Total enrolled 2009–2010 full-time, 54. Openings 2010–2011, 15. The median number of years required for completion of a degree in 2008–2009 were 3. The number of students enrolled full- and part-time who were dismissed or voluntarily withdrew from this program area in 2008–2009 were 2. Forensic Psychology MA/MS (Master of Arts/Science)—Applications 2009–2010, 50. Total applicants accepted 2009–2010, 10. Number full-time enrolled (new admits only) 2009–2010, 10. Number part-time enrolled (new admits only) 2009–2010, 0. Openings 2010–2011, 15. The median number of years required for completion of a degree in 2008–2009 were 2. The number of students enrolled full- and part-time who were dismissed or voluntarily withdrew from this program area in 2008–2009 were 1.

Scores: Entries appear in this order: required test or GPA, minimum score (if required), median score of students entering in 2009–2010. *General/Theoretical Psychology MA/MS (Master of Arts/Science)*: GRE-V no minimum stated, GRE-Q no minimum stated, GRE-Analytical no minimum stated, GRE-Subject (Psychology) no minimum stated; *Forensic Psychology MA/MS (Master of Arts/Science)*: GRE-V 500, GRE-Q 500, GRE-Analytical no minimum stated, GRE-Subject (Psychology) no minimum stated.

Other Criteria: (importance of criteria rated low, medium, or high): GRE scores—medium, research experience—high, work experience—medium, extracurricular activity—medium, clinically related public service—high, letters of recommendation—high, interview—high, statement of goals and objectives—high, These criteria are used for admission to PhD and PsyD programs. For PsyD program, research experience would be low and work experience would be medium-high. For additional information on admission requirements, go to http://www.fdu.edu/schoolofpsychology.

Student Characteristics: The following represents characteristics of students in 2009–2010 in all graduate psychology programs in the department: Female—full-time 169, part-time 46; Male—full-time 51, part-time 24; African American/Black—full-time 0, part-time 0; Hispanic/Latino(a)—full-time 0, part-time 0; Asian/Pacific Islander—full-time 0, part-time 0; American Indian/Alaska

Native—full-time 0, part-time 0; Caucasian/White—full-time 0, part-time 0; Multi-ethnic—full-time 0, part-time 0; students subject to the Americans With Disabilities Act—full-time 0, part-time 0; Unknown ethnicity—full-time 0, part-time 0; International students who hold an F-1 or J-1 Visa—full-time 0, part-time 0.

Financial Information/Assistance:
Tuition for Full-Time Study: *Master's:* State residents: $974 per credit hour; Nonstate residents: $974 per credit hour. *Doctoral:* State residents: per academic year $25,008; Nonstate residents: per academic year $25,008. Tuition is subject to change. See the following Web site for updates and changes in tuition costs: http://view.fdu.edu/default.aspx?id=438. Higher tuition cost for this program: Clinical Psychology: $30,970/academic year.

Financial Assistance:
First-Year Students: Research assistantships available for first year. Average amount paid per academic year: $16,644. Average number of hours worked per week: 8.
Advanced Students: Research assistantships available for advanced students. Average amount paid per academic year: $14,644. Average number of hours worked per week: 8.
Additional Information: Of all students currently enrolled full time, 33% benefited from one or more of the listed financial assistance programs. Application and information available online at: http://www.fdu.edu/schoolofpsychology.

Internships/Practica: Doctoral Degree (PhD Clinical Psychology): For those doctoral students for whom a professional internship was required in this program prior to graduation, (15) students applied for an internship in 2008–2009, with (15) students obtaining an internship. Of those students who obtained an internship, (15) were paid internships. Of those students who obtained an internship, (14) students placed in APA/CPA accredited internships, (1) students placed in internships not APA/CPA accredited, but listed with the Association of Psychology Postdoctoral and Internship Programs (APPIC), (0) students placed in internships conforming to guidelines of the Council of Directors of School Psychology Programs (CDSPP), (0) students placed in internships that were not APA/CPA accredited, APPIC or CDSPP listed. Doctoral Degree (PsyD School Psychology): For those doctoral students for whom a professional internship was required in this program prior to graduation, (9) students applied for an internship in 2008–2009, with (9) students obtaining an internship. Of those students who obtained an internship, (9) were paid internships. Of those students who obtained an internship, (0) students placed in APA/CPA accredited internships, (0) students placed in internships not APA/CPA accredited, but listed with the Association of Psychology Postdoctoral and Internship Programs (APPIC), (0) students placed in internships conforming to guidelines of the Council of Directors of School Psychology Programs (CDSPP), (9) students placed in internships that were not APA/CPA accredited, APPIC or CDSPP listed. Master's Degree (MA/MS Psychopharmacology): An internship experience, such as a final research project or "capstone" experience is required of graduates. Master's Degree (MA/MS School Psychology): An internship experience, such as a final research project or "capstone" experience is required of graduates. Master's Degree (MA/MS Forensic Psychology): An internship experience, such as a final research project or "capstone" experience is required of graduates. All PhD students are required to complete research and clinical practica during their first three years. Clinical practica may be completed on-campus at the University's Center for Psychological Services. Externships are required for the Forensic and School MA programs. PsyD students must complete a one-year internship.

Housing and Day Care: No on-campus housing is available. No on-campus day care facilities are available.

Employment of Department Graduates:
Master's Degree Graduates: Of those who graduated in the academic year 2008–2009, the following categories and numbers represent the postgraduate activities and employment of master's degree graduates: Enrolled in a postdoctoral residency/fellowship (n/a), employed in independent practice (n/a), total from the above (master's) (0).
Doctoral Degree Graduates: Of those who graduated in the academic year 2008–2009, the following categories and numbers represent the postgraduate activities and employment of doctoral degree graduates: Enrolled in a psychology doctoral program (n/a), total from the above (doctoral) (0).

Additional Information:
Orientation, Objectives, and Emphasis of Department: The orientation of the department is essentially based on the scientist–practitioner model. In terms of theoretical orientations, some faculty are dynamicists, some behaviorists, and some humanists, though there is a sense of eclecticism that pervades those who are practitioners. There is a considerable emphasis on empirical research as the preferred basis for developing a theoretical orientation.

Special Facilities or Resources: The department operates the Center for Psychological Services which provides students in the PhD and PsyD programs opportunities in therapy and assessment with adults, children, families, and couples. The department has research laboratories equipped for experiments with humans as well as with small animals. Equipment includes computer facilities (both micro- and mainframe), a four-channel physiograph, electrophysiological stimulating and recording equipment, operant equipment for programming and recording behavior, two- and four-channel tachistoscopes, various other sensory apparatuses, standard and computer-based EEG recorders, and equipment and supplies for psychopharmacological studies.

Application Information:
Send to School of Psychology (T-WH1-01), Fairleigh Dickinson University, 1000 River Road, Teaneck, NJ 07666. URL of online application: http://view.fdu.edu/default.aspx?id=1936. Students are admitted in the Fall, application deadline January 15; Spring, application deadline. Application deadline for Fall: January 15 for Clinical Psychology PhD; March 1 for School Psychology PsyD; March 15 for Master's degrees in School and Forensic Psychology. Spring admission is only for applicants to MA program in general/theoretical psychology. *Fee:* $40. The application fee is waived or deferred for Fairleigh Dickinson graduates. Fee is $40 for doctoral programs and $35 for MA programs.

Kean University
Department of Psychology; Department of Doctoral Programs in Psychology
Morris Avenue
Union, NJ 07083
Telephone: (908) 737-5870
Fax: (908) 737-5875
E-mail: *sbousque@kean.edu* and *fgardner@kean.edu*
Web: *http://www.kean.edu*

Department Information:
1969. Chairperson: Dr. Suzanne Bousquet; Dr. Frank Gardner. Number of faculty: total—full-time 18, part-time 60; women—full-time 13, part-time 40; total—minority—full-time 3, part-time 15; women minority—full-time 3, part-time 10; faculty subject to the Americans With Disabilities Act 1.

Programs and Degrees Offered:
Listed in the following order: Program area, degree type (T if terminal Master's), number awarded 7/08–6/09. Marriage and Family Therapy Diploma 7, Human Behavior and Organizational Psychology MA/MS (Master of Arts/Science) (T) 6, Psychological Services MA/MS (Master of Arts/Science) (T) 11, School Psychology Diploma 10, Educational Psychology MA/MS (Master of Arts/Science) (T) 8, School and Clinical Psychology PsyD (Doctor of Psychology).

Student Applications/Admissions:
Student Applications
Marriage and Family Therapy Diploma—Applications 2009–2010, 16. Total enrolled 2009–2010 full-time, 10, part-time, 40. Openings 2010–2011, 12. The median number of years required for completion of a degree in 2008–2009 were 3. The number of students enrolled full- and part-time who were dismissed or voluntarily withdrew from this program area in 2008–2009 were 0. *Human Behavior and Organizational Psychology MA/MS (Master of Arts/Science)*—Total enrolled 2009–2010 full-time, 4, part-time, 45. Openings 2010–2011, 20. The median number of years required for completion of a degree in 2008–2009 were 2. The number of students enrolled full- and part-time who were dismissed or voluntarily withdrew from this program area in 2008–2009 were 0. *Psychological Services MA/MS (Master of Arts/Science)*—Total enrolled 2009–2010 full-time, 7, part-time, 30. Openings 2010–2011, 15. The median number of years required for completion of a degree in 2008–2009 were 3. The number of students enrolled full- and part-time who were dismissed or voluntarily withdrew from this program area in 2008–2009 were 0. *School Psychology Diploma*—Total enrolled 2009–2010 full-time, 12, part-time, 12. Openings 2010–2011, 12. The number of students enrolled full- and part-time who were dismissed or voluntarily withdrew from this program area in 2008–2009 were 0. *Educational Psychology MA/MS (Master of Arts/Science)*—Total enrolled 2009–2010 full-time, 2, part-time, 12. Openings 2010–2011, 12. The median number of years required for completion of a degree in 2008–2009 were 3. The number of students enrolled full- and part-time who were dismissed or voluntarily withdrew from this program area in 2008–2009 were 0. *School and Clinical Psychology PsyD (Doctor of Psychology)*—Applications 2009–2010, 35. Total applicants accepted 2009–2010, 12. Number full-time enrolled (new admits only) 2009–2010, 10. Total enrolled 2009–2010 full-time, 10. Openings 2010–2011, 12.

Scores: Entries appear in this order: required test or GPA, minimum score (if required), median score of students entering in 2009–2010. *Marriage and Family Therapy Diploma:* GRE-V no minimum stated, GRE-Q no minimum stated, GRE-Analytical no minimum stated; *Human Behavior and Organizational Psychology MA/MS (Master of Arts/Science):* GRE-V no minimum stated, GRE-Q no minimum stated, GRE-Analytical no minimum stated; *Psychological Services MA/MS (Master of Arts/Science):* GRE-V no minimum stated, GRE-Q no minimum stated, GRE-Analytical no minimum stated; *School Psychology Diploma:* GRE-V no minimum stated, GRE-Q no minimum stated, GRE-Analytical no minimum stated; *Educational Psychology MA/MS (Master of Arts/Science):* GRE-V no minimum stated, GRE-Q no minimum stated, GRE-Analytical no minimum stated; *School and Clinical Psychology PsyD (Doctor of Psychology):* GRE-V no minimum stated, GRE-Q no minimum stated, GRE-Analytical no minimum stated, GRE-Subject (Psychology) 550, overall undergraduate GPA 3.30, Masters GPA 3.5.

Other Criteria: (importance of criteria rated low, medium, or high): GRE scores—high, research experience—high, work experience—medium, extracurricular activity—low, clinically related public service—high, GPA—high, letters of recommendation—high, interview—high, statement of goals and objectives—high, undergraduate major in psychology—high, specific undergraduate psychology courses taken—medium, Varies between Masters Programs, Professional Diploma Programs and PsyD Program. For additional information on admission requirements, go to http://www.kean.edu.

Student Characteristics: The following represents characteristics of students in 2009–2010 in all graduate psychology programs in the department: Female—full-time 11, part-time 73; Male—full-time 1, part-time 30; African American/Black—full-time 1, part-time 17; Hispanic/Latino(a)—full-time 0, part-time 11; Asian/Pacific Islander—full-time 0, part-time 4; American Indian/Alaska Native—full-time 0, part-time 0; Caucasian/White—full-time 11, part-time 65; Multi-ethnic—full-time 0, part-time 0; students subject to the Americans With Disabilities Act—full-time 0, part-time 0; Unknown ethnicity—full-time 0, part-time 5; International students who hold an F-1 or J-1 Visa—full-time 0, part-time 0.

Financial Information/Assistance:
Tuition for Full-Time Study: *Master's:* State residents: per academic year $6,541, $435 per credit hour; Nonstate residents: per academic year $8,401, $590 per credit hour. *Doctoral:* State residents: per academic year $13,630, $525 per credit hour; Nonstate residents: per academic year $16,966, $625 per credit hour. Tuition is subject to change. Additional fees are assessed to students beyond the costs of tuition for the following: Full-Time Clinic Fee/PsyD program is $500.00 per semester. See the following Web site for updates and changes in tuition costs: www.kean.edu.

Financial Assistance:
First-Year Students: Teaching assistantships available for first year. Average amount paid per academic year: $3,217. Average number of hours worked per week: 15. Apply by June 1.

Advanced Students: Teaching assistantships available for advanced students. Average amount paid per academic year: $3,217. Average number of hours worked per week: 15. Apply by June 1.

Additional Information: Of all students currently enrolled full time, 20% benefited from one or more of the listed financial assistance programs. Application and information available online at: http://www.kean.edu.

Internships/Practica: Master's Degree (School Psychology Diploma): An internship experience, such as a final research project or "capstone" experience is required of graduates. Master's Degree (MA/MS Educational Psychology): An internship experience, such as a final research project or "capstone" experience is required of graduates. Internships/practica in a variety of settings are available for students in the professional diploma programs in school psychology and marriage and family therapy. For doctoral students, internships are available in an on-site community psychology clinic.

Housing and Day Care: No on-campus housing is available. On-campus day care facilities are available. See the following Web site for more information: http://www.kean.edu/~kuccc.

Employment of Department Graduates:
Master's Degree Graduates: Of those who graduated in the academic year 2008–2009, the following categories and numbers represent the postgraduate activities and employment of master's degree graduates: Enrolled in a postdoctoral residency/fellowship (n/a), employed in independent practice (n/a), total from the above (master's) (0).
Doctoral Degree Graduates: Of those who graduated in the academic year 2008–2009, the following categories and numbers represent the postgraduate activities and employment of doctoral degree graduates: Enrolled in a psychology doctoral program (n/a), total from the above (doctoral) (0).

Additional Information:
Orientation, Objectives, and Emphasis of Department: Our academic emphasis is eclectic. All classes are small, which facilitates the opportunity for personal growth.

Special Facilities or Resources: Special resources include computer facilities that are integrated with statistics, measurements, and professional psychology testing courses.

Information for Students With Physical Disabilities: See the following Web site for more information: http://www.kean.edu/~disabsus.

Application Information:
Send to Office of Graduate Admissions, Kean University, Union, NJ 07083. Application available online. URL of online application: http://www.kean.edu/~keangrad/Application/Apply.online.html. Students are admitted in the Fall, application deadline May 1; Spring, application deadline November 1. For School Psychology, fall admission only with deadline of March 15. For PsyD, fall admission only with deadline of January 2. All other programs, fall and spring admissions. *Fee:* $60. $150 for international students.

Rowan University (2009 data)
Department of Psychology
College of Liberal Arts and Sciences
201 Mullica Hill Road
Glassboro, NJ 08028-1701
Telephone: (856) 256-4500 ext 3780
Fax: (856) 256-4892
E-mail: *Angeloned@rowan.edu*
Web: *http://www.rowan.edu/colleges/las_new/departments/psychology/maCounseling*

Department Information:
1969. Program Coordinator: D.J. Angelone, PhD. Number of faculty: total—full-time 19; women—full-time 13; total—minority—full-time 3; women minority—full-time 3.

Programs and Degrees Offered:
Listed in the following order: Program area, degree type (T if terminal Master's), number awarded 7/08–6/09. Clinical Mental Health Counseling MA/MS (Master of Arts/Science) (T) 12.

Student Applications/Admissions:
Student Applications
Clinical Mental Health Counseling MA/MS *(Master of Arts/Science)*—Applications 2009–2010, 55. Total applicants accepted 2009–2010, 15. Number full-time enrolled (new admits only) 2009–2010, 12. Number part-time enrolled (new admits only) 2009–2010, 3. Total enrolled 2009–2010 full-time, 24, part-time, 11. Openings 2010–2011, 15. The median number of years required for completion of a degree in 2008–2009 were 2. The number of students enrolled full- and part-time who were dismissed or voluntarily withdrew from this program area in 2008–2009 were 2.
Other Criteria: (importance of criteria rated low, medium, or high): GRE scores—medium, research experience—medium, work experience—medium, extracurricular activity—low, clinically related public service—high, GPA—high, letters of recommendation—high, interview—high, statement of goals and objectives—high, undergraduate major in psychology—high, specific undergraduate psychology courses taken—medium.

Student Characteristics: The following represents characteristics of students in 2009–2010 in all graduate psychology programs in the department: Female—full-time 11, part-time 21; Male—full-time 3, part-time 1; African American/Black—full-time 0, part-time 1; Hispanic/Latino(a)—full-time 0, part-time 0; Asian/Pacific Islander—full-time 0, part-time 0; American Indian/Alaska Native—full-time 0, part-time 0; Caucasian/White—full-time 0, part-time 0; Multi-ethnic—full-time 0, part-time 0; students subject to the Americans With Disabilities Act—full-time 0, part-time 0; Unknown ethnicity—full-time 0, part-time 0; International students who hold an F-1 or J-1 Visa—full-time 0, part-time 0.

Financial Information/Assistance:
Tuition for Full-Time Study: *Master's:* State residents: per academic year $5,312, $590 per credit hour; Nonstate residents: per academic year $5,312, $590 per credit hour. Tuition is subject to change. See the following Web site for updates and changes in

tuition costs: http://www.rowan.edu/adminfinance/bursar/tuitionfeesandrates.html.

Financial Assistance:
First-Year Students: Research assistantships available for first year. Average amount paid per academic year: $5,000. Average number of hours worked per week: 20. Fellowships and scholarships available for first year. Average amount paid per academic year: $5,000. Average number of hours worked per week: 20.
Advanced Students: Research assistantships available for advanced students. Average amount paid per academic year: $5,000. Fellowships and scholarships available for advanced students. Average amount paid per academic year: $5,000.
Additional Information: Of all students currently enrolled full time, 20% benefited from one or more of the listed financial assistance programs. Application and information available online at: http://www.rowan.edu/colleges/graduate/currentstudents/assistantships.html.

Internships/Practica: Master's Degree (MA/MS Clinical Mental Health Counseling): An internship experience, such as a final research project or "capstone" experience is required of graduates. Practica are available in a wide range of mental health settings.

Housing and Day Care: On-campus housing is available. See the following Web site for more information: http://www.rowan.edu/studentaffairs/reslife. On-campus day care facilities are available. See the following Web site for more information: http://www.rowan.edu/colleges/education/childcare/.

Employment of Department Graduates:
Master's Degree Graduates: Of those who graduated in the academic year 2008–2009, the following categories and numbers represent the postgraduate activities and employment of master's degree graduates: Enrolled in a postdoctoral residency/fellowship (n/a), employed in independent practice (n/a), total from the above (master's) (0).
Doctoral Degree Graduates: Of those who graduated in the academic year 2008–2009, the following categories and numbers represent the postgraduate activities and employment of doctoral degree graduates: Enrolled in a psychology doctoral program (n/a), total from the above (doctoral) (0).

Additional Information:
Orientation, Objectives, and Emphasis of Department: The program is designed to be consistent with an evidence based practice model. This 60 credit Master's program prepares students to become mental health counselors and is designed to meet the coursework and practicum requirements of the National Board of Certified Counselors. Students completing this program and additional supervised hours will be eligible to apply for the New Jersey Licensed Professional Counseling Certification. Graduate may also qualify for licensure in other states as well dependent upon specific state criteria and guidelines.

Special Facilities or Resources: Rowan's Child and Family Assessment Clinic provides opportunities for both clinical assessment and research. The clinic uses a broad range of assessment tools and techniques to evaluate the functioning and needs of children and families involved in the child welfare system.

Application Information:
Send to The Graduate School, Rowan University, 201 Mullica Hill Road, Glassboro, NJ 08028-1701. Application available online. URL of online application: http://www.rowan.edu/graduateschool. Students are admitted in the Fall, application deadline February 15. *Fee:* $50.

Rutgers University - New Brunswick
Graduate Program in Psychology
Faculty of Arts and Sciences
152 Frelinghuysen Road
Piscataway, NJ 08854-8020
Telephone: (732) 445-2556
Fax: (732) 445-2263
E-mail: *gradvc@rci.rutgers.edu*
Web: *http://psych.rutgers.edu/graduate/*

Department Information:
1942. Chair and Graduate Director: Gretchen Chapman. Number of faculty: total—full-time 46; women—full-time 15; total—minority—full-time 2; women minority—full-time 1; faculty subject to the Americans With Disabilities Act 1.

Programs and Degrees Offered:
Listed in the following order: Program area, degree type (T if terminal Master's), number awarded 7/08–6/09. Social Psychology PhD (Doctor of Philosophy) 2, Clinical Psychology PhD (Doctor of Philosophy) 7, Behavioral Neuroscience PhD (Doctor of Philosophy) 2, Cognitive Psychology PhD (Doctor of Philosophy) 1.

APA Accreditation: Clinical PhD (Doctor of Philosophy). Student Outcome Data Website: http://psych.rutgers.edu/graduate/clinical/index.html.

Student Applications/Admissions:
Student Applications
Social Psychology PhD (Doctor of Philosophy)—Applications 2009–2010, 86. Total applicants accepted 2009–2010, 8. Number full-time enrolled (new admits only) 2009–2010, 5. Total enrolled 2009–2010 full-time, 22. Openings 2010–2011, 5. The median number of years required for completion of a degree in 2008–2009 were 5. The number of students enrolled full- and part-time who were dismissed or voluntarily withdrew from this program area in 2008–2009 were 0. *Clinical Psychology PhD (Doctor of Philosophy)*—Applications 2009–2010, 296. Total applicants accepted 2009–2010, 7. Number full-time enrolled (new admits only) 2009–2010, 3. Total enrolled 2009–2010 full-time, 29. Openings 2010–2011, 5. The median number of years required for completion of a degree in 2008–2009 were 6. The number of students enrolled full- and part-time who were dismissed or voluntarily withdrew from this program area in 2008–2009 were 0. *Behavioral Neuroscience PhD (Doctor of Philosophy)*—Applications 2009–2010, 34. Total applicants accepted 2009–2010, 4. Number full-time enrolled (new admits only) 2009–2010, 3. Total enrolled 2009–2010 full-time, 16. Openings 2010–2011, 4. The median number of years required for completion of a degree in 2008–2009 were 6. The number of students enrolled full- and part-time who were dismissed or voluntarily withdrew from this program area in 2008–2009 were 1. *Cognitive Psychology PhD (Doctor*

of Philosophy)—Applications 2009–2010, 53. Total applicants accepted 2009–2010, 15. Number full-time enrolled (new admits only) 2009–2010, 5. Total enrolled 2009–2010 full-time, 22. Openings 2010–2011, 6. The median number of years required for completion of a degree in 2008–2009 were 5. The number of students enrolled full- and part-time who were dismissed or voluntarily withdrew from this program area in 2008–2009 were 0.

Scores: Entries appear in this order: required test or GPA, minimum score (if required), median score of students entering in 2009–2010. *Social Psychology PhD (Doctor of Philosophy):* GRE-V 550, 620, GRE-Q 550, 670, overall undergraduate GPA 3.2, 3.48; *Clinical Psychology PhD (Doctor of Philosophy):* GRE-V 550, 640, GRE-Q 550, 690, overall undergraduate GPA 3.2, 3.61; *Behavioral Neuroscience PhD (Doctor of Philosophy):* GRE-V 500, 540, GRE-Q 550, 670, overall undergraduate GPA 3.2, 3.50; *Cognitive Psychology PhD (Doctor of Philosophy):* GRE-V 550, 590, GRE-Q 550, 670, overall undergraduate GPA 3.2, 3.35.

Other Criteria: (importance of criteria rated low, medium, or high): GRE scores—high, research experience—high, clinically related public service—low, GPA—high, letters of recommendation—high, interview—medium, statement of goals and objectives—high. For additional information on admission requirements, go to http://psych.rutgers.edu/graduate/.

Student Characteristics: The following represents characteristics of students in 2009–2010 in all graduate psychology programs in the department: Female—full-time 65, part-time 0; Male—full-time 33, part-time 0; African American/Black—full-time 4, part-time 0; Hispanic/Latino(a)—full-time 4, part-time 0; Asian/Pacific Islander—full-time 16, part-time 0; American Indian/Alaska Native—full-time 0, part-time 0; Caucasian/White—full-time 0, part-time 0; Multi-ethnic—full-time 0, part-time 0; students subject to the Americans With Disabilities Act—full-time 0, part-time 0; Unknown ethnicity—full-time 0, part-time 0; International students who hold an F-1 or J-1 Visa—full-time 0, part-time 0.

Financial Information/Assistance:

Tuition for Full-Time Study: *Doctoral:* State residents: per academic year $13,848, $577 per credit hour; Nonstate residents: per academic year $21,264, $886 per credit hour. Tuition is subject to change. See the following Web site for updates and changes in tuition costs: http://gradstudy.rutgers.edu/funding.shtml.

Financial Assistance:

First-Year Students: Teaching assistantships available for first year. Average number of hours worked per week: 15. Apply by January 1. Research assistantships available for first year. Average number of hours worked per week: 15. Apply by January 1. Traineeships available for first year. Apply by January 1. Fellowships and scholarships available for first year. Apply by January 1.

Advanced Students: Teaching assistantships available for advanced students. Average number of hours worked per week: 15. Apply by January 1. Research assistantships available for advanced students. Average number of hours worked per week: 15. Apply by January 1. Traineeships available for advanced students. Apply by January 1. Fellowships and scholarships available for advanced students. Apply by January 1.

Additional Information: Of all students currently enrolled full time, 98% benefited from one or more of the listed financial assistance programs. Application and information available online at: http://studentaid.rutgers.edu/.

Internships/Practica: Doctoral Degree (PhD Clinical Psychology): For those doctoral students for whom a professional internship was required in this program prior to graduation, (7) students applied for an internship in 2008–2009, with (7) students obtaining an internship. Of those students who obtained an internship, (7) were paid internships. Of those students who obtained an internship, (7) students placed in APA/CPA accredited internships, (0) students placed in internships not APA/CPA accredited, but listed with the Association of Psychology Postdoctoral and Internship Programs (APPIC), (0) students placed in internships conforming to guidelines of the Council of Directors of School Psychology Programs (CDSPP), (0) students placed in internships that were not APA/CPA accredited, APPIC or CDSPP listed. Clinical students must complete an APA-approved clinical internship. None of these required internships are offered by our program. There are several university-based practica, including both general and specialty outpatient clinics, however, where clinical students do training before their internships.

Housing and Day Care: On-campus housing is available. See the following Web site for more information: http://housing.rutgers.edu/. On-campus day care facilities are available. See the following Web site for more information: http://nbweb.rutgers.edu/menus/childcare.shtml.

Employment of Department Graduates:

Master's Degree Graduates: Of those who graduated in the academic year 2008–2009, the following categories and numbers represent the postgraduate activities and employment of master's degree graduates: Enrolled in a postdoctoral residency/fellowship (n/a), employed in independent practice (n/a), total from the above (master's) (0).

Doctoral Degree Graduates: Of those who graduated in the academic year 2008–2009, the following categories and numbers represent the postgraduate activities and employment of doctoral degree graduates: Enrolled in a psychology doctoral program (n/a), enrolled in a postdoctoral residency/fellowship (8), employed in an academic position at a 2-year/4-year college (1), employed in a community mental health/counseling center (1), employed in a hospital/medical center (1), other employment position (1), total from the above (doctoral) (12).

Additional Information:

Orientation, Objectives, and Emphasis of Department: The Rutgers University Graduate Program in Psychology has one of the country's largest faculties, including fifty full-time professors of psychology. The graduate program trains students for careers as professors; researchers in government, corporate, and non-profit settings; and clinical researchers. There are four main areas (Behavioral Neuroscience, Cognitive Psychology, Clinical Psychology and Social Psychology) and two interdisciplinary programs: Health Psychology and Developmental Psychology (students with interdisciplinary interest must apply to one of the four main areas). Faculty advisors closely mentor students through a series of progressively more sophisticated research experiences. Basic courses and more advanced specialty seminars are available within each area of psychology. The clinical program is designed to develop clinical scientists.

Information for Students With Physical Disabilities: See the following Web site for more information: http://disabilityservices.rutgers.edu/.

Application Information:
Send to Office of Graduate and Professional Admissions, Rutgers, The State University of New Jersey, 18 Bishop Place, New Brunswick, NJ 08901-8530. Application available online. URL of online application: http://gradstudy.rutgers.edu/apply.shtml. Students are admitted in the Fall, application deadline January 1. *Fee:* $60. Fee waived for McNair Scholars.

Rutgers—The State University of New Jersey
Department of Applied Psychology
Graduate School of Applied and Professional Psychology
152 Frelinghuysen Road, Busch Campus, Psychology Building Addition
Piscataway, NJ 08854
Telephone: (732) 445-2000 Ext. 104
Fax: (732) 445-4888
E-mail: *sgforman@rci.rutgers.edu*
Web: *http://gsappweb.rutgers.edu*

Department Information:
1974. Chairperson: Susan G. Forman, PhD. Number of faculty: total—full-time 7, part-time 5; women—full-time 5, part-time 4; total—minority—full-time 1; women minority—full-time 1.

Programs and Degrees Offered:
Listed in the following order: Program area, degree type (T if terminal Master's), number awarded 7/08–6/09. School Psychology PsyD (Doctor of Psychology) 9.

APA Accreditation: School PsyD (Doctor of Psychology). Student Outcome Data Website: http://gsappweb.rutgers.edu/programs/school/index.php.

Student Applications/Admissions:
Student Applications
School Psychology PsyD (Doctor of Psychology)—Applications 2009–2010, 91. Total applicants accepted 2009–2010, 25. Number full-time enrolled (new admits only) 2009–2010, 19. Total enrolled 2009–2010 full-time, 78. Openings 2010–2011, 18. The median number of years required for completion of a degree in 2008–2009 were 5. The number of students enrolled full- and part-time who were dismissed or voluntarily withdrew from this program area in 2008–2009 were 1.
Scores: Entries appear in this order: required test or GPA, minimum score (if required), median score of students entering in 2009–2010. School Psychology PsyD (Doctor of Psychology): GRE-V no minimum stated, 560, GRE-Q no minimum stated, 630, GRE-Analytical no minimum stated, 4.0, GRE-Subject (Psychology) no minimum stated, 640, overall undergraduate GPA no minimum stated, 3.57.
Other Criteria: (importance of criteria rated low, medium, or high): GRE scores—high, research experience—medium, work experience—high, extracurricular activity—medium, clinically related public service—high, GPA—high, letters of recommendation—high, interview—high, statement of goals and objectives—high, undergraduate major in psychology—medium, specific undergraduate psychology courses taken—high. For additional information on admission requirements, go to http://gsappweb.rutgers.edu/pstudents/admissions.php.

Student Characteristics: The following represents characteristics of students in 2009–2010 in all graduate psychology programs in the department: Female—full-time 79, part-time 0; Male—full-time 15, part-time 0; African American/Black—full-time 12, part-time 0; Hispanic/Latino(a)—full-time 2, part-time 0; Asian/Pacific Islander—full-time 4, part-time 0; American Indian/Alaska Native—full-time 0, part-time 0; Caucasian/White—full-time 76, part-time 0; Multi-ethnic—full-time 0, part-time 0; students subject to the Americans With Disabilities Act—full-time 0, part-time 0; Unknown ethnicity—full-time 0, part-time 0; International students who hold an F-1 or J-1 Visa—full-time 0, part-time 0.

Financial Information/Assistance:
Tuition for Full-Time Study: Doctoral: State residents: per academic year $16,676, $699 per credit hour; Nonstate residents: per academic year $25,848, $1,077 per credit hour. Tuition is subject to change. Additional fees are assessed to students beyond the costs of tuition for the following: campus fee, computer fee, and student fee. See the following Web site for updates and changes in tuition costs: http://gradstudy.rutgers.edu/funding.shtml.

Financial Assistance:
First-Year Students: Fellowships and scholarships available for first year. Average amount paid per academic year: $12,500.
Advanced Students: Teaching assistantships available for advanced students. Average amount paid per academic year: $16,988. Traineeships available for advanced students. Average amount paid per academic year: $12,000. Fellowships and scholarships available for advanced students. Average amount paid per academic year: $12,500.
Additional Information: Of all students currently enrolled full time, 25% benefited from one or more of the listed financial assistance programs. Application and information available online at: http://studentaid.rutgers.edu.

Internships/Practica: Doctoral Degree (PsyD School Psychology): For those doctoral students for whom a professional internship was required in this program prior to graduation, (9) students applied for an internship in 2008–2009, with (9) students obtaining an internship. Of those students who obtained an internship, (9) were paid internships. Of those students who obtained an internship, (1) students placed in APA/CPA accredited internships, (0) students placed in internships not APA/CPA accredited, but listed with the Association of Psychology Postdoctoral and Internship Programs (APPIC), (8) students placed in internships conforming to guidelines of the Council of Directors of School Psychology Programs (CDSPP), (0) students placed in internships that were not APA/CPA accredited, APPIC or CDSPP listed. A special component of the student's training is the integration of practicum experiences with didactic courses from the second semester of the first year throughout the remaining semesters of training. These experiences begin by introducing the student to the roles and functions of a school psychologist, the functioning of child study teams, and a variety of schooling issues. For three consecutive semesters, students spend a minimum of one day per week in a public school with a doctoral level school psychologist supervisor/mentor. During the fifth and sixth semester, students may elect a different practicum experience from their first based upon their interests. These practica are supervised by on-site doctoral school psychologists and by on-campus faculty. The courses, the practica, and the supervision comprise the planned scaffold for educating students. In addition, there are numerous opportunities for learning and practice through colloquia, symposia, informal discussions, faculty projects, the psychological clinic and the Center for Applied Psychology.

Housing and Day Care: On-campus housing is available. See the following Web site for more information: http://housing.rutgers.edu. On-campus day care facilities are available. See the following Web site for more information: http://uhr.rutgers.edu/ben/ChildCare.htm.

Employment of Department Graduates:
Master's Degree Graduates: Of those who graduated in the academic year 2008–2009, the following categories and numbers represent the postgraduate activities and employment of master's degree graduates: Enrolled in a postdoctoral residency/fellowship (n/a), employed in independent practice (n/a), total from the above (master's) (0).
Doctoral Degree Graduates: Of those who graduated in the academic year 2008–2009, the following categories and numbers represent the postgraduate activities and employment of doctoral degree graduates: Enrolled in a psychology doctoral program (n/a), employed in a professional position in a school system (9), employed in business or industry (3), total from the above (doctoral) (12).

Additional Information:
Orientation, Objectives, and Emphasis of Department: The department of applied psychology is a unit dedicated (1) to enhancement of mental health and learning of children, adolescents, and adults in schools and related educational settings, and (2) to development of organizations that allow schooling to occur in effective and efficient ways. Three interrelated dimensions serve to structure the department. An applied research dimension signifies the important weight placed on generating new knowledge; an education and training dimension reflects concern for development of high-level practitioners and leaders of school psychology; an organizational and community services dimension is targeted at providing schools and related educational settings with consultation and technical assistance in areas of instruction and learning. A continuum of instruction ranges from observation and assessment through intervention models that include supervised experience as an essential component of didactic instruction. Core faculty are augmented by senior psychologists whose major professional involvement is in the schools or organizational and community settings.

Special Facilities or Resources: There are two special facilities that are an integrated part of the training program. One is an on-site psychological clinic which serves the university and state communities. Assessment and intervention programs are offered. The other is the Center for Applied Psychology, a division of GSAPP, that develops, implements, and evaluates projects involving faculty, students and others from the community. Included in these projects are the Eating Disorders Clinic, Foster Care Counseling, and a home-based intervention program for developmentally disabled individuals.

Information for Students With Physical Disabilities: See the following Web site for more information: http://disabilityservices.rutgers.edu/.

Application Information:
Send to Rutgers, The State University of New Jersey, Office of Graduate Admissions, 18 Bishop Place, New Brunswick, NJ 08901. Application available online. URL of online application: http://gradstudy.rutgers.edu/apply.shtml. Students are admitted in the Fall, application deadline January 5. *Fee:* $65. Project 1000 application fee is waived.

Rutgers—The State University of New Jersey
Department of Clinical Psychology
Graduate School of Applied and Professional Psychology, 152 Frelinghuysen Road
Piscataway, NJ 08854
Telephone: (732) 445-2000 x117
Fax: (732) 445-4888
E-mail: *bbry@rci.rutgers.edu*
Web: *http://gsappweb.rutgers.edu*

Department Information:
1974. Chair: Brenna H. Bry. Number of faculty: total—full-time 15, part-time 10; women—full-time 8, part-time 7; total—minority—full-time 3, part-time 1; women minority—full-time 2, part-time 2; faculty subject to the Americans With Disabilities Act 1.

Programs and Degrees Offered:
Listed in the following order: Program area, degree type (T if terminal Master's), number awarded 7/08–6/09. Clinical Psychology PsyD (Doctor of Psychology) 14.

APA Accreditation: Clinical PsyD (Doctor of Psychology).

Student Applications/Admissions:
Student Applications
Clinical Psychology PsyD (Doctor of Psychology)—Applications 2009–2010, 414. Total applicants accepted 2009–2010, 27. Number full-time enrolled (new admits only) 2009–2010, 17. Number part-time enrolled (new admits only) 2009–2010, 0. Openings 2010–2011, 18. The median number of years required for completion of a degree in 2008–2009 were 5. The number of students enrolled full- and part-time who were dismissed or voluntarily withdrew from this program area in 2008–2009 were 0.
Scores: Entries appear in this order: required test or GPA, minimum score (if required), median score of students entering in 2009–2010. *Clinical Psychology PsyD (Doctor of Psychology)*: GRE-V no minimum stated, GRE-Q no minimum stated, GRE-Analytical no minimum stated, GRE-Subject (Psychology) no minimum stated, overall undergraduate GPA no minimum stated.
Other Criteria: (importance of criteria rated low, medium, or high): GRE scores—medium, research experience—medium, work experience—high, extracurricular activity—high, clinically related public service—high, GPA—high, letters of recommendation—high, interview—high, statement of goals and objectives—high, undergraduate major in psychology—medium, specific undergraduate psychology courses taken—me-

dium. For additional information on admission requirements, go to http://gsappweb.rutgers.edu/programs/clinical.

Student Characteristics: The following represents characteristics of students in 2009–2010 in all graduate psychology programs in the department: Female—full-time 72, part-time 0; Male—full-time 32, part-time 0; African American/Black—full-time 12, part-time 0; Hispanic/Latino(a)—full-time 13, part-time 0; Asian/Pacific Islander—full-time 11, part-time 0; American Indian/Alaska Native—full-time 0, part-time 0; Caucasian/White—full-time 65, part-time 0; Multi-ethnic—full-time 0, part-time 0; students subject to the Americans With Disabilities Act—full-time 0, part-time 0; Unknown ethnicity—full-time 3, part-time 0; International students who hold an F-1 or J-1 Visa—full-time 3, part-time 0.

Financial Information/Assistance:

Tuition for Full-Time Study: *Doctoral:* State residents: per academic year $16,676, $699 per credit hour; Nonstate residents: per academic year $25,848, $1,077 per credit hour. Tuition is subject to change. Additional fees are assessed to students beyond the costs of tuition for the following: college fees and computer fees. See the following Web site for updates and changes in tuition costs: http://www.studentabc.rutgers.edu.

Financial Assistance:

First-Year Students: Fellowships and scholarships available for first year. Average amount paid per academic year: $13,500.

Advanced Students: Teaching assistantships available for advanced students. Average amount paid per academic year: $16,988. Research assistantships available for advanced students. Average amount paid per academic year: $16,988. Traineeships available for advanced students. Average amount paid per academic year: $20,772. Fellowships and scholarships available for advanced students. Average amount paid per academic year: $13,500.

Additional Information: Of all students currently enrolled full time, 25% benefited from one or more of the listed financial assistance programs. Application and information available online at: http://gradstudy.rutgers.edu/funding.shtml.

Internships/Practica: Doctoral Degree (PsyD Clinical Psychology): For those doctoral students for whom a professional internship was required in this program prior to graduation, (22) students applied for an internship in 2008–2009, with (22) students obtaining an internship. Of those students who obtained an internship, (22) were paid internships. Of those students who obtained an internship, (21) students placed in APA/CPA accredited internships, (0) students placed in internships not APA/CPA accredited, but listed with the Association of Psychology Postdoctoral and Internship Programs (APPIC), (0) students placed in internships conforming to guidelines of the Council of Directors of School Psychology Programs (CDSPP), (1) students placed in internships that were not APA/CPA accredited, APPIC or CDSPP listed. The PsyD program provides a broadly based practicum program which is structured around the needs and interests of our students. Students can choose placements in hospitals which include a hospice program, neuropsych testing, long and short term inpatient treatment programs for both adolescents and adults. They can choose to be placed in university-based specialty clinics, traditional community mental health centers, college counseling centers, specialized schools for children (autism, learning disabled, emotionally disturbed). Students can be placed in public school based mental health clinics, in programs which provide service to at-risk youth, those with serious mental illness, and those with addictive disorders. Our programs are selected for their attention to supervision but also for their balance regarding gender, race and socio-economic levels.

Housing and Day Care: On-campus housing is available. See the following Web site for more information: http://housing.rutgers.edu/ie/. On-campus day care facilities are available. See the following Web site for more information: http://ruinfo.rutgers.edu/.

Employment of Department Graduates:

Master's Degree Graduates: Of those who graduated in the academic year 2008–2009, the following categories and numbers represent the postgraduate activities and employment of master's degree graduates: Enrolled in a postdoctoral residency/fellowship (n/a), employed in independent practice (n/a), total from the above (master's) (0).

Doctoral Degree Graduates: Of those who graduated in the academic year 2008–2009, the following categories and numbers represent the postgraduate activities and employment of doctoral degree graduates: Enrolled in a psychology doctoral program (n/a), enrolled in another graduate/professional program (0), enrolled in a postdoctoral residency/fellowship (3), employed in independent practice (1), employed in an academic position at a university (0), employed in an academic position at a 2-year/4-year college (0), employed in other positions at a higher education institution (3), employed in a professional position in a school system (0), employed in business or industry (0), employed in government agency (0), employed in a community mental health/counseling center (2), employed in a hospital/medical center (2), not seeking employment (0), other employment position (0), do not know (2), total from the above (doctoral) (13).

Additional Information:

Orientation, Objectives, and Emphasis of Department: The PsyD program emphasizes pragmatic training in problem solving and planned change techniques. Didactic training in basic psychological principles is coupled with practical, graduate instruction in a range of assessment and intervention modes. The level of involvement becomes progressively more intense during the student's course of training. Most courses include (1) a seminar component oriented around case discussions and substantive theoretical issues of clinical import, (2) a practicum component during which students see clients in the intervention mode or problem area under study, and (3) a supervision component by which the student receives guidance from an experienced clinical instructor in a wide range of applied clinical settings. All three components are coordinated around a central conceptual issue, such as a mode of intervention or a clinical problem area. Instruction and supervision are offered by full-time faculty and senior psychologists whose primary professional involvement is in applied clinical settings throughout the state. In addition to required general core courses, students may emphasize training within any of three perspectives: psychodynamic, behavioral, or systems approaches. This last perspective focuses on family, organizational and community services.

Special Facilities or Resources: The Center for Applied Psychology at GSAPP is the focal point for the field experiences that are critical in the development of professional psychologists. The projects overseen by the Center are cornerstones of training for our students; the GSAPP Psychological Clinic, the Foster Care Counseling project, the Natural Setting Therapeutic Management program, the Anxiety Disorders Clinic, and our extensive network of practicum placements are all available to our students. Students are placed in community-based organizations where the recipients of the services we provide are often underserved. These placements include community mental health centers, hospitals, special schools, and other programs. All students are placed in a practicum setting for at least one full day per week during their years at GSAPP. All students see clients through our Clinic and receive one-hour of individual supervision for each hour of therapy. The Clinic has specialty sub-clinics which will allow students to gain experience and supervision in specific treatment approaches working with faculty experts.

Information for Students With Physical Disabilities: See the following Web site for more information: http://disabilityservices.rutgers.edu.

Application Information:
Send to Graduate and Professional Admissions, Rutgers, The State University of New Jersey, 18 Bishop Place, New Brunswick, NJ 08901-8530. Application available online. URL of online application: http://gradstudy.rutgers.edu. Students are admitted in the Fall, application deadline January 5. *Fee:* $65. Project 1000 - Fee waived.

Rutgers—The State University of New Jersey, New Brunswick (2009 data)
Department of Educational Psychology
Graduate School of Education
10 Seminary Place
New Brunswick, NJ 08901-1183
Telephone: (732) 932-7496 x8327
Fax: (732) 932-6829
E-mail: *mccune@rci.rutgers.edu*
Web: *http://www.gse.rutgers.edu*

Department Information:
1923. Chairperson: Lorraine McCune. Number of faculty: total—full-time 17; women—full-time 8; total—minority—full-time 3; women minority—full-time 1.

Programs and Degrees Offered:
Listed in the following order: Program area, degree type (T if terminal Master's), number awarded 7/08–6/09. Learning, Cognition, & Development MEd (Education) 4, Special Education MEd (Education) 39, Educational Psychology PhD (Doctor of Philosophy) 4, Educational Statistics & Measurement MEd (Education) 8, Counseling Psychology MEd (Education) 15.

Student Applications/Admissions:
Student Applications
Learning, Cognition, & Development MEd (Education)—Applications 2009–2010, 19. Total applicants accepted 2009–2010, 11. Openings 2010–2011, 10. The median number of years required for completion of a degree in 2008–2009 was 1. The number of students enrolled full- and part-time who were dismissed or voluntarily withdrew from this program area in 2008–2009 were 0. *Special Education MEd (Education)*—Applications 2009–2010, 43. Total applicants accepted 2009–2010, 31. Openings 2010–2011, 35. The median number of years required for completion of a degree in 2008–2009 were 2. The number of students enrolled full- and part-time who were dismissed or voluntarily withdrew from this program area in 2008–2009 were 0. *Educational Psychology PhD (Doctor of Philosophy)*—The median number of years required for completion of a degree in 2008–2009 were 5. *Educational Statistics & Measurement MEd (Education)*—Applications 2009–2010, 10. Total applicants accepted 2009–2010, 5. Openings 2010–2011, 10. The median number of years required for completion of a degree in 2008–2009 were 2. The number of students enrolled full- and part-time who were dismissed or voluntarily withdrew from this program area in 2008–2009 were 0. *Counseling Psychology MEd (Education)*—Applications 2009–2010, 82. Total applicants accepted 2009–2010, 59. Openings 2010–2011, 50. The median number of years required for completion of a degree in 2008–2009 were 2.

Other Criteria: (importance of criteria rated low, medium, or high): GRE scores—high, research experience—high, work experience—medium, GPA—high, letters of recommendation—high, statement of goals and objectives—high. For additional information on admission requirements, go to http://gse.rutgers.edu.

Student Characteristics: The following represents characteristics of students in 2009–2010 in all graduate psychology programs in the department: Female—full-time 122, part-time 156; Male—full-time 28, part-time 32; African American/Black—full-time 15, part-time 14; Hispanic/Latino(a)—full-time 8, part-time 12; Asian/Pacific Islander—full-time 20, part-time 33; American Indian/Alaska Native—full-time 0, part-time 1; Caucasian/White—full-time 76, part-time 118; Multi-ethnic—full-time 6, part-time 8; students subject to the Americans With Disabilities Act—full-time 0, part-time 0; Unknown ethnicity—full-time 0, part-time 0; International students who hold an F-1 or J-1 Visa—full-time 0, part-time 0.

Financial Information/Assistance:
Tuition for Full-Time Study: *Master's:* State residents: per academic year $13,440, $560 per credit hour; Nonstate residents: per academic year $20,256, $844 per credit hour. *Doctoral:* State residents: per academic year $13,440, $560 per credit hour; Nonstate residents: per academic year $20,256, $844 per credit hour. Tuition is subject to change. See the following Web site for updates and changes in tuition costs: http://www.studentabc.rutgers.edu.

Financial Assistance:
First-Year Students: Teaching assistantships available for first year. Average amount paid per academic year: $18,347. Average number of hours worked per week: 15. Apply by February 1. Research assistantships available for first year. Average amount paid per academic year: $18,347. Average number of hours worked per week: 15. Apply by February 1. Fellowships and scholarships available for first year. Average number of hours worked per week: 0. Apply by March 1.

Advanced Students: Teaching assistantships available for advanced students. Average amount paid per academic year: $18,347. Average number of hours worked per week: 15. Apply by February 1. Research assistantships available for advanced students. Average amount paid per academic year: $18,347. Average number of hours worked per week: 15. Apply by February 1. Fellowships and scholarships available for advanced students. Apply by March 1.

Additional Information: Application and information available online at: http://studentaid.rutgers.edu/.

Internships/Practica: No information provided.

Housing and Day Care: On-campus housing is available. See the following Web site for more information: http://housing.rutgers.edu/ie. On-campus day care facilities are available. See the following Web site for more information: http://nbpweb.rutgers.edu/menus/childcare.shtml.

Employment of Department Graduates:
Master's Degree Graduates: Of those who graduated in the academic year 2008–2009, the following categories and numbers represent the postgraduate activities and employment of master's degree graduates: Enrolled in a postdoctoral residency/fellowship (n/a), employed in independent practice (n/a), total from the above (master's) (0).
Doctoral Degree Graduates: Of those who graduated in the academic year 2008–2009, the following categories and numbers represent the postgraduate activities and employment of doctoral degree graduates: Enrolled in a psychology doctoral program (n/a), total from the above (doctoral) (0).

Additional Information:
Orientation, Objectives, and Emphasis of Department: The Department of Educational Psychology offers a PhD in Educational Psychology that seeks to prepare scholarly researchers in areas that include theory and methods of statistical analysis, evaluation, and measurement as applied to educational issues; and the psychology of human learning, cognition and development in schools, families, and communities. At the master's level, the Department offers graduate Masters in Education (Ed.M.) degree programs of study in (a) counseling psychology, (b) educational statistics, measurement and evaluation, (c) learning, cognition, & development, (d) special education, and (e) school counseling. Completion of these master's degree programs can also result in various professional credentials including certification as a Learning Disabilities Teacher Consultant and School Counselor. The Department also offers a certificate program in Interdisciplinary Infant Studies. All programs in the Department include research training and pertain to the description, explanation and optimization of human development in various contexts.

Special Facilities or Resources: We have all the resources normally associated with a major research university.

Information for Students With Physical Disabilities: See the following Web site for more information: http://disabilityservices.rutgers.edu.

Application Information:
Send to Office of Graduate and Professional Admissions, Rutgers, The State University of New Jersey, 18 Bishop Place, New Brunswick, NJ 08901-8530; Application available online. URL of online application: http://gradstudy.rutgers.edu. Students are admitted in the Fall, application deadline February 1. EdM in School Counseling has Fall admission only: February 1 deadline. PhD program has Fall admission only: February 1 deadline. *Fee:* $65. Contact the Office of Graduate and Professional Admissions about fee waivers or deferrals.

Seton Hall University
Professional Psychology and Family Therapy
Education and Human Services
400 South Orange Avenue
South Orange, NJ 07079
Telephone: (973) 761-9451
Fax: (973) 275-2188
E-mail: *Laura.Palmer@shu.edu*
Web: *http://www.shu.edu/academics/education/professional-psychology/*

Department Information:
1965. Chairperson: Laura Palmer, PhD. Number of faculty: total—full-time 14; women—full-time 6; total—minority—full-time 3; women minority—full-time 1.

Programs and Degrees Offered:
Listed in the following order: Program area, degree type (T if terminal Master's), number awarded 7/08–6/09. Counseling Psychology PhD (Doctor of Philosophy) 5, Marriage and Family Therapy EdS (School Psychology), Mental Health Counseling EdS (School Psychology), School Counseling MA/MS (Master of Arts/Science), Counseling (Online) MEd (Education), Psychological Studies MEd (Education), School Counseling (Online) MEd (Education), Marriage and Family Therapy MA/MS (Master of Arts/Science), Counseling/Professional Counseling MA/MS (Master of Arts/Science) 10, Professional Counseling EdS (School Psychology), School-Community Psychology EdS (School Psychology), Counseling MA/MS (Master of Arts/Science), Counseling (Online) MA/MS (Master of Arts/Science), Counseling and Psychological Studies MA/MS (Master of Arts/Science), Psychological Studies MA/MS (Master of Arts/Science), School Counseling (Online) MA/MS (Master of Arts/Science), Professional Counseling (Online) EdS (School Psychology).

APA Accreditation: Counseling PhD (Doctor of Philosophy).

Student Applications/Admissions:
Student Applications
Counseling Psychology PhD (Doctor of Philosophy)—Applications 2009–2010, 125. Total applicants accepted 2009–2010, 4. Number full-time enrolled (new admits only) 2009–2010, 3. Total enrolled 2009–2010 full-time, 25. Openings 2010–2011, 10. The median number of years required for completion of a degree in 2008–2009 were 5. The number of students enrolled full- and part-time who were dismissed or voluntarily withdrew from this program area in 2008–2009 were 0. *Marriage and Family Therapy EdS (School Psychology)*—Total enrolled 2009–2010 full-time, 10. *Mental Health Counseling EdS (School Psychology)*—Total enrolled 2009–2010 full-time, 1. *School Counseling MA/MS (Master of Arts/Science)*—Total enrolled 2009–2010 part-time, 14. *Counseling (Online) MEd (Education)*—Total enrolled 2009–2010 part-time, 4. *Psychological Studies MEd (Education)*—Total enrolled 2009–2010 full-time, 4. *School Counseling (Online) MEd (Education)*—Total enrolled 2009–2010 part-time, 2. *Marriage and Family Therapy MA/MS*

(*Master of Arts/Science*)—Total enrolled 2009–2010 full-time, 21. *Counseling/Professional Counseling MA/MS (Master of Arts/Science)*—Applications 2009–2010, 33. Total applicants accepted 2009–2010, 29. Number full-time enrolled (new admits only) 2009–2010, 17. Number part-time enrolled (new admits only) 2009–2010, 1. Openings 2010–2011, 11. The median number of years required for completion of a degree in 2008–2009 were 3. The number of students enrolled full- and part-time who were dismissed or voluntarily withdrew from this program area in 2008–2009 were 2. *Professional Counseling EdS (School Psychology)*—Total enrolled 2009–2010 full-time, 4. *School-Community Psychology EdS (School Psychology)*—Total enrolled 2009–2010 full-time, 26. *Counseling MA/MS (Master of Arts/Science)*—Total enrolled 2009–2010 full-time, 36. *Counseling (Online) MA/MS (Master of Arts/Science)*—Total enrolled 2009–2010 part-time, 87. *Counseling and Psychological Studies MA/MS (Master of Arts/Science)*—Total enrolled 2009–2010 full-time, 6. *Psychological Studies MA/MS (Master of Arts/Science)*—Total enrolled 2009–2010 full-time, 27. *School Counseling (Online) MA/MS (Master of Arts/Science)*—Total enrolled 2009–2010 part-time, 115. *Professional Counseling (Online) EdS (School Psychology)*—Total enrolled 2009–2010 full-time, 7.

Other Criteria: (importance of criteria rated low, medium, or high): GRE scores—medium, research experience—high, work experience—medium, extracurricular activity—medium, clinically related public service—medium, GPA—high, letters of recommendation—high, interview—high, statement of goals and objectives—high, undergraduate major in psychology—low, specific undergraduate psychology courses taken—low. For additional information on admission requirements, go to http://www.shu.edu/academics/education/graduate-programs.cfm.

Student Characteristics: The following represents characteristics of students in 2009–2010 in all graduate psychology programs in the department: Female—full-time 0, part-time 0; Male—full-time 0, part-time 0; African American/Black—full-time 0, part-time 0; Hispanic/Latino(a)—full-time 0, part-time 0; Asian/Pacific Islander—full-time 0, part-time 0; American Indian/Alaska Native—full-time 0, part-time 0; Caucasian/White—full-time 0, part-time 0; Multi-ethnic—full-time 0, part-time 0; students subject to the Americans With Disabilities Act—full-time 0, part-time 0; Unknown ethnicity—full-time 0, part-time 0; International students who hold an F-1 or J-1 Visa—full-time 0, part-time 0.

Financial Information/Assistance:
Tuition for Full-Time Study: *Master's:* State residents: $901 per credit hour; Nonstate residents: $901 per credit hour. *Doctoral:* State residents: $901 per credit hour; Nonstate residents: $901 per credit hour. Tuition is subject to change. There is a different fee structure for the online masters and EdS degrees. See the following Web site for updates and changes in tuition costs: http://www.shu.edu/applying/graduate/tuition-costs.cfm.

Financial Assistance:
First-Year Students: Research assistantships available for first year. Average amount paid per academic year: $4,500. Average number of hours worked per week: 20. Apply by Spring.
Advanced Students: Research assistantships available for advanced students. Average amount paid per academic year: $4,500. Average number of hours worked per week: 20. Apply by Spring.

Additional Information: Of all students currently enrolled full time, 75% benefited from one or more of the listed financial assistance programs. Application and information available online at: http://www.shu.edu/applying/graduate/grad-finaid.cfm.

Internships/Practica: Doctoral Degree (PhD Counseling Psychology): For those doctoral students for whom a professional internship was required in this program prior to graduation, (6) students applied for an internship in 2008–2009, with (5) students obtaining an internship. Of those students who obtained an internship, (5) were paid internships. Of those students who obtained an internship, (5) students placed in APA/CPA accredited internships, (0) students placed in internships not APA/CPA accredited, but listed with the Association of Psychology Postdoctoral and Internship Programs (APPIC), (0) students placed in internships conforming to guidelines of the Council of Directors of School Psychology Programs (CDSPP), (0) students placed in internships that were not APA/CPA accredited, APPIC or CDSPP listed. Master's Degree (MA/MS Counseling/Professional Counseling): An internship experience, such as a final research project or "capstone" experience is required of graduates. The Marriage and Family students follow the standards of the Commission on Accreditation for Marriage and Family Therapy Education. The doctoral students adhere to Psychology guidelines. The students in all MA and EdS programs (except Psychological Studies) complete a practicum sequence consistent with their professional training models.

Housing and Day Care: No on-campus housing is available. No on-campus day care facilities are available.

Employment of Department Graduates:
Master's Degree Graduates: Of those who graduated in the academic year 2008–2009, the following categories and numbers represent the postgraduate activities and employment of master's degree graduates: Enrolled in a psychology doctoral program (0), enrolled in another graduate/professional program (0), enrolled in a postdoctoral residency/fellowship (n/a), employed in independent practice (n/a), employed in an academic position at a university (0), employed in an academic position at a 2-year/4-year college (0), employed in other positions at a higher education institution (0), employed in a professional position in a school system (0), employed in business or industry (0), employed in government agency (0), employed in a community mental health/counseling center (0), employed in a hospital/medical center (0), still seeking employment (0), other employment position (0), total from the above (master's) (0).
Doctoral Degree Graduates: Of those who graduated in the academic year 2008–2009, the following categories and numbers represent the postgraduate activities and employment of doctoral degree graduates: Enrolled in a psychology doctoral program (n/a), enrolled in a postdoctoral residency/fellowship (4), employed in independent practice (5), employed in an academic position at a university (0), employed in an academic position at a 2-year/4-year college (0), employed in other positions at a higher education institution (0), employed in a professional position in a school system (0), employed in business or industry (0), employed in government agency (0), employed in a community mental health/counseling center (0), employed in a hospital/medical center (1),

still seeking employment (0), other employment position (0), total from the above (doctoral) (10).

Additional Information:
Orientation, Objectives, and Emphasis of Department: The Marriage and Family program is based on a systemic orientation to family psychology and family therapy. The goals of Counseling Psychology encompass knowledge of the science of psychology and counseling psychology as a specialty, integration of research and practice, and commitment to ongoing professional development. Professional counselors are mental health practitioners trained to help individual clients and groups address common developmental challenges and transitions as well as more severe emotional difficulties. School psychology students learn to specialize in assessment and evaluations in schools.

Special Facilities or Resources: The department has individual counseling/assessment rooms, family and couple laboratories, and group therapy rooms, all of which are wired with audiovisual equipment with centralized viewing in a control room. There are rooms for data analysis as well.

Information for Students With Physical Disabilities: See the following Web site for more information: http://www.shu.edu/offices/disability-support-services-index.cfm.

Application Information:
Send to Graduate Admissions, College of Education and Human Services, Seton Hall University, 400 South Orange Avenue, South Orange, NJ 07079. Application available online. URL of online application: http://www.shu.edu/academics/education/index.cfm. Students are admitted in the Fall. Counseling Psychology PhD (January 15), Counseling/ School Counseling MA/EdS (Spring: November 1 and Fall: June1); School and Community Psychology EdS (Spring: October 1 and Fall: February 1), and all other programs rolling admissions. *Fee:* $50.

Seton Hall University
Psychology/Experimental Psychology
Arts and Sciences
400 South Orange Avenue
South Orange, NJ 07079
Telephone: (973) 761-9484
Fax: (973) 275-5829
E-mail: *psych@shu.edu*
Web: *http://www.shu.edu/academics/artsci/psychology/*

Department Information:
1952. Chairperson: Susan A. Nolan, PhD Number of faculty: total—full-time 12, part-time 5; women—full-time 7, part-time 3; minority—part-time 1; women minority—part-time 1; faculty subject to the Americans With Disabilities Act 1.

Programs and Degrees Offered:
Listed in the following order: Program area, degree type (T if terminal Master's), number awarded 7/08–6/09. Experimental Psychology MA/MS (Master of Arts/Science) (T) 4.

Student Applications/Admissions:
Student Applications

Experimental Psychology MA/MS (Master of Arts/Science)—Applications 2009–2010, 22. Total applicants accepted 2009–2010, 20. Number full-time enrolled (new admits only) 2009–2010, 10. Number part-time enrolled (new admits only) 2009–2010, 0. Total enrolled 2009–2010 full-time, 15, part-time, 1. Openings 2010–2011, 12. The median number of years required for completion of a degree in 2008–2009 were 2. The number of students enrolled full- and part-time who were dismissed or voluntarily withdrew from this program area in 2008–2009 were 1.

Scores: Entries appear in this order: required test or GPA, minimum score (if required), median score of students entering in 2009–2010. *Experimental Psychology MA/MS (Master of Arts/Science):* GRE-V no minimum stated, GRE-Q no minimum stated, GRE-Analytical no minimum stated, overall undergraduate GPA 3.0.

Other Criteria: (importance of criteria rated low, medium, or high): GRE scores—medium, research experience—high, work experience—low, extracurricular activity—medium, GPA—high, letters of recommendation—high, statement of goals and objectives—high, undergraduate major in psychology—low, specific undergraduate psychology courses taken—high. If applying for a concentration in Behavioral Neuroscience track, demonstration of physiological, cognitive, learning types of courses is preferred. For additional information on admission requirements, go to http://www.shu.edu/academics/artsci/ms-psychology/admissions.cfm.

Student Characteristics: The following represents characteristics of students in 2009–2010 in all graduate psychology programs in the department: Female—full-time 7, part-time 1; Male—full-time 7, part-time 0; African American/Black—full-time 0, part-time 0; Hispanic/Latino(a)—full-time 0, part-time 0; Asian/Pacific Islander—full-time 1, part-time 0; American Indian/Alaska Native—full-time 0, part-time 0; Caucasian/White—full-time 0, part-time 0; Multi-ethnic—full-time 1, part-time 0; students subject to the Americans With Disabilities Act—full-time 0, part-time 0; Unknown ethnicity—full-time 0, part-time 0; International students who hold an F-1 or J-1 Visa—full-time 0, part-time 0.

Financial Information/Assistance:
Tuition for Full-Time Study: Master's: State residents: per academic year $16,218, $901 per credit hour. Tuition is subject to change. Additional fees are assessed to students beyond the costs of tuition for the following: university and technology Fees, $305 per semester. See the following Web site for updates and changes in tuition costs: http://www.shu.edu/applying/graduate/tuition-costs.cfm.

Financial Assistance:
First-Year Students: Teaching assistantships available for first year. Average amount paid per academic year: $8,500. Average number of hours worked per week: 20. Research assistantships available for first year. Average amount paid per academic year: $5,200. Average number of hours worked per week: 20.

Advanced Students: Teaching assistantships available for advanced students. Average amount paid per academic year: $8,500. Average number of hours worked per week: 20. Research assistantships available for advanced students. Average amount paid per academic year: $5,200. Average number of hours worked per week: 20.

Additional Information: Of all students currently enrolled full time, 50% benefited from one or more of the listed financial assistance programs. Application and information available online at: http://www.shu.edu/applying/graduate.

Internships/Practica: Master's Degree (MA/MS Experimental Psychology): An internship experience, such as a final research project or "capstone" experience is required of graduates.

Housing and Day Care: No on-campus housing is available. No on-campus day care facilities are available.

Employment of Department Graduates:
Master's Degree Graduates: Of those who graduated in the academic year 2008–2009, the following categories and numbers represent the postgraduate activities and employment of master's degree graduates: Enrolled in a psychology doctoral program (4), enrolled in a postdoctoral residency/fellowship (n/a), employed in independent practice (n/a), total from the above (master's) (4).
Doctoral Degree Graduates: Of those who graduated in the academic year 2008–2009, the following categories and numbers represent the postgraduate activities and employment of doctoral degree graduates: Enrolled in a psychology doctoral program (n/a), total from the above (doctoral) (0).

Additional Information:
Orientation, Objectives, and Emphasis of Department: The MS degree in experimental psychology is designed specifically for students seeking to gain a solid foundation in empirical research for eventual entry into PhD programs in scientific psychology or for students desiring to explore the field. The Experimental Psychology program consists of 36 credits to be completed in 2 years. All incoming students are required to participate in research each semester. The courses offered (including a research thesis) comprise traditional areas in experimental psychology with optional concentrations in General Psychology and Behavioral Neuroscience. The Behavioral Neuroscience concentration represents courses that are most directly relevant to behavioral studies of brain functioning.

Special Facilities or Resources: Faculty have private offices of approximately 150 square feet each. A suite of nine 8' X 8' cubicles are available for graduate student use. An Animal Conditioning Laboratory consists of eight test cubicles, each equipped with an operant chamber interfaced to an IBM desktop computer. A five room Physiological Psychology suite of approximately 400 square feet is used for surgical preparations, histology, and behavioral testing of rodents. Several mazes are also available for the study of learning and memory in rodents. The laboratories share access to two animal colony rooms for housing rodents. Research space for human experimental psychology investigations includes a corridor lined by eleven research cubicles, each one approximately 90 square feet, and a research participant reception area of approximately 200 square feet. Equipment for these cubicles includes desktop computers and associated equipment that allows them to function as laboratory control devices. Three of these machines have video capture cards permitting still frame capture and videoconferencing with Sony video camcorders. In addition, the department's Perceptual Laboratory consists of a three-room suite totaling 650 square feet. A one-way vision room is also available, as are additional suites for data collection.

Application Information:
Send to Office of the Provost, Attn: Graduate Admissions, Seton Hall University, 400 South Orange Avenue, South Orange, New Jersey 07079. Application available online. URL of online application: https://apply.embark.com/grad/setonhall/cas/. Students are admitted in the Fall, application deadline July 1. Strong applications submitted before April 1 have a greater chance of admittance and of receiving Graduate Assistantships. *Fee:* $50.

William Paterson University
Psychology/MA in Clinical and Counseling Psychology
Humanities & Social Sciences
300 Pompton Road
Wayne, NJ 07470
Telephone: (973) 720-3629
Fax: (973) 720-3392
E-mail: *Psychgrad@wpunj.edu*
Web: *http://www.wpunj.edu/cohss/psychology/Masters.htm*

Department Information:
1999. Graduate Director: Bruce J. Diamond, PhD. Number of faculty: total—full-time 8; women—full-time 5; total—minority—full-time 1; women minority—full-time 1.

Programs and Degrees Offered:
Listed in the following order: Program area, degree type (T if terminal Master's), number awarded 7/08–6/09. Clinical and Counseling Psychology MA/MS (Master of Arts/Science) (T) 11.

Student Applications/Admissions:
Student Applications

Clinical and Counseling Psychology MA/MS (Master of Arts/Science)—Applications 2009–2010, 45. Total applicants accepted 2009–2010, 23. Number full-time enrolled (new admits only) 2009–2010, 7. Number part-time enrolled (new admits only) 2009–2010, 2. Total enrolled 2009–2010 full-time, 13, part-time, 17. Openings 2010–2011, 20. The median number of years required for completion of a degree in 2008–2009 were 3. The number of students enrolled full- and part-time who were dismissed or voluntarily withdrew from this program area in 2008–2009 were 0.

Other Criteria: (importance of criteria rated low, medium, or high): GRE scores—high, research experience—high, work experience—medium, extracurricular activity—medium, clinically related public service—high, GPA—high, letters of recommendation—high, interview—medium, statement of goals and objectives—high, undergraduate major in psychology—medium, specific undergraduate psychology courses taken—high. For additional information on admission requirements, go to http://www.wpunj.edu/cohss/psychology/masters.htm.

Student Characteristics: The following represents characteristics of students in 2009–2010 in all graduate psychology programs in the department: Female—full-time 5, part-time 2; Male—full-time 2, part-time 0; African American/Black—full-time 1, part-time 0; Hispanic/Latino(a)—full-time 1, part-time 1; Asian/Pa-

cific Islander—full-time 2, part-time 0; American Indian/Alaska Native—full-time 0, part-time 0; Caucasian/White—full-time 3, part-time 1; students subject to the Americans With Disabilities Act—full-time 0, part-time 0; Unknown ethnicity—full-time 0, part-time 0; International students who hold an F-1 or J-1 Visa—full-time 0, part-time 0.

Financial Information/Assistance:
Tuition for Full-Time Study: Master's: State residents: per academic year $14,675, $587 per credit hour; Nonstate residents: per academic year $22,750, $910 per credit hour. See the following Web site for updates and changes in tuition costs: http://cms.wpunj.edu/studentaccounts/tuition-and-fees/graduate.dot.

Financial Assistance:
First-Year Students: Traineeships available for first year. Average amount paid per academic year: $6,000. Average number of hours worked per week: 20. Apply by April 1.
Advanced Students: Traineeships available for advanced students. Average amount paid per academic year: $6,000. Average number of hours worked per week: 20. Apply by April 1.
Additional Information: Of all students currently enrolled full time, 17% benefited from one or more of the listed financial assistance programs.

Internships/Practica: Master's Degree (MA/MS Clinical and Counseling Psychology): An internship experience, such as a final research project or "capstone" experience is required of graduates. Graduates and interns serve in a wide variety of inpatient and outpatient settings including hospitals, community mental health clinics, wellness centers, health maintenance facilities, local, regional, national and international health care organizations, group homes, drug treatment facilities, rehabilitation centers, correctional facilities and gerontology programs. Under proper licensed supervision, graduates of our program are able to conduct assessments; provide clinical and health-related services to individuals, groups and families using appropriate diagnostic and intervention techniques; participate in institutional and organizational research projects at the Master's level and work on an elective basis with a variety of populations (e.g., chronic and acute diseases and disorders, children, adolescents, the elderly, the severely mentally ill, substance abusers, and others).

Housing and Day Care: On-campus housing is available. See the following Web site for more information: http://www.wpunj.edu/reslife. On-campus day care facilities are available. See the following Web site for more information: http://ww2.wpunj.edu/childcare_center.

Employment of Department Graduates:
Master's Degree Graduates: Of those who graduated in the academic year 2008–2009, the following categories and numbers represent the postgraduate activities and employment of master's degree graduates: Enrolled in a psychology doctoral program (3), enrolled in another graduate/professional program (0), enrolled in a postdoctoral residency/fellowship (n/a), employed in independent practice (n/a), employed in an academic position at a 2-year/4-year college (3), employed in other positions at a higher education institution (0), employed in a professional position in a school system (0), employed in business or industry (0), employed in government agency (0), employed in a community mental health/counseling center (8), employed in a hospital/medical center (3), still seeking employment (0), not seeking employment (0), other employment position (0), do not know (0), total from the above (master's) (17).
Doctoral Degree Graduates: Of those who graduated in the academic year 2008–2009, the following categories and numbers represent the postgraduate activities and employment of doctoral degree graduates: Enrolled in a psychology doctoral program (n/a), total from the above (doctoral) (0).

Additional Information:
Orientation, Objectives, and Emphasis of Department: The Graduate program provides an ethically and cross-culturally sensitive program in clinical and counseling psychology with emphasis on theoretical and applied perspectives. Our focus is on understanding, preventing and treating disorders and diseases that compromise mental and physical health by fostering knowledge and understanding of the diagnosis, etiology and biopsychosocial factors that contribute to the onset, progression and consequences of these disorders. The purpose of the program is to prepare students who are knowledgeable in clinical theory, empiricism, assessment and in the application of clinical and research techniques and procedures and to provide a foundation for doctoral-level work. We anticipate offering a 49-credit program in Fall 2010 that requires completion of a comprehensive Master's Project involving a clinical case or a research thesis/project. Faculty The graduate faculty's ongoing research includes: clinical health psychology, mind-body approaches to well-being, lifespan issues, trauma, substance abuse and addiction, chronic illness in pediatric populations, relationships between personality, career choice and substance abuse, gerontology, serious and persistent psychiatric disorders, and neuropsychological performance (e.g., memory, information processing, executive function) in healthy individuals and those with organic brain disorders (e.g., stroke, Multiple Sclerosis, brain injury).

Special Facilities or Resources: The University has a modern library with numerous online databases, media and study areas. The new University Commons provides a food mall, recreation area, ballrooms and informal leisure spaces and lounges. The campus is wired and includes numerous labs equipped with a variety of software applications for teaching and research. The campus also has an active Instructional Research Technology Lab that helps support IT-related activities. The Graduate Program maintains a wide array of assessments, tests, videos and equipment which are available to faculty and students. Research and teaching facilities will be significantly enhanced in our soon-to-be renovated academic building which will include space for a clinical training suite/clinic. The 370 acre campus is 30 minutes from NYC, 45 minutes from scenic northern NJ and 90 minutes from the Pocono Mountains.

Information for Students With Physical Disabilities: See the following Web site for more information: http://ww2.wpunj.edu/studentservices/disability.

Application Information:
Send to Office of Graduate Studies, Raubinger Hall, Room 139, William Paterson University, 300 Pompton Road, Wayne, NJ 07470. Application available online. URL of online application: http://www.wpunj.edu/admissions/graduate/apply-now.dot. Students are admitted in the Fall, application deadline May 1. *Fee:* $50.

NEW MEXICO

New Mexico Highlands University
Department of Social and Behavioral Sciences
College of Sciences and Mathematics
Hewett Hall
Las Vegas, NM 87701-4073
Telephone: (505) 454-3343
Fax: (505) 454-3331
E-mail: *iwilliamson@nmhu.edu*
Web: *http://www.nmhu.edu/academics/graduate/ gscienceandmath/socialandbehavioral/psychology/index.aspx*

Department Information:
1946. Psychology Program Coordinator: Ian Williamson. Number of faculty: total—full-time 4, part-time 3; women—full-time 3, part-time 2; minority—part-time 1.

Programs and Degrees Offered:
Listed in the following order: Program area, degree type (T if terminal Master's), number awarded 7/08–6/09. General/Clinical/Counseling Psychology MA/MS (Master of Arts/Science) (T) 3.

Student Applications/Admissions:
Student Applications
General/Clinical/Counseling Psychology MA/MS (*Master of Arts/Science*)—Applications 2009–2010, 24. Total applicants accepted 2009–2010, 19. Number full-time enrolled (new admits only) 2009–2010, 11. Number part-time enrolled (new admits only) 2009–2010, 0. Total enrolled 2009–2010 full-time, 11, part-time, 16. Openings 2010–2011, 15. The median number of years required for completion of a degree in 2008–2009 were 4. The number of students enrolled full- and part-time who were dismissed or voluntarily withdrew from this program area in 2008–2009 were 3.
Other Criteria: (importance of criteria rated low, medium, or high): research experience—medium, work experience—medium, extracurricular activity—low, clinically related public service—medium, GPA—high, letters of recommendation—medium, statement of goals and objectives—high, undergraduate major in psychology—low, specific undergraduate psychology courses taken—medium.

Student Characteristics: The following represents characteristics of students in 2009–2010 in all graduate psychology programs in the department: Female—full-time 7, part-time 11; Male—full-time 4, part-time 5; African American/Black—full-time 1, part-time 1; Hispanic/Latino(a)—full-time 3, part-time 6; Asian/Pacific Islander—full-time 0, part-time 0; American Indian/Alaska Native—full-time 0, part-time 0; Caucasian/White—full-time 7, part-time 9; Multi-ethnic—full-time 0, part-time 0; students subject to the Americans With Disabilities Act—full-time 0, part-time 0; Unknown ethnicity—full-time 0, part-time 0; International students who hold an F-1 or J-1 Visa—full-time 0, part-time 1.

Financial Information/Assistance:
Tuition for Full-Time Study: Master's: State residents: per academic year $2,937, $122 per credit hour; Nonstate residents: per academic year $4,526, $122 per credit hour. Tuition is subject to change. See the following Web site for updates and changes in tuition costs: http://www.nmhu.edu/future/tuition/index.aspx.

Financial Assistance:
First-Year Students: Teaching assistantships available for first year. Average amount paid per academic year: $6,500. Average number of hours worked per week: 20. Research assistantships available for first year. Average amount paid per academic year: $6,500. Average number of hours worked per week: 20. Fellowships and scholarships available for first year. Average amount paid per academic year: $6,500. Average number of hours worked per week: 20.

Advanced Students: Teaching assistantships available for advanced students. Average amount paid per academic year: $6,500. Average number of hours worked per week: 20. Research assistantships available for advanced students. Average amount paid per academic year: $6,500. Average number of hours worked per week: 20. Fellowships and scholarships available for advanced students. Average amount paid per academic year: $6,500. Average number of hours worked per week: 20.

Additional Information: Of all students currently enrolled full time, 100% benefited from one or more of the listed financial assistance programs.

Internships/Practica: Students in the Clinical Psychology/Counseling track must complete 12 credit hours of Field Experience. Completion of the 12 credit hours ensures that each student in this track gains 720 hours of direct clinical experience while completing the program. Field Experience placements are arranged through cooperative planning by the student, the program, and the agency. Students from our program have been placed with the following agencies: the forensic, adolescent, and adult units of the state psychiatric hospital; the local community mental health center; the state juvenile correctional facility; local schools; an equine therapy program; and many others.

Housing and Day Care: On-campus housing is available. See the following Web site for more information: http://www.nmhu.edu/future/housing/index.aspx. On-campus day care facilities are available. See the following Web site for more information: http://www.nmhu.edu/parentsandcounselors/Parents/childdevelopment/index.aspx.

Employment of Department Graduates:
Master's Degree Graduates: Of those who graduated in the academic year 2008–2009, the following categories and numbers represent the postgraduate activities and employment of master's degree graduates: Enrolled in a postdoctoral residency/fellowship (n/a), employed in independent practice (n/a), total from the above (master's) (0).
Doctoral Degree Graduates: Of those who graduated in the academic year 2008–2009, the following categories and numbers represent the postgraduate activities and employment of doctoral degree graduates: Enrolled in a psychology doctoral program (n/a), total from the above (doctoral) (0).

Additional Information:
Orientation, Objectives, and Emphasis of Department: The department offers two tracks that lead to a Master of Science degree in psychology. The General Psychology track requires 36 credit hours and is intended to provide a background similar to that given in many PhD programs. This track is organized around a general core of courses designed to educate the student in all areas of psychology with the opportunity to further pursue an area of interest such as physiological, experimental, neuropsychological, or social psychology. This track is especially useful for those students whose goals include either entering a doctoral program or working in a non-clinical position (research, etc.) upon completing the master's degree. The Clinical Psychology/Counseling track is a 67-credit hour emphasis area that is unique because it is one of the only programs in the U.S. that provides comprehensive training in psychological training and assessment in four areas: neuropsychological, behavioral, intelligence, and personality. This track is designed to prepare students to continue their education at the doctoral level or to work as a master's level clinician. The student successfully completing this track will qualify for licensure as a master's level clinician in approximately 40 states.

Special Facilities or Resources: The department offers laboratories for human subjects research, and is in the process of building a cognitive psychology laboratory. In addition, the department has an extensive computer laboratory. We also have relationships with members of the state psychiatric hospital, which is located in the community.

Application Information:
Send to Psychology Program Coordinator. URL of online application: http://www.nmhu.edu/future/admissions/index.aspx. Students are admitted in the Programs have rolling admissions. Earlier applications receive preferential treatment for financial aid. *Fee:* $15.

New Mexico State University
Counseling and Educational Psychology
College of Education
Box 30001 MSC 3CEP
Las Cruces, NM 88003-8001
Telephone: (575) 646-2121
Fax: (575) 646-8035
E-mail: *eadams@nmsu.edu*
Web: *http://education.nmsu.edu/cep/*

Department Information:
1905. Department Head: Jonathan Schwartz, PhD. Number of faculty: total—full-time 9, part-time 3; women—full-time 7, part-time 1; total—minority—full-time 6; women minority—full-time 5.

Programs and Degrees Offered:
Listed in the following order: Program area, degree type (T if terminal Master's), number awarded 7/08–6/09. Counseling and Guidance MA/MS (Master of Arts/Science) (T) 10, School Psychology EdS (School Psychology) 3, Counseling Psychology PhD (Doctor of Philosophy) 6.

APA Accreditation: Counseling PhD (Doctor of Philosophy). Student Outcome Data Website: http://education.nmsu.edu/cep/phd/.

Student Applications/Admissions:
Student Applications
Counseling and Guidance MA/MS (Master of Arts/Science)—Applications 2009–2010, 28. Total applicants accepted 2009–2010, 13. Number full-time enrolled (new admits only) 2009–2010, 6. Number part-time enrolled (new admits only) 2009–2010, 7. Total enrolled 2009–2010 full-time, 15, part-time, 15. Openings 2010–2011, 13. The median number of years required for completion of a degree in 2008–2009 were 2. The number of students enrolled full- and part-time who were dismissed or voluntarily withdrew from this program area in 2008–2009 were 1. *School Psychology EdS (School Psychology)*—Applications 2009–2010, 18. Total applicants accepted 2009–2010, 12. Number full-time enrolled (new admits only) 2009–2010, 6. Number part-time enrolled (new admits only) 2009–2010, 6. Total enrolled 2009–2010 full-time, 15, part-time, 11. Openings 2010–2011, 12. The median number of years required for completion of a degree in 2008–2009 were 3. The number of students enrolled full- and part-time who were dismissed or voluntarily withdrew from this program area in 2008–2009 were 3. *Counseling Psychology PhD (Doctor of Philosophy)*—Applications 2009–2010, 51. Total applicants accepted 2009–2010, 7. Number full-time enrolled (new admits only) 2009–2010, 6. Number part-time enrolled (new admits only) 2009–2010, 0. Openings 2010–2011, 6. The median number of years required for completion of a degree in 2008–2009 were 4. The number of students enrolled full- and part-time who were dismissed or voluntarily withdrew from this program area in 2008–2009 were 1.

Scores: Entries appear in this order: required test or GPA, minimum score (if required), median score of students entering in 2009–2010. *Counseling and Guidance MA/MS (Master of Arts/Science):* GRE-V no minimum stated, GRE-Q no minimum stated.

Other Criteria: (importance of criteria rated low, medium, or high): GRE scores—medium, research experience—high, work experience—medium, extracurricular activity—medium, clinically related public service—high, GPA—high, letters of recommendation—high, interview—high, statement of goals and objectives—high, writing sample—medium, undergraduate major in psychology—low, specific undergraduate psychology courses taken—low. Criteria do vary for different programs. For additional information on admission requirements, go to http://education.nmsu.edu/cep/.

Student Characteristics: The following represents characteristics of students in 2009–2010 in all graduate psychology programs in the department: Female—full-time 11, part-time 6; Male—full-time 7, part-time 0; African American/Black—full-time 0, part-time 0; Hispanic/Latino(a)—full-time 6, part-time 1; Asian/Pacific Islander—full-time 0, part-time 0; American Indian/Alaska Native—full-time 1, part-time 0; Caucasian/White—full-time 0, part-time 0; Multi-ethnic—full-time 0, part-time 0; students subject to the Americans With Disabilities Act—full-time 0, part-time 0; Unknown ethnicity—full-time 0, part-time 0; International students who hold an F-1 or J-1 Visa—full-time 0, part-time 0.

GRADUATE STUDY IN PSYCHOLOGY

Financial Information/Assistance:
  Tuition for Full-Time Study: *Master's:* State residents: per academic year $6,308, $200 per credit hour; Nonstate residents: per academic year $16,334, $625 per credit hour. *Doctoral:* State residents: per academic year $6,308, $200 per credit hour; Nonstate residents: per academic year $16,334, $625 per credit hour. Tuition is subject to change. See the following Web site for updates and changes in tuition costs: http://www.nmsu.edu/~uar/schcosts.

  Financial Assistance:
    First-Year Students: Teaching assistantships available for first year. Average amount paid per academic year: $8,000. Average number of hours worked per week: 10. Research assistantships available for first year. Average amount paid per academic year: $8,000. Average number of hours worked per week: 10. Fellowships and scholarships available for first year. Average amount paid per academic year: $4,500.
    Advanced Students: Teaching assistantships available for advanced students. Average amount paid per academic year: $8,000. Average number of hours worked per week: 10. Research assistantships available for advanced students. Average amount paid per academic year: $8,000. Average number of hours worked per week: 10. Fellowships and scholarships available for advanced students. Average amount paid per academic year: $4,500.
    Additional Information: Of all students currently enrolled full time, 60% benefited from one or more of the listed financial assistance programs. Application and information available online at: http://education.nmsu.edu/departments/academic/cep/phd/assistantships.html.

Internships/Practica: Doctoral Degree (PhD Counseling Psychology): For those doctoral students for whom a professional internship was required in this program prior to graduation, (3) students applied for an internship in 2008–2009, with (3) students obtaining an internship. Of those students who obtained an internship, (3) were paid internships. Of those students who obtained an internship, (3) students placed in APA/CPA accredited internships, (0) students placed in internships not APA/CPA accredited, but listed with the Association of Psychology Postdoctoral and Internship Programs (APPIC), (0) students placed in internships conforming to guidelines of the Council of Directors of School Psychology Programs (CDSPP), (0) students placed in internships that were not APA/CPA accredited, APPIC or CDSPP listed. Master's Degree (MA/MS Counseling and Guidance): An internship experience, such as a final research project or "capstone" experience is required of graduates. Practicum placements include university counseling centers, public schools, a primary care setting, community mental health centers, hospitals, adolescent residential centers, the Department of Vocational Rehabilitation, military bases, substance abuse treatment centers, and nursing homes.

Housing and Day Care: On-campus housing is available. See the following Web site for more information: http://www.nmsu.edu/~housing/. On-campus day care facilities are available. http://education.nmsu.edu/ci/earlychildhood/mcrj.html.

Employment of Department Graduates:
  Master's Degree Graduates: Of those who graduated in the academic year 2008–2009, the following categories and numbers represent the postgraduate activities and employment of master's degree graduates: Enrolled in a psychology doctoral program (2), enrolled in another graduate/professional program (0), enrolled in a postdoctoral residency/fellowship (n/a), employed in independent practice (n/a), employed in an academic position at a university (0), employed in an academic position at a 2-year/4-year college (0), employed in other positions at a higher education institution (0), employed in a professional position in a school system (3), employed in business or industry (0), employed in government agency (0), employed in a community mental health/counseling center (6), employed in a hospital/medical center (0), still seeking employment (0), not seeking employment (0), other employment position (0), do not know (0), total from the above (master's) (11).
  Doctoral Degree Graduates: Of those who graduated in the academic year 2008–2009, the following categories and numbers represent the postgraduate activities and employment of doctoral degree graduates: Enrolled in a psychology doctoral program (n/a), enrolled in another graduate/professional program (0), enrolled in a postdoctoral residency/fellowship (0), employed in independent practice (1), employed in an academic position at a university (1), employed in an academic position at a 2-year/4-year college (0), employed in other positions at a higher education institution (2), employed in a professional position in a school system (0), employed in business or industry (0), employed in government agency (0), employed in a community mental health/counseling center (1), employed in a hospital/medical center (2), still seeking employment (0), not seeking employment (1), other employment position (0), do not know (0), total from the above (doctoral) (8).

Additional Information:
  Orientation, Objectives, and Emphasis of Department: The major thrust of the department is the preparation of professionals for licensure and positions in counseling psychology, mental health and school counseling, school psychology, and related areas. Three graduate degrees are available: (1) Doctor of Philosophy, (2) Masters of Arts, and (3) Specialist in Education. The PhD in Counseling Psychology, which is accredited by the American Psychological Association, is based on the scientist–practitioner model through which both research and service delivery skills are acquired. Graduates of the program are prepared to conduct research, provide services, teach, and supervise. Emphases in the Counseling Psychology program include cultural diversity, generalist training in a variety of modalities, supervision and consultation. The Master of Arts in Counseling and Guidance prepares professional counselors to offer individual, family, and group counseling in schools, agencies, hospitals, and private practice. The curriculum covers human development; appraisal; diagnosis; treatment planning; individual, and professional issues. The School Psychology Program (EdS) prepares professionals for positions in public schools and other organizations which require advanced assessment, counseling, consultation and supervision skills. A major research project (thesis) is a degree requirement.

  Special Facilities or Resources: The Counseling and School Psychology Training and Research Center is a training/service facility sponsored by the Department of Counseling and Educational Psychology which provides excellent opportunities for supervised counseling and supervision-of-supervision. Four rooms are available for videotaping, which have one-way mirrors, telephones, and microphone-speakers for live supervision of counseling and live supervision of supervision. The facility has a "state-of-the-art" bug in the ear system which helps facilitate live supervision for immediate feedback to the counselor in training. We also have extensive training with similar supervisory capabilities at the Family Medicine Center, a primary care center staffed by Family Medicine residents and Counseling Psychology students.

Information for Students With Physical Disabilities: See the following Web site for more information: http://www.nmsu.edu/~ssd/.

Application Information:
Send to Department of Counseling & Educational Psychology, MSC 3CEP/Box 30001, Las Cruces, NM 88003-8001. Application available online. http://prospective.nmsu.edu/graduate.apply. Students are admitted in the Fall, application deadline March 1; The PhD Program deadline is December 15. The EdS Program deadline is January 15. The MA Program deadline is March 1. *Fee:* $30. McNair scholars can have their fees waived.

New Mexico State University
Department of Psychology
Department 3452, P.O. Box 30001
Las Cruces, NM 88003
Telephone: (575) 646-2502
Fax: (575) 646-6212
E-mail: *lmadson@nmsu.edu*
Web: *http://www-psych.nmsu.edu*

Department Information:
1950. Head: James E. McDonald. Number of faculty: total—full-time 13; women—full-time 3; faculty subject to the Americans With Disabilities Act 1.

Programs and Degrees Offered:
Listed in the following order: Program area, degree type (T if terminal Master's), number awarded 7/08–6/09. Engineering PhD (Doctor of Philosophy) 1, Social Psychology PhD (Doctor of Philosophy) 3, Cognitive Psychology PhD (Doctor of Philosophy) 1, General Experimental Psychology MA/MS (Master of Arts/Science) 7.

Student Applications/Admissions:
Student Applications
Engineering PhD (Doctor of Philosophy)—Applications 2009–2010, 0. Total applicants accepted 2009–2010, 1. Number full-time enrolled (new admits only) 2009–2010, 1. Number part-time enrolled (new admits only) 2009–2010, 0. Openings 2010–2011, 2. The median number of years required for completion of a degree in 2008–2009 were 4. The number of students enrolled full- and part-time who were dismissed or voluntarily withdrew from this program area in 2008–2009 were 0. Social Psychology PhD (Doctor of Philosophy)—Applications 2009–2010, 1. Total applicants accepted 2009–2010, 2. Number full-time enrolled (new admits only) 2009–2010, 2. Number part-time enrolled (new admits only) 2009–2010, 0. Openings 2010–2011, 2. The median number of years required for completion of a degree in 2008–2009 were 4. The number of students enrolled full- and part-time who were dismissed or voluntarily withdrew from this program area in 2008–2009 were 0. Cognitive Psychology PhD (Doctor of Philosophy)—Applications 2009–2010, 0. Total applicants accepted 2009–2010, 1. Number full-time enrolled (new admits only) 2009–2010, 1. Number part-time enrolled (new admits only) 2009–2010, 0. Openings 2010–2011, 2. The median number of years required for completion of a degree in 2008–2009 were 4. The number of students enrolled full- and part-time who were dismissed or voluntarily withdrew from this program area in 2008–2009 were 0. *General Experimental Psychology MA/MS (Master of Arts/Science)*—Applications 2009–2010, 35. Total applicants accepted 2009–2010, 16. Number full-time enrolled (new admits only) 2009–2010, 14. Number part-time enrolled (new admits only) 2009–2010, 0. Openings 2010–2011, 2. The median number of years required for completion of a degree in 2008–2009 were 2. The number of students enrolled full- and part-time who were dismissed or voluntarily withdrew from this program area in 2008–2009 were 0.

Scores: Entries appear in this order: required test or GPA, minimum score (if required), median score of students entering in 2009–2010. *Engineering PhD (Doctor of Philosophy):* GRE-V 560, GRE-Q 720, GRE-Analytical 5.0, overall undergraduate GPA 3.0, Masters GPA 3.0; *Social Psychology PhD (Doctor of Philosophy):* GRE-V 560, GRE-Q 720, GRE-Analytical 5.0, overall undergraduate GPA 3.0, Masters GPA 3.0; *Cognitive Psychology PhD (Doctor of Philosophy):* GRE-V 560, GRE-Q 720, GRE-Analytical 5.0, overall undergraduate GPA 3.0, Masters GPA 3.0; *General Experimental Psychology MA/MS (Master of Arts/Science):* GRE-V 500, GRE-Q 600, GRE-Analytical 4.0, overall undergraduate GPA 3.0.

Other Criteria: (importance of criteria rated low, medium, or high): GRE scores—high, research experience—medium, work experience—low, GPA—high, letters of recommendation—high, statement of goals and objectives—high, undergraduate major in psychology—medium, specific undergraduate psychology courses taken—low. For additional information on admission requirements, go to http://www-psych.nmsu.edu.

Student Characteristics: The following represents characteristics of students in 2009–2010 in all graduate psychology programs in the department: Female—full-time 19, part-time 0; Male—full-time 21, part-time 0; African American/Black—full-time 0, part-time 0; Hispanic/Latino(a)—full-time 3, part-time 0; Asian/Pacific Islander—full-time 0, part-time 0; American Indian/Alaska Native—part-time 0; Caucasian/White—full-time 32, part-time 0; Multi-ethnic—full-time 0, part-time 0; students subject to the Americans With Disabilities Act—full-time 0, part-time 0; Unknown ethnicity—full-time 5, part-time 0; International students who hold an F-1 or J-1 Visa—full-time 5, part-time 0.

Financial Information/Assistance:
Tuition for Full-Time Study: Master's: State residents: per academic year $2,679, $223 per credit hour; Nonstate residents: per academic year $7,767, $647 per credit hour. Doctoral: State residents: per academic year $2,679, $223 per credit hour; Nonstate residents: per academic year $7,767, $647 per credit hour. Tuition is subject to change. Additional fees are assessed to students beyond the costs of tuition for the following: health/activity fees, Associated Students of NMSU fee,. See the following Web site for updates and changes in tuition costs: http://www.nmsu.edu/~uar/schcosts.htm.

Financial Assistance:
First-Year Students: Teaching assistantships available for first year. Average amount paid per academic year: $16,000. Aver-

age number of hours worked per week: 20. Apply by February 1. Research assistantships available for first year. Average amount paid per academic year: $16,000. Average number of hours worked per week: 20. Apply by February 1. Fellowships and scholarships available for first year. Apply by February 1.

Advanced Students: Teaching assistantships available for advanced students. Average amount paid per academic year: $16,000. Average number of hours worked per week: 20. Apply by February 1. Research assistantships available for advanced students. Average amount paid per academic year: $16,000. Average number of hours worked per week: 20. Apply by February 1. Fellowships and scholarships available for advanced students. Apply by February 1.

Additional Information: Of all students currently enrolled full time, 100% benefited from one or more of the listed financial assistance programs. Application and information available online at: http://gradschool.nmsu.edu/fellowships/.

Internships/Practica: For the PhD degree in Engineering Psychology, students must complete an internship in an industrial, government, or other laboratory setting of at least three months duration. Many master's students in Engineering Psychology and Cognitive Psychology spend a summer or half-year as an intern in industry, but it is not required for the MA degree.

Housing and Day Care: On-campus housing is available. On-campus day care facilities are available.

Employment of Department Graduates:

Master's Degree Graduates: Of those who graduated in the academic year 2008–2009, the following categories and numbers represent the postgraduate activities and employment of master's degree graduates: Enrolled in a psychology doctoral program (2), enrolled in another graduate/professional program (0), enrolled in a postdoctoral residency/fellowship (n/a), employed in independent practice (n/a), do not know (5), total from the above (master's) (7).

Doctoral Degree Graduates: Of those who graduated in the academic year 2008–2009, the following categories and numbers represent the postgraduate activities and employment of doctoral degree graduates: Enrolled in a psychology doctoral program (n/a), enrolled in another graduate/professional program (0), enrolled in a postdoctoral residency/fellowship (2), employed in independent practice (0), employed in an academic position at a university (0), employed in an academic position at a 2-year/4-year college (0), employed in other positions at a higher education institution (0), employed in a professional position in a school system (0), employed in business or industry (0), employed in government agency (1), employed in a community mental health/counseling center (0), employed in a hospital/medical center (0), still seeking employment (0), not seeking employment (0), other employment position (0), do not know (0), total from the above (doctoral) (3).

Additional Information:

Orientation, Objectives, and Emphasis of Department: The department offers an MA degree in general experimental psychology that allows an emphasis in cognitive, engineering, or social psychology. The PhD is offered in the major areas of cognitive, engineering, and social psychology. Students must earn an MA degree before being admitted to the doctoral program. All programs are experimentally oriented and have the distinctive characteristic of pursuing and extending basic research questions in applied settings.

Special Facilities or Resources: All faculty members have specialized laboratories with a wide variety of computer hardware and software. These include auditory perception and eye tracking labs used to study perceptual and cognitive issues, a biopsychology lab equipped to measure ERPs, an automation lab used to study human interactions with automated systems including unmanned aerial vehicles, and a developmental laboratory equipped with sophisticated equipment for recording, analyzing, and editing mother-infant interactions, etc.

Information for Students With Physical Disabilities: See the following Web site for more information: http://www.nmsu.edu/~ssd/.

Application Information:
Send to Chair of Graduate Committee, Department of Psychology, MSC 3452 New Mexico State University, Las Cruces, NM 88003-8001. Application available online. URL of online application: http://gradschool.nmsu.edu/admit-form.html. Students are admitted in the Fall, application deadline February 1. *Fee:* $30.

New Mexico, University of
Department of Psychology
Arts and Science
Logan Hall, MSC03 2220
Albuquerque, NM 87131-1161
Telephone: (505) 277-4121
Fax: (505) 277-1394
E-mail: *psych@unm.edu*
Web: *http://psych.unm.edu*

Department Information:
1960. Chairperson: Jane Ellen Smith. Number of faculty: total—full-time 25, part-time 2; women—full-time 9, part-time 2; total—minority—full-time 2, part-time 1; women minority—full-time 1, part-time 1.

Programs and Degrees Offered:
Listed in the following order: Program area, degree type (T if terminal Master's), number awarded 7/08–6/09. Clinical Psychology PhD (Doctor of Philosophy) 2, Developmental Psychology PhD (Doctor of Philosophy) 0, Evolutionary Psychology PhD (Doctor of Philosophy) 0, Cognition, Brain and Behavior PhD (Doctor of Philosophy) 1, Health Psychology PhD (Doctor of Philosophy) 0.

APA Accreditation: Clinical PhD (Doctor of Philosophy). Student Outcome Data Website: http://psych.unm.edu/clinical.html.

Student Applications/Admissions:
Student Applications
Clinical Psychology PhD (Doctor of Philosophy)—Applications 2009–2010, 133. Total applicants accepted 2009–2010, 11. Number full-time enrolled (new admits only) 2009–2010, 7. Number part-time enrolled (new admits only) 2009–2010, 0.

Openings 2010–2011, 7. The median number of years required for completion of a degree in 2008–2009 were 6. The number of students enrolled full- and part-time who were dismissed or voluntarily withdrew from this program area in 2008–2009 were 0. *Developmental Psychology PhD (Doctor of Philosophy)*— Applications 2009–2010, 2. Total applicants accepted 2009–2010, 0. Number full-time enrolled (new admits only) 2009–2010, 0. Number part-time enrolled (new admits only) 2009–2010, 0. Openings 2010–2011, 1. The number of students enrolled full- and part-time who were dismissed or voluntarily withdrew from this program area in 2008–2009 were 0. *Evolutionary Psychology PhD (Doctor of Philosophy)*—Applications 2009–2010, 19. Total applicants accepted 2009–2010, 0. Number full-time enrolled (new admits only) 2009–2010, 0. Number part-time enrolled (new admits only) 2009–2010, 0. Openings 2010–2011, 1. The number of students enrolled full- and part-time who were dismissed or voluntarily withdrew from this program area in 2008–2009 were 0. *Cognition, Brain and Behavior PhD (Doctor of Philosophy)*—Applications 2009–2010, 30. Total applicants accepted 2009–2010, 3. Number full-time enrolled (new admits only) 2009–2010, 3. Number part-time enrolled (new admits only) 2009–2010, 0. Openings 2010–2011, 3. The median number of years required for completion of a degree in 2008–2009 were 5. The number of students enrolled full- and part-time who were dismissed or voluntarily withdrew from this program area in 2008–2009 were 0. *Health Psychology PhD (Doctor of Philosophy)*—Applications 2009–2010, 17. Total applicants accepted 2009–2010, 1. Number full-time enrolled (new admits only) 2009–2010, 1. Total enrolled 2009–2010 full-time, 2. Openings 2010–2011, 1. The number of students enrolled full- and part-time who were dismissed or voluntarily withdrew from this program area in 2008–2009 were 0.

Scores: Entries appear in this order: required test or GPA, minimum score (if required), median score of students entering in 2009–2010. *Clinical Psychology PhD (Doctor of Philosophy):* GRE-V no minimum stated, 555, GRE-Q no minimum stated, 640, GRE-Analytical no minimum stated, 4.7, GRE-Subject (Psychology) no minimum stated, 648, overall undergraduate GPA no minimum stated, 3.55, Masters GPA no minimum stated, 3.76; *Developmental Psychology PhD (Doctor of Philosophy):* GRE-V no minimum stated, 555, GRE-Q no minimum stated, 640, GRE-Analytical no minimum stated, 4.7, GRE-Subject (Psychology) no minimum stated, 648, overall undergraduate GPA no minimum stated, 3.55, Masters GPA no minimum stated, 3.76; *Evolutionary Psychology PhD (Doctor of Philosophy):* GRE-V no minimum stated, 555, GRE-Q no minimum stated, 640, GRE-Analytical no minimum stated, 4.7, GRE-Subject (Psychology) no minimum stated, 648, overall undergraduate GPA no minimum stated, 3.55, Masters GPA no minimum stated, 3.76; *Cognition, Brain and Behavior PhD (Doctor of Philosophy):* GRE-V no minimum stated, 555, GRE-Q no minimum stated, 640, GRE-Analytical no minimum stated, 4.7, GRE-Subject (Psychology) no minimum stated, 648, overall undergraduate GPA no minimum stated, 3.55, Masters GPA no minimum stated, 3.76; *Health Psychology PhD (Doctor of Philosophy):* GRE-V no minimum stated, 555, GRE-Q no minimum stated, 640, GRE-Analytical no minimum stated, 4.7, GRE-Subject (Psychology) no minimum stated, 648, overall undergraduate GPA no minimum stated, 3.55, Masters GPA no minimum stated, 3.76.

Other Criteria: (importance of criteria rated low, medium, or high): GRE scores—high, research experience—high, work experience—medium, extracurricular activity—medium, clinically related public service—medium, GPA—high, letters of recommendation—high, interview—high, statement of goals and objectives—high, undergraduate major in psychology—high, specific undergraduate psychology courses taken—high. For additional information on admission requirements, go to http://psych.unm.edu/grad_welcome.html.

Student Characteristics: The following represents characteristics of students in 2009–2010 in all graduate psychology programs in the department: Female—full-time 58, part-time 0; Male—full-time 26, part-time 0; African American/Black—full-time 0, part-time 0; Hispanic/Latino(a)—full-time 11, part-time 0; Asian/Pacific Islander—full-time 6, part-time 0; American Indian/Alaska Native—full-time 0, part-time 0; Caucasian/White—full-time 63, part-time 0; Multi-ethnic—full-time 1, part-time 0; students subject to the Americans With Disabilities Act—full-time 0, part-time 0; Unknown ethnicity—full-time 3, part-time 0; International students who hold an F-1 or J-1 Visa—full-time 8, part-time 0.

Financial Information/Assistance:

Tuition for Full-Time Study: *Master's:* State residents: per academic year $5,546; Nonstate residents: per academic year $17,682. *Doctoral:* State residents: per academic year $5,546; Nonstate residents: per academic year $17,682. Tuition is subject to change. Additional fees are assessed to students beyond the costs of tuition for the following: GPSA, course fees. See the following Web site for updates and changes in tuition costs: http://www.unm.edu/~bursar/tuitionrates.html.

Financial Assistance:

First-Year Students: Teaching assistantships available for first year. Average amount paid per academic year: $12,467. Average number of hours worked per week: 20. Apply by January 15. Research assistantships available for first year. Average amount paid per academic year: $12,467. Average number of hours worked per week: 20. Apply by January 15.

Advanced Students: Teaching assistantships available for advanced students. Average amount paid per academic year: $14,791. Average number of hours worked per week: 20. Apply by January 15. Research assistantships available for advanced students. Average amount paid per academic year: $14,791. Average number of hours worked per week: 20. Apply by January 15.

Additional Information: Of all students currently enrolled full time, 80% benefited from one or more of the listed financial assistance programs. Application and information available online at: http://www.unm.edu/~grad/indices/index_funding.html.

Internships/Practica: Doctoral Degree (PhD Clinical Psychology): For those doctoral students for whom a professional internship was required in this program prior to graduation, (6) students applied for an internship in 2008–2009, with (6) students obtaining an internship. Of those students who obtained an internship, (6) were paid internships. Of those students who obtained an internship, (6) students placed in APA/CPA accredited internships, (0) students placed in internships not APA/CPA accredited, but listed with the Association of Psychology Postdoctoral and Internship Programs (APPIC), (0) students placed in internships conforming to guidelines of the Council of Directors of

School Psychology Programs (CDSPP), (0) students placed in internships that were not APA/CPA accredited, APPIC or CDSPP listed.

Housing and Day Care: On-campus housing is available. See the following Web site for more information: http://housing.unm.edu/home.htm. On-campus day care facilities are available. See the following Web site for more information: http://childcare.unm.edu/.

Employment of Department Graduates:
Master's Degree Graduates: Of those who graduated in the academic year 2008–2009, the following categories and numbers represent the postgraduate activities and employment of master's degree graduates: Enrolled in a postdoctoral residency/fellowship (n/a), employed in independent practice (n/a), total from the above (master's) (0).
Doctoral Degree Graduates: Of those who graduated in the academic year 2008–2009, the following categories and numbers represent the postgraduate activities and employment of doctoral degree graduates: Enrolled in a psychology doctoral program (n/a), total from the above (doctoral) (0).

Additional Information:
Orientation, Objectives, and Emphasis of Department: Founded in 1960, the doctoral training program in psychology is based on the premise that psychology, in all of its areas, is fundamentally an experimental discipline. For all students, the PhD degree is awarded in general experimental psychology, and students acquire a solid foundation in both scientific methodology and general psychology. Within this framework, students specialize in any of several competency areas. The well-trained psychologist, within this perspective, is one who combines competence in the general discipline of psychology with excellence in his or her chosen specialization.

Special Facilities or Resources: The department is housed in a building on the central campus. In addition to faculty and administrative offices and seminar rooms, the building is equipped for sophisticated research. There are soundproof chambers for conducting experiments, a variety of timing devices, computer terminals, and electromechanical measuring equipment. Laboratory facilities exist for research in human memory, learning, cognitive psychology, perception, information processing, attention, decision making, developmental, social, personality, neuropsychology, psychophysiology, and clinical psychology. The building also has a large animal research facility with primates and rodents. The campus animal research facility is equipped for surgery and for delicate measurements of brain activities as well as for tests of physical, cognitive, and emotional responses. Microcomputers are widely used in individual faculty laboratories and in a graduate student computer room. The Department of Psychology Clinic opened in 1982 and offers diagnostic and therapeutic services to the Albuquerque community while providing an excellent training facility for clinical students.

Information for Students With Physical Disabilities: See the following Web site for more information: http://as2.unm.edu/index.html.

Application Information:
Send to Graduate Admissions Coordinator, 1 University of New Mexico, Department of Psychology, MSC03 2220, Albuquerque, NM 87131. Application available online. URL of online application: http://psych.unm.edu/grad_welcome.html. Students are admitted in the Fall, application deadline January 15. The deadline for full financial consideration is January 15, we accept applications through May 1 ONLY IF positions remain. *Fee:* $50.

NEW YORK

Adelphi University (2009 data)
The Derner Institute of Advanced Psychological Studies,
 School of Professional Psychology
Adelphi University
158 Cambridge Avenue
Garden City, NY 11530
Telephone: (516) 877-4185
Fax: (516) 877-4805
E-mail: *chin@adelphi.edu*
Web: *http://derner.adelphi.edu*

Department Information:
1952. Dean: Jean Lau Chin. Number of faculty: total—full-time 25, part-time 172; women—full-time 11, part-time 95; total—minority—full-time 5, part-time 12; women minority—full-time 5, part-time 10.

Programs and Degrees Offered:
Listed in the following order: Program area, degree type (T if terminal Master's), number awarded 7/08–6/09. Clinical PhD (Doctor of Philosophy) 25, Psychoanalysis Other 28, Respecialization Diploma 0, General Psychology MA/MS (Master of Arts/Science) (T) 44, Mental Health Counseling MA/MS (Master of Arts/Science) (T) 17, School Psychology MA/MS (Master of Arts/Science) (T) 17.

APA Accreditation: Clinical PhD (Doctor of Philosophy).

Student Applications/Admissions:
Student Applications
Clinical PhD (Doctor of Philosophy)—Applications 2009–2010, 226. Total applicants accepted 2009–2010, 49. Number full-time enrolled (new admits only) 2009–2010, 20. Openings 2010–2011, 20. The median number of years required for completion of a degree in 2008–2009 were 6. The number of students enrolled full- and part-time who were dismissed or voluntarily withdrew from this program area in 2008–2009 were 1. *Psychoanalysis Other*—Applications 2009–2010, 50. Total applicants accepted 2009–2010, 48. Number full-time enrolled (new admits only) 2009–2010, 0. Number part-time enrolled (new admits only) 2009–2010, 47. Openings 2010–2011, 45. The median number of years required for completion of a degree in 2008–2009 were 3. The number of students enrolled full- and part-time who were dismissed or voluntarily withdrew from this program area in 2008–2009 were 8. *Respecialization Diploma*—Applications 2009–2010, 2. Total applicants accepted 2009–2010, 1. Number part-time enrolled (new admits only) 2009–2010, 1. Openings 2010–2011, 2. The number of students enrolled full- and part-time who were dismissed or voluntarily withdrew from this program area in 2008–2009 were 0. *General Psychology MA/MS (Master of Arts/Science)*—Applications 2009–2010, 128. Total applicants accepted 2009–2010, 60. Number full-time enrolled (new admits only) 2009–2010, 40. Number part-time enrolled (new admits only) 2009–2010, 20. Total enrolled 2009–2010 full-time, 75, part-time, 50. Openings 2010–2011, 60. The median number of years required for completion of a degree in 2008–2009 was 1. The number of students enrolled full- and part-time who were dismissed or voluntarily withdrew from this program area in 2008–2009 were 6. *Mental Health Counseling MA/MS (Master of Arts/Science)*—Applications 2009–2010, 43. Total applicants accepted 2009–2010, 22. Number full-time enrolled (new admits only) 2009–2010, 20. Total enrolled 2009–2010 full-time, 55. Openings 2010–2011, 20. The median number of years required for completion of a degree in 2008–2009 were 2. The number of students enrolled full- and part-time who were dismissed or voluntarily withdrew from this program area in 2008–2009 were 3. *School Psychology MA/MS (Master of Arts/Science)*—Applications 2009–2010, 120. Total applicants accepted 2009–2010, 60. Number full-time enrolled (new admits only) 2009–2010, 31. Number part-time enrolled (new admits only) 2009–2010, 0. Openings 2010–2011, 30. The median number of years required for completion of a degree in 2008–2009 were 3. The number of students enrolled full- and part-time who were dismissed or voluntarily withdrew from this program area in 2008–2009 were 1.

Other Criteria: (importance of criteria rated low, medium, or high): GRE scores—high, research experience—high, work experience—high, extracurricular activity—low, clinically related public service—high, GPA—high, letters of recommendation—high, interview—high, statement of goals and objectives—high, specific undergraduate psychology courses taken—high.

Student Characteristics: The following represents characteristics of students in 2009–2010 in all graduate psychology programs in the department: Female—full-time 171, part-time 91; Male—full-time 90, part-time 49; African American/Black—full-time 6, part-time 35; Hispanic/Latino(a)—full-time 6, part-time 8; Asian/Pacific Islander—full-time 10, part-time 5; American Indian/Alaska Native—full-time 0, part-time 0; Caucasian/White—full-time 0, part-time 0; Multi-ethnic—full-time 0, part-time 0; students subject to the Americans With Disabilities Act—full-time 0, part-time 0; Unknown ethnicity—full-time 0, part-time 0; International students who hold an F-1 or J-1 Visa—full-time 0, part-time 0.

Financial Information/Assistance:
Tuition for Full-Time Study: *Master's:* State residents: $755 per credit hour; Nonstate residents: $755 per credit hour. *Doctoral:* State residents: per academic year $30,000; Nonstate residents: per academic year $30,000.

Financial Assistance:
First-Year Students: Teaching assistantships available for first year. Average amount paid per academic year: $7,500. Average number of hours worked per week: 7. Apply by April 15. Research assistantships available for first year. Average amount paid per academic year: $7,500. Average number of hours worked per week: 7. Apply by April 15.

Advanced Students: Teaching assistantships available for advanced students. Average amount paid per academic year: $7,500. Average number of hours worked per week: 7. Apply by April 15. Research assistantships available for advanced students.

Average amount paid per academic year: $7,500. Average number of hours worked per week: 7. Apply by April 15.

Additional Information: Of all students currently enrolled full time, 85% benefited from one or more of the listed financial assistance programs.

Internships/Practica: Doctoral Degree (PhD Clinical): For those doctoral students for whom a professional internship was required in this program prior to graduation, (18) students applied for an internship in 2008–2009, with (17) students obtaining an internship. Of those students who obtained an internship, (17) were paid internships. Of those students who obtained an internship, (17) students placed in APA/CPA accredited internships, (0) students placed in internships not APA/CPA accredited, but listed with the Association of Psychology Postdoctoral and Internship Programs (APPIC), (0) students placed in internships conforming to guidelines of the Council of Directors of School Psychology Programs (CDSPP), (0) students placed in internships that were not APA/CPA accredited, APPIC or CDSPP listed. For the doctoral program, students are assigned to the Psychological Services Clinic, the training facility of the PhD Program. Beginning in the first year of the doctoral program, students are trained to perform intake evaluations. In the following years, students are to perform psychodiagnostic evaluations and psychotherapy. Students are also assigned to externships at full service mental health centers during their second year of training. During their fifth year, students complete a one-year internship in clinical psychology. For the postdoctoral program, students are assigned to the Postdoctoral Psychotherapy Center, the training facility of the postdoctoral program.

Housing and Day Care: On-campus housing is available. http://www.adelphi.edu/elc.

Employment of Department Graduates:
Master's Degree Graduates: Of those who graduated in the academic year 2008–2009, the following categories and numbers represent the postgraduate activities and employment of master's degree graduates: Enrolled in a psychology doctoral program (24), enrolled in another graduate/professional program (14), enrolled in a postdoctoral residency/fellowship (n/a), employed in independent practice (n/a), employed in a professional position in a school system (15), employed in business or industry (6), employed in a community mental health/counseling center (7), employed in a hospital/medical center (7), do not know (5), total from the above (master's) (78).
Doctoral Degree Graduates: Of those who graduated in the academic year 2008–2009, the following categories and numbers represent the postgraduate activities and employment of doctoral degree graduates: Enrolled in a psychology doctoral program (n/a), enrolled in a postdoctoral residency/fellowship (3), employed in independent practice (2), employed in an academic position at a university (2), employed in other positions at a higher education institution (2), employed in a community mental health/counseling center (5), employed in a hospital/medical center (9), total from the above (doctoral) (23).

Additional Information:
Orientation, Objectives, and Emphasis of Department: The Derner Institute of Advanced Psychological Studies is the first university-based professional school of psychology. The orientation is psychodynamic and scholar-professional. The doctoral program in clinical and the respecialization program are oriented toward community service and prepare the students for careers in clinical service; the postdoctoral programs prepare graduates for the practice of psychoanalysis and psychotherapy. All doctoral programs offer supervised experience in research and theory. The clinical program consists of four years of coursework, which includes at least one day a week of supervised practice each year and a fifth-year full-time internship; the respecialization program consists of two years of coursework, including at least one day a week of supervised practice each year and a third-year full-time internship; the postdoctoral programs consist of four years of seminars, case conferences, personal therapy, and supervised practice, the master's program consists of two years of course work, which includes a thesis or project. A new MA program in School Psychology was begun in Spring 2003; it is a three-year program, with a joint emphasis on didactic instruction and supervised practice. A new MA program in Mental Health Counseling, also with a joint emphasis on didactic instruction and supervised practice, was begun in Fall 2004.

Special Facilities or Resources: Facilities include a videotape recording studio and perception, learning, developmental, cognition, and applied research laboratories. The Institute has close interaction with two health-related professional schools, the Adelphi School of Nursing and the Adelphi School of Social Work, and with affiliated community school and clinical facilities. The Institute maintains two major clinical facilities, the Adelphi University Psychological Services Center and the Postdoctoral Psychotherapy Center. An APA-accredited continuing education program brings a series of distinguished workshops to the campus.

Application Information:
Send to Graduate Admissions. Application available online. URL of online application: https://www.applyweb.com/apply/adelphi/menu.html. Students are admitted in the Fall, application deadline January 15; Spring, application deadline. Applicants for the PhD program have a January 15 deadline. MA applicants may begin in either Fall or Spring semester. There is no application deadline for the MA in General Psychology. For School Psychology the application deadline March 1. For the MA program in Mental health Counseling the deadline is April 1. Postdoctoral applicants begin in Fall only, but there is no application deadline. *Fee:* $50. Graduate admissions will waive application fee if a request for waiver is completed.

Alfred University
Division of School Psychology
Graduate School
Saxon Drive
Alfred, NY 14802-1205
Telephone: (607) 871-2212
Fax: (607) 871-3422
E-mail: *fevangel@alfred.edu*
Web: *http://www.alfred.edu*

Department Information:
1953. Chairperson: Nancy J. Evangelista. Number of faculty: total—full-time 7, part-time 7; women—full-time 3, part-time 4; total—minority—full-time 1; faculty subject to the Americans With Disabilities Act 1.

Programs and Degrees Offered:
Listed in the following order: Program area, degree type (T if terminal Master's), number awarded 7/08–6/09. School Psychology EdS (School Psychology) 16, School Psychology PsyD (Doctor of Psychology) 3.

APA Accreditation: School PsyD (Doctor of Psychology). Student Outcome Data Website: http://www.alfred.edu/gradschool/school-psychology/psyd-specialization.cfm.

Student Applications/Admissions:

Student Applications

School Psychology EdS (School Psychology)—Applications 2009–2010, 50. Total applicants accepted 2009–2010, 27. Number full-time enrolled (new admits only) 2009–2010, 17. Number part-time enrolled (new admits only) 2009–2010, 0. Openings 2010–2011, 15. The median number of years required for completion of a degree in 2008–2009 were 3. The number of students enrolled full- and part-time who were dismissed or voluntarily withdrew from this program area in 2008–2009 were 0. School Psychology PsyD (Doctor of Psychology)—Applications 2009–2010, 32. Total applicants accepted 2009–2010, 12. Number full-time enrolled (new admits only) 2009–2010, 5. Number part-time enrolled (new admits only) 2009–2010, 0. Total enrolled 2009–2010 full-time, 26, part-time, 26. Openings 2010–2011, 7. The median number of years required for completion of a degree in 2008–2009 were 6. The number of students enrolled full- and part-time who were dismissed or voluntarily withdrew from this program area in 2008–2009 were 3.

Scores: Entries appear in this order: required test or GPA, minimum score (if required), median score of students entering in 2009–2010. School Psychology EdS (School Psychology): GRE-V no minimum stated, 460, GRE-Q no minimum stated, 530, GRE-Analytical no minimum stated, 4.5, overall undergraduate GPA no minimum stated, 3.48; School Psychology PsyD (Doctor of Psychology): GRE-V no minimum stated, 520, GRE-Q no minimum stated, 610, GRE-Analytical no minimum stated, 4.5, overall undergraduate GPA no minimum stated, 3.58.

Other Criteria: (importance of criteria rated low, medium, or high): GRE scores—medium, research experience—medium, work experience—medium, extracurricular activity—medium, clinically related public service—low, GPA—high, letters of recommendation—high, interview—high, statement of goals and objectives—high, undergraduate major in psychology—medium, specific undergraduate psychology courses taken—high. The PsyD program places a higher emphasis on research experience as an undergraduate, and requires a statement of research interests. For additional information on admission requirements, go to http://www.alfred.edu/gradschool/school-psychology/applying.cfm.

Student Characteristics: The following represents characteristics of students in 2009–2010 in all graduate psychology programs in the department: Female—full-time 54, part-time 22; Male—full-time 12, part-time 4; African American/Black—full-time 1, part-time 2; Hispanic/Latino(a)—full-time 2, part-time 1; Asian/Pacific Islander—full-time 0, part-time 0; American Indian/Alaska Native—full-time 0, part-time 0; Caucasian/White—full-time 62, part-time 22; Multi-ethnic—full-time 1, part-time 1; students subject to the Americans With Disabilities Act—full-time 1, part-time 0; Unknown ethnicity—full-time 0, part-time 0; International students who hold an F-1 or J-1 Visa—full-time 0, part-time 0.

Financial Information/Assistance:

Tuition for Full-Time Study: *Master's:* State residents: per academic year $34,294, $730 per credit hour; Nonstate residents: per academic year $34,294, $703 per credit hour. *Doctoral:* State residents: per academic year $34,294, $730 per credit hour; Nonstate residents: per academic year $34,294, $730 per credit hour. Tuition is subject to change. Additional fees are assessed to students beyond the costs of tuition for the following: student activity fee, lab fees for assessment courses. See the following Web site for updates and changes in tuition costs: http://www.alfred.edu/finaid/graduate/cost.cfm.

Financial Assistance:

First-Year Students: Research assistantships available for first year. Average amount paid per academic year: $17,147. Average number of hours worked per week: 7. Apply by None. Fellowships and scholarships available for first year. Average amount paid per academic year: $15,812. Average number of hours worked per week: 0. Apply by January 5.

Advanced Students: Teaching assistantships available for advanced students. Average amount paid per academic year: $16,648. Average number of hours worked per week: 7. Apply by None. Research assistantships available for advanced students. Average amount paid per academic year: $17,147. Average number of hours worked per week: 7. Apply by None. Traineeships available for advanced students. Average amount paid per academic year: $34,294. Average number of hours worked per week: 15. Apply by Variable.

Additional Information: Of all students currently enrolled full time, 100% benefited from one or more of the listed financial assistance programs.

Internships/Practica: Doctoral Degree (PsyD School Psychology): For those doctoral students for whom a professional internship was required in this program prior to graduation, (9) students applied for an internship in 2008–2009, with (9) students obtaining an internship. Of those students who obtained an internship, (9) were paid internships. Of those students who obtained an internship, (1) students placed in APA/CPA accredited internships, (0) students placed in internships not APA/CPA accredited, but listed with the Association of Psychology Postdoctoral and Internship Programs (APPIC), (8) students placed in internships conforming to guidelines of the Council of Directors of School Psychology Programs (CDSPP), (0) students placed in internships that were not APA/CPA accredited, APPIC or CDSPP listed. Master's and doctoral students may pursue internships anyplace in the United States. Most master's students choose sites at public schools across New York State and northern Pennsylvania. Doctoral students are required to complete a portion of their internship in a school setting, but many also choose sites and internship experiences in both school and clinical settings. A portion of doctoral students each year choose to intern at APPIC and APA accredited sites.

Housing and Day Care: On-campus housing is available. On-campus day care facilities are available.

Employment of Department Graduates:
Master's Degree Graduates: Of those who graduated in the academic year 2008–2009, the following categories and numbers represent the postgraduate activities and employment of master's degree graduates: Enrolled in a psychology doctoral program (1), enrolled in another graduate/professional program (0), enrolled in a postdoctoral residency/fellowship (n/a), employed in independent practice (n/a), employed in an academic position at a university (1), employed in an academic position at a 2-year/4-year college (0), employed in other positions at a higher education institution (0), employed in a professional position in a school system (13), employed in business or industry (0), employed in government agency (0), employed in a community mental health/counseling center (2), employed in a hospital/medical center (0), still seeking employment (0), not seeking employment (0), other employment position (0), do not know (0), total from the above (master's) (17).
Doctoral Degree Graduates: Of those who graduated in the academic year 2008–2009, the following categories and numbers represent the postgraduate activities and employment of doctoral degree graduates: Enrolled in a psychology doctoral program (n/a), enrolled in another graduate/professional program (0), enrolled in a postdoctoral residency/fellowship (0), employed in independent practice (0), employed in an academic position at a university (0), employed in an academic position at a 2-year/4-year college (0), employed in other positions at a higher education institution (0), employed in a professional position in a school system (2), employed in business or industry (0), employed in government agency (0), employed in a community mental health/counseling center (1), employed in a hospital/medical center (0), still seeking employment (0), not seeking employment (0), other employment position (0), do not know (0), total from the above (doctoral) (3).

Additional Information:
Orientation, Objectives, and Emphasis of Department: The Alfred School Psychology program emphasizes a field-centered, systems-oriented, practitioner-scientist approach. The primary goal of the program is the preparation of problem-solving psychologists with special concern for the application of psychological knowledge in a variety of child and family related settings. Students acquire knowledge in a wide variety of psychological theories and practices; skills are learned and then demonstrated in a number of different applied settings. They develop the personal characteristics and academic competencies necessary to work effectively with others in the identification, prevention and remediation of psychological and educational problems with children and adults. Training in school psychology at Alfred University offers extensive one-to-one contact between students and faculty members to encourage the personalized learning process. PsyD students are involved in field experience and research orientation from the first semester on. Training in the following areas is provided: knowledge base in psychology and education, assessment, intervention and remediation including counseling, play therapy and family work, consulting/training with teachers, administrators and parents, research methodology, program evaluation, and professional identification and functioning. Training at the doctoral level emphasizes applied research and the development of an area of specialization.

Special Facilities or Resources: Departmental resources include an extensive library of psychological and educational assessment materials, an audio-video tape library, and library of counseling and intervention materials. All students gain practicum experience in the on-campus Child and Family Services Center, operated by the Division of Counseling and School Psychology. The Center provides consultation, assessment, and counseling services to children and families of the region. The Center is a state of the art facility with all therapy and consultation rooms equipped with observation mirrors and remote audio-video recording equipment. The Center serves training, service and research functions for faculty and students. Graduate students have a work/computer room and a spacious lounge. Additionally, all graduate students have access to the mainframe computer and numerous PCs at no cost.

Information for Students With Physical Disabilities: See the following Web site for more information: http://www.alfred.edu/academics/disabled.cfm.

Application Information:
Send to Graduate Admissions, Alfred University, Saxon Drive, Alfred, NY 14802. Application available online. URL of online application: http://www.alfred.edu/admissions/gradapp. Students are admitted in the Fall, application deadline January 5. Deadline for fall admission to the PsyD program is January 5; for the MA/CAS program the deadline is January 15. Late applications may be considered if places in the class still exist for qualified applicants. *Fee:* $50.

City University of New York
Department of Psychology/Biopsychology and Behavioral Neuroscience PhD Subprogram
Hunter College
695 Park Avenue, Room 611 North Building
New York, NY 10021
Telephone: (212) 772-5621
Fax: (212) 772-5620
E-mail: *biopsychology@hunter.cuny.edu*
Web: *http://www.hunter.cuny.edu/biopsych/home*

Department Information:
1962. Program Head: Michael J. Lewis. Number of faculty: total—full-time 23; women—full-time 7; total—minority—full-time 3; women minority—full-time 1.

Programs and Degrees Offered:
Listed in the following order: Program area, degree type (T if terminal Master's), number awarded 7/08–6/09. Biopsychology and Behavioral Neuroscience PhD (Doctor of Philosophy) 4.

Student Applications/Admissions:
Student Applications
Biopsychology and Behavioral Neuroscience PhD (Doctor of Philosophy)—Applications 2009–2010, 24. Total applicants accepted 2009–2010, 6. Number full-time enrolled (new admits only) 2009–2010, 6. Openings 2010–2011, 7. The median

number of years required for completion of a degree in 2008–2009 were 5. The number of students enrolled full- and part-time who were dismissed or voluntarily withdrew from this program area in 2008–2009 were 0.

Other Criteria: (importance of criteria rated low, medium, or high): GRE scores—medium, research experience—high, extracurricular activity—low, GPA—high, letters of recommendation—high, interview—medium, statement of goals and objectives—high.

Student Characteristics: The following represents characteristics of students in 2009–2010 in all graduate psychology programs in the department: Female—full-time 26, part-time 0; Male—full-time 8, part-time 0; African American/Black—full-time 3, part-time 0; Hispanic/Latino(a)—full-time 2, part-time 0; Asian/Pacific Islander—full-time 1, part-time 0; American Indian/Alaska Native—full-time 0, part-time 0; Caucasian/White—full-time 27, part-time 0; Multi-ethnic—full-time 1, part-time 0; students subject to the Americans With Disabilities Act—full-time 0, part-time 0; Unknown ethnicity—full-time 0, part-time 0; International students who hold an F-1 or J-1 Visa—full-time 1, part-time 0.

Financial Information/Assistance:
Tuition for Full-Time Study: *Doctoral:* State residents: per academic year $6,580; Nonstate residents: $645 per credit hour. Tuition is subject to change. Additional fees are assessed to students beyond the costs of tuition for the following: student activities fee, consolidated services fee, and technology fee.

Financial Assistance:
First-Year Students: Teaching assistantships available for first year. Average amount paid per academic year: $20,801. Research assistantships available for first year. Average amount paid per academic year: $20,801. Fellowships and scholarships available for first year. Average amount paid per academic year: $24,000.

Advanced Students: Teaching assistantships available for advanced students. Average amount paid per academic year: $21,596. Fellowships and scholarships available for advanced students. Average amount paid per academic year: $24,000.

Additional Information: Of all students currently enrolled full time, 100% benefited from one or more of the listed financial assistance programs. Application and information available online at: http://www.gc.cuny.edu/admin_offices/finaid.

Housing and Day Care: On-campus housing is available. On-campus day care facilities are available.

Employment of Department Graduates:
Master's Degree Graduates: Of those who graduated in the academic year 2008–2009, the following categories and numbers represent the postgraduate activities and employment of master's degree graduates: Enrolled in a postdoctoral residency/fellowship (n/a), employed in independent practice (n/a), total from the above (master's) (0).

Doctoral Degree Graduates: Of those who graduated in the academic year 2008–2009, the following categories and numbers represent the postgraduate activities and employment of doctoral degree graduates: Enrolled in a psychology doctoral program (n/a), employed in an academic position at a 2-year/4-year college (1), employed in other positions at a higher education institution (1), employed in government agency (1), still seeking employment (1), total from the above (doctoral) (4).

Additional Information:
Orientation, Objectives, and Emphasis of Department: The doctoral program in biopsychology and behavioral neuroscience interrelates the concepts and methods of neuroscience, cognitive science, the biological disciplines, and behavior analysis to offer a comparative and ontogenetic perspective on species-typical behavior and behavior acquired and modified during the individual's life-cycle. Basic psychological processes are studied in conjunction with contributions from neurobiology, ethology, ecology, evolutionary biology, genetics, endocrinology, pharmacology, and other sciences to illuminate the many ways in which all species adapt, survive, reproduce, and evolve. Through diversified laboratory experiences plus core courses, electives, seminars, colloquia, and field studies, students develop an interdisciplinary perspective. Neuroscience and animal behavior are taught jointly with the biology faculty. Electives address a wide range of topics in basic and applied areas of traditional psychology, neuroscience, and cognitive science. The biopsychology program provides unique training for basic research and teaching in the field of animal and human behavior, and in the application of biobehavioral knowledge to problems in industrial, business, institutional, health, and environmental settings.

Special Facilities or Resources: Laboratories for research with human subjects and with a variety of animal species are located at Hunter College. The College has a modern animal-care facility. Facilities for field research in animal behavior are available at the Southwest Field Station of the American Museum of Natural History in the Chiricahua Mountains of Arizona. Additional research opportunities are available through minority programs such as RCMI, MBRS, MIDARP and also through the Center for the Study of Gene Structure and Function. There is also collaboration with programs such as Biology, Chemistry and Physiology and faculty affiliations with many other academic and research institutes in New York City, including a Clinical and Translational Science Award with the Weill Cornell Medical College, Memorial Sloan-Kettering Cancer Center, and Hospital for Special Surgery. Hunter College lab facilities include equipment for electrophysiology, phase-fluorescence, and transmission microscopy, electron- and scanning-electron microscopy, radio immunoassay, high-performance liquid chromatography, autoradiography and other radioreceptor techniques, human and animal psychophysiology, histology, operant and classical conditioning, and video/cinematographic analysis. Computer facilities include a variety of micro- and minicomputers as well as access to the University computer center. Doctoral students may register for specialized courses at any CUNY campus and have privileges at all CUNY libraries.

Application Information:
Send to Graduate Admissions, 695 Park Avenue, Hunter College, CUNY, New York, NY 10021. Students are admitted in the Fall, application deadline February 1.

GRADUATE STUDY IN PSYCHOLOGY

City University of New York: Brooklyn College
Department of Psychology
Brooklyn
2900 Bedford Avenue
Brooklyn, NY 11210
Telephone: (718) 951-5601
Fax: (718) 951-4814
E-mail: *AaronK@brooklyn.cuny.edu*
Web: *http://www.brooklyn.cuny.edu/pub/departments/psychology/index.htm*

Department Information:
1935. PhD Program Head or MA Program Head: Aaron Kozbelt or Benzion Chanowitz. Number of faculty: total—full-time 25; women—full-time 11; total—minority—full-time 2; women minority—full-time 1.

Programs and Degrees Offered:
Listed in the following order: Program area, degree type (T if terminal Master's), number awarded 7/08–6/09. Cognition, Brain, and Behavior PhD (Doctor of Philosophy) 4, Experimental Psychology MA/MS (Master of Arts/Science) (T) 10, Industrial/Organizational Psychology MA/MS (Master of Arts/Science) (T) 34, Mental Health Counseling MA/MS (Master of Arts/Science) (T) 15.

Student Applications/Admissions:

Student Applications

Cognition, Brain, and Behavior PhD (Doctor of Philosophy)—Applications 2009–2010, 32. Total applicants accepted 2009–2010, 5. Number full-time enrolled (new admits only) 2009–2010, 6. Number part-time enrolled (new admits only) 2009–2010, 0. Openings 2010–2011, 5. The median number of years required for completion of a degree in 2008–2009 were 5. The number of students enrolled full- and part-time who were dismissed or voluntarily withdrew from this program area in 2008–2009 were 0. *Experimental Psychology MA/MS (Master of Arts/Science)*—Applications 2009–2010, 67. Total applicants accepted 2009–2010, 16. Number full-time enrolled (new admits only) 2009–2010, 3. Number part-time enrolled (new admits only) 2009–2010, 12. Total enrolled 2009–2010 full-time, 2, part-time, 40. Openings 2010–2011, 15. The median number of years required for completion of a degree in 2008–2009 were 3. The number of students enrolled full- and part-time who were dismissed or voluntarily withdrew from this program area in 2008–2009 were 0. *Industrial/Organizational Psychology MA/MS (Master of Arts/Science)*—Applications 2009–2010, 141. Total applicants accepted 2009–2010, 74. Number full-time enrolled (new admits only) 2009–2010, 6. Number part-time enrolled (new admits only) 2009–2010, 47. Total enrolled 2009–2010 full-time, 6, part-time, 122. Openings 2010–2011, 50. The median number of years required for completion of a degree in 2008–2009 were 3. The number of students enrolled full- and part-time who were dismissed or voluntarily withdrew from this program area in 2008–2009 were 0. *Mental Health Counseling MA/MS (Master of Arts/Science)*—Applications 2009–2010, 140. Total applicants accepted 2009–2010, 55. Number full-time enrolled (new admits only) 2009–2010, 42. Number part-time enrolled (new admits only) 2009–2010, 0. Openings 2010–2011, 40.

The median number of years required for completion of a degree in 2008–2009 were 2. The number of students enrolled full- and part-time who were dismissed or voluntarily withdrew from this program area in 2008–2009 were 3.

Other Criteria: (importance of criteria rated low, medium, or high): GRE scores—medium, research experience—high, work experience—medium, extracurricular activity—low, clinically related public service—low, GPA—medium, letters of recommendation—high, interview—medium, statement of goals and objectives—high, psychology coursework—high, undergraduate major in psychology—medium, specific undergraduate psychology courses taken—high. For additional information on admission requirements, go to http://www.brooklyn.cuny.edu/courses/acad/info_doctoral.jsp?program_code=6.

Student Characteristics: The following represents characteristics of students in 2009–2010 in all graduate psychology programs in the department: Female—full-time 0, part-time 0; Male—full-time 0, part-time 0; African American/Black—full-time 0, part-time 0; Hispanic/Latino(a)—full-time 0, part-time 0; Asian/Pacific Islander—full-time 0, part-time 0; American Indian/Alaska Native—full-time 0, part-time 0; Caucasian/White—full-time 0, part-time 0; Multi-ethnic—full-time 0, part-time 0; students subject to the Americans With Disabilities Act—full-time 0, part-time 0; Unknown ethnicity—full-time 0, part-time 0; International students who hold an F-1 or J-1 Visa—full-time 0, part-time 0.

Financial Information/Assistance:

Tuition for Full-Time Study: *Master's:* State residents: per academic year $3,200, $270 per credit hour; Nonstate residents: per academic year $6,000, $500 per credit hour. *Doctoral:* State residents: per academic year $6,580, $325 per credit hour; Nonstate residents: per academic year $9,030, $560 per credit hour. Tuition is subject to change. Additional fees are assessed to students beyond the costs of tuition for the following: student technology fee, student activity fee, CUNY consolidation fee. Tuition costs vary by program. See the following Web site for updates and changes in tuition costs: http://www.gc.cuny.edu/current_students/tuition_curnt_stdnts.htm.

Financial Assistance:

First-Year Students: Teaching assistantships available for first year. Average amount paid per academic year: $12,000. Average number of hours worked per week: 20. Apply by January 15. Research assistantships available for first year. Average amount paid per academic year: $14,000. Average number of hours worked per week: 20. Apply by January 15. Fellowships and scholarships available for first year. Average amount paid per academic year: $2,000. Apply by January 1.

Advanced Students: Teaching assistantships available for advanced students. Average amount paid per academic year: $12,000. Average number of hours worked per week: 20. Apply by January 1. Research assistantships available for advanced students. Average amount paid per academic year: $14,000. Average number of hours worked per week: 20. Apply by January 1. Fellowships and scholarships available for advanced students. Average amount paid per academic year: $2,000. Apply by February 1.

Additional Information: Of all students currently enrolled full time, 65% benefited from one or more of the listed financial assistance programs. Application and information available online at: http://www.brooklyn.cuny.edu/pub/1186.htm.

Internships/Practica: Master's Degree (MA/MS Mental Health Counseling): An internship experience, such as a final research project or "capstone" experience is required of graduates. The MA program in Industrial/Organizational psychology has an internship component that most students avail themselves of. It functions as both training and as an opportunity to experience the hands-on application of principles in a work setting. The MA program in Mental Health Counseling requires two semesters of pre-degree supervised internships. An additional 3,000 hours of post-degree supervised internship is required for licensure.

Housing and Day Care: No on-campus housing is available. On-campus day care facilities are available. See the following Web site for more information: http://depthome.brooklyn.cuny.edu/schooled/ECC/ECC-index.htm.

Employment of Department Graduates:
Master's Degree Graduates: Of those who graduated in the academic year 2008–2009, the following categories and numbers represent the postgraduate activities and employment of master's degree graduates: Enrolled in a psychology doctoral program (6), enrolled in another graduate/professional program (3), enrolled in a postdoctoral residency/fellowship (n/a), employed in independent practice (n/a), employed in other positions at a higher education institution (1), employed in a professional position in a school system (1), employed in business or industry (6), employed in a community mental health/counseling center (4), do not know (1), total from the above (master's) (22).
Doctoral Degree Graduates: Of those who graduated in the academic year 2008–2009, the following categories and numbers represent the postgraduate activities and employment of doctoral degree graduates: Enrolled in a psychology doctoral program (n/a), enrolled in a postdoctoral residency/fellowship (3), employed in an academic position at a university (1), total from the above (doctoral) (4).

Additional Information:
Orientation, Objectives, and Emphasis of Department: The PhD program is broadly based, with concentrations in cognitive neuroscience, cognition, learning, social, and developmental psychology. These diverse areas are bound by a commitment to empirical methods and theory development; we train research scientists in basic and applied approaches using the apprenticeship model. The CUNY consortium allows students to collaborate with faculty at other CUNY campuses and research universities in New York. Students work with faculty in chosen areas of specialization and are encouraged to collaborate with other faculty and students. Historically, graduates have started careers in teaching and research as well as in applied fields. The MA program in Experimental Psychology mirrors the first two years of the PhD program. The Industrial/Organizational Psychology MA program offers training in two tracks: Human Relations, with focus on the group, and Organizational Behavior, with focus on the organization. Graduates from both tracks are prepared for entry-level executive positions in Human Resources and Personnel. The MA program in Mental Health Counseling provides experiential learning with counseling practicum experience in mental health settings, along with comprehensive course work that prepares students for practice in mental health counseling. Graduates are eligible to take the NYS licensing exam which permits private/independent practice of counseling.

Special Facilities or Resources: There are over a dozen active laboratories in the department focusing on topics such as the physiology of taste and preference formation, children's acquisition of spatial knowledge, transactive knowledge in organizations, implicit learning in cognitive disorders, visual functions in Down syndrome, creativity and cognition in the arts, comparative psychology in cephalopods, amphibians, and crustaceans, hippocampal atrophy in early Alzheimer's disease, implicit impression formation, Darwinian models of mate selection, biomemetic robotics, neurodegeneration in the aged, and parent-child communication. All labs are well equipped and some supported by grants from NSF, NIH, NASA, DARPA, and other organizations. Several faculty have appointments and working collaborations with research labs in city hospitals and medical schools with access to technologies such as fMRI.

Application Information:
Send to PhD Office of Graduate Admissions, Brooklyn College, 2900 Bedford Avenue, Brooklyn, NY 11210. Application available online. URL of online application: http://www.brooklyn.cuny.edu/pub/departments/psychology/programs.php. Students are admitted in the Fall, application deadline see below; Spring, application deadline November 1 (MA). MA application for Mental Health Counseling is February 1. All other MA applications deadline for Fall is March 1. Spring admissions are for the Experimental MA program only. PhD applications deadline is January 15. PhD Minority applicants should apply by January 1 to secure chance to apply for minority fellowships. Fee: $125. Requests for waivers can be made to Office of Admissions and contact the Head of the PhD program.

City University of New York: Brooklyn College
School Psychologist Graduate Program, School of Education
Brooklyn College
2900 Bedford Avenue, Room 1205 James
Brooklyn, NY 11210
Telephone: (718) 951-5876
Fax: (718) 951-4232
E-mail: *rubinson@brooklyn.cuny.edu*
Web: *http://www.depthome.brooklyn.cuny.edu/schooled/ed-psych.htm*

Department Information:
1968. Program Head: Florence Rubinson. Number of faculty: total—full-time 5, part-time 6; women—full-time 3, part-time 3; total—minority—full-time 2, part-time 2; women minority—full-time 1, part-time 1.

Programs and Degrees Offered:
Listed in the following order: Program area, degree type (T if terminal Master's), number awarded 7/08–6/09. School Psychology (Bilingual) MA/MS (Master of Arts/Science) 3, School Psychology MA/MS (Master of Arts/Science) 20.

Student Applications/Admissions:
Student Applications
School Psychology (Bilingual) MA/MS (Master of Arts/Science)—Applications 2009–2010, 25. Total applicants accepted 2009–2010, 8. Number full-time enrolled (new admits only) 2009–2010, 6. Number part-time enrolled (new admits only) 2009–

2010, 1. Total enrolled 2009–2010 full-time, 7, part-time, 3. Openings 2010–2011, 15. The median number of years required for completion of a degree in 2008–2009 were 3. The number of students enrolled full- and part-time who were dismissed or voluntarily withdrew from this program area in 2008–2009 were 1. *School Psychology MA/MS (Master of Arts/Science)*—Applications 2009–2010, 125. Total applicants accepted 2009–2010, 27. Number full-time enrolled (new admits only) 2009–2010, 20. Number part-time enrolled (new admits only) 2009–2010, 7. Total enrolled 2009–2010 full-time, 43, part-time, 48. The median number of years required for completion of a degree in 2008–2009 were 3. The number of students enrolled full- and part-time who were dismissed or voluntarily withdrew from this program area in 2008–2009 were 9.

Scores: Entries appear in this order: required test or GPA, minimum score (if required), median score of students entering in 2009–2010. *School Psychology (Bilingual) MA/MS (Master of Arts/Science)*: overall undergraduate GPA 3.0; *School Psychology MA/MS (Master of Arts/Science)*: overall undergraduate GPA 3.0.

Other Criteria: (importance of criteria rated low, medium, or high): GRE scores—low, research experience—medium, work experience—high, extracurricular activity—medium, clinically related public service—high, GPA—high, letters of recommendation—high, interview—high, statement of goals and objectives—high, Writing sample—high, undergraduate major in psychology—low, specific undergraduate psychology courses taken—low. For additional information on admission requirements, go to http://depthome.brooklyn.cuny.edu/schooled/edpsych.htm.

Student Characteristics: The following represents characteristics of students in 2009–2010 in all graduate psychology programs in the department: Female—full-time 44, part-time 35; Male—full-time 6, part-time 1; African American/Black—full-time 9, part-time 5; Hispanic/Latino(a)—full-time 6, part-time 3; Asian/Pacific Islander—full-time 1, part-time 3; American Indian/Alaska Native—full-time 0, part-time 0; Caucasian/White—full-time 33, part-time 25; Multi-ethnic—full-time 0, part-time 0; students subject to the Americans With Disabilities Act—full-time 0, part-time 0; Unknown ethnicity—full-time 1, part-time 0; International students who hold an F-1 or J-1 Visa—full-time 0, part-time 1.

Financial Information/Assistance:
Tuition for Full-Time Study: *Master's:* State residents: $310 per credit hour; Nonstate residents: $575 per credit hour. Additional fees are assessed to students beyond the costs of tuition for the following: student technology fee. See the following Web site for updates and changes in tuition costs: http://www.brooklyn.cuny.edu/pub/tuition.htm.

Financial Assistance:
First-Year Students: Fellowships and scholarships available for first year. Apply by March 15.
Advanced Students: Fellowships and scholarships available for advanced students. Apply by March 15.
Additional Information: Of all students currently enrolled full time, 10% benefited from one or more of the listed financial assistance programs. Application and information available online at: http://www.brooklyn.cuny.edu/pub/1186.htm.

Internships/Practica: Internships are available and coordinated through our program with various schools, both public and private, working with both the mainstream population, as well as special populations. In addition, internships are available in mental health clinics, agencies, and hospitals. Practica in assessment, intervention, consultation, and counseling are designed to reinforce students' course work.

Housing and Day Care: No on-campus housing is available. On-campus day care facilities are available. See the following Web site for more information: http://depthome.brooklyn.cuny.edu/schooled/ECC/ECC-index.htm.

Employment of Department Graduates:
Master's Degree Graduates: Of those who graduated in the academic year 2008–2009, the following categories and numbers represent the postgraduate activities and employment of master's degree graduates: Enrolled in a psychology doctoral program (4), enrolled in a postdoctoral residency/fellowship (n/a), employed in independent practice (n/a), employed in other positions at a higher education institution (1), employed in a professional position in a school system (15), employed in a community mental health/counseling center (4), total from the above (master's) (24).
Doctoral Degree Graduates: Of those who graduated in the academic year 2008–2009, the following categories and numbers represent the postgraduate activities and employment of doctoral degree graduates: Enrolled in a psychology doctoral program (n/a), total from the above (doctoral) (0).

Additional Information:
Orientation, Objectives, and Emphasis of Department: The aim of the school psychologists' training program is to meet the community needs for professionally competent personnel to function in the schools as consultants on psychological aspects of learning and mental health. Students are prepared to make assessments of situations involving children, parents, and school personnel to achieve the more optimal functioning of children in the school setting. Coursework will prepare students in the areas of measurement and evaluation, personality understanding, educational objectives and procedures, curriculum development, and research. Students will also be trained to achieve greater integration between school and community. Elements of the program will provide students with opportunities for self-reflection, collaboration with other professionals and families, and engagement in issues of diversity and social justice.

Special Facilities or Resources: In addition to the use of the Brooklyn College library, students are welcome to use all the libraries at other colleges within the CUNY system. The School Psychology Program also has a small library of texts and journals for the students' use.

Application Information:
Send to Brooklyn College, Admissions Office, 2900 Bedford Avenue, Brooklyn, NY 11210. Application available online. URL of online application: https://websql2.brooklyn.cuny.edu/graduate/. Students are admitted in the Fall, application deadline March 1. *Fee:* $125.

City University of New York: Graduate Center
Learning Processes and Behavior Analysis Doctoral Subprogram
Queens College
65-30 Kissena Boulevard
Flushing, NY 11367
Telephone: (718) 997-3630
Fax: (718) 997-3257
E-mail: *bruce.brown@qc.cuny.edu*
Web: *http://www.qcpages.qc.cuny.edu/Psychology/Grad/phd/lpba/index.html*

Department Information:
1967. Program Head: Bruce L. Brown. Number of faculty: total—full-time 9; women—full-time 3; total—minority—full-time 1; women minority—full-time 1.

Programs and Degrees Offered:
Listed in the following order: Program area, degree type (T if terminal Master's), number awarded 7/08–6/09. Learning Processes and Behavior Analysis PhD (Doctor of Philosophy) 6.

Student Applications/Admissions:
Student Applications
Learning Processes and Behavior Analysis PhD (Doctor of Philosophy)—Applications 2009–2010, 19. Total applicants accepted 2009–2010, 5. Number full-time enrolled (new admits only) 2009–2010, 4. Number part-time enrolled (new admits only) 2009–2010, 0. Openings 2010–2011, 8. The median number of years required for completion of a degree in 2008–2009 were 8. The number of students enrolled full- and part-time who were dismissed or voluntarily withdrew from this program area in 2008–2009 were 2.
Other Criteria: (importance of criteria rated low, medium, or high): GRE scores—medium, research experience—high, work experience—low, extracurricular activity—low, clinically related public service—low, GPA—high, letters of recommendation—high, interview—medium, statement of goals and objectives—high, undergraduate major in psychology—medium, specific undergraduate psychology courses taken—high.

Student Characteristics: The following represents characteristics of students in 2009–2010 in all graduate psychology programs in the department: Female—full-time 20, part-time 0; Male—full-time 14, part-time 0; African American/Black—full-time 0, part-time 0; Hispanic/Latino(a)—full-time 2, part-time 0; Asian/Pacific Islander—full-time 1, part-time 0; American Indian/Alaska Native—full-time 0, part-time 0; Caucasian/White—full-time 31, part-time 0; Multi-ethnic—full-time 0, part-time 0; students subject to the Americans With Disabilities Act—full-time 0, part-time 0; Unknown ethnicity—full-time 0, part-time 0; International students who hold an F-1 or J-1 Visa—full-time 2, part-time 0.

Financial Information/Assistance:
Tuition for Full-Time Study: *Doctoral:* State residents: per academic year $6,580; Nonstate residents: $645 per credit hour. Tuition is subject to change.

Financial Assistance:
First-Year Students: Fellowships and scholarships available for first year. Average amount paid per academic year: $18,000. Average number of hours worked per week: 20. Apply by January 1.
Advanced Students: Teaching assistantships available for advanced students. Average amount paid per academic year: $10,000. Average number of hours worked per week: 6.
Additional Information: Of all students currently enrolled full time, 50% benefited from one or more of the listed financial assistance programs. Application and information available online at: http://www.gc.cuny.edu/prospective_students/.

Internships/Practica: Information concerning practica and internships is available on request. Internships are available, but not required.

Housing and Day Care: On-campus housing is available. See the following Web site for more information: http://www.thesummitatqc.com/main.html. On-campus day care facilities are available. See the following Web site for more information: http://www.qc.cuny.edu/StudentLife/services/ChildDevelopment/Pages/default.aspx.

Employment of Department Graduates:
Master's Degree Graduates: Of those who graduated in the academic year 2008–2009, the following categories and numbers represent the postgraduate activities and employment of master's degree graduates: Enrolled in a psychology doctoral program (0), enrolled in another graduate/professional program (0), enrolled in a postdoctoral residency/fellowship (n/a), employed in independent practice (n/a), employed in an academic position at a university (0), employed in an academic position at a 2-year/4-year college (0), employed in other positions at a higher education institution (0), employed in a professional position in a school system (0), employed in business or industry (0), employed in government agency (0), employed in a community mental health/counseling center (0), employed in a hospital/medical center (0), still seeking employment (0), other employment position (0), total from the above (master's) (0).
Doctoral Degree Graduates: Of those who graduated in the academic year 2008–2009, the following categories and numbers represent the postgraduate activities and employment of doctoral degree graduates: Enrolled in a psychology doctoral program (n/a), enrolled in a postdoctoral residency/fellowship (1), employed in independent practice (0), employed in an academic position at a university (0), employed in an academic position at a 2-year/4-year college (0), employed in other positions at a higher education institution (0), employed in a professional position in a school system (2), employed in business or industry (1), employed in government agency (0), employed in a community mental health/counseling center (0), employed in a hospital/medical center (0), still seeking employment (0), not seeking employment (0), other employment position (1), do not know (1), total from the above (doctoral) (6).

Additional Information:
Orientation, Objectives, and Emphasis of Department: The Learning Processes and Behavior Analysis (LPBA) program offers doctoral students in psychology training in the experimental analysis of human and animal behavior and in applied behavior analysis. Students and faculty investigate a wide spectrum of behavioral

processes through lectures and experimental laboratory course work, advanced seminars, informal student-faculty discussions, practica, internships, and individual research projects. Faculty and students publish regularly in peer-reviewed journals and are strongly represented at major national and international conferences. Their current research interests include such topics as categorization and concept formation, language acquisition, affective behavior, behavioral assessment, human and animal timing, pattern recognition, stimulus control, behavioral community psychology, education and training of children with autism, and staff training in organizational settings. The LPBA program is accredited in behavior analysis by the Association for Behavior Analysis, and its curriculum is licensure-qualifying in New York State. In addition, the Behavior Analyst Certification Board, Inc. has approved a subset of the curriculum as a course sequence that meets the coursework requirements for eligibility to take the Board Certified Behavior Analyst Examination. Applicants will have to meet additional requirements to qualify.

Application Information:
Send to Office of Admissions, The Graduate School & University Center of the City University of New York, 365 Fifth Avenue, New York, NY 10016-4309. Application available online. URL of online application: http://www.gc.cuny.edu/admin_offices/admissions/index.htm. Students are admitted in the Fall, application deadline January 1. *Fee:* $125.

City University of New York: Graduate Center
Neuropsychology Doctoral Program
Queens College
65-30 Kissena Boulevard
Flushing, NY 11367
Telephone: (718) 997-3630
Fax: (718) 997-3257
E-mail: *joshua.brumberg@qc.cuny.edu*
Web: *http://www.qcneuropsychology.org/*

Department Information:
1968. Program Head: Joshua C. Brumberg, PhD. Number of faculty: total—full-time 26, part-time 3; women—full-time 12, part-time 2; total—minority—full-time 1.

Programs and Degrees Offered:
Listed in the following order: Program area, degree type (T if terminal Master's), number awarded 7/08–6/09. Clinical Neuropsychology PhD (Doctor of Philosophy) 4, Basic Neuropsychology PhD (Doctor of Philosophy) 0.

Student Applications/Admissions:
Student Applications
Clinical Neuropsychology PhD (Doctor of Philosophy)—Applications 2009–2010, 54. Total applicants accepted 2009–2010, 18. Number full-time enrolled (new admits only) 2009–2010, 6. Total enrolled 2009–2010 full-time, 53. The median number of years required for completion of a degree in 2008–2009 were 6. The number of students enrolled full- and part-time who were dismissed or voluntarily withdrew from this program area in 2008–2009 were 0. Basic Neuropsychology PhD (Doctor of Philosophy)—Applications 2009–2010, 20. Total applicants accepted 2009–2010, 8. Number full-time enrolled (new admits only) 2009–2010, 5. Total enrolled 2009–2010 full-time, 21. The median number of years required for completion of a degree in 2008–2009 were 4. The number of students enrolled full- and part-time who were dismissed or voluntarily withdrew from this program area in 2008–2009 were 0.

Scores: Entries appear in this order: required test or GPA, minimum score (if required), median score of students entering in 2009–2010. *Basic Neuropsychology PhD (Doctor of Philosophy):* GRE-V no minimum stated, GRE-Q no minimum stated, GRE-Analytical no minimum stated, overall undergraduate GPA no minimum stated, psychology GPA no minimum stated, Masters GPA no minimum stated.

Other Criteria: (importance of criteria rated low, medium, or high): GRE scores—medium, research experience—high, work experience—low, extracurricular activity—low, clinically related public service—low, GPA—high, letters of recommendation—high, interview—high, statement of goals and objectives—high, undergraduate major in psychology—low, Interviews will be carried out for the clinical track only. For additional information on admission requirements, go to http://www.qcneuropsychology.org/prospective_students.

Student Characteristics: The following represents characteristics of students in 2009–2010 in all graduate psychology programs in the department: Female—full-time 42, part-time 0; Male—full-time 13, part-time 0; African American/Black—full-time 2, part-time 0; Hispanic/Latino(a)—full-time 2, part-time 0; Asian/Pacific Islander—full-time 1, part-time 0; American Indian/Alaska Native—full-time 0, part-time 0; Caucasian/White—full-time 0, part-time 0; Multi-ethnic—full-time 0, part-time 0; students subject to the Americans With Disabilities Act—full-time 0, part-time 0; Unknown ethnicity—full-time 0, part-time 0; International students who hold an F-1 or J-1 Visa—full-time 0, part-time 0.

Financial Information/Assistance:
Tuition for Full-Time Study: *Doctoral:* State residents: per academic year $6,580; Nonstate residents: $645 per credit hour. Tuition is subject to change. Additional fees are assessed to students beyond the costs of tuition for the following: student activity fee, student technology fee, student health fee. See the following Web site for updates and changes in tuition costs: http://www.gc.cuny.edu/current_students/tuition_curnt_stdnts.htm.

Financial Assistance:
First-Year Students: Teaching assistantships available for first year. Average amount paid per academic year: $0. Average number of hours worked per week: 0. Research assistantships available for first year. Average amount paid per academic year: $0. Average number of hours worked per week: 0. Traineeships available for first year. Average amount paid per academic year: $0. Average number of hours worked per week: 0. Fellowships and scholarships available for first year. Average amount paid per academic year: $0. Average number of hours worked per week: 0.

Advanced Students: Teaching assistantships available for advanced students. Average number of hours worked per week: 0. Research assistantships available for advanced students. Average number of hours worked per week: 0. Fellowships and scholarships available for advanced students. Average number of hours worked per week: 0.

Additional Information: Of all students currently enrolled full time, 60% benefited from one or more of the listed financial assistance programs. Application and information available online at: http://www.gc.cuny.edu/admin_offices/finaid/index.htm.

Internships/Practica: Doctoral Degree (PhD Clinical Neuropsychology): For those doctoral students for whom a professional internship was required in this program prior to graduation, (8) students applied for an internship in 2008–2009, with (7) students obtaining an internship. Of those students who obtained an internship, (7) were paid internships. Of those students who obtained an internship, (5) students placed in APA/CPA accredited internships, (2) students placed in internships not APA/CPA accredited, but listed with the Association of Psychology Postdoctoral and Internship Programs (APPIC), (0) students placed in internships conforming to guidelines of the Council of Directors of School Psychology Programs (CDSPP), (0) students placed in internships that were not APA/CPA accredited, APPIC or CDSPP listed. Clinical track students experience at least three different clinical practica. Additionally, all clinical track students must complete a one year predoctoral internship.

Housing and Day Care: On-campus housing is available. See the following Web site for more information: http://www.thesummitatqc.com/. On-campus day care facilities are available. See the following Web site for more information: http://qcpages.qc.cuny.edu/qcchild/.

Employment of Department Graduates:
Master's Degree Graduates: Of those who graduated in the academic year 2008–2009, the following categories and numbers represent the postgraduate activities and employment of master's degree graduates: Enrolled in a postdoctoral residency/fellowship (n/a), employed in independent practice (n/a), total from the above (master's) (0).
Doctoral Degree Graduates: Of those who graduated in the academic year 2008–2009, the following categories and numbers represent the postgraduate activities and employment of doctoral degree graduates: Enrolled in a psychology doctoral program (n/a), enrolled in a postdoctoral residency/fellowship (10), employed in a hospital/medical center (2), total from the above (doctoral) (12).

Additional Information:
Orientation, Objectives, and Emphasis of Department: The Neuropsychology Subprogram is an academically-oriented PhD program with a core philosophy based on two premises. The first of these is that productive research, effective teaching, and responsible clinical practice are integrally interdependent. That is, effective teaching must include critical analysis of current research data, and clinical assessment and treatment procedures must be empirically validated. The second premise is that the understanding of impaired or disordered brain function in humans requires rigorous training in the neurosciences as well as in the traditional clinical topics. The Subprogram was designed to train professionals with competence in research and/or teaching in the area of brain-behavior relationships, and in the application of these competencies in clinical settings. There are two tracks within the program: the basic track requires 60 course credits; the clinical track requires 82 credits including at least two years of practicum training. Both tracks focus heavily on neuroscience topics, and provide intensive experience in human and animal experimentation. The clinical track also provides students the opportunity to acquire and apply the skills appropriate to the practice of clinical neuropsychology. Students in the clinical track thus receive training in the evaluation of psychological and neuropsychological function in various clinical populations, which may include children or adults, neurological, neurosurgical, rehabilitation medicine and psychiatric patients, as well as in the use of rehabilitative, psychotherapeutic, and remediative techniques. A full-year internship is required for graduation from the clinical track.

Special Facilities or Resources: The Neuropsychology program has well equipped laboratories for clinical and basic neuropsychology research. Equipment includes evoked potential recording set-ups, microscopy, histology and imaging cores.

Application Information:
Send to Office of Admissions, The Graduate School & University Center of the City University of New York, 365 Fifth Avenue, New York, NY 10016-4309. Application available online. URL of online application: http://www.gc.cuny.edu/admin_offices/admissions/index.htm. Students are admitted in the Fall, application deadline December 15. *Fee:* $150.

City University of New York: Graduate School and University Center
PhD Program in Educational Psychology
365 Fifth Avenue
New York, NY 10016-4309
Telephone: (212) 817-8285
Fax: (212) 817-1516
E-mail: *mkopala@gc.cuny.edu*
Web: *http://www.gc.cuny.edu*

Department Information:
1969. Executive Officer: Mary Kopala. Number of faculty: total—full-time 35, part-time 1; women—full-time 14; total—minority—full-time 4; women minority—full-time 1.

Programs and Degrees Offered:
Listed in the following order: Program area, degree type (T if terminal Master's), number awarded 7/08–6/09. Educational Psychology PhD (Doctor of Philosophy) 8.

APA Accreditation: School PhD (Doctor of Philosophy).

Student Applications/Admissions:
Student Applications
Educational Psychology PhD (Doctor of Philosophy)—Applications 2009–2010, 68. Total applicants accepted 2009–2010, 4. Number full-time enrolled (new admits only) 2009–2010, 11. Number part-time enrolled (new admits only) 2009–2010, 3. Total enrolled 2009–2010 full-time, 118, part-time, 13. Openings 2010–2011, 18. The median number of years required for completion of a degree in 2008–2009 were 6. The number of students enrolled full- and part-time who were dismissed or voluntarily withdrew from this program area in 2008–2009 were 0.
Other Criteria: (importance of criteria rated low, medium, or high): GRE scores—high, research experience—medium,

work experience—medium, extracurricular activity—low, clinically related public service—low, GPA—medium, letters of recommendation—high, interview—high, statement of goals and objectives—high, undergraduate major in psychology—low, specific undergraduate psychology courses taken—low. For additional information on admission requirements, go to http://web.gc.cuny.edu/content/edpsychology.

Student Characteristics: The following represents characteristics of students in 2009–2010 in all graduate psychology programs in the department: Female—full-time 98, part-time 9; Male—full-time 20, part-time 4; African American/Black—full-time 9, part-time 1; Hispanic/Latino(a)—full-time 3, part-time 0; Asian/Pacific Islander—full-time 7, part-time 0; American Indian/Alaska Native—full-time 0, part-time 0; Caucasian/White—full-time 94, part-time 10; Multi-ethnic—full-time 0, part-time 0; students subject to the Americans With Disabilities Act—full-time 0, part-time 0; Unknown ethnicity—full-time 5, part-time 2; International students who hold an F-1 or J-1 Visa—full-time 1, part-time 0.

Financial Information/Assistance:
Tuition for Full-Time Study: *Doctoral:* State residents: per academic year $6,580; Nonstate residents: $645 per credit hour. Additional fees are assessed to students beyond the costs of tuition for the following: student activities fee=$41.60/semester; technology fee=$100/semester. See the following Web site for updates and changes in tuition costs: http://www.gc.cuny.edu/current_students/tuition_curnt_stdnts.htm.

Financial Assistance:
First-Year Students: Teaching assistantships available for first year. Average amount paid per academic year: $18,000. Average number of hours worked per week: 5. Apply by February 1. Research assistantships available for first year. Average amount paid per academic year: $5,000. Average number of hours worked per week: 5. Apply by February 1. Fellowships and scholarships available for first year. Average amount paid per academic year: $5,000. Average number of hours worked per week: 5. Apply by February 1.

Advanced Students: Teaching assistantships available for advanced students. Average amount paid per academic year: $18,000. Average number of hours worked per week: 10. Apply by February 1. Research assistantships available for advanced students. Average amount paid per academic year: $4,000. Average number of hours worked per week: 4. Apply by February 1. Fellowships and scholarships available for advanced students. Average amount paid per academic year: $5,000. Average number of hours worked per week: 5. Apply by February 1.

Additional Information: Of all students currently enrolled full time, 50% benefited from one or more of the listed financial assistance programs. Application and information available online at: http://www.gc.cuny.edu/admin_offices/finaid.

Internships/Practica: Doctoral Degree (PhD Educational Psychology): For those doctoral students for whom a professional internship was required in this program prior to graduation, (3) students applied for an internship in 2008–2009, with (3) students obtaining an internship. Of those students who obtained an internship, (3) were paid internships. Of those students who obtained an internship, (0) students placed in APA/CPA accredited internships, (0) students placed in internships not APA/CPA accredited, but listed with the Association of Psychology Postdoctoral and Internship Programs (APPIC), (3) students placed in internships conforming to guidelines of the Council of Directors of School Psychology Programs (CDSPP), (0) students placed in internships that were not APA/CPA accredited, APPIC or CDSPP listed.

Housing and Day Care: No on-campus housing is available. On-campus day care facilities are available. Child Development & Learning Center: (212) 817-7032.

Employment of Department Graduates:
Master's Degree Graduates: Of those who graduated in the academic year 2008–2009, the following categories and numbers represent the postgraduate activities and employment of master's degree graduates: Enrolled in a psychology doctoral program (0), enrolled in another graduate/professional program (0), enrolled in a postdoctoral residency/fellowship (n/a), employed in independent practice (n/a), employed in an academic position at a university (0), employed in an academic position at a 2-year/4-year college (0), employed in other positions at a higher education institution (0), employed in a professional position in a school system (0), employed in business or industry (0), employed in government agency (0), employed in a community mental health/counseling center (0), employed in a hospital/medical center (0), still seeking employment (0), not seeking employment (0), other employment position (0), do not know (0), total from the above (master's) (0).

Doctoral Degree Graduates: Of those who graduated in the academic year 2008–2009, the following categories and numbers represent the postgraduate activities and employment of doctoral degree graduates: Enrolled in a psychology doctoral program (n/a), enrolled in another graduate/professional program (0), enrolled in a postdoctoral residency/fellowship (0), employed in independent practice (0), employed in an academic position at a university (0), employed in an academic position at a 2-year/4-year college (0), employed in other positions at a higher education institution (0), employed in a professional position in a school system (0), employed in business or industry (0), employed in government agency (0), employed in a community mental health/counseling center (0), employed in a hospital/medical center (0), still seeking employment (0), not seeking employment (0), other employment position (0), do not know (0), total from the above (doctoral) (0).

Additional Information:
Orientation, Objectives, and Emphasis of Department: The PhD program in Educational Psychology is research oriented, preparing students for teaching, research, and program development in various educational settings such as universities, school systems, research institutions, community agencies, as well as in educational publishing, television, and in other agencies with training programs.

Special Facilities or Resources: The Educational Psychology program is affiliated with a university based research institute, CASE (Center for Advanced Study in Education). CASE is heavily involved in the evaluation and implementation of various applied educational programs. Our faculty and students have worked as principal investigators and research assistants on CASE projects.

Application Information:
Send to Admissions Office, CUNY Graduate Center, 365 Fifth Avenue, New York City, New York 10016-4309. Application available

online. URL of online application: http://www.gc.cuny.edu/admin_offices/admissions. Students are admitted in the Fall, application deadline January 15. Deadline for financial aid applicants is February 1. *Fee:* $125.

City University of New York: Graduate School and University Center (2009 data)
PhD Program in Psychology
365 Fifth Avenue
New York, NY 10016-4309
Telephone: (212) 817-8705
Fax: (212) 817-1533
E-mail: *moconnor@gc.cuny.edu*
Web: *http://www.gc.cuny.edu*

Department Information:
1961. Executive Officer: Maureen O'Connor. Number of faculty: total—full-time 170, part-time 18; women—full-time 75, part-time 7; total—minority—full-time 18; women minority—full-time 8.

Programs and Degrees Offered:
Listed in the following order: Program area, degree type (T if terminal Master's), number awarded 7/08–6/09. Biopsychology and Behavioral Neuroscience PhD (Doctor of Philosophy) 4, Clinical PhD (Doctor of Philosophy) 17, Developmental PhD (Doctor of Philosophy) 4, Cognition, Brain and Behavior PhD (Doctor of Philosophy) 7, Cognitive Neuroscience PhD (Doctor of Philosophy) 1, Environmental PhD (Doctor of Philosophy) 4, Industrial/Organizational PhD (Doctor of Philosophy) 5, Learning Processes and Behavior Analysis PhD (Doctor of Philosophy) 2, Neuropsychology PhD (Doctor of Philosophy) 4, Social/Personality PhD (Doctor of Philosophy) 4, Forensic Psychology PhD (Doctor of Philosophy).

Student Applications/Admissions:
Student Applications
Biopsychology and Behavioral Neuroscience PhD (Doctor of Philosophy)—Applications 2009–2010, 27. Total applicants accepted 2009–2010, 6. Openings 2010–2011, 8. The median number of years required for completion of a degree in 2008–2009 were 6. *Clinical PhD (Doctor of Philosophy)*—Applications 2009–2010, 274. Total applicants accepted 2009–2010, 12. Openings 2010–2011, 12. The median number of years required for completion of a degree in 2008–2009 were 6. *Developmental PhD (Doctor of Philosophy)*—Applications 2009–2010, 38. Total applicants accepted 2009–2010, 12. Number full-time enrolled (new admits only) 2009–2010, 8. Openings 2010–2011, 8. The median number of years required for completion of a degree in 2008–2009 were 6. *Cognition, Brain and Behavior PhD (Doctor of Philosophy)*—Applications 2009–2010, 35. Total applicants accepted 2009–2010, 7. Number full-time enrolled (new admits only) 2009–2010, 6. Number part-time enrolled (new admits only) 2009–2010, 0. Openings 2010–2011, 6. The median number of years required for completion of a degree in 2008–2009 were 5. The number of students enrolled full- and part-time who were dismissed or voluntarily withdrew from this program area in 2008–2009 were 1. *Cognitive Neuroscience PhD (Doctor of Philosophy)*—Applications 2009–2010, 25. Total applicants accepted 2009–2010, 7. Openings 2010–2011, 5. The median number of years required for completion of a degree in 2008–2009 were 8. *Environmental PhD (Doctor of Philosophy)*—Applications 2009–2010, 22. Total applicants accepted 2009–2010, 10. Openings 2010–2011, 10. The median number of years required for completion of a degree in 2008–2009 were 7. *Industrial/Organizational PhD (Doctor of Philosophy)*—Applications 2009–2010, 25. Total applicants accepted 2009–2010, 5. Openings 2010–2011, 7. The median number of years required for completion of a degree in 2008–2009 were 7. *Learning Processes and Behavior Analysis PhD (Doctor of Philosophy)*—Applications 2009–2010, 38. Total applicants accepted 2009–2010, 7. Openings 2010–2011, 10. The median number of years required for completion of a degree in 2008–2009 were 6. *Neuropsychology PhD (Doctor of Philosophy)*—Applications 2009–2010, 68. Total applicants accepted 2009–2010, 9. Openings 2010–2011, 8. *Social/Personality PhD (Doctor of Philosophy)*—Applications 2009–2010, 62. Total applicants accepted 2009–2010, 8. Number full-time enrolled (new admits only) 2009–2010, 6. Openings 2010–2011, 79. *Forensic Psychology PhD (Doctor of Philosophy)*—Applications 2009–2010, 166. Total applicants accepted 2009–2010, 12. Number full-time enrolled (new admits only) 2009–2010, 10. Openings 2010–2011, 10.

Other Criteria: (importance of criteria rated low, medium, or high): GRE scores—medium, research experience—medium, work experience—low, extracurricular activity—low, clinically related public service—medium, GPA—medium, letters of recommendation—high, interview—high, statement of goals and objectives—high.

Student Characteristics: The following represents characteristics of students in 2009–2010 in all graduate psychology programs in the department: Female—full-time 335, part-time 2; Male—full-time 128, part-time 2; African American/Black—full-time 39, part-time 0; Hispanic/Latino(a)—full-time 72, part-time 0; Asian/Pacific Islander—full-time 20, part-time 0; American Indian/Alaska Native—full-time 1, part-time 0; Caucasian/White—full-time 0, part-time 0; Multi-ethnic—full-time 0, part-time 0; students subject to the Americans With Disabilities Act—full-time 0, part-time 0; Unknown ethnicity—full-time 0, part-time 0; International students who hold an F-1 or J-1 Visa—full-time 0, part-time 0.

Financial Information/Assistance:
Financial Assistance:
First-Year Students: Teaching assistantships available for first year. Average amount paid per academic year: $5,000. Average number of hours worked per week: 5. Research assistantships available for first year. Average amount paid per academic year: $9,000. Average number of hours worked per week: 15. Fellowships and scholarships available for first year. Average amount paid per academic year: $18,000. Average number of hours worked per week: 10.

Advanced Students: Teaching assistantships available for advanced students. Average amount paid per academic year: $11,000. Average number of hours worked per week: 12. Research assistantships available for advanced students. Fellowships and scholarships available for advanced students. Average amount paid per academic year: $18,000. Average number of hours worked per week: 15.

Additional Information: Of all students currently enrolled full time, 90% benefited from one or more of the listed financial assistance programs.

Internships/Practica: Clinical students are placed at agencies or hospitals. Neuropsychology students are placed at hospitals or clinics Learning Processes students are placed in service agencies and treatment facilities. Forensic students find placement in various justice system related positions.

Housing and Day Care: No on-campus housing is available. On-campus day care facilities are available.

Employment of Department Graduates:
Master's Degree Graduates: Of those who graduated in the academic year 2008–2009, the following categories and numbers represent the postgraduate activities and employment of master's degree graduates: Enrolled in a postdoctoral residency/fellowship (n/a), employed in independent practice (n/a), total from the above (master's) (0).
Doctoral Degree Graduates: Of those who graduated in the academic year 2008–2009, the following categories and numbers represent the postgraduate activities and employment of doctoral degree graduates: Enrolled in a psychology doctoral program (n/a), enrolled in a postdoctoral residency/fellowship (4), employed in an academic position at a university (16), employed in an academic position at a 2-year/4-year college (9), employed in a professional position in a school system (13), employed in business or industry (2), total from the above (doctoral) (44).

Additional Information:
Orientation, Objectives, and Emphasis of Department: The developmental subprogram offers training in all areas of developmental research, with emphasis on social, cognitive, and language development. The Environmental subprogram provides interdisciplinary training with relationships between the physical environment and behavior. Concepts and approaches of fields such as urban planning, psychology, architecture, geography, anthropology, landscape architecture, and sociology are learned in a context that emphasizes the integration of systematic research and applied work with the development of theory. The social-personality subprogram trains students in the theory and research methods of both social and personality psychology. A health psychology concentration is available to students in all subprograms. Through courses, research projects, and practica, the concentration seeks to train psychologists to be able to work in a variety of health-related settings. Industrial/Organizational psychology trains people to do research in organizations and in personnel issues. Neuropsychology trains students in both basic and clinical neuroscience. Learning processes offers training in Applied Behavior Analysis. Clinical offers training in psychodynamic approaches to mental health with particular attention paid to minority populations. Experimental psychology and Experimental Cognition focus on the experimental approach to a wide variety of phenomena. Forensic psychology has two tracks, clinical (90 credits) and experimental (60 credits); the clinical track prepares people to work within the criminal justice system in a variety of clinical roles, and the experimental track prepares people in basic research dealing with the interface of psychology and the law.

Special Facilities or Resources: Computers for student use are available in the library; computer hubs, on most academic floors; and student carrel spaces, in the academic program offices. An assortment of programming languages and statistical, graphical, wordprocessing, and specialty software applications are provided. Also available are laser printers, file format translation, image scanning, and optical character recognition facilities. Adaptive technology for students with disabilities is available and includes screen-access software and such peripheral devices as reading machines, a computer-linked closed-circuit TV, and a Braille printer. Most computers designated for students are 400Mhz Celeron processor systems with 6GB hard drives, 64 MB Ram, and 15-inch flat-screen monitors. Five special-purpose classrooms, with a total of more than 100 computers, are furnished with 450 Mhz Pentium III computers and 15-inch flat-screen monitors. Students may access UNIX-based academic software from home or via a telnet session upon request. The UNIX accounts provide access to statistical or other academic software but not e-mail support. Information Resources maintains an ongoing program of equipment, computer hardware, and software modernization and provides such client services as documentation, training, and lab consulting. Workshops are held throughout the year on a wide range of topics and include many hands-on training programs.

Application Information:
Send to Admissions Office, City University Graduate Center, 365 Fifth Avenue, New York, NY 10016-4309. URL of online application: http://www.gc.cuny.edu/prospective_students/index.htm. Students are admitted in the Fall. Deadline is January 1 for Clinical and Neuropsychology; December 15 for Social/Personality, January 15 for Developmental, Environmental, Forensic; February 1 for Cognitive Neuroscience, Industrial/Organizational, March 1 for Biopsychology and Behavioral Neuroscience; March 15 for Learning Processes and Behavior Analysis, Cognition, Brain and Behavior. *Fee:* $125.

City University of New York: John Jay College of Criminal Justice
Department of Psychology
John Jay College of Criminal Justice, CUNY
445 West 59th Street
New York, NY 10019
Telephone: (212) 237-8782
Fax: (212) 237-8742
E-mail: *Jwulach@jjay.cuny.edu*
Web: *http://www.jjay.cuny.edu*

Department Information:
1976. Director, MA Program: James S. Wulach, PhD, J.D. Number of faculty: total—full-time 46, part-time 14; women—full-time 25, part-time 6; total—minority—full-time 12, part-time 4; women minority—full-time 5, part-time 2; faculty subject to the Americans With Disabilities Act 16.

Programs and Degrees Offered:
Listed in the following order: Program area, degree type (T if terminal Master's), number awarded 7/08–6/09. Forensic Psychology MA/MS (Master of Arts/Science) (T) 137, Forensic Mental Health Counseling MA/MS (Master of Arts/Science) (T) 0.

Student Applications/Admissions:
Student Applications
Forensic Psychology MA/MS (Master of Arts/Science)—Applications 2009–2010, 307. Total applicants accepted 2009–2010, 254. Number full-time enrolled (new admits only) 2009–2010, 117. Number part-time enrolled (new admits only) 2009–2010, 103. Total enrolled 2009–2010 full-time, 157, part-time, 154. Openings 2010–2011, 115. The median number of years required for completion of a degree in 2008–2009 were 2. The number of students enrolled full- and part-time who were dismissed or voluntarily withdrew from this program area in 2008–2009 were 26. Forensic Mental Health Counseling MA/MS (Master of Arts/Science)—Applications 2009–2010, 156. Total applicants accepted 2009–2010, 124. Number full-time enrolled (new admits only) 2009–2010, 52. Number part-time enrolled (new admits only) 2009–2010, 72. Total enrolled 2009–2010 full-time, 52, part-time, 72. Openings 2010–2011, 35. The number of students enrolled full- and part-time who were dismissed or voluntarily withdrew from this program area in 2008–2009 were 0.

Scores: Entries appear in this order: required test or GPA, minimum score (if required), median score of students entering in 2009–2010. Forensic Psychology MA/MS (Master of Arts/Science): GRE-V no minimum stated, 520, GRE-Q no minimum stated, 500, GRE-Analytical no minimum stated, overall undergraduate GPA 3.00, 3.20; Forensic Mental Health Counseling MA/MS (Master of Arts/Science): GRE-V no minimum stated, 520, GRE-Q no minimum stated, 500, GRE-Analytical no minimum stated, overall undergraduate GPA 3.00, 3.20.

Other Criteria: (importance of criteria rated low, medium, or high): GRE scores—high, research experience—low, work experience—low, GPA—high, letters of recommendation—medium, statement of goals and objectives—low, undergraduate major in psychology—medium, specific undergraduate psychology courses taken—high. MA Program: GPA & GRE Scores weighted most heavily. For additional information on admission requirements, go to http://www.jjay.cuny.edu/451.php.

Student Characteristics: The following represents characteristics of students in 2009–2010 in all graduate psychology programs in the department: Female—full-time 150, part-time 146; Male—full-time 66, part-time 62; African American/Black—full-time 14, part-time 35; Hispanic/Latino(a)—full-time 17, part-time 26; Asian/Pacific Islander—full-time 2, part-time 9; American Indian/Alaska Native—full-time 1, part-time 0; Caucasian/White—full-time 0, part-time 0; Multi-ethnic—full-time 0, part-time 0; students subject to the Americans With Disabilities Act—full-time 0, part-time 0; Unknown ethnicity—full-time 0, part-time 0; International students who hold an F-1 or J-1 Visa—full-time 0, part-time 0.

Financial Information/Assistance:
Tuition for Full-Time Study: *Master's:* State residents: per academic year $7,360, $310 per credit hour; Nonstate residents: $575 per credit hour. Tuition is subject to change. See the following Web site for updates and changes in tuition costs: http://www.jjay.cuny.edu/501.php.

Financial Assistance:
First-Year Students: No information provided.
Advanced Students: No information provided.

Additional Information: No information provided.

Internships/Practica: Master's Degree (MA/MS Forensic Psychology): An internship experience, such as a final research project or "capstone" experience is required of graduates. Master's Degree (MA/MS Forensic Mental Health Counseling): An internship experience, such as a final research project or "capstone" experience is required of graduates. MA Program in Forensic Psychology: Most students complete a 300-hour externship in local forensic psychology settings, such as hospitals or prisons. MA Program in Forensic Mental Health Counseling: Most students complete a 600-hour externship in local forensic psychology settings, such as hospitals or prisons.

Housing and Day Care: No on-campus housing is available. On-campus day care facilities are available. See the following Web site for more information: http://www.jjay.cuny.edu/childrenscenter.

Employment of Department Graduates:
Master's Degree Graduates: Of those who graduated in the academic year 2008–2009, the following categories and numbers represent the postgraduate activities and employment of master's degree graduates: Enrolled in a postdoctoral residency/fellowship (n/a), employed in independent practice (n/a), total from the above (master's) (0).
Doctoral Degree Graduates: Of those who graduated in the academic year 2008–2009, the following categories and numbers represent the postgraduate activities and employment of doctoral degree graduates: Enrolled in a psychology doctoral program (n/a), total from the above (doctoral) (0).

Additional Information:
Orientation, Objectives, and Emphasis of Department: MA Program in Forensic Psychology: This 42-credit program is designed to train students to provide professional MA-level psychological services to, and within, the legal system—especially the criminal justice system; and to provide a background for psychology doctoral study in the future. In addition to offering (and requiring) traditional master's level clinical psychology courses, we offer specialized courses in psychology and the law; the psychology and treatment of juvenile and adult offenders and the victims of crime; forensic evaluation and testimony; jury research; eyewitness research; psychological profiles of homicidal offenders; psychology of terrorism; and forensic psychological research. There is a research track for advanced students to work on MA theses with professors. Courses are primarily offered in the afternoon and evening. Many of our full-time faculty members have postdoctoral psychological certifications; 6 are lawyers as well as psychologists; and many have extensive forensic experience as practitioners and/or researchers. In addition, the full educational resources of the John Jay College of Criminal Justice are available to our students. Some of our graduates become MA psychologists within the criminal justice system, working with offenders, delinquents, and victims. Other graduates enhance their present careers in law enforcement, probation, or parole by completing the program. Many of our graduates continue their education in psychology doctoral programs, or in law. MA Program in Forensic Mental Health Counseling: This is a new 60-credit program, sponsored by the Psychology Department, that has been approved by NY State as a "license eligible" program for NY Mental Health Counselors, with a forensic spcialization. Coursework is similar to the MA Program in Forensic Psychology, with less emphasis on research, and more

courses oriented towards becoming a NY licensed mental health counselor.

Special Facilities or Resources: The department maintains affiliations with the major forensic psychology institutions in the New York metropolitan area. The program is endowed for student-psychology research in the Forensic Psychology Research Institute. In addition, the full academic resources and educational milieu of John Jay College of Criminal Justice, CUNY, are available to our students.

Information for Students With Physical Disabilities: See the following Web site for more information: http://www.jjay.cuny.edu/2023.php.

Application Information:
Send to Graduate Admissions, John Jay College of Criminal Justice, CUNY, Room 4205N, 445 West 59th Street, New York, NY 10019. Students are admitted in the Fall, application deadline May 5; Spring, application deadline December 1. Fee: $125.

Columbia University
Health and Behavior Studies/School Psychology
Teachers College
525 West 120th Street, Box 120
New York, NY 10027
Telephone: (212) 678-3942
Fax: (212) 678-4034
E-mail: peverly@tc.edu
Web: http://www.tc.columbia.edu/hbs/schoolpsych/

Department Information:
1996. Chairperson: Stephen Peverly. Number of faculty: total—full-time 3, part-time 11; women—full-time 1, part-time 9.

Programs and Degrees Offered:
Listed in the following order: Program area, degree type (T if terminal Master's), number awarded 7/08–6/09. School Psychology PhD (Doctor of Philosophy) 5, School Psychology MEd (Education) 17.

APA Accreditation: School PhD (Doctor of Philosophy). Student Outcome Data Website: http://www.tc.columbia.edu/hbs/schoolpsych/index.asp?Id=Student+Handbook&Info=Student+Handbook.

Student Applications/Admissions:
Student Applications
School Psychology PhD (Doctor of Philosophy)—Applications 2009–2010, 67. Total applicants accepted 2009–2010, 6. Number full-time enrolled (new admits only) 2009–2010, 5. Number part-time enrolled (new admits only) 2009–2010, 0. Total enrolled 2009–2010 full-time, 19, part-time, 8. Openings 2010–2011, 4. The median number of years required for completion of a degree in 2008–2009 were 6. The number of students enrolled full- and part-time who were dismissed or voluntarily withdrew from this program area in 2008–2009 were 1. School Psychology MEd (Education)—Applications 2009–2010, 115. Total applicants accepted 2009–2010, 56. Number full-time enrolled (new admits only) 2009–2010, 23. Number part-time enrolled (new admits only) 2009–2010, 0. Openings 2010–2011, 23. The median number of years required for completion of a degree in 2008–2009 were 3. The number of students enrolled full- and part-time who were dismissed or voluntarily withdrew from this program area in 2008–2009 were 1.

Scores: Entries appear in this order: required test or GPA, minimum score (if required), median score of students entering in 2009–2010. School Psychology PhD (Doctor of Philosophy): GRE-V no minimum stated, 585, GRE-Q no minimum stated, 735, GRE-Analytical no minimum stated, 5.5, overall undergraduate GPA no minimum stated, 3.49, Masters GPA no minimum stated; School Psychology MEd (Education): GRE-V no minimum stated, 525, GRE-Q no minimum stated, 635, GRE-Analytical no minimum stated, 4.5, overall undergraduate GPA no minimum stated, 3.5.

Other Criteria: (importance of criteria rated low, medium, or high): GRE scores—high, research experience—high, work experience—medium, extracurricular activity—medium, clinically related public service—medium, GPA—high, letters of recommendation—high, interview—high, statement of goals and objectives—high. For additional information on admission requirements, go to http://www.tc.edu/hbs/SchoolPsych.

Student Characteristics: The following represents characteristics of students in 2009–2010 in all graduate psychology programs in the department: Female—full-time 76, part-time 7; Male—full-time 9, part-time 1; African American/Black—full-time 3, part-time 1; Hispanic/Latino(a)—full-time 3, part-time 0; Asian/Pacific Islander—full-time 10, part-time 1; American Indian/Alaska Native—full-time 0, part-time 0; Caucasian/White—full-time 67, part-time 6; Multi-ethnic—full-time 2, part-time 0; students subject to the Americans With Disabilities Act—full-time 0, part-time 0; Unknown ethnicity—full-time 0, part-time 0; International students who hold an F-1 or J-1 Visa—full-time 0, part-time 0.

Financial Information/Assistance:
Tuition for Full-Time Study: *Master's:* State residents: $1,127 per credit hour; Nonstate residents: $1,127 per credit hour. *Doctoral:* State residents: $1,127 per credit hour; Nonstate residents: $1,127 per credit hour. Additional fees are assessed to students beyond the costs of tuition for the following: College fee, Medical fee, research fee. See the following Web site for updates and changes in tuition costs: http://www.tc.columbia.edu/controller/.

Financial Assistance:
First-Year Students: Fellowships and scholarships available for first year. Average amount paid per academic year: $14,000.

Advanced Students: Teaching assistantships available for advanced students. Average amount paid per academic year: $1,830. Average number of hours worked per week: 5. Fellowships and scholarships available for advanced students. Average amount paid per academic year: $14,000.

Additional Information: Of all students currently enrolled full time, 25% benefited from one or more of the listed financial assistance programs. Application and information available online at: http://www.tc.columbia.edu/financialaid.

Internships/Practica: Doctoral Degree (PhD School Psychology): For those doctoral students for whom a professional internship was required in this program prior to graduation, (5) students applied for an internship in 2008–2009, with (5) students obtaining an internship. Of those students who obtained an internship, (5) were paid internships. Of those students who obtained an internship, (5) students placed in APA/CPA accredited internships, (0) students placed in internships not APA/CPA accredited, but listed with the Association of Psychology Postdoctoral and Internship Programs (APPIC), (0) students placed in internships conforming to guidelines of the Council of Directors of School Psychology Programs (CDSPP), (0) students placed in internships that were not APA/CPA accredited, APPIC or CDSPP listed. First year—Two practica in our Center for Educational and Psychological Services: (1) Practicum in Assessment of Reading and School Subject Difficulties (Fall); (2) Practicum in Psychoeducational Assessment with Culturally Diverse Students (Spring). Second year—students engage in (1) Fieldwork (2 days/week over the academic year in one of our cooperating inner-city schools) (2) a practicum in psychoeducational groups (the groups are run within students' fieldwork sites). Third year—Externship (2 days/week over an academic year; most students are required to do 2 externships: one in a school and one in a hospital or clinic); Fourth or Fifth year—Internship (full calendar year; students must have an approved dissertation proposal before they begin to do the internship after completing most or all of their dissertation).

Housing and Day Care: On-campus housing is available. See the following Web site for more information: http://www.tc.columbia.edu/housing/. No on-campus day care facilities are available.

Employment of Department Graduates:
Master's Degree Graduates: Of those who graduated in the academic year 2008–2009, the following categories and numbers represent the postgraduate activities and employment of master's degree graduates: Enrolled in a psychology doctoral program (2), enrolled in a postdoctoral residency/fellowship (n/a), employed in independent practice (n/a), employed in a professional position in a school system (17), total from the above (master's) (19).
Doctoral Degree Graduates: Of those who graduated in the academic year 2008–2009, the following categories and numbers represent the postgraduate activities and employment of doctoral degree graduates: Enrolled in a psychology doctoral program (n/a), enrolled in a postdoctoral residency/fellowship (2), employed in a professional position in a school system (2), employed in a community mental health/counseling center (1), total from the above (doctoral) (5).

Additional Information:
Orientation, Objectives, and Emphasis of Department: The primary theoretical orientation of our program is cognitive and developmental with strong applications to instruction and mental health. We place a particularly strong emphasis on prevention and intervention in these areas. Throughout the curriculum, there is a balance between science and practice, and we ensure that all students are well grounded in the theory and methods of psychological science. Most students opt to go through the general curriculum. However, some have adopted a specialization in the deaf and hearing impaired.

Special Facilities or Resources: The School Psychology program has strong collaborative relationships with several inner-city schools that serve as fieldwork sites for our master's and doctoral students.

Information for Students With Physical Disabilities: See the following Web site for more information: http://www.tc.columbia.edu/oasid/.

Application Information:
Send to Office of Admissions, Box 302, Teachers College, Columbia University, 525 West 120th Street, New York, NY 10027; 212-678-3710. Application available online. URL of online application: http://www.tc.columbia.edu/admissions/. Students are admitted in the Fall, application deadline December 15. January 15 for the Ed.M. Program. *Fee:* $65. Re-applicants—$35. Paper applications are not accepted.

Cornell University
Department of Human Development
The New York State College of Human Ecology
G77 Martha Van Rensselaer Hall
Ithaca, NY 14853-4401
Telephone: (607) 255-7620
Fax: (607) 255-9856
E-mail: *blb5@cornell.edu*
Web: *http://www.human.cornell.edu/che/HD/*

Department Information:
1925. Chairperson: Ritch Savin-Williams. Number of faculty: total—full-time 21; women—full-time 9; total—minority—full-time 3; women minority—full-time 2.

Programs and Degrees Offered:
Listed in the following order: Program area, degree type (T if terminal Master's), number awarded 7/08–6/09. Developmental Psychology PhD (Doctor of Philosophy) 3, Human Development and Family Studies PhD (Doctor of Philosophy) 2.

Student Applications/Admissions:
Student Applications
Developmental Psychology PhD (Doctor of Philosophy)—Applications 2009–2010, 82. Total applicants accepted 2009–2010, 11. Number full-time enrolled (new admits only) 2009–2010, 6. Number part-time enrolled (new admits only) 2009–2010, 0. Openings 2010–2011, 7. The median number of years required for completion of a degree in 2008–2009 were 5. The number of students enrolled full- and part-time who were dismissed or voluntarily withdrew from this program area in 2008–2009 were 0. Human Development and Family Studies PhD (Doctor of Philosophy)—Applications 2009–2010, 15. Total applicants accepted 2009–2010, 1. Number full-time enrolled (new admits only) 2009–2010, 1. Number part-time enrolled (new admits only) 2009–2010, 0. Openings 2010–2011, 1. The median number of years required for completion of a degree in 2008–2009 were 5. The number of students enrolled full- and part-time who were dismissed or voluntarily withdrew from this program area in 2008–2009 were 0.
Other Criteria: (importance of criteria rated low, medium, or high): GRE scores—high, research experience—high, work experience—low, extracurricular activity—low, clinically related public service—low, GPA—high, letters of recommenda-

tion—high, statement of goals and objectives—high, specific undergraduate psychology courses taken—medium. For additional information on admission requirements, go to http://www.human.cornell.edu/che/HD/graduate/Admissions-Funding.cfm.

Student Characteristics: The following represents characteristics of students in 2009–2010 in all graduate psychology programs in the department: Female—full-time 23, part-time 0; Male—full-time 10, part-time 0; African American/Black—full-time 1, part-time 0; Hispanic/Latino(a)—full-time 1, part-time 0; Asian/Pacific Islander—full-time 1, part-time 0; American Indian/Alaska Native—full-time 0, part-time 0; Caucasian/White—full-time 30, part-time 0; Multi-ethnic—full-time 0, part-time 0; students subject to the Americans With Disabilities Act—full-time 0, part-time 0; Unknown ethnicity—full-time 0, part-time 0; International students who hold an F-1 or J-1 Visa—full-time 11, part-time 0.

Financial Information/Assistance:
Tuition for Full-Time Study: Doctoral: State residents: per academic year $20,800; Nonstate residents: per academic year $20,800. Tuition is subject to change. See the following Web site for updates and changes in tuition costs: http://www.gradschool.cornell.edu/index.php?p=143.

Financial Assistance:
First-Year Students: Teaching assistantships available for first year. Average amount paid per academic year: $21,800. Average number of hours worked per week: 15. Apply by January 1. Research assistantships available for first year. Average amount paid per academic year: $21,800. Average number of hours worked per week: 15. Apply by January 1. Fellowships and scholarships available for first year. Average amount paid per academic year: $21,800. Average number of hours worked per week: 0. Apply by January 1.

Advanced Students: Teaching assistantships available for advanced students. Average amount paid per academic year: $21,800. Average number of hours worked per week: 15. Apply by January 1. Research assistantships available for advanced students. Average amount paid per academic year: $21,800. Average number of hours worked per week: 15. Apply by January 1. Fellowships and scholarships available for advanced students. Average amount paid per academic year: $21,800. Average number of hours worked per week: 0. Apply by January 1.

Additional Information: Of all students currently enrolled full time, 100% benefited from one or more of the listed financial assistance programs. Application and information available online at: http://www.gradschool.cornell.edu/index.php?p=131.

Housing and Day Care: On-campus housing is available. See the following Web site for more information: http://www.campuslife.cornell.edu/. On-campus day care facilities are available. See the following Web site for more information: http://www.hr.cornell.edu/life/support/child_care_center.html.

Employment of Department Graduates:
Master's Degree Graduates: Of those who graduated in the academic year 2008–2009, the following categories and numbers represent the postgraduate activities and employment of master's degree graduates: Enrolled in a postdoctoral residency/fellowship (n/a), employed in independent practice (n/a), total from the above (master's) (0).

Doctoral Degree Graduates: Of those who graduated in the academic year 2008–2009, the following categories and numbers represent the postgraduate activities and employment of doctoral degree graduates: Enrolled in a psychology doctoral program (n/a), employed in an academic position at a university (2), total from the above (doctoral) (2).

Additional Information:
Orientation, Objectives, and Emphasis of Department: The graduate program trains researchers and prepares students for research and teaching careers in academic life, work in government agencies, and careers as researchers on projects carried out in a variety of public and private sectors. We offer training in six broad categories: Aging and Health; Cognitive Development; Group Disparities in Development; Human Behavioral Neuroscience; and Law, Psychology, and Human Development. We do not offer training in counseling psychology, marriage counseling, or family therapy. The doctoral program in Human Development has 33 faculty; 21 are members of the Department of Human Development and 12 have primary appointments in the departments of Psychology, Design and Environmental Analysis, Policy Analysis and Management, the Law school, or in the Weill Cornell Medical College. The faculty includes psychologists and sociologists. There are approximately 35 graduate students in the program.

Special Facilities or Resources: The department houses a number of laboratories dedicated to individual projects as well as several non-dedicated laboratories, including rooms with audio and visual recording capability. Opportunities for research exist in area public schools, nursery schools and day care centers, and youth service agencies. The department also maintains graduate student computer facilities with statistical software and various programs such as E-prime and Noldus. In addition, the department has ties with several centers in the College including the Bronfenbrenner Life Course Institute (with its concentration on life course studies), the Family Life Development Center (which concentrates on families under stress), the Institute for Research on Children, and the Institute for Translational Research on Aging.

Information for Students With Physical Disabilities: See the following Web site for more information: http://sds.cornell.edu/.

Application Information:
Send to Bonnie Biata, Human Development, G77 Martha VanRensselaer Hall, Cornell University, Ithaca, NY 14853. Application available online. URL of online application: http://www.gradschool.cornell.edu/index.php?p=102. Students are admitted in the Fall, application deadline January 1. *Fee:* $70. In cases of extreme financial need, a fee waiver will be considered. A letter of request for a waiver and documentation of need such as a letter from the college financial aid office needs to be submitted.

Cornell University
Graduate Field of Psychology
Arts & Sciences
211 Uris Hall
Ithaca, NY 14853-7601
Telephone: (607) 255-3834
Fax: (607) 255-8433
E-mail: pac34@cornell.edu
Web: http://www.psych.cornell.edu/

Department Information:
1885. Director of Graduate Studies: Timothy J. DeVoogd. Number of faculty: total—full-time 24, part-time 1; women—full-time 8; total—minority—full-time 1; women minority—full-time 1.

Programs and Degrees Offered:
Listed in the following order: Program area, degree type (T if terminal Master's), number awarded 7/08–6/09. Behavioral and Evolutionary Neuroscience PhD (Doctor of Philosophy), Perception, Cognition and Development PhD (Doctor of Philosophy) 2, Social and Personality Psychology PhD (Doctor of Philosophy) 1.

Student Applications/Admissions:
Student Applications
Behavioral and Evolutionary Neuroscience PhD (Doctor of Philosophy)—Applications 2009–2010, 45. Total applicants accepted 2009–2010, 4. Number full-time enrolled (new admits only) 2009–2010, 3. Openings 2010–2011, 2. The median number of years required for completion of a degree in 2008–2009 were 5. *Perception, Cognition and Development PhD (Doctor of Philosophy)*—Applications 2009–2010, 78. Total applicants accepted 2009–2010, 3. Number full-time enrolled (new admits only) 2009–2010, 2. Openings 2010–2011, 2. The median number of years required for completion of a degree in 2008–2009 were 5. The number of students enrolled full- and part-time who were dismissed or voluntarily withdrew from this program area in 2008–2009 were 0. *Social and Personality Psychology PhD (Doctor of Philosophy)*—Applications 2009–2010, 143. Total applicants accepted 2009–2010, 3. Number full-time enrolled (new admits only) 2009–2010, 2. Openings 2010–2011, 2. The median number of years required for completion of a degree in 2008–2009 were 5.
Other Criteria: (importance of criteria rated low, medium, or high): GRE scores—high, research experience—high, work experience—low, extracurricular activity—low, GPA—high, letters of recommendation—high, statement of goals and objectives—high. For additional information on admission requirements, go to http://www.psych.cornell.edu/grad_howto_apply.

Student Characteristics: The following represents characteristics of students in 2009–2010 in all graduate psychology programs in the department: Female—full-time 26, part-time 0; Male—full-time 13, part-time 0; African American/Black—full-time 2, part-time 0; Hispanic/Latino(a)—full-time 3, part-time 0; Asian/Pacific Islander—full-time 5, part-time 0; American Indian/Alaska Native—full-time 0, part-time 0; Caucasian/White—full-time 28, part-time 0; Multi-ethnic—full-time 1, part-time 0; students subject to the Americans With Disabilities Act—full-time 0, part-time 0; Unknown ethnicity—full-time 0, part-time 0; International students who hold an F-1 or J-1 Visa—full-time 11, part-time 0.

Financial Information/Assistance:
Tuition for Full-Time Study: Doctoral: State residents: per academic year $29,500; Nonstate residents: per academic year $29,500. Tuition is subject to change. See the following Web site for updates and changes in tuition costs: http://www.gradschool.cornell.edu/index.php?p=143.

Financial Assistance:
First-Year Students: Teaching assistantships available for first year. Average amount paid per academic year: $21,800. Average number of hours worked per week: 20. Fellowships and scholarships available for first year. Average amount paid per academic year: $21,800.
Advanced Students: No information provided.
Additional Information: Of all students currently enrolled full time, 100% benefited from one or more of the listed financial assistance programs. Application and information available online at: http://www.gradschool.cornell.edu/index.php?p=143.

Housing and Day Care: On-campus housing is available. See the following Web site for more information: http://www.campuslife.cornell.edu/campuslife/housing/index.cfm. On-campus day care facilities are available. See the following Web site for more information: http://www.hr.cornell.edu/life/support/child_care.html.

Employment of Department Graduates:
Master's Degree Graduates: Of those who graduated in the academic year 2008–2009, the following categories and numbers represent the postgraduate activities and employment of master's degree graduates: Enrolled in a postdoctoral residency/fellowship (n/a), employed in independent practice (n/a), total from the above (master's) (0).
Doctoral Degree Graduates: Of those who graduated in the academic year 2008–2009, the following categories and numbers represent the postgraduate activities and employment of doctoral degree graduates: Enrolled in a psychology doctoral program (n/a), enrolled in a postdoctoral residency/fellowship (3), total from the above (doctoral) (3).

Additional Information:
Orientation, Objectives, and Emphasis of Department: The Psychology Department of the College of Arts and Sciences at Cornell has a faculty of 25 psychologists and is divided into three areas—perception, cognition and development (encompassing cognition, language, perception, and its developmental perspectives), behavioral and evolutionary neuroscience (focusing on hormones and behavior, neural development, and sensory systems), and social and personality psychology (social cognition, judgment, and decision making). We do not have clinical, community, or counseling programs. We have a strong research orientation, training our students to become professional academics or researchers. Our 39 students design their graduate programs under the supervision of their special committees. These committees consist of at least four members of the graduate faculty at Cornell; at least three are from within the department. The chair of the committee is a member of the Graduate Field of Psychology, which consists of the 26 members of our department plus 20 researchers in allied fields (human development, education, industrial and labor relations, and neurobiology and behavior). Two

other committee members serve as minor members, one of whom can be outside the Graduate Field of Psychology, and the fourth member oversees breadth requirements.

Special Facilities or Resources: The three areas of our program each have laboratories associated with them. Each of the members of the perception, cognition and development program has a separate laboratory, fully equipped with state-of-the-art computer equipment. In addition, the program has several computer-based teaching laboratories. The Behavioral Evolutionary Neuroscience group each has separate labs and computers, and animal housing facilities where relevant, but they share much of equipment and lab space. There is also a teaching lab associated with B.E.N.'s group labs. The social and personality psychologists share a large lab space with the sociology department.

Information for Students With Physical Disabilities: See the following Web site for more information: http://sds.cornell.edu/.

Application Information:
Send to Graduate School, Caldwell Hall, Cornell University, Ithaca, NY 14853. Application available online. URL of online application: http://gradschool.cornell.edu. Students are admitted in the Fall, application deadline December 15. *Fee:* $70.

Fordham University
Department of Psychology
Arts and Sciences
441 East Fordham Road
Bronx, NY 10458
Telephone: (718) 817-3775
Fax: (718) 817-3785
E-mail: *schiaffino@fordham.edu*
Web: *http://www.fordham.edu/psychology*

Department Information:
1933. Chairperson: Kathleen M. Schiaffino. Number of faculty: total—full-time 26; women—full-time 13; total—minority—full-time 4; women minority—full-time 3.

Programs and Degrees Offered:
Listed in the following order: Program area, degree type (T if terminal Master's), number awarded 7/08–6/09. Clinical Psychology PhD (Doctor of Philosophy) 8, Psychometrics PhD (Doctor of Philosophy) 2, Applied Developmental Psychology PhD (Doctor of Philosophy) 2.

APA Accreditation: Clinical PhD (Doctor of Philosophy).

Student Applications/Admissions:
Student Applications
Clinical Psychology PhD (Doctor of Philosophy)—Applications 2009–2010, 400. Total applicants accepted 2009–2010, 19. Number full-time enrolled (new admits only) 2009–2010, 11. Number part-time enrolled (new admits only) 2009–2010, 0. Openings 2010–2011, 12. The median number of years required for completion of a degree in 2008–2009 were 6. The number of students enrolled full- and part-time who were dismissed or voluntarily withdrew from this program area in 2008–2009 were 0. *Psychometrics PhD (Doctor of Philosophy)*—Applications 2009–2010, 23. Total applicants accepted 2009–2010, 9. Number full-time enrolled (new admits only) 2009–2010, 4. Number part-time enrolled (new admits only) 2009–2010, 0. Openings 2010–2011, 4. The median number of years required for completion of a degree in 2008–2009 were 6. The number of students enrolled full- and part-time who were dismissed or voluntarily withdrew from this program area in 2008–2009 were 1. *Applied Developmental Psychology PhD (Doctor of Philosophy)*—Applications 2009–2010, 40. Total applicants accepted 2009–2010, 12. Number full-time enrolled (new admits only) 2009–2010, 5. Number part-time enrolled (new admits only) 2009–2010, 0. Openings 2010–2011, 6. The median number of years required for completion of a degree in 2008–2009 were 5. The number of students enrolled full- and part-time who were dismissed or voluntarily withdrew from this program area in 2008–2009 were 1.

Scores: Entries appear in this order: required test or GPA, minimum score (if required), median score of students entering in 2009–2010. *Clinical Psychology PhD (Doctor of Philosophy)*: GRE-V no minimum stated, GRE-Q no minimum stated, GRE-Analytical no minimum stated, overall undergraduate GPA no minimum stated; *Applied Developmental Psychology PhD (Doctor of Philosophy)*: GRE-V no minimum stated, GRE-Q no minimum stated, GRE-Analytical no minimum stated, overall undergraduate GPA no minimum stated.

Other Criteria: (importance of criteria rated low, medium, or high): GRE scores—high, research experience—high, work experience—medium, extracurricular activity—medium, clinically related public service—medium, GPA—high, letters of recommendation—high, interview—high, statement of goals and objectives—high, undergraduate major in psychology—medium, specific undergraduate psychology courses taken—high.

Student Characteristics: The following represents characteristics of students in 2009–2010 in all graduate psychology programs in the department: Female—full-time 82, part-time 0; Male—full-time 42, part-time 0; African American/Black—full-time 5, part-time 0; Hispanic/Latino(a)—full-time 3, part-time 0; Asian/Pacific Islander—full-time 10, part-time 0; American Indian/Alaska Native—full-time 1, part-time 0; Caucasian/White—full-time 105, part-time 0; Multi-ethnic—full-time 0, part-time 0; students subject to the Americans With Disabilities Act—full-time 0, part-time 0; Unknown ethnicity—full-time 0, part-time 0; International students who hold an F-1 or J-1 Visa—full-time 5, part-time 0.

Financial Information/Assistance:
Tuition for Full-Time Study: *Doctoral:* State residents: $1,190 per credit hour; Nonstate residents: $1,190 per credit hour. Tuition is subject to change.

Financial Assistance:
First-Year Students: Teaching assistantships available for first year. Average amount paid per academic year: $19,900. Average number of hours worked per week: 15. Apply by December 9. Research assistantships available for first year. Average amount paid per academic year: $19,900. Average number of hours worked per week: 15. Apply by December 9. Fellowships and scholarships available for first year. Average amount paid per academic year:

$22,000. Average number of hours worked per week: 0. Apply by December 9.

Advanced Students: Teaching assistantships available for advanced students. Average amount paid per academic year: $19,700. Average number of hours worked per week: 15. Apply by January 4. Research assistantships available for advanced students. Average amount paid per academic year: $19,700. Average number of hours worked per week: 15. Apply by January 4. Fellowships and scholarships available for advanced students. Average amount paid per academic year: $21,000. Average number of hours worked per week: 15. Apply by January 4.

Additional Information: Of all students currently enrolled full time, 90% benefited from one or more of the listed financial assistance programs. Application and information available online at: http://www.fordham.edu/financialaid.

Internships/Practica: Doctoral Degree (PhD Clinical Psychology): For those doctoral students for whom a professional internship was required in this program prior to graduation, (11) students applied for an internship in 2008–2009, with (10) students obtaining an internship. Of those students who obtained an internship, (10) were paid internships. Of those students who obtained an internship, (10) students placed in APA/CPA accredited internships, (0) students placed in internships not APA/CPA accredited, but listed with the Association of Psychology Postdoctoral and Internship Programs (APPIC), (0) students placed in internships conforming to guidelines of the Council of Directors of School Psychology Programs (CDSPP), (0) students placed in internships that were not APA/CPA accredited, APPIC or CDSPP listed. Internships in a variety of public and private facilities are available for students after they have completed their coursework in the program.

Housing and Day Care: No on-campus housing is available. No on-campus day care facilities are available.

Employment of Department Graduates:
Master's Degree Graduates: Of those who graduated in the academic year 2008–2009, the following categories and numbers represent the postgraduate activities and employment of master's degree graduates: Enrolled in a postdoctoral residency/fellowship (n/a), employed in independent practice (n/a), total from the above (master's) (0).
Doctoral Degree Graduates: Of those who graduated in the academic year 2008–2009, the following categories and numbers represent the postgraduate activities and employment of doctoral degree graduates: Enrolled in a psychology doctoral program (n/a), enrolled in another graduate/professional program (0), enrolled in a postdoctoral residency/fellowship (3), employed in business or industry (2), employed in government agency (3), employed in a hospital/medical center (3), do not know (2), total from the above (doctoral) (13).

Additional Information:
Orientation, Objectives, and Emphasis of Department: Clinical psychology prepares students for practice, research, and teaching in the clinical field as both professionals and scientists. Courses can be grouped under four major areas: clinical theory and methodology, research topics and methods, behavioral classification and assessment, and treatment approaches. Specializations include Family and Child, Health/Neuropsychology, and Forensics. There is a full-time, one-year internship. Applied Developmental psychology (ADP) trains professionals who can conduct both basic and applied research in developmental processes across the lifespan and who can share their knowledge in academic and community-based settings. ADP focuses on the interplay between developmental processes and social contexts including design and evaluation of programs; consultation to courts, lawyers, and public policy makers; development and evaluation of programs and materials directed at children and families; and parent and family education. The Psychometrics program focuses on the quantitative and research-oriented commonalities relevant to most of the behavioral sciences, and their applications in industry, education, and the health services. Students in Psychometrics become familiar with statistics, psychological testing, use of computer systems, and other research techniques, as well as with the psychology of individual differences.

Application Information:
Send to Graduate Admissions Office, Keating 216. Students are admitted in the Fall, application deadline December 8. *Fee:* $70.

Fordham University
Division of Psychological and Educational Services
Graduate School of Education
113 West 60th Street, Room 1008
New York, NY 10023
Telephone: (212) 636-6646
Fax: (212) 636-6641
E-mail: *horisk@fordham.edu*
Web: *http://www.fordham.edu/gse*

Department Information:
1927. Chairperson: Mitchell Rabinowitz. Number of faculty: total—full-time 13, part-time 8; women—full-time 8, part-time 8; total—minority—full-time 4; women minority—full-time 3.

Programs and Degrees Offered:
Listed in the following order: Program area, degree type (T if terminal Master's), number awarded 7/08–6/09. Counseling Psychology PhD (Doctor of Philosophy) 16, Educational Psychology PhD (Doctor of Philosophy), School Psychology PhD (Doctor of Philosophy) 8, School Psychology Diploma 30, Bilingual School Psychology Diploma 3, Educational Psychology MEd (Education), Counseling and Personnel Services MEd (Education), Mental Health Counseling MEd (Education).

APA Accreditation: Counseling PhD (Doctor of Philosophy). School PhD (Doctor of Philosophy).

Student Applications/Admissions:
Student Applications
Counseling Psychology PhD (Doctor of Philosophy)—Applications 2009–2010, 121. Total applicants accepted 2009–2010, 9. Number full-time enrolled (new admits only) 2009–2010, 9. Total enrolled 2009–2010 full-time, 55. Openings 2010–2011, 12. The median number of years required for completion of a degree in 2008–2009 were 6. The number of students enrolled full- and part-time who were dismissed or voluntarily withdrew from this program area in 2008–2009 were 0. *Educational Psychology PhD (Doctor of Philosophy)*—Applications

2009–2010, 11. Total applicants accepted 2009–2010, 5. Number full-time enrolled (new admits only) 2009–2010, 6. Total enrolled 2009–2010 full-time, 16, part-time, 12. Openings 2010–2011, 8. The number of students enrolled full- and part-time who were dismissed or voluntarily withdrew from this program area in 2008–2009 were 0. *School Psychology PhD (Doctor of Philosophy)*—Applications 2009–2010, 80. Total applicants accepted 2009–2010, 25. Number full-time enrolled (new admits only) 2009–2010, 10. Total enrolled 2009–2010 full-time, 50, part-time, 30. Openings 2010–2011, 12. The median number of years required for completion of a degree in 2008–2009 were 7. The number of students enrolled full- and part-time who were dismissed or voluntarily withdrew from this program area in 2008–2009 were 2. *School Psychology Diploma*—Applications 2009–2010, 70. Total applicants accepted 2009–2010, 40. Number full-time enrolled (new admits only) 2009–2010, 22. Number part-time enrolled (new admits only) 2009–2010, 0. Total enrolled 2009–2010 full-time, 50, part-time, 25. Openings 2010–2011, 25. The median number of years required for completion of a degree in 2008–2009 were 3. The number of students enrolled full- and part-time who were dismissed or voluntarily withdrew from this program area in 2008–2009 were 0. *Bilingual School Psychology Diploma*—Applications 2009–2010, 8. Total applicants accepted 2009–2010, 6. Number full-time enrolled (new admits only) 2009–2010, 5. Total enrolled 2009–2010 full-time, 22. Openings 2010–2011, 8. The median number of years required for completion of a degree in 2008–2009 were 3. The number of students enrolled full- and part-time who were dismissed or voluntarily withdrew from this program area in 2008–2009 were 0. *Educational Psychology MEd (Education)*—Applications 2009–2010, 23. Total applicants accepted 2009–2010, 17. Number full-time enrolled (new admits only) 2009–2010, 5. Total enrolled 2009–2010 full-time, 10. Openings 2010–2011, 7. The median number of years required for completion of a degree in 2008–2009 were 2. The number of students enrolled full- and part-time who were dismissed or voluntarily withdrew from this program area in 2008–2009 were 0. *Counseling and Personnel Services MEd (Education)*—Applications 2009–2010, 90. Total applicants accepted 2009–2010, 55. Number full-time enrolled (new admits only) 2009–2010, 21. Total enrolled 2009–2010 full-time, 64. Openings 2010–2011, 25. The median number of years required for completion of a degree in 2008–2009 were 2. The number of students enrolled full- and part-time who were dismissed or voluntarily withdrew from this program area in 2008–2009 were 0. *Mental Health Counseling MEd (Education)*—Applications 2009–2010, 70. Total applicants accepted 2009–2010, 67. Number full-time enrolled (new admits only) 2009–2010, 21. Total enrolled 2009–2010 full-time, 52. Openings 2010–2011, 25. The median number of years required for completion of a degree in 2008–2009 were 2. The number of students enrolled full- and part-time who were dismissed or voluntarily withdrew from this program area in 2008–2009 were 0.

Scores: Entries appear in this order: required test or GPA, minimum score (if required), median score of students entering in 2009–2010. *School Psychology PhD (Doctor of Philosophy):* GRE-V 490, 550, GRE-Q 550, 660, GRE-Analytical 4, 5, overall undergraduate GPA 3.1, 3.49.

Other Criteria: (importance of criteria rated low, medium, or high): GRE scores—high, research experience—medium, work experience—medium, extracurricular activity—medium, clinically related public service—medium, GPA—high, letters of recommendation—high, interview—low, statement of goals and objectives—high.

Student Characteristics: The following represents characteristics of students in 2009–2010 in all graduate psychology programs in the department: Female—full-time 286, part-time 50; Male—full-time 33, part-time 17; African American/Black—full-time 18, part-time 2; Hispanic/Latino(a)—full-time 18, part-time 5; Asian/Pacific Islander—full-time 9, part-time 3; American Indian/Alaska Native—full-time 0, part-time 0; Caucasian/White—full-time 102, part-time 16; Multi-ethnic—full-time 0, part-time 0; students subject to the Americans With Disabilities Act—full-time 0, part-time 0; Unknown ethnicity—full-time 172, part-time 41; International students who hold an F-1 or J-1 Visa—full-time 0, part-time 0.

Financial Information/Assistance:

Tuition for Full-Time Study: *Master's:* State residents: $1,050 per credit hour; Nonstate residents: $1,050 per credit hour. *Doctoral:* State residents: $1,050 per credit hour; Nonstate residents: $1,050 per credit hour. Tuition is subject to change. Additional fees are assessed to students beyond the costs of tuition for the following: University Fees. See the following Web site for updates and changes in tuition costs: http://www.fordham.edu/academics/colleges__graduate_s/graduate__profession/education/financial_aid/t.

Financial Assistance:

First-Year Students: Research assistantships available for first year. Average number of hours worked per week: 7. Apply by March. Fellowships and scholarships available for first year.

Advanced Students: Research assistantships available for advanced students. Average number of hours worked per week: 12. Apply by March. Fellowships and scholarships available for advanced students.

Additional Information: Of all students currently enrolled full time, 60% benefited from one or more of the listed financial assistance programs.

Internships/Practica: Doctoral Degree (PhD Counseling Psychology): For those doctoral students for whom a professional internship was required in this program prior to graduation, (12) students applied for an internship in 2008–2009, with (11) students obtaining an internship. Of those students who obtained an internship, (11) were paid internships. Of those students who obtained an internship, (7) students placed in APA/CPA accredited internships, (4) students placed in internships not APA/CPA accredited, but listed with the Association of Psychology Postdoctoral and Internship Programs (APPIC), (0) students placed in internships conforming to guidelines of the Council of Directors of School Psychology Programs (CDSPP), (0) students placed in internships that were not APA/CPA accredited, APPIC or CDSPP listed. Doctoral Degree (PhD School Psychology): For those doctoral students for whom a professional internship was required in this program prior to graduation, (8) students applied for an internship in 2008–2009, with (8) students obtaining an internship. Of those students who obtained an internship, (6) were paid internships. Of those students who obtained an internship, (2) students placed in APA/CPA accredited internships, (0) students placed in internships not APA/CPA accredited, but listed with the Association of Psychology Postdoctoral and Internship Programs (APPIC), (6) students placed in internships conforming to guidelines of the Council of Directors of School Psychology Programs (CDSPP), (0) students placed in internships that were not APA/CPA accredited, APPIC or CDSPP listed. Students complete practica, field experiences, externships and internships in a wide variety of sites throughout the metropolitan NYC area. Sites such as P-12 schools, hospitals, mental health agencies and clinics and college counseling centers all vary by setting, type and diversity of the population served.

Housing and Day Care: No on-campus housing is available. No on-campus day care facilities are available.

Employment of Department Graduates:
Master's Degree Graduates: Of those who graduated in the academic year 2008–2009, the following categories and numbers represent the postgraduate activities and employment of master's degree graduates: Enrolled in a postdoctoral residency/fellowship (n/a), employed in independent practice (n/a), total from the above (master's) (0).
Doctoral Degree Graduates: Of those who graduated in the academic year 2008–2009, the following categories and numbers represent the postgraduate activities and employment of doctoral degree graduates: Enrolled in a psychology doctoral program (n/a), enrolled in a postdoctoral residency/fellowship (1), employed in other positions at a higher education institution (1), employed in government agency (1), employed in a community mental health/counseling center (1), employed in a hospital/medical center (3), total from the above (doctoral) (7).

Additional Information:
Orientation, Objectives, and Emphasis of Department: Prepares professionals for positions in PreK–12 schools, mental health settings; counseling services in higher education, adult education, business, industry, and independent psychological practice. Also provides advanced training for teachers and individuals interested in research or the development and evaluation of educational programs and materials.

Special Facilities or Resources: Fordham University's Graduate School of Education offers several higher learning and community based centers and institutes: The Center for Educational Partnerships, The Rosa A. Hagin School Consultation Center and Early Childhood Center, The Center for Catholic Leadership and Faith-Based Education, Center for Learning in Unsupervised Environment, Human Resiliency, Advancement Placement Summer Institute and the Psychological Services Institute.

Information for Students With Physical Disabilities: See the following Web site for more information: http://www.fordham.edu/campus_resources/student_services/disability_service.

Application Information:
Send to N/A. Application available online. URL of online application: www.fordham.edu/gse. Students are admitted in the Fall, application deadline. Counseling Psychology PhD - December 15 School Psychology PhD and PD - January 15 Counseling MSE - March 1 Educational Psychology programs have rolling admissions. *Fee:* $50.

Hofstra University (2009 data)
Department of Psychology
Hofstra College of Liberal Arts and Sciences
135 Hofstra University
Hempstead, NY 11549
Telephone: (516) 463-5624
Fax: (516) 463-6052
E-mail: *Charles.F.Levinthal@hofstra.edu*
Web: *http://www.hofstra.edu/Academics/HCLAS/Psychology/*

Department Information:
1948. Chairperson: Charles F. Levinthal, PhD. Number of faculty: total—full-time 34, part-time 19; women—full-time 12, part-time 8; total—minority—full-time 2, part-time 1; women minority—full-time 1; faculty subject to the Americans With Disabilities Act 1.

Programs and Degrees Offered:
Listed in the following order: Program area, degree type (T if terminal Master's), number awarded 7/08–6/09. Clinical PhD (Doctor of Philosophy) 16, Industrial-Organizational MA/MS (Master of Arts/Science) (T) 19, School-Community PsyD (Doctor of Psychology) 15, Applied Organizational Psychology PhD (Doctor of Philosophy) 2.

APA Accreditation: Clinical PhD (Doctor of Philosophy). School PsyD (Doctor of Psychology).

Student Applications/Admissions:
Student Applications
Clinical PhD (Doctor of Philosophy)—Applications 2009–2010, 221. Total applicants accepted 2009–2010, 23. Number full-time enrolled (new admits only) 2009–2010, 14. Openings 2010–2011, 15. The median number of years required for completion of a degree in 2008–2009 were 5. The number of students enrolled full- and part-time who were dismissed or voluntarily withdrew from this program area in 2008–2009 were 1. *Industrial-Organizational MA/MS (Master of Arts/Science)*—Applications 2009–2010, 94. Total applicants accepted 2009–2010, 55. Number full-time enrolled (new admits only) 2009–2010, 23. Number part-time enrolled (new admits only) 2009–2010, 4. Total enrolled 2009–2010 full-time, 49, part-time, 7. Openings 2010–2011, 24. The median number of years required for completion of a degree in 2008–2009 were 2. The number of students enrolled full- and part-time who were dismissed or voluntarily withdrew from this program area in 2008–2009 were 2. *School-Community PsyD (Doctor of Psychology)*—Applications 2009–2010, 100. Total applicants accepted 2009–2010, 22. Number full-time enrolled (new admits only) 2009–2010, 8. Number part-time enrolled (new admits only) 2009–2010, 4. Total enrolled 2009–2010 full-time, 46, part-time, 6. Openings 2010–2011, 12. The median number of years required for completion of a degree in 2008–2009 were 5. *Applied Organizational Psychology PhD (Doctor of Philosophy)*—Applications 2009–2010, 20. Total applicants accepted 2009–2010, 10. Number full-time enrolled (new admits only) 2009–2010, 6. Number part-time enrolled (new admits only) 2009–2010, 2. Total enrolled 2009–2010 full-time, 28, part-time, 2. Openings 2010–2011, 8. The median number of years required for completion of a degree in 2008–2009 were

3. The number of students enrolled full- and part-time who were dismissed or voluntarily withdrew from this program area in 2008–2009 were 0.

Other Criteria: (importance of criteria rated low, medium, or high): GRE scores—high, research experience—high, work experience—medium, extracurricular activity—medium, clinically related public service—medium, GPA—high, letters of recommendation—medium, interview—high, statement of goals and objectives—medium. For Clinical PhD program: research experience high, especially professional presentations and publications, clinically related public service high, statement of goals and objectives high. For PsyD program: research experience low, clinically related public service medium, statement of goals and objectives medium. For PhD in Applied Organizational Psychology, a master's degree in one of the social sciences or in business is required.

Student Characteristics: The following represents characteristics of students in 2009–2010 in all graduate psychology programs in the department: Female—full-time 0, part-time 0; Male—full-time 0, part-time 0; African American/Black—full-time 0, part-time 0; Hispanic/Latino(a)—full-time 0, part-time 0; Asian/Pacific Islander—full-time 0, part-time 0; American Indian/Alaska Native—full-time 0, part-time 0; Caucasian/White—full-time 0, part-time 0; Multi-ethnic—full-time 0, part-time 0; students subject to the Americans With Disabilities Act—full-time 0, part-time 0; Unknown ethnicity—full-time 0, part-time 0; International students who hold an F-1 or J-1 Visa—full-time 0, part-time 0.

Financial Information/Assistance:

Tuition for Full-Time Study: *Master's:* State residents: $900 per credit hour; Nonstate residents: $900 per credit hour. *Doctoral:* State residents: $900 per credit hour; Nonstate residents: $900 per credit hour. Tuition is subject to change. Tuition costs vary by program.

Financial Assistance:
First-Year Students: Teaching assistantships available for first year. Average number of hours worked per week: 6. Apply by variable. Research assistantships available for first year. Average number of hours worked per week: 5. Apply by variable. Fellowships and scholarships available for first year. Apply by variable.
Advanced Students: Teaching assistantships available for advanced students. Average number of hours worked per week: 6. Apply by variable. Research assistantships available for advanced students. Average number of hours worked per week: 5. Apply by variable. Fellowships and scholarships available for advanced students. Apply by varable.
Additional Information: Of all students currently enrolled full time, 33% benefited from one or more of the listed financial assistance programs.

Internships/Practica: Doctoral Degree (PsyD School-Community): For those doctoral students for whom a professional internship was required in this program prior to graduation, (22) students applied for an internship in 2008–2009, with (22) students obtaining an internship. Of those students who obtained an internship, (13) were paid internships. Of those students who obtained an internship, (0) students placed in APA/CPA accredited internships, (0) students placed in internships not APA/CPA accredited, but listed with the Association of Psychology Postdoctoral and Internship Programs (APPIC), (0) students placed in internships conforming to guidelines of the Council of Directors of School Psychology Programs (CDSPP), (22) students placed in internships that were not APA/CPA accredited, APPIC or CDSPP listed. In the clinical PhD and PsyD programs students complete a series of practica in which assessment, testing, and interviewing skills are developed. PhD students complete various courses and role playing experiences in adult psychotherapy. PhD students are required to apply for internships using the APPIC national match process following the completion of all coursework and the defense of a dissertation proposal. PsyD students complete a diversified and extended internship over a two-year period. The students are first placed in a school (three days per week) and then in a community agency (3 days per week). In the PhD program in Applied Organizational Psychology, a major part of the student's training, including a paid internship, research courses, and doctoral dissertation, will involve projects in organizations. The internship provides practical experience working for an organization for approximately 20 hours per week, under the supervision of a manager designated by the organization and approved by the program faculty. All research projects, including the dissertation, must serve the educational needs of the students and advance scientific knowledge in the field of organizational psychology; they cannot only serve the interests of the organization. Dissertation research may be conducted in the laboratory, the organization, or both. In addition to sound scientific methodology, the dissertation must have both practical and theoretical significance. This integration of science and practice is a major objective of the program. MA students in Industrial/Organizational Psychology, during their second year of training, complete an internship in a business setting.

Housing and Day Care: On-campus housing is available. On-campus day care facilities are available. Child care is available in the Saltzman Community Services Center.

Employment of Department Graduates:
Master's Degree Graduates: Of those who graduated in the academic year 2008–2009, the following categories and numbers represent the postgraduate activities and employment of master's degree graduates: Enrolled in a psychology doctoral program (11), enrolled in a postdoctoral residency/fellowship (n/a), employed in independent practice (n/a), employed in business or industry (13), total from the above (master's) (24).
Doctoral Degree Graduates: Of those who graduated in the academic year 2008–2009, the following categories and numbers represent the postgraduate activities and employment of doctoral degree graduates: Enrolled in a psychology doctoral program (n/a), employed in an academic position at a university (2), employed in an academic position at a 2-year/4-year college (3), employed in other positions at a higher education institution (1), employed in a professional position in a school system (12), employed in business or industry (1), employed in a community mental health/counseling center (3), employed in a hospital/medical center (2), total from the above (doctoral) (24).

Additional Information:
Orientation, Objectives, and Emphasis of Department: The PhD program in Clinical Psychology is designed to provide doctoral students with assessment and therapeutic skill competence along with a solid scientific foundation in order to have careers working with the wide variety of psychopathology found among the men-

tally ill. The program employs a scientist–practitioner model of education. Program graduates have readily found employment in a wide variety of mental health clinics, group practices, public and private agencies as well as hospitals and medical centers. Many have chosen academic paths by becoming college and university faculty members, medical school faculty, research scientists, expert consultants or editors for psychological publishers. The clinical psychology program is based upon cognitive-behavioral theory and represents the full psychotherapeutic spectrum of this orientation. The APA accredited PsyD program in School-Community Psychology trains practitioners who are skilled in providing psychological services to children, families, and schools. Schools are viewed as being part of the larger community. Thus, in addition to being trained in a school-based, direct service model, emphasis is placed upon training students whose subject of study is the educational or community system in which children develop. PsyD students are trained as consultants who may be involved in educational and mental health program implementation and evaluation in settings such as the judicial system, the schools, personnel agencies, police departments, immigration centers, etc. Most graduates of the PsyD program are employed in schools. The PhD program in Applied Organizational Psychology prepares students for careers as psychologists in business, industry, government, and other private and public organizations. Graduates of this program are trained to apply scientific methods to the solutions of problems related to individual and group behavior in organizations. They are also capable of teaching and researching these topics in higher education settings. The program's overall approach is based on a scientist–practitioner model in which students are exposed to research methodology, factual content, theory, and the application of these skills and knowledge to the solution of practical problems in organizations. The MA program in Industrial/Organizational Psychology prepares students for careers in human resources, training, management, and organizational development. It provides a background in statistics, research design, social psychology, cognition and perception, and learning. The courses in I/O Psychology include selection, training, performance appraisal, worker motivation, and organization development. The curriculum is strengthened by an internship sequence which provides on-site supervised experience working on applied projects in business. The types of work that graduates perform include employee selection, management development, survey research, training, organizational development, performance appraisal, career development and program evaluation.

Special Facilities or Resources: A community services center, the Psychological Evaluation, Research and Counseling Clinic (PERCC), provides practicum experiences for students in the areas of assessment, intervention, and research. A laboratory, instrumented for videotaping, is equipped to handle research in areas of interviewing, communication, problem solving, psychotherapy, and team building. An outstanding library and a computer center are also available, as are many department microcomputers and videotape equipment. The student workroom has six computers for exclusive doctoral student use and all major software programs are available for student use.

Information for Students With Physical Disabilities: See the following Web site for more information: http://www.hofstra.edu/StudentAffairs/stddis.

Application Information:
Send to Graduate Admissions, Bernon Hall, Hofstra University, Hempstead, NY 11549. Application available online. URL of online application: http://www.hofstra.edu/Academics/grad/grad_apply.html. Students are admitted in the Fall, application deadline January 15. Deadline for the PhD in Clinical Psychology is December 15. Deadline for the PsyD in School-Community Psychology is January 15. Applications for the MA in Industrial-Organizational Psychology are accepted on a rolling basis until the class is filled. Deadline for the PhD in Applied Organizational Psychology is February 1. *Fee:* $60.

Iona College
Department of Psychology/Masters of Arts in Psychology
715 North Avenue
New Rochelle, NY 10801
Telephone: (914) 637-7788
Fax: (914) 633-2528
E-mail: *agotlieb@iona.edu*
Web: *http://www.iona.edu/academic/artsscience/departments/Psychology*

Department Information:
1963. Chairperson: Paul Greene, PhD. Number of faculty: total—full-time 11, part-time 28; women—full-time 6, part-time 21; total—minority—full-time 2, part-time 3; women minority—full-time 1, part-time 3.

Programs and Degrees Offered:
Listed in the following order: Program area, degree type (T if terminal Master's), number awarded 7/08–6/09. School Psychology MA/MS (Master of Arts/Science) (T) 5, Industrial/Organizational Psychology MA/MS (Master of Arts/Science) (T) 12, Mental Health Counseling MA/MS (Master of Arts/Science) (T) 6, General-Experimental Psychology MA/MS (Master of Arts/Science) (T) 2.

Student Applications/Admissions:
Student Applications
School Psychology MA/MS (*Master of Arts/Science*)—Applications 2009–2010, 62. Total applicants accepted 2009–2010, 54. Number full-time enrolled (new admits only) 2009–2010, 19. Number part-time enrolled (new admits only) 2009–2010, 5. Total enrolled 2009–2010 full-time, 33, part-time, 10. Openings 2010–2011, 20. The median number of years required for completion of a degree in 2008–2009 were 3. The number of students enrolled full- and part-time who were dismissed or voluntarily withdrew from this program area in 2008–2009 were 7. *Industrial/Organizational Psychology MA/MS (Master of Arts/Science)*—Applications 2009–2010, 60. Total applicants accepted 2009–2010, 20. Number full-time enrolled (new admits only) 2009–2010, 8. Number part-time enrolled (new admits only) 2009–2010, 3. Total enrolled 2009–2010 full-time, 27, part-time, 3. Openings 2010–2011, 15. The median number of years required for completion of a degree in 2008–2009 were 2. The number of students enrolled full- and part-time who were dismissed or voluntarily withdrew from this program area in 2008–2009 were 0. *Mental Health Counseling MA/MS (Master of Arts/Science)*—Applications 2009–2010, 54. Total applicants accepted 2009–2010, 18. Number

full-time enrolled (new admits only) 2009–2010, 9. Number part-time enrolled (new admits only) 2009–2010, 9. Total enrolled 2009–2010 full-time, 35, part-time, 10. Openings 2010–2011, 20. The median number of years required for completion of a degree in 2008–2009 were 4. The number of students enrolled full- and part-time who were dismissed or voluntarily withdrew from this program area in 2008–2009 were 5. *General-Experimental Psychology MA/MS (Master of Arts/Science)*—Applications 2009–2010, 6. Total applicants accepted 2009–2010, 5. Number full-time enrolled (new admits only) 2009–2010, 2. Number part-time enrolled (new admits only) 2009–2010, 0. Total enrolled 2009–2010 full-time, 5, part-time, 2. Openings 2010–2011, 15. The median number of years required for completion of a degree in 2008–2009 were 3. The number of students enrolled full- and part-time who were dismissed or voluntarily withdrew from this program area in 2008–2009 were 0.

Other Criteria: (importance of criteria rated low, medium, or high): research experience—high, work experience—medium, extracurricular activity—medium, clinically related public service—medium, GPA—high, letters of recommendation—high, interview—low, undergraduate major in psychology—medium, specific undergraduate psychology courses taken—high. For additional information on admission requirements, go to http://www.iona.edu/ionagrad.

Student Characteristics: The following represents characteristics of students in 2009–2010 in all graduate psychology programs in the department: Female—full-time 80, part-time 18; Male—full-time 20, part-time 7; African American/Black—full-time 6, part-time 2; Hispanic/Latino(a)—full-time 10, part-time 3; Asian/Pacific Islander—full-time 4, part-time 0; American Indian/Alaska Native—full-time 0, part-time 0; Caucasian/White—full-time 77, part-time 20; Multi-ethnic—full-time 3, part-time 0; students subject to the Americans With Disabilities Act—full-time 0, part-time 0; Unknown ethnicity—full-time 0, part-time 0; International students who hold an F-1 or J-1 Visa—full-time 0, part-time 0.

Financial Information/Assistance:
Tuition for Full-Time Study: *Master's:* State residents: $830 per credit hour; Nonstate residents: $830 per credit hour. See the following Web site for updates and changes in tuition costs: http://www.iona.edu/admin/sfs/sa/tuition.

Financial Assistance:
First-Year Students: Fellowships and scholarships available for first year. Average amount paid per academic year: $14,600. Average number of hours worked per week: 20.
Advanced Students: Fellowships and scholarships available for advanced students. Average amount paid per academic year: $14,600. Average number of hours worked per week: 20.
Additional Information: Of all students currently enrolled full time, 10% benefited from one or more of the listed financial assistance programs. Application and information available online at: http://www.iona.edu/iongrad/financialaid.

Internships/Practica: Master's Degree (MA/MS School Psychology): An internship experience, such as a final research project or "capstone" experience is required of graduates. Master's Degree (MA/MS Industrial/Organizational Psychology): An internship experience, such as a final research project or "capstone" experience is required of graduates. Master's Degree (MA/MS Mental Health Counseling): An internship experience, such as a final research project or "capstone" experience is required of graduates. Master's Degree (MA/MS General-Experimental Psychology): An internship experience, such as a final research project or "capstone" experience is required of graduates. Students specializing in areas that may meet New York State requirements for employment, certification, or licensure, are required to take appropriate internship courses. While there is no guarantee that the student will get accepted by a site, the Department fully assists its students by providing instruction and personal guidance.

Housing and Day Care: No on-campus housing is available. No on-campus day care facilities are available.

Employment of Department Graduates:
Master's Degree Graduates: Of those who graduated in the academic year 2008–2009, the following categories and numbers represent the postgraduate activities and employment of master's degree graduates: Enrolled in a postdoctoral residency/fellowship (n/a), employed in independent practice (n/a), total from the above (master's) (0).
Doctoral Degree Graduates: Of those who graduated in the academic year 2008–2009, the following categories and numbers represent the postgraduate activities and employment of doctoral degree graduates: Enrolled in a psychology doctoral program (n/a), total from the above (doctoral) (0).

Additional Information:
Orientation, Objectives, and Emphasis of Department: The Psychology Department offers separate MA degrees in School Psychology, Mental Health Counseling, and one in Psychology with a specialization in either experimental psychology or industrial/organizational psychology. All degree programs have been approved by the Education Department of New York State. The School Psychology program has been approved by NCATE and gained provisional approved by NASP. The MA in Mental Health Counseling fulfills the academic requirements to take the licensing exam in New York. All programs have been designed for persons who are considering a career in psychology or who are en route to doctoral study in psychology, or are already employed in the field. The programs provide a balance of theoretical, methodological and practical expertise, as well as extensive training in written and oral expression. It is designed to provide pertinent new experiences, to enhance knowledge in substantive areas, and to facilitate maximum development of essential professional competencies and attitudes.

Special Facilities or Resources: The Department contains 2000 square feet of research space and supports research projects in specialties of psychology including social, perception, developmental, learning, treatment, and cognition. Extensive computer and software capabilities are available.

Application Information:
Send to Office of Graduate Admissions, School of Arts and Sciences, 715 North Avenue, New Rochelle, NY 10801. Application available online. URL of online application: http://www.iona.edu/admissions/applytoiona.cfm. Students are admitted in the Fall, application deadline; Winter, application deadline; Spring, application deadline; Summer, application deadline; Programs have rolling admissions. The

School Psychology Program admits new students in the Fall Semester only. *Fee:* $50.

Long Island University
Department of Psychology
C.W. Post
720 Northern Boulevard
Brookville, NY 11548
Telephone: (516) 299-2377
Fax: (516) 299-3105
E-mail: *gerald.lachter@liu.edu*
Web: *http://www.cwpost.liu.edu/cwis/cwp/clas/psych/index.html*

Department Information:
1954. Chairperson: Gerald D. Lachter. Number of faculty: total—full-time 18, part-time 8; women—full-time 8, part-time 6; total—minority—full-time 1, part-time 1; women minority—part-time 1.

Programs and Degrees Offered:
Listed in the following order: Program area, degree type (T if terminal Master's), number awarded 7/08–6/09. Experimental Psychology MA/MS (Master of Arts/Science) (T) 2, Clinical Psychology PsyD (Doctor of Psychology) 10, Certificate Applied Behavior Analysis 10.

APA Accreditation: Clinical PsyD (Doctor of Psychology). Student Outcome Data Website: http://www.cwpost.liu.edu/cwis/cwp/clas/psych/doctoral/students.html.

Student Applications/Admissions:
Student Applications
Experimental Psychology MA/MS (Master of Arts/Science)—Applications 2009–2010, 35. Total applicants accepted 2009–2010, 13. Number full-time enrolled (new admits only) 2009–2010, 4. Total enrolled 2009–2010 full-time, 6. Openings 2010–2011, 10. The median number of years required for completion of a degree in 2008–2009 were 2. The number of students enrolled full- and part-time who were dismissed or voluntarily withdrew from this program area in 2008–2009 were 0. Clinical Psychology PsyD (Doctor of Psychology)—Applications 2009–2010, 267. Total applicants accepted 2009–2010, 53. Number full-time enrolled (new admits only) 2009–2010, 25. Total enrolled 2009–2010 full-time, 95. Openings 2010–2011, 20. The median number of years required for completion of a degree in 2008–2009 were 5. The number of students enrolled full- and part-time who were dismissed or voluntarily withdrew from this program area in 2008–2009 were 0. Certificate Applied Behavior Analysis—Applications 2009–2010, 25. Total applicants accepted 2009–2010, 20. Number part-time enrolled (new admits only) 2009–2010, 18. Total enrolled 2009–2010 part-time, 18. Openings 2010–2011, 20. The median number of years required for completion of a degree in 2008–2009 was 1. The number of students enrolled full- and part-time who were dismissed or voluntarily withdrew from this program area in 2008–2009 were 0.
Scores: Entries appear in this order: required test or GPA, minimum score (if required), median score of students entering in 2009–2010. *Experimental Psychology MA/MS (Master of Arts/Science):* GRE-V no minimum stated, GRE-Q no minimum stated, overall undergraduate GPA no minimum stated, psychology GPA no minimum stated; *Clinical Psychology PsyD (Doctor of Psychology):* GRE-V no minimum stated, GRE-Q no minimum stated, GRE-Analytical no minimum stated, GRE-Subject (Psychology) no minimum stated.
Other Criteria: (importance of criteria rated low, medium, or high): GRE scores—medium, research experience—high, work experience—high, extracurricular activity—low, clinically related public service—high, GPA—high, letters of recommendation—high, interview—high, statement of goals and objectives—medium, undergraduate major in psychology—medium, specific undergraduate psychology courses taken—medium. For additional information on admission requirements, go to http://www.cwpost.liunet.edu/cwis/cwp/clas/psych/doctoral/.

Student Characteristics: The following represents characteristics of students in 2009–2010 in all graduate psychology programs in the department: Female—full-time 76, part-time 18; Male—full-time 25, part-time 0; African American/Black—full-time 3, part-time 1; Hispanic/Latino(a)—full-time 8, part-time 2; Asian/Pacific Islander—full-time 4, part-time 0; American Indian/Alaska Native—full-time 0, part-time 0; Caucasian/White—full-time 77, part-time 15; Multi-ethnic—full-time 0, part-time 0; students subject to the Americans With Disabilities Act—full-time 0, part-time 0; Unknown ethnicity—full-time 9, part-time 0; International students who hold an F-1 or J-1 Visa—full-time 0, part-time 0.

Financial Information/Assistance:
Tuition for Full-Time Study: *Master's:* State residents: $930 per credit hour; Nonstate residents: $930 per credit hour. *Doctoral:* State residents: per academic year $38,500; Nonstate residents: per academic year $38,500. Tuition is subject to change. Additional fees are assessed to students beyond the costs of tuition for the following: $100/semester activity fee. See the following Web site for updates and changes in tuition costs: http://www.cwpost.liu.edu/cwis/cwp/bursar/tuition/.

Financial Assistance:
First-Year Students: Teaching assistantships available for first year. Research assistantships available for first year. Fellowships and scholarships available for first year.
Advanced Students: Teaching assistantships available for advanced students. Research assistantships available for advanced students.
Additional Information: Of all students currently enrolled full time, 75% benefited from one or more of the listed financial assistance programs. Application and information available online at: http://www.cwpost.liu.edu/cwis/cwp/clas/psych/index.html.

Internships/Practica: Doctoral Degree (PsyD Clinical Psychology): For those doctoral students for whom a professional internship was required in this program prior to graduation, (16) students applied for an internship in 2008–2009, with (15) students obtaining an internship. Of those students who obtained an internship, (15) were paid internships. Of those students who obtained an internship, (14) students placed in APA/CPA accredited internships, (1) students placed in internships not APA/CPA accredited, but listed with the Association of Psychology Postdoctoral and Internship Programs (APPIC), (0) students placed in internships conforming to guidelines of the Council of Directors of School Psychology Programs (CDSPP), (0) students placed in internships that were not APA/CPA accredited, APPIC or CDSPP listed. Master's Degree (MA/MS Experimental Psychology): An internship experience, such as a final research project or "capstone" experience is required of graduates. A wide range of internship and practicum placements are available.

Housing and Day Care: On-campus housing is available. See the following Web site for more information: http://www.cwpost.liu.edu/cwis/cwp/stuact/housing/housing.html. No on-campus day care facilities are available.

Employment of Department Graduates:
Master's Degree Graduates: Of those who graduated in the academic year 2008–2009, the following categories and numbers represent the postgraduate activities and employment of master's degree graduates: Enrolled in a psychology doctoral program (2), enrolled in another graduate/professional program (0), enrolled in a postdoctoral residency/fellowship (n/a), employed in independent practice (n/a), total from the above (master's) (2).
Doctoral Degree Graduates: Of those who graduated in the academic year 2008–2009, the following categories and numbers represent the postgraduate activities and employment of doctoral degree graduates: Enrolled in a psychology doctoral program (n/a), employed in a community mental health/counseling center (12), employed in a hospital/medical center (2), total from the above (doctoral) (14).

Additional Information:
Orientation, Objectives, and Emphasis of Department: The Master's degree program gives students a broad background in Experimental Psychology. Faculty interests include Behavior Analysis, Cognition and Perception, and Neuroscience. The program is designed to prepare students for admission to doctoral programs, or to give them the skills necessary to obtain employment. The Clinical Psychology Doctoral program at the C.W. Post Campus of Long Island University offers a Doctor of Psychology (PsyD) degree and has as its basic purpose the training of doctoral level clinical psychologists who will exhibit professional attitudes and apply current knowledge and practice skills for the prevention and alleviation of psychological problems. The program is also committed to training students who will provide services in public sector settings to traditionally underserved groups. While the mission is to broadly train clinical psychologists, the program also seeks to provide each student with special competencies in one of three areas: family violence, developmental disabilities, or serious and persistent mental illness. The program also provides its graduates with clinical and theoretical training in two major orientations — cognitive-behavioral and psychoanalytic. The Clinical Psychology Doctoral program is fully accredited by the American Psychological Association. In 2009, the APA awarded the Program with accreditation until 2016, the longest possible period of accreditation. The program is also registered by the New York State Education Department and listed by the Association of State and Provincial Psychology Boards and the National Register of Health Service Providers in Psychology as a designated institution offering a doctoral program in psychology. The program is based on the practitioner-scholar model of clinical training.

Special Facilities or Resources: Laboratories exist for the study of animal and human learning, cognition and perception, and neuroscience. The PsyD program has its own Psychological Services Center that provides mental health services to the community as well as serving as a site for training students.

Information for Students With Physical Disabilities: See the following Web site for more information: http://www.cwpost.liu.edu/cwis/cwp/stuact/arc/learning.htm.

Application Information:
Send to Graduate Admissions, C.W. Post Campus of Long Island University, Brookville, NY 11548. Application available online. URL of online application: http://www.cwpost.liu.edu/cwis/cwp/admissions/graduate/howtoapplyg.html. Students are admitted in the Fall, application deadline February 1; February 1 for PsyD; June 1 for MA; August 1 for Advanced Certificate Program. *Fee:* $30.

Long Island University
Psychology/Clinical Psychology
Richard L. Conolly College
1 University Plaza
Brooklyn, NY 11201
Telephone: (718) 488-1164
Fax: (718) 488-1179
E-mail: *nicholas.papouchis@liu.edu*
Web: *http://www.brooklyn.liu.edu/psych*

Department Information:
1967. Director, PhD Program in Clinical Psychology: Nicholas Papouchis. Number of faculty: total—full-time 15, part-time 6; women—full-time 5, part-time 2; total—minority—full-time 5, part-time 2; women minority—full-time 2; faculty subject to the Americans With Disabilities Act 1.

Programs and Degrees Offered:
Listed in the following order: Program area, degree type (T if terminal Master's), number awarded 7/08–6/09. Clinical Psychology PhD (Doctor of Philosophy) 20, General Psychology MA/MS (Master of Arts/Science) (T) 9.

APA Accreditation: Clinical PhD (Doctor of Philosophy).

Student Applications/Admissions:
Student Applications
Clinical Psychology PhD (Doctor of Philosophy)—Applications 2009–2010, 235. Total applicants accepted 2009–2010, 25. Number full-time enrolled (new admits only) 2009–2010, 16. Number part-time enrolled (new admits only) 2009–2010, 0. Total enrolled 2009–2010 full-time, 89, part-time, 20. Openings 2010–2011, 16. The median number of years required for completion of a degree in 2008–2009 were 6. The number of students enrolled full- and part-time who were dismissed or voluntarily withdrew from this program area in 2008–2009 were 1. *General Psychology MA/MS (Master of Arts/Science)*— Applications 2009–2010, 16. Total applicants accepted 2009–2010, 9. Number full-time enrolled (new admits only) 2009–2010, 19. Number part-time enrolled (new admits only) 2009–2010, 13. Total enrolled 2009–2010 full-time, 29, part-time, 34. Openings 2010–2011, 20. The median number of years

required for completion of a degree in 2008–2009 were 4. The number of students enrolled full- and part-time who were dismissed or voluntarily withdrew from this program area in 2008–2009 were 0.

Scores: Entries appear in this order: required test or GPA, minimum score (if required), median score of students entering in 2009–2010. *Clinical Psychology PhD (Doctor of Philosophy):* GRE-V 550, 650, GRE-Q 550, 625, GRE-Analytical 4.0, 5.0, GRE-Subject (Psychology) 550, 660, overall undergraduate GPA 3.2, 3.5, last 2 years GPA 3.4, 3.5, psychology GPA 3.5, 3.75.

Other Criteria: (importance of criteria rated low, medium, or high): GRE scores—high, research experience—high, work experience—high, extracurricular activity—low, clinically related public service—medium, GPA—high, letters of recommendation—high, interview—high, statement of goals and objectives—high, undergraduate major in psychology—medium, specific undergraduate psychology courses taken—medium. The above requirements are for the PhD program in Clinical Psychology. requirements for the MA program require a GPA of 2.75 and good letters of recommendation and a committment pursue a scholarly foundation at the graduate level in psychology.

Student Characteristics: The following represents characteristics of students in 2009–2010 in all graduate psychology programs in the department: Female—full-time 91, part-time 40; Male—full-time 27, part-time 14; African American/Black—full-time 23, part-time 32; Hispanic/Latino(a)—full-time 14, part-time 7; Asian/Pacific Islander—full-time 7, part-time 1; American Indian/Alaska Native—full-time 1, part-time 0; Caucasian/White—full-time 73, part-time 15; Multi-ethnic—full-time 0, part-time 0; students subject to the Americans With Disabilities Act—full-time 0, part-time 0; Unknown ethnicity—full-time 0, part-time 0; International students who hold an F-1 or J-1 Visa—full-time 3, part-time 0.

Financial Information/Assistance:

Tuition for Full-Time Study: *Master's:* State residents: $930 per credit hour; Nonstate residents: $930 per credit hour. *Doctoral:* State residents: per academic year $37,997, $1,214 per credit hour; Nonstate residents: per academic year $37,997, $1,214 per credit hour. Tuition is subject to change. Tuition costs vary by program. See the following Web site for updates and changes in tuition costs: http://www.brooklyn.liu.edu/busar/graduate_tuition.html.

Financial Assistance:

First-Year Students: Research assistantships available for first year. Average amount paid per academic year: $100. Average number of hours worked per week: 10. Apply by April. Fellowships and scholarships available for first year. Average amount paid per academic year: $3,800. Average number of hours worked per week: 10. Apply by April 15.

Advanced Students: Teaching assistantships available for advanced students. Average amount paid per academic year: $2,500. Average number of hours worked per week: 10. Apply by April 15. Research assistantships available for advanced students. Average amount paid per academic year: $1,100. Average number of hours worked per week: 10. Apply by April 15. Fellowships and scholarships available for advanced students. Average amount paid per academic year: $3,800. Average number of hours worked per week: 10. Apply by April 15.

Additional Information: Of all students currently enrolled full time, 100% benefited from one or more of the listed financial assistance programs.

Internships/Practica: Doctoral Degree (PhD Clinical Psychology): For those doctoral students for whom a professional internship was required in this program prior to graduation, (13) students applied for an internship in 2008–2009, with (13) students obtaining an internship. Of those students who obtained an internship, (13) were paid internships. Of those students who obtained an internship, (13) students placed in APA/CPA accredited internships, (0) students placed in internships not APA/CPA accredited, but listed with the Association of Psychology Postdoctoral and Internship Programs (APPIC), (0) students placed in internships conforming to guidelines of the Council of Directors of School Psychology Programs (CDSPP), (0) students placed in internships that were not APA/CPA accredited, APPIC or CDSPP listed. Students in the Master's program have a variety of practica available to them. Doctoral practicum settings and internships in the New York City Metropolitan area are among the best in the country and offer training with a wide range of clinical patients and a number of specializations. Among these are child training, family training, neuropsychology and forensic training. Students in the PhD program regularly train in the best of these externship and practicum settings and over the three years from 2002 to 2005 doctoral students matched 100% with their internship choices. For 2005-2006 to 2009-2010 the percentage of doctoral students matching was 97%. This is an exceptional record of being accepted at the finest internship sites in the Northeast.

Housing and Day Care: On-campus housing is available. On-campus day care facilities are available.

Employment of Department Graduates:

Master's Degree Graduates: Of those who graduated in the academic year 2008–2009, the following categories and numbers represent the postgraduate activities and employment of master's degree graduates: Enrolled in a psychology doctoral program (4), enrolled in a postdoctoral residency/fellowship (n/a), employed in independent practice (n/a), employed in a professional position in a school system (5), employed in a community mental health/counseling center (7), employed in a hospital/medical center (2), other employment position (2), total from the above (master's) (20).

Doctoral Degree Graduates: Of those who graduated in the academic year 2008–2009, the following categories and numbers represent the postgraduate activities and employment of doctoral degree graduates: Enrolled in a psychology doctoral program (n/a), employed in an academic position at a university (1), employed in a professional position in a school system (3), employed in government agency (3), employed in a community mental health/counseling center (5), employed in a hospital/medical center (6), not seeking employment (2), total from the above (doctoral) (20).

Additional Information:

Orientation, Objectives, and Emphasis of Department: The PhD and master's programs are housed in an urban institution with a multicultural undergraduate student body. This diversity enriches the students' appreciation of the complexity of the clinical and theoretical issues relevant to work in psychology. The theoretical orientation of the clinical training sequence reflects the spectrum of psychodynamic approaches to treatment and familiarities students with cognitive-behavioral and family systems approaches as well. Clinical students are exposed, in a graded series of practicum experiences, to both short-term and longer term approaches to psychotherapy with the New York area's culturally diverse clinical populations. Students are also trained in a range of psychological assessment procedures including cognitive, projective, and neuropsychological testing. The program also seeks to train clinical psychologists who are competent in research and grounded in the science of psychology. To this end, doctoral students receive extensive training in research design and statistics early in their coursework and complete a second-year research project preparatory to beginning their dissertation. The final goal and emphasis of the department and the PhD program is to enable students to develop a broad base of knowledge in clinical psychology. Doctoral students are provided with opportunities for clinical training with adults, children and adolescents, training in family therapy, group therapy and research training in a range of topics relevant to psychology.

Special Facilities or Resources: The Department of Psychology has the following facilities and resources: An on-site Psychological Services Center where students' clinical work is carefully supervised by the doctoral faculty; an ongoing psychotherapy research group; research labs for the study of unconscious cognitive processes and personality and mood/anxiety disorders; training in child and adolescent clinical work at a number of New York area clinical training facilities; opportunity for specialized electives in neuropsychology; free access to computer training and computer facilities; full-tuition minority research fellowships for selected minority doctoral candidates. Students in the PhD program have the spectrum of New York City's clinical and educational facilities available for them to be trained in. The PhD program has also sponsored the development of the Center for Studies in Ethnicity and Human Development under the leadership of Dr. Carol Magai. This center is devoted to research with diverse ethnic groups and minorities.

Application Information:
Send to Admissions Office, Long Island University, Brooklyn Campus, 1 University Plaza, Brooklyn, NY 11201. Application available online. URL of online application: http://www.brooklyn.liu.edu/admissions. Students are admitted in the Fall, application deadline December 1. For MA program, deadline is one month before the beginning of the semester. *Fee:* $30. For MA program, deadline for applications is one month before the semester begins.

Marist College
Department of Psychology
Poughkeepsie, NY 12601
Telephone: (845) 575-3000
Fax: (845) 575-3965
E-mail: *james.regan@marist.edu*
Web: *http://www.marist.edu/admission/graduate/*

Department Information:
1972. Graduate Program Director: James Regan, PhD. Number of faculty: total—full-time 16, part-time 10; women—full-time 6, part-time 8; total—minority—full-time 4, part-time 3; women minority—full-time 2, part-time 3; faculty subject to the Americans With Disabilities Act 4.

Programs and Degrees Offered:
Listed in the following order: Program area, degree type (T if terminal Master's), number awarded 7/08–6/09. General Psychology MA/MS (Master of Arts/Science) (T) 12, School Psychology MA/MS (Master of Arts/Science) (T) 22, Educational Psychology MEd (Education), Mental Health Counseling MA/MS (Master of Arts/Science) (T) 15.

Student Applications/Admissions:
Student Applications
General Psychology MA/MS (Master of Arts/Science)—Applications 2009–2010, 28. Total applicants accepted 2009–2010, 24. Number full-time enrolled (new admits only) 2009–2010, 24. Number part-time enrolled (new admits only) 2009–2010, 0. Openings 2010–2011, 20. The median number of years required for completion of a degree in 2008–2009 were 2. The number of students enrolled full- and part-time who were dismissed or voluntarily withdrew from this program area in 2008–2009 were 0. *School Psychology MA/MS (Master of Arts/Science)*—Applications 2009–2010, 35. Total applicants accepted 2009–2010, 27. Number full-time enrolled (new admits only) 2009–2010, 16. Number part-time enrolled (new admits only) 2009–2010, 5. Total enrolled 2009–2010 full-time, 32, part-time, 7. Openings 2010–2011, 18. The median number of years required for completion of a degree in 2008–2009 were 3. The number of students enrolled full- and part-time who were dismissed or voluntarily withdrew from this program area in 2008–2009 were 2. *Educational Psychology MEd (Education)*—Number part-time enrolled (new admits only) 2009–2010, 20. Total enrolled 2009–2010 part-time, 77. *Mental Health Counseling MA/MS (Master of Arts/Science)*—Applications 2009–2010, 25. Total applicants accepted 2009–2010, 18. Number full-time enrolled (new admits only) 2009–2010, 15. Number part-time enrolled (new admits only) 2009–2010, 3. Total enrolled 2009–2010 full-time, 30, part-time, 10. Openings 2010–2011, 18. The median number of years required for completion of a degree in 2008–2009 were 2. The number of students enrolled full- and part-time who were dismissed or voluntarily withdrew from this program area in 2008–2009 were 2.

Other Criteria: (importance of criteria rated low, medium, or high): GRE scores—low, research experience—low, work experience—medium, extracurricular activity—low, clinically related public service—low, GPA—high, letters of recommendation—high, interview—high, statement of goals and objectives—low.

Student Characteristics: The following represents characteristics of students in 2009–2010 in all graduate psychology programs in the department: Female—full-time 45, part-time 72; Male—full-time 8, part-time 22; African American/Black—full-time 5, part-time 4; Hispanic/Latino(a)—full-time 4, part-time 9; Asian/Pacific Islander—full-time 1, part-time 3; American Indian/Alaska Native—full-time 0, part-time 3; Caucasian/White—full-time 43, part-time 72; Multi-ethnic—full-time 0, part-time 3; students subject to the Americans With Disabilities Act—full-time 1, part-time 2; Unknown ethnicity—full-time 0, part-time 0; International students who hold an F-1 or J-1 Visa—full-time 0, part-time 0.

NEW YORK

Financial Information/Assistance:
Tuition for Full-Time Study: *Master's:* State residents: per academic year $16,680, $695 per credit hour; Nonstate residents: per academic year $16,680, $695 per credit hour. Tuition is subject to change. See the following Web site for updates and changes in tuition costs: http://www.marist.edu/financialaid/tf.html.

Financial Assistance:
First-Year Students: Research assistantships available for first year. Average amount paid per academic year: $4,500. Average number of hours worked per week: 10. Apply by April 15.
Advanced Students: Research assistantships available for advanced students. Average amount paid per academic year: $4,500. Average number of hours worked per week: 10. Apply by April 15.
Additional Information: Of all students currently enrolled full time, 80% benefited from one or more of the listed financial assistance programs. Application and information available online at: http://www.marist.edu/financialaid/index.html.

Internships/Practica: Master's Degree (MA/MS General Psychology): An internship experience, such as a final research project or "capstone" experience is required of graduates. Master's Degree (MA/MS Mental Health Counseling): An internship experience, such as a final research project or "capstone" experience is required of graduates. The Mid-Hudson area has many public and private agencies dealing with mental health, developmental disabilities, criminal justice, and social services. In addition, numerous school districts participate with the school psychology program. Students choose their own placement site in consultation with faculty supervisor.

Housing and Day Care: No on-campus housing is available. No on-campus day care facilities are available.

Employment of Department Graduates:
Master's Degree Graduates: Of those who graduated in the academic year 2008–2009, the following categories and numbers represent the postgraduate activities and employment of master's degree graduates: Enrolled in a psychology doctoral program (10), enrolled in another graduate/professional program (5), enrolled in a postdoctoral residency/fellowship (n/a), employed in independent practice (n/a), employed in an academic position at a 2-year/4-year college (3), employed in other positions at a higher education institution (3), employed in a professional position in a school system (22), employed in business or industry (2), employed in government agency (2), employed in a community mental health/counseling center (8), employed in a hospital/medical center (2), still seeking employment (2), total from the above (master's) (59).
Doctoral Degree Graduates: Of those who graduated in the academic year 2008–2009, the following categories and numbers represent the postgraduate activities and employment of doctoral degree graduates: Enrolled in a psychology doctoral program (n/a), total from the above (doctoral) (0).

Additional Information:
Orientation, Objectives, and Emphasis of Department: The Master of Arts programs focus on either mental health counseling or school psychology. The program goals include providing students with the relevant theory, skills, and practical experience that will enable them to perform competently in assessing individual differences, in counseling, and in planning and implementing effective individual, group, and system level interventions. Students interested in working in community settings will find a variety of opportunities for "hands-on" experience. The mental health counseling program fulfills the academic component for students who want to be licensed in New York State as Mental Health Counselors and the school psychology program leads to New York certification as a school psychologist.

Special Facilities or Resources: Interested students can assist in research at facilities such as the Nathan Kline Research Institute, The Center for Advanced Brain Imaging, The Marist Institute for Community Research, Hudson River Psychiatric Center, Dutchess County Department of Mental Hygiene and Public Health, and the Montrose and Castlepoint Veterans Hospitals.

Information for Students With Physical Disabilities: See the following Web site for more information: http://www.marist.edu/specialservices/.

Application Information:
Send to Director of Graduate Admissions, Marist College, Poughkeepsie, NY 12601. Application available online. URL of online application: http://www.marist.edu/admission/graduate/. Students are admitted in the Fall, application deadline April 15; Spring, application deadline December 1; Summer, application deadline April 15. Students considered after deadlines as space allows. *Fee:* $50.

New York University
Department of Applied Psychology
The Steinhardt School of Education
246 Greene Street, Kimball Hall
New York, NY 10003
Telephone: (212) 998-5555
Fax: (212) 995-3654
E-mail: *arnold.grossman@nyu.edu*
Web: *http://steinhardt.nyu.edu/appsych*

Department Information:
1990. Chairperson: Dr. Jacqueline Mattis. Number of faculty: total—full-time 37, part-time 41; women—full-time 23, part-time 23; total—minority—full-time 9, part-time 7; women minority—full-time 8, part-time 5; faculty subject to the Americans With Disabilities Act 5.

Programs and Degrees Offered:
Listed in the following order: Program area, degree type (T if terminal Master's), number awarded 7/08–6/09. Counseling and Guidance MA/MS (Master of Arts/Science) (T) 80, Counseling Psychology PhD (Doctor of Philosophy) 4, Psychological Development PhD (Doctor of Philosophy) 1, Educational Psychology MA/MS (Master of Arts/Science) (T) 28, Psychology and Social Intervention PhD (Doctor of Philosophy) 0, Human Development and Social Intervention MA/MS (Master of Arts/Science) (T) 0.

APA Accreditation: Counseling PhD (Doctor of Philosophy).

GRADUATE STUDY IN PSYCHOLOGY

Student Applications/Admissions:

Student Applications

Counseling and Guidance MA/MS (Master of Arts/Science)—Applications 2009–2010, 587. Total applicants accepted 2009–2010, 199. Number full-time enrolled (new admits only) 2009–2010, 60. Number part-time enrolled (new admits only) 2009–2010, 16. Total enrolled 2009–2010 full-time, 106, part-time, 27. Openings 2010–2011, 105. The median number of years required for completion of a degree in 2008–2009 were 2. The number of students enrolled full- and part-time who were dismissed or voluntarily withdrew from this program area in 2008–2009 were 0. *Counseling Psychology PhD (Doctor of Philosophy)*—Applications 2009–2010, 179. Total applicants accepted 2009–2010, 3. Number full-time enrolled (new admits only) 2009–2010, 3. Total enrolled 2009–2010 full-time, 14, part-time, 26. Openings 2010–2011, 4. The median number of years required for completion of a degree in 2008–2009 were 8. The number of students enrolled full- and part-time who were dismissed or voluntarily withdrew from this program area in 2008–2009 were 1. *Psychological Development PhD (Doctor of Philosophy)*—Applications 2009–2010, 48. Total applicants accepted 2009–2010, 4. Number full-time enrolled (new admits only) 2009–2010, 2. Number part-time enrolled (new admits only) 2009–2010, 0. Total enrolled 2009–2010 full-time, 30, part-time, 5. Openings 2010–2011, 4. The median number of years required for completion of a degree in 2008–2009 were 6. The number of students enrolled full- and part-time who were dismissed or voluntarily withdrew from this program area in 2008–2009 were 0. *Educational Psychology MA/MS (Master of Arts/Science)*—Applications 2009–2010, 92. Total applicants accepted 2009–2010, 21. Number full-time enrolled (new admits only) 2009–2010, 19. Number part-time enrolled (new admits only) 2009–2010, 2. Total enrolled 2009–2010 full-time, 21, part-time, 26. The median number of years required for completion of a degree in 2008–2009 were 2. The number of students enrolled full- and part-time who were dismissed or voluntarily withdrew from this program area in 2008–2009 were 0. *Psychology and Social Intervention PhD (Doctor of Philosophy)*—Applications 2009–2010, 76. Total applicants accepted 2009–2010, 3. Number full-time enrolled (new admits only) 2009–2010, 3. Number part-time enrolled (new admits only) 2009–2010, 0. Openings 2010–2011, 5. The number of students enrolled full- and part-time who were dismissed or voluntarily withdrew from this program area in 2008–2009 were 0. *Human Development and Social Intervention MA/MS (Master of Arts/Science)*—Applications 2009–2010, 50. Total applicants accepted 2009–2010, 15. Number full-time enrolled (new admits only) 2009–2010, 12. Number part-time enrolled (new admits only) 2009–2010, 3. Total enrolled 2009–2010 full-time, 12, part-time, 3. Openings 2010–2011, 20.

Scores: Entries appear in this order: required test or GPA, minimum score (if required), median score of students entering in 2009–2010. *Counseling and Guidance MA/MS (Master of Arts/Science)*: overall undergraduate GPA 3.0, 3.5, last 2 years GPA 3.0, 3.5; *Counseling Psychology PhD (Doctor of Philosophy)*: GRE-V 500, 500, GRE-Q 500, 500, last 2 years GPA 3.0, 3.5, psychology GPA 3.0, 3.5; *Psychological Development PhD (Doctor of Philosophy)*: GRE-V 500, 500, GRE-Q 500, 500, overall undergraduate GPA 3.0, 3.0, last 2 years GPA 3.5, 3.5; *Educational Psychology MA/MS (Master of Arts/Science)*: overall undergraduate GPA 3.0, 3.5, last 2 years GPA 3.0, 3.5; *Psychology and Social Intervention PhD (Doctor of Philosophy)*: GRE-V 500, 500, GRE-Q 500, 500, overall undergraduate GPA 3.0, 3.0, last 2 years GPA 3.5, 3.5; *Human Development and Social Intervention MA/MS (Master of Arts/Science)*: GRE-V 500, 500, GRE-Q 500, 500, overall undergraduate GPA 3.0, 3.5, last 2 years GPA 3.0, 3.5.

Other Criteria: (importance of criteria rated low, medium, or high): GRE scores—medium, research experience—high, work experience—medium, extracurricular activity—low, clinically related public service—medium, GPA—medium, letters of recommendation—high, interview—high, statement of goals and objectives—high. The above criteria range from "medium" to "high" for admission into the doctoral programs. Masters programs primarily consider GPA, statement of goals and objectives, and letters of recommendation; interviews sometimes required for master's applicants.

Student Characteristics: The following represents characteristics of students in 2009–2010 in all graduate psychology programs in the department: Female—full-time 162, part-time 80; Male—full-time 32, part-time 19; African American/Black—full-time 15, part-time 11; Hispanic/Latino(a)—full-time 16, part-time 12; Asian/Pacific Islander—full-time 10, part-time 17; American Indian/Alaska Native—full-time 1, part-time 0; Caucasian/White—full-time 107, part-time 49; Multi-ethnic—full-time 35, part-time 1; students subject to the Americans With Disabilities Act—full-time 0, part-time 0; Unknown ethnicity—full-time 10, part-time 9; International students who hold an F-1 or J-1 Visa—full-time 0, part-time 0.

Financial Information/Assistance:

Tuition for Full-Time Study: **Master's:** State residents: per academic year $30,240, $1,260 per credit hour; Nonstate residents: per academic year $30,240, $1,260 per credit hour. *Doctoral:* State residents: per academic year $30,240, $1,260 per credit hour; Nonstate residents: per academic year $30,240, $1,260 per credit hour. Tuition is subject to change. Additional fees are assessed to students beyond the costs of tuition for the following: registration fee for 1st credit- $412 and $60 per additional credit. See the following Web site for updates and changes in tuition costs: http://steinhardt.nyu.edu/graduate_admissions/.

Financial Assistance:

First-Year Students: Research assistantships available for first year. Average amount paid per academic year: $30,240. Average number of hours worked per week: 20. Apply by December 1. Fellowships and scholarships available for first year. Average amount paid per academic year: $30,240. Apply by December 1.

Advanced Students: Research assistantships available for advanced students. Average amount paid per academic year: $30,240. Average number of hours worked per week: 20. Fellowships and scholarships available for advanced students. Average amount paid per academic year: $18,000.

Additional Information: Of all students currently enrolled full time, 100% benefited from one or more of the listed financial assistance programs. Application and information available online at: http://steinhardt.nyu.edu/financial_aid/.

Internships/Practica: Doctoral Degree (PhD Counseling Psychology): For those doctoral students for whom a professional internship was required in this program prior to graduation, (4) students applied for an internship in 2008–2009, with (3) students obtaining an internship. Of those students who obtained an internship, (3) were paid internships. Of those students who obtained an internship, (3) students placed in APA/CPA accredited internships, (0) students placed in internships not APA/CPA accredited, but listed with the Association of Psychology Postdoctoral and Internship Programs (APPIC), (0) students placed in internships conforming to guidelines of the Council of Directors of School Psychology Programs (CDSPP), (0) students placed in internships that were not APA/CPA accredited, APPIC or CDSPP listed. Master's Degree (MA/MS Counseling and Guidance): An internship experience, such as a final research project or "capstone" experience is required of graduates. Available in the following areas: school and university counseling; counseling in community agencies, hospitals, and business; school psychology; psychological development; measurement and evaluation.

Housing and Day Care: On-campus housing is available. See the following Web site for more information: http://www.nyu.edu/housing/. No on-campus day care facilities are available.

Employment of Department Graduates:

Master's Degree Graduates: Of those who graduated in the academic year 2008–2009, the following categories and numbers represent the postgraduate activities and employment of master's degree graduates: Enrolled in a postdoctoral residency/fellowship (n/a), employed in independent practice (n/a), do not know (108), total from the above (master's) (108).

Doctoral Degree Graduates: Of those who graduated in the academic year 2008–2009, the following categories and numbers represent the postgraduate activities and employment of doctoral degree graduates: Enrolled in a psychology doctoral program (n/a), do not know (10), total from the above (doctoral) (10).

Additional Information:

Orientation, Objectives, and Emphasis of Department: The cornerstone of our department is the marriage of theory and practice driven by the University's commitment to being a private university in the public service. To this end, the department's programs reflect both a concern for excellence in teaching and the opportunity to learn from involvement in community based data collection. Emphasis and specific core requirements differ somewhat from program to program, but include a solid foundation in the basic psychological disciplines. Departmental faculty have research projects in several areas, and students have the opportunity to participate in community based data collection. Departmental faculty have ongoing research projects in many areas, including: cognition; language; social and emotional development; health and human development; applied measurement and research methods; working people's lives; spirituality; multicultural assessment; group and organizational dynamics; psychopathology and personality; sexual and gender identity; communication and creative expression; trauma and resilience; parenting; immigration.

Special Facilities or Resources: The Infancy Studies Laboratory conducts research in infant temperament, perceptual development, learning and attention, parenting views and child rearing styles. The Measurement Laboratory contains educational and psychological tests and reference books. PC computers are available for data analysis and word processing. The Institute for Human Development and Social Change aims to break new intellectual ground through its support for interdisciplinary research and training across social, behavioral, health, and policy sciences. In the spirit of the common enterprise university, it brings together faculty, graduate students and undergraduate students from professional schools and the Faculty of Arts and Science. The Center for Research on Culture, Development and Education conducts longitudinal research on the pathways to educational success in early childhood and early adolescence, among New York City families of 5 ethnic groups. Center for Health, Identity, Behavior, & Prevention Studies (CHIBPS) conducts formative and intervention research on social and psychological factors that contribute to HIV transmission and the synergy between drug use, mental health, and HIV transmission. The Child and Family Policy Center conducts research, offers technical assistance and works to disseminate state-of-the-field knowledge to bring children's healthy development and school success to the forefront of policymaking, program design, and practice. The Arnold and Rosalie Weiss Resource Center in Applied Psychology provides a departmental library to assist students and researchers within the department.

Information for Students With Physical Disabilities: See the following Web site for more information: http://www.nyu.edu/osl/csd/.

Application Information:

Send to Office of Graduate Admissions, The Steinhardt School of Education, New York University, 82 Washington Sq. East, Floor 3, New York, NY 10003. Application available online. URL of online application: http://steinhardt.nyu.edu/graduate_admissions/. Students are admitted in the Fall, application deadline MA-Feb 1; Spring, application deadline MA-Dec 1. Fall deadline: doctoral -January 15; Ed Psych Master's has rolling admissions. *Fee:* $50. $60 for international students.

New York University, Graduate School of Arts and Science (2009 data)
Department of Psychology
6 Washington Place, Room 550
New York, NY 10003
Telephone: (212) 998-7900
Fax: (212) 995-4018
E-mail: *s.zoubok@nyu.edu*
Web: *http://www.psych.nyu.edu*

Department Information:

1950. Chairperson: Tom Tyler. Number of faculty: total—full-time 37; women—full-time 13; total—minority—full-time 1; women minority—full-time 1.

Programs and Degrees Offered:

Listed in the following order: Program area, degree type (T if terminal Master's), number awarded 7/08–6/09. General Psychology MA/MS (Master of Arts/Science) (T) 58, Industrial/Organizational MA/MS (Master of Arts/Science) (T) 25, Cognition and Perception PhD (Doctor of Philosophy) 8, Social PhD (Doctor of Philosophy) 7.

Student Applications/Admissions:
Student Applications

General Psychology MA/MS (Master of Arts/Science)—Applications 2009–2010, 336. Total applicants accepted 2009–2010,

185. Number part-time enrolled (new admits only) 2009–2010, 46. Total enrolled 2009–2010 part-time, 148. *Industrial/Organizational MA/MS (Master of Arts/Science)*—Applications 2009–2010, 239. Total applicants accepted 2009–2010, 83. Number part-time enrolled (new admits only) 2009–2010, 28. Total enrolled 2009–2010 part-time, 81. *Cognition and Perception PhD (Doctor of Philosophy)*—Applications 2009–2010, 165. Total applicants accepted 2009–2010, 13. Number full-time enrolled (new admits only) 2009–2010, 6. Total enrolled 2009–2010 full-time, 43. *Social PhD (Doctor of Philosophy)*—Applications 2009–2010, 216. Total applicants accepted 2009–2010, 8. Number full-time enrolled (new admits only) 2009–2010, 2. Total enrolled 2009–2010 full-time, 30. *Other Criteria:* (importance of criteria rated low, medium, or high): GRE scores—medium, research experience—high, work experience—low, extracurricular activity—low, clinically related public service—low, GPA—medium, letters of recommendation—high, statement of goals and objectives—high. These rankings are for the PhD only. For master's program, letters of recommendation and statement of goals and objectives have high importance; other criteria are low; no interviews are given.

Student Characteristics: The following represents characteristics of students in 2009–2010 in all graduate psychology programs in the department: Female—full-time 53, part-time 180; Male—full-time 23, part-time 61; African American/Black—full-time 4, part-time 11; Hispanic/Latino(a)—full-time 6, part-time 14; Asian/Pacific Islander—full-time 13, part-time 32; American Indian/Alaska Native—full-time 0, part-time 0; Caucasian/White—full-time 0, part-time 0; Multi-ethnic—full-time 0, part-time 5; students subject to the Americans With Disabilities Act—full-time 0, part-time 0; Unknown ethnicity—full-time 0, part-time 0; International students who hold an F-1 or J-1 Visa—full-time 0, part-time 0.

Financial Information/Assistance:
Financial Assistance:
First-Year Students: Teaching assistantships available for first year. Average amount paid per academic year: $22,440. Average number of hours worked per week: 20. Apply by December 18. Research assistantships available for first year. Average amount paid per academic year: $22,440. Average number of hours worked per week: 20. Apply by December 18. Traineeships available for first year. Fellowships and scholarships available for first year. Average amount paid per academic year: $22,440. Apply by December 18.

Advanced Students: Teaching assistantships available for advanced students. Average amount paid per academic year: $22,440. Average number of hours worked per week: 20. Apply by December 18. Research assistantships available for advanced students. Average amount paid per academic year: $22,440. Average number of hours worked per week: 20. Apply by December 18. Traineeships available for advanced students. Fellowships and scholarships available for advanced students. Average amount paid per academic year: $22,440. Apply by December 18.

Additional Information: Of all students currently enrolled full time, 100% benefited from one or more of the listed financial assistance programs. Application and information available online.

Internships/Practica: Master's students may opt to take Fieldwork, which would enable them to obtain supervised experience in selected agencies, clinics, and industrial and non-profit organizations relevant to the career or academic objectives of the student.

Housing and Day Care: On-campus housing is available. See the following Web site for more information: http://www.nyu.edu/housing/. No on-campus day care facilities are available.

Employment of Department Graduates:
Master's Degree Graduates: Of those who graduated in the academic year 2008–2009, the following categories and numbers represent the postgraduate activities and employment of master's degree graduates: Enrolled in a postdoctoral residency/fellowship (n/a), employed in independent practice (n/a), total from the above (master's) (0).
Doctoral Degree Graduates: Of those who graduated in the academic year 2008–2009, the following categories and numbers represent the postgraduate activities and employment of doctoral degree graduates: Enrolled in a psychology doctoral program (n/a), total from the above (doctoral) (0).

Additional Information:
Orientation, Objectives, and Emphasis of Department: The doctoral programs all emphasize research. The cognition-perception program has faculty whose research focuses on memory, emotion, psycholinguistics, categorization, cognitive neuroscience, visual perception and attention. The social program trains researchers in theory and methods for understanding individuals and groups in social and organizational contexts. Training is provided in subareas ranging from social cognition to motivation, personality, close relationships, groups and organizations. A doctoral concentration in developmental psychology emphasizes research training cutting across the traditional areas of psychology. Students may minor in quantitative psychology or in any of the above programs. The Master's program in General Psychology has the flexibility to suit students who wish to explore several areas of psychology to find the area that interests them most, as well as students who wish to shape their course of study to fit special interests and needs, including preparation for admission to a doctoral program. The Master's program in Industrial/Organizational Psychology is designed to prepare graduates to apply research and principles of human behavior to a variety of organizational settings, such as human resources departments and management consulting firms. The program can also be modified for students who are preparing for admission to doctoral programs in Industrial/Organizational and related fields. Students in the master's programs may opt for either full- or part-time status.

Special Facilities or Resources: The Department of Psychology maintains laboratories, classrooms, project rooms, and a magnetic resonance (MR) neuroimaging facility. Modern laboratories are continually improved through grants from foundations and federal agencies. The Center for Brain Imaging houses a research-dedicated 3 Tesla Siemens MR system for the use of faculty and students interested in research using functional brain imaging. The center includes faculty members from both the Department of Psychology and the Center for Neural Science, as well as individuals whose expertise is in MR physics and statistical methods for analysis. The Department also has an Magnetoencephalography (MEG) lab dedicated to Cognitive Neuroscience investigations, primarily of language but also of vision and other cognitive functions. Finally, the department maintains several computer classrooms and laboratories, and the University offers technical courses on emerging computational tools. Faculty laboratories are equipped with specialized computer equipment within each of the graduate programs. The department collaborates closely with the Center for Neural Science in maintaining a technical shop.

Application Information:
Send to New York University, Graduate School of Arts & Sciences, Graduate Enrollment Services, P.O. Box 907, New York, NY 10276-0907. Application available online. URL of online application: http://gsas.nyu.edu/page/grad.admissionsapplication.html. PhD students admitted only in the Fall (application deadline December 18). Master's in General Psychology: Fall deadline: May 15; Spring deadline: October 15; Summer deadline: March 15. Master's in Industrial/Organizational Psychology: Fall deadline: February 1; Spring deadline: October 1; Summer deadline: February 1. *Fee:* $85.

Pace University
Department of Psychology
Dyson College of Arts and Sciences
One Pace Plaza
New York, NY 10038
Telephone: (212) 346-1506
Fax: (212) 346-1618
E-mail: *bmowder@pace.edu*
Web: *http://www.pace.edu*

Department Information:
1961. Associate Chair: Barbara A. Mowder. Number of faculty: total—full-time 13, part-time 42; women—full-time 9, part-time 22; total—minority—full-time 4, part-time 6; women minority—full-time 3, part-time 4.

Programs and Degrees Offered:
Listed in the following order: Program area, degree type (T if terminal Master's), number awarded 7/08–6/09. General Psychology MA/MS (Master of Arts/Science) (T) 12, School-Clinical Child Psychology PsyD (Doctor of Psychology) 22, School Psychology EdS (School Psychology) 19.

APA Accreditation: Combination PsyD (Doctor of Psychology).

Student Applications/Admissions:
Student Applications
General Psychology MA/MS (Master of Arts/Science)—Applications 2009–2010, 93. Total applicants accepted 2009–2010, 66. Number full-time enrolled (new admits only) 2009–2010, 7. Number part-time enrolled (new admits only) 2009–2010, 7. Total enrolled 2009–2010 full-time, 18, part-time, 18. Openings 2010–2011, 25. The median number of years required for completion of a degree in 2008–2009 were 2. The number of students enrolled full- and part-time who were dismissed or voluntarily withdrew from this program area in 2008–2009 were 0. *School-Clinical Child Psychology PsyD (Doctor of Psychology)*—Applications 2009–2010, 247. Total applicants accepted 2009–2010, 77. Number full-time enrolled (new admits only) 2009–2010, 28. Number part-time enrolled (new admits only) 2009–2010, 0. Total enrolled 2009–2010 full-time, 130, part-time, 4. Openings 2010–2011, 20. The median number of years required for completion of a degree in 2008–2009 were 5. The number of students enrolled full- and part-time who were dismissed or voluntarily withdrew from this program area in 2008–2009 were 1. *School Psychology EdS (School Psychology)*—Applications 2009–2010, 45. Total applicants accepted 2009–2010, 3. Number full-time enrolled (new admits only) 2009–2010, 1. Openings 2010–2011, 5. The median number of years required for completion of a degree in 2008–2009 were 3. The number of students enrolled full- and part-time who were dismissed or voluntarily withdrew from this program area in 2008–2009 were 0.

Scores: Entries appear in this order: required test or GPA, minimum score (if required), median score of students entering in 2009–2010. *General Psychology MA/MS (Master of Arts/Science)*: GRE-V no minimum stated, GRE-Q no minimum stated, overall undergraduate GPA no minimum stated; *School-Clinical Child Psychology PsyD (Doctor of Psychology)*: GRE-V no minimum stated, GRE-Q no minimum stated, overall undergraduate GPA no minimum stated; *School Psychology EdS (School Psychology)*: GRE-V no minimum stated, GRE-Q no minimum stated, overall undergraduate GPA no minimum stated.

Other Criteria: (importance of criteria rated low, medium, or high): GRE scores—high, research experience—medium, work experience—medium, extracurricular activity—low, clinically related public service—medium, GPA—high, letters of recommendation—high, interview—high, statement of goals and objectives—high, undergraduate major in psychology—medium, specific undergraduate psychology courses taken—low. These criteria are used for the MSEd and PsyD programs only.

Student Characteristics: The following represents characteristics of students in 2009–2010 in all graduate psychology programs in the department: Female—full-time 139, part-time 9; Male—full-time 19, part-time 4; African American/Black—full-time 4, part-time 0; Hispanic/Latino(a)—full-time 16, part-time 1; Asian/Pacific Islander—full-time 13, part-time 2; American Indian/Alaska Native—full-time 0, part-time 0; Caucasian/White—full-time 108, part-time 6; Multi-ethnic—full-time 12, part-time 1; students subject to the Americans With Disabilities Act—full-time 0, part-time 0; Unknown ethnicity—full-time 12, part-time 2; International students who hold an F-1 or J-1 Visa—full-time 2, part-time 0.

Financial Information/Assistance:
Financial Assistance:
First-Year Students: Research assistantships available for first year. Average amount paid per academic year: $2,500. Average number of hours worked per week: 10. Apply by January 15. Fellowships and scholarships available for first year. Average amount paid per academic year: $5,000. Apply by January 15.

Advanced Students: Research assistantships available for advanced students. Average amount paid per academic year: $2,500. Average number of hours worked per week: 10. Apply by January 15. Fellowships and scholarships available for advanced students. Average amount paid per academic year: $5,000. Apply by January 15.

Additional Information: Of all students currently enrolled full time, 50% benefited from one or more of the listed financial assistance programs.

Internships/Practica: Doctoral Degree (PsyD School-Clinical Child Psychology): For those doctoral students for whom a professional internship was required in this program prior to graduation, (15) students applied for an internship in 2008–2009, with (15) students obtaining an internship. Of those students who obtained an internship, (15) were paid internships. Of those students who obtained an internship, (9) students placed in APA/CPA accredited internships, (5) students placed in internships not APA/CPA accredited, but listed with the Association of Psychology Postdoctoral and Internship Programs (APPIC), (1) students placed in internships conforming to guidelines of the Council of Directors of School Psychology Programs (CDSPP), (0) students placed in internships that were not APA/CPA accredited, APPIC or CDSPP listed. Most school psychology and bilingual school psychology internships occur in the New York metropolitan region, including Long Island, Westchester County, and school districts throughout northern and central New Jersey. Doctoral internships are typically secured through the APPIC system. Doctoral students typically secure internships in the New York metropolitan region.

Housing and Day Care: On-campus housing is available. No on-campus day care facilities are available.

Employment of Department Graduates:
Master's Degree Graduates: Of those who graduated in the academic year 2008–2009, the following categories and numbers represent the postgraduate activities and employment of master's degree graduates: Enrolled in a postdoctoral residency/fellowship (n/a), employed in independent practice (n/a), total from the above (master's) (0).
Doctoral Degree Graduates: Of those who graduated in the academic year 2008–2009, the following categories and numbers represent the postgraduate activities and employment of doctoral degree graduates: Enrolled in a psychology doctoral program (n/a), employed in independent practice (1), employed in other positions at a higher education institution (2), employed in a professional position in a school system (8), employed in a community mental health/counseling center (3), employed in a hospital/medical center (2), do not know (6), total from the above (doctoral) (22).

Additional Information:
Orientation, Objectives, and Emphasis of Department: The PsyD program in School-Clinical Child Psychology at Pace University is a professional practice training program that is dedicated to the training model of school/clinical child psychologists as practitioner-scholars. The focus is on developing individuals whose theoretical and research knowledge and professional skills enable them to deliver a broad array of direct and indirect psychological services to infants, children, adolescents, and families, and the personnel, organizations and institutions that serve them. The purpose of the program is to train school/clinical child psychology practitioners to possess broad knowledge about general psychological theoretical foundations, as well as more specific knowledge pertaining to the scientific foundations of psychological practice and professional School-Clinical Child Psychology practice competencies. School psychologists-in-training receive instruction and supervision related to following ethical guidelines and being sensitive to diversity and multicultural issues. The program coordinates placement in University-based and field-based supervised training experiences, which are carefully integrated with theoretical coursework and a seminar, enabling practitioners in training to compare key aspects of professional functioning across a wide variety of settings. There are sixteen specific training goals of the School-Clinical Child Psychology program. The goals include the following: 1. Psychoeducational assessment related to school difficulties and learning disorders. 2. Psychological assessment related to personality and mental disorders. 3. Delivery of psychological interventions aimed at ameliorating adjustment and personal difficulties experienced by children, adolescents, and families. 4. Delivery of psychoeducational interventions aimed at ameliorating learning difficulties experienced by children, adolescents, and families. 5. Providing psychological services with an awareness of and sensitivity to ethnic and cultural diversity. 6. Development and/or implementation of programmatic/preventive interventions. 7. Development and/or implementation of a broad range of consultation services. 8. Enlisting the aid of community agencies to secure services or prevent circumstances contributing to unsatisfactory adjustment or behavior problems. 9. Initiating and/or directing group interventions. 10. Initiating and/or directing family interventions. 11. Conducting in-service training sessions for parents and/or school personnel. 12. Coordinating interdisciplinary assessment and intervention strategies. 13. Providing psychotherapy to children, adolescents, and families. 14. Providing diagnoses related to mental disorders. 15. Carrying out applied research. 16. Supervising the provision of direct psychological services.

Special Facilities or Resources: The Psychology Department maintains the McShane Center for Psychological Services. This on-site training facility provides practicum training for students in the M.S.Ed., M.S.Ed. Bilingual, and PsyD programs. For example, training opportunities include biofeedback, interviewing, parent-infant observations, psychodiagnostics, and psychotherapy.

Application Information:
Send to Graduate Admissions, Pace University, 1 Pace Plaza, NY, NY 10038. Application available online. URL of online application: gradnyc@pace.edu. Students are admitted in the Fall, application deadline January 15; Winter, application deadline August 1; Spring, application deadline December 1; Summer, application deadline May 1. January 15 deadline for MS Ed and PsyD programs; this is the only application date for these two programs. Fall deadline for MA is August 1, spring deadline for MA is December 1, and summer deadline for MA is May 1. *Fee:* $65.

Rensselaer Polytechnic Institute
Cognitive Science
110 8th Street, Carnegie Building, Room #305
Troy, NY 12180-3590
Telephone: (518) 276-6473
Fax: (518) 276-8268
E-mail: *osgane@rpi.edu*
Web: *http://cogsci.rpi.edu/*

Department Information:
2000. Head: Selmer Bringsjord. Number of faculty: total—full-time 21, part-time 4; women—full-time 1, part-time 2; total—minority—full-time 1.

Programs and Degrees Offered:
Listed in the following order: Program area, degree type (T if terminal Master's), number awarded 7/08–6/09. Cognitive Science PhD (Doctor of Philosophy) 2.

Student Applications/Admissions:
Student Applications
Cognitive Science PhD (Doctor of Philosophy)—Applications 2009–2010, 30. Total applicants accepted 2009–2010, 8. Number full-time enrolled (new admits only) 2009–2010, 8. Total enrolled 2009–2010 full-time, 19, part-time, 3. Openings 2010–2011, 5.
Scores: Entries appear in this order: required test or GPA, minimum score (if required), median score of students entering in 2009–2010. Cognitive Science PhD (Doctor of Philosophy): GRE-V 550, 640, GRE-Q 550, 800, GRE-Analytical no minimum stated, overall undergraduate GPA 3.0, 3.4.
Other Criteria: (importance of criteria rated low, medium, or high): GRE scores—high, research experience—high, work experience—low, extracurricular activity—low, GPA—medium, letters of recommendation—high, interview—medium, statement of goals and objectives—high.

Student Characteristics: The following represents characteristics of students in 2009–2010 in all graduate psychology programs in the department: Female—full-time 4, part-time 2; Male—full-time 15, part-time 1; African American/Black—full-time 0, part-time 0; Hispanic/Latino(a)—full-time 3, part-time 0; Asian/Pacific Islander—full-time 2, part-time 2; American Indian/Alaska Native—full-time 0, part-time 0; Caucasian/White—full-time 14, part-time 1; Multi-ethnic—full-time 0, part-time 0; students subject to the Americans With Disabilities Act—full-time 0, part-time 0; Unknown ethnicity—full-time 0, part-time 0; International students who hold an F-1 or J-1 Visa—full-time 0, part-time 0.

Financial Information/Assistance:
Tuition for Full-Time Study: Doctoral: State residents: per academic year $38,100, $1,588 per credit hour; Nonstate residents: per academic year $38,100, $1,588 per credit hour. See the following Web site for updates and changes in tuition costs: http://gradoffice.rpi.edu/update.do?catcenterkey=17.

Financial Assistance:
First-Year Students: Teaching assistantships available for first year. Average amount paid per academic year: $22,000. Average number of hours worked per week: 20. Apply by January 15. Research assistantships available for first year. Average amount paid per academic year: $22,000. Average number of hours worked per week: 20. Apply by January 15. Fellowships and scholarships available for first year. Average amount paid per academic year: $22,000. Apply by January 15.
Advanced Students: No information provided.
Additional Information: Of all students currently enrolled full time, 100% benefited from one or more of the listed financial assistance programs. Application and information available online at: http://admissions.rpi.edu/graduate/index.html.

Housing and Day Care: On-campus housing is available. See the following Web site for more information: http://reslife.rpi.edu/setup.do. On-campus day care facilities are available. See the following Web site for more information: http://reslife.rpi.edu/update.do?artcenterkey=63.

Employment of Department Graduates:
Master's Degree Graduates: Of those who graduated in the academic year 2008–2009, the following categories and numbers represent the postgraduate activities and employment of master's degree graduates: Enrolled in a postdoctoral residency/fellowship (n/a), employed in independent practice (n/a), total from the above (master's) (0).
Doctoral Degree Graduates: Of those who graduated in the academic year 2008–2009, the following categories and numbers represent the postgraduate activities and employment of doctoral degree graduates: Enrolled in a psychology doctoral program (n/a), total from the above (doctoral) (0).

Additional Information:
Orientation, Objectives, and Emphasis of Department: The department is committed to the concept of integrated cognitive systems. Specifically, research and teaching falls into areas that together cover low- to high-level cognition, whether in minds or machines: reasoning (human and machine); computational cognitive modeling; cognitive engineering; perception and action.

Special Facilities or Resources: Modern research facilities, including the CogWorks Laboratory, Interactive and Distance Education Assessment (IDEA) Laboratory, Rensselaer Artificial Intelligence and Reasoning Laboratory (RAIR Lab), Perception and Action Lab (PandA Lab), Human-Level Intelligence Laboratory, the Cognitive Architecture Laboratory (CogArch Lab), and dedicated space in the Institute's new Social and Behavioral Research Laboratory, provide a new expression of the Department's interests in cognitive science that integrates the diverse research activities of the faculty in the Department.

Information for Students With Physical Disabilities: See the following Web site for more information: http://doso.rpi.edu/update.do?catcenterkey=5.

Application Information:
Send to Admissions, Rensselaer Polytechnic Institute, Troy, NY 12180. Application available online. URL of online application: http://admissions.rpi.edu/graduate/. Students are admitted in the Fall, application deadline January 15. *Fee:* $75.

Roberts Wesleyan College
Social Science Division/Graduate Psychology Program
2301 Westside Drive
Rochester, NY 14624
Telephone: (585) 594-6011
Fax: (585) 594-6124
E-mail: *repass_cheryl@roberts.edu*
Web: *http://www.roberts.edu/gradpsych*

Department Information:
2002. Department Chairperson: Cheryl L. Repass. Number of faculty: total—full-time 8; women—full-time 5.

GRADUATE STUDY IN PSYCHOLOGY

Programs and Degrees Offered:
Listed in the following order: Program area, degree type (T if terminal Master's), number awarded 7/08–6/09. School Psychology MA/MS (Master of Arts/Science) (T) 22, School Counseling MA/MS (Master of Arts/Science) (T) 14.

Student Applications/Admissions:
Student Applications
School Psychology MA/MS (Master of Arts/Science)—Applications 2009–2010, 50. Total applicants accepted 2009–2010, 37. Number full-time enrolled (new admits only) 2009–2010, 14. Number part-time enrolled (new admits only) 2009–2010, 2. Total enrolled 2009–2010 full-time, 44, part-time, 3. Openings 2010–2011, 15. The median number of years required for completion of a degree in 2008–2009 were 3. The number of students enrolled full- and part-time who were dismissed or voluntarily withdrew from this program area in 2008–2009 were 0. School Counseling MA/MS (Master of Arts/Science)—Applications 2009–2010, 25. Total applicants accepted 2009–2010, 18. Number full-time enrolled (new admits only) 2009–2010, 13. Number part-time enrolled (new admits only) 2009–2010, 0. Openings 2010–2011, 15. The median number of years required for completion of a degree in 2008–2009 were 2. The number of students enrolled full- and part-time who were dismissed or voluntarily withdrew from this program area in 2008–2009 were 1.
Scores: Entries appear in this order: required test or GPA, minimum score (if required), median score of students entering in 2009–2010. *School Psychology MA/MS (Master of Arts/Science)*: GRE-V no minimum stated, GRE-Q no minimum stated, overall undergraduate GPA 3.0; *School Counseling MA/MS (Master of Arts/Science)*: GRE-V no minimum stated, GRE-Q no minimum stated, overall undergraduate GPA 3.0.
Other Criteria: (importance of criteria rated low, medium, or high): GRE scores—medium, work experience—medium, extracurricular activity—low, clinically related public service—low, GPA—high, letters of recommendation—high, interview—high, statement of goals and objectives—high, fit w/ college's mission—high. For additional information on admission requirements, go to http://www.roberts.edu/gradpsych.

Student Characteristics: The following represents characteristics of students in 2009–2010 in all graduate psychology programs in the department: Female—full-time 58, part-time 3; Male—full-time 9, part-time 0; African American/Black—full-time 6, part-time 0; Hispanic/Latino(a)—full-time 0, part-time 0; Asian/Pacific Islander—full-time 1, part-time 0; American Indian/Alaska Native—full-time 1, part-time 0; Caucasian/White—full-time 59, part-time 3; Multi-ethnic—full-time 0, part-time 0; students subject to the Americans With Disabilities Act—full-time 0, part-time 0; Unknown ethnicity—full-time 0, part-time 0; International students who hold an F-1 or J-1 Visa—full-time 0, part-time 0.

Financial Information/Assistance:
Tuition for Full-Time Study: Master's: State residents: per academic year $17,580, $586 per credit hour; Nonstate residents: per academic year $17,580, $586 per credit hour. Tuition is subject to change.

Financial Assistance:
First-Year Students: No information provided.
Advanced Students: Teaching assistantships available for advanced students. Average amount paid per academic year: $500. Average number of hours worked per week: 8. Apply by None.
Additional Information: Of all students currently enrolled full time, 7% benefited from one or more of the listed financial assistance programs.

Internships/Practica: Master's Degree (MA/MS School Psychology): An internship experience, such as a final research project or "capstone" experience is required of graduates. Master's Degree (MA/MS School Counseling): An internship experience, such as a final research project or "capstone" experience is required of graduates. Students in school psychology complete a 1200-hour internship their third year which is typically paid by the school district in the form of a stipend. Out of state internships are also a possibility. These internships pay anywhere from 28K - 40K and are also contracted for 1200 hours. Students in school counseling secure local unpaid internships for 600 hours.

Housing and Day Care: No on-campus housing is available. No on-campus day care facilities are available.

Employment of Department Graduates:
Master's Degree Graduates: Of those who graduated in the academic year 2008–2009, the following categories and numbers represent the postgraduate activities and employment of master's degree graduates: Enrolled in a psychology doctoral program (0), enrolled in another graduate/professional program (0), enrolled in a postdoctoral residency/fellowship (n/a), employed in independent practice (n/a), employed in an academic position at a university (0), employed in an academic position at a 2-year/4-year college (0), employed in other positions at a higher education institution (0), employed in a professional position in a school system (27), employed in business or industry (0), employed in government agency (0), employed in a community mental health/counseling center (0), employed in a hospital/medical center (0), still seeking employment (0), not seeking employment (1), other employment position (0), do not know (8), total from the above (master's) (36).
Doctoral Degree Graduates: Of those who graduated in the academic year 2008–2009, the following categories and numbers represent the postgraduate activities and employment of doctoral degree graduates: Enrolled in a psychology doctoral program (n/a), total from the above (doctoral) (0).

Additional Information:
Orientation, Objectives, and Emphasis of Department: The mission of the School Psychology and School Counseling programs is to prepare students, in a Christian context, for effective, compassionate, professional practice. The programs aim to prepare students for exemplary service and leadership in private and public agencies/educational institutions, utilizing a scientist–practitioner approach, with special attention given to the Christian community, locally, nationally, and internationally.

Personal Behavior Statement: The full text of the statement is included in our application.

Information for Students With Physical Disabilities: Contact the Learning Center at (585) 594-6270 or (800) 777-4792 (ext. 6270).

Application Information:
Send to Division of Social Sciences Graduate Admissions Office, Roberts Wesleyan College 2301 Westside Drive Rochester, NY 14624-1997. Students are admitted in the Fall, application deadline February 15. After March 1, admissions will be handled on a rolling basis, as space in the program permits. *Fee:* $35. Application fee is waived for online applicants.

Sage Colleges, The
Department of Psychology
45 Ferry Street
Troy, NY 12180
Telephone: (518) 244-2221
Fax: (518) 244-4564
E-mail: *poppej@sage.edu*
Web: *http://www.sage.edu/academics/psychology/*

Department Information:
Chairperson: Dr. Jean E. Poppei. Number of faculty: total—full-time 10, part-time 9; women—full-time 9, part-time 4.

Programs and Degrees Offered:
Listed in the following order: Program area, degree type (T if terminal Master's), number awarded 7/08–6/09. Community Psychology MA/MS (Master of Arts/Science) (T) 10, Counseling and Community Psychology MA/MS (Master of Arts/Science) (T) 19, Forensic Mental Health Certificate 1.

Student Applications/Admissions:
Student Applications

Community Psychology MA/MS (Master of Arts/Science)—Applications 2009–2010, 12. Total applicants accepted 2009–2010, 8. Number full-time enrolled (new admits only) 2009–2010, 0. Number part-time enrolled (new admits only) 2009–2010, 7. Openings 2010–2011, 20. The median number of years required for completion of a degree in 2008–2009 were 3. The number of students enrolled full- and part-time who were dismissed or voluntarily withdrew from this program area in 2008–2009 were 1. Counseling and Community Psychology MA/MS (Master of Arts/Science)—Applications 2009–2010, 51. Total applicants accepted 2009–2010, 34. Number part-time enrolled (new admits only) 2009–2010, 30. Total enrolled 2009–2010 part-time, 96. Openings 2010–2011, 30. The median number of years required for completion of a degree in 2008–2009 were 4. The number of students enrolled full- and part-time who were dismissed or voluntarily withdrew from this program area in 2008–2009 were 6. Forensic Mental Health Certificate—Applications 2009–2010, 7. Total applicants accepted 2009–2010, 7. Number part-time enrolled (new admits only) 2009–2010, 7. Total enrolled 2009–2010 part-time, 24. Openings 2010–2011, 10. The median number of years required for completion of a degree in 2008–2009 were 3. The number of students enrolled full- and part-time who were dismissed or voluntarily withdrew from this program area in 2008–2009 were 1.

Scores: Entries appear in this order: required test or GPA, minimum score (if required), median score of students entering in 2009–2010. *Counseling and Community Psychology MA/MS (Master of Arts/Science):* overall undergraduate GPA 3.0.

Other Criteria: (importance of criteria rated low, medium, or high): research experience—low, work experience—high, extracurricular activity—low, clinically related public service—medium, GPA—high, letters of recommendation—high, interview—high, statement of goals and objectives—high, undergraduate major in psychology—medium, specific undergraduate psychology courses taken—high. For additional information on admission requirements, go to http://www.sage.edu/psychology.

Student Characteristics: The following represents characteristics of students in 2009–2010 in all graduate psychology programs in the department: Female—full-time 2, part-time 104; Male—full-time 1, part-time 7; African American/Black—full-time 0, part-time 11; Hispanic/Latino(a)—full-time 0, part-time 5; Asian/Pacific Islander—full-time 0, part-time 1; American Indian/Alaska Native—full-time 0, part-time 0; Caucasian/White—full-time 3, part-time 93; Multi-ethnic—full-time 0, part-time 1; students subject to the Americans With Disabilities Act—full-time 0, part-time 0; Unknown ethnicity—full-time 0, part-time 0; International students who hold an F-1 or J-1 Visa—full-time 0, part-time 0.

Financial Information/Assistance:
Tuition for Full-Time Study: *Master's:* State residents: $585 per credit hour; Nonstate residents: $585 per credit hour. Tuition is subject to change.

Financial Assistance:
First-Year Students: Research assistantships available for first year. Average amount paid per academic year: $2,000. Average number of hours worked per week: 10. Apply by June 1.

Advanced Students: Teaching assistantships available for advanced students. Average amount paid per academic year: $2,000. Average number of hours worked per week: 10. Apply by June 1. Research assistantships available for advanced students. Average amount paid per academic year: $2,000. Average number of hours worked per week: 10. Apply by June 1.

Additional Information: Of all students currently enrolled full time, 25% benefited from one or more of the listed financial assistance programs. Application and information available online at: http://www.sage.edu/sgs/costaid.

Internships/Practica: Master's Degree (MA/MS Counseling and Community Psychology): An internship experience, such as a final research project or "capstone" experience is required of graduates. As part of each degree, all students are required to complete an internship (direct services) and/or externship (not direct services) placement, depending upon the selected area of concentration. Internships comprise one year of counseling placements in a setting appropriate to the student's interests; externships are one semester projects in a setting of the student's choice.

Housing and Day Care: On-campus housing is available. See the following Web site for more information: http://www.sage.edu/sgs/studentlife. No on-campus day care facilities are available.

Employment of Department Graduates:
Master's Degree Graduates: Of those who graduated in the academic year 2008–2009, the following categories and numbers represent the postgraduate activities and employment of master's degree graduates: Enrolled in a psychology doctoral program (0), enrolled in another graduate/professional program (2), enrolled in a postdoctoral residency/fellowship (n/a), employed in independent practice (n/a), employed in an academic position at a university (0), employed in an academic position at a 2-year/4-year college (0), employed in government agency (1), employed in a community mental health/counseling center (8), other employment position (2), do not know (16), total from the above (master's) (29).
Doctoral Degree Graduates: Of those who graduated in the academic year 2008–2009, the following categories and numbers represent the postgraduate activities and employment of doctoral degree graduates: Enrolled in a psychology doctoral program (n/a), total from the above (doctoral) (0).

Additional Information:
Orientation, Objectives, and Emphasis of Department: Our two degrees (MA in Community Psychology, and MA in Counseling/Community Psychology) provide students with the academic and skills training to become practitioners at the master's level. The programs range in credits from 42 to 60, depending on degree. The emphasis is on developing and strengthening student skills for application (whether individual or systems level) in the context of strong theoretical foundations. Graduates of MA in Counseling/Community Psychology are eligible to sit for licensure as a mental health counselor in New York State.

Special Facilities or Resources: In addition to the faculty resources one would assume at the master's level, a particular advantage for psychology programs at Sage Graduate School is our prime location in the Capital District area of New York State. The geographic size, population density, and availability of widely varied populations make possible a wide variety of experiences.

Information for Students With Physical Disabilities: See the following Web site for more information: http://www.sage.edu/current/DisabilitiesServices.

Application Information:
Send to Graduate Admissions, The Sage Colleges, 45 Ferry Street, Troy, New York 12180. Application available online. URL of online application: http://www.sage.edu/sgs/admission. Students are admitted in the Fall, application deadline April 1; Winter, application deadline; Spring, application deadline November 1; Summer, application deadline April 1; Programs have rolling admissions. Community Psychology: rolling admissions. Counseling/Community Psychology: November 1 for Spring; April 1 for Summer and Fall-priority deadline Forensic Mental Health Certificate: November 1 for Spring; April 1 for Fall-priority deadline. *Fee:* $40. Fee waived for graduates of The Sage Colleges.

State University of New York at New Paltz
Department of Psychology
JFT 314, 600 Hawk Drive
New Paltz, NY 12561-2440
Telephone: (845) 257-3467
Fax: (845) 257-3474
E-mail: *gradpsych@newpaltz.edu*
Web: *http://www.newpaltz.edu/psychology/graduate*

Department Information:
1969. Chairperson: Glenn Geher. Number of faculty: total—full-time 17, part-time 12; women—full-time 9, part-time 10; total—minority—full-time 5, part-time 2; women minority—full-time 2, part-time 2.

Programs and Degrees Offered:
Listed in the following order: Program area, degree type (T if terminal Master's), number awarded 7/08–6/09. Mental Health Counseling MA/MS (Master of Arts/Science) (T) 10, Psychology MA/MS (Master of Arts/Science) (T) 8, School Counseling MA/MS (Master of Arts/Science) (T) 0.

Student Applications/Admissions:
Student Applications
Mental Health Counseling MA/MS (Master of Arts/Science)—Applications 2009–2010, 35. Total enrolled 2009–2010 full-time, 21. Openings 2010–2011, 15. *Psychology MA/MS (Master of Arts/Science)*—Applications 2009–2010, 23. Total applicants accepted 2009–2010, 4. Total enrolled 2009–2010 full-time, 19. Openings 2010–2011, 6. The number of students enrolled full- and part-time who were dismissed or voluntarily withdrew from this program area in 2008–2009 were 0. *School Counseling MA/MS (Master of Arts/Science)*—Applications 2009–2010, 21. Number full-time enrolled (new admits only) 2009–2010, 0. Number part-time enrolled (new admits only) 2009–2010, 0. Openings 2010–2011, 4. The number of students enrolled full- and part-time who were dismissed or voluntarily withdrew from this program area in 2008–2009 were 0.
Scores: Entries appear in this order: required test or GPA, minimum score (if required), median score of students entering in 2009–2010. *Mental Health Counseling MA/MS (Master of Arts/Science)*: GRE-V no minimum stated, GRE-Q no minimum stated, overall undergraduate GPA 3.0; *Psychology MA/MS (Master of Arts/Science)*: GRE-V no minimum stated, GRE-Q no minimum stated, overall undergraduate GPA 3.0, psychology GPA 3.0; *School Counseling MA/MS (Master of Arts/Science)*: GRE-V no minimum stated, GRE-Q no minimum stated, overall undergraduate GPA 3.0.
Other Criteria: (importance of criteria rated low, medium, or high): GRE scores—medium, research experience—high, work experience—low, extracurricular activity—low, clinically related public service—medium, GPA—high, letters of recommendation—high, interview—medium, statement of goals and objectives—high, Writing ability—high, undergraduate major in psychology—low, specific undergraduate psychology courses taken—high. For additional information on admission requirements, go to http://www.newpaltz.edu/psychology/graduate/.

Student Characteristics: The following represents characteristics of students in 2009–2010 in all graduate psychology programs in the department: Female—full-time 9, part-time 8; Male—full-time 8, part-time 3; African American/Black—full-time 1, part-time 0; Hispanic/Latino(a)—full-time 1, part-time 0; Asian/Pacific Islander—full-time 1, part-time 0; American Indian/Alaska Native—full-time 0, part-time 0; Caucasian/White—full-time 0, part-time 0; Multi-ethnic—full-time 0, part-time 0; students subject to the Americans With Disabilities Act—full-time 1, part-time 1; Unknown ethnicity—full-time 0, part-time 0; International students who hold an F-1 or J-1 Visa—full-time 0, part-time 0.

Financial Information/Assistance:
Tuition for Full-Time Study: *Master's:* State residents: per academic year $8,370, $349 per credit hour; Nonstate residents: per academic year $13,250, $552 per credit hour. Tuition is subject to change. See the following Web site for updates and changes in tuition costs: http://www.newpaltz.edu/financialaid/tuition.cfm.

Financial Assistance:
First-Year Students: Teaching assistantships available for first year. Average amount paid per academic year: $5,000. Average number of hours worked per week: 20. Research assistantships available for first year. Traineeships available for first year. Fellowships and scholarships available for first year. Average number of hours worked per week: 10.

Advanced Students: Teaching assistantships available for advanced students. Average amount paid per academic year: $5,000. Average number of hours worked per week: 20. Research assistantships available for advanced students. Fellowships and scholarships available for advanced students.

Additional Information: Of all students currently enrolled full time, 30% benefited from one or more of the listed financial assistance programs. Application and information available online at: http://www.newpaltz.edu/financialaid.

Internships/Practica: Master's Degree (MA/MS Psychology): An internship experience, such as a final research project or "capstone" experience is required of graduates. All students in the mental health counseling program complete a practicum at the college counseling center and the career advising center. Additional internship opportunities are available with regional public and private mental health agencies. In addition to practicum and internship requirements, mental health counseling students complete a curriculum of mental health counseling coursework. The program is registered with New York State as a program meeting the educational requirements for mental health counseling licensure. All students in the school counseling program must complete a practicum and an internship experience at one of several area school districts. The practicum and internship may be completed within an elementary, middle, or high school setting. Students will have the option of completing the practicum and internship within the same school/school district or to change the school, school district, and/or grade level to gain a wide range of experience.

Housing and Day Care: On-campus housing is available. See the following Web site for more information: http://www.newpaltz.edu/reslife/. On-campus day care facilities are available. See the following Web site for more information: http://www.newpaltz.edu/childrenscenter/.

Employment of Department Graduates:
Master's Degree Graduates: Of those who graduated in the academic year 2008–2009, the following categories and numbers represent the postgraduate activities and employment of master's degree graduates: Enrolled in a postdoctoral residency/fellowship (n/a), employed in independent practice (n/a), total from the above (master's) (0).

Doctoral Degree Graduates: Of those who graduated in the academic year 2008–2009, the following categories and numbers represent the postgraduate activities and employment of doctoral degree graduates: Enrolled in a psychology doctoral program (n/a), total from the above (doctoral) (0).

Additional Information:
Orientation, Objectives, and Emphasis of Department: Founded in 1828, America's 99th oldest university is an exciting blend of tradition and vision, providing students with the skills and knowledge needed to meet the challenges of the 21st century. SUNY New Paltz offers graduate training in psychology and mental health counseling. The 36-credit MA in psychology program offers general graduate training in psychology. The program provides students with the opportunity to select electives in a variety of fields including social, experimental, and organizational psychology as well as counseling. The program may serve as preparation for entry into a doctoral program or as additional training for those who plan to enter or are already involved in applied areas of psychology. The 48-credit MS in mental health counseling program serves both students looking to become licensed as mental health counselors and those seeking to eventually proceed into doctoral training programs. Degree requirements cover a core curriculum and specialization courses. Three fieldwork courses provide hands-on mental health counseling training experiences under supervision of licensed professionals. The program is registered with the State Education Department as meeting the educational requirements necessary for mental health counseling licensure in New York, making this a very marketable degree.

Special Facilities or Resources: Laboratory facilities and equipment (computers, videotaping equipment) are available to support student and faculty research in a variety of research areas. The department also maintains links to local and community organizations for research opportunities. In addition, the department has a computer lab for research and instruction with Internet access. All graduate students have access to word processing, SPSS, and the world-wide Web through the campus computer network.

Information for Students With Physical Disabilities: See the following Web site for more information: http://www.newpaltz.edu/drc.

Application Information:
Send to The Graduate School SUNY New Paltz 1 Hawk Drive New Paltz, NY 12561-2443. Application available online. URL of online application: http://www.newpaltz.edu/graduate/apply.html. Students are admitted in the Fall, application deadline February 15; Spring, application deadline November 15. Counseling programs have fall admissions only. The MA in Psychology program does have spring admissions. *Fee:* $50.

GRADUATE STUDY IN PSYCHOLOGY

State University of New York, Binghamton University

Psychology
Arts and Sciences
P.O. Box 6000
Binghamton, NY 13902-6000
Telephone: (607) 777-2334
Fax: (607) 777-4890
E-mail: rmiller@binghamton.edu
Web: http://psychology.binghamton.edu/

Department Information:
65. Chairperson: Celia Klin. Number of faculty: total—full-time 29, part-time 6; women—full-time 12, part-time 2; total—minority—full-time 2; women minority—full-time 2.

Programs and Degrees Offered:
Listed in the following order: Program area, degree type (T if terminal Master's), number awarded 7/08–6/09. Clinical Psychology PhD (Doctor of Philosophy) 5, Cognitive Psychology PhD (Doctor of Philosophy) 1, Behavioral Neuroscience PhD (Doctor of Philosophy) 4.

APA Accreditation: Clinical PhD (Doctor of Philosophy). Student Outcome Data Website: http://www2.binghamton.edu/psychology/graduate/clinical-psychology/applicant-data.html.

Student Applications/Admissions:

Student Applications

Clinical Psychology PhD (Doctor of Philosophy)—Applications 2009–2010, 291. Total applicants accepted 2009–2010, 7. Number full-time enrolled (new admits only) 2009–2010, 5. Number part-time enrolled (new admits only) 2009–2010, 0. Openings 2010–2011, 11. The median number of years required for completion of a degree in 2008–2009 were 7. The number of students enrolled full- and part-time who were dismissed or voluntarily withdrew from this program area in 2008–2009 were 1. *Cognitive Psychology PhD (Doctor of Philosophy)*—Applications 2009–2010, 23. Total applicants accepted 2009–2010, 3. Number full-time enrolled (new admits only) 2009–2010, 2. Number part-time enrolled (new admits only) 2009–2010, 0. Openings 2010–2011, 4. The median number of years required for completion of a degree in 2008–2009 were 5. The number of students enrolled full- and part-time who were dismissed or voluntarily withdrew from this program area in 2008–2009 were 1. *Behavioral Neuroscience PhD (Doctor of Philosophy)*—Applications 2009–2010, 30. Total applicants accepted 2009–2010, 5. Number full-time enrolled (new admits only) 2009–2010, 4. Number part-time enrolled (new admits only) 2009–2010, 0. Openings 2010–2011, 6. The median number of years required for completion of a degree in 2008–2009 were 7. The number of students enrolled full- and part-time who were dismissed or voluntarily withdrew from this program area in 2008–2009 were 4.

Scores: Entries appear in this order: required test or GPA, minimum score (if required), median score of students entering in 2009–2010. *Clinical Psychology PhD (Doctor of Philosophy):* GRE-V no minimum stated, GRE-Q no minimum stated, GRE-Analytical no minimum stated; *Cognitive Psychology PhD (Doctor of Philosophy):* GRE-V no minimum stated, GRE-Q no minimum stated, overall undergraduate GPA no minimum stated; *Behavioral Neuroscience PhD (Doctor of Philosophy):* GRE-V no minimum stated, GRE-Q no minimum stated, overall undergraduate GPA no minimum stated.

Other Criteria: (importance of criteria rated low, medium, or high): GRE scores—high, research experience—high, work experience—medium, extracurricular activity—low, clinically related public service—medium, GPA—high, letters of recommendation—high, interview—high, statement of goals and objectives—high, undergraduate major in psychology—low, specific undergraduate psychology courses taken—medium.

Student Characteristics: The following represents characteristics of students in 2009–2010 in all graduate psychology programs in the department: Female—full-time 57, part-time 0; Male—full-time 24, part-time 0; African American/Black—full-time 3, part-time 0; Hispanic/Latino(a)—full-time 5, part-time 0; Asian/Pacific Islander—full-time 1, part-time 0; American Indian/Alaska Native—full-time 0, part-time 0; Caucasian/White—full-time 0, part-time 0; Multi-ethnic—full-time 0, part-time 0; students subject to the Americans With Disabilities Act—full-time 0, part-time 0; Unknown ethnicity—full-time 0, part-time 0; International students who hold an F-1 or J-1 Visa—full-time 0, part-time 0.

Financial Information/Assistance:

Tuition for Full-Time Study: Doctoral: State residents: per academic year $8,310, $349 per credit hour; Nonstate residents: per academic year $13,250, $552 per credit hour. Tuition is subject to change. See the following Web site for updates and changes in tuition costs: http://studentaccounts.binghamton.edu/.

Financial Assistance:

First-Year Students: Teaching assistantships available for first year. Average amount paid per academic year: $16,500. Average number of hours worked per week: 10. Research assistantships available for first year. Average amount paid per academic year: $16,500. Fellowships and scholarships available for first year. Average amount paid per academic year: $16,500.

Advanced Students: Teaching assistantships available for advanced students. Average amount paid per academic year: $16,500. Average number of hours worked per week: 10. Research assistantships available for advanced students. Average amount paid per academic year: $16,500. Fellowships and scholarships available for advanced students. Average amount paid per academic year: $16,500.

Additional Information: Of all students currently enrolled full time, 96% benefited from one or more of the listed financial assistance programs. Application and information available online at: http://www2.binghamton.edu/grad-school/prospective-students/funding-graduate-studies/index.html.

Internships/Practica: Doctoral Degree (PhD Clinical Psychology): For those doctoral students for whom a professional internship was required in this program prior to graduation, (7) students applied for an internship in 2008–2009, with (7) students obtaining an internship. Of those students who obtained an internship, (7) were paid internships. Of those students who obtained an internship, (7) students placed in APA/CPA accredited internships, (0) students placed in internships not APA/CPA accredited, but listed with the Association of Psychology Postdoctoral and Internship Programs (APPIC), (0) students placed in internships conforming to guidelines of the Council of Directors of School Psychology Programs (CDSPP), (0) students placed in internships that were not APA/CPA accredited, APPIC or CDSPP listed. Students in the clinical area are required to complete two practica, a psychotherapy practicum and a community practicum. The psychotherapy practicum is conducted in the department clinic under the supervision of a faculty member and generally involves the joint treatment of a variety of problems across a broad range of ages and diagnoses. The community practicum consists of supervised clinical activity and/or research at one of a wide range of local agencies, hospitals, and clinics. Students in cognitive psychology are invited—but not required—to complete a research-related practicum in industry. Past internships included training at GE, IBM, Microsoft, Lockheed Martin, and others.

Housing and Day Care: No on-campus housing is available. On-campus day care facilities are available. See the following Web site for more information: http://www2.binghamton.edu/campus-pre-school/.

Employment of Department Graduates:

Master's Degree Graduates: Of those who graduated in the academic year 2008–2009, the following categories and numbers represent the postgraduate activities and employment of master's degree graduates: Enrolled in a postdoctoral residency/fellowship (n/a), employed in independent practice (n/a), total from the above (master's) (0).

Doctoral Degree Graduates: Of those who graduated in the academic year 2008–2009, the following categories and numbers represent the postgraduate activities and employment of doctoral degree graduates: Enrolled in a psychology doctoral program (n/a), enrolled in a postdoctoral residency/fellowship (10), employed in independent practice (0), employed in an academic position at a university (0), employed in an academic position at a 2-year/4-year college (0), employed in other positions at a higher education institution (0), employed in a professional position in a school system (0), employed in business or industry (0), employed in government agency (0), employed in a community mental health/counseling center (0), employed in a hospital/medical center (0), still seeking employment (0), other employment position (0), total from the above (doctoral) (10).

Additional Information:

Orientation, Objectives, and Emphasis of Department: The psychology department emphasizes basic and applied research in its three areas of specialization: clinical psychology, cognitive/behavioral psychology, and behavioral neuroscience. The goal of our APA-accredited clinical program is to develop scientists and practitioners. By virtue of ongoing research involvement, students are expected to contribute to knowledge about psychopathology, assessment, and treatment. Our cognitive program has two major research emphases, one focused on learning and memory and the other focused on perception and language (in both the visual and auditory domains). Researchers in this area also work in industrial settings and collaborate with local industry. Our behavioral neuroscience program emphasizes the study of neural and hormonal bases of normal and abnormal behavior and their developmental antecedents in preclinical animal models.

Special Facilities or Resources: All faculty have state-of-the-art, spacious laboratories. The clinical program supports an active in-house mental health clinic. Members of the cognitive area have access to sophisticated systems for the manipulation of auditory and visual stimuli and the online measurement of cognitive processes, and members of the behavioral neurosciences area share multi-user histology, microneuroimaging, and neurochemistry laboratories. A new building for animal research is currently being completed.

Information for Students With Physical Disabilities: See the following Web site for more information: http://www2.binghamton.edu/ssd/.

Application Information:
Send to Graduate Admissions Office. Application available online. URL of online application: http://gradschool.binghamton.edu/. Students are admitted in the Fall, application deadline December 15. Deadline for Clinical program is December 15. Deadline for Cognitive and Behavioral Neuroscience programs is January 15. *Fee:* $60.

State University of New York, College at Plattsburgh
Psychology Department
Beaumont Hall, 101 Broad Street
Plattsburgh, NY 12901
Telephone: (518) 564-3076
Fax: (518) 564-3397
E-mail: *renee.bator@plattsburgh.edu*
Web: *http://www.plattsburgh.edu/academics/psychology*

Department Information:
1970. Chairperson: Drs. Renee Bator and Stephen Mansfield, Co-Chairs. Number of faculty: total—full-time 13, part-time 5; women—full-time 6, part-time 4; total—minority—full-time 1, part-time 1; women minority—part-time 1.

Programs and Degrees Offered:
Listed in the following order: Program area, degree type (T if terminal Master's), number awarded 7/08–6/09. School Psychology MA/MS (Master of Arts/Science) (T) 11.

Student Applications/Admissions:
Student Applications
School Psychology MA/MS (Master of Arts/Science)—Applications 2009–2010, 30. Total applicants accepted 2009–2010, 11. Number full-time enrolled (new admits only) 2009–2010, 11. Number part-time enrolled (new admits only) 2009–2010, 0. Openings 2010–2011, 10. The median number of years required for completion of a degree in 2008–2009 were 4. The number of students enrolled full- and part-time who were dismissed or voluntarily withdrew from this program area in 2008–2009 were 0.

Other Criteria: (importance of criteria rated low, medium, or high): GRE scores—low, research experience—medium, work experience—high, extracurricular activity—low, clinically related public service—medium, GPA—high, letters of recommendation—medium, statement of goals and objectives—high, undergraduate major in psychology—low, specific undergraduate psychology courses taken—medium. For additional information on admission requirements, go to http://www.plattsburgh.edu/academics/psychology/graduateprogram.

Student Characteristics: The following represents characteristics of students in 2009–2010 in all graduate psychology programs in the department: Female—full-time 24, part-time 0; Male—full-time 4, part-time 0; African American/Black—full-time 1, part-time 0; Hispanic/Latino(a)—full-time 0, part-time 0; Asian/Pacific Islander—full-time 0, part-time 0; American Indian/Alaska Native—full-time 0, part-time 0; Caucasian/White—full-time 25, part-time 0; Multi-ethnic—full-time 2, part-time 0; students subject to the Americans With Disabilities Act—full-time 0, part-time 0; Unknown ethnicity—full-time 0, part-time 0; International students who hold an F-1 or J-1 Visa—full-time 0, part-time 0.

Financial Information/Assistance:
Financial Assistance:
First-Year Students: Research assistantships available for first year. Average amount paid per academic year: $4,600. Average number of hours worked per week: 10. Apply by February 15. Traineeships available for first year. Average amount paid per academic year: $5,000. Average number of hours worked per week: 15. Apply by February 15.

Advanced Students: Research assistantships available for advanced students. Average amount paid per academic year: $4,600. Average number of hours worked per week: 10. Apply by February 15. Traineeships available for advanced students. Average amount paid per academic year: $5,000. Average number of hours worked per week: 15. Apply by February 15.

Additional Information: Of all students currently enrolled full time, 40% benefited from one or more of the listed financial assistance programs.

Internships/Practica: Master's Degree (MA/MS School Psychology): An internship experience, such as a final research project or "capstone" experience is required of graduates. During the third and final year of graduate study, students are placed within school districts on a full-time basis. School districts sometimes offer a stipend under contractual agreement with the graduate student and the University. Stipends range from $7,000 to $14,000. Relocating to a school district in order to receive a stipend might be necessary.

Housing and Day Care: On-campus housing is available. On-campus day care facilities are available.

Employment of Department Graduates:
Master's Degree Graduates: Of those who graduated in the academic year 2008–2009, the following categories and numbers represent the postgraduate activities and employment of master's degree graduates: Enrolled in a psychology doctoral program (0), enrolled in a postdoctoral residency/fellowship (n/a), employed in independent practice (n/a), employed in a professional position in a school system (9), still seeking employment (0), total from the above (master's) (9).
Doctoral Degree Graduates: Of those who graduated in the academic year 2008–2009, the following categories and numbers represent the postgraduate activities and employment of doctoral degree graduates: Enrolled in a psychology doctoral program (n/a), total from the above (doctoral) (0).

Additional Information:
Orientation, Objectives, and Emphasis of Department: The curriculum is a three-year, 70 hour MA program in psychology. The program offers coursework in psychological theories and skill development and applied experiences in area schools and community agencies. The goal of the program is to enable students to work effectively with individuals and groups and to act as psychological resources in schools and the community. A unique feature of the program is that many courses, beginning in the first semester, combine theory and research with practicum experiences in school and clinical work. Students develop competencies in personality, research methods, psychological assessment, behavior modification, individual and group psychotherapy, and community mental health. An important aspect of graduate training is the internship served the third year of graduate study at area schools. The Psychology Department and the agencies involved provide extensive supervision of students' work.

Special Facilities or Resources: All students participate in off-site practicum experiences in local schools. The Neuropsychology Clinic and Psychoeducational Services center provide some graduate students with on-site practicum experiences. The Nexus program (an after school program for children diagnosed with Autism Spectrum Disorders) provides some graduate students with on-site practicum experiences.

Information for Students With Physical Disabilities: See the following Web site for more information: http://www.plattsburgh.edu/offices/support/sss.

Application Information:
Send to Graduate Admissions, Kehoe Hall, SUNY-Plattsburgh, 101 Broad Street, Plattsburgh, NY 12901. Application available online. URL of online application: http://www.plattsburgh.edu/admissions/graduate/apply.php. Students are admitted in the Fall, application deadline February 15. *Fee:* $75.

Stony Brook University
Department of Psychology
Stony Brook, NY 11794-2500
Telephone: (631) 632-7855
Fax: (631) 632-632-7876
E-mail: *mwollmuth@notes.cc.sunysb.edu*
Web: *http://www.psychology.sunysb.edu*

Department Information:
1961. Interim Chair: Arthur Samuel. Number of faculty: total—full-time 31; women—full-time 16; total—minority—full-time 3; women minority—full-time 2.

Programs and Degrees Offered:
Listed in the following order: Program area, degree type (T if terminal Master's), number awarded 7/08–6/09. Biopsychology PhD (Doctor of Philosophy) 2, Clinical Psychology PhD (Doctor of Philosophy) 5, Cognitive/Experimental Psychology PhD (Doctor of Philosophy) 1, Social/Health Psychology PhD (Doctor of Philosophy) 5.

APA Accreditation: Clinical PhD (Doctor of Philosophy). Student Outcome Data Website: http://www.psychology.sunysb.edu/psychology/graduate/areasofstudy/disclosuredata.htm.

Student Applications/Admissions:
Student Applications
Biopsychology PhD (Doctor of Philosophy)—Applications 2009–2010, 30. Total applicants accepted 2009–2010, 5. Number full-time enrolled (new admits only) 2009–2010, 4. Total enrolled 2009–2010 full-time, 16. Openings 2010–2011, 5. The median number of years required for completion of a degree in 2008–2009 were 5. The number of students enrolled full- and part-time who were dismissed or voluntarily withdrew from this program area in 2008–2009 were 0. *Clinical Psychology PhD (Doctor of Philosophy)*—Applications 2009–2010, 319. Total applicants accepted 2009–2010, 8. Number full-time enrolled (new admits only) 2009–2010, 5. Total enrolled 2009–2010 full-time, 37. Openings 2010–2011, 6. The median number of years required for completion of a degree in 2008–2009 were 6. The number of students enrolled full- and part-time who were dismissed or voluntarily withdrew from this program area in 2008–2009 were 1. *Cognitive/Experimental Psychology PhD (Doctor of Philosophy)*—Applications 2009–2010, 29. Total applicants accepted 2009–2010, 5. Number full-time enrolled (new admits only) 2009–2010, 2. Total enrolled 2009–2010 full-time, 16. Openings 2010–2011, 5. The median number of years required for completion of a degree in 2008–2009 were 5. The number of students enrolled full- and part-time who were dismissed or voluntarily withdrew from this program area in 2008–2009 were 0. *Social/Health Psychology PhD (Doctor of Philosophy)*—Applications 2009–2010, 95. Total applicants accepted 2009–2010, 5. Number full-time enrolled (new admits only) 2009–2010, 6. Total enrolled 2009–2010 full-time, 25. Openings 2010–2011, 5. The median number of years required for completion of a degree in 2008–2009 were 5. The number of students enrolled full- and part-time who were dismissed or voluntarily withdrew from this program area in 2008–2009 were 0.
Scores: Entries appear in this order: required test or GPA, minimum score (if required), median score of students entering in 2009–2010. *Clinical Psychology PhD (Doctor of Philosophy)*: GRE-V no minimum stated, 680, GRE-Q no minimum stated, 750, GRE-Analytical no minimum stated, 5.5, overall undergraduate GPA no minimum stated, 3.75.
Other Criteria: (importance of criteria rated low, medium, or high): GRE scores—high, research experience—high, work experience—low, extracurricular activity—low, clinically related public service—low, GPA—medium, letters of recommendation—high, interview—medium, statement of goals and objectives—high. For additional information on admission requirements, go to http://www.psychology.sunysb.edu/psychology/index.php?graduate/prospectivestudents.

Student Characteristics: The following represents characteristics of students in 2009–2010 in all graduate psychology programs in the department: Female—full-time 72, part-time 0; Male—full-time 30, part-time 0; African American/Black—full-time 3, part-time 0; Hispanic/Latino(a)—full-time 7, part-time 0; Asian/Pacific Islander—full-time 13, part-time 0; American Indian/Alaska Native—full-time 0, part-time 0; Caucasian/White—full-time 73, part-time 0; Multi-ethnic—full-time 6, part-time 0; students subject to the Americans With Disabilities Act—full-time 0, part-time 0; Unknown ethnicity—full-time 0, part-time 0; International students who hold an F-1 or J-1 Visa—full-time 12, part-time 0.

Financial Information/Assistance:
Tuition for Full-Time Study: *Master's:* State residents: per academic year $4,185, $349 per credit hour; Nonstate residents: per academic year $6,625, $552 per credit hour. *Doctoral:* State residents: per academic year $4,185, $349 per credit hour; Nonstate residents: per academic year $6,625, $552 per credit hour. Tuition is subject to change. See the following Web site for updates and changes in tuition costs: http://www.stonybrook.edu/bursar/tuition/grad.shtml.

Financial Assistance:
First-Year Students: Teaching assistantships available for first year. Average amount paid per academic year: $15,145. Average number of hours worked per week: 20. Apply by December 15. Research assistantships available for first year. Average amount paid per academic year: $15,145. Average number of hours worked per week: 20. Apply by December 15. Fellowships and scholarships available for first year. Average amount paid per academic year: $17,572. Average number of hours worked per week: 20. Apply by December 15.
Advanced Students: Teaching assistantships available for advanced students. Average amount paid per academic year: $15,145. Average number of hours worked per week: 20. Research assistantships available for advanced students. Average amount paid per academic year: $15,145. Average number of hours worked per week: 20. Fellowships and scholarships available for advanced students. Average amount paid per academic year: $17,572. Average number of hours worked per week: 20.
Additional Information: Of all students currently enrolled full time, 99% benefited from one or more of the listed financial assistance programs. Application and information available online at: http://www.grad.sunysb.edu/admissions/financial_aid.shtml.

Internships/Practica: Doctoral Degree (PhD Clinical Psychology): For those doctoral students for whom a professional internship was required in this program prior to graduation, (6) students applied for an internship in 2008–2009, with (6) students obtaining an internship. Of those students who obtained an internship, (6) were paid internships. Of those students who obtained an internship, (5) students placed in APA/CPA accredited internships, (1) students placed in internships not APA/CPA accredited, but listed with the Association of Psychology Postdoctoral and Internship Programs (APPIC), (0) students placed in internships conforming to guidelines of the Council of Directors of School Psychology Programs (CDSPP), (0) students placed in internships that were not APA/CPA accredited, APPIC or CDSPP listed.

Housing and Day Care: On-campus housing is available. See the following Web site for more information: http://studentaffairs.stonybrook.edu/res. On-campus day care facilities are available. See the following Web site for more information: http://ws.cc.stonybrook.edu/sb/childcare/.

GRADUATE STUDY IN PSYCHOLOGY

Employment of Department Graduates:
Master's Degree Graduates: Of those who graduated in the academic year 2008–2009, the following categories and numbers represent the postgraduate activities and employment of master's degree graduates: Enrolled in a postdoctoral residency/fellowship (n/a), employed in independent practice (n/a), total from the above (master's) (0).

Doctoral Degree Graduates: Of those who graduated in the academic year 2008–2009, the following categories and numbers represent the postgraduate activities and employment of doctoral degree graduates: Enrolled in a psychology doctoral program (n/a), enrolled in a postdoctoral residency/fellowship (7), employed in an academic position at a university (7), employed in other positions at a higher education institution (1), still seeking employment (1), total from the above (doctoral) (16).

Additional Information:
Orientation, Objectives, and Emphasis of Department: In all areas, the primary emphasis is on research training through research advisement and apprenticeship. Students are encouraged to become involved in ongoing research immediately and to engage in independent research when sufficient skills and knowledge permit, with the goal of becoming active and original contributors. As the first behavioral clinical curriculum in the country, Stony Brook has served as a model for a number of other behaviorally oriented clinical programs and continues to be a leader in that field. Research in the experimental area focuses on human perception and cognition and now includes visual cognition, psycholinguistics, memory, attention, and perception. The biopsychology research of core faculty spans the fields of behavioral neuroscience, molecular biology, cognitive neuroscience and affective neuroscience. Students obtain a broad foundation in neuroscience while developing expertise in a focused research program. Research in social and health psychology includes the study of close relationships in adults and children; prejudice, racism, and stereotyping; and the representation and processing of social experience, motivation, and self-regulation.

Special Facilities or Resources: Besides faculty laboratories for human, animal, and physiological research, and electronics and machine shops, other campus facilities for research and graduate training include: Psychological Center, the training, research, and service unit for clinical psychology; Point of Woods Laboratory School with a special education class for elementary students; University Preschool with children from 18 months to 5 years of age; University Marital Therapy Clinic; and Suffolk Child Development Center, a private school for autistic, retarded, aphasic, and developmentally delayed children. Clinical neuropsychology uses affiliations with the University Health Sciences Center, local schools, an agency for the mentally retarded, and a Veterans Administration hospital. Departmental CRT terminals and 12 additional terminals and two printers in the division's Social Science Data Laboratory are used with campus computers.

Application Information:
Send to Graduate Office-Department of Psychology, Stony Brook University, Stony Brook, NY 11794-2500. Application available online. URL of online application: http://www.grad.sunysb.edu/admissions/app_info.shtml. Students are admitted in the Fall, application deadline December 15. *Fee:* $70.

Syracuse University
Department of Psychology
Arts and Sciences
430 Huntington Hall, 150 Marshall Street
Syracuse, NY 13244-2340
Telephone: (315) 443-2354
Fax: (315) 443-4085
E-mail: *pvanable@syr.edu*
Web: *http://psychweb.syr.edu*

Department Information:
1952. Chairperson: Peter A. Vanable. Number of faculty: total—full-time 27, part-time 2; women—full-time 10, part-time 1; total—minority—full-time 3; women minority—full-time 3.

Programs and Degrees Offered:
Listed in the following order: Program area, degree type (T if terminal Master's), number awarded 7/08–6/09. Clinical Psychology PhD (Doctor of Philosophy) 4, Experimental Psychology PhD (Doctor of Philosophy) 1, School Psychology PhD (Doctor of Philosophy) 3, Social Psychology PhD (Doctor of Philosophy) 0.

APA Accreditation: Clinical PhD (Doctor of Philosophy). Student Outcome Data Website: http://psychweb.syr.edu/GPClinical.htm. School PhD (Doctor of Philosophy). Student Outcome Data Website: http://psychweb.syr.edu/GPSchool.htm.

Student Applications/Admissions:
Student Applications
Clinical Psychology PhD (Doctor of Philosophy)—Applications 2009–2010, 117. Total applicants accepted 2009–2010, 9. Number full-time enrolled (new admits only) 2009–2010, 3. Number part-time enrolled (new admits only) 2009–2010, 0. Openings 2010–2011, 4. The median number of years required for completion of a degree in 2008–2009 were 7. The number of students enrolled full- and part-time who were dismissed or voluntarily withdrew from this program area in 2008–2009 were 0. *Experimental Psychology PhD (Doctor of Philosophy)*— Applications 2009–2010, 13. Total applicants accepted 2009–2010, 6. Number full-time enrolled (new admits only) 2009–2010, 3. Number part-time enrolled (new admits only) 2009–2010, 0. Openings 2010–2011, 4. The median number of years required for completion of a degree in 2008–2009 were 5. The number of students enrolled full- and part-time who were dismissed or voluntarily withdrew from this program area in 2008–2009 were 0. *School Psychology PhD (Doctor of Philosophy)*—Applications 2009–2010, 39. Total applicants accepted 2009–2010, 3. Number full-time enrolled (new admits only) 2009–2010, 2. Number part-time enrolled (new admits only) 2009–2010, 0. Openings 2010–2011, 4. The median number of years required for completion of a degree in 2008–2009 were 5. The number of students enrolled full- and part-time who were dismissed or voluntarily withdrew from this program area in 2008–2009 were 0. *Social Psychology PhD (Doctor of Philosophy)*—Applications 2009–2010, 52. Total applicants accepted 2009–2010, 3. Number full-time enrolled (new admits

only) 2009–2010, 1. Number part-time enrolled (new admits only) 2009–2010, 0. Openings 2010–2011, 2. The number of students enrolled full- and part-time who were dismissed or voluntarily withdrew from this program area in 2008–2009 were 0.

Scores: Entries appear in this order: required test or GPA, minimum score (if required), median score of students entering in 2009–2010. *Clinical Psychology PhD (Doctor of Philosophy):* GRE-V 540, 560, GRE-Q 710, 720, GRE-Analytical 4.5, 5, overall undergraduate GPA 3.02, 3.45; *Experimental Psychology PhD (Doctor of Philosophy):* GRE-V 400, 420, GRE-Q 540, 550, GRE-Analytical 3.5, 4, overall undergraduate GPA 3.13, 3.56; *School Psychology PhD (Doctor of Philosophy):* GRE-V 510, 535, GRE-Q 600, 665, GRE-Analytical 4, 4.5, overall undergraduate GPA 3.1, 3.55; *Social Psychology PhD (Doctor of Philosophy):* GRE-V 590, 590, GRE-Q 760, 760, GRE-Analytical 5.5, 5.5, overall undergraduate GPA 3.98, 3.98.

Other Criteria: (importance of criteria rated low, medium, or high): GRE scores—high, research experience—high, work experience—medium, extracurricular activity—low, clinically related public service—medium, GPA—high, letters of recommendation—high, interview—high, statement of goals and objectives—high. Interview requirements vary from program to program. For additional information on admission requirements, go to http://psychweb.syr.edu.

Student Characteristics: The following represents characteristics of students in 2009–2010 in all graduate psychology programs in the department: Female—full-time 47, part-time 0; Male—full-time 10, part-time 0; African American/Black—full-time 0, part-time 0; Hispanic/Latino(a)—full-time 0, part-time 0; Asian/Pacific Islander—full-time 5, part-time 0; American Indian/Alaska Native—full-time 0, part-time 0; Caucasian/White—full-time 51, part-time 0; Multi-ethnic—full-time 1, part-time 0; students subject to the Americans With Disabilities Act—full-time 0, part-time 0; Unknown ethnicity—full-time 0, part-time 0; International students who hold an F-1 or J-1 Visa—full-time 8, part-time 0.

Financial Information/Assistance:

Tuition for Full-Time Study: *Doctoral:* State residents: per academic year $20,106, $1,117 per credit hour; Nonstate residents: per academic year $20,106, $1,117 per credit hour. Tuition is subject to change. See the following Web site for updates and changes in tuition costs: http://financialaid.syr.edu.

Financial Assistance:

First-Year Students: Teaching assistantships available for first year. Average amount paid per academic year: $12,703. Average number of hours worked per week: 20. Apply by January 1. Research assistantships available for first year. Average amount paid per academic year: $12,703. Average number of hours worked per week: 20. Apply by January 1. Fellowships and scholarships available for first year. Average amount paid per academic year: $21,170. Average number of hours worked per week: 0. Apply by January 1.

Advanced Students: Teaching assistantships available for advanced students. Average amount paid per academic year: $12,703. Average number of hours worked per week: 20. Research assistantships available for advanced students. Average amount paid per academic year: $12,703. Average number of hours worked per week: 20. Fellowships and scholarships available for advanced students. Average amount paid per academic year: $21,170. Average number of hours worked per week: 0.

Additional Information: Of all students currently enrolled full time, 61% benefited from one or more of the listed financial assistance programs.

Internships/Practica: Doctoral Degree (PhD Clinical Psychology): For those doctoral students for whom a professional internship was required in this program prior to graduation, (3) students applied for an internship in 2008–2009, with (3) students obtaining an internship. Of those students who obtained an internship, (3) were paid internships. Of those students who obtained an internship, (3) students placed in APA/CPA accredited internships, (0) students placed in internships not APA/CPA accredited, but listed with the Association of Psychology Postdoctoral and Internship Programs (APPIC), (0) students placed in internships conforming to guidelines of the Council of Directors of School Psychology Programs (CDSPP), (0) students placed in internships that were not APA/CPA accredited, APPIC or CDSPP listed. Doctoral Degree (PhD School Psychology): For those doctoral students for whom a professional internship was required in this program prior to graduation, (3) students applied for an internship in 2008–2009, with (3) students obtaining an internship. Of those students who obtained an internship, (3) were paid internships. Of those students who obtained an internship, (2) students placed in APA/CPA accredited internships, (0) students placed in internships not APA/CPA accredited, but listed with the Association of Psychology Postdoctoral and Internship Programs (APPIC), (1) students placed in internships conforming to guidelines of the Council of Directors of School Psychology Programs (CDSPP), (0) students placed in internships that were not APA/CPA accredited, APPIC or CDSPP listed. Students in the clinical and school psychology training programs have appropriate internship and practicum experiences available in hospitals, schools, and other community and University settings. Following completion of their coursework, clinical students complete APA approved internships as part of their required program of study.

Housing and Day Care: On-campus housing is available. See the following Web site for more information: http://housingmealplans.syr.edu. On-campus day care facilities are available.

Employment of Department Graduates:

Master's Degree Graduates: Of those who graduated in the academic year 2008–2009, the following categories and numbers represent the postgraduate activities and employment of master's degree graduates: Enrolled in a psychology doctoral program (0), enrolled in a postdoctoral residency/fellowship (n/a), employed in independent practice (n/a), total from the above (master's) (0).

Doctoral Degree Graduates: Of those who graduated in the academic year 2008–2009, the following categories and numbers represent the postgraduate activities and employment of doctoral degree graduates: Enrolled in a psychology doctoral program (n/a), enrolled in a postdoctoral residency/fellowship (5), employed in an academic position at a 2-year/4-year college (2), employed in a professional position in a school system (1), total from the above (doctoral) (8).

GRADUATE STUDY IN PSYCHOLOGY

Additional Information:

Orientation, Objectives, and Emphasis of Department: Our goal is to train high caliber scientists in psychology. Students work closely with a faculty advisor whose research interests are similar to the student's (one can change to a new advisor, however, if one's research interests change). Our APA-approved programs in clinical and school psychology are based on the Boulder scientist–practitioner model. There are four thematic foci in the department: Cognitive Aging; Health and Behavior; the Scholarship of the Causes, Consequences, and Remediation of Social Challenges; and the Psychology of Children in Home and School. Students can gain exposure to research in coping with chronic illness, HIV prevention, memory processes in older adults, school based intervention, substance abuse, stigma and group process, to name a few. A second goal is training future teachers of Psychology. Students typically engage in several semesters of teaching, beginning with sections of introductory psychology and moving on to teach more specialized courses. Entering students participate in the University's "Future Professoriate Program," a teaching practicum nationally known for helping new graduate students enter the profession. Other teaching opportunities are available in the Department's Allport Project, which involves undergraduates in faculty research activities. As part of this program, graduate students may offer supervised but essentially independent seminars for undergraduates in their specialty area. Students enrolled in the clinical and school psychology programs gain clinical experience through our university based psychological services center and placement in area schools and hospitals.

Special Facilities or Resources: The Department of Psychology is housed in Huntington Hall, an historic building that has been remodeled to provide offices and seminar rooms, as well as laboratories for the study of cognition, social psychology, behavioral medicine, family interaction, and group processes. Labs and offices are equipped with microcomputers for data collection and analysis. A separate wing houses the Department's Psychological Services Center, which offers facilities for clinical and school psychology practicum training and research. In addition, the Department has two facilities on campus and two facilities off campus that provide additional lab space. Other facilities are available through faculty collaborations with researchers at the Upstate Medical University, which is adjacent to Huntington Hall. The Department and its Center for Health and Behavior support two full-time computer technicians.

Information for Students With Physical Disabilities: See the following Web site for more information: http://syr.edu/disabilityservices/.

Application Information:
Send to Graduate School, Suite 303, Bowne Hall, Syracuse University, Syracuse, NY 13244-1200. Application available online. URL of online application: http://apply.embark.com/grad/Syracuse/37. Students are admitted in the Fall, application deadline January 1. To be considered for a University Fellowship, completed applications must be received by January 1. Due to APA requirements, all applications (fellowship and non-fellowship) for the School and Clinical Psychology Programs are due by January 1. *Fee:* $65.

Teachers College, Columbia University
Department of Counseling and Clinical Psychology
Teachers College, Columbia University
Box 303, 525 West 120th Street
New York, NY 10027-6696
Telephone: (212) 678-3257
Fax: (212) 678-3275
E-mail: *farber@exchange.tc.columbia.edu*
Web: *http://www.tc.edu/ccp*

Department Information:
1996. Chair: George Bonanno. Number of faculty: total—full-time 18, part-time 26; women—full-time 11, part-time 15; total—minority—full-time 9, part-time 2; women minority—full-time 6, part-time 1; faculty subject to the Americans With Disabilities Act 1.

Programs and Degrees Offered:
Listed in the following order: Program area, degree type (T if terminal Master's), number awarded 7/08–6/09. Psychological Counseling Other 89, Clinical Psychology PhD (Doctor of Philosophy) 7, Counseling Psychology PhD (Doctor of Philosophy) 12, Personality and Psychopathology MA/MS (Master of Arts/Science) (T) 70.

APA Accreditation: Clinical PhD (Doctor of Philosophy). Student Outcome Data Website: http://www.tc.edu/ccp/Clinical/. Counseling PhD (Doctor of Philosophy).

Student Applications/Admissions:
Student Applications
Psychological Counseling Other—Applications 2009–2010, 189. Total applicants accepted 2009–2010, 98. Number full-time enrolled (new admits only) 2009–2010, 75. Number part-time enrolled (new admits only) 2009–2010, 9. Total enrolled 2009–2010 full-time, 152, part-time, 68. Openings 2010–2011, 90. The median number of years required for completion of a degree in 2008–2009 were 2. The number of students enrolled full- and part-time who were dismissed or voluntarily withdrew from this program area in 2008–2009 were 0. *Clinical Psychology PhD (Doctor of Philosophy)*—Applications 2009–2010, 305. Total applicants accepted 2009–2010, 7. Number full-time enrolled (new admits only) 2009–2010, 6. Total enrolled 2009–2010 full-time, 29, part-time, 25. Openings 2010–2011, 7. The median number of years required for completion of a degree in 2008–2009 were 6. The number of students enrolled full- and part-time who were dismissed or voluntarily withdrew from this program area in 2008–2009 were 0. *Counseling Psychology PhD (Doctor of Philosophy)*—Applications 2009–2010, 275. Total applicants accepted 2009–2010, 8. Number full-time enrolled (new admits only) 2009–2010, 8. Number part-time enrolled (new admits only) 2009–2010, 0. Total enrolled 2009–2010 full-time, 39, part-time, 11. Openings 2010–2011, 8. The median number of years required for completion of a degree in 2008–2009 were 7. The number of students enrolled full- and part-time who were dismissed or voluntarily withdrew from this program area in 2008–2009 were 0. *Personality and Psychopathology MA/MS (Master of Arts/Science)*—Applications 2009–2010, 150. Total applicants accepted 2009–2010, 108. Number full-time enrolled (new admits only) 2009–2010,

93. Number part-time enrolled (new admits only) 2009–2010, 15. Total enrolled 2009–2010 full-time, 128, part-time, 55. Openings 2010–2011, 95. The median number of years required for completion of a degree in 2008–2009 were 2. The number of students enrolled full- and part-time who were dismissed or voluntarily withdrew from this program area in 2008–2009 were 0.

Scores: Entries appear in this order: required test or GPA, minimum score (if required), median score of students entering in 2009–2010. *Clinical Psychology PhD (Doctor of Philosophy):* GRE-V 640, 670, GRE-Q 640, 680, GRE-Analytical no minimum stated, GRE-Subject (Psychology) 640, 680, overall undergraduate GPA no minimum stated, last 2 years GPA no minimum stated, psychology GPA no minimum stated.

Other Criteria: (importance of criteria rated low, medium, or high): GRE scores—high, research experience—high, work experience—high, extracurricular activity—medium, clinically related public service—medium, GPA—medium, letters of recommendation—high, interview—high, statement of goals and objectives—medium, undergraduate major in psychology—medium, specific undergraduate psychology courses taken—medium. For additional information on admission requirements, go to http://www.tc.edu/ccp.

Student Characteristics: The following represents characteristics of students in 2009–2010 in all graduate psychology programs in the department: Female—full-time 200, part-time 102; Male—full-time 89, part-time 50; African American/Black—full-time 21, part-time 10; Hispanic/Latino(a)—full-time 17, part-time 6; Asian/Pacific Islander—full-time 33, part-time 4; American Indian/Alaska Native—full-time 1, part-time 0; Caucasian/White—full-time 199, part-time 118; Multi-ethnic—full-time 14, part-time 2; students subject to the Americans With Disabilities Act—full-time 3, part-time 0; Unknown ethnicity—full-time 0, part-time 0; International students who hold an F-1 or J-1 Visa—full-time 0, part-time 0.

Financial Information/Assistance:
Tuition for Full-Time Study: *Master's:* State residents: $1,127 per credit hour; Nonstate residents: $1,127 per credit hour. *Doctoral:* State residents: $1,127 per credit hour; Nonstate residents: $1,127 per credit hour. Tuition is subject to change.

Financial Assistance:
First-Year Students: Research assistantships available for first year. Apply by December 15. Fellowships and scholarships available for first year. Average amount paid per academic year: $12,000. Apply by December 15.
Advanced Students: Teaching assistantships available for advanced students. Average amount paid per academic year: $1,600. Average number of hours worked per week: 3. Research assistantships available for advanced students. Average amount paid per academic year: $4,000. Apply by December 15. Fellowships and scholarships available for advanced students. Average amount paid per academic year: $12,000.
Additional Information: Of all students currently enrolled full time, 20% benefited from one or more of the listed financial assistance programs. Application and information available online at: http://www.tc.edu/admissions/finaid.htm.

Internships/Practica: Doctoral Degree (PhD Clinical Psychology): For those doctoral students for whom a professional internship was required in this program prior to graduation, (9) students applied for an internship in 2008–2009, with (8) students obtaining an internship. Of those students who obtained an internship, (8) were paid internships. Of those students who obtained an internship, (8) students placed in APA/CPA accredited internships, (0) students placed in internships not APA/CPA accredited, but listed with the Association of Psychology Postdoctoral and Internship Programs (APPIC), (0) students placed in internships conforming to guidelines of the Council of Directors of School Psychology Programs (CDSPP), (0) students placed in internships that were not APA/CPA accredited, APPIC or CDSPP listed. Doctoral Degree (PhD Counseling Psychology): For those doctoral students for whom a professional internship was required in this program prior to graduation, (11) students applied for an internship in 2008–2009, with (9) students obtaining an internship. Of those students who obtained an internship, (9) were paid internships. Of those students who obtained an internship, (9) students placed in APA/CPA accredited internships, (0) students placed in internships not APA/CPA accredited, but listed with the Association of Psychology Postdoctoral and Internship Programs (APPIC), (0) students placed in internships conforming to guidelines of the Council of Directors of School Psychology Programs (CDSPP), (0) students placed in internships that were not APA/CPA accredited, APPIC or CDSPP listed. Master's students in the Department of Counseling and Clinical Psychology complete fieldwork appropriate to their track or area of interest in a variety of settings including schools, hospitals, diverse mental health clinics and rehabilitation centers. Doctoral students do externships in settings similar to the ones indicated above, in preparation for their required APA-approved internships. In addition, all PhD students as well as the MEd students engage in practicum experiences at the Center for Educational and Psychological Services at the College. The Center is a community resource that provides low-cost services for the public utilizing graduate students from several departments within the College. All students receive supervision provided by full-time and adjunct faculty. PhD students in the clinical and counseling programs complete a one-year (or equivalent) full-time internship.

Housing and Day Care: On-campus housing is available. See the following Web site for more information: http://www.tc.columbia.edu/housing/. On-campus day care facilities are available. See the following Web site for more information: http://www.tc.edu/ritagold/.

Employment of Department Graduates:
Master's Degree Graduates: Of those who graduated in the academic year 2008–2009, the following categories and numbers represent the postgraduate activities and employment of master's degree graduates: Enrolled in a psychology doctoral program (22), enrolled in a postdoctoral residency/fellowship (n/a), employed in independent practice (n/a), total from the above (master's) (22).
Doctoral Degree Graduates: Of those who graduated in the academic year 2008–2009, the following categories and numbers represent the postgraduate activities and employment of doctoral degree graduates: Enrolled in a psychology doctoral program (n/a), enrolled in another graduate/professional program (0), enrolled in a postdoctoral residency/fellowship (6), employed in independent practice (6), employed in an academic position at a university (2), employed in an academic position at a 2-year/4-year college

(2), employed in other positions at a higher education institution (1), employed in a community mental health/counseling center (2), employed in a hospital/medical center (4), still seeking employment (1), total from the above (doctoral) (24).

Additional Information:
Orientation, Objectives, and Emphasis of Department: This department prepares students to investigate and address the psychological needs of individuals, families, groups, organizations/institutions and communities. Counseling psychology focuses on normal and optimal development across the lifespan, with particular attention to expanding knowledge and skills in occupational choice and transitions, and multicultural and group counseling. Clinical Psychology primarily uses a broad-based psychodynamic perspective to study and treat a variety of psychological and psychoeducational problems. In addition to sharing an interest and appreciation for the critical role of culture in development and adaptation, both programs highly value the teaching of clinical and research skills. Thus, students in this department are trained to become knowledgeable and proficient researchers, to provide psychological and educational leadership, and to be effective practitioners. Specifically, graduates from these programs seek positions in teaching, research, policy, administration, psychotherapy, and counseling.

Special Facilities or Resources: The College provides academic/research support in several ways. Students of the College have access to all the libraries of Columbia University. Of particular interest in addition to the Milbank Memorial Library here at Teachers College, are the Psychology Library on the main Columbia campus and the library at the School of Social Work. Technology has transformed most libraries to computer-oriented environments with immediate access to information. The Library not only provides the access but instruction to students so they may avail themselves of the new technology. The ERIC system as well as Inter-Library Loan are also available. The Microcomputer Center provides students with access to PC and Mac computers, which allow for sharing disk, file and printer resources as well as email services to Columbia University and to the Internet. Other hardware includes CD-ROMs, zip drives, a color scanner, and a sound and video digitizer.

Information for Students With Physical Disabilities: See the following Web site for more information: http://www.tc.columbia.edu/administration/ossd/.

Application Information:
Send to Teachers College Office of Admission, Thorndike Hall, 3rd Floor 525 West 120th Street, New York, NY 10027-6696. Application available online. URL of online application: https://app.applyyourself.com/?id=col-tc. Students are admitted in the Fall, application deadline (see below). The Doctoral application deadline is December 15. For masters applications, all admissions materials must be received by January 15 for priority consideration or by April 15 for final consideration. *Fee:* $65. Waiver is available. Hardship verification is done via a letter from Financial Aid Officer at the applicant's previous academic institution.

The College at Brockport, State University of New York (2009 data)
Department of Psychology
350 New Campus Drive
Brockport, NY 14420
Telephone: (585) 395-2488
Fax: (585) 395-2116
E-mail: *psychdpt@brockport.edu*
Web: *http://www.brockport.edu/psh/grad/*

Department Information:
1965. Chairperson: Melissa M. Brown. Number of faculty: total—full-time 12, part-time 3; women—full-time 10, part-time 1.

Programs and Degrees Offered:
Listed in the following order: Program area, degree type (T if terminal Master's), number awarded 7/08–6/09. Clinical MA/MS (Master of Arts/Science) (T) 11.

Student Applications/Admissions:
Student Applications
Clinical MA/MS (Master of Arts/Science)—Applications 2009–2010, 28. Total applicants accepted 2009–2010, 14. Number full-time enrolled (new admits only) 2009–2010, 11. Number part-time enrolled (new admits only) 2009–2010, 3. Total enrolled 2009–2010 full-time, 20, part-time, 4. Openings 2010–2011, 15. The median number of years required for completion of a degree in 2008–2009 were 2. The number of students enrolled full- and part-time who were dismissed or voluntarily withdrew from this program area in 2008–2009 were 0.
Other Criteria: (importance of criteria rated low, medium, or high): GRE scores—medium, research experience—medium, work experience—medium, clinically related public service—medium, GPA—high, letters of recommendation—high, interview—high, statement of goals and objectives—high, Psychology GPA—high, undergraduate major in psychology—medium, specific undergraduate psychology courses taken—low. For additional information on admission requirements, go to http://www.brockport.edu/psh/grad/.

Student Characteristics: The following represents characteristics of students in 2009–2010 in all graduate psychology programs in the department: Female—full-time 4, part-time 13; Male—full-time 1, part-time 4; African American/Black—full-time 0, part-time 0; Hispanic/Latino(a)—full-time 1, part-time 0; Asian/Pacific Islander—full-time 0, part-time 0; American Indian/Alaska Native—full-time 0, part-time 0; Caucasian/White—full-time 4, part-time 17; Multi-ethnic—full-time 0, part-time 0; students subject to the Americans With Disabilities Act—full-time 0, part-time 0; Unknown ethnicity—full-time 0, part-time 0; International students who hold an F-1 or J-1 Visa—full-time 0, part-time 0.

Financial Information/Assistance:
Tuition for Full-Time Study: Master's: State residents: per academic year $7,880, $328 per credit hour; Nonstate residents: per academic year $14,250, $552 per credit hour. Tuition is subject to change.

Financial Assistance:

First-Year Students: Teaching assistantships available for first year. Average amount paid per academic year: $6,000. Average number of hours worked per week: 20. Apply by May 15.

Advanced Students: Teaching assistantships available for advanced students. Average amount paid per academic year: $6,000. Average number of hours worked per week: 20. Apply by May 15.

Additional Information: Of all students currently enrolled full time, 10% benefited from one or more of the listed financial assistance programs.

Internships/Practica: Master's Degree (MA/MS Clinical): An internship experience, such as a final research project or "capstone" experience is required of graduates. Practical experience is offered in one of nearly 50 human service agencies in western New York, including the college counseling center, VA and academic medical centers, and state and local mental health, developmental disability/autism centers, and other community service agencies. Each practicum placement is developed individually, based on the specific student and agency involved. Each practicum is supervised by an agency staff member as well as a faculty member from the Department of Psychology. Students must successfully complete all required coursework before beginning the practicum.

Housing and Day Care: No on-campus housing is available. On-campus day care facilities are available.

Employment of Department Graduates:

Master's Degree Graduates: Of those who graduated in the academic year 2008–2009, the following categories and numbers represent the postgraduate activities and employment of master's degree graduates: Enrolled in a psychology doctoral program (0), enrolled in another graduate/professional program (0), enrolled in a postdoctoral residency/fellowship (n/a), employed in independent practice (n/a), employed in an academic position at a university (0), employed in an academic position at a 2-year/4-year college (2), employed in other positions at a higher education institution (0), employed in a professional position in a school system (1), employed in business or industry (0), employed in government agency (0), employed in a community mental health/counseling center (7), employed in a hospital/medical center (1), still seeking employment (0), other employment position (0), total from the above (master's) (11).

Doctoral Degree Graduates: Of those who graduated in the academic year 2008–2009, the following categories and numbers represent the postgraduate activities and employment of doctoral degree graduates: Enrolled in a psychology doctoral program (n/a), total from the above (doctoral) (0).

Additional Information:

Orientation, Objectives, and Emphasis of Department: The MA in psychology program is designed to prepare students for both doctoral work and also careers in applied psychology and the helping professions. Students are trained as scientists and practitioners, concerned with the application of psychological principles to the treatment and prevention of behavior disorders. Courses provide theoretical and practical training in contemporary methods of assessment, behavioral and cognitive-behavioral clinical intervention, and program evaluation applicable to child, adolescent and adult populations. Faculty includes board-certified applied behavior analysts and licensed psychologists.

Special Facilities or Resources: The department has facilities for research in the biobehavioral sciences, as well as sensory-perceptual, clinical, developmental, and personality psychology topics; and assessment/intervention training. Laboratory space, computer equipment, and an extensive file of psychological assessment instruments are also available.

Application Information:
Send to Office of Graduate Studies, SUNY College at Brockport, 350 New Campus Dr., Brockport, NY 14420-2914. Students are admitted in the Fall, application deadline April 1. *Fee:* $50.

The New School for Social Research
Department of Psychology
80 Fifth Avenue, 7th Floor
New York, NY 10011
Telephone: (212) 229-5727
Fax: (212) 989-0846
E-mail: *gfpsych@newschool.edu*
Web: *http://www.newschool.edu/nssr/psychology/*

Department Information:
1936. Chairperson: McWelling Todman, PhD Number of faculty: total—full-time 15; women—full-time 5; total—minority—full-time 3; women minority—full-time 1.

Programs and Degrees Offered:
Listed in the following order: Program area, degree type (T if terminal Master's), number awarded 7/08–6/09. Mental Health and Substance Abuse Counseling MA/MS (Master of Arts/Science) (T) 20, Clinical Psychology PhD (Doctor of Philosophy) 13, Cognitive, Social, Developmental Psychology PhD (Doctor of Philosophy) 5, General Psychology MA/MS (Master of Arts/Science) (T) 54.

APA Accreditation: Clinical PhD (Doctor of Philosophy). Student Outcome Data Website: http://www.newschool.edu/nssr/subpage.aspx?id=9888.

Student Applications/Admissions:
Student Applications

Mental Health and Substance Abuse Counseling MA/MS (Master of Arts/Science)—Applications 2009–2010, 46. Total applicants accepted 2009–2010, 31. Number full-time enrolled (new admits only) 2009–2010, 10. Number part-time enrolled (new admits only) 2009–2010, 1. Total enrolled 2009–2010 full-time, 13, part-time, 7. Openings 2010–2011, 14. The median number of years required for completion of a degree in 2008–2009 were 2. The number of students enrolled full- and part-time who were dismissed or voluntarily withdrew from this program area in 2008–2009 were 0. *Clinical Psychology PhD (Doctor of Philosophy)*—Applications 2009–2010, 32. Total applicants accepted 2009–2010, 16. Number full-time enrolled (new admits only) 2009–2010, 16. Number part-time enrolled (new admits only) 2009–2010, 0. Openings 2010–2011, 16. The median number of years required for completion of a degree in 2008–2009 were 5. The number of students enrolled full- and part-time who were dismissed or voluntarily withdrew from this program area in 2008–2009 were 0. *Cognitive, Social,*

Developmental Psychology PhD (Doctor of Philosophy)—Applications 2009–2010, 10. Total applicants accepted 2009–2010, 8. Number full-time enrolled (new admits only) 2009–2010, 8. Number part-time enrolled (new admits only) 2009–2010, 0. Openings 2010–2011, 10. The median number of years required for completion of a degree in 2008–2009 were 5. The number of students enrolled full- and part-time who were dismissed or voluntarily withdrew from this program area in 2008–2009 were 0. *General Psychology MA/MS (Master of Arts/Science)*—Applications 2009–2010, 266. Total applicants accepted 2009–2010, 210. Number full-time enrolled (new admits only) 2009–2010, 58. Number part-time enrolled (new admits only) 2009–2010, 22. Total enrolled 2009–2010 full-time, 67, part-time, 111. Openings 2010–2011, 73. The median number of years required for completion of a degree in 2008–2009 were 2. The number of students enrolled full- and part-time who were dismissed or voluntarily withdrew from this program area in 2008–2009 were 11.

Other Criteria: (importance of criteria rated low, medium, or high): GRE scores—medium, research experience—medium, work experience—high, extracurricular activity—medium, clinically related public service—medium, GPA—high, letters of recommendation—high, statement of goals and objectives—high, writing sample—high, undergraduate major in psychology—medium, specific undergraduate psychology courses taken—medium. Only Master's students at The New School for Social Research are eligible to apply to our PhD Programs. Outside applicants with previous graduate credit must apply first to the MA program at The New School for Social Research, then once they complete 12 credits of course work here, they may transfer credits from a previous degree. For additional information on admission requirements, go to http://www.newschool.edu/nssr/subpage.aspx?id=9884.

Student Characteristics: The following represents characteristics of students in 2009–2010 in all graduate psychology programs in the department: Female—full-time 137, part-time 98; Male—full-time 43, part-time 20; African American/Black—full-time 6, part-time 7; Hispanic/Latino(a)—full-time 15, part-time 7; Asian/Pacific Islander—full-time 7, part-time 10; American Indian/Alaska Native—full-time 1, part-time 1; Caucasian/White—full-time 104, part-time 73; Multi-ethnic—full-time 15, part-time 6; students subject to the Americans With Disabilities Act—full-time 8, part-time 7; Unknown ethnicity—full-time 32, part-time 14; International students who hold an F-1 or J-1 Visa—full-time 34, part-time 8.

Financial Information/Assistance:
Tuition for Full-Time Study: *Master's:* State residents: $1,645 per credit hour; Nonstate residents: $1,645 per credit hour. *Doctoral:* State residents: $1,645 per credit hour; Nonstate residents: $1,645 per credit hour. Tuition is subject to change. See the following Web site for updates and changes in tuition costs: http://www.newschool.edu/tuition/index.html.

Financial Assistance:
First-Year Students: Fellowships and scholarships available for first year. Average amount paid per academic year: $7,800. Apply by December 15.

Advanced Students: Teaching assistantships available for advanced students. Average amount paid per academic year: $7,500. Average number of hours worked per week: 10. Apply by March 1. Research assistantships available for advanced students. Average amount paid per academic year: $6,000. Average number of hours worked per week: 15. Apply by March 1. Fellowships and scholarships available for advanced students. Average amount paid per academic year: $9,660. Apply by March 1.

Additional Information: Of all students currently enrolled full time, 56% benefited from one or more of the listed financial assistance programs. Application and information available online at: http://www.newschool.edu/nssr/subpage.aspx?id=14556.

Internships/Practica: Doctoral Degree (PhD Clinical Psychology): For those doctoral students for whom a professional internship was required in this program prior to graduation, (14) students applied for an internship in 2008–2009, with (13) students obtaining an internship. Of those students who obtained an internship, (13) were paid internships. Of those students who obtained an internship, (13) students placed in APA/CPA accredited internships, (0) students placed in internships not APA/CPA accredited, but listed with the Association of Psychology Postdoctoral and Internship Programs (APPIC), (0) students placed in internships conforming to guidelines of the Council of Directors of School Psychology Programs (CDSPP), (0) students placed in internships that were not APA/CPA accredited, APPIC or CDSPP listed. Depending on their research areas, students pursuing general psychology can gain internship and work experience in a range of applied settings, including industry research labs and non-profit organizations. Master's level psychology students who are interested in applying to the Clinical PhD program are strongly encouraged to pursue volunteer clinical positions available at local hospitals or institutes. First-year doctoral students in the clinical program participate in an integrated program designed to help them develop as scientist–practitioners. The practicum is based at Beth Israel Medical Center and involves supervised psychotherapy and Structured Clinical Interview for DSM-V-TR (SCID) training within the Brief Psychotherapy Research Program established at Beth Israel. Students also spend 4 hours per week on an inpatient rotation, co-leading groups and attending relevant unit meetings. Clinical supervision is provided by The New School faculty and by Beth Israel staff psychologists and psychiatrists. This experience provides strong preparation for the 16-20 hour per week externships in their second and third years of PhD level study at approved, affiliated sites. After completing their dissertation proposals, all Clinical PhD students are required to complete an APA-accredited predoctoral internship. During the internship application process, students receive administrative and academic support services from the Director of Clinical Training, Assistant Director of Clinical Training and the Director of Clinical Student Affairs.

Housing and Day Care: On-campus housing is available. See the following Web site for more information: http://www.newschool.edu/studentservices/housing/. No on-campus day care facilities are available.

Employment of Department Graduates:
Master's Degree Graduates: Of those who graduated in the academic year 2008–2009, the following categories and numbers represent the postgraduate activities and employment of master's degree graduates: Enrolled in a postdoctoral residency/fellowship (n/a), employed in independent practice (n/a), total from the above (master's) (0).

Doctoral Degree Graduates: Of those who graduated in the academic year 2008–2009, the following categories and numbers represent the postgraduate activities and employment of doctoral degree graduates: Enrolled in a psychology doctoral program (n/a), enrolled in a postdoctoral residency/fellowship (1), employed in independent practice (3), employed in business or industry (1), employed in a community mental health/counseling center (2), employed in a hospital/medical center (4), not seeking employment (1), do not know (1), total from the above (doctoral) (13).

Additional Information:
Orientation, Objectives, and Emphasis of Department: The Psychology Department provides a broad theoretical background emphasizing the scientific study of human behavior. The master's program accommodates both full- and part-time students, with courses in cognitive, developmental, social, and clinical psychology. All MA students design and carry out original individual research projects. At the PhD level, students may specialize either in research psychology or in clinical psychology. The doctoral program reflects an apprenticeship model in which students work closely with individual faculty on collaborative research. Admission to doctoral candidacy is based on students' academic performance in our master's program, interviews with faculty, a personal essay, and passing the psychology comprehensive examination. There is a strong emphasis on cultural psychology as a framework for understanding basic psychological theories, and on approaching psychology in ways that are sensitive to socio-cultural diversity. Students enrolled in the Ph.D program in Cognitive, Social, and Developmental Psychology (CSD) are prepared for careers in academics as well as in applied settings. Within the clinical psychology doctoral program, there is a strong emphasis on both theory and research. Clinical students have opportunities to gain clinical experience and are prepared as scientist–practitioners equally at home in clinical, research, and teaching settings.

Special Facilities or Resources: All students may participate in collaborative research projects with faculty in labs that feature equipment and software dedicated to the particular research carried out by department members. Students have library access not only at New School social science libraries but also at NYU's Bobst library, the Cooper Union Library, and other libraries within a New York consortium. Various state-of-the-art computing facilities are also available. For clinical PhD students, the New School-Beth Israel Center for Clinical Training and Research provides unusually broad training in outpatient clinics, inpatient units, and clinical research programs. First year clinical PhD students have access to the Psychology library at Beth Israel Medical Center, perform intake evaluations on Beth Israel's psychiatry outpatient clinic and provide group therapy on adult inpatient units. They also attend psychiatry grand rounds and training seminars on child abuse and assault prevention. Second and third-year clinical students may continue work at Beth Israel Medical Center conducting therapy through the Brief Psychotherapy Research Project. Psychotherapy sessions are videotaped with patients' consent, and students review these sessions in supervision with Beth Israel supervising psychologists. Cases are also discussed in externship seminars with New School faculty.

Information for Students With Physical Disabilities: See the following Web site for more information: http://www.newschool.edu/studentservices/disability/.

Application Information:
Send to Office of Admission, New School for Social Research, 72 Fifth Avenue, 3rd Fl., New York, NY 10011. Application available online. URL of online application: http://www.newschool.edu/nssr/admission/. Students are admitted in the Fall, application deadline August 1; Spring, application deadline December 1. Applications for fall admission completed by January 15 may be considered for full-funding fellowships. *Fee:* $50.

University at Albany, State University of New York
Department of Psychology
College of Arts and Sciences
1400 Washington Avenue
Albany, NY 12222
Telephone: (518) 442-4820
Fax: (518) 442-4867
E-mail: *cm949@albany.edu*
Web: *http://www.albany.edu/psy/*

Department Information:
1950. Chairperson: Kevin J. Williams. Number of faculty: total—full-time 31; women—full-time 13; total—minority—full-time 5; women minority—full-time 4.

Programs and Degrees Offered:
Listed in the following order: Program area, degree type (T if terminal Master's), number awarded 7/08–6/09. Biopsychology PhD (Doctor of Philosophy) 2, Clinical PhD (Doctor of Philosophy) 4, Cognitive PhD (Doctor of Philosophy) 0, Industrial/Organizational PhD (Doctor of Philosophy) 2, Social/Personality PhD (Doctor of Philosophy) 0, Industrial/Organizational MA/MS (Master of Arts/Science) (T) 2.

APA Accreditation: Clinical PhD (Doctor of Philosophy). Student Outcome Data Website: http://www.albany.edu/psy/gradclinical_Education_Training_Outcomes_Information.html.

Student Applications/Admissions:
Student Applications
Biopsychology PhD (Doctor of Philosophy)—Applications 2009–2010, 13. Total applicants accepted 2009–2010, 4. Number full-time enrolled (new admits only) 2009–2010, 3. Number part-time enrolled (new admits only) 2009–2010, 0. Openings 2010–2011, 3. The median number of years required for completion of a degree in 2008–2009 were 8. The number of students enrolled full- and part-time who were dismissed or voluntarily withdrew from this program area in 2008–2009 were 0. Clinical PhD (Doctor of Philosophy)—Applications 2009–2010, 137. Total applicants accepted 2009–2010, 13. Number full-time enrolled (new admits only) 2009–2010, 7. Number part-time enrolled (new admits only) 2009–2010, 0. Openings 2010–2011, 6. The median number of years required for completion of a degree in 2008–2009 were 6. The number of students enrolled full- and part-time who were dismissed or voluntarily withdrew from this program area in 2008–2009 were 0. Cognitive PhD (Doctor of Philosophy)—Applications 2009–2010, 14. Total applicants accepted 2009–2010, 6. Number full-time enrolled (new admits only) 2009–2010, 2. Number part-time enrolled (new admits only) 2009–2010, 0. Open-

ings 2010–2011, 3. The number of students enrolled full- and part-time who were dismissed or voluntarily withdrew from this program area in 2008–2009 were 0. *Industrial/Organizational PhD (Doctor of Philosophy)*—Applications 2009–2010, 29. Total applicants accepted 2009–2010, 7. Number full-time enrolled (new admits only) 2009–2010, 1. Number part-time enrolled (new admits only) 2009–2010, 0. Openings 2010–2011, 3. The median number of years required for completion of a degree in 2008–2009 were 5. The number of students enrolled full- and part-time who were dismissed or voluntarily withdrew from this program area in 2008–2009 were 0. *Social/Personality PhD (Doctor of Philosophy)*—Applications 2009–2010, 26. Total applicants accepted 2009–2010, 6. Number full-time enrolled (new admits only) 2009–2010, 3. Number part-time enrolled (new admits only) 2009–2010, 0. Openings 2010–2011, 3. The number of students enrolled full- and part-time who were dismissed or voluntarily withdrew from this program area in 2008–2009 were 0. *Industrial/Organizational MA/MS (Master of Arts/Science)*—Applications 2009–2010, 26. Total applicants accepted 2009–2010, 7. Number full-time enrolled (new admits only) 2009–2010, 4. Number part-time enrolled (new admits only) 2009–2010, 0. Total enrolled 2009–2010 full-time, 7, part-time, 1. Openings 2010–2011, 3. The median number of years required for completion of a degree in 2008–2009 were 2. The number of students enrolled full- and part-time who were dismissed or voluntarily withdrew from this program area in 2008–2009 were 0.

Scores: Entries appear in this order: required test or GPA, minimum score (if required), median score of students entering in 2009–2010. *Clinical PhD (Doctor of Philosophy)*: GRE-V no minimum stated, 645, GRE-Q no minimum stated, 677, GRE-Subject (Psychology) no minimum stated, 679, overall undergraduate GPA no minimum stated, 3.48, psychology GPA no minimum stated, 3.69; *Cognitive PhD (Doctor of Philosophy)*: GRE-V no minimum stated, 600, GRE-Q no minimum stated, 646, overall undergraduate GPA no minimum stated, 3.5; *Industrial/Organizational PhD (Doctor of Philosophy)*: GRE-V no minimum stated, 570, GRE-Q no minimum stated, 674, overall undergraduate GPA no minimum stated, 3.56; *Social/Personality PhD (Doctor of Philosophy)*: GRE-V no minimum stated, 660, GRE-Q no minimum stated, 715, overall undergraduate GPA no minimum stated, 3.6.

Other Criteria: (importance of criteria rated low, medium, or high): GRE scores—high, research experience—high, work experience—low, extracurricular activity—low, clinically related public service—medium, GPA—high, letters of recommendation—high, interview—high, statement of goals and objectives—high, undergraduate major in psychology—medium, specific undergraduate psychology courses taken—medium. The interview process and clinically related service are relevant for the clinical psychology program only. For additional information on admission requirements, go to http://www.albany.edu/psy.

Student Characteristics: The following represents characteristics of students in 2009–2010 in all graduate psychology programs in the department: Female—full-time 73, part-time 1; Male—full-time 32, part-time 0; African American/Black—full-time 5, part-time 0; Hispanic/Latino(a)—full-time 6, part-time 0; Asian/Pacific Islander—full-time 8, part-time 0; American Indian/Alaska Native—full-time 1, part-time 0; Caucasian/White—full-time 80, part-time 1; Multi-ethnic—full-time 3, part-time 0; students subject to the Americans With Disabilities Act—full-time 0, part-time 0; Unknown ethnicity—full-time 2, part-time 0; International students who hold an F-1 or J-1 Visa—full-time 9, part-time 0.

Financial Information/Assistance:
Tuition for Full-Time Study: *Master's:* State residents: per academic year $8,370, $349 per credit hour; Nonstate residents: per academic year $13,250, $552 per credit hour. *Doctoral:* State residents: per academic year $8,370, $349 per credit hour; Nonstate residents: per academic year $13,250, $552 per credit hour. Tuition is subject to change. Additional fees are assessed to students beyond the costs of tuition for the following: university fee, comprehensive service fee, grad student organization fee. See the following Web site for updates and changes in tuition costs: http://www.albany.edu/studentaccounts/costs.shtml.

Financial Assistance:
First-Year Students: Teaching assistantships available for first year. Average amount paid per academic year: $14,000. Average number of hours worked per week: 20. Research assistantships available for first year. Average amount paid per academic year: $14,000. Average number of hours worked per week: 20.

Advanced Students: Teaching assistantships available for advanced students. Average amount paid per academic year: $14,000. Average number of hours worked per week: 20. Research assistantships available for advanced students. Average amount paid per academic year: $14,000. Average number of hours worked per week: 20.

Additional Information: Of all students currently enrolled full time, 48% benefited from one or more of the listed financial assistance programs. Application and information available online at: http://www.albany.edu/grad.

Internships/Practica: Doctoral Degree (PhD Clinical): For those doctoral students for whom a professional internship was required in this program prior to graduation, (9) students applied for an internship in 2008–2009, with (7) students obtaining an internship. Of those students who obtained an internship, (7) were paid internships. Of those students who obtained an internship, (7) students placed in APA/CPA accredited internships, (0) students placed in internships not APA/CPA accredited, but listed with the Association of Psychology Postdoctoral and Internship Programs (APPIC), (0) students placed in internships conforming to guidelines of the Council of Directors of School Psychology Programs (CDSPP), (0) students placed in internships that were not APA/CPA accredited, APPIC or CDSPP listed. Master's Degree (MA/MS Industrial/Organizational): An internship experience, such as, a final research project or "capstone" experience is required of graduates. During the second year of our doctoral program in Clinical Psychology, students are placed at the Psychological Services Center, a University operated center that serves the general population of the city of Albany. During this placement students are supervised by members of the Clinical faculty. In their third year, students are required to participate in a community-based practicum. These practica include community mental health centers, VA inpatient and outpatient centers, inpatient and outpatient clinics in community hospitals and rehabilitation centers, residential facilities for youth, and the University's counseling center. Students may also elect to participate in an additional community-based practicum experience during their 4th year of training. Students are encouraged to attend APA accredited internships during their 5th year of study. Our students have attended internships in a variety of settings including children's hospitals, psychiatric hospitals, VA hospitals, university affiliated medical centers, general hospitals, and rehabilitation centers. Practicum and internship placements for doctoral students in the Industrial/Organizational Psychology specialization are possible with a number of local and national corporations and government agencies.

Housing and Day Care: On-campus housing is available. See the following Web site for more information: http://www.albany.edu/housing. On-campus day care facilities are available. U-Kids Child Care Center, (518) 442-2660.

Employment of Department Graduates:
Master's Degree Graduates: Of those who graduated in the academic year 2008–2009, the following categories and numbers represent the postgraduate activities and employment of master's degree graduates: Enrolled in a postdoctoral residency/fellowship (n/a), employed in independent practice (n/a), total from the above (master's) (0).
Doctoral Degree Graduates: Of those who graduated in the academic year 2008–2009, the following categories and numbers represent the postgraduate activities and employment of doctoral degree graduates: Enrolled in a psychology doctoral program (n/a), enrolled in another graduate/professional program (0), enrolled in a postdoctoral residency/fellowship (2), employed in independent practice (1), employed in an academic position at a 2-year/4-year college (1), employed in other positions at a higher education institution (1), employed in a professional position in a school system (0), employed in business or industry (1), employed in a community mental health/counseling center (0), employed in a hospital/medical center (1), still seeking employment (0), not seeking employment (0), do not know (1), total from the above (doctoral) (8).

Additional Information:
Orientation, Objectives, and Emphasis of Department: All facets of the graduate program reflect a commitment to the empirical tradition in psychology. Thus, involvement in research is stressed in all areas of study. Students begin an apprentice relationship with faculty members upon entry into the department and are expected to remain actively involved in research throughout their graduate careers. A major goal of the department is to train individuals who will make research contributions to the field. All areas of concentration train students for careers as teachers and research scientists. In addition, the social, clinical, and industrial/organizational areas prepare students for careers in applied settings. The orientation of the clinical program emphasizes cognitive and behavioral approaches. Admission is offered in five areas: biopsychology, clinical, cognitive, industrial/organizational, and social-personality.

Special Facilities or Resources: Resources and facilities include university- and grant-funded student stipends, plus stipends from other campus sources; a state-of-the-art animal facility and research laboratories in the Life Sciences Building; several human research laboratories; grant-supported research and treatment clinics; the Psychological Services Center for practicum training; and a variety of research equipment.

Information for Students With Physical Disabilities: See the following Web site for more information: www.albany.edu/studentlife.

Application Information:
Send to The Office of Graduate Admissions, University Administration Building 121, 1400 Washington Avenue, Albany, NY 12222. Application available online. URL of online application: http://www.albany.edu/graduate/. Students are admitted in the Fall, application deadline see below. PhD programs - December 1 for clinical psychology; January 15 for all other PhD programs. I/O MA program - March 1. *Fee:* $75. University guidelines permit waiver of this required fee only for those applicants who can evidence prior or current participation in a qualifying educational opportunity program. Typically, that would include but not be limited to Project 1000, EOP, HEOP or similar specially targeted higher education opportunity programs.

University at Buffalo, State University of New York
Department of Counseling, School, and Educational Psychology
Graduate School of Education
409 Baldy Hall
Buffalo, NY 14260-1000
Telephone: (716) 645-2484
Fax: (716) 645-6616
E-mail: *nmyers@buffalo.edu*
Web: *http://gse.buffalo.edu/cspp*

Department Information:
1949. Chairperson: Timothy P. Janikowski. Number of faculty: total—full-time 17, part-time 2; women—full-time 8, part-time 2; total—minority—full-time 3; women minority—full-time 2.

Programs and Degrees Offered:
Listed in the following order: Program area, degree type (T if terminal Master's), number awarded 7/08–6/09. Counselor Education PhD (Doctor of Philosophy) 3, Educational Psychology PhD (Doctor of Philosophy) 1, Rehabilitation Counseling MA/MS (Master of Arts/Science) (T) 7, School Counseling MEd (Education) 27, Educational Psychology MA/MS (Master of Arts/Science) (T) 5, Counseling/School Psychology PhD (Doctor of Philosophy) 8, Mental Health Counseling MA/MS (Master of Arts/Science) (T) 10, School Psychology MA/MS (Master of Arts/Science) (T) 10.

APA Accreditation: Combination PhD (Doctor of Philosophy).

Student Applications/Admissions:
Student Applications
Counselor Education PhD (Doctor of Philosophy)—Applications 2009–2010, 17. Total applicants accepted 2009–2010, 10. Number full-time enrolled (new admits only) 2009–2010, 0. Number part-time enrolled (new admits only) 2009–2010, 10. Total enrolled 2009–2010 full-time, 4, part-time, 22. Openings 2010–2011, 5. The median number of years required for completion of a degree in 2008–2009 were 6. The number of students enrolled full- and part-time who were dismissed or voluntarily withdrew from this program area in 2008–2009 were 2. *Educational Psychology PhD (Doctor of Philosophy)*—

Applications 2009–2010, 6. Total applicants accepted 2009–2010, 2. Number full-time enrolled (new admits only) 2009–2010, 1. Number part-time enrolled (new admits only) 2009–2010, 0. Total enrolled 2009–2010 full-time, 6, part-time, 5. Openings 2010–2011, 3. The median number of years required for completion of a degree in 2008–2009 were 5. The number of students enrolled full- and part-time who were dismissed or voluntarily withdrew from this program area in 2008–2009 were 0. *Rehabilitation Counseling MA/MS (Master of Arts/Science)*—Applications 2009–2010, 75. Total applicants accepted 2009–2010, 30. Number full-time enrolled (new admits only) 2009–2010, 13. Number part-time enrolled (new admits only) 2009–2010, 17. Total enrolled 2009–2010 full-time, 30, part-time, 22. Openings 2010–2011, 20. The median number of years required for completion of a degree in 2008–2009 were 2. The number of students enrolled full- and part-time who were dismissed or voluntarily withdrew from this program area in 2008–2009 were 0. *School Counseling MEd (Education)*—Applications 2009–2010, 66. Total applicants accepted 2009–2010, 34. Number full-time enrolled (new admits only) 2009–2010, 25. Number part-time enrolled (new admits only) 2009–2010, 4. Total enrolled 2009–2010 full-time, 28, part-time, 7. Openings 2010–2011, 25. The median number of years required for completion of a degree in 2008–2009 was 1. The number of students enrolled full- and part-time who were dismissed or voluntarily withdrew from this program area in 2008–2009 were 1. *Educational Psychology MA/MS (Master of Arts/Science)*—Applications 2009–2010, 22. Total applicants accepted 2009–2010, 4. Number full-time enrolled (new admits only) 2009–2010, 0. Number part-time enrolled (new admits only) 2009–2010, 0. Total enrolled 2009–2010 full-time, 4, part-time, 4. Openings 2010–2011, 4. The median number of years required for completion of a degree in 2008–2009 were 2. The number of students enrolled full- and part-time who were dismissed or voluntarily withdrew from this program area in 2008–2009 were 0. *Counseling/School Psychology PhD (Doctor of Philosophy)*—Applications 2009–2010, 105. Total applicants accepted 2009–2010, 10. Number full-time enrolled (new admits only) 2009–2010, 10. Number part-time enrolled (new admits only) 2009–2010, 0. Openings 2010–2011, 11. The median number of years required for completion of a degree in 2008–2009 were 5. The number of students enrolled full- and part-time who were dismissed or voluntarily withdrew from this program area in 2008–2009 were 0. *Mental Health Counseling MA/MS (Master of Arts/Science)*—Applications 2009–2010, 61. Total applicants accepted 2009–2010, 14. Number full-time enrolled (new admits only) 2009–2010, 12. Number part-time enrolled (new admits only) 2009–2010, 0. Total enrolled 2009–2010 full-time, 16, part-time, 2. Openings 2010–2011, 12. The median number of years required for completion of a degree in 2008–2009 were 2. The number of students enrolled full- and part-time who were dismissed or voluntarily withdrew from this program area in 2008–2009 were 1. *School Psychology MA/MS (Master of Arts/Science)*—Applications 2009–2010, 75. Total applicants accepted 2009–2010, 14. Number full-time enrolled (new admits only) 2009–2010, 10. Number part-time enrolled (new admits only) 2009–2010, 0. Openings 2010–2011, 10. The median number of years required for completion of a degree in 2008–2009 were 3. The number of students enrolled full- and part-time who were dismissed or voluntarily withdrew from this program area in 2008–2009 were 0.

Scores: Entries appear in this order: required test or GPA, minimum score (if required), median score of students entering in 2009–2010. *Counselor Education PhD (Doctor of Philosophy)*: GRE-V 400, 500, GRE-Q 400, 500, GRE-Analytical 4.0, 4.5, overall undergraduate GPA 3.0, 3.2, Masters GPA 3.0, 3.75; *Educational Psychology PhD (Doctor of Philosophy)*: GRE-V no minimum stated, GRE-Q no minimum stated, GRE-Analytical no minimum stated, overall undergraduate GPA no minimum stated, Masters GPA 3.0; *Rehabilitation Counseling MA/MS (Master of Arts/Science)*: overall undergraduate GPA 3.0, 3.15; *School Counseling MEd (Education)*: GRE-V no minimum stated, GRE-Q no minimum stated, GRE-Analytical no minimum stated, overall undergraduate GPA 3.0; *Educational Psychology MA/MS (Master of Arts/Science)*: GRE-V no minimum stated, GRE-Q no minimum stated, GRE-Analytical no minimum stated, overall undergraduate GPA no minimum stated; *Counseling/School Psychology PhD (Doctor of Philosophy)*: GRE-V no minimum stated, 530, GRE-Q no minimum stated, 630, GRE-Analytical no minimum stated, 5.0, overall undergraduate GPA 3.0, 3.58; *Mental Health Counseling MA/MS (Master of Arts/Science)*: GRE-V no minimum stated, 473, GRE-Q no minimum stated, 506, GRE-Analytical no minimum stated, 3.5, overall undergraduate GPA 3.0, 3.35; *School Psychology MA/MS (Master of Arts/Science)*: GRE-V 400, 514, GRE-Q 400, 621, GRE-Analytical 3.0, 4.75, overall undergraduate GPA 3.0, 3.59.

Other Criteria: (importance of criteria rated low, medium, or high): GRE scores—high, research experience—medium, work experience—low, extracurricular activity—low, clinically related public service—medium, GPA—high, letters of recommendation—medium, interview—high, statement of goals and objectives—high, undergraduate major in psychology—low, specific undergraduate psychology courses taken—low. Not all programs conduct personal interviews.

Student Characteristics: The following represents characteristics of students in 2009–2010 in all graduate psychology programs in the department: Female—full-time 138, part-time 47; Male—full-time 33, part-time 15; African American/Black—full-time 22, part-time 11; Hispanic/Latino(a)—full-time 7, part-time 1; Asian/Pacific Islander—full-time 14, part-time 0; American Indian/Alaska Native—full-time 0, part-time 2; Caucasian/White—full-time 135, part-time 57; Multi-ethnic—full-time 0, part-time 0; students subject to the Americans With Disabilities Act—full-time 0, part-time 0; Unknown ethnicity—full-time 0, part-time 0; International students who hold an F-1 or J-1 Visa—full-time 0, part-time 0.

Financial Information/Assistance:

Tuition for Full-Time Study: *Master's:* State residents: per academic year $8,370, $349 per credit hour; Nonstate residents: per academic year $13,250, $552 per credit hour. *Doctoral:* State residents: per academic year $8,370, $349 per credit hour; Nonstate residents: per academic year $13,250, $552 per credit hour. Tuition is subject to change. See the following Web site for updates and changes in tuition costs: http://src.buffalo.edu/studentaccount/tuition.shtml.

Financial Assistance:

First-Year Students: Research assistantships available for first year. Average amount paid per academic year: $9,000. Average number of hours worked per week: 20. Apply by April 15.

Advanced Students: Research assistantships available for advanced students. Average amount paid per academic year: $9,000. Average number of hours worked per week: 20. Apply by April 15.

Additional Information: Of all students currently enrolled full time, 10% benefited from one or more of the listed financial assistance programs. Application and information available online at: http://www.gse.buffalo.edu/admissions/scholarships.

Internships/Practica: Doctoral Degree (PhD Counseling/School Psychology): For those doctoral students for whom a professional internship was required in this program prior to graduation, (8) students applied for an internship in 2008–2009, with (8) students obtaining an internship. Of those students who obtained an internship, (8) were paid internships. Of those students who obtained an internship, (5) students placed in APA/CPA accredited internships, (0) students placed in internships not APA/CPA accredited, but listed with the Association of Psychology Postdoctoral and Internship Programs (APPIC), (2) students placed in internships conforming to guidelines of the Council of Directors of School Psychology Programs (CDSPP), (1) students placed in internships that were not APA/CPA accredited, APPIC or CDSPP listed. Master's Degree (MA/MS Rehabilitation Counseling): An internship experience, such as a final research project or "capstone" experience is required of graduates. Master's Degree (MA/MS Educational Psychology): An internship experience, such as a final research project or "capstone" experience is required of graduates. Master's Degree (MA/MS Mental Health Counseling): An internship experience, such as a final research project or "capstone" experience is required of graduates. Master's Degree (MA/MS School Psychology): An internship experience, such as a final research project or "capstone" experience is required of graduates. Practica and internships are available at area schools, community agencies, and hospitals. Experience with death and end of life issues, forensics, persons with disabilities, and assessment is available.

Housing and Day Care: On-campus housing is available. See the following Web site for more information: http://www.ub-housing.buffalo.edu/. On-campus day care facilities are available. See the following Web site for more information: http://www.ubccc.buffalo.edu/; http://ecrc.buffalo.edu/.

Employment of Department Graduates:

Master's Degree Graduates: Of those who graduated in the academic year 2008–2009, the following categories and numbers represent the postgraduate activities and employment of master's degree graduates: Enrolled in a psychology doctoral program (0), enrolled in another graduate/professional program (0), enrolled in a postdoctoral residency/fellowship (n/a), employed in independent practice (n/a), employed in an academic position at a university (0), employed in an academic position at a 2-year/4-year college (0), employed in other positions at a higher education institution (0), employed in a professional position in a school system (0), employed in business or industry (0), employed in government agency (0), employed in a community mental health/counseling center (0), employed in a hospital/medical center (0), still seeking employment (0), not seeking employment (0), other employment position (0), do not know (0), total from the above (master's) (0).

Doctoral Degree Graduates: Of those who graduated in the academic year 2008–2009, the following categories and numbers represent the postgraduate activities and employment of doctoral degree graduates: Enrolled in a psychology doctoral program (n/a), enrolled in another graduate/professional program (0), enrolled in a postdoctoral residency/fellowship (0), employed in independent practice (0), employed in an academic position at a university (1), employed in an academic position at a 2-year/4-year college (0), employed in other positions at a higher education institution (2), employed in a professional position in a school system (2), employed in business or industry (0), employed in government agency (1), employed in a community mental health/counseling center (0), employed in a hospital/medical center (2), still seeking employment (0), not seeking employment (0), other employment position (0), do not know (0), total from the above (doctoral) (8).

Additional Information:

Orientation, Objectives, and Emphasis of Department: Departmental emphasis is on research based counseling with adults, college students, adolescents, children, and persons with disabilities. Doctoral programs follow the scientist–practitioner model. Some focus on preparing college faculty. Increased integration of counseling, school, and educational psychology programs is developing. Field experience and research experience are continuous throughout the programs.

Special Facilities or Resources: Department offers training experiences in a wide variety of schools, agencies, and college in both urban and suburban settings.

Application Information:
Send to Office of Graduate Admissions, Graduate School of Education, 366 Baldy Hall University at Buffalo, The State University of New York, Buffalo, NY 14260-1000. Application available online. URL of online application: http://www.gse.buffalo.edu/admissions/apply. Students are admitted in the Fall, application deadline Counseling/School Psychology: February 1. Counselor Education and Rehabilitation Counseling: March 1 application deadline for fall admission. Mental Health Counseling: March 15 application deadline for fall admission. Educational Psychology has rolling admissions and applications are considered for both fall and spring admission. *Fee:* $50.

University at Buffalo, State University of New York
Department of Psychology
College of Arts and Sciences
206 Park Hall
Buffalo, NY 14260-4110
Telephone: (716) 645-3651
Fax: (716) 645-3801
E-mail: *ccolder@buffalo.edu*
Web: *http://www.psychology.buffalo.edu*

Department Information:
1921. Chairperson: Paul A. Luce. Number of faculty: total—full-time 27; women—full-time 8; total—minority—full-time 2; women minority—full-time 1.

Programs and Degrees Offered:
Listed in the following order: Program area, degree type (T if terminal Master's), number awarded 7/08–6/09. Clinical PhD (Doctor of Philosophy) 3, Cognitive PhD (Doctor of Philosophy)

GRADUATE STUDY IN PSYCHOLOGY

2, Social-Personality PhD (Doctor of Philosophy) 3, Behavioral Neuroscience PhD (Doctor of Philosophy) 0, General MA/MS (Master of Arts/Science) (T) 6.

APA Accreditation: Clinical PhD (Doctor of Philosophy). Student Outcome Data Website: http://www.psychology.buffalo.edu/graduate/phd/clinical/more/admissions/.

Student Applications/Admissions:
Student Applications

Clinical PhD (Doctor of Philosophy)—Applications 2009–2010, 172. Total applicants accepted 2009–2010, 9. Number full-time enrolled (new admits only) 2009–2010, 4. Number part-time enrolled (new admits only) 2009–2010, 0. Total enrolled 2009–2010 full-time, 45, part-time, 1. Openings 2010–2011, 6. The median number of years required for completion of a degree in 2008–2009 were 7. The number of students enrolled full- and part-time who were dismissed or voluntarily withdrew from this program area in 2008–2009 were 0. *Cognitive PhD (Doctor of Philosophy)*—Applications 2009–2010, 27. Total applicants accepted 2009–2010, 9. Number full-time enrolled (new admits only) 2009–2010, 3. Total enrolled 2009–2010 full-time, 19. Openings 2010–2011, 3. The median number of years required for completion of a degree in 2008–2009 were 5. The number of students enrolled full- and part-time who were dismissed or voluntarily withdrew from this program area in 2008–2009 were 0. *Social-Personality PhD (Doctor of Philosophy)*—Applications 2009–2010, 45. Total applicants accepted 2009–2010, 3. Number full-time enrolled (new admits only) 2009–2010, 3. Total enrolled 2009–2010 full-time, 11. Openings 2010–2011, 3. The median number of years required for completion of a degree in 2008–2009 were 5. The number of students enrolled full- and part-time who were dismissed or voluntarily withdrew from this program area in 2008–2009 were 0. *Behavioral Neuroscience PhD (Doctor of Philosophy)*—Applications 2009–2010, 27. Total applicants accepted 2009–2010, 3. Number full-time enrolled (new admits only) 2009–2010, 3. Total enrolled 2009–2010 full-time, 13. Openings 2010–2011, 3. The median number of years required for completion of a degree in 2008–2009 were 7. The number of students enrolled full- and part-time who were dismissed or voluntarily withdrew from this program area in 2008–2009 were 0. *General MA/MS (Master of Arts/Science)*—Applications 2009–2010, 70. Total applicants accepted 2009–2010, 11. Number full-time enrolled (new admits only) 2009–2010, 6. Total enrolled 2009–2010 full-time, 11, part-time, 2. Openings 2010–2011, 6. The median number of years required for completion of a degree in 2008–2009 were 2. The number of students enrolled full- and part-time who were dismissed or voluntarily withdrew from this program area in 2008–2009 were 0.

Scores: Entries appear in this order: required test or GPA, minimum score (if required), median score of students entering in 2009–2010. *Clinical PhD (Doctor of Philosophy)*: GRE-V no minimum stated, GRE-Q no minimum stated, GRE-Analytical no minimum stated, overall undergraduate GPA no minimum stated; *Cognitive PhD (Doctor of Philosophy)*: GRE-V no minimum stated, GRE-Q no minimum stated, GRE-Analytical no minimum stated, overall undergraduate GPA no minimum stated; *Social-Personality PhD (Doctor of Philosophy)*: GRE-V no minimum stated, GRE-Q no minimum stated, GRE-Analytical no minimum stated, overall undergraduate GPA no minimum stated; *Behavioral Neuroscience PhD (Doctor of Philosophy)*: GRE-V no minimum stated, GRE-Q no minimum stated, GRE-Analytical no minimum stated, overall undergraduate GPA no minimum stated; *General MA/MS (Master of Arts/Science)*: GRE-V no minimum stated, GRE-Q no minimum stated, GRE-Analytical no minimum stated, overall undergraduate GPA no minimum stated.

Other Criteria: (importance of criteria rated low, medium, or high): GRE scores—medium, research experience—high, work experience—low, extracurricular activity—low, clinically related public service—medium, GPA—high, letters of recommendation—high, interview—medium, statement of goals and objectives—high, undergraduate major in psychology—low, specific undergraduate psychology courses taken—low, Interview for clinical only. For additional information on admission requirements, go to http://www.psychology.buffalo.edu.

Student Characteristics: The following represents characteristics of students in 2009–2010 in all graduate psychology programs in the department: Female—full-time 69, part-time 1; Male—full-time 30, part-time 2; African American/Black—full-time 3, part-time 0; Hispanic/Latino(a)—full-time 8, part-time 0; Asian/Pacific Islander—full-time 8, part-time 0; American Indian/Alaska Native—full-time 2, part-time 0; Caucasian/White—full-time 77, part-time 3; Multi-ethnic—full-time 0, part-time 0; students subject to the Americans With Disabilities Act—full-time 0, part-time 0; Unknown ethnicity—full-time 1, part-time 0; International students who hold an F-1 or J-1 Visa—full-time 12, part-time 0.

Financial Information/Assistance:
Tuition for Full-Time Study: *Master's:* State residents: per academic year $9,882, $464 per credit hour; Nonstate residents: per academic year $14,762, $667 per credit hour. *Doctoral:* State residents: per academic year $9,882, $464 per credit hour; Nonstate residents: per academic year $14,762, $667 per credit hour. Tuition is subject to change. See the following Web site for updates and changes in tuition costs: http://src.buffalo.edu.

Financial Assistance:

First-Year Students: Teaching assistantships available for first year. Average amount paid per academic year: $13,500. Average number of hours worked per week: 20. Research assistantships available for first year. Average amount paid per academic year: $13,500. Average number of hours worked per week: 20. Fellowships and scholarships available for first year. Average amount paid per academic year: $6,000.

Advanced Students: Teaching assistantships available for advanced students. Average amount paid per academic year: $13,850. Average number of hours worked per week: 20. Research assistantships available for advanced students. Average amount paid per academic year: $13,850. Average number of hours worked per week: 20. Fellowships and scholarships available for advanced students. Average amount paid per academic year: $6,000.

Additional Information: Of all students currently enrolled full time, 69% benefited from one or more of the listed financial assistance programs. Application and information available online at: http://www.psychology.buffalo.edu.

Internships/Practica: Doctoral Degree (PhD Clinical): For those doctoral students for whom a professional internship was required in this program prior to graduation, (3) students applied for an internship in 2008–2009, with (3) students obtaining an internship. Of those students who obtained an internship, (3) were paid internships. Of those students who obtained an internship, (3) students placed in APA/CPA accredited internships, (0) students placed in internships not APA/CPA accredited, but listed with the Association of Psychology Postdoctoral and Internship Programs (APPIC), (0) students placed in internships conforming to guidelines of the Council of Directors of School Psychology Programs (CDSPP), (0) students placed in internships that were not APA/CPA accredited, APPIC or CDSPP listed. Several clinical practica are offered each year for students in the doctoral program in Clinical Psychology and for other doctoral students with permission of the instructor. In addition, there is a summer practicum focused on treatment of children with attention deficit/hyperactivity disorder.

Housing and Day Care: On-campus housing is available. See the following Web site for more information: http://www.grad.buffalo.edu/life/housing.php. On-campus day care facilities are available. See the following Web site for more information: http://www.ubccc.buffalo.edu/.

Employment of Department Graduates:
Master's Degree Graduates: Of those who graduated in the academic year 2008–2009, the following categories and numbers represent the postgraduate activities and employment of master's degree graduates: Enrolled in a postdoctoral residency/fellowship (n/a), employed in independent practice (n/a), total from the above (master's) (0).
Doctoral Degree Graduates: Of those who graduated in the academic year 2008–2009, the following categories and numbers represent the postgraduate activities and employment of doctoral degree graduates: Enrolled in a psychology doctoral program (n/a), enrolled in another graduate/professional program (0), enrolled in a postdoctoral residency/fellowship (4), employed in independent practice (1), employed in an academic position at a university (7), employed in an academic position at a 2-year/4-year college (0), employed in other positions at a higher education institution (0), employed in a professional position in a school system (0), employed in business or industry (0), employed in government agency (0), employed in a community mental health/counseling center (0), employed in a hospital/medical center (1), still seeking employment (0), not seeking employment (0), other employment position (0), do not know (1), total from the above (doctoral) (14).

Additional Information:
Orientation, Objectives, and Emphasis of Department: The Department of Psychology offers doctoral degrees in Behavioral Neuroscience, Clinical Psychology, Cognitive Psychology, and Social-Personality Psychology and a Master's degree in psychology with several specializations. The department has as its defining characteristic and distinguishing mission the conduct and communication of research and scholarship that contributes to the scientific understanding of psychology and the provision of high-quality graduate education and training. The department is dedicated to offering state-of-the-art education and training to its graduate students to prepare them to become leading researchers and to assume important positions in academic institutions or professional practice. We offer students a learning environment that is exciting and challenging, one that will allow them to follow their interests and fully develop their research skills. The research emphasis in the doctoral program in Behavioral Neuroscience is on the neural, endocrine, and molecular bases of behavior. Areas of specialization in Clinical Psychology include adult mood and anxiety disorders, relationship dysfunction, behavioral medicine, attention deficit/hyperactivity disorder, and child and adolescent aggression and substance abuse. The program in Cognitive Psychology focuses on the processes underlying perception, attention, memory, spoken and written language comprehension, language acquisition, categorization, problem solving, and thinking. Faculty research interests in the Social-Personality program include close relationships, social cognition, self-concept, and self-esteem.

Special Facilities or Resources: The Department of Psychology has specialized research facilities for the study of language comprehension, auditory and speech perception, memory, categorization, animal cognition, visual perception, attention, social interaction, small group processes, animal surgery research, behavior therapy, human psychophysiology and biofeedback, and neurochemical and electrophysiological investigations into the physiological bases of behavior. Many of these laboratories are computer-based. The department also has ample facilities for individual and group therapy, marriage counseling, and therapeutic work with children. One-way vision screens and videotape equipment are available for observation and supervision. Internships are available through the department's Psychological Services Center. Excellent facilities are available for working with animals. Students have liberal access to the University's computing services on the North Campus.

Information for Students With Physical Disabilities: See the following Web site for more information: http://www.student-affairs.buffalo.edu/ods/index.php.

Application Information:
Send to Director of Graduate Admissions, Department of Psychology, University at Buffalo—The State University of New York, Park Hall Room 210, Buffalo, NY 14260-4110. Application available online. URL of online application: http://www.psychology.buffalo.edu. Students are admitted in the Fall, application deadline December 1. MA application deadline for fall enrollment is April 1. *Fee:* $75. Fee is waived for McNair Scholar, Project 1000, EOP, HEOP or SEEK.

Yeshiva University
Ferkauf Graduate School of Psychology
Albert Einstein College of Medicine
1300 Morris Park Avenue
Bronx, NY 10461-1602
Telephone: (718) 430-3850
Fax: (718) 430-3960
E-mail: *gill@aecom.yu.edu*
Web: *http://www.yu.edu/ferkauf*

Department Information:
1957. Dean: Lawrence J. Siegel, PhD, ABPP. Number of faculty: total—full-time 30, part-time 28; women—full-time 14, part-time 17; total—minority—full-time 5, part-time 6; women minority—full-time 3, part-time 4; faculty subject to the Americans With Disabilities Act 1.

GRADUATE STUDY IN PSYCHOLOGY

Programs and Degrees Offered:
Listed in the following order: Program area, degree type (T if terminal Master's), number awarded 7/08–6/09. Clinical PsyD (Doctor of Psychology) 20, School/Clinical Child PsyD (Doctor of Psychology) 21, Clinical Health PhD (Doctor of Philosophy) 13, Mental Health Counseling MA/MS (Master of Arts/Science) (T) 10.

APA Accreditation: Clinical PsyD (Doctor of Psychology). Student Outcome Data Website: http://www.yu.edu/ferkauf/clinic.aspx?id=20912. Combination PsyD (Doctor of Psychology). Student Outcome Data Website: http://www.yu.edu/ferkauf/page.aspx?id=733. Clinical PhD (Doctor of Philosophy). Student Outcome Data Website: http://www.yu.edu/ferkauf/page.aspx?id=5206.

Student Applications/Admissions:
Student Applications
 Clinical PsyD (Doctor of Psychology)—Applications 2009–2010, 300. Total applicants accepted 2009–2010, 79. Number full-time enrolled (new admits only) 2009–2010, 21. Total enrolled 2009–2010 full-time, 115, part-time, 11. Openings 2010–2011, 21. The median number of years required for completion of a degree in 2008–2009 were 5. The number of students enrolled full- and part-time who were dismissed or voluntarily withdrew from this program area in 2008–2009 were 2. School/Clinical Child PsyD (Doctor of Psychology)—Applications 2009–2010, 200. Total applicants accepted 2009–2010, 43. Number full-time enrolled (new admits only) 2009–2010, 24. Total enrolled 2009–2010 full-time, 101, part-time, 9. Openings 2010–2011, 20. The median number of years required for completion of a degree in 2008–2009 were 5. The number of students enrolled full- and part-time who were dismissed or voluntarily withdrew from this program area in 2008–2009 were 1. Clinical Health PhD (Doctor of Philosophy)—Applications 2009–2010, 105. Total applicants accepted 2009–2010, 55. Number full-time enrolled (new admits only) 2009–2010, 15. Number part-time enrolled (new admits only) 2009–2010, 4. Total enrolled 2009–2010 full-time, 83, part-time, 11. Openings 2010–2011, 14. The median number of years required for completion of a degree in 2008–2009 were 5. The number of students enrolled full- and part-time who were dismissed or voluntarily withdrew from this program area in 2008–2009 were 1. Mental Health Counseling MA/MS (Master of Arts/Science)—Applications 2009–2010, 300. Total applicants accepted 2009–2010, 111. Number full-time enrolled (new admits only) 2009–2010, 20. Number part-time enrolled (new admits only) 2009–2010, 5. Total enrolled 2009–2010 full-time, 44, part-time, 6. Openings 2010–2011, 25. The median number of years required for completion of a degree in 2008–2009 were 2. The number of students enrolled full- and part-time who were dismissed or voluntarily withdrew from this program area in 2008–2009 were 1.
Scores: Entries appear in this order: required test or GPA, minimum score (if required), median score of students entering in 2009–2010. Clinical PsyD (Doctor of Psychology): GRE-V no minimum stated, GRE-Q no minimum stated.
Other Criteria: (importance of criteria rated low, medium, or high): GRE scores—high, research experience—high, work experience—high, extracurricular activity—high, clinically related public service—high, GPA—high, letters of recommendation—high, interview—high, statement of goals and objectives—high, undergraduate major in psychology—medium, specific undergraduate psychology courses taken—medium.

Student Characteristics: The following represents characteristics of students in 2009–2010 in all graduate psychology programs in the department: Female—full-time 247, part-time 17; Male—full-time 87, part-time 14; African American/Black—full-time 9, part-time 0; Hispanic/Latino(a)—full-time 21, part-time 1; Asian/Pacific Islander—full-time 9, part-time 1; American Indian/Alaska Native—full-time 0, part-time 0; Caucasian/White—full-time 0, part-time 0; Multi-ethnic—full-time 4, part-time 1; students subject to the Americans With Disabilities Act—full-time 1, part-time 1; Unknown ethnicity—full-time 0, part-time 0; International students who hold an F-1 or J-1 Visa—full-time 0, part-time 0.

Financial Information/Assistance:
Tuition for Full-Time Study: *Master's:* State residents: per academic year $31,440, $1,435 per credit hour; Nonstate residents: per academic year $31,440, $1,435 per credit hour. *Doctoral:* State residents: per academic year $31,440, $1,435 per credit hour; Nonstate residents: per academic year $31,440, $1,435 per credit hour. Tuition is subject to change. See the following Web site for updates and changes in tuition costs: http://www.yu.edu/student_aid/.

Financial Assistance:
 First-Year Students: Teaching assistantships available for first year. Average amount paid per academic year: $4,000. Average number of hours worked per week: 10. Research assistantships available for first year. Average amount paid per academic year: $1,000. Average number of hours worked per week: 20. Traineeships available for first year. Average amount paid per academic year: $15,000. Average number of hours worked per week: 20. Fellowships and scholarships available for first year. Average amount paid per academic year: $20,000. Average number of hours worked per week: 0.
 Advanced Students: Teaching assistantships available for advanced students. Average amount paid per academic year: $4,000. Average number of hours worked per week: 10. Research assistantships available for advanced students. Average amount paid per academic year: $10,000. Average number of hours worked per week: 20. Traineeships available for advanced students. Average amount paid per academic year: $15,000. Average number of hours worked per week: 20. Fellowships and scholarships available for advanced students. Average amount paid per academic year: $20,000. Average number of hours worked per week: 0.
 Additional Information: Of all students currently enrolled full time, 70% benefited from one or more of the listed financial assistance programs. Application and information available online at: http://www.yu.edu/student_aid/.

Internships/Practica: Doctoral Degree (PsyD Clinical): For those doctoral students for whom a professional internship was required in this program prior to graduation, (29) students applied for an internship in 2008–2009, with (29) students obtaining an internship. Of those students who obtained an internship, (27) were paid internships. Of those students who obtained an internship, (23) students placed in APA/CPA accredited internships, (4) students placed in internships not APA/CPA accredited, but listed with the Association of Psychology Postdoctoral and Internship Programs (APPIC), (0) students placed in internships conforming to guidelines of the Council of Directors of School Psychology Programs (CDSPP), (2) students placed in internships that were not APA/CPA accredited, APPIC or CDSPP listed. Doctoral Degree (PsyD School/Clinical Child): For those doctoral students for whom a professional internship was required in this program prior to graduation, (10) students applied for an internship in 2008–2009, with (10) students obtaining an internship. Of those students who obtained an internship, (10) were paid internships. Of those students who obtained an internship, (9) students placed in APA/CPA accredited internships, (0) students placed in internships not APA/CPA accredited, but listed with the Association of Psychology Postdoctoral and Internship Programs (APPIC), (1) students placed in internships conforming to guidelines of the Council of Directors of School Psychology Programs (CDSPP), (0) students placed in internships that were not APA/CPA accredited, APPIC or CDSPP listed. Doctoral Degree (PhD Clinical Health): For those doctoral students for whom a professional internship was required in this program prior to graduation, (13) students applied for an internship in 2008–2009, with (13) students obtaining an internship. Of those students who obtained an internship, (11) were paid internships. Of those students who obtained an internship, (11) students placed in APA/CPA accredited internships, (2) students placed in internships not APA/CPA accredited, but listed with the Association of Psychology Postdoctoral and Internship Programs (APPIC), (0) students placed in internships conforming to guidelines of the Council of Directors of School Psychology Programs (CDSPP), (0) students placed in internships that were not APA/CPA accredited, APPIC or CDSPP listed. Master's Degree (MA/MS Mental Health Counseling): An internship experience, such as, a final research project or "capstone" experience is required of graduates. Examples listed in catalog and on web-page: www.yu.edu/ferkauf.

Housing and Day Care: No on-campus housing is available. On-campus day care facilities are available.

Employment of Department Graduates:
Master's Degree Graduates: Of those who graduated in the academic year 2008–2009, the following categories and numbers represent the postgraduate activities and employment of master's degree graduates: Enrolled in a psychology doctoral program (65), enrolled in another graduate/professional program (5), enrolled in a postdoctoral residency/fellowship (n/a), employed in independent practice (n/a), total from the above (master's) (70).
Doctoral Degree Graduates: Of those who graduated in the academic year 2008–2009, the following categories and numbers represent the postgraduate activities and employment of doctoral degree graduates: Enrolled in a psychology doctoral program (n/a), enrolled in a postdoctoral residency/fellowship (3), employed in independent practice (7), employed in an academic position at a university (2), employed in an academic position at a 2-year/4-year college (2), employed in other positions at a higher education institution (1), employed in a professional position in a school system (15), employed in business or industry (3), employed in a community mental health/counseling center (11), employed in a hospital/medical center (20), still seeking employment (1), other employment position (2), do not know (1), total from the above (doctoral) (68).

Additional Information:
Orientation, Objectives, and Emphasis of Department: The objective of the Ferkauf Graduate School of Psychology is to promote a balance between the scientific-research orientation and the practitioner model. Clinical Psychology (Health Emphasis) program places greater emphasis upon applied and basic research, whereas the Clinical and School-Clinical Child psychology programs focus on the scientist–practitioner model with integrated clinical research and supervised practicum experiences. Further, Ferkauf offers PhD and PsyD degrees placing emphasis on research in the former and on application in the latter. A comprehensive theoretical orientation is offered with a psychodynamic focus and an applied behavioral emphasis. In all specialty areas, and at all levels of training, there is a strong commitment to the foundations of psychology, and a core of basic courses is required in all programs. Collaborations with the major NYC health and hospital institutions and schools are well established for all programs.

Special Facilities or Resources: All psychology programs offer practicum experience through Ferkauf's Center for Psychological and Psychoeducational Services. The Center provides a wide range of evaluation, remediation, and therapeutic services for children, adolescents, and adults in the neighboring communities, in addition to consultation services directly to the local schools. Ferkauf is located on Yeshiva University's campus of the Albert Einstein College of Medicine which has led to the development of cooperative programs and activities with various disciplines in medicine as well as added training opportunities for students at the various service delivery agencies affiliated with the medical college.

Application Information:
Send to Director of Admissions, Ferkauf Graduate School of Psychology, 1300 Morris Park Avenue, Bronx, NY 10461. Application available online. URL of online application: http://www.yu.edu/ferkauf/FGS03APP.pdf. Students are admitted in the Fall, application deadline January 1. Mental Health Counseling Psychology MA deadline is February 15. *Fee:* $50.

NORTH CAROLINA

Appalachian State University
Department of Psychology
Arts and Science
Smith-Wright Hall
Boone, NC 28608
Telephone: (828) 262-2272
Fax: (828) 262-2974
E-mail: dennistonjc@appstate.edu
Web: http://www.psych.appstate.edu

Department Information:
1966. Chairperson: James C. Denniston. Number of faculty: total—full-time 32, part-time 3; women—full-time 12, part-time 2; minority—part-time 1; women minority—part-time 1.

Programs and Degrees Offered:
Listed in the following order: Program area, degree type (T if terminal Master's), number awarded 7/08–6/09. General Experimental MA/MS (Master of Arts/Science) (T) 8, Industrial/Organizational MA/MS (Master of Arts/Science) (T) 7, Clinical Health Psychology MA/MS (Master of Arts/Science) (T) 8, School Psychology EdS (School Psychology) 7.

Student Applications/Admissions:

Student Applications

General Experimental MA/MS (Master of Arts/Science)—Applications 2009–2010, 20. Total applicants accepted 2009–2010, 5. Number full-time enrolled (new admits only) 2009–2010, 4. Number part-time enrolled (new admits only) 2009–2010, 0. Openings 2010–2011, 5. The median number of years required for completion of a degree in 2008–2009 were 3. *Industrial/Organizational MA/MS (Master of Arts/Science)*—Applications 2009–2010, 35. Total applicants accepted 2009–2010, 7. Number full-time enrolled (new admits only) 2009–2010, 6. Number part-time enrolled (new admits only) 2009–2010, 0. Openings 2010–2011, 8. The median number of years required for completion of a degree in 2008–2009 were 2. *Clinical Health Psychology MA/MS (Master of Arts/Science)*—Applications 2009–2010, 65. Total applicants accepted 2009–2010, 9. Number full-time enrolled (new admits only) 2009–2010, 8. Total enrolled 2009–2010 full-time, 20. Openings 2010–2011, 8. The median number of years required for completion of a degree in 2008–2009 were 3. The number of students enrolled full- and part-time who were dismissed or voluntarily withdrew from this program area in 2008–2009 were 2. *School Psychology EdS (School Psychology)*—Applications 2009–2010, 37. Total applicants accepted 2009–2010, 7. Number full-time enrolled (new admits only) 2009–2010, 7. Number part-time enrolled (new admits only) 2009–2010, 0. Openings 2010–2011, 8. The median number of years required for completion of a degree in 2008–2009 were 3. The number of students enrolled full- and part-time who were dismissed or voluntarily withdrew from this program area in 2008–2009 were 1.

Scores: Entries appear in this order: required test or GPA, minimum score (if required), median score of students entering in 2009–2010. *General Experimental MA/MS (Master of Arts/Science):* GRE-V 420, 435, GRE-Q 530, 580, GRE-Analytical 3.4, 4.5, overall undergraduate GPA 2.84, 3.64; *Industrial/Organizational MA/MS (Master of Arts/Science):* GRE-V 430, 515, GRE-Q 530, 655, GRE-Analytical 4.2, overall undergraduate GPA 2.92, 3.64; *Clinical Health Psychology MA/MS (Master of Arts/Science):* GRE-V 420, 570, GRE-Q 550, 625, GRE-Analytical 4, 5, overall undergraduate GPA 3.4, 3.85; *School Psychology EdS (School Psychology):* GRE-V 420, 425, GRE-Q 490, 530, GRE-Analytical 4, 4, overall undergraduate GPA 3.3, 3.73.

Other Criteria: (importance of criteria rated low, medium, or high): GRE scores—high, research experience—medium, work experience—low, extracurricular activity—low, clinically related public service—low, GPA—high, letters of recommendation—medium, interview—high, statement of goals and objectives—high, undergraduate major in psychology—medium, specific undergraduate psychology courses taken—medium. An interview is not required for Industrial/Organizational or Experimental Psychology. Interviews are given high importance for the Clinical Health and School Psychology programs. For additional information on admission requirements, go to http://www.psych.appstate.edu/gradprograms.html.

Student Characteristics: The following represents characteristics of students in 2009–2010 in all graduate psychology programs in the department: Female—full-time 57, part-time 0; Male—full-time 17, part-time 0; African American/Black—full-time 2, part-time 0; Hispanic/Latino(a)—part-time 0; Asian/Pacific Islander—full-time 0, part-time 0; American Indian/Alaska Native—full-time 0, part-time 0; Caucasian/White—full-time 70, part-time 0; Multi-ethnic—full-time 0, part-time 0; students subject to the Americans With Disabilities Act—full-time 1, part-time 0; Unknown ethnicity—full-time 2, part-time 0; International students who hold an F-1 or J-1 Visa—full-time 4, part-time 0.

Financial Information/Assistance:
Tuition for Full-Time Study: *Master's:* State residents: per academic year $4,959; Nonstate residents: per academic year $15,373. Tuition is subject to change. See the following Web site for updates and changes in tuition costs: http://www.studentaccounts.appstate.edu/tuition-and-fees.

Financial Assistance:

First-Year Students: Research assistantships available for first year. Average amount paid per academic year: $7,000. Average number of hours worked per week: 15. Fellowships and scholarships available for first year. Average amount paid per academic year: $8,000. Average number of hours worked per week: 20. Apply by March.

Advanced Students: Teaching assistantships available for advanced students. Average amount paid per academic year: $7,500. Average number of hours worked per week: 15. Research assistantships available for advanced students. Average amount paid per academic year: $5,000. Average number of hours worked per week: 10.

Additional Information: Of all students currently enrolled full time, 100% benefited from one or more of the listed financial

assistance programs. Application and information available online at: http://www.graduate.appstate.edu/admissions/index.html.

Internships/Practica: Master's Degree (MA/MS General Experimental): An internship experience, such as a final research project or "capstone" experience is required of graduates. Master's Degree (MA/MS Industrial/Organizational-HR Management): An internship experience, such as a final research project or "capstone" experience is required of graduates. Master's Degree (MA/MS Clinical Health Psychology): An internship experience, such as a final research project or "capstone" experience is required of graduates. Clinical Health students complete two semester-long practica. These are often at the University Counseling Center, the Psychology AD/HD Clinic, or at two other regional mental health institutes. Students complete a 1,000-hour internship at a medical or mental health setting. School students complete two semester-long practica in public schools and a 1200-hour internship, half of which must be in a public school setting. Industrial/Organizational students have the option of completing a 450-hour internship in human resources or organizational development.

Housing and Day Care: No on-campus housing is available. On-campus day care facilities are available. We offer two pre-schools each with select slots for student's children on a sliding scale fee.

Employment of Department Graduates:
Master's Degree Graduates: Of those who graduated in the academic year 2008–2009, the following categories and numbers represent the postgraduate activities and employment of master's degree graduates: Enrolled in a psychology doctoral program (2), enrolled in a postdoctoral residency/fellowship (n/a), employed in independent practice (n/a), employed in an academic position at a university (1), employed in an academic position at a 2-year/4-year college (4), employed in a professional position in a school system (7), employed in business or industry (5), employed in government agency (2), employed in a community mental health/counseling center (6), employed in a hospital/medical center (1), still seeking employment (0), do not know (2), total from the above (master's) (30).
Doctoral Degree Graduates: Of those who graduated in the academic year 2008–2009, the following categories and numbers represent the postgraduate activities and employment of doctoral degree graduates: Enrolled in a psychology doctoral program (n/a), total from the above (doctoral) (0).

Additional Information:
Orientation, Objectives, and Emphasis of Department: The department is student oriented, with a Program Director for each graduate program and a Graduate Programs Coordinator. The General-Experimental program is primarily predoctoral for experimental psychology, but one can structure an applied orientation. The Clinical Health program trains professionals for master's level licensure as LPAs and applied practice in mental health and medical settings or for doctoral study in clinical psychology. The School Psychology program is NCATE/NASP accredited and offers the master's and specialist degree. The Industrial/Organizational program integrates with Department of Management in the College of Business and trains professionals to work in business, industry, and government.

Special Facilities or Resources: Biofeedback facilities, student computer laboratory, neuroscience laboratory, an animal operant conditioning laboratory, and a Psychology Clinic at the Institute of Health & Human Services are available.

Information for Students With Physical Disabilities: See the following Web site for more information: http://www.ods.appstate.edu.

Application Information:
Send to The Dean, Cratis D. Williams Graduate School, John E. Thomas Building, Appalachian State University, Boone NC 28608. Application available online. URL of online application: http://www.appstate.edu. Students are admitted in the Fall, application deadline February 15. Clinical Health has a February 1, School Psychology programs has a February 15, and I/O and General Experimental programs have March 1 application deadlines. *Fee:* $50.

Duke University
Department of Psychology and Neuroscience
229 Psychology/Sociology Building, P.O. Box 90085
9 Flowers Drive
Durham, NC 27708
Telephone: (919) 660-5715
Fax: (919) 660-5726
E-mail: *morrell@duke.edu*
Web: *http://psychandneuro.duke.edu/*

Department Information:
1948. Chairperson: Dr. Harris Cooper. Number of faculty: total—full-time 37, part-time 11; women—full-time 15, part-time 3; total—minority—full-time 7; women minority—full-time 3.

Programs and Degrees Offered:
Listed in the following order: Program area, degree type (T if terminal Master's), number awarded 7/08–6/09. JD/MA Social and Health Sciences MA/MS (Master of Arts/Science) 4, Clinical Psychology PhD (Doctor of Philosophy) 5, Developmental Psychology PhD (Doctor of Philosophy) 1, Social Psychology PhD (Doctor of Philosophy) 1, Systems & Integrative Neuroscience PhD (Doctor of Philosophy) 1, Cognition & Cognitive Neuroscience PhD (Doctor of Philosophy) 2.

APA Accreditation: Clinical PhD (Doctor of Philosophy). Student Outcome Data Website: http://psychandneuro.duke.edu/graduate/training/clinical.

Student Applications/Admissions:
Student Applications
JD/MA Social and Health Sciences MA/MS (*Master of Arts/Science*)—Applications 2009–2010, 4. Total applicants accepted 2009–2010, 4. Number full-time enrolled (new admits only) 2009–2010, 2. Total enrolled 2009–2010 full-time, 4. Openings 2010–2011, 2. The median number of years required for completion of a degree in 2008–2009 were 3. *Clinical Psychology PhD (Doctor of Philosophy)*—Applications 2009–2010, 241. Total applicants accepted 2009–2010, 10. Number full-time enrolled (new admits only) 2009–2010, 6. Number part-time enrolled (new admits only) 2009–2010, 0. Openings 2010–2011, 4. The median number of years required for com-

pletion of a degree in 2008–2009 were 7. The number of students enrolled full- and part-time who were dismissed or voluntarily withdrew from this program area in 2008–2009 were 0. *Developmental Psychology PhD (Doctor of Philosophy)*—Applications 2009–2010, 43. Total applicants accepted 2009–2010, 5. Number full-time enrolled (new admits only) 2009–2010, 0. Number part-time enrolled (new admits only) 2009–2010, 0. Openings 2010–2011, 5. The median number of years required for completion of a degree in 2008–2009 were 6. The number of students enrolled full- and part-time who were dismissed or voluntarily withdrew from this program area in 2008–2009 were 0. *Social Psychology PhD (Doctor of Philosophy)*—Applications 2009–2010, 76. Total applicants accepted 2009–2010, 4. Number full-time enrolled (new admits only) 2009–2010, 2. Number part-time enrolled (new admits only) 2009–2010, 0. Openings 2010–2011, 4. The median number of years required for completion of a degree in 2008–2009 were 5. The number of students enrolled full- and part-time who were dismissed or voluntarily withdrew from this program area in 2008–2009 were 0. *Systems & Integrative Neuroscience PhD (Doctor of Philosophy)*—Applications 2009–2010, 25. Total applicants accepted 2009–2010, 6. Number full-time enrolled (new admits only) 2009–2010, 5. Number part-time enrolled (new admits only) 2009–2010, 0. Openings 2010–2011, 4. The median number of years required for completion of a degree in 2008–2009 were 6. The number of students enrolled full- and part-time who were dismissed or voluntarily withdrew from this program area in 2008–2009 were 0. *Cognition & Cognitive Neuroscience PhD (Doctor of Philosophy)*—Applications 2009–2010, 58. Total applicants accepted 2009–2010, 6. Number full-time enrolled (new admits only) 2009–2010, 6. Number part-time enrolled (new admits only) 2009–2010, 0. Openings 2010–2011, 8. The median number of years required for completion of a degree in 2008–2009 were 6. The number of students enrolled full- and part-time who were dismissed or voluntarily withdrew from this program area in 2008–2009 were 0.

Scores: Entries appear in this order: required test or GPA, minimum score (if required), median score of students entering in 2009–2010. *Clinical Psychology PhD (Doctor of Philosophy)*: GRE-V no minimum stated, 620, GRE-Q no minimum stated, 730, GRE-Analytical no minimum stated, 5.0, GRE-Subject (Psychology) no minimum stated, 700, overall undergraduate GPA no minimum stated, 3.8; *Developmental Psychology PhD (Doctor of Philosophy)*: GRE-V no minimum stated, 675, GRE-Q no minimum stated, 695, GRE-Analytical no minimum stated, 4.5, overall undergraduate GPA no minimum stated, 3.7; *Social Psychology PhD (Doctor of Philosophy)*: GRE-V no minimum stated, 703, GRE-Q no minimum stated, 743, GRE-Analytical no minimum stated, 5.6, overall undergraduate GPA no minimum stated, 3.9; *Systems & Integrative Neuroscience PhD (Doctor of Philosophy)*: GRE-V no minimum stated, 620, GRE-Q no minimum stated, 680, GRE-Analytical no minimum stated, 4.7, overall undergraduate GPA no minimum stated, 3.9; *Cognition & Cognitive Neuroscience PhD (Doctor of Philosophy)*: GRE-V no minimum stated, 720, GRE-Q no minimum stated, 800, GRE-Analytical no minimum stated, 6.0, overall undergraduate GPA no minimum stated, 3.9.

Other Criteria: (importance of criteria rated low, medium, or high): GRE scores—high, research experience—high, work experience—high, extracurricular activity—low, clinically related public service—medium, GPA—high, letters of recommendation—high, interview—high, statement of goals and objectives—high. Clinically Related Public Service is not required for Developmental, Social, Cognitive, or Neuro. For additional information on admission requirements, go to http://psychandneuro.duke.edu/graduate/apply.

Student Characteristics: The following represents characteristics of students in 2009–2010 in all graduate psychology programs in the department: Female—full-time 67, part-time 0; Male—full-time 20, part-time 0; African American/Black—full-time 5, part-time 0; Hispanic/Latino(a)—full-time 4, part-time 0; Asian/Pacific Islander—full-time 6, part-time 0; American Indian/Alaska Native—full-time 1, part-time 0; Caucasian/White—full-time 70, part-time 0; Multi-ethnic—full-time 1, part-time 0; students subject to the Americans With Disabilities Act—full-time 0, part-time 0; Unknown ethnicity—full-time 0, part-time 0; International students who hold an F-1 or J-1 Visa—full-time 7, part-time 0.

Financial Information/Assistance:

Tuition for Full-Time Study: *Doctoral:* State residents: per academic year $39,150; Nonstate residents: per academic year $39,150. Tuition is subject to change. See the following Web site for updates and changes in tuition costs: http://gradschool.duke.edu/financial_support/coa/.

Financial Assistance:

First-Year Students: Teaching assistantships available for first year. Average amount paid per academic year: $19,840. Average number of hours worked per week: 19. Apply by December 1. Research assistantships available for first year. Average amount paid per academic year: $19,840. Average number of hours worked per week: 19. Apply by December 1. Fellowships and scholarships available for first year. Average amount paid per academic year: $19,840. Apply by December 1.

Advanced Students: Teaching assistantships available for advanced students. Average amount paid per academic year: $19,840. Average number of hours worked per week: 19. Apply by December 1. Research assistantships available for advanced students. Average amount paid per academic year: $19,840. Average number of hours worked per week: 19. Apply by December 1. Fellowships and scholarships available for advanced students. Average amount paid per academic year: $19,840. Apply by December 1.

Additional Information: Of all students currently enrolled full time, 100% benefited from one or more of the listed financial assistance programs. Application and information available online at: http://gradschool.duke.edu/financial_support/.

Internships/Practica: Doctoral Degree (PhD Clinical Psychology): For those doctoral students for whom a professional internship was required in this program prior to graduation, (10) students applied for an internship in 2008–2009, with (10) students obtaining an internship. Of those students who obtained an internship, (10) were paid internships. Of those students who obtained an internship, (10) students placed in APA/CPA accredited internships, (0) students placed in internships not APA/CPA accredited, but listed with the Association of Psychology Postdoctoral and Internship Programs (APPIC), (0) students placed in internships conforming to guidelines of the Council of Directors of School Psychology Programs (CDSPP), (0) students placed in internships that were not APA/CPA accredited, APPIC or

CDSPP listed. Doctoral students in our clinical program receive experience in our own departmental clinic as well as a great number of local institutions and medical center facilities.

Housing and Day Care: On-campus housing is available. See the following Web site for more information: http://communityhousing.duke.edu. On-campus day care facilities are available. See the following Web site for more information: http://www.hr.duke.edu/dcc/.

Employment of Department Graduates:
Master's Degree Graduates: Of those who graduated in the academic year 2008–2009, the following categories and numbers represent the postgraduate activities and employment of master's degree graduates: Enrolled in a postdoctoral residency/fellowship (n/a), employed in independent practice (n/a), total from the above (master's) (0).
Doctoral Degree Graduates: Of those who graduated in the academic year 2008–2009, the following categories and numbers represent the postgraduate activities and employment of doctoral degree graduates: Enrolled in a psychology doctoral program (n/a), enrolled in another graduate/professional program (4), enrolled in a postdoctoral residency/fellowship (5), employed in an academic position at a university (1), total from the above (doctoral) (10).

Additional Information:
Orientation, Objectives, and Emphasis of Department: The department features a strong mentor-oriented training program with areas of specialization in clinical health, adult and child psychology, as well as programs in developmental and social psychology. Emphasis is placed on informal interaction among faculty and students; seminars and small groups of faculty and graduate students meet regularly.

Special Facilities or Resources: The department has collaborative ties with the Center for Child and Family Policy, the Center for Cognitive Neuroscience, the Center for the Study of Aging and Human Development, the Fuqua School of Business, Medical Psychology, the Center for Aging and Human Development, the Center for Child and Family Policy, and the Carolina Consortium on Human Development and UNC-Duke Collaborative Graduate Certificate Program in Developmental Psychology. State-of-the-art facilities, including specially equipped laboratories and clinics, are available for student use. These include computational facilities for word processing, data analysis, and experimental programming.

Information for Students With Physical Disabilities: See the following Web site for more information: http://www.access.duke.edu/.

Application Information:
Send to The Graduate School, 2127 Campus Drive, Box 90065, Durham, NC 27708. Application available online. URL of online application: http://gradschool.duke.edu/admissions/requirements/online_ap.php. Students are admitted in the Fall, application deadline December 1. Clinical deadline is December 1; deadline for all other programs is December 8. *Fee:* $75.

East Carolina University
Department of Psychology
Arts and Sciences
104 Rawl
Greenville, NC 27858-4353
Telephone: (252) 328-6800
Fax: (252) 328-6283
E-mail: *rowk@ecu.edu; ericsonj@ecu.edu*
Web: *http://www.ecu.edu/psyc*

Department Information:
1959. Chairperson: Kathleen A. Lawler Row. Number of faculty: total—full-time 40, part-time 5; women—full-time 22, part-time 3; total—minority—full-time 5; women minority—full-time 4.

Programs and Degrees Offered:
Listed in the following order: Program area, degree type (T if terminal Master's), number awarded 7/08–6/09. General MA/MS (Master of Arts/Science) (T) 7, School Psychology MA/MS (Master of Arts/Science) (T) 8, Health Psychology PhD (Doctor of Philosophy) 0.

Student Applications/Admissions:
Student Applications
General MA/MS (Master of Arts/Science)—Applications 2009–2010, 67. Total applicants accepted 2009–2010, 42. Number full-time enrolled (new admits only) 2009–2010, 20. Number part-time enrolled (new admits only) 2009–2010, 0. Total enrolled 2009–2010 full-time, 59. Openings 2010–2011, 20. The median number of years required for completion of a degree in 2008–2009 were 2. The number of students enrolled full- and part-time who were dismissed or voluntarily withdrew from this program area in 2008–2009 were 1. *School Psychology MA/MS (Master of Arts/Science)*—Applications 2009–2010, 45. Total applicants accepted 2009–2010, 14. Number full-time enrolled (new admits only) 2009–2010, 7. Number part-time enrolled (new admits only) 2009–2010, 0. Openings 2010–2011, 8. The median number of years required for completion of a degree in 2008–2009 were 3. The number of students enrolled full- and part-time who were dismissed or voluntarily withdrew from this program area in 2008–2009 were 1. *Health Psychology PhD (Doctor of Philosophy)*—Applications 2009–2010, 45. Total applicants accepted 2009–2010, 7. Number full-time enrolled (new admits only) 2009–2010, 7. Number part-time enrolled (new admits only) 2009–2010, 0. Openings 2010–2011, 8. The median number of years required for completion of a degree in 2008–2009 were 5. The number of students enrolled full- and part-time who were dismissed or voluntarily withdrew from this program area in 2008–2009 were 0.

Scores: Entries appear in this order: required test or GPA, minimum score (if required), median score of students entering in 2009–2010. *General MA/MS (Master of Arts/Science):* GRE-V no minimum stated, 500, GRE-Q no minimum stated, 600, overall undergraduate GPA 3.0, 3.25.

Other Criteria: (importance of criteria rated low, medium, or high): GRE scores—high, research experience—high, work experience—medium, extracurricular activity—low, clinically related public service—medium, GPA—high, letters of recommendation—high, interview—high, statement of goals and objectives—high, undergraduate major in psychology—medium, specific undergraduate psychology courses taken—medium, Doctoral programs strongly recommend interview. For additional information on admission requirements, go to http://www.ecu.edu/psyc.

Student Characteristics: The following represents characteristics of students in 2009–2010 in all graduate psychology programs in the department: Female—full-time 48, part-time 0; Male—full-time 8, part-time 0; African American/Black—full-time 2, part-time 0; Hispanic/Latino(a)—full-time 0, part-time 0; Asian/Pacific Islander—full-time 1, part-time 0; American Indian/Alaska Native—full-time 0, part-time 0; Caucasian/White—full-time 0, part-time 0; Multi-ethnic—full-time 0, part-time 0; students subject to the Americans With Disabilities Act—full-time 0, part-time 0; Unknown ethnicity—full-time 0, part-time 0; International students who hold an F-1 or J-1 Visa—full-time 0, part-time 0.

Financial Information/Assistance:
Tuition for Full-Time Study: *Master's:* State residents: per academic year $4,831; Nonstate residents: per academic year $15,147. *Doctoral:* State residents: per academic year $4,831; Nonstate residents: per academic year $15,147. Tuition is subject to change. See the following Web site for updates and changes in tuition costs: http://www.ecu.edu/gradschool/.

Financial Assistance:
First-Year Students: Teaching assistantships available for first year. Average amount paid per academic year: $3,750. Average number of hours worked per week: 10. Apply by Mar 1. Research assistantships available for first year. Average amount paid per academic year: $3,750. Average number of hours worked per week: 10. Apply by Mar 1. Fellowships and scholarships available for first year. Average amount paid per academic year: $7,500. Average number of hours worked per week: 20. Apply by Mar 1.
Advanced Students: Teaching assistantships available for advanced students. Average amount paid per academic year: $15,000. Average number of hours worked per week: 20. Apply by February 15. Research assistantships available for advanced students. Average amount paid per academic year: $13,000. Average number of hours worked per week: 20. Apply by February 15. Fellowships and scholarships available for advanced students. Average amount paid per academic year: $3,000. Average number of hours worked per week: 0. Apply by February 15.
Additional Information: Of all students currently enrolled full time, 60% benefited from one or more of the listed financial assistance programs.

Internships/Practica: Master's Degree (MA/MS General): An internship experience, such as a final research project or "capstone" experience is required of graduates. Master's Degree (MA/MS School Psychology): An internship experience, such as a final research project or "capstone" experience is required of graduates. School internships in area school systems offer stipends of up to $2,450 per month for 10 months. Paid I/O internships are usually available during the summer. Predoctoral internships are completed during the fifth year of the PhD Health Psychology program. We admitted our first doctoral class Fall 2007.

Housing and Day Care: On-campus housing is available. See the following Web site for more information: http://www.ecu.edu/campusliving/. No on-campus day care facilities are available.

Employment of Department Graduates:
Master's Degree Graduates: Of those who graduated in the academic year 2008–2009, the following categories and numbers represent the postgraduate activities and employment of master's degree graduates: Enrolled in a psychology doctoral program (6), enrolled in another graduate/professional program (1), enrolled in a postdoctoral residency/fellowship (n/a), employed in independent practice (n/a), employed in an academic position at a university (0), employed in an academic position at a 2-year/4-year college (0), employed in other positions at a higher education institution (0), employed in a professional position in a school system (7), employed in business or industry (6), employed in government agency (0), employed in a community mental health/counseling center (0), employed in a hospital/medical center (5), still seeking employment (0), other employment position (3), do not know (1), total from the above (master's) (29).
Doctoral Degree Graduates: Of those who graduated in the academic year 2008–2009, the following categories and numbers represent the postgraduate activities and employment of doctoral degree graduates: Enrolled in a psychology doctoral program (n/a), total from the above (doctoral) (0).

Additional Information:
Orientation, Objectives, and Emphasis of Department: The School Psychology MA/CAS program is approved by the National Association of School Psychologists and the NC Department of Public Instruction. The program provides training and experience in assessment, consultation, and intervention. The General Psychology program offers students the opportunity to specialize in three concentrations. The Academic concentration prepares students to teach psychology at the community/junior college level. The Industrial/Organizational concentration prepares students for careers involving the application of psychology and human resources in organizations. Students who complete the PhD in Health Psychology will be prepared for a number of practitioner, faculty, and research roles within various health care and academic settings. The clinical health concentration trains students to become members of primary health care teams in hospitals, health maintenance organizations, community mental health agencies, and private practice. The pediatric school psychology concentration prepares psychologists for practice within settings that serve children and adolescents with health-related problems. Clinical health graduates are eligible to apply for licensure as a Licensed Psychologist and Health Services Provider-Psychologist (HSP-P) and pediatric school psychology graduates are eligible to apply for licensure as a school psychologist as well as for licensure as a Licensed Psychologist and Health Services Provider-Psychologist (HSP-P) by the NC State Board of Psychology. The program will be eligible to seek accreditation by the American Psychological Association and the doctoral program requirements of the National Association of School Psychologists in 2012.

Special Facilities or Resources: The department has student computer facilities, interview and testing facilities, and an animal laboratory. The school program works closely with community schools and mental health agencies. The doctoral health psychology program works closely with the Brody School of Medicine, family care practices, state health agencies, as well as with the Sleep Disorders Center, the Heart Center and psychiatric medicine.

Information for Students With Physical Disabilities: See the following Web site for more information: http://www.ecu.edu/cs-studentlife/dss/.

Application Information:
Send to East Carolina University Graduate School, 131 Ragsdale Hall, Greenville, NC 27858-4353. Application available online. URL of online application: http://www.ecu.edu/cs-cas/psyc/Psychology-Graduate-Programs.cfm. Students are admitted in the Fall, application deadline February 15. March 1 deadline for all MA programs. February 15 deadline for PhD Health Psychology Program. *Fee:* $50.

North Carolina State University
Department of Psychology
College of Humanities and Social Sciences
640 Poe Hall, Box 7650
Raleigh, NC 27695-7650
Telephone: (919) 515-2251
Fax: (919) 515-1716
E-mail: *psych_graduate programs@ncsu.edu*
Web: *http://psychology.chass.ncsu.edu/*

Department Information:
1938. Department Head: Douglas J. Gillan. Number of faculty: total—full-time 36, part-time 1; women—full-time 14; total—minority—full-time 3; women minority—full-time 1.

Programs and Degrees Offered:
Listed in the following order: Program area, degree type (T if terminal Master's), number awarded 7/08–6/09. Human Factors & Ergonomics PhD (Doctor of Philosophy), Lifespan Developmental Psychology PhD (Doctor of Philosophy), Industrial/Organizational Psychology PhD (Doctor of Philosophy), Public Interest PhD (Doctor of Philosophy), School Psychology PhD (Doctor of Philosophy).

APA Accreditation: School PhD (Doctor of Philosophy).

Student Applications/Admissions:
Student Applications
Human Factors & Ergonomics PhD (Doctor of Philosophy)—Applications 2009–2010, 28. Total applicants accepted 2009–2010, 10. Number full-time enrolled (new admits only) 2009–2010, 2. Total enrolled 2009–2010 full-time, 16, part-time, 2. Openings 2010–2011, 4. Lifespan Developmental Psychology PhD (Doctor of Philosophy)—Applications 2009–2010, 39. Total applicants accepted 2009–2010, 13. Number full-time enrolled (new admits only) 2009–2010, 3. Total enrolled 2009–2010 full-time, 13, part-time, 2. Openings 2010–2011, 4. Industrial/Organizational Psychology PhD (Doctor of Philosophy)—Applications 2009–2010, 88. Total applicants accepted 2009–2010, 12. Number full-time enrolled (new admits only) 2009–2010, 5. Total enrolled 2009–2010 full-time, 22, part-time, 5. Openings 2010–2011, 5. Public Interest PhD (Doctor of Philosophy)—Applications 2009–2010, 26. Total applicants accepted 2009–2010, 8. Number full-time enrolled (new admits only) 2009–2010, 7. Total enrolled 2009–2010 full-time, 20, part-time, 8. Openings 2010–2011, 5. School Psychology PhD (Doctor of Philosophy)—Applications 2009–2010, 58. Total applicants accepted 2009–2010, 8. Number full-time enrolled (new admits only) 2009–2010, 3. Total enrolled 2009–2010 full-time, 17, part-time, 7. Openings 2010–2011, 5.

Other Criteria: (importance of criteria rated low, medium, or high): GRE scores—high, research experience—high, work experience—medium, extracurricular activity—low, GPA—high, letters of recommendation—high, interview—medium, statement of goals and objectives—high, Research Interests—high, Psychology in the Public Interest gives greater weight to work experience and public service than do other program areas. Human Factors and Ergonomics has a special interest in math and non-psychology-science backgrounds of applicants. For additional information on admission requirements, go to http://psychology.chass.ncsu.edu/graduate.

Student Characteristics: The following represents characteristics of students in 2009–2010 in all graduate psychology programs in the department: Female—full-time 68, part-time 18; Male—full-time 20, part-time 6; African American/Black—full-time 10, part-time 6; Hispanic/Latino(a)—full-time 1, part-time 0; Asian/Pacific Islander—full-time 10, part-time 1; American Indian/Alaska Native—full-time 0, part-time 0; Caucasian/White—full-time 62, part-time 17; Multi-ethnic—full-time 5, part-time 0; students subject to the Americans With Disabilities Act—full-time 1, part-time 0; Unknown ethnicity—full-time 0, part-time 0; International students who hold an F-1 or J-1 Visa—full-time 6, part-time 1.

Financial Information/Assistance:
Tuition for Full-Time Study: *Master's:* State residents: per academic year $4,408; Nonstate residents: per academic year $16,456. *Doctoral:* State residents: per academic year $4,408; Nonstate residents: per academic year $16,456. Tuition is subject to change. See the following Web site for updates and changes in tuition costs: http://www.fis.ncsu.edu/cashier/tuition/gradtuition.asp.

Financial Assistance:
First-Year Students: Teaching assistantships available for first year. Average amount paid per academic year: $12,500. Average number of hours worked per week: 20. Research assistantships available for first year. Average amount paid per academic year: $14,500. Average number of hours worked per week: 20.

Advanced Students: Teaching assistantships available for advanced students. Average amount paid per academic year: $12,500. Average number of hours worked per week: 20. Research assistantships available for advanced students. Average amount paid per academic year: $14,500. Average number of hours worked per week: 20.

Additional Information: Of all students currently enrolled full time, 60% benefited from one or more of the listed financial assistance programs.

Internships/Practica: Doctoral Degree (PhD School Psychology): For those doctoral students for whom a professional internship was required in this program prior to graduation, (3) students applied for an internship in 2008–2009, with (3) students obtaining an internship. Of those students who obtained an internship, (1) were paid internships. Of those students who obtained an internship, (0) students placed in APA/CPA accredited internships, (0) students placed in internships not APA/CPA accredited, but listed with the Association of Psychology Postdoctoral and Internship Programs (APPIC), (3) students placed in internships conforming to guidelines of the Council of Directors of School Psychology Programs (CDSPP), (0) students placed in internships that were not APA/CPA accredited, APPIC or CDSPP listed. Practica and internships are required for both master's and doctoral students in the School Psychology program. These include supervised experiences in assessment, consultation, intervention, research, and professional school psychology in a wide variety of school-related settings. Students in Human Factors and Ergonomics are also expected to obtain employment for at least one summer/semester in one of the many suitable companies located in the Research Triangle area.

Housing and Day Care: On-campus housing is available. See the following Web site for more information: http://www.ncsu.edu/housing/. No on-campus day care facilities are available.

Employment of Department Graduates:
Master's Degree Graduates: Of those who graduated in the academic year 2008–2009, the following categories and numbers represent the postgraduate activities and employment of master's degree graduates: Enrolled in a postdoctoral residency/fellowship (n/a), employed in independent practice (n/a), total from the above (master's) (0).
Doctoral Degree Graduates: Of those who graduated in the academic year 2008–2009, the following categories and numbers represent the postgraduate activities and employment of doctoral degree graduates: Enrolled in a psychology doctoral program (n/a), total from the above (doctoral) (0).

Additional Information:
Orientation, Objectives, and Emphasis of Department: The department trains in the scientist–practitioner model. Students are expected to become knowledgeable about both research and application within their area of study. There are five specialty areas with different emphases. Lifespan Developmental Psychology stresses a balance of conceptual, research-analytical, and application skills and encompasses social and cognitive development from infancy to old age. Human Factors and Ergonomics emphasizes the cognitive/perceptual aspects of human factors, including research on visual displays, visual/auditory spatial judgments, ergonomics for older adults and the effective information transfer for complex systems. This track has a cooperative relationship with the Ergonomics/Biomechanics Program in Industrial & Systems Engineering. The Psychology in the Public Interest program (formerly known as Human Resource Development/Community Psychology) is a problem-oriented program dealing with research and professional issues in communities and social systems. Industrial-Organizational (I-O) students may concentrate in areas such as performance appraisal, selection, training, job analysis, work motivation, organizational theory/development and the interface of technology with I-O issues. School Psychology develops behavioral scientists who apply psychological knowledge and techniques in school and family settings to help students, parents, and teachers.

Special Facilities or Resources: The department is housed primarily on two floors of a modern building. Teaching Assistants share office space; Research Assistants have space within faculty research areas. All programs have appropriate laboratory space and facilities. These include specialized lab facilities: Audition Laboratory, Cognitive-Development Laboratory, Ergonomics and Aging Laboratory, Human-Computer Interaction Laboratory, Social Development Laboratory, and Visual Performance Laboratory. Ergonomics, Public Interest, I/O, and School students may have opportunities to work in state government, industry, schools, and community agencies to gain practical and research experience. As the surrounding region continues to develop, more opportunities appear each year. Students are, however, required to maintain continuous registration and carry an adequate course load each semester. Students are permitted to enroll in courses at the University of North Carolina-Chapel Hill and at Duke University, as if the courses were offered on their home campus. Beyond basic research, statistics, and program/departmental course requirements, students have considerable flexibility in developing individually-tailored plans of study.

Information for Students With Physical Disabilities: See the following Web site for more information: http://www.ncsu.edu/dso.

Application Information:
Send to Director of Graduate Programs, Psychology Department, Box 7650, NCSU, Raleigh, NC 27695-7650. Application available online. URL of online application: http://www2.acs.ncsu.edu/grad/applygrad.htm. Students are admitted in the Fall, application deadline January 5. The program in School Psychology sets its deadline at December 15. Application Fee = $65 for U.S. citizens and permanent residents; $75 for non-resident (international) applicants. McNair Scholars, or other U.S. citizens with significant financial restrictions, may request waiver of the application fee; contact Graduate School, Room 240, Research Building III, 1005 Capability Drive, Box 7102, NCSU, Raleigh, NC 27695-7102 for details.

North Carolina, University of, Chapel Hill
Department of Psychology
Arts and Sciences
CB #3270
Chapel Hill, NC 27599-3270
Telephone: (919) 962-7149
Fax: (919) 962-2537
E-mail: *jenningj@email.unc.edu*
Web: *http://psychology.unc.edu/*

Department Information:
1921. Chairperson: Donald T. Lysle. Number of faculty: total—full-time 62; women—full-time 30; total—minority—full-time 11; women minority—full-time 7.

Programs and Degrees Offered:
Listed in the following order: Program area, degree type (T if terminal Master's), number awarded 7/08–6/09. Clinical PhD (Doctor of Philosophy) 11, Cognitive PhD (Doctor of Philosophy) 1, Developmental PhD (Doctor of Philosophy) 2, Behavioral Neuroscience PhD (Doctor of Philosophy) 2, Quantitative PhD (Doctor of Philosophy) 3, Social PhD (Doctor of Philosophy) 1.

APA Accreditation: Clinical PhD (Doctor of Philosophy).

Student Applications/Admissions:
Student Applications
Clinical PhD (Doctor of Philosophy)—Applications 2009–2010, 379. Total applicants accepted 2009–2010, 6. Number full-

time enrolled (new admits only) 2009–2010, 9. Number part-time enrolled (new admits only) 2009–2010, 0. Openings 2010–2011, 6. The median number of years required for completion of a degree in 2008–2009 were 5. *Cognitive PhD (Doctor of Philosophy)*—Applications 2009–2010, 38. Total applicants accepted 2009–2010, 4. Number full-time enrolled (new admits only) 2009–2010, 2. Number part-time enrolled (new admits only) 2009–2010, 0. Total enrolled 2009–2010 full-time, 13. Openings 2010–2011, 4. The median number of years required for completion of a degree in 2008–2009 were 5. *Developmental PhD (Doctor of Philosophy)*—Applications 2009–2010, 65. Total applicants accepted 2009–2010, 7. Number full-time enrolled (new admits only) 2009–2010, 2. Number part-time enrolled (new admits only) 2009–2010, 0. Openings 2010–2011, 4. The median number of years required for completion of a degree in 2008–2009 were 5. *Behavioral Neuroscience PhD (Doctor of Philosophy)*—Applications 2009–2010, 46. Total applicants accepted 2009–2010, 5. Number full-time enrolled (new admits only) 2009–2010, 3. Number part-time enrolled (new admits only) 2009–2010, 0. Openings 2010–2011, 4. The median number of years required for completion of a degree in 2008–2009 were 5. *Quantitative PhD (Doctor of Philosophy)*—Applications 2009–2010, 45. Total applicants accepted 2009–2010, 4. Number full-time enrolled (new admits only) 2009–2010, 4. Openings 2010–2011, 4. The median number of years required for completion of a degree in 2008–2009 were 5. *Social PhD (Doctor of Philosophy)*—Applications 2009–2010, 108. Total applicants accepted 2009–2010, 4. Number full-time enrolled (new admits only) 2009–2010, 3. Openings 2010–2011, 4. The median number of years required for completion of a degree in 2008–2009 were 5.

Scores: Entries appear in this order: required test or GPA, minimum score (if required), median score of students entering in 2009–2010. *Clinical PhD (Doctor of Philosophy)*: GRE-V 500, 639, GRE-Q 500, 700, overall undergraduate GPA 3.0, 3.72; *Cognitive PhD (Doctor of Philosophy)*: GRE-V 500, GRE-Q 500, overall undergraduate GPA 3.0; *Developmental PhD (Doctor of Philosophy)*: GRE-V 500, GRE-Q 500, overall undergraduate GPA 3.0; *Behavioral Neuroscience PhD (Doctor of Philosophy)*: GRE-V 500, GRE-Q 500, overall undergraduate GPA 3.0; *Quantitative PhD (Doctor of Philosophy)*: GRE-V 500, GRE-Q 500, overall undergraduate GPA 3.0; *Social PhD (Doctor of Philosophy)*: GRE-V 500, GRE-Q 500, overall undergraduate GPA 3.0.

Other Criteria: (importance of criteria rated low, medium, or high): GRE scores—high, research experience—high, work experience—medium, clinically related public service—medium, GPA—high, letters of recommendation—high, interview—medium, statement of goals and objectives—high. For additional information on admission requirements, go to http://psychology.unc.edu/graduate/admissions.html.

Student Characteristics: The following represents characteristics of students in 2009–2010 in all graduate psychology programs in the department: Female—full-time 78, part-time 0; Male—full-time 36, part-time 0; African American/Black—full-time 12, part-time 0; Hispanic/Latino(a)—full-time 4, part-time 0; Asian/Pacific Islander—full-time 11, part-time 0; American Indian/Alaska Native—full-time 0, part-time 0; Caucasian/White—full-time 83, part-time 0; Multi-ethnic—full-time 0, part-time 0; students subject to the Americans With Disabilities Act—full-time 0, part-time 0; Unknown ethnicity—full-time 4, part-time 0; International students who hold an F-1 or J-1 Visa—full-time 12, part-time 0.

Financial Information/Assistance:

Tuition for Full-Time Study: *Doctoral:* State residents: per academic year $7,162; Nonstate residents: per academic year $21,560. See the following Web site for updates and changes in tuition costs: http://finance.unc.edu/university-controller/student-account-services/student-billing.html.

Financial Assistance:

First-Year Students: Teaching assistantships available for first year. Average amount paid per academic year: $15,140. Average number of hours worked per week: 15. Research assistantships available for first year. Average amount paid per academic year: $15,140. Average number of hours worked per week: 15. Traineeships available for first year. Average amount paid per academic year: $20,996. Fellowships and scholarships available for first year. Average amount paid per academic year: $20,000.

Advanced Students: Teaching assistantships available for advanced students. Average amount paid per academic year: $16,200. Average number of hours worked per week: 15. Research assistantships available for advanced students. Average amount paid per academic year: $15,000. Average number of hours worked per week: 15. Traineeships available for advanced students. Average amount paid per academic year: $20,996. Fellowships and scholarships available for advanced students. Average amount paid per academic year: $20,000.

Additional Information: Of all students currently enrolled full time, 90% benefited from one or more of the listed financial assistance programs.

Internships/Practica: Doctoral Degree (PhD Clinical): For those doctoral students for whom a professional internship was required in this program prior to graduation, (6) students applied for an internship in 2008–2009, with (6) students obtaining an internship. Of those students who obtained an internship, (6) were paid internships. Of those students who obtained an internship, (4) students placed in APA/CPA accredited internships, (2) students placed in internships not APA/CPA accredited, but listed with the Association of Psychology Postdoctoral and Internship Programs (APPIC), (0) students placed in internships conforming to guidelines of the Council of Directors of School Psychology Programs (CDSPP), (0) students placed in internships that were not APA/CPA accredited, APPIC or CDSPP listed. Students within the doctoral program in clinical psychology engage in a wide range of clinical practicum activities beginning in the first year of doctoral study. A variety of sites are included in our practicum arrangements. One of these sites is the University of North Carolina Medical School, which includes opportunities in a number of areas including child, family, adolescent, and adults. There are also specialized opportunities at that site to work with children with developmental disabilities and college students in a university counseling setting. Students also receive training at John Umstead Hospital, a state psychiatric hospital; opportunities there range from child, adolescent, adult, and geriatric patients. Overall, Umstead Hospital emphasizes treatment of more disturbed individuals, but opportunities are available as well for outpatient treatment. Third, students are involved in our Psychology Department Psychological Services Center, our in-house outpatient treatment facility. Students work with a wide variety of clients within that context, with specialized opportunities in the anxiety disorders and marital therapy. Among other sites, students provide consultation to the local school system, to the Orange-Person-Chatham Mental Health Center, and a variety of other sites that are arranged on an as needed basis.

Housing and Day Care: On-campus housing is available. See the following Web site for more information: http://housing.unc.edu/. No on-campus day care facilities are available.

Employment of Department Graduates:
Master's Degree Graduates: Of those who graduated in the academic year 2008–2009, the following categories and numbers represent the postgraduate activities and employment of master's degree graduates: Enrolled in a postdoctoral residency/fellowship (n/a), employed in independent practice (n/a), total from the above (master's) (0).
Doctoral Degree Graduates: Of those who graduated in the academic year 2008–2009, the following categories and numbers represent the postgraduate activities and employment of doctoral degree graduates: Enrolled in a psychology doctoral program (n/a), total from the above (doctoral) (0).

Additional Information:
Orientation, Objectives, and Emphasis of Department: Each graduate training program is designed to acquaint students with the theoretical and research content of their specialty and to train them in the research and teaching skills needed to make contributions to science and society. In addition, certain programs (for example, the clinical program) include an emphasis on the development of competence in appropriate professional skills. Faculty members maintain a balance of commitment to research, teaching and service.

Special Facilities or Resources: Affiliated clinical and research facilities are: the Psychological Services Center, Psychology Department; John Umstead State Hospital, Butner, NC; North Carolina Memorial Hospital, Chapel Hill; Murdoch Center for the Retarded, Butner; Division for Disorders of Development and Learning, Chapel Hill; VA Hospital, Durham; Frank Porter Graham Child Development Center, Chapel Hill; Carolina Population Center, Chapel Hill; Alcoholic Rehabilitation Center, Butner; North Carolina Highway Safety Research Center, Chapel Hill; L.L. Thurstone Psychometric Laboratory, Chapel Hill; Human Psychophysiology Laboratory, Chapel Hill; Institute for Research in Social Sciences, Chapel Hill; Laboratory for Computing and Cognition, Chapel Hill; Neurobiology Curriculum, University of North Carolina; Research Laboratories of the U.S. Environmental Protection Agency, Research Triangle Park; and TEACCH Division, North Carolina Memorial Hospital, specializing in the treatment and education of victims of autism and related disorders of communication.

Information for Students With Physical Disabilities: See the following Web site for more information: http://disabilityservices.unc.edu/.

Application Information:
Send to Graduate Admissions, CB#3270, 203 Davie Hall, Department of Psychology, UNC-Chapel Hill, NC 27599-3270. Application available online. URL of online application: http://psychology.unc.edu/graduate/admissions.html. Students are admitted in the Fall, application deadline December 1. *Fee:* $77.

North Carolina, University of, Charlotte
Department of Psychology
Arts and Sciences
9201 University City Boulevard
Charlotte, NC 28223-0001
Telephone: (704) 687-4731
Fax: (704) 687-3096
E-mail: *rtedesch@email.uncc.edu*
Web: *http://psych.uncc.edu/*

Department Information:
1960. Graduate Coordinator: Dr. Richard Tedeschi. Number of faculty: total—full-time 29, part-time 6; women—full-time 12, part-time 2; total—minority—full-time 3; women minority—full-time 2.

Programs and Degrees Offered:
Listed in the following order: Program area, degree type (T if terminal Master's), number awarded 7/08–6/09. Clinical/Community MA/MS (Master of Arts/Science) (T) 3, Industrial/Organizational MA/MS (Master of Arts/Science) (T) 7, Organizational Science PhD (Doctor of Philosophy) 0, Health Psychology PhD (Doctor of Philosophy) 0.

Student Applications/Admissions:
Student Applications
Clinical/Community MA/MS (Master of Arts/Science)—Applications 2009–2010, 75. Total applicants accepted 2009–2010, 10. Number full-time enrolled (new admits only) 2009–2010, 4. Number part-time enrolled (new admits only) 2009–2010, 0. Total enrolled 2009–2010 full-time, 17, part-time, 20. Openings 2010–2011, 12. The median number of years required for completion of a degree in 2008–2009 were 2. The number of students enrolled full- and part-time who were dismissed or voluntarily withdrew from this program area in 2008–2009 were 2. *Industrial/Organizational MA/MS (Master of Arts/Science)*—Applications 2009–2010, 103. Total applicants accepted 2009–2010, 7. Number full-time enrolled (new admits only) 2009–2010, 7. Number part-time enrolled (new admits only) 2009–2010, 0. Total enrolled 2009–2010 full-time, 16, part-time, 3. Openings 2010–2011, 12. The median number of years required for completion of a degree in 2008–2009 were 2. The number of students enrolled full- and part-time who were dismissed or voluntarily withdrew from this program area in 2008–2009 were 0. *Organizational Science PhD (Doctor of Philosophy)*—Applications 2009–2010, 50. Total applicants accepted 2009–2010, 8. Number full-time enrolled (new admits only) 2009–2010, 8. Total enrolled 2009–2010 full-time, 15. Openings 2010–2011, 4. The median number of years required for completion of a degree in 2008–2009 were 2. The number of students enrolled full- and part-time who were dismissed or voluntarily withdrew from this program area in 2008–2009 were 0. *Health Psychology PhD (Doctor of Philosophy)*—Applications 2009–2010, 35. Total applicants accepted 2009–2010, 6. Number full-time enrolled (new admits only) 2009–2010, 3. Number part-time enrolled (new

admits only) 2009–2010, 0. Total enrolled 2009–2010 full-time, 23, part-time, 7. The number of students enrolled full- and part-time who were dismissed or voluntarily withdrew from this program area in 2008–2009 were 1.

Scores: Entries appear in this order: required test or GPA, minimum score (if required), median score of students entering in 2009–2010. *Clinical/Community MA/MS (Master of Arts/Science):* overall undergraduate GPA 2.8, psychology GPA 3.0; *Industrial/Organizational MA/MS (Master of Arts/Science):* GRE-V no minimum stated, GRE-Q no minimum stated, overall undergraduate GPA 3.0; *Organizational Science PhD (Doctor of Philosophy):* GRE-V no minimum stated, GRE-Q no minimum stated, GRE-Analytical no minimum stated, overall undergraduate GPA 3.0.

Other Criteria: (importance of criteria rated low, medium, or high): GRE scores—high, research experience—high, work experience—medium, extracurricular activity—low, clinically related public service—medium, GPA—high, letters of recommendation—high, interview—low, statement of goals and objectives—high, Community work important for clinical/community MA program only.

Student Characteristics: The following represents characteristics of students in 2009–2010 in all graduate psychology programs in the department: Female—full-time 51, part-time 13; Male—full-time 15, part-time 2; African American/Black—full-time 5, part-time 0; Hispanic/Latino(a)—full-time 1, part-time 0; Asian/Pacific Islander—full-time 3, part-time 0; American Indian/Alaska Native—full-time 0, part-time 0; Caucasian/White—full-time 57, part-time 15; Multi-ethnic—full-time 0, part-time 0; students subject to the Americans With Disabilities Act—full-time 0, part-time 0; Unknown ethnicity—full-time 0, part-time 0; International students who hold an F-1 or J-1 Visa—full-time 1, part-time 0.

Financial Information/Assistance:
Tuition for Full-Time Study: *Master's:* State residents: per academic year $4,830; Nonstate residents: per academic year $15,237. *Doctoral:* State residents: per academic year $4,830; Nonstate residents: per academic year $15,237. Tuition is subject to change.

Financial Assistance:
First-Year Students: Teaching assistantships available for first year. Average amount paid per academic year: $9,000. Average number of hours worked per week: 20. Apply by March 1. Research assistantships available for first year. Average amount paid per academic year: $8,500. Average number of hours worked per week: 20. Apply by March 1. Fellowships and scholarships available for first year. Average amount paid per academic year: $2,150. Apply by March 1.

Advanced Students: Teaching assistantships available for advanced students. Average amount paid per academic year: $9,000. Average number of hours worked per week: 20. Research assistantships available for advanced students. Average amount paid per academic year: $8,500. Average number of hours worked per week: 20.

Additional Information: Of all students currently enrolled full time, 60% benefited from one or more of the listed financial assistance programs. Application and information available online at: http://www.uncc.edu/finaid.

Internships/Practica: Clinical/Community: Students are required to enroll in 2 semesters of practicum, working 22 hrs/week in community agencies such as mental health centers, prisons, hospitals, and non-profit organizations. Industrial/Organizational: An extensive practicum component utilizes the Charlotte area as the setting for applied experience. All students must complete 3 hours of projects in I/O Psychology and they are strongly encouraged to take 6 hours.

Housing and Day Care: On-campus housing is available. No on-campus day care facilities are available.

Employment of Department Graduates:
Master's Degree Graduates: Of those who graduated in the academic year 2008–2009, the following categories and numbers represent the postgraduate activities and employment of master's degree graduates: Enrolled in a postdoctoral residency/fellowship (n/a), employed in independent practice (n/a), employed in other positions at a higher education institution (1), employed in business or industry (5), total from the above (master's) (6).

Doctoral Degree Graduates: Of those who graduated in the academic year 2008–2009, the following categories and numbers represent the postgraduate activities and employment of doctoral degree graduates: Enrolled in a psychology doctoral program (n/a), total from the above (doctoral) (0).

Additional Information:
Orientation, Objectives, and Emphasis of Department: The objective of the master's degree program is to train psychologists in the knowledge and skills necessary to address problems encountered in industry, organizations, and the community. The program has an applied emphasis. Graduates of the program are eligible to apply for licensing in North Carolina as psychological associates. Although our goals emphasize application of psychological principles in organizational, clinical, and community settings, the rigorous program allows students to prepare themselves well for further education in psychology.

Special Facilities or Resources: The psychology department is housed in a modern classroom office building that provides offices, demonstration rooms, a workshop, and specialty laboratories for research. Facilities include a computerized laboratory with 37 microcomputers; many small testing, training, and interview rooms with one-way mirrors for direct observation; audio intercommunications; and closed circuit television. There is extensive audio and video equipment available as well as a research trailer, tachistoscopes, programming and timing equipment, and microcomputers. The psychometric laboratory contains an extensive inventory of current tests of intelligence, personality, and interest, as well as calculators and microcomputers for testing, test score evaluation and data analysis. A well-equipped physiological laboratory is available for work including human electrophysiology.

Application Information:
Send to Graduate Admissions, UNC-Charlotte, 9201 University City Blvd., Charlotte, NC 28223. Application available online. URL of online application: https://app.applyyourself.com/?id=uncc-cob. Students are admitted in the Fall, application deadline March 1. January 15 is the deadline for Industrial/Organizational program. March 1 is the deadline for Clinical/Community MA program. December 1 is the deadline for Health PhD program. *Fee:* $35.

North Carolina, University of, Wilmington
Psychology
Arts and Sciences
601 South College Road
Wilmington, NC 28403-5612
Telephone: (910) 962-3370
Fax: (910) 962-7010
E-mail: ogler@uncw.edu
Web: http://www.uncw.edu/psy/

Department Information:
1972. Chairperson: J. Mark Galizio, PhD Number of faculty: total—full-time 32; women—full-time 16; total—minority—full-time 4; women minority—full-time 2; faculty subject to the Americans With Disabilities Act 1.

Programs and Degrees Offered:
Listed in the following order: Program area, degree type (T if terminal Master's), number awarded 7/08–6/09. General Psychology MA/MS (Master of Arts/Science) (T) 9, Applied Behavior Analysis MA/MS (Master of Arts/Science) (T) 1, Substance Abuse Treatment MA/MS (Master of Arts/Science) (T) 6.

Student Applications/Admissions:
Student Applications
General Psychology MA/MS (Master of Arts/Science)—Applications 2009–2010, 50. Total applicants accepted 2009–2010, 15. Number full-time enrolled (new admits only) 2009–2010, 10. Number part-time enrolled (new admits only) 2009–2010, 0. Total enrolled 2009–2010 full-time, 15, part-time, 7. Openings 2010–2011, 14. The median number of years required for completion of a degree in 2008–2009 were 2. The number of students enrolled full- and part-time who were dismissed or voluntarily withdrew from this program area in 2008–2009 were 0. Applied Behavior Analysis MA/MS (Master of Arts/Science)—Applications 2009–2010, 22. Total applicants accepted 2009–2010, 6. Number full-time enrolled (new admits only) 2009–2010, 5. Number part-time enrolled (new admits only) 2009–2010, 0. Openings 2010–2011, 6. The median number of years required for completion of a degree in 2008–2009 were 3. The number of students enrolled full- and part-time who were dismissed or voluntarily withdrew from this program area in 2008–2009 were 0. Substance Abuse Treatment MA/MS (Master of Arts/Science)—Applications 2009–2010, 35. Total applicants accepted 2009–2010, 9. Number full-time enrolled (new admits only) 2009–2010, 7. Number part-time enrolled (new admits only) 2009–2010, 0. Openings 2010–2011, 7. The median number of years required for completion of a degree in 2008–2009 were 3. The number of students enrolled full- and part-time who were dismissed or voluntarily withdrew from this program area in 2008–2009 were 0.
Other Criteria: (importance of criteria rated low, medium, or high): GRE scores—high, research experience—high, work experience—low, extracurricular activity—low, clinically related public service—medium, GPA—high, letters of recommendation—high, interview—high, statement of goals and objectives—high, In the Substance Abuse Treatment Psychology concentration, clinically related public service may be given more weight, since this concentration emphasizes the development of clinical as well as research skills. In the Applied Behavior Analysis concentration, previous experience—volunteer or paid—with people with disabilities is very important. For additional information on admission requirements, go to http://www.uncw.edu/psy/.

Student Characteristics: The following represents characteristics of students in 2009–2010 in all graduate psychology programs in the department: Female—full-time 20, part-time 4; Male—full-time 15, part-time 1; African American/Black—full-time 3, part-time 0; Hispanic/Latino(a)—full-time 2, part-time 1; Asian/Pacific Islander—full-time 1, part-time 0; American Indian/Alaska Native—full-time 0, part-time 0; Caucasian/White—full-time 29, part-time 4; Multi-ethnic—full-time 0, part-time 0; students subject to the Americans With Disabilities Act—full-time 0, part-time 0; Unknown ethnicity—full-time 0, part-time 0; International students who hold an F-1 or J-1 Visa—full-time 0, part-time 0.

Financial Information/Assistance:
Tuition for Full-Time Study: *Master's:* State residents: per academic year $5,094; Nonstate residents: per academic year $15,808. Tuition is subject to change. See the following Web site for updates and changes in tuition costs: http://www.uncw.edu/ba/finance/StudentAccounts/tuition_fees.html.

Financial Assistance:
First-Year Students: Teaching assistantships available for first year. Average amount paid per academic year: $9,500. Average number of hours worked per week: 20. Apply by January 15. Research assistantships available for first year. Average amount paid per academic year: $9,500. Average number of hours worked per week: 20. Apply by January 15. Traineeships available for first year. Apply by January 15.
Advanced Students: Teaching assistantships available for advanced students. Average amount paid per academic year: $9,500. Average number of hours worked per week: 20. Apply by January 15. Research assistantships available for advanced students. Average amount paid per academic year: $9,500. Average number of hours worked per week: 20. Apply by January 15.
Additional Information: Of all students currently enrolled full time, 83% benefited from one or more of the listed financial assistance programs.

Internships/Practica: Master's Degree (MA/MS Applied Behavior Analysis): An internship experience, such as, a final research project or "capstone" experience is required of graduates. Master's Degree (MA/MS Substance Abuse Treatment): An internship experience, such as, a final research project or "capstone" experience is required of graduates. In the Substance Abuse Treatment Psychology concentration and our new Applied Behavior Analysis Concentration, students are prepared for work with dual diagnosis clients or with developmentally disabled clients through the completion of a required practicum and internship. The required internship and practicum consist of at least 1500 hours total of supervised experience working with substance abuse, autism, mental retardation and other psychological and behavioral problems. Training sites include: community mental health centers, correctional Institutions, university counseling centers, Inpatient and outpatient substance abuse treatment centers, and residential centers for autistic and mentally retarded individuals.

Housing and Day Care: On-campus housing is available. See the following Web site for more information: http://www.uncw.edu/stuaff/housing/. No on-campus day care facilities are available.

Employment of Department Graduates:
Master's Degree Graduates: Of those who graduated in the academic year 2008–2009, the following categories and numbers represent the postgraduate activities and employment of master's degree graduates: Enrolled in a psychology doctoral program (4), enrolled in another graduate/professional program (1), enrolled in a postdoctoral residency/fellowship (n/a), employed in independent practice (n/a), employed in an academic position at a 2-year/4-year college (2), employed in other positions at a higher education institution (1), employed in business or industry (2), employed in government agency (1), employed in a community mental health/counseling center (4), not seeking employment (1), other employment position (2), total from the above (master's) (18).
Doctoral Degree Graduates: Of those who graduated in the academic year 2008–2009, the following categories and numbers represent the postgraduate activities and employment of doctoral degree graduates: Enrolled in a psychology doctoral program (n/a), total from the above (doctoral) (0).

Additional Information:
Orientation, Objectives, and Emphasis of Department: The department is committed to fostering an understanding of psychological research and stresses the relationship between students and professors in this process. Research methodology and application are emphasized for all students. Students in the General Psychology concentration are prepared to continue to the PhD in a variety of content areas. Students completing the clinical concentration in Substance Abuse Treatment are prepared to work with dual diagnosis clients in mental health clinics and other public service agencies. The clinical Applied Behavior Analysis concentration prepares students for work primarily with autistic and mentally retarded individuals. The SATP and ABA graduates meet all academic requirements to apply for North Carolina state licensure as a Psychological Associate and either North Carolina state certification as a Licensed Clinical Addictions Specialist (SATP concentration) or national Board Certification as a Behavior Analyst (BCBA concentration).

Special Facilities or Resources: Special facilities or resources include research laboratories (behavioral pharmacology, human, and animal) videotape and digital recording equipment. All students have access to word processing, SAS, and SPSS on the university computer system.

Information for Students With Physical Disabilities: See the following Web site for more information: http://www.uncw.edu/stuaff/disability/.

Application Information:
Send to Graduate School, University of North Carolina Wilmington, 601 South College Road, Wilmington, NC 28403-5955. Application available online. URL of online application: http://uncw.edu/grad_info/prospectivestudents.htm. Students are admitted in the Fall, application deadline January 15. *Fee:* $45. Fee waived for McNair Scholars.

Wake Forest University
Department of Psychology
Arts and Sciences
P.O. Box 7778
Winston-Salem, NC 27109
Telephone: (336) 758-5424
Fax: (336) 758-4733
E-mail: *seta@wfu.edu*
Web: *http://www.wfu.edu/psychology*

Department Information:
1958. Chairperson: Dale Dagenbach. Number of faculty: total—full-time 16, part-time 13; women—full-time 6, part-time 5; total—minority—full-time 1; women minority—full-time 1.

Programs and Degrees Offered:
Listed in the following order: Program area, degree type (T if terminal Master's), number awarded 7/08–6/09. General Psychology MA/MS (Master of Arts/Science) (T) 11.

Student Applications/Admissions:
Student Applications
General Psychology MA/MS (*Master of Arts/Science*)—Applications 2009–2010, 108. Total applicants accepted 2009–2010, 11. Number full-time enrolled (new admits only) 2009–2010, 11. Number part-time enrolled (new admits only) 2009–2010, 0. Openings 2010–2011, 13. The median number of years required for completion of a degree in 2008–2009 were 2. The number of students enrolled full- and part-time who were dismissed or voluntarily withdrew from this program area in 2008–2009 were 1.
Scores: Entries appear in this order: required test or GPA, minimum score (if required), median score of students entering in 2009–2010. *General Psychology MA/MS (Master of Arts/Science):* GRE-V no minimum stated, 550, GRE-Q no minimum stated, 695, GRE-Analytical no minimum stated, overall undergraduate GPA no minimum stated, 3.57, last 2 years GPA no minimum stated, psychology GPA no minimum stated.
Other Criteria: (importance of criteria rated low, medium, or high): GRE scores—medium, research experience—high, GPA—medium, letters of recommendation—high, interview—medium, statement of goals and objectives—high, undergraduate major in psychology—low, specific undergraduate psychology courses taken—medium. For additional information on admission requirements, go to http://www.wfu.edu/psychology/grad/index.html.

Student Characteristics: The following represents characteristics of students in 2009–2010 in all graduate psychology programs in the department: Female—full-time 14, part-time 0; Male—full-time 7, part-time 0; African American/Black—part-time 0; Hispanic/Latino(a)—full-time 0, part-time 0; Asian/Pacific Islander—full-time 1, part-time 0; American Indian/Alaska Native—full-time 0, part-time 0; Caucasian/White—full-time 19, part-time 0; Multi-ethnic—full-time 1, part-time 0; students subject to the Americans With Disabilities Act—full-time 0, part-time 0; Unknown ethnicity—full-time 0, part-time 0; International students who hold an F-1 or J-1 Visa—full-time 0, part-time 0.

Financial Information/Assistance:

Tuition for Full-Time Study: *Master's:* State residents: per academic year $29,190, $1,040 per credit hour; Nonstate residents: per academic year $29,190, $1,040 per credit hour. Tuition is subject to change. See the following Web site for updates and changes in tuition costs: http://graduate.wfu.edu/.

Financial Assistance:

First-Year Students: Teaching assistantships available for first year. Average amount paid per academic year: $9,000. Average number of hours worked per week: 15. Apply by January 15. Research assistantships available for first year. Average amount paid per academic year: $9,000. Average number of hours worked per week: 15. Apply by January 15.

Advanced Students: Teaching assistantships available for advanced students. Average amount paid per academic year: $9,000. Average number of hours worked per week: 15. Apply by January 15. Research assistantships available for advanced students. Average amount paid per academic year: $9,000. Average number of hours worked per week: 15. Apply by January 15.

Additional Information: Of all students currently enrolled full time, 100% benefited from one or more of the listed financial assistance programs. Application and information available online at: http://graduate.wfu.edu/admissions/index.html.

Internships/Practica: Master's Degree (MA/MS General Psychology): An internship experience, such as, a final research project or "capstone" experience is required of graduates.

Housing and Day Care: No on-campus housing is available. No on-campus day care facilities are available.

Employment of Department Graduates:

Master's Degree Graduates: Of those who graduated in the academic year 2008–2009, the following categories and numbers represent the postgraduate activities and employment of master's degree graduates: Enrolled in a psychology doctoral program (8), enrolled in another graduate/professional program (0), enrolled in a postdoctoral residency/fellowship (n/a), employed in independent practice (n/a), employed in other positions at a higher education institution (1), total from the above (master's) (9).

Doctoral Degree Graduates: Of those who graduated in the academic year 2008–2009, the following categories and numbers represent the postgraduate activities and employment of doctoral degree graduates: Enrolled in a psychology doctoral program (n/a), total from the above (doctoral) (0).

Additional Information:

Orientation, Objectives, and Emphasis of Department: The department aims to provide rigorous master's level training, with an emphasis on mastery of theory, research methodology, and content in the basic areas of psychology. This is a general, research-oriented MA program for capable students, most of whom will continue to the PhD.

Special Facilities or Resources: The department of psychology occupies a beautiful and spacious building that is equipped with state-of-the art teaching and laboratory facilities. Learning resources include in-class multimedia instruction equipment, departmental mini- and microcomputers, departmental and university libraries, and information technology centers. Ample research space is available, including social, developmental, cognitive, perception, physiological, and animal behavior laboratories. Office space is available for graduate students. The department has links with the Wake Forest University School of Medicine (e.g., Neuroscience) which can provide opportunities for students. All students work closely with individual faculty on research during both years (2:1 student/faculty ratio). Wake Forest University offers the academic and technological resources, facilities, and Division I athletic programs, music, theater, and art associated with a larger university, with the individual attention that a smaller university can provide.

Information for Students With Physical Disabilities: See the following Web site for more information: http://www.wfu.edu/lac/disability-svcs.html.

Application Information:

Send to Dean of Graduate School, Wake Forest University, PO 7487, Winston-Salem, NC 27109. Application available online. URL of online application: http://graduate.wfu.edu/admissions/onlineapp.html. Students are admitted in the Fall, application deadline January 15. *Fee:* $60. Upon request to the Graduate School, application fee can be waived for reasons of financial hardship.

NORTH DAKOTA

North Dakota State University
Department of Psychology
Science and Mathematics
115 Minard Hall
Fargo, ND 58105
Telephone: (701) 231-8622
Fax: (701) 231-8426
E-mail: NDSU.psych@ndsu.edu
Web: http://www.psych.ndsu.nodak.edu/

Department Information:
1965. Chairperson: Paul D. Rokke. Number of faculty: total—full-time 20, part-time 5; women—full-time 5, part-time 4.

Programs and Degrees Offered:
Listed in the following order: Program area, degree type (T if terminal Master's), number awarded 7/08–6/09. Clinical Psychology MA/MS (Master of Arts/Science) (T) 1, Cognitive and Visual Neuroscience PhD (Doctor of Philosophy) 0, Health/Social Psychology PhD (Doctor of Philosophy) 1.

Student Applications/Admissions:
Student Applications
Clinical Psychology MA/MS (Master of Arts/Science)—Applications 2009–2010, 25. Total applicants accepted 2009–2010, 7. Number full-time enrolled (new admits only) 2009–2010, 4. Openings 2010–2011, 6. The median number of years required for completion of a degree in 2008–2009 were 2. The number of students enrolled full- and part-time who were dismissed or voluntarily withdrew from this program area in 2008–2009 were 1. Cognitive and Visual Neuroscience PhD (Doctor of Philosophy)—Applications 2009–2010, 3. Total applicants accepted 2009–2010, 1. Number full-time enrolled (new admits only) 2009–2010, 0. Total enrolled 2009–2010 full-time, 8. Openings 2010–2011, 3. The number of students enrolled full- and part-time who were dismissed or voluntarily withdrew from this program area in 2008–2009 were 2. Health/Social Psychology PhD (Doctor of Philosophy)—Applications 2009–2010, 13. Total applicants accepted 2009–2010, 3. Number full-time enrolled (new admits only) 2009–2010, 1. Total enrolled 2009–2010 full-time, 12. Openings 2010–2011, 3. The median number of years required for completion of a degree in 2008–2009 were 4. The number of students enrolled full- and part-time who were dismissed or voluntarily withdrew from this program area in 2008–2009 were 1.
Other Criteria: (importance of criteria rated low, medium, or high): GRE scores—high, research experience—high, extracurricular activity—low, GPA—high, letters of recommendation—high, statement of goals and objectives—high, undergraduate major in psychology—low, specific undergraduate psychology courses taken—medium.

Student Characteristics: The following represents characteristics of students in 2009–2010 in all graduate psychology programs in the department: Female—full-time 20, part-time 0; Male—full-time 10, part-time 1; African American/Black—full-time 0, part-time 0; Hispanic/Latino(a)—full-time 1, part-time 0; Asian/Pacific Islander—full-time 1, part-time 0; American Indian/Alaska Native—full-time 0, part-time 0; Caucasian/White—full-time 0, part-time 0; Multi-ethnic—full-time 0, part-time 0; students subject to the Americans With Disabilities Act—full-time 0, part-time 0; Unknown ethnicity—full-time 0, part-time 0; International students who hold an F-1 or J-1 Visa—full-time 2, part-time 0.

Financial Information/Assistance:
Tuition for Full-Time Study: *Master's:* State residents: per academic year $5,995, $236 per credit hour; Nonstate residents: per academic year $14,354, $628 per credit hour. *Doctoral:* State residents: per academic year $5,995, $236 per credit hour; Nonstate residents: per academic year $14,354, $628 per credit hour. Additional fees are assessed to students beyond the costs of tuition for the following: Student fees cover cost of wellness center, technology access, athletic events. See the following Web site for updates and changes in tuition costs: http://www.ndsu.edu/bisonconnection/accounts/tuition/.

Financial Assistance:
First-Year Students: Teaching assistantships available for first year. Average amount paid per academic year: $5,800. Average number of hours worked per week: 10. Apply by February 15. Research assistantships available for first year. Average amount paid per academic year: $5,800. Average number of hours worked per week: 10. Apply by February 15.

Advanced Students: Teaching assistantships available for advanced students. Average amount paid per academic year: $16,000. Average number of hours worked per week: 20. Apply by February 15. Research assistantships available for advanced students. Average amount paid per academic year: $16,000. Average number of hours worked per week: 20. Apply by February 15. Fellowships and scholarships available for advanced students. Average amount paid per academic year: $16,000. Average number of hours worked per week: 20. Apply by February 15.

Additional Information: Of all students currently enrolled full time, 100% benefited from one or more of the listed financial assistance programs. Application and information available online at: http://www.ndsu.edu/bisonconnection/finaid/.

Internships/Practica: Master's Degree (MA/MS Clinical Psychology): An internship experience, such as a final research project or "capstone" experience is required of graduates. Our master's program in clinical psychology has a number of clinical practica that provide a variety of experiences. These include work with traditional one-on-one counseling, chronic pain, eating disorders, behavior analysis, developmental disabilities, child and adolescent psychotherapy, community mental health, and clinical neuropsychology. Research practica are available for doctoral students who wish to develop applied research skills and experiences. Sites include a private foundation for research on addictions and eating disorders, a nationally prominent organization for clinical drug trials, a chronic pain treatment program, a community mental health center, and several sites devoted to survey research.

Housing and Day Care: On-campus housing is available. See the following Web site for more information: http://www.ndsu.edu/

reslife/. On-campus day care facilities are available. See the following Web site for more information: http://www.ndsu.edu/hdfs/center_for_child_development/.

Employment of Department Graduates:
Master's Degree Graduates: Of those who graduated in the academic year 2008–2009, the following categories and numbers represent the postgraduate activities and employment of master's degree graduates: Enrolled in a psychology doctoral program (4), enrolled in a postdoctoral residency/fellowship (n/a), employed in independent practice (n/a), employed in a community mental health/counseling center (1), employed in a hospital/medical center (1), do not know (1), total from the above (master's) (7).
Doctoral Degree Graduates: Of those who graduated in the academic year 2008–2009, the following categories and numbers represent the postgraduate activities and employment of doctoral degree graduates: Enrolled in a psychology doctoral program (n/a), employed in an academic position at a university (1), total from the above (doctoral) (1).

Additional Information:
Orientation, Objectives, and Emphasis of Department: Our strong research tradition has earned us a reputation as one of the best small psychology departments in the nation. Our clinical master's program is over 30 years old, and many of our alumni have gone on to earn PhDs at top institutions. Our doctoral program emphasizes our strengths in health psychology and neuroscience. PhD training is designed to produce graduates with records in research and teaching, which will make them highly competitive for employment in both traditional academic and nontraditional government and private sector settings. Our programs are based on a mentoring model, in which students work closely with specific faculty members who match their research interests.

Special Facilities or Resources: The department has state-of-the-art facilities for research in electrophysiology (including EEG), vision, and cognition, as well as ample space for other research projects. A center for research on virtual reality, multi-sensory integration, and driving simulation is very active. As the largest population center in the region, Fargo-Moorhead serves as a center for medical services for a large geographic area. There are 3 major hospitals (including a VA), a medical school Department of Neuroscience, a psychiatric hospital, a neuroscience research institute, and a private pharmaceutical research institute, which offer opportunities for collaboration. NDSU also has a Research and Technology Park which may offer research experiences involving advanced technology.

Information for Students With Physical Disabilities: See the following Web site for more information: http://www.ndsu.edu/disabilityservices/.

Application Information:
Send to Office of Graduate Studies, PO Box 5790, NDSU, Fargo, ND 58105-5790. Application available online. URL of online application: http://www.ndsu.edu/gradschool/. Students are admitted in the Fall, application deadline February 15. Applications arriving after deadlines will be considered until positions are filled. *Fee:* $50.

North Dakota, University of
Department of Psychology
Arts and Science
P.O. Box 8380
Grand Forks, ND 58202-8380
Telephone: (701) 777-3451
Fax: (701) 777-3454
E-mail: *alan.king@und.edu*
Web: *http://www.und.edu/dept/psych/*

Department Information:
1921. Chairperson: Mark Grabe. Number of faculty: total—full-time 21; women—full-time 8; total—minority—full-time 1; faculty subject to the Americans With Disabilities Act 1.

Programs and Degrees Offered:
Listed in the following order: Program area, degree type (T if terminal Master's), number awarded 7/08–6/09. Clinical Psychology PhD (Doctor of Philosophy) 7, General Experimental Psychology PhD (Doctor of Philosophy) 1.

APA Accreditation: Clinical PhD (Doctor of Philosophy). Student Outcome Data Website: http://www.und.edu/dept/psych/clinical.html.

Student Applications/Admissions:
Student Applications
Clinical Psychology PhD (Doctor of Philosophy)—Applications 2009–2010, 111. Total applicants accepted 2009–2010, 7. Number full-time enrolled (new admits only) 2009–2010, 7. Number part-time enrolled (new admits only) 2009–2010, 0. Openings 2010–2011, 7. The median number of years required for completion of a degree in 2008–2009 were 6. The number of students enrolled full- and part-time who were dismissed or voluntarily withdrew from this program area in 2008–2009 were 2. *General Experimental Psychology PhD (Doctor of Philosophy)*—Applications 2009–2010, 12. Total applicants accepted 2009–2010, 2. Number full-time enrolled (new admits only) 2009–2010, 2. Number part-time enrolled (new admits only) 2009–2010, 0. Openings 2010–2011, 3. The median number of years required for completion of a degree in 2008–2009 were 5. The number of students enrolled full- and part-time who were dismissed or voluntarily withdrew from this program area in 2008–2009 were 0.
Scores: Entries appear in this order: required test or GPA, minimum score (if required), median score of students entering in 2009–2010. *Clinical Psychology PhD (Doctor of Philosophy):* GRE-V no minimum stated, 606, GRE-Q no minimum stated, 650, GRE-Analytical no minimum stated, 4.7, GRE-Subject (Psychology) no minimum stated, 691, overall undergraduate GPA no minimum stated, 3.73, last 2 years GPA no minimum stated, Masters GPA no minimum stated.
Other Criteria: (importance of criteria rated low, medium, or high): GRE scores—medium, research experience—high, work experience—medium, extracurricular activity—low, clinically related public service—medium, GPA—high, letters of recommendation—medium, interview—low, statement of goals and objectives—medium, specific undergraduate psychology courses taken—medium. For additional information on admission requirements, go to http://www.und.edu/dept/psych/clinicaladmission.html.

Student Characteristics: The following represents characteristics of students in 2009–2010 in all graduate psychology programs in the department: Female—full-time 46, part-time 0; Male—full-time 11, part-time 0; African American/Black—full-time 1, part-time 0; Hispanic/Latino(a)—full-time 0, part-time 0; Asian/Pacific Islander—full-time 1, part-time 0; American Indian/Alaska Native—full-time 11, part-time 0; Caucasian/White—full-time 0, part-time 0; Multi-ethnic—full-time 0, part-time 0; students subject to the Americans With Disabilities Act—full-time 0, part-time 0; Unknown ethnicity—full-time 0, part-time 0; International students who hold an F-1 or J-1 Visa—full-time 0, part-time 0.

Financial Information/Assistance:

Tuition for Full-Time Study: *Master's:* State residents: per academic year $7,565, $298 per credit hour; Nonstate residents: per academic year $17,810, $706 per credit hour. *Doctoral:* State residents: per academic year $7,565, $298 per credit hour; Nonstate residents: per academic year $17,810, $706 per credit hour. Tuition is subject to change. See the following Web site for updates and changes in tuition costs: http://www.und.edu/dept/studentaccounts/html/tuitionrates.htm. Higher tuition cost for this program: Tuition rates apply only to students not supported by tuition waivers.

Financial Assistance:

First-Year Students: Teaching assistantships available for first year. Average amount paid per academic year: $11,241. Average number of hours worked per week: 15. Apply by none.

Advanced Students: Teaching assistantships available for advanced students. Average amount paid per academic year: $15,581. Average number of hours worked per week: 15.

Additional Information: Of all students currently enrolled full time, 100% benefited from one or more of the listed financial assistance programs.

Internships/Practica: Doctoral Degree (PhD Clinical Psychology): For those doctoral students for whom a professional internship was required in this program prior to graduation, (9) students applied for an internship in 2008–2009, with (9) students obtaining an internship. Of those students who obtained an internship, (9) were paid internships. Of those students who obtained an internship, (7) students placed in APA/CPA accredited internships, (2) students placed in internships not APA/CPA accredited, but listed with the Association of Psychology Postdoctoral and Internship Programs (APPIC), (0) students placed in internships conforming to guidelines of the Council of Directors of School Psychology Programs (CDSPP), (0) students placed in internships that were not APA/CPA accredited, APPIC or CDSPP listed. Psychological Services Center (PSC): each year you will be assigned to one of the four PSC supervision teams. These teams are primarily supervised by program faculty, and students typically plan to work with as many different PSC supervisors as possible during their time in the program. You will be assigned to a team during your first year, but in subsequent years your preferences will be taken into consideration during team assignments. This process usually occurs late in the Spring semester. PSC teams typically consist of one or two students from each class. Student responsibilities, duties, and opportunities will vary from team to team. The clinical curriculum provides requirements regarding the number of Clinical Practice (PSY 580) credit hours in which you should enroll each semester. External Placements: the clinical program also maintains agreements with over a dozen institutions within and beyond the Grand Forks community to provide more extensive training opportunities. Upper-level students compete for these positions in April and May of each year. Clinical students typically complete two full years (one full year at 16-20 hrs/wk) of external placement prior to internship. Our rate of success in attaining accredited internships on APPIC match day has been 29/32 over the past five years (91%).

Housing and Day Care: On-campus housing is available. On-campus day care facilities are available.

Employment of Department Graduates:

Master's Degree Graduates: Of those who graduated in the academic year 2008–2009, the following categories and numbers represent the postgraduate activities and employment of master's degree graduates: Enrolled in a postdoctoral residency/fellowship (n/a), employed in independent practice (n/a), total from the above (master's) (0).

Doctoral Degree Graduates: Of those who graduated in the academic year 2008–2009, the following categories and numbers represent the postgraduate activities and employment of doctoral degree graduates: Enrolled in a psychology doctoral program (n/a), enrolled in a postdoctoral residency/fellowship (3), employed in a community mental health/counseling center (4), employed in a hospital/medical center (2), total from the above (doctoral) (9).

Additional Information:

Orientation, Objectives, and Emphasis of Department: The Psychology Department has a multidimensional mission to provide quality undergraduate and graduate education, student advisement at both the baccalaureate and post-baccalaureate levels, teacher education for graduate students pursuing higher education positions, and a high level of faculty and student scholarship. The department also commits to efforts to enhance mental health care service delivery in underserved populations by underrepresented emerging professionals via our Indians in Psychology Doctoral Education (INPSYDE) clinical training program. We maintain large graduate training commitments to our clinical PhD (n = 38), experimental PhD (n = 5), forensic M.S. (n = 8), and forensic MA (n > 60) doctoral and master's students. The department presently has 23 full-time faculty positions. Students are admitted into one of four different training tracks in the Department of Psychology: Clinical PhD program, General-Experimental PhD program, Forensic M.S. program, or Forensic MA distance program. The department awards an MA degree in general psychology after completion of the thesis (and remaining curriculum requirements) for students enrolled in one of our two PhD programs. UND does not offer a terminal master's degree in clinical or general experimental psychology. The department's graduate programs are designed for residential students who are enrolled full-time (part-time students are not admitted). The PhD programs are scientifically-oriented and offer intensive training in the scholarly research and applied aspects of their areas. They are designed to produce respected scholars in the field as manifested in the generation of high quality research which is disseminated in lecturing, writing, and presentations. We also expect students to apply scientific findings in their respective area of specialization and to integrate scientific and applied activities as a method of further enhancing the quality of each.

Special Facilities or Resources: The Psychology Department is housed in Corwin-Larimore Hall, a four-story building remodeled to provide a facility for study and research. The department was also fortunate to occupy about a third of the Northern Plains Center for Behavioral Research Building next to Corwin-Larimore and the Nursing College. This four-story building is provides additional research space for a number of our faculty as well as our INPSYDE program. The department also utilizes space in Montgomery Hall across the street to house our Psychological Services Center (PSC) which serves as a community training clinic for the clinical psychology PhD program.

Information for Students With Physical Disabilities: See the following Web site for more information: http://www.und.edu/dept/dss.

Application Information:
Send to Graduate School University of North Dakota Box 8178 Grand Forks, ND 58202. Application available online. URL of online application: http://www.graduateschool.und.edu. Students are admitted in the Fall, application deadline January 15. *Fee:* $35.

OHIO

Akron, University of
Department of Counseling, Collaborative Program in Counseling Psychology
The College of Education
27 Fir Hill
Akron, OH 44325-5007
Telephone: (330) 972-7777
Fax: (330) 972-5292
E-mail: kj25@uakron.edu
Web: http://www.uakron.edu/colleges/educ/Counseling/

Department Information:
1968. Chairperson: Dr. Karin Jordan. Number of faculty: total—full-time 14, part-time 4; women—full-time 8, part-time 1; total—minority—full-time 3; women minority—full-time 1.

Programs and Degrees Offered:
Listed in the following order: Program area, degree type (T if terminal Master's), number awarded 7/08–6/09. Collaborative Program in Counseling Psychology PhD (Doctor of Philosophy) 6.

APA Accreditation: Counseling PhD (Doctor of Philosophy). Student Outcome Data Website: http://www3.uakron.edu/psychology/counseling/outcome_data.html.

Student Applications/Admissions:

Student Applications

Collaborative Program in Counseling Psychology PhD (Doctor of Philosophy)—Applications 2009–2010, 35. Total applicants accepted 2009–2010, 4. Number full-time enrolled (new admits only) 2009–2010, 4. Number part-time enrolled (new admits only) 2009–2010, 0. Total enrolled 2009–2010 full-time, 11, part-time, 14. Openings 2010–2011, 4. The median number of years required for completion of a degree in 2008–2009 were 7. The number of students enrolled full- and part-time who were dismissed or voluntarily withdrew from this program area in 2008–2009 were 0.

Scores: Entries appear in this order: required test or GPA, minimum score (if required), median score of students entering in 2009–2010. *Collaborative Program in Counseling Psychology PhD (Doctor of Philosophy):* GRE-V 550, GRE-Q 550, GRE-Subject (Psychology) no minimum stated, overall undergraduate GPA 2.75, last 2 years GPA 3.0, Masters GPA 3.25.

Other Criteria: (importance of criteria rated low, medium, or high): GRE scores—high, research experience—high, work experience—medium, extracurricular activity—low, clinically related public service—low, GPA—high, letters of recommendation—high, interview—high, statement of goals and objectives—high. For additional information on admission requirements, go to http://www3.uakron.edu/psychology/counseling/.

Student Characteristics: The following represents characteristics of students in 2009–2010 in all graduate psychology programs in the department: Female—full-time 16, part-time 7; Male—full-time 1, part-time 4; African American/Black—full-time 0, part-time 0; Hispanic/Latino(a)—full-time 0, part-time 0; Asian/Pacific Islander—full-time 0, part-time 0; American Indian/Alaska Native—full-time 0, part-time 0; Caucasian/White—full-time 0, part-time 0; Multi-ethnic—full-time 0, part-time 0; students subject to the Americans With Disabilities Act—full-time 0, part-time 1; Unknown ethnicity—full-time 0, part-time 0; International students who hold an F-1 or J-1 Visa—full-time 0, part-time 0.

Financial Information/Assistance:

Tuition for Full-Time Study: *Doctoral:* State residents: $387 per credit hour; Nonstate residents: $657 per credit hour. Tuition is subject to change. See the following Web site for updates and changes in tuition costs: http://www.uakron.edu/busfin/studentfin/tuition.php.

Financial Assistance:

First-Year Students: Teaching assistantships available for first year. Average amount paid per academic year: $10,500. Average number of hours worked per week: 20. Apply by April 15th. Research assistantships available for first year. Average amount paid per academic year: $10,500. Average number of hours worked per week: 20. Apply by April 15th.

Advanced Students: Teaching assistantships available for advanced students. Average amount paid per academic year: $10,500. Average number of hours worked per week: 20. Apply by April 15th. Research assistantships available for advanced students. Average amount paid per academic year: $10,500. Average number of hours worked per week: 20. Apply by April 15th.

Additional Information: Of all students currently enrolled full time, 92% benefited from one or more of the listed financial assistance programs. Application and information available online at: http://www.uakron.edu/admissions/graduate/financial_aid/graduate_assistantships.dot.

Internships/Practica: Doctoral Degree (PhD Collaborative Program in Counseling Psychology): For those doctoral students for whom a professional internship was required in this program prior to graduation, (5) students applied for an internship in 2008–2009, with (3) students obtaining an internship. Of those students who obtained an internship, (3) were paid internships. Of those students who obtained an internship, (3) students placed in APA/CPA accredited internships, (0) students placed in internships not APA/CPA accredited, but listed with the Association of Psychology Postdoctoral and Internship Programs (APPIC), (0) students placed in internships conforming to guidelines of the Council of Directors of School Psychology Programs (CDSPP), (0) students placed in internships that were not APA/CPA accredited, APPIC or CDSPP listed. Practica are offered in the department's clinic, the counseling center on campus, and a broad range of settings in the community.

Housing and Day Care: On-campus housing is available. See the following Web site for more information: Limited housing is available. For more information contact: http://www.uakron.edu/college_life/housing_dining. On-campus day care facilities are available. See the following Web site for more information: http://www.uakron.edu/colleges/educ/CCD/index.php.

Employment of Department Graduates:
Master's Degree Graduates: Of those who graduated in the academic year 2008–2009, the following categories and numbers represent the postgraduate activities and employment of master's degree graduates: Enrolled in a postdoctoral residency/fellowship (n/a), employed in independent practice (n/a), total from the above (master's) (0).
Doctoral Degree Graduates: Of those who graduated in the academic year 2008–2009, the following categories and numbers represent the postgraduate activities and employment of doctoral degree graduates: Enrolled in a psychology doctoral program (n/a), enrolled in another graduate/professional program (0), employed in independent practice (0), employed in an academic position at a university (0), employed in an academic position at a 2-year/4-year college (0), employed in other positions at a higher education institution (2), employed in a professional position in a school system (0), employed in business or industry (0), employed in government agency (1), employed in a community mental health/counseling center (3), employed in a hospital/medical center (0), still seeking employment (0), not seeking employment (0), other employment position (0), total from the above (doctoral) (6).

Additional Information:
Orientation, Objectives, and Emphasis of Department: The department subscribes to a scientist–practitioner model of training. Its objective is to provide a core of courses in general psychology and courses in the specialty of counseling psychology. The emphasis is on preparation for teaching, research, and practice career paths.

Special Facilities or Resources: The department has its own computer lab and houses the College of Education Clinic for Individual and Family Counseling.

Information for Students With Physical Disabilities: See the following Web site for more information: http://www3.uakron.edu/access/.

Application Information:
Send to The Graduate School, Polsky Building, Room 469, The University of Akron Akron, OH 44325-2101. Application available online. URL of online application: http://www.uakron.edu/gradsch/. Students are admitted in the Fall, application deadline December 1. Prospective students with Masters degrees in a related field should indicate that they are applying to the Collaborative Program in Counseling Psychology (PhD) through the Department of Counseling. Prospective students with Bachelor's degrees should indicate that they are applying to the Collaborative Program in Counseling Psychology (MA/PhD) through the Department of Psychology.

Akron, University of
Department of Psychology
Buchtel College of Arts and Sciences
Arts and Sciences Building, 290 East Buchtel Avenue
Akron, OH 44325-4301
Telephone: (330) 972-7280
Fax: (330) 972-5174
E-mail: *plevy@uakron.edu*
Web: *http://www.uakron.edu/psychology*

Department Information:
1921. Chairperson: Paul E. Levy. Number of faculty: total—full-time 21; women—full-time 9; total—minority—full-time 2; women minority—full-time 2.

Programs and Degrees Offered:
Listed in the following order: Program area, degree type (T if terminal Master's), number awarded 7/08–6/09. Industrial/Organizational Psychology MA/MS (Master of Arts/Science) (T) 3, Industrial/Organizational Psychology PhD (Doctor of Philosophy) 8, Counseling Psychology PhD (Doctor of Philosophy) 2, Applied Cognitive Aging PhD (Doctor of Philosophy) 0, Adult Development and Aging PhD (Doctor of Philosophy) 0.

APA Accreditation: Counseling PhD (Doctor of Philosophy). Student Outcome Data Website: http://www3.uakron.edu/psychology/counseling/outcome_data.html.

Student Applications/Admissions:
Student Applications
Industrial/Organizational Psychology MA/MS (Master of Arts/Science)—Applications 2009–2010, 8. Total applicants accepted 2009–2010, 5. Number full-time enrolled (new admits only) 2009–2010, 5. Number part-time enrolled (new admits only) 2009–2010, 0. Total enrolled 2009–2010 full-time, 7, part-time, 2. The median number of years required for completion of a degree in 2008–2009 were 2. The number of students enrolled full- and part-time who were dismissed or voluntarily withdrew from this program area in 2008–2009 were 0. *Industrial/Organizational Psychology PhD (Doctor of Philosophy)*—Applications 2009–2010, 45. Total applicants accepted 2009–2010, 4. Number full-time enrolled (new admits only) 2009–2010, 4. Number part-time enrolled (new admits only) 2009–2010, 0. Total enrolled 2009–2010 full-time, 29, part-time, 13. Openings 2010–2011, 5. The median number of years required for completion of a degree in 2008–2009 were 5. The number of students enrolled full- and part-time who were dismissed or voluntarily withdrew from this program area in 2008–2009 were 0. *Counseling Psychology PhD (Doctor of Philosophy)*—Applications 2009–2010, 42. Total applicants accepted 2009–2010, 6. Number full-time enrolled (new admits only) 2009–2010, 6. Number part-time enrolled (new admits only) 2009–2010, 0. Total enrolled 2009–2010 full-time, 21, part-time, 12. Openings 2010–2011, 4. The median number of years required for completion of a degree in 2008–2009 were 7. The number of students enrolled full- and part-time who were dismissed or voluntarily withdrew from this program area in 2008–2009 were 0. *Applied Cognitive Aging PhD (Doctor of Philosophy)*—Applications 2009–2010, 0. Total applicants accepted 2009–2010, 0. Number full-time enrolled (new

admits only) 2009–2010, 0. Number part-time enrolled (new admits only) 2009–2010, 0. The number of students enrolled full- and part-time who were dismissed or voluntarily withdrew from this program area in 2008–2009 were 0. *Adult Development and Aging PhD (Doctor of Philosophy)*—Applications 2009–2010, 6. Total applicants accepted 2009–2010, 2. Number full-time enrolled (new admits only) 2009–2010, 2. Number part-time enrolled (new admits only) 2009–2010, 0. Openings 2010–2011, 2. The number of students enrolled full- and part-time who were dismissed or voluntarily withdrew from this program area in 2008–2009 were 0.

Scores: Entries appear in this order: required test or GPA, minimum score (if required), median score of students entering in 2009–2010. *Industrial/Organizational Psychology MA/MS (Master of Arts/Science):* GRE-V 410, 460, GRE-Q 480, 590, GRE-Analytical 3.5, 4.5, overall undergraduate GPA 3.50, 3.80, psychology GPA 3.70, 3.80; *Industrial/Organizational Psychology PhD (Doctor of Philosophy):* GRE-V 550, 590, GRE-Q 650, 710, GRE-Analytical 4.0, 5.0, overall undergraduate GPA 3.50, 3.60, psychology GPA 3.60, 3.70; *Counseling Psychology PhD (Doctor of Philosophy):* GRE-V 460, 520, GRE-Q 510, 630, GRE-Analytical 4.0, 5.0, GRE-Subject (Psychology) 520, 660, overall undergraduate GPA 3.30, 3.60, psychology GPA 3.40, 3.70; *Adult Development and Aging PhD (Doctor of Philosophy):* GRE-V 430, 485, GRE-Q 610, 620, GRE-Analytical 4.5, 5.25, GRE-Subject (Psychology) 610, 610, overall undergraduate GPA 3.70, 3.80, psychology GPA 4.00, 4.00.

Other Criteria: (importance of criteria rated low, medium, or high): GRE scores—high, research experience—high, work experience—low, extracurricular activity—low, clinically related public service—low, GPA—high, letters of recommendation—medium, interview—medium, statement of goals and objectives—high. Telephone interviews are used as a selection criterion only in the Counseling Psychology program. Clinical service may be considered more heavily for admissions to the Counseling Psychology MA-PhD program. The I/O program does telephone screening of those that it intends to accept. For additional information on admission requirements, go to http://www3.uakron.edu/psychology/gradschool/minreq.html.

Student Characteristics: The following represents characteristics of students in 2009–2010 in all graduate psychology programs in the department: Female—full-time 46, part-time 23; Male—full-time 13, part-time 6; African American/Black—full-time 4, part-time 4; Hispanic/Latino(a)—full-time 2, part-time 0; Asian/Pacific Islander—full-time 6, part-time 2; American Indian/Alaska Native—full-time 0, part-time 0; Caucasian/White—full-time 47, part-time 23; Multi-ethnic—full-time 0, part-time 0; students subject to the Americans With Disabilities Act—full-time 0, part-time 0; Unknown ethnicity—full-time 0, part-time 0; International students who hold an F-1 or J-1 Visa—full-time 0, part-time 0.

Financial Information/Assistance:
Tuition for Full-Time Study: *Master's:* State residents: per academic year $10,756, $343 per credit hour; Nonstate residents: per academic year $18,246, $588 per credit hour. *Doctoral:* State residents: per academic year $10,756, $343 per credit hour; Nonstate residents: per academic year $18,246, $588 per credit hour. Tuition is subject to change. See the following Web site for updates and changes in tuition costs: http://www.uakron.edu/busfin/studentfin/tuition.php.

Financial Assistance:
First-Year Students: Teaching assistantships available for first year. Average amount paid per academic year: $12,500. Average number of hours worked per week: 20. Apply by January 15. Fellowships and scholarships available for first year. Average amount paid per academic year: $0. Average number of hours worked per week: 0. Apply by January 15.

Advanced Students: Teaching assistantships available for advanced students. Average amount paid per academic year: $12,200. Average number of hours worked per week: 20. Apply by April 15. Research assistantships available for advanced students. Average amount paid per academic year: $12,200. Average number of hours worked per week: 20. Apply by April 15.

Additional Information: Of all students currently enrolled full time, 100% benefited from one or more of the listed financial assistance programs. Application and information available online at: http://www.uakron.edu/admissions/graduate/financial_aid.

Internships/Practica: Doctoral Degree (PhD Counseling Psychology): For those doctoral students for whom a professional internship was required in this program prior to graduation, (6) students applied for an internship in 2008–2009, with (6) students obtaining an internship. Of those students who obtained an internship, (6) were paid internships. Of those students who obtained an internship, (6) students placed in APA/CPA accredited internships, (0) students placed in internships not APA/CPA accredited, but listed with the Association of Psychology Postdoctoral and Internship Programs (APPIC), (0) students placed in internships conforming to guidelines of the Council of Directors of School Psychology Programs (CDSPP), (0) students placed in internships that were not APA/CPA accredited, APPIC or CDSPP listed. Practica are offered in the department's own Counseling Training Clinic and Center for Organizational Research. Students also have access to a wide variety of community-based practica in industrial and public settings, hospitals, the University's Counseling Testing and Careers Center, and community mental health centers.

Housing and Day Care: On-campus housing is available. See the following Web site for more information: http://www.uakron.edu/college_life/housing_dining. On-campus day care facilities are available. See the following Web site for more information: http://www.uakron.edu/colleges/educ/CCD.

Employment of Department Graduates:
Master's Degree Graduates: Of those who graduated in the academic year 2008–2009, the following categories and numbers represent the postgraduate activities and employment of master's degree graduates: Enrolled in a psychology doctoral program (12), enrolled in another graduate/professional program (0), enrolled in a postdoctoral residency/fellowship (n/a), employed in independent practice (n/a), employed in an academic position at a university (0), employed in an academic position at a 2-year/4-year college (0), employed in other positions at a higher education institution (0), employed in a professional position in a school system (0), employed in business or industry (3), employed in government agency (0), employed in a community mental health/counseling center (0), employed in a hospital/medical center (0), still seeking employment (0), not seeking employment (0), other employment position (0), do not know (0), total from the above (master's) (15).

Doctoral Degree Graduates: Of those who graduated in the academic year 2008–2009, the following categories and numbers represent the postgraduate activities and employment of doctoral degree graduates: Enrolled in a psychology doctoral program (n/a), enrolled in another graduate/professional program (0), enrolled in a postdoctoral residency/fellowship (0), employed in independent practice (0), employed in an academic position at a university (7), employed in an academic position at a 2-year/4-year college (0), employed in other positions at a higher education institution (0), employed in a professional position in a school system (0), employed in business or industry (5), employed in government agency (0), employed in a community mental health/counseling center (0), employed in a hospital/medical center (0), still seeking employment (0), not seeking employment (0), other employment position (0), do not know (0), total from the above (doctoral) (12).

Additional Information:
Orientation, Objectives, and Emphasis of Department: The department's goals are to: (1) increase and diffuse psychological knowledge by advancing the discipline both as a science and as a means of promoting human welfare; (2) promote psychology in all its branches in the broadest and most liberal manner; (3) encourage research in psychology; and (4) advance high standards of education, achievement, professional ethics and conduct. The department subscribes to a scientist–practitioner model of training. Graduate students take a common set of courses in foundational areas of psychology in addition to their specialty coursework, with study in the specialty area beginning early in graduate training. The emphasis is on preparation for teaching as well as for research, industrial, or mental health services career paths. Industrial/organizational, industrial gerontological, and counseling psychology are the specialty emphases at the MA and PhD level.

Special Facilities or Resources: To enhance research and instruction, we maintain a number of psychological research laboratories designed for individual and group studies, and equipped with computers, one-way viewing mirrors, video equipment, etc. Over 60 computers are available to faculty and students for word processing, statistical analysis, classroom instruction, e-mail correspondence, and web access. A programmer/technician provides full-time support for the hardware and software for the department and writes custom software for experimental control, stimulus display, and data collection. We maintain an in-house library of teaching resources for graduate teaching assistants, as well as a test library with over 100 tests and manuals for assessment of a broad range of constructs. We are affiliated with the university's Institute for Life-Span Development and Gerontology and the Archives of the History of American Psychology.

Information for Students With Physical Disabilities: See the following Web site for more information: http://www3.uakron.edu/access/.

Application Information:
Send to Graduate School, The University of Akron, Polsky Building Room 469 Akron, OH 44325-2101. Application available online. URL of online application: http://www.uakron.edu/gradsch/apply-online. Students are admitted in the Fall, application deadline January 15. Fee: $30. International student's fee is $40.

Bowling Green State University
Department of Psychology
Bowling Green, OH 43403
Telephone: (419) 372-2301
Fax: (419) 372-6013
E-mail: pwatson@bgsu.edu
Web: http://www.bgsu.edu/departments/psych/

Department Information:
1947. Chairperson: Michael Zickar. Number of faculty: total—full-time 26; women—full-time 10; total—minority—full-time 2.

Programs and Degrees Offered:
Listed in the following order: Program area, degree type (T if terminal Master's), number awarded 7/08–6/09. Industrial/Organizational Psychology PhD (Doctor of Philosophy) 1, Clinical Psychology PhD (Doctor of Philosophy) 11, Developmental Psychology PhD (Doctor of Philosophy) 0, Neural & Cognitive Sciences PhD (Doctor of Philosophy) 2.

APA Accreditation: Clinical PhD (Doctor of Philosophy). Student Outcome Data Website: http://www.bgsu.edu/departments/psych/page36679.html.

Student Applications/Admissions:
Student Applications

Industrial/Organizational Psychology PhD (Doctor of Philosophy)—Applications 2009–2010, 78. Total applicants accepted 2009–2010, 12. Number full-time enrolled (new admits only) 2009–2010, 4. Total enrolled 2009–2010 full-time, 25. Openings 2010–2011, 5. The median number of years required for completion of a degree in 2008–2009 were 4. The number of students enrolled full- and part-time who were dismissed or voluntarily withdrew from this program area in 2008–2009 were 0. *Clinical Psychology PhD (Doctor of Philosophy)*—Applications 2009–2010, 107. Total applicants accepted 2009–2010, 19. Number full-time enrolled (new admits only) 2009–2010, 10. Openings 2010–2011, 8. The median number of years required for completion of a degree in 2008–2009 were 7. The number of students enrolled full- and part-time who were dismissed or voluntarily withdrew from this program area in 2008–2009 were 0. *Developmental Psychology PhD (Doctor of Philosophy)*—Applications 2009–2010, 7. Total applicants accepted 2009–2010, 2. Number full-time enrolled (new admits only) 2009–2010, 1. Total enrolled 2009–2010 full-time, 6. Openings 2010–2011, 3. The number of students enrolled full- and part-time who were dismissed or voluntarily withdrew from this program area in 2008–2009 were 0. *Neural & Cognitive Sciences PhD (Doctor of Philosophy)*—Applications 2009–2010, 24. Total applicants accepted 2009–2010, 6. Number full-time enrolled (new admits only) 2009–2010, 2. Total enrolled 2009–2010 full-time, 22. Openings 2010–2011, 4. The median number of years required for completion of a degree in 2008–2009 were 6. The number of students enrolled full- and part-time who were dismissed or voluntarily withdrew from this program area in 2008–2009 were 0.

Scores: Entries appear in this order: required test or GPA, minimum score (if required), median score of students entering in 2009–2010. *Clinical Psychology PhD (Doctor of Philosophy):* GRE-V no minimum stated, 520, GRE-Q no minimum stated,

675, GRE-Subject (Psychology) no minimum stated, 715, overall undergraduate GPA no minimum stated, 3.86.

Other Criteria: (importance of criteria rated low, medium, or high): GRE scores—high, research experience—high, work experience—medium, extracurricular activity—medium, clinically related public service—high, GPA—high, letters of recommendation—high, interview—high, statement of goals and objectives—high. Clinically related public service and interview are high for Clinical program only. For additional information on admission requirements, go to http://www.bgsu.edu/departments/psych/page31038.html.

Student Characteristics: The following represents characteristics of students in 2009–2010 in all graduate psychology programs in the department: Female—full-time 84, part-time 0; Male—full-time 33, part-time 0; African American/Black—full-time 1, part-time 0; Hispanic/Latino(a)—full-time 1, part-time 0; Asian/Pacific Islander—full-time 3, part-time 0; American Indian/Alaska Native—full-time 1, part-time 0; Caucasian/White—full-time 83, part-time 0; Multi-ethnic—full-time 1, part-time 0; students subject to the Americans With Disabilities Act—full-time 0, part-time 0; Unknown ethnicity—full-time 27, part-time 0; International students who hold an F-1 or J-1 Visa—full-time 5, part-time 0.

Financial Information/Assistance:

Tuition for Full-Time Study: *Doctoral:* State residents: per academic year $11,488; Nonstate residents: per academic year $18,796. Tuition is subject to change. See the following Web site for updates and changes in tuition costs: http://www.bgsu.edu/offices/bursar/index.html.

Financial Assistance:

First-Year Students: Teaching assistantships available for first year. Average amount paid per academic year: $11,302. Average number of hours worked per week: 20. Apply by December 15. Research assistantships available for first year. Average amount paid per academic year: $11,302. Average number of hours worked per week: 20. Apply by December 15.

Advanced Students: Teaching assistantships available for advanced students. Average amount paid per academic year: $13,538. Average number of hours worked per week: 20. Apply by December 15. Research assistantships available for advanced students. Average amount paid per academic year: $13,538. Average number of hours worked per week: 20. Apply by December 15. Traineeships available for advanced students. Average amount paid per academic year: $13,538. Average number of hours worked per week: 20. Apply by December 15. Fellowships and scholarships available for advanced students. Average amount paid per academic year: $16,923. Average number of hours worked per week: 0. Apply by March.

Additional Information: Of all students currently enrolled full time, 100% benefited from one or more of the listed financial assistance programs. Application and information available online at: http://www.bgsu.edu/departments/psych/.

Internships/Practica: Doctoral Degree (PhD Clinical Psychology): For those doctoral students for whom a professional internship was required in this program prior to graduation, (14) students applied for an internship in 2008–2009, with (13) students obtaining an internship. Of those students who obtained an internship, (13) were paid internships. Of those students who obtained an internship, (12) students placed in APA/CPA accredited internships, (1) students placed in internships not APA/CPA accredited, but listed with the Association of Psychology Postdoctoral and Internship Programs (APPIC), (0) students placed in internships conforming to guidelines of the Council of Directors of School Psychology Programs (CDSPP), (0) students placed in internships that were not APA/CPA accredited, APPIC or CDSPP listed. In their beginning years, clinical students are placed on Basic Clinical Skills practicum teams through the Department's Psychological Services Center (PSC) that provide experience with a broad range of clients and clinical problems. Students focus on the application of such basic clinical skills as psychological assessment and interventions, the integration of science and practice, case conceptualization, clinical judgment and decision-making report writing. In their second year students begin receiving in-house training in psychotherapy through the PSC. As clinical students progress through the program they are placed on Advanced Clinical Skills teams that involve them in current projects providing "hands-on" experience with the integration of research and practice as it applies to individuals, health/behavioral medicine, the community, or special populations (e.g., children; problem drinkers). More advanced clinical students are provided practicum opportunities consistent with their interest through a number of outside placements, such as community mental health centers, a nearby medical college, the university counseling center and health service, an inpatient child and adolescent facility, hospital-based rehabilitation centers, treatment centers for children and families, and programs for individuals with severe mental disabilities and emotional disorders. Industrial/Organizational students are strongly encouraged to apply for a formal internship after completion of their Master's project. Although such experiences are encouraged and typically followed, internships are not required of I/O students for completion of the doctoral degree. Other experiences through coursework activities and Institute for Psychological Research and Application (IPRA) projects can collectively serve the same function as an internship.

Housing and Day Care: No on-campus housing is available. No on-campus day care facilities are available.

Employment of Department Graduates:

Master's Degree Graduates: Of those who graduated in the academic year 2008–2009, the following categories and numbers represent the postgraduate activities and employment of master's degree graduates: Enrolled in a postdoctoral residency/fellowship (n/a), employed in independent practice (n/a), total from the above (master's) (0).

Doctoral Degree Graduates: Of those who graduated in the academic year 2008–2009, the following categories and numbers represent the postgraduate activities and employment of doctoral degree graduates: Enrolled in a psychology doctoral program (n/a), total from the above (doctoral) (0).

Additional Information:

Orientation, Objectives, and Emphasis of Department: The primary goal of the PhD program is the development of scientists capable of advancing psychological knowledge. The program is characterized by both an emphasis on extensive academic training in general psychology and an early and continuing commitment to research. Although each graduate student will seek an area in which to develop his or her own expertise, students will be expected to be knowledgeable about many areas and will be encouraged to pursue interests that cross conventional specialty lines. The program is research-oriented. Each student normally works in close association with a sponsor or chairperson whose special competence matches the student's interest, but students are free to pursue research interests with any faculty member and in any area(s) they choose. Both basic and applied research are well represented within the department. The clinical program has concentrations in clinical child, behavioral medicine, and community, as well as general clinical.

Special Facilities or Resources: The department is located in the psychology building with excellent facilities for all forms of research. The building houses all faculty and graduate students. The department operates a community-oriented Psychological Services Center and the Institute for Psychological Research and Application. The department operates its own computer facility with terminals to the mainframe computer available in the building, as well as a microcomputer facility.

Information for Students With Physical Disabilities: See the following Web site for more information: http://www.bgsu.edu/offices/sa/disability/.

Application Information:
Send to Graduate Secretary, 206 Psychology Building, 822 E. Merry Street, Bowling Green, OH 43403. Application available online. URL of online application: http://www.bgsu.edu/colleges/gradcol/page24959.html. Students are admitted in the Fall, application deadline December 15. December 15 deadline for Clinical and January 1 deadline for Industrial/Organizational, Developmental, Neural & Cognitive. *Fee:* $30.

Case Western Reserve University
Department of Psychology
Arts and Sciences
Mather Memorial Building, 11220 Bellflower Road, Room 103
Cleveland, OH 44106-7123
Telephone: (216) 368-2686
Fax: (216) 368-4891
E-mail: *rlg2@case.edu*
Web: *http://psychology.case.edu/*

Department Information:
1928. Chairperson: Robert L. Greene. Number of faculty: total—full-time 16; women—full-time 8; total—minority—full-time 1.

Programs and Degrees Offered:
Listed in the following order: Program area, degree type (T if terminal Master's), number awarded 7/08–6/09. Clinical Psychology PhD (Doctor of Philosophy) 3, Experimental Psychology PhD (Doctor of Philosophy) 1.

APA Accreditation: Clinical PhD (Doctor of Philosophy).

Student Applications/Admissions:
Student Applications
Clinical Psychology PhD (Doctor of Philosophy)—Applications 2009–2010, 181. Total applicants accepted 2009–2010, 6. Number full-time enrolled (new admits only) 2009–2010, 5. Number part-time enrolled (new admits only) 2009–2010, 0. Openings 2010–2011, 5. The median number of years required for completion of a degree in 2008–2009 were 6. The number of students enrolled full- and part-time who were dismissed or voluntarily withdrew from this program area in 2008–2009 were 0. *Experimental Psychology PhD (Doctor of Philosophy)*—Applications 2009–2010, 12. Total applicants accepted 2009–2010, 1. Number full-time enrolled (new admits only) 2009–2010, 3. Number part-time enrolled (new admits only) 2009–2010, 0. Openings 2010–2011, 2. The median number of years required for completion of a degree in 2008–2009 were 4. The number of students enrolled full- and part-time who were dismissed or voluntarily withdrew from this program area in 2008–2009 were 0.

Other Criteria: (importance of criteria rated low, medium, or high): GRE scores—high, research experience—high, work experience—low, extracurricular activity—low, clinically related public service—medium, GPA—high, letters of recommendation—medium, interview—medium, statement of goals and objectives—medium, undergraduate major in psychology—low, specific undergraduate psychology courses taken—low.

Student Characteristics: The following represents characteristics of students in 2009–2010 in all graduate psychology programs in the department: Female—full-time 33, part-time 0; Male—full-time 7, part-time 0; African American/Black—full-time 1, part-time 0; Hispanic/Latino(a)—full-time 2, part-time 0; Asian/Pacific Islander—full-time 6, part-time 0; American Indian/Alaska Native—full-time 0, part-time 0; Caucasian/White—full-time 31, part-time 0; Multi-ethnic—full-time 0, part-time 0; students subject to the Americans With Disabilities Act—full-time 0, part-time 0; Unknown ethnicity—full-time 0, part-time 0; International students who hold an F-1 or J-1 Visa—full-time 1, part-time 0.

Financial Information/Assistance:
Tuition for Full-Time Study: *Master's:* State residents: per academic year $34,320, $1,430 per credit hour; Nonstate residents: per academic year $34,320, $1,430 per credit hour. *Doctoral:* State residents: per academic year $34,320, $1,430 per credit hour; Nonstate residents: per academic year $34,320, $1,430 per credit hour. Tuition is subject to change.

Financial Assistance:
First-Year Students: Research assistantships available for first year. Average amount paid per academic year: $20,000. Traineeships available for first year. Average amount paid per academic year: $20,772.

Advanced Students: Research assistantships available for advanced students. Average amount paid per academic year: $20,000. Traineeships available for advanced students. Average amount paid per academic year: $20,722. Fellowships and scholarships available for advanced students. Average amount paid per academic year: $20,000.

Additional Information: Of all students currently enrolled full time, 100% benefited from one or more of the listed financial assistance programs. Application and information available online at: http://finaid.case.edu.

Internships/Practica: Doctoral Degree (PhD Clinical Psychology): For those doctoral students for whom a professional internship was required in this program prior to graduation, (6) students applied for an internship in 2008–2009, with (6) students obtaining an internship. Of those students who obtained an internship, (6) were paid internships. Of those students who obtained an internship, (6) students placed in APA/CPA accredited internships, (0) students placed in internships not APA/CPA accredited, but listed with the Association of Psychology Postdoctoral and Internship Programs (APPIC), (0) students placed in internships conforming to guidelines of the Council of Directors of School Psychology Programs (CDSPP), (0) students placed in internships that were not APA/CPA accredited, APPIC or CDSPP listed. The clinical psychology graduate program has a number of practicum placements in the Cleveland area. Students spend time in different settings during their second, third, and fourth years. In addition, the department requires two in-house practica in different types of psychotherapy.

Housing and Day Care: On-campus housing is available. No on-campus day care facilities are available.

Employment of Department Graduates:
Master's Degree Graduates: Of those who graduated in the academic year 2008–2009, the following categories and numbers represent the postgraduate activities and employment of master's degree graduates: Enrolled in a postdoctoral residency/fellowship (n/a), employed in independent practice (n/a), total from the above (master's) (0).
Doctoral Degree Graduates: Of those who graduated in the academic year 2008–2009, the following categories and numbers represent the postgraduate activities and employment of doctoral degree graduates: Enrolled in a psychology doctoral program (n/a), enrolled in another graduate/professional program (0), enrolled in a postdoctoral residency/fellowship (3), employed in independent practice (0), employed in an academic position at a university (0), employed in an academic position at a 2-year/4-year college (0), employed in other positions at a higher education institution (1), employed in a professional position in a school system (0), employed in business or industry (0), employed in government agency (0), employed in a community mental health/counseling center (0), employed in a hospital/medical center (0), still seeking employment (0), other employment position (0), do not know (0), total from the above (doctoral) (4).

Additional Information:
Orientation, Objectives, and Emphasis of Department: The graduate program seeks to give students a thorough grounding in basic areas of fact and theory in psychology, to train them in research methods by which knowledge in the behavioral sciences is advanced, and to prepare them for careers as teachers and researchers. During the first year, students begin a research clerkship under the tutelage of a faculty member. A variety of facilities and subject populations are available for the study of developmental processes, and a number of well-equipped laboratories are used for research in perception, memory, cognition, learning, physiological psychology, and individual differences. The department offers programs in experimental and clinical psychology. Within each of these major areas of concentration, a number of sub-specializations are available. For clinical psychology, these include adult, child, and pediatric psychology. For experimental psychology, the areas of specialization are determined by the faculty member with whom the student works. These include, but are not limited to, cognition, human intelligence, aging, social, and physiological psychology.

Special Facilities or Resources: A number of excellent facilities for clinical training and research are available on campus and in the surrounding community, such as the Student Counseling Center of Case Western Reserve, University Hospitals, the Cleveland Veterans Administration Hospital, and MetroHealth Medical Center. The department also maintains an extensive perceptual development laboratory to study the developmental aspects of learning, cognition, and language acquisition, and several experimental laboratories for the study of learning, perception, cognition, physiological psychology, and social psychology.

Application Information:
Send to Department of Psychology, Case Western Reserve University, 10900 Euclid Avenue, Cleveland, OH 44106-7123. Students are admitted in the Fall, application deadline January 8. Deadline is January 8 for Clinical and February 15 for Experimental. Fee: $50.

Cincinnati, University of
Department of Psychology
Arts and Sciences
4130 Edwards I
Cincinnati, OH 45221-0376
Telephone: (513) 556-5539
Fax: (513) 556-1904
E-mail: *steven.howe@uc.edu*
Web: *http://www.artsci.uc.edu/psychology/*

Department Information:
1901. Head: Steven R. Howe, PhD. Number of faculty: total—full-time 31, part-time 8; women—full-time 16, part-time 3; total—minority—full-time 6, part-time 2; women minority—full-time 4, part-time 2.

Programs and Degrees Offered:
Listed in the following order: Program area, degree type (T if terminal Master's), number awarded 7/08–6/09. Clinical Psychology PhD (Doctor of Philosophy) 7, Experimental Psychology PhD (Doctor of Philosophy) 3.

APA Accreditation: Clinical PhD (Doctor of Philosophy). Student Outcome Data Website: http://www.artsci.uc.edu/psychology/grad/clinical.cfm.

Student Applications/Admissions:
Student Applications
Clinical Psychology PhD (Doctor of Philosophy)—Applications 2009–2010, 261. Total applicants accepted 2009–2010, 7. Number full-time enrolled (new admits only) 2009–2010, 7. Number part-time enrolled (new admits only) 2009–2010, 0. Total enrolled 2009–2010 full-time, 39, part-time, 5. Openings 2010–2011, 8. The median number of years required for completion of a degree in 2008–2009 were 6. The number of

students enrolled full- and part-time who were dismissed or voluntarily withdrew from this program area in 2008–2009 were 0. *Experimental Psychology PhD (Doctor of Philosophy)*— Applications 2009–2010, 30. Total applicants accepted 2009–2010, 8. Number full-time enrolled (new admits only) 2009–2010, 8. Number part-time enrolled (new admits only) 2009–2010, 0. Total enrolled 2009–2010 full-time, 23, part-time, 5. Openings 2010–2011, 7. The median number of years required for completion of a degree in 2008–2009 were 6. The number of students enrolled full- and part-time who were dismissed or voluntarily withdrew from this program area in 2008–2009 were 1.

Scores: Entries appear in this order: required test or GPA, minimum score (if required), median score of students entering in 2009–2010. *Clinical Psychology PhD (Doctor of Philosophy)*: GRE-V 430, 530, GRE-Q 560, 610, GRE-Analytical 4, 4.5, overall undergraduate GPA 3.6, 3.79; *Experimental Psychology PhD (Doctor of Philosophy)*: GRE-V 470, 570, GRE-Q 540, 635, GRE-Analytical 4.5, 4, overall undergraduate GPA 3.2, 3.55.

Other Criteria: (importance of criteria rated low, medium, or high): GRE scores—medium, research experience—high, work experience—high, extracurricular activity—low, clinically related public service—medium, GPA—high, letters of recommendation—high, interview—high, statement of goals and objectives—high, Fit w/ faculty mentor—high, undergraduate major in psychology—medium, specific undergraduate psychology courses taken—high, Clinically related public service is only considered strongly for students applying for clinical training. For additional information on admission requirements, go to http://www.artsci.uc.edu/psychology/.

Student Characteristics: The following represents characteristics of students in 2009–2010 in all graduate psychology programs in the department: Female—full-time 67, part-time 0; Male—full-time 19, part-time 0; African American/Black—full-time 11, part-time 0; Hispanic/Latino(a)—full-time 1, part-time 0; Asian/Pacific Islander—full-time 3, part-time 0; American Indian/Alaska Native—full-time 0, part-time 0; Caucasian/White—full-time 71, part-time 0; Multi-ethnic—full-time 0, part-time 0; students subject to the Americans With Disabilities Act—full-time 0, part-time 0; Unknown ethnicity—full-time 0, part-time 0; International students who hold an F-1 or J-1 Visa—full-time 0, part-time 0.

Financial Information/Assistance:

Tuition for Full-Time Study: *Doctoral:* State residents: per academic year $16,944, $415 per credit hour; Nonstate residents: per academic year $30,320, $759 per credit hour. Tuition is subject to change. See the following Web site for updates and changes in tuition costs: http://www.financialaid.uc.edu/costs.html.

Financial Assistance:

First-Year Students: Teaching assistantships available for first year. Research assistantships available for first year. Fellowships and scholarships available for first year.

Advanced Students: Teaching assistantships available for advanced students. Research assistantships available for advanced students. Traineeships available for advanced students. Fellowships and scholarships available for advanced students.

Additional Information: Of all students currently enrolled full time, 99% benefited from one or more of the listed financial assistance programs. Application and information available online at: http://www.financialaid.uc.edu/gradstudent.html.

Internships/Practica: Doctoral Degree (PhD Clinical Psychology): For those doctoral students for whom a professional internship was required in this program prior to graduation, (4) students applied for an internship in 2008–2009, with (4) students obtaining an internship. Of those students who obtained an internship, (4) were paid internships. Of those students who obtained an internship, (4) students placed in APA/CPA accredited internships, (0) students placed in internships not APA/CPA accredited, but listed with the Association of Psychology Postdoctoral and Internship Programs (APPIC), (0) students placed in internships conforming to guidelines of the Council of Directors of School Psychology Programs (CDSPP), (0) students placed in internships that were not APA/CPA accredited, APPIC or CDSPP listed. All clinical students in years three and four typically perform a paid, 20-hour/week clinical (or clinical research) training placement at an external site in the Greater Cincinnati area. Often these placements are at the University of Cincinnati Medical Center, the Cincinnati Children's Hospital Medical Center, or a variety of community agencies. If students need a fifth year of support prior to beginning an APA-accredited clinical internship, we can generally arrange a clinical training opportunity, although priority for placements goes to students in years 1 through 4. While most of our experimental students do their paid training assignments within the department, there are also paid external training slots available for some of our students in private industry or with the federal government.

Housing and Day Care: No on-campus housing is available. On-campus day care facilities are available. See the following Web site for more information: http://www.ucchildcare.org/.

Employment of Department Graduates:

Master's Degree Graduates: Of those who graduated in the academic year 2008–2009, the following categories and numbers represent the postgraduate activities and employment of master's degree graduates: Enrolled in a postdoctoral residency/fellowship (n/a), employed in independent practice (n/a), total from the above (master's) (0).

Doctoral Degree Graduates: Of those who graduated in the academic year 2008–2009, the following categories and numbers represent the postgraduate activities and employment of doctoral degree graduates: Enrolled in a psychology doctoral program (n/a), enrolled in a postdoctoral residency/fellowship (5), employed in other positions at a higher education institution (1), employed in a hospital/medical center (3), not seeking employment (1), total from the above (doctoral) (10).

Additional Information:

Orientation, Objectives, and Emphasis of Department: The University of Cincinnati offers the PhD in Psychology, including an APA-accredited training program in Clinical Psychology. Clinical students must specify a specialty training area, which may include health, neuropsychology or general training. For students who are seeking Experimental training, we offer training primarily in Cognition, Action and Perception; Human Factors and Experimental Neuropsychology. The doctoral program is limited to full-time students who show outstanding promise. Students are admitted to the doctoral program to work with a faculty research mentor. Faculty mentors are responsible for ensuring that students are actively engaged in doing research from the very start of their graduate school career, and that this work leads successfully to a master's thesis and a dissertation.

Special Facilities or Resources: The department's clinical program has close ties to the UC College of Medicine, Cincinnati Children's Hospital Medical Center, and a wide range of community agencies. The experimental program has close collaborations with the UC College of Medicine, the College of Engineering, and agencies including Wright Patterson Air Force Base and NIOSH.

Information for Students With Physical Disabilities: See the following Web site for more information: http://www.uc.edu/sas/disability/.

Application Information:
Send to Graduate Secretary, Department of Psychology, University of Cincinnati, P.O. Box 210376, Cincinnati, OH 45221-0376. Application available online. URL of online application: http://www.grad.uc.edu/admissions.aspx. Students are admitted in the Fall, application deadline January 5. *Fee:* $50.

Cincinnati, University of
Human Services/School Psychology
Education, Criminal Justice, and Human Services
P.O. Box 210068
Cincinnati, OH 45221-0068
Telephone: (513) 556-3335
Fax: (513) 556-3898
E-mail: janet.graden@uc.edu
Web: http://www.uc.edu/schoolpsychology/

Department Information:
1992. School Director: Janet Graden. Number of faculty: total—full-time 5, part-time 2; women—full-time 3, part-time 1.

Programs and Degrees Offered:
Listed in the following order: Program area, degree type (T if terminal Master's), number awarded 7/08–6/09. School Psychology PhD (Doctor of Philosophy) 2, School Psychology EdS (School Psychology) 13.

Student Applications/Admissions:
Student Applications
School Psychology PhD (Doctor of Philosophy)—Applications 2009–2010, 9. Total applicants accepted 2009–2010, 5. Number full-time enrolled (new admits only) 2009–2010, 4. Number part-time enrolled (new admits only) 2009–2010, 0. Total enrolled 2009–2010 full-time, 12, part-time, 9. Openings 2010–2011, 4. The median number of years required for completion of a degree in 2008–2009 were 7. The number of students enrolled full- and part-time who were dismissed or voluntarily withdrew from this program area in 2008–2009 were 1. School Psychology EdS (School Psychology)—Applications 2009–2010, 64. Total applicants accepted 2009–2010, 19. Number full-time enrolled (new admits only) 2009–2010, 12. Number part-time enrolled (new admits only) 2009–2010, 0. Openings 2010–2011, 15. The median number of years required for completion of a degree in 2008–2009 were 3. The number of students enrolled full- and part-time who were dismissed or voluntarily withdrew from this program area in 2008–2009 were 1.

Scores: Entries appear in this order: required test or GPA, minimum score (if required), median score of students entering in 2009–2010. School Psychology PhD (Doctor of Philosophy): GRE-V no minimum stated, 520, GRE-Q no minimum stated, 620, GRE-Analytical no minimum stated, 4.5, GRE-Subject (Psychology) no minimum stated, 600, overall undergraduate GPA no minimum stated, 3.5, last 2 years GPA no minimum stated, 3.6, psychology GPA no minimum stated, 3.75; School Psychology EdS (School Psychology): GRE-V no minimum stated, 520, GRE-Q no minimum stated, 550, GRE-Analytical no minimum stated, 4, overall undergraduate GPA no minimum stated, 3.6, last 2 years GPA no minimum stated, 3.8, psychology GPA no minimum stated, 3.6.

Other Criteria: (importance of criteria rated low, medium, or high): GRE scores—high, research experience—medium, work experience—medium, extracurricular activity—medium, clinically related public service—high, GPA—high, letters of recommendation—high, interview—high, statement of goals and objectives—high. Specific, focused goals aligned with doctoral study (including research) are expected for doctoral program. For additional information on admission requirements, go to http://www.uc.edu/schoolpsychology/.

Student Characteristics: The following represents characteristics of students in 2009–2010 in all graduate psychology programs in the department: Female—full-time 40, part-time 9; Male—full-time 6, part-time 0; African American/Black—full-time 1, part-time 1; Hispanic/Latino(a)—full-time 0, part-time 1; Asian/Pacific Islander—full-time 0, part-time 0; American Indian/Alaska Native—full-time 0, part-time 0; Caucasian/White—full-time 45, part-time 6; Multi-ethnic—full-time 0, part-time 1; students subject to the Americans With Disabilities Act—full-time 0, part-time 0; Unknown ethnicity—full-time 0, part-time 0; International students who hold an F-1 or J-1 Visa—full-time 0, part-time 0.

Financial Information/Assistance:
Tuition for Full-Time Study: *Master's:* State residents: per academic year $12,723, $425 per credit hour; Nonstate residents: per academic year $23,055, $769 per credit hour. *Doctoral:* State residents: per academic year $12,723, $425 per credit hour; Nonstate residents: per academic year $23,055, $769 per credit hour. Tuition is subject to change. See the following Web site for updates and changes in tuition costs: http://www.financialaid.uc.edu/costs.html.

Financial Assistance:
First-Year Students: Research assistantships available for first year. Average amount paid per academic year: $10,200. Average number of hours worked per week: 20. Fellowships and scholarships available for first year. Average amount paid per academic year: $15,000. Average number of hours worked per week: 20.

Advanced Students: Teaching assistantships available for advanced students. Average number of hours worked per week: 20. Research assistantships available for advanced students. Average amount paid per academic year: $10,944. Average number of hours worked per week: 20. Traineeships available for advanced students. Average amount paid per academic year: $25,000. Average number of hours worked per week: 40. Fellowships and scholarships available for advanced students. Average amount paid per academic year: $15,000. Average number of hours worked per week: 20.

Additional Information: Of all students currently enrolled full time, 100% benefited from one or more of the listed financial assistance programs. Application and information available online at: http://www.financialaid.uc.edu/gradstudent.html.

Internships/Practica: All students, specialist and doctoral level, complete extensive practica experiences prior to internship in field settings that include local school districts and educational agencies. In the first year, students are enrolled in Externship, in which they are placed in schools (urban settings, K-12) to learn about schooling, educational issues, effective instruction, and roles and responsibilities of various personnel. Field experiences also occur to support foundation skills in applied behavior analysis and academic and behavioral intervention. Doctoral students also participate as research team members in schools in Years 1 through 3. Throughout the second year, students are enrolled each quarter in an integrated Practicum experience, in which students obtain extensive supervised experience in delivery of services from a consultative, intervention-based tiered services delivery model. Students collaborate to design, implement, and evaluate prevention and intervention plans in the practicum, incorporating elements of their learning from across course work. In addition, they complete field experiences in behavioral counseling and functional assessment. Third-year doctoral students complete advanced field-based work in research and facilitating systems change. Specialist-level students complete a 10-month, 1500 hour school-based internship. These internships are arranged through the program and are paid. In the internship, students provide a full range of comprehensive school psychological services, with supervision from a licensed school psychologist and from university faculty. Doctoral students complete an Advanced School Experience in Year 3, participating in leadership, staff development, supervision, and research activities. Doctoral students complete a 1500 hour internship consistent with CDSPP, APA, and NASP internship requirements.

Housing and Day Care: On-campus housing is available. See the following Web site for more information: http://www.uc.edu/housing/. On-campus day care facilities are available. See the following Web site for more information: http://www.ucchildcare.org.

Employment of Department Graduates:
Master's Degree Graduates: Of those who graduated in the academic year 2008–2009, the following categories and numbers represent the postgraduate activities and employment of master's degree graduates: Enrolled in a postdoctoral residency/fellowship (n/a), employed in independent practice (n/a), employed in a professional position in a school system (13), total from the above (master's) (13).
Doctoral Degree Graduates: Of those who graduated in the academic year 2008–2009, the following categories and numbers represent the postgraduate activities and employment of doctoral degree graduates: Enrolled in a psychology doctoral program (n/a), employed in an academic position at a university (0), employed in a professional position in a school system (2), total from the above (doctoral) (2).

Additional Information:
Orientation, Objectives, and Emphasis of Department: The School Psychology program at the University of Cincinnati is dedicated to preparing highly competent professional school psychologists, at the specialist (EdS) and doctoral (PhD) levels, according to the scientist–practitioner model. The program builds on foundations in psychology and education, and fosters a special sensitivity to cultural diversity of all people and respect for the uniqueness and human dignity of each person. The program emphasizes the delivery of school psychological services within a tiered services delivery model (prevention to targeted intervention) using a collaborative consultation model from an ecological/behavioral orientation. Students learn to view problems from an ecological/systems perspective focusing on child, family, school and community and to provide comprehensive intervention-based services utilizing data-based decision making to design, implement, and evaluate strategies for preventing and resolving learning and adjustment problem situations across a tiered service delivery model. A child advocacy perspective, built on a scientist–practitioner foundation, provides a framework for guiding decisions and practices to support positive outcomes for all children. Both theoretical and empirical bases of professional practice are emphasized and a diverse range of practical experiences are provided throughout all preparation (preschool to high school, in urban, suburban, and rural settings). The program is noted for its intervention emphasis, focusing on data-based decision making across all tiers of service delivery (prevention/school-wide intervention, target and supplemental intervention, and intensive, individualized intervention). In addition to these program themes, training at the doctoral level emphasizes advanced research and evaluation training, leadership supervision and systems-level change facilitation. Doctoral students participate as research team members in schools in Years 1 through 3.

Special Facilities or Resources: The program has access to excellent field-based training and research partnerships through collaborative relationships with several local school districts, educational agencies, and Head Start programs. Research facilities include statistical consultation for students, a college evaluation services center, and support for student research through college-sponsored mentoring grants.

Information for Students With Physical Disabilities: http://www.uc.edu/sas/disability.

Application Information:
Send to Applications are online through the Graduate School. Application available online. URL of online application: http://www.grad.uc.edu. Students are admitted in the Fall, application deadline January 15. *Fee:* $45.

Cleveland State University
Counseling Psychology Specialization of Urban Education Doctoral Program
Education and Human Services
2121 Euclid Avenue
Cleveland, OH 44115
Telephone: (216) 687-4697
Fax: (216) 875-9697
E-mail: *w.pruett-butler@csuohio.edu*
Web: *http://www.csuohio.edu/cehs/departments/phd/counseling-psychology*

Department Information:
1986. Co-Directors of Training: Donna Schultheiss / Elizabeth Welfel. Number of faculty: total—full-time 7; women—full-time 5; total—minority—full-time 2; women minority—full-time 1.

Programs and Degrees Offered:
Listed in the following order: Program area, degree type (T if terminal Master's), number awarded 7/08–6/09. Counseling Psychology PhD (Doctor of Philosophy) 0, Community Agency Counseling MEd (Education) 20, School Counseling MEd (Education) 30.

Student Applications/Admissions:
Student Applications
Counseling Psychology PhD (Doctor of Philosophy)—Applications 2009–2010, 15. Total applicants accepted 2009–2010, 6. Number full-time enrolled (new admits only) 2009–2010, 6. Number part-time enrolled (new admits only) 2009–2010, 0. Openings 2010–2011, 7. The number of students enrolled full- and part-time who were dismissed or voluntarily withdrew from this program area in 2008–2009 were 0. Community Agency Counseling MEd (Education)—Applications 2009–2010, 34. Total applicants accepted 2009–2010, 11. Total enrolled 2009–2010 full-time, 26, part-time, 40. Openings 2010–2011, 35. The median number of years required for completion of a degree in 2008–2009 were 3. The number of students enrolled full- and part-time who were dismissed or voluntarily withdrew from this program area in 2008–2009 were 0. School Counseling MEd (Education)—Applications 2009–2010, 25. Total applicants accepted 2009–2010, 18. Total enrolled 2009–2010 full-time, 10, part-time, 72. Openings 2010–2011, 35. The median number of years required for completion of a degree in 2008–2009 were 2.
Scores: Entries appear in this order: required test or GPA, minimum score (if required), median score of students entering in 2009–2010. Counseling Psychology PhD (Doctor of Philosophy): GRE-V no minimum stated, 510, GRE-Q no minimum stated, 530, overall undergraduate GPA no minimum stated, 3.27, Masters GPA no minimum stated, 3.88; Community Agency Counseling MEd (Education): GRE-V no minimum stated, 470, GRE-Q no minimum stated, 490, overall undergraduate GPA no minimum stated, 3.3; School Counseling MEd (Education): GRE-V no minimum stated, 390, GRE-Q no minimum stated, 480, overall undergraduate GPA no minimum stated, 3.2.
Other Criteria: (importance of criteria rated low, medium, or high): GRE scores—high, research experience—high, work experience—medium, extracurricular activity—low, clinically related public service—medium, GPA—high, letters of recommendation—high, interview—high, statement of goals and objectives—high, undergraduate major in psychology—low, specific undergraduate psychology courses taken—low. Criteria vary for masters programs. For additional information on admission requirements, go to http://www.csuohio.edu/cehs/departments/phd/admission-requirements.html.

Student Characteristics: The following represents characteristics of students in 2009–2010 in all graduate psychology programs in the department: Female—full-time 0, part-time 0; Male—full-time 0, part-time 0; African American/Black—full-time 11, part-time 27; Hispanic/Latino(a)—full-time 1, part-time 4; Asian/Pacific Islander—full-time 1, part-time 0; American Indian/Alaska Native—full-time 0, part-time 0; Caucasian/White—full-time 37, part-time 74; Multi-ethnic—full-time 0, part-time 0; students subject to the Americans With Disabilities Act—full-time 0, part-time 0; Unknown ethnicity—full-time 9, part-time 7; International students who hold an F-1 or J-1 Visa—full-time 4, part-time 0.

Financial Information/Assistance:
Tuition for Full-Time Study: *Master's:* State residents: per academic year $5,909, $454 per credit hour; Nonstate residents: per academic year $8,029, $617 per credit hour. *Doctoral:* State residents: per academic year $5,909, $454 per credit hour; Nonstate residents: per academic year $8,029, $617 per credit hour. Tuition is subject to change. See the following Web site for updates and changes in tuition costs: http://www.csuohio.edu/offices/treasuryservices/tuition/.

Financial Assistance:
First-Year Students: Teaching assistantships available for first year. Average amount paid per academic year: $7,800. Average number of hours worked per week: 20. Apply by April 15. Research assistantships available for first year. Average amount paid per academic year: $7,800. Average number of hours worked per week: 20. Apply by April 15.
Advanced Students: Teaching assistantships available for advanced students. Average amount paid per academic year: $7,800. Average number of hours worked per week: 20. Apply by April 15. Research assistantships available for advanced students. Average amount paid per academic year: $7,800. Average number of hours worked per week: 20. Apply by April 15.
Additional Information: Of all students currently enrolled full time, 59% benefited from one or more of the listed financial assistance programs. Application and information available online at: http://graduatestudies.csuohio.edu/catalog/?CategoryID=88.

Internships/Practica: Consistent with the program's focus on serving diverse urban populations, all practicum sites are situated in Northeast Ohio, and most are located in the heart of the greater Cleveland area. Our sites include mental health agencies, hospitals, residential centers, schools, and college counseling centers. As such, students have a rich opportunity to gain exposure to clients from a variety of backgrounds. This also ensures that students have ample opportunity to be trained across the spectrum of functioning and in a wide continuum of roles, including testing, treatment, community outreach and prevention.

Housing and Day Care: On-campus housing is available. See the following Web site for more information: http://www.csuohio.edu/services/reslife/. On-campus day care facilities are available. See the following Web site for more information: http://www.csuohio.edu/services/childcare/.

Employment of Department Graduates:
Master's Degree Graduates: Of those who graduated in the academic year 2008–2009, the following categories and numbers represent the postgraduate activities and employment of master's degree graduates: Enrolled in a postdoctoral residency/fellowship (n/a), employed in independent practice (n/a), total from the above (master's) (0).
Doctoral Degree Graduates: Of those who graduated in the academic year 2008–2009, the following categories and numbers represent the postgraduate activities and employment of doctoral degree graduates: Enrolled in a psychology doctoral program (n/a), employed in a community mental health/counseling center (1), employed in a hospital/medical center (1), total from the above (doctoral) (2).

Additional Information:
Orientation, Objectives, and Emphasis of Department: The Counseling Psychology program at Cleveland State University is based on a scientist–practitioner model of training and practice. The program emphasizes counseling psychology as a scientific discipline that is based in the tradition of studying individual differences and the social and cultural context of human behavior. It provides extensive study of multicultural aspects of human behavior with particular emphasis on the impact of urban environments. Its mission is to educate counseling psychologists with strong professional identification with the discipline and with the knowledge, skills, and attitudes to work effectively with diverse populations of clients. In the tradition of counseling psychology, the program's mission is also to educate students who are skilled not only to intervene with clients experiencing psychological dysfunction, but also to facilitate healthy development. Its training model is largely interdisciplinary, integrating knowledge in urban studies, educational psychology, organizational development, and educational policy with core content in research design, foundations of psychology, and counseling psychology courses. Counseling psychology students are enrolled in Urban Education courses with doctoral students in related disciplines in several courses to foster an interdisciplinary understanding of human behavior in urban contexts.

Information for Students With Physical Disabilities: See the following Web site for more information: http://www.csuohio.edu/offices/disability/.

Application Information:
Send to Graduate Admissions Parker Hannifan 227 Cleveland State University 2121 Euclid Avenue Cleveland, Ohio 44115. Application available online. URL of online application: http://www.csuohio.edu/gradcollege/admissions/degree.html. Students are admitted in the fall, application deadline January 15. Doctoral applications for Counseling Psychology accepted January 15 only. *Fee:* $30.

Dayton, University of
Department of Psychology
300 College Park Avenue
Dayton, OH 45469-1430
Telephone: (937) 229-2713
Fax: (937) 229-3900
E-mail: *carolyn.roecker-phelps@notes.udayton.edu*
Web: *http://campus.udayton.edu/~psych*

Department Information:
1937. Chairperson: Carolyn Roecker Phelps. Number of faculty: total—full-time 17, part-time 6; women—full-time 5, part-time 3.

Programs and Degrees Offered:
Listed in the following order: Program area, degree type (T if terminal Master's), number awarded 7/08–6/09. Clinical Psychology MA/MS (Master of Arts/Science) (T) 7, General Psychology MA/MS (Master of Arts/Science) (T) 4.

Student Applications/Admissions:
Student Applications
Clinical Psychology MA/MS (Master of Arts/Science)—Applications 2009–2010, 76. Total applicants accepted 2009–2010, 13. Number full-time enrolled (new admits only) 2009–2010, 8. Number part-time enrolled (new admits only) 2009–2010, 0. Openings 2010–2011, 10. General Psychology MA/MS (Master of Arts/Science)—Applications 2009–2010, 26. Total applicants accepted 2009–2010, 13. Number full-time enrolled (new admits only) 2009–2010, 5. Number part-time enrolled (new admits only) 2009–2010, 0. Openings 2010–2011, 8.
Other Criteria: (importance of criteria rated low, medium, or high): GRE scores—high, research experience—high, work experience—medium, extracurricular activity—low, clinically related public service—medium, GPA—high, letters of recommendation—high, interview—low, statement of goals and objectives—high, undergraduate major in psychology—medium, specific undergraduate psychology courses taken—high.

Student Characteristics: The following represents characteristics of students in 2009–2010 in all graduate psychology programs in the department: Female—full-time 22, part-time 0; Male—full-time 5, part-time 0; African American/Black—full-time 3, part-time 0; Hispanic/Latino(a)—full-time 1, part-time 0; Asian/Pacific Islander—full-time 2, part-time 0; American Indian/Alaska Native—full-time 1, part-time 0; Caucasian/White—full-time 20, part-time 0; Multi-ethnic—full-time 0, part-time 0; students subject to the Americans With Disabilities Act—full-time 0, part-time 0; Unknown ethnicity—full-time 0, part-time 0; International students who hold an F-1 or J-1 Visa—full-time 0, part-time 0.

Financial Information/Assistance:
Tuition for Full-Time Study: Master's: State residents: $729 per credit hour; Nonstate residents: $729 per credit hour.

Financial Assistance:
First-Year Students: Teaching assistantships available for first year. Average amount paid per academic year: $10,298. Average number of hours worked per week: 20. Apply by March 1. Research assistantships available for first year. Average amount

paid per academic year: $10,298. Average number of hours worked per week: 20. Apply by March 1. Traineeships available for first year. Average amount paid per academic year: $6,000. Average number of hours worked per week: 17. Apply by March 1.

Advanced Students: Teaching assistantships available for advanced students. Average amount paid per academic year: $10,606. Average number of hours worked per week: 20. Apply by March 1. Research assistantships available for advanced students. Average amount paid per academic year: $10,606. Average number of hours worked per week: 20. Apply by March 1.

Additional Information: Of all students currently enrolled full time, 72% benefited from one or more of the listed financial assistance programs.

Internships/Practica: A limited number of paid traineeship placements at local mental health agencies are available for both first and second year clinical students. These traineeships satisfy the programs's practicum requirements and include partial tuition remission. The human factors practicum is required of all program students and enables the student to gain practical experience working for governmental agencies or industrial firms during the summer between their first and second years.

Housing and Day Care: No on-campus housing is available. On-campus day care facilities are available.

Employment of Department Graduates:

Master's Degree Graduates: Of those who graduated in the academic year 2008–2009, the following categories and numbers represent the postgraduate activities and employment of master's degree graduates: Enrolled in a psychology doctoral program (7), enrolled in a postdoctoral residency/fellowship (n/a), employed in independent practice (n/a), employed in business or industry (1), employed in a community mental health/counseling center (1), employed in a hospital/medical center (1), other employment position (1), total from the above (master's) (11).

Doctoral Degree Graduates: Of those who graduated in the academic year 2008–2009, the following categories and numbers represent the postgraduate activities and employment of doctoral degree graduates: Enrolled in a psychology doctoral program (n/a), total from the above (doctoral) (0).

Additional Information:

Orientation, Objectives, and Emphasis of Department: The Department of Psychology offers graduate programs leading to the MA degree in clinical and general psychology. Emphasis is placed on integrating theory and literature with appropriate applied experience and on competence in the development of relevant research. This is the product of individual supervision and a low student-to-faculty ratio. The aim of the department is to prepare the student for doctoral training or employment at the MA level in an applied/community setting, in research, or in teaching. A recent survey has shown that over 86% of our MA graduates who applied for doctoral programs in the last 6 years were accepted. Also, 98% of our MA graduates seeking employment have found jobs in psychologically related areas.

Special Facilities or Resources: Laboratory and computer facilities are available to support student and faculty research. These include computer-based facilities for research in cognitive science, human factors, social psychology, and clinical psychology as well as a state-of-the-art Information Science Research Laboratory for multidisciplinary research in human-computer interaction. In addition, research opportunities are available through the University's Research Institute, the Fitz Center for Leadership in Community, and local community agencies.

Application Information:
Application available online. URL of online application: http://gradadmission.udayton.edu. Students are admitted in the Fall, application deadline March 1. *Fee:* $50. Fee waived if apply online.

Kent State University (2009 data)
Department of Psychology
Arts and Sciences
Kent, OH 44242
Telephone: (330) 672-2166
Fax: (330) 672-3786
E-mail: *gradpsych@kent.edu*
Web: *http://www.kent.edu/cas/psychology/*

Department Information:
1936. Chairperson: Mary Ann Stephens. Number of faculty: total—full-time 28; women—full-time 11; total—minority—full-time 4; women minority—full-time 3; faculty subject to the Americans With Disabilities Act 2.

Programs and Degrees Offered:
Listed in the following order: Program area, degree type (T if terminal Master's), number awarded 7/08–6/09. Experimental PhD (Doctor of Philosophy) 11, Clinical PhD (Doctor of Philosophy) 13.

APA Accreditation: Clinical PhD (Doctor of Philosophy).

Student Applications/Admissions:
Student Applications
Experimental PhD (Doctor of Philosophy)—Applications 2009–2010, 56. Total applicants accepted 2009–2010, 12. Number full-time enrolled (new admits only) 2009–2010, 7. Number part-time enrolled (new admits only) 2009–2010, 0. Openings 2010–2011, 12. The median number of years required for completion of a degree in 2008–2009 were 5. The number of students enrolled full- and part-time who were dismissed or voluntarily withdrew from this program area in 2008–2009 were 1. *Clinical PhD (Doctor of Philosophy)*—Applications 2009–2010, 245. Total applicants accepted 2009–2010, 18. Number full-time enrolled (new admits only) 2009–2010, 12. Number part-time enrolled (new admits only) 2009–2010, 0. Openings 2010–2011, 12. The median number of years required for completion of a degree in 2008–2009 were 6. The number of students enrolled full- and part-time who were dismissed or voluntarily withdrew from this program area in 2008–2009 were 1.

Other Criteria: (importance of criteria rated low, medium, or high): GRE scores—high, research experience—high, work experience—low, extracurricular activity—low, clinically related public service—low, GPA—high, letters of recommendation—high, interview—high, statement of goals and objectives—high, specific undergraduate psychology courses taken—medium. For additional information on admission requirements, go to http://www.kent.edu/cas/psychology/.

Student Characteristics: The following represents characteristics of students in 2009–2010 in all graduate psychology programs in the department: Female—full-time 83, part-time 0; Male—full-time 33, part-time 0; African American/Black—full-time 3, part-time 0; Hispanic/Latino(a)—full-time 8, part-time 0; Asian/Pacific Islander—full-time 4, part-time 0; American Indian/Alaska Native—full-time 1, part-time 0; Caucasian/White—full-time 100, part-time 0; Multi-ethnic—full-time 0, part-time 0; students subject to the Americans With Disabilities Act—full-time 0, part-time 0; Unknown ethnicity—full-time 0, part-time 0; International students who hold an F-1 or J-1 Visa—full-time 0, part-time 0.

Financial Information/Assistance:
Tuition for Full-Time Study: *Master's:* State residents: per academic year $8,968, $408 per credit hour. *Doctoral:* State residents: per academic year $8,968, $408 per credit hour. Tuition is subject to change.

Financial Assistance:
First-Year Students: Teaching assistantships available for first year. Average amount paid per academic year: $12,863. Average number of hours worked per week: 20. Apply by January 1. Research assistantships available for first year. Average amount paid per academic year: $12,863. Average number of hours worked per week: 20. Apply by January 1.

Advanced Students: Teaching assistantships available for advanced students. Average amount paid per academic year: $12,863. Average number of hours worked per week: 20. Apply by January 1. Research assistantships available for advanced students. Average amount paid per academic year: $12,863. Average number of hours worked per week: 20. Apply by January 1. Traineeships available for advanced students. Average amount paid per academic year: $12,863. Average number of hours worked per week: 20. Apply by January 1. Fellowships and scholarships available for advanced students. Average amount paid per academic year: $6,000. Average number of hours worked per week: 10. Apply by January 1.

Additional Information: Of all students currently enrolled full time, 100% benefited from one or more of the listed financial assistance programs. Application and information available online at: http://www.sfa.kent.edu.

Internships/Practica: Doctoral Degree (PhD Clinical): For those doctoral students for whom a professional internship was required in this program prior to graduation, (6) students applied for an internship in 2008–2009, with (6) students obtaining an internship. Of those students who obtained an internship, (6) were paid internships. Of those students who obtained an internship, (6) students placed in APA/CPA accredited internships, (0) students placed in internships not APA/CPA accredited, but listed with the Association of Psychology Postdoctoral and Internship Programs (APPIC), (0) students placed in internships conforming to guidelines of the Council of Directors of School Psychology Programs (CDSPP), (0) students placed in internships that were not APA/CPA accredited, APPIC or CDSPP listed. Seven semesters of clinical practica are required through the department's Psychological Clinic; 1,000 hours of supervised clinical experience at local field placement sites are provided with additional hours sometimes available; 2,000 hours of supervised internship experience in a program accredited by the American Psychological Association (these are competitive internships) are required.

Housing and Day Care: On-campus housing is available. See the following Web site for more information: http://www.kent.edu/childdevelopmentcenter. On-campus day care facilities are available. See the following Web site for more information: http://www.kent.edu/housing. (330) 672-2559.

Employment of Department Graduates:
Master's Degree Graduates: Of those who graduated in the academic year 2008–2009, the following categories and numbers represent the postgraduate activities and employment of master's degree graduates: Enrolled in a psychology doctoral program (15), enrolled in another graduate/professional program (0), enrolled in a postdoctoral residency/fellowship (n/a), employed in independent practice (n/a), employed in an academic position at a university (0), employed in an academic position at a 2-year/4-year college (0), employed in other positions at a higher education institution (0), employed in a professional position in a school system (0), employed in business or industry (0), employed in government agency (0), employed in a community mental health/counseling center (0), employed in a hospital/medical center (0), still seeking employment (0), not seeking employment (0), other employment position (0), do not know (0), total from the above (master's) (15).

Doctoral Degree Graduates: Of those who graduated in the academic year 2008–2009, the following categories and numbers represent the postgraduate activities and employment of doctoral degree graduates: Enrolled in a psychology doctoral program (n/a), enrolled in a postdoctoral residency/fellowship (7), employed in independent practice (0), employed in an academic position at a university (0), employed in an academic position at a 2-year/4-year college (7), employed in other positions at a higher education institution (1), employed in a professional position in a school system (0), employed in business or industry (0), employed in government agency (2), employed in a community mental health/counseling center (0), employed in a hospital/medical center (2), still seeking employment (1), other employment position (0), do not know (4), total from the above (doctoral) (24).

Additional Information:
Orientation, Objectives, and Emphasis of Department: Doctoral training is provided in clinical and in various experimental areas. The doctoral program requires full-time, continuous enrollment and is strongly research oriented. Students in clinical may specialize in adult psychopathology, assessment, child, or health. Students in experimental may specialize in biopsychology, child, cognitive, health or social psychology. Students in both programs can obtain a minor in Quantitative Methods. A common program of basic core courses is required of all students. Training facilities and laboratories are freely available to graduate students. The program's objective is to train those who can contribute through research, teaching, service, innovation, and administration.

Special Facilities or Resources: The department has well-equipped laboratories available for human and animal experimentation. Research opportunities are also available in various mental health and hospital settings in the area and at the SUMMA/KSU Center for the Treatment and Study of Traumatic Stress. Clinical training opportunities are available in the Psychological Clinic, which is staffed by clinical faculty and graduate students. The Applied Psychology Center supports research focused on psychological problems of social significance.

Information for Students With Physical Disabilities: See the following Web site for more information: http://www.kent.edu/sas.

Application Information:
Send to Chair, Graduate Admissions; Department of Psychology, Kent State University, Kent, OH 44242. Application available online. URL of online application: http://www.admissions.kent.edu/apply/Graduate/. Students are admitted in the Fall, application deadline January 1. *Fee:* $30.

Kent State University
School Psychology Program
College of Education, Health, and Human Services
405 White Hall
Kent, OH 44242
Telephone: (330) 672-2294
Fax: (330) 672-2512
E-mail: rcowan1@kent.edu
Web: http://www.kent.edu/ehhs/spsy

Department Information:
1964. School Director: Dr. Mary Dellmann-Jenkins. Number of faculty: total—full-time 4, part-time 2; women—full-time 1, part-time 2; total—minority—full-time 1; women minority—full-time 1.

Programs and Degrees Offered:
Listed in the following order: Program area, degree type (T if terminal Master's), number awarded 7/08–6/09. School Psychology EdS (School Psychology) 17, School Psychology PhD (Doctor of Philosophy) 1.

APA Accreditation: School PhD (Doctor of Philosophy). Student Outcome Data Website: http://www.kent.edu/ehhs/spsy/doctorate/index.cfm.

Student Applications/Admissions:
Student Applications
School Psychology EdS (School Psychology)—Applications 2009–2010, 42. Total applicants accepted 2009–2010, 19. Number full-time enrolled (new admits only) 2009–2010, 19. Number part-time enrolled (new admits only) 2009–2010, 0. Total enrolled 2009–2010 full-time, 49, part-time, 1. Openings 2010–2011, 16. The median number of years required for completion of a degree in 2008–2009 were 3. The number of students enrolled full- and part-time who were dismissed or voluntarily withdrew from this program area in 2008–2009 were 2. School Psychology PhD (Doctor of Philosophy)—Applications 2009–2010, 15. Total applicants accepted 2009–2010, 3. Number full-time enrolled (new admits only) 2009–2010, 2. Number part-time enrolled (new admits only) 2009–2010, 0. Total enrolled 2009–2010 full-time, 14, part-time, 4. Openings 2010–2011, 4. The median number of years required for completion of a degree in 2008–2009 were 7. The number of students enrolled full- and part-time who were dismissed or voluntarily withdrew from this program area in 2008–2009 were 2.

Scores: Entries appear in this order: required test or GPA, minimum score (if required), median score of students entering in 2009–2010. *School Psychology EdS (School Psychology):* GRE-V no minimum stated, GRE-Q no minimum stated; *School Psychology PhD (Doctor of Philosophy):* GRE-V no minimum stated, GRE-Q no minimum stated.

Other Criteria: (importance of criteria rated low, medium, or high): GRE scores—medium, research experience—high, work experience—high, extracurricular activity—medium, clinically related public service—high, GPA—high, letters of recommendation—high, interview—high, statement of goals and objectives—high. For additional information on admission requirements, go to http://www.kent.edu/ehhs/spsy/masters/apply-now.cfm.

Student Characteristics: The following represents characteristics of students in 2009–2010 in all graduate psychology programs in the department: Female—full-time 56, part-time 4; Male—full-time 7, part-time 1; African American/Black—full-time 5, part-time 0; Hispanic/Latino(a)—full-time 3, part-time 0; Asian/Pacific Islander—full-time 0, part-time 0; American Indian/Alaska Native—full-time 0, part-time 0; Caucasian/White—full-time 53, part-time 5; Multi-ethnic—full-time 2, part-time 0; students subject to the Americans With Disabilities Act—full-time 1, part-time 2; Unknown ethnicity—full-time 0, part-time 0; International students who hold an F-1 or J-1 Visa—full-time 0, part-time 0.

Financial Information/Assistance:
Tuition for Full-Time Study: Master's: State residents: per academic year $8,968, $408 per credit hour; Nonstate residents: per academic year $15,980, $728 per credit hour. *Doctoral:* State residents: per academic year $8,968, $408 per credit hour; Nonstate residents: per academic year $15,980, $728 per credit hour. Tuition is subject to change. See the following Web site for updates and changes in tuition costs: http://www.kent.edu/bursar/.

Financial Assistance:
First-Year Students: Teaching assistantships available for first year. Average amount paid per academic year: $8,313. Average number of hours worked per week: 20. Apply by May 1. Research assistantships available for first year. Average amount paid per academic year: $8,313. Average number of hours worked per week: 20. Apply by May 1.

Advanced Students: Teaching assistantships available for advanced students. Average amount paid per academic year: $10,952. Average number of hours worked per week: 20. Apply by May 1. Research assistantships available for advanced students. Average amount paid per academic year: $10,952. Average number of hours worked per week: 20. Apply by May 1.

Additional Information: Of all students currently enrolled full time, 60% benefited from one or more of the listed financial assistance programs. Application and information available online at: http://www.kent.edu/financialaid/.

Internships/Practica: Doctoral Degree (PhD School Psychology): For those doctoral students for whom a professional internship was required in this program prior to graduation, (2) students applied for an internship in 2008–2009, with (2) students obtaining an internship. Of those students who obtained an internship, (2) were paid internships. Of those students who obtained an internship, (0) students placed in APA/CPA accredited internships, (0) students placed in internships not APA/CPA accredited, but listed with the Association of Psychology Postdoctoral and Internship Programs (APPIC), (0) students placed in internships conforming to guidelines of the Council of Directors of School Psychology Programs (CDSPP), (2) students placed in internships that were not APA/CPA accredited, APPIC or CDSPP listed. Practica occur in educational and mental health settings that are chosen to provide: (a) comprehensive experiences that complement previous and current preparation; (b) appropriate supervision and mentorship; and (c) applied experiences to address individual and program objectives. EdS students take two years of practica prior to internship. Doctoral students who enter without specialist-level training in school psychology participate in three years of practica. Both the Specialist Level and Doctoral internships in school psychology follow the completion of all course work and practica. Specialist level internships are full-time for an academic year, and must occur in school settings. If completed in Ohio, the internship must conform to the Ohio Internship in School Psychology Guidelines. These internships have historically been state supported, and students receive a generous training stipend. A variety of approved settings may be appropriate for the doctoral internship, including educational settings, hospitals, and mental health centers.

Housing and Day Care: On-campus housing is available. See the following Web site for more information: http://www.kent.edu/housing/index.cfm. On-campus day care facilities are available. See the following Web site for more information: http://www.kent.edu/childdevelopmentcenter/.

Employment of Department Graduates:
Master's Degree Graduates: Of those who graduated in the academic year 2008–2009, the following categories and numbers represent the postgraduate activities and employment of master's degree graduates: Enrolled in a postdoctoral residency/fellowship (n/a), employed in independent practice (n/a), employed in a professional position in a school system (18), total from the above (master's) (18).
Doctoral Degree Graduates: Of those who graduated in the academic year 2008–2009, the following categories and numbers represent the postgraduate activities and employment of doctoral degree graduates: Enrolled in a psychology doctoral program (n/a), total from the above (doctoral) (0).

Additional Information:
Orientation, Objectives, and Emphasis of Department: The KSU school psychology program embraces a preventive mental health model as a context for the study of psychological and educational principles that influence the adjustment of individuals and systems. A commitment to using the science of psychology to promote human welfare is emphasized. In addition, recognizing the pluralistic nature of our society, the program is committed to fostering in its students sensitivity to, appreciation for, and understanding of all individual differences. A scientist–practitioner model of training, which conceptualizes school psychologists as data-oriented problem-solvers and transmitters of psychological knowledge and skill, provides another organizing theme of training. The program emphasizes the provision of services to individual schools and children, in addition to attaining a functional understanding of systems-consultation and the ability to promote and implement primary and secondary prevention programs to optimize adjustment. Since the program's emphasis is on the application of psychology in applied educational and mental health settings, students are required to demonstrate competence in the substantive content areas of psychological and educational theory and practice. Other related areas outside the school psychology core include coursework in the biological, cognitive/perceptual, social, and developmental bases of behavior, as well as in the areas of curriculum and instruction, educational foundations, and research.

Special Facilities or Resources: The Center for Disability Studies provides interdisciplinary research support for faculty and graduate students engaged in research on disability issues. The Child Development Center, an early childhood model laboratory school, provides opportunities for faculty and student research and practice. The Family Child Learning Center, which offers early intervention services to infants and toddlers with disabilities and their families, offers a training location for grant-funded school psychology students and for faculty research. The Bureau of Educational Research provides a source of support for students who are engaged in research activities, including data entry and analysis.

Information for Students With Physical Disabilities: See the following Web site for more information: http://www.registrars.kent.edu/disability/.

Application Information:
Send to Office of Graduate Student Services 418 White Hall Kent State University Kent, OH 44242. Application available online. URL of online application: http://www.kent.edu/admissions/apply/graduate/index.cfm. Students are admitted in the Fall, application deadline June 15; Spring, application deadline October 15; Summer, application deadline January 10. The preferred admission cycle is the January 10 deadline in order to begin the program in June. *Fee:* $30.

Marietta College
Department of Psychology
215 Fifth Street
Marietta, OH 45750
Telephone: (740) 376-4762
Fax: (740) 376-4459
E-mail: *sibickym@marietta.edu*
Web: *http://www.marietta.edu/departments/Psychology/*

Department Information:
1940. Director of the MAP Program: Mark E. Sibicky. Number of faculty: total—full-time 5, part-time 3; women—full-time 2, part-time 1.

Programs and Degrees Offered:
Listed in the following order: Program area, degree type (T if terminal Master's), number awarded 7/08–6/09. General Psychology MA/MS (Master of Arts/Science) (T) 12.

Student Applications/Admissions:
Student Applications
General Psychology MA/MS *(Master of Arts/Science)*—Applications 2009–2010, 24. Total applicants accepted 2009–2010,

8. Number full-time enrolled (new admits only) 2009–2010, 8. Number part-time enrolled (new admits only) 2009–2010, 0. Openings 2010–2011, 8. The median number of years required for completion of a degree in 2008–2009 were 2. The number of students enrolled full- and part-time who were dismissed or voluntarily withdrew from this program area in 2008–2009 were 1.

Scores: Entries appear in this order: required test or GPA, minimum score (if required), median score of students entering in 2009–2010. *General Psychology MA/MS (Master of Arts/Science):* GRE-V 450, GRE-Q 500, GRE-Analytical 3.75, overall undergraduate GPA 3.0.

Other Criteria: (importance of criteria rated low, medium, or high): GRE scores—medium, research experience—medium, work experience—low, extracurricular activity—low, GPA—medium, letters of recommendation—high, statement of goals and objectives—high, course work in psychology—high, undergraduate major in psychology—high, specific undergraduate psychology courses taken—high. For additional information on admission requirements, go to http://www.marietta.edu/Academics/graduate_degrees/Master_of_Arts_in_Psychology.html.

Student Characteristics: The following represents characteristics of students in 2009–2010 in all graduate psychology programs in the department: Female—full-time 17, part-time 0; Male—full-time 3, part-time 0; African American/Black—full-time 0, part-time 0; Hispanic/Latino(a)—full-time 1, part-time 0; Asian/Pacific Islander—full-time 0, part-time 0; American Indian/Alaska Native—full-time 0, part-time 0; Caucasian/White—full-time 18, part-time 0; Multi-ethnic—full-time 0, part-time 0; students subject to the Americans With Disabilities Act—full-time 0, part-time 0; Unknown ethnicity—full-time 1, part-time 0; International students who hold an F-1 or J-1 Visa—full-time 0, part-time 0.

Financial Information/Assistance:
Tuition for Full-Time Study: *Master's:* State residents: $565 per credit hour; Nonstate residents: $565 per credit hour. Tuition is subject to change. See the following Web site for updates and changes in tuition costs: http://www.marietta.edu/.

Financial Assistance:
First-Year Students: No information provided.
Advanced Students: Research assistantships available for advanced students. Average amount paid per academic year: $5,000. Average number of hours worked per week: 20. Apply by March.
Additional Information: Of all students currently enrolled full time, 2% benefited from one or more of the listed financial assistance programs.

Internships/Practica: Master's Degree (MA/MS General Psychology): An internship experience, such as a final research project or "capstone" experience is required of graduates. Students select two three-credit electives in an applied professional practicum experience. The practicum is designed to provide students with an applied experience relating to their career interests in psychology. Students choose electives from the following areas: The Teaching of Psychology - designed to train students to be effective instructors of psychology; Supervised Internship - internships in the area of clinical, developmental, or applied psychology (e.g. business/law); Directed Independent Research - students pursue their own research interests under the direction of a faculty member.

Housing and Day Care: No on-campus housing is available. No on-campus day care facilities are available.

Employment of Department Graduates:
Master's Degree Graduates: Of those who graduated in the academic year 2008–2009, the following categories and numbers represent the postgraduate activities and employment of master's degree graduates: Enrolled in a psychology doctoral program (3), enrolled in another graduate/professional program (1), enrolled in a postdoctoral residency/fellowship (n/a), employed in independent practice (n/a), employed in government agency (2), employed in a community mental health/counseling center (5), still seeking employment (1), total from the above (master's) (12).
Doctoral Degree Graduates: Of those who graduated in the academic year 2008–2009, the following categories and numbers represent the postgraduate activities and employment of doctoral degree graduates: Enrolled in a psychology doctoral program (n/a), total from the above (doctoral) (0).

Additional Information:
Orientation, Objectives, and Emphasis of Department: The Psychology Department at Marietta College offers a two-year Master of Arts degree in General Psychology. The program is designed to give students a strong graduate level foundation in psychology so students may pursue further education in psychology at the PhD level or to aid students in securing employment in a field related to psychology. The orientation of the department faculty is that psychology is a science, and that psychological research and knowledge can be applied to improving people's lives. The two year program consists of 24 core content hours in psychology, six hours of applied practicum electives in an area of professional psychology (e.g., clinical internship, developmental internship, teaching of psychology), and six hours of supervised thesis research. The program offers the opportunity for students to focus their research interest in the area of clinical, social, developmental, cognitive, and bio-psychology. Faculty have high expectations for student's academic performance, yet are committed to mentoring students and helping students achieve their educational and professional goals.

Special Facilities or Resources: The Psychology Department at Marietta College has a newly remodeled human research laboratory equipped with several research cubicles, video equipment, one way observational windows, and specialized cognitive and physiological equipment and software. Students interested in children and families have internship and research opportunities at the Marietta College Center for Families and Children on campus and in grant funded programs for children in the community. The department also maintains its own computer lab for instruction and research equipped with (SPSS) and other software. Students have access to graduate research and conference travel funds. There is also a designated graduate conference room, graduate student office and lounge area.

Information for Students With Physical Disabilities: See the following Web site for more information: http://www.marietta.edu/departments/Psychology/.

GRADUATE STUDY IN PSYCHOLOGY

Application Information:
Send to Office of Admissions, Master of Arts in Psychology, Marietta College, 215 Fifth Street, Marietta, Ohio 45750 1-800-331-7896. Students are admitted in the Fall, application deadline March 1. *Fee:* $25.

Miami University of Ohio
Department of Psychology
Oxford, OH 45056
Telephone: (513) 529-2400
Fax: (513) 529-2420
E-mail: hugenbk@muohio.edu
Web: http://www.units.muohio.edu/psychology/

Department Information:
1888. Chairperson: Carl E. Paternite. Number of faculty: total—full-time 37, part-time 1; women—full-time 20; total—minority—full-time 3; women minority—full-time 2.

Programs and Degrees Offered:
Listed in the following order: Program area, degree type (T if terminal Master's), number awarded 7/08–6/09. Clinical Psychology PhD (Doctor of Philosophy) 7, Brain and Cognitive Science PhD (Doctor of Philosophy) 3, Social Psychology PhD (Doctor of Philosophy) 4.

APA Accreditation: Clinical PhD (Doctor of Philosophy).

Student Applications/Admissions:
Student Applications
Clinical Psychology PhD (Doctor of Philosophy)—Applications 2009–2010, 100. Total applicants accepted 2009–2010, 6. Number full-time enrolled (new admits only) 2009–2010, 6. Number part-time enrolled (new admits only) 2009–2010, 0. Openings 2010–2011, 6. The median number of years required for completion of a degree in 2008–2009 were 7. The number of students enrolled full- and part-time who were dismissed or voluntarily withdrew from this program area in 2008–2009 were 0. *Brain and Cognitive Science PhD (Doctor of Philosophy)*—Applications 2009–2010, 18. Total applicants accepted 2009–2010, 8. Number full-time enrolled (new admits only) 2009–2010, 8. Number part-time enrolled (new admits only) 2009–2010, 0. Openings 2010–2011, 3. The median number of years required for completion of a degree in 2008–2009 were 6. The number of students enrolled full- and part-time who were dismissed or voluntarily withdrew from this program area in 2008–2009 were 1. *Social Psychology PhD (Doctor of Philosophy)*—Applications 2009–2010, 49. Total applicants accepted 2009–2010, 4. Number full-time enrolled (new admits only) 2009–2010, 4. Number part-time enrolled (new admits only) 2009–2010, 0. Openings 2010–2011, 2. The median number of years required for completion of a degree in 2008–2009 were 5. The number of students enrolled full- and part-time who were dismissed or voluntarily withdrew from this program area in 2008–2009 were 0.

Other Criteria: (importance of criteria rated low, medium, or high): GRE scores—medium, research experience—high, work experience—low, extracurricular activity—medium, clinically related public service—medium, GPA—high, letters of recommendation—high, interview—medium, statement of goals and objectives—high.

Student Characteristics: The following represents characteristics of students in 2009–2010 in all graduate psychology programs in the department: Female—full-time 45, part-time 0; Male—full-time 31, part-time 0; African American/Black—full-time 6, part-time 0; Hispanic/Latino(a)—full-time 1, part-time 0; Asian/Pacific Islander—full-time 5, part-time 0; American Indian/Alaska Native—full-time 1, part-time 0; Caucasian/White—full-time 63, part-time 0; Multi-ethnic—full-time 0, part-time 0; students subject to the Americans With Disabilities Act—full-time 1, part-time 0; Unknown ethnicity—full-time 0, part-time 0; International students who hold an F-1 or J-1 Visa—full-time 0, part-time 0.

Financial Information/Assistance:

Tuition for Full-Time Study: *Doctoral:* State residents: per academic year $11,759, $435 per credit hour; Nonstate residents: per academic year $25,390, $970 per credit hour. Tuition is subject to change. See the following Web site for updates and changes in tuition costs: http://www.miami.muohio.edu/graduate/fees.cfm.

Financial Assistance:
First-Year Students: Teaching assistantships available for first year. Average amount paid per academic year: $18,000. Average number of hours worked per week: 20. Apply by December 1. Research assistantships available for first year. Average amount paid per academic year: $14,800. Average number of hours worked per week: 20. Apply by December 1.

Advanced Students: Teaching assistantships available for advanced students. Average amount paid per academic year: $18,000. Average number of hours worked per week: 20. Research assistantships available for advanced students. Average amount paid per academic year: $14,800. Average number of hours worked per week: 20. Fellowships and scholarships available for advanced students. Average amount paid per academic year: $18,000. Average number of hours worked per week: 20.

Additional Information: Of all students currently enrolled full time, 100% benefited from one or more of the listed financial assistance programs. Application and information available online at: http://www.units.muohio.edu/sfa.

Internships/Practica: Doctoral Degree (PhD Clinical Psychology): For those doctoral students for whom a professional internship was required in this program prior to graduation, (6) students applied for an internship in 2008–2009, with (5) students obtaining an internship. Of those students who obtained an internship, (5) were paid internships. Of those students who obtained an internship, (4) students placed in APA/CPA accredited internships, (0) students placed in internships not APA/CPA accredited, but listed with the Association of Psychology Postdoctoral and Internship Programs (APPIC), (0) students placed in internships conforming to guidelines of the Council of Directors of School Psychology Programs (CDSPP), (1) students placed in internships that were not APA/CPA accredited, APPIC or CDSPP listed. There are opportunities for students to engage in practica and internships as well as conduct applied research.

Traineeships for advanced clinical students are available in a wide range of settings including community mental health centers, hospitals, and school systems.

Housing and Day Care: On-campus housing is available. See the following Web site for more information: http://www.miami.muohio.edu/housing/. On-campus day care facilities are available. See the following Web site for more information: http://www.childcare.muohio.edu/.

Employment of Department Graduates:
Master's Degree Graduates: Of those who graduated in the academic year 2008–2009, the following categories and numbers represent the postgraduate activities and employment of master's degree graduates: Enrolled in a postdoctoral residency/fellowship (n/a), employed in independent practice (n/a), total from the above (master's) (0).
Doctoral Degree Graduates: Of those who graduated in the academic year 2008–2009, the following categories and numbers represent the postgraduate activities and employment of doctoral degree graduates: Enrolled in a psychology doctoral program (n/a), enrolled in another graduate/professional program (0), enrolled in a postdoctoral residency/fellowship (3), employed in independent practice (0), employed in an academic position at a university (6), employed in an academic position at a 2-year/4-year college (0), employed in other positions at a higher education institution (0), employed in a professional position in a school system (0), employed in business or industry (1), employed in government agency (0), employed in a community mental health/counseling center (1), employed in a hospital/medical center (0), still seeking employment (0), not seeking employment (0), other employment position (1), do not know (2), total from the above (doctoral) (14).

Additional Information:
Orientation, Objectives, and Emphasis of Department: The goal of the department is to provide an environment in which students thrive intellectually. We strive for a balance between enough structure to gauge student progress and provide grounding in the breadth of psychology and enough freedom for students to design programs optimal to their own professional goals. The department provides training and experience in research, teaching, and application of psychology. The department offers basic and applied research orientations in all programs. The clinical program emphasizes a theory-research-practicum combination, so that graduates will be able to function in a variety of academic and service settings. The objective of the department is to produce skilled, informed, and enthusiastic psychologists, capable of contributing to their field in a variety of ways.

Special Facilities or Resources: The department has laboratories dedicated to the study of social cognition, group processes and social interaction as well as the fundamental cognitive processes of perception, categorization, decision making and choice, spatial cognition and motor control. Two laboratories use virtual environments to study spatial cognition and posture. One of these laboratories has created one of the largest virtual environments in the world. Two psychobiology laboratories offer advanced facilities for neurological recording, drug delivery, and pharmacological and histological analyses. The Psychology Clinic includes group and child therapy rooms, individual assessment and therapy rooms, a test library, conference room, and offices for the clinic director and a full-time secretary. Clinical services are offered in a training or research context to university students and the Oxford community, including a school-based mental health program. Research with children is facilitated by a good relationship with local public school systems and child-care facilities. Access to clinical populations is available through the Psychology Clinic and through cooperative arrangements with mental health centers in nearby communities. Several clinical faculty are engaged in community action projects related to mental health needs in local communities.

Information for Students With Physical Disabilities: See the following Web site for more information: http://www.units.muohio.edu/oeeo/odr/.

Application Information:
Send to The Graduate School, 102 Roudebush, Miami University, Oxford, Ohio 45056. Application available online. URL of online application: http://www.miami.muohio.edu/graduate/. Students are admitted in the Fall, application deadline. December 1 for Clinical applicants. January 1 for Social & B&C applicants. *Fee:* $35.

Ohio State University
School of Physical Activity and Educational Services
Education
100A PAES Building, 305 West 17th Avenue
Columbus, OH 43210
Telephone: (614) 292-5909
Fax: (614) 292-4255
E-mail: *joseph.21@osu.edu*
Web: *http://ehe.osu.edu/paes/*

Department Information:
1996. Director: Donna Pastore. Number of faculty: total—full-time 3; women—full-time 3; total—minority—full-time 2; women minority—full-time 2.

Programs and Degrees Offered:
Listed in the following order: Program area, degree type (T if terminal Master's), number awarded 7/08–6/09. School Psychology MA/MS (Master of Arts/Science) (T) 16, School Psychology PhD (Doctor of Philosophy) 2.

Student Applications/Admissions:
Student Applications
School Psychology MA/MS (Master of Arts/Science)—Applications 2009–2010, 89. Total applicants accepted 2009–2010, 12. Number full-time enrolled (new admits only) 2009–2010, 11. Openings 2010–2011, 10. The median number of years required for completion of a degree in 2008–2009 were 3. The number of students enrolled full- and part-time who were dismissed or voluntarily withdrew from this program area in 2008–2009 were 1. School Psychology PhD (Doctor of Philosophy)—Applications 2009–2010, 15. Total applicants accepted 2009–2010, 5. Number full-time enrolled (new admits only) 2009–2010, 2. Total enrolled 2009–2010 full-time, 19. Openings 2010–2011, 5. The median number of years required for completion of a degree in 2008–2009 were 5. The number of students enrolled full- and part-time who were dismissed or

voluntarily withdrew from this program area in 2008–2009 were 0.

Scores: Entries appear in this order: required test or GPA, minimum score (if required), median score of students entering in 2009–2010. *School Psychology MA/MS (Master of Arts/Science):* GRE-V no minimum stated, GRE-Q no minimum stated, overall undergraduate GPA 3.0; *School Psychology PhD (Doctor of Philosophy):* GRE-V no minimum stated, GRE-Q no minimum stated, overall undergraduate GPA 3.0.

Other Criteria: (importance of criteria rated low, medium, or high): GRE scores—high, research experience—high, work experience—medium, extracurricular activity—medium, clinically related public service—medium, GPA—high, letters of recommendation—high, interview—high, statement of goals and objectives—high, undergraduate major in psychology—medium, specific undergraduate psychology courses taken—medium.

Student Characteristics: The following represents characteristics of students in 2009–2010 in all graduate psychology programs in the department: Female—full-time 27, part-time 0; Male—full-time 6, part-time 0; African American/Black—full-time 4, part-time 0; Hispanic/Latino(a)—full-time 3, part-time 0; Asian/Pacific Islander—full-time 0, part-time 0; American Indian/Alaska Native—full-time 0, part-time 0; Caucasian/White—full-time 0, part-time 0; Multi-ethnic—full-time 0, part-time 0; students subject to the Americans With Disabilities Act—full-time 1, part-time 0; Unknown ethnicity—full-time 0, part-time 0; International students who hold an F-1 or J-1 Visa—full-time 0, part-time 0.

Financial Information/Assistance:
 Tuition for Full-Time Study: *Master's:* State residents: per academic year $9,000; Nonstate residents: per academic year $21,000. *Doctoral:* State residents: per academic year $9,000; Nonstate residents: per academic year $21,000. Tuition is subject to change.

 Financial Assistance:
  First-Year Students: Fellowships and scholarships available for first year. Average amount paid per academic year: $10,000. Apply by January 1.
  Advanced Students: Fellowships and scholarships available for advanced students. Average amount paid per academic year: $10,000. Apply by January 1.
  Additional Information: Of all students currently enrolled full time, 40% benefited from one or more of the listed financial assistance programs.

Internships/Practica: Doctoral Degree (PhD School Psychology): For those doctoral students for whom a professional internship was required in this program prior to graduation, (1) students applied for an internship in 2008–2009, with (1) students obtaining an internship. Of those students who obtained an internship, (1) were paid internships. Of those students who obtained an internship, (0) students placed in APA/CPA accredited internships, (0) students placed in internships not APA/CPA accredited, but listed with the Association of Psychology Postdoctoral and Internship Programs (APPIC), (0) students placed in internships conforming to guidelines of the Council of Directors of School Psychology Programs (CDSPP), (1) students placed in internships that were not APA/CPA accredited, APPIC or CDSPP listed. Master's Degree (MA/MS School Psychology): An internship experience, such as, a final research project or "capstone" experience is required of graduates. Master's students are engaged in practica during their two years of study. All students gain experience in an urban school district as well as either a rural or suburban setting. Students are involved in a 9-month school-based internship in the Central Ohio area. Internships are paid.

Housing and Day Care: On-campus housing is available. See the following Web site for more information: http://www.osuhousing.com/. On-campus day care facilities are available. See the following Web site for more information: http://hr.osu.edu/childcare/index.aspx.

Employment of Department Graduates:
 Master's Degree Graduates: Of those who graduated in the academic year 2008–2009, the following categories and numbers represent the postgraduate activities and employment of master's degree graduates: Enrolled in a postdoctoral residency/fellowship (n/a), employed in independent practice (n/a), employed in an academic position at a 2-year/4-year college (1), employed in a professional position in a school system (10), total from the above (master's) (11).
 Doctoral Degree Graduates: Of those who graduated in the academic year 2008–2009, the following categories and numbers represent the postgraduate activities and employment of doctoral degree graduates: Enrolled in a psychology doctoral program (n/a), total from the above (doctoral) (0).

Additional Information:
 Orientation, Objectives, and Emphasis of Department: The Counselor Education, Rehabilitation Services, and School Psychology Section in the School of Physical Activity and Educational Services emphasizes the preparation of individuals who can function in human services settings such as public and private schools and universities, social agencies, state and federal government agencies, business and industry, hospitals and health care facilities, and rehabilitation agencies. Emphasizing primary prevention, the program will help students, learners, and clients achieve optimal levels of human functioning and advocate for organizations and systems that promote optimal levels of human functioning. Students in the program may undertake course work to emphasize one or more of the three areas: (a) counselor education; (b) rehabilitation services; (c) school psychology.

 Special Facilities or Resources: The School of Physical Activities and Educational Services moved into a new building Spring of 2007. The Counselor Education and School Psychology Programs have a state of the art clinic facility.

Application Information:
Send to School of Physical Activity and Educational Services, Student Services and Academic Programs, 100A PAES Building, 305 W. 17th Avenue, Columbus, OH 43210. Students are admitted in the Fall, application deadline December 15. *Fee:* $40.

Ohio State University, The
Department of Psychology
College of Social and Behavioral Sciences
225 Psychology Building, 1835 Neil Avenue
Columbus, OH 43210
Telephone: (614) 292-4112
Fax: (614) 292-4537
E-mail: sexton.3@osu.edu
Web: http://www.psy.ohio-state.edu

Department Information:
1907. Chairperson: Richard E. Petty, PhD. Number of faculty: total—full-time 42, part-time 26; women—full-time 9, part-time 13; total—minority—full-time 5, part-time 3; women minority—full-time 1, part-time 1.

Programs and Degrees Offered:
Listed in the following order: Program area, degree type (T if terminal Master's), number awarded 7/08–6/09. Intellectual and Developmental Disabilities PhD (Doctor of Philosophy) 1, Behavioral Neuroscience PhD (Doctor of Philosophy) 1, Quantitative Psychology PhD (Doctor of Philosophy) 1, Social Psychology PhD (Doctor of Philosophy) 3, Cognitive Psychology PhD (Doctor of Philosophy) 1, Counseling Psychology PhD (Doctor of Philosophy) 6, Developmental Psychology PhD (Doctor of Philosophy) 2, Clinical Psychology PhD (Doctor of Philosophy) 5.

APA Accreditation: Counseling PhD (Doctor of Philosophy). Clinical PhD (Doctor of Philosophy). Student Outcome Data Website: http://www.psy.ohio-state.edu/programs/clinical/html/admin.htm.

Student Applications/Admissions:
Student Applications

Intellectual and Developmental Disabilities PhD (Doctor of Philosophy)—Applications 2009–2010, 23. Total applicants accepted 2009–2010, 4. Number full-time enrolled (new admits only) 2009–2010, 2. Number part-time enrolled (new admits only) 2009–2010, 0. Openings 2010–2011, 2. The median number of years required for completion of a degree in 2008–2009 were 5. The number of students enrolled full- and part-time who were dismissed or voluntarily withdrew from this program area in 2008–2009 were 0. *Behavioral Neuroscience PhD (Doctor of Philosophy)*—Applications 2009–2010, 21. Total applicants accepted 2009–2010, 4. Number full-time enrolled (new admits only) 2009–2010, 2. Number part-time enrolled (new admits only) 2009–2010, 0. Openings 2010–2011, 5. The median number of years required for completion of a degree in 2008–2009 were 5. The number of students enrolled full- and part-time who were dismissed or voluntarily withdrew from this program area in 2008–2009 were 0. *Quantitative Psychology PhD (Doctor of Philosophy)*—Applications 2009–2010, 23. Total applicants accepted 2009–2010, 7. Number full-time enrolled (new admits only) 2009–2010, 3. Number part-time enrolled (new admits only) 2009–2010, 0. Openings 2010–2011, 3. The median number of years required for completion of a degree in 2008–2009 were 4. The number of students enrolled full- and part-time who were dismissed or voluntarily withdrew from this program area in 2008–2009 were 1. *Social Psychology PhD (Doctor of Philosophy)*—Applications 2009–2010, 105. Total applicants accepted 2009–2010, 13. Number full-time enrolled (new admits only) 2009–2010, 7. Number part-time enrolled (new admits only) 2009–2010, 0. Openings 2010–2011, 5. The median number of years required for completion of a degree in 2008–2009 were 6. The number of students enrolled full- and part-time who were dismissed or voluntarily withdrew from this program area in 2008–2009 were 0. *Cognitive Psychology PhD (Doctor of Philosophy)*—Applications 2009–2010, 37. Total applicants accepted 2009–2010, 9. Number full-time enrolled (new admits only) 2009–2010, 4. Number part-time enrolled (new admits only) 2009–2010, 0. Openings 2010–2011, 5. The median number of years required for completion of a degree in 2008–2009 were 6. The number of students enrolled full- and part-time who were dismissed or voluntarily withdrew from this program area in 2008–2009 were 2. *Counseling Psychology PhD (Doctor of Philosophy)*—Applications 2009–2010, 0. Total applicants accepted 2009–2010, 0. Number full-time enrolled (new admits only) 2009–2010, 0. Number part-time enrolled (new admits only) 2009–2010, 0. The median number of years required for completion of a degree in 2008–2009 were 5. The number of students enrolled full- and part-time who were dismissed or voluntarily withdrew from this program area in 2008–2009 were 0. *Developmental Psychology PhD (Doctor of Philosophy)*—Applications 2009–2010, 22. Total applicants accepted 2009–2010, 8. Number full-time enrolled (new admits only) 2009–2010, 3. Number part-time enrolled (new admits only) 2009–2010, 0. Openings 2010–2011, 3. The median number of years required for completion of a degree in 2008–2009 were 5. The number of students enrolled full- and part-time who were dismissed or voluntarily withdrew from this program area in 2008–2009 were 0. *Clinical Psychology PhD (Doctor of Philosophy)*—Applications 2009–2010, 222. Total applicants accepted 2009–2010, 20. Number full-time enrolled (new admits only) 2009–2010, 11. Number part-time enrolled (new admits only) 2009–2010, 0. Openings 2010–2011, 8. The median number of years required for completion of a degree in 2008–2009 were 5. The number of students enrolled full- and part-time who were dismissed or voluntarily withdrew from this program area in 2008–2009 were 0.

Scores: Entries appear in this order: required test or GPA, minimum score (if required), median score of students entering in 2009–2010. *Intellectual and Developmental Disabilities PhD (Doctor of Philosophy)*: GRE-V no minimum stated, GRE-Q no minimum stated, GRE-Analytical no minimum stated, overall undergraduate GPA 3.2; *Behavioral Neuroscience PhD (Doctor of Philosophy)*: GRE-V no minimum stated, GRE-Q no minimum stated, GRE-Analytical no minimum stated, overall undergraduate GPA 3.2; *Quantitative Psychology PhD (Doctor of Philosophy)*: GRE-V no minimum stated, GRE-Q no minimum stated, GRE-Analytical no minimum stated, overall undergraduate GPA 3.2; *Social Psychology PhD (Doctor of Philosophy)*: GRE-V no minimum stated, GRE-Q no minimum stated, GRE-Analytical no minimum stated, overall undergraduate GPA 3.2; *Cognitive Psychology PhD (Doctor of Philosophy)*: GRE-V no minimum stated, GRE-Q no minimum stated, GRE-Analytical no minimum stated, overall undergraduate GPA 3.2; *Developmental Psychology PhD (Doctor of Philosophy)*: GRE-V no minimum stated, GRE-Q no minimum stated, GRE-Analytical no minimum stated, overall undergraduate GPA 3.2; *Clinical Psychology PhD (Doctor of Philosophy)*: GRE-V no minimum stated, GRE-Q no minimum stated, GRE-

Analytical no minimum stated, overall undergraduate GPA 3.2.

Other Criteria: (importance of criteria rated low, medium, or high): research experience—high, work experience—low, extracurricular activity—low, clinically related public service—low, letters of recommendation—high, statement of goals and objectives—high. Clinical area ranks interview as high.

Student Characteristics: The following represents characteristics of students in 2009–2010 in all graduate psychology programs in the department: Female—full-time 91, part-time 0; Male—full-time 45, part-time 0; African American/Black—full-time 7, part-time 0; Hispanic/Latino(a)—full-time 7, part-time 0; Asian/Pacific Islander—full-time 5, part-time 0; American Indian/Alaska Native—full-time 1, part-time 0; Caucasian/White—full-time 86, part-time 0; Multi-ethnic—full-time 0, part-time 0; students subject to the Americans With Disabilities Act—full-time 1, part-time 0; Unknown ethnicity—full-time 10, part-time 0; International students who hold an F-1 or J-1 Visa—full-time 20, part-time 0.

Financial Information/Assistance:

Tuition for Full-Time Study: *Doctoral:* State residents: per academic year $14,244, $356 per credit hour; Nonstate residents: per academic year $34,564, $864 per credit hour. Tuition is subject to change. See the following Web site for updates and changes in tuition costs: http://gradapply.osu.edu/BufferCosts.htm.

Financial Assistance:

First-Year Students: Teaching assistantships available for first year. Average amount paid per academic year: $14,400. Average number of hours worked per week: 20. Apply by December 1. Research assistantships available for first year. Average amount paid per academic year: $14,400. Average number of hours worked per week: 20. Apply by December 1. Fellowships and scholarships available for first year. Average amount paid per academic year: $20,220. Average number of hours worked per week: 0. Apply by December 1.

Advanced Students: Teaching assistantships available for advanced students. Average amount paid per academic year: $16,200. Average number of hours worked per week: 20. Apply by December 1. Research assistantships available for advanced students. Average amount paid per academic year: $16,200. Average number of hours worked per week: 20. Apply by December 1. Traineeships available for advanced students. Average amount paid per academic year: $16,200. Average number of hours worked per week: 20. Apply by December 1.

Additional Information: Of all students currently enrolled full time, 100% benefited from one or more of the listed financial assistance programs. Application and information available online at: http://www.psy.ohio-state.edu/graduate/.

Internships/Practica: Doctoral Degree (PhD Intellectual and Developmental Disabilities): For those doctoral students for whom a professional internship was required in this program prior to graduation, (1) students applied for an internship in 2008–2009, with (1) students obtaining an internship. Of those students who obtained an internship, (1) were paid internships. Of those students who obtained an internship, (1) students placed in APA/CPA accredited internships, (0) students placed in internships not APA/CPA accredited, but listed with the Association of Psychology Postdoctoral and Internship Programs (APPIC), (0) students placed in internships conforming to guidelines of the Council of Directors of School Psychology Programs (CDSPP), (0) students placed in internships that were not APA/CPA accredited, APPIC or CDSPP listed. Doctoral Degree (PhD Counseling Psychology): For those doctoral students for whom a professional internship was required in this program prior to graduation, (1) students applied for an internship in 2008–2009, with (1) students obtaining an internship. Of those students who obtained an internship, (1) were paid internships. Of those students who obtained an internship, (0) students placed in APA/CPA accredited internships, (1) students placed in internships not APA/CPA accredited, but listed with the Association of Psychology Postdoctoral and Internship Programs (APPIC), (0) students placed in internships conforming to guidelines of the Council of Directors of School Psychology Programs (CDSPP), (0) students placed in internships that were not APA/CPA accredited, APPIC or CDSPP listed. Doctoral Degree (PhD Clinical Psychology): For those doctoral students for whom a professional internship was required in this program prior to graduation, (8) students applied for an internship in 2008–2009, with (7) students obtaining an internship. Of those students who obtained an internship, (7) were paid internships. Of those students who obtained an internship, (7) students placed in APA/CPA accredited internships, (0) students placed in internships not APA/CPA accredited, but listed with the Association of Psychology Postdoctoral and Internship Programs (APPIC), (0) students placed in internships conforming to guidelines of the Council of Directors of School Psychology Programs (CDSPP), (0) students placed in internships that were not APA/CPA accredited, APPIC or CDSPP listed. For students in the clinical training program, initial practica are conducted at the in-house Psychological Services Center (PSC), supervised by core clinical faculty. Following one year of in-house training, students progress to advanced clinical experiences at program-approved externship sites throughout the community, where students gain clinical assessment and treatment experiences in a variety of settings consistent with the program's three training tracks: Adult Psychopathology, Health Psychology, and Child-Clinical Psychology. Advanced students also have the opportunity to continue treating clients in the in-house PSC while receiving supervision from adjunct faculty in the community. Additionally, all students must complete a one-year full-time internship in clinical psychology prior to the awarding of the doctoral degree.

Housing and Day Care: On-campus housing is available. See the following Web site for more information: http://housing.osu.edu/gradpro.asp. On-campus day care facilities are available. See the following Web site for more information: http://hr.osu.edu/ccc/home.htm.

Employment of Department Graduates:

Master's Degree Graduates: Of those who graduated in the academic year 2008–2009, the following categories and numbers represent the postgraduate activities and employment of master's degree graduates: Enrolled in a postdoctoral residency/fellowship (n/a), employed in independent practice (n/a), total from the above (master's) (0).

Doctoral Degree Graduates: Of those who graduated in the academic year 2008–2009, the following categories and numbers represent the postgraduate activities and employment of doctoral degree graduates: Enrolled in a psychology doctoral program (n/a), enrolled in a postdoctoral residency/fellowship (5), employed in an academic position at a university (5), employed in a professional position in a school system (1), employed in business or industry (3), employed in government agency (2), do not know (4), total from the above (doctoral) (20).

Additional Information:
Orientation, Objectives, and Emphasis of Department: The department is comprehensive in nature, with PhD programs in nearly all the major fields of study in psychology. The programs all strive to educate psychological scientists, and there is consequently a strong emphasis on research training in the doctoral programs, even in the applied areas. Our objective is to prepare theoretically sophisticated psychologists who leave us with effective skills to build upon in their later careers and with the ability to grow as psychology develops as a science and profession.

Special Facilities or Resources: There are several research labs specializing in the various programs of the OSU psychology department. In addition, since The Ohio State University is a well-known and well-established research institution, there are several non-department labs located throughout the campus that would be of possible interest to psychology graduate students.

Information for Students With Physical Disabilities: See the following Web site for more information: http://www.ods.ohio-state.edu/.

Application Information:
Application available online. URL of online application: http://www.psy.ohio-state.edu/graduate/html/application.htm. Students are admitted in the Fall, application deadline December 1. Deadline for all international applicants—November 30. Deadline for domestic applicants (except Clinical)—December 15. *Fee:* $40. International applications $50.

Ohio University
Department of Psychology
Arts and Sciences
200 Porter Hall
Athens, OH 45701-2979
Telephone: (740) 593-1707
Fax: (740) 593-0579
E-mail: *carlsonb@ohiou.edu*
Web: *http://www.psych.ohiou.edu*

Department Information:
1922. Chairperson: Bruce Carlson, PhD Number of faculty: total—full-time 29; women—full-time 12; total—minority—full-time 4; women minority—full-time 3.

Programs and Degrees Offered:
Listed in the following order: Program area, degree type (T if terminal Master's), number awarded 7/08–6/09. Clinical Psychology PhD (Doctor of Philosophy) 7, Industrial/Organizational Psychology PhD (Doctor of Philosophy) 2, Social Psychology PhD (Doctor of Philosophy) 1, Cognitive Psychology PhD (Doctor of Philosophy) 0, Health Psychology PhD (Doctor of Philosophy), Applied Quantitative Psychology PhD (Doctor of Philosophy) 0.

APA Accreditation: Clinical PhD (Doctor of Philosophy).

Student Applications/Admissions:
Student Applications
Clinical Psychology PhD (Doctor of Philosophy)—Applications 2009–2010, 154. Total applicants accepted 2009–2010, 12. Number full-time enrolled (new admits only) 2009–2010, 8. Total enrolled 2009–2010 full-time, 58. Openings 2010–2011, 9. The median number of years required for completion of a degree in 2008–2009 were 8. The number of students enrolled full- and part-time who were dismissed or voluntarily withdrew from this program area in 2008–2009 were 0. *Industrial/Organizational Psychology PhD (Doctor of Philosophy)*—Applications 2009–2010, 24. Total applicants accepted 2009–2010, 4. Number full-time enrolled (new admits only) 2009–2010, 3. Openings 2010–2011, 3. The median number of years required for completion of a degree in 2008–2009 were 6. The number of students enrolled full- and part-time who were dismissed or voluntarily withdrew from this program area in 2008–2009 were 0. *Social Psychology PhD (Doctor of Philosophy)*—Applications 2009–2010, 20. Total applicants accepted 2009–2010, 4. Number full-time enrolled (new admits only) 2009–2010, 2. Total enrolled 2009–2010 full-time, 11. Openings 2010–2011, 3. The median number of years required for completion of a degree in 2008–2009 were 8. The number of students enrolled full- and part-time who were dismissed or voluntarily withdrew from this program area in 2008–2009 were 0. *Cognitive Psychology PhD (Doctor of Philosophy)*—Applications 2009–2010, 13. Total applicants accepted 2009–2010, 3. Number full-time enrolled (new admits only) 2009–2010, 2. Total enrolled 2009–2010 full-time, 8. Openings 2010–2011, 2. The number of students enrolled full- and part-time who were dismissed or voluntarily withdrew from this program area in 2008–2009 were 1. *Health Psychology PhD (Doctor of Philosophy)*—Applications 2009–2010, 10. Total applicants accepted 2009–2010, 3. Number full-time enrolled (new admits only) 2009–2010, 1. Total enrolled 2009–2010 full-time, 5. Openings 2010–2011, 2. The number of students enrolled full- and part-time who were dismissed or voluntarily withdrew from this program area in 2008–2009 were 1. *Applied Quantitative Psychology PhD (Doctor of Philosophy)*—Applications 2009–2010, 3. Total applicants accepted 2009–2010, 2. Total enrolled 2009–2010 full-time, 5. Openings 2010–2011, 2.

Other Criteria: (importance of criteria rated low, medium, or high): GRE scores—high, research experience—high, work experience—low, extracurricular activity—low, clinically related public service—medium, GPA—high, letters of recommendation—high, interview—medium, statement of goals and objectives—medium, undergraduate major in psychology—low, specific undergraduate psychology courses taken—low. For additional information on admission requirements, go to http://www.psych.ohiou.edu/academics/grad_studies/grad_studies.html.

Student Characteristics: The following represents characteristics of students in 2009–2010 in all graduate psychology programs in the department: Female—full-time 64, part-time 0; Male—full-time 34, part-time 0; African American/Black—full-time 3, part-time 0; Hispanic/Latino(a)—full-time 2, part-time 0; Asian/Pa-

cific Islander—full-time 5, part-time 0; American Indian/Alaska Native—full-time 0, part-time 0; Caucasian/White—full-time 88, part-time 0; Multi-ethnic—full-time 0, part-time 0; students subject to the Americans With Disabilities Act—full-time 0, part-time 0; Unknown ethnicity—full-time 0, part-time 0; International students who hold an F-1 or J-1 Visa—full-time 10, part-time 0.

Financial Information/Assistance:
Tuition for Full-Time Study: *Master's:* State residents: per academic year $7,839; Nonstate residents: per academic year $15,831. *Doctoral:* State residents: per academic year $7,839; Nonstate residents: per academic year $15,831. Tuition is subject to change. Additional fees are assessed to students beyond the costs of tuition for the following: general, technology, medical (optional), and legal (optional) fees. See the following Web site for updates and changes in tuition costs: http://www.ohio.edu/finance/bursar/athenstuition.cfm.

Financial Assistance:
First-Year Students: Teaching assistantships available for first year. Average amount paid per academic year: $13,600. Average number of hours worked per week: 15. Research assistantships available for first year. Average amount paid per academic year: $13,600. Average number of hours worked per week: 15. Fellowships and scholarships available for first year. Average amount paid per academic year: $17,600. Average number of hours worked per week: 12.

Advanced Students: Teaching assistantships available for advanced students. Average amount paid per academic year: $13,600. Average number of hours worked per week: 15. Research assistantships available for advanced students. Average amount paid per academic year: $13,600. Average number of hours worked per week: 15. Traineeships available for advanced students. Average amount paid per academic year: $13,600. Average number of hours worked per week: 15. Fellowships and scholarships available for advanced students. Average amount paid per academic year: $17,600. Average number of hours worked per week: 12.

Additional Information: Of all students currently enrolled full time, 100% benefited from one or more of the listed financial assistance programs. Application and information available online at: http://www.psych.ohiou.edu/.

Internships/Practica: Doctoral Degree (PhD Clinical Psychology): For those doctoral students for whom a professional internship was required in this program prior to graduation, (7) students applied for an internship in 2008–2009, with (6) students obtaining an internship. Of those students who obtained an internship, (6) were paid internships. Of those students who obtained an internship, (6) students placed in APA/CPA accredited internships, (0) students placed in internships not APA/CPA accredited, but listed with the Association of Psychology Postdoctoral and Internship Programs (APPIC), (0) students placed in internships conforming to guidelines of the Council of Directors of School Psychology Programs (CDSPP), (0) students placed in internships that were not APA/CPA accredited, APPIC or CDSPP listed. Clinical doctoral interns are placed in APA-approved, one-year internships throughout the country. Supervised training in clinical skills is provided for all clinical students in area mental health agencies, clinics, and the departmental psychology clinic. Such training is in addition to traineeships and internships. Supervised practicum experience is provided for organizational students in area industries and organizations.

Housing and Day Care: On-campus housing is available. See the following Web site for more information: http://www.ohio.edu/graduate/housing.cfm. On-campus day care facilities are available. See the following Web site for more information: http://www.ohio.edu/childdevcenter/.

Employment of Department Graduates:
Master's Degree Graduates: Of those who graduated in the academic year 2008–2009, the following categories and numbers represent the postgraduate activities and employment of master's degree graduates: Enrolled in a postdoctoral residency/fellowship (n/a), employed in independent practice (n/a), total from the above (master's) (0).

Doctoral Degree Graduates: Of those who graduated in the academic year 2008–2009, the following categories and numbers represent the postgraduate activities and employment of doctoral degree graduates: Enrolled in a psychology doctoral program (n/a), enrolled in a postdoctoral residency/fellowship (1), employed in other positions at a higher education institution (1), employed in business or industry (1), employed in a community mental health/counseling center (3), other employment position (1), total from the above (doctoral) (7).

Additional Information:
Orientation, Objectives, and Emphasis of Department: The clinical doctoral program is a scientist/practitioner program, offering balanced training in research and clinical skills. Practicum training is offered in intellectual and personality assessment. Therapy sequences are offered in health psychology, individual and group psychotherapy, behavior modification, and child psychology. Traineeships are available at the university counseling center and area mental health agencies and clinics. The department has a psychology training clinic. The doctoral program in experimental psychology provides intensive training in scholarly and research activities, preparing the student for positions in academic and research settings. The department offers an applied quantitative psychology track. This track offers advanced training in quantitative methods to graduate students who are concurrently studying in one of the other experimental or clinical psychology programs. Besides the usual coursework in psychology, students who select this track receive extensive training in mathematics, computer science, and statistics.

Special Facilities or Resources: A new addition to Porter Hall, where the Department of Psychology is housed, was completed in the Fall of 2008. This addition contains numerous research labs equipped for a wide variety of human research activities, including psychophysiology, cognitive, social, and health. The department has its own clinic, which is used to train clinical doctoral students. Two computer laboratories in the Psychology Department, one with 30 computers and one with 4 computers, are also available for student research. All computer services are free of charge. Ohio University recently awarded the Psychology Department selective investment funds, which represent a major increase in funding for the department.

Information for Students With Physical Disabilities: See the following Web site for more information: http://www.ohio.edu/disabilities/.

Application Information:
Send to Graduate College Ohio University 2nd Floor, Room 220 Research and Technology Center Athens, OH 45701-2979 USA. Application available online. URL of online application: http://www.ohio.edu/graduate/apply.cfm. Students are admitted in the Fall, application deadline January 1. *Fee:* $50. The fee is waived or deferred with a statement of need from the financial aid office of the applicant's college.

Toledo, University of
Department of Psychology
Arts and Science
Department of Psychology, The University of Toledo, MS#948
Toledo, OH 43606
Telephone: (419) 530-2717
Fax: (419) 530-8479
E-mail: mark.denham@utoledo.edu
Web: http://www.utoledo.edu/psychology/

Department Information:
1913. Interim Chair: Dr. Mark Denham. Number of faculty: total—full-time 18; women—full-time 8; total—minority—full-time 3; women minority—full-time 1.

Programs and Degrees Offered:
Listed in the following order: Program area, degree type (T if terminal Master's), number awarded 7/08–6/09. Experimental Psychology PhD (Doctor of Philosophy) 6, Clinical Psychology PhD (Doctor of Philosophy) 5.

APA Accreditation: Clinical PhD (Doctor of Philosophy). Student Outcome Data Website: http://psychology.utoledo.edu/showpage.asp?name=statistics.

Student Applications/Admissions:
Student Applications
Experimental Psychology PhD (Doctor of Philosophy)—Applications 2009–2010, 45. Total applicants accepted 2009–2010, 8. Number full-time enrolled (new admits only) 2009–2010, 2. Number part-time enrolled (new admits only) 2009–2010, 0. Openings 2010–2011, 6. The median number of years required for completion of a degree in 2008–2009 were 5. The number of students enrolled full- and part-time who were dismissed or voluntarily withdrew from this program area in 2008–2009 were 0. Clinical Psychology PhD (Doctor of Philosophy)—Applications 2009–2010, 123. Total applicants accepted 2009–2010, 7. Number full-time enrolled (new admits only) 2009–2010, 7. Number part-time enrolled (new admits only) 2009–2010, 0. Openings 2010–2011, 7. The median number of years required for completion of a degree in 2008–2009 were 5. The number of students enrolled full- and part-time who were dismissed or voluntarily withdrew from this program area in 2008–2009 were 1.
Scores: Entries appear in this order: required test or GPA, minimum score (if required), median score of students entering in 2009–2010. Clinical Psychology PhD (Doctor of Philosophy): GRE-V no minimum stated, 560, GRE-Q no minimum stated, 640, GRE-Analytical no minimum stated, 4.9, overall undergraduate GPA no minimum stated, 3.65.

Other Criteria: (importance of criteria rated low, medium, or high): GRE scores—high, research experience—high, work experience—medium, extracurricular activity—medium, clinically related public service—low, GPA—high, letters of recommendation—high, interview—medium, statement of goals and objectives—high, undergraduate major in psychology—medium. For additional information on admission requirements, go to http://www.utoledo.edu/psychology.

Student Characteristics: The following represents characteristics of students in 2009–2010 in all graduate psychology programs in the department: Female—full-time 32, part-time 0; Male—full-time 11, part-time 3; African American/Black—full-time 0, part-time 0; Hispanic/Latino(a)—full-time 0, part-time 0; Asian/Pacific Islander—full-time 6, part-time 0; American Indian/Alaska Native—full-time 0, part-time 0; Caucasian/White—full-time 36, part-time 0; Multi-ethnic—full-time 1, part-time 0; students subject to the Americans With Disabilities Act—full-time 0, part-time 0; Unknown ethnicity—full-time 0, part-time 0; International students who hold an F-1 or J-1 Visa—full-time 7, part-time 0.

Financial Information/Assistance:
Financial Assistance:
First-Year Students: Teaching assistantships available for first year. Average amount paid per academic year: $11,000. Average number of hours worked per week: 20. Research assistantships available for first year. Average amount paid per academic year: $11,000. Average number of hours worked per week: 20.
Advanced Students: Teaching assistantships available for advanced students. Average amount paid per academic year: $11,000. Average number of hours worked per week: 20. Research assistantships available for advanced students. Average amount paid per academic year: $11,000. Average number of hours worked per week: 20. Traineeships available for advanced students. Average amount paid per academic year: $11,000. Average number of hours worked per week: 20.
Additional Information: Of all students currently enrolled full time, 100% benefited from one or more of the listed financial assistance programs. Application and information available online at: http://www.utoledo.edu/psychology.

Internships/Practica: Doctoral Degree (PhD Clinical Psychology): For those doctoral students for whom a professional internship was required in this program prior to graduation, (9) students applied for an internship in 2008–2009, with (9) students obtaining an internship. Of those students who obtained an internship, (9) were paid internships. Of those students who obtained an internship, (9) students placed in APA/CPA accredited internships, (0) students placed in internships not APA/CPA accredited, but listed with the Association of Psychology Postdoctoral and Internship Programs (APPIC), (0) students placed in internships conforming to guidelines of the Council of Directors of School Psychology Programs (CDSPP), (0) students placed in internships that were not APA/CPA accredited, APPIC or CDSPP listed.

Housing and Day Care: On-campus housing is available. See the following Web site for more information: http://www.utoledo.edu/studentaffairs/reslife. On-campus day care facilities are available.

GRADUATE STUDY IN PSYCHOLOGY

Employment of Department Graduates:
Master's Degree Graduates: Of those who graduated in the academic year 2008–2009, the following categories and numbers represent the postgraduate activities and employment of master's degree graduates: Enrolled in a psychology doctoral program (4), enrolled in a postdoctoral residency/fellowship (n/a), employed in independent practice (n/a), total from the above (master's) (4).
Doctoral Degree Graduates: Of those who graduated in the academic year 2008–2009, the following categories and numbers represent the postgraduate activities and employment of doctoral degree graduates: Enrolled in a psychology doctoral program (n/a), enrolled in a postdoctoral residency/fellowship (5), employed in an academic position at a 2-year/4-year college (1), employed in a hospital/medical center (1), total from the above (doctoral) (7).

Additional Information:
Orientation, Objectives, and Emphasis of Department: Our department features an APA accredited Clinical Psychology PhD program as well as a Behavioral Science PhD program, offering specializations in Social Psychology, Developmental Psychology, Cognitive Psychology, and Behavioral Neuroscience and Learning. Although these programs differ in many respects, the purpose of both programs is to provide superior training in psychological research methods, statistical procedures, clinical practice, and theoretical comprehension. Our doctoral training emphasizes the inculcation of scientific attitudes with regard to (a) the gathering and evaluation of information, (b) the solving of basic and applied research problems, and in the clinical area, (c) clinical assessment and psychotherapy.

Information for Students With Physical Disabilities: See the following Web site for more information: http://www.student-services.utoledo.edu/accessibility/index.html.

Application Information:
Send to Graduate School, University of Toledo, Toledo, OH 43606. Application available online. URL of online application: http://www.utoledo.edu/graduate. Students are admitted in the Fall, application deadline December 15. *Fee:* $35.

Wright State University
Department of Psychology
College of Science and Mathematics
335 Fawcett Hall, 3640 Colonel Glenn Highway
Dayton, OH 45435-0001
Telephone: (937) 775-3348
Fax: (937) 775-3347
E-mail: *john.flach@wright.edu*
Web: *http://www.psych.wright.edu*

Department Information:
1979. Chairperson: John M. Flach. Number of faculty: total—full-time 26, part-time 31; women—full-time 9, part-time 12; total—minority—full-time 2, part-time 2; women minority—full-time 1, part-time 1; faculty subject to the Americans With Disabilities Act 1.

Programs and Degrees Offered:
Listed in the following order: Program area, degree type (T if terminal Master's), number awarded 7/08–6/09. Industrial/Organizational Psychology PhD (Doctor of Philosophy) 2, Human Factors PhD (Doctor of Philosophy) 6.

Student Applications/Admissions:
Student Applications
Industrial/Organizational Psychology PhD (Doctor of Philosophy)—Applications 2009–2010, 44. Total applicants accepted 2009–2010, 3. Number full-time enrolled (new admits only) 2009–2010, 4. Number part-time enrolled (new admits only) 2009–2010, 0. Total enrolled 2009–2010 full-time, 21, part-time, 2. Openings 2010–2011, 4. The median number of years required for completion of a degree in 2008–2009 were 8. The number of students enrolled full- and part-time who were dismissed or voluntarily withdrew from this program area in 2008–2009 were 0. *Human Factors PhD (Doctor of Philosophy)*—Applications 2009–2010, 27. Total applicants accepted 2009–2010, 5. Number full-time enrolled (new admits only) 2009–2010, 4. Number part-time enrolled (new admits only) 2009–2010, 0. Total enrolled 2009–2010 full-time, 28, part-time, 7. Openings 2010–2011, 4. The median number of years required for completion of a degree in 2008–2009 were 6. The number of students enrolled full- and part-time who were dismissed or voluntarily withdrew from this program area in 2008–2009 were 1.

Other Criteria: (importance of criteria rated low, medium, or high): GRE scores—high, research experience—high, work experience—medium, extracurricular activity—low, GPA—high, letters of recommendation—high, interview—medium, statement of goals and objectives—high. For additional information on admission requirements, go to http://www.psych.wright.edu.

Student Characteristics: The following represents characteristics of students in 2009–2010 in all graduate psychology programs in the department: Female—full-time 21, part-time 4; Male—full-time 27, part-time 5; African American/Black—full-time 2, part-time 0; Hispanic/Latino(a)—full-time 2, part-time 2; Asian/Pacific Islander—full-time 4, part-time 0; American Indian/Alaska Native—full-time 0, part-time 0; Caucasian/White—full-time 40, part-time 6; Multi-ethnic—full-time 0, part-time 0; students subject to the Americans With Disabilities Act—full-time 1, part-time 0; Unknown ethnicity—full-time 1, part-time 0; International students who hold an F-1 or J-1 Visa—full-time 0, part-time 0.

Financial Information/Assistance:
Tuition for Full-Time Study: *Doctoral:* State residents: per academic year $3,644, $335 per credit hour; Nonstate residents: per academic year $6,190, $631 per credit hour. Tuition is subject to change.

Financial Assistance:
First-Year Students: Teaching assistantships available for first year. Average amount paid per academic year: $12,793. Average number of hours worked per week: 20. Apply by January 1. Research assistantships available for first year. Average amount paid per academic year: $12,793. Average number of hours worked per week: 20. Apply by January 1. Fellowships and scholarships

available for first year. Average amount paid per academic year: $13,000. Average number of hours worked per week: 20. Apply by January 1.

Advanced Students: Teaching assistantships available for advanced students. Average amount paid per academic year: $12,793. Average number of hours worked per week: 20. Apply by January 1. Research assistantships available for advanced students. Average amount paid per academic year: $12,793. Average number of hours worked per week: 20. Apply by January 1.

Additional Information: Of all students currently enrolled full time, 100% benefited from one or more of the listed financial assistance programs.

Internships/Practica: Students participate in internships and practica with local businesses and Wright Patterson Air Force Base. Students working at the base can receive support.

Housing and Day Care: No on-campus housing is available. On-campus day care facilities are available. Mini University, Inc., (937) 775-4070.

Employment of Department Graduates:

Master's Degree Graduates: Of those who graduated in the academic year 2008–2009, the following categories and numbers represent the postgraduate activities and employment of master's degree graduates: Enrolled in a psychology doctoral program (7), enrolled in another graduate/professional program (0), enrolled in a postdoctoral residency/fellowship (n/a), employed in independent practice (n/a), employed in an academic position at a university (0), employed in an academic position at a 2-year/4-year college (0), employed in other positions at a higher education institution (0), employed in a professional position in a school system (0), employed in business or industry (0), employed in government agency (0), employed in a community mental health/counseling center (0), employed in a hospital/medical center (0), still seeking employment (0), other employment position (0), do not know (3), total from the above (master's) (10).

Doctoral Degree Graduates: Of those who graduated in the academic year 2008–2009, the following categories and numbers represent the postgraduate activities and employment of doctoral degree graduates: Enrolled in a psychology doctoral program (n/a), enrolled in another graduate/professional program (0), enrolled in a postdoctoral residency/fellowship (0), employed in independent practice (0), employed in an academic position at a university (0), employed in an academic position at a 2-year/4-year college (0), employed in other positions at a higher education institution (0), employed in a professional position in a school system (0), employed in business or industry (0), employed in government agency (0), employed in a community mental health/counseling center (0), employed in a hospital/medical center (0), still seeking employment (0), other employment position (0), do not know (1), total from the above (doctoral) (1).

Additional Information:

Orientation, Objectives, and Emphasis of Department: The Department offers MS and PhD degrees in Human Factors and Industrial/Organizational Psychology. Students specialize in one of these areas, but the program is designed to foster an understanding of both areas and the importance of considering both aspects in the design of industrial, aerospace, health care, and other systems. The program prepares students for careers in research, teaching, design and practice in government, consulting, business, or industry. It includes course work, research training, and experience with system design and applications. Students work closely with faculty beginning early in the program. Human factors, including cognitive engineering, deals with the characteristics of human beings that are applicable to the design of systems and devices of all kinds while industrial/organizational deals with individual or group behaviors in work settings (macrosystem variables). The department has a critical mass of students and faculty in these areas and is unique because its focus on applied psychology does not include students in clinical psychology. Both majors are strengthened by being located in the Dayton, Ohio metropolitan region, which is a rapidly developing high technology sector, a major human factors and cognitive engineering research and development center, and a region of considerable industrial and corporate strength.

Special Facilities or Resources: The Department of Psychology has modern state-of-the-art research laboratories, well-equipped teaching laboratories, and office space for faculty and graduate assistants. Specialized equipment in dedicated research laboratories supports research on sensory processes, motor control, spatial orientation, human computer interaction and display design, flight simulation, cultural cognition, naturalistic decision making, memory, aging, expertise, teamwork, assessment, training, and stress in the workplace. In addition, faculty and student share a number of individual and group testing rooms. Computer facilities include over 350 UNIX workstations, PCs, and Macintoshes. The Department works cooperatively with research laboratories, research and development organizations, and corporations in the region. These include facilities for virtual environment generation, including 3-D visual displays, 3-D auditory displays, and tactile/haptic displays. The Virtual Environment Research, Interactive Technology, and Simulation (VERITAS) facility, which is owned and operated by Wright State University but housed at Wright Patterson Air Force Base, is unique in the world. The facility includes a room-size display that surrounds the user with interactive 3-D auditory and visual images. The Department of Psychology has a Memorandum of Agreement with the U.S. Air Force Research Laboratory that facilitates utilization of its sophisticated behavioral laboratories such as flight simulators and the Auditory Localization Facility. The Air Force Research Laboratory supports multi-nation research on complex cognition. The department has two well equipped laboratories for the study of the performance and training for complex team tasks.

Information for Students With Physical Disabilities: http://www.wright.edu/students/dis_services.

Application Information:
Send to School of Graduate Studies, Wright State University, E344 Student Union, 3640 Colonel Glenn Highway, Dayton, OH 45435-0001. Application available online. URL of online application: http://www.wright.edu/sogs. Students are admitted in the Fall, application deadline January 1. Send 3 letters of recommendation on letterhead (no form required) to the School of Graduate Studies at the address listed above. *Fee:* $25.

GRADUATE STUDY IN PSYCHOLOGY

Wright State University
School of Professional Psychology
3640 Colonel Glenn Highway
Dayton, OH 45435
Telephone: (937) 775-3490
Fax: (937) 775-3434
E-mail: *eve.wolf@wright.edu*
Web: *http://www.wright.edu/sopp/*

Department Information:
1979. Dean: Larry C. James, PhD. Number of faculty: total—full-time 16, part-time 10; women—full-time 9, part-time 3; total—minority—full-time 5; women minority—full-time 2; faculty subject to the Americans With Disabilities Act 1.

Programs and Degrees Offered:
Listed in the following order: Program area, degree type (T if terminal Master's), number awarded 7/08–6/09. Clinical Psychology PsyD (Doctor of Psychology) 21.

APA Accreditation: Clinical PsyD (Doctor of Psychology).

Student Applications/Admissions:
Student Applications
Clinical Psychology PsyD (Doctor of Psychology)—Applications 2009–2010, 125. Total applicants accepted 2009–2010, 25. Number full-time enrolled (new admits only) 2009–2010, 25. Number part-time enrolled (new admits only) 2009–2010, 0. Total enrolled 2009–2010 full-time, 108, part-time, 7. Openings 2010–2011, 25. The median number of years required for completion of a degree in 2008–2009 were 5. The number of students enrolled full- and part-time who were dismissed or voluntarily withdrew from this program area in 2008–2009 were 3.
Scores: Entries appear in this order: required test or GPA, minimum score (if required), median score of students entering in 2009–2010. Clinical Psychology PsyD (Doctor of Psychology): GRE-V 500, GRE-Q 500, GRE-Analytical 4, GRE-Subject (Psychology) 500, overall undergraduate GPA 3.0, psychology GPA 3.0.
Other Criteria: (importance of criteria rated low, medium, or high): GRE scores—medium, research experience—low, work experience—medium, extracurricular activity—medium, clinically related public service—high, GPA—high, letters of recommendation—high, interview—high, statement of goals and objectives—high, Resume—high, undergraduate major in psychology—medium, specific undergraduate psychology courses taken—medium. For additional information on admission requirements, go to www.wright.edu/sopp.

Student Characteristics: The following represents characteristics of students in 2009–2010 in all graduate psychology programs in the department: Female—full-time 81, part-time 5; Male—full-time 27, part-time 2; African American/Black—full-time 18, part-time 1; Hispanic/Latino(a)—full-time 6, part-time 0; Asian/Pacific Islander—full-time 7, part-time 1; American Indian/Alaska Native—full-time 1, part-time 0; Caucasian/White—full-time 72, part-time 5; Multi-ethnic—full-time 3, part-time 0; students subject to the Americans With Disabilities Act—full-time 2, part-time 1; Unknown ethnicity—full-time 1, part-time 0; International students who hold an F-1 or J-1 Visa—full-time 6, part-time 1.

Financial Information/Assistance:
Tuition for Full-Time Study: Doctoral: State residents: per academic year $17,032, $394 per credit hour; Nonstate residents: per academic year $27,216, $631 per credit hour. Tuition is subject to change.

Financial Assistance:
First-Year Students: Fellowships and scholarships available for first year. Average amount paid per academic year: $9,726.
Advanced Students: Traineeships available for advanced students. Average amount paid per academic year: $7,000. Average number of hours worked per week: 16. Fellowships and scholarships available for advanced students. Average amount paid per academic year: $13,000. Average number of hours worked per week: 0.
Additional Information: Of all students currently enrolled full time, 100% benefited from one or more of the listed financial assistance programs. Application and information available online at: http://www.wright/sopp/apply.

Internships/Practica: Doctoral Degree (PsyD Clinical Psychology): For those doctoral students for whom a professional internship was required in this program prior to graduation, (24) students applied for an internship in 2008–2009, with (21) students obtaining an internship. Of those students who obtained an internship, (21) were paid internships. Of those students who obtained an internship, (19) students placed in APA/CPA accredited internships, (0) students placed in internships not APA/CPA accredited, but listed with the Association of Psychology Postdoctoral and Internship Programs (APPIC), (0) students placed in internships conforming to guidelines of the Council of Directors of School Psychology Programs (CDSPP), (2) students placed in internships that were not APA/CPA accredited, APPIC or CDSPP listed. During years two, three, and four of the doctoral program, students are assigned to yearlong practicum placements for 2 days (16-20 hours) per week. Most practicum placements carry a stipend of $7,000 per year. Approximately half the practicum placements are in the two clinical/teaching facilities operated by the school. These include Counseling and Wellness Services on WSU's campus, which provides psychological services for the university's student body, and the Ellis Human Development Institute, which is located in Dayton, Ohio and provides a broad range of psychological services and special treatment programs developed in response to the needs of the Dayton community. The remaining practicum placements are located in a broad array of service settings located primarily in Dayton and southwestern Ohio. These practicum settings include public agencies, correctional settings, hospitals, health and mental health clinics.

Housing and Day Care: On-campus housing is available. See the following Web site for more information: http://www.wright.edu/students/housing. On-campus day care facilities are available. http://www.miniuniversity.net/Wright-State-University.asp.

Employment of Department Graduates:
Master's Degree Graduates: Of those who graduated in the academic year 2008–2009, the following categories and numbers represent the postgraduate activities and employment of master's degree graduates: Enrolled in a postdoctoral residency/fellowship

(n/a), employed in independent practice (n/a), total from the above (master's) (0).

Doctoral Degree Graduates: Of those who graduated in the academic year 2008–2009, the following categories and numbers represent the postgraduate activities and employment of doctoral degree graduates: Enrolled in a psychology doctoral program (n/a), enrolled in another graduate/professional program (0), enrolled in a postdoctoral residency/fellowship (0), employed in independent practice (2), employed in an academic position at a university (0), employed in an academic position at a 2-year/4-year college (0), employed in other positions at a higher education institution (2), employed in a professional position in a school system (0), employed in business or industry (0), employed in government agency (5), employed in a community mental health/counseling center (2), employed in a hospital/medical center (4), still seeking employment (0), not seeking employment (0), other employment position (4), do not know (2), total from the above (doctoral) (21).

Additional Information:

Orientation, Objectives, and Emphasis of Department: The School of Professional Psychology is committed to a practitioner model of professional education that educates students at the doctoral level for the eclectic, general practice of psychology. As a part of its educational mission, the school emphasizes cultural and other aspects of diversity in the composition of its student body, faculty and curriculum. The curriculum is organized around seven core competency areas that are fundamental to the practice of psychology currently and in the future, including diversity, research and evaluation, assessment, intervention, relationship, management- supervision, and consultation-education. In years 1 and 2 the curriculum is designed around foundation coursework and the development of basic competencies. Years 3 and 4 are devoted to the development of advanced competency levels. Year 5 is dedicated to a predoctoral internship.

Special Facilities or Resources: The program operates two large clinical service centers that are designed to accommodate academic teaching, clinical training, clinical program development and research. Counseling and Wellness Services is located in the Student Union along with other student health and wellness services. This service center provides assessment and group and individual therapy services to the university student body which numbers approximately 18,000. Opportunities are available for trainees to participate in crisis intervention, prevention programs, outreach to residence halls, and multidisciplinary training with medical and nursing students. The second service center, the Ellis Human Development Institute, is located in an urban, primarily African-American section of Dayton. The Ellis Human Development Institute provides assessment and group and individual therapy to children, adolescents and adults from the Dayton community. Several special treatment programs provide unique opportunities for trainees. These include violence prevention programs for minority adolescents, treatment programs addressing perpetrators and victims of domestic violence, and an assessment/intervention program for persons with dementia. Both service centers house trainee and faculty offices and computers for student use in research and training activities; both facilities are equipped with state-of-the-art equipment for videotaped and live clinical supervision.

Information for Students With Physical Disabilities: See the following Web site for more information: www.wright.edu/students/dis_services/.

Application Information:
Send to Office of Admissions/Alumni Relations, 110 Health Sciences Building, Wright State University, Dayton, OH 45435. Application available online. URL of online application: http://www.wright.edu/sopp. Students are admitted in the Fall, application deadline January 15. *Fee:* $50. Application fee can be waived if applicant provides data of financial hardship.

Xavier University
Department of Psychology
College of Social Sciences, Health and Education
Elet Hall
Cincinnati, OH 45207-6511
Telephone: (513) 745-3533
Fax: (513) 745-3327
E-mail: *dacey@xavier.edu*
Web: *http://www.xavier.edu/psychology-grad*

Department Information:
1962. Chairperson: Christine M. Dacey, PhD, ABPP. Number of faculty: total—full-time 16, part-time 11; women—full-time 8, part-time 6; total—minority—full-time 2, part-time 1; women minority—full-time 2, part-time 1.

Programs and Degrees Offered:
Listed in the following order: Program area, degree type (T if terminal Master's), number awarded 7/08–6/09. Clinical Psychology PsyD (Doctor of Psychology) 14, Experimental Psychology MA/MS (Master of Arts/Science) (T) 0, Industrial/Organizational Psychology MA/MS (Master of Arts/Science) (T) 6.

APA Accreditation: Clinical PsyD (Doctor of Psychology).

Student Applications/Admissions:
Student Applications

Clinical Psychology PsyD (Doctor of Psychology)—Applications 2009–2010, 219. Total applicants accepted 2009–2010, 44. Number full-time enrolled (new admits only) 2009–2010, 28. Number part-time enrolled (new admits only) 2009–2010, 0. Total enrolled 2009–2010 full-time, 90, part-time, 7. Openings 2010–2011, 16. The median number of years required for completion of a degree in 2008–2009 were 6. The number of students enrolled full- and part-time who were dismissed or voluntarily withdrew from this program area in 2008–2009 were 2. *Experimental Psychology MA/MS (Master of Arts/Science)*—Applications 2009–2010, 8. Total applicants accepted 2009–2010, 0. Number full-time enrolled (new admits only) 2009–2010, 0. Number part-time enrolled (new admits only) 2009–2010, 0. The number of students enrolled full- and part-time who were dismissed or voluntarily withdrew from this program area in 2008–2009 were 0. *Industrial/Organizational Psychology MA/MS (Master of Arts/Science)*—Applications 2009–2010, 45. Total applicants accepted 2009–2010, 21. Number full-time enrolled (new admits only) 2009–2010, 11. Number part-time enrolled (new admits only) 2009–2010, 0.

Total enrolled 2009–2010 full-time, 20, part-time, 1. Openings 2010–2011, 10. The median number of years required for completion of a degree in 2008–2009 were 2. The number of students enrolled full- and part-time who were dismissed or voluntarily withdrew from this program area in 2008–2009 were 1.

Scores: Entries appear in this order: required test or GPA, minimum score (if required), median score of students entering in 2009–2010. *Clinical Psychology PsyD (Doctor of Psychology)*: GRE-V no minimum stated, GRE-Q no minimum stated, GRE-Analytical no minimum stated, overall undergraduate GPA 3.0, psychology GPA 3.0; *Experimental Psychology MA/MS (Master of Arts/Science)*: GRE-V no minimum stated, GRE-Q no minimum stated, GRE-Analytical no minimum stated, overall undergraduate GPA 3.0, psychology GPA 3.0; *Industrial/Organizational Psychology MA/MS (Master of Arts/Science)*: GRE-V no minimum stated, GRE-Q no minimum stated, GRE-Analytical no minimum stated, overall undergraduate GPA 3.0, psychology GPA 3.0.

Other Criteria: (importance of criteria rated low, medium, or high): GRE scores—high, research experience—medium, work experience—medium, extracurricular activity—low, clinically related public service—medium, GPA—high, letters of recommendation—high, interview—low, statement of goals and objectives—high. For additional information on admission requirements, go to http://www.xavier.edu/psychology.

Student Characteristics: The following represents characteristics of students in 2009–2010 in all graduate psychology programs in the department: Female—full-time 85, part-time 4; Male—full-time 25, part-time 4; African American/Black—full-time 4, part-time 1; Hispanic/Latino(a)—full-time 3, part-time 0; Asian/Pacific Islander—full-time 2, part-time 1; American Indian/Alaska Native—full-time 0, part-time 0; Caucasian/White—full-time 101, part-time 6; Multi-ethnic—full-time 0, part-time 0; students subject to the Americans With Disabilities Act—full-time 0, part-time 0; Unknown ethnicity—full-time 0, part-time 0; International students who hold an F-1 or J-1 Visa—full-time 2, part-time 0.

Financial Information/Assistance:

Tuition for Full-Time Study: *Master's:* State residents: $566 per credit hour; Nonstate residents: $566 per credit hour. *Doctoral:* State residents: $720 per credit hour; Nonstate residents: $720 per credit hour. Additional fees are assessed to students beyond the costs of tuition for the following: assessment course materials, diversity course fee, APAGS dues. Tuition costs vary by program.

Financial Assistance:

First-Year Students: Teaching assistantships available for first year. Average number of hours worked per week: 20. Apply by December 15. Research assistantships available for first year. Average number of hours worked per week: 10. Apply by December 15. Fellowships and scholarships available for first year. Apply by December 15.

Advanced Students: Teaching assistantships available for advanced students. Average number of hours worked per week: 10. Apply by March 1. Traineeships available for advanced students. Apply by March 1. Fellowships and scholarships available for advanced students. Apply by March 1.

Additional Information: Application and information available online at: http://www.xavier.edu/financial-aid/graduate-aid.

Internships/Practica: Doctoral Degree (PsyD Clinical Psychology): For those doctoral students for whom a professional internship was required in this program prior to graduation, (16) students applied for an internship in 2008–2009, with (16) students obtaining an internship. Of those students who obtained an internship, (16) were paid internships. Of those students who obtained an internship, (14) students placed in APA/CPA accredited internships, (0) students placed in internships not APA/CPA accredited, but listed with the Association of Psychology Postdoctoral and Internship Programs (APPIC), (0) students placed in internships conforming to guidelines of the Council of Directors of School Psychology Programs (CDSPP), (2) students placed in internships that were not APA/CPA accredited, APPIC or CDSPP listed. Master's Degree (MA/MS Industrial/Organizational Psychology): An internship experience, such as a final research project or "capstone" experience is required of graduates. In an urban setting, the university has established relationships with a number of private and public agencies, businesses, hospitals, and mental health care centers. PsyD students are given the opportunity to work with underserved populations within the three areas of interest in our PsyD program— child/adolescent, older adults and severe mental illness.

Housing and Day Care: No on-campus housing is available. No on-campus day care facilities are available.

Employment of Department Graduates:

Master's Degree Graduates: Of those who graduated in the academic year 2008–2009, the following categories and numbers represent the postgraduate activities and employment of master's degree graduates: Enrolled in a psychology doctoral program (2), enrolled in a postdoctoral residency/fellowship (n/a), employed in independent practice (n/a), employed in business or industry (3), employed in government agency (1), total from the above (master's) (6).

Doctoral Degree Graduates: Of those who graduated in the academic year 2008–2009, the following categories and numbers represent the postgraduate activities and employment of doctoral degree graduates: Enrolled in a psychology doctoral program (n/a), enrolled in a postdoctoral residency/fellowship (6), employed in independent practice (0), employed in an academic position at a university (0), employed in an academic position at a 2-year/4-year college (0), employed in a professional position in a school system (0), employed in business or industry (1), employed in government agency (1), employed in a community mental health/counseling center (6), still seeking employment (0), not seeking employment (0), other employment position (0), do not know (0), total from the above (doctoral) (14).

Additional Information:

Orientation, Objectives, and Emphasis of Department: Both the master's and doctoral programs provide students with the knowledge and range of skills necessary to provide psychological services in today's changing professional climate. Our objective for the master's students is to prepare them for immediate employment or entry into a doctoral program in their field. Our objective for the doctoral program is to prepare students to serve as clinical psychologists in their communities. The basic philosophy of the PsyD program is to educate skilled practitioners who have a solid appreciation of the role of science in all aspects of professional activity. It is based on a practitioner-scientist model of training.

Special Facilities or Resources: The department has an affiliation with the Psychological Services Center on campus, which provides psychological services to both the university population and the Greater Cincinnati community. The Center provides the opportunity for training, service, and research. There are opportunities to work in various other areas (e.g., student development) in the university. The department also has established contact with care providers in the community, which provides the opportunity to learn the delivery of service and research that occurs in such organizations.

Information for Students With Physical Disabilities: See the following Web site for more information: http://www.xavier.edu/lac.

Application Information:
Send to Margaret Maybury, Assistant Director Enrollment and Student Services Psychology Department Xavier University 3800 Victory Parkway Cincinnati, OH 45207-6511. Application available online. URL of online application: http://www.xavier.edu/psychology-grad. Students are admitted in the Fall, application deadline December 15. February 1 deadline for master's applicants. *Fee:* $35.

OKLAHOMA

Central Oklahoma, University of (2009 data)
Department of Psychology
100 North University Drive
Edmond, OK 73034
Telephone: (405) 974-5707
Fax: (405) 974-3822
E-mail: *mknight@uco.edu*
Web: *http://ceps.uco.edu*

Department Information:
1968. Chairperson: Mike Knight. Number of faculty: total—full-time 13, part-time 5; women—full-time 7, part-time 4; total—minority—full-time 1; women minority—full-time 1.

Programs and Degrees Offered:
Listed in the following order: Program area, degree type (T if terminal Master's), number awarded 7/08–6/09. Counseling Psychology MA/MS (Master of Arts/Science) (T) 38, General Psychology MA/MS (Master of Arts/Science) (T) 12, Experimental Psychology MA/MS (Master of Arts/Science) 6.

Student Applications/Admissions:
Student Applications
Counseling Psychology MA/MS (Master of Arts/Science)—Applications 2009–2010, 88. Total applicants accepted 2009–2010, 85. Total enrolled 2009–2010 full-time, 88, part-time, 23. Openings 2010–2011, 25. The median number of years required for completion of a degree in 2008–2009 were 2. The number of students enrolled full- and part-time who were dismissed or voluntarily withdrew from this program area in 2008–2009 were 22. *General Psychology MA/MS (Master of Arts/Science)*—Applications 2009–2010, 30. Total applicants accepted 2009–2010, 30. Total enrolled 2009–2010 full-time, 20, part-time, 10. Openings 2010–2011, 25. The median number of years required for completion of a degree in 2008–2009 were 2. The number of students enrolled full- and part-time who were dismissed or voluntarily withdrew from this program area in 2008–2009 were 0. *Experimental Psychology MA/MS (Master of Arts/Science)*—Applications 2009–2010, 28. Total applicants accepted 2009–2010, 22. Total enrolled 2009–2010 full-time, 20, part-time, 10. Openings 2010–2011, 10. The median number of years required for completion of a degree in 2008–2009 were 2. The number of students enrolled full- and part-time who were dismissed or voluntarily withdrew from this program area in 2008–2009 were 5.
Other Criteria: (importance of criteria rated low, medium, or high): GRE scores—medium, research experience—high, work experience—medium, extracurricular activity—medium, clinically related public service—high, letters of recommendation—high.

Student Characteristics: The following represents characteristics of students in 2009–2010 in all graduate psychology programs in the department: Female—full-time 50, part-time 10; Male—full-time 30, part-time 6; African American/Black—full-time 15, part-time 4; Hispanic/Latino(a)—full-time 7, part-time 1; Asian/Pacific Islander—full-time 7, part-time 0; American Indian/Alaska Native—full-time 4, part-time 0; Caucasian/White—full-time 0, part-time 0; Multi-ethnic—full-time 0, part-time 0; students subject to the Americans With Disabilities Act—full-time 0, part-time 0; Unknown ethnicity—full-time 0, part-time 0; International students who hold an F-1 or J-1 Visa—full-time 0, part-time 0.

Financial Information/Assistance:
Tuition for Full-Time Study: Master's: State residents: $88 per credit hour; Nonstate residents: $247 per credit hour.

Financial Assistance:
First-Year Students: No information provided.
Advanced Students: No information provided.
Additional Information: Of all students currently enrolled full time, 0% benefited from one or more of the listed financial assistance programs.

Internships/Practica: Practica and internships are available through our program in Counseling Psychology. Students initially work in our departmental clinic and then are placed off-campus in community mental health clinics in our area.

Housing and Day Care: No on-campus housing is available. No on-campus day care facilities are available.

Employment of Department Graduates:
Master's Degree Graduates: Of those who graduated in the academic year 2008–2009, the following categories and numbers represent the postgraduate activities and employment of master's degree graduates: Enrolled in a postdoctoral residency/fellowship (n/a), employed in independent practice (n/a), total from the above (master's) (0).
Doctoral Degree Graduates: Of those who graduated in the academic year 2008–2009, the following categories and numbers represent the postgraduate activities and employment of doctoral degree graduates: Enrolled in a psychology doctoral program (n/a), total from the above (doctoral) (0).

Additional Information:
Orientation, Objectives, and Emphasis of Department: Excellent training to pursue doctoral work. General experimental option - or Licensed Professional Counselor (LPC), or Licensed Behavioral Practitioner (LPB) - Counseling Psychology Option.

Special Facilities or Resources: The department has excellent computer facilities. It also has excellent clinic facilities with audio/visual equipment to train students in community counseling.

Application Information:
Send to Dean of the Graduate College, 100 North University Drive, University of Central OK, Edmund, OK 73034. Students are admitted in the Fall, application deadline November 1; Spring, application deadline March 1. These deadlines are for the Counseling option only. Experimental and General are open enrollment. *Fee:* $50.

Oklahoma State University
Department of Psychology
Arts and Sciences
116 North Murray Hall
Stillwater, OK 74078-3064
Telephone: (405) 744-6027
Fax: (405) 744-8067
E-mail: *larry.mullins@okstate.edu*
Web: *http://psychology.okstate.edu*

Department Information:
1920. Head: Larry L. Mullins. Number of faculty: total—full-time 20; women—full-time 8; total—minority—full-time 5; women minority—full-time 1.

Programs and Degrees Offered:
Listed in the following order: Program area, degree type (T if terminal Master's), number awarded 7/08–6/09. Clinical Psychology PhD (Doctor of Philosophy) 1, Lifespan Developmental Psychology PhD (Doctor of Philosophy) 1.

APA Accreditation: Clinical PhD (Doctor of Philosophy). Student Outcome Data Website: http://psychology.okstate.edu/templates/o-state/files/disclosure08.pdf.

Student Applications/Admissions:
Student Applications
Clinical Psychology PhD (Doctor of Philosophy)—Applications 2009–2010, 112. Total applicants accepted 2009–2010, 4. Number full-time enrolled (new admits only) 2009–2010, 4. Number part-time enrolled (new admits only) 2009–2010, 0. Openings 2010–2011, 7. The median number of years required for completion of a degree in 2008–2009 were 6. The number of students enrolled full- and part-time who were dismissed or voluntarily withdrew from this program area in 2008–2009 were 1. Lifespan Developmental Psychology PhD (Doctor of Philosophy)—Applications 2009–2010, 24. Total applicants accepted 2009–2010, 3. Number full-time enrolled (new admits only) 2009–2010, 3. Number part-time enrolled (new admits only) 2009–2010, 0. Openings 2010–2011, 5. The median number of years required for completion of a degree in 2008–2009 were 5. The number of students enrolled full- and part-time who were dismissed or voluntarily withdrew from this program area in 2008–2009 were 0.
Other Criteria: (importance of criteria rated low, medium, or high): GRE scores—high, research experience—high, work experience—low, extracurricular activity—low, clinically related public service—low, GPA—high, letters of recommendation—high, interview—high, statement of goals and objectives—high. For additional information on admission requirements, go to http://psychology.okstate.edu/.

Student Characteristics: The following represents characteristics of students in 2009–2010 in all graduate psychology programs in the department: Female—full-time 29, part-time 0; Male—full-time 20, part-time 0; African American/Black—full-time 2, part-time 0; Hispanic/Latino(a)—full-time 4, part-time 0; Asian/Pacific Islander—full-time 0, part-time 0; American Indian/Alaska Native—full-time 3, part-time 0; Caucasian/White—full-time 39, part-time 0; Multi-ethnic—full-time 1, part-time 0; students subject to the Americans With Disabilities Act—full-time 1, part-time 0; Unknown ethnicity—full-time 0, part-time 0; International students who hold an F-1 or J-1 Visa—full-time 1, part-time 0.

Financial Information/Assistance:
Tuition for Full-Time Study: *Master's:* State residents: $155 per credit hour; Nonstate residents: $602 per credit hour. *Doctoral:* State residents: $155 per credit hour; Nonstate residents: $602 per credit hour. Tuition is subject to change. Additional fees are assessed to students beyond the costs of tuition for the following: Health services, activities, technology. See the following Web site for updates and changes in tuition costs: http://bursar.okstate.edu/tuitionestimate.asp.

Financial Assistance:
First-Year Students: Teaching assistantships available for first year. Average amount paid per academic year: $9,805. Average number of hours worked per week: 20. Research assistantships available for first year. Average amount paid per academic year: $9,805. Average number of hours worked per week: 20. Traineeships available for first year. Average amount paid per academic year: $12,540. Average number of hours worked per week: 20. Fellowships and scholarships available for first year. Average amount paid per academic year: $3,000. Average number of hours worked per week: 0.
Advanced Students: Teaching assistantships available for advanced students. Average amount paid per academic year: $11,727. Average number of hours worked per week: 20. Research assistantships available for advanced students. Average amount paid per academic year: $11,727. Average number of hours worked per week: 20. Traineeships available for advanced students. Average amount paid per academic year: $12,540. Average number of hours worked per week: 20. Fellowships and scholarships available for advanced students. Average amount paid per academic year: $3,000. Average number of hours worked per week: 0.
Additional Information: Of all students currently enrolled full time, 100% benefited from one or more of the listed financial assistance programs. Application and information available online at: http://psychology.okstate.edu/.

Internships/Practica: Doctoral Degree (PhD Clinical Psychology): For those doctoral students for whom a professional internship was required in this program prior to graduation, (7) students applied for an internship in 2008–2009, with (7) students obtaining an internship. Of those students who obtained an internship, (7) were paid internships. Of those students who obtained an internship, (7) students placed in APA/CPA accredited internships, (0) students placed in internships not APA/CPA accredited, but listed with the Association of Psychology Postdoctoral and Internship Programs (APPIC), (0) students placed in internships conforming to guidelines of the Council of Directors of School Psychology Programs (CDSPP), (0) students placed in internships that were not APA/CPA accredited, APPIC or CDSPP listed. For clinical students, the first 2 years of practicum experience are through our on-site clinic. Advanced students are eligible to participate in external supervised practica at affiliated agencies.

Housing and Day Care: On-campus housing is available. See the following Web site for more information: http://www.reslife.okstate.edu. No on-campus day care facilities are available.

Employment of Department Graduates:
Master's Degree Graduates: Of those who graduated in the academic year 2008–2009, the following categories and numbers represent the postgraduate activities and employment of master's degree graduates: Enrolled in a postdoctoral residency/fellowship (n/a), employed in independent practice (n/a), total from the above (master's) (0).

Doctoral Degree Graduates: Of those who graduated in the academic year 2008–2009, the following categories and numbers represent the postgraduate activities and employment of doctoral degree graduates: Enrolled in a psychology doctoral program (n/a), enrolled in a postdoctoral residency/fellowship (7), employed in an academic position at a university (1), employed in a community mental health/counseling center (1), employed in a hospital/medical center (1), total from the above (doctoral) (10).

Additional Information:
Orientation, Objectives, and Emphasis of Department: The doctoral program in clinical psychology is based on the scientist–practitioner model. The program emphasizes the development of knowledge and skills in basic psychology, clinical theory, assessment and treatment procedures, and research. Practica, coursework, and internships are selected to enhance the student's interests. Students are expected, through additional coursework, specialized practica, and research, to develop a subspecialty in general clinical, clinical child, or health psychology. The program in Lifespan Developmental Psychology is a true lifespan program that has three primary goals: instruction in content areas of developmental psychology, training in research methodology and quantitative analysis, and preparation for teaching and/or research on applied topics. Students with interests in animal behavior, personality, psycholinguistics, social psychology, and quantitative methods are also encouraged to apply.

Special Facilities or Resources: The Department of Psychology is located in North Murray Hall near the center of the OSU campus. All students are provided office space that they share with 2-4 others. Offices are equipped with personal computers with access to SPSS, MS Office, the Internet, and printers. Wireless internet access is available in North Murray Hall. Every student is also provided a free email account. Graduate students also share a common room with a refrigerator, microwave oven, 2 additional computers with Adobe Professional, and a color printer. In addition, the Department of Psychology maintains a 24-station computer lab for student research, teaching, and other endeavors. The department operates the Psychological Services Center, an on-campus facility for clinical work and research. The center has equipment and facilities to accommodate a number of specialized services and functions, including videotaping, direct observation of clinical work using one-way mirrors, and direct supervision through telephones placed in therapy rooms. The department maintains liaisons with many off-campus organizations and agencies which provide the student with access to special populations for research as well as clinical activities. The department offers a variety of support services through the Psychology Diversified Students Program and the Psychology Graduate Students Association. Students are provided preadmission and postadmission assistance.

Information for Students With Physical Disabilities: See the following Web site for more information: http://sds.okstate.edu/.

Application Information:
Send to Department Head, Department of Psychology, OSU, 116 N Murray Hall, Stillwater, OK 74078-3064. Application available online. URL of online application: http://psychology.okstate.edu/. Students are admitted in the Fall, application deadline December 1. December 1 deadline for Clinical; January 15 for Lifespan Developmental. *Fee:* $40.

Oklahoma State University
School of Applied Health and Educational Psychology
College of Education
434 Willard Hall
Stillwater, OK 74078
Telephone: (405) 744-6040
Fax: (405) 744-6756
E-mail: *john.romans@okstate.edu*
Web: *http://www.okstate.edu/education/*

Department Information:
1997. School Head: Dr. John S.C. Romans, PhD Number of faculty: total—full-time 37, part-time 31; women—full-time 17, part-time 18; total—minority—full-time 5; women minority—full-time 3; faculty subject to the Americans With Disabilities Act 1.

Programs and Degrees Offered:
Listed in the following order: Program area, degree type (T if terminal Master's), number awarded 7/08–6/09. Counseling Psychology PhD (Doctor of Philosophy) 6, School Psychology PhD (Doctor of Philosophy) 6, School Psychology EdS (School Psychology) 5, Educational Psychology PhD (Doctor of Philosophy) 7.

APA Accreditation: Counseling PhD (Doctor of Philosophy). School PhD (Doctor of Philosophy).

Student Applications/Admissions:
Student Applications
Counseling Psychology PhD (Doctor of Philosophy)—Applications 2009–2010, 64. Total applicants accepted 2009–2010, 9. Number full-time enrolled (new admits only) 2009–2010, 9. Number part-time enrolled (new admits only) 2009–2010, 0. Total enrolled 2009–2010 full-time, 42, part-time, 15. Openings 2010–2011, 9. The median number of years required for completion of a degree in 2008–2009 were 5. The number of students enrolled full- and part-time who were dismissed or voluntarily withdrew from this program area in 2008–2009 were 1. School Psychology PhD (Doctor of Philosophy)—Applications 2009–2010, 23. Total applicants accepted 2009–2010, 8. Number full-time enrolled (new admits only) 2009–2010, 8. Number part-time enrolled (new admits only) 2009–2010, 0. Total enrolled 2009–2010 full-time, 41, part-time, 6. Openings 2010–2011, 8. The median number of years required for completion of a degree in 2008–2009 were 5. The number of students enrolled full- and part-time who were dismissed or voluntarily withdrew from this program area in 2008–2009 were 0. School Psychology EdS (School Psychology)—Applications 2009–2010, 18. Total applicants accepted 2009–2010, 4. Number full-time enrolled (new admits only) 2009–2010, 4. Number part-time enrolled (new admits only) 2009–2010,

0. Openings 2010–2011, 8. The median number of years required for completion of a degree in 2008–2009 were 4. *Educational Psychology PhD (Doctor of Philosophy)*—Applications 2009–2010, 13. Total applicants accepted 2009–2010, 10. Number full-time enrolled (new admits only) 2009–2010, 4. Number part-time enrolled (new admits only) 2009–2010, 6. Total enrolled 2009–2010 full-time, 8, part-time, 13. Openings 2010–2011, 6. The median number of years required for completion of a degree in 2008–2009 were 5. The number of students enrolled full- and part-time who were dismissed or voluntarily withdrew from this program area in 2008–2009 were 0.

Other Criteria: (importance of criteria rated low, medium, or high): GRE scores—high, research experience—high, work experience—medium, extracurricular activity—medium, clinically related public service—medium, GPA—high, letters of recommendation—high, interview—high, statement of goals and objectives—high. School Psychology: work experience and clinically related public service low, letters and interview are high, statement of goals—high. For additional information on admission requirements, go to http://education.okstate.edu/.

Student Characteristics: The following represents characteristics of students in 2009–2010 in all graduate psychology programs in the department: Female—full-time 97, part-time 17; Male—full-time 14, part-time 17; African American/Black—full-time 8, part-time 0; Hispanic/Latino(a)—full-time 4, part-time 2; Asian/Pacific Islander—full-time 4, part-time 1; American Indian/Alaska Native—full-time 5, part-time 1; Caucasian/White—full-time 89, part-time 28; Multi-ethnic—full-time 1, part-time 2; students subject to the Americans With Disabilities Act—full-time 0, part-time 0; Unknown ethnicity—full-time 0, part-time 0; International students who hold an F-1 or J-1 Visa—full-time 0, part-time 0.

Financial Information/Assistance:

Tuition for Full-Time Study: *Master's:* State residents: per academic year $2,664, $148 per credit hour; Nonstate residents: per academic year $9,985, $554 per credit hour. *Doctoral:* State residents: per academic year $2,664, $148 per credit hour; Nonstate residents: per academic year $9,985, $554 per credit hour. Tuition is subject to change. See the following Web site for updates and changes in tuition costs: http://bursar.okstate.edu/tuition.html.

Financial Assistance:

First-Year Students: Teaching assistantships available for first year. Average amount paid per academic year: $4,005. Average number of hours worked per week: 10. Apply by April 15. Research assistantships available for first year. Average amount paid per academic year: $8,010. Average number of hours worked per week: 20. Apply by April 15. Traineeships available for first year.

Advanced Students: Teaching assistantships available for advanced students. Average amount paid per academic year: $4,635. Average number of hours worked per week: 10. Apply by April 15. Research assistantships available for advanced students. Average amount paid per academic year: $4,635. Average number of hours worked per week: 10. Apply by April 15. Traineeships available for advanced students. Average amount paid per academic year: $9,270. Average number of hours worked per week: 20. Fellowships and scholarships available for advanced students. Average amount paid per academic year: $250.

Additional Information: Of all students currently enrolled full time, 84% benefited from one or more of the listed financial assistance programs. Application and information available online at: http://okstate.edu/education/gradcollege/.

Internships/Practica: Doctoral Degree (PhD Counseling Psychology): For those doctoral students for whom a professional internship was required in this program prior to graduation, (7) students applied for an internship in 2008–2009, with (7) students obtaining an internship. Of those students who obtained an internship, (6) were paid internships. Of those students who obtained an internship, (6) students placed in APA/CPA accredited internships, (0) students placed in internships not APA/CPA accredited, but listed with the Association of Psychology Postdoctoral and Internship Programs (APPIC), (0) students placed in internships conforming to guidelines of the Council of Directors of School Psychology Programs (CDSPP), (1) students placed in internships that were not APA/CPA accredited, APPIC or CDSPP listed. Doctoral Degree (PhD School Psychology): For those doctoral students for whom a professional internship was required in this program prior to graduation, (8) students applied for an internship in 2008–2009, with (8) students obtaining an internship. Of those students who obtained an internship, (8) were paid internships. Of those students who obtained an internship, (8) students placed in APA/CPA accredited internships, (0) students placed in internships not APA/CPA accredited, but listed with the Association of Psychology Postdoctoral and Internship Programs (APPIC), (0) students placed in internships conforming to guidelines of the Council of Directors of School Psychology Programs (CDSPP), (0) students placed in internships that were not APA/CPA accredited, APPIC or CDSPP listed. Multiple settings for internship experiences are available nationally on a competitive basis, faculty must approve site selection. Students have obtained internships in a wide variety of settings (i.e., health centers, hospital settings). Internships must meet established standards for predoctoral internships in counseling psychology. Practica are available at on-campus agencies, including a university counseling service, a mental health clinic at the student hospital, a career information center, and a marriage and family counseling service. Several off-campus placements are within a 75-mile radius of Stillwater, particularly in and around Tulsa and Oklahoma City. School Psychology PhD students are required to compete for internships through APPIC. There has been a 100% match for school psychology students. School Psychology EdS students complete the internship in approved public school settings. Practica are completed in public school settings and in the School Psychology Center.

Housing and Day Care: On-campus housing is available. See the following Web site for more information: http://www.reslife.okstate.edu. No on-campus day care facilities are available.

Employment of Department Graduates:

Master's Degree Graduates: Of those who graduated in the academic year 2008–2009, the following categories and numbers represent the postgraduate activities and employment of master's degree graduates: Enrolled in a psychology doctoral program (0), enrolled in a postdoctoral residency/fellowship (n/a), employed in independent practice (n/a), total from the above (master's) (0).

Doctoral Degree Graduates: Of those who graduated in the academic year 2008–2009, the following categories and numbers represent the postgraduate activities and employment of doctoral degree graduates: Enrolled in a psychology doctoral program (n/a), enrolled in a postdoctoral residency/fellowship (3), employed in independent practice (3), employed in an academic position at a university (2), employed in other positions at a higher education institution (2), total from the above (doctoral) (10).

Additional Information:
Orientation, Objectives, and Emphasis of Department: The orientation of the Counseling Psychology program is consistent both with the historical development of counseling psychology and with the current roles and functions of counseling psychology. We give major emphasis to prevention/developmental/educational interventions, and to remediation of problems that arise in the normal development of relatively well functioning people. The focus on prevention and developmental change brings us to seek knowledge and skills related to facilitation of growth, such as training in education, consultation, environmental change and self-help. It is the focus upon the assets, skills and strengths, and possibilities for further development of persons that is most reflective of the general philosophical orientation, of counseling psychology and of this program. The School Psychology program is based on the scientist–practitioner model, which emphasizes the application of the scientific knowledge base and methodological rigor in the delivery of school psychology services and in conducting research. Training in the scientist–practitioner model at OSU is for the purpose of developing a Science-Based Learner Success (SBLS) orientation in our students. Our philosophy is that all children and youth have the right to be successful and that school psychologists are important agents who assist children, families, and others to be successful. Success refers not only to accomplishment of immediate goals but also to long range goals of adulthood such as contributing to society, social integration, meaningful work, and maximizing personal potential. The SBLS orientation focuses on prevention and intervention services related to children's psychoeducational and mental health and wellness needs. School Specialist and Doctoral programs are also approved by the National Association of School Psychologists. Educational Psychology is concerned with all aspects of psychology that are relevant to education, in particular, focal areas in the professions of Human Development, Education of the Gifted and Talented, and Instructional Psychology. The Educational Psychology program aims to bring together theory and research from psychology and related disciplines in order to facilitate healthy human development and effective learning and teaching in any educational setting. The program is designed to prepare graduates to teach in college or university settings, public education, and/or to do research in university, business, and government settings.

Special Facilities or Resources: Community/School Services, Counseling Psychology Clinic and the School Psychology Clinic.

Information for Students With Physical Disabilities: See the following Web site for more information: http://okstate.edu/sds.

Application Information:
Send to College of Education, Graduate Studies Records, Oklahoma State University, 325 Willard, Stillwater, OK 74078. Application available online. URL of online application: http://gradcollege.okstate.edu/apply/. Counseling Psychology application deadlines: PhD: December 1, Master's: March 15 & October 15. School Psychology application deadline: PhD: February 1. Educational Psychology application deadline: PhD: February 1, Master's: Rolling. *Fee:* $40. The international application fee is $75.00.

Oklahoma, University of
Department of Educational Psychology
College of Education
820 Van Vleet Oval, Room 321
Norman, OK 73019-2041
Telephone: (405) 325-5974
Fax: (405) 325-6655
E-mail: *edpsych@ou.edu*
Web: *http://education.ou.edu/departments_1/edpy/*

Department Information:
1986. Chairperson: Dr. Teresa K. DeBacker. Number of faculty: total—full-time 24, part-time 2; women—full-time 16, part-time 1; total—minority—full-time 5; women minority—full-time 4.

Programs and Degrees Offered:
Listed in the following order: Program area, degree type (T if terminal Master's), number awarded 7/08–6/09. Counseling Psychology PhD (Doctor of Philosophy) 5, Community Counseling MEd (Education) 17, Special Education MEd (Education) 10, Special Education PhD (Doctor of Philosophy) 2, Instructional Psychology and Technology MEd (Education) 6, Instructional Psychology and Technology PhD (Doctor of Philosophy) 1.

APA Accreditation: Counseling PhD (Doctor of Philosophy).

Student Applications/Admissions:
Student Applications
Counseling Psychology PhD (Doctor of Philosophy)—Applications 2009–2010, 70. Total applicants accepted 2009–2010, 7. Number full-time enrolled (new admits only) 2009–2010, 7. Number part-time enrolled (new admits only) 2009–2010, 0. Total enrolled 2009–2010 full-time, 23, part-time, 21. Openings 2010–2011, 6. The median number of years required for completion of a degree in 2008–2009 were 4. The number of students enrolled full- and part-time who were dismissed or voluntarily withdrew from this program area in 2008–2009 were 1. *Community Counseling MEd (Education)*—Applications 2009–2010, 53. Total applicants accepted 2009–2010, 17. Number full-time enrolled (new admits only) 2009–2010, 17. Number part-time enrolled (new admits only) 2009–2010, 0. Openings 2010–2011, 20. The median number of years required for completion of a degree in 2008–2009 were 2. The number of students enrolled full- and part-time who

were dismissed or voluntarily withdrew from this program area in 2008–2009 were 0. *Special Education MEd (Education)*—Applications 2009–2010, 5. Total applicants accepted 2009–2010, 5. Number full-time enrolled (new admits only) 2009–2010, 5. Number part-time enrolled (new admits only) 2009–2010, 0. Total enrolled 2009–2010 full-time, 13, part-time, 11. Openings 2010–2011, 20. The median number of years required for completion of a degree in 2008–2009 were 2. The number of students enrolled full- and part-time who were dismissed or voluntarily withdrew from this program area in 2008–2009 were 0. *Special Education PhD (Doctor of Philosophy)*—Applications 2009–2010, 1. Total applicants accepted 2009–2010, 1. Number full-time enrolled (new admits only) 2009–2010, 1. Total enrolled 2009–2010 full-time, 17, part-time, 12. Openings 2010–2011, 10. The median number of years required for completion of a degree in 2008–2009 were 3. The number of students enrolled full- and part-time who were dismissed or voluntarily withdrew from this program area in 2008–2009 were 1. *Instructional Psychology and Technology MEd (Education)*—Applications 2009–2010, 12. Total enrolled 2009–2010 full-time, 9, part-time, 25. Openings 2010–2011, 15. The median number of years required for completion of a degree in 2008–2009 were 3. The number of students enrolled full- and part-time who were dismissed or voluntarily withdrew from this program area in 2008–2009 were 5. *Instructional Psychology and Technology PhD (Doctor of Philosophy)*—Applications 2009–2010, 16. Total applicants accepted 2009–2010, 6. Number full-time enrolled (new admits only) 2009–2010, 6. Number part-time enrolled (new admits only) 2009–2010, 0. Total enrolled 2009–2010 full-time, 14, part-time, 11. Openings 2010–2011, 10. The median number of years required for completion of a degree in 2008–2009 were 4. The number of students enrolled full- and part-time who were dismissed or voluntarily withdrew from this program area in 2008–2009 were 0.

Scores: Entries appear in this order: required test or GPA, minimum score (if required), median score of students entering in 2009–2010. *Community Counseling MEd (Education):* GRE-V no minimum stated, 550, GRE-Q no minimum stated, 550, GRE-Analytical no minimum stated, 4.0, overall undergraduate GPA 3.0, last 2 years GPA 3.0.

Other Criteria: (importance of criteria rated low, medium, or high): GRE scores—medium, research experience—medium, work experience—medium, extracurricular activity—medium, clinically related public service—medium, GPA—medium, letters of recommendation—medium, interview—high, statement of goals and objectives—medium. The Instructional Psychology and Technology programs do not require interviews for all applicants. However, the Admissions Committee may require some students to interview in order to make final decisions regarding admission. For additional information on admission requirements, go to http://www.ou.edu/education/edpsy.

Student Characteristics: The following represents characteristics of students in 2009–2010 in all graduate psychology programs in the department: Female—full-time 29, part-time 0; Male—full-time 16, part-time 0; African American/Black—full-time 3, part-time 0; Hispanic/Latino(a)—full-time 2, part-time 0; Asian/Pacific Islander—full-time 3, part-time 0; American Indian/Alaska Native—full-time 4, part-time 0; Caucasian/White—full-time 0, part-time 0; Multi-ethnic—full-time 0, part-time 0; students subject to the Americans With Disabilities Act—full-time 1, part-time 0; Unknown ethnicity—full-time 0, part-time 0; International students who hold an F-1 or J-1 Visa—full-time 0, part-time 0.

Financial Information/Assistance:
Tuition for Full-Time Study: *Master's:* State residents: per academic year $5,492, $277 per credit hour; Nonstate residents: per academic year $12,866, $686 per credit hour. *Doctoral:* State residents: per academic year $5,492, $277 per credit hour; Nonstate residents: per academic year $12,866, $686 per credit hour. Tuition is subject to change. Additional fees are assessed to students beyond the costs of tuition for the following: university services, course materials, and technology. Tuition costs vary by program. See the following Web site for updates and changes in tuition costs: https://bursar.ou.edu/.

Financial Assistance:
First-Year Students: Teaching assistantships available for first year. Average amount paid per academic year: $9,900. Average number of hours worked per week: 20. Research assistantships available for first year. Average amount paid per academic year: $9,900. Average number of hours worked per week: 20. Fellowships and scholarships available for first year.

Advanced Students: Teaching assistantships available for advanced students. Average amount paid per academic year: $9,900. Average number of hours worked per week: 20. Research assistantships available for advanced students. Average amount paid per academic year: $9,900. Average number of hours worked per week: 20. Fellowships and scholarships available for advanced students.

Additional Information: Of all students currently enrolled full time, 25% benefited from one or more of the listed financial assistance programs. Application and information available online at: http://ou.edu/gradweb/funding.

Internships/Practica: Doctoral Degree (PhD Counseling Psychology): For those doctoral students for whom a professional internship was required in this program prior to graduation, (9) students applied for an internship in 2008–2009, with (8) students obtaining an internship. Of those students who obtained an internship, (8) were paid internships. Of those students who obtained an internship, (8) students placed in APA/CPA accredited internships, (0) students placed in internships not APA/CPA accredited, but listed with the Association of Psychology Postdoctoral and Internship Programs (APPIC), (0) students placed in internships conforming to guidelines of the Council of Directors of School Psychology Programs (CDSPP), (0) students placed in internships that were not APA/CPA accredited, APPIC or CDSPP listed. Master's: Numerous hospitals and clinics in the local area. Doctoral: Students choose from APA-accredited sites (two in the local area, and others across the nation).

Housing and Day Care: On-campus housing is available. See the following Web site for more information: http://www.housing.ou.edu. On-campus day care facilities are available. See the following Web site for more information: http://kindercare.com/.

Employment of Department Graduates:
Master's Degree Graduates: Of those who graduated in the academic year 2008–2009, the following categories and numbers represent the postgraduate activities and employment of master's

degree graduates: Enrolled in a psychology doctoral program (4), enrolled in another graduate/professional program (0), enrolled in a postdoctoral residency/fellowship (n/a), employed in independent practice (n/a), employed in an academic position at a university (0), employed in an academic position at a 2-year/4-year college (0), employed in other positions at a higher education institution (1), employed in a professional position in a school system (3), employed in business or industry (0), employed in government agency (1), employed in a community mental health/counseling center (0), employed in a hospital/medical center (0), still seeking employment (0), not seeking employment (0), other employment position (1), do not know (15), total from the above (master's) (25).

Doctoral Degree Graduates: Of those who graduated in the academic year 2008–2009, the following categories and numbers represent the postgraduate activities and employment of doctoral degree graduates: Enrolled in a psychology doctoral program (n/a), enrolled in another graduate/professional program (0), enrolled in a postdoctoral residency/fellowship (0), employed in independent practice (1), employed in an academic position at a university (2), employed in an academic position at a 2-year/4-year college (0), employed in other positions at a higher education institution (0), employed in a professional position in a school system (0), employed in business or industry (0), employed in government agency (0), employed in a community mental health/counseling center (2), employed in a hospital/medical center (0), still seeking employment (0), not seeking employment (0), other employment position (0), do not know (3), total from the above (doctoral) (8).

Additional Information:
Orientation, Objectives, and Emphasis of Department: The Counseling Psychology program emphasizes training in working with couples and families with children. The program has a scientist–practitioner orientation designed to encourage the professional development of the students. Minority applications are encouraged for all of our programs.

Special Facilities or Resources: The Counseling Psychology Clinic is a community-based training site for our students. The clientele reflects diverse diagnostic classifications with some cultural diversity. Couples, children, and families make up a large proportion of the population served by the clinic.

Information for Students With Physical Disabilities: See the following Web site for more information: http://drc.ou.edu/.

Application Information:
Send to Graduate Programs Officer, Department of Educational Psychology, University of Oklahoma, 820 Van Vleet Oval, Room 321, Norman, OK 73019-2041. Application available online. URL of online application: http://www.ou.edu/education/edpsy. Deadline for Counseling PhD is January 10 (Begins in fall semester). Deadline for Community Counseling MEd is January 31 (Begins in summer semester). Deadlines for Instructional Psychology & Technology MEd: Spring - October 15; Fall - March 15 and July 1. Deadline for Instructional Psychology & Technology PhD: Fall only - February 1. Special Education PhD - Spring - October 1; Fall - March 1. Special Education MEd - Spring - November 1; Fall - April 1. *Fee:* $40 for U.S., $90 for international.

Oklahoma, University of
Department of Psychology
Arts and Sciences
455 West Lindsey
Norman, OK 73019-2007
Telephone: (405) 325-4511
Fax: (405) 325-4737
E-mail: *KPaine@ou.edu*
Web: *http://www.ou.edu/cas/psychology/*

Department Information:
1928. Chairperson: Jorge Mendoza. Number of faculty: total—full-time 21, part-time 1; women—full-time 9, part-time 1; total—minority—full-time 3; women minority—full-time 2.

Programs and Degrees Offered:
Listed in the following order: Program area, degree type (T if terminal Master's), number awarded 7/08–6/09. Industrial/Organizational Psychology MA/MS (Master of Arts/Science) (T) 1, Developmental Psychology PhD (Doctor of Philosophy) 0, Experimental Personality PhD (Doctor of Philosophy) 1, Social Psychology PhD (Doctor of Philosophy) 2, Animal Cognition PhD (Doctor of Philosophy) 0, Cognitive Psychology PhD (Doctor of Philosophy) 1, Quantitative/Measurement PhD (Doctor of Philosophy) 1, Industrial/Organizational Psychology PhD (Doctor of Philosophy) 4.

Student Applications/Admissions:
Student Applications
Industrial/Organizational Psychology MA/MS (Master of Arts/Science)—Applications 2009–2010, 5. Total applicants accepted 2009–2010, 1. Number full-time enrolled (new admits only) 2009–2010, 0. Number part-time enrolled (new admits only) 2009–2010, 0. Openings 2010–2011, 2. *Developmental Psychology PhD (Doctor of Philosophy)*—Applications 2009–2010, 9. Total applicants accepted 2009–2010, 1. Number full-time enrolled (new admits only) 2009–2010, 1. Number part-time enrolled (new admits only) 2009–2010, 0. Openings 2010–2011, 2. *Experimental Personality PhD (Doctor of Philosophy)*—Applications 2009–2010, 3. Total applicants accepted 2009–2010, 0. Number full-time enrolled (new admits only) 2009–2010, 0. Number part-time enrolled (new admits only) 2009–2010, 0. Openings 2010–2011, 2. *Social Psychology PhD (Doctor of Philosophy)*—Applications 2009–2010, 20. Total applicants accepted 2009–2010, 1. Number full-time enrolled (new admits only) 2009–2010, 6. Number part-time enrolled (new admits only) 2009–2010, 0. Openings 2010–2011, 4. The median number of years required for completion of a degree in 2008–2009 were 5. The number of students enrolled full- and part-time who were dismissed or voluntarily withdrew from this program area in 2008–2009 were 0. *Animal Cognition PhD (Doctor of Philosophy)*—Applications 2009–2010, 7. Total applicants accepted 2009–2010, 0. Number full-time enrolled (new admits only) 2009–2010, 0. Number part-time enrolled (new admits only) 2009–2010, 0. Openings 2010–2011, 1. *Cognitive Psychology PhD (Doctor of Philosophy)*—Applications 2009–2010, 11. Total applicants accepted 2009–2010, 1. Number full-time enrolled (new admits only) 2009–2010, 3. Number part-time enrolled (new admits only) 2009–2010, 0. Total enrolled 2009–2010 full-time, 13, part-time, 1. Openings

2010–2011, 4. *Quantitative/Measurement PhD (Doctor of Philosophy)*—Applications 2009–2010, 9. Total applicants accepted 2009–2010, 3. Number full-time enrolled (new admits only) 2009–2010, 1. Openings 2010–2011, 3. The number of students enrolled full- and part-time who were dismissed or voluntarily withdrew from this program area in 2008–2009 were 0. *Industrial/Organizational Psychology PhD (Doctor of Philosophy)*—Applications 2009–2010, 44. Total applicants accepted 2009–2010, 16. Number full-time enrolled (new admits only) 2009–2010, 4. Number part-time enrolled (new admits only) 2009–2010, 0. Total enrolled 2009–2010 full-time, 25. Openings 2010–2011, 8. The median number of years required for completion of a degree in 2008–2009 were 5. The number of students enrolled full- and part-time who were dismissed or voluntarily withdrew from this program area in 2008–2009 were 1.

Other Criteria: (importance of criteria rated low, medium, or high): GRE scores—high, research experience—high, work experience—low, extracurricular activity—low, GPA—high, letters of recommendation—high, interview—low, statement of goals and objectives—high, undergraduate major in psychology—low, specific undergraduate psychology courses taken—medium, Work experience is more important to the I/O program.

Student Characteristics: The following represents characteristics of students in 2009–2010 in all graduate psychology programs in the department: Female—full-time 34, part-time 0; Male—full-time 40, part-time 0; African American/Black—full-time 2, part-time 0; Hispanic/Latino(a)—full-time 1, part-time 0; Asian/Pacific Islander—full-time 5, part-time 0; American Indian/Alaska Native—full-time 2, part-time 0; Caucasian/White—full-time 64, part-time 0; Multi-ethnic—full-time 0, part-time 0; students subject to the Americans With Disabilities Act—full-time 0, part-time 0; Unknown ethnicity—full-time 0, part-time 0; International students who hold an F-1 or J-1 Visa—full-time 5, part-time 0.

Financial Information/Assistance:

Tuition for Full-Time Study: *Master's:* State residents: $156 per credit hour; Nonstate residents: $565 per credit hour. *Doctoral:* State residents: $156 per credit hour; Nonstate residents: $565 per credit hour. Tuition is subject to change. Additional fees are assessed to students beyond the costs of tuition for the following: Note: all areas have additional fees which cannot be waived. See the following Web site for updates and changes in tuition costs: https://bursar.ou.edu/tuition_fees.cfm.

Financial Assistance:

First-Year Students: Teaching assistantships available for first year. Average amount paid per academic year: $12,587. Average number of hours worked per week: 20. Apply by January 1. Research assistantships available for first year. Average amount paid per academic year: $12,587. Average number of hours worked per week: 20. Apply by January 1. Fellowships and scholarships available for first year. Average amount paid per academic year: $19,587. Average number of hours worked per week: 20.

Advanced Students: Teaching assistantships available for advanced students. Average amount paid per academic year: $13,530. Average number of hours worked per week: 20. Research assistantships available for advanced students. Average amount paid per academic year: $13,530. Average number of hours worked per week: 20.

Additional Information: Of all students currently enrolled full time, 95% benefited from one or more of the listed financial assistance programs. Application and information available online at: http://www.ou.edu/cas/psychology/grad/fund.htm.

Housing and Day Care: On-campus housing is available. See the following Web site for more information: http://www.housing.ou.edu/. No on-campus day care facilities are available.

Employment of Department Graduates:

Master's Degree Graduates: Of those who graduated in the academic year 2008–2009, the following categories and numbers represent the postgraduate activities and employment of master's degree graduates: Enrolled in a postdoctoral residency/fellowship (n/a), employed in independent practice (n/a), total from the above (master's) (0).

Doctoral Degree Graduates: Of those who graduated in the academic year 2008–2009, the following categories and numbers represent the postgraduate activities and employment of doctoral degree graduates: Enrolled in a psychology doctoral program (n/a), employed in an academic position at a university (1), employed in an academic position at a 2-year/4-year college (1), employed in business or industry (5), employed in government agency (2), do not know (1), total from the above (doctoral) (10).

Additional Information:

Orientation, Objectives, and Emphasis of Department: All programs are highly research oriented within the broad framework of experimental psychology. The department aims to produce creative and productive psychologists to function in academic and research settings, and toward this end emphasizes early and continuing involvement in research. Achievement of orientation and objectives is demonstrated by the excellent placement record of doctoral graduates, and by the department's recent rating as ninth in the nation in percent of publishing faculty. An excellent program in Quantitative Methods in Psychology is an especially attractive feature of the quality graduate training offered.

Special Facilities or Resources: The department offers modern research facilities with microprocessor-controlled laboratories, instrumentation shops with a full-time engineer, a small animal colony, a university computing center, a departmental computing center for graduate students, and graduate offices located near faculty and departmental offices.

Application Information:

Send to Graduate Admissions Committee, Department of Psychology, University of Oklahoma, 455 W. Lindsey, Room 705, Norman, OK 73019-2007. Application available online. URL of online application: http://www.ou.edu/cas/psychology/grad/application.htm. Students are admitted in the Fall, application deadline January 1. *Fee:* $40. fee is $90 for international students.

Tulsa, University of
Department of Psychology
Henry Kendall College of Arts and Sciences
800 South Tucker Drive
Tulsa, OK 74104-3189
Telephone: (918) 631-2248
Fax: (918) 631-2833
E-mail: sandra-barney@utulsa.edu
Web: http://www.cas.utulsa.edu/psych

Department Information:
1926. Chairperson: Dr. Judy Berry. Number of faculty: total—full-time 12, part-time 6; women—full-time 6, part-time 5; total—minority—full-time 1; women minority—full-time 1.

Programs and Degrees Offered:
Listed in the following order: Program area, degree type (T if terminal Master's), number awarded 7/08–6/09. Industrial/Organizational Psychology MA/MS (Master of Arts/Science) (T) 7, Industrial/Organizational Psychology PhD (Doctor of Philosophy) 2, Clinical Psychology MA/MS (Master of Arts/Science) (T) 2, Clinical Psychology PhD (Doctor of Philosophy) 6, Clinical Psychology MA/JD MA/MS (Master of Arts/Science) (T) 0, Industrial/Organizational Psychology MA/JD MA/MS (Master of Arts/Science) 0.

APA Accreditation: Clinical PhD (Doctor of Philosophy). Student Outcome Data Website: http://www.utulsa.edu/academics/colleges/Henry-Kendall-College-of-Arts-and-Sciences/Departments-and-Schools/Department-of-Psychology/Programs-of-Study.

Student Applications/Admissions:
Student Applications
Industrial/Organizational Psychology MA/MS (Master of Arts/Science)—Applications 2009–2010, 23. Total applicants accepted 2009–2010, 12. Number full-time enrolled (new admits only) 2009–2010, 9. Number part-time enrolled (new admits only) 2009–2010, 0. Openings 2010–2011, 6. The median number of years required for completion of a degree in 2008–2009 were 2. The number of students enrolled full- and part-time who were dismissed or voluntarily withdrew from this program area in 2008–2009 were 1. Industrial/Organizational Psychology PhD (Doctor of Philosophy)—Applications 2009–2010, 32. Total applicants accepted 2009–2010, 3. Number full-time enrolled (new admits only) 2009–2010, 1. Number part-time enrolled (new admits only) 2009–2010, 0. Openings 2010–2011, 3. The median number of years required for completion of a degree in 2008–2009 were 6. The number of students enrolled full- and part-time who were dismissed or voluntarily withdrew from this program area in 2008–2009 were 0. Clinical Psychology MA/MS (Master of Arts/Science)—Applications 2009–2010, 11. Total applicants accepted 2009–2010, 3. Number full-time enrolled (new admits only) 2009–2010, 2. Openings 2010–2011, 5. The median number of years required for completion of a degree in 2008–2009 were 2. The number of students enrolled full- and part-time who were dismissed or voluntarily withdrew from this program area in 2008–2009 were 0. Clinical Psychology PhD (Doctor of Philosophy)—Applications 2009–2010, 47. Total applicants accepted 2009–2010, 12. Number full-time enrolled (new admits only) 2009–2010, 6. Number part-time enrolled (new admits only) 2009–2010, 0. Openings 2010–2011, 5. The median number of years required for completion of a degree in 2008–2009 were 5. The number of students enrolled full- and part-time who were dismissed or voluntarily withdrew from this program area in 2008–2009 were 1. Clinical Psychology MA/JD MA/MS (Master of Arts/Science)—Applications 2009–2010, 1. Total applicants accepted 2009–2010, 0. Number full-time enrolled (new admits only) 2009–2010, 0. Number part-time enrolled (new admits only) 2009–2010, 0. Openings 2010–2011, 1. The median number of years required for completion of a degree in 2008–2009 were 5. The number of students enrolled full- and part-time who were dismissed or voluntarily withdrew from this program area in 2008–2009 were 0. Industrial/Organizational Psychology MA/JD MA/MS (Master of Arts/Science)—Applications 2009–2010, 0. Total applicants accepted 2009–2010, 0. Number full-time enrolled (new admits only) 2009–2010, 0. Number part-time enrolled (new admits only) 2009–2010, 0. Openings 2010–2011, 1. The median number of years required for completion of a degree in 2008–2009 were 5. The number of students enrolled full- and part-time who were dismissed or voluntarily withdrew from this program area in 2008–2009 were 0.

Scores: Entries appear in this order: required test or GPA, minimum score (if required), median score of students entering in 2009–2010. *Industrial/Organizational Psychology MA/MS (Master of Arts/Science):* GRE-V no minimum stated, 520, GRE-Q no minimum stated, 620, GRE-Analytical no minimum stated, 4.5, overall undergraduate GPA 3.0, 3.5; *Industrial/Organizational Psychology PhD (Doctor of Philosophy):* GRE-V no minimum stated, 570, GRE-Q no minimum stated, 630, GRE-Analytical no minimum stated, 5.0, overall undergraduate GPA 3.0, 3.66; *Clinical Psychology MA/MS (Master of Arts/Science):* GRE-V no minimum stated, 600, GRE-Q no minimum stated, 588, GRE-Analytical no minimum stated, 4.8, overall undergraduate GPA 3.0, 3.5; *Clinical Psychology PhD (Doctor of Philosophy):* GRE-V no minimum stated, 570, GRE-Q no minimum stated, 630, GRE-Analytical no minimum stated, 5.0, overall undergraduate GPA 3.0, 3.75, Masters GRE no minimum stated, 3.6; *Clinical Psychology MA/JD MA/MS (Master of Arts/Science):* GRE-V no minimum stated, 600, GRE-Q no minimum stated, 588, GRE-Analytical no minimum stated, 4.8, overall undergraduate GPA 3.0; *Industrial/Organizational Psychology MA/JD MA/MS (Master of Arts/Science):* GRE-V no minimum stated, 520, GRE-Q no minimum stated, 620, GRE-Analytical no minimum stated, 4.5, overall undergraduate GPA 3.0, 3.5.

Other Criteria: (importance of criteria rated low, medium, or high): GRE scores—high, research experience—high, work experience—low, extracurricular activity—low, clinically related public service—medium, GPA—high, letters of recommendation—high, interview—high, statement of goals and objectives—high, quality of undergrad inst—medium, undergraduate major in psychology—medium, specific undergraduate psychology courses taken—medium. Resume or CV required for clinical program applicants. Interview for clinical PhD only. For additional information on admission requirements, go to http://www.cas.utulsa.edu/psych.

Student Characteristics: The following represents characteristics of students in 2009–2010 in all graduate psychology programs in the department: Female—full-time 57, part-time 0; Male—full-

time 18, part-time 0; African American/Black—full-time 2, part-time 0; Hispanic/Latino(a)—full-time 3, part-time 0; Asian/Pacific Islander—full-time 1, part-time 0; American Indian/Alaska Native—full-time 1, part-time 0; Caucasian/White—full-time 68, part-time 0; Multi-ethnic—full-time 0, part-time 0; students subject to the Americans With Disabilities Act—full-time 0, part-time 0; Unknown ethnicity—full-time 0, part-time 0; International students who hold an F-1 or J-1 Visa—full-time 3, part-time 0.

Financial Information/Assistance:
Tuition for Full-Time Study: *Master's:* State residents: $939 per credit hour; Nonstate residents: $939 per credit hour. *Doctoral:* State residents: $939 per credit hour; Nonstate residents: $939 per credit hour. Tuition is subject to change. See the following Web site for updates and changes in tuition costs: http://www.utulsa.edu/academics/colleges/Graduate-School/About-the-School/Tuition-and-Living-Expenses.aspx.

Financial Assistance:
First-Year Students: Teaching assistantships available for first year. Average amount paid per academic year: $11,942. Average number of hours worked per week: 20. Apply by February 1. Research assistantships available for first year. Average amount paid per academic year: $11,942. Average number of hours worked per week: 20. Apply by February 1. Fellowships and scholarships available for first year. Average number of hours worked per week: 20. Apply by varies.

Advanced Students: Teaching assistantships available for advanced students. Average amount paid per academic year: $12,382. Average number of hours worked per week: 20. Apply by February 1. Research assistantships available for advanced students. Average amount paid per academic year: $12,382. Average number of hours worked per week: 20. Apply by February 1. Fellowships and scholarships available for advanced students. Average number of hours worked per week: 20. Apply by varies.

Additional Information: Of all students currently enrolled full time, 70% benefited from one or more of the listed financial assistance programs. Application and information available online at: http://www.utulsa.edu/academics/colleges/Graduate-School/Graduate-Financial-Assistance.aspx.

Internships/Practica: Doctoral Degree (PhD Clinical Psychology): For those doctoral students for whom a professional internship was required in this program prior to graduation, (4) students applied for an internship in 2008–2009, with (4) students obtaining an internship. Of those students who obtained an internship, (4) were paid internships. Of those students who obtained an internship, (4) students placed in APA/CPA accredited internships, (0) students placed in internships not APA/CPA accredited, but listed with the Association of Psychology Postdoctoral and Internship Programs (APPIC), (0) students placed in internships conforming to guidelines of the Council of Directors of School Psychology Programs (CDSPP), (0) students placed in internships that were not APA/CPA accredited, APPIC or CDSPP listed. Master's Degree (MA/MS Industrial/Organizational Psychology): An internship experience, such as a final research project or "capstone" experience is required of graduates. In the clinical program, supervised applied training begins early in the program. Practicum experiences occur primarily in community settings, utilizing the wide variety of agencies with which the department has relationships and allowing the student to interact with various mental health professionals. Placements include the university health center, community mental health centers, hospitals, community service agencies, and private practice groups. Attempts are made to allow students to choose practicum activities that are most consistent with their professional goals, although it is recognized that a diversity of experiences can provide a strong foundation for professional development. Practicum activities are supervised by an on-site professional, and the practicum experience is organized and monitored by the Coordinator of Practicum Training in conjunction with the Clinical Program Committee.

Housing and Day Care: On-campus housing is available. See the following Web site for more information: http://www.utulsa.edu/student-life/Living-and-Dining-on-Campus.aspx. On-campus day care facilities are available.

Employment of Department Graduates:
Master's Degree Graduates: Of those who graduated in the academic year 2008–2009, the following categories and numbers represent the postgraduate activities and employment of master's degree graduates: Enrolled in a psychology doctoral program (4), enrolled in a postdoctoral residency/fellowship (n/a), employed in independent practice (n/a), employed in business or industry (3), employed in government agency (1), employed in a community mental health/counseling center (1), total from the above (master's) (9).

Doctoral Degree Graduates: Of those who graduated in the academic year 2008–2009, the following categories and numbers represent the postgraduate activities and employment of doctoral degree graduates: Enrolled in a psychology doctoral program (n/a), enrolled in a postdoctoral residency/fellowship (5), employed in business or industry (1), employed in government agency (1), employed in a community mental health/counseling center (1), total from the above (doctoral) (8).

Additional Information:
Orientation, Objectives, and Emphasis of Department: Our graduate programs in applied psychology are central to the departmental mission, which is: to generate new psychological knowledge to help individuals, organizations, and communities make decisions and solve problems; to offer a future-oriented, intellectually challenging, and socially relevant curriculum; and to equip students to make a difference through their work by providing them with an extensive knowledge base as well as the analytical and practical skills needed to apply knowledge wisely. Our programs train students to do what applied psychologists actually do in today's society. The programs in I/O psychology emphasize personnel psychology and organizational development, theory and behavior, with a special focus on individual assessment. The doctoral program in clinical psychology develops scientist–practitioners using the following training components. First, coursework is distributed across clinical core, general psychology, methodology core, and elective offerings. Second, research mentoring is experienced in the precandidacy and dissertation projects. Third, procedural knowledge is developed in clinical practicum and internship training. Fourth, declarative knowledge is developed through comprehensive written and oral examinations covering general psychological knowledge and methods, and clinical psychology.

Special Facilities or Resources: The Department of Psychology is located in Lorton Hall, a building located near the center of the TU campus. The building contains faculty offices, classrooms, offices for graduate students on assistantships, a graduate student lounge, research space, and clinical training space. McFarlin Library, a two-minute walk from Lorton Hall, contains more than three million items and more than 6,000 periodical subscriptions. The library's catalogue is computerized and is accessible from terminals across campus. Computer searches of the major information databases in psychology are available to students at no charge. Major computer application suites and statistical packages (e.g., SPSS) are available for word processing, data analysis, test interpretation, and other tasks. The university has several computer labs with a variety of hardware configurations and software packages for student use. Visiting scholars and professionals often join the graduate faculty in presenting special courses, workshops, and seminars. Each year, colloquium speakers offer opinions, ideas, and research on topics of current interest in psychology.

Information for Students With Physical Disabilities: See the following Web site for more information: http://www.utulsa.edu/student-life/Student-Academic-Support/.

Application Information:
Send to Graduate School, University of Tulsa, 800 S. Tucker Dr., Tulsa, OK 74104. Application available online. URL of online application: http://www.utulsa.edu/graduate/. Students are admitted in the Fall, application deadline December 1. For the Clinical psychology program, the application due date is December 1. For the Industrial/Organizational psychology program, the application due date is January 15. *Fee:* $40.

OREGON

George Fox University
Graduate Department of Clinical Psychology
School of Behavioral and Health Sciences
414 North Meridian Street, V104
Newberg, OR 97132-2697
Telephone: (503) 554-2371
Fax: (503) 554-3110
E-mail: *psyd@georgefox.edu*
Web: *http://psyd.georgefox.edu*

Department Information:
1981. Chairperson: Wayne Adams. Number of faculty: total—full-time 8, part-time 5; women—full-time 3, part-time 2; total—minority—full-time 1, part-time 1; women minority—part-time 1.

Programs and Degrees Offered:
Listed in the following order: Program area, degree type (T if terminal Master's), number awarded 7/08–6/09. Clinical Psychology PsyD (Doctor of Psychology) 15.

APA Accreditation: Clinical PsyD (Doctor of Psychology).

Student Applications/Admissions:
Student Applications
Clinical Psychology PsyD (Doctor of Psychology)—Applications 2009–2010, 84. Total applicants accepted 2009–2010, 28. Number full-time enrolled (new admits only) 2009–2010, 23. Number part-time enrolled (new admits only) 2009–2010, 0. Openings 2010–2011, 20. The median number of years required for completion of a degree in 2008–2009 were 5. The number of students enrolled full- and part-time who were dismissed or voluntarily withdrew from this program area in 2008–2009 were 2.
Scores: Entries appear in this order: required test or GPA, minimum score (if required), median score of students entering in 2009–2010. *Clinical Psychology PsyD (Doctor of Psychology):* GRE-V 500, GRE-Q 500, overall undergraduate GPA 3.0.
Other Criteria: (importance of criteria rated low, medium, or high): GRE scores—medium, research experience—medium, work experience—medium, extracurricular activity—low, clinically related public service—medium, GPA—high, letters of recommendation—high, interview—high, statement of goals and objectives—high, Christian worldview—high, undergraduate major in psychology—medium, specific undergraduate psychology courses taken—medium. For additional information on admission requirements, go to http://psyd.georgefox.edu.

Student Characteristics: The following represents characteristics of students in 2009–2010 in all graduate psychology programs in the department: Female—full-time 46, part-time 0; Male—full-time 41, part-time 0; African American/Black—full-time 0, part-time 0; Hispanic/Latino(a)—full-time 2, part-time 0; Asian/Pacific Islander—full-time 4, part-time 0; American Indian/Alaska Native—full-time 3, part-time 0; Caucasian/White—full-time 77, part-time 0; Multi-ethnic—full-time 1, part-time 0; students subject to the Americans With Disabilities Act—full-time 1, part-time 0; Unknown ethnicity—full-time 0, part-time 0; International students who hold an F-1 or J-1 Visa—full-time 0, part-time 0.

Financial Information/Assistance:
Tuition for Full-Time Study: *Doctoral:* State residents: $740 per credit hour; Nonstate residents: $740 per credit hour. Tuition is subject to change. Additional fees are assessed to students beyond the costs of tuition for the following: $70/sem student fee. See the following Web site for updates and changes in tuition costs: http://www.georgefox.edu/offices/stu_fin_srv/cost_psyd.html.

Financial Assistance:
First-Year Students: Fellowships and scholarships available for first year. Average amount paid per academic year: $4,000. Average number of hours worked per week: 0. Apply by March 30.
Advanced Students: Teaching assistantships available for advanced students. Average amount paid per academic year: $3,000. Average number of hours worked per week: 5. Research assistantships available for advanced students. Average amount paid per academic year: $2,100. Average number of hours worked per week: 5. Fellowships and scholarships available for advanced students. Average amount paid per academic year: $4,000. Average number of hours worked per week: 0. Apply by March 30.
Additional Information: Of all students currently enrolled full time, 40% benefited from one or more of the listed financial assistance programs. Application and information available online at: http://www.georgefox.edu/offices/stu_fin_serv.

Internships/Practica: Doctoral Degree (PsyD Clinical Psychology): For those doctoral students for whom a professional internship was required in this program prior to graduation, (12) students applied for an internship in 2008–2009, with (12) students obtaining an internship. Of those students who obtained an internship, (12) were paid internships. Of those students who obtained an internship, (8) students placed in APA/CPA accredited internships, (4) students placed in internships not APA/CPA accredited, but listed with the Association of Psychology Postdoctoral and Internship Programs (APPIC), (0) students placed in internships conforming to guidelines of the Council of Directors of School Psychology Programs (CDSPP), (0) students placed in internships that were not APA/CPA accredited, APPIC or CDSPP listed. Students are required to complete four years of practicum (minimum of 1500 hours) in a variety of settings in the greater Portland metropolitan area. Practicum settings include hospitals, community mental health agencies, drug and alcohol programs, behavioral medicine clinics, schools, and prisons. Inpatient and out-patient experiences are available. All practicum experience is gained under the careful supervision of licensed psychologists at the practicum sites. Additionally, students receive weekly clinical oversight on campus by core faculty. Students apply for internships within the system developed by the Association of Psychology Postdoctoral and Internship Centers (APPIC). Students complete a one-year full-time internship (2000 hours) at an approved internship site during their fifth year in the program. Usually, 90% of applicants obtain an APA- and/or APPIC-approved internships.

Housing and Day Care: No on-campus housing is available. No on-campus day care facilities are available.

Employment of Department Graduates:
Master's Degree Graduates: Of those who graduated in the academic year 2008–2009, the following categories and numbers represent the postgraduate activities and employment of master's degree graduates: Enrolled in a postdoctoral residency/fellowship (n/a), employed in independent practice (n/a), total from the above (master's) (0).
Doctoral Degree Graduates: Of those who graduated in the academic year 2008–2009, the following categories and numbers represent the postgraduate activities and employment of doctoral degree graduates: Enrolled in a psychology doctoral program (n/a), enrolled in another graduate/professional program (0), enrolled in a postdoctoral residency/fellowship (8), employed in independent practice (0), employed in an academic position at a university (0), employed in an academic position at a 2-year/4-year college (0), employed in other positions at a higher education institution (0), employed in a professional position in a school system (0), employed in business or industry (0), employed in government agency (1), employed in a community mental health/counseling center (2), employed in a hospital/medical center (0), still seeking employment (0), other employment position (0), do not know (1), total from the above (doctoral) (12).

Additional Information:
Orientation, Objectives, and Emphasis of Department: The goal of the Graduate Department of Clinical Psychology (GDCP) is to prepare professional psychologists who are competent to provide psychological services in a wide variety of clinical settings, who are knowledgeable in critical evaluation and application of psychological research, and who are committed to the highest standards of professional ethics. The central distinctive feature of the program is the integration of a Christian worldview and the science of psychology at philosophical, practical and personal levels. Graduates are trained broadly but also as specialists in meeting the unique psychological needs of the Christian community and others who wish a spiritual dimension to be included in their treatment. Other distinctive aspects of the program include close mentoring using clinical and research team models, and an option for training emphases in Assessment, Rural and Health Psychology. Graduates are prepared for licensure as clinical psychologists. Alumni of the GDCP are licensed in numerous states throughout the U.S. They engage in practice in a variety of settings, including independent and group practice, hospitals, community mental health clinics, government, corrections, public health agencies, and church and para-church organizations. Graduates also teach in a variety of settings, including colleges and seminaries.

Personal Behavior Statement: http://www.georgefox.edu/psyd/aboutgdcp/life.html.

Special Facilities or Resources: High-speed microcomputers, laser printers, and complete statistical (SPSS PC+) and graphics software are provided in a computer lab. The Murdock Learning Resource Center provides library support for the psychology program. The library has excellent access to materials important to contemporary clinical and empirical work in most areas of clinical psychology. In addition, the library receives more than 140 periodicals in psychology and related disciplines, most available electronically. Students also have online access to major computerized databases through library services, including PsycInfo, DIALOG, ERIC, and many others. In addition to full-text access to many psychology journals, George Fox University maintains cooperative arrangements with other local educational institutions providing psychology students with a full range of user services, including interlibrary loans and direct borrowing privileges. A full range of traditional campus facilities are also available such as athletic, arts outlets, student lounge and meal service. A newly remodeled building is the campus location for the PsyD program. The new quarters include all PsyD classrooms, faculty offices, student lounge area, computer lab, cafe, conference rooms, clinical demonstration and videotaping rooms, and student parking.

Information for Students With Physical Disabilities: See the following Web site for more information: http://www.georgefox.edu/offices/disab_services.

Application Information:
Send to Adina McConaughey, Graduate Admissions, George Fox University, 414 N Meridian St # 6149, Newberg, OR 97132. Phone: (503) 554-2263. Application available online. URL of online application: http://www.georgefox.edu/psyd/admission. Students are admitted in the Fall, application deadline January 15. Special circumstances for delayed or late applications will be considered. Especially strong applicants will be considered after deadline, on a space-available basis. *Fee:* $40. Fee waiver for McNairs Scholars and Act Six Leadership & Scholars.

Lewis & Clark College, Graduate School of Education and Counseling (2009 data)
Counseling Psychology Department
Graduate School of Education and Counseling
0615 SW Palatine Hill Road, Box 86
Portland, OR 97219-7899
Telephone: (503) 768-6060
Fax: (503) 768-6065
E-mail: *cpsy@lclark.edu*
Web: *http://education.lclark.edu/dept/cpsy/*

Department Information:
1972. Department Chair: Tod Sloan, PhD. Number of faculty: total—full-time 12, part-time 1; women—full-time 7, part-time 1; total—minority—full-time 2; women minority—full-time 1.

Programs and Degrees Offered:
Listed in the following order: Program area, degree type (T if terminal Master's), number awarded 7/08–6/09. School Psychology EdS (School Psychology) 13, Addictions Treatment MA/MS (Master of Arts/Science) (T) 17, Community Counseling MA/MS (Master of Arts/Science) (T) 21, Marriage, Couple and Family Therapy MA/MS (Master of Arts/Science) (T) 7, Psychological and Cultural Studies MA/MS (Master of Arts/Science) (T) 2.

Student Applications/Admissions:
Student Applications
School Psychology EdS (School Psychology)—Applications 2009–2010, 41. Total applicants accepted 2009–2010, 29. Number full-time enrolled (new admits only) 2009–2010, 15. Number part-time enrolled (new admits only) 2009–2010, 3. Total

enrolled 2009–2010 full-time, 35, part-time, 21. Openings 2010–2011, 22. The median number of years required for completion of a degree in 2008–2009 were 3. The number of students enrolled full- and part-time who were dismissed or voluntarily withdrew from this program area in 2008–2009 were 0. *Addictions Treatment MA/MS (Master of Arts/Science)*—Applications 2009–2010, 15. Total applicants accepted 2009–2010, 9. Number full-time enrolled (new admits only) 2009–2010, 4. Number part-time enrolled (new admits only) 2009–2010, 1. Total enrolled 2009–2010 full-time, 32, part-time, 4. Openings 2010–2011, 15. The median number of years required for completion of a degree in 2008–2009 were 3. The number of students enrolled full- and part-time who were dismissed or voluntarily withdrew from this program area in 2008–2009 were 0. *Community Counseling MA/MS (Master of Arts/Science)*—Applications 2009–2010, 67. Total applicants accepted 2009–2010, 53. Number full-time enrolled (new admits only) 2009–2010, 26. Number part-time enrolled (new admits only) 2009–2010, 3. Total enrolled 2009–2010 full-time, 92, part-time, 22. Openings 2010–2011, 40. The median number of years required for completion of a degree in 2008–2009 were 3. The number of students enrolled full- and part-time who were dismissed or voluntarily withdrew from this program area in 2008–2009 were 0. *Marriage, Couple and Family Therapy MA/MS (Master of Arts/Science)*—Applications 2009–2010, 62. Total applicants accepted 2009–2010, 37. Number full-time enrolled (new admits only) 2009–2010, 20. Number part-time enrolled (new admits only) 2009–2010, 1. Total enrolled 2009–2010 full-time, 52, part-time, 8. Openings 2010–2011, 20. The median number of years required for completion of a degree in 2008–2009 were 3. The number of students enrolled full- and part-time who were dismissed or voluntarily withdrew from this program area in 2008–2009 were 0. *Psychological and Cultural Studies MA/MS (Master of Arts/Science)*—Applications 2009–2010, 6. Total applicants accepted 2009–2010, 5. Number full-time enrolled (new admits only) 2009–2010, 3. Number part-time enrolled (new admits only) 2009–2010, 0. Total enrolled 2009–2010 full-time, 4, part-time, 3. Openings 2010–2011, 10. The median number of years required for completion of a degree in 2008–2009 were 2. The number of students enrolled full- and part-time who were dismissed or voluntarily withdrew from this program area in 2008–2009 were 0.

Other Criteria: (importance of criteria rated low, medium, or high): GRE scores—low, research experience—low, work experience—medium, extracurricular activity—medium, clinically related public service—low, GPA—medium, letters of recommendation—medium, interview—medium, statement of goals and objectives—high, undergraduate major in psychology—low, specific undergraduate psychology courses taken—low. For additional information on admission requirements, go to http://education.lclark.edu/dept/gseadmit/.

Student Characteristics: The following represents characteristics of students in 2009–2010 in all graduate psychology programs in the department: Female—full-time 186, part-time 0; Male—full-time 46, part-time 0; African American/Black—full-time 0, part-time 0; Hispanic/Latino(a)—full-time 3, part-time 2; Asian/Pacific Islander—full-time 5, part-time 3; American Indian/Alaska Native—full-time 1, part-time 0; Caucasian/White—full-time 0, part-time 0; Multi-ethnic—full-time 2, part-time 2; students subject to the Americans With Disabilities Act—full-time 2, part-time 1; Unknown ethnicity—full-time 0, part-time 0; International students who hold an F-1 or J-1 Visa—full-time 0, part-time 0.

Financial Information/Assistance:
Tuition for Full-Time Study: *Master's:* State residents: $677 per credit hour; Nonstate residents: $677 per credit hour. Tuition is subject to change.

Financial Assistance:
First-Year Students: No information provided.
Advanced Students: Fellowships and scholarships available for advanced students.
Additional Information: Application and information available online at: http://www.lclark.edu/dept/sfs/.

Internships/Practica: Master's Degree (MA/MS Addictions Treatment): An internship experience, such as a final research project or "capstone" experience is required of graduates. Master's Degree (MA/MS Community Counseling): An internship experience, such as a final research project or "capstone" experience is required of graduates. Master's Degree (MA/MS Marriage, Couple and Family Therapy): An internship experience, such as a final research project or "capstone" experience is required of graduates. Internship and practicum placements in community agencies and schools provide students with opportunities for supervised professional practice. As part of each placement, students receive supervision from qualified professionals in their community or school setting. Students also receive weekly instruction and supervision from on-campus instructors throughout their internship and practicum placements. Required hours, supervision, and activities meet standards set by licensing bodies for students in their respective specialty areas. This ensures that students will be qualified to pursue licensing after completing their degree program. Internships in marriage and family therapy, community counseling and addictions counseling involve part-time placements. Internships in school psychology are full-time for one academic year and usually involve a stipend to the student.

Housing and Day Care: No on-campus housing is available. No on-campus day care facilities are available.

Employment of Department Graduates:
Master's Degree Graduates: Of those who graduated in the academic year 2008–2009, the following categories and numbers represent the postgraduate activities and employment of master's degree graduates: Enrolled in a postdoctoral residency/fellowship (n/a), employed in independent practice (n/a), total from the above (master's) (0).
Doctoral Degree Graduates: Of those who graduated in the academic year 2008–2009, the following categories and numbers represent the postgraduate activities and employment of doctoral degree graduates: Enrolled in a psychology doctoral program (n/a), total from the above (doctoral) (0).

Additional Information:
Orientation, Objectives, and Emphasis of Department: Lewis & Clark College's Department of Counseling Psychology prepares professional counselors, therapists, and school psychologists to lead, serve, and work for social justice in community and school settings. Faculty and students are committed to disseminating and expanding the knowledge base relevant to this mission, promoting

the use of evidence-based treatment and prevention procedures, and adhering to the highest ethical standards as practitioners and researchers. The programs in counseling psychology prepare highly qualified mental health professionals for employment in public agencies, community-based programs, and schools. Curricular options also exist for those who would like to concentrate on research and establish a foundation in pursuit of doctoral training. We are especially interested in preparing students for multicultural competence and social justice advocacy.

Special Facilities or Resources: The program has established collaborative relationships with community schools and agencies which provide students opportunities to participate in ongoing research and program evaluation. These opportunities are open to students planning to complete a thesis and also to students who wish to secure increased training and experience without doing a full thesis.

Information for Students With Physical Disabilities: See the following Web site for more information: http://www.lclark.edu/dept/access.

Application Information:
Send to Counseling Psychology Department Lewis & Clark College Graduate School of Education and Counseling Admissions, MSC 87 0615 SW Palatine Hill Road Portland, OR 97219-7899. Application available online. URL of online application: http://www.lclark.edu/dept/gseadmit/. Students are admitted in the Fall, application deadline February 1; Spring, application deadline October 1. Fee: $50.

Oregon, University of
Counseling Psychology
College of Education
5251 University of Oregon
Eugene, OR 97403-5251
Telephone: (541) 346-2456
Fax: (541) 346-6778
E-mail: *cpsy@uoregon.edu*
Web: *http://www.counpsych.uoregon.edu*

Department Information:
1954. Area Head: Benedict McWhirter. Number of faculty: total—full-time 4, part-time 2; women—full-time 3, part-time 2; total—minority—full-time 1; women minority—full-time 1; faculty subject to the Americans With Disabilities Act 1.

Programs and Degrees Offered:
Listed in the following order: Program area, degree type (T if terminal Master's), number awarded 7/08–6/09. Counseling Psychology PhD (Doctor of Philosophy) 6.

APA Accreditation: Counseling PhD (Doctor of Philosophy). Student Outcome Data Website: http://counpsych.uoregon.edu/C-20.htm.

Student Applications/Admissions:
Student Applications
Counseling Psychology PhD (Doctor of Philosophy)—Applications 2009–2010, 203. Total applicants accepted 2009–2010, 10. Number full-time enrolled (new admits only) 2009–2010, 8. Number part-time enrolled (new admits only) 2009–2010, 0. Openings 2010–2011, 8. The median number of years required for completion of a degree in 2008–2009 were 6. The number of students enrolled full- and part-time who were dismissed or voluntarily withdrew from this program area in 2008–2009 were 1.

Scores: Entries appear in this order: required test or GPA, minimum score (if required), median score of students entering in 2009–2010. *Counseling Psychology PhD (Doctor of Philosophy)*: GRE-V no minimum stated, 610, GRE-Q no minimum stated, 645, GRE-Analytical no minimum stated, 4.7, overall undergraduate GPA no minimum stated, 3.52.

Other Criteria: (importance of criteria rated low, medium, or high): GRE scores—medium, research experience—high, work experience—medium, extracurricular activity—medium, clinically related public service—medium, GPA—high, letters of recommendation—high, interview—high, statement of goals and objectives—high, Second language skills—medium, undergraduate major in psychology—medium, specific undergraduate psychology courses taken—medium. For additional information on admission requirements, go to http://counpsych.uoregon.edu/admissions.htm.

Student Characteristics: The following represents characteristics of students in 2009–2010 in all graduate psychology programs in the department: Female—full-time 43, part-time 0; Male—full-time 6, part-time 0; African American/Black—full-time 5, part-time 0; Hispanic/Latino(a)—full-time 9, part-time 0; Asian/Pacific Islander—full-time 8, part-time 0; American Indian/Alaska Native—full-time 0, part-time 0; Caucasian/White—full-time 23, part-time 0; Multi-ethnic—full-time 3, part-time 0; students subject to the Americans With Disabilities Act—full-time 1, part-time 0; Unknown ethnicity—full-time 1, part-time 0; International students who hold an F-1 or J-1 Visa—full-time 2, part-time 0.

Financial Information/Assistance:
Tuition for Full-Time Study: *Doctoral:* State residents: per academic year $16,930, $470 per credit hour; Nonstate residents: per academic year $23,986, $666 per credit hour. Tuition is subject to change. See the following Web site for updates and changes in tuition costs: http://registrar.uoregon.edu/costs/tuition_fee_structure/graduate.

Financial Assistance:
First-Year Students: Teaching assistantships available for first year. Average amount paid per academic year: $6,937. Average number of hours worked per week: 12. Apply by March. Fellowships and scholarships available for first year. Average amount paid per academic year: $3,000. Average number of hours worked per week: 0. Apply by February.

Advanced Students: Teaching assistantships available for advanced students. Average amount paid per academic year: $10,445. Average number of hours worked per week: 16. Apply by March. Fellowships and scholarships available for advanced students. Average amount paid per academic year: $1,000. Average number of hours worked per week: 0. Apply by February.

Additional Information: Of all students currently enrolled full time, 100% benefited from one or more of the listed financial assistance programs. Application and information available online at: http://financialaid.uoregon.edu/.

Internships/Practica: Doctoral Degree (PhD Counseling Psychology): For those doctoral students for whom a professional internship was required in this program prior to graduation, (8) students applied for an internship in 2008–2009, with (8) students obtaining an internship. Of those students who obtained an internship, (8) were paid internships. Of those students who obtained an internship, (8) students placed in APA/CPA accredited internships, (0) students placed in internships not APA/CPA accredited, but listed with the Association of Psychology Postdoctoral and Internship Programs (APPIC), (0) students placed in internships conforming to guidelines of the Council of Directors of School Psychology Programs (CDSPP), (0) students placed in internships that were not APA/CPA accredited, APPIC or CDSPP listed. All students are required to participate in both adult and child/family practica. Numerous externship opportunities exist throughout the community.

Housing and Day Care: On-campus housing is available. See the following Web site for more information: http://housing.uoregon.edu/. On-campus day care facilities are available. See the following Web site for more information: http://housing.uoregon.edu/apartments/childcare.php.

Employment of Department Graduates:
Master's Degree Graduates: Of those who graduated in the academic year 2008–2009, the following categories and numbers represent the postgraduate activities and employment of master's degree graduates: Enrolled in a postdoctoral residency/fellowship (n/a), employed in independent practice (n/a), total from the above (master's) (0).
Doctoral Degree Graduates: Of those who graduated in the academic year 2008–2009, the following categories and numbers represent the postgraduate activities and employment of doctoral degree graduates: Enrolled in a psychology doctoral program (n/a), enrolled in a postdoctoral residency/fellowship (2), employed in independent practice (1), employed in an academic position at a university (1), employed in other positions at a higher education institution (1), employed in government agency (2), total from the above (doctoral) (7).

Additional Information:
Orientation, Objectives, and Emphasis of Department: Accredited by the American Psychological Association (APA) since 1955, the UO doctoral program in Counseling Psychology emphasizes an ecological model of training, research, and practice. Students focus research and training in prevention and treatment relevant to work with children, adolescents, families, and adults. The ecological model holds that human behavior occurs within a context of multiple interacting systems, influenced by unique social, historical, political, and cultural factors. Students in the CPSY program are trained to view assessment, intervention, and research within the contexts of these systems. Development of multicultural competencies is emphasized throughout the curriculum.

Special Facilities or Resources: Students work cooperatively in research areas at Oregon Social Learning Center, the Oregon Research Institute and the Child and Family Center.

Information for Students With Physical Disabilities: See the following Web site for more information: http://ds.uoregon.edu/.

Application Information:
Send to Academic Secretary, Counseling Psychology, 5251 University of Oregon, Eugene, OR, 97403-5251. Application available online. URL of online application: http://counpsych.uoregon.edu/admissions.htm. Students are admitted in the Fall, application deadline December 15. *Fee:* $50. Contact UO Graduate School Admissions regarding conditions for waiver or deferral of fee.

Oregon, University of
Department of Psychology
College of Arts and Sciences
1227 University of Oregon
Eugene, OR 97403-1227
Telephone: (541) 346-5060
Fax: (541) 346-4911
E-mail: *gradsec@psych.uoregon.edu*
Web: *http://psychweb.uoregon.edu*

Department Information:
1895. Department Head: Louis J. Moses, PhD. Number of faculty: total—full-time 26, part-time 2; women—full-time 10, part-time 1; total—minority—full-time 5; women minority—full-time 1.

Programs and Degrees Offered:
Listed in the following order: Program area, degree type (T if terminal Master's), number awarded 7/08–6/09. Clinical Psychology PhD (Doctor of Philosophy) 2, Cognitive/ Neuroscience/ Systems PhD (Doctor of Philosophy) 1, Developmental Psychology PhD (Doctor of Philosophy) 1, Individualized Master's MA/MS (Master of Arts/Science) (T) 5, Social/Personality Psychology PhD (Doctor of Philosophy) 5.

APA Accreditation: Clinical PhD (Doctor of Philosophy). Student Outcome Data Website: http://psychweb.uoregon.edu/graduates/intellectualcommunities/clinical.

Student Applications/Admissions:
Student Applications
Clinical Psychology PhD (Doctor of Philosophy)—Applications 2009–2010, 239. Total applicants accepted 2009–2010, 9. Number full-time enrolled (new admits only) 2009–2010, 0. Total enrolled 2009–2010 full-time, 19. Openings 2010–2011, 4. *Cognitive/ Neuroscience/Systems PhD (Doctor of Philosophy)*—Applications 2009–2010, 66. Total applicants accepted 2009–2010, 12. Number full-time enrolled (new admits only) 2009–2010, 0. Total enrolled 2009–2010 full-time, 15. Openings 2010–2011, 2. The number of students enrolled full- and part-time who were dismissed or voluntarily withdrew from this program area in 2008–2009 were 1. *Developmental Psychology PhD (Doctor of Philosophy)*—Applications 2009–2010, 26. Total applicants accepted 2009–2010, 5. Total enrolled 2009–2010 full-time, 10. Openings 2010–2011, 2. *Individualized Master's MA/MS (Master of Arts/Science)*—Total enrolled 2009–2010 full-time, 27. Openings 2010–2011, 10. *Social/Personality Psychology PhD (Doctor of Philosophy)*—Applications 2009–2010, 56. Total applicants accepted 2009–2010, 6. Total enrolled 2009–2010 full-time, 12. Openings 2010–2011, 2.
Scores: Entries appear in this order: required test or GPA, minimum score (if required), median score of students entering

in 2009–2010. *Clinical Psychology PhD (Doctor of Philosophy)*: GRE-V no minimum stated, GRE-Q no minimum stated, GRE-Analytical no minimum stated, overall undergraduate GPA no minimum stated, last 2 years GPA no minimum stated, psychology GPA no minimum stated; *Cognitive/Neuroscience/Systems PhD (Doctor of Philosophy)*: GRE-V no minimum stated, GRE-Q no minimum stated, GRE-Analytical no minimum stated, overall undergraduate GPA no minimum stated, last 2 years GPA no minimum stated, psychology GPA no minimum stated; *Developmental Psychology PhD (Doctor of Philosophy)*: GRE-V no minimum stated, GRE-Q no minimum stated, GRE-Analytical no minimum stated, overall undergraduate GPA no minimum stated, last 2 years GPA no minimum stated, psychology GPA no minimum stated; *Individualized Master's MA/MS (Master of Arts/Science)*: overall undergraduate GPA no minimum stated, last 2 years GPA no minimum stated, psychology GPA no minimum stated; *Social/Personality Psychology PhD (Doctor of Philosophy)*: GRE-V no minimum stated, GRE-Q no minimum stated, GRE-Analytical no minimum stated, overall undergraduate GPA no minimum stated, last 2 years GPA no minimum stated, psychology GPA no minimum stated.

Other Criteria: (importance of criteria rated low, medium, or high): GRE scores—high, research experience—high, work experience—low, extracurricular activity—low, clinically related public service—medium, GPA—high, letters of recommendation—high, interview—high, statement of goals and objectives—high. Please check with department regarding interviews. For additional information on admission requirements, go to http://psychweb.uoregon.edu.

Student Characteristics: The following represents characteristics of students in 2009–2010 in all graduate psychology programs in the department: Female—full-time 54, part-time 0; Male—full-time 29, part-time 0; African American/Black—full-time 1, part-time 0; Hispanic/Latino(a)—full-time 2, part-time 0; Asian/Pacific Islander—full-time 5, part-time 0; American Indian/Alaska Native—full-time 0, part-time 0; Caucasian/White—full-time 68, part-time 0; Multi-ethnic—full-time 6, part-time 0; students subject to the Americans With Disabilities Act—full-time 0, part-time 0; Unknown ethnicity—full-time 1, part-time 0; International students who hold an F-1 or J-1 Visa—full-time 13, part-time 0.

Financial Information/Assistance:
Tuition for Full-Time Study: *Master's:* State residents: $424 per credit hour; Nonstate residents: $620 per credit hour. *Doctoral:* State residents: $424 per credit hour; Nonstate residents: $620 per credit hour. Tuition is subject to change. See the following Web site for updates and changes in tuition costs: http://registrar.uoregon.edu/costs.

Financial Assistance:
First-Year Students: Teaching assistantships available for first year. Research assistantships available for first year. Fellowships and scholarships available for first year.

Advanced Students: Teaching assistantships available for advanced students. Research assistantships available for advanced students. Fellowships and scholarships available for advanced students.

Additional Information: Of all students currently enrolled full time, 95% benefited from one or more of the listed financial assistance programs.

Internships/Practica: Doctoral Degree (PhD Clinical Psychology): For those doctoral students for whom a professional internship was required in this program prior to graduation, (5) students applied for an internship in 2008–2009, with (5) students obtaining an internship. Of those students who obtained an internship, (5) were paid internships. Of those students who obtained an internship, (5) students placed in APA/CPA accredited internships, (0) students placed in internships not APA/CPA accredited, but listed with the Association of Psychology Postdoctoral and Internship Programs (APPIC), (0) students placed in internships conforming to guidelines of the Council of Directors of School Psychology Programs (CDSPP), (0) students placed in internships that were not APA/CPA accredited, APPIC or CDSPP listed. Master's Degree (MA/MS Individualized Master's): An internship experience, such as a final research project or "capstone" experience is required of graduates.

Housing and Day Care: On-campus housing is available. See the following Web site for more information: http://housing.uoregon.edu. On-campus day care facilities are available. See the following Web site for more information: http://housing.uoregon.edu/apartments/childcare.php.

Employment of Department Graduates:
Master's Degree Graduates: Of those who graduated in the academic year 2008–2009, the following categories and numbers represent the postgraduate activities and employment of master's degree graduates: Enrolled in a postdoctoral residency/fellowship (n/a), employed in independent practice (n/a), total from the above (master's) (0).

Doctoral Degree Graduates: Of those who graduated in the academic year 2008–2009, the following categories and numbers represent the postgraduate activities and employment of doctoral degree graduates: Enrolled in a psychology doctoral program (n/a), total from the above (doctoral) (0).

Additional Information:
Orientation, Objectives, and Emphasis of Department: The course of study is tailored largely to the student's particular needs. There are minimal formal requirements for the doctorate, which include three course sequences (contemporary issues in psychology, statistics, and a first-year research practicum); a supporting area requirement, consisting of at least two graduate-level, graded courses, and a major project, such as a paper or teaching an original course; a major preliminary examination; and, of course, the doctoral dissertation. Clinical students engage in several practica beginning in the first year. All programs require and are organized to facilitate student research from the first year.

Special Facilities or Resources: Straub Hall houses the psychology clinic, equipment for psychophysiological research, specialized facilities for research in child and social psychology, and experimental laboratories for human research. Numerous microcomputers are available for research and teaching. A short distance from the main psychology building are well-equipped animal labs for research in physiological psychology. Graduate students and faculty participate in interdisciplinary programs in cognitive science, neuroscience, and developmental psychopathology. Local nonprofit research groups including Oregon Research Institute, Oregon Social Learning Center and Decision Research provide unusual auspices and opportunities for students.

Information for Students With Physical Disabilities: See the following Web site for more information: http://ds.uoregon.edu/.

Application Information:
Send to Graduate Secretary, Department of Psychology, 1227 University of Oregon, Eugene, OR 97403-1227. Application available online. URL of online application: http://admissions.uoregon.edu/graduate/graduate. Students are admitted in the Fall, application deadline December 1. Individualized master's deadline for fall admission is May 15. *Fee:* $50.

Pacific University
School of Professional Psychology
College of Health Professions
Pacific University
222 Southeast 8th Avenue, Suite 563
Hillsboro, OR 97123-4218
Telephone: (503) 352-7277
Fax: (503) 352-7320
E-mail: *waldronk@pacificu.edu*
Web: *http://www.pacificu.edu/spp/*

Department Information:
1979. Dean: Michel Hersen. Number of faculty: total—full-time 24, part-time 29; women—full-time 14, part-time 16; total—minority—full-time 6; women minority—full-time 5; faculty subject to the Americans With Disabilities Act 1.

Programs and Degrees Offered:
Listed in the following order: Program area, degree type (T if terminal Master's), number awarded 7/08–6/09. Clinical Psychology PsyD (Doctor of Psychology) 31, Counseling Psychology MA/MS (Master of Arts/Science) (T) 35.

APA Accreditation: Clinical PsyD (Doctor of Psychology). Student Outcome Data Website: http://www.pacificu.edu/spp/program_stats.cfm.

Student Applications/Admissions:
Student Applications
Clinical Psychology PsyD (Doctor of Psychology)—Applications 2009–2010, 197. Total applicants accepted 2009–2010, 104. Number full-time enrolled (new admits only) 2009–2010, 52. Number part-time enrolled (new admits only) 2009–2010, 0. Total enrolled 2009–2010 full-time, 189, part-time, 81. Openings 2010–2011, 50. The median number of years required for completion of a degree in 2008–2009 were 6. The number of students enrolled full- and part-time who were dismissed or voluntarily withdrew from this program area in 2008–2009 were 2. *Counseling Psychology MA/MS (Master of Arts/Science)*—Applications 2009–2010, 114. Total applicants accepted 2009–2010, 64. Number full-time enrolled (new admits only) 2009–2010, 41. Number part-time enrolled (new admits only) 2009–2010, 3. Total enrolled 2009–2010 full-time, 72, part-time, 6. Openings 2010–2011, 40. The median number of years required for completion of a degree in 2008–2009 were 2. The number of students enrolled full- and part-time who were dismissed or voluntarily withdrew from this program area in 2008–2009 were 0.

Scores: Entries appear in this order: required test or GPA, minimum score (if required), median score of students entering in 2009–2010. *Clinical Psychology PsyD (Doctor of Psychology):* GRE-V no minimum stated, 511, GRE-Q no minimum stated, 567, GRE-Analytical no minimum stated, 4.5, overall undergraduate GPA no minimum stated, 3.53, last 2 years GPA 3.4.
Other Criteria: (importance of criteria rated low, medium, or high): GRE scores—medium, research experience—medium, work experience—medium, extracurricular activity—low, clinically related public service—low, GPA—medium, letters of recommendation—high, interview—high, statement of goals and objectives—medium, undergraduate major in psychology—low, specific undergraduate psychology courses taken—medium. GRE scores required for PsyD program only. For additional information on admission requirements, go to http://www.pacificu.edu/spp/admissions/index.cfm.

Student Characteristics: The following represents characteristics of students in 2009–2010 in all graduate psychology programs in the department: Female—full-time 200, part-time 56; Male—full-time 61, part-time 31; African American/Black—full-time 2, part-time 1; Hispanic/Latino(a)—full-time 10, part-time 0; Asian/Pacific Islander—full-time 13, part-time 1; American Indian/Alaska Native—full-time 2, part-time 0; Caucasian/White—full-time 161, part-time 2; Multi-ethnic—full-time 5, part-time 1; students subject to the Americans With Disabilities Act—full-time 9, part-time 7; Unknown ethnicity—full-time 67, part-time 0; International students who hold an F-1 or J-1 Visa—full-time 0, part-time 0.

Financial Information/Assistance:
Tuition for Full-Time Study: *Master's:* State residents: per academic year $19,728, $803 per credit hour; Nonstate residents: per academic year $19,728, $803 per credit hour. *Doctoral:* State residents: per academic year $27,750, $841 per credit hour; Nonstate residents: per academic year $27,750, $841 per credit hour. Tuition is subject to change. See the following Web site for updates and changes in tuition costs: http://www.pacificu.edu/spp/admissions/index.cfm.

Financial Assistance:
First-Year Students: Research assistantships available for first year. Average amount paid per academic year: $3,000. Average number of hours worked per week: 7. Apply by January 10. Fellowships and scholarships available for first year. Average amount paid per academic year: $3,000. Apply by January 10.

Advanced Students: Teaching assistantships available for advanced students. Average amount paid per academic year: $3,600. Average number of hours worked per week: 7. Apply by April 1. Research assistantships available for advanced students. Average amount paid per academic year: $3,000. Average number of hours worked per week: 7. Apply by April 1. Fellowships and scholarships available for advanced students. Average amount paid per academic year: $3,000. Apply by April 1.

Additional Information: Of all students currently enrolled full time, 30% benefited from one or more of the listed financial assistance programs. Application and information available online at: http://www.pacificu.edu/financialaid/.

Internships/Practica: Doctoral Degree (PsyD Clinical Psychology): For those doctoral students for whom a professional internship was required in this program prior to graduation, (45) students applied for an internship in 2008–2009, with (42) students obtaining an internship. Of those students who obtained an internship, (42) were paid internships. Of those students who obtained an internship, (17) students placed in APA/CPA accredited internships, (20) students placed in internships not APA/CPA accredited, but listed with the Association of Psychology Postdoctoral and Internship Programs (APPIC), (0) students placed in internships conforming to guidelines of the Council of Directors of School Psychology Programs (CDSPP), (5) students placed in internships that were not APA/CPA accredited, APPIC or CDSPP listed. Master's Degree (MA/MS Counseling Psychology): An internship experience, such as, a final research project or "capstone" experience is required of graduates. Each PsyD student is required to complete 6 terms (24 credits, two years) of practica. The practicum experience includes a minimum of 500 training hours per year, approximately one third to one half of which are in direct service, one fourth in supervisory and training activities, and the remainder in administrative/clerical duties related to the above. Training entails the integration of theoretical knowledge through its application in clinical practice. The experience includes supervised practice in the application of professional psychological competencies with a range of client populations, age groups, problems and service settings. The initial year of practicum is typically served at the Psychological Service Center. Later experiences are usually taken at community placements. Upon successful completion of practicum training, required coursework, and Competency Examination, the student is ready to begin an internship. Internship requires one calendar year of full-time experience, or two years half time, at an approved site. MA in Counseling Psychology students complete 700 hours (15 credits, 3 terms) of internship in their second year. Students who elect to complete the yearlong sequence of organizational behavior courses also complete a 100 hour OB practicum in addition.

Housing and Day Care: No on-campus housing is available. No on-campus day care facilities are available.

Employment of Department Graduates:
Master's Degree Graduates: Of those who graduated in the academic year 2008–2009, the following categories and numbers represent the postgraduate activities and employment of master's degree graduates: Enrolled in a postdoctoral residency/fellowship (n/a), employed in independent practice (n/a), total from the above (master's) (0).
Doctoral Degree Graduates: Of those who graduated in the academic year 2008–2009, the following categories and numbers represent the postgraduate activities and employment of doctoral degree graduates: Enrolled in a psychology doctoral program (n/a), employed in independent practice (2), employed in other positions at a higher education institution (3), employed in government agency (5), employed in a community mental health/counseling center (1), employed in a hospital/medical center (4), do not know (16), total from the above (doctoral) (31).

Additional Information:
Orientation, Objectives, and Emphasis of Department: The School of Professional Psychology at Pacific University educates informed practitioners of scientifically based professional psychology who are responsive to the latest empirical findings in the field. We strive to maintain a facilitative academic community based on collaborative inquiry. Faculty and students work together in multiple roles in program development, clinical research, and governance. We underscore provision of services to diverse populations at the individual, family, group, and community levels.

Special Facilities or Resources: The two internal training clinics of the Pacific University School of Professional Psychology provide a full range of quality outpatient psychological services to residents of the Portland Metropolitan area while providing intensive training for doctoral level clinical psychology students and providing a setting for on-going clinical research. The Psychological Service Center in Portland provides the full range of psychodiagnostic and treatment services to a variety of client populations, including intellectual, personality, and neuropsychological assessment, individual therapy, family therapy, group therapy, and consultation. The Iris Clinic in Hillsboro provides the opportunity to provide services in Spanish as well as English.

Information for Students With Physical Disabilities: See the following Web site for more information: http://www.pacificu.edu/studentlife/department/lss.cfm.

Application Information:
Send to Office of Admissions, Pacific University, 222 SE 8th Avenue, Ste 212, Hillsboro, OR 97123. Application available online. URL of online application: http://www.pacificu.edu/spp/admissions/howtoapply.cfm. Students are admitted in the Fall, application deadline January 8. MA Counseling Psychology - March 5. *Fee:* $40.

Portland State University
Psychology Department
College of Liberal Arts and Sciences
P.O. Box 751
Portland, OR 97207-0751
Telephone: (503) 725-3923
Fax: (503) 725-3904
E-mail: *mankowskie@pdx.edu*
Web: *http://www.pdx.edu/psy*

Department Information:
1955. Chairperson: Sherwin Davidson, Ph. D. Number of faculty: total—full-time 18; women—full-time 8; total—minority—full-time 4; women minority—full-time 2.

Programs and Degrees Offered:
Listed in the following order: Program area, degree type (T if terminal Master's), number awarded 7/08–6/09. Applied Developmental PhD (Doctor of Philosophy) 1, Applied Social & Community PhD (Doctor of Philosophy) 5, Industrial/Organizational PhD (Doctor of Philosophy) 5.

Student Applications/Admissions:
Student Applications
Applied Developmental PhD (Doctor of Philosophy)—Applications 2009–2010, 20. Total applicants accepted 2009–2010, 4. Number full-time enrolled (new admits only) 2009–2010, 3. Openings 2010–2011, 4. The median number of years required for completion of a degree in 2008–2009 were 6. The number of students enrolled full- and part-time who were dismissed or voluntarily withdrew from this program area in

2008–2009 were 1. *Applied Social & Community PhD (Doctor of Philosophy)*—Applications 2009–2010, 62. Total applicants accepted 2009–2010, 5. Number full-time enrolled (new admits only) 2009–2010, 3. Number part-time enrolled (new admits only) 2009–2010, 0. Openings 2010–2011, 5. The median number of years required for completion of a degree in 2008–2009 were 6. The number of students enrolled full- and part-time who were dismissed or voluntarily withdrew from this program area in 2008–2009 were 1. *Industrial/Organizational PhD (Doctor of Philosophy)*—Applications 2009–2010, 50. Total applicants accepted 2009–2010, 6. Number full-time enrolled (new admits only) 2009–2010, 4. Number part-time enrolled (new admits only) 2009–2010, 0. Openings 2010–2011, 6. The median number of years required for completion of a degree in 2008–2009 were 6. The number of students enrolled full- and part-time who were dismissed or voluntarily withdrew from this program area in 2008–2009 were 1.

Scores: Entries appear in this order: required test or GPA, minimum score (if required), median score of students entering in 2009–2010. *Applied Developmental PhD (Doctor of Philosophy)*: GRE-V no minimum stated, GRE-Q no minimum stated, GRE-Analytical no minimum stated, overall undergraduate GPA no minimum stated, last 2 years GPA no minimum stated; *Applied Social & Community PhD (Doctor of Philosophy)*: GRE-V no minimum stated, GRE-Q no minimum stated, GRE-Analytical no minimum stated, overall undergraduate GPA no minimum stated, last 2 years GPA no minimum stated; *Industrial/Organizational PhD (Doctor of Philosophy)*: GRE-V no minimum stated, GRE-Q no minimum stated, GRE-Analytical no minimum stated, overall undergraduate GPA no minimum stated, last 2 years GPA no minimum stated.

Other Criteria: (importance of criteria rated low, medium, or high): GRE scores—high, research experience—high, work experience—medium, extracurricular activity—medium, clinically related public service—low, GPA—high, letters of recommendation—high, statement of goals and objectives—high, undergraduate major in psychology—medium, specific undergraduate psychology courses taken—medium. For additional information on admission requirements, go to http://www.pdx.edu/psy/application-instructions.

Student Characteristics: The following represents characteristics of students in 2009–2010 in all graduate psychology programs in the department: Female—full-time 45, part-time 0; Male—full-time 18, part-time 0; African American/Black—full-time 0, part-time 0; Hispanic/Latino(a)—full-time 0, part-time 0; Asian/Pacific Islander—full-time 0, part-time 0; American Indian/Alaska Native—full-time 0, part-time 0; Caucasian/White—full-time 0, part-time 0; Multi-ethnic—full-time 0, part-time 0; students subject to the Americans With Disabilities Act—full-time 0, part-time 0; Unknown ethnicity—full-time 0, part-time 0; International students who hold an F-1 or J-1 Visa—full-time 0, part-time 0.

Financial Information/Assistance:
Tuition for Full-Time Study: *Master's:* State residents: per academic year $8,424, $312 per credit hour; Nonstate residents: per academic year $13,149, $487 per credit hour. *Doctoral:* State residents: per academic year $8,424, $312 per credit hour; Nonstate residents: per academic year $13,149, $487 per credit hour. Tuition is subject to change. Additional fees are assessed to students beyond the costs of tuition for the following: Health services, Building, Campus Recreation. See the following Web site for updates and changes in tuition costs: http://www.pdx.edu/bao/tuition-estimator.

Financial Assistance:
First-Year Students: Teaching assistantships available for first year. Average amount paid per academic year: $10,350. Average number of hours worked per week: 19. Research assistantships available for first year. Average amount paid per academic year: $10,350. Average number of hours worked per week: 19. Fellowships and scholarships available for first year. Average amount paid per academic year: $10,350. Average number of hours worked per week: 19.

Advanced Students: Teaching assistantships available for advanced students. Average amount paid per academic year: $12,000. Average number of hours worked per week: 19. Research assistantships available for advanced students. Average amount paid per academic year: $12,000. Average number of hours worked per week: 19. Fellowships and scholarships available for advanced students. Average amount paid per academic year: $12,000. Average number of hours worked per week: 19.

Additional Information: Of all students currently enrolled full time, 100% benefited from one or more of the listed financial assistance programs.

Internships/Practica: The university is located in downtown Portland, the major metropolitan area in the state of Oregon. Consequently, internships are readily available in a variety of applied settings. Placements are also available through the ongoing research activities of the faculty. The program is structured to provide everyone with (1) training in the basics of applied psychology and research methods, and (2) expertise in the psychological theories and research methods in their area of specialty. The basic training is provided by three advanced applied courses in the three areas we consider central to the understanding of social issues: social and group processes and interventions (referred to as Applied Social & Community); organizational and institutional processes (referred to as Industrial-Organizational); and process of change (referred to as Applied Developmental). Training in research methods is provided via a sequence of quantitative methods courses, three of which are required. The department offers a number of additional quantitative and qualitative methods courses which include: Factor Analysis, Structural Equation Modeling, HLM and Psychometrics and Scale Construction. Since the program emphasizes applied psychology, students receive training in their area of specialty not only through close work with faculty but also through structured participation in community organizations. Graduate students work in close collaboration with their faculty advisors and other members of the faculty who serve in a mentor role. Student experiences include seminars on special topics, individual reading and conference arrangements, research practica, and collaboration on joint projects. The primary vehicles for interactions with community organizations are practica and internships. To ensure relevant learning, these are supervised by departmental faculty. The program culminates for students in their own independent research (i.e., thesis and/or dissertation).

Housing and Day Care: On-campus housing is available. See the following Web site for more information: http://www.pdx.edu/housing/. On-campus day care facilities are available. See the

GRADUATE STUDY IN PSYCHOLOGY

following Web site for more information: http://www.tcc.pdx.edu/; http://www.hgcdc.pdx.edu/.

Employment of Department Graduates:
Master's Degree Graduates: Of those who graduated in the academic year 2008–2009, the following categories and numbers represent the postgraduate activities and employment of master's degree graduates: Enrolled in a psychology doctoral program (1), enrolled in a postdoctoral residency/fellowship (n/a), employed in independent practice (n/a), employed in business or industry (1), total from the above (master's) (2).
Doctoral Degree Graduates: Of those who graduated in the academic year 2008–2009, the following categories and numbers represent the postgraduate activities and employment of doctoral degree graduates: Enrolled in a psychology doctoral program (n/a), employed in an academic position at a university (2), employed in government agency (2), do not know (1), total from the above (doctoral) (5).

Additional Information:
Orientation, Objectives, and Emphasis of Department: The department accepts applicants to both the MA/M.S. (initiated fall 1969) and PhD (initiated fall 1986) programs. The master's program is fully integrated into the doctoral program. Those who are admitted to the master's program may later apply for admission to the doctoral program, conditional upon demonstrated competence at the master's level. The aim of the program is to prepare graduates for a university career and/or a research/service career in a variety of settings, such as governmental agencies, manufacturing and service industries, health organizations and labor organizations. Students are given a broad background in applied psychology. Doctoral students major in one of three specialty areas and select a minor in a second. Applied Developmental focuses on educational settings, family studies, and aging processes, providing training in family development (i.e., the processes of change that families as systems of member relationships experience), family and work (i.e., the interactive relationships between the two domains of family and work life), family and school, family processes in adult life, as well as cultural issues. Industrial-Organizational covers areas of theory, research methods, and social issues relevant to organizational and occupational life. Areas of study include leadership, work motivation, job stress, organizational development, etc. Applied Social & Community deals with how social psychological and community research methods, findings, and theories are applied to: a) social issues (e.g., prejudice, violence, AIDS, disabilities, problem behavior, child safety, and energy conservation); b) professions and institutions (e.g., health and law); and c) the design and evaluation of social interventions.

Special Facilities or Resources: The Department of Psychology's location in the heart of downtown Portland offers unique academic and research opportunities in the service of the department's applied mission. Strong collaborative relationships with local industry, organizations, and community agencies offer venues for course related projects, faculty research initiatives, practicum placements, and required student research. A number of University-based resources also enhance our students' skills and experiences. For example, the University's writing center allows faculty and students to hone technical writing skills. The Instructional Development Support Center provides training in computer and media-based applications to foster improved teaching and more sophisticated research approaches.

Information for Students With Physical Disabilities: See the following Web site for more information: http://www.drc.pdx.edu.

Application Information:
Send to Portland State University, Department of Psychology, P.O. Box 751, Portland, OR 97207-0751. Application available online. URL of online application: http://www.pdx.edu/psy/graduate. Students are admitted in the Fall, application deadline December 15. *Fee:* $50.

Southern Oregon University
Master in Mental Health Counseling
1250 Siskiyou Boulevard
Ashland, OR 97520
Telephone: (541) 552-6947
Fax: (541) 552-6988
E-mail: *MHC@sou.edu*
Web: *http://www.sou.edu/psychology/mhc/*

Department Information:
2000. Chairperson: Daniel DeNeui, PhD. Number of faculty: total—full-time 5, part-time 1; women—full-time 4; total—minority—full-time 1; women minority—full-time 1.

Programs and Degrees Offered:
Listed in the following order: Program area, degree type (T if terminal Master's), number awarded 7/08–6/09. Mental Health Counseling MA/MS (Master of Arts/Science) (T) 21.

Student Applications/Admissions:
Student Applications
Mental Health Counseling MA/MS (Master of Arts/Science)—Applications 2009–2010, 60. Total applicants accepted 2009–2010, 22. Number full-time enrolled (new admits only) 2009–2010, 22. Number part-time enrolled (new admits only) 2009–2010, 0. Total enrolled 2009–2010 full-time, 35, part-time, 4. Openings 2010–2011, 21. The median number of years required for completion of a degree in 2008–2009 were 2. The number of students enrolled full- and part-time who were dismissed or voluntarily withdrew from this program area in 2008–2009 were 0.

Scores: Entries appear in this order: required test or GPA, minimum score (if required), median score of students entering in 2009–2010. *Mental Health Counseling MA/MS (Master of Arts/Science)*: GRE-V 400, GRE-Q 400, GRE-Analytical 3.0, overall undergraduate GPA 3.0, last 2 years GPA 3.0, psychology GPA 3.0.

Other Criteria: (importance of criteria rated low, medium, or high): GRE scores—high, research experience—low, work experience—low, extracurricular activity—low, clinically related public service—low, GPA—high, letters of recommendation—high, statement of goals and objectives—high, specific undergraduate psychology courses taken—high. For additional information on admission requirements, go to http://www.sou.edu/psychology/mhc/.

Student Characteristics: The following represents characteristics of students in 2009–2010 in all graduate psychology programs in the department: Female—full-time 26, part-time 3; Male—full-time 9, part-time 1; African American/Black—full-time 0, part-time 0; Hispanic/Latino(a)—full-time 3, part-time 0; Asian/Pacific Islander—full-time 2, part-time 0; American Indian/Alaska Native—full-time 0, part-time 0; Caucasian/White—full-time 29, part-time 4; Multi-ethnic—full-time 0, part-time 0; students subject to the Americans With Disabilities Act—full-time 0, part-time 0; Unknown ethnicity—full-time 1, part-time 0; International students who hold an F-1 or J-1 Visa—full-time 0, part-time 0.

Financial Information/Assistance:
Tuition for Full-Time Study: *Master's:* State residents: per academic year $15,000; Nonstate residents: per academic year $20,000. Tuition is subject to change. See the following Web site for updates and changes in tuition costs: http://sou.edu/enrollment/financial-services/tuition-fees-schedule.html.

Financial Assistance:
First-Year Students: Teaching assistantships available for first year. Average amount paid per academic year: $2,400. Average number of hours worked per week: 12.

Advanced Students: Teaching assistantships available for advanced students. Average amount paid per academic year: $2,400. Average number of hours worked per week: 12.

Additional Information: Of all students currently enrolled full time, 10% benefited from one or more of the listed financial assistance programs. Application and information available online at: http://www.sou.edu/psychology/mhc/.

Internships/Practica: Master's Degree (MA/MS Mental Health Counseling): An internship experience, such as, a final research project or "capstone" experience is required of graduates. The Mental Health Counseling program requires practicum during the first year of courses. Internship placement in the community for students in the second year is required to help fulfill state license requirements. MHC students are trained to become Licensed Professional Counselors in the State of Oregon.

Housing and Day Care: On-campus housing is available. See the following Web site for more information: http://www.sou.edu/housing/. On-campus day care facilities are available. See the following Web site for more information: http://www.sou.edu/scc/.

Employment of Department Graduates:
Master's Degree Graduates: Of those who graduated in the academic year 2008–2009, the following categories and numbers represent the postgraduate activities and employment of master's degree graduates: Enrolled in a psychology doctoral program (1), enrolled in another graduate/professional program (0), enrolled in a postdoctoral residency/fellowship (n/a), employed in independent practice (n/a), employed in a community mental health/counseling center (20), total from the above (master's) (21).

Doctoral Degree Graduates: Of those who graduated in the academic year 2008–2009, the following categories and numbers represent the postgraduate activities and employment of doctoral degree graduates: Enrolled in a psychology doctoral program (n/a), total from the above (doctoral) (0).

Additional Information:
Orientation, Objectives, and Emphasis of Department: The principle objective of the Master's degree in Mental Health Counseling is to provide professional training in the application of psychological principles and methodologies in order to increase functioning and service delivery in public and private agencies, organizations, and communities. The Mental Health Counseling program is based on a common integrated core of courses. The central goal of this core is to train masters' level practitioners who are grounded in professional ethics and values, well-versed in the empirical nature of their professions, and sensitive to and supportive of the increasing multicultural diversity of our communities.

Special Facilities or Resources: The Mental Health Counseling track is accredited by the Council for Accreditation of Counseling and Related Educational Programs (CACREP). This track is also recognized by the Oregon Board of Licensed Professional Counselors and Therapists (OBLPCT) as meeting the educational requirements for application for licensure at a Licensed Professional Counselor in Oregon. The MHC track is also designed to meet the majority of requirement for licensure as a Marriage and Family therapist in California.

Information for Students With Physical Disabilities: See the following Web site for more information: http://www.sou.edu/access/dss/.

Application Information:
Send to Master in Mental Health Counseling Southern Oregon University 1250 Siskiyou Blvd Ashland, OR 97520. Application available online. URL of online application: http://www.sou.edu/psychology/mhc/. Students are admitted in the Fall, application deadline February 15. *Fee:* $50.

PENNSYLVANIA

Arcadia University
Department of Psychology
450 South Easton Road
Glenside, PA 19038-3295
Telephone: (267) 620-4130
Fax: (215) 881-8758
E-mail: *bartolie@arcadia.edu*
Web: *http://www.arcadia.edu/academic/default.aspx?id=559*

Department Information:
1986. Chairperson: Les Sdorow, PhD Number of faculty: total—full-time 9, part-time 9; women—full-time 4, part-time 5; total—minority—full-time 2, part-time 2; women minority—full-time 2, part-time 2.

Programs and Degrees Offered:
Listed in the following order: Program area, degree type (T if terminal Master's), number awarded 7/08–6/09. Elementary School Counseling MA/MS (Master of Arts/Science) (T), Secondary School Counseling MA/MS (Master of Arts/Science) (T), Public Health and Counseling Psychology MA/MS (Master of Arts/Science) (T), Community Counseling: Child and Family Therapy MA/MS (Master of Arts/Science) (T), Community Counseling: Trauma MA/MS (Master of Arts/Science) (T), Community Counseling: General MA/MS (Master of Arts/Science) (T).

Student Applications/Admissions:
Student Applications
Elementary School Counseling MA/MS (Master of Arts/Science)—Secondary School Counseling MA/MS (Master of Arts/Science)—Public Health and Counseling Psychology MA/MS (Master of Arts/Science)—Community Counseling: Child and Family Therapy MA/MS (Master of Arts/Science)—Community Counseling: Trauma MA/MS (Master of Arts/Science)—Community Counseling: General MA/MS (Master of Arts/Science)—
Other Criteria: (importance of criteria rated low, medium, or high): GRE scores—medium, research experience—medium, work experience—medium, extracurricular activity—medium, clinically related public service—medium, GPA—high, letters of recommendation—high, interview—high, statement of goals and objectives—high, undergraduate major in psychology—low, specific undergraduate psychology courses taken—high. For additional information on admission requirements, go to http://www.arcadia.edu/academic/default.aspx?id=3859.

Student Characteristics: The following represents characteristics of students in 2009–2010 in all graduate psychology programs in the department: Female—full-time 30, part-time 31; Male—full-time 4, part-time 7; African American/Black—full-time 5, part-time 4; Hispanic/Latino(a)—full-time 1, part-time 3; Asian/Pacific Islander—full-time 1, part-time 0; American Indian/Alaska Native—full-time 0, part-time 0; Caucasian/White—full-time 23, part-time 29; Multi-ethnic—full-time 0, part-time 0; students subject to the Americans With Disabilities Act—full-time 4, part-time 1; Unknown ethnicity—full-time 0, part-time 2; International students who hold an F-1 or J-1 Visa—full-time 0, part-time 1.

Financial Information/Assistance:
Tuition for Full-Time Study: *Master's:* State residents: $620 per credit hour; Nonstate residents: $620 per credit hour. See the following Web site for updates and changes in tuition costs: http://www.arcadia.edu/admissions/default.aspx?id=2395.

Financial Assistance:
First-Year Students: Traineeships available for first year. Average amount paid per academic year: $750. Average number of hours worked per week: 4.
Advanced Students: Traineeships available for advanced students. Average amount paid per academic year: $750. Average number of hours worked per week: 4.
Additional Information: Application and information available online at: http://www.arcadia.edu/admissions/default.aspx?id=609.

Internships/Practica: Master's Degree (MA/MS Elementary School Counseling): An internship experience, such as a final research project or "capstone" experience is required of graduates. Master's Degree (MA/MS Secondary School Counseling): An internship experience, such as a final research project or "capstone" experience is required of graduates. Master's Degree (MA/MS Public Health and Counseling Psychology): An internship experience, such as a final research project or "capstone" experience is required of graduates. Master's Degree (MA/MS Community Counseling: Child and Family Therapy): An internship experience, such as a final research project or "capstone" experience is required of graduates. Master's Degree (MA/MS Community Counseling: Trauma): An internship experience, such as a final research project or "capstone" experience is required of graduates. Master's Degree (MA/MS Community Counseling: General): An internship experience, such as a final research project or "capstone" experience is required of graduates. A practicum and an internship are required. Students have access to a variety of mental health agencies throughout the Philadelphia area.

Housing and Day Care: On-campus housing is available. See the following Web site for more information: http://www.arcadia.edu/student/default.aspx?id=4184. No on-campus day care facilities are available.

Employment of Department Graduates:
Master's Degree Graduates: Of those who graduated in the academic year 2008–2009, the following categories and numbers represent the postgraduate activities and employment of master's degree graduates: Enrolled in a postdoctoral residency/fellowship (n/a), employed in independent practice (n/a), total from the above (master's) (0).
Doctoral Degree Graduates: Of those who graduated in the academic year 2008–2009, the following categories and numbers represent the postgraduate activities and employment of doctoral degree graduates: Enrolled in a psychology doctoral program (n/a), total from the above (doctoral) (0).

Additional Information:
Orientation, Objectives, and Emphasis of Department: The Graduate Programs in Counseling Psychology prepares master's level students for professional positions in schools, social service, rehabilitation, industrial, health, and mental health settings. Graduates will be able to work as community mental health specialists, mental health counselors, crisis counselors, drug and alcohol counselors, illness and wellness counselors, geriatric counselors, employee-assistance counselors, school counselors, and staff developers or trainers. The program is designed on a part-time basis for the working professional. The orientation of the program is integrative with a strong emphasis on multicultural and evidence-based practices. Pennsylvania now licenses master's level counselors as Licensed Professional Counselors (LPC). Arcadia University's Master of Arts in Counseling Psychology provides the academic background to apply for licensure once 3,600 hours of mandated experience are acquired and the National Counselors Exam is taken.

Information for Students With Physical Disabilities: See the following Web site for more information: http://www.arcadia.edu/academic/default.aspx?id=15850.

Application Information:
Send to Office of Enrollment Management, Arcadia University, Glenside, PA 19038-3295. Application available online. URL of online application: http://www.arcadia.edu/admissions/default.aspx?id=644. Students are admitted in the Programs have rolling admissions. *Fee:* $40. The fee for online applications is only $20; the fee is waived for applications submitted by individuals who attended one of the Graduate Open House programs organized by the Office of Graduate Studies.

Bryn Mawr College
Department of Psychology
101 North Merion Avenue
Bryn Mawr, PA 19010-2899
Telephone: (610) 526-5010
Fax: (610) 526-7476
E-mail: aogle@brynmawr.edu
Web: http://www.brynmawr.edu/psychology/cdpp/

Department Information:
1890. Chairperson: Anjali Thapar. Number of faculty: total—full-time 7, part-time 6; women—full-time 3, part-time 5; total—minority—full-time 1; women minority—full-time 1.

Programs and Degrees Offered:
Listed in the following order: Program area, degree type (T if terminal Master's), number awarded 7/08–6/09. Clinical Developmental Psychology PhD (Doctor of Philosophy) 6.

Student Applications/Admissions:
Student Applications
Clinical Developmental Psychology PhD (Doctor of Philosophy)—Applications 2009–2010, 30. Total applicants accepted 2009–2010, 3. Number full-time enrolled (new admits only) 2009–2010, 3. Total enrolled 2009–2010 full-time, 28. Openings 2010–2011, 3. The median number of years required for completion of a degree in 2008–2009 were 7. The number of students enrolled full- and part-time who were dismissed or voluntarily withdrew from this program area in 2008–2009 were 0.

Scores: Entries appear in this order: required test or GPA, minimum score (if required), median score of students entering in 2009–2010. Clinical Developmental Psychology PhD (Doctor of Philosophy): GRE-V no minimum stated, 650, GRE-Q no minimum stated, 660, GRE-Analytical no minimum stated, 4.5, overall undergraduate GPA no minimum stated, 3.48.

Other Criteria: (importance of criteria rated low, medium, or high): GRE scores—medium, research experience—high, work experience—medium, extracurricular activity—low, clinically related public service—medium, GPA—high, letters of recommendation—high, interview—high, statement of goals and objectives—high, undergraduate major in psychology—medium, specific undergraduate psychology courses taken—low. For additional information on admission requirements, go to http://www.brynmawr.edu/psychology/cdpp/applying/.

Student Characteristics: The following represents characteristics of students in 2009–2010 in all graduate psychology programs in the department: Female—full-time 26, part-time 0; Male—full-time 2, part-time 0; African American/Black—full-time 0, part-time 0; Hispanic/Latino(a)—full-time 0, part-time 0; Asian/Pacific Islander—full-time 3, part-time 0; American Indian/Alaska Native—full-time 0, part-time 0; Caucasian/White—full-time 25, part-time 0; Multi-ethnic—full-time 0, part-time 0; students subject to the Americans With Disabilities Act—full-time 0, part-time 0; Unknown ethnicity—full-time 0, part-time 0; International students who hold an F-1 or J-1 Visa—full-time 2, part-time 0.

Financial Information/Assistance:
Tuition for Full-Time Study: Doctoral: State residents: per academic year $26,910; Nonstate residents: per academic year $26,910. Tuition is subject to change. See the following Web site for updates and changes in tuition costs: http://www.brynmawr.edu/gsas/Admissions/tuition_costs.html.

Financial Assistance:
First-Year Students: Teaching assistantships available for first year. Average amount paid per academic year: $14,000. Average number of hours worked per week: 17. Apply by 1/4. Fellowships and scholarships available for first year. Average amount paid per academic year: $13,500.

Advanced Students: Teaching assistantships available for advanced students. Average amount paid per academic year: $14,000. Average number of hours worked per week: 17. Fellowships and scholarships available for advanced students. Average amount paid per academic year: $13,500.

Additional Information: Of all students currently enrolled full time, 100% benefited from one or more of the listed financial assistance programs. Application and information available online at: http://www.brynmawr.edu/gsas/Resources/financial_support.html.

Internships/Practica: Doctoral Degree (PhD Clinical Developmental Psychology): For those doctoral students for whom a professional internship was required in this program prior to graduation, (1) students applied for an internship in 2008–2009, with

(1) students obtaining an internship. Of those students who obtained an internship, (1) were paid internships. Of those students who obtained an internship, (1) students placed in APA/CPA accredited internships, (0) students placed in internships not APA/CPA accredited, but listed with the Association of Psychology Postdoctoral and Internship Programs (APPIC), (0) students placed in internships conforming to guidelines of the Council of Directors of School Psychology Programs (CDSPP), (0) students placed in internships that were not APA/CPA accredited, APPIC or CDSPP listed. All students complete a sequence of clinical practica. During the third year of the program students complete a half time assessment/clinical practicum, typically in a school setting. In their fourth year, they complete a half-time clinical placement in local community mental health settings, university counseling centers, residential treatment facilities, university-affiliated training specialty clinics (e.g., specializing in anxiety disorders or eating disorders) or other clinically intensive settings. Many students complete additional part-time practica, and all students complete a year long clinical internship (6th year).

Housing and Day Care: No on-campus housing is available. On-campus day care facilities are available.

Employment of Department Graduates:
Master's Degree Graduates: Of those who graduated in the academic year 2008–2009, the following categories and numbers represent the postgraduate activities and employment of master's degree graduates: Enrolled in a postdoctoral residency/fellowship (n/a), employed in independent practice (n/a), total from the above (master's) (0).
Doctoral Degree Graduates: Of those who graduated in the academic year 2008–2009, the following categories and numbers represent the postgraduate activities and employment of doctoral degree graduates: Enrolled in a psychology doctoral program (n/a), enrolled in another graduate/professional program (0), enrolled in a postdoctoral residency/fellowship (0), employed in independent practice (0), employed in an academic position at a university (0), employed in an academic position at a 2-year/4-year college (0), employed in other positions at a higher education institution (4), employed in a professional position in a school system (2), employed in business or industry (0), employed in government agency (0), employed in a community mental health/counseling center (1), still seeking employment (0), other employment position (0), total from the above (doctoral) (7).

Additional Information:
Orientation, Objectives, and Emphasis of Department: The program integrates research and practice within a framework that views the developing individual in changing family, school, and societal contexts. Students enrolled in the clinical developmental psychology doctoral program obtain an understanding of basic psychological processes across the life-span and acquire the requisite skills to conduct effective research on these processes. The clinical developmental psychology program adheres to the scientist–practitioner model and offers clinical training that is informed by research. The focus of the program is on children and families within the larger social contexts of school and community.

Special Facilities or Resources: Each faculty member has a state-of-the-art lab with space and computers for students. The Child Study Institute (CSI) is the clinical training facility of the Department of Psychology. Staffed by licensed psychologists (including members of the department faculty), reading and math specialists, and predoctoral trainees in the clinical developmental program, CSI offers diagnostic assessment, school admission testing, individual, family, and group psychotherapy, and reading, math, and study skills tutoring. All students in the program receive family therapy training with live supervision at CSI. The Phebe Anna Thorne School is a nursery school and preschool research laboratory for the Department of Psychology and includes programs for both normally developing children and language-delayed preschoolers. Two first-year doctoral students in the Department of Psychology serve as teaching assistants in the Thorne School each year. The greater Philadelphia area features a very large and diverse community of psychologists, as well as many medical schools, teaching hospitals, mental health facilities, and research settings.

Information for Students With Physical Disabilities: See the following Web site for more information: http://www.brynmawr.edu/access_services/.

Application Information:
Send to The Graduate School of Arts and Sciences, Bryn Mawr College, 101 N. Merion Avenue, Bryn Mawr, PA 19010. Application available online. URL of online application: http://www.brynmawr.edu/gsas/Admissions/. Students are admitted in the Fall, application deadline January 4. *Fee:* $50.

Carnegie Mellon University
Department of Psychology
Humanities and Social Sciences
Baker Hall 332D
Pittsburgh, PA 15213
Telephone: (412) 268-6026
Fax: (412) 268-2798
E-mail: *donahoe@andrew.cmu.edu*
Web: *http://www.psy.cmu.edu/*

Department Information:
1948. Head: Michael Scheier. Number of faculty: total—full-time 27, part-time 5; women—full-time 11, part-time 1; total—minority—full-time 1; women minority—full-time 1.

Programs and Degrees Offered:
Listed in the following order: Program area, degree type (T if terminal Master's), number awarded 7/08–6/09. Cognitive/Cognitive Neuroscience PhD (Doctor of Philosophy) 2, Developmental Psychology PhD (Doctor of Philosophy) 2, Social/Health/Personality Psychology PhD (Doctor of Philosophy) 0, Psychology and Behavioral Decision Research PhD (Doctor of Philosophy) 0.

Student Applications/Admissions:
Student Applications
Cognitive/Cognitive Neuroscience PhD (Doctor of Philosophy)—Applications 2009–2010, 102. Total applicants accepted 2009–2010, 5. Number full-time enrolled (new admits only) 2009–2010, 3. Number part-time enrolled (new admits only) 2009–2010, 0. Openings 2010–2011, 3. The median number of years required for completion of a degree in 2008–2009 were 5. The number of students enrolled full- and part-time

who were dismissed or voluntarily withdrew from this program area in 2008–2009 were 1. *Developmental Psychology PhD (Doctor of Philosophy)*—Applications 2009–2010, 22. Total applicants accepted 2009–2010, 1. Number full-time enrolled (new admits only) 2009–2010, 1. Number part-time enrolled (new admits only) 2009–2010, 0. Openings 2010–2011, 1. The median number of years required for completion of a degree in 2008–2009 were 5. The number of students enrolled full- and part-time who were dismissed or voluntarily withdrew from this program area in 2008–2009 were 0. *Social/Health/Personality Psychology PhD (Doctor of Philosophy)*—Applications 2009–2010, 44. Total applicants accepted 2009–2010, 0. Number full-time enrolled (new admits only) 2009–2010, 2. Number part-time enrolled (new admits only) 2009–2010, 0. Openings 2010–2011, 2. The median number of years required for completion of a degree in 2008–2009 were 5. The number of students enrolled full- and part-time who were dismissed or voluntarily withdrew from this program area in 2008–2009 were 0. *Psychology and Behavioral Decision Research PhD (Doctor of Philosophy)*—Applications 2009–2010, 0. Total applicants accepted 2009–2010, 0. Number full-time enrolled (new admits only) 2009–2010, 0. Number part-time enrolled (new admits only) 2009–2010, 0. The number of students enrolled full- and part-time who were dismissed or voluntarily withdrew from this program area in 2008–2009 were 0.

Other Criteria: (importance of criteria rated low, medium, or high): GRE scores—high, research experience—high, work experience—low, GPA—high, letters of recommendation—high, interview—high, statement of goals and objectives—high. For additional information on admission requirements, go to http://www.psy.cmu.edu/grad_program/applying.html.

Student Characteristics: The following represents characteristics of students in 2009–2010 in all graduate psychology programs in the department: Female—full-time 30, part-time 0; Male—full-time 11, part-time 0; African American/Black—full-time 1, part-time 0; Hispanic/Latino(a)—full-time 1, part-time 0; Asian/Pacific Islander—full-time 2, part-time 0; American Indian/Alaska Native—full-time 1, part-time 0; Caucasian/White—full-time 23, part-time 0; Multi-ethnic—full-time 0, part-time 0; students subject to the Americans With Disabilities Act—full-time 0, part-time 0; Unknown ethnicity—full-time 13, part-time 0; International students who hold an F-1 or J-1 Visa—full-time 8, part-time 0.

Financial Information/Assistance:
  Tuition for Full-Time Study: **Doctoral:** State residents: per academic year $36,164; Nonstate residents: per academic year $36,164. Tuition is subject to change. See the following Web site for updates and changes in tuition costs: http://www.cmu.edu/hub/sa/sa_grad_tuition.html.

  Financial Assistance:
  First-Year Students: Fellowships and scholarships available for first year. Average amount paid per academic year: $20,976.
  Advanced Students: Fellowships and scholarships available for advanced students. Average amount paid per academic year: $20,976.
  Additional Information: Of all students currently enrolled full time, 100% benefited from one or more of the listed financial assistance programs. Application and information available online at: http://www.cmu.edu/hub/fa/fa_grad.html.

Housing and Day Care: On-campus housing is available. See the following Web site for more information: http://www.housing.cmu.edu. On-campus day care facilities are available. http://www.cmu.edu/hr/benefits/benefit_programs/child_care.

Employment of Department Graduates:
  Master's Degree Graduates: Of those who graduated in the academic year 2008–2009, the following categories and numbers represent the postgraduate activities and employment of master's degree graduates: Enrolled in a postdoctoral residency/fellowship (n/a), employed in independent practice (n/a), total from the above (master's) (0).
  Doctoral Degree Graduates: Of those who graduated in the academic year 2008–2009, the following categories and numbers represent the postgraduate activities and employment of doctoral degree graduates: Enrolled in a psychology doctoral program (n/a), enrolled in a postdoctoral residency/fellowship (2), employed in government agency (1), do not know (1), total from the above (doctoral) (4).

Additional Information:
  Orientation, Objectives, and Emphasis of Department: The department offers doctoral programs in the areas of cognitive psychology, cognitive neuroscience, social-personality psychology, and developmental psychology. Because the graduate program is small, the student's course of study can be tailored to meet individual needs and interests. Further, students have many opportunities to work closely with faculty members on research projects of mutual interest. Carnegie Mellon University has a strong tradition of interdisciplinary research, and it is easy for students to interact with faculty and students from other graduate programs on campus. Many of our students take courses or engage in research with people from the Departments of Computer Science, Statistics, Social Science, English, Philosophy, and the Graduate School of Industrial Administration.

Application Information:
Send to Graduate Program Coordinator, Department of Psychology, Carnegie Mellon University, Pittsburgh, PA 15213. Application available online. URL of online application: http://www.psy.cmu.edu/grad_program/applying.html. Students are admitted in the Fall, application deadline December 5. *Fee:* $45.

Carnegie Mellon University
Tepper School of Business
Schenley Park
Pittsburgh, PA 15213
Telephone: (412) 268-1319
Fax: (412) 268-7064
E-mail: *pg14@andrew.cmu.edu*
Web: *http://tepper.cmu.edu*

Department Information:
  OB PhD Coordinator: Paul S. Goodman. Number of faculty: total—full-time 7; women—full-time 5; total—minority—full-time 1.

GRADUATE STUDY IN PSYCHOLOGY

Programs and Degrees Offered:
Listed in the following order: Program area, degree type (T if terminal Master's), number awarded 7/08–6/09. Organizational Behavior and Theory PhD (Doctor of Philosophy) 1.

Student Applications/Admissions:
Student Applications
Organizational Behavior and Theory PhD (Doctor of Philosophy)—Applications 2009–2010, 88. Total applicants accepted 2009–2010, 7. Number full-time enrolled (new admits only) 2009–2010, 2. Total enrolled 2009–2010 full-time, 12. Openings 2010–2011, 3. The number of students enrolled full- and part-time who were dismissed or voluntarily withdrew from this program area in 2008–2009 were 0.
Other Criteria: (importance of criteria rated low, medium, or high): GRE scores—high, research experience—medium, GPA—high, letters of recommendation—high, statement of goals and objectives—high.

Student Characteristics: The following represents characteristics of students in 2009–2010 in all graduate psychology programs in the department: Female—full-time 6, part-time 0; Male—full-time 6, part-time 0; African American/Black—full-time 1, part-time 0; Hispanic/Latino(a)—full-time 0, part-time 0; Asian/Pacific Islander—full-time 4, part-time 0; American Indian/Alaska Native—full-time 0, part-time 0; Caucasian/White—full-time 7, part-time 0; Multi-ethnic—full-time 0, part-time 0; students subject to the Americans With Disabilities Act—full-time 0, part-time 0; Unknown ethnicity—full-time 0, part-time 0; International students who hold an F-1 or J-1 Visa—full-time 7, part-time 0.

Financial Information/Assistance:
Financial Assistance:
First-Year Students: Fellowships and scholarships available for first year. Average amount paid per academic year: $30,000. Apply by January 2.
Advanced Students: Fellowships and scholarships available for advanced students. Average amount paid per academic year: $25,000.
Additional Information: Of all students currently enrolled full time, 100% benefited from one or more of the listed financial assistance programs.

Housing and Day Care: No on-campus housing is available. No on-campus day care facilities are available.

Employment of Department Graduates:
Master's Degree Graduates: Of those who graduated in the academic year 2008–2009, the following categories and numbers represent the postgraduate activities and employment of master's degree graduates: Enrolled in a postdoctoral residency/fellowship (n/a), employed in independent practice (n/a), total from the above (master's) (0).
Doctoral Degree Graduates: Of those who graduated in the academic year 2008–2009, the following categories and numbers represent the postgraduate activities and employment of doctoral degree graduates: Enrolled in a psychology doctoral program (n/a), enrolled in a postdoctoral residency/fellowship (2), employed in an academic position at a 2-year/4-year college (1), total from the above (doctoral) (3).

Additional Information:
Orientation, Objectives, and Emphasis of Department: The goal of the doctoral program in organizational psychology and theory at the Tepper School of Business is to produce scientists who will make significant research contributions to our understanding of the structure and functioning of organizations. To achieve this goal the student is placed in a learning environment where a unique set of quantitative and discipline-based skills can be acquired. The opportunities for interdisciplinary work at Tepper provide new avenues for approaching organizational problems. The program attempts to combine structure and flexibility. Structure is achieved by identifying a set of core areas in which the student should become competent. These are quantitative methods, design and measurement, organization theory, and a selected specialty area. Flexibility in the program is achieved by having students and their advisers work out a combination of learning activities consistent with the students' interests and needs. Courses, participation in research projects, summer papers, and special tutorials with individual faculty are some of these learning activities.

Application Information:
Send to Doctoral Program Applications, 247 Posner Hall, Tepper School of Business, Carnegie Mellon University, Pittsburgh, PA 15213-3890. Application available online. URL of online application: https://app.applyyourself.com/?id=cmu-phd. Students are admitted in the Fall, application deadline January 15. *Fee:* $70.

Chestnut Hill College
Department of Professional Psychology
9601 Germantown Avenue
Philadelphia, PA 19118-2693
Telephone: (215) 248-7077
Fax: (215) 248-7155
E-mail: *profpsyc@chc.edu*
Web: *http://www.chc.edu*

Department Information:
1987. Chairperson: Joseph A. Micucci, PhD, ABPP. Number of faculty: total—full-time 10, part-time 44; women—full-time 4, part-time 29; total—minority—full-time 2, part-time 2; women minority—full-time 2, part-time 2.

Programs and Degrees Offered:
Listed in the following order: Program area, degree type (T if terminal Master's), number awarded 7/08–6/09. Clinical Psychology PsyD (Doctor of Psychology) 12, Clinical and Counseling Psychology MA/MS (Master of Arts/Science) (T) 64.

APA Accreditation: Clinical PsyD (Doctor of Psychology). Student Outcome Data Website: http://www.chc.edu/psyd/.

Student Applications/Admissions:
Student Applications
Clinical Psychology PsyD (Doctor of Psychology)—Applications 2009–2010, 159. Total applicants accepted 2009–2010, 44. Number full-time enrolled (new admits only) 2009–2010, 23. Number part-time enrolled (new admits only) 2009–2010, 0. Total enrolled 2009–2010 full-time, 69, part-time, 44. Open-

ings 2010–2011, 20. The median number of years required for completion of a degree in 2008–2009 were 6. The number of students enrolled full- and part-time who were dismissed or voluntarily withdrew from this program area in 2008–2009 were 5. *Clinical and Counseling Psychology MA/MS (Master of Arts/Science)*—Applications 2009–2010, 199. Total applicants accepted 2009–2010, 107. Number full-time enrolled (new admits only) 2009–2010, 37. Number part-time enrolled (new admits only) 2009–2010, 48. Total enrolled 2009–2010 full-time, 83, part-time, 157. The median number of years required for completion of a degree in 2008–2009 were 3.

Scores: Entries appear in this order: required test or GPA, minimum score (if required), median score of students entering in 2009–2010. *Clinical Psychology PsyD (Doctor of Psychology):* GRE-V no minimum stated, 550, GRE-Q no minimum stated, 645, GRE-Analytical no minimum stated, 4.5, overall undergraduate GPA no minimum stated, 3.6.

Other Criteria: (importance of criteria rated low, medium, or high): GRE scores—high, research experience—low, work experience—low, extracurricular activity—low, clinically related public service—low, GPA—high, letters of recommendation—high, interview—high, statement of goals and objectives—high, Writing Ability—high, undergraduate major in psychology—medium, specific undergraduate psychology courses taken—high, Writing ability is a criterion for the PsyD program. For additional information on admission requirements, go to http://www.chc.edu/sgs_admissions.aspx.

Student Characteristics: The following represents characteristics of students in 2009–2010 in all graduate psychology programs in the department: Female—full-time 126, part-time 157; Male—full-time 26, part-time 44; African American/Black—full-time 11, part-time 31; Hispanic/Latino(a)—full-time 3, part-time 4; Asian/Pacific Islander—full-time 7, part-time 4; American Indian/Alaska Native—full-time 0, part-time 0; Caucasian/White—full-time 114, part-time 149; Multi-ethnic—full-time 0, part-time 0; students subject to the Americans With Disabilities Act—full-time 0, part-time 0; Unknown ethnicity—full-time 17, part-time 13; International students who hold an F-1 or J-1 Visa—full-time 0, part-time 0.

Financial Information/Assistance:
Tuition for Full-Time Study: Master's: State residents: $560 per credit hour; Nonstate residents: $560 per credit hour. *Doctoral:* State residents: $825 per credit hour; Nonstate residents: $825 per credit hour. Tuition is subject to change. See the following Web site for updates and changes in tuition costs: http://www.chc.edu/sgs_admissions.aspx?id=305.

Financial Assistance:
First-Year Students: Teaching assistantships available for first year. Average number of hours worked per week: 12. Research assistantships available for first year. Average number of hours worked per week: 12.
Advanced Students: Teaching assistantships available for advanced students. Average number of hours worked per week: 12. Research assistantships available for advanced students. Average number of hours worked per week: 12.
Additional Information: No information provided.

Internships/Practica: Doctoral Degree (PsyD Clinical Psychology): For those doctoral students for whom a professional internship was required in this program prior to graduation, (11) students applied for an internship in 2008–2009, with (11) students obtaining an internship. Of those students who obtained an internship, (11) were paid internships. Of those students who obtained an internship, (0) students placed in APA/CPA accredited internships, (6) students placed in internships not APA/CPA accredited, but listed with the Association of Psychology Postdoctoral and Internship Programs (APPIC), (0) students placed in internships conforming to guidelines of the Council of Directors of School Psychology Programs (CDSPP), (5) students placed in internships that were not APA/CPA accredited, APPIC or CDSPP listed. Master's Degree (MA/MS Clinical and Counseling Psychology): An internship experience, such as a final research project or "capstone" experience is required of graduates. Students in the master's program must complete three semesters of practicum. Students in the doctoral program are required to complete three years of practicum (one of which may be waived if the student completed a practicum prior to admission as part of their master's program) and a full-time internship. Doctoral students have the option of completing an APA-accredited, APPIC, or other program approved internship. At the present time, there are over 50 mental health facilities that the program has approved as sites for practica and internships. Two faculty members are dedicated to assisting students in securing the most appropriate site for their practicum and internship experiences.

Housing and Day Care: No on-campus housing is available. No on-campus day care facilities are available.

Employment of Department Graduates:
Master's Degree Graduates: Of those who graduated in the academic year 2008–2009, the following categories and numbers represent the postgraduate activities and employment of master's degree graduates: Enrolled in a postdoctoral residency/fellowship (n/a), employed in independent practice (n/a), total from the above (master's) (0).
Doctoral Degree Graduates: Of those who graduated in the academic year 2008–2009, the following categories and numbers represent the postgraduate activities and employment of doctoral degree graduates: Enrolled in a psychology doctoral program (n/a), enrolled in a postdoctoral residency/fellowship (1), employed in independent practice (3), employed in an academic position at a 2-year/4-year college (1), employed in a community mental health/counseling center (4), employed in a hospital/medical center (3), total from the above (doctoral) (12).

Additional Information:
Orientation, Objectives, and Emphasis of Department: The theoretical base of the Department of Professional Psychology at Chestnut Hill College is a complementary blend of psychodynamic and systems theories. The insights of psychodynamic theory, including modern object relations theory, serve as a method for understanding the individual. Likewise, the perspective of systems theory addresses ways individuals, families and communities influence one another. This synergistic blend of psychodynamic and systems theories promotes a holistic understanding of human behavior within family and social contexts.

Special Facilities or Resources: All classrooms are fully equipped for Power Point and multi-media presentations. Observation rooms are available for recording and observing clinical sessions. An extensive library of psychological testing equipment is avail-

GRADUATE STUDY IN PSYCHOLOGY

able for student use. The college is part of a library consortium that increases available lending privileges offered to each student. Doctoral students have free interlibrary loan privileges. Students have access to statistical software and test scoring/interpretation software. Advanced doctoral students may teach a master's level course under the direct supervision of a faculty member.

Application Information:
Send to Director of Graduate Admissions, Chestnut Hill College, 9601 Germantown Avenue, Philadelphia, PA 19118-2693. Application available online. URL of online application: http://www.chc.edu/psyd/admissions. All students in the PsyD Program begin classes in the fall semester. Students in the terminal master's program may begin classes in the fall, spring or summer semester. Master's program has rolling admissions. The PsyD Program accepts applicants to Year I on a rolling admission basis until the entering class is filled. All applicants whose applications are complete by January 15 will be notified of their status by April 15. The application deadline for Year II is January 15. *Fee:* $80. PsyD application fee is $80. Master's application fee is $55.

Drexel University
Department of Psychology
College of Arts and Sciences
MS 626, 245 North 15th Street
Philadelphia, PA 19102
Telephone: (215) 762-7249
Fax: (215) 762-8625
E-mail: *kirk.heilbrun@drexel.edu*
Web: *http://psychology.drexel.edu*

Department Information:
2002. Chairperson: Kirk Heilbrun. Number of faculty: total—full-time 24, part-time 7; women—full-time 11, part-time 7; total—minority—full-time 2, part-time 2; women minority—full-time 1, part-time 2.

Programs and Degrees Offered:
Listed in the following order: Program area, degree type (T if terminal Master's), number awarded 7/08–6/09. Clinical PhD (Doctor of Philosophy) 10, Psychology MA/MS (Master of Arts/Science) (T) 8, Law-Psychology PhD (Doctor of Philosophy) 2, Applied Cognitive and Brain Science PhD (Doctor of Philosophy) 0.

APA Accreditation: Clinical PhD (Doctor of Philosophy). Student Outcome Data Website: http://www.drexel.edu/psychology/phd/overview.html. Clinical PhD (Doctor of Philosophy).

Student Applications/Admissions:
Student Applications
Clinical PhD (Doctor of Philosophy)—Applications 2009–2010, 440. Total applicants accepted 2009–2010, 14. Number full-time enrolled (new admits only) 2009–2010, 9. Number part-time enrolled (new admits only) 2009–2010, 0. Openings 2010–2011, 10. The median number of years required for completion of a degree in 2008–2009 were 5. The number of students enrolled full- and part-time who were dismissed or voluntarily withdrew from this program area in 2008–2009 were 0. *Psychology MA/MS (Master of Arts/Science)*—Applications 2009–2010, 28. Total applicants accepted 2009–2010, 16. Number full-time enrolled (new admits only) 2009–2010, 8. Total enrolled 2009–2010 full-time, 17. Openings 2010–2011, 10. The median number of years required for completion of a degree in 2008–2009 were 2. The number of students enrolled full- and part-time who were dismissed or voluntarily withdrew from this program area in 2008–2009 were 0. *Law-Psychology PhD (Doctor of Philosophy)*—Applications 2009–2010, 14. Total applicants accepted 2009–2010, 2. Number full-time enrolled (new admits only) 2009–2010, 2. Total enrolled 2009–2010 full-time, 13. Openings 2010–2011, 2. The median number of years required for completion of a degree in 2008–2009 were 7. The number of students enrolled full- and part-time who were dismissed or voluntarily withdrew from this program area in 2008–2009 were 0. *Applied Cognitive and Brain Science PhD (Doctor of Philosophy)*—Applications 2009–2010, 0. Total applicants accepted 2009–2010, 0. Number full-time enrolled (new admits only) 2009–2010, 0. Number part-time enrolled (new admits only) 2009–2010, 0. The number of students enrolled full- and part-time who were dismissed or voluntarily withdrew from this program area in 2008–2009 were 0.

Scores: Entries appear in this order: required test or GPA, minimum score (if required), median score of students entering in 2009–2010. *Clinical PhD (Doctor of Philosophy):* GRE-V 600, 680, GRE-Q 600, 670, GRE-Subject (Psychology) 600, 690, overall undergraduate GPA 3.4, 3.7, last 2 years GPA 3.5, 3.8, psychology GPA 3.5, 3.8; *Psychology MA/MS (Master of Arts/Science):* GRE-V 500, 540, GRE-Q 500, 590, GRE-Subject (Psychology) 500, 610, overall undergraduate GPA 3.0, 3.2, last 2 years GPA 3.2, 3.4, psychology GPA 3.2, 3.4; *Law-Psychology PhD (Doctor of Philosophy):* GRE-V 600, 650, GRE-Q 600, 670, GRE-Subject (Psychology) 600, 670, overall undergraduate GPA 3.2, 3.8, last 2 years GPA 3.4, 3.8, psychology GPA 3.5, 3.9; *Applied Cognitive and Brain Science PhD (Doctor of Philosophy):* GRE-V 600, GRE-Q 600, GRE-Subject (Psychology) 600, overall undergraduate GPA 3.2, last 2 years GPA 3.4, psychology GPA 3.5.

Other Criteria: (importance of criteria rated low, medium, or high): GRE scores—high, research experience—high, work experience—low, extracurricular activity—low, clinically related public service—medium, GPA—high, letters of recommendation—high, interview—high, statement of goals and objectives—high, Fit with faculty mentor—high, undergraduate major in psychology—medium, specific undergraduate psychology courses taken—medium, Research experience is weighted less heavily for applicants for the MS program. For additional information on admission requirements, go to http://psychology.drexel.edu.

Student Characteristics: The following represents characteristics of students in 2009–2010 in all graduate psychology programs in the department: Female—full-time 69, part-time 0; Male—full-time 12, part-time 0; African American/Black—full-time 4, part-time 0; Hispanic/Latino(a)—full-time 3, part-time 0; Asian/Pacific Islander—full-time 2, part-time 0; American Indian/Alaska Native—full-time 0, part-time 0; Caucasian/White—full-time 72, part-time 0; Multi-ethnic—full-time 0, part-time 0; students subject to the Americans With Disabilities Act—full-time 4, part-time 0; Unknown ethnicity—full-time 0, part-time 0; International students who hold an F-1 or J-1 Visa—full-time 1, part-time 0.

Financial Information/Assistance:
Tuition for Full-Time Study: *Master's:* State residents: $915 per credit hour; Nonstate residents: $915 per credit hour. *Doctoral:* State residents: $915 per credit hour; Nonstate residents: $915 per credit hour. Tuition is subject to change. Additional fees are assessed to students beyond the costs of tuition for the following: general fee of $240 per quarter. See the following Web site for updates and changes in tuition costs: http://www.drexel.edu/em/grad/coas/financialaid/tuition.html.

Financial Assistance:
First-Year Students: Teaching assistantships available for first year. Average amount paid per academic year: $9,000. Average number of hours worked per week: 15. Research assistantships available for first year. Average amount paid per academic year: $11,000. Fellowships and scholarships available for first year. Average amount paid per academic year: $5,000.
Advanced Students: Research assistantships available for advanced students. Average amount paid per academic year: $9,000. Average number of hours worked per week: 10. Traineeships available for advanced students. Average amount paid per academic year: $9,000. Average number of hours worked per week: 20. Fellowships and scholarships available for advanced students. Average amount paid per academic year: $5,000.
Additional Information: Of all students currently enrolled full time, 80% benefited from one or more of the listed financial assistance programs.

Internships/Practica: Doctoral Degree (PhD Clinical): For those doctoral students for whom a professional internship was required in this program prior to graduation, (10) students applied for an internship in 2008–2009, with (10) students obtaining an internship. Of those students who obtained an internship, (10) were paid internships. Of those students who obtained an internship, (9) students placed in APA/CPA accredited internships, (1) students placed in internships not APA/CPA accredited, but listed with the Association of Psychology Postdoctoral and Internship Programs (APPIC), (0) students placed in internships conforming to guidelines of the Council of Directors of School Psychology Programs (CDSPP), (0) students placed in internships that were not APA/CPA accredited, APPIC or CDSPP listed. Doctoral Degree (PhD Law-Psychology): For those doctoral students for whom a professional internship was required in this program prior to graduation, (2) students applied for an internship in 2008–2009, with (2) students obtaining an internship. Of those students who obtained an internship, (2) were paid internships. Of those students who obtained an internship, (2) students placed in APA/CPA accredited internships, (0) students placed in internships not APA/CPA accredited, but listed with the Association of Psychology Postdoctoral and Internship Programs (APPIC), (0) students placed in internships conforming to guidelines of the Council of Directors of School Psychology Programs (CDSPP), (0) students placed in internships that were not APA/CPA accredited, APPIC or CDSPP listed. Master's Degree (MA/MS Psychology): An internship experience, such as, a final research project or "capstone" experience is required of graduates. On-campus practicum sites include the Student Counseling and Development Center, the Forensic Clinic, and the Heart Failure/Cardiac Transplant Center. Off-campus practicum sites include a variety of in-/outpatient psychiatric units, Children's Hospital of Philadelphia and approximately sixty other practicum sites.

Housing and Day Care: On-campus housing is available: http://www.drexel.edu.dbs/universityHousing. No on-campus day care facilities are available.

Employment of Department Graduates:
Master's Degree Graduates: Of those who graduated in the academic year 2008–2009, the following categories and numbers represent the postgraduate activities and employment of master's degree graduates: Enrolled in a psychology doctoral program (3), enrolled in a postdoctoral residency/fellowship (n/a), employed in independent practice (n/a), employed in business or industry (1), employed in government agency (2), employed in a hospital/medical center (1), other employment position (2), total from the above (master's) (9).
Doctoral Degree Graduates: Of those who graduated in the academic year 2008–2009, the following categories and numbers represent the postgraduate activities and employment of doctoral degree graduates: Enrolled in a psychology doctoral program (n/a), enrolled in a postdoctoral residency/fellowship (4), employed in an academic position at a university (2), employed in government agency (1), employed in a hospital/medical center (1), other employment position (2), total from the above (doctoral) (10).

Additional Information:
Orientation, Objectives, and Emphasis of Department: The Drexel University Department of Psychology has doctoral programs based heavily upon a scientist–practitioner model of training in clinical psychology and has been designed to place emphasis on both components, but somewhat greater emphasis on research. The theoretical orientation is based largely on Social Learning Theory, in which students gain proficiency in the theory and practice of broad-spectrum behavioral approaches to assessment and intervention. The clinical PhD program offers concentrations in health psychology, neuropsychology, and forensic psychology. The new program in Applied Cognitive and Brain Sciences is focused primarily on cognitive psychology and cognitive neuroscience, although the research emphasis is of an applied nature. The MS program (non-clinical) is designed to provide students with research skills in preparation for application for doctoral training, or employment with researchers in academia, industry, or public sector settings.

Special Facilities or Resources: The graduate psychology programs at Drexel University have space on both the Drexel Main Campus in West Philadelphia and the center city campus. Drexel has a major tertiary care medical center that provides exceptional opportunities in health related areas for psychology. In addition, a Division of Behavioral Neurobiology and the University Neurobiology program, as well as the University Neurosciences program, provide opportunities for learning and collaboration on research at neuropharmacologic and neurophysiologic levels to complement our neuropsychological training.

Application Information:
Send to Graduate Admission, Drexel University, 3141 Chestnut Street, Suite 212, Philadelphia, PA 19104. Telephone: (215) 895-2000. Application available online. URL of online application: http://psychology.drexel.edu. Students are admitted in the Fall, application deadline December 1. Deadline for MS is February 15, for JD-PhD and PhD in Applied Cognitive and Brain Sciences is December 15. *Fee:* $50.

Duquesne University
Department of Counseling, Psychology and Special Education,
School Psychology Program
School of Education
G3 Canevin Hall
Pittsburgh, PA 15282
Telephone: (412) 396-1058
Fax: (412) 396-1340
E-mail: czwalgaa@duq.edu
Web: http://www.duq.edu/school-psychology/

Department Information:
1969. Program Director: Laura M. Crothers, PhD. Number of faculty: total—full-time 6, part-time 1; women—full-time 4.

Programs and Degrees Offered:
Listed in the following order: Program area, degree type (T if terminal Master's), number awarded 7/08–6/09. Child Psychology MEd (Education) 20, School Psychology Certificate Other 7, School Psychology PhD (Doctor of Philosophy) 4.

APA Accreditation: School PhD (Doctor of Philosophy). Student Outcome Data Website: http://www.duq.edu/school-psychology-phd/faq.cfm.

Student Applications/Admissions:
Student Applications
Child Psychology MEd (Education)—Applications 2009–2010, 18. Total applicants accepted 2009–2010, 17. Number full-time enrolled (new admits only) 2009–2010, 9. Number part-time enrolled (new admits only) 2009–2010, 0. Openings 2010–2011, 15. The median number of years required for completion of a degree in 2008–2009 were 2. The number of students enrolled full- and part-time who were dismissed or voluntarily withdrew from this program area in 2008–2009 were 0. School Psychology Certificate Other—Applications 2009–2010, 59. Total applicants accepted 2009–2010, 13. Number full-time enrolled (new admits only) 2009–2010, 13. Number part-time enrolled (new admits only) 2009–2010, 0. Openings 2010–2011, 10. The median number of years required for completion of a degree in 2008–2009 were 3. The number of students enrolled full- and part-time who were dismissed or voluntarily withdrew from this program area in 2008–2009 were 1. School Psychology PhD (Doctor of Philosophy)—Applications 2009–2010, 37. Total applicants accepted 2009–2010, 16. Number full-time enrolled (new admits only) 2009–2010, 5. Number part-time enrolled (new admits only) 2009–2010, 0. Openings 2010–2011, 11. The median number of years required for completion of a degree in 2008–2009 were 5. The number of students enrolled full- and part-time who were dismissed or voluntarily withdrew from this program area in 2008–2009 were 0.
Scores: Entries appear in this order: required test or GPA, minimum score (if required), median score of students entering in 2009–2010. Child Psychology MEd (Education): overall undergraduate GPA 3.0; School Psychology Certificate Other: GRE-V no minimum stated, 480, GRE-Q no minimum stated, 540, GRE-Analytical no minimum stated, 4.0, overall undergraduate GPA no minimum stated, 3.47; School Psychology PhD (Doctor of Philosophy): GRE-V no minimum stated, 490, GRE-Q no minimum stated, 580, GRE-Analytical no minimum stated, 4.0, overall undergraduate GPA no minimum stated, 3.5.
Other Criteria: (importance of criteria rated low, medium, or high): GRE scores—high, research experience—medium, work experience—medium, extracurricular activity—low, clinically related public service—low, GPA—high, letters of recommendation—medium, interview—high, statement of goals and objectives—high, undergraduate major in psychology—low, specific undergraduate psychology courses taken—low. For additional information on admission requirements, go to http://www.duq.edu/school-psychology/.

Student Characteristics: The following represents characteristics of students in 2009–2010 in all graduate psychology programs in the department: Female—full-time 74, part-time 0; Male—full-time 16, part-time 0; African American/Black—full-time 3, part-time 0; Hispanic/Latino(a)—full-time 1, part-time 0; Asian/Pacific Islander—full-time 1, part-time 0; American Indian/Alaska Native—full-time 0, part-time 0; Caucasian/White—full-time 98, part-time 0; Multi-ethnic—full-time 1, part-time 0; students subject to the Americans With Disabilities Act—full-time 0, part-time 0; Unknown ethnicity—full-time 0, part-time 0; International students who hold an F-1 or J-1 Visa—full-time 2, part-time 0.

Financial Information/Assistance:
Tuition for Full-Time Study: *Master's:* State residents: per academic year $27,960, $932 per credit hour; Nonstate residents: per academic year $27,960, $932 per credit hour. *Doctoral:* State residents: per academic year $27,960, $932 per credit hour; Nonstate residents: per academic year $27,960, $932 per credit hour. Tuition is subject to change. See the following Web site for updates and changes in tuition costs: http://www.duq.edu/student-accounts/tuition/grad.cfm.

Financial Assistance:
First-Year Students: Research assistantships available for first year. Average number of hours worked per week: 20. Apply by March 1.
Advanced Students: Research assistantships available for advanced students. Average number of hours worked per week: 20. Apply by March 1.
Additional Information: Of all students currently enrolled full time, 5% benefited from one or more of the listed financial assistance programs. Application and information available online at: http://www.duq.edu/financial-aid/.

Internships/Practica: Doctoral Degree (PhD School Psychology): For those doctoral students for whom a professional internship was required in this program prior to graduation, (8) students applied for an internship in 2008–2009, with (8) students obtaining an internship. Of those students who obtained an internship, (8) were paid internships. Of those students who obtained an internship, (1) students placed in APA/CPA accredited internships, (7) students placed in internships not APA/CPA accredited, but listed with the Association of Psychology Postdoctoral and Internship Programs (APPIC), (0) students placed in internships conforming to guidelines of the Council of Directors of School Psychology Programs (CDSPP), (0) students placed in internships that were not APA/CPA accredited, APPIC or CDSPP listed. Certification program requires 2 practica and 1 internship; Doctoral program requires 2 practica, 1 doctoral practicum and 1 internship.

Housing and Day Care: On-campus housing is available. See the following Web site for more information: http://www.duq.edu/residence-life/. On-campus day care facilities are available. See the following Web site for more information: http://www.duq.edu/hr/benefits/child-care.cfm.

Employment of Department Graduates:
Master's Degree Graduates: Of those who graduated in the academic year 2008–2009, the following categories and numbers represent the postgraduate activities and employment of master's degree graduates: Enrolled in a postdoctoral residency/fellowship (n/a), employed in independent practice (n/a), employed in a professional position in a school system (5), total from the above (master's) (5).
Doctoral Degree Graduates: Of those who graduated in the academic year 2008–2009, the following categories and numbers represent the postgraduate activities and employment of doctoral degree graduates: Enrolled in a psychology doctoral program (n/a), employed in a professional position in a school system (6), total from the above (doctoral) (6).

Additional Information:
Orientation, Objectives, and Emphasis of Department: The Duquesne University School Psychology program, guided by the belief that all children can learn, is dedicated to providing both breadth and depth of professional training in a theoretically-integrated, research-based learning environment. The program prepares ethical practitioners, scientists and scholars who are life-long learners committed to enhancing the well-being of youth, their families, and the systems that serve them. The program achieves this by engaging in scholarly activities that advance the field of school psychology, maintaining a modern curriculum that employs aspects of multiculturalism and diversity, examining emerging trends in the profession, conducting continuous outcome assessment for program improvement, and providing support to our graduates.

Special Facilities or Resources: The program has a curriculum library of current psychological and educational tests for training and research purposes.

Information for Students With Physical Disabilities: See the following Web site for more information: http://www.duq.edu/special-students/.

Application Information:
Send to Dr. Laura M. Crothers, School Psychology Program, G3B Canevin Hall, Pittsburgh, PA 15282. Application available online. URL of online application: http://www.duq.edu/school-psychology-cags/application-requirements.cfm. Students are admitted in the Fall, application deadline January 15. Masters program has rolling admissions. *Fee:* $50. The $50 fee is waived if application is completed online.

Duquesne University
Department of Psychology
McAnulty College and Graduate School of Liberal Arts
600 Forbes Avenue
Pittsburgh, PA 15282
Telephone: (412) 396-6520
Fax: (412) 396-1368
E-mail: *psychology@duq.edu*
Web: *http://www.duq.edu/psychology/graduate/index.cfm*

Department Information:
1959. Chairperson: Daniel Burston, PhD Number of faculty: total—full-time 16; women—full-time 6; total—minority—full-time 1.

Programs and Degrees Offered:
Listed in the following order: Program area, degree type (T if terminal Master's), number awarded 7/08–6/09. Clinical Psychology PhD (Doctor of Philosophy) 9.

APA Accreditation: Clinical PhD (Doctor of Philosophy). Student Outcome Data Website: http://www.duq.edu/psychology/_pdf/outcomes2008.pdf.

Student Applications/Admissions:
Student Applications
Clinical Psychology PhD (Doctor of Philosophy)—Applications 2009–2010, 128. Total applicants accepted 2009–2010, 7. Number full-time enrolled (new admits only) 2009–2010, 6. Number part-time enrolled (new admits only) 2009–2010, 0. Openings 2010–2011, 7. The median number of years required for completion of a degree in 2008–2009 were 8. The number of students enrolled full- and part-time who were dismissed or voluntarily withdrew from this program area in 2008–2009 were 3.
Other Criteria: (importance of criteria rated low, medium, or high): GRE scores—medium, research experience—medium, work experience—medium, extracurricular activity—medium, clinically related public service—medium, GPA—medium, letters of recommendation—high, interview—high, statement of goals and objectives—high. For additional information on admission requirements, go to http://www.duq.edu/psychology/graduate/apply.cfm.

Student Characteristics: The following represents characteristics of students in 2009–2010 in all graduate psychology programs in the department: Female—full-time 28, part-time 0; Male—full-time 26, part-time 0; African American/Black—full-time 0, part-time 0; Hispanic/Latino(a)—full-time 2, part-time 0; Asian/Pacific Islander—full-time 3, part-time 0; American Indian/Alaska Native—full-time 1, part-time 0; Caucasian/White—full-time 44, part-time 0; Multi-ethnic—full-time 4, part-time 0; students subject to the Americans With Disabilities Act—full-time 0, part-time 0; Unknown ethnicity—full-time 0, part-time 0; International students who hold an F-1 or J-1 Visa—full-time 10, part-time 0.

Financial Information/Assistance:
Tuition for Full-Time Study: *Doctoral:* State residents: $851 per credit hour; Nonstate residents: $851 per credit hour. Tuition is

subject to change. See the following Web site for updates and changes in tuition costs: http://www.duq.edu/student-accounts/tuition/grad.cfm.

Financial Assistance:
First-Year Students: Research assistantships available for first year. Average amount paid per academic year: $15,000. Average number of hours worked per week: 15. Apply by December 15.

Advanced Students: Teaching assistantships available for advanced students. Average amount paid per academic year: $15,000. Average number of hours worked per week: 15. Apply by December 15. Research assistantships available for advanced students. Average amount paid per academic year: $15,000. Average number of hours worked per week: 15. Apply by December 15.

Additional Information: Of all students currently enrolled full time, 100% benefited from one or more of the listed financial assistance programs. Application and information available online at: http://www.duq.edu/financial-aid/.

Internships/Practica: Doctoral Degree (PhD Clinical Psychology): For those doctoral students for whom a professional internship was required in this program prior to graduation, (5) students applied for an internship in 2008–2009, with (4) students obtaining an internship. Of those students who obtained an internship, (4) were paid internships. Of those students who obtained an internship, (4) students placed in APA/CPA accredited internships, (0) students placed in internships not APA/CPA accredited, but listed with the Association of Psychology Postdoctoral and Internship Programs (APPIC), (0) students placed in internships conforming to guidelines of the Council of Directors of School Psychology Programs (CDSPP), (0) students placed in internships that were not APA/CPA accredited, APPIC or CDSPP listed. The Duquesne University Psychology Clinic, which serves more than 70 clients weekly, is the primary training facility for the doctoral students. All services, including assessment and psychotherapy for Duquesne University students, employees, and members of the greater Pittsburgh communities, are provided by the doctoral students. Licensed clinical faculty members and selected licensed adjunct faculty psychologists in the community are involved in the supervision of all doctoral students. The first four years of the doctoral program typically involve case work at the Clinic. Additionally, students attend at least one academic year of external practicum placement in settings such as hospitals, university counseling centers, and VA centers. External practica are typically completed during the third year of the program. A second year of external practicum training, taken in the fourth year, is strongly recommended.

Housing and Day Care: On-campus housing is available. See the following Web site for more information: http://www.duq.edu/residence-life/. On-campus day care facilities are available. See the following Web site for more information: http://www.duq.edu/hr/benefits/child-care.cfm.

Employment of Department Graduates:
Master's Degree Graduates: Of those who graduated in the academic year 2008–2009, the following categories and numbers represent the postgraduate activities and employment of master's degree graduates: Enrolled in a postdoctoral residency/fellowship (n/a), employed in independent practice (n/a), total from the above (master's) (0).

Doctoral Degree Graduates: Of those who graduated in the academic year 2008–2009, the following categories and numbers represent the postgraduate activities and employment of doctoral degree graduates: Enrolled in a psychology doctoral program (n/a), total from the above (doctoral) (0).

Additional Information:
Orientation, Objectives, and Emphasis of Department: Internationally recognized for over three decades, the Psychology Department at Duquesne University engages in the systematic and rigorous articulation of psychology as a human science. The department understands psychology as a positive response to the challenges of the 21st century—one which includes existentialism, phenomenology, hermeneutics, psychoanalysis and depth psychology, feminism, critical theory, post-structuralism, and a sensitivity to the diverse cultural contexts within which this response may find expression. Psychology as a human science pursues collaborative, qualitative research methods that pay special attention to what is particular to human beings and their worlds. Accordingly, the department educates psychologists who are sensitive to the multiple meanings of human life and who work toward the liberation and well-being of persons individually as well as in the community.

Special Facilities or Resources: The psychology clinic provides the opportunity for supervised training in personal counseling and for research in the field of counseling and psychotherapy. Field placements are available in clinical psychology. The Silverman Center is a research center containing a comprehensive collection of world literature in phenomenology.

Information for Students With Physical Disabilities: See the following Web site for more information: http://www.duq.edu/special-students/index.cfm.

Application Information:
Send to Duquesne University, McAnulty College and Graduate School of Liberals Arts, Graduate Office, 600 Forbes Avenue, Pittsburgh, PA 15282. Application available online. URL of online application: http://www.duq.edu/psychology/graduate/apply.cfm. Students are admitted in the Fall, application deadline December 15. *Fee:* $0. There is no fee to apply online.

Geneva College
Master of Arts in Counseling
3200 College Avenue
Beaver Falls, PA 15010
Telephone: (724) 847-6697
Fax: (724) 847-6101
E-mail: *counseling@geneva.edu*
Web: *http://www.geneva.edu*

Department Information:
1987. MA in Counseling Program Director: Carol B. Luce, PhD. Number of faculty: total—full-time 4, part-time 3; women—full-time 1, part-time 1; faculty subject to the Americans With Disabilities Act 1.

Programs and Degrees Offered:
Listed in the following order: Program area, degree type (T if terminal Master's), number awarded 7/08–6/09. Marriage and Family Counseling MA/MS (Master of Arts/Science) 8, Mental Health Counseling MA/MS (Master of Arts/Science) 3, School Counseling MA/MS (Master of Arts/Science) 8.

Student Applications/Admissions:
Student Applications
Marriage and Family Counseling MA/MS (Master of Arts/Science)—Applications 2009–2010, 12. Total applicants accepted 2009–2010, 6. Number full-time enrolled (new admits only) 2009–2010, 4. Number part-time enrolled (new admits only) 2009–2010, 2. Total enrolled 2009–2010 full-time, 6, part-time, 10. Openings 2010–2011, 10. The median number of years required for completion of a degree in 2008–2009 were 2. The number of students enrolled full- and part-time who were dismissed or voluntarily withdrew from this program area in 2008–2009 were 0. Mental Health Counseling MA/MS (Master of Arts/Science)—Applications 2009–2010, 15. Total applicants accepted 2009–2010, 11. Number full-time enrolled (new admits only) 2009–2010, 5. Number part-time enrolled (new admits only) 2009–2010, 3. Total enrolled 2009–2010 full-time, 9, part-time, 9. Openings 2010–2011, 5. The median number of years required for completion of a degree in 2008–2009 were 2. The number of students enrolled full- and part-time who were dismissed or voluntarily withdrew from this program area in 2008–2009 were 2. School Counseling MA/MS (Master of Arts/Science)—Applications 2009–2010, 11. Total applicants accepted 2009–2010, 2. Number full-time enrolled (new admits only) 2009–2010, 2. Number part-time enrolled (new admits only) 2009–2010, 1. Total enrolled 2009–2010 full-time, 3, part-time, 5. Openings 2010–2011, 6. The median number of years required for completion of a degree in 2008–2009 were 3. The number of students enrolled full- and part-time who were dismissed or voluntarily withdrew from this program area in 2008–2009 were 1.

Other Criteria: (importance of criteria rated low, medium, or high): GRE scores—medium, research experience—low, work experience—medium, extracurricular activity—medium, clinically related public service—medium, GPA—medium, letters of recommendation—high, interview—medium, statement of goals and objectives—high, specific undergraduate psychology courses taken—medium. For additional information on admission requirements, go to http://www.geneva.edu/counseling_admissions.

Student Characteristics: The following represents characteristics of students in 2009–2010 in all graduate psychology programs in the department: Female—full-time 17, part-time 17; Male—full-time 4, part-time 4; African American/Black—full-time 0, part-time 3; Hispanic/Latino(a)—full-time 1, part-time 0; Asian/Pacific Islander—full-time 0, part-time 0; American Indian/Alaska Native—full-time 0, part-time 0; Caucasian/White—full-time 20, part-time 18; Multi-ethnic—full-time 0, part-time 0; students subject to the Americans With Disabilities Act—full-time 0, part-time 0; Unknown ethnicity—full-time 0, part-time 0; International students who hold an F-1 or J-1 Visa—full-time 0, part-time 0.

Financial Information/Assistance:
Tuition for Full-Time Study: Master's: State residents: $625 per credit hour; Nonstate residents: $625 per credit hour. Tuition is subject to change.

Financial Assistance:
First-Year Students: No information provided.
Advanced Students: No information provided.
Additional Information: Application and information available online at: http://www.geneva.edu/counseling_fin_aid.html.

Internships/Practica: A practicum and internship program is in place. This practicum and internship experience is in line with the CACREP standards for master's level counseling programs. Details are as follows: practica are 100 hours in length with individual and group supervision and direct client contact; marriage and family internships are 600 hours in length with direct client contact included; mental health internships are 900 hours in length with direct client contact hours included; school internships are 600 hours in length with 300 hours being on the elementary level and 300 hours on the secondary level. All internships will involve site placements typically in the Beaver County and Pittsburgh area, supervision via qualified master's and/or doctoral prepared practitioners, and onsite as well as college supervision. Practica and internship experiences are arranged by the faculty coordinators.

Housing and Day Care: No on-campus housing is available. No on-campus day care facilities are available.

Employment of Department Graduates:
Master's Degree Graduates: Of those who graduated in the academic year 2008–2009, the following categories and numbers represent the postgraduate activities and employment of master's degree graduates: Enrolled in a psychology doctoral program (0), enrolled in another graduate/professional program (0), enrolled in a postdoctoral residency/fellowship (n/a), employed in independent practice (n/a), employed in an academic position at a university (0), employed in an academic position at a 2-year/4-year college (0), employed in other positions at a higher education institution (0), employed in a professional position in a school system (1), employed in business or industry (0), employed in government agency (0), employed in a community mental health/counseling center (7), employed in a hospital/medical center (1), still seeking employment (1), not seeking employment (0), other employment position (1), do not know (1), total from the above (master's) (12).

Doctoral Degree Graduates: Of those who graduated in the academic year 2008–2009, the following categories and numbers represent the postgraduate activities and employment of doctoral degree graduates: Enrolled in a psychology doctoral program (n/a), total from the above (doctoral) (0).

Additional Information:
Orientation, Objectives, and Emphasis of Department: The philosophies of counseling in the MA in Counseling program at Geneva College are embedded in a Christian view of human nature and God's created world. A growing body of research literature affirms that Christian faith establishes a basis for healthy personality development, interpersonal relations, and mental health. A multidimensional holistic view of persons examines the interweaving of physical, emotional, social, cognitive, behavioral,

and spiritual aspects of life. Integrative psychotherapeutic conceptualizations based on this multidimensionality promote healing and change. Counseling students and faculty engage in Christian spiritual growth thus modeling adherence to the faith and values they profess and facilitating academic learning, counseling, effectiveness, and ability to consult in the larger church community and beyond. The MA in Counseling Program at Geneva College provides academic training in the development of knowledge, skills, and personal awareness pertinent to the counseling profession, and encourages students to integrate Christian faith and Biblical knowledge with the training and practice of counseling. The program is designed so that post-baccalaureate students who complete this degree and acquire the required postgraduate supervised experience in the practice of counseling will be eligible to become Licensed Professional Counselors.

Special Facilities or Resources: Department facilities include a computer lab and a modern clinical counseling facility. The computer lab is equipped with WordPerfect for Windows, SPSS for Windows, and various experimental and clinical software resources. The lab is also connected to Internet.

Information for Students With Physical Disabilities: See the following Web site for more information: http://www.geneva.edu/object/access_disability_serv.html.

Application Information:
Send to MA in Counseling Program Manager, Geneva College, 3200 College Avenue, Beaver Falls, PA 15010. Application available online. URL of online application: http://www.geneva.edu/counseling. Geneva College's MA in Counseling Program accepts applications on a rolling basis. There is no deadline. *Fee:* $50. Application fee will be waived for online application.

Immaculata University
Department of Graduate Psychology
College of Graduate Studies
Box 500, Loyola Hall
Immaculata, PA 19345-0500
Telephone: (215) 647-4400 Ext. 3509
Fax: (610) 647-2324
E-mail: *jyalof@immaculata.edu*
Web: *http://www.immaculata.edu/academics/departments/graduatepsychology*

Department Information:
1983. Chairperson: Jed Yalof. Number of faculty: total—full-time 10, part-time 23; women—full-time 8, part-time 13; total—minority—full-time 1; women minority—full-time 1.

Programs and Degrees Offered:
Listed in the following order: Program area, degree type (T if terminal Master's), number awarded 7/08–6/09. Clinical Psychology PsyD (Doctor of Psychology) 14, Counseling Psychology MA/MS (Master of Arts/Science) (T) 21, Elementary School Counseling MA/MS (Master of Arts/Science) (T) 6, School Psychology MA/MS (Master of Arts/Science) (T) 10, Secondary School Counseling MA/MS (Master of Arts/Science) 7, School Psychology PsyD (Doctor of Psychology) 3, Elementary/Secondary Counseling MA/MS (Master of Arts/Science) 1.

APA Accreditation: Clinical PsyD (Doctor of Psychology). Student Outcome Data Website: http://www.immaculata.edu/academics/departments/graduatepsychology/outcomes.

Student Applications/Admissions:
Student Applications
Clinical Psychology PsyD (Doctor of Psychology)—Applications 2009–2010, 102. Total applicants accepted 2009–2010, 43. Number full-time enrolled (new admits only) 2009–2010, 22. Total enrolled 2009–2010 full-time, 84, part-time, 42. Openings 2010–2011, 25. The median number of years required for completion of a degree in 2008–2009 were 6. The number of students enrolled full- and part-time who were dismissed or voluntarily withdrew from this program area in 2008–2009 were 5. *Counseling Psychology MA/MS (Master of Arts/Science)*—Applications 2009–2010, 90. Total applicants accepted 2009–2010, 76. Total enrolled 2009–2010 full-time, 25, part-time, 91. The number of students enrolled full- and part-time who were dismissed or voluntarily withdrew from this program area in 2008–2009 were 13. *Elementary School Counseling MA/MS (Master of Arts/Science)*—Total enrolled 2009–2010 full-time, 3, part-time, 6. The number of students enrolled full- and part-time who were dismissed or voluntarily withdrew from this program area in 2008–2009 were 0. *School Psychology MA/MS (Master of Arts/Science)*—Total enrolled 2009–2010 full-time, 13, part-time, 11. The number of students enrolled full- and part-time who were dismissed or voluntarily withdrew from this program area in 2008–2009 were 0. *Secondary School Counseling MA/MS (Master of Arts/Science)*—Total enrolled 2009–2010 full-time, 9, part-time, 4. The number of students enrolled full- and part-time who were dismissed or voluntarily withdrew from this program area in 2008–2009 were 1. *School Psychology PsyD (Doctor of Psychology)*—Total enrolled 2009–2010 full-time, 1, part-time, 4. The number of students enrolled full- and part-time who were dismissed or voluntarily withdrew from this program area in 2008–2009 were 0. *Elementary/Secondary Counseling MA/MS (Master of Arts/Science)*—Total enrolled 2009–2010 full-time, 3, part-time, 8. The number of students enrolled full- and part-time who were dismissed or voluntarily withdrew from this program area in 2008–2009 were 0.

Other Criteria: (importance of criteria rated low, medium, or high): GRE scores—medium, GPA—medium, letters of recommendation—medium, interview—high, statement of goals and objectives—medium. For additional information on admission requirements, go to http://www.immaculata.edu/admissions/graduate.

Student Characteristics: The following represents characteristics of students in 2009–2010 in all graduate psychology programs in the department: Female—full-time 109, part-time 139; Male—full-time 24, part-time 32; African American/Black—full-time 13, part-time 11; Hispanic/Latino(a)—full-time 5, part-time 3; Asian/Pacific Islander—full-time 6, part-time 2; American Indian/Alaska Native—full-time 0, part-time 0; Caucasian/White—full-time 101, part-time 142; Multi-ethnic—full-time 0, part-time 1; students subject to the Americans With Disabilities Act—full-time 0, part-time 0; Unknown ethnicity—full-time 8, part-time

12; International students who hold an F-1 or J-1 Visa—full-time 0, part-time 0.

Financial Information/Assistance:
Tuition for Full-Time Study: *Master's:* State residents: $570 per credit hour; Nonstate residents: $570 per credit hour. *Doctoral:* State residents: $780 per credit hour; Nonstate residents: $780 per credit hour. Tuition is subject to change. See the following Web site for updates and changes in tuition costs: http://www.immaculata.edu/cgs/tuition.

Financial Assistance:
First-Year Students: No information provided.
Advanced Students: Traineeships available for advanced students. Average amount paid per academic year: $22,000. Apply by May. Fellowships and scholarships available for advanced students. Average amount paid per academic year: $4,700. Apply by April.
Additional Information: Application and information available online at: http://www.immaculata.edu/FinAid.

Internships/Practica: Doctoral Degree (PsyD Clinical Psychology): For those doctoral students for whom a professional internship was required in this program prior to graduation, (14) students applied for an internship in 2008–2009, with (12) students obtaining an internship. Of those students who obtained an internship, (12) were paid internships. Of those students who obtained an internship, (3) students placed in APA/CPA accredited internships, (9) students placed in internships not APA/CPA accredited, but listed with the Association of Psychology Postdoctoral and Internship Programs (APPIC), (0) students placed in internships conforming to guidelines of the Council of Directors of School Psychology Programs (CDSPP), (0) students placed in internships that were not APA/CPA accredited, APPIC or CDSPP listed. Doctoral Degree (PsyD School Psychology): For those doctoral students for whom a professional internship was required in this program prior to graduation, (1) students applied for an internship in 2008–2009, with (1) students obtaining an internship. Of those students who obtained an internship, (1) were paid internships. Of those students who obtained an internship, (0) students placed in APA/CPA accredited internships, (1) students placed in internships not APA/CPA accredited, but listed with the Association of Psychology Postdoctoral and Internship Programs (APPIC), (0) students placed in internships conforming to guidelines of the Council of Directors of School Psychology Programs (CDSPP), (0) students placed in internships that were not APA/CPA accredited, APPIC or CDSPP listed. Master's Degree (MA/MS Counseling Psychology): An internship experience, such as, a final research project or "capstone" experience is required of graduates. Master's Degree (MA/MS Elementary School Counseling): An internship experience, such as a final research project or "capstone" experience is required of graduates. Master's Degree (MA/MS School Psychology): An internship experience, such as a final research project or "capstone" experience is required of graduates. The Graduate Psychology Department places counseling psychology, school psychology, and clinical psychology students at sites throughout the Philadelphia and tri-county area and with supervisors with qualifications specific to student and program requirements. The department has an APPIC consortium for predoctoral internship training to which its students are encouraged to apply, in addition to applying to APA-accredited sites and other APPIC internships both locally and nationally. Clinical doctoral students complete diagnostic and therapy placements prior to internship. Elective field placements are available and encouraged for clinical psychology doctoral students. Students entering the PsyD program with a BA or equivalent are required to complete a field placement early in their program of study as one of their electives. School doctoral students complete a practicum prior to internship. Students work with either the Master's field site coordinator or doctoral field site and predoctoral internship coordinator to identify prospective field placements for their different programs of study.

Housing and Day Care: On-campus housing is available. See the following Web site for more information: http://www.immaculata.edu/ResidenceLifeandHousing. No on-campus day care facilities are available.

Employment of Department Graduates:
Master's Degree Graduates: Of those who graduated in the academic year 2008–2009, the following categories and numbers represent the postgraduate activities and employment of master's degree graduates: Enrolled in a postdoctoral residency/fellowship (n/a), employed in independent practice (n/a), total from the above (master's) (0).
Doctoral Degree Graduates: Of those who graduated in the academic year 2008–2009, the following categories and numbers represent the postgraduate activities and employment of doctoral degree graduates: Enrolled in a psychology doctoral program (n/a), total from the above (doctoral) (0).

Additional Information:
Orientation, Objectives, and Emphasis of Department: At the master's level, the department's orientation is the professional preparation of the master's counselor in relation to counselor licensure in PA. The department also prepares students for elementary school counseling, secondary school counseling, combined elementary and secondary school counseling, and school psychology certification. There are also certification only programs for students with the MA degree; these programs are lower enrollment. In all cases, training emphasizes knowledge, skill and competency through classroom, practicum and internship. The department's orientation is the preparation of doctoral-level clinical psychologists within the practitioner-scholar model of professional psychology. This preparation entails a generalist curriculum emphasizing theory, therapy, diagnostics and clinical training, with doctoral dissertation research aligned with a practitioner model. The department's preparation of doctoral-level school psychologists is practitioner-oriented, focusing on advanced assessment and intervention, human diversity, biological bases, school-neuropsychological application, research and consultation within the context of school settings. Traineeships and scholarships are competitive and for MA and PsyD level students. There is also a Professional Development Award to support student attendance at conferences at which they present academic research and/or papers.

Special Facilities or Resources: The college has a comprehensive center for academic computing and modern technology available for student computer needs and utilization. The Gabrielle Library was opened in 1993 and houses journals and texts and has online search available to students.

Information for Students With Physical Disabilities: See the following Web site for more information: http://www.immaculata.edu/node/1141.

Application Information:
Send to Director of Graduate Admission, Immaculata University, 1145 King Road, Box 500, Immaculata, PA 19345. Students are admitted in the Fall, application deadline rolling; Winter, application deadline rolling; Spring, application deadline rolling; Summer, application deadline rolling. PsyD Clinical: January 15 application deadline. Application fee is $40 for master's, $55 for doctoral programs.

Indiana University of Pennsylvania (2009 data)
Department of Psychology/Clinical Psychology Doctoral Program
Natural Sciences and Mathematics
201 Uhler Hall
Indiana, PA 15705
Telephone: (724) 357-4519
Fax: (724) 357-4087
E-mail: *goodwin@iup.edu*
Web: *http://www.iup.edu/psychology*

Department Information:
1984. Chairperson: Mary Lou Zanich, PhD. Number of faculty: total—full-time 25, part-time 3; women—full-time 15, part-time 2; total—minority—full-time 2; women minority—full-time 1.

Programs and Degrees Offered:
Listed in the following order: Program area, degree type (T if terminal Master's), number awarded 7/08–6/09. Clinical Psychology PsyD (Doctor of Psychology) 11.

APA Accreditation: Clinical PsyD (Doctor of Psychology).

Student Applications/Admissions:
Student Applications
Clinical Psychology PsyD (Doctor of Psychology)—Applications 2009–2010, 83. Total applicants accepted 2009–2010, 11. Number full-time enrolled (new admits only) 2009–2010, 11. Total enrolled 2009–2010 full-time, 63, part-time, 5. Openings 2010–2011, 13. The median number of years required for completion of a degree in 2008–2009 were 6. The number of students enrolled full- and part-time who were dismissed or voluntarily withdrew from this program area in 2008–2009 were 1.
Other Criteria: (importance of criteria rated low, medium, or high): GRE scores—high, research experience—medium, work experience—medium, clinically related public service—high, GPA—high, letters of recommendation—high, interview—high, statement of goals and objectives—high, specific undergraduate psychology courses taken—medium. For additional information on admission requirements, go to http://www.iup.edu/psychology.

Student Characteristics: The following represents characteristics of students in 2009–2010 in all graduate psychology programs in the department: Female—full-time 36, part-time 0; Male—full-time 12, part-time 0; African American/Black—full-time 1, part-time 0; Hispanic/Latino(a)—full-time 1, part-time 0; Asian/Pacific Islander—full-time 1, part-time 0; American Indian/Alaska Native—full-time 1, part-time 0; Caucasian/White—full-time 44, part-time 0; Multi-ethnic—full-time 0, part-time 0; students subject to the Americans With Disabilities Act—full-time 1, part-time 0; Unknown ethnicity—full-time 0, part-time 0; International students who hold an F-1 or J-1 Visa—full-time 0, part-time 0.

Financial Information/Assistance:
Tuition for Full-Time Study: *Doctoral:* State residents: per academic year $6,430, $357 per credit hour; Nonstate residents: per academic year $1,028, $572 per credit hour. Tuition is subject to change. Additional fees are assessed to students beyond the costs of tuition for the following: technology fee, activity fee, instructional fee, registration fee.

Financial Assistance:
First-Year Students: Research assistantships available for first year. Average amount paid per academic year: $3,265. Average number of hours worked per week: 10. Apply by March 15. Fellowships and scholarships available for first year. Average amount paid per academic year: $5,000. Average number of hours worked per week: 0. Apply by March 15.

Advanced Students: Teaching assistantships available for advanced students. Average amount paid per academic year: $20,299. Average number of hours worked per week: 15. Apply by March 15. Research assistantships available for advanced students. Average amount paid per academic year: $3,265. Average number of hours worked per week: 10. Apply by March 15. Fellowships and scholarships available for advanced students. Average amount paid per academic year: $1,000. Average number of hours worked per week: 0. Apply by April 15.

Additional Information: Of all students currently enrolled full time, 100% benefited from one or more of the listed financial assistance programs. Application and information available online at: http://www.iup.edu/psychology.

Internships/Practica: Doctoral Degree (PsyD Clinical Psychology): For those doctoral students for whom a professional internship was required in this program prior to graduation, (10) students applied for an internship in 2008–2009, with (10) students obtaining an internship. Of those students who obtained an internship, (10) were paid internships. Of those students who obtained an internship, (7) students placed in APA/CPA accredited internships, (3) students placed in internships not APA/CPA accredited, but listed with the Association of Psychology Postdoctoral and Internship Programs (APPIC), (0) students placed in internships conforming to guidelines of the Council of Directors of School Psychology Programs (CDSPP), (0) students placed in internships that were not APA/CPA accredited, APPIC or CDSPP listed. Students begin clinical experiences in the first year through course-based practica. During the second and later years, students enroll in the department-sponsored Center for Applied Psychology (CAP) training clinics. These clinics employ a real-time supervision model. Training in the CAP clinics is supplemented with required external practica, currently available in approximately 30 different sites.

Housing and Day Care: No on-campus housing is available. On-campus day care facilities are available.

Employment of Department Graduates:
Master's Degree Graduates: Of those who graduated in the academic year 2008–2009, the following categories and numbers represent the postgraduate activities and employment of master's degree graduates: Enrolled in a postdoctoral residency/fellowship (n/a), employed in independent practice (n/a), total from the above (master's) (0).
Doctoral Degree Graduates: Of those who graduated in the academic year 2008–2009, the following categories and numbers represent the postgraduate activities and employment of doctoral degree graduates: Enrolled in a psychology doctoral program (n/a), enrolled in a postdoctoral residency/fellowship (2), employed in a community mental health/counseling center (7), employed in a hospital/medical center (2), total from the above (doctoral) (11).

Additional Information:
Orientation, Objectives, and Emphasis of Department: The Psychology Department offers a Doctor of Psychology degree in Clinical Psychology (PsyD) that places emphasis upon professional applications of psychology based on a solid grounding in the scientific knowledge base of psychology. Training follows a generalist model with opportunities to develop advanced competencies during the last two years through courses and special practica. The core curriculum consists of seven areas including elective coursework. Heavy emphasis is placed on integrating psychological knowledge with treatment, evaluation, consultation and service delivery program design. The program is designed to meet the academic requirements of licensure and provide the background to assume responsibilities in appropriate professional settings.

Special Facilities or Resources: The Department of Psychology includes two 16-computer laboratories, individual research space with audio/DVD capabilities, seminar rooms and a graduate student lounge. Each graduate student office is provided with computer access to the department server and the Internet. The facilities for the CAP include 12 treatment rooms as well as one seminar room, all connected with a master DVD system. The CAP also houses computer facilities for test administration and scoring.

Information for Students With Physical Disabilities: See the following Web site for more information: http://www.iup.edu/disabilitysupport.

Application Information:
Send to Graduate School Admissions, Indiana University of Pennsylvania, Stright Hall, Indiana, PA 15705. Application available online. URL of online application: http://www.iup.edu/graduate. Students are admitted in the Fall, application deadline December 15. *Fee:* $30.

La Salle University
Department of Psychology
1900 West Olney Avenue
Philadelphia, PA 19141
Telephone: (215) 951-1767
Fax: (215) 991-3585
E-mail: *rooney@lasalle.edu*
Web: *http://www.lasalle.edu*

Department Information:
1948. Chairperson: Joseph Burke, PhD. Number of faculty: total—full-time 16, part-time 19; women—full-time 10, part-time 8; total—minority—full-time 2, part-time 4; women minority—full-time 1, part-time 1.

Programs and Degrees Offered:
Listed in the following order: Program area, degree type (T if terminal Master's), number awarded 7/08–6/09. Clinical Counseling Psychology MA/MS (Master of Arts/Science) 102.

Student Applications/Admissions:
Student Applications
Clinical Counseling Psychology MA/MS (Master of Arts/Science)—Applications 2009–2010, 410. Total applicants accepted 2009–2010, 350. Number full-time enrolled (new admits only) 2009–2010, 150. Number part-time enrolled (new admits only) 2009–2010, 50. Total enrolled 2009–2010 full-time, 145, part-time, 285. Openings 2010–2011, 200. The median number of years required for completion of a degree in 2008–2009 were 3. The number of students enrolled full- and part-time who were dismissed or voluntarily withdrew from this program area in 2008–2009 were 6.
Other Criteria: (importance of criteria rated low, medium, or high): GRE scores—medium, research experience—medium, work experience—medium, extracurricular activity—medium, clinically related public service—medium, GPA—high, letters of recommendation—high, statement of goals and objectives—medium, statement of intent—high, undergraduate major in psychology—high. For additional information on admission requirements, go to http://www.lasalle.edu/admiss/grad/psych/.

Student Characteristics: The following represents characteristics of students in 2009–2010 in all graduate psychology programs in the department: Female—full-time 45, part-time 133; Male—full-time 15, part-time 45; African American/Black—full-time 5, part-time 36; Hispanic/Latino(a)—full-time 1, part-time 4; Asian/Pacific Islander—full-time 1, part-time 4; American Indian/Alaska Native—full-time 0, part-time 0; Caucasian/White—full-time 51, part-time 120; Multi-ethnic—full-time 2, part-time 24; students subject to the Americans With Disabilities Act—full-time 1, part-time 0; Unknown ethnicity—full-time 0, part-time 0; International students who hold an F-1 or J-1 Visa—full-time 0, part-time 0.

Financial Information/Assistance:
Tuition for Full-Time Study: Master's: State residents: $600 per credit hour; Nonstate residents: $600 per credit hour. Tuition is subject to change. Additional fees are assessed to students beyond

the costs of tuition for the following: $95.00 university fee assessed each semester.

Financial Assistance:
First-Year Students: Fellowships and scholarships available for first year. Average amount paid per academic year: $1,250.
Advanced Students: Teaching assistantships available for advanced students. Average amount paid per academic year: $4,500. Average number of hours worked per week: 10. Research assistantships available for advanced students. Average amount paid per academic year: $4,500. Average number of hours worked per week: 10. Traineeships available for advanced students. Fellowships and scholarships available for advanced students. Average amount paid per academic year: $2,500.
Additional Information: Of all students currently enrolled full time, 25% benefited from one or more of the listed financial assistance programs. Application and information available online at: http://www.lasalle.edu.

Internships/Practica: 125 Students are placed in sites, located throughout the Tri-State area. The internship placements are specific to the areas of concentrations and supervised by professionals highly qualified in particular realms of expertise.

Housing and Day Care: On-campus housing is available. See the following Web site for more information: http://www.lasalle.edu/students/dean/admin/housing/gradhousing.htm. On-campus day care facilities are available. Building Blocks Child Development Center. (215) 951-1572.

Employment of Department Graduates:
Master's Degree Graduates: Of those who graduated in the academic year 2008–2009, the following categories and numbers represent the postgraduate activities and employment of master's degree graduates: Enrolled in a postdoctoral residency/fellowship (n/a), employed in independent practice (n/a), total from the above (master's) (0).
Doctoral Degree Graduates: Of those who graduated in the academic year 2008–2009, the following categories and numbers represent the postgraduate activities and employment of doctoral degree graduates: Enrolled in a psychology doctoral program (n/a), total from the above (doctoral) (0).

Additional Information:
Orientation, Objectives, and Emphasis of Department: Four areas of concentration are available within the program: psychological counseling, marriage and family therapy, addictions counseling and industrial/organizational psychology. The program stresses skills training and clinical preparation for these concentrations, including preparation for Licensed Professional Counselor or Licensed Marriage and Family Therapist. It also prepares students for doctoral studies. The program is based on a holistic view of the person, which stresses the integration of the psychological, systemic, cultural, and spiritual dimensions of experience.

Special Facilities or Resources: Counselor training facilities include room and equipment for videotaping counseling sessions with individuals and families. A clinic for supervised training of students was opened in 1985. It has all the resources, equipment, and staff needed in such a facility.

Application Information:
Send to Dr. John Rooney, La Salle University, MA Clinical Counseling Psychology, Box 828, 1900 West Olney Avenue, Philadelphia, PA 19141. Application available online. URL of online application: http://www.lasalle.edu/admiss/grad/apply_nowgrad.php. Although there are no formal application deadlines, we recommend that all information necessary be received by August 1, December 1, and April 1, for the Fall, Spring, and Summer terms, respectively. International student applications should be completed at least two months prior to the dates listed above. *Fee:* $35. Fee waived for online application (which is recommended).

Lehigh University
Department of Education and Human Services
Education
Mountain Top Campus, 111 Research Drive
Bethlehem, PA 18015
Telephone: (610) 758-3241
Fax: (610) 758-6223
E-mail: *gjd3@lehigh.edu*
Web: *http://www.lehigh.edu/education/*

Department Information:
1995. Chairperson: George DuPaul. Number of faculty: total—full-time 30; women—full-time 19; total—minority—full-time 6; women minority—full-time 4.

Programs and Degrees Offered:
Listed in the following order: Program area, degree type (T if terminal Master's), number awarded 7/08–6/09. Counseling Psychology PhD (Doctor of Philosophy) 2, School Psychology EdS (School Psychology) 4, Counseling and Human Services MEd (Education) 12, Elementary School Counseling MEd (Education) 2, School Psychology PhD (Doctor of Philosophy) 8, Secondary School Counseling MEd (Education) 1, International Counseling MEd (Education) 0.

APA Accreditation: Counseling PhD (Doctor of Philosophy). Student Outcome Data Website: http://www.lehigh.edu/education/cp/apa/index.htm. School PhD (Doctor of Philosophy). Student Outcome Data Website: http://www.lehigh.edu/education/sp/phd_sp.html.

Student Applications/Admissions:
Student Applications
Counseling Psychology PhD (Doctor of Philosophy)—Applications 2009–2010, 105. Total applicants accepted 2009–2010, 10. Number full-time enrolled (new admits only) 2009–2010, 6. Number part-time enrolled (new admits only) 2009–2010, 0. Total enrolled 2009–2010 full-time, 25, part-time, 11. Openings 2010–2011, 7. The median number of years required for completion of a degree in 2008–2009 were 6. The number of students enrolled full- and part-time who were dismissed or voluntarily withdrew from this program area in 2008–2009 were 0. *School Psychology EdS (School Psychology)*—Applications 2009–2010, 56. Total applicants accepted 2009–2010, 9. Number full-time enrolled (new admits only) 2009–2010, 5. Number part-time enrolled (new admits only) 2009–2010, 0. Total enrolled 2009–2010 full-time, 11, part-time, 3. Openings 2010–2011, 5. The median number of years required for com-

pletion of a degree in 2008–2009 were 3. The number of students enrolled full- and part-time who were dismissed or voluntarily withdrew from this program area in 2008–2009 were 0. *Counseling and Human Services MEd (Education)*—Applications 2009–2010, 41. Total applicants accepted 2009–2010, 24. Number full-time enrolled (new admits only) 2009–2010, 9. Number part-time enrolled (new admits only) 2009–2010, 4. Total enrolled 2009–2010 full-time, 22, part-time, 14. Openings 2010–2011, 40. The median number of years required for completion of a degree in 2008–2009 were 2. The number of students enrolled full- and part-time who were dismissed or voluntarily withdrew from this program area in 2008–2009 were 0. *Elementary School Counseling MEd (Education)*—Applications 2009–2010, 13. Total applicants accepted 2009–2010, 11. Number full-time enrolled (new admits only) 2009–2010, 7. Number part-time enrolled (new admits only) 2009–2010, 2. Total enrolled 2009–2010 full-time, 5, part-time, 5. Openings 2010–2011, 10. The median number of years required for completion of a degree in 2008–2009 were 2. The number of students enrolled full- and part-time who were dismissed or voluntarily withdrew from this program area in 2008–2009 were 0. *School Psychology PhD (Doctor of Philosophy)*—Applications 2009–2010, 47. Total applicants accepted 2009–2010, 13. Number full-time enrolled (new admits only) 2009–2010, 7. Number part-time enrolled (new admits only) 2009–2010, 0. Total enrolled 2009–2010 full-time, 26, part-time, 12. Openings 2010–2011, 5. The median number of years required for completion of a degree in 2008–2009 were 6. The number of students enrolled full- and part-time who were dismissed or voluntarily withdrew from this program area in 2008–2009 were 3. *Secondary School Counseling MEd (Education)*—Applications 2009–2010, 16. Total applicants accepted 2009–2010, 10. Number full-time enrolled (new admits only) 2009–2010, 9. Number part-time enrolled (new admits only) 2009–2010, 3. Total enrolled 2009–2010 full-time, 6, part-time, 9. Openings 2010–2011, 10. The median number of years required for completion of a degree in 2008–2009 were 2. The number of students enrolled full- and part-time who were dismissed or voluntarily withdrew from this program area in 2008–2009 were 0. *International Counseling MEd (Education)*—Applications 2009–2010, 2. Total applicants accepted 2009–2010, 2. Number full-time enrolled (new admits only) 2009–2010, 2. Number part-time enrolled (new admits only) 2009–2010, 0. Total enrolled 2009–2010 full-time, 2. Openings 2010–2011, 10. The number of students enrolled full- and part-time who were dismissed or voluntarily withdrew from this program area in 2008–2009 were 0.

Scores: Entries appear in this order: required test or GPA, minimum score (if required), median score of students entering in 2009–2010. *Counseling Psychology PhD (Doctor of Philosophy)*: GRE-V no minimum stated, 490, GRE-Q no minimum stated, 583, overall undergraduate GPA no minimum stated, 3.70; *School Psychology EdS (School Psychology)*: GRE-V 520, 600, GRE-Q 520, 620, GRE-Analytical 4.0, 4.5, overall undergraduate GPA 3.27, 3.56, psychology GPA 3.08, 3.95; *School Psychology PhD (Doctor of Philosophy)*: GRE-V 520, 600, GRE-Q 520, 620, GRE-Analytical 4.0, 4.5, overall undergraduate GPA 3.27, 3.56, psychology GPA 3.08, 3.95, Masters GPA 3.97, 3.97.

Other Criteria: (importance of criteria rated low, medium, or high): GRE scores—medium, research experience—high, work experience—medium, extracurricular activity—medium, clinically related public service—medium, GPA—high, letters of recommendation—medium, interview—medium, statement of goals and objectives—high, Criteria vary by program.

Student Characteristics: The following represents characteristics of students in 2009–2010 in all graduate psychology programs in the department: Female—full-time 31, part-time 14; Male—full-time 6, part-time 1; African American/Black—full-time 2, part-time 1; Hispanic/Latino(a)—full-time 0, part-time 0; Asian/Pacific Islander—full-time 2, part-time 0; American Indian/Alaska Native—full-time 0, part-time 0; Caucasian/White—full-time 29, part-time 14; Multi-ethnic—full-time 1, part-time 0; students subject to the Americans With Disabilities Act—full-time 2, part-time 0; Unknown ethnicity—full-time 3, part-time 0; International students who hold an F-1 or J-1 Visa—full-time 0, part-time 0.

Financial Information/Assistance:

Tuition for Full-Time Study: *Master's:* State residents: $525 per credit hour; Nonstate residents: $525 per credit hour. *Doctoral:* State residents: $525 per credit hour; Nonstate residents: $525 per credit hour.

Financial Assistance:

First-Year Students: Research assistantships available for first year. Average amount paid per academic year: $14,000. Average number of hours worked per week: 20. Apply by January 1. Traineeships available for first year. Average amount paid per academic year: $14,000. Average number of hours worked per week: 20. Apply by January 1. Fellowships and scholarships available for first year. Average amount paid per academic year: $17,000. Average number of hours worked per week: 20. Apply by January 1.

Advanced Students: Research assistantships available for advanced students. Average amount paid per academic year: $14,000. Average number of hours worked per week: 20. Traineeships available for advanced students. Average amount paid per academic year: $14,000. Average number of hours worked per week: 20. Fellowships and scholarships available for advanced students. Average amount paid per academic year: $17,000. Average number of hours worked per week: 20.

Additional Information: Of all students currently enrolled full time, 80% benefited from one or more of the listed financial assistance programs.

Internships/Practica: Doctoral Degree (PhD Counseling Psychology): For those doctoral students for whom a professional internship was required in this program prior to graduation, (9) students applied for an internship in 2008–2009, with (9) students obtaining an internship. Of those students who obtained an internship, (9) were paid internships. Of those students who obtained an internship, (9) students placed in APA/CPA accredited internships, (0) students placed in internships not APA/CPA accredited, but listed with the Association of Psychology Postdoctoral and Internship Programs (APPIC), (0) students placed in internships conforming to guidelines of the Council of Directors of School Psychology Programs (CDSPP), (0) students placed in internships that were not APA/CPA accredited, APPIC or CDSPP listed. Doctoral Degree (PhD School Psychology): For those doctoral students for whom a professional internship was required in this program prior to graduation, (3) students applied for an internship in 2008–2009, with (3) students obtaining an internship. Of those students who obtained an internship, (3) were paid internships. Of those students who obtained an internship, (2) students placed in APA/CPA accredited internships, (0) students placed in internships not APA/CPA accredited, but listed with the Association of Psychology Postdoctoral and Internship Programs (APPIC), (1) students placed in internships conforming to guidelines of the Council of Directors of School Psychology Programs (CDSPP), (0) students placed in internships that were not APA/CPA accredited, APPIC or CDSPP listed. The Counseling Psychology program maintains contracts with a variety of practicum settings. Training in individual, group, couples, and family counseling is readily available. Students receive at least two hours of individual and two hours group supervision per week. Many sites provide additional training on specific issues in counseling. The Counseling Psychology programs have established a partnership with a local urban school district to provide enhanced in-school psychological services in elementary and middle schools. The School Psychology program, in cooperation with Centennial School, the University-affiliated school for students with emotional/behavioral disorders, supports a predoctoral internship opportunity in school psychology.

Housing and Day Care: On-campus housing is available. See the following Web site for more information: http://www.lehigh.edu/gradlife/housing_needs.html. On-campus day care facilities are available. See the following Web site for more information: http://www.lehigh.edu/~inluccc/.

Employment of Department Graduates:
Master's Degree Graduates: Of those who graduated in the academic year 2008–2009, the following categories and numbers represent the postgraduate activities and employment of master's degree graduates: Enrolled in a postdoctoral residency/fellowship (n/a), employed in independent practice (n/a), employed in a professional position in a school system (4), total from the above (master's) (4).
Doctoral Degree Graduates: Of those who graduated in the academic year 2008–2009, the following categories and numbers represent the postgraduate activities and employment of doctoral degree graduates: Enrolled in a psychology doctoral program (n/a), enrolled in a postdoctoral residency/fellowship (2), employed in an academic position at a university (3), employed in a professional position in a school system (3), not seeking employment (1), total from the above (doctoral) (9).

Additional Information:
Orientation, Objectives, and Emphasis of Department: The College of Education offers degree programs in counseling and school psychology. The program in school psychology offers training at both educational specialist (NASP approved) and doctoral (PhD) levels (NASP approved and APA accredited). Within the PhD program, subspecializations in Health/Pediatric School Psychology and in Counseling Psychology/Special Education are offered. The program at all levels is behaviorally oriented, emphasizing problem-solving based research, consultation, behavioral assessment and intervention in the implementation of school psychology services. The program in counseling psychology emphasizes a scientist–practitioner model and trains professional psychologists for employment in educational, industrial, and community settings. The counseling psychology program also offers training at the master's level.

Special Facilities or Resources: The school psychology program has a number of research and training projects that are focused on students with behavior and cognitive disabilities. The department has recently established the Center for Promoting Research to Practice, a unit that houses several major research grants involved in bringing known research findings into school and community settings. The department also has university-affiliated training and research programs that provide living arrangements and day treatment programs for adults with developmental disabilities. The department also operates a laboratory school for children and adolescents with emotional disturbances. All facilities are integrated into the training of students primarily in the school psychology programs. The counseling psychology program has a lab for video taping and editing. Both programs have established partnerships with urban school districts. School psychology has recently established a national internship in the University laboratory school for students with emotional/behavior disorders.

Application Information:
Send to Ms. Donna Johnson, College of Education, Lehigh University, 111 Research Dr., Bethlehem, PA 18015. Application available online. URL of online application: https://lewisweb.cc.lehigh.edu:448/pls/prod/bwskalog.P_DispLoginNon. Students are admitted in the Fall, application deadline January 1. Counseling Psychology (Master's)- March 1. Fall admission for Counseling Psychology and School Psychology doctoral programs is January 1. *Fee:* $65.

Lehigh University
Department of Psychology
Arts and Sciences
17 Memorial Drive East
Bethlehem, PA 18015
Telephone: (610) 758-3630
Fax: (610) 758-6277
E-mail: m.gill@lehigh.edu
Web: http://www.lehigh.edu/~inpsy/gradprogram.html

Department Information:
1931. Chairperson: Diane Hyland. Number of faculty: total—full-time 13, part-time 1; women—full-time 7.

Programs and Degrees Offered:
Listed in the following order: Program area, degree type (T if terminal Master's), number awarded 7/08–6/09. Human Cognition and Development PhD (Doctor of Philosophy) 5.

Student Applications/Admissions:
Student Applications
Human Cognition and Development PhD (Doctor of Philosophy)— Applications 2009–2010, 68. Total applicants accepted 2009–2010, 4. Number full-time enrolled (new admits only) 2009–

2010, 4. Number part-time enrolled (new admits only) 2009–2010, 0. Openings 2010–2011, 6. The median number of years required for completion of a degree in 2008–2009 were 5. The number of students enrolled full- and part-time who were dismissed or voluntarily withdrew from this program area in 2008–2009 were 0.

Other Criteria: (importance of criteria rated low, medium, or high): GRE scores—medium, research experience—high, work experience—low, GPA—medium, letters of recommendation—high, interview—medium, statement of goals and objectives—high, undergraduate major in psychology—low. For additional information on admission requirements, go to http://www.lehigh.edu/~inpsy/gradprogram.html.

Student Characteristics: The following represents characteristics of students in 2009–2010 in all graduate psychology programs in the department: Female—full-time 13, part-time 0; Male—full-time 3, part-time 0; African American/Black—full-time 0, part-time 0; Hispanic/Latino(a)—full-time 0, part-time 0; Asian/Pacific Islander—full-time 1, part-time 0; American Indian/Alaska Native—full-time 0, part-time 0; Caucasian/White—full-time 15, part-time 0; Multi-ethnic—full-time 0, part-time 0; students subject to the Americans With Disabilities Act—full-time 0, part-time 0; Unknown ethnicity—full-time 0, part-time 0; International students who hold an F-1 or J-1 Visa—full-time 4, part-time 0.

Financial Information/Assistance:
  Tuition for Full-Time Study: *Master's:* State residents: $1,185 per credit hour; Nonstate residents: $1,185 per credit hour. *Doctoral:* State residents: $1,185 per credit hour; Nonstate residents: $1,185 per credit hour. Tuition is subject to change. See the following Web site for updates and changes in tuition costs: http://cas.lehigh.edu/casweb/Content/default.aspx?pageid=57.

  Financial Assistance:
    First-Year Students: Teaching assistantships available for first year. Average amount paid per academic year: $16,900. Average number of hours worked per week: 15. Apply by January 15. Research assistantships available for first year. Average amount paid per academic year: $16,900. Average number of hours worked per week: 15. Apply by January 15. Fellowships and scholarships available for first year. Average amount paid per academic year: $22,000. Average number of hours worked per week: 0. Apply by January 15.
    Advanced Students: Teaching assistantships available for advanced students. Average amount paid per academic year: $17,400. Average number of hours worked per week: 15. Research assistantships available for advanced students. Average amount paid per academic year: $17,400. Average number of hours worked per week: 15. Fellowships and scholarships available for advanced students. Average amount paid per academic year: $22,000. Average number of hours worked per week: 0.
    Additional Information: Of all students currently enrolled full time, 100% benefited from one or more of the listed financial assistance programs. Application and information available online at: http://cas.lehigh.edu/casweb/Content/default.aspx?pageid=58.

Housing and Day Care: On-campus housing is available. See the following Web site for more information: http://www3.lehigh.edu/studentlife/housing/graduatetransfer.asp. On-campus day care facilities are available. See the following Web site for more information: http://www.lehigh.edu/~inluccc/.

Employment of Department Graduates:
  Master's Degree Graduates: Of those who graduated in the academic year 2008–2009, the following categories and numbers represent the postgraduate activities and employment of master's degree graduates: Enrolled in a postdoctoral residency/fellowship (n/a), employed in independent practice (n/a), total from the above (master's) (0).
  Doctoral Degree Graduates: Of those who graduated in the academic year 2008–2009, the following categories and numbers represent the postgraduate activities and employment of doctoral degree graduates: Enrolled in a psychology doctoral program (n/a), total from the above (doctoral) (0).

Additional Information:
  Orientation, Objectives, and Emphasis of Department: The Doctoral Program in Psychology is a research-intensive program that combines focus with flexibility. Focus is provided by the program emphasis on Human Cognition and Development and by a core curriculum. Flexibility is provided by the ability to tailor a research specialization in an area of Cognition and Language, Developmental Psychology, or Social Cognition and Personality. Graduate students define an area of specialization through their selection of graduate seminars and through their research experiences. All students are actively engaged in research throughout their residence in the program, and they work in collaboration with faculty members and student colleagues. Departmental faculty conduct research on basic cognitive, linguistic, and social-cognitive processes, and the development of these processes across the lifespan. In addition to research within the psychology department, the psychology faculty and students partake in interdisciplinary endeavors with researchers from other university departments and programs, including the Cognitive Science program.

  Special Facilities or Resources: The department's well-equipped laboratories provide an excellent setting for research. The department has extensive facilities available for graduate student research, including a child study center, and cognitive, developmental, and social laboratories. Lehigh has a sophisticated network system that connects all campus computers and servers and provides easy access to the Internet.

  Information for Students With Physical Disabilities: See the following Web site for more information: http://www.lehigh.edu/~inacsup/disabilities/.

Application Information:
Send to Graduate Programs Office, Lehigh University, 9 West Packer Avenue, Bethlehem, PA 18015-3075. Application available online. URL of online application: http://cas.lehigh.edu/casweb/Content/default.aspx?pageid=54. Students are admitted in the Fall, application deadline January 15. *Fee:* $75. Application fee waived for those who attend College of Arts and Sciences Open House for Prospective Graduate Students (typically in the fall).

Marywood University (2009 data)
Department of Psychology and Counseling
McGowan Center for Graduate and Professional Studies, 2300 Adams Avenue
Scranton, PA 18509
Telephone: (570) 348-6226
Fax: (570) 340-6040
E-mail: Crawley@Marywood.edu
Web: http://www.marywood.edu/Departments/psychology/index.html

Department Information:
1940. Chairperson: Edward J. Crawley, PhD Number of faculty: total—full-time 14, part-time 27; women—full-time 5, part-time 17; total—minority—full-time 1, part-time 2; women minority—full-time 1, part-time 1.

Programs and Degrees Offered:
Listed in the following order: Program area, degree type (T if terminal Master's), number awarded 7/08–6/09. School Psychology EdS (School Psychology) 7, Clinical Psychology PsyD (Doctor of Psychology) 6, Clinical Services MA/MS (Master of Arts/Science) (T) 4, Elementary School Counseling MA/MS (Master of Arts/Science) (T) 4, Mental Health Counseling MA/MS (Master of Arts/Science) (T) 5, Secondary School Counseling MA/MS (Master of Arts/Science) (T) 8, General Theoretical MA/MS (Master of Arts/Science) (T) 16, Child Clinical Services MA/MS (Master of Arts/Science) (T) 2.

APA Accreditation: Clinical PsyD (Doctor of Psychology).

Student Applications/Admissions:
Student Applications
School Psychology EdS (School Psychology)—Applications 2009–2010, 23. Total applicants accepted 2009–2010, 17. Number full-time enrolled (new admits only) 2009–2010, 6. Number part-time enrolled (new admits only) 2009–2010, 2. Total enrolled 2009–2010 full-time, 13, part-time, 14. Openings 2010–2011, 15. The median number of years required for completion of a degree in 2008–2009 were 3. The number of students enrolled full- and part-time who were dismissed or voluntarily withdrew from this program area in 2008–2009 were 0. Clinical Psychology PsyD (Doctor of Psychology)—Applications 2009–2010, 66. Total applicants accepted 2009–2010, 8. Number full-time enrolled (new admits only) 2009–2010, 8. Total enrolled 2009–2010 full-time, 26, part-time, 16. Openings 2010–2011, 8. The median number of years required for completion of a degree in 2008–2009 were 5. The number of students enrolled full- and part-time who were dismissed or voluntarily withdrew from this program area in 2008–2009 were 2. Clinical Services MA/MS (Master of Arts/Science)—Applications 2009–2010, 2. Total applicants accepted 2009–2010, 2. Number full-time enrolled (new admits only) 2009–2010, 1. Number part-time enrolled (new admits only) 2009–2010, 0. Openings 2010–2011, 10. The median number of years required for completion of a degree in 2008–2009 were 3. The number of students enrolled full- and part-time who were dismissed or voluntarily withdrew from this program area in 2008–2009 were 0. Elementary School Counseling MA/MS (Master of Arts/Science)—Applications 2009–2010, 11. Total applicants accepted 2009–2010, 10. Number full-time enrolled (new admits only) 2009–2010, 3. Number part-time enrolled (new admits only) 2009–2010, 4. Total enrolled 2009–2010 full-time, 8, part-time, 7. Openings 2010–2011, 10. The median number of years required for completion of a degree in 2008–2009 were 3. The number of students enrolled full- and part-time who were dismissed or voluntarily withdrew from this program area in 2008–2009 were 4. Mental Health Counseling MA/MS (Master of Arts/Science)—Applications 2009–2010, 22. Total applicants accepted 2009–2010, 15. Number full-time enrolled (new admits only) 2009–2010, 8. Number part-time enrolled (new admits only) 2009–2010, 1. Total enrolled 2009–2010 full-time, 10, part-time, 11. Openings 2010–2011, 10. The median number of years required for completion of a degree in 2008–2009 were 3. The number of students enrolled full- and part-time who were dismissed or voluntarily withdrew from this program area in 2008–2009 were 5. Secondary School Counseling MA/MS (Master of Arts/Science)—Applications 2009–2010, 11. Total applicants accepted 2009–2010, 8. Number full-time enrolled (new admits only) 2009–2010, 4. Number part-time enrolled (new admits only) 2009–2010, 2. Total enrolled 2009–2010 full-time, 12, part-time, 17. Openings 2010–2011, 10. The median number of years required for completion of a degree in 2008–2009 were 3. The number of students enrolled full- and part-time who were dismissed or voluntarily withdrew from this program area in 2008–2009 were 6. General Theoretical MA/MS (Master of Arts/Science)—Applications 2009–2010, 59. Total applicants accepted 2009–2010, 42. Number full-time enrolled (new admits only) 2009–2010, 22. Number part-time enrolled (new admits only) 2009–2010, 2. Total enrolled 2009–2010 full-time, 32, part-time, 15. Openings 2010–2011, 15. The median number of years required for completion of a degree in 2008–2009 were 3. The number of students enrolled full- and part-time who were dismissed or voluntarily withdrew from this program area in 2008–2009 were 18. Child Clinical Services MA/MS (Master of Arts/Science)—Applications 2009–2010, 1. Total applicants accepted 2009–2010, 1. Number full-time enrolled (new admits only) 2009–2010, 1. Number part-time enrolled (new admits only) 2009–2010, 0. Total enrolled 2009–2010 full-time, 1, part-time, 5. Openings 2010–2011, 8. The median number of years required for completion of a degree in 2008–2009 were 3. The number of students enrolled full- and part-time who were dismissed or voluntarily withdrew from this program area in 2008–2009 were 0.

Other Criteria: (importance of criteria rated low, medium, or high): GRE scores—medium, research experience—medium, work experience—medium, extracurricular activity—low, clinically related public service—medium, GPA—high, letters of recommendation—high, interview—low, statement of goals and objectives—medium, undergraduate major in psychology—medium, specific undergraduate psychology courses taken—medium. PsyD program prefers psychology major an interview is required. For additional information on admission requirements, go to http://gograduatemarywood.com.

Student Characteristics: The following represents characteristics of students in 2009–2010 in all graduate psychology programs in the department: Female—full-time 55, part-time 68; Male—full-time 15, part-time 22; African American/Black—full-time 0, part-time 0; Hispanic/Latino(a)—full-time 1, part-time 1; Asian/Pacific Islander—full-time 3, part-time 0; American Indian/Alaska

Native—full-time 1, part-time 0; Caucasian/White—full-time 64, part-time 90; Multi-ethnic—full-time 0, part-time 0; students subject to the Americans With Disabilities Act—full-time 0, part-time 1; Unknown ethnicity—full-time 0, part-time 0; International students who hold an F-1 or J-1 Visa—full-time 0, part-time 0.

Financial Information/Assistance:
Tuition for Full-Time Study: *Master's:* State residents: $695 per credit hour; Nonstate residents: $695 per credit hour. *Doctoral:* State residents: $785 per credit hour; Nonstate residents: $785 per credit hour. See the following Web site for updates and changes in tuition costs: http://www.marywood.edu/fin_aid/.

Financial Assistance:
First-Year Students: Research assistantships available for first year. Average amount paid per academic year: $5,405. Average number of hours worked per week: 20. Apply by February 15. Fellowships and scholarships available for first year. Average amount paid per academic year: $4,830. Average number of hours worked per week: 0. Apply by February 15.

Advanced Students: Research assistantships available for advanced students. Average amount paid per academic year: $5,405. Average number of hours worked per week: 20. Apply by February 15. Fellowships and scholarships available for advanced students. Average amount paid per academic year: $4,830. Average number of hours worked per week: 0. Apply by February 15.

Additional Information: Of all students currently enrolled full time, 60% benefited from one or more of the listed financial assistance programs. Application and information available online at: http://www.marywood.edu/grad_finaid/.

Internships/Practica: Doctoral Degree (PsyD Clinical Psychology): For those doctoral students for whom a professional internship was required in this program prior to graduation, (8) students applied for an internship in 2008–2009, with (8) students obtaining an internship. Of those students who obtained an internship, (8) were paid internships. Of those students who obtained an internship, (2) students placed in APA/CPA accredited internships, (6) students placed in internships not APA/CPA accredited, but listed with the Association of Psychology Postdoctoral and Internship Programs (APPIC), (0) students placed in internships conforming to guidelines of the Council of Directors of School Psychology Programs (CDSPP), (0) students placed in internships that were not APA/CPA accredited, APPIC or CDSPP listed. Master's Degree (MA/MS Elementary School Counseling): An internship experience, such as a final research project or "capstone" experience is required of graduates. Master's Degree (MA/MS Mental Health Counseling): An internship experience, such as a final research project or "capstone" experience is required of graduates. Master's Degree (MA/MS Secondary School Counseling): An internship experience, such as a final research project or "capstone" experience is required of graduates. Master's Degree (MA/MS General Theoretical): An internship experience, such as a final research project or "capstone" experience is required of graduates. Students have access to training at many schools, psychiatric hospitals, rehabilitation programs, community mental health programs, and prisons in the region of Northeastern Pennsylvania. The long history (we have been providing graduate-level training for over 60 years) and size of our programs have provided us with the opportunity to develop close working relationships with most schools, social services, and mental health agencies in the region. The PsyD program (initiated in 2001) places students in both internal and external practicum sites and regional/national placements in internship sites. The department houses a community-based mental health clinic, the Psychological Services Center, that provides training opportunities for master's and doctoral students in the program while providing significant clinical and school psychology services to children, adolescents and adults in the area.

Housing and Day Care: No on-campus housing is available. On-campus day care facilities are available.

Employment of Department Graduates:
Master's Degree Graduates: Of those who graduated in the academic year 2008–2009, the following categories and numbers represent the postgraduate activities and employment of master's degree graduates: Enrolled in a postdoctoral residency/fellowship (n/a), employed in independent practice (n/a), total from the above (master's) (0).

Doctoral Degree Graduates: Of those who graduated in the academic year 2008–2009, the following categories and numbers represent the postgraduate activities and employment of doctoral degree graduates: Enrolled in a psychology doctoral program (n/a), total from the above (doctoral) (0).

Additional Information:
Orientation, Objectives, and Emphasis of Department: The department provides students with a variety of coherent training experiences that lead to diverse career paths in school counseling, agency mental health work, school psychology, and doctoral-level training in clinical psychology. Master's students in psychology all enter initially in the General Theoretical program and then apply for the clinical services or child clinical services after completing 12 credits (candidacy). Ethical and professional practice issues are considered extensively. Professional guidelines are emphasized that increase students' awareness of their developing expertise and the limits of this expertise. Professional standards for practice, certification, and licensing guidelines are integrated into courses and advisement. Licensing of master's graduates in Counseling and Psychology in Pennsylvania is now possible with the implementation of the Professional Counseling Act. The Counseling Programs are accredited by the Council for the Accreditation of Counseling and Related Educational Programs (CACREP). The PsyD program follows the Vail model, training students to be scholar-practitioners and is a designee of the Association of State and Provincial Psychology Boards (ASPPB) and accredited by the American Psychological Association. The PsyD program includes both foundation courses in psychology and applied training. The use of empirically-supported assessments and intervention techniques is emphasized along with a focus on outcomes assessment. There are opportunities for work with children, adolescents, and adults. The PsyD program primarily is cognitive-behavioral in focus, with additional training provided in interpersonal and other approaches to psychotherapy.

Special Facilities or Resources: The department moved into the McGowan Center for Graduate and Professional Studies in the Fall, 1998 semester. This building more than doubled the research and clinical training facilities available to students and faculty in the department. Research facilities include three state-of-the-art computer laboratories that provide for group and individual instruction, computer-equipped research cubicles that provide for online data collection, psychophysiological monitoring equipment, video taping and editing facilities, digital video and CD-ROM/DVD creation capabilities, and an extensive testing laboratory. The department operates a clinic, the Psychological Services Center, that provides treatment and observation rooms for practicum training, individual therapy, play therapy, family, and group therapy.

Information for Students With Physical Disabilities: See the following Web site for more information: http://www.marywood.edu/Disabilities/disabilityservices.html.

Application Information:
Send to Graduate Admissions Office, Marywood University. Application available online. URL of online application: http://gograduatemarywood.com. Students are admitted in the Fall, application deadline April 1; Spring, application deadline November 15. Applications for the PsyD program are due January 8. *Fee:* $35.

Millersville University
Department of Psychology
Byerly Hall
Millersville, PA 17551
Telephone: (717) 872-3093
Fax: (717) 871-2480
E-mail: *claudia.haferkamp@millersville.edu*
Web: *http://www.millersville.edu/psychology/*

Department Information:
1967. Chairperson: Helena Tuleya-Payne. Number of faculty: total—full-time 18, part-time 11; women—full-time 12, part-time 8; total—minority—full-time 4; women minority—full-time 4.

Programs and Degrees Offered:
Listed in the following order: Program area, degree type (T if terminal Master's), number awarded 7/08–6/09. Clinical Psychology MA/MS (Master of Arts/Science) (T) 17, School Counseling MEd (Education) 12, School Psychology MA/MS (Master of Arts/Science) 12, Supervision Of School Guidance MEd (Education), Supervision Of School Psychology MA/MS (Master of Arts/Science) 0.

Student Applications/Admissions:
Student Applications
Clinical Psychology MA/MS (Master of Arts/Science)—Applications 2009–2010, 42. Total applicants accepted 2009–2010, 24. Number full-time enrolled (new admits only) 2009–2010, 23. Number part-time enrolled (new admits only) 2009–2010, 26. Total enrolled 2009–2010 full-time, 23, part-time, 26. Openings 2010–2011, 25. The median number of years required for completion of a degree in 2008–2009 were 2. *School Counseling MEd (Education)*—Applications 2009–2010, 46. Total applicants accepted 2009–2010, 25. Number full-time enrolled (new admits only) 2009–2010, 12. Number part-time enrolled (new admits only) 2009–2010, 45. Total enrolled 2009–2010 full-time, 12, part-time, 45. Openings 2010–2011, 25. The median number of years required for completion of a degree in 2008–2009 were 2. *School Psychology MA/MS (Master of Arts/Science)*—Applications 2009–2010, 47. Total applicants accepted 2009–2010, 29. Number full-time enrolled (new admits only) 2009–2010, 25. Number part-time enrolled (new admits only) 2009–2010, 20. Total enrolled 2009–2010 full-time, 25, part-time, 20. Openings 2010–2011, 25. The median number of years required for completion of a degree in 2008–2009 were 3. *Supervision Of School Guidance MEd (Education)*—Applications 2009–2010, 4. Total applicants accepted 2009–2010, 4. Number full-time enrolled (new admits only) 2009–2010, 6. Number part-time enrolled (new admits only) 2009–2010, 6. Total enrolled 2009–2010 full-time, 6, part-time, 6. Openings 2010–2011, 5. *Supervision Of School Psychology MA/MS (Master of Arts/Science)*—Applications 2009–2010, 1. Total applicants accepted 2009–2010, 1. Number full-time enrolled (new admits only) 2009–2010, 0. Number part-time enrolled (new admits only) 2009–2010, 1. Openings 2010–2011, 5.

Scores: Entries appear in this order: required test or GPA, minimum score (if required), median score of students entering in 2009–2010. *School Psychology MA/MS (Master of Arts/Science):* GRE-V 450, GRE-Q 450, GRE-Analytical 3.5, overall undergraduate GPA 2.75.

Other Criteria: (importance of criteria rated low, medium, or high): GRE scores—medium, research experience—low, work experience—high, extracurricular activity—low, clinically related public service—high, GPA—high, letters of recommendation—high, interview—high, statement of goals and objectives—medium, undergraduate major in psychology—high, specific undergraduate psychology courses taken—high.

Student Characteristics: The following represents characteristics of students in 2009–2010 in all graduate psychology programs in the department: Female—full-time 50, part-time 79; Male—full-time 10, part-time 13; African American/Black—full-time 1, part-time 3; Hispanic/Latino(a)—full-time 3, part-time 2; Asian/Pacific Islander—full-time 1, part-time 0; American Indian/Alaska Native—full-time 0, part-time 0; Caucasian/White—full-time 51, part-time 79; Multi-ethnic—full-time 0, part-time 0; students subject to the Americans With Disabilities Act—full-time 0, part-time 0; Unknown ethnicity—full-time 4, part-time 8; International students who hold an F-1 or J-1 Visa—full-time 1, part-time 0.

Financial Information/Assistance:
Tuition for Full-Time Study: *Master's:* State residents: per academic year $3,967, $357 per credit hour; Nonstate residents: per academic year $5,942, $572 per credit hour. Tuition is subject to change. Additional fees are assessed to students beyond the costs of tuition for the following: general fee (supports student organizations) and technology fee. See the following Web site for updates and changes in tuition costs: http://www.millersville.edu/admissions/graduate/tuition.php.

Financial Assistance:
First-Year Students: Teaching assistantships available for first year. Average amount paid per academic year: $5,000. Research assistantships available for first year. Average amount paid per academic year: $5,000.
Advanced Students: Teaching assistantships available for advanced students. Average amount paid per academic year: $5,400. Research assistantships available for advanced students. Average amount paid per academic year: $5,400.
Additional Information: No information provided.

Internships/Practica: Master's Degree (MA/MS Clinical Psychology): An internship experience, such as, a final research project or "capstone" experience is required of graduates. Field experiences are required of all students in clinical, school counseling, and school psychology programs. Students in the Certification Program in School Psychology are required to complete a full-time internship over one academic year (minimum 1200 hours). Students in the Clinical program complete a 600 hour practicum in inpatient or outpatient mental health settings. Students in School Counseling complete their practica as counselors working in K-12 schools.

Housing and Day Care: No on-campus housing is available. No on-campus day care facilities are available.

Employment of Department Graduates:
Master's Degree Graduates: Of those who graduated in the academic year 2008–2009, the following categories and numbers represent the postgraduate activities and employment of master's degree graduates: Enrolled in a postdoctoral residency/fellowship (n/a), employed in independent practice (n/a), total from the above (master's) (0).
Doctoral Degree Graduates: Of those who graduated in the academic year 2008–2009, the following categories and numbers represent the postgraduate activities and employment of doctoral degree graduates: Enrolled in a psychology doctoral program (n/a), total from the above (doctoral) (0).

Additional Information:
Orientation, Objectives, and Emphasis of Department: All programs emphasize theory, research skills, and applied practical experience combined with a high degree of self-awareness and interpersonal relationship skills. The MS program in Clinical Psychology prepares clinicians with skills in psychological assessment/diagnosis, and an eclectic/cognitive-behavioral repertoire of skills in individual, group and family therapies. Graduates may obtain PA licensure as "professional counselors" and work in a wide range of inpatient and outpatient mental health settings with children and adults. The Certification Program in School Psychology is approved by the National Association of School Psychologists (NASP) and prepares students for entry level positions as school psychologists. Knowledge about the educational process, psychological and emotional growth, and data-based decision-making are central to the training program and enable students as problem-solvers to promote effective learning in children. The MEd and Certification in School Counseling programs prepare students as school counselors for grades K-12. Operating under a prevention/intervention and solution-focused model, students develop into professionals who are responsive to the needs of the school setting.

Special Facilities or Resources: A microcomputer lab with access to the university's mainframe is available in the department. Millersville's campus is fully wireless. The Department has a clinic with one-way observation and videotaping facilities. Ganser Library houses approximately half a million books and provides access to nearly 3500 periodical titles. Electronic resources available via the World Wide Web, as well as the Millersville University library catalog, are accessible from the University home page. The research and information needs of faculty, staff, and students, are met by subject specialists who provide extensive reference service within the library, at off-site locations, and electronically. Scholarly research is supported by a comprehensive and well-developed library collection that is continuously being augmented by the most current and up-to-date resources available, both in print and electronic format. The Library belongs to several statewide and regional library consortia that allows for resource sharing, reciprocal borrowing, and collaborative purchasing.

Application Information:
Send to Graduate Studies Office, Millersville University, P.O. Box 1002, Millersville, PA 17551-0302. URL of online application: http://www.millersville.edu/admissions/graduate/apply/index.php. Students are admitted in the Fall, application deadline January 15; Spring, application deadline October 1. *Fee:* $40.

Penn State Harrisburg
Psychology Program
777 West Harrisburg Pike
Middletown, PA 17057-4898
Telephone: (717) 948-6040
Fax: (717) 948-6519
E-mail: *poyrazli@psu.edu*
Web: *http://www.hbg.psu.edu*

Department Information:
1992. Coordinator: Senel Poyrazli. Number of faculty: total—full-time 10; women—full-time 6.

Programs and Degrees Offered:
Listed in the following order: Program area, degree type (T if terminal Master's), number awarded 7/08–6/09. Applied Clinical Psychology MA/MS (Master of Arts/Science) (T) 12, Applied Psychological Research MA/MS (Master of Arts/Science) (T) 2.

Student Applications/Admissions:
Student Applications
Applied Clinical Psychology MA/MS (Master of Arts/Science)—Applications 2009–2010, 52. Total applicants accepted 2009–2010, 25. Number full-time enrolled (new admits only) 2009–2010, 13. Number part-time enrolled (new admits only) 2009–2010, 3. Total enrolled 2009–2010 full-time, 34, part-time, 26. Openings 2010–2011, 15. The median number of years required for completion of a degree in 2008–2009 were 4. The number of students enrolled full- and part-time who were dismissed or voluntarily withdrew from this program area in 2008–2009 were 0. Applied Psychological Research MA/MS (Master of Arts/Science)—Applications 2009–2010, 3. Total applicants accepted 2009–2010, 2. Number full-time enrolled (new admits only) 2009–2010, 1. Number part-time enrolled (new admits only) 2009–2010, 0. Total enrolled 2009–2010 full-time, 2, part-time, 14. Openings 2010–2011, 5. The median number of years required for completion of a degree in 2008–2009 were 3. The number of students enrolled full- and part-time who were dismissed or voluntarily withdrew from this program area in 2008–2009 were 0.

Scores: Entries appear in this order: required test or GPA, minimum score (if required), median score of students entering in 2009–2010. Applied Clinical Psychology MA/MS (Master of Arts/Science): overall undergraduate GPA no minimum stated,

last 2 years GPA 3.00; *Applied Psychological Research MA/MS (Master of Arts/Science)*: last 2 years GPA 3.00.
Other Criteria: (importance of criteria rated low, medium, or high): GRE scores—high, research experience—medium, work experience—low, extracurricular activity—low, clinically related public service—low, GPA—high, letters of recommendation—high, interview—high, statement of goals and objectives—high, undergraduate major in psychology—low, specific undergraduate psychology courses taken—high. For additional information on admission requirements, go to http://php.scripts.psu.edu/dept/iit/hbg/Programs/Graduate/MastersDegrees.php.

Student Characteristics: The following represents characteristics of students in 2009–2010 in all graduate psychology programs in the department: Female—full-time 27, part-time 33; Male—full-time 9, part-time 7; African American/Black—full-time 2, part-time 2; Hispanic/Latino(a)—full-time 1, part-time 1; Asian/Pacific Islander—full-time 0, part-time 0; American Indian/Alaska Native—full-time 0, part-time 0; Caucasian/White—full-time 30, part-time 37; Multi-ethnic—full-time 0, part-time 0; students subject to the Americans With Disabilities Act—full-time 0, part-time 2; Unknown ethnicity—full-time 3, part-time 0; International students who hold an F-1 or J-1 Visa—full-time 1, part-time 0.

Financial Information/Assistance:
Tuition for Full-Time Study: *Master's:* State residents: per academic year $15,446, $644 per credit hour; Nonstate residents: per academic year $21,494, $896 per credit hour. Tuition is subject to change. See the following Web site for updates and changes in tuition costs: http://tuition.psu.edu/.

Financial Assistance:
First-Year Students: Research assistantships available for first year. Average amount paid per academic year: $13,600. Average number of hours worked per week: 20. Apply by February 1. Fellowships and scholarships available for first year. Average amount paid per academic year: $13,365. Average number of hours worked per week: 20. Apply by February 1.
Advanced Students: Fellowships and scholarships available for advanced students.
Additional Information: Of all students currently enrolled full time, 10% benefited from one or more of the listed financial assistance programs. Application and information available online at: www.hbg.psu.edu.

Internships/Practica: Master's Degree (MA/MS Applied Clinical Psychology): An internship experience, such as a final research project or "capstone" experience is required of graduates. Master's Degree (MA/MS Applied Psychological Research): An internship experience, such as a final research project or "capstone" experience is required of graduates. Students in the Applied Clinical Psychology program are required to complete 7 credits of supervised clinical internships. Students in the Applied Psychological Research program are required to complete 6 credits of research in collaboration with the program faculty.

Housing and Day Care: On-campus housing is available. See the following Web site for more information: http://www.hfs.psu.edu/harrisburg/housing. On-campus day care facilities are available. http://hbg.psu.edu/facultystaff/childcare.php.

Employment of Department Graduates:
Master's Degree Graduates: Of those who graduated in the academic year 2008–2009, the following categories and numbers represent the postgraduate activities and employment of master's degree graduates: Enrolled in a postdoctoral residency/fellowship (n/a), employed in independent practice (n/a), total from the above (master's) (0).
Doctoral Degree Graduates: Of those who graduated in the academic year 2008–2009, the following categories and numbers represent the postgraduate activities and employment of doctoral degree graduates: Enrolled in a psychology doctoral program (n/a), total from the above (doctoral) (0).

Additional Information:
Orientation, Objectives, and Emphasis of Department: The Applied Clinical Psychology program prepares students to work as mental health professionals in a variety of settings and is intended to provide the academic training necessary for graduates to apply for master's-level licensing for mental health professionals in the Commonwealth of Pennsylvania. The overall model emphasizes the scientific bases of behavior, including biological, social, and individual difference factors. The training model is health-oriented rather than pathology-oriented and emphasizes the development of helping skills, including both assessment and intervention. The Applied Psychological Research program focuses on the development of research skills within the context of scientific training in psychology. The program is designed to meet the needs of students who plan careers in research or administration within human services or similar organizations, who plan to conduct research in other settings, or who plan to pursue doctoral study. Students can select electives and research experiences to reflect their individual interests in consultation with their advisor.

Special Facilities or Resources: The Psychology program maintains a small on-site clinic for the assessment of specific learning disorders in college students. This clinic provides advanced Applied Clinical Psychology students the opportunity to assist with psychological testing, report writing, diagnosis, and treatment recommendations under the supervision of the program faculty. Most students avail themselves of the resources in community hospitals, residential, and out-patient institiutions for hands-on clinical and research experience. The department maintains an on-campus research facility which is available for use by graduate students working with faculty on research projects.

Information for Students With Physical Disabilities: Contact Alan Babcock, Disability Services Coordinator: (717) 948-6025.

Application Information:
Send to Graduate Admissions, Penn State Harrisburg, 777 W. Harrisburg Pike, Middletown, PA 17057-4898. Application available online. URL of online application: http://www.hbg.psu.edu/admissions/graduate.php. Students are admitted in the Fall, application deadline April 30. January 10 application deadline for University fellowships and assistantships. We review applications on a rolling basis. Early applications are encouraged. *Fee:* $45.

Pennsylvania State University (2009 data)
Counseling Psychology Program
Education
327 Cedar Building
University Park, PA 16802
Telephone: (814) 865-8304
Fax: (814) 863-7750
E-mail: jxh34@psu.edu
Web: http://www.ed.psu.edu/educ/cecprs/counseling-psychology

Department Information:
1982. Head of Department: Dr. Spencer G. Niles. Number of faculty: total—full-time 4; women—full-time 3.

Programs and Degrees Offered:
Listed in the following order: Program area, degree type (T if terminal Master's), number awarded 7/08–6/09. Counseling Psychology PhD (Doctor of Philosophy) 4.

APA Accreditation: Counseling PhD (Doctor of Philosophy).

Student Applications/Admissions:
Student Applications
Counseling Psychology PhD (Doctor of Philosophy)—Applications 2009–2010, 65. Total applicants accepted 2009–2010, 5. Number full-time enrolled (new admits only) 2009–2010, 6. Number part-time enrolled (new admits only) 2009–2010, 0. Total enrolled 2009–2010 full-time, 36, part-time, 2. Openings 2010–2011, 6. The median number of years required for completion of a degree in 2008–2009 were 5. The number of students enrolled full- and part-time who were dismissed or voluntarily withdrew from this program area in 2008–2009 were 0.
Other Criteria: (importance of criteria rated low, medium, or high): GRE scores—high, research experience—high, work experience—medium, extracurricular activity—medium, clinically related public service—medium, GPA—high, letters of recommendation—high, interview—high, statement of goals and objectives—high, master's degree—high, undergraduate major in psychology—medium. For additional information on admission requirements, go to http://www.ed.psu.edu/educ/cecprs/counseling-psychology/resourcesforprospectivestudents.

Student Characteristics: The following represents characteristics of students in 2009–2010 in all graduate psychology programs in the department: Female—full-time 27, part-time 0; Male—full-time 10, part-time 0; African American/Black—full-time 7, part-time 0; Hispanic/Latino(a)—full-time 4, part-time 0; Asian/Pacific Islander—full-time 4, part-time 0; American Indian/Alaska Native—full-time 0, part-time 0; Caucasian/White—full-time 22, part-time 0; Multi-ethnic—full-time 0, part-time 0; students subject to the Americans With Disabilities Act—full-time 1, part-time 0; Unknown ethnicity—full-time 0, part-time 0; International students who hold an F-1 or J-1 Visa—full-time 0, part-time 0.

Financial Information/Assistance:
Tuition for Full-Time Study: Doctoral: State residents: per academic year $14,776, $616 per credit hour; Nonstate residents: per academic year $26,392, $1,100 per credit hour. Tuition is subject to change. See the following Web site for updates and changes in tuition costs: http://www.tuition.psu.edu.

Financial Assistance:
First-Year Students: Teaching assistantships available for first year. Average amount paid per academic year: $12,600. Average number of hours worked per week: 20. Research assistantships available for first year. Average amount paid per academic year: $12,600. Average number of hours worked per week: 20. Fellowships and scholarships available for first year. Average amount paid per academic year: $16,100.

Advanced Students: Teaching assistantships available for advanced students. Average amount paid per academic year: $12,600. Average number of hours worked per week: 20. Research assistantships available for advanced students. Average amount paid per academic year: $12,600. Average number of hours worked per week: 20.

Additional Information: Of all students currently enrolled full time, 73% benefited from one or more of the listed financial assistance programs.

Internships/Practica: Doctoral Degree (PhD Counseling Psychology): For those doctoral students for whom a professional internship was required in this program prior to graduation, (6) students applied for an internship in 2008–2009, with (6) students obtaining an internship. Of those students who obtained an internship, (6) were paid internships. Of those students who obtained an internship, (6) students placed in APA/CPA accredited internships, (0) students placed in internships not APA/CPA accredited, but listed with the Association of Psychology Postdoctoral and Internship Programs (APPIC), (0) students placed in internships conforming to guidelines of the Council of Directors of School Psychology Programs (CDSPP), (0) students placed in internships that were not APA/CPA accredited, APPIC or CDSPP listed. Students are placed in practica in the College of Education Counseling Service in their first semester. Supervision consists of 1 and 1/2 hours of individual supervision and a two-hour seminar. The same supervision and seminar arrangements are provided for the second practicum at Penn State's Career Services. A counseling psychology faculty member conducts the seminar and coordinates the interaction of students with the staff at Career Services. Although the program does not require students to be on campus during the summer, most students continue their practicum work at Penn State's Counseling and Psychological Services (CAPS) during the summer of their first year and for Fall and Spring of their second year. At CAPS, in addition to a two-hour seminar for case discussion and presentation, individual supervision is provided by the members of the CAPS staff and interns from their APA-approved internship program. Students must also take an additional 1-semester practicum in their third year either at Centre Volunteers in Medicine or an inpatient psychiatric hospital, both in town. Students typically apply for internships in their third or fourth year and go on internship in their fourth or fifth year. The program specifies that students apply to and accept only APA-approved internship positions.

Housing and Day Care: On-campus housing is available. See the following Web site for more information: http://www.hfs.psu.edu/universitypark/. On-campus day care facilities are available: http://www.ohr.psu.edu/WorkLife/childsub.cfm.

GRADUATE STUDY IN PSYCHOLOGY

Employment of Department Graduates:
Master's Degree Graduates: Of those who graduated in the academic year 2008–2009, the following categories and numbers represent the postgraduate activities and employment of master's degree graduates: Enrolled in a postdoctoral residency/fellowship (n/a), employed in independent practice (n/a), total from the above (master's) (0).
Doctoral Degree Graduates: Of those who graduated in the academic year 2008–2009, the following categories and numbers represent the postgraduate activities and employment of doctoral degree graduates: Enrolled in a psychology doctoral program (n/a), employed in other positions at a higher education institution (6), employed in a community mental health/counseling center (1), total from the above (doctoral) (7).

Additional Information:
Orientation, Objectives, and Emphasis of Department: The Counseling Psychology program at The Pennsylvania State University endorses the scientist–practitioner model of training. Psychological training is provided within this model with equal emphasis and value placed on both scholarly and clinical work as well as their integration. A primary goal of the program is the preparation of counseling psychologists for professional roles as academics, researchers, or practitioners who are concerned with interventions involving individual behavior and institutional settings which are focused on relational, multicultural, career, and psychosocial issues. More specifically, the primary objective of Penn State's Counseling Psychology program is to train carefully selected and promising graduate students to function as thoughtful, ethical, caring, and competent professional psychologists. Whereas the Counseling Psychology program is fully accredited by the American Psychological Association, our faculty and students strive to exceed the standards required for accreditation. One particular area in which we attempt to do so is in engendering a multicultural perspective in our students. At Penn State, we do not merely recognize the diversity represented in our faculty, students, and clients, we actively affirm the richness of our cultures and we embrace the continual challenge of examining ourselves to determine how to more effectively serve a pluralistic society.

Special Facilities or Resources: The department maintains a Resource Center that includes many of the professional journals, reference, and testing materials pertinent to the curriculum. Doctoral students are provided offices, when available, with access to personal computers. The university provides each student with an e-mail account. The College of Education Counseling Service is located in the building and provides practicum experiences for graduate students. The Service is coordinated by a licensed psychologist and serves clients from the campus, providing personal, academic, and vocational counseling. The Service has individual counseling rooms equipped for video recording and live observation through one-way mirrors.

Information for Students With Physical Disabilities: See the following Web site for more information: http://www.equity.psu.edu/ods/.

Application Information:
Send to Counseling Psychology Doctoral Program, 327 Cedar Bldg., Penn State, University Park, PA 16802. Application available online. URL of online application: http://www.ed.psu.edu/educ/cecprs/counseling-psychology/admissionsinfo/. Students are admitted in the Fall, application deadline December 15. *Fee:* $65.

Pennsylvania State University
Department of Psychology
111 Bruce V. Moore Building
University Park, PA 16802-3104
Telephone: (814) 863-1721
Fax: (814) 863-7002
E-mail: *sbg4@psu.edu*
Web: *http://psych.la.psu.edu*

Department Information:
1933. Department of Psychology: Melvin M. Mark. Number of faculty: total—full-time 56, part-time 4; women—full-time 24, part-time 2; total—minority—full-time 8; women minority—full-time 4, part-time 2.

Programs and Degrees Offered:
Listed in the following order: Program area, degree type (T if terminal Master's), number awarded 7/08–6/09. Clinical Psychology PhD (Doctor of Philosophy) 2, Clinical Child Psychology PhD (Doctor of Philosophy) 4, Cognitive Psychology PhD (Doctor of Philosophy) 5, Developmental Psychology PhD (Doctor of Philosophy) 0, Industrial/Organizational Psychology PhD (Doctor of Philosophy) 11, Social Psychology PhD (Doctor of Philosophy) 1.

APA Accreditation: Clinical PhD (Doctor of Philosophy).

Student Applications/Admissions:
Student Applications
Clinical Psychology PhD (Doctor of Philosophy)—Applications 2009–2010, 170. Total applicants accepted 2009–2010, 5. Number full-time enrolled (new admits only) 2009–2010, 5. Total enrolled 2009–2010 full-time, 30, part-time, 1. Openings 2010–2011, 5. The median number of years required for completion of a degree in 2008–2009 were 7. The number of students enrolled full- and part-time who were dismissed or voluntarily withdrew from this program area in 2008–2009 were 1. Clinical Child Psychology PhD (Doctor of Philosophy)—Applications 2009–2010, 140. Total applicants accepted 2009–2010, 4. Number full-time enrolled (new admits only) 2009–2010, 4. Total enrolled 2009–2010 full-time, 22, part-time, 1. Openings 2010–2011, 4. The median number of years required for completion of a degree in 2008–2009 were 7. The number of students enrolled full- and part-time who were dismissed or voluntarily withdrew from this program area in 2008–2009 were 2. Cognitive Psychology PhD (Doctor of Philosophy)—Applications 2009–2010, 34. Total applicants accepted 2009–2010, 4. Number full-time enrolled (new admits only) 2009–2010, 4. Openings 2010–2011, 4. The median number of years required for completion of a degree in 2008–2009 were 5. The number of students enrolled full- and part-time who were dismissed or voluntarily withdrew from this program area in 2008–2009 were 1. Developmental Psychology PhD (Doctor of Philosophy)—Applications 2009–2010, 20. Total applicants accepted 2009–2010, 3. Number full-time enrolled (new admits only) 2009–2010, 3. Total enrolled 2009–2010 full-

time, 12. Openings 2010–2011, 3. The number of students enrolled full- and part-time who were dismissed or voluntarily withdrew from this program area in 2008–2009 were 1. *Industrial/Organizational Psychology PhD (Doctor of Philosophy)*—Applications 2009–2010, 88. Total applicants accepted 2009–2010, 4. Number full-time enrolled (new admits only) 2009–2010, 4. Openings 2010–2011, 4. The median number of years required for completion of a degree in 2008–2009 were 5. The number of students enrolled full- and part-time who were dismissed or voluntarily withdrew from this program area in 2008–2009 were 0. *Social Psychology PhD (Doctor of Philosophy)*—Applications 2009–2010, 48. Total applicants accepted 2009–2010, 2. Number full-time enrolled (new admits only) 2009–2010, 2. Openings 2010–2011, 3. The median number of years required for completion of a degree in 2008–2009 were 5. The number of students enrolled full- and part-time who were dismissed or voluntarily withdrew from this program area in 2008–2009 were 0.

Other Criteria: (importance of criteria rated low, medium, or high): GRE scores—high, research experience—high, work experience—medium, extracurricular activity—low, clinically related public service—medium, GPA—high, letters of recommendation—high, interview—high, statement of goals and objectives—high, undergraduate major in psychology—medium, specific undergraduate psychology courses taken—medium. Clinical weighs work, clinical experience, and interviews heavily; other areas do not weight these factors strongly. For additional information on admission requirements, go to http://psych.la.psu.edu.

Student Characteristics: The following represents characteristics of students in 2009–2010 in all graduate psychology programs in the department: Female—full-time 80, part-time 3; Male—full-time 38, part-time 0; African American/Black—full-time 5, part-time 2; Hispanic/Latino(a)—full-time 6, part-time 1; Asian/Pacific Islander—full-time 7, part-time 1; American Indian/Alaska Native—full-time 1, part-time 0; Caucasian/White—full-time 90, part-time 1; Multi-ethnic—full-time 0, part-time 0; students subject to the Americans With Disabilities Act—full-time 0, part-time 0; Unknown ethnicity—full-time 0, part-time 0; International students who hold an F-1 or J-1 Visa—full-time 5, part-time 1.

Financial Information/Assistance:
Tuition for Full-Time Study: *Doctoral*: State residents: per academic year $15,705; Nonstate residents: per academic year $15,705. Tuition is subject to change. See the following Web site for updates and changes in tuition costs: http://www.tuition.psu.edu.

Financial Assistance:
First-Year Students: Teaching assistantships available for first year. Average amount paid per academic year: $15,705. Average number of hours worked per week: 20. Apply by December 1. Research assistantships available for first year. Average amount paid per academic year: $15,705. Average number of hours worked per week: 20. Apply by December 1. Fellowships and scholarships available for first year. Average amount paid per academic year: $20,000. Average number of hours worked per week: 0. Apply by December 1.

Advanced Students: Teaching assistantships available for advanced students. Average amount paid per academic year: $15,705. Average number of hours worked per week: 20. Research assistantships available for advanced students. Average amount paid per academic year: $15,705. Average number of hours worked per week: 20. Fellowships and scholarships available for advanced students. Average amount paid per academic year: $20,000. Average number of hours worked per week: 0.

Additional Information: Of all students currently enrolled full time, 85% benefited from one or more of the listed financial assistance programs.

Internships/Practica: Doctoral Degree (PhD Clinical Psychology): For those doctoral students for whom a professional internship was required in this program prior to graduation, (2) students applied for an internship in 2008–2009, with (2) students obtaining an internship. Of those students who obtained an internship, (2) were paid internships. Of those students who obtained an internship, (2) students placed in APA/CPA accredited internships, (0) students placed in internships not APA/CPA accredited, but listed with the Association of Psychology Postdoctoral and Internship Programs (APPIC), (0) students placed in internships conforming to guidelines of the Council of Directors of School Psychology Programs (CDSPP), (0) students placed in internships that were not APA/CPA accredited, APPIC or CDSPP listed. Doctoral Degree (PhD Clinical Child Psychology): For those doctoral students for whom a professional internship was required in this program prior to graduation, (3) students applied for an internship in 2008–2009, with (3) students obtaining an internship. Of those students who obtained an internship, (3) were paid internships. Of those students who obtained an internship, (3) students placed in APA/CPA accredited internships, (0) students placed in internships not APA/CPA accredited, but listed with the Association of Psychology Postdoctoral and Internship Programs (APPIC), (0) students placed in internships conforming to guidelines of the Council of Directors of School Psychology Programs (CDSPP), (0) students placed in internships that were not APA/CPA accredited, APPIC or CDSPP listed.

Housing and Day Care: On-campus housing is available. See the following Web site for more information: http://www.hfs.psu.edu/universitypark. On-campus day care facilities are available.

Employment of Department Graduates:
Master's Degree Graduates: Of those who graduated in the academic year 2008–2009, the following categories and numbers represent the postgraduate activities and employment of master's degree graduates: Enrolled in a postdoctoral residency/fellowship (n/a), employed in independent practice (n/a), total from the above (master's) (0).

Doctoral Degree Graduates: Of those who graduated in the academic year 2008–2009, the following categories and numbers represent the postgraduate activities and employment of doctoral degree graduates: Enrolled in a psychology doctoral program (n/a), enrolled in a postdoctoral residency/fellowship (11), employed in independent practice (0), employed in an academic position at a university (11), employed in an academic position at a 2-year/4-year college (0), employed in business or industry (4), employed in a community mental health/counseling center (6), still seeking employment (3), total from the above (doctoral) (35).

Additional Information:
Orientation, Objectives, and Emphasis of Department: Graduate study in psychology at Penn State is characterized by highly

flexible, individualized programs leading to the PhD in Psychology. Each student is associated with one of the five program areas offered in the department: clinical (including child clinical); cognitive; developmental; industrial/organizational; and social. Students in any program area may combine their program of study with a specialization in behavioral neuroscience by choosing appropriate courses and seminars. Students choosing this specialization may pursue the integration of neuroscience methods and theories by applying these approaches to research topics within their program areas. Within each area, certain courses are usually suggested for all students. The details of a student's program, however, are worked out on an individual basis with a faculty advisor. A major specialization and breadth outside the major are required. The major is selected from among the six specialty areas of the department listed above; breadth requirements are flexible and individualized to career goals. Depending upon the individual student's particular program of study, graduates may be employed in academic departments, research institutes, industry, governmental agencies, or various service delivery settings.

Special Facilities or Resources: The department has clinical, learning-cognition, perception, physiological, psychophysiology, developmental and social laboratories; microcomputer laboratories; access to the University's mainframe and electronic communication system (e-mail and Internet) and computer laboratories; clinical practica in local mental health centers and hospitals in addition to the department's Psychological Clinic, which functions as a mental health center for the catchment area of central Pennsylvania; industrial/organizational practica in industrial and government organizations; developmental practica and research opportunities in day care and preschool settings. A number of centers or institutes are housed within or affiliated with the department, including a new Child Study Center.

Application Information:
Send to Graduate Admissions, Department of Psychology, Penn State University, 110 Moore Building, University Park, PA 16802. Application available online. URL of online application: http://psych.la.psu.edu. Students are admitted in the Fall, application deadline December 1. *Fee:* $65.

Pennsylvania State University (2009 data)
Program in School Psychology
College of Education
125 Cedar Building
University Park, PA 16802
Telephone: (814) 865-1881
Fax: (814) 865-7066
E-mail: jcd12@psu.edu
Web: http://espse.ed.psu.edu/schoolpsych/

Department Information:
1965. Professor-in-Charge: James C. DiPerna. Number of faculty: total—full-time 4, part-time 1; women—full-time 3; total—minority—full-time 1; women minority—full-time 1.

Programs and Degrees Offered:
Listed in the following order: Program area, degree type (T if terminal Master's), number awarded 7/08–6/09. School PhD (Doctor of Philosophy) 7.

APA Accreditation: School PhD (Doctor of Philosophy).

Student Applications/Admissions:
Student Applications
School PhD (Doctor of Philosophy)—Applications 2009–2010, 87. Total applicants accepted 2009–2010, 22. Number full-time enrolled (new admits only) 2009–2010, 8. Number part-time enrolled (new admits only) 2009–2010, 0. Openings 2010–2011, 6. The median number of years required for completion of a degree in 2008–2009 were 8. The number of students enrolled full- and part-time who were dismissed or voluntarily withdrew from this program area in 2008–2009 were 0.
Other Criteria: (importance of criteria rated low, medium, or high): GRE scores—medium, research experience—medium, work experience—medium, clinically related public service—low, GPA—medium, letters of recommendation—high, interview—high, statement of goals and objectives—high.

Student Characteristics: The following represents characteristics of students in 2009–2010 in all graduate psychology programs in the department: Female—full-time 24, part-time 0; Male—full-time 2, part-time 0; African American/Black—full-time 1, part-time 0; Hispanic/Latino(a)—full-time 0, part-time 0; Asian/Pacific Islander—full-time 1, part-time 0; American Indian/Alaska Native—full-time 0, part-time 0; Caucasian/White—full-time 24, part-time 0; Multi-ethnic—full-time 0, part-time 0; students subject to the Americans With Disabilities Act—full-time 0, part-time 0; Unknown ethnicity—full-time 0, part-time 0; International students who hold an F-1 or J-1 Visa—full-time 0, part-time 0.

Financial Information/Assistance:
Tuition for Full-Time Study: *Doctoral:* State residents: per academic year $14,776; Nonstate residents: per academic year $26,392. Tuition is subject to change. Additional fees are assessed to students beyond the costs of tuition for the following: technology, facility, and activities. See the following Web site for updates and changes in tuition costs: http://www.bursar.psu.edu/.

Financial Assistance:
First-Year Students: Teaching assistantships available for first year. Average amount paid per academic year: $13,150. Average number of hours worked per week: 20. Apply by December 15. Research assistantships available for first year. Average amount paid per academic year: $13,150. Average number of hours worked per week: 20. Apply by December 15. Fellowships and scholarships available for first year. Average amount paid per academic year: $16,000. Average number of hours worked per week: 0. Apply by December 15.

Advanced Students: Teaching assistantships available for advanced students. Average amount paid per academic year: $13,150. Average number of hours worked per week: 20. Research assistantships available for advanced students. Average amount paid per academic year: $13,150. Average number of hours worked per week: 20. Fellowships and scholarships available for advanced

students. Average amount paid per academic year: $16,000. Average number of hours worked per week: 0. Apply by April 1.

Additional Information: Of all students currently enrolled full time, 100% benefited from one or more of the listed financial assistance programs. Application and information available online at: http://www.psu.edu/dept/studentaid.

Internships/Practica: All students complete a minimum of 1,000 practicum hours devoted to assessment, intervention, consultation, and supervision activities. Students also complete a 1,500 hour internship under the supervision of a psychologist licensed for professional practice and certified as a school psychologist. All students obtain paid internships, and at least half of their internship hours must be completed in a school setting.

Housing and Day Care: On-campus housing is available. See the following Web site for more information: http://www.hfs.psu.edu/housing/graduates/. On-campus day care facilities are available. See the following Web site for more information: http://www.hhdev.psu.edu/hdfs/cp/.

Employment of Department Graduates:
Master's Degree Graduates: Of those who graduated in the academic year 2008–2009, the following categories and numbers represent the postgraduate activities and employment of master's degree graduates: Enrolled in a psychology doctoral program (0), enrolled in another graduate/professional program (0), enrolled in a postdoctoral residency/fellowship (n/a), employed in independent practice (n/a), employed in an academic position at a university (0), employed in an academic position at a 2-year/4-year college (0), employed in other positions at a higher education institution (0), employed in a professional position in a school system (0), employed in business or industry (0), employed in government agency (0), employed in a community mental health/counseling center (0), employed in a hospital/medical center (0), still seeking employment (0), not seeking employment (0), other employment position (0), do not know (0), total from the above (master's) (0).
Doctoral Degree Graduates: Of those who graduated in the academic year 2008–2009, the following categories and numbers represent the postgraduate activities and employment of doctoral degree graduates: Enrolled in a psychology doctoral program (n/a), enrolled in another graduate/professional program (0), enrolled in a postdoctoral residency/fellowship (0), employed in independent practice (0), employed in an academic position at a university (0), employed in an academic position at a 2-year/4-year college (0), employed in other positions at a higher education institution (0), employed in a professional position in a school system (7), employed in business or industry (0), employed in government agency (0), employed in a community mental health/counseling center (0), employed in a hospital/medical center (0), still seeking employment (0), other employment position (0), do not know (0), total from the above (doctoral) (7).

Additional Information:
Orientation, Objectives, and Emphasis of Department: School psychologists from Penn State are exemplary scientist/practitioners, firmly grounded in both psychology and education. Our graduates are professional school psychologists who provide solutions for the many problems facing children. They contribute to the practice and knowledge base of psychology as it relates to education. Penn State school psychologists become leaders in the field as well as in academia. In conjunction with providing psychological services, school psychologists will be life-long learners who sustain an interest in maintaining and developing sound practices, which derive from up-to-date, research-based information. Psychologists will thoughtfully and critically evaluate their practices and remain informed consumers of available literature, assessment tools, and intervention strategies. School psychologists will help to provide a bridge to integrate research with professional practice along with other educators, systems, and institutions.

Special Facilities or Resources: The School Psychology program operates the CEDAR School Psychology Clinic. The CEDAR Clinic contains well appointed clinic rooms with direct observation facilities and a closed-circuit video system, which facilitate practicum supervision. Computers are available to students within the program, department, and university. Access to e-mail and the Internet are provided to all students and use of technology is encouraged by faculty. The Pattee and Paterno Libraries house an impressive array of scholarly resources. As a major research university, Penn State sponsors a number of research institutes and centers in education, psychology, and human development.

Information for Students With Physical Disabilities: See the following Web site for more information: http://www.equity.psu.edu/ods/index.html.

Application Information:
Send to Graduate Programs in School Psychology, Admissions Committee, 125C Cedar Bldg., Pennsylvania State University, University Park, PA 16802. Application available online. URL of online application: http://espse.ed.psu.edu. Students are admitted in the Fall, application deadline December 15. *Fee:* $60.

Pennsylvania State University, The
Department of Human Development and Family Studies, Graduate Program in Human Development and Family Studies
College of Health and Human Development
S-211 Henderson Building
University Park, PA 16802
Telephone: (814) 863-8000
Fax: (814) 863-7963
E-mail: *dmt16@psu.edu*
Web: *http://www.hhdev.psu.edu/hdfs/grad/index.html*

Department Information:
1974. Professor in Charge of Graduate Program: Douglas Teti. Number of faculty: total—full-time 34; women—full-time 16; total—minority—full-time 5; women minority—full-time 5.

Programs and Degrees Offered:
Listed in the following order: Program area, degree type (T if terminal Master's), number awarded 7/08–6/09. Human Development and Family Studies PhD (Doctor of Philosophy) 6.

Student Applications/Admissions:
Student Applications
Human Development and Family Studies PhD (Doctor of Philosophy)—Applications 2009–2010, 65. Total applicants accepted

2009–2010, 20. Number full-time enrolled (new admits only) 2009–2010, 15. Number part-time enrolled (new admits only) 2009–2010, 0. Openings 2010–2011, 10. The median number of years required for completion of a degree in 2008–2009 were 5. The number of students enrolled full- and part-time who were dismissed or voluntarily withdrew from this program area in 2008–2009 were 0.

Other Criteria: (importance of criteria rated low, medium, or high): GRE scores—high, research experience—high, work experience—low, extracurricular activity—low, GPA—high, letters of recommendation—high, interview—low, statement of goals and objectives—high, writing sample—high.

Student Characteristics: The following represents characteristics of students in 2009–2010 in all graduate psychology programs in the department: Female—full-time 66, part-time 0; Male—full-time 13, part-time 0; African American/Black—full-time 3, part-time 0; Hispanic/Latino(a)—full-time 3, part-time 0; Asian/Pacific Islander—full-time 8, part-time 0; American Indian/Alaska Native—full-time 0, part-time 0; Caucasian/White—full-time 0, part-time 0; Multi-ethnic—full-time 0, part-time 0; students subject to the Americans With Disabilities Act—full-time 0, part-time 0; Unknown ethnicity—full-time 0, part-time 0; International students who hold an F-1 or J-1 Visa—full-time 0, part-time 0.

Financial Information/Assistance:
Tuition for Full-Time Study: Doctoral: State residents: per academic year $19,937, $616 per credit hour; Nonstate residents: per academic year $26,738, $1,100 per credit hour. Tuition is subject to change. See the following Web site for updates and changes in tuition costs: http://tuition.psu.edu.

Financial Assistance:
First-Year Students: Teaching assistantships available for first year. Average amount paid per academic year: $15,705. Average number of hours worked per week: 20. Apply by January 5. Research assistantships available for first year. Average amount paid per academic year: $15,705. Average number of hours worked per week: 20. Apply by January 5. Fellowships and scholarships available for first year. Average amount paid per academic year: $16,100. Average number of hours worked per week: 10. Apply by January 5.

Advanced Students: Teaching assistantships available for advanced students. Average amount paid per academic year: $15,705. Average number of hours worked per week: 20. Apply by September. Research assistantships available for advanced students. Average amount paid per academic year: $15,705. Average number of hours worked per week: 20. Apply by September.

Additional Information: Of all students currently enrolled full time, 100% benefited from one or more of the listed financial assistance programs. Application and information available online at: http://www.hhdev.psu.edu/hdfs/grad/aid.html.

Housing and Day Care: On-campus housing is available. On-campus day care facilities are available. http://www.hhdev.psu.edu/hdfs/cp/cdl/.

Employment of Department Graduates:
Master's Degree Graduates: Of those who graduated in the academic year 2008–2009, the following categories and numbers represent the postgraduate activities and employment of master's degree graduates: Enrolled in a postdoctoral residency/fellowship (n/a), employed in independent practice (n/a), total from the above (master's) (0).

Doctoral Degree Graduates: Of those who graduated in the academic year 2008–2009, the following categories and numbers represent the postgraduate activities and employment of doctoral degree graduates: Enrolled in a psychology doctoral program (n/a), enrolled in another graduate/professional program (0), enrolled in a postdoctoral residency/fellowship (7), employed in independent practice (0), employed in an academic position at a university (2), employed in an academic position at a 2-year/4-year college (0), employed in other positions at a higher education institution (2), employed in a professional position in a school system (0), employed in business or industry (1), employed in government agency (0), employed in a community mental health/counseling center (0), employed in a hospital/medical center (0), still seeking employment (0), not seeking employment (0), other employment position (0), do not know (1), total from the above (doctoral) (13).

Additional Information:
Orientation, Objectives, and Emphasis of Department: The basic objectives of the human development and family studies (HDFS) program are the following: to expand knowledge about the development and functioning of individuals, small groups, and families; to improve methods for studying processes of human development and change; and to create and disseminate improved techniques and strategies for enhancing individual and family functioning, helping people learn to cope more effectively with problems of living, and preventing normal life problems from becoming serious difficulties. The program takes a life-span perspective, recognizing that the most important aspects of development and types of life tasks and situations vary from infancy and childhood through maturity and old age, as well as through the life cycle of the family, and that each phase of development is a precursor to the next. There is a firm commitment to an interdisciplinary and multiprofessional approach to these objectives and to the development of competence in applying rigorous methods of empirical inquiry. All students are expected to acquire a broad interdisciplinary base of knowledge and to develop competence in depth in one of four primary program areas: family development, individual development, human development intervention, or methodology.

Special Facilities or Resources: Several additional facilities are associated with the College of Health and Human Development that provide significant resources to our Department, in terms of graduate training opportunities and student funding. These include the Child Development Laboratory and Bennett Family Center, which are high quality early child care programs providing care to children from early infancy through kindergarten. Each unit has observational rooms for the study of individual and group behavior of children and adults. Our students also avail themselves of the resources provided by several College-based centers, including the Prevention Research Center for the Promotion of

Human Development, the Methodology Center, the Methodology Consulting Center, the Center for Childhood Obesity, the Center for Human Development and Family Research in Diverse Contexts, and the Gerontology Center. All of these centers are directed by HDFS faculty and provide a variety of funding and training opportunities for our graduate students. The Centers are direct outgrowths of our program's four core areas: Individual Development, Prevention/Intervention, Methodology, and Family Development.

Application Information:
Send to Graduate Admissions c/o Mary Jo Spicer, Penn State University, Department of Human Development and Family Studies, S211Henderson Building, University Park, PA 16802. Application available online. URL of online application: http://www.gradsch.psu.edu/portal. Students are admitted in the Fall, application deadline January 5. *Fee:* $65.

Pennsylvania, University of
Applied Psychology-Human Development Division
Graduate School of Education
3700 Walnut Street
Philadelphia, PA 19104-6216
Telephone: (215) 898-4176
Fax: (215) 573-2115
E-mail: *evelynj@gse.upenn.edu*
Web: *http://www.gse.upenn.edu/aphd/*

Department Information:
1975. Chair, Applied Psychology-Human Development Division: Michael J. Nakkula, Ed.D. Number of faculty: total—full-time 8, part-time 17; women—full-time 3, part-time 9; total—minority—full-time 3, part-time 8; women minority—full-time 1, part-time 2.

Programs and Degrees Offered:
Listed in the following order: Program area, degree type (T if terminal Master's), number awarded 7/08–6/09. Counseling and Psychological Services MEd (Education) 42, Interdisciplinary Studies in Human Development MA/MS (Master of Arts/Science) 11, Interdisciplinary Studies in Human Development PhD (Doctor of Philosophy) 6, Professional Counseling and Psychology Other 12, School Counseling Certification Other 0, School & Mental Health Counseling MEd (Education) 19.

Student Applications/Admissions:
Student Applications
Counseling and Psychological Services MEd (Education)—Applications 2009–2010, 122. Total applicants accepted 2009–2010, 60. Number full-time enrolled (new admits only) 2009–2010, 33. Number part-time enrolled (new admits only) 2009–2010, 9. Total enrolled 2009–2010 full-time, 40, part-time, 4. Openings 2010–2011, 35. The median number of years required for completion of a degree in 2008–2009 was 1. The number of students enrolled full- and part-time who were dismissed or voluntarily withdrew from this program area in 2008–2009 were 0. *Interdisciplinary Studies in Human Development MA/MS (Master of Arts/Science)*—Applications 2009–2010, 45. Total applicants accepted 2009–2010, 23. Number full-time enrolled (new admits only) 2009–2010, 17. Number part-time enrolled (new admits only) 2009–2010, 2. Total enrolled 2009–2010 full-time, 17, part-time, 13. Openings 2010–2011, 25. The median number of years required for completion of a degree in 2008–2009 was 1. *Interdisciplinary Studies in Human Development PhD (Doctor of Philosophy)*—Applications 2009–2010, 50. Total applicants accepted 2009–2010, 4. Number full-time enrolled (new admits only) 2009–2010, 1. Number part-time enrolled (new admits only) 2009–2010, 0. Openings 2010–2011, 4. The median number of years required for completion of a degree in 2008–2009 were 5. *Professional Counseling and Psychology Other*—Applications 2009–2010, 15. Total applicants accepted 2009–2010, 13. Number full-time enrolled (new admits only) 2009–2010, 10. Number part-time enrolled (new admits only) 2009–2010, 3. Total enrolled 2009–2010 full-time, 10, part-time, 3. Openings 2010–2011, 25. The median number of years required for completion of a degree in 2008–2009 were 2. The number of students enrolled full- and part-time who were dismissed or voluntarily withdrew from this program area in 2008–2009 were 0. *School Counseling Certification Other*—Applications 2009–2010, 13. Total applicants accepted 2009–2010, 12. Number full-time enrolled (new admits only) 2009–2010, 12. Number part-time enrolled (new admits only) 2009–2010, 0. Openings 2010–2011, 20. The median number of years required for completion of a degree in 2008–2009 were 2. *School & Mental Health Counseling MEd (Education)*—Applications 2009–2010, 40. Total applicants accepted 2009–2010, 25. Number full-time enrolled (new admits only) 2009–2010, 22. Number part-time enrolled (new admits only) 2009–2010, 0. Openings 2010–2011, 25. The median number of years required for completion of a degree in 2008–2009 were 2. The number of students enrolled full- and part-time who were dismissed or voluntarily withdrew from this program area in 2008–2009 were 1.

Scores: Entries appear in this order: required test or GPA, minimum score (if required), median score of students entering in 2009–2010. *Counseling and Psychological Services MEd (Education):* GRE-V no minimum stated, GRE-Q no minimum stated, GRE-Analytical no minimum stated; *Interdisciplinary Studies in Human Development MA/MS (Master of Arts/Science):* GRE-V no minimum stated, GRE-Q no minimum stated, GRE-Analytical no minimum stated; *Interdisciplinary Studies in Human Development PhD (Doctor of Philosophy):* GRE-V no minimum stated, GRE-Q no minimum stated, GRE-Analytical no minimum stated, GRE-Subject (Psychology) no minimum stated; *Professional Counseling and Psychology Other:* GRE-V no minimum stated, GRE-Q no minimum stated, GRE-Analytical no minimum stated; *School Counseling Certification Other:* GRE-V no minimum stated, GRE-Q no minimum stated, GRE-Analytical no minimum stated.

Other Criteria: (importance of criteria rated low, medium, or high): GRE scores—high, research experience—medium, work experience—medium, extracurricular activity—medium, clinically related public service—medium, GPA—high, letters of recommendation—high, interview—high, statement of goals and objectives—high, undergraduate major in psychology—medium, specific undergraduate psychology courses taken—medium. For additional information on admission requirements, go to http://www.gse.upenn.edu/admissions_financial/howtoapply.

GRADUATE STUDY IN PSYCHOLOGY

Student Characteristics: The following represents characteristics of students in 2009–2010 in all graduate psychology programs in the department: Female—full-time 110, part-time 17; Male—full-time 14, part-time 3; African American/Black—full-time 19, part-time 1; Hispanic/Latino(a)—full-time 7, part-time 0; Asian/Pacific Islander—full-time 16, part-time 7; American Indian/Alaska Native—full-time 0, part-time 0; Caucasian/White—full-time 72, part-time 12; Multi-ethnic—full-time 6, part-time 0; students subject to the Americans With Disabilities Act—full-time 4, part-time 0; Unknown ethnicity—full-time 4, part-time 0; International students who hold an F-1 or J-1 Visa—full-time 8, part-time 3.

Financial Information/Assistance:
Tuition for Full-Time Study: *Master's:* State residents: per academic year $35,144, $4,450 per credit hour; Nonstate residents: per academic year $35,144, $4,450 per credit hour. Tuition costs vary by program. See the following Web site for updates and changes in tuition costs: http://www.gse.upenn.edu/admissions_financial/tuition.

Financial Assistance:
First-Year Students: Teaching assistantships available for first year. Average number of hours worked per week: 20. Apply by December 15. Research assistantships available for first year. Average number of hours worked per week: 20. Apply by December 15. Fellowships and scholarships available for first year. Average number of hours worked per week: 20. Apply by December 15.
Advanced Students: Teaching assistantships available for advanced students. Average number of hours worked per week: 20. Research assistantships available for advanced students. Average number of hours worked per week: 20. Fellowships and scholarships available for advanced students. Average number of hours worked per week: 20.
Additional Information: Of all students currently enrolled full time, 85% benefited from one or more of the listed financial assistance programs. Application and information available online at: http://www.gse.upenn.edu/admissions_financial/finaid.

Internships/Practica: Master's students in Counseling and Psychological Services engage in supervised practica for 8 hours a week for two semesters. Placements include schools, community colleges, career services, clinics, and community agencies. MPhil students are required to complete a supervised two-semester, 20-hour per week internship. The Executive Program in School and Mental Health Counseling is an executive-style master's-degree program for working educators and professionals interested in working as school counselors or Licensed Professional Counselors. The program requires a practicum and an internship.

Housing and Day Care: On-campus housing is available. See the following Web site for more information: http://www.business-services.upenn.edu/housing/. On-campus day care facilities are available. See the following Web site for more information: http://www.business-services.upenn.edu/childcare/.

Employment of Department Graduates:
Master's Degree Graduates: Of those who graduated in the academic year 2008–2009, the following categories and numbers represent the postgraduate activities and employment of master's degree graduates: Enrolled in a postdoctoral residency/fellowship (n/a), employed in independent practice (n/a), total from the above (master's) (0).
Doctoral Degree Graduates: Of those who graduated in the academic year 2008–2009, the following categories and numbers represent the postgraduate activities and employment of doctoral degree graduates: Enrolled in a psychology doctoral program (n/a); total from the above (doctoral) (0).

Additional Information:
Orientation, Objectives, and Emphasis of Department: Our programs provide a foundation in the core concepts of applied psychology: intervention, prevention, assessment, learning/development, and applied practice and/or research, for careers in counseling, mental health, teaching, and research in various settings. The one-year Counseling and Psychological Services (CAPS) master's program prepares students in the foundations of providing supportive services. The MPhil Program in Professional Counseling and Psychology is a continuation for current CAPS students. The Executive Program in School & Mental Health Counseling (SMHC) enables students with full time careers to earn their degree in two years through one-weekend-a-month and one-week-in-summer sessions. The MPhil and SMHC programs prepare students for guidance counseling certification and/or licensure as a professional counselor. The Interdisciplinary Studies in Human Development PhD and MS.Ed. programs combine the study of social, emotional, cognitive, and physical aspects of human development that are focused on urban populations, considered within eco-cultural contexts, and relevant to social policies. Students create a specialized program of study of human development across the lifespan. Career interests: traditional academic appointment; youth programming/services; urban/ethnic studies; adult development/learning; corporate human resources development; international programming (e.g., work with NGOs); foundation administration/program development; collaborative efforts/health care facilities.

Special Facilities or Resources: Penn GSE houses state-of-the-art computer labs and classrooms, student lounges, and offers wireless access. Many opportunities exist for students to participate in the Faculty's new and ongoing research that addresses issues of local, national and international populations.

Information for Students With Physical Disabilities: See the following Web site for more information: http://www.college.upenn.edu/support/sds.php.

Application Information:
Send to Admissions Office, Graduate School of Education, Univ. of Pennsylvania, 3700 Walnut St. Philadelphia, PA 19104-6216. Application available online. URL of online application: https://app.applyyourself.com; Summer, application deadline See below; Programs have rolling admissions. Deadline for applications to the PhD program in Interdisciplinary Studies in Human Development is December 15. Executive Program in School and Mental Health Counseling M.S.Ed. deadline is June 15. Counseling and Psychological Services, M.S.Ed., Interdisciplinary Studies in Human Development M.S.Ed. and Professional Counseling and Psychology M.Phil. applications are accepted on a rolling basis for Fall Admission only. *Fee:* $0.

Pennsylvania, University of
Department of Psychology
3720 Walnut Street
Philadelphia, PA 19104
Telephone: (215) 898-7300
Fax: (215) 898-7301
E-mail: *greermb@psych.upenn.edu*
Web: *http://www.psych.upenn.edu/graduate*

Department Information:
1887. Chairperson: Dr. Robert DeRubeis. Number of faculty: total—full-time 29; women—full-time 10; total—minority—full-time 2; women minority—full-time 2.

Programs and Degrees Offered:
Listed in the following order: Program area, degree type (T if terminal Master's), number awarded 7/08–6/09. Psychology PhD (Doctor of Philosophy) 6, Clinical Psychology PhD (Doctor of Philosophy) 4.

APA Accreditation: Clinical PhD (Doctor of Philosophy).

Student Applications/Admissions:
Student Applications
Psychology PhD (Doctor of Philosophy)—Applications 2009–2010, 195. Total applicants accepted 2009–2010, 15. Number full-time enrolled (new admits only) 2009–2010, 6. Total enrolled 2009–2010 full-time, 28. Openings 2010–2011, 6. The median number of years required for completion of a degree in 2008–2009 were 6. The number of students enrolled full- and part-time who were dismissed or voluntarily withdrew from this program area in 2008–2009 were 0. *Clinical Psychology PhD (Doctor of Philosophy)*—Applications 2009–2010, 246. Total applicants accepted 2009–2010, 7. Number full-time enrolled (new admits only) 2009–2010, 2. Total enrolled 2009–2010 full-time, 26. Openings 2010–2011, 4. The median number of years required for completion of a degree in 2008–2009 were 6. The number of students enrolled full- and part-time who were dismissed or voluntarily withdrew from this program area in 2008–2009 were 0.
Scores: Entries appear in this order: required test or GPA, minimum score (if required), median score of students entering in 2009–2010. *Psychology PhD (Doctor of Philosophy)*: GRE-V no minimum stated, GRE-Q no minimum stated, GRE-Analytical no minimum stated; *Clinical Psychology PhD (Doctor of Philosophy)*: GRE-V no minimum stated, GRE-Q no minimum stated, GRE-Analytical no minimum stated.
Other Criteria: (importance of criteria rated low, medium, or high): GRE scores—medium, research experience—high, work experience—low, clinically related public service—low, GPA—medium, letters of recommendation—high, interview—medium, statement of goals and objectives—high. For additional information on admission requirements, go to http://www.psych.upenn.edu.

Student Characteristics: The following represents characteristics of students in 2009–2010 in all graduate psychology programs in the department: Female—full-time 34, part-time 0; Male—full-time 20, part-time 0; African American/Black—full-time 0, part-time 0; Hispanic/Latino(a)—full-time 1, part-time 0; Asian/Pacific Islander—full-time 8, part-time 0; American Indian/Alaska Native—full-time 0, part-time 0; Caucasian/White—full-time 41, part-time 0; Multi-ethnic—full-time 0, part-time 0; students subject to the Americans With Disabilities Act—full-time 0, part-time 0; Unknown ethnicity—full-time 4, part-time 0; International students who hold an F-1 or J-1 Visa—full-time 13, part-time 0.

Financial Information/Assistance:
Financial Assistance:
First-Year Students: Traineeships available for first year. Average number of hours worked per week: 12. Apply by December 15. Fellowships and scholarships available for first year. Average number of hours worked per week: 12. Apply by December 15.
Advanced Students: Teaching assistantships available for advanced students. Average number of hours worked per week: 12. Apply by December 15. Research assistantships available for advanced students. Average number of hours worked per week: 12. Apply by December 15. Traineeships available for advanced students. Average number of hours worked per week: 12. Apply by December 15. Fellowships and scholarships available for advanced students. Average number of hours worked per week: 12. Apply by December 15.
Additional Information: Of all students currently enrolled full time, 100% benefited from one or more of the listed financial assistance programs.

Internships/Practica: Doctoral Degree (PhD Clinical Psychology): For those doctoral students for whom a professional internship was required in this program prior to graduation, (6) students applied for an internship in 2008–2009, with (6) students obtaining an internship. Of those students who obtained an internship, (6) were paid internships. Of those students who obtained an internship, (6) students placed in APA/CPA accredited internships, (0) students placed in internships not APA/CPA accredited, but listed with the Association of Psychology Postdoctoral and Internship Programs (APPIC), (0) students placed in internships conforming to guidelines of the Council of Directors of School Psychology Programs (CDSPP), (0) students placed in internships that were not APA/CPA accredited, APPIC or CDSPP listed. Because of the wealth of opportunities for clinical training in the Philadelphia area, Penn does not run an in-house psychological services clinic. Rather, Penn's clinical students have the opportunity to participate in practica at local hospitals, clinics and research facilities staffed and run by world-renowned clinical scientists. The Associate Director of Clinical Training helps students decide which practicum experiences best suit the student's needs and interests, and arranges for placements at the appropriate sites.

Housing and Day Care: On-campus housing is available. See the following Web site for more information: http://www.upenn.edu/campus/housing.php. On-campus day care facilities are available.

Employment of Department Graduates:
Master's Degree Graduates: Of those who graduated in the academic year 2008–2009, the following categories and numbers represent the postgraduate activities and employment of master's degree graduates: Enrolled in a postdoctoral residency/fellowship (n/a), employed in independent practice (n/a), total from the above (master's) (0).

Doctoral Degree Graduates: Of those who graduated in the academic year 2008–2009, the following categories and numbers represent the postgraduate activities and employment of doctoral degree graduates: Enrolled in a psychology doctoral program (n/a), enrolled in a postdoctoral residency/fellowship (6), employed in an academic position at a university (1), total from the above (doctoral) (7).

Additional Information:
Orientation, Objectives, and Emphasis of Department: The Department of Psychology at the University of Pennsylvania offers curricular and research opportunities for the study of sensation, perception, cognition, cognitive neuroscience, decision-making, language, learning, motivation, emotion, motor control, psychopathology, and social processes. Biological, cultural, developmental, comparative, experimental, and mathematical approaches to these areas are used in ongoing teaching and research. The department has an APA-accredited clinical program that is designed to prepare students for research careers in interventions, psychopathology and personality. The interests of the faculty and students in the department cover the entire field of research-oriented psychology. Still, the Department of Psychology at Pennsylvania functions as a single unit whose guiding principle is scientific excellence. The primary determinant of acceptance is academic promise rather than specific area of interest. Faculty join together from different subdisciplines for teaching and research purposes so that students become conversant with issues in a number of different areas. A high level of interaction among department members (students and faculty), within and across disciplines, helps generate both a shared set of interests in the theoretical, historical, and philosophical foundations of psychology and active collaboration in research projects. The first-year program is divided between courses that introduce various areas of psychology and a focused research experience. A deep involvement in research continues throughout the graduate program, and is supplemented by participation in seminars, the weekly departmental colloquium, teaching, and general intellectual give and take.

Special Facilities or Resources: The department has facilities for functional magnetic resonance imaging, transcranial magnetic stimulation, high density electroencephalograhy and magneto encephalography, high speed computing capabilities, and high frequency electrophysiology recording. In addition, the department supports a fully equipped wood, metal, and electronics shop. Also readily available for research in the near environs of the department are 4 major University-affiliated hospitals, and urban public and private schools.

Information for Students With Physical Disabilities: See the following Web site for more information: http://www.vpul.upenn.edu/lrc/sds/.

Application Information:
Send to Graduate School of Arts and Sciences, 3401 Walnut Street, Suite 322A, Philadelphia, PA 19104. Application available online. URL of online application: https://app.applyyourself.com/?id=upenn-g. Students are admitted in the Fall, application deadline December 15. *Fee:* $70.

Philadelphia College of Osteopathic Medicine
Psychology Department
4190 City Avenue
Philadelphia, PA 19131-1693
Telephone: (215) 871-6442
Fax: (215) 871-6458
E-mail: *RobertD@pcom.edu*
Web: *http://www.pcom.edu*

Department Information:
1995. Chairperson: Robert A. DiTomasso, PhD, ABPP. Number of faculty: total—full-time 18, part-time 61; women—full-time 11, part-time 36; total—minority—full-time 2, part-time 7; women minority—full-time 1, part-time 4.

Programs and Degrees Offered:
Listed in the following order: Program area, degree type (T if terminal Master's), number awarded 7/08–6/09. Organizational Development and Leadership MA/MS (Master of Arts/Science) (T) 16, School Psychology MA/MS (Master of Arts/Science) (T) 23, School Psychology EdS (School Psychology) 18, Psychology CAGS Other 22, Counseling & Clinical Health Psychology MA/MS (Master of Arts/Science) (T) 32, Clinical Psychology Respecialization Diploma 0, Clinical Psychology PsyD (Doctor of Psychology) 31, School Psychology PsyD (Doctor of Psychology) 18, Clinical Health Psychology Certificate Other 0, Clinical Neuropsychology Certificate Other 0, School Psychology Respecialization Diploma 0.

APA Accreditation: Clinical PsyD (Doctor of Psychology). Student Outcome Data Website: http://www.pcom.edu/Academic_Programs/aca_psych/PsyD_in_Clinical_Psychology/APA_Disclosure_Statements.html. Clinical PsyD (Doctor of Psychology).

Student Applications/Admissions:
Student Applications

Organizational Development and Leadership MA/MS (Master of Arts/Science)—Applications 2009–2010, 45. Total applicants accepted 2009–2010, 22. Number full-time enrolled (new admits only) 2009–2010, 9. Number part-time enrolled (new admits only) 2009–2010, 11. Total enrolled 2009–2010 full-time, 27, part-time, 30. Openings 2010–2011, 25. The median number of years required for completion of a degree in 2008–2009 were 2. The number of students enrolled full- and part-time who were dismissed or voluntarily withdrew from this program area in 2008–2009 were 2. *School Psychology MA/MS (Master of Arts/Science)*—Applications 2009–2010, 51. Total applicants accepted 2009–2010, 31. Number full-time enrolled (new admits only) 2009–2010, 20. Number part-time enrolled (new admits only) 2009–2010, 0. Openings 2010–2011, 20. The median number of years required for completion of a degree in 2008–2009 was 1. The number of students enrolled full- and part-time who were dismissed or voluntarily withdrew from this program area in 2008–2009 were 0. *School Psychology EdS (School Psychology)*—Applications 2009–2010, 37. Total applicants accepted 2009–2010, 26. Number full-time enrolled (new admits only) 2009–2010, 24. Number part-time enrolled (new admits only) 2009–2010, 0. Openings 2010–2011, 20. The median number of years required for completion of a degree in 2008–2009 were 3. The number of students enrolled full- and part-time who were dismissed or voluntarily withdrew from this program area in 2008–2009 were 2. *Psychology CAGS Other*—Applications 2009–2010, 32. Total applicants accepted 2009–2010, 12. Number part-time enrolled (new admits only) 2009–2010, 9. Openings 2010–2011, 15. The median number of years required for completion of a degree in 2008–2009 was 1. The number of students enrolled full- and part-time who were dismissed or voluntarily withdrew from this program area in 2008–2009 were 0. *Counseling & Clinical Health Psychology MA/MS (Master of Arts/Science)*—Applications 2009–2010, 149. Total applicants accepted 2009–2010, 61. Number full-time enrolled (new admits only) 2009–2010, 37. Number part-time enrolled (new admits only) 2009–2010, 3. Total enrolled 2009–2010 full-time, 67, part-time, 9. Openings 2010–2011, 33. The median number of years required for completion of a degree in 2008–2009 were 2. The number of students enrolled full- and part-time who were dismissed or voluntarily withdrew from this program area in 2008–2009 were 1. *Clinical Psychology Respecialization Diploma*—Applications 2009–2010, 0. Total applicants accepted 2009–2010, 0. Number full-time enrolled (new admits only) 2009–2010, 0. Number part-time enrolled (new admits only) 2009–2010, 0. Openings 2010–2011, 2. The number of students enrolled full- and part-time who were dismissed or voluntarily withdrew from this program area in 2008–2009 were 0. *Clinical Psychology PsyD (Doctor of Psychology)*—Applications 2009–2010, 126. Total applicants accepted 2009–2010, 46. Number full-time enrolled (new admits only) 2009–2010, 31. Number part-time enrolled (new admits only) 2009–2010, 0. Openings 2010–2011, 28. The median number of years required for completion of a degree in 2008–2009 were 6. The number of students enrolled full- and part-time who were dismissed or voluntarily withdrew from this program area in 2008–2009 were 1. *School Psychology PsyD (Doctor of Psychology)*—Applications 2009–2010, 29. Total applicants accepted 2009–2010, 21. Number full-time enrolled (new admits only) 2009–2010, 16. Number part-time enrolled (new admits only) 2009–2010, 0. Openings 2010–2011, 15. The median number of years required for completion of a degree in 2008–2009 were 4. The number of students enrolled full- and part-time who were dismissed or voluntarily withdrew from this program area in 2008–2009 were 0. *Clinical Health Psychology Certificate Other*—Applications 2009–2010, 0. Total applicants accepted 2009–2010, 0. Number full-time enrolled (new admits only) 2009–2010, 0. Number part-time enrolled (new admits only) 2009–2010, 0. Openings 2010–2011, 6. The number of students enrolled full- and part-time who were dismissed or voluntarily withdrew from this program area in 2008–2009 were 0. *Clinical Neuropsychology Certificate Other*—Applications 2009–2010, 6. Total applicants accepted 2009–2010, 4. Number full-time enrolled (new admits only) 2009–2010, 0. Number part-time enrolled (new admits only) 2009–2010, 3. Openings 2010–2011, 6. The number of students enrolled full- and part-time who were dismissed or voluntarily withdrew from this program area in 2008–2009 were 2. *School Psychology Respecialization Diploma*—Applications 2009–2010, 0. Total applicants accepted 2009–2010, 0. Number full-time enrolled (new admits only) 2009–2010, 0. Number part-time enrolled (new admits only) 2009–2010, 0. Openings 2010–2011, 3. The number of students enrolled full- and part-time who were dismissed or voluntarily withdrew from this program area in 2008–2009 were 0.

Scores: Entries appear in this order: required test or GPA, minimum score (if required), median score of students entering in 2009–2010. *Organizational Development and Leadership MA/MS (Master of Arts/Science)*: overall undergraduate GPA 3.0; *School Psychology MA/MS (Master of Arts/Science)*: overall undergraduate GPA 3.0; *School Psychology EdS (School Psychology)*: overall undergraduate GPA 3.0; *Counseling & Clinical Health Psychology MA/MS (Master of Arts/Science)*: overall undergraduate GPA 3.0; *Clinical Psychology Respecialization Diploma*: overall undergraduate GPA 3.0; *Clinical Psychology PsyD (Doctor of Psychology)*: overall undergraduate GPA 3.0, Masters GPA 3.3; *School Psychology PsyD (Doctor of Psychology)*: overall undergraduate GPA 3.0, Masters GPA 3.0; *Clinical Health Psychology Certificate Other*: overall undergraduate GPA no minimum stated; *Clinical Neuropsychology Certificate Other*: overall undergraduate GPA no minimum stated; *School Psychology Respecialization Diploma*: overall undergraduate GPA no minimum stated.

Other Criteria: (importance of criteria rated low, medium, or high): GRE scores—medium, research experience—low, work experience—high, extracurricular activity—medium, clinically related public service—high, GPA—high, letters of recommendation—high, interview—high, statement of goals and objectives—high, graded writing sample—high, undergraduate major in psychology—medium, specific undergraduate psychology courses taken—medium. A master's degree in psychology or a related field is required for admissions to the Clinical PsyD program. Master's and EdS degrees are admissions requirements for the PsyD in School Psychology program. For additional information on admission requirements, go to http://www.pcom.edu.

Student Characteristics: The following represents characteristics of students in 2009–2010 in all graduate psychology programs in the department: Female—full-time 291, part-time 42; Male—full-time 81, part-time 14; African American/Black—full-time 59, part-time 16; Hispanic/Latino(a)—full-time 11, part-time 3; Asian/Pacific Islander—full-time 13, part-time 2; American Indian/Alaska Native—full-time 1, part-time 0; Caucasian/White—full-time 284, part-time 34; Multi-ethnic—full-time 1, part-time 0; students subject to the Americans With Disabilities Act—full-time 5, part-time 0; Unknown ethnicity—full-time 3, part-time 1; International students who hold an F-1 or J-1 Visa—full-time 2, part-time 0.

Financial Information/Assistance:

Tuition for Full-Time Study: *Master's:* State residents: $667 per credit hour; Nonstate residents: $667 per credit hour. *Doctoral:* State residents: $920 per credit hour; Nonstate residents: $920 per credit hour. Tuition is subject to change. Additional fees are assessed to students beyond the costs of tuition for the following: Comprehensive fee (each term): $117. Tuition costs vary by program. See the following Web site for updates and changes in tuition costs: http://www.pcom.edu/Administration/Administrative_Departments/Bursar_s_Office/do_tuition.html. Higher tuition cost for this program: EdS: $721/credit hour.

Financial Assistance:

First-Year Students: Research assistantships available for first year. Average amount paid per academic year: $6,000. Average number of hours worked per week: 12. Apply by late summer.

Fellowships and scholarships available for first year. Average amount paid per academic year: $1,000.

Advanced Students: Teaching assistantships available for advanced students. Average amount paid per academic year: $1,500. Average number of hours worked per week: 5. Research assistantships available for advanced students. Average amount paid per academic year: $7,200. Average number of hours worked per week: 12. Apply by late summer.

Additional Information: Of all students currently enrolled full time, 7% benefited from one or more of the listed financial assistance programs. Application and information available online at: http://www.pcom.edu.

Internships/Practica: Doctoral Degree (PsyD Clinical Psychology): For those doctoral students for whom a professional internship was required in this program prior to graduation, (18) students applied for an internship in 2008–2009, with (18) students obtaining an internship. Of those students who obtained an internship, (18) were paid internships. Of those students who obtained an internship, (6) students placed in APA/CPA accredited internships, (12) students placed in internships not APA/CPA accredited, but listed with the Association of Psychology Postdoctoral and Internship Programs (APPIC), (0) students placed in internships conforming to guidelines of the Council of Directors of School Psychology Programs (CDSPP), (0) students placed in internships that were not APA/CPA accredited, APPIC or CDSPP listed. Doctoral Degree (PsyD School Psychology): For those doctoral students for whom a professional internship was required in this program prior to graduation, (13) students applied for an internship in 2008–2009, with (13) students obtaining an internship. Of those students who obtained an internship, (5) were paid internships. Of those students who obtained an internship, (2) students placed in APA/CPA accredited internships, (2) students placed in internships not APA/CPA accredited, but listed with the Association of Psychology Postdoctoral and Internship Programs (APPIC), (9) students placed in internships conforming to guidelines of the Council of Directors of School Psychology Programs (CDSPP), (0) students placed in internships that were not APA/CPA accredited, APPIC or CDSPP listed. Master's Degree (MA/MS Organizational Development and Leadership): An internship experience, such as a final research project or "capstone" experience is required of graduates. Practica are fieldwork experiences completed by master's level and doctoral students at a PCOM-approved clinical training site. The minimum weekly hour requirements vary from program to program. Practicum sites are committed to excellence in the training of professionals, and provide extensive supervision and formative clinical experiences. They offer a wide range of training, including the use of empirically supported interventions, brief treatment models, cognitive behavioral therapy, and treatment of psychological/medical problems. Students engage in evaluation, psychological testing (PsyD only), psychotherapy, and professional clinical work. Practica include seminars taught by faculty that provide a place for students to discuss their experiences and help them integrate coursework with on-site training. Students participate in praticum at the Psychology Department's Center for Brief Therapy, a multi-faceted clinical training center, as well as sites including community agencies, hospitals, university counseling centers, prisons, schools, and specialized treatment centers. The department has a broad network of practicum sites in Pennsylvania, New Jersey, Maryland, and Delaware. Students apply for internships through the APPIC matching program.

Housing and Day Care: No on-campus housing is available. No on-campus day care facilities are available.

Employment of Department Graduates:
Master's Degree Graduates: Of those who graduated in the academic year 2008–2009, the following categories and numbers represent the postgraduate activities and employment of master's degree graduates: Enrolled in a psychology doctoral program (5), enrolled in another graduate/professional program (22), enrolled in a postdoctoral residency/fellowship (n/a), employed in independent practice (n/a), employed in other positions at a higher education institution (4), employed in a professional position in a school system (1), employed in business or industry (10), employed in government agency (3), employed in a community mental health/counseling center (19), employed in a hospital/medical center (7), total from the above (master's) (71).

Doctoral Degree Graduates: Of those who graduated in the academic year 2008–2009, the following categories and numbers represent the postgraduate activities and employment of doctoral degree graduates: Enrolled in a psychology doctoral program (n/a), enrolled in a postdoctoral residency/fellowship (19), employed in an academic position at a university (3), employed in an academic position at a 2-year/4-year college (1), employed in a professional position in a school system (17), employed in business or industry (1), employed in a community mental health/counseling center (7), employed in a hospital/medical center (1), total from the above (doctoral) (49).

Additional Information:
Orientation, Objectives, and Emphasis of Department: The mission of the Department of Psychology at PCOM is to prepare highly-skilled, compassionate psychologists and master's level psychological specialists to provide empirically-based, active, focused, and collaborative assessments and treatments with sensitivity to cultural and ethnic diversity and the underserved. Grounded in the cognitive-behavioral tradition, the graduate programs in psychology train practitioner-scholars to offer assessment, intervention, consultation, management, and leadership as local clinical scientists, and to engage in scholarly activities, advocacy, and life-long learning in the field of psychology. The PCOM Department of Psychology offers graduate programs in psychology at several levels to suit a variety of professional needs and interests.

Special Facilities or Resources: The academic facilities at PCOM include state-of-the-art amphitheaters and classroom facilities, computer laboratories with extensive software including PsycLIT and SPSS, a recently renovated library that includes sophisticated online resources, and the HealthNet teleconferencing system. The Center for Brief Therapy, a mental health clinic housed in the Department of Psychology, provides multi-faceted clinical training and research opportunities for students. PCOM also has three neighborhood health care centers in Philadelphia and one in LaPorte, Pennsylvania.

Information for Students With Physical Disabilities: See the following Web site for more information: http://www.pcom.edu/Student_Life/Student_Affairs_Main/Academic_Personal.htm.

Application Information:
Send to Philadelphia College of Osteopathic Medicine, Department of Admissions, 4170 City Avenue, Philadelphia, PA 19131. Application available online. URL of online application: http://www.pcom.edu/

General_Information/apply_now.html. The PsyD in Clinical Psychology, EdS in School Psychology, MS in Counseling & Clinical Health Psychology, and CAGS programs admit students in the fall term only. The MS in School Psychology and PsyD in School Psychology programs admit students in the summer term only. The MS in ODL program admits during all terms. *Fee:* $50.

Pittsburgh, University of
Department of Psychology in Education
School of Education
5930 Posvar Hall
Pittsburgh, PA 15260
Telephone: (412) 624-7230
Fax: (412) 624-7231
E-mail: *johnson@pitt.edu*
Web: *http://www.education.pitt.edu*

Department Information:
1986. Chairman: Carl Johnson. Number of faculty: total—full-time 6, part-time 4; women—full-time 3, part-time 3.

Programs and Degrees Offered:
Listed in the following order: Program area, degree type (T if terminal Master's), number awarded 7/08–6/09. Applied Developmental Psychology MA/MS (Master of Arts/Science) 38, Applied Developmental Psychology PhD (Doctor of Philosophy) 5.

Student Applications/Admissions:
Student Applications
Applied Developmental Psychology MA/MS (Master of Arts/Science)—Applications 2009–2010, 99. Total applicants accepted 2009–2010, 84. Number full-time enrolled (new admits only) 2009–2010, 7. Number part-time enrolled (new admits only) 2009–2010, 53. Total enrolled 2009–2010 full-time, 42, part-time, 42. Openings 2010–2011, 40. The median number of years required for completion of a degree in 2008–2009 were 2.
Applied Developmental Psychology PhD (Doctor of Philosophy)—Applications 2009–2010, 31. Total applicants accepted 2009–2010, 5. Number full-time enrolled (new admits only) 2009–2010, 0. Number part-time enrolled (new admits only) 2009–2010, 0. Total enrolled 2009–2010 full-time, 18, part-time, 6. Openings 2010–2011, 6.
Other Criteria: (importance of criteria rated low, medium, or high): GRE scores—medium, research experience—medium, work experience—medium, extracurricular activity—low, clinically related public service—medium, GPA—medium, letters of recommendation—medium, statement of goals and objectives—high, specific undergraduate psychology courses taken—high. For additional information on admission requirements, go to http://www.education.pitt.edu/.

Student Characteristics: The following represents characteristics of students in 2009–2010 in all graduate psychology programs in the department: Female—full-time 44, part-time 32; Male—full-time 1, part-time 5; African American/Black—full-time 7, part-time 12; Hispanic/Latino(a)—full-time 0, part-time 1; Asian/Pacific Islander—full-time 9, part-time 1; American Indian/Alaska Native—full-time 0, part-time 0; Caucasian/White—full-time 35, part-time 40; Multi-ethnic—full-time 0, part-time 0; students subject to the Americans With Disabilities Act—full-time 0, part-time 0; Unknown ethnicity—full-time 0, part-time 0; International students who hold an F-1 or J-1 Visa—full-time 0, part-time 0.

Financial Information/Assistance:
Tuition for Full-Time Study: *Master's:* State residents: per academic year $16,462, $640 per credit hour; Nonstate residents: per academic year $28,686, $1,147 per credit hour. *Doctoral:* State residents: per academic year $16,462, $640 per credit hour; Nonstate residents: per academic year $28,686, $1,147 per credit hour. See the following Web site for updates and changes in tuition costs: http://www.is.pitt.edu/tuition.

Financial Assistance:
First-Year Students: Teaching assistantships available for first year. Average amount paid per academic year: $7,532. Average number of hours worked per week: 10. Research assistantships available for first year. Average amount paid per academic year: $15,065. Average number of hours worked per week: 20.
Advanced Students: Teaching assistantships available for advanced students. Average amount paid per academic year: $7,532. Average number of hours worked per week: 10. Research assistantships available for advanced students. Average amount paid per academic year: $15,065. Average number of hours worked per week: 20.
Additional Information: Of all students currently enrolled full time, 20% benefited from one or more of the listed financial assistance programs. Application and information available online at: http://www.oafa.pitt.edu/fahome.aspx.

Internships/Practica: The Applied Developmental Program maintains extensive connections with community organizations that provide opportunities for internships in programs that serve children, youth and families in many different capacities.

Housing and Day Care: No on-campus housing is available. On-campus day care facilities are available. http://www.hr.pitt.edu/ucdc.

Employment of Department Graduates:
Master's Degree Graduates: Of those who graduated in the academic year 2008–2009, the following categories and numbers represent the postgraduate activities and employment of master's degree graduates: Enrolled in a postdoctoral residency/fellowship (n/a), employed in independent practice (n/a), total from the above (master's) (0).
Doctoral Degree Graduates: Of those who graduated in the academic year 2008–2009, the following categories and numbers represent the postgraduate activities and employment of doctoral degree graduates: Enrolled in a psychology doctoral program (n/a), total from the above (doctoral) (0).

Additional Information:
Orientation, Objectives, and Emphasis of Department: The Master of Science degree in Applied Developmental Psychology emphasizes the integration of knowledge of human development with the skills and expertise essential for developing, implementing and evaluating effective programs for children, youth and families. Graduates of the program pursue professional careers as program administrators and child development specialists in areas such as teaching, research and professional practice.

GRADUATE STUDY IN PSYCHOLOGY

Special Facilities or Resources: The Applied Developmental Program is closely allied with several leading research, policy and service organizations in the University including the Learning Policy Center, the Office of Child Development and the University, Community, Leaders, and Individuals with Disabilities (UCLID) Center.

Information for Students With Physical Disabilities: See the following Web site for more information: http://www.drs.pitt.edu/.

Application Information:
Send to University of Pittsburgh School of Education, Student Service Center, 5500 Wesley W. Posvar Hall, Pittsburgh, PA 15260. Application available online. URL of online application: http://www.education.pitt.edu/. Students are admitted in the Fall, application deadline March 1. Applications after the deadlines are seriously considered if all the places are not filled. *Fee:* $50.

Pittsburgh, University of
Psychology
Arts and Sciences
3129 Sennott Square, 210 South Bouquet Street
Pittsburgh, PA 15260
Telephone: (412) 624-4502
Fax: (412) 624-4428
E-mail: *psygrad@pitt.edu*
Web: *http://www.psychology.pitt.edu*

Department Information:
1904. Chairperson: Daniel Shaw. Number of faculty: total—full-time 39, part-time 8; women—full-time 16, part-time 4; total—minority—full-time 3; women minority—full-time 2.

Programs and Degrees Offered:
Listed in the following order: Program area, degree type (T if terminal Master's), number awarded 7/08–6/09. Clinical Psychology PhD (Doctor of Philosophy) 5, Cognitive Psychology PhD (Doctor of Philosophy) 1, Developmental Psychology PhD (Doctor of Philosophy) 0, Biological and Health Psychology PhD (Doctor of Philosophy) 0, Individualized PhD (Doctor of Philosophy) 1, Social Psychology PhD (Doctor of Philosophy) 0.

APA Accreditation: Clinical PhD (Doctor of Philosophy). Student Outcome Data Website: http://www.psychology.pitt.edu/graduate/clinical/index.php.

Student Applications/Admissions:
Student Applications
Clinical Psychology PhD (Doctor of Philosophy)—Applications 2009–2010, 312. Total applicants accepted 2009–2010, 8. Number full-time enrolled (new admits only) 2009–2010, 4. Openings 2010–2011, 5. The median number of years required for completion of a degree in 2008–2009 were 8. The number of students enrolled full- and part-time who were dismissed or voluntarily withdrew from this program area in 2008–2009 were 0. Cognitive Psychology PhD (Doctor of Philosophy)—Applications 2009–2010, 61. Total applicants accepted 2009–2010, 8. Number full-time enrolled (new admits only) 2009–2010, 5. Openings 2010–2011, 4. The median number of years required for completion of a degree in 2008–2009 were 6. The number of students enrolled full- and part-time who were dismissed or voluntarily withdrew from this program area in 2008–2009 were 1. Developmental Psychology PhD (Doctor of Philosophy)—Applications 2009–2010, 30. Total applicants accepted 2009–2010, 2. Number full-time enrolled (new admits only) 2009–2010, 1. Openings 2010–2011, 2. The number of students enrolled full- and part-time who were dismissed or voluntarily withdrew from this program area in 2008–2009 were 1. Biological and Health Psychology PhD (Doctor of Philosophy)—Applications 2009–2010, 27. Total applicants accepted 2009–2010, 2. Number full-time enrolled (new admits only) 2009–2010, 1. Total enrolled 2009–2010 full-time, 4. Openings 2010–2011, 3. The number of students enrolled full- and part-time who were dismissed or voluntarily withdrew from this program area in 2008–2009 were 0. Individualized PhD (Doctor of Philosophy)—Applications 2009–2010, 8. Total applicants accepted 2009–2010, 1. Number full-time enrolled (new admits only) 2009–2010, 1. Openings 2010–2011, 1. The median number of years required for completion of a degree in 2008–2009 were 10. The number of students enrolled full- and part-time who were dismissed or voluntarily withdrew from this program area in 2008–2009 were 0. Social Psychology PhD (Doctor of Philosophy)—Applications 2009–2010, 17. Total applicants accepted 2009–2010, 0. Number full-time enrolled (new admits only) 2009–2010, 0. Openings 2010–2011, 2. The number of students enrolled full- and part-time who were dismissed or voluntarily withdrew from this program area in 2008–2009 were 1.

Other Criteria: (importance of criteria rated low, medium, or high): GRE scores—high, research experience—high, work experience—medium, extracurricular activity—low, clinically related public service—low, GPA—high, letters of recommendation—high, interview—high, statement of goals and objectives—medium. For additional information on admission requirements, go to http://www.psychology.pitt.edu.

Student Characteristics: The following represents characteristics of students in 2009–2010 in all graduate psychology programs in the department: Female—full-time 87, part-time 0; Male—full-time 13, part-time 0; African American/Black—full-time 3, part-time 0; Hispanic/Latino(a)—full-time 6, part-time 0; Asian/Pacific Islander—full-time 7, part-time 0; American Indian/Alaska Native—full-time 0, part-time 0; Caucasian/White—full-time 84, part-time 0; Multi-ethnic—full-time 0, part-time 0; students subject to the Americans With Disabilities Act—full-time 1, part-time 0; Unknown ethnicity—full-time 0, part-time 0; International students who hold an F-1 or J-1 Visa—full-time 10, part-time 0.

Financial Information/Assistance:
Tuition for Full-Time Study: *Doctoral:* State residents: per academic year $17,052, $665 per credit hour; Nonstate residents: per academic year $29,344, $1,175 per credit hour. Tuition is subject to change. See the following Web site for updates and changes in tuition costs: http://www.ir.pitt.edu/tuition.

Financial Assistance:
First-Year Students: Teaching assistantships available for first year. Average amount paid per academic year: $15,065. Average number of hours worked per week: 20. Apply by December

1. Research assistantships available for first year. Average amount paid per academic year: $13,600. Average number of hours worked per week: 20. Apply by December 1. Traineeships available for first year. Average amount paid per academic year: $20,000. Apply by December 1. Fellowships and scholarships available for first year. Average amount paid per academic year: $17,972. Apply by December 1.

Advanced Students: Teaching assistantships available for advanced students. Average amount paid per academic year: $15,675. Average number of hours worked per week: 20. Research assistantships available for advanced students. Average amount paid per academic year: $13,600. Average number of hours worked per week: 20. Traineeships available for advanced students. Average amount paid per academic year: $20,000. Fellowships and scholarships available for advanced students. Average amount paid per academic year: $17,972.

Additional Information: Of all students currently enrolled full time, 100% benefited from one or more of the listed financial assistance programs. Application and information available online at: http://www.oafa.pitt.edu/fahome.aspx.

Internships/Practica: Doctoral Degree (PhD Clinical Psychology): For those doctoral students for whom a professional internship was required in this program prior to graduation, (9) students applied for an internship in 2008–2009, with (9) students obtaining an internship. Of those students who obtained an internship, (9) were paid internships. Of those students who obtained an internship, (9) students placed in APA/CPA accredited internships, (0) students placed in internships not APA/CPA accredited, but listed with the Association of Psychology Postdoctoral and Internship Programs (APPIC), (0) students placed in internships conforming to guidelines of the Council of Directors of School Psychology Programs (CDSPP), (0) students placed in internships that were not APA/CPA accredited, APPIC or CDSPP listed.

Housing and Day Care: No on-campus housing is available. On-campus day care facilities are available. See the following Web site for more information: http://www.hr.pitt.edu/ucdc/.

Employment of Department Graduates:
Master's Degree Graduates: Of those who graduated in the academic year 2008–2009, the following categories and numbers represent the postgraduate activities and employment of master's degree graduates: Enrolled in a postdoctoral residency/fellowship (n/a), employed in independent practice (n/a), total from the above (master's) (0).
Doctoral Degree Graduates: Of those who graduated in the academic year 2008–2009, the following categories and numbers represent the postgraduate activities and employment of doctoral degree graduates: Enrolled in a psychology doctoral program (n/a), enrolled in a postdoctoral residency/fellowship (4), employed in an academic position at a university (1), employed in business or industry (1), employed in a hospital/medical center (1), total from the above (doctoral) (7).

Additional Information:
Orientation, Objectives, and Emphasis of Department: Basic research training is emphasized, and most projects involve research with important practical implications. The graduate programs include Clinical Psychology, Cognitive Psychology and Cognitive Neuroscience, Developmental Psychology, Biological and Health Psychology, Social Psychology, and joint programs in Clinical-Developmental and Clinical-Health Psychology. Some examples of training opportunities are projects on infant socialization, cognitive, language and social development of children, psychological stress on the cardiovascular and immune systems, nicotine and alcohol use, decision making in groups, stereotyping, reading processes, school and non-school learning, and brain models of attention and reading. Seminars are small (5-12 students), and close working relationships are encouraged with faculty, especially the student's advisor. Excellent relationships with other departments and schools offer unusually flexible opportunities to carry out interdisciplinary work and gain access to scholars in the Pittsburgh community. All students are expected to teach at least one course, and carry out an original research dissertation. Financial support is available for students through teaching, research, and fellowships.

Special Facilities or Resources: The facilities of the department include experimental laboratories, extensive computer facilities, a small-group laboratory, the Clinical Psychology Center, and the laboratories of the Learning Research and Development Center. These services offer the advanced graduate student opportunities for supervised practicum and research experience. The department also maintains cooperative arrangements with many organizations in Pittsburgh engaged in various kinds of psychological work. These include the Brain Imaging Research Center, Children's Hospital, Pittsburgh Cancer Institute, the Western Psychiatric Institute and Clinic, and several local agencies of the Veterans Administration Medical Centers. Collaboration with these organizations consists of part-time instruction by the staff of these agencies, the sharing of laboratory and clinical facilities, and the appointment in those organizations of graduate students in psychology as clinical or research assistants.

Information for Students With Physical Disabilities: See the following Web site for more information: http://www.drs.pitt.edu/.

Application Information:
Application available online. URL of online application: http://www.psychology.pitt.edu. Students are admitted in the Fall, application deadline December 1. *Fee:* $50. Fees deferred for McNair Scholars.

Saint Joseph's University
Department of Psychology
5600 City Avenue
Philadelphia, PA 19131-1395
Telephone: (610) 660-1800
Fax: (610) 660-1819
E-mail: *jmindell@sju.edu*
Web: *http://www.sju.edu/psychology*

Department Information:
1960. Director, Graduate Psychology Program: Jodi A. Mindell, PhD Number of faculty: total—full-time 12; women—full-time 6; total—minority—full-time 1; women minority—full-time 1.

Programs and Degrees Offered:
Listed in the following order: Program area, degree type (T if terminal Master's), number awarded 7/08–6/09. Experimental MA/MS (Master of Arts/Science) (T) 19.

GRADUATE STUDY IN PSYCHOLOGY

Student Applications/Admissions:
Student Applications
Experimental MA/MS (Master of Arts/Science)—Applications 2009–2010, 52. Total applicants accepted 2009–2010, 20. Number full-time enrolled (new admits only) 2009–2010, 20. Openings 2010–2011, 18. The median number of years required for completion of a degree in 2008–2009 were 2. The number of students enrolled full- and part-time who were dismissed or voluntarily withdrew from this program area in 2008–2009 were 1.
Other Criteria: (importance of criteria rated low, medium, or high): GRE scores—medium, research experience—high, work experience—low, extracurricular activity—medium, clinically related public service—low, GPA—high, letters of recommendation—high, statement of goals and objectives—medium, undergraduate major in psychology—medium, specific undergraduate psychology courses taken—high.

Student Characteristics: The following represents characteristics of students in 2009–2010 in all graduate psychology programs in the department: Female—full-time 27, part-time 0; Male—full-time 7, part-time 0; African American/Black—full-time 3, part-time 0; Hispanic/Latino(a)—full-time 0, part-time 0; Asian/Pacific Islander—full-time 0, part-time 0; American Indian/Alaska Native—full-time 0, part-time 0; Caucasian/White—full-time 31, part-time 0; Multi-ethnic—full-time 0, part-time 0; students subject to the Americans With Disabilities Act—full-time 0, part-time 0; Unknown ethnicity—full-time 0, part-time 0; International students who hold an F-1 or J-1 Visa—full-time 0, part-time 0.

Financial Information/Assistance:
Tuition for Full-Time Study: *Master's:* State residents: $768 per credit hour; Nonstate residents: $768 per credit hour.

Financial Assistance:
First-Year Students: No information provided.
Advanced Students: Teaching assistantships available for advanced students. Average amount paid per academic year: $7,200. Average number of hours worked per week: 20. Research assistantships available for advanced students. Average amount paid per academic year: $7,200. Average number of hours worked per week: 20.
Additional Information: Of all students currently enrolled full time, 30% benefited from one or more of the listed financial assistance programs.

Internships/Practica: Master's Degree (MA/MS Experimental): An internship experience, such as a final research project or "capstone" experience is required of graduates.

Housing and Day Care: No on-campus housing is available. On-campus day care facilities are available. See the following Web site for more information: Children's School at St. John's at http://www.stjohnlm.org/address.html.

Employment of Department Graduates:
Master's Degree Graduates: Of those who graduated in the academic year 2008–2009, the following categories and numbers represent the postgraduate activities and employment of master's degree graduates: Enrolled in a psychology doctoral program (9), enrolled in a postdoctoral residency/fellowship (n/a), employed in independent practice (n/a), employed in business or industry (4), employed in a hospital/medical center (5), total from the above (master's) (18).
Doctoral Degree Graduates: Of those who graduated in the academic year 2008–2009, the following categories and numbers represent the postgraduate activities and employment of doctoral degree graduates: Enrolled in a psychology doctoral program (n/a), total from the above (doctoral) (0).

Additional Information:
Orientation, Objectives, and Emphasis of Department: The Saint Joseph's University graduate program in Experimental Psychology is designed to provide students with a solid grounding in the scientific study of psychology. Graduates of the program will have a firm foundation in the scientific method and the skills with which to pursue the scientific study of psychological questions. The program offers a traditional and academically oriented 36-credit curriculum, which requires a qualifying comprehensive examination and an empirical thesis project. The program is designed for successful completion over two academic years. Additionally, a five-year combined Bachelor/Master of Science degree in psychology is offered. The Saint Joseph's University psychology graduate program has been constructed to complement the strengths and interests of the present psychology faculty and facilities and to reflect the current state of the discipline of psychology. The curriculum is composed of three major components: an 8-credit common core required of all students; 24 credits of content based courses; and a 16-credit research component in which students complete the comprehensive examination and research thesis.

Special Facilities or Resources: All psychology faculty have equipped and active research laboratories in which graduate students pursue independent research projects for completion of their thesis requirement. Support facilities for graduate-level research and education are impressive. A vivarium, certifiable by the United States Public Health Service, for the housing of animal subjects is in operation and is fully staffed. For research involving human subjects, the department coordinates a subject pool consisting of approximately 300 subjects per semester. Additionally, the Psychology Department at Saint Joseph's operates PsyNet, a state-of-the-art Macintosh-AppleShare local area network which is attached to a campus-wide computer network through an EtherNet connection. PsyNet consists of 35 Macintosh computers and peripherals for all faculty and staff plus fileservers and laser printers. Two student computer classrooms/laboratories which include an additional 20 computers are also available within the department. PsyNet software includes various word processing, statistical, spreadsheet, database, graphics, and simulation packages.

Application Information:
Send to Graduate Admissions Office, Saint Joseph's University, 5600 City Avenue, Philadelphia, PA 19131-1395. Students are admitted in the Fall, application deadline March 1. *Fee:* $35.

Temple University (2009 data)
Department of Psychological Studies in Education
Education
Ritter Hall Annex, 2nd Floor, 1301 Cecil B. Moore Avenue
Philadelphia, PA 19122
Telephone: (215) 204-6009
Fax: (215) 204-6013
E-mail: *joseph.ducette@temple.edu*
Web: *http://www.temple.edu/education*

Department Information:
1984. Chairperson, Psychological studies in Ed.: Joseph P. DuCette. Number of faculty: total—full-time 19, part-time 119; women—full-time 8, part-time 108; total—minority—full-time 1, part-time 10; women minority—full-time 1, part-time 5.

Programs and Degrees Offered:
Listed in the following order: Program area, degree type (T if terminal Master's), number awarded 7/08–6/09. School Psychology PhD (Doctor of Philosophy) 8, Educational Psychology PhD (Doctor of Philosophy) 9, Adult & Organizational Development MA/MS (Master of Arts/Science) (T) 10, Counseling Psychology MA/MS (Master of Arts/Science) (T) 30, School Psychology (Master of Arts/Science) 3.

APA Accreditation: School PhD (Doctor of Philosophy).

Student Applications/Admissions:
Student Applications
School Psychology PhD (Doctor of Philosophy)—Applications 2009–2010, 40. Total applicants accepted 2009–2010, 6. Number full-time enrolled (new admits only) 2009–2010, 3. Total enrolled 2009–2010 full-time, 56, part-time, 7. Openings 2010–2011, 4. The median number of years required for completion of a degree in 2008–2009 were 7. The number of students enrolled full- and part-time who were dismissed or voluntarily withdrew from this program area in 2008–2009 were 2. *Educational Psychology PhD (Doctor of Philosophy)*—Applications 2009–2010, 23. Total applicants accepted 2009–2010, 10. Number full-time enrolled (new admits only) 2009–2010, 3. Number part-time enrolled (new admits only) 2009–2010, 3. Total enrolled 2009–2010 full-time, 20, part-time, 34. Openings 2010–2011, 8. The median number of years required for completion of a degree in 2008–2009 were 7. The number of students enrolled full- and part-time who were dismissed or voluntarily withdrew from this program area in 2008–2009 were 3. *Adult & Organizational Development MA/MS (Master of Arts/Science)*—Applications 2009–2010, 20. Total applicants accepted 2009–2010, 15. Number full-time enrolled (new admits only) 2009–2010, 5. Number part-time enrolled (new admits only) 2009–2010, 15. Total enrolled 2009–2010 full-time, 10, part-time, 20. Openings 2010–2011, 15. The median number of years required for completion of a degree in 2008–2009 were 2. The number of students enrolled full- and part-time who were dismissed or voluntarily withdrew from this program area in 2008–2009 were 0. *Counseling Psychology MA/MS (Master of Arts/Science)*—Applications 2009–2010, 60. Total applicants accepted 2009–2010, 30. Number full-time enrolled (new admits only) 2009–2010, 20. Number part-time enrolled (new admits only) 2009–2010, 10. Total enrolled 2009–2010 full-time, 40, part-time, 20. Openings 2010–2011, 30. The median number of years required for completion of a degree in 2008–2009 were 2. The number of students enrolled full- and part-time who were dismissed or voluntarily withdrew from this program area in 2008–2009 were 3. *School Psychology MA/MS (Master of Arts/Science)*—Applications 2009–2010, 25. Number full-time enrolled (new admits only) 2009–2010, 5. Number part-time enrolled (new admits only) 2009–2010, 2. Total enrolled 2009–2010 full-time, 7, part-time, 4. Openings 2010–2011, 10. The median number of years required for completion of a degree in 2008–2009 were 3. The number of students enrolled full- and part-time who were dismissed or voluntarily withdrew from this program area in 2008–2009 were 0.

Other Criteria: (importance of criteria rated low, medium, or high): GRE scores—medium, research experience—medium, work experience—medium, extracurricular activity—medium, clinically related public service—low, GPA—high, letters of recommendation—high, interview—high, statement of goals and objectives—high.

Student Characteristics: The following represents characteristics of students in 2009–2010 in all graduate psychology programs in the department: Female—full-time 100, part-time 75; Male—full-time 49, part-time 75; African American/Black—full-time 20, part-time 20; Hispanic/Latino(a)—full-time 4, part-time 4; Asian/Pacific Islander—full-time 3, part-time 3; American Indian/Alaska Native—full-time 0, part-time 0; Caucasian/White—full-time 0, part-time 0; Multi-ethnic—full-time 0, part-time 0; students subject to the Americans With Disabilities Act—full-time 3, part-time 2; Unknown ethnicity—full-time 0, part-time 0; International students who hold an F-1 or J-1 Visa—full-time 0, part-time 0.

Financial Information/Assistance:
Tuition for Full-Time Study: *Master's:* State residents: $590 per credit hour; Nonstate residents: $861 per credit hour. *Doctoral:* State residents: $590 per credit hour; Nonstate residents: $861 per credit hour. Tuition is subject to change. See the following Web site for updates and changes in tuition costs: http://www.temple.edu/bursar/about/tuitionrates.htm.

Financial Assistance:
First-Year Students: Fellowships and scholarships available for first year. Average amount paid per academic year: $18,000. Average number of hours worked per week: 0. Apply by January 2.
Advanced Students: Teaching assistantships available for advanced students. Average amount paid per academic year: $18,000. Average number of hours worked per week: 20. Apply by March 15. Research assistantships available for advanced students. Average amount paid per academic year: $18,000. Average number of hours worked per week: 20. Apply by March 15. Fellowships and scholarships available for advanced students. Average amount paid per academic year: $18,000. Average number of hours worked per week: 0. Apply by January 2.
Additional Information: Of all students currently enrolled full time, 30% benefited from one or more of the listed financial assistance programs.

Internships/Practica: For a master's degree and certification as a school psychologist, students are placed in an internship for one academic year. The average remuneration is $12,000. Practicum sites include public, private, and parochial schools and community mental health centers. Internships are supervised by department faculty and doctoral level school psychologists. For the doctoral program, one-year internships are available. Remuneration is highly variable for $8,750 to $22,000. Counseling Internships are also paid. Practicum experiences are part of coursework and are not paid.

Housing and Day Care: On-campus housing is available. No on-campus day care facilities are available.

Employment of Department Graduates:
Master's Degree Graduates: Of those who graduated in the academic year 2008–2009, the following categories and numbers represent the postgraduate activities and employment of master's degree graduates: Enrolled in a psychology doctoral program (8), enrolled in a postdoctoral residency/fellowship (n/a), employed in independent practice (n/a), employed in a professional position in a school system (15), employed in a community mental health/counseling center (20), employed in a hospital/medical center (4), do not know (23), total from the above (master's) (70).
Doctoral Degree Graduates: Of those who graduated in the academic year 2008–2009, the following categories and numbers represent the postgraduate activities and employment of doctoral degree graduates: Enrolled in a psychology doctoral program (n/a), employed in an academic position at a university (4), employed in an academic position at a 2-year/4-year college (2), employed in other positions at a higher education institution (1), employed in a professional position in a school system (8), employed in a community mental health/counseling center (8), do not know (3), total from the above (doctoral) (29).

Additional Information:
Orientation, Objectives, and Emphasis of Department: PSE is a graduate level department offering master's and doctoral programs in four areas: Adult and Organizational Development, Counseling Psychology, Educational Psychology and Educational Psychology-Instructional Learning Technology, and School Psychology. Certification is also offered in School Psychology and Counseling Psychology. Counseling Psychology and the School Psychology doctoral programs are APA-accredited. The AOD program offers only the Master's Degree at this time.

Special Facilities or Resources: The department conducts a psychoeducational clinic with observation and recording facilities. Counseling Psychology runs clinics in Family and Community Counseling and Vocational and Educational Guidance School Psychology also has a low incidence disabilities practicum.

Information for Students With Physical Disabilities: See the following Web site for more information: http://www.temple.edu/disability.

Application Information:
Send to Office of Student Services (R-A 238), 1301 Cecil B. Moore, Philadelphia, PA 19122. URL of online application: http://www.temple.edu/grad/admissions. Students are admitted in the Fall, application deadline January 2; Spring, application deadline October 2. Counseling Psychology and School Psychology: January 2. AOD and Educational Psychology have rolling admissions and will admit for each session. *Fee:* $40.

Temple University
Department of Psychology
College of Liberal Arts
1701 North 13th Street, Room 668
Philadelphia, PA 19122-6085
Telephone: (215) 204-7321
Fax: (215) 204-5539
E-mail: *marsha.weinraub@temple.edu*
Web: *http://www.temple.edu/psychology*

Department Information:
1924. Chairperson: Marsha Weinraub. Number of faculty: total—full-time 32; women—full-time 16; total—minority—full-time 3; women minority—full-time 2.

Programs and Degrees Offered:
Listed in the following order: Program area, degree type (T if terminal Master's), number awarded 7/08–6/09. Clinical Psychology PhD (Doctor of Philosophy) 7, Developmental Psychology PhD (Doctor of Philosophy) 2, Brain and Cognitive Sciences PhD (Doctor of Philosophy) 5, Social Psychology PhD (Doctor of Philosophy) 3, Developmental Psychopathology PhD (Doctor of Philosophy) 0.

APA Accreditation: Clinical PhD (Doctor of Philosophy).

Student Applications/Admissions:
Student Applications
Clinical Psychology PhD (Doctor of Philosophy)—Applications 2009–2010, 350. Total applicants accepted 2009–2010, 11. Number full-time enrolled (new admits only) 2009–2010, 12. Openings 2010–2011, 12. The median number of years required for completion of a degree in 2008–2009 were 6. The number of students enrolled full- and part-time who were dismissed or voluntarily withdrew from this program area in 2008–2009 were 0. *Developmental Psychology PhD (Doctor of Philosophy)*—Applications 2009–2010, 55. Total applicants accepted 2009–2010, 10. Number full-time enrolled (new admits only) 2009–2010, 5. Openings 2010–2011, 5. The median number of years required for completion of a degree in 2008–2009 were 5. The number of students enrolled full- and part-time who were dismissed or voluntarily withdrew from this program area in 2008–2009 were 1. *Brain and Cognitive Sciences PhD (Doctor of Philosophy)*—Applications 2009–2010, 52. Total applicants accepted 2009–2010, 5. Number full-time enrolled (new admits only) 2009–2010, 5. Openings 2010–2011, 5. The median number of years required for completion of a degree in 2008–2009 were 5. The number of students enrolled full- and part-time who were dismissed or voluntarily withdrew from this program area in 2008–2009 were 2. *Social Psychology PhD (Doctor of Philosophy)*—Applications 2009–2010, 47. Total applicants accepted 2009–2010, 2. Number full-time enrolled (new admits only) 2009–2010, 2. Openings 2010–2011, 2. The median number of years required for completion of a degree in 2008–2009 were 5. The number of students enrolled full- and part-time who were dismissed or voluntarily withdrew

from this program area in 2008–2009 were 0. *Developmental Psychopathology PhD (Doctor of Philosophy)*—Applications 2009–2010, 25. Total applicants accepted 2009–2010, 4. Number full-time enrolled (new admits only) 2009–2010, 2. Openings 2010–2011, 2.

Scores: Entries appear in this order: required test or GPA, minimum score (if required), median score of students entering in 2009–2010. *Clinical Psychology PhD (Doctor of Philosophy):* GRE-V no minimum stated, GRE-Q no minimum stated, GRE-Analytical no minimum stated, overall undergraduate GPA no minimum stated; *Developmental Psychology PhD (Doctor of Philosophy):* GRE-V no minimum stated, GRE-Q no minimum stated, GRE-Analytical no minimum stated, overall undergraduate GPA no minimum stated; *Brain and Cognitive Sciences PhD (Doctor of Philosophy):* GRE-V no minimum stated, GRE-Q no minimum stated, GRE-Analytical no minimum stated, overall undergraduate GPA no minimum stated; *Social Psychology PhD (Doctor of Philosophy):* GRE-V no minimum stated, GRE-Q no minimum stated, GRE-Analytical no minimum stated, overall undergraduate GPA no minimum stated; *Developmental Psychopathology PhD (Doctor of Philosophy):* GRE-V no minimum stated, GRE-Q no minimum stated, GRE-Analytical no minimum stated, overall undergraduate GPA no minimum stated.

Other Criteria: (importance of criteria rated low, medium, or high): GRE scores—high, research experience—high, work experience—low, extracurricular activity—low, clinically related public service—low, GPA—high, letters of recommendation—high, interview—high, statement of goals and objectives—high, undergraduate major in psychology—low, specific undergraduate psychology courses taken—medium.

Student Characteristics: The following represents characteristics of students in 2009–2010 in all graduate psychology programs in the department: Female—full-time 56, part-time 0; Male—full-time 33, part-time 0; African American/Black—full-time 5, part-time 0; Hispanic/Latino(a)—full-time 0, part-time 0; Asian/Pacific Islander—full-time 5, part-time 0; American Indian/Alaska Native—full-time 0, part-time 0; Caucasian/White—full-time 0, part-time 0; Multi-ethnic—full-time 0, part-time 0; students subject to the Americans With Disabilities Act—full-time 0, part-time 0; Unknown ethnicity—full-time 0, part-time 0; International students who hold an F-1 or J-1 Visa—full-time 0, part-time 0.

Financial Information/Assistance:

Tuition for Full-Time Study: *Doctoral:* State residents: $590 per credit hour; Nonstate residents: $861 per credit hour. Tuition is subject to change. See the following Web site for updates and changes in tuition costs: http://www.temple.edu/bursar/about/tuitionrates.htm.

Financial Assistance:

First-Year Students: Teaching assistantships available for first year. Average amount paid per academic year: $14,455. Average number of hours worked per week: 20. Research assistantships available for first year. Average amount paid per academic year: $14,455. Average number of hours worked per week: 20. Fellowships and scholarships available for first year. Average amount paid per academic year: $20,000. Average number of hours worked per week: 0.

Advanced Students: Teaching assistantships available for advanced students. Average amount paid per academic year: $14,455. Average number of hours worked per week: 20. Research assistantships available for advanced students. Average amount paid per academic year: $14,455. Average number of hours worked per week: 20. Fellowships and scholarships available for advanced students. Average amount paid per academic year: $20,000. Average number of hours worked per week: 0.

Additional Information: Of all students currently enrolled full time, 100% benefited from one or more of the listed financial assistance programs. Application and information available online at: http://www.temple.edu/grad/finances.

Internships/Practica: Doctoral Degree (PhD Clinical Psychology): For those doctoral students for whom a professional internship was required in this program prior to graduation, (10) students applied for an internship in 2008–2009, with (10) students obtaining an internship. Of those students who obtained an internship, (0) were paid internships. Of those students who obtained an internship, (10) students placed in APA/CPA accredited internships, (10) students placed in internships not APA/CPA accredited, but listed with the Association of Psychology Postdoctoral and Internship Programs (APPIC), (0) students placed in internships conforming to guidelines of the Council of Directors of School Psychology Programs (CDSPP), (0) students placed in internships that were not APA/CPA accredited, APPIC or CDSPP listed. Clinical students complete a 2,000-hour predoctoral internship at an agency or hospital typically in the Philadelphia metropolitan area.

Housing and Day Care: No on-campus housing is available. No on-campus day care facilities are available.

Employment of Department Graduates:

Master's Degree Graduates: Of those who graduated in the academic year 2008–2009, the following categories and numbers represent the postgraduate activities and employment of master's degree graduates: Enrolled in a postdoctoral residency/fellowship (n/a), employed in independent practice (n/a), total from the above (master's) (0).

Doctoral Degree Graduates: Of those who graduated in the academic year 2008–2009, the following categories and numbers represent the postgraduate activities and employment of doctoral degree graduates: Enrolled in a psychology doctoral program (n/a), enrolled in a postdoctoral residency/fellowship (2), employed in an academic position at a 2-year/4-year college (1), total from the above (doctoral) (3).

Additional Information:

Orientation, Objectives, and Emphasis of Department: The psychology department offers graduate training in: brain and cognitive sciences; clinical; developmental; developmental psychopathology; and social decision making and emotions. All doctoral programs are designed to prepare students for teaching in universities and colleges, conducting research in field and laboratory settings, and providing consultation in applied settings. The clinical program trains scientist–practitioners and provides students with research and clinical experience.

Special Facilities or Resources: The psychology department occupies eight floors of a high-rise building. The physical resources housed in the building include the Psychological Services Center (an in-house mental health facility where clinical students obtain practicum experience in psychotherapy), extensive laboratory space for human research, a human electrophysiology lab, an infant behavior lab, numerous observation rooms with one-way mirrors, audiovisual equipment (including mobile video equipment), and excellent computer facilities, including numerous micro- and minicomputers.

Information for Students With Physical Disabilities: See the following Web site for more information: http://www.temple.edu/disability.

Application Information:
Send to Graduate Administrator. Application available online. URL of online application: http://www.temple.edu/grad/admissions. Students are admitted in the Fall, application deadline December 1. *Fee:* $60.

Villanova University
Department of Psychology
800 Lancaster Avenue
Villanova, PA 19085
Telephone: (610) 519-4720
Fax: (610) 519-4269
E-mail: *psychologyinformation@villanova.edu*
Web: *http://www.villanova.edu/artsci/psychology/*

Department Information:
1962. Chairperson: Thomas Toppino. Number of faculty: total—full-time 16, part-time 6; women—full-time 5, part-time 3; total—minority—full-time 1, part-time 1; women minority—part-time 1.

Programs and Degrees Offered:
Listed in the following order: Program area, degree type (T if terminal Master's), number awarded 7/08–6/09. General Psychology MA/MS (Master of Arts/Science) (T) 21.

Student Applications/Admissions:
Student Applications
General Psychology MA/MS (Master of Arts/Science)—Applications 2009–2010, 125. Total applicants accepted 2009–2010, 36. Number full-time enrolled (new admits only) 2009–2010, 20. Openings 2010–2011, 21. The median number of years required for completion of a degree in 2008–2009 were 2. The number of students enrolled full- and part-time who were dismissed or voluntarily withdrew from this program area in 2008–2009 were 0.
Scores: Entries appear in this order: required test or GPA, minimum score (if required), median score of students entering in 2009–2010. *General Psychology MA/MS (Master of Arts/Science):* GRE-V no minimum stated, 570, GRE-Q no minimum stated, 660, GRE-Analytical no minimum stated, 5, overall undergraduate GPA no minimum stated, 3.7, psychology GPA no minimum stated, 3.8.
Other Criteria: (importance of criteria rated low, medium, or high): GRE scores—high, research experience—medium, work experience—low, extracurricular activity—low, clinically related public service—low, GPA—high, letters of recommendation—high, interview—medium, statement of goals and objectives—medium, undergraduate major in psychology—medium, specific undergraduate psychology courses taken—high. For additional information on admission requirements, go to http://www.villanova.edu/artsci/psychology/graduate/admission/.

Student Characteristics: The following represents characteristics of students in 2009–2010 in all graduate psychology programs in the department: Female—full-time 26, part-time 0; Male—full-time 13, part-time 0; African American/Black—full-time 0, part-time 0; Hispanic/Latino(a)—full-time 1, part-time 0; Asian/Pacific Islander—full-time 0, part-time 0; American Indian/Alaska Native—full-time 0, part-time 0; Caucasian/White—full-time 38, part-time 0; Multi-ethnic—full-time 0, part-time 0; students subject to the Americans With Disabilities Act—full-time 0, part-time 0; Unknown ethnicity—full-time 0, part-time 0; International students who hold an F-1 or J-1 Visa—full-time 0, part-time 0.

Financial Information/Assistance:
Tuition for Full-Time Study: Master's: State residents: $650 per credit hour; Nonstate residents: $650 per credit hour. Tuition is subject to change. See the following Web site for updates and changes in tuition costs: http://www.villanova.edu/artsci/psychology/graduate/admission/cost.htm.

Financial Assistance:
First-Year Students: Research assistantships available for first year. Average amount paid per academic year: $13,500. Average number of hours worked per week: 20. Apply by March 15. Traineeships available for first year. Average amount paid per academic year: $6,750. Average number of hours worked per week: 14. Apply by March 15. Fellowships and scholarships available for first year. Average amount paid per academic year: $0. Average number of hours worked per week: 7. Apply by March 15.
Advanced Students: Research assistantships available for advanced students. Average amount paid per academic year: $13,500. Average number of hours worked per week: 20. Apply by March 15. Traineeships available for advanced students. Average amount paid per academic year: $6,750. Average number of hours worked per week: 14. Apply by March 15. Fellowships and scholarships available for advanced students. Average amount paid per academic year: $0. Average number of hours worked per week: 7. Apply by March 15.
Additional Information: Of all students currently enrolled full time, 55% benefited from one or more of the listed financial assistance programs. Application and information available online at: http://www.villanova.edu/artsci/college/academics/graduate/policies/index.htm?page=gradasst.htm.

Internships/Practica: Master's Degree (MA/MS General Psychology): An internship experience, such as a final research project or "capstone" experience is required of graduates.

Housing and Day Care: No on-campus housing is available. No on-campus day care facilities are available.

Employment of Department Graduates:
Master's Degree Graduates: Of those who graduated in the academic year 2008–2009, the following categories and numbers

represent the postgraduate activities and employment of master's degree graduates: Enrolled in a psychology doctoral program (9), enrolled in another graduate/professional program (1), enrolled in a postdoctoral residency/fellowship (n/a), employed in independent practice (n/a), employed in business or industry (2), employed in a community mental health/counseling center (2), still seeking employment (2), total from the above (master's) (16).
Doctoral Degree Graduates: Of those who graduated in the academic year 2008–2009, the following categories and numbers represent the postgraduate activities and employment of doctoral degree graduates: Enrolled in a psychology doctoral program (n/a), total from the above (doctoral) (0).

Additional Information:
Orientation, Objectives, and Emphasis of Department: The department offers a program of study leading to the Master of Science in psychology. Individually tailored to meet each student's career interests and needs, the program provides a solid foundation in psychology with special emphasis on preparation for doctoral work. All incoming students are required to take a seminar in the foundations of research and a statistics course. All students also take laboratory courses in Cognition & Learning and Biopsychology. Depending upon the student's interest, he or she selects four elective courses from a reasonably broad range of course offerings such as psychopathology, psychological testing, developmental psychology, social psychology, personality, theories of psychotherapy, behavior modification, special topics, and individual research. During the second year, student efforts are concentrated on the thesis project, which is an intensive, empirically-based project, done under the supervision of a faculty mentor. The student/faculty ratio approaches 2:1, allowing close interaction, careful advisement, and individual attention. The department has an active, research-oriented faculty.

Special Facilities or Resources: In addition to office space for faculty and all graduate assistants, the department has approximately 5800-square feet available for research. Equipment of particular interest to the graduate student includes: electronic and computer-controlled tachistoscopes; animal conditioning chambers; cognitive/computer labs; complete facilities for surgery and histology, including stereotaxic equipment for brain implantation; environmental chambers and rooms equipped for observation and automated recording of animal behavior; radial mazes; well-equipped vision labs; one-way vision rooms; audio/video recording and playback facilities; facilities for the design and development of experiments; and computer-based teaching labs. University computing facilities are all networked, with hundreds of remote terminals available.

Application Information:
Send to Dean, Graduate School, Villanova University, 800 Lancaster Avenue, Villanova, PA 19085. Application available online. URL of online application: http://www.gradartsci.villanova.edu/. Students are admitted in the Fall. Strong applications received by March 15 have a better chance of acceptance. Completed applications must be received by March 15 to ensure full consideration for financial aid. *Fee:* $50.

West Chester University of Pennsylvania
Department of Psychology
West Chester, PA 19383
Telephone: (610) 436-2945
Fax: (610) 436-2846
E-mail: SYorges@wcupa.edu
Web: http://www.wcupa.edu/_academics/sch_cas.psy/

Department Information:
1967. Chairperson: Loretta Rieser-Danner. Number of faculty: total—full-time 20, part-time 8; women—full-time 13, part-time 6; total—minority—full-time 3; women minority—full-time 1.

Programs and Degrees Offered:
Listed in the following order: Program area, degree type (T if terminal Master's), number awarded 7/08–6/09. Clinical MA/MS (Master of Arts/Science) (T) 13, General MA/MS (Master of Arts/Science) (T) 2, Industrial/Organizational MA/MS (Master of Arts/Science) (T) 7.

Student Applications/Admissions:
Student Applications
Clinical MA/MS (Master of Arts/Science)—Applications 2009–2010, 93. Total applicants accepted 2009–2010, 70. Number full-time enrolled (new admits only) 2009–2010, 24. Number part-time enrolled (new admits only) 2009–2010, 2. Total enrolled 2009–2010 full-time, 59, part-time, 15. Openings 2010–2011, 25. The median number of years required for completion of a degree in 2008–2009 were 2. The number of students enrolled full- and part-time who were dismissed or voluntarily withdrew from this program area in 2008–2009 were 0. *General MA/MS (Master of Arts/Science)*—Applications 2009–2010, 12. Total applicants accepted 2009–2010, 3. Number full-time enrolled (new admits only) 2009–2010, 2. Number part-time enrolled (new admits only) 2009–2010, 1. Total enrolled 2009–2010 full-time, 5, part-time, 4. Openings 2010–2011, 4. The median number of years required for completion of a degree in 2008–2009 were 2. The number of students enrolled full- and part-time who were dismissed or voluntarily withdrew from this program area in 2008–2009 were 1. *Industrial/Organizational MA/MS (Master of Arts/Science)*—Applications 2009–2010, 48. Total applicants accepted 2009–2010, 33. Number full-time enrolled (new admits only) 2009–2010, 16. Number part-time enrolled (new admits only) 2009–2010, 2. Total enrolled 2009–2010 full-time, 28, part-time, 15. Openings 2010–2011, 15. The median number of years required for completion of a degree in 2008–2009 were 2.
Scores: Entries appear in this order: required test or GPA, minimum score (if required), median score of students entering in 2009–2010. *Clinical MA/MS (Master of Arts/Science)*: GRE-V 500, GRE-Q 500, overall undergraduate GPA 3.0, psychology GPA 3.25; *General MA/MS (Master of Arts/Science)*: GRE-V 500, GRE-Q 500, overall undergraduate GPA 3.0, psychology GPA 3.25; *Industrial/Organizational MA/MS (Master of Arts/Science)*: GRE-V 500, GRE-Q 500, overall undergraduate GPA 3.0, psychology GPA 3.25.
Other Criteria: (importance of criteria rated low, medium, or high): GRE scores—high, research experience—medium, work experience—medium, extracurricular activity—medium, clinically related public service—medium, GPA—high, letters

of recommendation—high, statement of goals and objectives—high, undergraduate major in psychology—low, specific undergraduate psychology courses taken—medium.

Student Characteristics: The following represents characteristics of students in 2009–2010 in all graduate psychology programs in the department: Female—full-time 33, part-time 22; Male—full-time 10, part-time 10; African American/Black—full-time 2, part-time 3; Hispanic/Latino(a)—full-time 0, part-time 0; Asian/Pacific Islander—full-time 0, part-time 0; American Indian/Alaska Native—full-time 0, part-time 0; Caucasian/White—full-time 0, part-time 0; Multi-ethnic—full-time 0, part-time 0; students subject to the Americans With Disabilities Act—full-time 0, part-time 2; Unknown ethnicity—full-time 0, part-time 0; International students who hold an F-1 or J-1 Visa—full-time 0, part-time 0.

Financial Information/Assistance:
Tuition for Full-Time Study: *Master's:* State residents: per academic year $3,215, $370 per credit hour; Nonstate residents: per academic year $5,144, $593 per credit hour. Tuition is subject to change.

Financial Assistance:
 First-Year Students: Research assistantships available for first year. Average amount paid per academic year: $2,500. Average number of hours worked per week: 10. Apply by March 1.
 Advanced Students: Research assistantships available for advanced students. Average amount paid per academic year: $2,500. Average number of hours worked per week: 10. Apply by March 1.
 Additional Information: Of all students currently enrolled full time, 40% benefited from one or more of the listed financial assistance programs.

Internships/Practica: Master's Degree (MA/MS Clinical): An internship experience, such as a final research project or "capstone" experience is required of graduates. Master's Degree (MA/MS General): An internship experience, such as a final research project or "capstone" experience is required of graduates. Master's Degree (MA/MS Industrial/Organizational): An internship experience, such as a final research project or "capstone" experience is required of graduates. Clinical students are required to complete 6 credit hours of practicum and internship in a mental health setting. I/O students are required to complete a 3 credit hour internship in business or industry.

Housing and Day Care: No on-campus housing is available. On-campus day care facilities are available. See the following Web site for more information: http://www.wcupa.edu/_services/stu.chi/.

Employment of Department Graduates:
 Master's Degree Graduates: Of those who graduated in the academic year 2008–2009, the following categories and numbers represent the postgraduate activities and employment of master's degree graduates: Enrolled in a postdoctoral residency/fellowship (n/a), employed in independent practice (n/a), total from the above (master's) (0).
 Doctoral Degree Graduates: Of those who graduated in the academic year 2008–2009, the following categories and numbers represent the postgraduate activities and employment of doctoral degree graduates: Enrolled in a psychology doctoral program (n/a), total from the above (doctoral) (0).

Additional Information:
 Orientation, Objectives, and Emphasis of Department: The concentration in clinical psychology is designed for students who wish to work in applied settings such as community mental health facilities, hospitals, counseling centers, and other social and rehabilitation agencies, or who wish to continue their education at the doctoral level. Students with the latter goal in mind are strongly encouraged to engage in research in the course of their master's degree training by participating in faculty members' ongoing research programs or conducting their own research under faculty supervision for research report or thesis credit. The industrial/organizational concentration is appropriate for students interested in employment in business or industry, or for those who wish to continue their education at the doctoral level in a related area. A 3-credit internship and 3- to 6-credit research report or thesis are required. With careful selection of electives, internship placement, and research focus, students are able to develop specialization in human factors, personnel evaluation and placement, or group and organizational processes. The concentration in general psychology, in addition to exposing students to the major traditional subject matter of psychology, also provides the opportunity to explore particular areas of psychology in depth through the appropriate selection of elective coursework and research. The general concentration is appropriate for students interested in continuing their education at the doctoral level, as well as those interested in employment, particularly in research positions, upon the receipt of their master's degree.

Special Facilities or Resources: The department has laboratory space and equipment to support a variety of animal and human research.

Application Information:
Send to Office of Graduate Studies and Sponsored Research, West Chester University, West Chester, PA 19383. Application available online. URL of online application: https://www.applyweb.com/apply/wcgrad/menu.html. Students are admitted in the Fall, application deadline March 1. Late applications will be reviewed if space remains in the program. *Fee:* $35.

Widener University
Institute for Graduate Clinical Psychology
One University Place
Chester, PA 19013
Telephone: (610) 499-1206
Fax: (610) 499-4625
E-mail: *VMBrabender@widener.edu*
Web: *http://www.widener.edu/igcp/*

Department Information:
 1970. Associate Dean and Director: Virginia Brabender. Number of faculty: total—full-time 15, part-time 32; women—full-time 4, part-time 18; total—minority—full-time 2, part-time 3; women minority—part-time 1.

Programs and Degrees Offered:
Listed in the following order: Program area, degree type (T if terminal Master's), number awarded 7/08–6/09. Clinical Psychology PsyD (Doctor of Psychology) 29.

APA Accreditation: Clinical PsyD (Doctor of Psychology). Student Outcome Data Website: http://www.widener.edu/academics/collegesandschools/humanserviceprofessions/clinicalpsychology/graduatestudentinformation.

Student Applications/Admissions:
Student Applications
Clinical Psychology PsyD (Doctor of Psychology)—Applications 2009–2010, 282. Total applicants accepted 2009–2010, 53. Number full-time enrolled (new admits only) 2009–2010, 33. Number part-time enrolled (new admits only) 2009–2010, 0. Openings 2010–2011, 33. The median number of years required for completion of a degree in 2008–2009 were 5. The number of students enrolled full- and part-time who were dismissed or voluntarily withdrew from this program area in 2008–2009 were 1.

Other Criteria: (importance of criteria rated low, medium, or high): GRE scores—high, work experience—medium, extracurricular activity—medium, clinically related public service—medium, GPA—high, letters of recommendation—high, interview—high, statement of goals and objectives—high, specific undergraduate psychology courses taken—low. An undergraduate major in psychology is not required for admission; however, some basic psychology courses are required before enrollment. We encourage applications from individuals from various disciplines and with a wide range of experiences. For additional information on admission requirements, go to http://www.widener.edu/admissions/graduate/apply/graduaterequirements.

Student Characteristics: The following represents characteristics of students in 2009–2010 in all graduate psychology programs in the department: Female—full-time 138, part-time 0; Male—full-time 47, part-time 0; African American/Black—full-time 12, part-time 0; Hispanic/Latino(a)—full-time 5, part-time 0; Asian/Pacific Islander—full-time 10, part-time 0; American Indian/Alaska Native—full-time 1, part-time 0; Caucasian/White—full-time 154, part-time 0; Multi-ethnic—full-time 3, part-time 0; students subject to the Americans With Disabilities Act—full-time 1, part-time 0; Unknown ethnicity—full-time 0, part-time 0; International students who hold an F-1 or J-1 Visa—full-time 6, part-time 0.

Financial Information/Assistance:
Tuition for Full-Time Study: *Doctoral:* State residents: per academic year $22,886; Nonstate residents: per academic year $22,886. Tuition is subject to change. See the following Web site for updates and changes in tuition costs: http://www.widener.edu/about/administration/enrollmentservices/studentfinancialservices.

Financial Assistance:
First-Year Students: Fellowships and scholarships available for first year. Average amount paid per academic year: $18,300. Average number of hours worked per week: 0. Apply by March 1.
Advanced Students: Fellowships and scholarships available for advanced students. Average amount paid per academic year: $1,500. Average number of hours worked per week: 0. Apply by April 15.

Additional Information: Of all students currently enrolled full time, 33% benefited from one or more of the listed financial assistance programs. Application and information available online at: http://www.widener.edu/about/administration/enrollmentservices/studentfinancialservices.

Internships/Practica: The program has an exclusively affiliated internship that is a half-time over a two-year period. The APA-accredited internship is housed at Widener University, but placements are within a 50-mile radius of the campus. 100% of fourth- and fifth-year students are placed.

Housing and Day Care: On-campus housing is available. See the following Web site for more information: http://www.widener.edu/campuslife/residencelife. On-campus day care facilities are available. See the following Web site for more information: http://cdc.widener.edu/.

Employment of Department Graduates:
Master's Degree Graduates: Of those who graduated in the academic year 2008–2009, the following categories and numbers represent the postgraduate activities and employment of master's degree graduates: Enrolled in a postdoctoral residency/fellowship (n/a), employed in independent practice (n/a), total from the above (master's) (0).
Doctoral Degree Graduates: Of those who graduated in the academic year 2008–2009, the following categories and numbers represent the postgraduate activities and employment of doctoral degree graduates: Enrolled in a psychology doctoral program (n/a), enrolled in a postdoctoral residency/fellowship (5), employed in independent practice (2), employed in an academic position at a university (1), employed in other positions at a higher education institution (2), employed in a professional position in a school system (3), employed in business or industry (2), employed in government agency (4), employed in a community mental health/counseling center (7), employed in a hospital/medical center (3), total from the above (doctoral) (29).

Additional Information:
Orientation, Objectives, and Emphasis of Department: The PsyD program retains the basic skills and knowledge traditional to clinical psychology, such as psychodiagnostic testing and psychotherapy, while simultaneously exposing the individual to new ideas and practices in the field. The law-psychology (JD/PsyD) program presumes that every law and court decision is in part based upon psychological assumptions about how people act and how their actions can be controlled. It is designed to train lawyer-clinical psychologists to identify and evaluate these assumptions and apply their psychological knowledge to improve the law, legal process, and legal system. Students earn a law degree from the Widener University School of Law, and a doctorate in psychology from Widener's Institute for Graduate Clinical Psychology. The PsyD/MBA program is based on the premise that health care organizations as well as the mental health and health care fields at large are in need of well-trained leaders and advocates who integrate psychological and business-organizational knowledge.

Special Facilities or Resources: One of the hallmarks of our program is the variety of internship and practicum opportunities available to students, all of which are within driving distance of the university. A corollary resource is the availability of practicing clinicians to teach in the program, a factor that provides breadth, relevance, and enrichment to the curriculum. Widener University is situated near Philadelphia and in the middle of the Eastern corridor between New York and Washington, DC. As a result, our students enjoy a rich diversity of educational resources, field experiences, and employment opportunities. Here is a place where you can enjoy big cities or the beauty of the countryside, a vast array of cultural events and historical opportunities, and all forms of sports, arts, and entertainment. It is a wonderful place to live, learn and work.

Information for Students With Physical Disabilities: See the following Web site for more information: http://www.widener.edu/disabilitiesserv/default.asp.

Application Information:
Send to Director of Admissions, The Institute for Graduate Clinical Psychology, Widener University, One University Place, Chester, PA 19013. Application available online. URL of online application: http://www.widener.edu/admissions/graduate. Students are admitted in the Fall, application deadline December 31. *Fee:* $75.

Widener University
Law-Psychology (JD-PsyD) Graduate Training Program
Institute for Graduate Clinical Psychology & School of Law
One University Place
Chester, PA 19013-5792
Telephone: (610) 499-1206
Fax: (610) 499-4625
E-mail: *aelwork@widener.edu*
Web: *http://www.widener.edu/jdpsyd*

Department Information:
1989. Director: Amiram Elwork, PhD. Number of faculty: total—full-time 13, part-time 15; women—full-time 5, part-time 10; total—minority—full-time 2, part-time 4; women minority—full-time 1, part-time 2.

Programs and Degrees Offered:
Listed in the following order: Program area, degree type (T if terminal Master's), number awarded 7/08–6/09. Law-Psychology (JD/ PsyD) Other 2.

Student Applications/Admissions:
Student Applications
Law-Psychology (JD/ PsyD) Other—Applications 2009–2010, 12. Total applicants accepted 2009–2010, 2. Number full-time enrolled (new admits only) 2009–2010, 2. Openings 2010–2011, 3. The median number of years required for completion of a degree in 2008–2009 were 6. The number of students enrolled full- and part-time who were dismissed or voluntarily withdrew from this program area in 2008–2009 were 0.
Other Criteria: (importance of criteria rated low, medium, or high): GRE scores—high, research experience—low, work experience—medium, extracurricular activity—medium, clinically related public service—medium, GPA—high, letters of recommendation—medium, interview—high, statement of goals and objectives—high, LSAT—high.

Student Characteristics: The following represents characteristics of students in 2009–2010 in all graduate psychology programs in the department: Female—full-time 12, part-time 0; Male—full-time 4, part-time 0; African American/Black—full-time 0, part-time 0; Hispanic/Latino(a)—full-time 1, part-time 0; Asian/Pacific Islander—full-time 0, part-time 0; American Indian/Alaska Native—full-time 0, part-time 0; Caucasian/White—full-time 15, part-time 0; Multi-ethnic—full-time 0, part-time 0; students subject to the Americans With Disabilities Act—full-time 0, part-time 0; Unknown ethnicity—full-time 0, part-time 0; International students who hold an F-1 or J-1 Visa—full-time 0, part-time 0.

Financial Information/Assistance:
Tuition for Full-Time Study: Doctoral: State residents: per academic year $25,500; Nonstate residents: per academic year $25,500. Tuition is subject to change.

Financial Assistance:
First-Year Students: Fellowships and scholarships available for first year. Average amount paid per academic year: $0. Average number of hours worked per week: 0.
Advanced Students: Traineeships available for advanced students. Average amount paid per academic year: $0. Average number of hours worked per week: 0. Fellowships and scholarships available for advanced students. Average amount paid per academic year: $0. Average number of hours worked per week: 0.
Additional Information: Of all students currently enrolled full time, 80% benefited from one or more of the listed financial assistance programs.

Internships/Practica: Students are in field placements during five of the six years of training. During two of the first three years, students are assigned to clinical psychology practica. These are introductory experiences designed to acquaint the students with a variety of settings in which they can develop fundamental psychological skills in testing/assessment and psychotherapy/intervention. Fourth year field experiences are in a legal setting (law firm, court, legal agency) where they are given an opportunity to practice their legal skills. Fifth and sixth year experiences are internship rotations that allow students the opportunity to sharpen their clinical and forensic psychology skills. Widener's APA accredited integrated clinical internship with its various rotations (including forensic rotations) is highly unusual. In most programs, students participate in internships that are independent of their graduate programs. Our internship is embedded in the program. While continuing to take their coursework, students complete their internship rotations over a two-year period at various clinical sites affiliated with Widener. This allows for better integration between coursework and practical experience and relieves the student of the inconveniences associated with finding a separate internship and/or relocating.

Housing and Day Care: On-campus housing is available. See the following Web site for more information: http://www.widener.edu/campuslife/residencelife. On-campus day care facilities are available.

Employment of Department Graduates:
Master's Degree Graduates: Of those who graduated in the academic year 2008–2009, the following categories and numbers represent the postgraduate activities and employment of master's

degree graduates: Enrolled in a psychology doctoral program (0), enrolled in another graduate/professional program (0), enrolled in a postdoctoral residency/fellowship (n/a), employed in independent practice (n/a), employed in an academic position at a university (0), employed in an academic position at a 2-year/4-year college (0), employed in other positions at a higher education institution (0), employed in a professional position in a school system (0), employed in business or industry (0), employed in government agency (0), employed in a community mental health/counseling center (0), employed in a hospital/medical center (0), still seeking employment (0), other employment position (0), total from the above (master's) (0).

Doctoral Degree Graduates: Of those who graduated in the academic year 2008–2009, the following categories and numbers represent the postgraduate activities and employment of doctoral degree graduates: Enrolled in a psychology doctoral program (n/a), enrolled in a postdoctoral residency/fellowship (0), employed in independent practice (0), employed in an academic position at a university (0), employed in an academic position at a 2-year/4-year college (0), employed in other positions at a higher education institution (0), employed in a professional position in a school system (0), employed in business or industry (0), employed in government agency (0), employed in a community mental health/counseling center (0), employed in a hospital/medical center (0), still seeking employment (0), other employment position (0), total from the above (doctoral) (0).

Additional Information:

Orientation, Objectives, and Emphasis of Department: Widener University's Law-Psychology Graduate Program is based on the idea that many legal issues involve underlying psychological questions. It trains graduates to combine their knowledge of psychology and law and bring fresh insights to the process of understanding, evaluating and correcting important psycholegal problems. While a large portion of the curriculum is similar to that required of all students in the PsyD and JD programs, it includes a number of courses and requirements (e.g., dissertation) designed specifically to help students acquire an integration of psychology and law and to develop specialized skills. In addition, students are given opportunities to put their integrated skills into practice within their field placements. Students develop special expertise on many issues at the interface of law and clinical psychology and are prepared to play diverse roles in society, including: lawyer, forensic psychologist, professor, consultant, administrator, policy maker, judge, legislator, etc. This six-year program offers several benefits: (1) It allows students to pursue clinical psychology and law simultaneously; (2) It saves students the equivalent of two years of tuition and time; (3) It trains graduates to integrate the two fields conceptually and offers them a significant way of differentiating themselves in the job market.

Special Facilities or Resources: Widener University is situated near Philadelphia and in the middle of the eastern corridor between New York and Washington, DC As a result, our students enjoy a rich diversity of educational resources, field experiences, and employment opportunities. Whether you enjoy big cities or beautiful scenery, cultural events and history, all forms of entertainment and sports, our location is an ideal place to live, learn and work.

Information for Students With Physical Disabilities: See the following Web site for more information: http://www.widener.edu/disabilitiesserv.

Application Information:
Send to Law-Psychology Graduate Program - Admissions Institute for Graduate Clinical Psychology One University Place, Chester, PA 19013-5792. Application available online. URL of online application: http://www.widener.edu/admissions/graduate/. Students are admitted in the Fall, application deadline February 1. *Fee:* $60.

PUERTO RICO

Puerto Rico, University of
Department of Psychology
College of Social Sciences
P.O. Box 23345
San Juan, PR 00931-3345
Telephone: (787) 764-0000 ext 3164
Fax: (787) 763-4599
E-mail: *psic@uprrp.edu*
Web: *http://psic.uprrp.edu*

Department Information:
1963. Chairperson: Dolores Miranda-Gierbolini, PhD. Number of faculty: total—full-time 26, part-time 4; women—full-time 19, part-time 3; total—minority—full-time 26, part-time 4; women minority—full-time 19, part-time 3.

Programs and Degrees Offered:
Listed in the following order: Program area, degree type (T if terminal Master's), number awarded 7/08–6/09. Clinical Psychology PhD (Doctor of Philosophy) 6, Academic-Research Psychology PhD (Doctor of Philosophy) 2, Industrial/Organizational Psychology PhD (Doctor of Philosophy) 4, Social-Community Psychology PhD (Doctor of Philosophy) 3.

Student Applications/Admissions:

Student Applications

Clinical Psychology PhD (Doctor of Philosophy)—Applications 2009–2010, 100. Total applicants accepted 2009–2010, 18. Number full-time enrolled (new admits only) 2009–2010, 16. Number part-time enrolled (new admits only) 2009–2010, 1. Total enrolled 2009–2010 full-time, 91, part-time, 4. Openings 2010–2011, 12. The median number of years required for completion of a degree in 2008–2009 were 8. The number of students enrolled full- and part-time who were dismissed or voluntarily withdrew from this program area in 2008–2009 were 1. *Academic-Research Psychology PhD (Doctor of Philosophy)*—Applications 2009–2010, 10. Total applicants accepted 2009–2010, 5. Number full-time enrolled (new admits only) 2009–2010, 5. Number part-time enrolled (new admits only) 2009–2010, 0. Total enrolled 2009–2010 full-time, 29, part-time, 7. Openings 2010–2011, 9. The median number of years required for completion of a degree in 2008–2009 were 12. The number of students enrolled full- and part-time who were dismissed or voluntarily withdrew from this program area in 2008–2009 were 1. *Industrial/Organizational Psychology PhD (Doctor of Philosophy)*—Applications 2009–2010, 20. Total applicants accepted 2009–2010, 8. Number full-time enrolled (new admits only) 2009–2010, 6. Number part-time enrolled (new admits only) 2009–2010, 0. Total enrolled 2009–2010 full-time, 36, part-time, 7. Openings 2010–2011, 10. The median number of years required for completion of a degree in 2008–2009 were 8. The number of students enrolled full- and part-time who were dismissed or voluntarily withdrew from this program area in 2008–2009 were 2. *Social-Community Psychology PhD (Doctor of Philosophy)*—Applications 2009–2010, 24. Total applicants accepted 2009–2010, 12. Number full-time enrolled (new admits only) 2009–2010, 8. Number part-time enrolled (new admits only) 2009–2010, 3. Total enrolled 2009–2010 full-time, 31, part-time, 7. Openings 2010–2011, 11. The median number of years required for completion of a degree in 2008–2009 were 6. The number of students enrolled full- and part-time who were dismissed or voluntarily withdrew from this program area in 2008–2009 were 1.

Scores: Entries appear in this order: required test or GPA, minimum score (if required), median score of students entering in 2009–2010. Clinical Psychology PhD (Doctor of Philosophy): GRE-V no minimum stated, GRE-Q no minimum stated, GRE-Analytical no minimum stated, overall undergraduate GPA 3.00, 3.84, psychology GPA 3.00; *Academic-Research Psychology PhD (Doctor of Philosophy)*: GRE-V no minimum stated, GRE-Q no minimum stated, GRE-Analytical no minimum stated, overall undergraduate GPA 3.00, 3.42, psychology GPA 3.00; *Industrial/Organizational Psychology PhD (Doctor of Philosophy)*: GRE-V no minimum stated, GRE-Q no minimum stated, GRE-Analytical no minimum stated, overall undergraduate GPA 3.00, 3.68, psychology GPA 3.00; *Social-Community Psychology PhD (Doctor of Philosophy)*: GRE-V no minimum stated, GRE-Q no minimum stated, GRE-Analytical no minimum stated, overall undergraduate GPA 3.00, 3.67, psychology GPA 3.00.

Other Criteria: (importance of criteria rated low, medium, or high): GRE scores—high, research experience—medium, work experience—low, extracurricular activity—low, clinically related public service—medium, GPA—high, interview—high, statement of goals and objectives—high, undergraduate major in psychology—medium, specific undergraduate psychology courses taken—high. Students may present GRE scores instead of the Spanish version (known as EXADEP) for all graduate programs. For additional information on admission requirements, go to http://psic.uprrp.edu/aplicargradu.htm.

Student Characteristics: The following represents characteristics of students in 2009–2010 in all graduate psychology programs in the department: Female—full-time 155, part-time 23; Male—full-time 42, part-time 6; African American/Black—full-time 0, part-time 0; Hispanic/Latino(a)—full-time 197, part-time 29; Asian/Pacific Islander—full-time 0, part-time 0; American Indian/Alaska Native—full-time 0, part-time 0; Caucasian/White—full-time 0, part-time 0; Multi-ethnic—full-time 0, part-time 0; Unknown ethnicity—full-time 0, part-time 0; International students who hold an F-1 or J-1 Visa—full-time 15, part-time 0.

Financial Information/Assistance:
Tuition for Full-Time Study: *Master's:* State residents: $132 per credit hour; Nonstate residents: per academic year $6,126. *Doctoral:* State residents: $132 per credit hour; Nonstate residents: per academic year $6,126. Tuition is subject to change. Additional fees are assessed to students beyond the costs of tuition for the following: technology fee: $25; maintenance fee: $47. See the following Web site for updates and changes in tuition costs: http://graduados.uprrp.edu/admisiones/.

Financial Assistance:

First-Year Students: Teaching assistantships available for first year. Average amount paid per academic year: $8,000. Average number of hours worked per week: 18. Research assistantships available for first year. Average amount paid per academic year: $8,000. Average number of hours worked per week: 18. Fellowships and scholarships available for first year. Average amount paid per academic year: $1,000. Average number of hours worked per week: 0.

Advanced Students: Teaching assistantships available for advanced students. Average amount paid per academic year: $10,000. Average number of hours worked per week: 18. Research assistantships available for advanced students. Average amount paid per academic year: $10,000. Average number of hours worked per week: 18. Fellowships and scholarships available for advanced students. Average amount paid per academic year: $10,000. Average number of hours worked per week: 0. Apply by March 31.

Additional Information: Of all students currently enrolled full time, 29% benefited from one or more of the listed financial assistance programs. Application and information available online at: http://graduados.uprrp.edu/asuntos_estudiantiles/becas.htm.

Internships/Practica: Doctoral Degree (PhD Clinical Psychology): For those doctoral students for whom a professional internship was required in this program prior to graduation, (14) students applied for an internship in 2008–2009, with (14) students obtaining an internship. Of those students who obtained an internship, (14) were paid internships. Of those students who obtained an internship, (0) students placed in APA/CPA accredited internships, (0) students placed in internships not APA/CPA accredited, but listed with the Association of Psychology Postdoctoral and Internship Programs (APPIC), (0) students placed in internships conforming to guidelines of the Council of Directors of School Psychology Programs (CDSPP), (14) students placed in internships that were not APA/CPA accredited, APPIC or CDSPP listed. All programs require at least two semesters of practica; a 2000 hour internship is also required to complete the clinical psychology specialty. The settings for practica and internships include the University Center for Psychological Services and Research; public and private mental health clinics and hospitals, community-based organizations, government agencies, private businesses, educational institutions and other settings according to the specialty. Some internship sites are located outside of Puerto Rico, in Florida, New York and other continental U.S. locations. In their practica, students perform tasks that include clinical, organizational and community services; teaching undergraduate psychology courses, coordinating community interventions, research on problems such as learning disabilities, eating disorders, violence, depression, promotion of tolerance in ethnically diverse communities, computer based teaching, behavioral effects of brain damage, ecological issues of urban areas, homelessness, social problems in Caribbean nations, standardizing and developing culturally relevant testing instruments, public policy issues and others.

Housing and Day Care: On-campus housing is available. See the following Web site for more information: http://graduados.uprrp.edu/asuntos_estudiantiles/vivienda.htm. On-campus day care facilities are available. See the following Web site for more information: http://graduados.uprrp.edu/asuntos_estudiantiles/cuido_hijos.htm.

Employment of Department Graduates:

Master's Degree Graduates: Of those who graduated in the academic year 2008–2009, the following categories and numbers represent the postgraduate activities and employment of master's degree graduates: Enrolled in a psychology doctoral program (3), enrolled in another graduate/professional program (1), enrolled in a postdoctoral residency/fellowship (n/a), employed in independent practice (n/a), total from the above (master's) (4).

Doctoral Degree Graduates: Of those who graduated in the academic year 2008–2009, the following categories and numbers represent the postgraduate activities and employment of doctoral degree graduates: Enrolled in a psychology doctoral program (n/a), employed in an academic position at a 2-year/4-year college (7), employed in other positions at a higher education institution (2), employed in a hospital/medical center (1), still seeking employment (1), not seeking employment (1), do not know (3), total from the above (doctoral) (15).

Additional Information:

Orientation, Objectives, and Emphasis of Department: The Psychology Graduate Program of the University of Puerto Rico was established in 1963, when the Master's degree in Psychology was offered for the first time in Puerto Rico. In 1986, the doctoral program was established, with four specialties: clinical, social/community, academic/research and industrial/organizational. The program adheres to the scientist–practitioner Model and its vision is to be the foremost graduate program in psychology in the Caribbean. The program's objectives are: 1. To develop a critical approach to the study of psychology and the capacity to contribute to the understanding of Puerto Ricans and others; 2. To develop psychologists who are competent researchers, with profound knowledge of Puerto Rican reality, who may increase knowledge for the psychological understanding of behavior in general and Puerto Rican society in particular; 3. To prepare competent professionals who respond conscientiously and with social responsibility to the needs of psychological services for individuals, families, groups, organizations and communities; 4. To reinforce the development of undergraduate programs through a constant exchange of ideas and activities with graduate students; and 5. To provide the opportunity to prepare and improve professional competencies in psychology professors. The program's curriculum provides opportunities to learn and apply diverse theoretical orientations and research modalities.

Special Facilities or Resources: Founded in 1986 as part of the Department of Psychology Graduate Program, the University Center for Psychological Services and Research (CUSEP, for its Spanish acronym) is intended to facilitate student and faculty research as well as training and psychological services. CUSEP offers a unique context in which faculty and students can integrate professional practice, theory, and research. The research unit, one of the principal components of the Center, promotes, supports, and develops quality bio-psycho-social studies by training students and developing the faculty members' research skills. In this way, the unit aims to generate and extend knowledge, and form responsible researchers who will help satisfy the needs of the Puerto Rican population. The Center for Urban Action, Community and Economical Development (CAUCE, for its initials in Spanish) was established by the University of Puerto Rico to promote revitalization of the urban communities of Rio Piedras, which surround the UPR Campus. Psychology Department faculty and students share projects and interventions with other Departments, such as Social Work and Rehabilitation Counseling. Social/Community workshops are carried out to support grassroots organizations in communities in the San Juan Metropolitan area.

Information for Students With Physical Disabilities: See the following Web site for more information: http://graduados.uprrp.edu/asuntos_estudiantiles/personas_con_impedimentos.

Application Information:
Send to Department of Psychology, University of Puerto Rico Río Piedras Campus, P.O. Box 23345, San Juan, PR 00931-3345. Application available online. URL of online application: https://app.applyyourself.com/?id=upr-grad. Students are admitted in the Fall, application deadline January 19. Deadline for international students is December 3. *Fee:* $20.

RHODE ISLAND

Rhode Island College
Psychology Department
Faculty of Arts and Sciences
600 Mount Pleasant Avenue
Providence, RI 02908
Telephone: (401) 863-2727
Fax: (401) 863-1300
E-mail: *psychgradprgm@ric.edu*
Web: *http://www.ric.edu/psychology/index.php*

Department Information:
Director, Graduate Psychology Program: Christine A. Marco, PhD. Number of faculty: total—full-time 17; women—full-time 9; total—minority—full-time 1; women minority—full-time 1; faculty subject to the Americans With Disabilities Act 3.

Programs and Degrees Offered:
Listed in the following order: Program area, degree type (T if terminal Master's), number awarded 7/08–6/09. Psychology MA/MS (Master of Arts/Science) (T) 1.

Student Applications/Admissions:
Student Applications
Psychology MA/MS (Master of Arts/Science)—Applications 2009–2010, 14. Total applicants accepted 2009–2010, 9. Number full-time enrolled (new admits only) 2009–2010, 4. Number part-time enrolled (new admits only) 2009–2010, 3. Total enrolled 2009–2010 full-time, 6, part-time, 12. Openings 2010–2011, 12. The median number of years required for completion of a degree in 2008–2009 were 2. The number of students enrolled full- and part-time who were dismissed or voluntarily withdrew from this program area in 2008–2009 were 2.
Scores: Entries appear in this order: required test or GPA, minimum score (if required), median score of students entering in 2009–2010. *Psychology MA/MS (Master of Arts/Science):* GRE-V no minimum stated, GRE-Q no minimum stated, overall undergraduate GPA 3.0, last 2 years GPA 3.0, psychology GPA 3.0.
Other Criteria: (importance of criteria rated low, medium, or high): GRE scores—high, research experience—high, GPA—high, letters of recommendation—high, interview—high, statement of goals and objectives—high, undergraduate major in psychology—high, specific undergraduate psychology courses taken—high. For additional information on admission requirements, go to http://www.ric.edu/psychology/degreeList_psycMA.php.

Student Characteristics: The following represents characteristics of students in 2009–2010 in all graduate psychology programs in the department: Female—full-time 0, part-time 0; Male—full-time 0, part-time 0; African American/Black—full-time 0, part-time 0; Hispanic/Latino(a)—full-time 0, part-time 0; Asian/Pacific Islander—full-time 0, part-time 0; American Indian/Alaska Native—full-time 0, part-time 0; Caucasian/White—full-time 0, part-time 0; Multi-ethnic—full-time 0, part-time 0; students subject to the Americans With Disabilities Act—full-time 0, part-time 0; Unknown ethnicity—full-time 0, part-time 0; International students who hold an F-1 or J-1 Visa—full-time 0, part-time 0.

Financial Information/Assistance:
Tuition for Full-Time Study: *Master's:* State residents: $342 per credit hour; Nonstate residents: $670 per credit hour. Tuition is subject to change. See the following Web site for updates and changes in tuition costs: http://www.ric.edu/bursar/tuition.php. Higher tuition cost for this program: MA and CT students within a 50-mile radius receive a discounted tuition rate.

Financial Assistance:
First-Year Students: Teaching assistantships available for first year. Average amount paid per academic year: $4,000. Apply by April 1. Fellowships and scholarships available for first year. Average amount paid per academic year: $1,000. Apply by April 1.
Advanced Students: Teaching assistantships available for advanced students. Average amount paid per academic year: $4,000. Apply by April 1.
Additional Information: Application and information available online at: http://www.ric.edu/psychology/degreeList_psycMA.php.

Internships/Practica: Master's Degree (MA/MS Psychology): An internship experience, such as a final research project or "capstone" experience is required of graduates.

Housing and Day Care: No on-campus housing is available. On-campus day care facilities are available. See the following Web site for more information: http://www.riccoop.org/.

Employment of Department Graduates:
Master's Degree Graduates: Of those who graduated in the academic year 2008–2009, the following categories and numbers represent the postgraduate activities and employment of master's degree graduates: Enrolled in a postdoctoral residency/fellowship (n/a), employed in independent practice (n/a), total from the above (master's) (0).
Doctoral Degree Graduates: Of those who graduated in the academic year 2008–2009, the following categories and numbers represent the postgraduate activities and employment of doctoral degree graduates: Enrolled in a psychology doctoral program (n/a), total from the above (doctoral) (0).

Additional Information:
Orientation, Objectives, and Emphasis of Department: The MA program in Psychology at Rhode Island College provides a basic graduate education in psychology with a core curriculum in research methods and statistics, and the main content areas of personality, cognitive, developmental and social psychology. The MA in psychology prepares students for doctoral study and has applications for careers in such areas as business, education, and human services.

Information for Students With Physical Disabilities: See the following Web site for more information: http://www.ric.edu/disabilityservices/.

GRADUATE STUDY IN PSYCHOLOGY

Application Information:
Send to Graduate Program Admissions, c/o Dean of the Faculty of Arts and Sciences, 150 Gaige Hall, Rhode Island College, 600 Mt. Pleasant Avenue, Providence, RI 02908. Application available online. URL of online application: http://www.ric.edu/facultyArtsSciences/graduate_requirements.php. Students are admitted in the Fall, application deadline April 1; Spring, application deadline November 1. Applications received after these deadlines will be considered for admission on a space-available basis. *Fee:* $50. Requests for deferral of the application fee must be made directly to the Dean of Arts and Sciences.

Rhode Island, University of, Chafee Social Sciences Center
Department of Psychology
Arts and Sciences
10 Chafee Road, Room 313 Chafee Building
Kingston, RI 02881
Telephone: (401) 874-2193
Fax: (401) 874-2157
E-mail: *morokoff@uri.edu*
Web: *http://www.uri.edu/artsci/psy*

Department Information:
1961. Chairperson: Patricia J. Morokoff. Number of faculty: total—full-time 28; women—full-time 12; total—minority—full-time 1; women minority—full-time 1.

Programs and Degrees Offered:
Listed in the following order: Program area, degree type (T if terminal Master's), number awarded 7/08–6/09. School Psychology MA/MS (Master of Arts/Science) (T) 4, Clinical Psychology PhD (Doctor of Philosophy) 3, School Psychology PhD (Doctor of Philosophy) 3, Behavioral Science PhD (Doctor of Philosophy) 7.

APA Accreditation: Clinical PhD (Doctor of Philosophy). Student Outcome Data Website: http://www.uri.edu/artsci/psy/clinical_stats. School PhD (Doctor of Philosophy). Student Outcome Data Website: http://www.uri.edu/artsci/psy/school_prospectivestudent.

Student Applications/Admissions:
Student Applications
School Psychology MA/MS (Master of Arts/Science)—Applications 2009–2010, 20. Total applicants accepted 2009–2010, 12. Number full-time enrolled (new admits only) 2009–2010, 5. Number part-time enrolled (new admits only) 2009–2010, 0. Openings 2010–2011, 6. The median number of years required for completion of a degree in 2008–2009 were 3. The number of students enrolled full- and part-time who were dismissed or voluntarily withdrew from this program area in 2008–2009 were 0. *Clinical Psychology PhD (Doctor of Philosophy)*—Applications 2009–2010, 202. Total applicants accepted 2009–2010, 10. Number full-time enrolled (new admits only) 2009–2010, 6. Number part-time enrolled (new admits only) 2009–2010, 0. Openings 2010–2011, 6. The median number of years required for completion of a degree in 2008–2009 were 8. The number of students enrolled full- and part-time who were dismissed or voluntarily withdrew from this program area in 2008–2009 were 1. *School Psychology PhD (Doctor of Philosophy)*—Applications 2009–2010, 16. Total applicants accepted 2009–2010, 9. Number full-time enrolled (new admits only) 2009–2010, 5. Number part-time enrolled (new admits only) 2009–2010, 0. Openings 2010–2011, 6. The median number of years required for completion of a degree in 2008–2009 were 5. The number of students enrolled full- and part-time who were dismissed or voluntarily withdrew from this program area in 2008–2009 were 1. *Behavioral Science PhD (Doctor of Philosophy)*—Applications 2009–2010, 31. Total applicants accepted 2009–2010, 13. Number full-time enrolled (new admits only) 2009–2010, 8. Number part-time enrolled (new admits only) 2009–2010, 0. Openings 2010–2011, 6. The median number of years required for completion of a degree in 2008–2009 were 5. The number of students enrolled full- and part-time who were dismissed or voluntarily withdrew from this program area in 2008–2009 were 1.

Scores: Entries appear in this order: required test or GPA, minimum score (if required), median score of students entering in 2009–2010. *School Psychology MA/MS (Master of Arts/Science):* GRE-V no minimum stated, 540, GRE-Q no minimum stated, 600, GRE-Analytical no minimum stated, 4, overall undergraduate GPA no minimum stated, 3.70; *Clinical Psychology PhD (Doctor of Philosophy):* GRE-V no minimum stated, 530, GRE-Q no minimum stated, 640, overall undergraduate GPA no minimum stated, 3.52; *School Psychology PhD (Doctor of Philosophy):* GRE-V no minimum stated, 550, GRE-Q no minimum stated, 520, GRE-Analytical no minimum stated, 4.0, overall undergraduate GPA no minimum stated, 3.83; *Behavioral Science PhD (Doctor of Philosophy):* GRE-V no minimum stated, 530, GRE-Q no minimum stated, 570, overall undergraduate GPA no minimum stated, 3.88.

Other Criteria: (importance of criteria rated low, medium, or high): GRE scores—medium, research experience—high, work experience—medium, extracurricular activity—low, clinically related public service—medium, GPA—high, letters of recommendation—high, interview—high, statement of goals and objectives—high, Program match—high, undergraduate major in psychology—medium, specific undergraduate psychology courses taken—medium. Importance of criteria varies by program. Behavioral Science: High emphasis on research interest and experience; no required interview; we also look at GPA, GRE, focus and quality of personal statement, teaching experience, multicultural interests, reference letters, and program-applicant fit. Clinical program: Factors we look at are: GRE, GPA, program/applicant match, research experience, letters of recommendation, and overall evaluation. Interview required. School program: Academic aptitude (GRE+GPA); quality of personal statement; research and applied experience; letters of recommendation; fit between applicant goals and program offerings. For additional information on admission requirements, go to http://www.uri.edu/artsci/psy/all_admissions.

Student Characteristics: The following represents characteristics of students in 2009–2010 in all graduate psychology programs in the department: Female—full-time 87, part-time 0; Male—full-time 25, part-time 0; African American/Black—full-time 8, part-time 0; Hispanic/Latino(a)—full-time 9, part-time 0; Asian/Pacific Islander—full-time 11, part-time 0; American Indian/Alaska Native—full-time 1, part-time 0; Caucasian/White—full-time 83, part-time 0; Multi-ethnic—full-time 0, part-time 0; students subject to the Americans With Disabilities Act—full-time 4, part-time 0; Unknown ethnicity—full-time 0, part-time 0; Interna-

tional students who hold an F-1 or J-1 Visa—full-time 5, part-time 0.

Financial Information/Assistance:
Tuition for Full-Time Study: *Master's:* State residents: per academic year $8,828, $490 per credit hour; Nonstate residents: per academic year $22,100, $1,228 per credit hour. *Doctoral:* State residents: per academic year $8,828, $490 per credit hour; Nonstate residents: per academic year $22,100, $1,228 per credit hour. Tuition is subject to change. Additional fees are assessed to students beyond the costs of tuition for the following: health, student services, accident/sick insurance, one-time registration. See the following Web site for updates and changes in tuition costs: http://www.uri.edu/es/acadinfo/acadyear/tuition.html.

Financial Assistance:
First-Year Students: Teaching assistantships available for first year. Average amount paid per academic year: $13,894. Average number of hours worked per week: 20. Apply by March 31. Research assistantships available for first year. Average amount paid per academic year: $13,894. Average number of hours worked per week: 20. Apply by varies. Fellowships and scholarships available for first year. Average amount paid per academic year: $13,894. Average number of hours worked per week: 0. Apply by March 10.

Advanced Students: Teaching assistantships available for advanced students. Average amount paid per academic year: $14,806. Average number of hours worked per week: 20. Apply by March 31. Research assistantships available for advanced students. Average amount paid per academic year: $14,806. Average number of hours worked per week: 20. Apply by varies. Fellowships and scholarships available for advanced students. Average amount paid per academic year: $14,806. Average number of hours worked per week: 0. Apply by March 10.

Additional Information: Of all students currently enrolled full time, 64% benefited from one or more of the listed financial assistance programs. Application and information available online at: http://www.uri.edu/artsci/psy.

Internships/Practica: Doctoral Degree (PhD Clinical Psychology): For those doctoral students for whom a professional internship was required in this program prior to graduation, (6) students applied for an internship in 2008–2009, with (6) students obtaining an internship. Of those students who obtained an internship, (6) were paid internships. Of those students who obtained an internship, (6) students placed in APA/CPA accredited internships, (0) students placed in internships not APA/CPA accredited, but listed with the Association of Psychology Postdoctoral and Internship Programs (APPIC), (0) students placed in internships conforming to guidelines of the Council of Directors of School Psychology Programs (CDSPP), (0) students placed in internships that were not APA/CPA accredited, APPIC or CDSPP listed. Doctoral Degree (PhD School Psychology): For those doctoral students for whom a professional internship was required in this program prior to graduation, (3) students applied for an internship in 2008–2009, with (3) students obtaining an internship. Of those students who obtained an internship, (3) were paid internships. Of those students who obtained an internship, (1) students placed in APA/CPA accredited internships, (0) students placed in internships not APA/CPA accredited, but listed with the Association of Psychology Postdoctoral and Internship Programs (APPIC), (2) students placed in internships conforming to guidelines of the Council of Directors of School Psychology Programs (CDSPP), (0) students placed in internships that were not APA/CPA accredited, APPIC or CDSPP listed. Master's Degree (MA/MS School Psychology): An internship experience, such as a final research project or "capstone" experience is required of graduates. The Clinical Psychology program has a 94% record of matching students to internships in the past 9 years (52/55 who applied were matched). Our students attend top New England and national internship programs. School Psychology students who choose to apply for APPIC internships have had similar success in internship placements. The Clinical program requires 5 semesters of practicum placement in our on-campus training clinic in cognitive behavior therapy, family therapy, and interpersonal process therapy. Students also receive training in working with ethnically diverse clients. From the third year on, clinical students may be placed in off campus externships that include training in neuropsychological assessment, structured diagnostic interviewing, psychotherapy, university counseling, and pediatric psychology. School students complete school-based practica in Years 1 and 2 of the program, with advanced practica in Years 3 and 4 in school settings as well as a variety of other child and adolescent service delivery settings (e.g., pediatric hospitals). The School program adheres to the internship guidelines of the Council of Directors of School Psychology Programs.

Housing and Day Care: On-campus housing is available. See the following Web site for more information: http://housing.uri.edu/grad.html. On-campus day care facilities are available. See the following Web site for more information: http://www.uri.edu/hss/hdf/cdc/.

Employment of Department Graduates:
Master's Degree Graduates: Of those who graduated in the academic year 2008–2009, the following categories and numbers represent the postgraduate activities and employment of master's degree graduates: Enrolled in a psychology doctoral program (0), enrolled in another graduate/professional program (0), enrolled in a postdoctoral residency/fellowship (n/a), employed in independent practice (n/a), employed in an academic position at a university (0), employed in an academic position at a 2-year/4-year college (0), employed in other positions at a higher education institution (0), employed in a professional position in a school system (4), employed in business or industry (0), employed in government agency (0), employed in a community mental health/counseling center (0), employed in a hospital/medical center (0), still seeking employment (0), not seeking employment (0), other employment position (0), do not know (0), total from the above (master's) (4).

Doctoral Degree Graduates: Of those who graduated in the academic year 2008–2009, the following categories and numbers represent the postgraduate activities and employment of doctoral degree graduates: Enrolled in a psychology doctoral program (n/a), enrolled in another graduate/professional program (0), enrolled in a postdoctoral residency/fellowship (1), employed in independent practice (0), employed in an academic position at a university (2), employed in an academic position at a 2-year/4-year college (0), employed in other positions at a higher education institution (4), employed in a professional position in a school system (3), employed in business or industry (0), employed in government agency (0), employed in a community mental health/counseling center (1), employed in a hospital/medical center (1), still seeking employment (1), not seeking employment (0), other employment position (0), do not know (0), total from the above (doctoral) (13).

Additional Information:
Orientation, Objectives, and Emphasis of Department: Both the Clinical and School Psychology programs of the URI Psychology Department identify as scientist–practitioner programs and both are accredited by the American Psychological Association. The Behavior Science program has an applied quantitative emphasis. The department has a strong commitment to diversity and multicultural competence. There is a lively interaction among the programs and access to training in advanced statistical and methodological approaches. The research and professional interests of the faculty fall into these areas: (1) health psychology with an emphasis on health promotion/disease prevention; (2) research methodology; (3) gender, diversity, and multicultural psychology; (4) family, child, and developmental psychology; (5) neuropsychology; and (6) school psychology practice. Graduates of our programs have developed diverse careers in academia, government service, schools, private industry, the nonprofit sector, and private consulting and practice.

Special Facilities or Resources: The Department operates an on-campus training facility, the Psychological Consultation Center, where students train under direct faculty supervision for professional practice service roles with individual clients, families, and children. The department is closely allied with the Cancer Prevention Research Center, one of the nation's leading centers for behavioral health promotion and disease prevention. Students also participate in research and training activities with the Department's Community Research and Services Team, the URI Family Resource Partnership, the Feinstein Hunger Center, as well as with several training partnerships with medical centers and community mental health service agencies.

Information for Students With Physical Disabilities: See the following Web site for more information: http://www.uri.edu/disability/.

Application Information:
Send to Department of Psychology, 10 Chafee Road, 313 Chafee Bldg., Kingston, RI 02881. Application available online. URL of online application: http://www.uri.edu/artsci/psy. Students are admitted in the Fall, application deadline Clinical - December 1; School - January 15; Behavioral Science - January 6. Fee: $65.

Roger Williams University
Department of Psychology
Arts and Sciences
One Old Ferry Road
Bristol, RI 02809-2921
Telephone: (401) 254-3509
Fax: (401) 254-3286
E-mail: *dwhitworth@rwu.edu*
Web: *http://www.rwu.edu*

Department Information:
1969. Chairperson: Laura Turner, PhD. Number of faculty: total—full-time 13, part-time 13; women—full-time 7, part-time 9; total—minority—full-time 3, part-time 2; women minority—full-time 1, part-time 1.

Programs and Degrees Offered:
Listed in the following order: Program area, degree type (T if terminal Master's), number awarded 7/08–6/09. Forensic Psychology MA/MS (Master of Arts/Science) (T).

Student Applications/Admissions:
Student Applications
Forensic Psychology MA/MS (Master of Arts/Science)—Applications 2009–2010, 70. Total applicants accepted 2009–2010, 43. Number full-time enrolled (new admits only) 2009–2010, 14. Number part-time enrolled (new admits only) 2009–2010, 0. Openings 2010–2011, 20. The number of students enrolled full- and part-time who were dismissed or voluntarily withdrew from this program area in 2008–2009 were 0.

Scores: Entries appear in this order: required test or GPA, minimum score (if required), median score of students entering in 2009–2010. *Forensic Psychology MA/MS (Master of Arts/Science)*: GRE-V 500, GRE-Q 500, overall undergraduate GPA 3.0, 3.2.

Other Criteria: (importance of criteria rated low, medium, or high): GRE scores—high, research experience—high, work experience—medium, extracurricular activity—low, clinically related public service—medium, GPA—high, letters of recommendation—high, statement of goals and objectives—high, undergraduate major in psychology—medium, specific undergraduate psychology courses taken—high.

Student Characteristics: The following represents characteristics of students in 2009–2010 in all graduate psychology programs in the department: Female—full-time 23, part-time 0; Male—full-time 3, part-time 0; African American/Black—full-time 0, part-time 0; Hispanic/Latino(a)—full-time 0, part-time 0; Asian/Pacific Islander—full-time 0, part-time 0; American Indian/Alaska Native—full-time 0, part-time 0; Caucasian/White—full-time 26, part-time 0; Multi-ethnic—full-time 0, part-time 0; students subject to the Americans With Disabilities Act—full-time 0, part-time 0; Unknown ethnicity—full-time 0, part-time 0; International students who hold an F-1 or J-1 Visa—full-time 0, part-time 0.

Financial Information/Assistance:
Tuition for Full-Time Study: Master's: State residents: per academic year $16,104, $671 per credit hour; Nonstate residents: per academic year $16,104, $671 per credit hour. Tuition is subject to change. See the following Web site for updates and changes in tuition costs: http://www.rwu.edu/admission/grad/mafp/.

Financial Assistance:
First-Year Students: Research assistantships available for first year. Average amount paid per academic year: $1,000. Apply by March 15. Fellowships and scholarships available for first year. Average amount paid per academic year: $1,500. Apply by March 15.

Advanced Students: Research assistantships available for advanced students. Average amount paid per academic year: $1,000. Fellowships and scholarships available for advanced students. Average amount paid per academic year: $1,500.

Additional Information: Of all students currently enrolled full time, 70% benefited from one or more of the listed financial

assistance programs. Application and information available online at: http://www.rwu.edu/admission/financialaid/.

Internships/Practica: The clinical training program for the Master of Arts in Forensic Psychology at Roger Williams University offers a wide range of practicum placement sites in Massachusetts and Rhode Island with opportunities to work clinically with a diversity of forensic populations. We currently have practicum placements within adult and juvenile correctional settings, adult inpatient forensic hospitals and state hospitals, juvenile court clinics, juvenile treatment programs, state and federal correctional programs for the evaluation and treatment of adult sex offenders, community mental health programs, and outpatient substance abuse programs. There are also a few research practicum placements available. Students receive comprehensive training and clinical supervision on-site from practicing forensic psychologists and forensic mental health practitioners in the assessment and treatment of forensic mental health patients and clients. The focus of the clinical practicum placements is to provide the student with an opportunity to apply clinical skills and techniques learned in clinical course work. Students are encouraged to examine case studies, training issues, ethical dilemmas and conflicts within their continued course work on campus. The practicum placements function as a vital place for students to form professional relationships in the field and to network with allied forensic mental health professionals, a key to later opportunities for employment in the forensic mental health field. Practicum placements also provide a valuable enhancement of a student's application for continued graduate education toward a doctorate in psychology.

Housing and Day Care: On-campus housing is available. See the following Web site for more information: http://www.rwu.edu/studentlife/residencelife/universityhousing/. No on-campus day care facilities are available.

Employment of Department Graduates:

Master's Degree Graduates: Of those who graduated in the academic year 2008–2009, the following categories and numbers represent the postgraduate activities and employment of master's degree graduates: Enrolled in a psychology doctoral program (2), enrolled in a postdoctoral residency/fellowship (n/a), employed in independent practice (n/a), employed in a community mental health/counseling center (12), employed in a hospital/medical center (3), total from the above (master's) (17).

Doctoral Degree Graduates: Of those who graduated in the academic year 2008–2009, the following categories and numbers represent the postgraduate activities and employment of doctoral degree graduates: Enrolled in a psychology doctoral program (n/a), total from the above (doctoral) (0).

Additional Information:

Orientation, Objectives, and Emphasis of Department: The Psychology Department strives to provide assessment and treatment skills for students interested in employment in a forensic setting or further training at the doctoral level. Faculty members work closely with students to help them develop an understanding and appreciation of the role of psychologists in legal proceedings and the law. Students are prepared to apply these skills to the problems of community and of the larger society. The department stresses tolerance for the views of others and an appreciation of the value of diversity. Other departmental objectives include preparing students to evaluate published research and think critically about their own ideas and the ideas of others.

Information for Students With Physical Disabilities: See the following Web site for more information: http://www.rwu.edu/academics/centyers/cad/dss.

Application Information:
Send to Office of Graduate Admission, One Old Ferry Road, Bristol, RI 02809. Application available online. URL of online application: http://www.rwu.edu/admission/. Students are admitted in the Fall, application deadline March 15. *Fee:* $50.

SOUTH CAROLINA

Citadel, The
Department of Psychology
171 Moultrie Street
Charleston, SC 29409
Telephone: (843) 953-5320
Fax: (843) 953-6797
E-mail: *politanom@citadel.edu*
Web: *http://www.citadel.edu/psyc/*

Department Information:
1976. Department Head: P. Michael Politano. Number of faculty: total—full-time 12, part-time 5; women—full-time 4, part-time 3; total—minority—full-time 1; faculty subject to the Americans With Disabilities Act 1.

Programs and Degrees Offered:
Listed in the following order: Program area, degree type (T if terminal Master's), number awarded 7/08–6/09. School Psychology EdS (School Psychology) 13, Clinical Counseling Psychology MA/MS (Master of Arts/Science) (T) 14.

Student Applications/Admissions:
Student Applications
School Psychology EdS (School Psychology)—Applications 2009–2010, 44. Total applicants accepted 2009–2010, 14. Number full-time enrolled (new admits only) 2009–2010, 14. Number part-time enrolled (new admits only) 2009–2010, 0. Total enrolled 2009–2010 full-time, 53, part-time, 2. Openings 2010–2011, 14. The median number of years required for completion of a degree in 2008–2009 were 3. The number of students enrolled full- and part-time who were dismissed or voluntarily withdrew from this program area in 2008–2009 were 1. *Clinical Counseling Psychology MA/MS (Master of Arts/Science)*—Applications 2009–2010, 62. Total applicants accepted 2009–2010, 43. Number full-time enrolled (new admits only) 2009–2010, 17. Number part-time enrolled (new admits only) 2009–2010, 15. Total enrolled 2009–2010 full-time, 40, part-time, 32. Openings 2010–2011, 40. The median number of years required for completion of a degree in 2008–2009 were 3. The number of students enrolled full- and part-time who were dismissed or voluntarily withdrew from this program area in 2008–2009 were 5.
Scores: Entries appear in this order: required test or GPA, minimum score (if required), median score of students entering in 2009–2010. *School Psychology EdS (School Psychology):* GRE-V 450, 470, GRE-Q 450, 590, overall undergraduate GPA 3.00, 3.39; *Clinical Counseling Psychology MA/MS (Master of Arts/Science):* GRE-V 450, 470, GRE-Q 450, 550, overall undergraduate GPA 3.00, 3.3.
Other Criteria: (importance of criteria rated low, medium, or high): GRE scores—high, research experience—medium, work experience—medium, extracurricular activity—low, clinically related public service—medium, GPA—high, letters of recommendation—high, interview—high, statement of goals and objectives—high, undergraduate major in psychology—low. For additional information on admission requirements, go to http://www.citadel.edu/psyc/.

Student Characteristics: The following represents characteristics of students in 2009–2010 in all graduate psychology programs in the department: Female—full-time 29, part-time 14; Male—full-time 2, part-time 1; African American/Black—full-time 11, part-time 7; Hispanic/Latino(a)—full-time 0, part-time 0; Asian/Pacific Islander—full-time 0, part-time 3; American Indian/Alaska Native—full-time 0, part-time 0; Caucasian/White—full-time 82, part-time 24; Multi-ethnic—full-time 0, part-time 0; students subject to the Americans With Disabilities Act—full-time 4, part-time 1; Unknown ethnicity—full-time 0, part-time 0; International students who hold an F-1 or J-1 Visa—full-time 0, part-time 0.

Financial Information/Assistance:
Tuition for Full-Time Study: Master's: State residents: $400 per credit hour; Nonstate residents: $657 per credit hour. Tuition is subject to change. See the following Web site for updates and changes in tuition costs: http://www.citadel.edu/graduatecollege/fees.html.

Financial Assistance:
First-Year Students: Teaching assistantships available for first year. Average amount paid per academic year: $7,000. Average number of hours worked per week: 20. Research assistantships available for first year. Average amount paid per academic year: $7,000. Average number of hours worked per week: 20.
Advanced Students: Teaching assistantships available for advanced students. Average amount paid per academic year: $7,000. Average number of hours worked per week: 20. Research assistantships available for advanced students. Average amount paid per academic year: $7,000. Average number of hours worked per week: 20.
Additional Information: Of all students currently enrolled full time, 25% benefited from one or more of the listed financial assistance programs. Application and information available online at: http://www.citadel.edu/finaid/g/index.shtml.

Internships/Practica: The EdS program in School Psychology requires two practica courses where students provide services in the public school systems (40 and 125 hours, respectively) and a 1200-hour internship (some are paid), at least 600 of which involve direct services within the public school system. The MA in Clinical Counseling Psychology requires one practicum (150 hours) and one internship (600 hours) where students provide clinical/counseling services in public mental health/substance abuse treatment facilities. These are unpaid field experiences.

Housing and Day Care: No on-campus housing is available. No on-campus day care facilities are available.

Employment of Department Graduates:

Master's Degree Graduates: Of those who graduated in the academic year 2008–2009, the following categories and numbers represent the postgraduate activities and employment of master's degree graduates: Enrolled in a psychology doctoral program (1), enrolled in a postdoctoral residency/fellowship (n/a), employed in independent practice (n/a), employed in a professional position in a school system (12), employed in government agency (1), employed in a community mental health/counseling center (7), employed in a hospital/medical center (4), do not know (6), total from the above (master's) (31).

Doctoral Degree Graduates: Of those who graduated in the academic year 2008–2009, the following categories and numbers represent the postgraduate activities and employment of doctoral degree graduates: Enrolled in a psychology doctoral program (n/a), total from the above (doctoral) (0).

Additional Information:

Orientation, Objectives, and Emphasis of Department: The School Psychology program is based on the scientist–practitioner model and emphasizes the school psychologist as a data-based problem-solver who applies psychological principles, knowledge and skill to processes and problems of education and schooling. Students are trained to provide a range of psychological assessment, consultation, intervention, prevention, program development and evaluation services with the goal of maximizing student learning and development. The School Psychology program has been accredited by the National Association of School Psychologists (NASP) since 1988. Students in the Master of Arts in Psychology: Clinical Counseling program are prepared to become scholarly practitioners of psychosocial counseling in community agencies, including college counseling centers, hospitals, mental health centers, and social services agencies. The program's model blends didactic and experience-based training to facilitate students' ability to utilize an empirical approach to assessment, goal development, intervention, and evaluation of services for a wide range of individuals and families experiencing a variety of psychosocial difficulties. The program is accredited by the Master's in Psychology Accreditation Council and is a member of the Council of Applied Master's Programs in Psychology.

Special Facilities or Resources: The Citadel's Department of Psychology enjoys a strong working relationship with the area school districts and agencies which provide mental health/substance abuse services. In addition, the nearby Medical University of South Carolina provides internship opportunities.

Information for Students With Physical Disabilities: See the following Web site for more information: http://www.citadel.edu/academicsupportcenter/.

Application Information:
Send to College of Graduate and Professional Studies, The Citadel, 171 Moultrie Street, Charleston, SC 29409. Application available online. URL of online application: http://www.citadel.edu/graduatecollege/apply/graduate.html. Students are admitted in the Fall, application deadline March 15. *Fee:* $30.

Clemson University
Department of Psychology
418 Brackett Hall
Clemson, SC 29634-1355
Telephone: (864) 656-3210
Fax: (864) 656-0358
E-mail: *praymar@clemson.edu*
Web: *http://www.clemson.edu/psych/*

Department Information:
1976. Interim Department Chair: Patrick Raymark. Number of faculty: total—full-time 27; women—full-time 8; total—minority—full-time 3.

Programs and Degrees Offered:
Listed in the following order: Program area, degree type (T if terminal Master's), number awarded 7/08–6/09. Human Factors PhD (Doctor of Philosophy) 0, Industrial/Organizational PhD (Doctor of Philosophy) 3.

Student Applications/Admissions:
Student Applications

Human Factors PhD (Doctor of Philosophy)—Applications 2009–2010, 50. Total applicants accepted 2009–2010, 4. Number full-time enrolled (new admits only) 2009–2010, 4. Number part-time enrolled (new admits only) 2009–2010, 0. Total enrolled 2009–2010 full-time, 17, part-time, 2. Openings 2010–2011, 6. The number of students enrolled full- and part-time who were dismissed or voluntarily withdrew from this program area in 2008–2009 were 0. Industrial/Organizational PhD (Doctor of Philosophy)—Applications 2009–2010, 140. Total applicants accepted 2009–2010, 3. Number full-time enrolled (new admits only) 2009–2010, 3. Total enrolled 2009–2010 full-time, 23, part-time, 5. Openings 2010–2011, 6. The median number of years required for completion of a degree in 2008–2009 were 4. The number of students enrolled full- and part-time who were dismissed or voluntarily withdrew from this program area in 2008–2009 were 0.

Scores: Entries appear in this order: required test or GPA, minimum score (if required), median score of students entering in 2009–2010. Human Factors PhD (Doctor of Philosophy): GRE-V no minimum stated, 540, GRE-Q no minimum stated, 650, GRE-Analytical no minimum stated, 4, overall undergraduate GPA no minimum stated, 2.9; *Industrial/Organizational PhD (Doctor of Philosophy)*: GRE-V no minimum stated, 560, GRE-Q no minimum stated, 610, GRE-Analytical no minimum stated, 4.5, overall undergraduate GPA no minimum stated, 3.7.

Other Criteria: (importance of criteria rated low, medium, or high): GRE scores—high, research experience—high, work experience—medium, extracurricular activity—low, GPA—high, letters of recommendation—high, interview—medium, statement of goals and objectives—high, undergraduate major in psychology—medium, specific undergraduate psychology courses taken—low. For additional information on admission requirements, go to http://www.clemson.edu/psych/.

Student Characteristics: The following represents characteristics of students in 2009–2010 in all graduate psychology programs in the department: Female—full-time 25, part-time 3; Male—full-time 15, part-time 4; African American/Black—full-time 2, part-time 0; Hispanic/Latino(a)—full-time 1, part-time 0; Asian/Pacific Islander—full-time 0, part-time 0; American Indian/Alaska Native—full-time 0, part-time 0; Caucasian/White—full-time 37, part-time 7; Multi-ethnic—full-time 0, part-time 0; students subject to the Americans With Disabilities Act—full-time 0, part-time 0; Unknown ethnicity—full-time 0, part-time 0; International students who hold an F-1 or J-1 Visa—full-time 1, part-time 0.

Financial Information/Assistance:

Tuition for Full-Time Study: *Master's:* State residents: per academic year $4,710; Nonstate residents: per academic year $9,382. *Doctoral:* State residents: per academic year $4,710; Nonstate residents: per academic year $9,382. Tuition is subject to change. See the following Web site for updates and changes in tuition costs: http://www.grad.clemson.edu/Financial.php.

Financial Assistance:

First-Year Students: Teaching assistantships available for first year. Average amount paid per academic year: $12,000. Average number of hours worked per week: 20. Apply by December 15. Research assistantships available for first year. Average amount paid per academic year: $16,000. Average number of hours worked per week: 20. Apply by December 15. Fellowships and scholarships available for first year. Average amount paid per academic year: $10,000. Average number of hours worked per week: 0. Apply by December 15.

Advanced Students: Teaching assistantships available for advanced students. Average amount paid per academic year: $13,000. Average number of hours worked per week: 20. Apply by December 15. Research assistantships available for advanced students. Average amount paid per academic year: $18,000. Average number of hours worked per week: 20. Apply by December 15. Fellowships and scholarships available for advanced students. Average amount paid per academic year: $10,000. Average number of hours worked per week: 0. Apply by December 15.

Additional Information: Of all students currently enrolled full time, 95% benefited from one or more of the listed financial assistance programs.

Internships/Practica: Students are expected to complete a summer internship during either their first or second year of study.

Housing and Day Care: On-campus housing is available. See the following Web site for more information: http://www.housing.clemson.edu/. No on-campus day care facilities are available.

Employment of Department Graduates:

Master's Degree Graduates: Of those who graduated in the academic year 2008–2009, the following categories and numbers represent the postgraduate activities and employment of master's degree graduates: Enrolled in a psychology doctoral program (4), enrolled in a postdoctoral residency/fellowship (n/a), employed in independent practice (n/a), employed in business or industry (3), total from the above (master's) (7).

Doctoral Degree Graduates: Of those who graduated in the academic year 2008–2009, the following categories and numbers represent the postgraduate activities and employment of doctoral degree graduates: Enrolled in a psychology doctoral program (n/a), employed in an academic position at a university (1), employed in business or industry (2), total from the above (doctoral) (3).

Additional Information:

Orientation, Objectives, and Emphasis of Department: The faculty of the Psychology Department are committed to excellence in teaching and research. The primary goals of the Master of Science program are to provide students with an essential core of knowledge in applied psychology and to develop applied research skills. The program is specifically designed to provide the student with the requisite theoretical foundations, skills in quantitative techniques and experimental design, and the practical problem-solving skills necessary to address real world problems in industry, business, and government. The emphasis is on the direct application of acquired training upon completion of the program. All of our graduate programs have a heavy out of the classroom research component with a required empirical thesis. The PhD programs prepare the student to generate and use knowledge in accordance with the scientist–practitioner model. In addition to the traditional areas of study in Industrial-Organizational Psychology and Human Factors (Engineering) Psychology, a new emphasis area in Occupational Health Psychology has been added to both the MS and PhD degree programs.

Special Facilities or Resources: The Psychology Department is housed on 4 floors of Brackett Hall. Students have access to several laboratories, including a Process Control Simulator Lab, Task Performance Lab, Psychophysiology Research Lab, Sleep Research Lab, Perception & Action Lab, Motion Sciences & Uncoupled Motion Simulation Lab, Visual Performance Lab, Driving Simulator Lab, Usability Testing Lab, Personnel Selection and Performance Appraisal Lab, I-O Research Lab, I-O Quant Lab, Social Psychology Lab, Residential Research Facility, Cognitive Aging & Technology Lab, as well as Virtual Reality and Robotics & Teleoperation facilities. To date, nearly 100% of our graduates have either gained employment in their chosen field or have been accepted into PhD programs (in many cases they have had one or more job offers before the completion of their degree). Our Human Factors program is one of only eight Psychology programs accredited by the Human Factors and Ergonomics Society.

Information for Students With Physical Disabilities: See the following Web site for more information: http://www.clemson.edu/sds/.

Application Information:

Application available online. URL of online application: http://www.grad.clemson.edu/Admission.php. Students are admitted in the Fall, application deadline December 15. *Fee:* $75.

Francis Marion University
Master's of Science in Applied Psychology
P.O. Box 100547
Florence, SC 29502
Telephone: (843) 661-1641
Fax: (843) 661-1628
E-mail: jhester@fmarion.edu
Web: http://www.fmarion.edu/academics/psychology

Department Information:
1970. Chair: John R. Hester, PhD. Number of faculty: total—full-time 11, part-time 6; women—full-time 5, part-time 4; minority—part-time 1.

Programs and Degrees Offered:
Listed in the following order: Program area, degree type (T if terminal Master's), number awarded 7/08–6/09. Clinical/Counseling Psychology MA/MS (Master of Arts/Science) (T) 8, School Psychology MA/MS (Master of Arts/Science) (T) 7.

Student Applications/Admissions:
Student Applications
Clinical/Counseling Psychology MA/MS (Master of Arts/Science)—Applications 2009–2010, 30. Total applicants accepted 2009–2010, 15. Number full-time enrolled (new admits only) 2009–2010, 9. Number part-time enrolled (new admits only) 2009–2010, 0. Total enrolled 2009–2010 full-time, 23. Openings 2010–2011, 10. The median number of years required for completion of a degree in 2008–2009 were 3. The number of students enrolled full- and part-time who were dismissed or voluntarily withdrew from this program area in 2008–2009 were 0. School Psychology MA/MS (Master of Arts/Science)—Applications 2009–2010, 30. Total applicants accepted 2009–2010, 17. Number full-time enrolled (new admits only) 2009–2010, 7. Number part-time enrolled (new admits only) 2009–2010, 0. Openings 2010–2011, 10. The median number of years required for completion of a degree in 2008–2009 were 3. The number of students enrolled full- and part-time who were dismissed or voluntarily withdrew from this program area in 2008–2009 were 0.
Other Criteria: (importance of criteria rated low, medium, or high): GRE scores—high, research experience—medium, work experience—medium, extracurricular activity—low, clinically related public service—medium, GPA—high, letters of recommendation—high, statement of goals and objectives—high, specific undergraduate psychology courses taken—medium. For additional information on admission requirements, go to http://www.fmarion.edu/academics/psy_msap/.

Student Characteristics: The following represents characteristics of students in 2009–2010 in all graduate psychology programs in the department: Female—full-time 41, part-time 0; Male—full-time 3, part-time 0; African American/Black—full-time 6, part-time 0; Hispanic/Latino(a)—full-time 0, part-time 0; Asian/Pacific Islander—full-time 0, part-time 0; American Indian/Alaska Native—full-time 0, part-time 0; Caucasian/White—full-time 37, part-time 0; Multi-ethnic—full-time 1, part-time 0; students subject to the Americans With Disabilities Act—full-time 0, part-time 0; Unknown ethnicity—full-time 0, part-time 0; International students who hold an F-1 or J-1 Visa—full-time 1, part-time 0.

Financial Information/Assistance:
Tuition for Full-Time Study: Master's: State residents: per academic year $7,825, $391 per credit hour; Nonstate residents: per academic year $15,650, $782 per credit hour. Tuition is subject to change. See the following Web site for updates and changes in tuition costs: http://www.fmarion.edu/about/fees/.

Financial Assistance:
First-Year Students: Teaching assistantships available for first year. Average amount paid per academic year: $8,000. Average number of hours worked per week: 20. Research assistantships available for first year. Average amount paid per academic year: $7,000. Average number of hours worked per week: 20. Fellowships and scholarships available for first year. Average amount paid per academic year: $500.
Advanced Students: Teaching assistantships available for advanced students. Average amount paid per academic year: $8,000. Average number of hours worked per week: 20. Research assistantships available for advanced students. Average amount paid per academic year: $7,000. Average number of hours worked per week: 20. Fellowships and scholarships available for advanced students. Average amount paid per academic year: $500.
Additional Information: Of all students currently enrolled full time, 35% benefited from one or more of the listed financial assistance programs. Application and information available online at: http://www.fmarion.edu/academics/psy_msap.

Internships/Practica: Master's Degree (MA/MS Clinical/Counseling Psychology): An internship experience, such as a final research project or "capstone" experience is required of graduates. Master's Degree (MA/MS School Psychology): An internship experience, such as a final research project or "capstone" experience is required of graduates. Internships occur in a variety of community settings. Typically Clinical/Counseling students complete a full-time, six-month internship in state human service agencies. The School Psychology Internship is a full-time experience as a school psychologist during Fall and Spring semester. All interns develop a broad array of skills under supervision.

Housing and Day Care: On-campus housing is available. See the following Web site for more information: http://www.fmuhousing.com. On-campus day care facilities are available. http://www.centerforthechild.org.

Employment of Department Graduates:
Master's Degree Graduates: Of those who graduated in the academic year 2008–2009, the following categories and numbers represent the postgraduate activities and employment of master's degree graduates: Enrolled in a psychology doctoral program (0), enrolled in another graduate/professional program (0), enrolled in a postdoctoral residency/fellowship (n/a), employed in independent practice (n/a), employed in an academic position at a university (0), employed in an academic position at a 2-year/4-year college (1), employed in other positions at a higher education institution (0), employed in a professional position in a school system (7), employed in government agency (1), employed in a community mental health/counseling center (6), total from the above (master's) (15).

GRADUATE STUDY IN PSYCHOLOGY

Doctoral Degree Graduates: Of those who graduated in the academic year 2008–2009, the following categories and numbers represent the postgraduate activities and employment of doctoral degree graduates: Enrolled in a psychology doctoral program (n/a), do not know (0), total from the above (doctoral) (0).

Additional Information:
Orientation, Objectives, and Emphasis of Department: The primary purpose of the program is to prepare professionals for employment in human services agencies, schools, or similar settings. The program also provides for the continuing education of those individuals currently employed in the helping professions and prepares students for further graduate study.

Special Facilities or Resources: The department has excellent laboratory facilities on campus including a computer laboratory. Regional human services facilities, community agencies, and school districts are accessible off campus. In addition, the Richardson Center for the Child is located on campus and provides opportunities for observation as well as training of graduate students.

Information for Students With Physical Disabilities: See the following Web site for more information: http://www.fmarion.edu/students/disabilityservices.

Application Information:
Send to Graduate Office, Francis Marion University, P.O. Box 100547, Florence, SC 29502-0547. Application available online. URL of online application: http://www.fmarion.edu/academics/GraduatePrograms. Students are admitted in the Fall, application deadline March 15; Spring, application deadline October 15. The School Psychology option only has Fall admissions. *Fee:* $30.

South Carolina, University of
Department of Psychology
College of Arts and Sciences
1512 Pendleton Street
Columbia, SC 29208
Telephone: (803) 777-4137
Fax: (803) 777-9558
E-mail: *martibrown@sc.edu*
Web: *http://www.psych.sc.edu*

Department Information:
1912. Interim Department Chair: John E. Richards. Number of faculty: total—full-time 40, part-time 8; women—full-time 24, part-time 5; total—minority—full-time 4, part-time 1; women minority—full-time 7, part-time 2.

Programs and Degrees Offered:
Listed in the following order: Program area, degree type (T if terminal Master's), number awarded 7/08–6/09. Clinical-Community Psychology PhD (Doctor of Philosophy) 10, Experimental Psychology PhD (Doctor of Philosophy) 2, School Psychology PhD (Doctor of Philosophy) 6.

APA Accreditation: Clinical PhD (Doctor of Philosophy). School PhD (Doctor of Philosophy).

Student Applications/Admissions:
Student Applications
Clinical-Community Psychology PhD (Doctor of Philosophy)—Applications 2009–2010, 106. Total applicants accepted 2009–2010, 11. Number full-time enrolled (new admits only) 2009–2010, 8. Number part-time enrolled (new admits only) 2009–2010, 0. Total enrolled 2009–2010 full-time, 42, part-time, 7. Openings 2010–2011, 8. The median number of years required for completion of a degree in 2008–2009 were 6. The number of students enrolled full- and part-time who were dismissed or voluntarily withdrew from this program area in 2008–2009 were 2. *Experimental Psychology PhD (Doctor of Philosophy)*—Applications 2009–2010, 32. Total applicants accepted 2009–2010, 10. Number full-time enrolled (new admits only) 2009–2010, 5. Number part-time enrolled (new admits only) 2009–2010, 0. Total enrolled 2009–2010 full-time, 21, part-time, 1. Openings 2010–2011, 7. The median number of years required for completion of a degree in 2008–2009 were 5. The number of students enrolled full- and part-time who were dismissed or voluntarily withdrew from this program area in 2008–2009 were 1. *School Psychology PhD (Doctor of Philosophy)*—Applications 2009–2010, 53. Total applicants accepted 2009–2010, 10. Number full-time enrolled (new admits only) 2009–2010, 8. Number part-time enrolled (new admits only) 2009–2010, 0. Total enrolled 2009–2010 full-time, 27, part-time, 1. Openings 2010–2011, 4. The median number of years required for completion of a degree in 2008–2009 were 5. The number of students enrolled full- and part-time who were dismissed or voluntarily withdrew from this program area in 2008–2009 were 0.

Scores: Entries appear in this order: required test or GPA, minimum score (if required), median score of students entering in 2009–2010. *Clinical-Community Psychology PhD (Doctor of Philosophy):* GRE-V no minimum stated, 590, GRE-Q no minimum stated, 660, GRE-Analytical no minimum stated, 4.5, GRE-Subject (Psychology) no minimum stated, 660, overall undergraduate GPA no minimum stated, 3.75, last 2 years GPA no minimum stated, 3.98, psychology GPA no minimum stated, 4.0; *Experimental Psychology PhD (Doctor of Philosophy):* GRE-V no minimum stated, 610, GRE-Q no minimum stated, 700, GRE-Analytical no minimum stated, 4.0, overall undergraduate GPA no minimum stated, 3.7, last 2 years GPA no minimum stated, 3.7, psychology GPA no minimum stated, 3.9; *School Psychology PhD (Doctor of Philosophy):* GRE-V no minimum stated, 480, GRE-Q no minimum stated, 720, GRE-Analytical no minimum stated, 4.5, overall undergraduate GPA no minimum stated, 3.57, last 2 years GPA no minimum stated, 3.73, psychology GPA no minimum stated, 3.95.

Other Criteria: (importance of criteria rated low, medium, or high): GRE scores—medium, research experience—high, work experience—medium, extracurricular activity—medium, clinically related public service—medium, GPA—high, letters of recommendation—high, interview—high, statement of goals and objectives—high, undergraduate major in psychology—medium, specific undergraduate psychology courses taken—medium. Criteria vary for different programs. For additional information on admission requirements, go to http://www.psych.sc.edu.

Student Characteristics: The following represents characteristics of students in 2009–2010 in all graduate psychology programs in the department: Female—full-time 55, part-time 17; Male—full-

time 20, part-time 6; African American/Black—full-time 8, part-time 2; Hispanic/Latino(a)—full-time 3, part-time 0; Asian/Pacific Islander—full-time 5, part-time 2; American Indian/Alaska Native—full-time 0, part-time 0; Caucasian/White—full-time 52, part-time 18; Multi-ethnic—full-time 0, part-time 0; students subject to the Americans With Disabilities Act—full-time 1, part-time 0; Unknown ethnicity—full-time 7, part-time 1; International students who hold an F-1 or J-1 Visa—full-time 5, part-time 0.

Financial Information/Assistance:
Tuition for Full-Time Study: *Doctoral:* State residents: per academic year $9,788, $484 per credit hour; Nonstate residents: per academic year $21,080, $1,028 per credit hour. Tuition is subject to change. Additional fees are assessed to students beyond the costs of tuition for the following: one time matriculation fee, technology & lab fees, international student fees & taxes, health insurance. See the following Web site for updates and changes in tuition costs: http://www.sc.edu/bursar/schedule.html.

Financial Assistance:
First-Year Students: Teaching assistantships available for first year. Average amount paid per academic year: $15,000. Average number of hours worked per week: 20. Research assistantships available for first year. Average amount paid per academic year: $15,000. Average number of hours worked per week: 20. Traineeships available for first year. Fellowships and scholarships available for first year.

Advanced Students: Teaching assistantships available for advanced students. Average amount paid per academic year: $15,000. Average number of hours worked per week: 20. Research assistantships available for advanced students. Average amount paid per academic year: $15,000. Average number of hours worked per week: 20. Traineeships available for advanced students. Fellowships and scholarships available for advanced students.

Additional Information: Of all students currently enrolled full time, 100% benefited from one or more of the listed financial assistance programs.

Internships/Practica: Doctoral Degree (PhD Clinical-Community Psychology): For those doctoral students for whom a professional internship was required in this program prior to graduation, (6) students applied for an internship in 2008–2009, with (6) students obtaining an internship. Of those students who obtained an internship, (6) were paid internships. Of those students who obtained an internship, (4) students placed in APA/CPA accredited internships, (0) students placed in internships not APA/CPA accredited, but listed with the Association of Psychology Postdoctoral and Internship Programs (APPIC), (0) students placed in internships conforming to guidelines of the Council of Directors of School Psychology Programs (CDSPP), (2) students placed in internships that were not APA/CPA accredited, APPIC or CDSPP listed. Doctoral Degree (PhD School Psychology): For those doctoral students for whom a professional internship was required in this program prior to graduation, (7) students applied for an internship in 2008–2009, with (7) students obtaining an internship. Of those students who obtained an internship, (6) were paid internships. Of those students who obtained an internship, (2) students placed in APA/CPA accredited internships, (0) students placed in internships not APA/CPA accredited, but listed with the Association of Psychology Postdoctoral and Internship Programs (APPIC), (5) students placed in internships conforming to guidelines of the Council of Directors of School Psychology Programs (CDSPP), (0) students placed in internships that were not APA/CPA accredited, APPIC or CDSPP listed. Students in school psychology and clinical-community psychology complete at least one year of half-time placement in a community service agency expanding their experience with a diverse client population and multidisciplinary service providers.

Housing and Day Care: On-campus housing is available. See the following Web site for more information: http://www.housing.sc.edu/famgrad.asp. On-campus day care facilities are available. See the following Web site for more information: http://www.sc.edu/childrenscenter/.

Employment of Department Graduates:
Master's Degree Graduates: Of those who graduated in the academic year 2008–2009, the following categories and numbers represent the postgraduate activities and employment of master's degree graduates: Enrolled in a psychology doctoral program (7), enrolled in another graduate/professional program (0), enrolled in a postdoctoral residency/fellowship (n/a), employed in independent practice (n/a), total from the above (master's) (7).

Doctoral Degree Graduates: Of those who graduated in the academic year 2008–2009, the following categories and numbers represent the postgraduate activities and employment of doctoral degree graduates: Enrolled in a psychology doctoral program (n/a), enrolled in a postdoctoral residency/fellowship (4), employed in other positions at a higher education institution (1), employed in a professional position in a school system (1), employed in a community mental health/counseling center (2), employed in a hospital/medical center (2), other employment position (1), total from the above (doctoral) (11).

Additional Information:
Orientation, Objectives, and Emphasis of Department: The department has interdisciplinary research emphases in developmental cognitive neuroscience/neurodevelopmental disorders, prevention science, reading and language, and ethnic minority health and mental health. The experimental program offers concentrations in behavioral neuroscience, cognitive neuroscience, cognitive, developmental, and quantitative psychology built on broad scientific training in experimental psychology. The school psychology program includes emphasis in child assessment, individual and group consultation, educational research, and professional roles. In clinical-community, there is a wide latitude of choices: assessment, psychotherapy and behavioral interventions, community psychology, and consultation. Regular clinical-community training includes both adults and children, with an option of special emphasis on children or community settings.

Special Facilities or Resources: The special facilities and resources of the department include the university-directed psychological service center, the medical school, the VA hospital, the department-directed outpatient psychological services center, mental health centers and other educational and mental health service settings. Other laboratories include Behavioral Pharmacology Lab; Behavioral Neuroscience Lab with high density EEG and MRI; Developmental Sensory Neuroscience Lab; Experimental and Cognitive Processes Lab; Infant Attention Lab; Judgment and Decision Making Lab; and Attention and Perception Lab. We are actively involved in community agencies, the psychiatric training institution, and the psychopharmacology laboratory.

Information for Students With Physical Disabilities: See the following Web site for more information: http://www.sa.sc.edu/sds/.

Application Information:
Send to Graduate Admissions Coordinator, Department of Psychology, University of South Carolina, Columbia, SC 29208. Application available online. URL of online application: http://www.gradschool.sc.edu/apply.htm. Students are admitted in the Fall, application deadline December 1. The application deadline for fall admission in Clinical-Community Psychology and School Psychology is December 1 and for Experimental Psychology is January 1. *Fee:* $50.

South Carolina, University of, Aiken
Department of Psychology/Applied Clinical Psychology Graduate Program
College of Sciences
471 University Parkway
Aiken, SC 29801
Telephone: (803) 641-3358
Fax: (803) 641-3726
E-mail: *jstafford@usca.edu*
Web: *http://www.web.usca.edu/psychology/*

Department Information:
1976. Chairperson: Dr. Ed Callen. Number of faculty: total—full-time 9; women—full-time 7.

Programs and Degrees Offered:
Listed in the following order: Program area, degree type (T if terminal Master's), number awarded 7/08–6/09. Applied Clinical Psychology MA/MS (Master of Arts/Science) (T) 7.

Student Applications/Admissions:
Student Applications
Applied Clinical Psychology MA/MS (Master of Arts/Science)—Applications 2009–2010, 43. Total applicants accepted 2009–2010, 25. Number full-time enrolled (new admits only) 2009–2010, 13. Number part-time enrolled (new admits only) 2009–2010, 0. Total enrolled 2009–2010 full-time, 19, part-time, 6. Openings 2010–2011, 13. The median number of years required for completion of a degree in 2008–2009 were 2. The number of students enrolled full- and part-time who were dismissed or voluntarily withdrew from this program area in 2008–2009 were 3.
Scores: Entries appear in this order: required test or GPA, minimum score (if required), median score of students entering in 2009–2010. *Applied Clinical Psychology MA/MS (Master of Arts/Science):* GRE-V no minimum stated, GRE-Q no minimum stated, overall undergraduate GPA no minimum stated, psychology GPA no minimum stated.
Other Criteria: (importance of criteria rated low, medium, or high): GRE scores—high, research experience—high, work experience—low, extracurricular activity—low, clinically related public service—low, GPA—high, letters of recommendation—high, statement of goals and objectives—medium, undergraduate major in psychology—medium, specific undergraduate psychology courses taken—medium. For additional information on admission requirements, go to http://web.usca.edu/psychology/programs-and-courses/master-of-science.dot?

Student Characteristics: The following represents characteristics of students in 2009–2010 in all graduate psychology programs in the department: Female—full-time 16, part-time 6; Male—full-time 3, part-time 1; African American/Black—full-time 2, part-time 0; Hispanic/Latino(a)—full-time 0, part-time 0; Asian/Pacific Islander—full-time 0, part-time 0; American Indian/Alaska Native—full-time 0, part-time 0; Caucasian/White—full-time 17, part-time 7; Multi-ethnic—full-time 0, part-time 0; students subject to the Americans With Disabilities Act—full-time 0, part-time 1; Unknown ethnicity—full-time 0, part-time 0; International students who hold an F-1 or J-1 Visa—full-time 1, part-time 0.

Financial Information/Assistance:
Tuition for Full-Time Study: *Master's:* State residents: per academic year $9,788; Nonstate residents: per academic year $21,080. Tuition is subject to change. See the following Web site for updates and changes in tuition costs: http://web.usca.edu/admissions/cost_attendance.dot.

Financial Assistance:
First-Year Students: Research assistantships available for first year. Average amount paid per academic year: $6,667. Average number of hours worked per week: 15. Traineeships available for first year. Average amount paid per academic year: $6,667. Average number of hours worked per week: 15.
Advanced Students: Research assistantships available for advanced students. Average amount paid per academic year: $6,667. Average number of hours worked per week: 15. Traineeships available for advanced students. Average amount paid per academic year: $6,667. Average number of hours worked per week: 15.
Additional Information: Of all students currently enrolled full time, 90% benefited from one or more of the listed financial assistance programs. Application and information available online at: http://web.usca.edu/financialaid/.

Internships/Practica: Master's Degree (MA/MS Applied Clinical Psychology): An internship experience, such as a final research project or "capstone" experience is required of graduates. Students are required to take two semesters of practica during which they will have the opportunity to provide assessment and treatment to a variety of types of clients (e.g., children, adults, couples, families) with a variety of diagnoses or difficulties. Students will also gain experience providing group therapy (e.g., anger management, parenting) during practica. These cases are seen in the departmental clinic, which services the community, and practicum students are supervised by clinical faculty. Most students are also given the opportunity to have a paid assistantship, however, this is not a program requirement and assistantships are not always available for all students. Students with an assistantship work 15 hours a week and receive several benefits in addition to gaining clinical experience. Assistantships are offered in a variety of settings including a private psychiatric hospital, the student counseling center, an emergency shelter for children, and a community mental health agency. A large majority of students graduate with over 1000 hours of applied clinical experience.

Housing and Day Care: On-campus housing is available. See the following Web site for more information: http://web.usca.edu/

housing. On-campus day care facilities are available. See the following Web site for more information: http://www.usca.edu/childcenter/.

Employment of Department Graduates:
Master's Degree Graduates: Of those who graduated in the academic year 2008–2009, the following categories and numbers represent the postgraduate activities and employment of master's degree graduates: Enrolled in a psychology doctoral program (1), enrolled in another graduate/professional program (0), enrolled in a postdoctoral residency/fellowship (n/a), employed in independent practice (n/a), employed in an academic position at a university (0), employed in an academic position at a 2-year/4-year college (0), employed in other positions at a higher education institution (0), employed in a professional position in a school system (0), employed in business or industry (0), employed in government agency (0), employed in a community mental health/counseling center (5), employed in a hospital/medical center (0), still seeking employment (0), not seeking employment (1), other employment position (0), do not know (2), total from the above (master's) (9).
Doctoral Degree Graduates: Of those who graduated in the academic year 2008–2009, the following categories and numbers represent the postgraduate activities and employment of doctoral degree graduates: Enrolled in a psychology doctoral program (n/a), total from the above (doctoral) (0).

Additional Information:
Orientation, Objectives, and Emphasis of Department: Our program provides graduate study and clinical experience in preparation for careers in applied clinical and counseling settings and as a foundation for students interested in pursuing advanced doctoral studies. Students enrolled in this program are expected to pursue a plan of study to ensure increased professional competence and breadth of knowledge in the field of clinical and counseling psychology. The degree objectives are designed to enable the student to: understand principles of psychology and how they are applied; understand a diversity of theoretical perspectives; interpret and apply statistical and research techniques; understand professional, legal and ethical principles as they pertain to professional conduct and responsibility; and understand and develop skills in assessment procedures and intervention strategies. A strong emphasis has been placed on the need to train students within the tradition of the scientist–practitioner model. It is the belief of faculty that the master's-level practitioner is well-served by participation in this process and that the critical-thinking skills so essential to sound clinical decision-making are enhanced through research experience. The clinical faculty are all of a cognitive behavioral orientation but support student training and therapeutic practice in various orientations as long as they have empirical support.

Special Facilities or Resources: The Psychology Department has its own computer laboratory for use by graduate and undergraduate Psychology students. The lab contains 20 new computers, LCD projector, scanner, and network printer. All of the machines have standard software as well as copies of SPSS, which is the department's statistics software standard. Additionally, computers are located in all laboratory research rooms, and LCD computer setups are available for use in all of the psychology classrooms. The Psychology Clinic is currently housed in an area that includes a graduate student office, waiting area, the Program Director's office, two individual therapy/assessment rooms with observation decks, a storage area for testing and library material, and a separate group therapy room with observation deck. The Psychology Department also has a laboratory facility to support the research activities of the faculty and students, comprised of an office for the lab director, an animal vivarium, 7 individual human research rooms, a large experimental room for group testing, and separate research cubicles with state of the art equipment to support animal research. The total square footage of psychology laboratory space is 3400 feet.

Information for Students With Physical Disabilities: See the following Web site for more information: http://www.usca.edu/ds/.

Application Information:
Send to Ms. Karen Morris, Coordinator for Office of Graduate Admissions, 471 University Parkway, Aiken, South Carolina, 29801. Application available online. URL of online application: http://web.usca.edu/graduate-admissions/index.dot. Students are admitted in the Fall, application deadline April 1. Admission for terms other than Fall are considered on a rolling basis and are dependent upon space availability. *Fee:* $45.

Winthrop University
Department of Psychology
Arts and Sciences
135 Kinard
Rock Hill, SC 29733
Telephone: (803) 323-2117
Fax: (803) 323-2371
E-mail: *prusj@winthrop.edu*
Web: *http://www.winthrop.edu/psychology*

Department Information:
1923. Chairperson: Dr. Joe Prus. Number of faculty: total—full-time 15, part-time 4; women—full-time 8, part-time 4; total—minority—full-time 2, part-time 1; women minority—full-time 2, part-time 1.

Programs and Degrees Offered:
Listed in the following order: Program area, degree type (T if terminal Master's), number awarded 7/08–6/09. School Psychology Other 11.

Student Applications/Admissions:
Student Applications
School Psychology Other—Applications 2009–2010, 55. Total applicants accepted 2009–2010, 10. Number full-time enrolled (new admits only) 2009–2010, 10. Number part-time enrolled (new admits only) 2009–2010, 0. Openings 2010–2011, 10. The median number of years required for completion of a degree in 2008–2009 were 3. The number of students enrolled full- and part-time who were dismissed or voluntarily withdrew from this program area in 2008–2009 were 0.
Scores: Entries appear in this order: required test or GPA, minimum score (if required), median score of students entering in 2009–2010. School Psychology Other: GRE-V no minimum stated, 490, GRE-Q no minimum stated, 560, GRE-Analytical no minimum stated, 4.5, overall undergraduate GPA no mini-

mum stated, 3.6, last 2 years GPA no minimum stated, 3.7, psychology GPA no minimum stated, 3.7.

Other Criteria: (importance of criteria rated low, medium, or high): GRE scores—medium, research experience—low, work experience—medium, extracurricular activity—low, clinically related public service—medium, GPA—high, letters of recommendation—medium, interview—high, statement of goals and objectives—medium, experience with children—high, undergraduate major in psychology—medium, specific undergraduate psychology courses taken—medium. For additional information on admission requirements, go to http://www2.winthrop.edu/psychology/.

Student Characteristics: The following represents characteristics of students in 2009–2010 in all graduate psychology programs in the department: Female—full-time 28, part-time 0; Male—full-time 3, part-time 0; African American/Black—full-time 2, part-time 0; Hispanic/Latino(a)—full-time 0, part-time 0; Asian/Pacific Islander—full-time 0, part-time 0; American Indian/Alaska Native—full-time 0, part-time 0; Caucasian/White—full-time 29, part-time 0; Multi-ethnic—full-time 0, part-time 0; students subject to the Americans With Disabilities Act—full-time 0, part-time 0; Unknown ethnicity—full-time 0, part-time 0; International students who hold an F-1 or J-1 Visa—full-time 0, part-time 0.

Financial Information/Assistance:
Tuition for Full-Time Study: *Master's:* State residents: per academic year $11,180, $469 per credit hour; Nonstate residents: per academic year $16,244, $676 per credit hour. Tuition is subject to change. See the following Web site for updates and changes in tuition costs: http://www.winthrop.edu/cashiers/.

Financial Assistance:
First-Year Students: Teaching assistantships available for first year. Average amount paid per academic year: $3,600. Average number of hours worked per week: 20. Apply by April 15. Research assistantships available for first year. Average amount paid per academic year: $3,600. Average number of hours worked per week: 20. Apply by April 15. Fellowships and scholarships available for first year. Average amount paid per academic year: $1,000. Apply by April 15.

Advanced Students: Traineeships available for advanced students. Average amount paid per academic year: $4,500. Average number of hours worked per week: 15.

Additional Information: Of all students currently enrolled full time, 95% benefited from one or more of the listed financial assistance programs. Application and information available online at: http://www.winthrop.edu/graduateschool/.

Internships/Practica: The program provides paid traineeships during the second year and internships during the third year in area school districts and agencies. Rural, suburban, and urban field settings include diverse student/client populations. The internship includes a full range of school psychological services. Each intern receives weekly supervision from both a faculty member and a field-based, credentialed supervisor.

Housing and Day Care: On-campus housing is available. See the following Web site for more information: http://www.winthrop.edu/reslife/default.aspx. On-campus day care facilities are available. See the following Web site for more information: http://coe.winthrop.edu/macfeat/.

Employment of Department Graduates:
Master's Degree Graduates: Of those who graduated in the academic year 2008–2009, the following categories and numbers represent the postgraduate activities and employment of master's degree graduates: Enrolled in a postdoctoral residency/fellowship (n/a), employed in independent practice (n/a), employed in a professional position in a school system (10), still seeking employment (1), total from the above (master's) (11).

Doctoral Degree Graduates: Of those who graduated in the academic year 2008–2009, the following categories and numbers represent the postgraduate activities and employment of doctoral degree graduates: Enrolled in a psychology doctoral program (n/a), total from the above (doctoral) (0).

Additional Information:
Orientation, Objectives, and Emphasis of Department: The Winthrop School Psychology program is designed to prepare practitioners who are competent to provide a full range of school psychological services, including consultation, behavioral intervention, psychoeducational assessment, research and evaluation, and counseling. The three-year, full-time program leading to both MS and Specialist in School Psychology degrees qualifies graduates for state and national certification as a school psychologist pending attainment of a passing score on the Praxis II exam in school psychology. The program emphasizes evidenced-based psychological and psychoeducational methods. Students are prepared to work with diverse clients from birth to adulthood, and with families, teachers, and others in the schools and community. The program includes an applied, competency-based approach to training that progresses sequentially from foundations and practicum courses to a 450 hour traineeship to a 1200-hour internship, and affords maximum individualized supervision. Program faculty represent considerable ethnic and experiential diversity. All have advanced degrees and credentials in school psychology, are active in the profession at local, state, and national levels, and view teaching and supervision as their primary roles. Faculty encourage a collaborative approach to learning and close cooperation and support among students.

Special Facilities or Resources: Winthrop University is a state-supported institution of about 6,500 students which provides students with access to an academic computer center, state-of-the-art health center, university library with nearly 500,000 volumes and 4,000 periodicals and serials, and a variety of other resources. Access to such department resources as a graduate student workroom and school psychology mini-library and assessment resource center are available. Winthrop's 418-acre campus is located in the greater Charlotte, NC area, which includes a great variety of resources which may be of personal or professional interest to graduate students in school psychology.

Information for Students With Physical Disabilities: See the following Web site for more information: http://www2.winthrop.edu/hcs/DS.htm.

Application Information:
Send to The Graduate School, Winthrop University, Rock Hill, SC 29733. Application available online. URL of online application: http://www.winthrop.edu/graduateschool/. Students are admitted in the Fall, application deadline February 1. *Fee:* $50. Application fee may be waived by program director in cases of financial hardship.

SOUTH DAKOTA

South Dakota, University of
Department of Psychology
414 East Clark Street
Vermillion, SD 57069
Telephone: (605) 677-5351
Fax: (605) 677-3195
E-mail: *Randy.Quevillon@usd.edu*
Web: *http://www.usd.edu/psyc*

Department Information:
1926. Chairperson: Randal Quevillon. Number of faculty: total—full-time 15, part-time 1; women—full-time 7; total—minority—full-time 3; women minority—full-time 2.

Programs and Degrees Offered:
Listed in the following order: Program area, degree type (T if terminal Master's), number awarded 7/08–6/09. Human Factors PhD (Doctor of Philosophy) 4, Clinical Psychology PhD (Doctor of Philosophy) 7.

APA Accreditation: Clinical PhD (Doctor of Philosophy). Student Outcome Data Website: http://www.usd.edu/arts-and-sciences/psychology/clinical-psychology/student-admissions-outcomes-data.cfm.

Student Applications/Admissions:
Student Applications
Human Factors PhD (Doctor of Philosophy)—Applications 2009–2010, 8. Total applicants accepted 2009–2010, 3. Number full-time enrolled (new admits only) 2009–2010, 2. Openings 2010–2011, 3. The median number of years required for completion of a degree in 2008–2009 were 6. The number of students enrolled full- and part-time who were dismissed or voluntarily withdrew from this program area in 2008–2009 were 0. Clinical Psychology PhD (Doctor of Philosophy)—Applications 2009–2010, 47. Total applicants accepted 2009–2010, 6. Number full-time enrolled (new admits only) 2009–2010, 6. Openings 2010–2011, 7. The median number of years required for completion of a degree in 2008–2009 were 6. The number of students enrolled full- and part-time who were dismissed or voluntarily withdrew from this program area in 2008–2009 were 0.
Scores: Entries appear in this order: required test or GPA, minimum score (if required), median score of students entering in 2009–2010. Human Factors PhD (Doctor of Philosophy): GRE-V no minimum stated, GRE-Q no minimum stated, overall undergraduate GPA 3.0; Clinical Psychology PhD (Doctor of Philosophy): GRE-V no minimum stated, 550, GRE-Q no minimum stated, 530, GRE-Analytical no minimum stated, GRE-Subject (Psychology) no minimum stated, 665, overall undergraduate GPA no minimum stated, 3.7.
Other Criteria: (importance of criteria rated low, medium, or high): GRE scores—medium, research experience—high, work experience—medium, extracurricular activity—medium, clinically related public service—medium, GPA—medium, letters of recommendation—high, interview—high, statement of goals and objectives—medium, match with program—high, Applicant's responses to the Supplemental Application questions are highly weighted in the Clinical program admissions process. The Clinical program requires an interview and the Human Factors program does not. For additional information on admission requirements, go to http://www.usd.edu/arts-and-sciences/psychology/graduate.cfm.

Student Characteristics: The following represents characteristics of students in 2009–2010 in all graduate psychology programs in the department: Female—full-time 35, part-time 0; Male—full-time 17, part-time 0; African American/Black—full-time 1, part-time 0; Hispanic/Latino(a)—full-time 2, part-time 0; Asian/Pacific Islander—full-time 5, part-time 0; American Indian/Alaska Native—full-time 2, part-time 0; Caucasian/White—full-time 42, part-time 0; Multi-ethnic—full-time 0, part-time 0; students subject to the Americans With Disabilities Act—full-time 0, part-time 0; Unknown ethnicity—full-time 0, part-time 0; International students who hold an F-1 or J-1 Visa—full-time 0, part-time 0.

Financial Information/Assistance:
Tuition for Full-Time Study: *Doctoral:* State residents: $139 per credit hour; Nonstate residents: $294 per credit hour. Tuition is subject to change. See the following Web site for updates and changes in tuition costs: http://www.usd.edu/finance-and-administration/business-office/graduate-tuition.cfm.

Financial Assistance:
First-Year Students: Teaching assistantships available for first year. Average amount paid per academic year: $5,750. Average number of hours worked per week: 16. Research assistantships available for first year. Average amount paid per academic year: $5,750. Average number of hours worked per week: 16. Fellowships and scholarships available for first year. Average amount paid per academic year: $9,000. Average number of hours worked per week: 16.
Advanced Students: Teaching assistantships available for advanced students. Average amount paid per academic year: $6,000. Average number of hours worked per week: 16. Research assistantships available for advanced students. Average amount paid per academic year: $8,000. Average number of hours worked per week: 16. Traineeships available for advanced students. Average amount paid per academic year: $10,000. Average number of hours worked per week: 16. Fellowships and scholarships available for advanced students. Average amount paid per academic year: $10,000. Average number of hours worked per week: 16.
Additional Information: Of all students currently enrolled full time, 100% benefited from one or more of the listed financial assistance programs. Application and information available online at: http://www.usd.edu/finaid.

Internships/Practica: Doctoral Degree (PhD Clinical Psychology): For those doctoral students for whom a professional internship was required in this program prior to graduation, (11) students applied for an internship in 2008–2009, with (9) students obtaining an internship. Of those students who obtained an internship, (9) were paid internships. Of those students who obtained

an internship, (9) students placed in APA/CPA accredited internships, (0) students placed in internships not APA/CPA accredited, but listed with the Association of Psychology Postdoctoral and Internship Programs (APPIC), (0) students placed in internships conforming to guidelines of the Council of Directors of School Psychology Programs (CDSPP), (0) students placed in internships that were not APA/CPA accredited, APPIC or CDSPP listed. Several internships are available in Human Factors: placements with IBM, Lockheed, Hewlett-Packard, and Intel have been recent examples. In Clinical, a twelve month internship is required in the final year, and we are proud of the record our students have achieved in obtaining top placements. We also have available a series of paid clinical placements. In addition, many graduate courses include practicum components, and clinical students are placed on practicum teams through the Psychological Services Center each semester.

Housing and Day Care: On-campus housing is available. See the following Web site for more information: http://www.usd.edu/campus-life/student-services/university-housing/. On-campus day care facilities are available. See the following Web site for more information: http://www.usd.edu/childcare.

Employment of Department Graduates:
Master's Degree Graduates: Of those who graduated in the academic year 2008–2009, the following categories and numbers represent the postgraduate activities and employment of master's degree graduates: Enrolled in a postdoctoral residency/fellowship (n/a), employed in independent practice (n/a), total from the above (master's) (0).
Doctoral Degree Graduates: Of those who graduated in the academic year 2008–2009, the following categories and numbers represent the postgraduate activities and employment of doctoral degree graduates: Enrolled in a psychology doctoral program (n/a), employed in an academic position at a 2-year/4-year college (1), employed in government agency (3), employed in a community mental health/counseling center (3), total from the above (doctoral) (7).

Additional Information:
Orientation, Objectives, and Emphasis of Department: The department seeks to develop scholars who can contribute to the expansion of psychological information. The major goals of the theoretically eclectic program in clinical psychology are to increase students' knowledge of and identification with psychology as a method of inquiry about human behavior and to provide students with the theory, skills, and experience to function in a professional, research, or academic capacity. Training is provided in traditional areas as well as disaster psychology, rural community psychology, cross-cultural issues (particularly work with American Indian populations), program evaluation, neuropsychology, family therapy, and women's issues. The experience thus provided serves to broaden professional competencies and increase the versatility of the program's graduates. The overall mission of Human Factors psychology is to improve living and working through knowledge of the abilities and limitations of the person part of human-machine or socio-technical systems. The program's goal is to train doctoral-level professionals qualified to do research in industry, government, and universities. As an element of their training, all graduate students conduct empirical investigations. In recent years, the Human Factors Laboratory has supported studies of information processing, human-computer interfaces, motor performance, program evaluation and testing, traffic safety, transportation systems, and the effects of chemical agents and stress on human efficiency.

Special Facilities or Resources: Available to all psychology graduate students are computer lab facilities including word processing and statistical analysis software. Microcomputers are also easily accessible within the department for personal computing and research purposes. Much general purpose, highly adaptable research equipment is available to both Clinical and Human Factors students. The Human Factors Laboratory is particularly well-equipped for experimentation within the specialty areas of current interest to associated faculty. The Department houses the Disaster Mental Health Institute, a South Dakota Board of Regents Center of Excellence, which provides unique research and service opportunities for graduate students as well as specialized coursework and assistantships. The Psychological Services Center, which supplies clinical services for both University students and the general public, accepts referrals from physicians, schools, and other community and state agencies. The Center has offices equipped for a variety of diagnostic and therapeutic activities, including neuropsychological work. The Department's students take full advantage of training and experience available at local, state, and regional mental health facilities.

Information for Students With Physical Disabilities: See the following Web site for more information: http://www.usd.edu/academics/disability-services/index.cfm.

Application Information:
Send to Dean, Graduate School, University of South Dakota, 414 E Clark Street, Vermilion, SD 57069-2390. Application available online. URL of online application: http://www.usd.edu/gradsch/gradapp.cfm. Students are admitted in the Fall, application deadline January 5. Clinical Program due January 5, Human Factors Program due February 15. *Fee:* $35.

TENNESSEE

Austin Peay State University
Department of Psychology
601 College Street
Clarksville, TN 37044
Telephone: (931) 221-7233
Fax: (931) 221-6267
E-mail: *Fungs@apsu.edu*
Web: *http://www.apsu.edu/psychology/*

Department Information:
1968. Chairperson: Dr. Samuel Fung. Number of faculty: total—full-time 14; women—full-time 6; total—minority—full-time 3; women minority—full-time 2; faculty subject to the Americans With Disabilities Act 1.

Programs and Degrees Offered:
Listed in the following order: Program area, degree type (T if terminal Master's), number awarded 7/08–6/09. Community Counseling MA/MS (Master of Arts/Science) (T), Industrial/Organizational Psychology MA/MS (Master of Arts/Science) (T), School Counseling MA/MS (Master of Arts/Science) (T).

Student Applications/Admissions:
Student Applications
Community Counseling MA/MS (Master of Arts/Science)—Applications 2009–2010, 30. Total applicants accepted 2009–2010, 11. Number full-time enrolled (new admits only) 2009–2010, 11. Total enrolled 2009–2010 full-time, 26. Openings 2010–2011, 10. The number of students enrolled full- and part-time who were dismissed or voluntarily withdrew from this program area in 2008–2009 were 0. *Industrial/Organizational Psychology MA/MS (Master of Arts/Science)*—Applications 2009–2010, 44. Total applicants accepted 2009–2010, 13. Number full-time enrolled (new admits only) 2009–2010, 13. Total enrolled 2009–2010 full-time, 35. Openings 2010–2011, 15. The number of students enrolled full- and part-time who were dismissed or voluntarily withdrew from this program area in 2008–2009 were 0. *School Counseling MA/MS (Master of Arts/Science)*—Applications 2009–2010, 28. Total applicants accepted 2009–2010, 13. Number full-time enrolled (new admits only) 2009–2010, 13. Total enrolled 2009–2010 full-time, 33. Openings 2010–2011, 10.
Scores: Entries appear in this order: required test or GPA, minimum score (if required), median score of students entering in 2009–2010. *Community Counseling MA/MS (Master of Arts/Science)*: GRE-V 350, GRE-Q 350, overall undergraduate GPA 3.0; *Industrial/Organizational Psychology MA/MS (Master of Arts/Science)*: GRE-V 350, GRE-Q 350, overall undergraduate GPA 3.0; *School Counseling MA/MS (Master of Arts/Science)*: GRE-V 350, GRE-Q 350, overall undergraduate GPA 3.0.
Other Criteria: (importance of criteria rated low, medium, or high): GRE scores—medium, research experience—low, GPA—medium, letters of recommendation—high, statement of goals and objectives—high, undergraduate major in psychology—high, specific undergraduate psychology courses taken—medium. For additional information on admission requirements, go to http://www.apsu.edu/psychology/grad.aspx.

Student Characteristics: The following represents characteristics of students in 2009–2010 in all graduate psychology programs in the department: Female—part-time 0; Male—part-time 0; African American/Black—part-time 0; Hispanic/Latino(a)—full-time 0, part-time 0; Asian/Pacific Islander—full-time 0, part-time 0; American Indian/Alaska Native—full-time 0, part-time 0; Caucasian/White—full-time 0, part-time 0; Multi-ethnic—full-time 0, part-time 0; students subject to the Americans With Disabilities Act—full-time 0, part-time 0; Unknown ethnicity—full-time 0, part-time 0; International students who hold an F-1 or J-1 Visa—full-time 0, part-time 0.

Financial Information/Assistance:
Tuition for Full-Time Study: *Master's:* State residents: per academic year $6,600, $369 per credit hour; Nonstate residents: per academic year $16,400, $915 per credit hour. Tuition is subject to change. Additional fees are assessed to students beyond the costs of tuition for the following: technology access fee, general access fee. See the following Web site for updates and changes in tuition costs: http://www.apsu.edu/BUSINESSOFFICE/ACCTREC/tuition_fees.htm.

Financial Assistance:
First-Year Students: Teaching assistantships available for first year. Average number of hours worked per week: 20.
Advanced Students: Teaching assistantships available for advanced students.
Additional Information: Of all students currently enrolled full time, 11% benefited from one or more of the listed financial assistance programs. Application and information available online at: http://www.apsu.edu/financialaid/.

Internships/Practica: Master's Degree (MA/MS Community Counseling): An internship experience, such as a final research project or "capstone" experience is required of graduates. Master's Degree (MA/MS School Counseling): An internship experience, such as a final research project or "capstone" experience is required of graduates. There are some paid internships available at the present. A variety of unpaid internships are available in mental health agencies, schools, or community agencies.

Housing and Day Care: On-campus housing is available. See the following Web site for more information: http://www.apsu.edu/housing/. On-campus day care facilities are available. See the following Web site for more information: http://www.apsu.edu/clc/.

Employment of Department Graduates:
Master's Degree Graduates: Of those who graduated in the academic year 2008–2009, the following categories and numbers represent the postgraduate activities and employment of master's degree graduates: Enrolled in a postdoctoral residency/fellowship (n/a), employed in independent practice (n/a), total from the above (master's) (0).
Doctoral Degree Graduates: Of those who graduated in the academic year 2008–2009, the following categories and numbers represent the postgraduate activities and employment of doctoral degree graduates: Enrolled in a psychology doctoral program (n/a), total from the above (doctoral) (0).

Additional Information:
Orientation, Objectives, and Emphasis of Department: The programs in the department are based on the concept that both a strong foundation in theoretical principles and the development of skills in the application of these principles and techniques is necessary in the training of psychologists or counselors. The Master of Arts (MA) with a major in Industrial/Organizational Psychology is an online degree program. The program educates students to design, develop, implement, and evaluate psychologically-based human resources, interventions in organizations. The Master of Science (MS) in Counseling program has two concentrations: Community Counseling and School Counseling. The community counseling concentration prepares students to work in a variety of community agency settings and/or eventual private practice. Students completing this concentration will have met the educational requirements for licensure in Tennessee as a Licensed Professional Counselor with Mental Health Service provider status. The school counseling program is designed to prepare graduates for school counseling positions at elementary, middle/junior high and high school levels. Graduates will meet the current licensing requirements for the Tennessee Board of Education.

Special Facilities or Resources: The department of psychology has a variety of facilities to provide learning and research opportunities. Rooms equipped with one-way observation windows, video and other monitoring equipment are available for counseling, testing and human research. The department has arranged for internship and practicum experiences with a variety of community agencies. Laboratories for vision, infant development, animal learning, and behavioral physiology are available for faculty and student research. The department has numerous microcomputers connected to the University's high-speed fiber-optic network for data collection, analysis, and the preparation of manuscripts.

Information for Students With Physical Disabilities: See the following Web site for more information: http://www.apsu.edu/disability/.

Application Information:
Send to Office of Graduate Studies, Austin Peay State University, Clarksville, TN 37044. Application available online. URL of online application: http://www.apsu.edu/Admissions/apply.aspx. Students are admitted in the Fall, application deadline March 1. We begin to review applications beginning March 1, but continue to accept applications and admit students until program capacity is reached. *Fee:* $25.

East Tennessee State University
Department of Psychology
College of Arts and Sciences
Box 70649 (Psychology)
Johnson City, TN 37614-0649
Telephone: (423) 439-4424
Fax: (423) 439-5695
E-mail: *dixonw@etsu.edu*
Web: *http://www.etsu.edu/cas/psychology*

Department Information:
1966. Chairperson: Wallace E. Dixon, Jr. Number of faculty: total—full-time 15, part-time 4; women—full-time 6, part-time 2; minority—part-time 1.

Programs and Degrees Offered:
Listed in the following order: Program area, degree type (T if terminal Master's), number awarded 7/08–6/09. General Psychology MA/MS (Master of Arts/Science) (T) 2, Clinical Psychology PhD (Doctor of Philosophy) 0.

Student Applications/Admissions:
Student Applications
General Psychology MA/MS (Master of Arts/Science)—Applications 2009–2010, 15. Total applicants accepted 2009–2010, 7. Number full-time enrolled (new admits only) 2009–2010, 6. Number part-time enrolled (new admits only) 2009–2010, 1. Total enrolled 2009–2010 full-time, 11, part-time, 3. Openings 2010–2011, 8. The median number of years required for completion of a degree in 2008–2009 were 2. The number of students enrolled full- and part-time who were dismissed or voluntarily withdrew from this program area in 2008–2009 were 1. *Clinical Psychology PhD (Doctor of Philosophy)*—Applications 2009–2010, 43. Total applicants accepted 2009–2010, 6. Number full-time enrolled (new admits only) 2009–2010, 6. Number part-time enrolled (new admits only) 2009–2010, 0. Total enrolled 2009–2010 full-time, 19, part-time, 2. Openings 2010–2011, 6.

Scores: Entries appear in this order: required test or GPA, minimum score (if required), median score of students entering in 2009–2010. *General Psychology MA/MS (Master of Arts/Science):* GRE-V 450, 450, GRE-Q 450, 510, GRE-Analytical 3.5, 3.5, overall undergraduate GPA 3.0, psychology GPA 3.0; *Clinical Psychology PhD (Doctor of Philosophy):* GRE-V 480, 610, GRE-Q 610, 670, GRE-Analytical 4, 5, overall undergraduate GPA 3.0, 3.78.

Other Criteria: (importance of criteria rated low, medium, or high): GRE scores—high, research experience—high, work experience—medium, extracurricular activity—low, clinically related public service—low, GPA—high, letters of recommendation—high, interview—medium, statement of goals and objectives—high, undergraduate major in psychology—high, specific undergraduate psychology courses taken—medium. Interview is none to low for the general program. For additional information on admission requirements, go to http://www.etsu.edu/cas/psychology.

Student Characteristics: The following represents characteristics of students in 2009–2010 in all graduate psychology programs in the department: Female—full-time 19, part-time 4; Male—full-

time 11, part-time 1; African American/Black—full-time 0, part-time 0; Hispanic/Latino(a)—full-time 0, part-time 0; Asian/Pacific Islander—full-time 0, part-time 0; American Indian/Alaska Native—full-time 0, part-time 0; Caucasian/White—full-time 30, part-time 5; Multi-ethnic—full-time 0, part-time 0; students subject to the Americans With Disabilities Act—full-time 1, part-time 0; Unknown ethnicity—full-time 0, part-time 0; International students who hold an F-1 or J-1 Visa—full-time 0, part-time 0.

Financial Information/Assistance:
Tuition for Full-Time Study: *Master's:* State residents: per academic year $7,169, $367 per credit hour; Nonstate residents: per academic year $18,201, $913 per credit hour. *Doctoral:* State residents: per academic year $7,169, $367 per credit hour; Nonstate residents: per academic year $18,201, $913 per credit hour. Tuition is subject to change. See the following Web site for updates and changes in tuition costs: http://www.etsu.edu/fa/fs/bursar/.

Financial Assistance:
First-Year Students: Research assistantships available for first year. Average amount paid per academic year: $12,000. Average number of hours worked per week: 20. Apply by February 1.
Advanced Students: Traineeships available for advanced students. Average amount paid per academic year: $12,000. Average number of hours worked per week: 20. Apply by February 1.
Additional Information: Of all students currently enrolled full time, 100% benefited from one or more of the listed financial assistance programs. Application and information available online at: http://www.etsu.edu/finaid.

Internships/Practica: Doctoral Degree (PhD Clinical Psychology): For those doctoral students for whom a professional internship was required in this program prior to graduation, (1) students applied for an internship in 2008–2009, with (1) students obtaining an internship. Of those students who obtained an internship, (1) were paid internships. Of those students who obtained an internship, (1) students placed in APA/CPA accredited internships, (0) students placed in internships not APA/CPA accredited, but listed with the Association of Psychology Postdoctoral and Internship Programs (APPIC), (0) students placed in internships conforming to guidelines of the Council of Directors of School Psychology Programs (CDSPP), (0) students placed in internships that were not APA/CPA accredited, APPIC or CDSPP listed. Internships and practica in assessment and therapy are available to students enrolled in the clinical psychology program. They are conducted in the area mental health, behavioral health and primary care facilities under the joint supervision of departmental faculty and adjunct faculty located in the facilities. Students also participate in intensive clinical training in the department's training clinic.

Housing and Day Care: On-campus housing is available. See the following Web site for more information: http://www.etsu.edu/students/housing. On-campus day care facilities are available. See the following Web site for more information: http://www.etsu.edu/students/acts/students/childcareservices.aspx.

Employment of Department Graduates:
Master's Degree Graduates: Of those who graduated in the academic year 2008–2009, the following categories and numbers represent the postgraduate activities and employment of master's degree graduates: Enrolled in a postdoctoral residency/fellowship (n/a), employed in independent practice (n/a), total from the above (master's) (0).
Doctoral Degree Graduates: Of those who graduated in the academic year 2008–2009, the following categories and numbers represent the postgraduate activities and employment of doctoral degree graduates: Enrolled in a psychology doctoral program (n/a), total from the above (doctoral) (0).

Additional Information:
Orientation, Objectives, and Emphasis of Department: The Department of Psychology, College of Arts and Sciences, offers a Master of Arts degree in general psychology and a new Doctor of Philosophy in clinical psychology. The general psychology option prepares students for various endeavors, such as teaching at the community college level and doctoral study in psychology. The clinical psychology option provides students with training in clinical psychology with an emphasis in integrated rural primary care psychology.

Special Facilities or Resources: The psychology department maintains general experimental psychology, physiological psychology, and clinical psychology laboratory facilities. All laboratories are used for undergraduate and graduate instructional research and for student and faculty research. Assistantships/employment are available outside of the department, including the medical school.

Information for Students With Physical Disabilities: See the following Web site for more information: http://www.etsu.edu/students/disable/.

Application Information:
Send to School of Graduate Studies, East Tennessee State University, P. O. Box 70720, Johnson City, TN 37614-1710. Application available online. URL of online application: http://www.etsu.edu/gradstud/. Students are admitted in the Fall, application deadline February 1. The Clinical Program deadline is February 1; the General program is March 1. Students are normally admitted only in the Fall term, although exceptions for students in the General Option can sometimes be made. Fee: $25.

Memphis, University of
Department of Counseling, Educational Psychology and Research, Program in Counseling Psychology
Education
100 Ball Building
Memphis, TN 38152
Telephone: (901) 678-2841
Fax: (901) 678-5114
E-mail: *slease@memphis.edu*
Web: *http://cpsy.memphis.edu*

Department Information:
1972. Chairperson: Douglas Strohmer. Number of faculty: total—full-time 24, part-time 1; women—full-time 13, part-time 1; total—minority—full-time 6, part-time 1; women minority—full-

time 2, part-time 1; faculty subject to the Americans With Disabilities Act 2.

Programs and Degrees Offered:
Listed in the following order: Program area, degree type (T if terminal Master's), number awarded 7/08–6/09. Counseling Psychology PhD (Doctor of Philosophy) 12.

APA Accreditation: Counseling PhD (Doctor of Philosophy). Student Outcome Data Website: http://www.memphis.edu/cepr/counseling-psychology-information.htm.

Student Applications/Admissions:
Student Applications
Counseling Psychology PhD (Doctor of Philosophy)—Applications 2009–2010, 44. Total applicants accepted 2009–2010, 12. Number full-time enrolled (new admits only) 2009–2010, 8. Number part-time enrolled (new admits only) 2009–2010, 0. Total enrolled 2009–2010 full-time, 31, part-time, 4. Openings 2010–2011, 8. The median number of years required for completion of a degree in 2008–2009 were 4. The number of students enrolled full- and part-time who were dismissed or voluntarily withdrew from this program area in 2008–2009 were 0.
Scores: Entries appear in this order: required test or GPA, minimum score (if required), median score of students entering in 2009–2010. Counseling Psychology PhD (Doctor of Philosophy): GRE-V 500, 530, GRE-Q 500, 600, Masters GPA 3.5, 3.85.
Other Criteria: (importance of criteria rated low, medium, or high): GRE scores—high, research experience—medium, work experience—medium, clinically related public service—low, GPA—high, letters of recommendation—high, interview—medium, statement of goals and objectives—high, Fit with program philosophy—high. For additional information on admission requirements, go to http://cpsy.memphis.edu.

Student Characteristics: The following represents characteristics of students in 2009–2010 in all graduate psychology programs in the department: Female—full-time 21, part-time 0; Male—full-time 10, part-time 4; African American/Black—full-time 3, part-time 0; Hispanic/Latino(a)—full-time 0, part-time 0; Asian/Pacific Islander—full-time 1, part-time 0; American Indian/Alaska Native—full-time 0, part-time 0; Caucasian/White—full-time 25, part-time 4; Multi-ethnic—full-time 2, part-time 0; students subject to the Americans With Disabilities Act—full-time 1, part-time 0; Unknown ethnicity—full-time 0, part-time 0; International students who hold an F-1 or J-1 Visa—full-time 3, part-time 0.

Financial Information/Assistance:
Tuition for Full-Time Study: Master's: State residents: per academic year $11,871, $417 per credit hour; Nonstate residents: per academic year $27,531, $953 per credit hour. *Doctoral:* State residents: per academic year $11,871, $417 per credit hour; Nonstate residents: per academic year $27,531, $953 per credit hour. Tuition is subject to change. See the following Web site for updates and changes in tuition costs: http://bf.memphis.edu/finance/bursar/feepayment.php.

Financial Assistance:
First-Year Students: Teaching assistantships available for first year. Average amount paid per academic year: $6,000. Average number of hours worked per week: 20. Apply by April 1. Research assistantships available for first year. Average amount paid per academic year: $6,000. Average number of hours worked per week: 20. Apply by April 1. Fellowships and scholarships available for first year.
Advanced Students: Teaching assistantships available for advanced students. Average amount paid per academic year: $6,000. Average number of hours worked per week: 20. Apply by April 1. Research assistantships available for advanced students. Average amount paid per academic year: $6,000. Average number of hours worked per week: 20. Apply by April 1. Traineeships available for advanced students. Average amount paid per academic year: $10,000. Average number of hours worked per week: 20. Fellowships and scholarships available for advanced students. Average amount paid per academic year: $10,000. Average number of hours worked per week: 20.
Additional Information: Of all students currently enrolled full time, 100% benefited from one or more of the listed financial assistance programs. Application and information available online at: http://www.memphis.edu/gradschool/ga_awards_fellowships/gainfo.php.

Internships/Practica: Doctoral Degree (PhD Counseling Psychology): For those doctoral students for whom a professional internship was required in this program prior to graduation, (5) students applied for an internship in 2008–2009, with (5) students obtaining an internship. Of those students who obtained an internship, (5) were paid internships. Of those students who obtained an internship, (5) students placed in APA/CPA accredited internships, (0) students placed in internships not APA/CPA accredited, but listed with the Association of Psychology Postdoctoral and Internship Programs (APPIC), (0) students placed in internships conforming to guidelines of the Council of Directors of School Psychology Programs (CDSPP), (0) students placed in internships that were not APA/CPA accredited, APPIC or CDSPP listed. Doctoral students complete a minimum of two practica during their three years of coursework; many students complete up to five practica. The department has an extensive network of relationships with community agencies for providing practicum placements for students. These placements include: university and college counseling centers, VAs/hospitals, community mental health centers, private practice, pediatric neuroassessment, and correctional services.

Housing and Day Care: On-campus housing is available. See the following Web site for more information: http://www.memphis.edu/reslife/. On-campus day care facilities are available. See the following Web site for more information: http://www.memphis.edu/childcareweb/.

Employment of Department Graduates:
Master's Degree Graduates: Of those who graduated in the academic year 2008–2009, the following categories and numbers represent the postgraduate activities and employment of master's degree graduates: Enrolled in a postdoctoral residency/fellowship

(n/a), employed in independent practice (n/a), total from the above (master's) (0).

Doctoral Degree Graduates: Of those who graduated in the academic year 2008–2009, the following categories and numbers represent the postgraduate activities and employment of doctoral degree graduates: Enrolled in a psychology doctoral program (n/a), enrolled in a postdoctoral residency/fellowship (0), employed in independent practice (3), employed in an academic position at a university (1), employed in an academic position at a 2-year/4-year college (0), employed in other positions at a higher education institution (3), employed in a professional position in a school system (0), employed in business or industry (0), employed in government agency (1), employed in a hospital/medical center (4), not seeking employment (0), do not know (0), total from the above (doctoral) (12).

Additional Information:
Orientation, Objectives, and Emphasis of Department: The PhD in Counseling Psychology at the University of Memphis is designed to train psychologists who promote human development in the areas of mental health, career development, emotional and social learning, and decision-making in a rapidly changing global environment. Training is organized around the scientist–practitioner model of critical thinking and emphasizes multicultural competency and responsibility and commitment to human welfare. Didactic and experiential activities are designed to anchor persons firmly within the discipline of psychology. The program emphasizes research, development, prevention, and remediation in the context of social justice as vehicles for helping individuals, families, and groups achieve competence and a sense of well-being. The department has a strong commitment to training professionals to work with diverse populations in urban settings. Within the context of the University mission, students are expected to develop the critical thinking skills necessary for lifelong learning and to contribute to the global community. Students are expected to acquire: (1) an identity as a counseling psychologist; (2) a knowledge foundation in psychology, research, counseling, psychological evaluation, and professional standards; and (3) competencies in research, practice, and teaching. The program is individualized to meet the student's goals. Graduates are prepared for positions in various settings, including counseling centers, mental health centers, hospitals, private practice, or academia.

Special Facilities or Resources: Department faculty have research teams that provide opportunities for faculty and students to collaborate on research and consultation products. Many students are also involved in cross-disciplinary research with Psychology and Women's Studies faculty.

Information for Students With Physical Disabilities: See the following Web site for more information: http://www.memphis.edu/sds/.

Application Information:
Send to Suzanne Lease, Counseling Psychology Admissions, 100 Ball Building, The University of Memphis, Memphis, TN 38152. Application available online. URL of online application: http://cpsy.memphis.edu. Students are admitted in the Fall, application deadline January 15. *Fee:* $35. The fee is $60 for international students.

Memphis, University of
Department of Psychology
College of Arts and Sciences
202 Psychology Building
Memphis, TN 38152-3230
Telephone: (901) 678-2145
Fax: (901) 678-2579
E-mail: *dconnabl@memphis.edu*
Web: *http://www.memphis.edu/psychology*

Department Information:
1957. Interim Chair: William H. Zachry. Number of faculty: total—full-time 36; women—full-time 9; total—minority—full-time 5; women minority—full-time 2; faculty subject to the Americans With Disabilities Act 1.

Programs and Degrees Offered:
Listed in the following order: Program area, degree type (T if terminal Master's), number awarded 7/08–6/09. Clinical Psychology PhD (Doctor of Philosophy) 4, School Psychology MA/MS (Master of Arts/Science) (T) 12, General Psychology MA/MS (Master of Arts/Science) (T) 10, School Psychology PhD (Doctor of Philosophy) 2, Experimental Psychology PhD (Doctor of Philosophy) 6.

APA Accreditation: Clinical PhD (Doctor of Philosophy).

Student Applications/Admissions:
Student Applications
Clinical Psychology PhD (Doctor of Philosophy)—Applications 2009–2010, 135. Total applicants accepted 2009–2010, 7. Number full-time enrolled (new admits only) 2009–2010, 7. Number part-time enrolled (new admits only) 2009–2010, 0. Openings 2010–2011, 8. The median number of years required for completion of a degree in 2008–2009 were 6. The number of students enrolled full- and part-time who were dismissed or voluntarily withdrew from this program area in 2008–2009 were 1. *School Psychology MA/MS (Master of Arts/Science)*—Applications 2009–2010, 15. Total applicants accepted 2009–2010, 11. Number full-time enrolled (new admits only) 2009–2010, 9. Number part-time enrolled (new admits only) 2009–2010, 0. Openings 2010–2011, 12. The median number of years required for completion of a degree in 2008–2009 were 3. The number of students enrolled full- and part-time who were dismissed or voluntarily withdrew from this program area in 2008–2009 were 1. *General Psychology MA/MS (Master of Arts/Science)*—Applications 2009–2010, 48. Total applicants accepted 2009–2010, 17. Number full-time enrolled (new admits only) 2009–2010, 12. Number part-time enrolled (new admits only) 2009–2010, 0. Total enrolled 2009–2010 full-time, 18, part-time, 24. Openings 2010–2011, 15. The median number of years required for completion of a degree in 2008–2009 were 3. The number of students enrolled full- and part-time who were dismissed or voluntarily withdrew from this program area in 2008–2009 were 0. *School Psychology PhD (Doctor of Philosophy)*—Applications 2009–2010, 6. Total applicants accepted 2009–2010, 2. Number full-time enrolled (new admits only) 2009–2010, 2. Number part-time enrolled (new admits only) 2009–2010, 0. Openings 2010–2011, 2. The median number of years required for completion of a

degree in 2008–2009 were 5. The number of students enrolled full- and part-time who were dismissed or voluntarily withdrew from this program area in 2008–2009 were 0. *Experimental Psychology PhD (Doctor of Philosophy)*—Applications 2009–2010, 41. Total applicants accepted 2009–2010, 6. Number full-time enrolled (new admits only) 2009–2010, 6. Number part-time enrolled (new admits only) 2009–2010, 0. Openings 2010–2011, 6. The median number of years required for completion of a degree in 2008–2009 were 5. The number of students enrolled full- and part-time who were dismissed or voluntarily withdrew from this program area in 2008–2009 were 1.

Scores: Entries appear in this order: required test or GPA, minimum score (if required), median score of students entering in 2009–2010. *Clinical Psychology PhD (Doctor of Philosophy):* GRE-V no minimum stated, 540, GRE-Q no minimum stated, 650, GRE-Analytical no minimum stated, overall undergraduate GPA no minimum stated, 3.67.

Other Criteria: (importance of criteria rated low, medium, or high): GRE scores—high, research experience—high, work experience—medium, extracurricular activity—low, clinically related public service—low, GPA—high, letters of recommendation—high, interview—medium, statement of goals and objectives—high, undergraduate major in psychology—high, specific undergraduate psychology courses taken—medium.

Student Characteristics: The following represents characteristics of students in 2009–2010 in all graduate psychology programs in the department: Female—full-time 89, part-time 16; Male—full-time 36, part-time 8; African American/Black—full-time 10, part-time 5; Hispanic/Latino(a)—full-time 0, part-time 0; Asian/Pacific Islander—full-time 11, part-time 1; American Indian/Alaska Native—full-time 1, part-time 0; Caucasian/White—full-time 103, part-time 18; Multi-ethnic—full-time 0, part-time 0; students subject to the Americans With Disabilities Act—full-time 0, part-time 0; Unknown ethnicity—full-time 0, part-time 0; International students who hold an F-1 or J-1 Visa—full-time 3, part-time 0.

Financial Information/Assistance:

Tuition for Full-Time Study: *Master's:* State residents: per academic year $11,871, $417 per credit hour; Nonstate residents: per academic year $27,531, $953 per credit hour. *Doctoral:* State residents: per academic year $11,871, $417 per credit hour; Nonstate residents: per academic year $27,531, $953 per credit hour. Tuition is subject to change. See the following Web site for updates and changes in tuition costs: http://bf.memphis.edu/finance/bursar/.

Financial Assistance:

First-Year Students: Teaching assistantships available for first year. Average amount paid per academic year: $12,000. Average number of hours worked per week: 20. Research assistantships available for first year. Average amount paid per academic year: $12,000. Average number of hours worked per week: 20.

Advanced Students: Teaching assistantships available for advanced students. Average amount paid per academic year: $13,000. Average number of hours worked per week: 20. Research assistantships available for advanced students. Average amount paid per academic year: $13,000. Average number of hours worked per week: 20. Traineeships available for advanced students. Average amount paid per academic year: $13,000. Average number of hours worked per week: 20.

Additional Information: Of all students currently enrolled full time, 65% benefited from one or more of the listed financial assistance programs. Application and information available online at: http://www.memphis.edu/psychology.

Internships/Practica: Doctoral Degree (PhD Clinical Psychology): For those doctoral students for whom a professional internship was required in this program prior to graduation, (3) students applied for an internship in 2008–2009, with (3) students obtaining an internship. Of those students who obtained an internship, (3) were paid internships. Of those students who obtained an internship, (3) students placed in APA/CPA accredited internships, (0) students placed in internships not APA/CPA accredited, but listed with the Association of Psychology Postdoctoral and Internship Programs (APPIC), (0) students placed in internships conforming to guidelines of the Council of Directors of School Psychology Programs (CDSPP), (0) students placed in internships that were not APA/CPA accredited, APPIC or CDSPP listed. Doctoral Degree (PhD School Psychology): For those doctoral students for whom a professional internship was required in this program prior to graduation, (1) students applied for an internship in 2008–2009, with (1) students obtaining an internship. Of those students who obtained an internship, (1) were paid internships. Of those students who obtained an internship, (1) students placed in APA/CPA accredited internships, (0) students placed in internships not APA/CPA accredited, but listed with the Association of Psychology Postdoctoral and Internship Programs (APPIC), (0) students placed in internships conforming to guidelines of the Council of Directors of School Psychology Programs (CDSPP), (0) students placed in internships that were not APA/CPA accredited, APPIC or CDSPP listed. Master's Degree (MA/MS General Psychology): An internship experience, such as a final research project or "capstone" experience is required of graduates. The department has an extensive network of relationships with local agencies for providing practicum experiences for students. PhD clinical students work 20 hours per week at several of these practicum sites for a minimum of one year. All students can use these sites for other forms of practicum experience and research as the need arises. The department has no in-house internships. Students complete internships during the fifth or sixth year at sites nationwide.

Housing and Day Care: On-campus housing is available. See the following Web site for more information: http://www.memphis.edu/reslife/. On-campus day care facilities are available. See the following Web site for more information: http://www.memphis.edu/childcareweb/.

Employment of Department Graduates:

Master's Degree Graduates: Of those who graduated in the academic year 2008–2009, the following categories and numbers represent the postgraduate activities and employment of master's degree graduates: Enrolled in a psychology doctoral program (4), enrolled in another graduate/professional program (8), enrolled in a postdoctoral residency/fellowship (n/a), employed in independent practice (n/a), employed in an academic position at a university (0), employed in an academic position at a 2-year/4-year college (0), employed in other positions at a higher education institution (0), employed in business or industry (2), employed in government agency (0), employed in a community mental health/counseling center (0), employed in a hospital/medical center (0), still seeking employment (0), other employment position (0), do not know (5), total from the above (master's) (19).

Doctoral Degree Graduates: Of those who graduated in the academic year 2008–2009, the following categories and numbers represent the postgraduate activities and employment of doctoral degree graduates: Enrolled in a psychology doctoral program (n/a), enrolled in a postdoctoral residency/fellowship (2), employed in independent practice (0), employed in an academic position at a university (1), employed in an academic position at a 2-year/4-year college (1), employed in other positions at a higher education institution (1), employed in a professional position in a school system (5), employed in business or industry (1), employed in government agency (0), employed in a community mental health/counseling center (2), employed in a hospital/medical center (0), still seeking employment (0), other employment position (0), do not know (2), total from the above (doctoral) (15).

Additional Information:

Orientation, Objectives, and Emphasis of Department: The department philosophy emphasizes the training of experimentally sophisticated research scientists and practitioners. All programs have a strong research emphasis. Professional training is based upon a research foundation and students are exposed to a broad range of theoretical perspectives. Diversity of professional training activities and collaborative research activities is emphasized. Students are afforded maximum freedom to pursue their own interests and tailor programs to their needs. All PhD and master's programs are serviced by six research areas within the department: Clinical Health Psychology, Behavioral Neuroscience, Child and Family Studies, Cognitive and Social Processes, Industrial/Organizational and Applied Psychology, and Psychopathology/Psychotherapy.

Special Facilities or Resources: The department as a whole has a strong research orientation, ranking high among psychology departments across the nation in total research and development expenditures. The department is housed in a modern, well-equipped barrier-free building, providing offices and laboratory space for all students. The department includes the Center for Applied Psychological Research (CAPR), the Institute for Intelligent Systems (IIS), and the Psychological Services Center (PSC). The CAPR is a state-sponsored center of excellence that has provided the department with approximately $1 million per year for the past 20 years. The IIS is an interdisciplinary enterprise comprised of researchers and students from the fields of cognitive psychology, computer science, mathematics, physics, neuroscience, education, linguistics, philosophy, anthropology, engineering, and business. The Psychological Services Center is a fee-for-service outpatient mental health clinic located in the psychology building. In this clinic, doctoral students receive intensive supervision as they learn to provide a wide range of assessment and intervention services. In addition, the PSC provides an invaluable resource for the conduct of a variety of research projects. The clients are referred from the greater Memphis area.

Information for Students With Physical Disabilities: See the following Web site for more information: http://www.memphis.edu/sds/.

Application Information:
Send to Graduate Admissions / Department of Psychology / 202 Psychology Building / University of Memphis / Memphis, TN 38152. Application available online. URL of online application: http://www.memphis.edu/psychology/graduate/Apply/index.php. Students are admitted in the Fall, application deadline. The application deadline for the clinical PhD program is December 5. The application deadline for all other PhD programs is January 15. The application deadline for the Master's program in General Psychology is May 15. The application deadline for the MA/EdS in School Psychology is June 15. *Fee:* $50. The application fee for the graduate school is $35 for domestic students and $60 for international students. There is an additional fee of $15 for the Department of Psychology application.

Middle Tennessee State University
Department of Psychology
Education and Behavioral Science
Box 87
Murfreesboro, TN 37132
Telephone: (615) 898-2706
Fax: (615) 898-5027
E-mail: *gschmidt@mtsu.edu*
Web: *http://www.mtsu.edu/psychology/*

Department Information:
1967. Chairperson: Dennis R. Papini. Number of faculty: total—full-time 42, part-time 16; women—full-time 18, part-time 10; total—minority—full-time 4, part-time 1; women minority—full-time 2.

Programs and Degrees Offered:
Listed in the following order: Program area, degree type (T if terminal Master's), number awarded 7/08–6/09. Clinical Psychology MA/MS (Master of Arts/Science) (T) 10, Experimental Psychology MA/MS (Master of Arts/Science) (T) 4, Industrial/Organizational Psychology MA/MS (Master of Arts/Science) (T) 15, Quantitative Psychology MA/MS (Master of Arts/Science) (T) 4, School Psychology EdS (School Psychology) 10, Professional Counseling MEd (Education) 12.

Student Applications/Admissions:
Student Applications
Clinical Psychology MA/MS (Master of Arts/Science)—Applications 2009–2010, 40. Total applicants accepted 2009–2010, 18. Number full-time enrolled (new admits only) 2009–2010, 15. Number part-time enrolled (new admits only) 2009–2010, 0. Total enrolled 2009–2010 full-time, 26, part-time, 4. Openings 2010–2011, 14. The median number of years required for completion of a degree in 2008–2009 were 2. The number of students enrolled full- and part-time who were dismissed or voluntarily withdrew from this program area in 2008–2009 were 1. *Experimental Psychology MA/MS (Master of Arts/Science)*—Applications 2009–2010, 15. Total applicants accepted 2009–2010, 8. Number full-time enrolled (new admits only) 2009–2010, 5. Openings 2010–2011, 8. The median number of years required for completion of a degree in 2008–2009 were 2. The number of students enrolled full- and part-time who were dismissed or voluntarily withdrew from this program area in 2008–2009 were 0. *Industrial/Organizational Psychology MA/MS (Master of Arts/Science)*—Applications 2009–2010, 45. Total applicants accepted 2009–2010, 20. Number full-time enrolled (new admits only) 2009–2010, 14. Total enrolled

2009–2010 full-time, 25, part-time, 2. Openings 2010–2011, 12. The median number of years required for completion of a degree in 2008–2009 were 2. The number of students enrolled full- and part-time who were dismissed or voluntarily withdrew from this program area in 2008–2009 were 1. *Quantitative Psychology MA/MS (Master of Arts/Science)*—Applications 2009–2010, 9. Total applicants accepted 2009–2010, 7. Number full-time enrolled (new admits only) 2009–2010, 6. Total enrolled 2009–2010 full-time, 12, part-time, 1. Openings 2010–2011, 6. The median number of years required for completion of a degree in 2008–2009 were 2. The number of students enrolled full- and part-time who were dismissed or voluntarily withdrew from this program area in 2008–2009 were 1. *School Psychology EdS (School Psychology)*—Applications 2009–2010, 32. Total applicants accepted 2009–2010, 25. Number full-time enrolled (new admits only) 2009–2010, 12. Number part-time enrolled (new admits only) 2009–2010, 1. Total enrolled 2009–2010 full-time, 27, part-time, 2. Openings 2010–2011, 12. The median number of years required for completion of a degree in 2008–2009 were 3. The number of students enrolled full- and part-time who were dismissed or voluntarily withdrew from this program area in 2008–2009 were 1. *Professional Counseling MEd (Education)*—Applications 2009–2010, 40. Total applicants accepted 2009–2010, 18. Number full-time enrolled (new admits only) 2009–2010, 12. Number part-time enrolled (new admits only) 2009–2010, 6. Total enrolled 2009–2010 full-time, 30, part-time, 16. Openings 2010–2011, 25. The median number of years required for completion of a degree in 2008–2009 were 3. The number of students enrolled full- and part-time who were dismissed or voluntarily withdrew from this program area in 2008–2009 were 4.

Scores: Entries appear in this order: required test or GPA, minimum score (if required), median score of students entering in 2009–2010. *Experimental Psychology MA/MS (Master of Arts/Science)*: GRE-V 450, 500, GRE-Q 450, 560, overall undergraduate GPA 300, 3.7; *School Psychology EdS (School Psychology)*: GRE-V 450, 510, GRE-Q 450, 530, GRE-Analytical no minimum stated, 4.1, overall undergraduate GPA no minimum stated.

Other Criteria: (importance of criteria rated low, medium, or high): GRE scores—high, research experience—high, work experience—low, extracurricular activity—low, clinically related public service—medium, GPA—high, letters of recommendation—high, interview—high, statement of goals and objectives—high. Interview: School Counseling and Mental Health Counseling. Statement of Goals & Objectives for Experimental & School Psychology only. For additional information on admission requirements, go to http://www.mtsu.edu/psychology/grad.shtml.

Student Characteristics: The following represents characteristics of students in 2009–2010 in all graduate psychology programs in the department: Female—full-time 144, part-time 0; Male—full-time 38, part-time 0; African American/Black—full-time 7, part-time 0; Hispanic/Latino(a)—full-time 1, part-time 0; Asian/Pacific Islander—full-time 7, part-time 0; American Indian/Alaska Native—full-time 1, part-time 0; Caucasian/White—full-time 165, part-time 0; Multi-ethnic—full-time 0, part-time 0; students subject to the Americans With Disabilities Act—full-time 0, part-time 0; Unknown ethnicity—full-time 1, part-time 0; International students who hold an F-1 or J-1 Visa—full-time 7, part-time 0.

Financial Information/Assistance:
  Tuition for Full-Time Study: *Master's:* State residents: per academic year $7,340, $367 per credit hour; Nonstate residents: per academic year $18,260, $913 per credit hour. Tuition is subject to change. See the following Web site for updates and changes in tuition costs: http://www.mtsu.edu/bursar.

Financial Assistance:
  First-Year Students: Research assistantships available for first year. Average amount paid per academic year: $3,000. Average number of hours worked per week: 10. Apply by March/Oct 1.
  Advanced Students: Research assistantships available for advanced students. Average amount paid per academic year: $3,000. Average number of hours worked per week: 10. Apply by March/Oct 1.
  Additional Information: Of all students currently enrolled full time, 20% benefited from one or more of the listed financial assistance programs. Application and information available online at: http://www.mtsu.edu/graduate/student/gtas.shtml.

Internships/Practica: Master's Degree (MA/MS Clinical Psychology): An internship experience, such as a final research project or "capstone" experience is required of graduates. Master's Degree (MA/MS Experimental Psychology): An internship experience, such as a final research project or "capstone" experience is required of graduates. Master's Degree (MA/MS Industrial/Organizational Psychology): An internship experience, such as a final research project or "capstone" experience is required of graduates. Field placements are available in a variety of mental health facilities, inpatient facilities, the VA hospital, drug abuse facilities, K-12 school settings, and industrial sites.

Housing and Day Care: On-campus housing is available. See the following Web site for more information: http://www.mtsu.edu/housing/. On-campus day care facilities are available. See the following Web site for more information: http://www.mtsu.edu/pcsw/childcare_Dir/childcare.shtml.

Employment of Department Graduates:
  Master's Degree Graduates: Of those who graduated in the academic year 2008–2009, the following categories and numbers represent the postgraduate activities and employment of master's degree graduates: Enrolled in a psychology doctoral program (2), enrolled in a postdoctoral residency/fellowship (n/a), employed in independent practice (n/a), employed in a professional position in a school system (11), employed in business or industry (4), total from the above (master's) (17).
  Doctoral Degree Graduates: Of those who graduated in the academic year 2008–2009, the following categories and numbers represent the postgraduate activities and employment of doctoral degree graduates: Enrolled in a psychology doctoral program (n/a), total from the above (doctoral) (0).

Additional Information:
  Orientation, Objectives, and Emphasis of Department: We have an applied department with research and service priorities. A strong academic program is available for students seeking to improve their backgrounds in core areas of psychology for admission to doctoral programs. Applied programs lead to certification and/

or licensure in school psychology, school counseling, and clinical. Our Industrial/Organizational program is nationally acclaimed.

Information for Students With Physical Disabilities: See the following Web site for more information: http://www.mtsu.edu/dssemail/.

Application Information:
Send to Office of Graduate Studies, Cope Administration Building, 114 Middle Tennessee State University, Murfreesboro, TN 37132. Application available online. URL of online application: http://www.mtsu.edu/graduate/apply.shtml. Students are admitted in the Spring, application deadline October 1; Fall, application deadline March 1. Fee: $25. $30 for international applicants.

Tennessee, University of, Chattanooga
Department of Psychology
College of Arts and Sciences
350 Holt Hall
Chattanooga, TN 37403
Telephone: (423) 425-4262
Fax: (423) 425-4284
E-mail: *boleary@utc.edu*
Web: *http://www.utc.edu/ioprog*

Department Information:
1969. Head: Paul J. Watson. Number of faculty: total—full-time 10, part-time 6; women—full-time 3, part-time 3; total—minority—full-time 1; women minority—full-time 1.

Programs and Degrees Offered:
Listed in the following order: Program area, degree type (T if terminal Master's), number awarded 7/08–6/09. Industrial/Organizational Psychology MA/MS (Master of Arts/Science) (T) 20, Research MA/MS (Master of Arts/Science) (T) 4.

Student Applications/Admissions:
Student Applications
Industrial/Organizational Psychology MA/MS (Master of Arts/Science)—Applications 2009–2010, 45. Total applicants accepted 2009–2010, 36. Number full-time enrolled (new admits only) 2009–2010, 15. Openings 2010–2011, 18. The median number of years required for completion of a degree in 2008–2009 were 2. The number of students enrolled full- and part-time who were dismissed or voluntarily withdrew from this program area in 2008–2009 were 2. *Research MA/MS (Master of Arts/Science)*—Applications 2009–2010, 10. Total applicants accepted 2009–2010, 6. Number full-time enrolled (new admits only) 2009–2010, 5. Openings 2010–2011, 8. The median number of years required for completion of a degree in 2008–2009 were 2. The number of students enrolled full- and part-time who were dismissed or voluntarily withdrew from this program area in 2008–2009 were 0.
Other Criteria: (importance of criteria rated low, medium, or high): GRE scores—high, research experience—medium, work experience—medium, extracurricular activity—low, clinically related public service—low, GPA—high, letters of recommendation—medium, interview—low, statement of goals and objectives—medium, undergraduate major in psychology—low, specific undergraduate psychology courses taken—low. Admission to the Research program requires sponsorship of a faculty member. For additional information on admission requirements, go to http://www.utc.edu/Academic/.

Student Characteristics: The following represents characteristics of students in 2009–2010 in all graduate psychology programs in the department: Female—full-time 36, part-time 0; Male—full-time 10, part-time 0; African American/Black—full-time 4, part-time 0; Hispanic/Latino(a)—full-time 0, part-time 0; Asian/Pacific Islander—full-time 0, part-time 0; American Indian/Alaska Native—full-time 0, part-time 0; Caucasian/White—full-time 42, part-time 0; Multi-ethnic—full-time 0, part-time 0; students subject to the Americans With Disabilities Act—full-time 1, part-time 0; Unknown ethnicity—full-time 0, part-time 0; International students who hold an F-1 or J-1 Visa—full-time 1, part-time 0.

Financial Information/Assistance:
Tuition for Full-Time Study: Master's: State residents: per academic year $6,554; Nonstate residents: per academic year $17,852. Tuition is subject to change. See the following Web site for updates and changes in tuition costs: http://www.utc.edu/Administration/Bursar.

Financial Assistance:
First-Year Students: Teaching assistantships available for first year. Average amount paid per academic year: $1,600. Average number of hours worked per week: 5. Apply by August 20. Research assistantships available for first year. Average amount paid per academic year: $2,750. Average number of hours worked per week: 10. Apply by July 1.
Advanced Students: Teaching assistantships available for advanced students. Average amount paid per academic year: $1,600. Average number of hours worked per week: 5. Apply by August 20. Research assistantships available for advanced students. Average amount paid per academic year: $2,750. Average number of hours worked per week: 10. Apply by July 1.
Additional Information: Of all students currently enrolled full time, 50% benefited from one or more of the listed financial assistance programs. Application and information available online at: http://www.utc.edu/Administration/GraduateSchool/index.php.

Internships/Practica: The integration of course work and practice throughout the students' graduate academic program is essential to prepare I/O students for applied professional careers. To achieve this end, I/O students become involved in a variety of real life work organization activities through completion of a practicum program. They are encouraged to start this practicum after their second semester of academic work. Six semester hours of practicum credit are required (involving at least 300 hours of actual work time), and an additional three semester hours may be taken as a part of the elective portion of the program. The practicum is carried out in private and public work organizations in which the students engage in a wide variety of projects under the guidance of field supervisors, coordinated by the I/O faculty.

Housing and Day Care: On-campus housing is available. See the following Web site for more information: http://www.utc.edu/

Administration/StudentHousing. On-campus day care facilities are available.

Employment of Department Graduates:
Master's Degree Graduates: Of those who graduated in the academic year 2008–2009, the following categories and numbers represent the postgraduate activities and employment of master's degree graduates: Enrolled in a psychology doctoral program (3), enrolled in a postdoctoral residency/fellowship (n/a), employed in independent practice (n/a), employed in business or industry (13), employed in government agency (0), do not know (2), total from the above (master's) (18).
Doctoral Degree Graduates: Of those who graduated in the academic year 2008–2009, the following categories and numbers represent the postgraduate activities and employment of doctoral degree graduates: Enrolled in a psychology doctoral program (n/a), total from the above (doctoral) (0).

Additional Information:
Orientation, Objectives, and Emphasis of Department: The goal of the I/O program is to provide students with the training necessary to pursue a variety of I/O related fields. These include, but are not limited to, positions in human resources, industrial/organizational consulting, training, and organization development. The I/O program can be used as a preparation for the pursuit of doctoral training in I/O related fields of study. The curriculum is organized around specific core knowledge domains particular to I/O psychology. The industrial domain includes content such as job analysis, selection, and training. The organizational domain includes content such as work motivation, attitudes, leadership, organizational development, and group processes. The third domain, research methodology, includes experimental design and univariate and multivariate statistical analysis. The research program is designed primarily to prepare students to pursue doctoral level training. Students work in an apprenticeship model with faculty to develop strong design and analysis skills.

Special Facilities or Resources: The Center for Applied Social Research conducts surveys and other applied research in the community. We have a close relationship with SHRM Chattanooga, the local SHRM chapter, and with several local work organizations.

Information for Students With Physical Disabilities: See the following Web site for more information: www.utc.edu/Administration/OfficeForStudentsWithDisabilities/.

Application Information:
Send to Graduate School, 5305 University of Tennessee—Chattanooga, Chattanooga, TN 37403. Application available online. URL of online application: http://www.utc.edu/ioprog. Students are admitted in the Fall, application deadline March 15; Spring, application deadline December 15. Students may be admitted after the March deadline if space permits. Programs are designed to begin in the fall semester. Spring and summer admissions are possible although students admitted in spring or summer will likely require more than two years to complete the program. *Fee:* $30. $35 for international students.

Tennessee, University of, Knoxville
Department of Educational Psychology and Counseling
Education, Health, and Human Sciences
525 Jane and David Bailey Education Complex
Knoxville, TN 37996-3452
Telephone: (865) 974-8145
Fax: (865) 974-0135
E-mail: *mccallum@utk.edu*
Web: *http://web.utk.edu/~edpsych/*

Department Information:
1956. Head: R. Steve McCallum. Number of faculty: total—full-time 27, part-time 2; women—full-time 12; total—minority—full-time 2; women minority—full-time 1.

Programs and Degrees Offered:
Listed in the following order: Program area, degree type (T if terminal Master's), number awarded 7/08–6/09. School Psychology PhD (Doctor of Philosophy) 7, Educational Psychology and Research PhD (Doctor of Philosophy) 8, Counselor Education PhD (Doctor of Philosophy) 6, Evaluation and Assessment PhD (Doctor of Philosophy) 3, Instructional Technology PhD (Doctor of Philosophy), Learning Environments and Educational Studies PhD (Doctor of Philosophy) 2.

APA Accreditation: School PhD (Doctor of Philosophy). Student Outcome Data Website: http://web.utk.edu/~edpsych/school_psychology/APA_info.html.

Student Applications/Admissions:
Student Applications
School Psychology PhD (Doctor of Philosophy)—Applications 2009–2010, 44. Total applicants accepted 2009–2010, 7. Number full-time enrolled (new admits only) 2009–2010, 7. Openings 2010–2011, 7. The median number of years required for completion of a degree in 2008–2009 were 5. The number of students enrolled full- and part-time who were dismissed or voluntarily withdrew from this program area in 2008–2009 were 0. *Educational Psychology and Research PhD (Doctor of Philosophy)*—Applications 2009–2010, 21. Total applicants accepted 2009–2010, 9. Number full-time enrolled (new admits only) 2009–2010, 8. Number part-time enrolled (new admits only) 2009–2010, 2. Total enrolled 2009–2010 full-time, 35, part-time, 4. The median number of years required for completion of a degree in 2008–2009 were 4. The number of students enrolled full- and part-time who were dismissed or voluntarily withdrew from this program area in 2008–2009 were 1. *Counselor Education PhD (Doctor of Philosophy)*—Applications 2009–2010, 12. Total applicants accepted 2009–2010, 5. Number full-time enrolled (new admits only) 2009–2010, 5. Number part-time enrolled (new admits only) 2009–2010, 0. Openings 2010–2011, 4. The median number of years required for completion of a degree in 2008–2009 were 4. The number of students enrolled full- and part-time who were dismissed or voluntarily withdrew from this program area in 2008–2009 were 1. *Evaluation and Assessment PhD (Doctor of Philosophy)*—Applications 2009–2010, 10. Total applicants accepted 2009–2010, 3. Number full-time enrolled (new admits only) 2009–2010, 3. Number part-time enrolled (new admits only) 2009–2010, 2. Total enrolled 2009–2010 full-time, 6, part-time, 6.

Openings 2010–2011, 4. The median number of years required for completion of a degree in 2008–2009 were 4. The number of students enrolled full- and part-time who were dismissed or voluntarily withdrew from this program area in 2008–2009 were 0. *Instructional Technology PhD (Doctor of Philosophy)*— Applications 2009–2010, 8. Total applicants accepted 2009–2010, 4. Number full-time enrolled (new admits only) 2009–2010, 3. Total enrolled 2009–2010 full-time, 19. Openings 2010–2011, 8. The number of students enrolled full- and part-time who were dismissed or voluntarily withdrew from this program area in 2008–2009 were 0. *Learning Environments and Educational Studies PhD (Doctor of Philosophy)*—Applications 2009–2010, 3. Total applicants accepted 2009–2010, 2. Number full-time enrolled (new admits only) 2009–2010, 2. Total enrolled 2009–2010 full-time, 8. Openings 2010–2011, 3. The median number of years required for completion of a degree in 2008–2009 were 3.

Other Criteria: (importance of criteria rated low, medium, or high): GRE scores—medium, research experience—low, work experience—low, extracurricular activity—medium, clinically related public service—medium, GPA—high, letters of recommendation—medium, interview—low, statement of goals and objectives—medium. For additional information on admission requirements, go to http://web.utk.edu/~edpsych/admissions_US.html.

Student Characteristics: The following represents characteristics of students in 2009–2010 in all graduate psychology programs in the department: Female—full-time 210, part-time 5; Male—full-time 90, part-time 9; African American/Black—full-time 6, part-time 0; Hispanic/Latino(a)—full-time 0, part-time 0; Asian/Pacific Islander—full-time 2, part-time 0; American Indian/Alaska Native—full-time 0, part-time 0; Caucasian/White—full-time 0, part-time 0; Multi-ethnic—full-time 2, part-time 0; students subject to the Americans With Disabilities Act—full-time 2, part-time 0; Unknown ethnicity—full-time 0, part-time 0; International students who hold an F-1 or J-1 Visa—full-time 0, part-time 0.

Financial Information/Assistance:

Tuition for Full-Time Study: Nonstate residents: $1,147 per credit hour. *Doctoral:* State residents: per academic year $7,748, $380 per credit hour; Nonstate residents: per academic year $21,844, $1,147 per credit hour. Tuition is subject to change. See the following Web site for updates and changes in tuition costs: http://web.utk.edu/~bursar/tuition.html.

Financial Assistance:

First-Year Students: Teaching assistantships available for first year. Average amount paid per academic year: $6,000. Average number of hours worked per week: 10. Apply by January 31. Research assistantships available for first year. Average amount paid per academic year: $4,000. Average number of hours worked per week: 10. Apply by January 31.

Advanced Students: Teaching assistantships available for advanced students. Average amount paid per academic year: $6,000. Average number of hours worked per week: 10. Apply by January 31. Research assistantships available for advanced students. Average amount paid per academic year: $5,000. Average number of hours worked per week: 10. Apply by January 31.

Additional Information: Of all students currently enrolled full time, 25% benefited from one or more of the listed financial assistance programs. Application and information available online at: http://finaid.utk.edu/.

Internships/Practica: Doctoral Degree (PhD School Psychology): For those doctoral students for whom a professional internship was required in this program prior to graduation, (6) students applied for an internship in 2008–2009, with (6) students obtaining an internship. Of those students who obtained an internship, (6) were paid internships. Of those students who obtained an internship, (5) students placed in APA/CPA accredited internships, (0) students placed in internships not APA/CPA accredited, but listed with the Association of Psychology Postdoctoral and Internship Programs (APPIC), (0) students placed in internships conforming to guidelines of the Council of Directors of School Psychology Programs (CDSPP), (1) students placed in internships that were not APA/CPA accredited, APPIC or CDSPP listed. Assessment, counseling, and consultation practica are required of all school psychology/counseling students. In addition, a 1,500-hour internship is required for EdS students and a 2000-hour internship is required for PhD students. The Department is a member of an APA-approved internship consortium.

Housing and Day Care: On-campus housing is available. See the following Web site for more information: http://uthousing.utk.edu/. On-campus day care facilities are available. See the following Web site for more information: http://elc.utk.edu/.

Employment of Department Graduates:

Master's Degree Graduates: Of those who graduated in the academic year 2008–2009, the following categories and numbers represent the postgraduate activities and employment of master's degree graduates: Enrolled in a postdoctoral residency/fellowship (n/a), employed in independent practice (n/a), total from the above (master's) (0).

Doctoral Degree Graduates: Of those who graduated in the academic year 2008–2009, the following categories and numbers represent the postgraduate activities and employment of doctoral degree graduates: Enrolled in a psychology doctoral program (n/a), total from the above (doctoral) (0).

Additional Information:

Orientation, Objectives, and Emphasis of Department: Members of the Educational Psychology and Counseling Department envision playing an instrumental role in the creation of contextually linked learning environments that promote and enhance success for all learners. We expect these environments to exemplify a spirit of collaboration and cooperation, respect for diversity, concern for mental and physical health, positive attitudes toward constructive and meaningful change, and a commitment to lifelong learning. Faculty and students in the Psychoeducational Studies Unit are expected to model the behaviors and reflect the values that are necessary to achieve this vision. The Psychoeducational Studies Unit will provide national leadership in creating learning environments that: (1) foster psychological health, (2) address authentic educational needs, and (3) promote lifelong learning. Unit faculty and students will draw upon a growing body of knowledge about the psychology, biology, and social/cultural contexts of learning in promoting systematic change that leads to the enhancement of the learner. Specifically, the Unit will seek opportunities in a diversity of contexts for learners to apply information-based problem solving, engage in critical thinking, provide counseling services, and implement the structures and processes necessary for effective collaboration.

Information for Students With Physical Disabilities: See the following Web site for more information: http://ods.utk.edu/.

Application Information:
Send to Julie Harden, Educational Psychology and Counseling, 453 Claxton Complex, The University of Tennessee, Knoxville, TN 37996-3452. Application available online. URL of online application: http://admissions.utk.edu/graduate/apply.shtml. Students are admitted in the Fall, application deadline January 15. Program deadline is January 15 for School Psychology program, February 1 for Counselor Education and Learning Environments and Educational Studies programs. Fee: $35.

Tennessee, University of, Knoxville (2009 data)
Department of Psychology
Arts and Sciences
312 Austin Peay Building
Knoxville, TN 37996-0900
Telephone: (865) 974-3328
Fax: (865) 974-3330
E-mail: *cjogle@utk.edu*
Web: *http://psychology.utk.edu/*

Department Information:
1957. Department Head: James E. Lawler. Number of faculty: total—full-time 31, part-time 17; women—full-time 12, part-time 7; total—minority—full-time 1; women minority—full-time 1.

Programs and Degrees Offered:
Listed in the following order: Program area, degree type (T if terminal Master's), number awarded 7/08–6/09. Clinical PhD (Doctor of Philosophy) 5, Experimental MA/MS (Master of Arts/Science) (T) 1, Counseling PhD (Doctor of Philosophy) 2, Experimental PhD (Doctor of Philosophy) 9.

APA Accreditation: Clinical PhD (Doctor of Philosophy). Counseling PhD (Doctor of Philosophy).

Student Applications/Admissions:
Student Applications
Clinical PhD (Doctor of Philosophy)—Applications 2009–2010, 80. Total applicants accepted 2009–2010, 7. Number full-time enrolled (new admits only) 2009–2010, 7. Openings 2010–2011, 8. The number of students enrolled full- and part-time who were dismissed or voluntarily withdrew from this program area in 2008–2009 were 0. *Experimental MA/MS (Master of Arts/Science)*—Applications 2009–2010, 11. Total applicants accepted 2009–2010, 2. Number full-time enrolled (new admits only) 2009–2010, 2. Openings 2010–2011, 4. The median number of years required for completion of a degree in 2008–2009 were 2. The number of students enrolled full- and part-time who were dismissed or voluntarily withdrew from this program area in 2008–2009 were 0. *Counseling PhD (Doctor of Philosophy)*—Applications 2009–2010, 49. Total applicants accepted 2009–2010, 5. Number full-time enrolled (new admits only) 2009–2010, 5. Total enrolled 2009–2010 full-time, 28. Openings 2010–2011, 6. The median number of years required for completion of a degree in 2008–2009 were 5. The number of students enrolled full- and part-time who were dismissed or voluntarily withdrew from this program area in 2008–2009 were 0. *Experimental PhD (Doctor of Philosophy)*—Applications 2009–2010, 24. Total applicants accepted 2009–2010, 7. Number full-time enrolled (new admits only) 2009–2010, 6. Total enrolled 2009–2010 full-time, 29. Openings 2010–2011, 7. The median number of years required for completion of a degree in 2008–2009 were 4. The number of students enrolled full- and part-time who were dismissed or voluntarily withdrew from this program area in 2008–2009 were 1.

Other Criteria: (importance of criteria rated low, medium, or high): GRE scores—medium, research experience—high, work experience—low, extracurricular activity—low, clinically related public service—low, GPA—high, letters of recommendation—high, interview—high, statement of goals and objectives—high.

Student Characteristics: The following represents characteristics of students in 2009–2010 in all graduate psychology programs in the department: Female—full-time 60, part-time 0; Male—full-time 39, part-time 0; African American/Black—full-time 9, part-time 0; Hispanic/Latino(a)—full-time 1, part-time 0; Asian/Pacific Islander—full-time 4, part-time 0; American Indian/Alaska Native—full-time 0, part-time 0; Caucasian/White—full-time 0, part-time 0; Multi-ethnic—full-time 1, part-time 0; students subject to the Americans With Disabilities Act—full-time 0, part-time 0; Unknown ethnicity—full-time 0, part-time 0; International students who hold an F-1 or J-1 Visa—full-time 0, part-time 0.

Financial Information/Assistance:
Tuition for Full-Time Study: *Master's:* State residents: per academic year $6,366, $310 per credit hour; Nonstate residents: per academic year $17,932, $937 per credit hour. *Doctoral:* State residents: per academic year $6,366, $310 per credit hour; Nonstate residents: per academic year $17,932, $937 per credit hour. Tuition is subject to change. See the following Web site for updates and changes in tuition costs: http://web.utk.edu/~bursar/.

Financial Assistance:
First-Year Students: Research assistantships available for first year. Fellowships and scholarships available for first year.
Advanced Students: Teaching assistantships available for advanced students. Research assistantships available for advanced students. Fellowships and scholarships available for advanced students.
Additional Information: Of all students currently enrolled full time, 100% benefited from one or more of the listed financial assistance programs.

Internships/Practica: All Clinical students are required to participate in two 12-month practica, one in our Departmental Psychological Clinic and the other in a community mental health facility. Both practica are supervised by doctoral degreed clinical psychologists, and the clientele are children, adolescents, and adults who seek help for their emotional and behavioral problems. In addition, Clinical and Counseling students are required to serve a one-year internship.

Housing and Day Care: On-campus housing is available. See the following Web site for more information: http://uthousing.utk.edu. On-campus day care facilities are available. See the following Web site for more information: http://elc.utk.edu.

Employment of Department Graduates:
Master's Degree Graduates: Of those who graduated in the academic year 2008–2009, the following categories and numbers represent the postgraduate activities and employment of master's degree graduates: Enrolled in a postdoctoral residency/fellowship (n/a), employed in independent practice (n/a), total from the above (master's) (0).
Doctoral Degree Graduates: Of those who graduated in the academic year 2008–2009, the following categories and numbers represent the postgraduate activities and employment of doctoral degree graduates: Enrolled in a psychology doctoral program (n/a), total from the above (doctoral) (0).

Additional Information:
Orientation, Objectives, and Emphasis of Department: The graduate faculty maintain active research programs in cognition, developmental, ethology, gender, health, organizational, personality, phenomenology, psychobiology, psychometrics, sensation/perception, and social psychology. The MA program is appropriate for students wanting a master's degree as part of progress toward a doctorate, or for those who wish to complement a degree in a different field. The Experimental PhD program prepares students for academic/research careers and for careers involving the application of psychological principles as practitioners in industrial, forensic, organizational, and community settings. Areas of concentration include applied psychology, child development, cognition and consciousness, health psychology, phenomenology, and social/personality. The Clinical PhD program combines psychodynamic and research components, requiring exposure to a wide range of theoretical views and technical practices. Minors available are child development, health psychology, and social psychology. In order to foster appropriate breadth and interdisciplinary training, some cognate work outside the department of psychology is required of all doctoral students. The Counseling program is designed to enable students to become behavioral scientists, skilled in psychological research and its application. Students are trained to provide services to a wide variety of clients in numerous settings. Program objectives are to train doctoral-level counseling psychologists who have knowledge of, and competence in, (a) the foundation and discipline of psychology, (b) social science research and methodology, and (c) specific therapeutic and intervention skills related to being a counseling psychologist.

Special Facilities or Resources: Facilities include computer support in equipment and staff, human and animal laboratories, a psychology clinic for training and research, and a new university library with expanded serial holdings.

Information for Students With Physical Disabilities: See the following Web site for more information: http://ods.utk.edu/.

Application Information:
Send to Ms. Connie J. Ogle, 312C Austin Peay Building, University of Tennessee, Knoxville, TN 37996-0900. Students are admitted in the Fall, application deadline December 10 for Clinical PhD and Counseling PhD; January 15 for Experimental PhD; March 15 for Experimental MA. *Fee:* $35.

Tennessee, University of, Knoxville
Industrial and Organizational Psychology Program
Business Administration
408 Stokely Management Center
Knoxville, TN 37996-0545
Telephone: (865) 974-4843
Fax: (865) 974-2048
E-mail: *ghurst@utk.edu*
Web: *http://bus.utk.edu/iopsyc*

Department Information:
1964. Department Head: Donde Plowman. Number of faculty: total—full-time 4; women—full-time 1.

Programs and Degrees Offered:
Listed in the following order: Program area, degree type (T if terminal Master's), number awarded 7/08–6/09. Industrial/Organizational Psychology PhD (Doctor of Philosophy) 6.

Student Applications/Admissions:
Student Applications
Industrial/Organizational Psychology PhD (Doctor of Philosophy)—Applications 2009–2010, 0. Total applicants accepted 2009–2010, 0. Number full-time enrolled (new admits only) 2009–2010, 0. Number part-time enrolled (new admits only) 2009–2010, 0. The median number of years required for completion of a degree in 2008–2009 were 5. The number of students enrolled full- and part-time who were dismissed or voluntarily withdrew from this program area in 2008–2009 were 0.

Scores: Entries appear in this order: required test or GPA, minimum score (if required), median score of students entering in 2009–2010. *Industrial/Organizational Psychology PhD (Doctor of Philosophy):* GRE-V 500, 568, GRE-Q 580, 652, GRE-Analytical no minimum stated, overall undergraduate GPA 3.7, 3.85, last 2 years GPA no minimum stated, 3.9.

Other Criteria: (importance of criteria rated low, medium, or high): GRE scores—high, research experience—high, work experience—medium, extracurricular activity—low, GPA—high, letters of recommendation—high, statement of goals and objectives—high. For additional information on admission requirements, go to http://bus.utk.edu/iopsyc/Admissions/index.html.

Student Characteristics: The following represents characteristics of students in 2009–2010 in all graduate psychology programs in the department: Female—full-time 6, part-time 0; Male—full-time 2, part-time 0; African American/Black—full-time 0, part-time 0; Hispanic/Latino(a)—full-time 0, part-time 0; Asian/Pacific Islander—full-time 1, part-time 0; American Indian/Alaska Native—full-time 0, part-time 0; Caucasian/White—full-time 7, part-time 0; Multi-ethnic—full-time 0, part-time 0; students subject to the Americans With Disabilities Act—full-time 0, part-time 0; Unknown ethnicity—full-time 0, part-time 0; International students who hold an F-1 or J-1 Visa—full-time 0, part-time 0.

Financial Information/Assistance:
Tuition for Full-Time Study: *Doctoral:* State residents: per academic year $6,826, $380 per credit hour; Nonstate residents: per

academic year $20,622, $1,147 per credit hour. Tuition is subject to change. See the following Web site for updates and changes in tuition costs: http://web.utk.edu/~bursar/tuition.html.

Financial Assistance:
First-Year Students: Teaching assistantships available for first year. Average amount paid per academic year: $15,000. Average number of hours worked per week: 15. Research assistantships available for first year. Average amount paid per academic year: $15,000. Average number of hours worked per week: 15. Fellowships and scholarships available for first year. Average amount paid per academic year: $15,000. Average number of hours worked per week: 15.

Advanced Students: Teaching assistantships available for advanced students. Average amount paid per academic year: $15,000. Average number of hours worked per week: 15. Research assistantships available for advanced students. Average amount paid per academic year: $15,000. Average number of hours worked per week: 15. Traineeships available for advanced students. Fellowships and scholarships available for advanced students.

Additional Information: Of all students currently enrolled full time, 100% benefited from one or more of the listed financial assistance programs. Application and information available online at: http://gradschool.utk.edu/CurrentStudents.shtml.

Internships/Practica: An internship or practicum is required but these vary considerably.

Housing and Day Care: No on-campus housing is available. No on-campus day care facilities are available.

Employment of Department Graduates:
Master's Degree Graduates: Of those who graduated in the academic year 2008–2009, the following categories and numbers represent the postgraduate activities and employment of master's degree graduates: Enrolled in a postdoctoral residency/fellowship (n/a), employed in independent practice (n/a), total from the above (master's) (0).
Doctoral Degree Graduates: Of those who graduated in the academic year 2008–2009, the following categories and numbers represent the postgraduate activities and employment of doctoral degree graduates: Enrolled in a psychology doctoral program (n/a), employed in an academic position at a university (2), employed in business or industry (4), total from the above (doctoral) (6).

Additional Information:
Orientation, Objectives, and Emphasis of Department: The industrial/organizational program is designed to prepare students for personnel, managerial, and organizational research; for university teaching; and for consulting relationships with industry. The program emphasizes a scientist–practitioner model in applying and conducting research based on accepted theory found in classical and modern organization theory, organizational behavior, psychology, management, and statistics.

Special Facilities or Resources: Computing and Academic Services (CAS) provides computing facilities, services, and support for the university's teaching, research, public service, and administrative activities. Individual UNIX and Lotus Notes accounts are provided for students, faculty and staff for the duration of their affiliation with UTK at no charge. CAS maintains six staffed computing labs, 15 unstaffed labs, and supports computing installations in all residence halls. Training and documentation are also available through CAS. Statistical and mathematical consulting is available to all students, faculty, and staff. CAS operates the core mainframe and large-scale servers; equipment includes multiple systems from SUN, SGI, and IBM systems. In addition to university computing services and facilities, the Department of Management and the College of Business Administration provide students with microcomputers in student offices, which are networked to departmental printers and the Internet. The University Libraries own approximately 2 million volumes and subscribe to more than 11,000 periodicals and other serial titles. The Libraries' membership in the Association of Research Libraries reflects the University's emphasis on graduate instruction and research and the support of comprehensive collections of library materials on a permanent basis.

Information for Students With Physical Disabilities: See the following Web site for more information: http://ods.utk.edu/.

Application Information:
Application available online. URL of online application: http://admissions.utk.edu/graduate/apply.shtml. Students are admitted in the Fall, application deadline February 1. *Fee:* $35.

Vanderbilt University
Human and Organizational Development
Peabody College of Education & Human Development
Peabody #90, 230 Appleton Place
Nashville, TN 37203-5721
Telephone: (615) 322-8484
Fax: (615) 343-2661
E-mail: *joe.cunningham@vanderbilt.edu*
Web: *http://peabody.vanderbilt.edu/hod/*

Department Information:
1999. Chairperson: Joseph Cunningham, EdD. Number of faculty: total—full-time 19, part-time 17; women—full-time 10, part-time 12; total—minority—full-time 5; women minority—full-time 3.

Programs and Degrees Offered:
Listed in the following order: Program area, degree type (T if terminal Master's), number awarded 7/08–6/09. Human Development Counseling MEd (Education) 21, Community Research & Action PhD (Doctor of Philosophy) 5, Community Research & Action MA/MS (Master of Arts/Science) (T) 5, Community Development & Action MEd (Education) 10.

Student Applications/Admissions:
Student Applications
Human Development Counseling MEd (Education)—Applications 2009–2010, 117. Total applicants accepted 2009–2010, 41. Number full-time enrolled (new admits only) 2009–2010, 29. Number part-time enrolled (new admits only) 2009–2010, 6. Total enrolled 2009–2010 full-time, 56, part-time, 9. Openings 2010–2011, 35. The median number of years required for completion of a degree in 2008–2009 were 2. The number of students enrolled full- and part-time who were dismissed or voluntarily withdrew from this program area in 2008–2009 were 0. *Community Research & Action PhD (Doctor of Philoso-*

phy)—Applications 2009–2010, 91. Total applicants accepted 2009–2010, 10. Number full-time enrolled (new admits only) 2009–2010, 6. Number part-time enrolled (new admits only) 2009–2010, 0. Total enrolled 2009–2010 full-time, 24, part-time, 3. Openings 2010–2011, 10. The median number of years required for completion of a degree in 2008–2009 were 2. The number of students enrolled full- and part-time who were dismissed or voluntarily withdrew from this program area in 2008–2009 were 1. *Community Research & Action MA/MS (Master of Arts/Science)*—The median number of years required for completion of a degree in 2008–2009 was 1. *Community Development & Action MEd (Education)*—Applications 2009–2010, 50. Total applicants accepted 2009–2010, 22. Number full-time enrolled (new admits only) 2009–2010, 12. Number part-time enrolled (new admits only) 2009–2010, 1. Total enrolled 2009–2010 full-time, 26, part-time, 5. Openings 2010–2011, 25. The median number of years required for completion of a degree in 2008–2009 was 1. The number of students enrolled full- and part-time who were dismissed or voluntarily withdrew from this program area in 2008–2009 were 2.

Scores: Entries appear in this order: required test or GPA, minimum score (if required), median score of students entering in 2009–2010. *Human Development Counseling MEd (Education):* GRE-V 500, 550, GRE-Q 500, 640, GRE-Analytical 3.5, 5.0, overall undergraduate GPA 3.0, 3.5; *Community Research & Action PhD (Doctor of Philosophy):* GRE-V 600, 630, GRE-Q 700, 700, GRE-Analytical 4.0, 5.0, overall undergraduate GPA 3.2, 3.3, Masters GPA 3.6, 3.6; *Community Research & Action MA/MS (Master of Arts/Science):* GRE-V 600, 630, GRE-Q 700, 700, GRE-Analytical 4.0, 5.0, overall undergraduate GPA 3.2, 3.3, last 2 years GPA 3.6, 3.6; *Community Development & Action MEd (Education):* GRE-V 500, 550, GRE-Q 500, 600, GRE-Analytical 3.5, 4.4, overall undergraduate GPA 3.0, 3.3.

Other Criteria: (importance of criteria rated low, medium, or high): GRE scores—high, research experience—medium, work experience—low, extracurricular activity—low, clinically related public service—medium, GPA—high, letters of recommendation—high, interview—high, statement of goals and objectives—high, writing samples—high, undergraduate major in psychology—low, specific undergraduate psychology courses taken—low. Research experience less important for Master's programs than for the PhD program. Clinically related public service helpful for all programs. For additional information on admission requirements, go to http://peabody.vanderbilt.edu/Prospective_Students.xml.

Student Characteristics: The following represents characteristics of students in 2009–2010 in all graduate psychology programs in the department: Female—full-time 86, part-time 15; Male—full-time 20, part-time 2; African American/Black—full-time 8, part-time 4; Hispanic/Latino(a)—full-time 4, part-time 0; Asian/Pacific Islander—full-time 2, part-time 0; American Indian/Alaska Native—full-time 0, part-time 0; Caucasian/White—full-time 92, part-time 13; Multi-ethnic—full-time 0, part-time 0; students subject to the Americans With Disabilities Act—full-time 0, part-time 0; Unknown ethnicity—full-time 0, part-time 0; International students who hold an F-1 or J-1 Visa—full-time 3, part-time 0.

Financial Information/Assistance:
Tuition for Full-Time Study: *Master's:* State residents: per academic year $27,500, $1,125 per credit hour; Nonstate residents: per academic year $27,500, $1,125 per credit hour. *Doctoral:* State residents: per academic year $27,500, $1,125 per credit hour; Nonstate residents: per academic year $27,500, $1,125 per credit hour. Tuition is subject to change. Additional fees are assessed to students beyond the costs of tuition for the following: student health insurance, student activities and recreation. See the following Web site for updates and changes in tuition costs: http://www.vanderbilt.edu/stuaccts/.

Financial Assistance:
First-Year Students: Teaching assistantships available for first year. Average amount paid per academic year: $14,000. Average number of hours worked per week: 20. Apply by February 1. Research assistantships available for first year. Average amount paid per academic year: $14,000. Average number of hours worked per week: 20. Apply by February 1. Fellowships and scholarships available for first year. Average amount paid per academic year: $24,000. Average number of hours worked per week: 20. Apply by February 1.

Advanced Students: Teaching assistantships available for advanced students. Average amount paid per academic year: $14,000. Average number of hours worked per week: 20. Apply by February 1. Research assistantships available for advanced students. Average amount paid per academic year: $14,000. Average number of hours worked per week: 20. Apply by February 1. Fellowships and scholarships available for advanced students. Average amount paid per academic year: $24,000. Average number of hours worked per week: 20. Apply by February 1.

Additional Information: Of all students currently enrolled full time, 70% benefited from one or more of the listed financial assistance programs. Application and information available online at: http://peabody.vanderbilt.edu/x3006.xml.

Internships/Practica: Master's Degree (MA/MS Community Research & Action): An internship experience, such as a final research project or "capstone" experience is required of graduates. The CDA and CRA programs require a 15-week internship. Possible sites include: Mayor's Office/Metro Council/Planning Commission; local community development organization; regional planning or civic design center; youth development center; healthcare corporation; neighborhood health clinic; alcohol and drug treatment center; welfare or housing agency; state health and human service agencies; Vanderbilt Institute for Public Policy Studies (Centers for Mental Health Policy, Evaluation Research and Methodology, Child and Family Policy, Crime and Justice Policy, Environmental Management Studies, Health Policy, Psychotherapy Research and Policy, State and Local Policy). The HDC Program requires a one-year internship that provides opportunities to apply knowledge and skills primarily in the areas of: social service agencies; mental health centers; schools (K-12); employee assistance programs; and other human services delivery programs.

Housing and Day Care: No on-campus housing is available. On-campus day care facilities are available. See the following Web site for more information: http://childandfamilycenter.vanderbilt.edu/.

Employment of Department Graduates:
Master's Degree Graduates: Of those who graduated in the academic year 2008–2009, the following categories and numbers represent the postgraduate activities and employment of master's degree graduates: Enrolled in another graduate/professional program (7), enrolled in a postdoctoral residency/fellowship (n/a), employed in independent practice (n/a), employed in a professional position in a school system (11), employed in a community mental health/counseling center (18), total from the above (master's) (36).
Doctoral Degree Graduates: Of those who graduated in the academic year 2008–2009, the following categories and numbers represent the postgraduate activities and employment of doctoral degree graduates: Enrolled in a psychology doctoral program (n/a), enrolled in a postdoctoral residency/fellowship (1), employed in an academic position at a university (3), other employment position (1), total from the above (doctoral) (5).

Additional Information:
Orientation, Objectives, and Emphasis of Department: Although the vast majority of faculty in the department are psychologists, our orientation is interdisciplinary. There are three graduate programs, all oriented to helping diverse communities and individuals identify and develop their strengths: a long-standing Master's in Human Development Counseling (HDC), a Master's in Community Development & Action (CDA), and a PhD in Community Research & Action (CRA, with a terminal masters degree included). The latter two started in 2001. The HDC Program prepares students to meet the psychological needs of the normally developing population, who sometimes require professional help. Through a humanistic training model and a two-year curriculum, students develop a strong theoretical grounding in life-span human development, and school or community counseling. The CDA program is for those who desire training for program administration/evaluation work in public or private, international or domestic, community service, planning, or development organizations. The Doctoral Degree in Community Research and Action is designed to train action-researchers for academic or program/policy-related careers in applied community studies: i.e., community psychology, community development, prevention, community health/mental health, organizational change, and ethics. Coursework in qualitative and quantitative methods and evaluation research is required. The program builds on the one in Community Psychology previously in the Department of Psychology and Human Development and reflects the move in the field to become interdisciplinary.

Special Facilities or Resources: Peabody College has its own library, several computer centers, and nationally known research centers, including the Learning Sciences Institute and the Kennedy Center for Research on Human Development, mental retardation and other disabilities. Also on the beautiful and historic Peabody campus is the Vanderbilt Institute for Public Policy Studies (Centers for Mental Health Policy, Evaluation Research and Methodology, Child and Family Policy, Crime and Justice Policy, Environmental Management Studies, Health Policy, Psychotherapy Research and Policy, State and Local Policy). Our department in Human & Organizational Development has its own center, the Center for Community Studies. Located in Nashville, the Tennessee state capital, opportunities abound for research and internships in state and local health and human service agencies and schools.

Information for Students With Physical Disabilities: See the following Web site for more information: http://www.vanderbilt.edu/ead/.

Application Information:
Send to Office of Graduate Admissions, Peabody College at Vanderbilt University, 230 Appleton Place, Peabody #327, Nashville, TN 37203-5721. Application available online. URL of online application: http://peabody.vanderbilt.edu/x3006.xml. Students are admitted in the Fall, application deadline December 1; Spring, application deadline November 1. The deadline for the PhD program in Community Research and Action is December 1, and the deadline for the MEd in Human Development Counseling is December 31. The Community Development & Action MEd Program has a rolling admissions process and also admits for the spring semester. November 1 is the preferred deadline for spring admissions. *Fee:* $40. Application fee is waived when applying online.

Vanderbilt University
Psychological Sciences
111 21st Avenue South
Nashville, TN 37240
Telephone: (615) 322-2874
Fax: (615) 343-8449
E-mail: *vay.welch@vanderbilt.edu*
Web: *http://www.vanderbilt.edu/psychological_sciences/home*

Department Information:
1925. Chairs: Andrew J. Tomarken & David Cole. Number of faculty: total—full-time 65, part-time 6; women—full-time 28, part-time 4; total—minority—full-time 5, part-time 1; women minority—full-time 3, part-time 1.

Programs and Degrees Offered:
Listed in the following order: Program area, degree type (T if terminal Master's), number awarded 7/08–6/09. Clinical Science PhD (Doctor of Philosophy) 8, Neuroscience PhD (Doctor of Philosophy) 5, Cognition and Cognitive Neuroscience PhD (Doctor of Philosophy) 4, Developmental Science PhD (Doctor of Philosophy) 0, Quantitative Methods and Evaluation PhD (Doctor of Philosophy) 0.

APA Accreditation: Clinical PhD (Doctor of Philosophy).

Student Applications/Admissions:
Student Applications
Clinical Science PhD (Doctor of Philosophy)—Applications 2009–2010, 286. Total applicants accepted 2009–2010, 12. Number full-time enrolled (new admits only) 2009–2010, 6. Number part-time enrolled (new admits only) 2009–2010, 0. Openings 2010–2011, 10. The median number of years required for completion of a degree in 2008–2009 were 7. The number of students enrolled full- and part-time who were dismissed or voluntarily withdrew from this program area in 2008–2009 were 1. *Neuroscience PhD (Doctor of Philosophy)*—Applications 2009–2010, 47. Total applicants accepted 2009–2010, 5. Number full-time enrolled (new admits only) 2009–2010, 4. Number part-time enrolled (new admits only) 2009–2010, 0. Openings 2010–2011, 3. The median number of years

required for completion of a degree in 2008–2009 were 6. The number of students enrolled full- and part-time who were dismissed or voluntarily withdrew from this program area in 2008–2009 were 0. *Cognition and Cognitive Neuroscience PhD (Doctor of Philosophy)*—Applications 2009–2010, 99. Total applicants accepted 2009–2010, 7. Number full-time enrolled (new admits only) 2009–2010, 8. Total enrolled 2009–2010 full-time, 25. Openings 2010–2011, 6. The median number of years required for completion of a degree in 2008–2009 were 6. The number of students enrolled full- and part-time who were dismissed or voluntarily withdrew from this program area in 2008–2009 were 0. *Developmental Science PhD (Doctor of Philosophy)*—Applications 2009–2010, 74. Total applicants accepted 2009–2010, 5. Number full-time enrolled (new admits only) 2009–2010, 0. Total enrolled 2009–2010 full-time, 11. Openings 2010–2011, 5. The number of students enrolled full- and part-time who were dismissed or voluntarily withdrew from this program area in 2008–2009 were 1. *Quantitative Methods and Evaluation PhD (Doctor of Philosophy)*—Applications 2009–2010, 28. Total applicants accepted 2009–2010, 1. Number full-time enrolled (new admits only) 2009–2010, 1. Total enrolled 2009–2010 full-time, 9. Openings 2010–2011, 4. The number of students enrolled full- and part-time who were dismissed or voluntarily withdrew from this program area in 2008–2009 were 0.

Scores: Entries appear in this order: required test or GPA, minimum score (if required), median score of students entering in 2009–2010. *Clinical Science PhD (Doctor of Philosophy)*: GRE-V no minimum stated, 650, GRE-Q no minimum stated, 720, overall undergraduate GPA no minimum stated, 3.7, psychology GPA no minimum stated, 3.79; *Neuroscience PhD (Doctor of Philosophy)*: GRE-V no minimum stated, 650, GRE-Q no minimum stated, 740, overall undergraduate GPA no minimum stated, 3.55, psychology GPA no minimum stated, 3.64; *Cognition and Cognitive Neuroscience PhD (Doctor of Philosophy)*: GRE-V no minimum stated, 620, GRE-Q no minimum stated, 760, overall undergraduate GPA no minimum stated, 3.56, psychology GPA no minimum stated, 3.62; *Developmental Science PhD (Doctor of Philosophy)*: GRE-V no minimum stated, 650, GRE-Q no minimum stated, 720, overall undergraduate GPA no minimum stated, 3.63, psychology GPA no minimum stated, 3.7; *Quantitative Methods and Evaluation PhD (Doctor of Philosophy)*: GRE-V no minimum stated, 640, GRE-Q no minimum stated, 750, overall undergraduate GPA no minimum stated, 3.73, psychology GPA no minimum stated, 3.75.

Other Criteria: (importance of criteria rated low, medium, or high): GRE scores—high, research experience—high, work experience—low, extracurricular activity—low, clinically related public service—low, GPA—high, letters of recommendation—high, interview—high, statement of goals and objectives—high, undergraduate major in psychology—low, specific undergraduate psychology courses taken—low. For additional information on admission requirements, go to http://www.vanderbilt.edu/psychological_sciences/home.

Student Characteristics: The following represents characteristics of students in 2009–2010 in all graduate psychology programs in the department: Female—full-time 67, part-time 0; Male—full-time 29, part-time 0; African American/Black—full-time 7, part-time 0; Hispanic/Latino(a)—full-time 5, part-time 0; Asian/Pacific Islander—full-time 17, part-time 0; American Indian/Alaska Native—full-time 0, part-time 0; Caucasian/White—full-time 67, part-time 0; Multi-ethnic—full-time 0, part-time 0; students subject to the Americans With Disabilities Act—full-time 0, part-time 0; Unknown ethnicity—full-time 0, part-time 0; International students who hold an F-1 or J-1 Visa—full-time 19, part-time 0.

Financial Information/Assistance:
Tuition for Full-Time Study: *Doctoral:* State residents: per academic year $37,632, $1,568 per credit hour; Nonstate residents: per academic year $37,632, $1,568 per credit hour. Tuition is subject to change. Additional fees are assessed to students beyond the costs of tuition for the following: student activity and recreation fees, one-time transcript fee.

Financial Assistance:
First-Year Students: Teaching assistantships available for first year. Average amount paid per academic year: $20,200. Average number of hours worked per week: 20. Apply by December 15. Research assistantships available for first year. Average amount paid per academic year: $20,200. Average number of hours worked per week: 20. Apply by December 15. Fellowships and scholarships available for first year. Average amount paid per academic year: $20,200. Average number of hours worked per week: 20. Apply by December 15.

Advanced Students: Teaching assistantships available for advanced students. Average amount paid per academic year: $20,200. Average number of hours worked per week: 20. Apply by December 15. Research assistantships available for advanced students. Average amount paid per academic year: $20,200. Average number of hours worked per week: 20. Apply by December 15. Traineeships available for advanced students. Average amount paid per academic year: $20,976. Average number of hours worked per week: 20. Apply by December 15. Fellowships and scholarships available for advanced students. Average amount paid per academic year: $20,200. Average number of hours worked per week: 20. Apply by December 15.

Additional Information: Of all students currently enrolled full time, 100% benefited from one or more of the listed financial assistance programs. Application and information available online at: http://www.vanderbilt.edu/financialaid.

Internships/Practica: Doctoral Degree (PhD Clinical Science): For those doctoral students for whom a professional internship was required in this program prior to graduation, (5) students applied for an internship in 2008–2009, with (5) students obtaining an internship. Of those students who obtained an internship, (5) were paid internships. Of those students who obtained an internship, (5) students placed in APA/CPA accredited internships, (0) students placed in internships not APA/CPA accredited, but listed with the Association of Psychology Postdoctoral and Internship Programs (APPIC), (0) students placed in internships conforming to guidelines of the Council of Directors of School Psychology Programs (CDSPP), (0) students placed in internships that were not APA/CPA accredited, APPIC or CDSPP listed. We offer up to two dozen different placements for students to do their practica. These include two VA Medical Centers, VU Child and Adolescent Psychiatric Hospital, VU Diabetes Center, VU Psychological and Counseling Center, Mobile Crisis Response Service, public school systems, state prison, and mental health facilities for both children and adults.

Housing and Day Care: No on-campus housing is available. On-campus day care facilities are available. See the following Web site for more information: http://childandfamilycenter.vanderbilt.edu/.

Employment of Department Graduates:

Master's Degree Graduates: Of those who graduated in the academic year 2008–2009, the following categories and numbers represent the postgraduate activities and employment of master's degree graduates: Enrolled in a postdoctoral residency/fellowship (n/a), employed in independent practice (n/a), total from the above (master's) (0).

Doctoral Degree Graduates: Of those who graduated in the academic year 2008–2009, the following categories and numbers represent the postgraduate activities and employment of doctoral degree graduates: Enrolled in a psychology doctoral program (n/a), enrolled in a postdoctoral residency/fellowship (11), employed in an academic position at a university (1), employed in a hospital/medical center (2), still seeking employment (1), other employment position (1), do not know (1), total from the above (doctoral) (17).

Additional Information:

Orientation, Objectives, and Emphasis of Department: The doctoral program in Psychological Sciences is offered jointly by the Department of Psychology in the College of Arts and Science and the Department of Psychology and Human Development in the Peabody College at Vanderbilt University. The program focuses on psychological theory and the development of original empirical research. Students are admitted to work toward the PhD in these areas: Clinical Science, Cognition and Cognitive Neuroscience, Developmental Science, Neuroscience, or Quantitative Methods and Evaluation. A major goal is the placement of students in academic settings. The curriculum is designed to: (a) familiarize students with major areas of psychology; (b) provide specialized training in at least one of the five specific areas; and (c) provide students flexibility to enroll in classes consistent with their research interests. Students take core courses in quantitative methods and substantive area, enroll in advanced seminars, and attend weekly area group colloquia. In addition to coursework, we expect students to be continually involved in research throughout their tenure in our program. We use a one-on-one mentoring model as a primary, though not exclusive, means of advisement for the acquisition of scientific skills by students.

Special Facilities or Resources: Psychological Sciences is housed in Wilson Hall, Jesup Psychological Laboratory, and Hobbs Laboratory of Human Development. We have state-of-the-art laboratories for carrying out basic research with humans and animals that include computer stimulus presentation and response collection capabilities, computers for data analysis and computational modeling, and specialized research equipment (including eyetracking environments, virtual reality, and custom experimental hardware and electronics). Research with humans, including both adults and children, and including those with brain damage and mental illness, is conducted in laboratories at Wilson, Hobbs and at laboratories in the Kennedy Center and the Vanderbilt Medical Center. Wilson Hall contains an AAALAC-accredited animal care facility with dedicated and experienced staff to support husbandry, enrichment, and surgery for species used in basic research. Faculty members have their own dedicated laboratory space for conducting clinical, cognition and cognitive neuroscience, developmental, neuroscience, and quantitative research. Research in Psychological Sciences is enhanced by a number of research centers that support a variety of shared research equipment and services: Advanced Computing Center for Research and Education, Center for Integrative and Cognitive Neuroscience, Institute for Imaging Science, Kennedy Center, Learning Sciences Institute, Vanderbilt Vision Research Center.

Information for Students With Physical Disabilities: See the following Web site for more information: http://www.vanderbilt.edu/ead/.

Application Information:
Send to Psychological Sciences Program, Vanderbilt University GPC #324, 230 Appleton Place, Nashville, TN 37203-5721 U.S.A. Application available online. URL of online application: https://graduateapplications.vanderbilt.edu/. Students are admitted in the Fall, application deadline December 15. *Fee:* $40. Application fees are waived with online application.

TEXAS

Angelo State University
Department of Psychology, Sociology, and Social Work
College of Liberal and Fine Arts
2601 West Avenue North
San Angelo, TX 76909
Telephone: (325) 942-2068
Fax: (325) 942-2290
E-mail: Bill.Davidson@angelo.edu
Web: http://www.angelo.edu/dept/psychology_sociology/

Department Information:
1983. Department Head: William B. Davidson. Number of faculty: total—full-time 13, part-time 8; women—full-time 4, part-time 6; total—minority—full-time 2, part-time 1; women minority—full-time 2, part-time 1.

Programs and Degrees Offered:
Listed in the following order: Program area, degree type (T if terminal Master's), number awarded 7/08–6/09. Counseling Psychology MA/MS (Master of Arts/Science) (T) 7, Applied Psychology MA/MS (Master of Arts/Science) (T) 4, Industrial/Organizational Psychology MA/MS (Master of Arts/Science) (T) 5.

Student Applications/Admissions:
Student Applications
   Counseling Psychology MA/MS (Master of Arts/Science)—Applications 2009–2010, 35. Total applicants accepted 2009–2010, 25. Number full-time enrolled (new admits only) 2009–2010, 13. Number part-time enrolled (new admits only) 2009–2010, 4. Total enrolled 2009–2010 full-time, 15, part-time, 10. Openings 2010–2011, 10. The median number of years required for completion of a degree in 2008–2009 were 2. The number of students enrolled full- and part-time who were dismissed or voluntarily withdrew from this program area in 2008–2009 were 1. *Applied Psychology MA/MS (Master of Arts/Science)*—Applications 2009–2010, 7. Total applicants accepted 2009–2010, 5. Number full-time enrolled (new admits only) 2009–2010, 4. Number part-time enrolled (new admits only) 2009–2010, 0. Openings 2010–2011, 10. The median number of years required for completion of a degree in 2008–2009 were 2. The number of students enrolled full- and part-time who were dismissed or voluntarily withdrew from this program area in 2008–2009 were 0. *Industrial/Organizational Psychology MA/MS (Master of Arts/Science)*—Applications 2009–2010, 18. Total applicants accepted 2009–2010, 14. Number full-time enrolled (new admits only) 2009–2010, 7. Number part-time enrolled (new admits only) 2009–2010, 0. Openings 2010–2011, 10. The median number of years required for completion of a degree in 2008–2009 were 2. The number of students enrolled full- and part-time who were dismissed or voluntarily withdrew from this program area in 2008–2009 were 0.
   Other Criteria: (importance of criteria rated low, medium, or high): GRE scores—high, research experience—low, work experience—low, GPA—high, letters of recommendation—medium, statement of goals and objectives—medium, undergraduate major in psychology—low, specific undergraduate psychology courses taken—low. The criteria do vary for different programs. For additional information on admission requirements, go to http://www.angelo.edu/dept/psychology_sociology/grad_programs.

Student Characteristics: The following represents characteristics of students in 2009–2010 in all graduate psychology programs in the department: Female—full-time 23, part-time 10; Male—full-time 11, part-time 0; African American/Black—full-time 0, part-time 0; Hispanic/Latino(a)—full-time 3, part-time 2; Asian/Pacific Islander—full-time 1, part-time 0; American Indian/Alaska Native—full-time 0, part-time 0; Caucasian/White—full-time 30, part-time 8; Multi-ethnic—full-time 0, part-time 0; students subject to the Americans With Disabilities Act—full-time 0, part-time 0; Unknown ethnicity—full-time 0, part-time 0; International students who hold an F-1 or J-1 Visa—full-time 0, part-time 0.

Financial Information/Assistance:
   Tuition for Full-Time Study: *Master's:* State residents: per academic year $2,339, $260 per credit hour; Nonstate residents: per academic year $4,832, $537 per credit hour. Tuition is subject to change. See the following Web site for updates and changes in tuition costs: http://www.angelo.edu/cstudent/tuition_and_fees.html.

Financial Assistance:
   First-Year Students: Research assistantships available for first year. Average amount paid per academic year: $7,490. Average number of hours worked per week: 17. Apply by April 15. Fellowships and scholarships available for first year. Average amount paid per academic year: $2,300. Apply by March 1.
   Advanced Students: Teaching assistantships available for advanced students. Average amount paid per academic year: $11,095. Average number of hours worked per week: 20. Apply by April 15. Research assistantships available for advanced students. Average amount paid per academic year: $7,490. Average number of hours worked per week: 17. Apply by April 15. Fellowships and scholarships available for advanced students. Average amount paid per academic year: $2,300. Apply by March 1.
   Additional Information: Of all students currently enrolled full time, 36% benefited from one or more of the listed financial assistance programs. Application and information available online at: http://www.angelo.edu/dept/grad_school/financial_aid.html.

Internships/Practica: Practicum opportunities are available in many local public and private mental health facilities and also in local corporate entities.

Housing and Day Care: On-campus housing is available. See the following Web site for more information: http://www.angelo.edu/dept/residential_programs. No on-campus day care facilities are available.

Employment of Department Graduates:
   Master's Degree Graduates: Of those who graduated in the academic year 2008–2009, the following categories and numbers

represent the postgraduate activities and employment of master's degree graduates: Enrolled in a postdoctoral residency/fellowship (n/a), employed in independent practice (n/a), total from the above (master's) (0).

Doctoral Degree Graduates: Of those who graduated in the academic year 2008–2009, the following categories and numbers represent the postgraduate activities and employment of doctoral degree graduates: Enrolled in a psychology doctoral program (n/a), total from the above (doctoral) (0).

Additional Information:
Orientation, Objectives, and Emphasis of Department: The department emphasizes personalized training, small class sizes, and a balance between research skills and practitioner skills. We offer the Applied Psychology program completely online.

Special Facilities or Resources: The department is equipped with state-of-the-art psychology and computer laboratories. Training also occurs in local agencies and hospitals, private companies and university administration offices.

Information for Students With Physical Disabilities: See the following Web site for more information: http://www.angelo.edu/services/student_life/disability.html.

Application Information:
Send to Office of the Graduate Dean, Angelo State University, ASU Station #11025, San Angelo, TX 76909-1025. Application available online. URL of online application: http://www.angelo.edu/dept/grad_school/index.html. Students are admitted in the Fall, application deadline July 15; Spring, application deadline December 1; Summer, application deadline April 30. Summer I Application Deadline is April 30 Summer II Application Deadline is May 31. *Fee:* $40.

Baylor University
Department of Psychology and Neuroscience, PhD Program in Psychology
Arts and Sciences
One Bear Place 97334
Waco, TX 76798-7334
Telephone: (254) 710-2961
Fax: (254) 710-3033
E-mail: *Matthew_Stanford@baylor.edu*
Web: *http://www.baylor.edu/psychologyneuroscience*

Department Information:
1950. Chairperson: J.L. Diaz-Granados, PhD. Number of faculty: total—full-time 20; women—full-time 6; total—minority—full-time 2; women minority—full-time 1.

Programs and Degrees Offered:
Listed in the following order: Program area, degree type (T if terminal Master's), number awarded 7/08–6/09. Clinical Psychology PsyD (Doctor of Psychology) 12, Psychology PhD (Doctor of Philosophy) 0.

APA Accreditation: Clinical PsyD (Doctor of Psychology). Student Outcome Data Website: http://www.baylor.edu/psychologyneuroscience/index.php?id=21427.

Student Applications/Admissions:
Student Applications
Clinical Psychology PsyD (Doctor of Psychology)—Applications 2009–2010, 156. Total applicants accepted 2009–2010, 7. Number full-time enrolled (new admits only) 2009–2010, 7. Openings 2010–2011, 7. The median number of years required for completion of a degree in 2008–2009 were 5. The number of students enrolled full- and part-time who were dismissed or voluntarily withdrew from this program area in 2008–2009 were 1. *Psychology PhD (Doctor of Philosophy)*—Applications 2009–2010, 58. Total applicants accepted 2009–2010, 3. Number full-time enrolled (new admits only) 2009–2010, 3. Total enrolled 2009–2010 full-time, 16. Openings 2010–2011, 6. The number of students enrolled full- and part-time who were dismissed or voluntarily withdrew from this program area in 2008–2009 were 1.

Scores: Entries appear in this order: required test or GPA, minimum score (if required), median score of students entering in 2009–2010. *Clinical Psychology PsyD (Doctor of Psychology)*: GRE-V 587, GRE-Q 587, overall undergraduate GPA 2.7, psychology GPA 3.0; *Psychology PhD (Doctor of Philosophy)*: GRE-V 500, GRE-Q 500.

Other Criteria: (importance of criteria rated low, medium, or high): GRE scores—high, research experience—high, work experience—medium, extracurricular activity—medium, clinically related public service—medium, GPA—high, letters of recommendation—high, interview—high, statement of goals and objectives—medium, undergraduate major in psychology—low.

Student Characteristics: The following represents characteristics of students in 2009–2010 in all graduate psychology programs in the department: Female—full-time 34, part-time 0; Male—full-time 15, part-time 0; African American/Black—full-time 2, part-time 0; Hispanic/Latino(a)—full-time 4, part-time 0; Asian/Pacific Islander—full-time 1, part-time 0; American Indian/Alaska Native—full-time 0, part-time 0; Caucasian/White—full-time 0, part-time 0; Multi-ethnic—full-time 0, part-time 0; students subject to the Americans With Disabilities Act—full-time 0, part-time 0; Unknown ethnicity—full-time 0, part-time 0; International students who hold an F-1 or J-1 Visa—full-time 0, part-time 0.

Financial Information/Assistance:
Tuition for Full-Time Study: *Doctoral:* State residents: $1,124 per credit hour; Nonstate residents: $1,124 per credit hour. Tuition is subject to change. See the following Web site for updates and changes in tuition costs: http://www.baylor.edu/graduate/index.php?id=42277.

Financial Assistance:
First-Year Students: Teaching assistantships available for first year. Average amount paid per academic year: $19,000. Average number of hours worked per week: 20. Apply by January 2. Research assistantships available for first year. Average amount paid per academic year: $19,000. Average number of hours worked per week: 20. Apply by January 2. Traineeships available for first year. Average amount paid per academic year: $19,000. Average number of hours worked per week: 20. Apply by January 2. Fellowships and scholarships available for first year.

Advanced Students: Teaching assistantships available for advanced students. Average amount paid per academic year:

$19,000. Average number of hours worked per week: 20. Apply by January 2. Research assistantships available for advanced students. Average amount paid per academic year: $19,000. Average number of hours worked per week: 20. Apply by January 2. Traineeships available for advanced students. Average amount paid per academic year: $19,000. Average number of hours worked per week: 20. Apply by January 2. Fellowships and scholarships available for advanced students.

Additional Information: Of all students currently enrolled full time, 100% benefited from one or more of the listed financial assistance programs. Application and information available online at: http://www.baylor.edu/psychologyneuroscience.

Internships/Practica: Doctoral Degree (PsyD Clinical Psychology): For those doctoral students for whom a professional internship was required in this program prior to graduation, (5) students applied for an internship in 2008–2009, with (4) students obtaining an internship. Of those students who obtained an internship, (4) were paid internships. Of those students who obtained an internship, (3) students placed in APA/CPA accredited internships, (1) students placed in internships not APA/CPA accredited, but listed with the Association of Psychology Postdoctoral and Internship Programs (APPIC), (0) students placed in internships conforming to guidelines of the Council of Directors of School Psychology Programs (CDSPP), (0) students placed in internships that were not APA/CPA accredited, APPIC or CDSPP listed. The PsyD Program incorporates an extensive practicum program with placements available in 16 community agencies and treatment facilities. Of our graduates over the last 11 years, 105 of 107 have obtained APA-accredited internships.

Housing and Day Care: No on-campus housing is available. On-campus day care facilities are available. http://www.baylor.edu/pipercdc.

Employment of Department Graduates:
Master's Degree Graduates: Of those who graduated in the academic year 2008–2009, the following categories and numbers represent the postgraduate activities and employment of master's degree graduates: Enrolled in a postdoctoral residency/fellowship (n/a), employed in independent practice (n/a), total from the above (master's) (0).
Doctoral Degree Graduates: Of those who graduated in the academic year 2008–2009, the following categories and numbers represent the postgraduate activities and employment of doctoral degree graduates: Enrolled in a psychology doctoral program (n/a), employed in independent practice (6), employed in an academic position at a university (0), employed in an academic position at a 2-year/4-year college (1), employed in a community mental health/counseling center (2), employed in a hospital/medical center (2), still seeking employment (0), total from the above (doctoral) (11).

Additional Information:
Orientation, Objectives, and Emphasis of Department: The department offers a broad range of courses in the areas of clinical psychology, behavioral neuroscience, social psychology and general experimental psychology. The Doctor of Psychology (PsyD) program has the longest history of accreditation by the American Psychological Association. The PsyD program emphasizes a professional-scholar model with a goal of developing competencies based on current research and scholarship in clinical psychology. Extensive practicum experience is integrated with concurrent coursework. A formal dissertation involving applied clinical research is also required. The goal of Baylor's PsyD Program is to develop professional psychologists with the conceptual and clinical competencies necessary to deliver psychological services in a manner that is effective and responsive to individual and societal needs both now and in the future. The doctoral program in Psychology (PhD) has three training tracks; Behavioral Neuroscience, Social Psychology and General Experimental. Doctoral students are expected to acquire sufficient knowledge and expertise to permit them to work as independent scholars at the frontier of their field upon graduation. Extensive training is provided in laboratory research and experimental design for social psychology and behavioral neuroscience students. The Doctor of Philosophy (PhD) degree is ultimately awarded to those individuals who have attained a high level of scholarship in a selected field through independent study, research, and creative thought.

Special Facilities or Resources: The department has a number of well-equipped research laboratories. PhD program: Computer-controlled programmable laboratory in memory and cognition; complete facilities for research on animal learning and behavior (including animal colony); developmental psychobiology laboratory, with facilities for behavioral and pharmacological research, including teratological studies; inhalation chambers for administration of ethanol (and other substances). Single-subject brain-recording (EEG) and electron microscopy facilities are available. The Department also houses a community clinic that facilitates the clinical training and related research activities for PsyD students.

Application Information:
Send to Baylor University; Graduate Admissions; One Bear Place 97264; Waco, TX 76798. Application available online. URL of online application: http://www.baylor.edu/graduate/. Students are admitted in the Fall, application deadline February 15; Summer, application deadline January 2. Psychology (PhD), February 15; only accept applications for Fall admission Clinical Psychology (PsyD), January 2; only accept applications for Summer admission. *Fee:* $40.

Houston Baptist University
Psychology Department
College of Arts and Humanities
7502 Fondren Road
Houston, TX 77074
Telephone: (281) 649-3171
Fax: (281) 649-3361
E-mail: *rnero@hbu.edu*
Web: *http://www.hbu.edu*

Department Information:
1985. Chairperson: Renata Nero, PhD. Number of faculty: total—full-time 6, part-time 6; women—full-time 3, part-time 5; total—minority—full-time 2; women minority—full-time 1.

Programs and Degrees Offered:
Listed in the following order: Program area, degree type (T if terminal Master's), number awarded 7/08–6/09. Psychology MA/MS (Master of Arts/Science) (T) 18, Christian Counseling MA/MS (Master of Arts/Science) (T) 1.

Student Applications/Admissions:
Student Applications
Psychology MA/MS (Master of Arts/Science)—Applications 2009–2010, 32. Total applicants accepted 2009–2010, 13. Number full-time enrolled (new admits only) 2009–2010, 11. Number part-time enrolled (new admits only) 2009–2010, 2. Total enrolled 2009–2010 full-time, 52, part-time, 9. Openings 2010–2011, 45. The median number of years required for completion of a degree in 2008–2009 were 2. The number of students enrolled full- and part-time who were dismissed or voluntarily withdrew from this program area in 2008–2009 were 1. *Christian Counseling MA/MS (Master of Arts/Science)*—Applications 2009–2010, 6. Total applicants accepted 2009–2010, 2. Number full-time enrolled (new admits only) 2009–2010, 2. Number part-time enrolled (new admits only) 2009–2010, 0. Total enrolled 2009–2010 full-time, 14, part-time, 1. Openings 2010–2011, 30. The median number of years required for completion of a degree in 2008–2009 were 2. The number of students enrolled full- and part-time who were dismissed or voluntarily withdrew from this program area in 2008–2009 were 1.
Other Criteria: (importance of criteria rated low, medium, or high): GRE scores—high, clinically related public service—low, GPA—high, letters of recommendation—medium, interview—medium, statement of goals and objectives—medium. For additional information on admission requirements, go to http://www.hbu.edu.

Student Characteristics: The following represents characteristics of students in 2009–2010 in all graduate psychology programs in the department: Female—full-time 58, part-time 7; Male—full-time 11, part-time 0; African American/Black—full-time 8, part-time 7; Hispanic/Latino(a)—full-time 8, part-time 0; Asian/Pacific Islander—full-time 3, part-time 0; American Indian/Alaska Native—full-time 1, part-time 0; Caucasian/White—full-time 49, part-time 0; Multi-ethnic—full-time 0, part-time 0; students subject to the Americans With Disabilities Act—full-time 0, part-time 0; Unknown ethnicity—full-time 0, part-time 0; International students who hold an F-1 or J-1 Visa—full-time 1, part-time 0.

Financial Information/Assistance:
Tuition for Full-Time Study: *Master's:* State residents: $500 per credit hour; Nonstate residents: $500 per credit hour. Tuition is subject to change. See the following Web site for updates and changes in tuition costs: http://www.hbu.edu.

Financial Assistance:
First-Year Students: No information provided.
Advanced Students: No information provided.

Additional Information: Of all students currently enrolled full time, 0% benefited from one or more of the listed financial assistance programs. Application and information available online at: http://www.hbu.edu.

Internships/Practica: Students complete their practicum requirements (450 clock hours supervised by a licensed psychologist or licensed professional counselor-supervisor) in area hospitals, social service agencies, schools and counseling centers. MACC students complete their practica in church or Christian counseling centers. LSSP students complete a 1,200-hour internship in a school setting.

Housing and Day Care: On-campus housing is available. Husky Village, (281) 649-3100. No on-campus day care facilities are available.

Employment of Department Graduates:
Master's Degree Graduates: Of those who graduated in the academic year 2008–2009, the following categories and numbers represent the postgraduate activities and employment of master's degree graduates: Enrolled in a postdoctoral residency/fellowship (n/a), employed in independent practice (n/a), total from the above (master's) (0).
Doctoral Degree Graduates: Of those who graduated in the academic year 2008–2009, the following categories and numbers represent the postgraduate activities and employment of doctoral degree graduates: Enrolled in a psychology doctoral program (n/a), total from the above (doctoral) (0).

Additional Information:
Orientation, Objectives, and Emphasis of Department: The master's program follows the scientist–practitioner model of training. Some students become psychological associates, some seek doctoral training, and a large number add the 12 hours required to become licensed specialists in school psychology. The majority pursue licensure as professional counselors.

Special Facilities or Resources: The department has a full-time faculty of dedicated teaching professionals. All graduate faculty hold terminal degrees. Two are licensed psychologists, one is a licensed professional counselor-supervisor, and two are social psychologists. All adjuncts have terminal degrees and are practicing clinicians. Computer facilities are available for use in research and statistical analyses.

Information for Students With Physical Disabilities: See the following Web site for more information: www.hbu.edu/hbu/Academic_Accommodations_for_students_with_Learning.asp.

Application Information:
Send to Houston Baptist University, 7502 Fondren, Houston, TX 77074. Application available online. URL of online application: http://www.hbu.edu. Students are admitted in the Fall, application deadline August 1; Spring, application deadline December 1; Summer, application deadline May 1. Deadlines are flexible. *Fee:* $0.

Houston, University of
Department of Educational Psychology
College of Education
491 Farish Hall
Houston, TX 77204-5029
Telephone: (713) 743-5019
Fax: (713) 743-4996
E-mail: tkubiszyn@uh.edu
Web: http://www.coe.uh.edu/academic-department/espy/

Department Information:
1980. Chairperson: Dr. Thomas Kubiszyn. Number of faculty: total—full-time 25, part-time 20; women—full-time 14, part-time 13; total—minority—full-time 6, part-time 5; women minority—full-time 4, part-time 4.

Programs and Degrees Offered:
Listed in the following order: Program area, degree type (T if terminal Master's), number awarded 7/08–6/09. Counseling Psychology PhD (Doctor of Philosophy) 5, Educational Psychology & Individual Differences PhD (Doctor of Philosophy) 1, Counseling MEd (Education) 24, Educational Psychology MEd (Education) 5, School Psychology PhD (Doctor of Philosophy) 1.

APA Accreditation: Counseling PhD (Doctor of Philosophy). School PhD (Doctor of Philosophy).

Student Applications/Admissions:
Student Applications

Counseling Psychology PhD (Doctor of Philosophy)—Applications 2009–2010, 83. Total applicants accepted 2009–2010, 8. Number full-time enrolled (new admits only) 2009–2010, 7. Total enrolled 2009–2010 full-time, 31, part-time, 18. Openings 2010–2011, 9. The median number of years required for completion of a degree in 2008–2009 were 6. The number of students enrolled full- and part-time who were dismissed or voluntarily withdrew from this program area in 2008–2009 were 0. *Educational Psychology & Individual Differences PhD (Doctor of Philosophy)*—Applications 2009–2010, 18. Total applicants accepted 2009–2010, 6. Number full-time enrolled (new admits only) 2009–2010, 1. Number part-time enrolled (new admits only) 2009–2010, 1. Total enrolled 2009–2010 full-time, 9, part-time, 15. The median number of years required for completion of a degree in 2008–2009 were 4. The number of students enrolled full- and part-time who were dismissed or voluntarily withdrew from this program area in 2008–2009 were 0. *Counseling MEd (Education)*—Applications 2009–2010, 162. Total applicants accepted 2009–2010, 81. Number full-time enrolled (new admits only) 2009–2010, 34. Number part-time enrolled (new admits only) 2009–2010, 24. Total enrolled 2009–2010 full-time, 61, part-time, 43. The median number of years required for completion of a degree in 2008–2009 were 2. The number of students enrolled full- and part-time who were dismissed or voluntarily withdrew from this program area in 2008–2009 were 0. *Educational Psychology MEd (Education)*—Applications 2009–2010, 58. Total applicants accepted 2009–2010, 16. Number full-time enrolled (new admits only) 2009–2010, 5. Number part-time enrolled (new admits only) 2009–2010, 7. Total enrolled 2009–2010 full-time, 10, part-time, 20. The median number of years required for completion of a degree in 2008–2009 were 2. The number of students enrolled full- and part-time who were dismissed or voluntarily withdrew from this program area in 2008–2009 were 0. *School Psychology PhD (Doctor of Philosophy)*—Applications 2009–2010, 20. Total applicants accepted 2009–2010, 11. Number full-time enrolled (new admits only) 2009–2010, 6. Total enrolled 2009–2010 full-time, 16, part-time, 7. Openings 2010–2011, 68. The median number of years required for completion of a degree in 2008–2009 were 4. The number of students enrolled full- and part-time who were dismissed or voluntarily withdrew from this program area in 2008–2009 were 3.

Scores: Entries appear in this order: required test or GPA, minimum score (if required), median score of students entering in 2009–2010. *Counseling Psychology PhD (Doctor of Philosophy):* GRE-V no minimum stated, GRE-Q no minimum stated, GRE-Analytical no minimum stated, overall undergraduate GPA no minimum stated; *Educational Psychology & Individual Differences PhD (Doctor of Philosophy):* GRE-V no minimum stated, GRE-Q no minimum stated, GRE-Analytical no minimum stated; *Counseling MEd (Education):* GRE-V no minimum stated, GRE-Q no minimum stated, GRE-Analytical no minimum stated, overall undergraduate GPA no minimum stated; *Educational Psychology MEd (Education):* GRE-V no minimum stated, GRE-Q no minimum stated, GRE-Analytical no minimum stated, overall undergraduate GPA no minimum stated; *School Psychology PhD (Doctor of Philosophy):* GRE-V no minimum stated, GRE-Q no minimum stated, GRE-Analytical no minimum stated, overall undergraduate GPA no minimum stated.

Other Criteria: (importance of criteria rated low, medium, or high): GRE scores—high, research experience—high, work experience—medium, extracurricular activity—high, clinically related public service—medium, GPA—high, letters of recommendation—high, interview—high, statement of goals and objectives—high, undergraduate major in psychology—medium, specific undergraduate psychology courses taken—medium. PhD programs emphasize research experience and research interests more than do the master's programs. For additional information on admission requirements, go to http://www.coe.uh.edu/future-students/how-to-apply/graduate.

Student Characteristics: The following represents characteristics of students in 2009–2010 in all graduate psychology programs in the department: Female—full-time 109, part-time 85; Male—full-time 18, part-time 18; African American/Black—full-time 16, part-time 7; Hispanic/Latino(a)—full-time 19, part-time 17; Asian/Pacific Islander—full-time 11, part-time 13; American Indian/Alaska Native—full-time 3, part-time 1; Caucasian/White—full-time 78, part-time 65; Multi-ethnic—full-time 0, part-time 0; students subject to the Americans With Disabilities Act—full-time 0, part-time 0; Unknown ethnicity—full-time 0, part-time 0; International students who hold an F-1 or J-1 Visa—full-time 0, part-time 0.

Financial Information/Assistance:
Tuition for Full-Time Study: *Master's:* State residents: per academic year $4,716, $262 per credit hour; Nonstate residents: per academic year $9,720, $540 per credit hour. *Doctoral:* State residents: per academic year $4,716, $262 per credit hour; Nonstate residents: per academic year $9,720, $540 per credit hour. Tuition is subject to change. Additional fees are assessed to stu-

dents beyond the costs of tuition for the following: various fees are required, please review the website for details. See the following Web site for updates and changes in tuition costs: http://www.uh.edu/financial/graduate/tuition-fees/tuition/.

Financial Assistance:

First-Year Students: Teaching assistantships available for first year. Average amount paid per academic year: $12,732. Average number of hours worked per week: 20. Apply by April 15. Research assistantships available for first year. Average amount paid per academic year: $12,732. Average number of hours worked per week: 20. Apply by April 15. Fellowships and scholarships available for first year. Average amount paid per academic year: $3,000. Apply by March 1.

Advanced Students: Teaching assistantships available for advanced students. Average amount paid per academic year: $15,132. Average number of hours worked per week: 20. Apply by Aptil 15. Research assistantships available for advanced students. Average amount paid per academic year: $15,132. Average number of hours worked per week: 20. Apply by April 15.

Additional Information: Of all students currently enrolled full time, 33% benefited from one or more of the listed financial assistance programs. Application and information available online at: http://www.uh.edu/financial/graduate/.

Internships/Practica: Doctoral Degree (PhD Counseling Psychology): For those doctoral students for whom a professional internship was required in this program prior to graduation, (10) students applied for an internship in 2008–2009, with (10) students obtaining an internship. Of those students who obtained an internship, (10) were paid internships. Of those students who obtained an internship, (9) students placed in APA/CPA accredited internships, (0) students placed in internships not APA/CPA accredited, but listed with the Association of Psychology Postdoctoral and Internship Programs (APPIC), (0) students placed in internships conforming to guidelines of the Council of Directors of School Psychology Programs (CDSPP), (1) students placed in internships that were not APA/CPA accredited, APPIC or CDSPP listed. Doctoral Degree (PhD School Psychology): For those doctoral students for whom a professional internship was required in this program prior to graduation, (3) students applied for an internship in 2008–2009, with (3) students obtaining an internship. Of those students who obtained an internship, (3) were paid internships. Of those students who obtained an internship, (3) students placed in APA/CPA accredited internships, (0) students placed in internships not APA/CPA accredited, but listed with the Association of Psychology Postdoctoral and Internship Programs (APPIC), (0) students placed in internships conforming to guidelines of the Council of Directors of School Psychology Programs (CDSPP), (0) students placed in internships that were not APA/CPA accredited, APPIC or CDSPP listed. All counseling psychology doctoral students and counseling master's students participate in supervised practica at numerous sites throughout the Houston area. Examples of the types of sites at which students have completed practica include veteran's and children's hospitals, counseling centers and school districts. In addition, doctoral counseling psychology students are required to complete a one year, full-time internship approved by the faculty. These sites range widely in orientation, focus and geographic location. All school psychology doctoral students must complete two years of advanced practicum (half-time) as well as a one year, full-time predoctoral internship. A supervised school psychology practicum may also be required (waived for those in possession of the Texas Licensed Specialist in School Psychology [LSSP] credential, or its equivalent). Practica are arranged for students, and are available at various sites around the Houston area, including school districts, Texas Children's Hospital, M.D. Anderson Children's Cancer Hospital, Harris County Juvenile Probation, and the Mental Retardation and Autism Unit of the Harris County Mental Health and Mental Retardation Department. Internship sites are available in a variety of settings in the Houston area and around the country. All School Psychology students who have applied for APA accredited internships have obtained one.

Housing and Day Care: On-campus housing is available. See the following Web site for more information: http://www.housing.uh.edu/. On-campus day care facilities are available. See the following Web site for more information: http://www.uh.edu/ccc/.

Employment of Department Graduates:

Master's Degree Graduates: Of those who graduated in the academic year 2008–2009, the following categories and numbers represent the postgraduate activities and employment of master's degree graduates: Enrolled in a postdoctoral residency/fellowship (n/a), employed in independent practice (n/a), total from the above (master's) (0).

Doctoral Degree Graduates: Of those who graduated in the academic year 2008–2009, the following categories and numbers represent the postgraduate activities and employment of doctoral degree graduates: Enrolled in a psychology doctoral program (n/a), enrolled in a postdoctoral residency/fellowship (1), employed in independent practice (2), employed in an academic position at a university (1), employed in other positions at a higher education institution (1), employed in a professional position in a school system (4), employed in a community mental health/counseling center (1), employed in a hospital/medical center (2), total from the above (doctoral) (12).

Additional Information:

Orientation, Objectives, and Emphasis of Department: Graduates of the Educational Psychology Department have made significant contributions to many university faculties, state and national boards, in private practice, in government agencies, and in leadership roles in public and private schools. Students choose the Educational Psychology Department in order to study with our nationally recognized faculty and to participate in innovative research in one of the most diverse research institutions in the country. The Counseling Psychology PhD program prepares highly skilled scientist–practitioners. Counseling psychologists can assume several roles in a variety of settings including personal, educational and career counseling services; college and university teaching; research; and consultation to organizations concerned with psychological and interpersonal development. The Educational Psychology and Individual Differences PhD program is dedicated to the advancement and application of knowledge relevant to human learning, development, and psychological functioning, especially within academic contexts. Graduates pursue careers as faculty members, researchers, and other leadership positions in a variety of organizations. The PhD program in School Psychology prepares professional psychologists in the scientist–practitioner tradition. Graduates are trained to assume leadership, direct service and consultative roles and careers in public and private PK-12 schools, health and mental health related settings, colleges and universities, research institutions, and in independent practice. The Master's of Education (MEd) in Counseling program prepares counselors to assume positions in education and mental health settings, such as public schools, junior colleges, university counseling and advisement centers, and community mental health agencies. The major objective of the Masters of Education (MEd) program in Educational Psychology is to offer students preparation in psychological theories and their application to teaching and learning in school and other educational settings, and research, measurement, and evaluation.

Special Facilities or Resources: Located in the heart of a highly diverse metropolitan area with almost 5 million inhabitants, the Department has access to a wealth of community research facilities and resources (e.g., 56 school districts, a range of community-based mental health and specialty clinics and agencies, a large VA Hospital, 20 hospitals within the Texas Medical Center). Within the College of Education, the Center for Information Technology in Education (CITE) Laboratory, with a full-time staff of ten, provides faculty, staff, and students with computing and multimedia environments, technology resources, and timely service-oriented user support. Several faculty have active funded and unfunded research teams that provide students with a range of research options, often in collaboration with major facilities (i.e., medical faciulities, schools, community/state organizations) in the Houston community.

Information for Students With Physical Disabilities: See the following Web site for more information: http://www.uh.edu/csd/.

Application Information:

Send to Kimberly Zainfeld, Dept. of Educational Psychology, University of Houston, 491 Farish Hall, Houston, TX 77204-5871. Application available online. URL of online application: http://www.uh.edu/admissions/graduate/how-apply/. Students are admitted in the Fall, application deadline December 1; Spring, application deadline August 15. Application deadline for Counseling Psychology PhD and School Psychology PhD is December 1. Deadline for PhD in Educational Psychology and Individual Differences is February 1. Counseling MEd deadlines are January 15 (fall) and August 15 (spring); Educational Psychology MEd is March 15 (fall) and October 15 (spring). *Fee:* $45.

Houston, University of
Department of Psychology
College of Liberal Arts and Social Sciences
126 Heyne Building
Houston, TX 77204-5022
Telephone: (713) 743-8508
Fax: (713) 743-8588
E-mail: ptolar@uh.edu
Web: http://www.psychology.uh.edu

Department Information:
1939. Chairperson: David J. Francis. Number of faculty: total—full-time 33, part-time 3; women—full-time 14; total—minority—full-time 6; women minority—full-time 4.

Programs and Degrees Offered:
Listed in the following order: Program area, degree type (T if terminal Master's), number awarded 7/08–6/09. Industrial/Organizational PhD (Doctor of Philosophy) 4, Social PhD (Doctor of Philosophy) 4, Clinical PhD (Doctor of Philosophy) 8, Developmental PhD (Doctor of Philosophy) 0.

APA Accreditation: Clinical PhD (Doctor of Philosophy). Student Outcome Data Website: http://www.psychology.uh.edu/GraduatePrograms/Clinical/about/index.html.

Student Applications/Admissions:
Student Applications
Industrial/Organizational PhD (Doctor of Philosophy)—Applications 2009–2010, 89. Total applicants accepted 2009–2010, 13. Number full-time enrolled (new admits only) 2009–2010, 7. Number part-time enrolled (new admits only) 2009–2010, 0. Openings 2010–2011, 6. The median number of years required for completion of a degree in 2008–2009 were 5. The number of students enrolled full- and part-time who were dismissed or voluntarily withdrew from this program area in 2008–2009 were 1. *Social PhD (Doctor of Philosophy)*—Applications 2009–2010, 37. Total applicants accepted 2009–2010, 9. Number full-time enrolled (new admits only) 2009–2010, 5. Number part-time enrolled (new admits only) 2009–2010, 0. Openings 2010–2011, 4. The median number of years required for completion of a degree in 2008–2009 were 6. The number of students enrolled full- and part-time who were dismissed or voluntarily withdrew from this program area in 2008–2009 were 0. *Clinical PhD (Doctor of Philosophy)*—Applications 2009–2010, 270. Total applicants accepted 2009–2010, 21. Number full-time enrolled (new admits only) 2009–2010, 14. Number part-time enrolled (new admits only) 2009–2010, 0. Openings 2010–2011, 12. The median number of years required for completion of a degree in 2008–2009 were 5. The number of students enrolled full- and part-time who were dismissed or voluntarily withdrew from this program area in 2008–2009 were 0. *Developmental PhD (Doctor of Philosophy)*—Applications 2009–2010, 28. Total applicants accepted 2009–2010, 7. Number full-time enrolled (new admits only) 2009–2010, 4. Total enrolled 2009–2010 full-time, 12. Openings 2010–2011, 4. The number of students enrolled full- and part-time who were dismissed or voluntarily withdrew from this program area in 2008–2009 were 0.

Scores: Entries appear in this order: required test or GPA, minimum score (if required), median score of students entering in 2009–2010. *Industrial/Organizational PhD (Doctor of Philosophy):* GRE-V no minimum stated, GRE-Q no minimum stated, GRE-Analytical no minimum stated, overall undergraduate GPA no minimum stated, psychology GPA no minimum stated; *Social PhD (Doctor of Philosophy):* GRE-V no minimum stated, GRE-Q no minimum stated, GRE-Analytical no minimum stated, overall undergraduate GPA no minimum stated, psychology GPA no minimum stated; *Clinical PhD (Doctor of Philosophy):* GRE-V no minimum stated, GRE-Q no minimum stated, GRE-Analytical no minimum stated, overall undergraduate GPA no minimum stated, psychology GPA no minimum stated; *Developmental PhD (Doctor of Philosophy):* GRE-V no minimum stated, GRE-Q no minimum stated, GRE-Analytical no minimum stated, overall undergraduate GPA no minimum stated, psychology GPA no minimum stated.

Other Criteria: (importance of criteria rated low, medium, or high): GRE scores—medium, research experience—high, work experience—medium, extracurricular activity—medium, clinically related public service—medium, GPA—medium, letters of recommendation—high, interview—high, statement of goals and objectives—high. The clinical program requires an interview. For additional information on admission requirements, go to http://www.psych.uh.edu/GraduatePrograms/ApplicationInformation/.

Student Characteristics: The following represents characteristics of students in 2009–2010 in all graduate psychology programs in the department: Female—full-time 111, part-time 0; Male—full-time 31, part-time 0; African American/Black—full-time 4, part-time 0; Hispanic/Latino(a)—full-time 10, part-time 0; Asian/Pacific Islander—full-time 15, part-time 0; American Indian/Alaska Native—full-time 0, part-time 0; Caucasian/White—full-time 113, part-time 0; Multi-ethnic—full-time 0, part-time 0; students subject to the Americans With Disabilities Act—full-time 1, part-time 0; Unknown ethnicity—full-time 0, part-time 0; International students who hold an F-1 or J-1 Visa—full-time 14, part-time 0.

Financial Information/Assistance:
  Tuition for Full-Time Study: *Doctoral:* State residents: per academic year $6,990, $233 per credit hour; Nonstate residents: per academic year $15,420, $514 per credit hour. Tuition is subject to change. See the following Web site for updates and changes in tuition costs: http://www.uh.edu/financial/graduate/tuition-fees/index.php.

  Financial Assistance:
  First-Year Students: Teaching assistantships available for first year. Average amount paid per academic year: $11,580. Average number of hours worked per week: 20. Research assistantships available for first year. Average amount paid per academic year: $14,400. Average number of hours worked per week: 20. Fellowships and scholarships available for first year. Average amount paid per academic year: $3,000.
  Advanced Students: Teaching assistantships available for advanced students. Average amount paid per academic year: $13,200. Average number of hours worked per week: 20. Research assistantships available for advanced students. Average amount paid per academic year: $16,800. Average number of hours worked per week: 20. Fellowships and scholarships available for advanced students. Average amount paid per academic year: $3,000.
  Additional Information: Of all students currently enrolled full time, 85% benefited from one or more of the listed financial assistance programs. Application and information available online at: http://www.uh.edu/financial/graduate/index.php.

Internships/Practica: Doctoral Degree (PhD Clinical): For those doctoral students for whom a professional internship was required in this program prior to graduation, (11) students applied for an internship in 2008–2009, with (10) students obtaining an internship. Of those students who obtained an internship, (10) were paid internships. Of those students who obtained an internship, (10) students placed in APA/CPA accredited internships, (0) students placed in internships not APA/CPA accredited, but listed with the Association of Psychology Postdoctoral and Internship Programs (APPIC), (0) students placed in internships conforming to guidelines of the Council of Directors of School Psychology Programs (CDSPP), (0) students placed in internships that were not APA/CPA accredited, APPIC or CDSPP listed. Internships are available for advanced students at a number of sites that include private industry, medical centers, state hospitals, and private practices.

Housing and Day Care: On-campus housing is available. See the following Web site for more information: http://www.housing.uh.edu. On-campus day care facilities are available. See the following Web site for more information: http://www.uh.edu/ccc/.

Employment of Department Graduates:
  Master's Degree Graduates: Of those who graduated in the academic year 2008–2009, the following categories and numbers represent the postgraduate activities and employment of master's degree graduates: Enrolled in a postdoctoral residency/fellowship (n/a), employed in independent practice (n/a), total from the above (master's) (0).
  Doctoral Degree Graduates: Of those who graduated in the academic year 2008–2009, the following categories and numbers represent the postgraduate activities and employment of doctoral degree graduates: Enrolled in a psychology doctoral program (n/a), total from the above (doctoral) (0).

Additional Information:
  Orientation, Objectives, and Emphasis of Department: Clinical offers APA-approved training in research, assessment, intervention, and consultation related to complex human problems, including behavioral problems having a neurological basis. Industrial/Organizational offers broad training in industrial/organizational psychology with options for specialization in either the personnel or organizational subfields. Social emphasizes research careers in behavioral and preventive medicine; interpersonal interaction processes, with an emphasis on close relationships and motivation; and social cognition. Developmental focuses on experimental research in developmental cognitive neuroscience, including perception, speech, language, reading, attention, decision-making, memory, and emotion, using imaging, electrophysiological, and neurochemical techniques in human and animal models.

  Special Facilities or Resources: The facilities of the department are comparable to those of any major department in a large university. A variety of community settings are available for applied research in all areas of specialization. Specialized laboratories have modern equipment for research in family and couple interaction, biofeedback, personnel interviewing, electrophysiology, and animal studies, as well as access to an fMRI scanner. Several research and clinical practica are available within the community and at several hospitals (the Texas Medical Center is one of the largest in the world). The department has over 150 computer work stations.

  Information for Students With Physical Disabilities: See the following Web site for more information: http://www.uh.edu/csd/.

Application Information:
Send to Academic Affairs Office, Department of Psychology, 126 Heyne Building, University of Houston, Houston, TX 77204-5022. Application available online. URL of online application: http://www.uh.edu/admissions/graduate/. Students are admitted in the Fall, application deadline December 15. Deadline for Clinical is December 15. Deadline for Developmental, I/O, and Social is January 15. *Fee:* $40. In cases of financial hardship, a waiver of the application fee may be requested by writing to: Dr. Roy Lachman, Director of Graduate

Education, University of Houston, Department of Psychology, 126 Heyne Building, Houston, TX 77204-5022.

Lamar University-Beaumont
Department of Psychology
Arts and Sciences
P.O. Box 10036
Beaumont, TX 77710
Telephone: (409) 880-8285
Fax: (409) 880-1779
E-mail: RANDOLPH.SMITH@lamar.edu
Web: http://dept.lamar.edu/psychology/

Department Information:
1964. Chairperson: Randolph A. Smith. Number of faculty: total—full-time 10, part-time 3; women—full-time 7, part-time 2; total—minority—full-time 1, part-time 1; women minority—full-time 1.

Programs and Degrees Offered:
Listed in the following order: Program area, degree type (T if terminal Master's), number awarded 7/08–6/09. Community-Clinical Psychology MA/MS (Master of Arts/Science) (T) 3, Industrial/Organizational Psychology MA/MS (Master of Arts/Science) (T) 1.

Student Applications/Admissions:
Student Applications
Community-Clinical Psychology MA/MS (Master of Arts/Science)—Applications 2009–2010, 12. Total applicants accepted 2009–2010, 6. Number full-time enrolled (new admits only) 2009–2010, 6. Number part-time enrolled (new admits only) 2009–2010, 0. Total enrolled 2009–2010 full-time, 14, part-time, 4. Openings 2010–2011, 6. The median number of years required for completion of a degree in 2008–2009 were 2. The number of students enrolled full- and part-time who were dismissed or voluntarily withdrew from this program area in 2008–2009 were 3. Industrial/Organizational Psychology MA/MS (Master of Arts/Science)—Applications 2009–2010, 6. Total applicants accepted 2009–2010, 3. Number full-time enrolled (new admits only) 2009–2010, 0. Number part-time enrolled (new admits only) 2009–2010, 0. Total enrolled 2009–2010 full-time, 6, part-time, 1. Openings 2010–2011, 6. The median number of years required for completion of a degree in 2008–2009 were 2. The number of students enrolled full- and part-time who were dismissed or voluntarily withdrew from this program area in 2008–2009 were 2.
Scores: Entries appear in this order: required test or GPA, minimum score (if required), median score of students entering in 2009–2010. Community-Clinical Psychology MA/MS (Master of Arts/Science): GRE-V 500, GRE-Q 500, overall undergraduate GPA 2.75, last 2 years GPA 3.00, psychology GPA 3.00; Industrial/Organizational Psychology MA/MS (Master of Arts/Science): GRE-V 500, GRE-Q 500, overall undergraduate GPA 2.75, last 2 years GPA 3.00, psychology GPA 3.00.
Other Criteria: (importance of criteria rated low, medium, or high): GRE scores—high, research experience—medium, work experience—low, extracurricular activity—low, clinically related public service—low, GPA—medium, letters of recommendation—low, statement of goals and objectives—low, undergraduate major in psychology—low, specific undergraduate psychology courses taken—high.

Student Characteristics: The following represents characteristics of students in 2009–2010 in all graduate psychology programs in the department: Female—full-time 9, part-time 2; Male—full-time 4, part-time 0; African American/Black—full-time 0, part-time 0; Hispanic/Latino(a)—full-time 0, part-time 0; Asian/Pacific Islander—full-time 0, part-time 0; American Indian/Alaska Native—full-time 0, part-time 0; Caucasian/White—full-time 0, part-time 0; Multi-ethnic—full-time 0, part-time 0; students subject to the Americans With Disabilities Act—full-time 0, part-time 0; Unknown ethnicity—full-time 0, part-time 0; International students who hold an F-1 or J-1 Visa—full-time 0, part-time 0.

Financial Information/Assistance:
Tuition for Full-Time Study: Master's: State residents: $200 per credit hour; Nonstate residents: $477 per credit hour. Tuition is subject to change. Additional fees are assessed to students beyond the costs of tuition for the following: health center, technology, library, student services. See the following Web site for updates and changes in tuition costs: http://www.lamar.edu.

Financial Assistance:
First-Year Students: Teaching assistantships available for first year. Average amount paid per academic year: $4,500. Average number of hours worked per week: 20. Fellowships and scholarships available for first year. Average amount paid per academic year: $1,000.
Advanced Students: Teaching assistantships available for advanced students. Average amount paid per academic year: $4,500. Average number of hours worked per week: 20. Fellowships and scholarships available for advanced students. Average amount paid per academic year: $1,000.
Additional Information: Of all students currently enrolled full time, 100% benefited from one or more of the listed financial assistance programs.

Internships/Practica: Master's Degree (MA/MS Community-Clinical Psychology): An internship experience, such as a final research project or "capstone" experience is required of graduates. Master's Degree (MA/MS Industrial/Organizational Psychology): An internship experience, such as a final research project or "capstone" experience is required of graduates. A variety of community health settings provide useful practicum experiences for Community-Clinical students in child, adolescent and adult counseling and assessment. There is also a clinic in the Psychology Department where students practice counseling under supervision. Practicum experiences for the Industrial/Organizational students place them in a variety of organizational and industrial work environments.

Housing and Day Care: On-campus housing is available. Lamar University, Office of Residence Life, Box 10041, Beaumont, TX 77710. No on-campus day care facilities are available.

Employment of Department Graduates:
Master's Degree Graduates: Of those who graduated in the academic year 2008–2009, the following categories and numbers represent the postgraduate activities and employment of master's

degree graduates: Enrolled in a psychology doctoral program (2), enrolled in a postdoctoral residency/fellowship (n/a), employed in independent practice (n/a), employed in other positions at a higher education institution (1), employed in a community mental health/counseling center (2), do not know (2), total from the above (master's) (7).

Doctoral Degree Graduates: Of those who graduated in the academic year 2008–2009, the following categories and numbers represent the postgraduate activities and employment of doctoral degree graduates: Enrolled in a psychology doctoral program (n/a), total from the above (doctoral) (0).

Additional Information:
Orientation, Objectives, and Emphasis of Department: The Department of Psychology offers a program of study leading to the Master of Science degree in applied psychology. It is designed to prepare professional personnel for employment in business, industry, or community mental health agencies. The MS in Community-Clinical Psychology includes training in assessment and therapy techniques for individuals, groups, and families. The MS in Industrial/Organizational Psychology integrates the traditional areas of industrial psychology with the more contemporary areas of organizational development and analysis. Both programs also prepare graduates for entry to doctoral programs.

Special Facilities or Resources: The Department currently maintains a psychological clinic that is used for training and research. It is available to both the student population as well as those in the surrounding community. The department also has a computer lab and research space.

Information for Students With Physical Disabilities: See the following Web site for more information: http://dept.lamar.edu/sfswd/.

Application Information:
Send to Graduate Admissions, Lamar University, Box 10078, Beaumont, TX 77710. Application available online. URL of online application: http://www.lamar.edu. Students are admitted in the Fall, application deadline March 15. *Fee:* $30.

Midwestern State University
Department of Psychology
Prothro-Yeager College of Humanities and Social Sciences
3410 Taft Boulevard
Wichita Falls, TX 76308
Telephone: (940) 397-4340
Fax: (940) 397-4682
E-mail: *david.carlston@mwsu.edu*
Web: *http://libarts.mwsu.edu/psychology/ma/*

Department Information:
1975. Psychology Graduate Coordinator: Dave Carlston. Number of faculty: total—full-time 7; women—full-time 2; total—minority—full-time 1; women minority—full-time 1.

Programs and Degrees Offered:
Listed in the following order: Program area, degree type (T if terminal Master's), number awarded 7/08–6/09. Clinical/Counseling Psychology MA/MS (Master of Arts/Science) (T) 7.

Student Applications/Admissions:
Student Applications
Clinical/Counseling Psychology MA/MS (Master of Arts/Science)—Applications 2009–2010, 15. Total applicants accepted 2009–2010, 7. Number full-time enrolled (new admits only) 2009–2010, 7. Number part-time enrolled (new admits only) 2009–2010, 0. Openings 2010–2011, 9. The median number of years required for completion of a degree in 2008–2009 were 2. The number of students enrolled full- and part-time who were dismissed or voluntarily withdrew from this program area in 2008–2009 were 0.

Scores: Entries appear in this order: required test or GPA, minimum score (if required), median score of students entering in 2009–2010. Clinical/Counseling Psychology MA/MS (Master of Arts/Science): GRE-V no minimum stated, GRE-Q no minimum stated, GRE-Analytical no minimum stated, overall undergraduate GPA no minimum stated, last 2 years GPA no minimum stated, psychology GPA no minimum stated.

Other Criteria: (importance of criteria rated low, medium, or high): GRE scores—high, research experience—medium, work experience—low, extracurricular activity—low, clinically related public service—low, GPA—high, letters of recommendation—medium, statement of goals and objectives—medium, undergraduate major in psychology—medium, specific undergraduate psychology courses taken—high. For additional information on admission requirements, go to http://libarts.mwsu.edu/psychology/ma/Prospective_Students_index.asp.

Student Characteristics: The following represents characteristics of students in 2009–2010 in all graduate psychology programs in the department: Female—full-time 14, part-time 0; Male—full-time 3, part-time 0; African American/Black—full-time 2, part-time 0; Hispanic/Latino(a)—full-time 1, part-time 0; Asian/Pacific Islander—full-time 0, part-time 0; American Indian/Alaska Native—full-time 0, part-time 0; Caucasian/White—full-time 14, part-time 0; Multi-ethnic—full-time 0, part-time 0; students subject to the Americans With Disabilities Act—full-time 0, part-time 0; Unknown ethnicity—full-time 0, part-time 0; International students who hold an F-1 or J-1 Visa—full-time 1, part-time 0.

Financial Information/Assistance:
Tuition for Full-Time Study: Master's: State residents: per academic year $5,892, $245 per credit hour; Nonstate residents: per academic year $6,612, $275 per credit hour. Tuition is subject to change. See the following Web site for updates and changes in tuition costs: http://admissions.mwsu.edu/fees.asp.

Financial Assistance:
First-Year Students: Research assistantships available for first year. Average amount paid per academic year: $3,750. Average number of hours worked per week: 5. Apply by July 1. Fellowships and scholarships available for first year. Average amount paid per academic year: $1,000. Average number of hours worked per week: 0. Apply by July 1.

Advanced Students: Teaching assistantships available for advanced students. Average amount paid per academic year: $3,750. Average number of hours worked per week: 5. Apply by July 1. Research assistantships available for advanced students. Average amount paid per academic year: $3,750. Average number of hours worked per week: 5. Apply by July 1. Fellowships and scholarships available for advanced students. Average amount paid per academic year: $1,000. Average number of hours worked per week: 0. Apply by July 1.

Additional Information: Of all students currently enrolled full time, 100% benefited from one or more of the listed financial assistance programs.

Internships/Practica: Master's Degree (MA/MS Clinical/Counseling Psychology): An internship experience, such as a final research project or "capstone" experience is required of graduates. Students completing the clinical/counseling program complete 9 credit hours of practicum for a total of 450 clock-hours of work and study in an applied clinical/counseling setting.

Housing and Day Care: On-campus housing is available. See the following Web site for more information: http://housing.mwsu.edu/. No on-campus day care facilities are available.

Employment of Department Graduates:
Master's Degree Graduates: Of those who graduated in the academic year 2008–2009, the following categories and numbers represent the postgraduate activities and employment of master's degree graduates: Enrolled in a psychology doctoral program (1), enrolled in a postdoctoral residency/fellowship (n/a), employed in independent practice (n/a), employed in a community mental health/counseling center (2), not seeking employment (1), do not know (2), total from the above (master's) (6).
Doctoral Degree Graduates: Of those who graduated in the academic year 2008–2009, the following categories and numbers represent the postgraduate activities and employment of doctoral degree graduates: Enrolled in a psychology doctoral program (n/a), total from the above (doctoral) (0).

Additional Information:
Orientation, Objectives, and Emphasis of Department: The clinical/counseling psychology graduate program is available in either a 50-hour or 60-hour curriculum option and is designed to lead to certification as a Licensed Professional Counselor (LPC) or Licensed Psychological Associate (LPA). Students may pursue thesis or non-thesis options. Although our emphasis is on training the master's level practitioner, we actively encourage our students to pursue doctoral training, and we see the training we provide as a first step toward that goal.

Special Facilities or Resources: Midwestern State University is located near two state hospitals, a regional community mental health and mental retardation center, and two private psychiatric hospitals. A newly remodeled clinic and computer lab are available for student use, and Graduate Research and Teaching Assistants are provided with office space. Financial assistance to Texas nonresidents includes waiver of the nonresident tuition differential.

Information for Students With Physical Disabilities: See the following Web site for more information: http://students.mwsu.edu/disability/.

Application Information:
Send to Dr. David Carlston, Graduate Coordinator Department of Psychology, Midwestern State University, 3410 Taft, Wichita Falls, TX 76308. Application available online. URL of online application: http://admissions.mwsu.edu/apply.asp. Students are admitted in the Fall, application deadline May 15; Spring, application deadline November 15. *Fee:* $35.

North Texas, University of (2009 data)
Department of Psychology
College of Arts and Sciences
P.O. Box 311280
Denton, TX 76203-1280
Telephone: (940) 565-2671
Fax: (940) 565-4682
E-mail: *amym@unt.edu*
Web: *http://www.psyc.unt.edu*

Department Information:
1968. Chairperson: Linda L. Marshall. Number of faculty: total—full-time 26, part-time 4; women—full-time 8, part-time 3; total—minority—full-time 2; faculty subject to the Americans With Disabilities Act 2.

Programs and Degrees Offered:
Listed in the following order: Program area, degree type (T if terminal Master's), number awarded 7/08–6/09. Clinical Psychology: Health & Behavioral Medicine PhD (Doctor of Philosophy) 5, Experimental Psychology PhD (Doctor of Philosophy) 0, Counseling Psychology PhD (Doctor of Philosophy) 7, Clinical Psychology PhD (Doctor of Philosophy) 3.

APA Accreditation: Clinical PhD (Doctor of Philosophy). Counseling PhD (Doctor of Philosophy). Clinical PhD (Doctor of Philosophy).

Student Applications/Admissions:
Student Applications
Clinical Psychology: Health & Behavioral Medicine PhD (Doctor of Philosophy)—Applications 2009–2010, 27. Total applicants accepted 2009–2010, 5. Number full-time enrolled (new admits only) 2009–2010, 5. Number part-time enrolled (new admits only) 2009–2010, 0. Openings 2010–2011, 8. The median number of years required for completion of a degree in 2008–2009 were 6. The number of students enrolled full- and part-time who were dismissed or voluntarily withdrew from this program area in 2008–2009 were 0. *Experimental Psychology PhD (Doctor of Philosophy)*—Applications 2009–2010, 20. Total applicants accepted 2009–2010, 3. Number full-time enrolled (new admits only) 2009–2010, 3. Number part-time enrolled (new admits only) 2009–2010, 0. Openings 2010–2011, 5. The median number of years required for completion of a degree in 2008–2009 were 6. The number of students enrolled full- and part-time who were dismissed or voluntarily withdrew from this program area in 2008–2009 were 0. *Counseling Psychology PhD (Doctor of Philosophy)*—Applications 2009–2010, 101. Total applicants accepted 2009–2010, 8. Number full-time enrolled (new admits only) 2009–2010, 8. Number part-time enrolled (new admits only) 2009–2010, 0. Openings 2010–2011, 8. The median number of years required for completion of a degree in 2008–2009 were 6. The number of students enrolled full- and part-time who were dismissed or voluntarily withdrew from this program area in 2008–2009 were 1. *Clinical Psychology PhD (Doctor of Philosophy)*—Applications 2009–2010, 70. Total applicants accepted 2009–2010,

8. Number full-time enrolled (new admits only) 2009–2010, 8. Number part-time enrolled (new admits only) 2009–2010, 0. Openings 2010–2011, 8. The median number of years required for completion of a degree in 2008–2009 were 6. The number of students enrolled full- and part-time who were dismissed or voluntarily withdrew from this program area in 2008–2009 were 0.

Other Criteria: (importance of criteria rated low, medium, or high): GRE scores—medium, research experience—high, work experience—medium, extracurricular activity—medium, clinically related public service—high, GPA—medium, letters of recommendation—medium, interview—medium, statement of goals and objectives—high, undergraduate major in psychology—medium, specific undergraduate psychology courses taken—high.

Student Characteristics: The following represents characteristics of students in 2009–2010 in all graduate psychology programs in the department: Female—full-time 139, part-time 24; Male—full-time 54, part-time 9; African American/Black—full-time 5, part-time 0; Hispanic/Latino(a)—full-time 1, part-time 0; Asian/Pacific Islander—full-time 3, part-time 0; American Indian/Alaska Native—full-time 1, part-time 0; Caucasian/White—full-time 0, part-time 0; Multi-ethnic—full-time 0, part-time 0; students subject to the Americans With Disabilities Act—full-time 4, part-time 0; Unknown ethnicity—full-time 0, part-time 0; International students who hold an F-1 or J-1 Visa—full-time 0, part-time 0.

Financial Information/Assistance:

Tuition for Full-Time Study: *Master's:* State residents: per academic year $6,622, $473 per credit hour; Nonstate residents: per academic year $13,294, $752 per credit hour. *Doctoral:* State residents: per academic year $6,622, $473 per credit hour; Nonstate residents: per academic year $13,294, $752 per credit hour. Tuition is subject to change. See the following Web site for updates and changes in tuition costs: http://essc.unt.edu/saucs/tuition.htm.

Financial Assistance:

First-Year Students: Teaching assistantships available for first year. Average amount paid per academic year: $6,500. Average number of hours worked per week: 20. Apply by April 15. Research assistantships available for first year. Average amount paid per academic year: $6,800. Average number of hours worked per week: 20. Traineeships available for first year. Average amount paid per academic year: $5,000. Average number of hours worked per week: 10. Fellowships and scholarships available for first year. Average amount paid per academic year: $1,000. Apply by April 15.

Advanced Students: Teaching assistantships available for advanced students. Average amount paid per academic year: $7,200. Average number of hours worked per week: 20. Apply by April 15. Research assistantships available for advanced students. Average amount paid per academic year: $6,800. Average number of hours worked per week: 20. Traineeships available for advanced students. Average amount paid per academic year: $12,000. Average number of hours worked per week: 20. Fellowships and scholarships available for advanced students. Average amount paid per academic year: $12,000. Apply by January 15.

Additional Information: Of all students currently enrolled full time, 73% benefited from one or more of the listed financial assistance programs.

Internships/Practica: Doctoral Degree (PhD Clinical Psychology: Health & Behavioral Medicine): For those doctoral students for whom a professional internship was required in this program prior to graduation, (6) students applied for an internship in 2008–2009, with (5) students obtaining an internship. Of those students who obtained an internship, (5) were paid internships. Of those students who obtained an internship, (3) students placed in APA/CPA accredited internships, (1) students placed in internships not APA/CPA accredited, but listed with the Association of Psychology Postdoctoral and Internship Programs (APPIC), (0) students placed in internships conforming to guidelines of the Council of Directors of School Psychology Programs (CDSPP), (1) students placed in internships that were not APA/CPA accredited, APPIC or CDSPP listed. Doctoral Degree (PhD Counseling Psychology): For those doctoral students for whom a professional internship was required in this program prior to graduation, (6) students applied for an internship in 2008–2009, with (6) students obtaining an internship. Of those students who obtained an internship, (6) were paid internships. Of those students who obtained an internship, (6) students placed in APA/CPA accredited internships, (0) students placed in internships not APA/CPA accredited, but listed with the Association of Psychology Postdoctoral and Internship Programs (APPIC), (0) students placed in internships conforming to guidelines of the Council of Directors of School Psychology Programs (CDSPP), (0) students placed in internships that were not APA/CPA accredited, APPIC or CDSPP listed. Doctoral Degree (PhD Clinical Psychology): For those doctoral students for whom a professional internship was required in this program prior to graduation, (9) students applied for an internship in 2008–2009, with (8) students obtaining an internship. Of those students who obtained an internship, (8) were paid internships. Of those students who obtained an internship, (8) students placed in APA/CPA accredited internships, (0) students placed in internships not APA/CPA accredited, but listed with the Association of Psychology Postdoctoral and Internship Programs (APPIC), (0) students placed in internships conforming to guidelines of the Council of Directors of School Psychology Programs (CDSPP), (0) students placed in internships that were not APA/CPA accredited, APPIC or CDSPP listed.

Housing and Day Care: On-campus housing is available. See the following Web site for more information: http://www.unt.edu/housing/. No on-campus day care facilities are available.

Employment of Department Graduates:

Master's Degree Graduates: Of those who graduated in the academic year 2008–2009, the following categories and numbers represent the postgraduate activities and employment of master's degree graduates: Enrolled in a psychology doctoral program (4), enrolled in a postdoctoral residency/fellowship (n/a), employed in independent practice (n/a), employed in a community mental health/counseling center (1), total from the above (master's) (5).

Doctoral Degree Graduates: Of those who graduated in the academic year 2008–2009, the following categories and numbers represent the postgraduate activities and employment of doctoral degree graduates: Enrolled in a psychology doctoral program (n/a), enrolled in a postdoctoral residency/fellowship (5), employed in independent practice (1), employed in an academic position at a university (2), employed in other positions at a higher education institution (2), employed in business or industry (1), employed in government agency (1), employed in a community mental health/counseling center (2), employed in a hospital/medical center (6), other employment position (1), total from the above (doctoral) (21).

Additional Information:
Orientation, Objectives, and Emphasis of Department: Our department adopts the scientist–practitioner model, fostering an appreciation of psychology as a science and as a profession. We embrace a multiplicity of theoretical viewpoints and research interests. Students are involved in graded research and/or clinical practicum experiences by integrating experiential with didactic instruction. Experimental psychology provides a highly individualized program for the student interested in study and research in one of several specialized areas. Clinical and Counseling Psychology programs support the development of a well-rounded professional psychologist. These purposes include a thorough grounding in scientific methodology and an orientation to the profession, development of competency in psychological assessment and evaluation, and training in various psychotherapeutic and counseling techniques and skills. Clinical Psychology: Health & Behavioral Medicine involves a joint program with UNT Health Science Center which emphasizes mind/body interaction as students focus on the matrix of biopsychosocial and environmental processes in understanding etiological and diagnostic factors of illness, prevention, and recovery in order to meet the holistic needs of the individual.

Special Facilities or Resources: The Psychology Clinic at the University of North Texas was founded in 1972 with the purpose of providing professional training, scientific research and community service. Professional competent training in clinical services and research is offered to graduate students in the APA-accredited Clinical, Counseling and Clinical Health/Behavior Medicine Psychology PhD programs in the Department of Psychology. The Clinic staff is comprised of teams of licensed psychologists and doctoral-level psychology students who provide therapy and psychological testing to adults, adolescents, children, couples and families. All clients receive the benefits of a licensed psychologist's supervisory expertise and oversight. As a non-profit training clinic, we can provide clients with professional, confidential psychological services based on a reduced - cost sliding scale. We provide services to a wide range of people, with problems ranging from everyday stress and relationship issues to more serious problems like depression, anxiety, bipolar disorder, ADHD, and chronic medical conditions. The research and service activities of the Clinic involve members of the entire Psychology Department and are directed toward prevention, evaluation, and intervention. The center for sport psychology and performance excellence (CSPPE) provides interdisciplinary training for students in psychology and kinesiology who are interested in specializing in sport psychology. Through the Center, students work with Psychology and KHPR faculty in coursework, research, and applied experiences. The Center for Psychosocial Health Research is an interdisciplinary center that conducts research on wellness in a chronic illness context. Our research focuses on exploring stigma and forgiveness as a stressor and coping strategy for people living with HIV/AIDS and for the LGBT community. The Sleep and Health Research Lab focuses on the epidemiology of sleep and health and explores the role insomnia plays as a risk factor for psychological and medical disorders in various populations. At the University of North Texas Health Science Center, practicum and research experiences are available through Departments of Pediatrics, Family Medicine, Internal Medicine, Gerontology, and Rehabilitation Medicine. Labs: Brain-mapping Facility, Applied Psychophysiology & Biofeedback Lab, Neurofeedback Lab, Psychoneuroimmunology Lab, Computer/Statistics Lab, Neuropsychology Lab.

Information for Students With Physical Disabilities: See the following Web site for more information: http://www.unt.edu/oda/.

Application Information:
Send to Psychology Department, Graduate Admissions, University of North Texas, BOX 311280, Denton, TX 76203-1280. Application available online. URL of online application: http://www.psyc.unt.edu. Students are admitted in the Fall, application deadline December 1.

Our Lady of the Lake University
Psychology
School of Professional Studies
411 Southwest 24th Street
San Antonio, TX 78207
Telephone: (210) 431-3914
Fax: (210) 431-3927
E-mail: *jbiever@ollusa.edu*
Web: *http://www.ollusa.edu*

Department Information:
1983. Chairperson: Joan Biever, PhD. Number of faculty: total—full-time 12, part-time 12; women—full-time 9, part-time 9; total—minority—full-time 4, part-time 6; women minority—full-time 2, part-time 5.

Programs and Degrees Offered:
Listed in the following order: Program area, degree type (T if terminal Master's), number awarded 7/08–6/09. Counseling Psychology PsyD (Doctor of Psychology) 4, School Psychology MA/MS (Master of Arts/Science) (T) 10, Marriage and Family Therapy MA/MS (Master of Arts/Science) (T) 11, Counseling Psychology MA/MS (Master of Arts/Science) (T) 10.

APA Accreditation: Counseling PsyD (Doctor of Psychology). Student Outcome Data Website: http://www.ollusa.edu/s/1190/ollu.aspx?sid=1190&gid=1&pgid=2319.

Student Applications/Admissions:
Student Applications
Counseling Psychology PsyD (Doctor of Psychology)—Applications 2009–2010, 25. Total applicants accepted 2009–2010, 12. Number full-time enrolled (new admits only) 2009–2010, 4. Number part-time enrolled (new admits only) 2009–2010, 4. Total enrolled 2009–2010 full-time, 22, part-time, 26. Openings 2010–2011, 8. The median number of years required for completion of a degree in 2008–2009 were 6. The number of students enrolled full- and part-time who were dismissed or voluntarily withdrew from this program area in 2008–2009 were 2. School Psychology MA/MS (Master of Arts/Science)—Applications 2009–2010, 30. Total applicants accepted 2009–2010, 18. Number full-time enrolled (new admits only) 2009–

2010, 7. Number part-time enrolled (new admits only) 2009–2010, 1. Total enrolled 2009–2010 full-time, 17, part-time, 15. Openings 2010–2011, 10. The median number of years required for completion of a degree in 2008–2009 were 2. The number of students enrolled full- and part-time who were dismissed or voluntarily withdrew from this program area in 2008–2009 were 0. *Marriage and Family Therapy MA/MS (Master of Arts/Science)*—Applications 2009–2010, 30. Total applicants accepted 2009–2010, 28. Number full-time enrolled (new admits only) 2009–2010, 10. Number part-time enrolled (new admits only) 2009–2010, 5. Total enrolled 2009–2010 full-time, 42, part-time, 26. Openings 2010–2011, 10. The median number of years required for completion of a degree in 2008–2009 were 2. The number of students enrolled full- and part-time who were dismissed or voluntarily withdrew from this program area in 2008–2009 were 2. *Counseling Psychology MA/MS (Master of Arts/Science)*—Applications 2009–2010, 42. Total applicants accepted 2009–2010, 31. Number full-time enrolled (new admits only) 2009–2010, 7. Number part-time enrolled (new admits only) 2009–2010, 3. Total enrolled 2009–2010 full-time, 34, part-time, 19. Openings 2010–2011, 10. The median number of years required for completion of a degree in 2008–2009 were 2. The number of students enrolled full- and part-time who were dismissed or voluntarily withdrew from this program area in 2008–2009 were 2.

Scores: Entries appear in this order: required test or GPA, minimum score (if required), median score of students entering in 2009–2010. *Counseling Psychology PsyD (Doctor of Psychology):* GRE-V no minimum stated, GRE-Q no minimum stated, GRE-Analytical no minimum stated, GRE-Subject (Psychology) 520, Masters GPA 3.5; *Counseling Psychology MA/MS (Master of Arts/Science):* GRE-V no minimum stated, GRE-Q no minimum stated, overall undergraduate GPA 2.5, last 2 years GPA 3.0.

Other Criteria: (importance of criteria rated low, medium, or high): GRE scores—medium, research experience—low, work experience—high, extracurricular activity—low, clinically related public service—medium, GPA—high, letters of recommendation—high, interview—high, statement of goals and objectives—high.

Student Characteristics: The following represents characteristics of students in 2009–2010 in all graduate psychology programs in the department: Female—full-time 100, part-time 70; Male—full-time 15, part-time 16; African American/Black—full-time 9, part-time 12; Hispanic/Latino(a)—full-time 58, part-time 40; Asian/Pacific Islander—full-time 2, part-time 1; American Indian/Alaska Native—full-time 0, part-time 1; Caucasian/White—full-time 35, part-time 23; Multi-ethnic—full-time 4, part-time 1; students subject to the Americans With Disabilities Act—full-time 0, part-time 0; Unknown ethnicity—full-time 7, part-time 8; International students who hold an F-1 or J-1 Visa—full-time 4, part-time 1.

Financial Information/Assistance:
Tuition for Full-Time Study: *Master's:* State residents: $685 per credit hour; Nonstate residents: $685 per credit hour. *Doctoral:* State residents: $795 per credit hour; Nonstate residents: $795 per credit hour. Tuition is subject to change. See the following Web site for updates and changes in tuition costs: http://www.ollusa.edu/s/346/ollu.aspx?sid=346&gid=1&pgid=909.

Financial Assistance:
First-Year Students: Teaching assistantships available for first year. Average amount paid per academic year: $7,980. Average number of hours worked per week: 12. Research assistantships available for first year. Average amount paid per academic year: $7,980. Average number of hours worked per week: 12. Fellowships and scholarships available for first year. Average amount paid per academic year: $11,000. Average number of hours worked per week: 0.

Advanced Students: Teaching assistantships available for advanced students. Average amount paid per academic year: $7,980. Average number of hours worked per week: 12. Research assistantships available for advanced students. Average amount paid per academic year: $7,980. Average number of hours worked per week: 12. Fellowships and scholarships available for advanced students. Average amount paid per academic year: $11,000.

Additional Information: Of all students currently enrolled full time, 20% benefited from one or more of the listed financial assistance programs.

Internships/Practica: Doctoral Degree (PsyD Counseling Psychology): For those doctoral students for whom a professional internship was required in this program prior to graduation, (5) students applied for an internship in 2008–2009, with (4) students obtaining an internship. Of those students who obtained an internship, (4) were paid internships. Of those students who obtained an internship, (4) students placed in APA/CPA accredited internships, (0) students placed in internships not APA/CPA accredited, but listed with the Association of Psychology Postdoctoral and Internship Programs (APPIC), (0) students placed in internships conforming to guidelines of the Council of Directors of School Psychology Programs (CDSPP), (0) students placed in internships that were not APA/CPA accredited, APPIC or CDSPP listed. The psychology department operates a training clinic, the Community Counseling Service (CCS), which serves as the initial practicum site for all master's and doctoral students. At the CCS, practicum students work in teams of up to six students under the live supervision of psychology faculty. The CCS is located in and serves a low-income, predominantly Mexican-American community. Supervision of Spanish-language psychotherapy is available. A variety of off-campus sites are available to students in their second and subsequent semesters of practica. Students are placed at off-campus sites according to their career interests and training needs. Available practicum sites include public and private schools, hospitals, and community agencies.

Housing and Day Care: On-campus housing is available. See the following Web site for more information: http://www.ollusa.edu/housing. No on-campus day care facilities are available.

Employment of Department Graduates:
Master's Degree Graduates: Of those who graduated in the academic year 2008–2009, the following categories and numbers represent the postgraduate activities and employment of master's degree graduates: Enrolled in a postdoctoral residency/fellowship (n/a), employed in independent practice (n/a), total from the above (master's) (0).

Doctoral Degree Graduates: Of those who graduated in the academic year 2008–2009, the following categories and numbers represent the postgraduate activities and employment of doctoral degree graduates: Enrolled in a psychology doctoral program (n/a), enrolled in a postdoctoral residency/fellowship (2), employed in independent practice (20), employed in a professional position in a school system (2), employed in a community mental health/counseling center (2), employed in a hospital/medical center (5), total from the above (doctoral) (31).

Additional Information:
Orientation, Objectives, and Emphasis of Department: Graduate psychology programs at OLLU adhere to the practitioner-scholar model of training and emphasize brief, systemic approaches to psychotherapy. Postmodern and multicultural perspectives are infused throughout the curriculum, including practica. A certificate in psychological services for Spanish-speaking populations is available.

Special Facilities or Resources: The department's training clinic serves as both a training and research facility. Research facilities are also available in the building which houses the psychology department.

Information for Students With Physical Disabilities: See the following Web site for more information: http://www.ollusa.edu/s/1190/ollu.aspx?sid=1190&gid=1&pgid=4619.

Application Information:
Send to Graduate Admissions Office, Our Lady of the Lake University, 411 SW 24th Street, San Antonio, TX 78207. Application available online. URL of online application: http://admissions.ollusa.edu/s/1190/ollu.aspx?sid=1190&gid=1&pgid=257. Students are admitted in the Fall, application deadline January 15. January 15 for PsyD program; March 1 for MS programs. Fee: $25.

Rice University
Department of Psychology
6100 Main Street - MS 25
Houston, TX 77005-1892
Telephone: (713) 348-4856
Fax: (713) 348-5221
E-mail: psyc@rice.edu
Web: http://www.psychology.rice.edu/

Department Information:
1966. Chairperson: Jim Dannemiller. Number of faculty: total—full-time 18; women—full-time 8.

Programs and Degrees Offered:
Listed in the following order: Program area, degree type (T if terminal Master's), number awarded 7/08–6/09. Industrial/Organizational Psychology PhD (Doctor of Philosophy) 3, Cognitive Psychology PhD (Doctor of Philosophy) 1, Human-Computer Interaction/Human Factors PhD (Doctor of Philosophy) 2, Training PhD (Doctor of Philosophy) 1, Cognitive Neuroscience PhD (Doctor of Philosophy) 1.

Student Applications/Admissions:
Student Applications
Industrial/Organizational Psychology PhD (Doctor of Philosophy)—Applications 2009–2010, 70. Total applicants accepted 2009–2010, 3. Number full-time enrolled (new admits only) 2009–2010, 3. Total enrolled 2009–2010 full-time, 12. Openings 2010–2011, 4. The median number of years required for completion of a degree in 2008–2009 were 4. The number of students enrolled full- and part-time who were dismissed or voluntarily withdrew from this program area in 2008–2009 were 1. *Cognitive Psychology PhD (Doctor of Philosophy)*—Applications 2009–2010, 16. Total applicants accepted 2009–2010, 4. Number full-time enrolled (new admits only) 2009–2010, 0. Number part-time enrolled (new admits only) 2009–2010, 0. Openings 2010–2011, 4. The median number of years required for completion of a degree in 2008–2009 were 5. The number of students enrolled full- and part-time who were dismissed or voluntarily withdrew from this program area in 2008–2009 were 0. *Human-Computer Interaction/Human Factors PhD (Doctor of Philosophy)*—Applications 2009–2010, 14. Total applicants accepted 2009–2010, 1. Number full-time enrolled (new admits only) 2009–2010, 4. Number part-time enrolled (new admits only) 2009–2010, 0. Openings 2010–2011, 3. The median number of years required for completion of a degree in 2008–2009 were 5. The number of students enrolled full- and part-time who were dismissed or voluntarily withdrew from this program area in 2008–2009 were 0. *Training PhD (Doctor of Philosophy)*—Applications 2009–2010, 34. Total applicants accepted 2009–2010, 4. Number full-time enrolled (new admits only) 2009–2010, 0. Number part-time enrolled (new admits only) 2009–2010, 0. Openings 2010–2011, 4. The median number of years required for completion of a degree in 2008–2009 were 5. The number of students enrolled full- and part-time who were dismissed or voluntarily withdrew from this program area in 2008–2009 were 0. *Cognitive Neuroscience PhD (Doctor of Philosophy)*—Applications 2009–2010, 20. Total applicants accepted 2009–2010, 3. Number full-time enrolled (new admits only) 2009–2010, 0. Total enrolled 2009–2010 full-time, 7. Openings 2010–2011, 3. The median number of years required for completion of a degree in 2008–2009 were 5.

Scores: Entries appear in this order: required test or GPA, minimum score (if required), median score of students entering in 2009–2010. *Industrial/Organizational Psychology PhD (Doctor of Philosophy)*: GRE-V no minimum stated, 620, GRE-Q no minimum stated, 700, overall undergraduate GPA no minimum stated, 3.8, last 2 years GPA no minimum stated, 3.8, psychology GPA no minimum stated, 3.8; *Training PhD (Doctor of Philosophy)*: GRE-V no minimum stated, 600, GRE-Q no minimum stated, 620, overall undergraduate GPA no minimum stated, 3.8, last 2 years GPA no minimum stated, 3.8.

Other Criteria: (importance of criteria rated low, medium, or high): GRE scores—high, research experience—high, work experience—low, extracurricular activity—low, GPA—high, letters of recommendation—high, statement of goals and objectives—high, undergraduate major in psychology—medium, specific undergraduate psychology courses taken—medium. For additional information on admission requirements, go to http://psychology.rice.edu/Content.aspx?id=173.

Student Characteristics: The following represents characteristics of students in 2009–2010 in all graduate psychology programs in the department: Female—full-time 26, part-time 0; Male—full-time 12, part-time 0; African American/Black—full-time 4, part-time 0; Hispanic/Latino(a)—full-time 4, part-time 0; Asian/Pacific Islander—full-time 1, part-time 0; American Indian/Alaska Native—full-time 0, part-time 0; Caucasian/White—full-time 28,

part-time 0; Multi-ethnic—full-time 1, part-time 0; students subject to the Americans With Disabilities Act—full-time 0, part-time 0; Unknown ethnicity—full-time 0, part-time 0; International students who hold an F-1 or J-1 Visa—full-time 0, part-time 0.

Financial Information/Assistance:
Tuition for Full-Time Study: *Master's:* State residents: per academic year $31,430; Nonstate residents: per academic year $31,430. *Doctoral:* State residents: per academic year $31,430; Nonstate residents: per academic year $31,430. Tuition is subject to change. See the following Web site for updates and changes in tuition costs: http://www.students.rice.edu/students/Tuition_Fees.asp.

Financial Assistance:
First-Year Students: Research assistantships available for first year. Average amount paid per academic year: $19,500. Average number of hours worked per week: 18. Fellowships and scholarships available for first year. Average amount paid per academic year: $18,500. Average number of hours worked per week: 0. Apply by January 15.

Advanced Students: Research assistantships available for advanced students. Average amount paid per academic year: $19,500. Average number of hours worked per week: 18. Apply by January 15. Fellowships and scholarships available for advanced students. Average amount paid per academic year: $18,500. Average number of hours worked per week: 0. Apply by January 15.

Additional Information: Of all students currently enrolled full time, 100% benefited from one or more of the listed financial assistance programs. Application and information available online at: http://psychology.rice.edu/Content.aspx?id=173.

Internships/Practica: Graduate students beyond their third year have the opportunity to work in internships in the Houston area. Although not required, many of our students work part-time in local organizations including NASA, the Texas Medical Center, Hewlett Packard, and a variety of consulting firms. Other students work in summer internships around the country.

Housing and Day Care: On-campus housing is available. See the following Web site for more information: http://campushousing.rice.edu/graduate. No on-campus day care facilities are available.

Employment of Department Graduates:
Master's Degree Graduates: Of those who graduated in the academic year 2008–2009, the following categories and numbers represent the postgraduate activities and employment of master's degree graduates: Enrolled in a psychology doctoral program (0), enrolled in another graduate/professional program (0), enrolled in a postdoctoral residency/fellowship (n/a), employed in independent practice (n/a), total from the above (master's) (0).
Doctoral Degree Graduates: Of those who graduated in the academic year 2008–2009, the following categories and numbers represent the postgraduate activities and employment of doctoral degree graduates: Enrolled in a psychology doctoral program (n/a), enrolled in another graduate/professional program (0), enrolled in a postdoctoral residency/fellowship (0), employed in independent practice (0), employed in an academic position at a university (4), employed in an academic position at a 2-year/4-year college (0), employed in other positions at a higher education institution (0), employed in a professional position in a school system (0), employed in business or industry (2), employed in government agency (0), employed in a community mental health/counseling center (0), employed in a hospital/medical center (0), still seeking employment (0), not seeking employment (0), other employment position (0), do not know (0), total from the above (doctoral) (6).

Additional Information:
Orientation, Objectives, and Emphasis of Department: The Rice program emphasizes training in basic and applied research and in the skills necessary to conduct research. The content areas to which this emphasis is applied are cognitive psychology (including cognitive neuroscience), industrial/organizational, and human-computer interaction. We believe that training in research and research skills generalizes very broadly to the kinds of tasks that professional psychologists will be asked to perform both in the university laboratory and in addressing such diverse applied questions as organizational management, system design, or program evaluation. Students in the cognitive neuroscience program are encouraged to participate in courses and research opportunities available from our joint program in Neuroscience with Baylor College of Medicine. Students in the other areas are encouraged to develop research interests that combine content areas across the department. Industrial/organizational and human factors psychologists, for example, might collaborate on research dealing with organizational communication via electronic mail. Cognitive and industrial/organizational psychologists might, for instance, investigate cognitive processes underlying performance appraisal; and human factors and cognitive psychologists might collaborate on studies of risk perception and the perceptual and attentional properties of computer displays. Although some of our students prefer to devote their energies to laboratory research in preparation for academic positions in basic areas, many students take advantage of the opportunities we provide for "real world" experience. The department arranges internships or practica in a wide variety of settings for interested advanced students.

Special Facilities or Resources: Graduate students in the Rice Psychology programs benefit from their access to a large and vital Houston business community, NASA, and over 40 teaching and research centers in the Texas Medical Center. Within the department, graduate students in all programs have ready access to a variety of powerful Macintosh and Windows-based computers that more than meet the needs of students for data collection, simulation, instruction, word processing, and computation. The department contains facilities for the study of dyadic and small group interaction, social judgment, decision making, and computer-interface design. In addition to the facilities physically located in the Psychology Department, Rice University has a state-of-the-art computer laboratory for research in the social sciences that has been constructed with support from the National Science Foundation. The cognitive neuroscience area has benefitted from the recent acquisition of a transcranial magnetic stimulation (TMS) device for investigating brain function, two eye tracking devices, a Silicon Graphics workstation for neuroimaging data analysis and 3D rendering of brains from MRI scans, and a dense-sensor array (128 channel) event-related potential (ERP) recording system that allows the detailed description of neural systems. Collaborations with institutions in the nearby Texas Medical Center provide access to functional neuroimaging facilities, which include the new Houston Neuroimaging Laboratory at Baylor College of Medicine that has two 3T research-dedicated scanners.

Information for Students With Physical Disabilities: See the following Web site for more information: http://dss.rice.edu/.

Application Information:
Send to Graduate Chair, Psychology Department, Rice University - MS 25, 6100 Main Street, Houston, TX 77005. Application available online. URL of online application: https://www.applyweb.com/apply/ricegrad/index.html. Students are admitted in the Fall, application deadline January 15. *Fee:* $70. Conditions for waiver of fee: Hardship.

Sam Houston State University (2009 data)
Department of Psychology
Humanities and Social Sciences
Box 2447
Huntsville, TX 77341-2447
Telephone: (936) 294-1174
Fax: (936) 294-3798
E-mail: *psychology@shsu.edu*
Web: *http://www.shsu.edu/~psy_www/*

Department Information:
1970. Chairperson: Christopher Wilson. Number of faculty: total—full-time 18, part-time 4; women—full-time 5, part-time 1; total—minority—full-time 2; faculty subject to the Americans With Disabilities Act 1.

Programs and Degrees Offered:
Listed in the following order: Program area, degree type (T if terminal Master's), number awarded 7/08–6/09. Clinical MA/MS (Master of Arts/Science) (T) 13, General MA/MS (Master of Arts/Science) (T) 4, School MA/MS (Master of Arts/Science) (T) 6, Clinical (Forensic Emphasis) PhD (Doctor of Philosophy) 8.

APA Accreditation: Clinical PhD (Doctor of Philosophy).

Student Applications/Admissions:
Student Applications
Clinical MA/MS *(Master of Arts/Science)*—Applications 2009–2010, 47. Total applicants accepted 2009–2010, 20. Number full-time enrolled (new admits only) 2009–2010, 15. Number part-time enrolled (new admits only) 2009–2010, 0. Openings 2010–2011, 20. The median number of years required for completion of a degree in 2008–2009 were 2. The number of students enrolled full- and part-time who were dismissed or voluntarily withdrew from this program area in 2008–2009 were 0. General MA/MS *(Master of Arts/Science)*—Applications 2009–2010, 15. Total applicants accepted 2009–2010, 5. Number full-time enrolled (new admits only) 2009–2010, 3. Number part-time enrolled (new admits only) 2009–2010, 1. Total enrolled 2009–2010 full-time, 11, part-time, 1. Openings 2010–2011, 10. The median number of years required for completion of a degree in 2008–2009 were 2. The number of students enrolled full- and part-time who were dismissed or voluntarily withdrew from this program area in 2008–2009 were 0. School MA/MS *(Master of Arts/Science)*—Applications 2009–2010, 21. Total applicants accepted 2009–2010, 11. Number full-time enrolled (new admits only) 2009–2010, 9. Number part-time enrolled (new admits only) 2009–2010, 0. Openings 2010–2011, 15. The median number of years required for completion of a degree in 2008–2009 were 3. The number of students enrolled full- and part-time who were dismissed or voluntarily withdrew from this program area in 2008–2009 were 0. Clinical (Forensic Emphasis) PhD *(Doctor of Philosophy)*—Applications 2009–2010, 89. Total applicants accepted 2009–2010, 8. Number full-time enrolled (new admits only) 2009–2010, 8. Number part-time enrolled (new admits only) 2009–2010, 0. Openings 2010–2011, 8. The median number of years required for completion of a degree in 2008–2009 were 7. The number of students enrolled full- and part-time who were dismissed or voluntarily withdrew from this program area in 2008–2009 were 1.

Other Criteria: (importance of criteria rated low, medium, or high): GRE scores—high, research experience—high, work experience—low, extracurricular activity—low, clinically related public service—medium, GPA—high, letters of recommendation—high, interview—high, statement of goals and objectives—high, fit with the program—high, specific undergraduate psychology courses taken—medium. No interview is required for admission to our Master's program. For additional information on admission requirements, go to http://www.shsu.edu/~psy_www.

Student Characteristics: The following represents characteristics of students in 2009–2010 in all graduate psychology programs in the department: Female—full-time 75, part-time 2; Male—full-time 14, part-time 1; African American/Black—full-time 3, part-time 0; Hispanic/Latino(a)—full-time 6, part-time 0; Asian/Pacific Islander—full-time 1, part-time 0; American Indian/Alaska Native—full-time 1, part-time 0; Caucasian/White—full-time 0, part-time 0; Multi-ethnic—full-time 0, part-time 0; students subject to the Americans With Disabilities Act—full-time 0, part-time 0; Unknown ethnicity—full-time 0, part-time 0; International students who hold an F-1 or J-1 Visa—full-time 0, part-time 0.

Financial Information/Assistance:
Tuition for Full-Time Study: *Master's:* State residents: per academic year $4,920, $205 per credit hour; Nonstate residents: per academic year $11,568, $482 per credit hour. *Doctoral:* State residents: per academic year $4,920, $205 per credit hour. Tuition is subject to change. Additional fees are assessed to students beyond the costs of tuition for the following: student service, student center, computer use, library, rec sports, advisement, and records. See the following Web site for updates and changes in tuition costs: http://www.shsu.edu/schedule/.

Financial Assistance:
First-Year Students: Teaching assistantships available for first year. Average amount paid per academic year: $10,000. Average number of hours worked per week: 20. Research assistantships available for first year. Average amount paid per academic year: $10,000. Average number of hours worked per week: 20. Fellowships and scholarships available for first year. Average amount paid per academic year: $10,000.

Advanced Students: Teaching assistantships available for advanced students. Average amount paid per academic year: $10,000. Average number of hours worked per week: 20. Research assistantships available for advanced students. Average amount paid per academic year: $10,000. Average number of hours worked per week: 20. Traineeships available for advanced students. Average amount paid per academic year: $10,000. Average number of hours worked per week: 20. Fellowships and scholarships available for advanced students. Average amount paid per academic year: $10,000.

Additional Information: Of all students currently enrolled full time, 100% benefited from one or more of the listed financial assistance programs. Application and information available online at: http://www.shsu.edu/~fao_www.

Internships/Practica: Doctoral Degree (PhD Clinical (Forensic Emphasis)): For those doctoral students for whom a professional internship was required in this program prior to graduation, (5) students applied for an internship in 2008–2009, with (5) students obtaining an internship. Of those students who obtained an internship, (5) were paid internships. Of those students who obtained an internship, (5) students placed in APA/CPA accredited internships, (0) students placed in internships not APA/CPA accredited, but listed with the Association of Psychology Postdoctoral and Internship Programs (APPIC), (0) students placed in internships conforming to guidelines of the Council of Directors of School Psychology Programs (CDSPP), (0) students placed in internships that were not APA/CPA accredited, APPIC or CDSPP listed. Master's Degree (MA/MS School): An internship experience, such as a final research project or "capstone" experience is required of graduates. We offer a variety of internships and practica for each of the applied tracks. Students in the School psychology program complete a one-year internship in schools. There are a variety of practicum placements for students in the Clinical psychology master's program, including the University Counseling Center, area community mental health centers, and the psychological services centers of the Texas Department of Criminal Justice (TDCJ). Students in the clinical doctoral program are assigned to a variety of practica, including Ben Taub General Hospital in Houston, ADAPT Counseling, various private facilities and practices, probation departments, and the Institute for Rehabilitation and Research (neuropsychology). These students also work at our on-campus Psychological Services Center, which provides both general mental health services (e.g., individual psychotherapy, couples counseling, psychological assessment), and forensic services (e.g., treatment programs for offender populations and evaluations for the courts).

Housing and Day Care: On-campus housing is available. See the following Web site for more information: http://www.shsu.edu/~hou_www/. No on-campus day care facilities are available.

Employment of Department Graduates:
Master's Degree Graduates: Of those who graduated in the academic year 2008–2009, the following categories and numbers represent the postgraduate activities and employment of master's degree graduates: Enrolled in a postdoctoral residency/fellowship (n/a), employed in independent practice (n/a), total from the above (master's) (0).
Doctoral Degree Graduates: Of those who graduated in the academic year 2008–2009, the following categories and numbers represent the postgraduate activities and employment of doctoral degree graduates: Enrolled in a psychology doctoral program (n/a), enrolled in a postdoctoral residency/fellowship (0), employed in independent practice (0), employed in an academic position at a university (1), employed in an academic position at a 2-year/4-year college (1), employed in other positions at a higher education institution (0), employed in a professional position in a school system (0), employed in business or industry (0), employed in government agency (2), employed in a community mental health/counseling center (1), employed in a hospital/medical center (3), still seeking employment (0), not seeking employment (0), other employment position (0), do not know (0), total from the above (doctoral) (8).

Additional Information:
Orientation, Objectives, and Emphasis of Department: The Clinical and School Master's programs are applied training programs that develop effective Master's-level practitioners. Students in these programs receive extensive and eclectic training in both psychotherapy and psychometrics and conclude their training with extensive supervised practicum experience. Graduates can seek licensure as psychological associates through Texas State Board of Examiners of Psychologists. Graduates of the School program can seek national certification from National Association of School Psychologists and licensure as specialists in school psychology in Texas. Other licensures within the state of Texas such as professional counselor licensure may be available with additional course work. The General track involves broader exposure to psychology's core disciplines and allows the student more elective flexibility to craft an individual specialty. The focus within the General Program is on developing research skills. Graduates of all three programs often progress to doctoral training here or elsewhere. Our clinical doctoral program is a scientist–practitioner program that provides broad and general training in clinical psychology with an emphasis on forensic psychology and the training of legally informed clinicians. In addition to extensive training in general psychological assessment and treatment, students participate in conducting a variety of forensic evaluations for the courts (e.g., risk assessment, competence, and sanity evaluations). Students will have the basic preparation they need to pursue postdoctoral specialty training and conduct legally-relevant clinical psychology research.

Special Facilities or Resources: The department enjoys ample testing and observation space, including a live animal facility. The university's computing facilities offer extensive access to personal computers complete with the latest software. The area provides access to a wide variety of clinical and research populations. These include persons housed in medical and mental health facilities located in the Texas Medical Center, as well as juvenile and adult offender populations. The town of Huntsville (population 35,078) is located in southeastern Texas with Houston only one hour away.

Information for Students With Physical Disabilities: See the following Web site for more information: http://www.shsu.edu/~counsel/sswd.html.

Application Information:
Send to Mary Alice Conroy. All applications should all be sent to Office of Graduate Studies, Sam Houston State University, PO Box 2478, Huntsville, TX 77341-2478. Department of Psychology, Sam Houston State University, PO Box 2447, Huntsville, TX 77341-2447. Application available online. URL of online application: http://www.shsu.edu/~grs_www/application/. Students are admitted in the Fall, application deadline May 1st (MA). This deadline is for our Master's programs. December 15 is the deadline for the doctoral program. Both programs admit students only in the fall. The fee for the Master's program is $20. $40 is the application fee for the doctoral program

(includes $20 Graduate School application fee and $20 Doctoral Program application fee).

Southern Methodist University
Department of Psychology
Dedman College
6424 Hilltop Lane, P.O. Box 750442
Dallas, TX 75275-0442
Telephone: (214) 768-4924
Fax: (214) 768-3910
E-mail: aconner@smu.edu
Web: http://www.smu.edu/psychology/

Department Information:
1925. Chairperson: Ernest Jouriles, PhD. Number of faculty: total—full-time 13; women—full-time 5; total—minority—full-time 1; women minority—full-time 1.

Programs and Degrees Offered:
Listed in the following order: Program area, degree type (T if terminal Master's), number awarded 7/08–6/09. Clinical Psychology PhD (Doctor of Philosophy) 0.

APA Accreditation: Clinical PhD (Doctor of Philosophy). Student Outcome Data Website: http://smu.edu/psychology/html/graduateStudentStats.html.

Student Applications/Admissions:
Student Applications
Clinical Psychology PhD (Doctor of Philosophy)—Applications 2009–2010, 91. Total applicants accepted 2009–2010, 5. Number full-time enrolled (new admits only) 2009–2010, 5. Total enrolled 2009–2010 full-time, 24. Openings 2010–2011, 5. The number of students enrolled full- and part-time who were dismissed or voluntarily withdrew from this program area in 2008–2009 were 0.
Scores: Entries appear in this order: required test or GPA, minimum score (if required), median score of students entering in 2009–2010. Clinical Psychology PhD (Doctor of Philosophy): GRE-V 500, 550, GRE-Q 500, 610, GRE-Analytical 4.5, 4.5, overall undergraduate GPA 3.0, 3.4, Masters GPA no minimum stated.
Other Criteria: (importance of criteria rated low, medium, or high): GRE scores—high, research experience—high, work experience—low, extracurricular activity—low, clinically related public service—medium, GPA—high, letters of recommendation—high, interview—high, statement of goals and objectives—high, research interests—high, undergraduate major in psychology—low, specific undergraduate psychology courses taken—low. For additional information on admission requirements, go to http://smu.edu/psychology/html/graduate.html.

Student Characteristics The following represents characteristics of students in 2009–2010 in all graduate psychology programs in the department: Female—full-time 21, part-time 0; Male—full-time 3, part-time 0; African American/Black—full-time 0, part-time 0; Hispanic/Latino(a)—full-time 3, part-time 0; Asian/Pacific Islander—full-time 0, part-time 0; American Indian/Alaska Native—full-time 1, part-time 0; Caucasian/White—full-time 19, part-time 0; Multi-ethnic—full-time 1, part-time 0; students subject to the Americans With Disabilities Act—full-time 0, part-time 0; Unknown ethnicity—full-time 0, part-time 0; International students who hold an F-1 or J-1 Visa—full-time 1, part-time 0.

Financial Information/Assistance:
Tuition for Full-Time Study: Doctoral: State residents: per academic year $28,026, $1,557 per credit hour; Nonstate residents: per academic year $28,026, $1,557 per credit hour. Tuition is subject to change. See the following Web site for updates and changes in tuition costs: http://smu.edu/bursar/gradtuit.asp.

Financial Assistance:
First-Year Students: Research assistantships available for first year. Average amount paid per academic year: $14,000. Average number of hours worked per week: 20. Apply by December 1.
Advanced Students: Research assistantships available for advanced students. Average amount paid per academic year: $14,000. Average number of hours worked per week: 20. Apply by June 1.
Additional Information: Of all students currently enrolled full time, 100% benefited from one or more of the listed financial assistance programs. Application and information available online at: http://smu.edu/psychology/html/graduateStudentSupport.html.

Internships/Practica: Doctoral Degree (PhD Clinical Psychology): For those doctoral students for whom a professional internship was required in this program prior to graduation, (4) students applied for an internship in 2008–2009, with (4) students obtaining an internship. Of those students who obtained an internship, (4) were paid internships. Of those students who obtained an internship, (4) students placed in APA/CPA accredited internships, (0) students placed in internships not APA/CPA accredited, but listed with the Association of Psychology Postdoctoral and Internship Programs (APPIC), (0) students placed in internships conforming to guidelines of the Council of Directors of School Psychology Programs (CDSPP), (0) students placed in internships that were not APA/CPA accredited, APPIC or CDSPP listed. Internal practica include Assessment, Dating Violence Prevention, Social Anxiety Disorders Treatment, and Project Support (which involves parent training and family support for victims of domestic violence). External practica include a variety of supervised experiences in correctional facilities, hospitals, wellness centers, counseling centers, and couples/family therapy settings.

Housing and Day Care: On-campus housing is available. See the following Web site for more information: http://smu.edu/housing/. On-campus day care facilities are available. See the following Web site for more information: http://smu.edu/childcare/.

Employment of Department Graduates:
Master's Degree Graduates: Of those who graduated in the academic year 2008–2009, the following categories and numbers represent the postgraduate activities and employment of master's degree graduates: Enrolled in a postdoctoral residency/fellowship (n/a), employed in independent practice (n/a), total from the above (master's) (0).

Doctoral Degree Graduates: Of those who graduated in the academic year 2008–2009, the following categories and numbers represent the postgraduate activities and employment of doctoral degree graduates: Enrolled in a psychology doctoral program (n/a), enrolled in a postdoctoral residency/fellowship (1), total from the above (doctoral) (1).

Additional Information:
Orientation, Objectives, and Emphasis of Department: The mission of SMU's 70 hour doctoral program in clinical psychology is to train psychologists whose professional activities are based on scientific knowledge and methods. The program integrates rigorous research training with state-of the-art, evidence-based clinical training. Thus, our program emphasizes the development of conceptual and research skills as well as scientifically-based clinical practice skills. The overarching goal is for our graduates to use empirical methods to advance psychological knowledge and whose approach to clinical phenomena is consistent with scientific evidence.

Special Facilities or Resources: The department houses a Family Research Center and has a number of well-equipped laboratories for research on various topics in clinical psychology.

Information for Students With Physical Disabilities: See the following Web site for more information: http://smu.edu/studentlife/SSD/.

Application Information:
Send to The Office of Graduate Studies, Southern Methodist University, PO Box 750240, Dallas, TX 75275-0240. Application available online. URL of online application: http://smu.edu/graduate/apply.asp. Students are admitted in the Fall, application deadline December 1. *Fee:* $75.

Stephen F. Austin State University
Department of Psychology
Liberal and Applied Arts and Sciences
Box 13046, SFA Station
Nacogdoches, TX 75962
Telephone: (936) 468-4402
Fax: (936) 468-4015
E-mail: *heiderj@sfasu.edu*
Web: *http://www.sfasu.edu/sfapsych/*

Department Information:
1962. Chairperson: Dr. Kandy Stahl. Number of faculty: total—full-time 11, part-time 4; women—full-time 7, part-time 3; total—minority—full-time 1; women minority—full-time 1.

Programs and Degrees Offered:
Listed in the following order: Program area, degree type (T if terminal Master's), number awarded 7/08–6/09. General Psychology MA/MS (Master of Arts/Science) (T) 5.

Student Applications/Admissions:
Student Applications
General Psychology MA/MS (Master of Arts/Science)—Applications 2009–2010, 30. Total applicants accepted 2009–2010, 10. Number full-time enrolled (new admits only) 2009–2010, 6. Number part-time enrolled (new admits only) 2009–2010, 0. Total enrolled 2009–2010 full-time, 14, part-time, 2. Openings 2010–2011, 15. The median number of years required for completion of a degree in 2008–2009 was 1. The number of students enrolled full- and part-time who were dismissed or voluntarily withdrew from this program area in 2008–2009 were 1.

Scores: Entries appear in this order: required test or GPA, minimum score (if required), median score of students entering in 2009–2010. *General Psychology MA/MS (Master of Arts/Science)*: GRE-V no minimum stated, GRE-Q no minimum stated, overall undergraduate GPA 3.0.

Other Criteria: (importance of criteria rated low, medium, or high): GRE scores—high, research experience—low, work experience—low, extracurricular activity—low, clinically related public service—low, GPA—high, letters of recommendation—medium, statement of goals and objectives—medium, undergraduate major in psychology—low, specific undergraduate psychology courses taken—high. For additional information on admission requirements, go to http://www2.sfasu.edu/sfapsych/graduate/admissions/.

Student Characteristics: The following represents characteristics of students in 2009–2010 in all graduate psychology programs in the department: Female—full-time 9, part-time 2; Male—full-time 5, part-time 0; African American/Black—full-time 1, part-time 0; Hispanic/Latino(a)—full-time 1, part-time 0; Asian/Pacific Islander—full-time 0, part-time 0; American Indian/Alaska Native—full-time 0, part-time 0; Caucasian/White—full-time 12, part-time 2; Multi-ethnic—full-time 0, part-time 0; students subject to the Americans With Disabilities Act—full-time 0, part-time 0; Unknown ethnicity—full-time 0, part-time 0; International students who hold an F-1 or J-1 Visa—part-time 1.

Financial Information/Assistance:
Tuition for Full-Time Study: Master's: State residents: per academic year $4,536, $126 per credit hour; Nonstate residents: per academic year $14,472, $402 per credit hour. Tuition is subject to change. Additional fees are assessed to students beyond the costs of tuition for the following: student service, student center, computer use, library use, publication, recreation center use.

Financial Assistance:
First-Year Students: Teaching assistantships available for first year. Average amount paid per academic year: $9,225. Average number of hours worked per week: 20. Apply by May 15. Research assistantships available for first year. Average amount paid per academic year: $9,225. Average number of hours worked per week: 20. Apply by May 15.

Advanced Students: Teaching assistantships available for advanced students. Average amount paid per academic year: $9,225. Average number of hours worked per week: 20. Research assistantships available for advanced students. Average amount paid per academic year: $9,225. Average number of hours worked per week: 20.

Additional Information: Of all students currently enrolled full time, 70% benefited from one or more of the listed financial assistance programs. Application and information available online at: http://www.sfasu.edu/sfapsych/.

Housing and Day Care: On-campus housing is available. See the following Web site for more information: http://www.sfasu.edu/

housing/. On-campus day care facilities are available. See the following Web site for more information: http://www.sfasu.edu/echl/.

Employment of Department Graduates:
Master's Degree Graduates: Of those who graduated in the academic year 2008–2009 the following categories and numbers represent the postgraduate activities and employment of master's degree graduates: Enrolled in a postdoctoral residency/fellowship (n/a), employed in independent practice (n/a), total from the above (master's) (0).
Doctoral Degree Graduates: Of those who graduated in the academic year 2008–2009, the following categories and numbers represent the postgraduate activities and employment of doctoral degree graduates: Enrolled in a psychology doctoral program (n/a), total from the above (doctoral) (0).

Additional Information:
Orientation, Objectives, and Emphasis of Department: The primary goal of this one-year, 36-hour, General Psychology MA program is to prepare students for admission to doctoral training programs in psychology by enabling them to earn graduate course credit and gain valuable research and teaching experience. Our degree program would also be of interest to persons who would like to earn an MA in psychology as a means of furthering their professional goals (e.g., by augmenting their research skills), even if those goals have no explicit connection to psychology. This is a non-thesis master's program. However, students can elect to continue for a second year in order to conduct a formal thesis research project. Students interested in a career in teaching psychology have the option of enrolling in a Teaching Seminar; excellent performance in this course could lead to an opportunity to teach a freshman-level course, should the student elect to remain in the program for a second year. Applications for Spring admission will be considered; however, students entering in Spring should recognize that, due to course prerequisites, they will not be able to complete the program in one year. Completion of the program would require an additional Spring semester.

Special Facilities or Resources: The department's facilities occupy more than 20,000 square feet. An extensive research suite and other research spaces permit data collection either with individual participants or groups. The spaces include 50 PC microcomputers for various programs in the department. There are also laboratories for human research in sensory psychophysics, learning, cognition, social, developmental, personality, and industrial/organizational psychology. Supplemental technical assistance from facilities in other departments on campus is available. All department classrooms are supplied with multimedia equipment. The department has an instructional computing laboratory consisting of 21 networked PC microcomputers and extensive supporting hardware and software for computing across the psychology curriculum. Most laboratory areas, classrooms, and graduate assistant offices contain both PC and Macintosh microcomputers, many of which are networked and support research and instruction.

Information for Students With Physical Disabilities: See the following Web site for more information: http://www.sfasu.edu/disabilityservices/.

Application Information:
Send to Dr. Gary G. Ford, Graduate Program Coordinator, Department of Psychology, Stephen F. Austin State University, Box 13046, SFA Station, Nacogdoches, TX 75962. Application available online. URL of online application: http://www.sfasu.edu/sfapsych/. Students are admitted in the Fall, application deadline August 1; Spring, application deadline December 1; Summer, application deadline May 1. The earlier the submission, the greater the likelihood of receiving an assistantship. We recommend applications be received by July 15 (Fall), November 15 (Spring), or April 15 (Summer), although we will accept them later. *Fee:* $25.

Texas A&M International University
Department of Behavioral, Applied Sciences and Criminal Justice
College of Arts and Sciences
5201 University Boulevard
Laredo, TX 78041-1900
Telephone: (956) 326-2475
Fax: (956) 326-2474
E-mail: *brudolph@tamiu.edu*
Web: *http://www.tamiu.edu/coas/psy*

Department Information:
1994. Director of Master's Program in Counseling Psychology: Bonnie A. Rudolph. Number of faculty: total—full-time 7, part-time 5; women—full-time 4, part-time 3; total—minority—full-time 4, part-time 5; women minority—full-time 2, part-time 3.

Programs and Degrees Offered:
Listed in the following order: Program area, degree type (T if terminal Master's), number awarded 7/08–6/09. Counseling Psychology MA/MS (Master of Arts/Science) (T) 15, Psychology MA/MS (Master of Arts/Science) (T) 0.

Student Applications/Admissions:
Student Applications
Counseling Psychology MA/MS (Master of Arts/Science)—Applications 2009–2010, 23. Total applicants accepted 2009–2010, 23. Number full-time enrolled (new admits only) 2009–2010, 23. Total enrolled 2009–2010 full-time, 23. Openings 2010–2011, 15. The median number of years required for completion of a degree in 2008–2009 were 2. The number of students enrolled full- and part-time who were dismissed or voluntarily withdrew from this program area in 2008–2009 were 1. *Psychology MA/MS (Master of Arts/Science)*—Applications 2009–2010, 6. Total applicants accepted 2009–2010, 6. Number full-time enrolled (new admits only) 2009–2010, 6. Total enrolled 2009–2010 full-time, 6. Openings 2010–2011, 6. The number of students enrolled full- and part-time who were dismissed or voluntarily withdrew from this program area in 2008–2009 were 0.

Other Criteria: (importance of criteria rated low, medium, or high): GRE scores—medium, research experience—medium, work experience—medium, extracurricular activity—medium, clinically related public service—high, GPA—medium, letters of recommendation—medium, interview—high, statement of goals and objectives—medium, specific undergraduate psychology courses taken—high.

Student Characteristics: The following represents characteristics of students in 2009–2010 in all graduate psychology programs in the department: Female—full-time 22, part-time 0; Male—full-time 7, part-time 0; African American/Black—full-time 0, part-time 0; Hispanic/Latino(a)—full-time 28, part-time 0; Asian/Pacific Islander—full-time 0, part-time 0; American Indian/Alaska Native—full-time 0, part-time 0; Caucasian/White—full-time 1, part-time 0; Multi-ethnic—full-time 0, part-time 0; students subject to the Americans With Disabilities Act—full-time 0, part-time 0; Unknown ethnicity—full-time 0, part-time 0; International students who hold an F-1 or J-1 Visa—full-time 0, part-time 0.

Financial Information/Assistance:
Tuition for Full-Time Study: *Master's:* State residents: per academic year $3,690; Nonstate residents: per academic year $8,670. Tuition is subject to change. Tuition costs vary by program.

Financial Assistance:
First-Year Students: Teaching assistantships available for first year. Average number of hours worked per week: 20. Apply by May 1. Research assistantships available for first year. Average amount paid per academic year: $9,000. Average number of hours worked per week: 20. Apply by May 1. Fellowships and scholarships available for first year. Average amount paid per academic year: $1,500. Average number of hours worked per week: 0. Apply by May 2.

Advanced Students: Teaching assistantships available for advanced students. Average amount paid per academic year: $9,000. Average number of hours worked per week: 20. Apply by May 1. Research assistantships available for advanced students. Average amount paid per academic year: $9,000. Average number of hours worked per week: 20. Apply by May 1.

Additional Information: Of all students currently enrolled full time, 15% benefited from one or more of the listed financial assistance programs.

Internships/Practica: Master's Degree (MA/MS Counseling Psychology): An internship experience, such as a final research project or "capstone" experience is required of graduates. Master's Degree (MA/MS Psychology): An internship experience, such as a final research project or "capstone" experience is required of graduates. The practicum and internships offer unique training opportunities to prepare competent counselors. Competence exercises include alliance and outcome measurement as well as session process analyses, in addition to more conventional training in documentation and treatment planning. Practica and internships consist of working at settings such as college counseling centers, forensic settings, drug and alcohol counseling/prevention agencies, domestic violence/battered women shelters, child advocacy centers, and professional counseling clinics. On-site supervisors provide thirty-minute supervision sessions. Psychologists on campus provide an additional 2.5 hours of supervision in individual, triadic, and group formats. Peer feedback and group cohesiveness are also vital parts of training. All graduates complete Practicum and Counseling Internship I. Students who choose the non-thesis (clinical) track also complete Internship II. The clinical track provides a total of 3 semesters of practical experience in counseling (600 hours), with a minimum of 240 hours of face-to-face counseling activities.

Housing and Day Care: On-campus housing is available. See the following Web site for more information: http://housing.tamiu.edu. No on-campus day care facilities are available.

Employment of Department Graduates:
Master's Degree Graduates: Of those who graduated in the academic year 2008–2009, the following categories and numbers represent the postgraduate activities and employment of master's degree graduates: Enrolled in a postdoctoral residency/fellowship (n/a), employed in independent practice (n/a), employed in an academic position at a university (4), employed in an academic position at a 2-year/4-year college (2), employed in other positions at a higher education institution (2), employed in a professional position in a school system (2), employed in government agency (5), employed in a community mental health/counseling center (6), employed in a hospital/medical center (2), total from the above (master's) (23).

Doctoral Degree Graduates: Of those who graduated in the academic year 2008–2009, the following categories and numbers represent the postgraduate activities and employment of doctoral degree graduates: Enrolled in a psychology doctoral program (n/a), total from the above (doctoral) (0).

Additional Information:
Orientation, Objectives, and Emphasis of Department: The Master of Arts in Counseling Psychology provides training for counselors with strong foundations in eclectic, humanistic, multicultural and community perspectives. Students in our international campus and community are self-reflective active learners. The excellent student-faculty ratio (average class=11) provides extra attention for its students to identify and achieve their own individual goals. There is an advisory board composed of student and faculty representatives as well as community leaders, which strives to expand the counseling program to improve the quality of life in South Texas. Students complete courses in counseling theories, techniques, and attitudes, multicultural counseling, human development, psychopathology, ethical and legal issues, group counseling, career counseling, assessment, and statistical research design. Electives include coursework in crisis counseling, brief collaborative therapy, community interventions, play therapy, elderly mental health, Latino mental health, alcohol and drug counseling, and bilingualism. Faculty are specialists in brief collaborative therapy, crisis intervention, psycholinguistics, memory, multicultural counseling, psychotherapy research, and counselor professional development. Graduates are eligible to sit for the Licensed Professional Counselor (LPC-Texas) Examination. Students can select a thesis track if they are interested in research and further study at the doctoral level. Our program meets every recommendation of the Multicultural Competency Checklist. The new MS in Psychology is designed to prepare the student for PhD work. The focus of preparation is methodology and research.

Special Facilities or Resources: The international flavor of the University and Texas/Mexico border community provide a rich milieu for multicultural and community counseling exploration and education. This is one of the program's greatest resources. Texas A&M International is one of the fastest growing university communities in the United States. Additionally, an off-campus community-counseling center, the Texas A&M International University Community Stress Center, offers free bilingual counseling and psycho-educational services. At this center student-counselors complete practica and internships in direct and indirect community and client interventions with faculty supervision. The Master of Arts in Counseling Psychology (MACP) program works closely with Career Services, Student Counseling, and Academic Support and Enrichment to provide training and employment opportunities for student-counselors. A departmental computer lab exists that is currently used for cognitive and language research. It is equipped for detailed analysis of research in memory, cognition, psycholinguistics, bilingualism, as well as other research. A Counseling/Research lab is equipped with digital and video recording, internet video conferencing and standard computer programs. It is available for student use in recording counseling sessions and conducting research.

Application Information:
Send to Texas A & M International University, Office of Graduate Studies & Research, 5201 University Boulevard, Laredo, TX 78041-1900. Application available online. URL of online application: http://www.tamiu.edu/gradschool/. Students are admitted in the Fall, application deadline April 30; Spring, application deadline November 30; Summer, application deadline April 30. *Fee:* $25. $10.00 late fee if submitted after the dealine.

Texas A&M University
Department of Psychology
Liberal Arts
Psychology Department
College Station, TX 77843-4235
Telephone: (979) 845-2581
Fax: (979) 845-4727
E-mail: *sstarr@psych.tamu.edu*
Web: *http://psychology.tamu.edu*

Department Information:
1968. Department Head: Les Morey. Number of faculty: total—full-time 46, part-time 2; women—full-time 18, part-time 1; total—minority—full-time 7, part-time 1; women minority—full-time 4, part-time 1.

Programs and Degrees Offered:
Listed in the following order: Program area, degree type (T if terminal Master's), number awarded 7/08–6/09. Clinical Psychology PhD (Doctor of Philosophy) 3, Cognitive Psychology PhD (Doctor of Philosophy) 1, Developmental Psychology PhD (Doctor of Philosophy) 0, Industrial/Organizational Psychology PhD (Doctor of Philosophy) 7, Social Psychology PhD (Doctor of Philosophy) 1, Behavioral and Cellular Neuroscience PhD (Doctor of Philosophy) 0.

APA Accreditation: Clinical PhD (Doctor of Philosophy).

Student Applications/Admissions:
Student Applications
Clinical Psychology PhD (Doctor of Philosophy)—Applications 2009–2010, 141. Total applicants accepted 2009–2010, 7. Number full-time enrolled (new admits only) 2009–2010, 4. Number part-time enrolled (new admits only) 2009–2010, 0. Total enrolled 2009–2010 full-time, 19, part-time, 4. Openings 2010–2011, 7. The median number of years required for completion of a degree in 2008–2009 were 6. The number of students enrolled full- and part-time who were dismissed or voluntarily withdrew from this program area in 2008–2009 were 0. *Cognitive Psychology PhD (Doctor of Philosophy)*—Applications 2009–2010, 16. Total applicants accepted 2009–2010, 7. Number full-time enrolled (new admits only) 2009–2010, 5. Number part-time enrolled (new admits only) 2009–2010, 0. Total enrolled 2009–2010 full-time, 9, part-time, 1. Openings 2010–2011, 3. The median number of years required for completion of a degree in 2008–2009 were 5. The number of students enrolled full- and part-time who were dismissed or voluntarily withdrew from this program area in 2008–2009 were 0. *Developmental Psychology PhD (Doctor of Philosophy)*—Applications 2009–2010, 5. Total applicants accepted 2009–2010, 2. Number full-time enrolled (new admits only) 2009–2010, 2. Total enrolled 2009–2010 full-time, 3. The number of students enrolled full- and part-time who were dismissed or voluntarily withdrew from this program area in 2008–2009 were 0. *Industrial/Organizational Psychology PhD (Doctor of Philosophy)*—Applications 2009–2010, 46. Total applicants accepted 2009–2010, 12. Number full-time enrolled (new admits only) 2009–2010, 6. Total enrolled 2009–2010 full-time, 19, part-time, 4. Openings 2010–2011, 3. The median number of years required for completion of a degree in 2008–2009 were 6. The number of students enrolled full- and part-time who were dismissed or voluntarily withdrew from this program area in 2008–2009 were 0. *Social Psychology PhD (Doctor of Philosophy)*—Applications 2009–2010, 33. Total applicants accepted 2009–2010, 6. Number full-time enrolled (new admits only) 2009–2010, 2. Total enrolled 2009–2010 full-time, 9, part-time, 1. Openings 2010–2011, 7. The median number of years required for completion of a degree in 2008–2009 were 5. The number of students enrolled full- and part-time who were dismissed or voluntarily withdrew from this program area in 2008–2009 were 0. *Behavioral and Cellular Neuroscience PhD (Doctor of Philosophy)*—Applications 2009–2010, 18. Total applicants accepted 2009–2010, 7. Number full-time enrolled (new admits only) 2009–2010, 5. Number part-time enrolled (new admits only) 2009–2010, 0. Openings 2010–2011, 5.

Other Criteria: (importance of criteria rated low, medium, or high): GRE scores—high, research experience—high, work experience—high, extracurricular activity—high, clinically related public service—high, GPA—high, letters of recommendation—high, interview—high, statement of goals and objectives—high.

Student Characteristics: The following represents characteristics of students in 2009–2010 in all graduate psychology programs in the department: Female—full-time 54, part-time 9; Male—full-time 26, part-time 1; African American/Black—full-time 5, part-time 1; Hispanic/Latino(a)—full-time 15, part-time 3; Asian/Pacific Islander—full-time 6, part-time 2; American Indian/Alaska Native—full-time 0, part-time 0; Caucasian/White—full-time 54, part-time 4; Multi-ethnic—full-time 0, part-time 0; students subject to the Americans With Disabilities Act—full-time 0, part-time 0; Unknown ethnicity—full-time 0, part-time 0; International students who hold an F-1 or J-1 Visa—full-time 4, part-time 0.

Financial Information/Assistance:
Tuition for Full-Time Study: *Doctoral:* State residents: $222 per credit hour; Nonstate residents: $503 per credit hour. Tuition is subject to change.

Financial Assistance:

First-Year Students: Teaching assistantships available for first year. Average amount paid per academic year: $10,867. Average number of hours worked per week: 20. Apply by December 15. Research assistantships available for first year. Average amount paid per academic year: $10,867. Average number of hours worked per week: 20. Apply by December 15. Fellowships and scholarships available for first year. Average amount paid per academic year: $25,000. Apply by December 15.

Advanced Students: Teaching assistantships available for advanced students. Average amount paid per academic year: $10,867. Average number of hours worked per week: 20. Research assistantships available for advanced students. Average amount paid per academic year: $10,867. Average number of hours worked per week: 20.

Additional Information: Of all students currently enrolled full time, 95% benefited from one or more of the listed financial assistance programs. Application and information available online at: http://psychology.tamu.edu.

Internships/Practica: Doctoral Degree (PhD Clinical Psychology): For those doctoral students for whom a professional internship was required in this program prior to graduation, (7) students applied for an internship in 2008–2009, with (7) students obtaining an internship. Of those students who obtained an internship, (7) were paid internships. Of those students who obtained an internship, (7) students placed in APA/CPA accredited internships, (0) students placed in internships not APA/CPA accredited, but listed with the Association of Psychology Postdoctoral and Internship Programs (APPIC), (0) students placed in internships conforming to guidelines of the Council of Directors of School Psychology Programs (CDSPP), (0) students placed in internships that were not APA/CPA accredited, APPIC or CDSPP listed.

Housing and Day Care: On-campus housing is available. On-campus day care facilities are available.

Employment of Department Graduates:

Master's Degree Graduates: Of those who graduated in the academic year 2008–2009, the following categories and numbers represent the postgraduate activities and employment of master's degree graduates: Enrolled in a postdoctoral residency/fellowship (n/a), employed in independent practice (n/a), total from the above (master's) (0).

Doctoral Degree Graduates: Of those who graduated in the academic year 2008–2009, the following categories and numbers represent the postgraduate activities and employment of doctoral degree graduates: Enrolled in a psychology doctoral program (n/a), enrolled in a postdoctoral residency/fellowship (7), employed in an academic position at a university (6), employed in a hospital/medical center (1), other employment position (1), total from the above (doctoral) (15).

Additional Information:

Orientation, Objectives, and Emphasis of Department: The goals of the PhD program in Psychology are: 1) to prepare students for careers as researchers and teachers at colleges and universities, and 2) to prepare students for careers as scientist–practitioners in clinical psychology and industrial/organizational psychology. The Department offers a PhD in six areas of specialization: Behavioral Neuroscience, Clinical (accredited by the APA), Cognitive, Developmental, Social, and Industrial/Organizational Psychology. The Department enrolls approximately 100 graduate students and offers numerous opportunities for student collaboration with faculty. The student-faculty ratio is approximately 3:1, which allows individualized attention to develop research and/or professional skills. Over the last decade, all graduates have obtained full-time employment as researchers, teachers, or practitioners. Faculty members are heavily involved in the placement of graduate students.

Special Facilities or Resources: The Department is housed in an attractive four-story building that contains faculty and graduate student offices, research laboratories, administrative offices, and classrooms. Laboratory facilities are excellent, including labs designated for faculty and student research in behavioral neuroscience, cognitive, developmental, industrial/organizational, and social psychology. The Department also maintains a Psychology Clinic in which clinical students are trained to provide a range of psychological services and conduct applied research under supervision from the clinical faculty.

Information for Students With Physical Disabilities: http://disability.tamu.edu.

Application Information:
Send to Texas A & M University, Graduate Adm. Supv., Dept. of Psyc, College Station, TX 77843-4235. Application available online. Students are admitted in the Fall, application deadline December 15. *Fee:* $50.

Texas A&M University
Educational Psychology
College of Education and Human Development
704 Harrington Tower, MS 4225
College Station, TX 77843-4225
Telephone: (979) 845-1831
Fax: (979) 862-1256
E-mail: *v-willson@tamu.edu*
Web: *http://epsy.tamu.edu/*

Department Information:
Department Head: Victor Willson. Number of faculty: total—full-time 44, part-time 3; women—full-time 25, part-time 2; total—minority—full-time 17; women minority—full-time 11.

Programs and Degrees Offered:
Listed in the following order: Program area, degree type (T if terminal Master's), number awarded 7/08–6/09. Educational Psychology PhD (Doctor of Philosophy) 15, Counseling Psychology PhD (Doctor of Philosophy) 9, School Psychology PhD (Doctor of Philosophy) 9.

APA Accreditation: Counseling PhD (Doctor of Philosophy). Student Outcome Data Website: http://cpsy.tamu.edu/program_statistics/disclosure.pdf. School PhD (Doctor of Philosophy). Student Outcome Data Website: http://epsy.tamu.edu/articles/school_psychology.

GRADUATE STUDY IN PSYCHOLOGY

Student Applications/Admissions:
 Student Applications
  Educational Psychology PhD (Doctor of Philosophy)—Applications 2009–2010, 26. Total applicants accepted 2009–2010, 15. Number full-time enrolled (new admits only) 2009–2010, 15. Total enrolled 2009–2010 full-time, 26, part-time, 66. Openings 2010–2011, 18. The median number of years required for completion of a degree in 2008–2009 were 4. The number of students enrolled full- and part-time who were dismissed or voluntarily withdrew from this program area in 2008–2009 were 0. *Counseling Psychology PhD (Doctor of Philosophy)*—Applications 2009–2010, 83. Total applicants accepted 2009–2010, 11. Number full-time enrolled (new admits only) 2009–2010, 7. Total enrolled 2009–2010 full-time, 49. Openings 2010–2011, 8. The median number of years required for completion of a degree in 2008–2009 were 6. The number of students enrolled full- and part-time who were dismissed or voluntarily withdrew from this program area in 2008–2009 were 0. *School Psychology PhD (Doctor of Philosophy)*—Applications 2009–2010, 43. Total applicants accepted 2009–2010, 20. Number full-time enrolled (new admits only) 2009–2010, 8. Number part-time enrolled (new admits only) 2009–2010, 0. Openings 2010–2011, 10. The median number of years required for completion of a degree in 2008–2009 were 6. The number of students enrolled full- and part-time who were dismissed or voluntarily withdrew from this program area in 2008–2009 were 0.

 Scores: Entries appear in this order: required test or GPA, minimum score (if required), median score of students entering in 2009–2010. *School Psychology PhD (Doctor of Philosophy)*: GRE-V no minimum stated, GRE-Q no minimum stated, overall undergraduate GPA no minimum stated.

 Other Criteria: (importance of criteria rated low, medium, or high): GRE scores—medium, research experience—high, work experience—medium, extracurricular activity—medium, clinically related public service—high, GPA—medium, letters of recommendation—high, interview—high, statement of goals and objectives—high, Fit with program—high, undergraduate major in psychology—low, specific undergraduate psychology courses taken—low. For additional information on admission requirements, go to http://epsy.tamu.edu/articles/graduate_admissions.

Student Characteristics: The following represents characteristics of students in 2009–2010 in all graduate psychology programs in the department: Female—full-time 166, part-time 76; Male—full-time 38, part-time 11; African American/Black—full-time 21, part-time 2; Hispanic/Latino(a)—full-time 34, part-time 14; Asian/Pacific Islander—full-time 3, part-time 9; American Indian/Alaska Native—full-time 0, part-time 0; Caucasian/White—full-time 111, part-time 53; Multi-ethnic—full-time 0, part-time 0; students subject to the Americans With Disabilities Act—full-time 0, part-time 0; Unknown ethnicity—full-time 35, part-time 9; International students who hold an F-1 or J-1 Visa—full-time 30, part-time 4.

Financial Information/Assistance:
 Tuition for Full-Time Study: *Doctoral:* State residents: $221 per credit hour; Nonstate residents: $698 per credit hour. Tuition is subject to change. See the following Web site for updates and changes in tuition costs: http://finance.tamu.edu/sbs/tuition/fee_information.asp.

Financial Assistance:
 First-Year Students: Research assistantships available for first year. Average amount paid per academic year: $13,500. Average number of hours worked per week: 20. Fellowships and scholarships available for first year. Average amount paid per academic year: $20,000. Average number of hours worked per week: 20. Apply by January 18.
 Advanced Students: Teaching assistantships available for advanced students. Average amount paid per academic year: $7,500. Average number of hours worked per week: 10. Research assistantships available for advanced students. Average amount paid per academic year: $13,500. Average number of hours worked per week: 20. Fellowships and scholarships available for advanced students. Average amount paid per academic year: $12,000.
 Additional Information: Of all students currently enrolled full time, 82% benefited from one or more of the listed financial assistance programs. Application and information available online at: http://epsy.tamu.edu/articles/assistantships.

Internships/Practica: Doctoral Degree (PhD Counseling Psychology): For those doctoral students for whom a professional internship was required in this program prior to graduation, (10) students applied for an internship in 2008–2009, with (10) students obtaining an internship. Of those students who obtained an internship, (9) were paid internships. Of those students who obtained an internship, (9) students placed in APA/CPA accredited internships, (0) students placed in internships not APA/CPA accredited, but listed with the Association of Psychology Postdoctoral and Internship Programs (APPIC), (0) students placed in internships conforming to guidelines of the Council of Directors of School Psychology Programs (CDSPP), (1) students placed in internships that were not APA/CPA accredited, APPIC or CDSPP listed. Doctoral Degree (PhD School Psychology): For those doctoral students for whom a professional internship was required in this program prior to graduation, (12) students applied for an internship in 2008–2009, with (12) students obtaining an internship. Of those students who obtained an internship, (12) were paid internships. Of those students who obtained an internship, (9) students placed in APA/CPA accredited internships, (0) students placed in internships not APA/CPA accredited, but listed with the Association of Psychology Postdoctoral and Internship Programs (APPIC), (3) students placed in internships conforming to guidelines of the Council of Directors of School Psychology Programs (CDSPP), (0) students placed in internships that were not APA/CPA accredited, APPIC or CDSPP listed. Students in the School Psychology and Counseling Psychology participate in the APPIC match program.

Housing and Day Care: On-campus housing is available. See the following Web site for more information: http://reslife.tamu.edu/. On-campus day care facilities are available. See the following Web site for more information: http://childrens-center.tamu.edu/.

Employment of Department Graduates:
 Master's Degree Graduates: Of those who graduated in the academic year 2008–2009, the following categories and numbers represent the postgraduate activities and employment of master's degree graduates: Enrolled in a postdoctoral residency/fellowship (n/a), employed in independent practice (n/a), total from the above (master's) (0).
 Doctoral Degree Graduates: Of those who graduated in the academic year 2008–2009, the following categories and numbers

represent the postgraduate activities and employment of doctoral degree graduates: Enrolled in a psychology doctoral program (n/a), enrolled in a postdoctoral residency/fellowship (1), employed in an academic position at a university (6), employed in other positions at a higher education institution (3), total from the above (doctoral) (10).

Additional Information:
Orientation, Objectives, and Emphasis of Department: We are among the top-ranked Educational Psychology departments in the nation. We are committed to making a difference through excellence in our research, education and community outreach activities.

Special Facilities or Resources: Education Research Evaluation Laboratory (EREL) and Counseling and Assessment Clinic (CAC) on campus and in Bryan, TX.

Information for Students With Physical Disabilities: See the following Web site for more information: http://disability.tamu.edu/.

Application Information:
All applications are processed online. Application available online. URL of online application: http://epsy.tamu.edu/articles/graduate_admissions. Students are admitted in the Fall, application deadline December 1. *Fee:* $50. $75.00 for international applicants.

Texas A&M University-Commerce
Department of Psychology and Special Education
College of Education and Human Services
Henderson Hall
Commerce, TX 75429
Telephone: (903) 886-5594
Fax: (903) 886-5510
E-mail: *thenley@tamu-commerce.edu*
Web: *http://web.tamu-commerce.edu/academics/colleges/educationHumanServices/departments/psychologySpecialEducation/*

Department Information:
1962. Department Head: Dr. Tracy Henley. Number of faculty: total—full-time 18, part-time 4; women—full-time 10, part-time 2; total—minority—full-time 3; women minority—full-time 3.

Programs and Degrees Offered:
Listed in the following order: Program area, degree type (T if terminal Master's), number awarded 7/08–6/09. Applied MA/MS (Master of Arts/Science) (T) 6, Educational Psychology PhD (Doctor of Philosophy) 3, School Psychology EdS (School Psychology) 7, General Experimental MA/MS (Master of Arts/Science) (T) 2.

Student Applications/Admissions:
Student Applications
Applied MA/MS (Master of Arts/Science)—Applications 2009–2010, 15. Total applicants accepted 2009–2010, 9. Number full-time enrolled (new admits only) 2009–2010, 9. Number part-time enrolled (new admits only) 2009–2010, 0. Total enrolled 2009–2010 full-time, 27, part-time, 13. Openings 2010–2011, 10. The median number of years required for completion of a degree in 2008–2009 were 2. The number of students enrolled full- and part-time who were dismissed or voluntarily withdrew from this program area in 2008–2009 were 0. *Educational Psychology PhD (Doctor of Philosophy)*—Applications 2009–2010, 22. Total applicants accepted 2009–2010, 6. Number full-time enrolled (new admits only) 2009–2010, 8. Number part-time enrolled (new admits only) 2009–2010, 4. Total enrolled 2009–2010 full-time, 39, part-time, 20. Openings 2010–2011, 10. The median number of years required for completion of a degree in 2008–2009 were 6. The number of students enrolled full- and part-time who were dismissed or voluntarily withdrew from this program area in 2008–2009 were 6. *School Psychology EdS (School Psychology)*—Applications 2009–2010, 20. Total applicants accepted 2009–2010, 10. Number full-time enrolled (new admits only) 2009–2010, 4. Number part-time enrolled (new admits only) 2009–2010, 6. Total enrolled 2009–2010 full-time, 20, part-time, 15. Openings 2010–2011, 10. The median number of years required for completion of a degree in 2008–2009 were 4. The number of students enrolled full- and part-time who were dismissed or voluntarily withdrew from this program area in 2008–2009 were 1. *General Experimental MA/MS (Master of Arts/Science)*—Applications 2009–2010, 3. Total applicants accepted 2009–2010, 3. Number full-time enrolled (new admits only) 2009–2010, 3. Number part-time enrolled (new admits only) 2009–2010, 0. Openings 2010–2011, 10. The median number of years required for completion of a degree in 2008–2009 were 3. The number of students enrolled full- and part-time who were dismissed or voluntarily withdrew from this program area in 2008–2009 were 0.

Scores: Entries appear in this order: required test or GPA, minimum score (if required), median score of students entering in 2009–2010. *Applied MA/MS (Master of Arts/Science):* GRE-V no minimum stated, GRE-Q no minimum stated, overall undergraduate GPA no minimum stated; *Educational Psychology PhD (Doctor of Philosophy):* GRE-V no minimum stated, 500, GRE-Q no minimum stated, 550, GRE-Analytical no minimum stated, 4.5; *General Experimental MA/MS (Master of Arts/Science):* GRE-V no minimum stated, 500, GRE-Q no minimum stated, 550, GRE-Analytical no minimum stated, 4.5.

Other Criteria: (importance of criteria rated low, medium, or high): GRE scores—medium, research experience—medium, work experience—medium, GPA—medium, letters of recommendation—medium, statement of goals and objectives—high, undergraduate major in psychology—low. Greater importance would be assigned to prior research experience, graduate education, and publications/scholarly activity for the doctoral program. For additional information on admission requirements, go to http://www.tamu-commerce.edu/psychology/.

Student Characteristics: The following represents characteristics of students in 2009–2010 in all graduate psychology programs in the department: Female—full-time 52, part-time 38; Male—full-time 37, part-time 10; African American/Black—full-time 11, part-time 5; Hispanic/Latino(a)—full-time 4, part-time 1; Asian/Pacific Islander—full-time 2, part-time 0; American Indian/Alaska Native—full-time 0, part-time 0; Caucasian/White—full-time 69, part-time 42; Multi-ethnic—full-time 0, part-time 0;

students subject to the Americans With Disabilities Act—full-time 0, part-time 0; Unknown ethnicity—full-time 3, part-time 0; International students who hold an F-1 or J-1 Visa—full-time 6, part-time 0.

Financial Information/Assistance:
Tuition for Full-Time Study: *Master's:* State residents: $363 per credit hour; Nonstate residents: $640 per credit hour. *Doctoral:* State residents: $363 per credit hour; Nonstate residents: $640 per credit hour. Tuition is subject to change. Additional fees are assessed to students beyond the costs of tuition for the following: Lab fees. See the following Web site for updates and changes in tuition costs: http://web.tamu-commerce.edu/admissions/tuitionCosts/default.aspx.

Financial Assistance:
First-Year Students: Teaching assistantships available for first year. Average amount paid per academic year: $8,000. Average number of hours worked per week: 20. Apply by Fall/Spring. Research assistantships available for first year. Average amount paid per academic year: $8,000. Average number of hours worked per week: 20. Apply by Fall/Spring. Fellowships and scholarships available for first year. Average amount paid per academic year: $1,000. Apply by Fall.

Advanced Students: Teaching assistantships available for advanced students. Average amount paid per academic year: $10,000. Average number of hours worked per week: 20. Apply by Fall/Spring. Research assistantships available for advanced students. Average amount paid per academic year: $10,000. Average number of hours worked per week: 20. Apply by Fall/Spring. Fellowships and scholarships available for advanced students. Average amount paid per academic year: $1,000. Apply by Fall.

Additional Information: Of all students currently enrolled full time, 10% benefited from one or more of the listed financial assistance programs. Application and information available online at: http://web.tamu-commerce.edu/academics/graduateSchool/funding/default.aspx.

Internships/Practica: Master's Degree (EdS School Psychology): An internship experience, such as a final research project or "capstone" experience is required of graduates. There are on-site university clinic practica for school and applied programs. The school psychology program requires a 1200-hour internship in the public schools.

Housing and Day Care: On-campus housing is available. See the following Web site for more information: http://www.tamu-commerce.edu/housing/. On-campus day care facilities are available. See the following Web site for more information: http://web.tamu-commerce.edu/studentLife/campusServices/childrensLearningCenter/aboutUs.aspx.

Employment of Department Graduates:
Master's Degree Graduates: Of those who graduated in the academic year 2008–2009, the following categories and numbers represent the postgraduate activities and employment of master's degree graduates: Enrolled in a psychology doctoral program (2), enrolled in another graduate/professional program (1), enrolled in a postdoctoral residency/fellowship (n/a), employed in independent practice (n/a), employed in an academic position at a university (0), employed in an academic position at a 2-year/4-year college (1), employed in other positions at a higher education institution (0), employed in a professional position in a school system (7), employed in business or industry (0), employed in government agency (0), employed in a community mental health/counseling center (3), employed in a hospital/medical center (0), still seeking employment (0), other employment position (1), total from the above (master's) (15).

Doctoral Degree Graduates: Of those who graduated in the academic year 2008–2009, the following categories and numbers represent the postgraduate activities and employment of doctoral degree graduates: Enrolled in a psychology doctoral program (n/a), enrolled in another graduate/professional program (0), enrolled in a postdoctoral residency/fellowship (0), employed in independent practice (0), employed in an academic position at a university (1), employed in an academic position at a 2-year/4-year college (0), employed in other positions at a higher education institution (1), employed in a professional position in a school system (1), employed in business or industry (0), employed in government agency (0), employed in a community mental health/counseling center (0), employed in a hospital/medical center (0), still seeking employment (0), other employment position (0), total from the above (doctoral) (3).

Additional Information:
Orientation, Objectives, and Emphasis of Department: The focus of the educational psychology program is human interventions (direct and indirect), statistics and research design, and cognition and instruction. Students will acquire an in-depth knowledge of human learning and cognition, instructional strategies, and research and evaluation. This emphasis will prepare students to integrate knowledge of human cognition and instructional practice across a variety of occupational, educational and content matter domains, with emphasis on applications of learning technologies. The applied master's program is fully accredited by the Interorganizational Board of Accreditation for Master's in Psychology Programs (IBAMPP). The applied master's program is designed to prepare students to meet the requirements for certification as an associate psychologist in the State of Texas. Associate psychologists are employed in a variety of governmental and private organizations, such as mental health centers, clinics, and hospitals. The school psychology program has been conditionally approved by the National Association of School Psychologists (NASP) and includes coursework in psychological foundations, educational foundations, assessment, professional school psychology, practica and internship.

Special Facilities or Resources: Multimedia Instructional Lab, multimedia classrooms, on-site Integrated University Clinic, research partnerships with business industry, Center for excellence-learning technologies, support for online learning, Cognitive Developmental Lab, Cognitive Science Lab, Cognition Lab, Health Psychology Lab, Social Cognition Lab, and School Psychology Resource Center.

Application Information:
Send to Graduate School, PO Box 3011, Texas A&M-Commerce, Commerce, TX 75429-3011. Application available online. URL of online application: http://web.tamu-commerce.edu/academics/graduateSchool/applyOnline.aspx. Students are admitted in the Fall, application deadline April; Spring, application deadline November; Summer, application deadline July. *Fee:* $35.

Texas Christian University
Department of Psychology
College of Science and Engineering
TCU Box 298920
Fort Worth, TX 76129
Telephone: (817) 257-7410
Fax: (817) 257-7681
E-mail: *m.eudaly@tcu.edu*
Web: *http://www.psy.tcu.edu/*

Department Information:
1959. Chairperson: Timothy Barth. Number of faculty: total—full-time 17, part-time 3; women—full-time 7, part-time 2; total—minority—full-time 1.

Programs and Degrees Offered:
Listed in the following order: Program area, degree type (T if terminal Master's), number awarded 7/08–6/09. Experimental Psychology PhD (Doctor of Philosophy) 3.

Student Applications/Admissions:
Student Applications
Experimental Psychology PhD (Doctor of Philosophy)—Applications 2009–2010, 19. Total applicants accepted 2009–2010, 13. Number full-time enrolled (new admits only) 2009–2010, 6. Number part-time enrolled (new admits only) 2009–2010, 0. Openings 2010–2011, 2. The median number of years required for completion of a degree in 2008–2009 were 4. The number of students enrolled full- and part-time who were dismissed or voluntarily withdrew from this program area in 2008–2009 were 0.
Scores: Entries appear in this order: required test or GPA, minimum score (if required), median score of students entering in 2009–2010. *Experimental Psychology PhD (Doctor of Philosophy):* GRE-V 390, 550, GRE-Q 520, 640, GRE-Analytical 3.0, 4.5, overall undergraduate GPA 3.2, 3.73, last 2 years GPA 3.26, 3.67, psychology GPA 3.2, 3.87.
Other Criteria: (importance of criteria rated low, medium, or high): GRE scores—low, research experience—high, GPA—medium, letters of recommendation—high, statement of goals and objectives—high. For additional information on admission requirements, go to http://www.psy.tcu.edu.

Student Characteristics: The following represents characteristics of students in 2009–2010 in all graduate psychology programs in the department: Female—full-time 21, part-time 0; Male—full-time 8, part-time 0; African American/Black—full-time 1, part-time 0; Hispanic/Latino(a)—full-time 1, part-time 0; Asian/Pacific Islander—full-time 2, part-time 0; American Indian/Alaska Native—full-time 0, part-time 0; Caucasian/White—full-time 25, part-time 0; Multi-ethnic—full-time 0, part-time 0; students subject to the Americans With Disabilities Act—full-time 0, part-time 0; Unknown ethnicity—full-time 0, part-time 0; International students who hold an F-1 or J-1 Visa—full-time 5, part-time 0.

Financial Information/Assistance:
Tuition for Full-Time Study: Doctoral: State residents: $980 per credit hour; Nonstate residents: $980 per credit hour. See the following Web site for updates and changes in tuition costs: http://www.graduate.tcu.edu/.

Financial Assistance:
First-Year Students: Fellowships and scholarships available for first year. Average amount paid per academic year: $0. Average number of hours worked per week: 0.
Advanced Students: Teaching assistantships available for advanced students. Average amount paid per academic year: $16,450. Average number of hours worked per week: 10. Apply by February 15.
Additional Information: Of all students currently enrolled full time, 96% benefited from one or more of the listed financial assistance programs. Application and information available online at: http://www.psy.tcu.edu/gradpro.html.

Housing and Day Care: On-campus housing is available. See the following Web site for more information: http://www.rlh.tcu.edu/. No on-campus day care facilities are available.

Employment of Department Graduates:
Master's Degree Graduates: Of those who graduated in the academic year 2008–2009, the following categories and numbers represent the postgraduate activities and employment of master's degree graduates: Enrolled in a psychology doctoral program (5), enrolled in a postdoctoral residency/fellowship (n/a), employed in independent practice (n/a), employed in business or industry (1), not seeking employment (1), total from the above (master's) (7).
Doctoral Degree Graduates: Of those who graduated in the academic year 2008–2009, the following categories and numbers represent the postgraduate activities and employment of doctoral degree graduates: Enrolled in a psychology doctoral program (n/a), employed in an academic position at a university (1), employed in other positions at a higher education institution (2), employed in business or industry (1), total from the above (doctoral) (4).

Additional Information:
Orientation, Objectives, and Emphasis of Department: The psychology graduate program at Texas Christian University leads to a predoctoral master's in experimental psychology and a PhD in general experimental psychology. The program is not limited to traditional experimental psychology, nor is it committed solely to laboratory-based methods. The department has long held that a measure of specialized knowledge—built upon a firm but broad base of psychological principles and methods—constitutes the best plan for most of its students. Within this plan, the student may study diverse areas of interest with emphasis possible in the following: learning-comparative, perception-cognition, social, personality, applied quantitative methods, and behavioral neuroscience. All graduate students receive training in both teaching and research. The environment is stimulating, informal, and conducive to close student-faculty relations.

Special Facilities or Resources: Assuming that physical proximity is conducive to more interdisciplinary work of substance, TCU has located all its science-related activities in or near the Science Research Center, dedicated in 1971. The Department of Psychology occupies two floors of the center's Winton-Scott Hall. The university library, containing over one million volumes, is located next to the science facilities. About 140 periodicals of psychological interest are available, plus online access to almost all journals.

Full-time personnel skilled in electronics, glass blowing, woodworking, and metalworking aid in construction and maintenance of special equipment or instruments. TCU has 10 open computer labs equipped with Windows-based PCs and Macintosh computers (over 100 Windows-based machines and 39 Mac-based machines). All of the labs provide full Internet access and laser printing. Additionally, some of the labs have scanners, zip drives, CD burners, and web cams. The Psychology department also has a computer lab with 6 Windows-based PCs, all of which are connected to the Internet, and a networked laser printer. Additionally, all of the research laboratories in the department have networked computers. From the various labs, students have access to a variety of software including SPSS, SAS, SYSTAT, and Microsoft Office. Also, the University provides e-mail accounts and storage space on the University server.

Information for Students With Physical Disabilities: See the following Web site for more information: http://www.acs.tcu.edu/disability.htm.

Application Information:
Send to Charles G. Lord, Coordinator of Graduate Studies, TCU Box 298920, Fort Worth, TX 76129. Application available online. URL of online application: http://www.psy.tcu.edu/gradpro.html. Students are admitted in the Fall, application deadline February 15. No deadline for admission; however, February 15 is recommended to be considered for funding. *Fee:* $50. Fees can be waived for exceptional or needy applicants. Contact the Graduate Director.

Texas of the Permian Basin, The University of
(2009 data)
Psychology Department
College of Arts and Sciences
4901 East University Boulevard
Odessa, TX 79762
Telephone: (432) 552-2325
Fax: (432) 552-3325
E-mail: *thompson_s@utpb.edu*
Web: *http://www.utpb.edu*

Department Information:
1973. Chairperson: Spencer Thompson. Number of faculty: total—full-time 6, part-time 1; women—full-time 4, part-time 1.

Programs and Degrees Offered:
Listed in the following order: Program area, degree type (T if terminal Master's), number awarded 7/08–6/09. Clinical Psychology MA/MS (Master of Arts/Science) (T) 6, Applied Research MA/MS (Master of Arts/Science) (T) 3.

Student Applications/Admissions:
Student Applications
Clinical Psychology MA/MS (*Master of Arts/Science*)—Applications 2009–2010, 12. Total applicants accepted 2009–2010, 10. Number full-time enrolled (new admits only) 2009–2010, 10. Total enrolled 2009–2010 full-time, 10, part-time, 20. Openings 2010–2011, 10. The median number of years required for completion of a degree in 2008–2009 were 3. The number of students enrolled full- and part-time who were dismissed or voluntarily withdrew from this program area in 2008–2009 were 1. *Applied Research MA/MS (Master of Arts/Science)*—Applications 2009–2010, 5. Total applicants accepted 2009–2010, 5. Number full-time enrolled (new admits only) 2009–2010, 5. Total enrolled 2009–2010 full-time, 5, part-time, 5. Openings 2010–2011, 5. The median number of years required for completion of a degree in 2008–2009 were 3. The number of students enrolled full- and part-time who were dismissed or voluntarily withdrew from this program area in 2008–2009 were 0.

Other Criteria: (importance of criteria rated low, medium, or high): GRE scores—high, research experience—low, work experience—low, extracurricular activity—low, clinically related public service—low, GPA—high, letters of recommendation—high, statement of goals and objectives—high, undergraduate major in psychology—low, specific undergraduate psychology courses taken—low.

Student Characteristics: The following represents characteristics of students in 2009–2010 in all graduate psychology programs in the department: Female—full-time 20, part-time 15; Male—full-time 15, part-time 10; African American/Black—full-time 0, part-time 0; Hispanic/Latino(a)—full-time 10, part-time 0; Asian/Pacific Islander—full-time 0, part-time 0; American Indian/Alaska Native—full-time 0, part-time 0; Caucasian/White—full-time 0, part-time 0; Multi-ethnic—full-time 0, part-time 0; students subject to the Americans With Disabilities Act—full-time 0, part-time 0; Unknown ethnicity—full-time 0, part-time 0; International students who hold an F-1 or J-1 Visa—full-time 0, part-time 0.

Financial Information/Assistance:
Tuition for Full-Time Study: *Master's:* State residents: per academic year $2,200, $122 per credit hour; Nonstate residents: per academic year $6,200, $342 per credit hour. Tuition is subject to change.

Financial Assistance:
First-Year Students: Research assistantships available for first year. Average amount paid per academic year: $12,000. Average number of hours worked per week: 19. Apply by April 15. Fellowships and scholarships available for first year. Average amount paid per academic year: $500. Apply by July 15.

Advanced Students: Teaching assistantships available for advanced students. Apply by April 15. Fellowships and scholarships available for advanced students. Average amount paid per academic year: $500.

Additional Information: Of all students currently enrolled full time, 20% benefited from one or more of the listed financial assistance programs. Application and information available online at: http://ss.utpb.edu/financial-aid.

Internships/Practica: Master's Degree (MA/MS Clinical Psychology): An internship experience, such as a final research project or "capstone" experience is required of graduates. Master's Degree (MA/MS Applied Research): An internship experience, such as a final research project or "capstone" experience is required of graduates. The University Counseling Center has opportunities for supervised clinical practica. Other practica are available in the community. Most students accumulate hours leading to Licensed Professional Counselor (LPC) certification in the State of Texas.

Students also qualify for certification as Psychological Associates in the State of Texas.

Housing and Day Care: On-campus housing is available. See the following Web site for more information: http://ss.utpb.edu/student-housing. No on-campus day care facilities are available.

Employment of Department Graduates:
Master's Degree Graduates: Of those who graduated in the academic year 2008–2009, the following categories and numbers represent the postgraduate activities and employment of master's degree graduates: Enrolled in a postdoctoral residency/fellowship (n/a), employed in independent practice (n/a), employed in a community mental health/counseling center (3), employed in a hospital/medical center (1), total from the above (master's) (4).
Doctoral Degree Graduates: Of those who graduated in the academic year 2008–2009, the following categories and numbers represent the postgraduate activities and employment of doctoral degree graduates: Enrolled in a psychology doctoral program (n/a), total from the above (doctoral) (0).

Additional Information:
Orientation, Objectives, and Emphasis of Department: The Master of Arts program in Psychology offers concentrations in both Clinical and Applied Research. The program offers students the opportunity to prepare themselves to work in mental health centers, juvenile detention centers, child service agencies, specialized school services, residential treatment facilities, family counseling agencies, teach in community colleges, or study at the doctoral level (PhD). The Clinical Psychology concentration is aimed at training students in the assessment and treatment of mental disorders, through individual, family, and group therapies. The program offers instruction in child, adolescent, and adult disorders. Successful completion of the Clinical Psychology concentration is designed to provide students with the opportunity to become eligible to take the state examinations for certification as a Psychological Associate (45 hours) or Licensed Professional Counselor (51 hours). The Licensed Professional Counselor certification requires an additional 2,000 supervised hours after the MA degree. The Applied Research concentration focuses on advanced psychological theory (i.e., developmental, personality, social, etc.), research methods, statistics, and manuscript preparation. The Applied Research concentration offers students the opportunity to prepare themselves to serve in governmental and community college or to pursue additional graduate study at the doctoral level. All students in the Applied Research concentration are expected to be involved in research activities throughout their graduate program.

Special Facilities or Resources: We have a newly remodeled on-campus center that has a counseling area for clinical practica and research space for applied research and thesis projects. In addition, cooperative arrangements are made with community health centers, schools, governmental agencies, and mental health practitioners for research and practicum opportunities.

Information for Students With Physical Disabilities: http://ss.utpb.edu/pass-office.

Application Information:
Send to Graduate Studies, The University of Texas of the Permian Basin, 4901 E. University, Odessa, TX 79762. Application available online. URL of online application: http://ss.utpb.edu/admissions/apply-now/graduate graduate. Students are admitted in the Fall, application deadline May 1; Spring, application deadline November 1. *Fee:* $0.

Texas Southwestern Medical Center at Dallas, The University of
Division of Psychology, Graduate Program in Clinical Psychology
5323 Harry Hines Boulevard
Dallas, TX 75390-9044
Telephone: (214) 648-5277
Fax: (214) 648-5297
E-mail: hm.evans@utsouthwestern.edu
Web: *http://www.utsouthwestern.edu/graduateschool/clinicalpsychology.html*

Department Information:
1956. Chairperson: C. Munro Cullum, PhD. Number of faculty: total—full-time 88, part-time 2; women—full-time 41; total—minority—full-time 10; women minority—full-time 5; faculty subject to the Americans With Disabilities Act 1.

Programs and Degrees Offered:
Listed in the following order: Program area, degree type (T if terminal Master's), number awarded 7/08–6/09. Clinical Psychology PhD (Doctor of Philosophy) 5.

APA Accreditation: Clinical PhD (Doctor of Philosophy). Student Outcome Data Website: http://www8.utsouthwestern.edu/utsw/cda/dept23139/files/85923.html.

Student Applications/Admissions:
Student Applications
Clinical Psychology PhD (Doctor of Philosophy)—Applications 2009–2010, 214. Total applicants accepted 2009–2010, 8. Number full-time enrolled (new admits only) 2009–2010, 7. The median number of years required for completion of a degree in 2008–2009 were 4. The number of students enrolled full- and part-time who were dismissed or voluntarily withdrew from this program area in 2008–2009 were 0.
Scores: Entries appear in this order: required test or GPA, minimum score (if required), median score of students entering in 2009–2010. *Clinical Psychology PhD (Doctor of Philosophy):* GRE-V 500, GRE-Q 500.
Other Criteria: (importance of criteria rated low, medium, or high): GRE scores—high, research experience—high, work experience—high, extracurricular activity—low, clinically related public service—medium, GPA—high, letters of recommendation—high, interview—high, statement of goals and objectives—high, undergraduate major in psychology—medium, specific undergraduate psychology courses taken—medium. For additional information on admission requirements, go to http://www8.utsouthwestern.edu/utsw/cda/dept23139/files/82507.html.

Student Characteristics: The following represents characteristics of students in 2009–2010 in all graduate psychology programs in the department: Female—full-time 31, part-time 0; Male—full-time 13, part-time 0; African American/Black—full-time 2, part-time 0; Hispanic/Latino(a)—full-time 3, part-time 0; Asian/Pacific Islander—full-time 6, part-time 0; American Indian/Alaska Native—full-time 0, part-time 0; Caucasian/White—full-time 33, part-time 0; Multi-ethnic—full-time 0, part-time 0; students subject to the Americans With Disabilities Act—full-time 0, part-time 0; Unknown ethnicity—full-time 0, part-time 0; International students who hold an F-1 or J-1 Visa—full-time 1, part-time 0.

Financial Information/Assistance:
Tuition for Full-Time Study: *Doctoral:* State residents: per academic year $4,569; Nonstate residents: per academic year $11,241. Tuition is subject to change. See the following Web site for updates and changes in tuition costs: http://www.utsouthwestern.edu/utsw/cda/dept315605/files/401638.html.

Financial Assistance:
First-Year Students: Teaching assistantships available for first year. Apply by January 1. Research assistantships available for first year. Apply by January 1.
Advanced Students: Teaching assistantships available for advanced students. Research assistantships available for advanced students. Traineeships available for advanced students. Average number of hours worked per week: 20.
Additional Information: Of all students currently enrolled full time, 77% benefited from one or more of the listed financial assistance programs. Application and information available online at: http://www.utsouthwestern.edu/utsw/home/financialaid/index.html.

Internships/Practica: Doctoral Degree (PhD Clinical Psychology): For those doctoral students for whom a professional internship was required in this program prior to graduation, (20) students applied for an internship in 2008–2009, with (20) students obtaining an internship. Of those students who obtained an internship, (20) were paid internships. Of those students who obtained an internship, (20) students placed in APA/CPA accredited internships, (0) students placed in internships not APA/CPA accredited, but listed with the Association of Psychology Postdoctoral and Internship Programs (APPIC), (0) students placed in internships conforming to guidelines of the Council of Directors of School Psychology Programs (CDSPP), (0) students placed in internships that were not APA/CPA accredited, APPIC or CDSPP listed. The program provides more than 1000 hours of clinical practica, followed by an APA-accredited captive internship. These clinical experiences are closely supervised. In order to achieve the goal of broad professional preparation, students will have a number of different clinical placements over the course of their practicum and internship assignments. These assignments are carried out at UT Southwestern facilities, agencies, regional medical centers, area schools, university counseling centers, and rehabilitation institutes. These clinical training sites include the following: Parkland Memorial Hospital [PMH]; Parkland Community Oriented Care Clinic [PMH]; Neuropsychology Service [UTSWMC]; McDermott Pain Management Center [UTSWMC]; University Rehabilitation Center [UTSWMC]; Children's Medical Center [CMC]; Cystic Fibrosis Center [CMC]; Episcopal School of Dallas [CMC]; Sleep Disorder Center [CMC]; the Mental Health Service of Southern Methodist University; Student Counseling Center at the University of Texas at Arlington; Terrell State Hospital; Dallas County Juvenile Department; Baylor University Medical Center; Baylor Institute for Rehabilitation; Presbyterian Hospital of Dallas; Shelton School; Fairhill School.

Housing and Day Care: On-campus housing is available. See the following Web site for more information: http://www.utsouthwestern.edu/utsw/home/facultyadministration/auxiliaryservices/campushousing/. On-campus day care facilities are available. See the following Web site for more information: http://www8.utsouthwestern.edu/utsw/home/research/WISMAC/index.html.

Employment of Department Graduates:
Master's Degree Graduates: Of those who graduated in the academic year 2008–2009, the following categories and numbers represent the postgraduate activities and employment of master's degree graduates: Enrolled in a postdoctoral residency/fellowship (n/a), employed in independent practice (n/a), total from the above (master's) (0).
Doctoral Degree Graduates: Of those who graduated in the academic year 2008–2009, the following categories and numbers represent the postgraduate activities and employment of doctoral degree graduates: Enrolled in a psychology doctoral program (n/a), enrolled in a postdoctoral residency/fellowship (5), total from the above (doctoral) (5).

Additional Information:
Orientation, Objectives, and Emphasis of Department: The Graduate Program in Clinical Psychology is a four-year doctoral program with an affiliated predoctoral internship program in clinical psychology, which is separately accredited by the APA. The program provides a combination of experiences in both clinical and research settings reflecting our basic training philosophy, which is a clinician-researcher model. Our specific objectives include offering the student the opportunity to acquire, experience, or develop the following: 1. A closely knit integration between basic psychological knowledge (both theoretical and empirical) and responsible professional services; 2. A wide variety of supervised and broadly conceived clinical and consulting experiences; 3. A sensitivity to professional responsibilities in the context of significant social needs; 4. An understanding of research principles, methodology, and skill in formulating, designing, and implementing psychological research; and 5. A competence and confidence in the role of psychology in multidisciplinary settings.

Special Facilities or Resources: UT Southwestern has a number of laboratories and clinical settings investigating the brain/behavior relationship, as well as many projects focusing on the psychosocial aspects of various medical and psychiatric disorders. Disorders studied include affective illness, anxiety, schizophrenia, sleep-wake dysfunctions, and medical conditions such as Alzheimer's disease, epilepsy, temporomandibular disorder, cystic fibrosis, and organ transplantation. Notable examples of comprehensive clinical research programs at UT Southwestern include the following: an affective disorders research program; a sleep disorders research laboratory; an Alzheimer's Disease Center; a neuropsychology laboratory; a pain management program; a schizophrenia research program that includes translational research; and research programs in basic neuroscience.

Application Information:
Application available online. URL of online application: http://www.utsouthwestern.edu/gradapp. Students are admitted in the Fall, application deadline January 1. *Fee:* $0.

Texas State University-San Marcos
Psychology Department/Master of Arts in Health Psychology Program
College of Liberal Arts
601 University Drive
San Marcos, TX 78666-4616
Telephone: (512) 245-2526
Fax: (512) 245-3153
E-mail: *so01@txstate.edu*
Web: *http://www.psych.txstate.edu*

Department Information:
1969. Chairperson: Shirley Ogletree, PhD. Number of faculty: total—full-time 27, part-time 3; women—full-time 13, part-time 1; total—minority—full-time 3; women minority—full-time 2.

Programs and Degrees Offered:
Listed in the following order: Program area, degree type (T if terminal Master's), number awarded 7/08–6/09. Health Psychology MA/MS (Master of Arts/Science) (T) 16.

Student Applications/Admissions:
Student Applications
Health Psychology MA/MS (Master of Arts/Science)—Applications 2009–2010, 47. Total applicants accepted 2009–2010, 24. Number full-time enrolled (new admits only) 2009–2010, 15. Number part-time enrolled (new admits only) 2009–2010, 0. Total enrolled 2009–2010 full-time, 32, part-time, 11. Openings 2010–2011, 20. The median number of years required for completion of a degree in 2008–2009 were 2. The number of students enrolled full- and part-time who were dismissed or voluntarily withdrew from this program area in 2008–2009 were 1.
Scores: Entries appear in this order: required test or GPA, minimum score (if required), median score of students entering in 2009–2010. Health Psychology MA/MS (Master of Arts/Science): GRE-V no minimum stated, GRE-Q no minimum stated, last 2 years GPA 3.0.
Other Criteria: (importance of criteria rated low, medium, or high): GRE scores—medium, research experience—medium, work experience—medium, extracurricular activity—low, clinically related public service—medium, GPA—high, letters of recommendation—high, statement of goals and objectives—high, undergraduate major in psychology—medium, specific undergraduate psychology courses taken—high. For additional information on admission requirements, go to http://www.psych.txstate.edu/graduate/gradreq.php.

Student Characteristics: The following represents characteristics of students in 2009–2010 in all graduate psychology programs in the department: Female—full-time 26, part-time 9; Male—full-time 6, part-time 2; African American/Black—full-time 0, part-time 0; Hispanic/Latino(a)—full-time 9, part-time 3; Asian/Pacific Islander—full-time 2, part-time 0; American Indian/Alaska Native—full-time 0, part-time 0; Caucasian/White—full-time 20, part-time 8; Multi-ethnic—full-time 0, part-time 0; students subject to the Americans With Disabilities Act—full-time 0, part-time 0; Unknown ethnicity—full-time 1, part-time 0; International students who hold an F-1 or J-1 Visa—full-time 0, part-time 0.

Financial Information/Assistance:
Tuition for Full-Time Study: *Master's:* State residents: per academic year $7,248, $302 per credit hour; Nonstate residents: per academic year $13,896, $579 per credit hour. Tuition is subject to change. See the following Web site for updates and changes in tuition costs: http://catsweb.txstate.edu/catsweb/sa/index.htm.

Financial Assistance:
First-Year Students: Teaching assistantships available for first year. Average amount paid per academic year: $5,076. Average number of hours worked per week: 10. Apply by February 1. Fellowships and scholarships available for first year. Average amount paid per academic year: $5,000. Average number of hours worked per week: 0.
Advanced Students: Teaching assistantships available for advanced students. Average amount paid per academic year: $5,202. Average number of hours worked per week: 10. Apply by February 1. Fellowships and scholarships available for advanced students. Average amount paid per academic year: $5,000. Average number of hours worked per week: 0.
Additional Information: Of all students currently enrolled full time, 50% benefited from one or more of the listed financial assistance programs. Application and information available online at: http://www.gradcollege.txstate.edu.

Internships/Practica: Multiple practicum sites are available and students in the clinical track must complete two semesters of practicum. Practicum sites include rehabilitation centers, behavioral health clinics, medical centers, pain clinics, juvenile forensic sites, state hospitals and facilities for persons with developmental disabilities, and offices of private practitioners.

Housing and Day Care: On-campus housing is available. See the following Web site for more information: http://www.reslife.txstate.edu. On-campus day care facilities are available. See the following Web site for more information: http://www.fcs.txstate.edu/cdc.htm.

Employment of Department Graduates:
Master's Degree Graduates: Of those who graduated in the academic year 2008–2009, the following categories and numbers represent the postgraduate activities and employment of master's degree graduates: Enrolled in a psychology doctoral program (2), enrolled in another graduate/professional program (3), enrolled in a postdoctoral residency/fellowship (n/a), employed in independent practice (n/a), employed in other positions at a higher education institution (1), employed in business or industry (1), employed in a hospital/medical center (2), still seeking employment (3), other employment position (3), do not know (1), total from the above (master's) (16).
Doctoral Degree Graduates: Of those who graduated in the academic year 2008–2009, the following categories and numbers represent the postgraduate activities and employment of doctoral degree graduates: Enrolled in a psychology doctoral program (n/a), total from the above (doctoral) (0).

GRADUATE STUDY IN PSYCHOLOGY

Additional Information:

Orientation, Objectives, and Emphasis of Department: The Master's program is intended to provide Master's level students with specific clinical skills, cognitive behavioral intervention techniques, and research skills for entry into PhD programs and direct employment in a variety of medical and health care settings. The program has been revised to offer 2 tracks, clinical approaches and applied research.

Special Facilities or Resources: The Psychology Department at Texas State University is currently developing relationships with the surrounding area's medical communities such as San Antonio's and Austin's major medical centers. We are also in the process of developing relationships with community health centers and private clinics.

Information for Students With Physical Disabilities: See the following Web site for more information: http://www.ods.txstate.edu/.

Application Information:
Send to The Graduate College, Texas State University, 601 University Drive, San Marcos, TX 78666-4605. Application available online. URL of online application: https://www.applytexas.org/adappc/gen/c_start.WBX. Students are admitted in the Fall, application deadline March 15. It should be noted that the deadline for many scholarships (including those administered by the Graduate College and Liberal Arts Graduate Scholarships) is March 1, and students who have complete application packets by February 1 will be given priority for departmental assistantships. *Fee:* $40.

Texas Tech University
Department of Psychology
Arts and Sciences
Box 42051
Lubbock, TX 79409-2051
Telephone: (806) 742-3711, ext. 222
Fax: (806) 742-0818
E-mail: *kay.hill@ttu.edu*
Web: *http://www.psychology.ttu.edu*

Department Information:
1950. Chairperson: Susan S. Hendrick, PhD Number of faculty: total—full-time 28; women—full-time 13; total—minority—full-time 1; faculty subject to the Americans With Disabilities Act 1.

Programs and Degrees Offered:
Listed in the following order: Program area, degree type (T if terminal Master's), number awarded 7/08–6/09. Clinical Psychology PhD (Doctor of Philosophy) 5, Applied Cognitive Psychology PhD (Doctor of Philosophy) 1, Counseling Psychology PhD (Doctor of Philosophy) 6, General Experimental Psychology PhD (Doctor of Philosophy) 1, Human Factors PhD (Doctor of Philosophy) 1, Social Psychology PhD (Doctor of Philosophy) 3.

APA Accreditation: Clinical PhD (Doctor of Philosophy). Student Outcome Data Website: http://www.depts.ttu.edu/psy/graduate/clinical/disclosuredata.php. Counseling PhD (Doctor of Philosophy). Student Outcome Data Website: http://www.depts.ttu.edu/psy/graduate/counseling/disclosuredata.php.

Student Applications/Admissions:
Student Applications
Clinical Psychology PhD (Doctor of Philosophy)—Applications 2009–2010, 131. Total applicants accepted 2009–2010, 7. Number full-time enrolled (new admits only) 2009–2010, 5. Number part-time enrolled (new admits only) 2009–2010, 0. Openings 2010–2011, 7. The median number of years required for completion of a degree in 2008–2009 were 5. The number of students enrolled full- and part-time who were dismissed or voluntarily withdrew from this program area in 2008–2009 were 0. *Applied Cognitive Psychology PhD (Doctor of Philosophy)*—Applications 2009–2010, 10. Total applicants accepted 2009–2010, 2. Number full-time enrolled (new admits only) 2009–2010, 2. Number part-time enrolled (new admits only) 2009–2010, 0. Openings 2010–2011, 4. The median number of years required for completion of a degree in 2008–2009 were 5. The number of students enrolled full- and part-time who were dismissed or voluntarily withdrew from this program area in 2008–2009 were 0. *Counseling Psychology PhD (Doctor of Philosophy)*—Applications 2009–2010, 91. Total applicants accepted 2009–2010, 7. Number full-time enrolled (new admits only) 2009–2010, 6. Number part-time enrolled (new admits only) 2009–2010, 0. Openings 2010–2011, 7. The median number of years required for completion of a degree in 2008–2009 were 5. The number of students enrolled full- and part-time who were dismissed or voluntarily withdrew from this program area in 2008–2009 were 0. *General Experimental Psychology PhD (Doctor of Philosophy)*—Applications 2009–2010, 3. Total applicants accepted 2009–2010, 1. Number full-time enrolled (new admits only) 2009–2010, 1. Number part-time enrolled (new admits only) 2009–2010, 0. Openings 2010–2011, 1. The median number of years required for completion of a degree in 2008–2009 were 5. The number of students enrolled full- and part-time who were dismissed or voluntarily withdrew from this program area in 2008–2009 were 0. *Human Factors PhD (Doctor of Philosophy)*—Applications 2009–2010, 25. Total applicants accepted 2009–2010, 3. Number full-time enrolled (new admits only) 2009–2010, 3. Number part-time enrolled (new admits only) 2009–2010, 0. Openings 2010–2011, 4. The median number of years required for completion of a degree in 2008–2009 were 5. The number of students enrolled full- and part-time who were dismissed or voluntarily withdrew from this program area in 2008–2009 were 0. *Social Psychology PhD (Doctor of Philosophy)*—Applications 2009–2010, 20. Total applicants accepted 2009–2010, 3. Number full-time enrolled (new admits only) 2009–2010, 3. Number part-time enrolled (new admits only) 2009–2010, 0. Openings 2010–2011, 4. The median number of years required for completion of a degree in 2008–2009 were 5. The number of students enrolled full- and part-time who were dismissed or voluntarily withdrew from this program area in 2008–2009 were 0.

Scores: Entries appear in this order: required test or GPA, minimum score (if required), median score of students entering in 2009–2010. *Clinical Psychology PhD (Doctor of Philosophy):*

GRE-V no minimum stated, 600, GRE-Q no minimum stated, 680, GRE-Analytical no minimum stated; *Applied Cognitive Psychology PhD (Doctor of Philosophy)*: GRE-V no minimum stated, 600, GRE-Q no minimum stated, 680, GRE-Analytical no minimum stated; *Counseling Psychology PhD (Doctor of Philosophy)*: GRE-V no minimum stated, 600, GRE-Q no minimum stated, 680, GRE-Analytical no minimum stated; *General Experimental Psychology PhD (Doctor of Philosophy)*: GRE-V no minimum stated, 600, GRE-Q no minimum stated, 680.

Other Criteria: (importance of criteria rated low, medium, or high): GRE scores—medium, research experience—high, work experience—medium, extracurricular activity—low, clinically related public service—medium, GPA—medium, letters of recommendation—high, interview—medium, statement of goals and objectives—high, undergraduate major in psychology—low. Work experience for experimental-low, counseling-medium, clinical-high; extracurricular activity for experimental-low, counseling-low; interview for clinical-high, counseling-medium, experimental-low. For additional information on admission requirements, go to http://www.psychology.ttu.edu.

Student Characteristics: The following represents characteristics of students in 2009–2010 in all graduate psychology programs in the department: Female—full-time 75, part-time 0; Male—full-time 36, part-time 0; African American/Black—full-time 8, part-time 0; Hispanic/Latino(a)—full-time 18, part-time 0; Asian/Pacific Islander—full-time 5, part-time 0; American Indian/Alaska Native—full-time 1, part-time 0; Caucasian/White—full-time 68, part-time 0; Multi-ethnic—full-time 3, part-time 0; students subject to the Americans With Disabilities Act—full-time 2, part-time 0; Unknown ethnicity—full-time 3, part-time 0; International students who hold an F-1 or J-1 Visa—full-time 7, part-time 0.

Financial Information/Assistance:

Tuition for Full-Time Study: *Doctoral:* State residents: per academic year $4,648, $212 per credit hour; Nonstate residents: per academic year $11,392, $474 per credit hour. Tuition is subject to change. See the following Web site for updates and changes in tuition costs: http://www.depts.ttu.edu/studentbusinessservices/tuitionfees/.

Financial Assistance:

First-Year Students: Teaching assistantships available for first year. Average amount paid per academic year: $11,500. Average number of hours worked per week: 20. Research assistantships available for first year. Average amount paid per academic year: $11,500. Average number of hours worked per week: 20. Fellowships and scholarships available for first year. Average amount paid per academic year: $1,000. Average number of hours worked per week: 0.

Advanced Students: Teaching assistantships available for advanced students. Average amount paid per academic year: $12,500. Average number of hours worked per week: 20. Research assistantships available for advanced students. Average amount paid per academic year: $12,500. Average number of hours worked per week: 20. Fellowships and scholarships available for advanced students. Average amount paid per academic year: $1,000. Average number of hours worked per week: 0.

Additional Information: Of all students currently enrolled full time, 95% benefited from one or more of the listed financial assistance programs. Application and information available online at: http://www.financialaid.ttu.edu/.

Internships/Practica: Doctoral Degree (PhD Clinical Psychology): For those doctoral students for whom a professional internship was required in this program prior to graduation, (7) students applied for an internship in 2008–2009, with (6) students obtaining an internship. Of those students who obtained an internship, (6) were paid internships. Of those students who obtained an internship, (6) students placed in APA/CPA accredited internships, (0) students placed in internships not APA/CPA accredited, but listed with the Association of Psychology Postdoctoral and Internship Programs (APPIC), (0) students placed in internships conforming to guidelines of the Council of Directors of School Psychology Programs (CDSPP), (0) students placed in internships that were not APA/CPA accredited, APPIC or CDSPP listed. Doctoral Degree (PhD Counseling Psychology): For those doctoral students for whom a professional internship was required in this program prior to graduation, (7) students applied for an internship in 2008–2009, with (7) students obtaining an internship. Of those students who obtained an internship, (7) were paid internships. Of those students who obtained an internship, (7) students placed in APA/CPA accredited internships, (0) students placed in internships not APA/CPA accredited, but listed with the Association of Psychology Postdoctoral and Internship Programs (APPIC), (0) students placed in internships conforming to guidelines of the Council of Directors of School Psychology Programs (CDSPP), (0) students placed in internships that were not APA/CPA accredited, APPIC or CDSPP listed. Practica are available in our Psychology Clinic and the Texas Tech University Counseling Center. Paid practica are available in the community. Such placements include a psychiatric prison, the pain clinic and Neuropsychiatry Department in the TTU Health Sciences Center, the local school district, a community mental health center, and conducting assessments at the state school and with local psychologists.

Housing and Day Care: On-campus housing is available. See the following Web site for more information: http://www.housing.ttu.edu/. On-campus day care facilities are available. See the following Web site for more information: http://www.depts.ttu.edu/hs/cdrc/.

Employment of Department Graduates:

Master's Degree Graduates: Of those who graduated in the academic year 2008–2009, the following categories and numbers represent the postgraduate activities and employment of master's degree graduates: Enrolled in a postdoctoral residency/fellowship (n/a), employed in independent practice (n/a), total from the above (master's) (0).

Doctoral Degree Graduates: Of those who graduated in the academic year 2008–2009, the following categories and numbers represent the postgraduate activities and employment of doctoral degree graduates: Enrolled in a psychology doctoral program (n/a), employed in independent practice (2), employed in an academic position at a university (4), employed in an academic position at a 2-year/4-year college (1), employed in government agency (3), employed in a community mental health/counseling center (2), employed in a hospital/medical center (2), do not know (2), total from the above (doctoral) (16).

Additional Information:
Orientation, Objectives, and Emphasis of Department: The clinical program adheres to a basic scientist–practitioner model with equal emphasis given to these components of clinical training. The program strives to develop student competencies in the following areas: psychotherapy and other major patterns of psychological treatment, clinical research, psychodiagnostic assessment, psychopathology, personality, and general psychology. The doctoral specialization in counseling psychology is also firmly committed to a concept of balanced scientist–practitioner training and is designed to foster the development of competence in basic psychology, counseling and psychotherapy, psychological assessment, psychological research, and professional ethics. Programs in experimental psychology (cognitive/applied cognitive, social, human factors) encompass a variety of research interests, both basic and applied. Students in these programs are exposed to the data, methods and theories and a wide variety of basic areas of psychology while at the same time developing a commitment to an area of special interest through research with a faculty mentor. Collaborative work across departmental programs is encouraged, and the department also collaborates with colleagues in management, industrial engineering, neuroscience, neuropsychiatry, and the Health Sciences Center.

Special Facilities or Resources: The department is housed in its own four-story building, which includes a large, well-equipped psychology clinic for practicum training, numerous laboratories equipped for human research activities, and sufficient student workspace and offices The university maintains constantly expanding computing support systems that can be accessed from computers in the psychology building. The Psychology Department has a number of microcomputers and software available for student use. The university enjoys an unusually good relationship with the local metropolitan community of over 250,000 residents. Major medical facilities, a private psychiatric hospital, a psychiatric prison and a state school for the developmentally disabled are located within the city, and APA-accredited internship training is available in the University Counseling Center. The cost of living is quite low and the climate is excellent. Texas Tech University (and the Lubbock region) was recently identified as having the most inexpensive housing market of surveyed university towns in the United States.

Information for Students With Physical Disabilities: See the following Web site for more information: http://www.depts.ttu.edu/students/sds/.

Application Information:
Send to Texas Tech University, Admissions, Psychology Department, Box 42051, Lubbock, TX 79409-2051. Application available online. URL of online application: http://www.depts.ttu.edu/gradschool/admissions/How.php. Students are admitted in the Fall, application deadline December 1. Deadlines for application: Clinical: December 1, Counseling: January 1, Experimental: January 15. *Fee:* $50.

Texas Tech University
Educational Psychology and Leadership
College of Education
Box 41071
Lubbock, TX 79409-1071
Telephone: (806) 742-1997
Fax: (806) 742-2179
E-mail: *tara.stevens@ttu.edu*
Web: *http://www.educ.ttu.edu*

Department Information:
1963. Program Coordinator: Tara Stevens, Ed.D. Number of faculty: total—full-time 9; women—full-time 3; total—minority—full-time 4.

Programs and Degrees Offered:
Listed in the following order: Program area, degree type (T if terminal Master's), number awarded 7/08–6/09. Educational Psychology PhD (Doctor of Philosophy) 1, Educational Psychology MA/MS (Master of Arts/Science) 2.

Student Applications/Admissions:
Student Applications
Educational Psychology PhD (Doctor of Philosophy)—Applications 2009–2010, 20. Total applicants accepted 2009–2010, 8. Number full-time enrolled (new admits only) 2009–2010, 4. Total enrolled 2009–2010 full-time, 16, part-time, 10. Openings 2010–2011, 15. The median number of years required for completion of a degree in 2008–2009 were 4. The number of students enrolled full- and part-time who were dismissed or voluntarily withdrew from this program area in 2008–2009 were 0. Educational Psychology MA/MS (Master of Arts/Science)—Applications 2009–2010, 14. Total applicants accepted 2009–2010, 4. Number full-time enrolled (new admits only) 2009–2010, 0. Total enrolled 2009–2010 full-time, 5. Openings 2010–2011, 10. The median number of years required for completion of a degree in 2008–2009 were 2. The number of students enrolled full- and part-time who were dismissed or voluntarily withdrew from this program area in 2008–2009 were 0.

Scores: Entries appear in this order: required test or GPA, minimum score (if required), median score of students entering in 2009–2010. Educational Psychology PhD (Doctor of Philosophy): GRE-V no minimum stated, GRE-Q no minimum stated, overall undergraduate GPA no minimum stated, Masters GPA no minimum stated.

Other Criteria: (importance of criteria rated low, medium, or high): GRE scores—low, research experience—high, work experience—medium, extracurricular activity—medium, clinically related public service—low, GPA—medium, letters of recommendation—high, interview—medium, statement of goals and objectives—high. For additional information on admission requirements, go to http://www.educ.ttu.edu/epsy/.

Student Characteristics: The following represents characteristics of students in 2009–2010 in all graduate psychology programs in the department: Female—full-time 14, part-time 8; Male—full-time 7, part-time 2; African American/Black—full-time 3, part-time 0; Hispanic/Latino(a)—full-time 0, part-time 1; Asian/Pacific Islander—full-time 2, part-time 1; American Indian/Alaska

Native—full-time 0, part-time 0; Caucasian/White—full-time 16, part-time 8; Multi-ethnic—full-time 0, part-time 0; students subject to the Americans With Disabilities Act—full-time 0, part-time 0; Unknown ethnicity—full-time 0, part-time 0; International students who hold an F-1 or J-1 Visa—full-time 7, part-time 0.

Financial Information/Assistance:
Tuition for Full-Time Study: *Master's:* State residents: per academic year $5,100, $212 per credit hour; Nonstate residents: per academic year $11,748, $489 per credit hour. *Doctoral:* State residents: per academic year $5,100, $212 per credit hour; Nonstate residents: per academic year $11,748, $489 per credit hour. See the following Web site for updates and changes in tuition costs: http://www.depts.ttu.edu/studentbusinessservices/.

Financial Assistance:
First-Year Students: Teaching assistantships available for first year. Average amount paid per academic year: $10,000. Average number of hours worked per week: 20. Apply by March 15. Research assistantships available for first year. Average amount paid per academic year: $10,000. Average number of hours worked per week: 20. Apply by March 15. Fellowships and scholarships available for first year.
Advanced Students: Teaching assistantships available for advanced students. Average amount paid per academic year: $9,450. Average number of hours worked per week: 20. Apply by March 15. Research assistantships available for advanced students. Average amount paid per academic year: $9,450. Average number of hours worked per week: 20. Apply by March 15.
Additional Information: Of all students currently enrolled full time, 60% benefited from one or more of the listed financial assistance programs. Application and information available online at: http://www.educ.ttu.edu.

Internships/Practica: Doctoral students are typically allowed to team teach with faculty who have graduate status. They may also teach an undergraduate course in educational psychology.

Housing and Day Care: On-campus housing is available. See the following Web site for more information: http://www.housing.ttu.edu/. On-campus day care facilities are available. See the following Web site for more information: http://www.depts.ttu.edu/hs/cdrc/.

Employment of Department Graduates:
Master's Degree Graduates: Of those who graduated in the academic year 2008–2009, the following categories and numbers represent the postgraduate activities and employment of master's degree graduates: Enrolled in a psychology doctoral program (2), enrolled in a postdoctoral residency/fellowship (n/a), employed in independent practice (n/a), total from the above (master's) (2).
Doctoral Degree Graduates: Of those who graduated in the academic year 2008–2009, the following categories and numbers represent the postgraduate activities and employment of doctoral degree graduates: Enrolled in a psychology doctoral program (n/a), enrolled in a postdoctoral residency/fellowship (0), employed in independent practice (0), total from the above (doctoral) (0).

Additional Information:
Orientation, Objectives, and Emphasis of Department: Educational Psychology is an academic program in the Department of Educational Psychology and Leadership. The program equips students with a comprehensive knowledge of learning, motivation, development, and educational foundations. Additionally, students learn to apply quantitative and qualitative research skills in a manner that promotes educational improvement while valuing diversity. Thus, educational psychology attracts students from various educational and professional backgrounds including education; psychology; human sciences; business; sports sciences; and health sciences. Students may seek either a Doctoral (PhD) or Master's degree (MEd) in Educational Psychology. The doctoral program emphasizes research and teaching and prepares students for career positions in academia. Additionally, Educational Psychology prepares students for careers in educational research and measurement, such as those found in universities (e.g., institutional research), government agencies, and testing companies. However, students may also choose a practitioner-oriented emphasis or specialization, such as school psychology or sport psychology, by crafting an individualized, interdisciplinary degree plan. The master's program is designed to provide students with content knowledge that facilitates the application of research in educational psychology to educational settings. Teachers are especially encouraged to select the applied master's degree plan that is designed to prepare highly effective, culturally sensitive educators.

Special Facilities or Resources: Educational Psychology students have access to focused research teams that facilitate inquiry through the support of data collection, availability of specialized statistical software, and consultation.

Information for Students With Physical Disabilities: See the following Web site for more information: http://www.depts.ttu.edu/studentaffairs/sds/.

Application Information:
Send to Office of Graduate Admissions, Texas Tech University, P.O. Box 41030, Lubbock, TX 79409-1070 Phone: (806) 742-2787. Application available online. URL of online application: http://www.educ.ttu.edu. Students are admitted in the Fall, application deadline June 1; Spring, application deadline October 1; Summer, application deadline March 1. Application should be complete at least three months prior to the date of intended enrollment. *Fee:* $50. Fee waived or deferred for full-time Texas Tech employees, spouses, and dependents less than 25 years.

Texas Woman's University
Department of Psychology and Philosophy
Arts and Sciences
P.O. Box 425470
Denton, TX 76204
Telephone: (940) 898-2303
Fax: (940) 898-2301
E-mail: *dmiller@twu.edu*
Web: *http://www.twu.edu/psychology-philosophy/*

Department Information:
1942. Chairperson: Daniel C. Miller, PhD, ABPP. Number of faculty: total—full-time 16; women—full-time 9; total—minority—full-time 3; women minority—full-time 2.

GRADUATE STUDY IN PSYCHOLOGY

Programs and Degrees Offered:
Listed in the following order: Program area, degree type (T if terminal Master's), number awarded 7/08–6/09. Counseling Psychology PhD (Doctor of Philosophy) 1, School Psychology PhD (Doctor of Philosophy) 3, Counseling MA/MS (Master of Arts/Science) (T) 11, School Psychology EdS (School Psychology) 6.

APA Accreditation: Counseling PhD (Doctor of Philosophy).

Student Applications/Admissions:
Student Applications
Counseling Psychology PhD (Doctor of Philosophy)—Applications 2009–2010, 74. Total applicants accepted 2009–2010, 7. Number full-time enrolled (new admits only) 2009–2010, 7. Number part-time enrolled (new admits only) 2009–2010, 0. Openings 2010–2011, 8. The median number of years required for completion of a degree in 2008–2009 were 10. The number of students enrolled full- and part-time who were dismissed or voluntarily withdrew from this program area in 2008–2009 were 1. *School Psychology PhD (Doctor of Philosophy)*—Applications 2009–2010, 19. Total applicants accepted 2009–2010, 7. Number full-time enrolled (new admits only) 2009–2010, 5. Number part-time enrolled (new admits only) 2009–2010, 0. Total enrolled 2009–2010 full-time, 27, part-time, 6. Openings 2010–2011, 10. The median number of years required for completion of a degree in 2008–2009 were 5. The number of students enrolled full- and part-time who were dismissed or voluntarily withdrew from this program area in 2008–2009 were 3. *Counseling MA/MS (Master of Arts/Science)*—Applications 2009–2010, 55. Total applicants accepted 2009–2010, 21. Number full-time enrolled (new admits only) 2009–2010, 9. Number part-time enrolled (new admits only) 2009–2010, 0. Openings 2010–2011, 12. The median number of years required for completion of a degree in 2008–2009 were 3. The number of students enrolled full- and part-time who were dismissed or voluntarily withdrew from this program area in 2008–2009 were 1. *School Psychology EdS (School Psychology)*—Applications 2009–2010, 21. Total applicants accepted 2009–2010, 12. Number full-time enrolled (new admits only) 2009–2010, 4. Number part-time enrolled (new admits only) 2009–2010, 1. Total enrolled 2009–2010 full-time, 20, part-time, 2. Openings 2010–2011, 12. The median number of years required for completion of a degree in 2008–2009 were 3. The number of students enrolled full- and part-time who were dismissed or voluntarily withdrew from this program area in 2008–2009 were 1.

Other Criteria: (importance of criteria rated low, medium, or high): GRE scores—medium, research experience—medium, work experience—high, extracurricular activity—medium, clinically related public service—medium, GPA—high, letters of recommendation—high, interview—high, statement of goals and objectives—high, writing skills—high.

Student Characteristics: The following represents characteristics of students in 2009–2010 in all graduate psychology programs in the department: Female—full-time 102, part-time 10; Male—full-time 12, part-time 0; African American/Black—full-time 7, part-time 2; Hispanic/Latino(a)—full-time 7, part-time 1; Asian/Pacific Islander—full-time 5, part-time 0; American Indian/Alaska Native—full-time 0, part-time 0; Caucasian/White—full-time 0, part-time 0; Multi-ethnic—full-time 0, part-time 0; students subject to the Americans With Disabilities Act—full-time 0, part-time 0; Unknown ethnicity—full-time 0, part-time 0; International students who hold an F-1 or J-1 Visa—full-time 0, part-time 0.

Financial Information/Assistance:
Tuition for Full-Time Study: *Master's:* State residents: $464 per credit hour; Nonstate residents: $705 per credit hour. *Doctoral:* State residents: $464 per credit hour; Nonstate residents: $705 per credit hour. Tuition is subject to change. Additional fees are assessed to students beyond the costs of tuition for the following: extra fees including library fee, student union fee, etc. See the following Web site for updates and changes in tuition costs: http://www.twu.edu/bursar.

Financial Assistance:
First-Year Students: Teaching assistantships available for first year. Average amount paid per academic year: $11,808. Average number of hours worked per week: 20. Apply by April. Research assistantships available for first year.

Advanced Students: Teaching assistantships available for advanced students. Average amount paid per academic year: $11,808. Average number of hours worked per week: 20. Apply by April. Research assistantships available for advanced students.

Additional Information: Of all students currently enrolled full time, 20% benefited from one or more of the listed financial assistance programs. Application and information available online at: http://www.twu.edu/finaid.

Internships/Practica: Doctoral Degree (PhD Counseling Psychology): For those doctoral students for whom a professional internship was required in this program prior to graduation, (10) students applied for an internship in 2008–2009, with (9) students obtaining an internship. Of those students who obtained an internship, (9) were paid internships. Of those students who obtained an internship, (9) students placed in APA/CPA accredited internships, (0) students placed in internships not APA/CPA accredited, but listed with the Association of Psychology Postdoctoral and Internship Programs (APPIC), (0) students placed in internships conforming to guidelines of the Council of Directors of School Psychology Programs (CDSPP), (0) students placed in internships that were not APA/CPA accredited, APPIC or CDSPP listed. Doctoral Degree (PhD School Psychology): For those doctoral students for whom a professional internship was required in this program prior to graduation, (6) students applied for an internship in 2008–2009, with (6) students obtaining an internship. Of those students who obtained an internship, (6) were paid internships. Of those students who obtained an internship, (0) students placed in APA/CPA accredited internships, (0) students placed in internships not APA/CPA accredited, but listed with the Association of Psychology Postdoctoral and Internship Programs (APPIC), (6) students placed in internships conforming to guidelines of the Council of Directors of School Psychology Programs (CDSPP), (0) students placed in internships that were not APA/CPA accredited, APPIC or CDSPP listed. Master's Degree (MA/MS Counseling): An internship experience, such as a final research project or "capstone" experience is required of graduates. There are numerous placements in the Dallas - Fort Worth metropolitan area. Doctoral students are expected to use the APPIC Directory for internship placement.

Housing and Day Care: On-campus housing is available. htp://www.twu.edu/housing. No on-campus day care facilities are available.

Employment of Department Graduates:

Master's Degree Graduates: Of those who graduated in the academic year 2008–2009, the following categories and numbers represent the postgraduate activities and employment of master's degree graduates: Enrolled in a psychology doctoral program (1), enrolled in another graduate/professional program (1), enrolled in a postdoctoral residency/fellowship (n/a), employed in independent practice (n/a), employed in an academic position at a university (1), employed in a professional position in a school system (6), employed in a community mental health/counseling center (6), do not know (2), total from the above (master's) (17).

Doctoral Degree Graduates: Of those who graduated in the academic year 2008–2009, the following categories and numbers represent the postgraduate activities and employment of doctoral degree graduates: Enrolled in a psychology doctoral program (n/a), employed in independent practice (2), employed in an academic position at a university (0), employed in an academic position at a 2-year/4-year college (0), employed in other positions at a higher education institution (0), employed in a professional position in a school system (2), employed in business or industry (0), employed in government agency (0), employed in a community mental health/counseling center (0), employed in a hospital/medical center (0), still seeking employment (0), not seeking employment (0), other employment position (0), do not know (0), total from the above (doctoral) (4).

Additional Information:

Orientation, Objectives, and Emphasis of Department: Both the APA-accredited Counseling Psychology doctoral program and the Counseling Psychology master's program prepare students in the practitioner-scientist model for counseling practice with particular emphasis on family systems, gender issues, assessment, and psychotherapeutic work with individuals and families in their contextual systems. The model provides clear training in both practice and science, but emphasizes practice, practice that is informed by science. The programs' philosophy, curricula, faculty, and students, situated within the unique context of the TWU mission, attempt to create an atmosphere that is supportive, open, and flexible. Graduate training in school psychology at the master's level provides a program emphasizing direct service to school settings. Specific competencies and areas of specialization stressed in coursework and field-based training include child development, psychopathology, theories and principles of learning, behavioral intervention and prevention strategies, diagnostic assessment, and evaluation techniques. Doctoral level training in school psychology focuses on applied preparation and training experiences in professional school psychology. This program prepares students in skills required in direct-to-client services (for example, diagnostic assessment and evaluation skills, therapeutic and intervention techniques, and competencies in the application of learning principles). This program also provides training and supervised experiences in the consultation model, emphasizing such competencies as systems and organizational analysis, supervision of programs and services, diagnostic team leadership, grant proposal writing, in-service education, and general coordination of school-based services in a consultative capacity.

Special Facilities or Resources: The University Counseling Center is an APA-approved internship site.

Information for Students With Physical Disabilities: See the following Web site for more information: http://www.twu.edu/dss/.

Application Information:
Send to Admissions Coordinator, Department of Psychology and Philosophy, Texas Woman's University, P.O. Box 425470, Denton, TX 76204-5470. Application available online. URL of online application: http://www.twu.edu/admissions/. Students are admitted in the Fall, application deadline February 1. March 1 for MA counseling psychology program. December 15 for PhD Counseling Program. *Fee:* $30.

Texas, University of, Arlington
Department of Psychology
College of Science
Department of Psychology, UTA Box 19528
Arlington, TX 76019-0528
Telephone: (817) 272-2281
Fax: (817) 272-2364
E-mail: *gatchel@uta.edu*
Web: *http://www.uta.edu/psychology*

Department Information:
1959. Chairperson: Robert J. Gatchel. Number of faculty: total—full-time 20, part-time 3; women—full-time 8, part-time 1; total—minority—full-time 4; women minority—full-time 3.

Programs and Degrees Offered:
Listed in the following order: Program area, degree type (T if terminal Master's), number awarded 7/08–6/09. Experimental Psychology PhD (Doctor of Philosophy) 11, Health Psychology PhD (Doctor of Philosophy) 1, Industrial/Organizational Psychology MA/MS (Master of Arts/Science) (T) 2.

Student Applications/Admissions:

Student Applications

Experimental Psychology PhD (Doctor of Philosophy)—Applications 2009–2010, 49. Total applicants accepted 2009–2010, 3. Number full-time enrolled (new admits only) 2009–2010, 3. Number part-time enrolled (new admits only) 2009–2010, 0. Openings 2010–2011, 7. The median number of years required for completion of a degree in 2008–2009 were 6. The number of students enrolled full- and part-time who were dismissed or voluntarily withdrew from this program area in 2008–2009 were 1. *Health Psychology PhD (Doctor of Philosophy)*—Applications 2009–2010, 20. Total applicants accepted 2009–2010, 6. Number full-time enrolled (new admits only) 2009–2010, 6. Number part-time enrolled (new admits only) 2009–2010, 0. Openings 2010–2011, 7. The number of students enrolled full- and part-time who were dismissed or voluntarily withdrew from this program area in 2008–2009 were 0. *Industrial/Organizational Psychology MA/MS (Master of Arts/Science)*—Applications 2009–2010, 32. Total applicants accepted 2009–2010, 5. Number full-time enrolled (new admits only) 2009–2010, 5. Number part-time enrolled (new admits only) 2009–2010, 0. Openings 2010–2011, 5. The median number of years required for completion of a degree in 2008–2009 were 2. The number of students enrolled full- and part-time who were dismissed or voluntarily withdrew from this program area in 2008–2009 were 2.

Scores: Entries appear in this order: required test or GPA, minimum score (if required), median score of students entering in 2009–2010. *Experimental Psychology PhD (Doctor of Philoso-*

phy): GRE-V no minimum stated, 517, GRE-Q no minimum stated, 577, GRE-Analytical no minimum stated, 4.33, overall undergraduate GPA no minimum stated, 3.42; *Health Psychology PhD (Doctor of Philosophy)*: GRE-V no minimum stated, 501, GRE-Q no minimum stated, 606, GRE-Analytical no minimum stated, 3.9, overall undergraduate GPA no minimum stated, 3.42; *Industrial/Organizational Psychology MA/MS (Master of Arts/Science)*: GRE-V no minimum stated, 520, GRE-Q no minimum stated, 600, GRE-Analytical no minimum stated, 4.0, overall undergraduate GPA no minimum stated, 3.36.
Other Criteria: (importance of criteria rated low, medium, or high): GRE scores—medium, research experience—high, extracurricular activity—low, clinically related public service—low, GPA—medium, letters of recommendation—high, statement of goals and objectives—high, undergraduate major in psychology—low, specific undergraduate psychology courses taken—medium. For additional information on admission requirements, go to http://www.uta.edu/psychology.

Student Characteristics: The following represents characteristics of students in 2009–2010 in all graduate psychology programs in the department: Female—full-time 38, part-time 3; Male—full-time 15, part-time 2; African American/Black—full-time 3, part-time 0; Hispanic/Latino(a)—full-time 3, part-time 0; Asian/Pacific Islander—full-time 13, part-time 0; American Indian/Alaska Native—full-time 0, part-time 0; Caucasian/White—full-time 0, part-time 0; Multi-ethnic—full-time 0, part-time 0; students subject to the Americans With Disabilities Act—full-time 1, part-time 0; Unknown ethnicity—full-time 0, part-time 0; International students who hold an F-1 or J-1 Visa—full-time 0, part-time 0.

Financial Information/Assistance:
Tuition for Full-Time Study: *Master's*: State residents: per academic year $7,200; *Doctoral*: State residents: per academic year $7,200. Tuition is subject to change. See the following Web site for updates and changes in tuition costs: http://grad.uta.edu/students/tuition.

Financial Assistance:
First-Year Students: Teaching assistantships available for first year. Average amount paid per academic year: $21,600. Average number of hours worked per week: 20. Research assistantships available for first year. Average amount paid per academic year: $21,600. Average number of hours worked per week: 20. Fellowships and scholarships available for first year. Average amount paid per academic year: $1,000.
Advanced Students: Teaching assistantships available for advanced students. Average amount paid per academic year: $21,600. Average number of hours worked per week: 20. Research assistantships available for advanced students. Average amount paid per academic year: $21,600. Average number of hours worked per week: 20. Fellowships and scholarships available for advanced students. Average amount paid per academic year: $1,000.
Additional Information: Of all students currently enrolled full time, 70% benefited from one or more of the listed financial assistance programs.

Internships/Practica: The Arlington-Dallas-Fort Worth area is a major center of business and industrial growth in Texas and offers diverse practical opportunities in consulting firms, corporations, government and private agencies, as well as health and health care agencies, social agencies and the like.

Housing and Day Care: On-campus housing is available. See the following Web site for more information: See http://www2.uta.edu/housing/. No on-campus day care facilities are available.

Employment of Department Graduates:
Master's Degree Graduates: Of those who graduated in the academic year 2008–2009, the following categories and numbers represent the postgraduate activities and employment of master's degree graduates: Enrolled in a psychology doctoral program (9), enrolled in another graduate/professional program (1), enrolled in a postdoctoral residency/fellowship (n/a), employed in independent practice (n/a), employed in an academic position at a university (3), employed in an academic position at a 2-year/4-year college (1), employed in other positions at a higher education institution (0), employed in a professional position in a school system (0), employed in business or industry (1), employed in government agency (0), employed in a community mental health/counseling center (1), employed in a hospital/medical center (0), still seeking employment (0), not seeking employment (0), other employment position (0), do not know (0), total from the above (master's) (16).
Doctoral Degree Graduates: Of those who graduated in the academic year 2008–2009, the following categories and numbers represent the postgraduate activities and employment of doctoral degree graduates: Enrolled in a psychology doctoral program (n/a), enrolled in another graduate/professional program (0), enrolled in a postdoctoral residency/fellowship (0), employed in independent practice (0), employed in an academic position at a university (1), employed in an academic position at a 2-year/4-year college (0), employed in other positions at a higher education institution (0), employed in a professional position in a school system (0), employed in business or industry (1), employed in government agency (0), employed in a community mental health/counseling center (0), employed in a hospital/medical center (1), still seeking employment (0), not seeking employment (1), other employment position (0), do not know (0), total from the above (doctoral) (4).

Additional Information:
Orientation, Objectives, and Emphasis of Department: The objective of graduate work in psychology is to educate the student in the methods and basic content of the discipline and to provide an apprenticeship in the execution of creative research in laboratory and/or field settings. The graduate programs provide comprehensive interdisciplinary training in Experimental Psychology, Health Psychology, and Industrial/Organizational Psychology. All students in the graduate program are broadly trained in statistical and experimental design. The concentration in Experimental Psychology is designed to form a basis for the doctoral program but is open to those seeking a terminal master's degree. The experimental program trains students to be research scientists in areas of interest that include animal behavior, animal learning, cognitive, developmental, evolutionary, neuroscience, quantitative, and social/personality psychology. The concentration in Health Psychology is designed to train researchers in health and behavior, working at the cutting edge of interdisciplinary, biomedical, and biobehavioral investigation in areas such as pain, stress,

psychoimmunology, cancer, and aging. The Master of Science in Industrial/Organizational Psychology combines rigorous course work in experimental design, quantitative methods, and management with practicum experience enabling students to perform effectively in the workplace.

Special Facilities or Resources: Each faculty member who is active in research in the Psychology Department is fortunate to have ample space. The department has approximately 18,000 total square feet of research space; 7,000 square feet for human subject research and 11,000 square feet for animal research. Graduate students work in faculty labs and use their research facilities. The department is able to utilize modern audiovisual technology in the classroom and is equipped with computer facilities for graduate research. Graduate students have in-office network connections as well as computer access in research laboratories and departmental computer labs. In addition to the departmental computer labs, the university academic computing services operate seven on-campus computing facilities and serve the academic and research needs of the university. The University Libraries include the Central Library, the Architecture and Fine Arts Library, and the Science and Engineering Library. Library resources include a full array of modern technological access to print electronic information, Internet access and an extensive interlibrary loan network in addition to the 2,430,000 books, periodicals, documents, technical reports, etc. on hand.

Information for Students With Physical Disabilities: See the following Web site for more information: http://www.uta.edu/disability/.

Application Information:
Send to Department of Psychology, Box 19528, The University of Texas at Arlington, Arlington, TX 76019-0528. Application available online. URL of online application: https://www.applytexas.org/adappc/gen/c_start.WBX. Students are admitted in the Fall, application deadline February 1; Spring, application deadline October 17. These deadlines are for U.S. student applications. International student application deadlines are in April, and September. *Fee:* $30. Application fee for international students is $60.

Texas, University of, Austin
Department of Educational Psychology
College of Education
1 University Station, D5800
Austin, TX 78712-1296
Telephone: (512) 471-4155
Fax: (512) 471-1288
E-mail: *emmer@mail.utexas.edu*
Web: *http://www.edb.utexas.edu/education/departments/edp/*

Department Information:
1923. Chairperson: Edmund T. Emmer. Number of faculty: total—full-time 31, part-time 8; women—full-time 18, part-time 5; total—minority—full-time 4, part-time 2; women minority—full-time 2, part-time 1; faculty subject to the Americans With Disabilities Act 1.

Programs and Degrees Offered:
Listed in the following order: Program area, degree type (T if terminal Master's), number awarded 7/08–6/09. Counseling Psychology PhD (Doctor of Philosophy) 10, Counselor Education MEd (Education) 11, Human Development and Culture PhD (Doctor of Philosophy) 1, Learning, Cognition, and Instruction PhD (Doctor of Philosophy) 6, Quantitative Methods PhD (Doctor of Philosophy) 4, School Psychology PhD (Doctor of Philosophy) 11, Academic Educational Psychology MEd (Education) 2, Academic Educational Psychology MA/MS (Master of Arts/Science) (T) 3.

APA Accreditation: Counseling PhD (Doctor of Philosophy). Student Outcome Data Website: http://www.edb.utexas.edu/education/departments/edp/admissions/programs/doctoral/counseling/. School PhD (Doctor of Philosophy). Student Outcome Data Website: http://www.edb.utexas.edu/education/departments/edp/admissions/programs/doctoral/school/.

Student Applications/Admissions:
Student Applications
Counseling Psychology PhD (Doctor of Philosophy)—Applications 2009–2010, 142. Total applicants accepted 2009–2010, 12. Number full-time enrolled (new admits only) 2009–2010, 9. Number part-time enrolled (new admits only) 2009–2010, 0. Total enrolled 2009–2010 full-time, 42, part-time, 17. Openings 2010–2011, 12. The median number of years required for completion of a degree in 2008–2009 were 6. The number of students enrolled full- and part-time who were dismissed or voluntarily withdrew from this program area in 2008–2009 were 0. *Counselor Education MEd (Education)*—Applications 2009–2010, 50. Total applicants accepted 2009–2010, 17. Number full-time enrolled (new admits only) 2009–2010, 12. Number part-time enrolled (new admits only) 2009–2010, 2. Total enrolled 2009–2010 full-time, 26, part-time, 3. Openings 2010–2011, 15. The median number of years required for completion of a degree in 2008–2009 were 2. The number of students enrolled full- and part-time who were dismissed or voluntarily withdrew from this program area in 2008–2009 were 1. *Human Development and Culture PhD (Doctor of Philosophy)*—Applications 2009–2010, 11. Total applicants accepted 2009–2010, 8. Number full-time enrolled (new admits only) 2009–2010, 3. Number part-time enrolled (new admits only) 2009–2010, 0. Total enrolled 2009–2010 full-time, 16, part-time, 4. Openings 2010–2011, 6. The median number of years required for completion of a degree in 2008–2009 were 6. The number of students enrolled full- and part-time who were dismissed or voluntarily withdrew from this program area in 2008–2009 were 1. *Learning, Cognition, and Instruction PhD (Doctor of Philosophy)*—Applications 2009–2010, 19. Total applicants accepted 2009–2010, 7. Number full-time enrolled (new admits only) 2009–2010, 4. Number part-time enrolled (new admits only) 2009–2010, 0. Total enrolled 2009–2010 full-time, 34, part-time, 9. Openings 2010–2011, 6. The median number of years required for completion of a degree in 2008–2009 were 5. The number of students enrolled full- and part-time who were dismissed or voluntarily withdrew from this program area in 2008–2009

were 0. *Quantitative Methods PhD (Doctor of Philosophy)*—Applications 2009–2010, 16. Total applicants accepted 2009–2010, 8. Number full-time enrolled (new admits only) 2009–2010, 8. Number part-time enrolled (new admits only) 2009–2010, 0. Total enrolled 2009–2010 full-time, 26, part-time, 4. Openings 2010–2011, 6. The median number of years required for completion of a degree in 2008–2009 were 7. The number of students enrolled full- and part-time who were dismissed or voluntarily withdrew from this program area in 2008–2009 were 3. *School Psychology PhD (Doctor of Philosophy)*—Applications 2009–2010, 48. Total applicants accepted 2009–2010, 14. Number full-time enrolled (new admits only) 2009–2010, 11. Number part-time enrolled (new admits only) 2009–2010, 0. Total enrolled 2009–2010 full-time, 51, part-time, 17. Openings 2010–2011, 12. The median number of years required for completion of a degree in 2008–2009 were 6. The number of students enrolled full- and part-time who were dismissed or voluntarily withdrew from this program area in 2008–2009 were 0. *Academic Educational Psychology MEd (Education)*—Applications 2009–2010, 15. Total applicants accepted 2009–2010, 7. Number full-time enrolled (new admits only) 2009–2010, 3. Number part-time enrolled (new admits only) 2009–2010, 1. Total enrolled 2009–2010 full-time, 5, part-time, 4. Openings 2010–2011, 5. The median number of years required for completion of a degree in 2008–2009 were 2. The number of students enrolled full- and part-time who were dismissed or voluntarily withdrew from this program area in 2008–2009 were 0. *Academic Educational Psychology MA/MS (Master of Arts/Science)*—Applications 2009–2010, 14. Total applicants accepted 2009–2010, 6. Number full-time enrolled (new admits only) 2009–2010, 1. Number part-time enrolled (new admits only) 2009–2010, 0. Total enrolled 2009–2010 full-time, 3, part-time, 3. Openings 2010–2011, 5. The median number of years required for completion of a degree in 2008–2009 were 2. The number of students enrolled full- and part-time who were dismissed or voluntarily withdrew from this program area in 2008–2009 were 2.

Scores: Entries appear in this order: required test or GPA, minimum score (if required), median score of students entering in 2009–2010. *Counseling Psychology PhD (Doctor of Philosophy)*: GRE-V no minimum stated, 640, GRE-Q no minimum stated, 630, GRE-Analytical no minimum stated, 5.0, last 2 years GPA no minimum stated, 3.92; *Counselor Education MEd (Education)*: GRE-V no minimum stated, 630, GRE-Q no minimum stated, 520, GRE-Analytical no minimum stated, 4.0, last 2 years GPA no minimum stated, 3.61; *Human Development and Culture PhD (Doctor of Philosophy)*: GRE-V no minimum stated, 760, GRE-Q no minimum stated, 620, GRE-Analytical no minimum stated, 5.75, last 2 years GPA no minimum stated, 3.92; *Learning, Cognition, and Instruction PhD (Doctor of Philosophy)*: GRE-V no minimum stated, 600, GRE-Q no minimum stated, 510, GRE-Analytical no minimum stated, 4.25, last 2 years GPA no minimum stated, 3.71; *Quantitative Methods PhD (Doctor of Philosophy)*: GRE-V no minimum stated, 735, GRE-Q no minimum stated, 540, GRE-Analytical no minimum stated, 4.5, last 2 years GPA no minimum stated, 3.44; *School Psychology PhD (Doctor of Philosophy)*: GRE-V no minimum stated, 700, GRE-Q no minimum stated, 600, GRE-Analytical no minimum stated, 4.5, last 2 years GPA no minimum stated, 3.71; *Academic Educational Psychology MEd (Education)*: GRE-V no minimum stated, 635, GRE-Q no minimum stated, 530, GRE-Analytical no minimum stated, 4.0, last 2 years GPA no minimum stated, 3.95; *Academic Educational Psychology MA/MS (Master of Arts/Science)*: GRE-V no minimum stated, 600, GRE-Q no minimum stated, 580, GRE-Analytical no minimum stated, 3.5, last 2 years GPA no minimum stated, 3.56.

Other Criteria: (importance of criteria rated low, medium, or high): GRE scores—high, research experience—medium, work experience—medium, extracurricular activity—medium, clinically related public service—medium, GPA—high, letters of recommendation—high, interview—medium, statement of goals and objectives—high. Different areas may consider criteria somewhat differently upon occasion. For additional information on admission requirements, go to http://www.edb.utexas.edu/education/departments/edp/prospective/.

Student Characteristics: The following represents characteristics of students in 2009–2010 in all graduate psychology programs in the department: Female—full-time 156, part-time 41; Male—full-time 47, part-time 20; African American/Black—full-time 12, part-time 0; Hispanic/Latino(a)—full-time 30, part-time 6; Asian/Pacific Islander—full-time 41, part-time 10; American Indian/Alaska Native—full-time 1, part-time 0; Caucasian/White—full-time 119, part-time 45; Multi-ethnic—full-time 0, part-time 0; students subject to the Americans With Disabilities Act—full-time 1, part-time 3; Unknown ethnicity—full-time 0, part-time 0; International students who hold an F-1 or J-1 Visa—full-time 22, part-time 4.

Financial Information/Assistance:
Tuition for Full-Time Study: *Master's:* State residents: $410 per credit hour; Nonstate residents: $803 per credit hour. *Doctoral:* State residents: $410 per credit hour; Nonstate residents: $803 per credit hour. Tuition is subject to change. See the following Web site for updates and changes in tuition costs: http://www.utexas.edu/business/accounting/sar/t_f_rates.html.

Financial Assistance:
First-Year Students: Teaching assistantships available for first year. Average amount paid per academic year: $12,849. Average number of hours worked per week: 20. Apply by April 1. Research assistantships available for first year. Average amount paid per academic year: $14,000. Average number of hours worked per week: 20. Apply by April 1. Fellowships and scholarships available for first year. Average amount paid per academic year: $1,000. Average number of hours worked per week: 0. Apply by December 1.

Advanced Students: Teaching assistantships available for advanced students. Average amount paid per academic year: $12,849. Average number of hours worked per week: 20. Apply by April 1. Research assistantships available for advanced students. Average amount paid per academic year: $14,000. Average number of hours worked per week: 20. Apply by April 1. Fellowships and scholarships available for advanced students. Average amount paid per academic year: $1,000. Average number of hours worked per week: 0. Apply by December 1.

Additional Information: Of all students currently enrolled full time, 70% benefited from one or more of the listed financial assistance programs. Application and information available online at: http://www.edb.utexas.edu/education/departments/edp/admissions/financial/.

Internships/Practica: Doctoral Degree (PhD Counseling Psychology): For those doctoral students for whom a professional internship was required in this program prior to graduation, (4) students applied for an internship in 2008–2009, with (4) students obtaining an internship. Of those students who obtained an internship, (4) were paid internships. Of those students who obtained an internship, (4) students placed in APA/CPA accredited internships, (0) students placed in internships not APA/CPA accredited, but listed with the Association of Psychology Postdoctoral and Internship Programs (APPIC), (0) students placed in internships conforming to guidelines of the Council of Directors of School Psychology Programs (CDSPP), (0) students placed in internships that were not APA/CPA accredited, APPIC or CDSPP listed. Doctoral Degree (PhD School Psychology): For those doctoral students for whom a professional internship was required in this program prior to graduation, (10) students applied for an internship in 2008–2009, with (10) students obtaining an internship. Of those students who obtained an internship, (10) were paid internships. Of those students who obtained an internship, (9) students placed in APA/CPA accredited internships, (1) students placed in internships not APA/CPA accredited, but listed with the Association of Psychology Postdoctoral and Internship Programs (APPIC), (0) students placed in internships conforming to guidelines of the Council of Directors of School Psychology Programs (CDSPP), (0) students placed in internships that were not APA/CPA accredited, APPIC or CDSPP listed. Master's Degree (MA/MS Academic Educational Psychology): An internship experience, such as, a final research project or "capstone" experience is required of graduates. In the Counseling Psychology program, internships are generally available in APA-approved counseling and mental health centers, other university counseling centers, and community/hospital settings that provide in-depth supervision. In the School Psychology program, internship sites are often in APA-approved school systems and hospital/community settings that have an educational component. Other programs coordinate a variety of practicum settings to provide both research and applied experiences.

Housing and Day Care: On-campus housing is available. See the following Web site for more information: http://www.utexas.edu/student/housing/. On-campus day care facilities are available. See the following Web site for more information: http://www.utexas.edu/childcenter/.

Employment of Department Graduates:

Master's Degree Graduates: Of those who graduated in the academic year 2008–2009, the following categories and numbers represent the postgraduate activities and employment of master's degree graduates: Enrolled in a psychology doctoral program (1), enrolled in another graduate/professional program (1), enrolled in a postdoctoral residency/fellowship (n/a), employed in independent practice (n/a), employed in an academic position at a university (1), employed in an academic position at a 2-year/4-year college (1), employed in other positions at a higher education institution (4), employed in a professional position in a school system (5), employed in business or industry (0), employed in government agency (0), employed in a community mental health/counseling center (2), employed in a hospital/medical center (0), still seeking employment (0), not seeking employment (0), other employment position (0), do not know (1), total from the above (master's) (16).

Doctoral Degree Graduates: Of those who graduated in the academic year 2008–2009, the following categories and numbers represent the postgraduate activities and employment of doctoral degree graduates: Enrolled in a psychology doctoral program (n/a), enrolled in a postdoctoral residency/fellowship (16), employed in an academic position at a university (3), employed in an academic position at a 2-year/4-year college (2), employed in other positions at a higher education institution (5), employed in a professional position in a school system (1), employed in business or industry (3), employed in government agency (1), employed in a community mental health/counseling center (0), employed in a hospital/medical center (0), still seeking employment (1), not seeking employment (0), other employment position (1), do not know (0), total from the above (doctoral) (33).

Additional Information:

Orientation, Objectives, and Emphasis of Department: Training in educational psychology relates human behavior to the educational process as it occurs in the home, in peer groups, in nursery school through graduate school, in business and industry, in the military, in institutions for persons with physical or mental disabilities, and in myriad other settings. In so doing, it includes study in the following areas: the biological bases of behavior; history and systems of psychology and of education; the psychology of learning, motivation, cognition, and instruction; developmental, social, and personality psychology; psychological and educational measurement, statistics, evaluation, and research methodology; the professional areas of school psychology and counseling psychology; and general academic educational psychology.

Special Facilities or Resources: The University of Texas at Austin has the fifth largest academic library in the United States and also provides online access to hundreds of electronic databases. Our department also has access, through our college's Learning Technology Center, to several microcomputer and multimedia laboratories, technical assistance, resource materials, and audiovisual equipment and services. Academic computing facilities are extensive, ranging from mainframes to microcomputers. Additional resources include several university-wide centers with which our faculty are associated, including UT's Counseling and Mental Health Center.

Information for Students With Physical Disabilities: See the following Web site for more information: http://deanofstudents.utexas.edu/ssd/.

Application Information:
Send to Graduate Advisor, Educational Psychology, 1 University Station, D5800 Austin, TX 78712-1296. Application available online. URL of online application: http://www.utexas.edu/ogs/admissions/. Students are admitted in the Fall, application deadline December 1. The deadline for Counseling Psychology and School Psychology is December 1. The priority deadline for other PhD areas is February 1 (although students who want to be considered for fellowships must have completed applications by December 1). The priority deadline for the master's specializations is March 1 for summer or fall admissions. *Fee:* $50. Fee may be waived, at the discretion of Graduate Admissions (GIAC), in cases of demonstrated financial need.

Texas, University of, Austin
Department of Human Development and Family Sciences
School of Human Ecology
1 University Station A2702
Austin, TX 78712-0141
Telephone: (512) 475-8800
Fax: (512) 475-8662
E-mail: *gsbaker@austin.utexas.edu*
Web: *http://www.he.utexas.edu/hdfs/hdfsgrad.php*

Department Information:
1962. Chairperson: Deborah Jacobvitz, PhD Number of faculty: total—full-time 14; women—full-time 10; total—minority—full-time 1; women minority—full-time 1.

Programs and Degrees Offered:
Listed in the following order: Program area, degree type (T if terminal Master's), number awarded 7/08–6/09. Human Development & Family Sciences PhD (Doctor of Philosophy) 5.

Student Applications/Admissions:
Student Applications
Human Development & Family Sciences PhD (Doctor of Philosophy)—Applications 2009–2010, 39. Total applicants accepted 2009–2010, 9. Number full-time enrolled (new admits only) 2009–2010, 7. Openings 2010–2011, 6. The median number of years required for completion of a degree in 2008–2009 were 5. The number of students enrolled full- and part-time who were dismissed or voluntarily withdrew from this program area in 2008–2009 were 0.
Scores: Entries appear in this order: required test or GPA, minimum score (if required), median score of students entering in 2009–2010. *Human Development & Family Sciences PhD (Doctor of Philosophy):* GRE-V no minimum stated, GRE-Q no minimum stated, last 2 years GPA 3.0.
Other Criteria: (importance of criteria rated low, medium, or high): GRE scores—medium, research experience—high, work experience—low, extracurricular activity—low, clinically related public service—low, GPA—medium, letters of recommendation—high, statement of goals and objectives—high. For additional information on admission requirements, go to http://www.he.utexas.edu/hdfs/hdfsgradadmit.php.

Student Characteristics: The following represents characteristics of students in 2009–2010 in all graduate psychology programs in the department: Female—full-time 25, part-time 1; Male—full-time 7, part-time 0; African American/Black—full-time 4, part-time 0; Hispanic/Latino(a)—full-time 0, part-time 0; Asian/Pacific Islander—full-time 7, part-time 0; American Indian/Alaska Native—full-time 0, part-time 0; Caucasian/White—full-time 27, part-time 0; Multi-ethnic—full-time 0, part-time 0; students subject to the Americans With Disabilities Act—full-time 0, part-time 0; Unknown ethnicity—full-time 0, part-time 0; International students who hold an F-1 or J-1 Visa—full-time 0, part-time 0.

Financial Information/Assistance:
Tuition for Full-Time Study: *Doctoral:* State residents: per academic year $7,376; Nonstate residents: per academic year $14,464. Tuition is subject to change. See the following Web site for updates and changes in tuition costs: http://www.utexas.edu/tuition/costs.html.

Financial Assistance:
First-Year Students: Teaching assistantships available for first year. Average amount paid per academic year: $15,600. Average number of hours worked per week: 20. Apply by January 15. Research assistantships available for first year. Average amount paid per academic year: $15,600. Average number of hours worked per week: 20. Apply by January 15. Fellowships and scholarships available for first year. Average amount paid per academic year: $15,600. Apply by January 15.
Advanced Students: Teaching assistantships available for advanced students. Average amount paid per academic year: $16,140. Average number of hours worked per week: 20. Apply by January 15. Research assistantships available for advanced students. Average amount paid per academic year: $16,140. Average number of hours worked per week: 20. Apply by January 15. Fellowships and scholarships available for advanced students. Average amount paid per academic year: $16,000. Apply by January 15.
Additional Information: Of all students currently enrolled full time, 92% benefited from one or more of the listed financial assistance programs.

Internships/Practica: A variety of practicum experiences may be arranged to meet students' individual needs.

Housing and Day Care: On-campus housing is available. See the following Web site for more information: http://www.utexas.edu/student/housing/. On-campus day care facilities are available. See the following Web site for more information: http://www.utexas.edu/services/childcare/.

Employment of Department Graduates:
Master's Degree Graduates: Of those who graduated in the academic year 2008–2009, the following categories and numbers represent the postgraduate activities and employment of master's degree graduates: Enrolled in a postdoctoral residency/fellowship (n/a), employed in independent practice (n/a), total from the above (master's) (0).
Doctoral Degree Graduates: Of those who graduated in the academic year 2008–2009, the following categories and numbers represent the postgraduate activities and employment of doctoral degree graduates: Enrolled in a psychology doctoral program (n/a), total from the above (doctoral) (0).

Additional Information:
Orientation, Objectives, and Emphasis of Department: The program leading to the PhD in Human Development and Family Sciences is designed to prepare individuals for research, teaching, and administrative positions in colleges and universities and for positions in research, government, and other public and private settings. The focus of the program is research concerning the interplay between individual development and family relationships. Development of the individual is considered within the context of the family, peer group, community, and culture. The family is studied as a system of relationships, with attention given

to roles, communication, conflict resolution and negotiation, socialization, and family members' perceptions and emotions during interactions with one another. The program emphasizes the investigation of the family and other social processes that contribute to competence and optimal development in individuals from birth to maturity and on how such competencies, once developed, are reflected in interpersonal relationships and family interactions. The MA program in Human Development and Family Sciences is designed to deepen the student's knowledge of normal development within the context of the family, peer group, community, and culture, and to develop the student's skill in generating new knowledge in the field through basic or applied research.

Special Facilities or Resources: The graduate program is housed in the Sarah and Charles Seay Building, supporting wireless internet service with access to the university's extensive library collection and statistical software packages, and a computer lab reserved for graduate student research. The Seay Building contains a number of facilities for data collection, including five rooms in which children, couples, or families can be observed unobtrusively behind a one-way mirror in an observation booth. Students in the program may become involved in the university child and family laboratory, a laboratory preschool with about 80 three- to five-year-old children enrolled each semester. The school contains research rooms and observation facilities. In addition to the departmental resources, the multicultural population of Austin constitutes a rich resource for both research and practicum experiences. The library, computation center, and support services of the University of Texas at Austin are among the best in the nation. Free services available to students include the Learning Skills Center, Career Choice Information Center, and Counseling Center.

Information for Students With Physical Disabilities: See the following Web site for more information: http://www.utexas.edu/diversity/ddce/ssd/index.php.

Application Information:
Send to Graduate Coordinator, The University of Texas at Austin, Department of Human Development and Family Sciences, 1 University Station, A2702 Seay Building - Rm 1.432A, Austin, TX 78712-0141. Application available online. URL of online application: http://www.utexas.edu/student/admissions/grad/. Students are admitted in the Fall, application deadline January 15. *Fee:* $50.

Texas, University of, Austin
Department of Psychology
College of Liberal Arts
1 University Station A8000
Austin, TX 78712
Telephone: (512) 471-6398
Fax: (512) 471-5935
E-mail: *mazzucco@psy.utexas.edu*
Web: *http://www.psy.utexas.edu*

Department Information:
1910. Chairperson: James Pennebaker. Number of faculty: total—full-time 63; women—full-time 24; total—minority—full-time 7; women minority—full-time 3.

Programs and Degrees Offered:
Listed in the following order: Program area, degree type (T if terminal Master's), number awarded 7/08–6/09. Clinical Psychology PhD (Doctor of Philosophy) 7, Developmental Psychology PhD (Doctor of Philosophy) 4, Individual Differences and Evolutionary Psychology PhD (Doctor of Philosophy) 2, Behavioral Neuroscience PhD (Doctor of Philosophy) 2, Social and Personality Psychology PhD (Doctor of Philosophy) 2, Cognitive Systems PhD (Doctor of Philosophy) 3, Perceptual Systems PhD (Doctor of Philosophy) 0.

APA Accreditation: Clinical PhD (Doctor of Philosophy). Student Outcome Data Website: http://www.psy.utexas.edu/psy/clinical/progstats.html.

Student Applications/Admissions:
Student Applications

Clinical Psychology PhD (Doctor of Philosophy)—Applications 2009–2010, 324. Total applicants accepted 2009–2010, 4. Number full-time enrolled (new admits only) 2009–2010, 4. Openings 2010–2011, 4. The median number of years required for completion of a degree in 2008–2009 were 6. The number of students enrolled full- and part-time who were dismissed or voluntarily withdrew from this program area in 2008–2009 were 2. *Developmental Psychology PhD (Doctor of Philosophy)*—Applications 2009–2010, 32. Total applicants accepted 2009–2010, 0. Number full-time enrolled (new admits only) 2009–2010, 0. Openings 2010–2011, 4. The median number of years required for completion of a degree in 2008–2009 were 5. The number of students enrolled full- and part-time who were dismissed or voluntarily withdrew from this program area in 2008–2009 were 2. *Individual Differences and Evolutionary Psychology PhD (Doctor of Philosophy)*—Applications 2009–2010, 35. Total applicants accepted 2009–2010, 1. Number full-time enrolled (new admits only) 2009–2010, 1. Openings 2010–2011, 1. The median number of years required for completion of a degree in 2008–2009 were 6. The number of students enrolled full- and part-time who were dismissed or voluntarily withdrew from this program area in 2008–2009 were 0. *Behavioral Neuroscience PhD (Doctor of Philosophy)*—Applications 2009–2010, 49. Total applicants accepted 2009–2010, 6. Number full-time enrolled (new admits only) 2009–2010, 4. Openings 2010–2011, 4. The median number of years required for completion of a degree in 2008–2009 were 7. The number of students enrolled full- and part-time who were dismissed or voluntarily withdrew from this program area in 2008–2009 were 1. *Social and Personality Psychology PhD (Doctor of Philosophy)*—Applications 2009–2010, 124. Total applicants accepted 2009–2010, 3. Number full-time enrolled (new admits only) 2009–2010, 2. Openings 2010–2011, 3. The median number of years required for completion of a degree in 2008–2009 were 5. The number of students enrolled full- and part-time who were dismissed or voluntarily withdrew from this program area in 2008–2009 were 0. *Cognitive Systems PhD (Doctor of Philosophy)*—Applications 2009–2010, 103. Total applicants accepted 2009–2010, 6. Number full-time enrolled (new admits only) 2009–2010, 5. Total enrolled 2009–2010 full-time, 18. Openings 2010–2011, 5. The median number of years required for completion of a degree in 2008–2009 were 6. The number of students enrolled full- and part-time who were dismissed or voluntarily withdrew from this program area in 2008–2009 were 3. *Perceptual Systems PhD (Doctor of Philosophy)*—Applications 2009–2010, 11. Total applicants accepted 2009–2010, 1. Number full-time enrolled (new admits only) 2009–2010, 1. Total enrolled 2009–2010 full-time, 8. Openings 2010–2011, 2. The number of students enrolled full- and part-time who were dismissed or voluntarily withdrew from this program area in 2008–2009 were 1.

Scores: Entries appear in this order: required test or GPA, minimum score (if required), median score of students entering in 2009–2010. *Clinical Psychology PhD (Doctor of Philosophy):* GRE-V no minimum stated, 576, GRE-Q no minimum stated, 649, GRE-Analytical no minimum stated, 4.48, last 2 years GPA no minimum stated, 3.77; *Developmental Psychology PhD (Doctor of Philosophy):* GRE-V no minimum stated, 532, GRE-Q no minimum stated, 640, GRE-Analytical no minimum stated, 3.96, last 2 years GPA no minimum stated, 3.67; *Individual Differences and Evolutionary Psychology PhD (Doctor of Philosophy):* GRE-V no minimum stated, 563, GRE-Q no minimum stated, 692, GRE-Analytical no minimum stated, 4.47, last 2 years GPA no minimum stated, 3.91; *Behavioral Neuroscience PhD (Doctor of Philosophy):* GRE-V no minimum stated, 527, GRE-Q no minimum stated, 639, GRE-Analytical no minimum stated, 4.26, last 2 years GPA no minimum stated, 3.43; *Social and Personality Psychology PhD (Doctor of Philosophy):* GRE-V no minimum stated, 575, GRE-Q no minimum stated, 656, GRE-Analytical no minimum stated, 4.33, last 2 years GPA no minimum stated, 3.85, Masters GPA no minimum stated; *Cognitive Systems PhD (Doctor of Philosophy):* GRE-V no minimum stated, 578, GRE-Q no minimum stated, 710, GRE-Analytical no minimum stated, 4.40, last 2 years GPA no minimum stated, 3.55; *Perceptual Systems PhD (Doctor of Philosophy):* GRE-V no minimum stated, 601, GRE-Q no minimum stated, 731, GRE-Analytical no minimum stated, 4.05, last 2 years GPA no minimum stated, 3.93.

Other Criteria: (importance of criteria rated low, medium, or high): GRE scores—high, research experience—high, work experience—medium, extracurricular activity—low, clinically related public service—medium, GPA—high, letters of recommendation—high, interview—high, statement of goals and objectives—high, undergraduate major in psychology—medium, specific undergraduate psychology courses taken—medium. For additional information on admission requirements, go to http://www.psy.utexas.edu/psy/GradProgram/application.html.

Student Characteristics: The following represents characteristics of students in 2009–2010 in all graduate psychology programs in the department: Female—full-time 43, part-time 0; Male—full-time 59, part-time 0; African American/Black—full-time 4, part-time 0; Hispanic/Latino(a)—full-time 9, part-time 0; Asian/Pacific Islander—full-time 4, part-time 0; American Indian/Alaska Native—full-time 1, part-time 0; Caucasian/White—full-time 68, part-time 0; Multi-ethnic—full-time 0, part-time 0; students subject to the Americans With Disabilities Act—full-time 0, part-time 0; Unknown ethnicity—full-time 16, part-time 0; International students who hold an F-1 or J-1 Visa—full-time 0, part-time 0.

Financial Information/Assistance:
 Tuition for Full-Time Study: *Doctoral:* State residents: per academic year $7,377; Nonstate residents: per academic year $14,759. Tuition is subject to change. See the following Web site for updates and changes in tuition costs: http://www.utexas.edu/business/accounting/sar/t_f_rates.html.

Financial Assistance:
 First-Year Students: Teaching assistantships available for first year. Average amount paid per academic year: $14,994. Average number of hours worked per week: 20. Research assistantships available for first year. Average amount paid per academic year: $14,994. Average number of hours worked per week: 20. Fellowships and scholarships available for first year. Average amount paid per academic year: $5,200.

 Advanced Students: Teaching assistantships available for advanced students. Average amount paid per academic year: $16,306. Average number of hours worked per week: 20. Research assistantships available for advanced students. Average amount paid per academic year: $16,306. Average number of hours worked per week: 20. Fellowships and scholarships available for advanced students. Average amount paid per academic year: $20,000.

 Additional Information: Of all students currently enrolled full time, 100% benefited from one or more of the listed financial assistance programs. Application and information available online at: http://www.psy.utexas.edu/psy/GradProgram/financial.html.

Internships/Practica: Doctoral Degree (PhD Clinical Psychology): For those doctoral students for whom a professional internship was required in this program prior to graduation, (5) students applied for an internship in 2008–2009, with (5) students obtaining an internship. Of those students who obtained an internship, (5) were paid internships. Of those students who obtained an internship, (5) students placed in APA/CPA accredited internships, (0) students placed in internships not APA/CPA accredited, but listed with the Association of Psychology Postdoctoral and Internship Programs (APPIC), (0) students placed in internships conforming to guidelines of the Council of Directors of School Psychology Programs (CDSPP), (0) students placed in internships that were not APA/CPA accredited, APPIC or CDSPP listed. Clinical students participate in practica at agencies in the Austin area, including the Austin State Hospital, Austin Child Guidance Center, Brown Schools, and the UT Counseling-Psychological Services Center. Most students select an internship at nationally recognized clinical settings such as the Langley Porter Neuropsychiatric Institute, or the University of California at San Diego Psychological Internship Consortium. Local settings are also available.

Housing and Day Care: No on-campus housing is available. On-campus day care facilities are available. See the following Web site for more information: http://www.utexas.edu/childcenter/.

Employment of Department Graduates:
 Master's Degree Graduates: Of those who graduated in the academic year 2008–2009, the following categories and numbers represent the postgraduate activities and employment of master's degree graduates: Enrolled in a postdoctoral residency/fellowship (n/a), employed in independent practice (n/a), total from the above (master's) (0).

 Doctoral Degree Graduates: Of those who graduated in the academic year 2008–2009, the following categories and numbers

represent the postgraduate activities and employment of doctoral degree graduates: Enrolled in a psychology doctoral program (n/a), enrolled in a postdoctoral residency/fellowship (6), employed in an academic position at a university (6), employed in an academic position at a 2-year/4-year college (1), employed in business or industry (1), employed in a hospital/medical center (5), do not know (1), total from the above (doctoral) (20).

Additional Information:
Orientation, Objectives, and Emphasis of Department: The major goal of graduate training in the Department of Psychology is to aid in developing the competence and professional commitment that are essential to scholarly contributions in the field of psychology. All students, upon completing the program, are expected to be well informed about general psychology, well qualified to conduct independent research, and prepared to teach in their area of interest. Within certain specialized areas, they will be prepared for professional practice. The program culminates in the PhD degree, and it is designed for the person committed to psychological research and an academic career. All of the graduate study areas have a strong academic research emphasis. All of the areas also recognize the necessity of developing knowledge and skills for applied research positions and, in the clinical area, for professional competence.

Special Facilities or Resources: The Department of Psychology moved into the Seay Building in May of 2002. This building houses seminar rooms, offices, and research laboratories. The research space includes small rooms for individual testing and larger rooms for group experiments. Some rooms have adjacent observation rooms. An anechoic testing chamber is available for auditory research. All of the departmental laboratories have computers associated with them. Departmental computers are available for student use. Facilities for research with children include the Children's Research Laboratory with numerous experimental suites. The facilities of the Animal Resource Center support research with animals. The support resources of the department include two well-equipped shops with full-time technicians and staff for computer assistance. The support resources of the university include the Computation Center, one of the finest academic computation facilities in the United States, and the Perry-Castaneda Library, one of the largest academic libraries in the country. Faculty members in the department of Psychology are affiliated with the Center for Perceptual Systems, the Institute for Cognitive Science, and the Institute for Neuroscience.

Information for Students With Physical Disabilities: See the following Web site for more information: http://deanofstudents.utexas.edu/ssd/.

Application Information:
Send to The University of Texas at Austin, Graduate and International Admissions Center, P.O. Box 7608, Austin, TX 78713-7608. Application available online. URL of online application: http://www.applytexas.org. Students are admitted in the Fall, application deadline January 1. The deadline for the Clinical Area only is December 1. *Fee:* $50. McNair Scholars will have application fee waived. International students pay a $75 application fee.

Texas, University of, Dallas
Psychological Sciences
School of Behavioral and Brain Sciences
800 West Campbell Road, GR 41
Richardson, TX 75080-3021
Telephone: (972) 883-2355
Fax: (972) 883-2491
E-mail: *mary.felipe@utdallas.edu;*
  adrienne.barnett@utdallas.edu
Web: *http://www.utdallas.edu/bbs/*

Department Information:
1976. Program Heads: Dr. Melanie Spence and Dr. Marion Underwood. Number of faculty: total—full-time 33; women—full-time 17.

Programs and Degrees Offered:
Listed in the following order: Program area, degree type (T if terminal Master's), number awarded 7/08–6/09. M.S. Psychological Sciences MA/MS (Master of Arts/Science) (T) 1, Phd Psychological Sciences PhD (Doctor of Philosophy) 3.

Student Applications/Admissions:
Student Applications
M.S. *Psychological Sciences MA/MS (Master of Arts/Science)*—Applications 2009–2010, 55. Total applicants accepted 2009–2010, 8. Number full-time enrolled (new admits only) 2009–2010, 8. Total enrolled 2009–2010 full-time, 22. Openings 2010–2011, 30. The median number of years required for completion of a degree in 2008–2009 were 2. The number of students enrolled full- and part-time who were dismissed or voluntarily withdrew from this program area in 2008–2009 were 0. *Phd Psychological Sciences PhD (Doctor of Philosophy)*—Applications 2009–2010, 56. Total applicants accepted 2009–2010, 11. Number full-time enrolled (new admits only) 2009–2010, 3. Number part-time enrolled (new admits only) 2009–2010, 2. Total enrolled 2009–2010 full-time, 17, part-time, 8. Openings 2010–2011, 5. The median number of years required for completion of a degree in 2008–2009 were 6. The number of students enrolled full- and part-time who were dismissed or voluntarily withdrew from this program area in 2008–2009 were 1.
Scores: Entries appear in this order: required test or GPA, minimum score (if required), median score of students entering in 2009–2010. M.S. *Psychological Sciences MA/MS (Master of Arts/Science):* GRE-V no minimum stated, GRE-Q no minimum stated, overall undergraduate GPA 3.0; *PhD Psychological Sciences PhD (Doctor of Philosophy):* GRE-V no minimum stated, GRE-Q no minimum stated, overall undergraduate GPA 3.0.
Other Criteria: (importance of criteria rated low, medium, or high): GRE scores—high, research experience—high, work experience—medium, extracurricular activity—medium, GPA—high, letters of recommendation—high, interview—medium, statement of goals and objectives—high, fit w/ faculty mentor—high, undergraduate major in psychology—high, specific undergraduate psychology courses taken—high. For additional information on admission requirements, go to http://bbs.utdallas.edu/students/graduate/prosp_psy_sciences.html.

GRADUATE STUDY IN PSYCHOLOGY

Student Characteristics: The following represents characteristics of students in 2009–2010 in all graduate psychology programs in the department: Female—full-time 29, part-time 6; Male—full-time 10, part-time 2; African American/Black—full-time 4, part-time 0; Hispanic/Latino(a)—full-time 2, part-time 2; Asian/Pacific Islander—full-time 6, part-time 2; American Indian/Alaska Native—full-time 0, part-time 0; Caucasian/White—full-time 27, part-time 4; Multi-ethnic—full-time 0, part-time 0; students subject to the Americans With Disabilities Act—full-time 0, part-time 0; Unknown ethnicity—full-time 0, part-time 0; International students who hold an F-1 or J-1 Visa—full-time 7, part-time 0.

Financial Information/Assistance:

Tuition for Full-Time Study: *Master's:* State residents: per academic year $10,248; Nonstate residents: per academic year $18,500. *Doctoral:* State residents: per academic year $10,248; Nonstate residents: per academic year $18,500. Tuition is subject to change. See the following Web site for updates and changes in tuition costs: http://www.utdallas.edu/finance/bursar/.

Financial Assistance:

First-Year Students: Teaching assistantships available for first year. Average amount paid per academic year: $13,656. Average number of hours worked per week: 20. Apply by February 1. Research assistantships available for first year. Average amount paid per academic year: $13,656. Average number of hours worked per week: 20. Apply by February 1.

Advanced Students: Teaching assistantships available for advanced students. Average amount paid per academic year: $16,224. Average number of hours worked per week: 20. Apply by February 1. Research assistantships available for advanced students. Average amount paid per academic year: $16,224. Average number of hours worked per week: 20. Apply by February 1.

Additional Information: Of all students currently enrolled full time, 98% benefited from one or more of the listed financial assistance programs. Application and information available online at: http://www.utdallas.edu/student/finaid/.

Internships/Practica: Master's Degree (MA/MS M.S. Psychological Sciences): An internship experience, such as a final research project or "capstone" experience is required of graduates. Students in the MS program have the opportunity to gain applied experiences through the internship program in the School of Behavioral and Brain Sciences, which facilitates networking with a variety of community agencies and programs.

Housing and Day Care: On-campus housing is available. See the following Web site for more information: http://www.utdallas.edu/housing/. No on-campus day care facilities are available.

Employment of Department Graduates:

Master's Degree Graduates: Of those who graduated in the academic year 2008–2009, the following categories and numbers represent the postgraduate activities and employment of master's degree graduates: Enrolled in a postdoctoral residency/fellowship (n/a), employed in independent practice (n/a), total from the above (master's) (0).

Doctoral Degree Graduates: Of those who graduated in the academic year 2008–2009, the following categories and numbers represent the postgraduate activities and employment of doctoral degree graduates: Enrolled in a psychology doctoral program (n/a), employed in an academic position at a university (2), do not know (1), total from the above (doctoral) (3).

Additional Information:

Orientation, Objectives, and Emphasis of Department: The Psychological Sciences PhD program is an experimental psychology program that prepares students for leadership roles in research and teaching. Students benefit from the high quality of faculty research, small classes and seminars, extensive professional development, and a rich array of interdisciplinary opportunities within the School of Behavioral and Brain Sciences. Students can major in developmental psychology or cognitive psychology. The University requires a minimum of 90 hours of coursework. The specific program requirements include: six credit hours of a doctoral proseminar, nine hours of core research methods courses, 12 hours of core psychological sciences courses, six hours of advanced electives, and independent study research hours each semester enrolled. From the start of training, students are actively engaged in research laboratories with a faculty mentor. The research requirements include a qualifying thesis research project and a dissertation research project. Students are expected to complete the program coursework and research requirements in four years. Professional development is facilitated through School colloquia, regular brown bag series, presentations at professional meetings, and guidance in the development of teaching skills. The Master of Science program, which began in Fall 2008, provides advanced training to prepare serious student scholars for nationally prominent doctoral programs in clinical and experimental psychology. This research-focused program requires active involvement with a research mentor and at least one laboratory throughout the two-year training. Students complete advanced coursework and have the opportunity to gain applied experiences through the internship program. The program does not provide clinical training or lead to licensure as a counselor or psychologist. The M.S. curriculum offers opportunities for specialization in the following core fields: developmental, cognitive, social and personality, and neuroscience. Masters students take mostly doctoral-level coursework. The degree requires 36 graduate credit hours: six hours of core courses in the student's area of specialization, six hours of core courses from an area other than the student's specialization, six hours of core courses in research methods, twelve hours of advanced electives and six hours of independent research or a practical internship.

Special Facilities or Resources: The Psychological Sciences program is a part of the U.T. Dallas School of Behavioral and Brain Sciences, which offers exceptional research facilities, including an on-site laboratory preschool, infant research labs, and video observation laboratories. The Psychological Sciences faculty has strong expertise in development from infancy through the lifespan, social relationships at all stages of life, and cognition and neuroscience, including an emerging emphasis on brain imaging. Many of the Psychological Sciences faculty work collaboratively across our doctoral programs in Cognition and Neuroscience, Communication Sciences and Disorders, and Audiology. The doctoral programs are complemented by four research centers: the Center for Brain Health, the Callier Center, the Center for Children and Families, and the Center for Vital Longevity.

Information for Students With Physical Disabilities: See the following Web site for more information: http://www.utdallas.edu/disability/.

Application Information:
Send to The University of Texas at Dallas Office of Enrollment Services, HH10 800 West Campbell Road Richardson, TX 75080-3021. Application available online. URL of online application: http://bbs.utdallas.edu/students/admissions/graduate.html. Students are admitted in the Fall, application deadline February 1. *Fee:* $50.

Texas, University of, El Paso
Department of Psychology
500 West University Avenue
El Paso, TX 79968-0553
Telephone: (915) 747-5551
Fax: (915) 747-6553
E-mail: *Lcohn@utep.edu*
Web: *http://academics.utep.edu/psychology*

Department Information:
1965. Chairperson: Edward Castaneda. Number of faculty: total—full-time 17; women—full-time 5; total—minority—full-time 4; women minority—full-time 1.

Programs and Degrees Offered:
Listed in the following order: Program area, degree type (T if terminal Master's), number awarded 7/08–6/09. Clinical Psychology MA/MS (Master of Arts/Science) (T) 4, Psychology PhD (Doctor of Philosophy) 5.

Student Applications/Admissions:
Student Applications
Clinical Psychology MA/MS (*Master of Arts/Science*)—Applications 2009–2010, 19. Total applicants accepted 2009–2010, 8. Number full-time enrolled (new admits only) 2009–2010, 3. Number part-time enrolled (new admits only) 2009–2010, 0. Openings 2010–2011, 5. The number of students enrolled full- and part-time who were dismissed or voluntarily withdrew from this program area in 2008–2009 were 1. *Psychology PhD (Doctor of Philosophy)*—Applications 2009–2010, 57. Total applicants accepted 2009–2010, 27. Number full-time enrolled (new admits only) 2009–2010, 6. Number part-time enrolled (new admits only) 2009–2010, 0. Openings 2010–2011, 17. The median number of years required for completion of a degree in 2008–2009 were 4. The number of students enrolled full- and part-time who were dismissed or voluntarily withdrew from this program area in 2008–2009 were 1.
Scores: Entries appear in this order: required test or GPA, minimum score (if required), median score of students entering in 2009–2010. *Clinical Psychology MA/MS (Master of Arts/Science):* GRE-V no minimum stated, GRE-Q no minimum stated, overall undergraduate GPA no minimum stated, 3.7; *Psychology PhD (Doctor of Philosophy):* GRE-V no minimum stated, GRE-Q no minimum stated, overall undergraduate GPA no minimum stated, 3.4.
Other Criteria: (importance of criteria rated low, medium, or high): GRE scores—high, research experience—high, work experience—low, extracurricular activity—low, clinically related public service—low, GPA—high, letters of recommendation—high, statement of goals and objectives—high, Applicants who did not major or minor in psychology need to take several leveling courses before their application will be considered competitive. For additional information on admission requirements, go to http://academics.utep.edu/Default.aspx?tabid=26639.

Student Characteristics: The following represents characteristics of students in 2009–2010 in all graduate psychology programs in the department: Female—full-time 28, part-time 0; Male—full-time 19, part-time 0; African American/Black—full-time 0, part-time 0; Hispanic/Latino(a)—full-time 19, part-time 0; Asian/Pacific Islander—full-time 1, part-time 0; American Indian/Alaska Native—part-time 0; Caucasian/White—full-time 21, part-time 0; Multi-ethnic—full-time 0, part-time 0; students subject to the Americans With Disabilities Act—full-time 0, part-time 0; Unknown ethnicity—full-time 6, part-time 0; International students who hold an F-1 or J-1 Visa—full-time 6, part-time 0.

Financial Information/Assistance:
Tuition for Full-Time Study: Master's: State residents: per academic year $4,547, $198 per credit hour; Nonstate residents: per academic year $9,583, $475 per credit hour. *Doctoral:* State residents: per academic year $4,547, $198 per credit hour; Nonstate residents: per academic year $4,547, $198 per credit hour. Tuition is subject to change. See the following Web site for updates and changes in tuition costs: http://academics.utep.edu/Default.aspx?tabid=44130.

Financial Assistance:
First-Year Students: Teaching assistantships available for first year. Average amount paid per academic year: $15,000. Average number of hours worked per week: 20. Apply by December 15. Research assistantships available for first year. Average amount paid per academic year: $15,000. Average number of hours worked per week: 20. Apply by December 15.
Advanced Students: Teaching assistantships available for advanced students. Average amount paid per academic year: $15,000. Average number of hours worked per week: 20. Apply by December 15. Research assistantships available for advanced students. Average amount paid per academic year: $15,000. Average number of hours worked per week: 20. Apply by December 15.
Additional Information: Of all students currently enrolled full time, 100% benefited from one or more of the listed financial assistance programs. Application and information available online at: http://academics.utep.edu/finaid.

Internships/Practica: Master's Degree (MA/MS Clinical Psychology): An internship experience, such as, a final research project or "capstone" experience is required of graduates. The Clinical MA program requires three hours of internship.

Housing and Day Care: On-campus housing is available. See the following Web site for more information: http://studentaffairs.utep.edu/minervillage. On-campus day care facilities are available. See the following Web site for more information: http://studentaffairs.utep.edu/childcare.

Employment of Department Graduates:
Master's Degree Graduates: Of those who graduated in the academic year 2008–2009, the following categories and numbers represent the postgraduate activities and employment of master's degree graduates: Enrolled in a psychology doctoral program (1), enrolled in another graduate/professional program (1), enrolled in a postdoctoral residency/fellowship (n/a), employed in indepen-

dent practice (n/a), employed in an academic position at a 2-year/4-year college (0), employed in a professional position in a school system (0), employed in business or industry (0), employed in government agency (0), employed in a community mental health/counseling center (0), employed in a hospital/medical center (0), still seeking employment (0), not seeking employment (0), other employment position (0), do not know (0), total from the above (master's) (2).

Doctoral Degree Graduates: Of those who graduated in the academic year 2008–2009, the following categories and numbers represent the postgraduate activities and employment of doctoral degree graduates: Enrolled in a psychology doctoral program (n/a), enrolled in another graduate/professional program (0), enrolled in a postdoctoral residency/fellowship (1), employed in independent practice (0), employed in an academic position at a university (2), employed in an academic position at a 2-year/4-year college (0), employed in other positions at a higher education institution (1), employed in a professional position in a school system (0), employed in business or industry (0), employed in government agency (1), employed in a community mental health/counseling center (0), employed in a hospital/medical center (0), still seeking employment (0), not seeking employment (0), other employment position (0), do not know (0), total from the above (doctoral) (5).

Additional Information:
Orientation, Objectives, and Emphasis of Department: The PhD program is designed to train research psychologists and offers four areas of concentration: (1) Health, (2) Legal, (3) Language Acquisition and Bilingualism, and (4) Social, Cognitive, & Neuroscience. The general experimental MA program, intended for students who will pursue a PhD degree, emphasizes research methodology and experimental design, and focuses on a variety of substantive areas in psychology. The clinical MA program is designed as a terminal master's degree and emphasizes all applied skills in psychological assessment. A special focus is directed toward bilingual, bicultural issues.

Special Facilities or Resources: The Psychology Department occupies a three story, 24,000 square foot building that contains state-of-the-art equipment for investigating a wide range of cognitive, behavioral, and neuro-chemical processes and phenomena. Laboratories contain virtual reality equipment for studies of aggression, reaction time equipment for studies of stereotyping and language processing, EEG equipment for studies of attitudes, stereotypes, and deception, picturing morphing equipment for studies of eyewitness identification, and eye-tracking equipment for studies of cognitive processes that guide bilingual reading. Neuroscience labs contain neurochemistry equipment for quantifying brain neurotransmitter levels, and behavioral equipment for assessing addictive behavior, anxiety-like properties, memory function, and fine motor movements. The neuroscience space also contains a recently renovated animal vivarium. Additional labs contain sound-proofed interview rooms equipped with covert digital audio-video recording devices, carbon monoxide monitors for assessing short term smoking status, blood alcohol level monitors for studies of intoxication, and psychophysiological instruments for monitoring heart rate, eye blinks, the startle reflex, and inhibitory control. The Psychology Department has also established numerous community-based participatory research projects. Off-campus sites include clinics, schools, hospitals, medical centers, and a large military base, as well as other community settings in a bi-cultural environment.

Information for Students With Physical Disabilities: See the following Web site for more information: http://www.utep.edu/.

Application Information:
Send to Graduate School Academic Services Building, Room 223, University of Texas at El Paso, 500 W. University Avenue, El Paso, TX 79968-0566. Application available online. URL of online application: http://academics.utep.edu/Default.aspx?tabid=25001. Students are admitted in the Fall, application deadline December 15. *Fee:* $45. The fee for Mexican applicants is $45; the fee for all other international applicants is $80.

Texas, University of, Pan American
Department of Psychology and Anthropology
College of Social and Behavioral Sciences
1201 West University Drive, SBSC 358
Edinburg, TX 78541
Telephone: (956) 381-3329
Fax: (956) 381-3333
E-mail: *pgasquoine@panam.edu*
Web: *http://www.utpa.edu/dept/psych-anth*

Department Information:
1972. Graduate Program Director: Philip Gasquoine, PhD. Number of faculty: total—full-time 14; women—full-time 6; total—minority—full-time 6; women minority—full-time 4.

Programs and Degrees Offered:
Listed in the following order: Program area, degree type (T if terminal Master's), number awarded 7/08–6/09. Clinical MA/MS (Master of Arts/Science) (T) 8, Experimental MA/MS (Master of Arts/Science) (T) 2, Experimental (Board Certified Behavior Analyst) MA/MS (Master of Arts/Science) 0.

Student Applications/Admissions:
Student Applications
Clinical MA/MS (Master of Arts/Science)—Applications 2009–2010, 56. Total applicants accepted 2009–2010, 14. Number full-time enrolled (new admits only) 2009–2010, 11. Number part-time enrolled (new admits only) 2009–2010, 3. Total enrolled 2009–2010 full-time, 28, part-time, 20. Openings 2010–2011, 20. The median number of years required for completion of a degree in 2008–2009 were 3. The number of students enrolled full- and part-time who were dismissed or voluntarily withdrew from this program area in 2008–2009 were 2. *Experimental MA/MS (Master of Arts/Science)*—Applications 2009–2010, 3. Total applicants accepted 2009–2010, 1. Number part-time enrolled (new admits only) 2009–2010, 0. Openings 2010–2011, 1. The median number of years required for completion of a degree in 2008–2009 were 2. The number of students enrolled full- and part-time who were dismissed or voluntarily withdrew from this program area in 2008–2009 were 0. *Experimental (Board Certified Behavior Analyst) MA/MS (Master of Arts/Science)*—Applications 2009–2010, 10. Total applicants accepted 2009–2010, 10. Number full-time enrolled (new admits only) 2009–2010, 10. Number part-time enrolled (new admits only) 2009–2010, 0. Openings 2010–2011, 10. The median number of years required for completion of a degree in 2008–2009 were 2. The number of

students enrolled full- and part-time who were dismissed or voluntarily withdrew from this program area in 2008–2009 were 1.

Scores: Entries appear in this order: required test or GPA, minimum score (if required), median score of students entering in 2009–2010. *Clinical MA/MS (Master of Arts/Science):* GRE-V no minimum stated, GRE-Q no minimum stated, last 2 years GPA 3.0, psychology GPA 3.0; *Experimental MA/MS (Master of Arts/Science):* GRE-V no minimum stated, GRE-Q no minimum stated, last 2 years GPA 3.0, psychology GPA 3.0; *Experimental (Board Certified Behavior Analyst) MA/MS (Master of Arts/Science):* GRE-V no minimum stated, GRE-Q no minimum stated, last 2 years GPA 3.0, psychology GPA 3.0.

Other Criteria: (importance of criteria rated low, medium, or high): GRE scores—low, research experience—high, work experience—high, extracurricular activity—medium, clinically related public service—medium, GPA—high, letters of recommendation—high, statement of goals and objectives—medium, undergraduate major in psychology—medium, specific undergraduate psychology courses taken—medium.

Student Characteristics: The following represents characteristics of students in 2009–2010 in all graduate psychology programs in the department: Female—full-time 41, part-time 13; Male—full-time 10, part-time 7; African American/Black—full-time 0, part-time 0; Hispanic/Latino(a)—full-time 45, part-time 17; Asian/Pacific Islander—full-time 0, part-time 0; American Indian/Alaska Native—full-time 0, part-time 0; Caucasian/White—full-time 6, part-time 3; Multi-ethnic—full-time 0, part-time 0; students subject to the Americans With Disabilities Act—full-time 1, part-time 0; Unknown ethnicity—full-time 0, part-time 0; International students who hold an F-1 or J-1 Visa—full-time 0, part-time 0.

Financial Information/Assistance:
Tuition for Full-Time Study: *Master's:* State residents: $277 per credit hour; Nonstate residents: $554 per credit hour. Tuition is subject to change. Additional fees are assessed to students beyond the costs of tuition for the following: $75 course fee per semester.

Financial Assistance:
First-Year Students: Teaching assistantships available for first year. Average amount paid per academic year: $7,000. Average number of hours worked per week: 19. Research assistantships available for first year. Average amount paid per academic year: $10,000. Average number of hours worked per week: 19.

Advanced Students: Teaching assistantships available for advanced students. Average amount paid per academic year: $7,000. Average number of hours worked per week: 19.

Additional Information: Of all students currently enrolled full time, 7% benefited from one or more of the listed financial assistance programs.

Internships/Practica: Master's Degree (MA/MS Clinical): An internship experience, such as a final research project or "capstone" experience is required of graduates. Internships in clinical psychology are for 480 clock hours, at least 100 of which must involve direct patient contact. Internship sites include independent licensed psychologists, public and private mental health clinics and hospitals. Practica for the Experimental BCBA program allow for completion of enough hours to become eligible to sit for the national certification exam.

Housing and Day Care: On-campus housing is available. See the following Web site for more information: Phone: (956) 381-3439; http://www.utpa.edu/reslife. On-campus day care facilities are available. See the following Web site for more information: http://www.utpa.edu/ess/childcare/.

Employment of Department Graduates:
Master's Degree Graduates: Of those who graduated in the academic year 2008–2009, the following categories and numbers represent the postgraduate activities and employment of master's degree graduates: Enrolled in a postdoctoral residency/fellowship (n/a), employed in independent practice (n/a), total from the above (master's) (0).

Doctoral Degree Graduates: Of those who graduated in the academic year 2008–2009, the following categories and numbers represent the postgraduate activities and employment of doctoral degree graduates: Enrolled in a psychology doctoral program (n/a), total from the above (doctoral) (0).

Additional Information:
Orientation, Objectives, and Emphasis of Department: The Masters degree in Clinical Psychology is designed to provide research-based assessment and intervention strategies, skills training, diagnostic assessment skills, clinical experience, and supervision of professional practices in the field of applied psychology. The program is designed to fulfill academic requirements for taking the Texas State Board Exam as a Licensed Psychological Associate (LPA) and/or a Licensed Professional Counselor (LPC). There are thesis and non-thesis tracks. The Masters degree in Experimental Psychology has two tracks, general and BCBA. All students must complete a thesis. The general track prepares students for admission to research PhD programs and the BCBA track satisfies requirements for taking the national Board Certification exam as a Behavior Analyst.

Special Facilities or Resources: The graduate psychology clinic has four consultation rooms, including monitoring equipment (A/V) for individual and group sessions and supervision.

Application Information:
Send to Office of Graduate Studies, Administration Building Rm 116, University of Texas - Pan American, 1201 West University Drive, Edinburg, TX 78541. Application available online. URL of online application: http://www.utpa.edu/gradschool. Students are admitted in the Fall, application deadline July 1; Spring, application deadline November 1. Experimental BCBA students are only admitted in the Fall. *Fee:* $50.

Texas, University of, Tyler
Department of Psychology
3900 University Boulevard
Tyler, TX 75799
Telephone: (903) 566-7130
Fax: (903) 565-5923
E-mail: *cbarke@uttyler.edu*
Web: *http://www.uttyler.edu/psychology/*

Department Information:
1973. Chairperson: Charles Barke. Number of faculty: total—full-time 13, part-time 6; women—full-time 5, part-time 4.

GRADUATE STUDY IN PSYCHOLOGY

Programs and Degrees Offered:
Listed in the following order: Program area, degree type (T if terminal Master's), number awarded 7/08–6/09. Counseling Psychology MA/MS (Master of Arts/Science) (T) 4, School Counseling MA/MS (Master of Arts/Science) (T) 10, Clinical MA/MS (Master of Arts/Science) (T) 11.

Student Applications/Admissions:

Student Applications
Counseling Psychology MA/MS (Master of Arts/Science)—Applications 2009–2010, 22. Total applicants accepted 2009–2010, 15. Number full-time enrolled (new admits only) 2009–2010, 9. Number part-time enrolled (new admits only) 2009–2010, 6. Total enrolled 2009–2010 full-time, 25, part-time, 22. Openings 2010–2011, 20. The median number of years required for completion of a degree in 2008–2009 were 2. The number of students enrolled full- and part-time who were dismissed or voluntarily withdrew from this program area in 2008–2009 were 5. *School Counseling MA/MS (Master of Arts/Science)*—Applications 2009–2010, 18. Total applicants accepted 2009–2010, 14. Number full-time enrolled (new admits only) 2009–2010, 2. Number part-time enrolled (new admits only) 2009–2010, 12. Total enrolled 2009–2010 full-time, 18, part-time, 32. Openings 2010–2011, 15. The median number of years required for completion of a degree in 2008–2009 were 2. The number of students enrolled full- and part-time who were dismissed or voluntarily withdrew from this program area in 2008–2009 were 3. *Clinical MA/MS (Master of Arts/Science)*—Applications 2009–2010, 30. Total applicants accepted 2009–2010, 14. Number full-time enrolled (new admits only) 2009–2010, 8. Number part-time enrolled (new admits only) 2009–2010, 6. Total enrolled 2009–2010 full-time, 30, part-time, 10. Openings 2010–2011, 15. The median number of years required for completion of a degree in 2008–2009 were 2. The number of students enrolled full- and part-time who were dismissed or voluntarily withdrew from this program area in 2008–2009 were 4.

Scores: Entries appear in this order: required test or GPA, minimum score (if required), median score of students entering in 2009–2010. *Counseling Psychology MA/MS (Master of Arts/Science)*: GRE-V 450, GRE-Q 450, overall undergraduate GPA 2.75; *School Counseling MA/MS (Master of Arts/Science)*: GRE-V 450, GRE-Q 450, overall undergraduate GPA 2.75; *Clinical MA/MS (Master of Arts/Science)*: GRE-V 450, GRE-Q 450, overall undergraduate GPA 2.75, last 2 years GPA 3.00.

Other Criteria: (importance of criteria rated low, medium, or high): GRE scores—high, research experience—low, work experience—low, extracurricular activity—low, clinically related public service—low, GPA—high, letters of recommendation—high, interview—low, statement of goals and objectives—medium.

Student Characteristics: The following represents characteristics of students in 2009–2010 in all graduate psychology programs in the department: Female—full-time 28, part-time 29; Male—full-time 8, part-time 9; African American/Black—full-time 3, part-time 0; Hispanic/Latino(a)—full-time 3, part-time 1; Asian/Pacific Islander—full-time 2, part-time 0; American Indian/Alaska Native—full-time 0, part-time 0; Caucasian/White—full-time 0, part-time 0; Multi-ethnic—full-time 0, part-time 0; students subject to the Americans With Disabilities Act—full-time 0, part-time 0; Unknown ethnicity—full-time 0, part-time 0; International students who hold an F-1 or J-1 Visa—full-time 0, part-time 0.

Financial Information/Assistance:
Tuition for Full-Time Study: *Master's:* State residents: per academic year $6,468; Nonstate residents: per academic year $13,116. Tuition is subject to change. See the following Web site for updates and changes in tuition costs: http://www.uttyler.edu/catalog/tuition.

Financial Assistance:
First-Year Students: Research assistantships available for first year. Fellowships and scholarships available for first year. Average amount paid per academic year: $1,000. Apply by October 1, February 1.

Advanced Students: Research assistantships available for advanced students. Average amount paid per academic year: $5,000. Average number of hours worked per week: 20. Apply by October 1, February 1. Fellowships and scholarships available for advanced students. Average amount paid per academic year: $1,000. Apply by October 1, February 1.

Additional Information: Of all students currently enrolled full time, 20% benefited from one or more of the listed financial assistance programs. Application and information available online at: http://www.uttyler.edu/financialaid.

Internships/Practica: Available practicum sites include nearby private psychiatric hospitals, MHMR facilities, children's therapy facilities, crisis centers and safe houses for abused women, neuropsychology rehabilitation hospitals, prisons, and schools.

Housing and Day Care: On-campus housing is available. See the following Web site for more information: http://www.uttyler.edu/housing/. No on-campus day care facilities are available.

Employment of Department Graduates:
Master's Degree Graduates: Of those who graduated in the academic year 2008–2009, the following categories and numbers represent the postgraduate activities and employment of master's degree graduates: Enrolled in a psychology doctoral program (3), enrolled in a postdoctoral residency/fellowship (n/a), employed in independent practice (n/a), employed in an academic position at a 2-year/4-year college (1), employed in a professional position in a school system (8), employed in a community mental health/counseling center (5), employed in a hospital/medical center (2), still seeking employment (2), total from the above (master's) (21).
Doctoral Degree Graduates: Of those who graduated in the academic year 2008–2009, the following categories and numbers represent the postgraduate activities and employment of doctoral degree graduates: Enrolled in a psychology doctoral program (n/a), total from the above (doctoral) (0).

Additional Information:
Orientation, Objectives, and Emphasis of Department: The purpose of our program is to prepare competent, applied practitioners at the master's level. The curriculum is very practical, stressing clinical assessment and intervention, and hands-on experience in relevant areas. Our students have been very successful in finding employment in mental health settings and in gaining admission to clinical and counseling doctoral programs. Special opportunities are provided for training in clinical neuropsychological assessment and psychopharmacology, for training in marital and family

counseling, school counseling or for training to become a licensed specialist in school psychology.

Information for Students With Physical Disabilities: See the following Web site for more information: http://www.uttyler.edu/disabilityservices.

Application Information:
Send to Psychology Graduate Coordinator, Department of Psychology, University of Texas at Tyler, 3900 University Blvd.,Tyler, TX 75799. Application available online. URL of online application: http://www.go2uttyler.com/apply.html. Students are admitted in the Fall, application deadline February 1; Spring, application deadline October 1. *Fee:* $25.

UTAH

Brigham Young University
Department of Counseling Psychology and Special Education
David O. McKay School of Education
340 MCKB
Provo, UT 84602
Telephone: (801) 422-3857
Fax: (801) 422-0198
E-mail: aaron_jackson@byu.edu
Web: http://education.byu.edu/cpse/

Department Information:
1969. Department Chair: Mary Anne Prater. Number of faculty: total—full-time 7, part-time 5; women—full-time 3, part-time 1; minority—part-time 1.

Programs and Degrees Offered:
Listed in the following order: Program area, degree type (T if terminal Master's), number awarded 7/08–6/09. School Psychology EdS (School Psychology) 12, Counseling Psychology PhD (Doctor of Philosophy) 6.

APA Accreditation: Counseling PhD (Doctor of Philosophy). Student Outcome Data Website: http://education.byu.edu/cpse/phd.

Student Applications/Admissions:
Student Applications
School Psychology EdS (School Psychology)—Applications 2009–2010, 34. Total applicants accepted 2009–2010, 12. Number full-time enrolled (new admits only) 2009–2010, 12. Total enrolled 2009–2010 full-time, 34. Openings 2010–2011, 12. The median number of years required for completion of a degree in 2008–2009 were 3. The number of students enrolled full- and part-time who were dismissed or voluntarily withdrew from this program area in 2008–2009 were 1. *Counseling Psychology PhD (Doctor of Philosophy)*—Applications 2009–2010, 58. Total applicants accepted 2009–2010, 7. Number full-time enrolled (new admits only) 2009–2010, 7. Number part-time enrolled (new admits only) 2009–2010, 0. Total enrolled 2009–2010 full-time, 30. Openings 2010–2011, 6. The median number of years required for completion of a degree in 2008–2009 were 5. The number of students enrolled full- and part-time who were dismissed or voluntarily withdrew from this program area in 2008–2009 were 0.

Scores: Entries appear in this order: required test or GPA, minimum score (if required), median score of students entering in 2009–2010. *Counseling Psychology PhD (Doctor of Philosophy):* GRE-V no minimum stated, 590, GRE-Q no minimum stated, 650, GRE-Analytical no minimum stated, 4.9, overall undergraduate GPA no minimum stated, last 2 years GPA no minimum stated, 3.64.

Other Criteria: (importance of criteria rated low, medium, or high): GRE scores—medium, research experience—medium, work experience—medium, extracurricular activity—low, clinically related public service—medium, GPA—high, letters of recommendation—medium, interview—high, statement of goals and objectives—high, undergraduate major in psychology—low, specific undergraduate psychology courses taken—medium.

Student Characteristics: The following represents characteristics of students in 2009–2010 in all graduate psychology programs in the department: Female—full-time 37, part-time 10; Male—full-time 23, part-time 11; African American/Black—full-time 0, part-time 0; Hispanic/Latino(a)—full-time 2, part-time 0; Asian/Pacific Islander—full-time 5, part-time 0; American Indian/Alaska Native—full-time 2, part-time 0; Caucasian/White—full-time 51, part-time 0; Multi-ethnic—full-time 0, part-time 0; students subject to the Americans With Disabilities Act—full-time 0, part-time 0; Unknown ethnicity—full-time 0, part-time 0; International students who hold an F-1 or J-1 Visa—full-time 1, part-time 0.

Financial Information/Assistance:
Tuition for Full-Time Study: *Master's:* State residents: per academic year $5,420, $301 per credit hour; Nonstate residents: per academic year $10,840, $602 per credit hour. *Doctoral:* State residents: per academic year $5,420, $301 per credit hour; Nonstate residents: per academic year $10,840, $602 per credit hour. Tuition is subject to change. See the following Web site for updates and changes in tuition costs: http://home.byu.edu/webapp/finserve/content/page/Tuition.html.

Financial Assistance:
First-Year Students: Teaching assistantships available for first year. Average amount paid per academic year: $7,800. Average number of hours worked per week: 15. Research assistantships available for first year. Average amount paid per academic year: $7,800. Average number of hours worked per week: 15. Fellowships and scholarships available for first year. Average amount paid per academic year: $1,200.

Advanced Students: Teaching assistantships available for advanced students. Average amount paid per academic year: $8,600. Average number of hours worked per week: 15. Research assistantships available for advanced students. Average amount paid per academic year: $8,600. Average number of hours worked per week: 15. Fellowships and scholarships available for advanced students. Average amount paid per academic year: $1,200.

Additional Information: Of all students currently enrolled full time, 100% benefited from one or more of the listed financial assistance programs.

Internships/Practica: Doctoral Degree (PhD Counseling Psychology): For those doctoral students for whom a professional internship was required in this program prior to graduation, (5) students applied for an internship in 2008–2009, with (5) students obtaining an internship. Of those students who obtained an internship, (5) were paid internships. Of those students who obtained an internship, (4) students placed in APA/CPA accredited internships, (1) students placed in internships not APA/CPA accredited, but listed with the Association of Psychology Postdoctoral and Internship Programs (APPIC), (0) students placed in internships conforming to guidelines of the Council of Directors of School Psychology Programs (CDSPP), (0) students placed in internships that were not APA/CPA accredited, APPIC or

CDSPP listed. Master's students complete practica for 5 hours per week during the first and second years of study and a full-time internship (5/8 of teacher pay) the third year. Doctoral students admitted at the bachelor's level complete 2 semesters of introductory practicum. All doctoral students complete 4 semesters of practicum in BYU's counseling center. They also complete 1 teaching practicum and 2 community-based practica. A full-year internship is required. Assistance is given for placements.

Housing and Day Care: On-campus housing is available. See the following Web site for more information: http://www.byu.edu/housing/. No on-campus day care facilities are available.

Employment of Department Graduates:
Master's Degree Graduates: Of those who graduated in the academic year 2008–2009, the following categories and numbers represent the postgraduate activities and employment of master's degree graduates: Enrolled in a postdoctoral residency/fellowship (n/a), employed in independent practice (n/a), total from the above (master's) (0).
Doctoral Degree Graduates: Of those who graduated in the academic year 2008–2009, the following categories and numbers represent the postgraduate activities and employment of doctoral degree graduates: Enrolled in a psychology doctoral program (n/a), employed in independent practice (2), employed in other positions at a higher education institution (3), employed in business or industry (1), total from the above (doctoral) (6).

Additional Information:
Orientation, Objectives, and Emphasis of Department: The Department of Counseling Psychology and Special Education offers master's programs in Special Education, an EdS degree in School Psychology, and a PhD program in Counseling Psychology. The School Psychology program prepares students for certification as school psychologists. The Counseling Psychology program prepares individuals for licensure as psychologists. The program is both broad-based and specific in nature; that is, one is expected to take certain courses that could be required for licensure or for certification and graduation, but the program encourages students to take coursework in varied disciplines such as marriage and family therapy, organizational behavior, and other fields allied with psychology and education. The focus of the School Psychology EdS program is to prepare graduates for K-12 school settings. The doctoral program prepares counseling psychologists to work in counseling centers, academic positions, and other mental health settings.

Personal Behavior Statement: http://honorcode.byu.edu/.

Special Facilities or Resources: The department has a Counseling Psychology Center (clinic) with five individual counseling rooms and one large group room available for the observation and videotaping of students in counseling and assessment. These are assigned specifically to the department, while an abundance of other media-related facilities for the teaching and learning experience are available on campus as well as off campus. The department also provides spacious study and work carrels. The Counseling and Career Center has eight offices for practicum students. All of these offices have videotaping capabilities and are equipped for live supervision.

Information for Students With Physical Disabilities: See the following Web site for more information: http://uac.byu.edu.

Application Information:
Send to Office of Graduate Studies, B-356 ASB, BYU, Provo, UT 84602. On-line applications are preferred. Application available online. URL of online application: http://www.byu.edu/gradstudies/. Students are admitted in the Fall, application deadline January 15. *Fee:* $50.

Brigham Young University
Department of Psychology
Family, Home and Social Sciences
1001 SWKT
Provo, UT 84602-5543
Telephone: (801) 422-4287
Fax: (801) 422-0602
E-mail: lisa_norton@byu.edu
Web: http://www.psychology.byu.edu

Department Information:
1921. Chairperson: Ramona O. Hopkins. Number of faculty: total—full-time 30, part-time 4; women—full-time 6, part-time 3; total—minority—full-time 1; women minority—full-time 1.

Programs and Degrees Offered:
Listed in the following order: Program area, degree type (T if terminal Master's), number awarded 7/08–6/09. General Psychology PhD (Doctor of Philosophy) 2, Clinical Psychology PhD (Doctor of Philosophy) 10, General Psychology MA/MS (Master of Arts/Science) (T) 7.

APA Accreditation: Clinical PhD (Doctor of Philosophy). Student Outcome Data Website: http://psychology.byu.edu/Clinical/Outcomes.dhtml.

Student Applications/Admissions:
Student Applications
General Psychology PhD (Doctor of Philosophy)—Applications 2009–2010, 14. Total applicants accepted 2009–2010, 1. Number full-time enrolled (new admits only) 2009–2010, 0. Total enrolled 2009–2010 full-time, 15. Openings 2010–2011, 5. The median number of years required for completion of a degree in 2008–2009 were 2. The number of students enrolled full- and part-time who were dismissed or voluntarily withdrew from this program area in 2008–2009 were 0. *Clinical Psychology PhD (Doctor of Philosophy)*—Applications 2009–2010, 58. Total applicants accepted 2009–2010, 10. Number full-time enrolled (new admits only) 2009–2010, 9. Total enrolled 2009–2010 full-time, 55. Openings 2010–2011, 10. The median number of years required for completion of a degree in 2008–2009 were 5. The number of students enrolled full- and part-time who were dismissed or voluntarily withdrew from this program area in 2008–2009 were 0. *General Psychology MA/MS (Master of Arts/Science)*—Applications 2009–2010, 25. Total applicants accepted 2009–2010, 9. Number full-time enrolled (new admits only) 2009–2010, 9. Total enrolled 2009–2010 full-time, 22. Openings 2010–2011, 10. The median number of years required for completion of a degree in 2008–2009 were 3. The number of students enrolled full- and part-time who were dismissed or voluntarily withdrew from this program area in 2008–2009 were 1.

Scores: Entries appear in this order: required test or GPA, minimum score (if required), median score of students entering in 2009–2010. *General Psychology PhD (Doctor of Philosophy):* GRE-V no minimum stated, GRE-Q no minimum stated, GRE-Analytical no minimum stated, overall undergraduate GPA no minimum stated, last 2 years GPA no minimum stated, Masters GPA no minimum stated; *Clinical Psychology PhD (Doctor of Philosophy):* GRE-V 480, 570, GRE-Q 500, 620, GRE-Analytical 3.5, 4.5, overall undergraduate GPA no minimum stated, last 2 years GPA 3.48, 3.82; *General Psychology MA/MS (Master of Arts/Science):* GRE-V 490, 590, GRE-Q 620, 650, GRE-Analytical 4.0, 4.5, overall undergraduate GPA no minimum stated, last 2 years GPA 3.43, 3.73.

Other Criteria: (importance of criteria rated low, medium, or high): GRE scores—high, research experience—high, work experience—medium, extracurricular activity—low, clinically related public service—medium, GPA—high, letters of recommendation—high, interview—high, statement of goals and objectives—high, undergraduate major in psychology—medium, specific undergraduate psychology courses taken—medium. Clinically related public service relevant to clinical PhD applicants only. For additional information on admission requirements, go to http://www.byu.edu/gradstudies/catalog/programs.php.

Student Characteristics: The following represents characteristics of students in 2009–2010 in all graduate psychology programs in the department: Female—full-time 31, part-time 0; Male—full-time 61, part-time 0; African American/Black—full-time 3, part-time 0; Hispanic/Latino(a)—full-time 4, part-time 0; Asian/Pacific Islander—full-time 9, part-time 0; American Indian/Alaska Native—full-time 0, part-time 0; Caucasian/White—full-time 76, part-time 0; Multi-ethnic—full-time 0, part-time 0; students subject to the Americans With Disabilities Act—full-time 1, part-time 0; Unknown ethnicity—full-time 0, part-time 0; International students who hold an F-1 or J-1 Visa—full-time 11, part-time 0.

Financial Information/Assistance:

Tuition for Full-Time Study: *Master's:* State residents: per academic year $5,420, $301 per credit hour; Nonstate residents: per academic year $10,840, $602 per credit hour. *Doctoral:* State residents: per academic year $5,420, $301 per credit hour; Nonstate residents: per academic year $10,840, $602 per credit hour. Tuition is subject to change. Resident tuition given to members of the sponsoring institution regardless of state of origin.

Financial Assistance:

First-Year Students: Teaching assistantships available for first year. Average amount paid per academic year: $9,000. Average number of hours worked per week: 13. Research assistantships available for first year. Average amount paid per academic year: $9,000. Average number of hours worked per week: 13.

Advanced Students: Teaching assistantships available for advanced students. Average amount paid per academic year: $9,500. Average number of hours worked per week: 13. Research assistantships available for advanced students. Average amount paid per academic year: $9,500. Average number of hours worked per week: 13. Traineeships available for advanced students. Average amount paid per academic year: $14,000. Average number of hours worked per week: 20.

Additional Information: Of all students currently enrolled full time, 96% benefited from one or more of the listed financial assistance programs.

Internships/Practica: Doctoral Degree (PhD Clinical Psychology): For those doctoral students for whom a professional internship was required in this program prior to graduation, (17) students applied for an internship in 2008–2009, with (16) students obtaining an internship. Of those students who obtained an internship, (15) were paid internships. Of those students who obtained an internship, (14) students placed in APA/CPA accredited internships, (0) students placed in internships not APA/CPA accredited, but listed with the Association of Psychology Postdoctoral and Internship Programs (APPIC), (0) students placed in internships conforming to guidelines of the Council of Directors of School Psychology Programs (CDSPP), (2) students placed in internships that were not APA/CPA accredited, APPIC or CDSPP listed. Students in the General PhD and General MS programs have the opportunity for internships in a wide variety of community settings, ranging from mental health to business. Clinical PhD students complete three types of practica: 1) BYU Comprehensive Clinic Integrative Practicum: Students see clients from the community in their first three years under the supervision of full-time clinical faculty. The clinic is a unique interdisciplinary training and research facility housing state-of-the-art audiovisual and computer resources for BYU's Clinical Psychology, Marriage and Family Therapy, Social Work, and Communication Disorders programs. 2) Clerkships: Students are required to complete two unpaid clerkships of 60 hours each. The clerkships allow students to work with different service agencies dealing with different focus groups: examples include prison, state hospital, residential treatment centers, private practice with a variety of age groups and presenting problems, developmentally disabled/autistic classrooms, and rehabilitation centers. 3) Externships: The clinical program arranges reimbursed training placements for students in over 25 community agencies where students are supervised by onsite licensed professionals, who typically hold adjunct appointments in the Psychology Department. These opportunities provide an excellent foundation for the integration of classroom experiences with practical work applications.

Housing and Day Care: On-campus housing is available. See the following Web site for more information: http://www.byu.edu/housing/. No on-campus day care facilities are available.

Employment of Department Graduates:

Master's Degree Graduates: Of those who graduated in the academic year 2008–2009, the following categories and numbers represent the postgraduate activities and employment of master's degree graduates: Enrolled in a psychology doctoral program (3), enrolled in another graduate/professional program (1), enrolled in a postdoctoral residency/fellowship (n/a), employed in independent practice (n/a), employed in an academic position at a 2-year/4-year college (1), employed in a professional position in a school system (1), employed in business or industry (1), total from the above (master's) (7).

Doctoral Degree Graduates: Of those who graduated in the academic year 2008–2009, the following categories and numbers represent the postgraduate activities and employment of doctoral degree graduates: Enrolled in a psychology doctoral program (n/a), employed in independent practice (3), employed in an academic position at a university (1), employed in a professional position in a school system (1), employed in business or industry (2), employed in a community mental health/counseling center (1), employed in a hospital/medical center (4), total from the above (doctoral) (12).

Additional Information:
Orientation, Objectives, and Emphasis of Department: The mission of the Psychology Department is to discover, disseminate, and apply principles of psychology within a scholarly framework that is compatible with the values and purposes of Brigham Young University and its sponsor. Three degrees are offered: Clinical Psychology PhD, General Psychology PhD (emphasis areas in Applied Social Psychology and Behavioral Neuroscience), and General MS. For the General PhD, students complete a common core of course work during the first three semesters. By the end of the second year students complete the requirements for an MS degree, including a master's thesis, if the degree has not been previously received. For the Clinical PhD, students do not complete a master's thesis. The philosophy of the clinical psychology program adheres to the scientist-professional model. Training focuses on academic and research competence as well as on theory and practicum experiences necessary to develop strong clinical skills. The program is eclectic in its theoretical approach, drawing from a wide range of orientations in an attempt to give broad exposure to a diversity of traditional and innovative approaches. If they wish, students may elect to complete an emphasis in 1) Child, Adolescent, and Family, 2) Clinical Neuropsychology, 3) Clinical Research.

Personal Behavior Statement: While the university is sponsored by the LDS (Mormon) Church, non-LDS students are welcome and considered without bias. The university does expect that all students, regardless of religion, maintain the behavioral standards of the university. These include high standards of honor, integrity, and morality; graciousness in personal behavior; and abstinence from such things as tobacco, alcohol, and the nonmedical use of drugs. The text of this agreement can be viewed at http://honorcode.byu.edu.

Special Facilities or Resources: 1) Computer Facilities: Extensive computer facilities are available throughout the department, college, and university. 2) Psychobiology Research Laboratories: These laboratories are equipped with facilities for brain-behavior analysis. Full histology and electrophysiology laboratories, along with the necessary surgical facilities, are available. 3) Neuroimaging and Behavior Laboratory: Research and training in the area of neuroimaging and cognitive neuroscience are supported by a laboratory consisting of multiple computers, video, data storage, and printer workstations. These are supported by software that allows for the capture, processing, isolation, and imaging output of specific areas of the brain from MRI and CT images and from metabolic imaging studies. 4) Multivariate Data Visualization Laboratory: Faculty and students interested in multivariate visualization of data and large-scale data analysis are supported by a mathematical psychology laboratory consisting of a network of NT workstations and laboratories for behavior analysis. Three laboratories feature online control of experimental procedures and data recording. 5) Comprehensive Clinic: The university maintains a large clinic for training and research purposes, serving 200-250 clients each week.

Information for Students With Physical Disabilities: See the following Web site for more information: http://uac.byu.edu.

Application Information:
Send to Graduate Studies Office, FPH, Brigham Young University, Provo, UT 84602. Application available online. URL of online application: https://app.applyyourself.com/?id=byugrad. Students are admitted in the Fall, application deadline January 3. *Fee:* $50.

Utah State University
Department of Psychology
Education and Human Services
2810 Old Main Hill
Logan, UT 84322-2810
Telephone: (435) 797-1460
Fax: (435) 797-1448
E-mail: *psydept@usu.edu*
Web: *http://www.usu.edu/psychology/*

Department Information:
1938. Chairperson: Gretchen Peacock, PhD Number of faculty: total—full-time 22, part-time 1; women—full-time 9, part-time 1; total—minority—full-time 3, part-time 1; women minority—full-time 3, part-time 1.

Programs and Degrees Offered:
Listed in the following order: Program area, degree type (T if terminal Master's), number awarded 7/08–6/09. Combined Clinical/Counseling/School Psychology PhD (Doctor of Philosophy) 3, Experimental and Applied Psychological Science PhD (Doctor of Philosophy) 4, School Psychology EdS (School Psychology) 8, School Counseling MA/MS (Master of Arts/Science) (T) 19.

APA Accreditation: Combination PhD (Doctor of Philosophy). Student Outcome Data Website: http://www.usu.edu/psychology/programs/combined/index.php.

Student Applications/Admissions:
Student Applications
Combined Clinical/Counseling/School Psychology PhD (Doctor of Philosophy)—Applications 2009–2010, 99. Total applicants accepted 2009–2010, 11. Number full-time enrolled (new admits only) 2009–2010, 7. Number part-time enrolled (new admits only) 2009–2010, 0. Openings 2010–2011, 8. The median number of years required for completion of a degree in 2008–2009 were 6. The number of students enrolled full- and part-time who were dismissed or voluntarily withdrew from this program area in 2008–2009 were 0. *Experimental and Applied Psychological Science PhD (Doctor of Philosophy)*—Applications 2009–2010, 28. Total applicants accepted 2009–2010, 10. Number full-time enrolled (new admits only) 2009–2010, 6. Number part-time enrolled (new admits only) 2009–2010, 0. Openings 2010–2011, 5. The number of students enrolled full- and part-time who were dismissed or voluntarily withdrew from this program area in 2008–2009 were 0. *School Psychology EdS (School Psychology)*—Applications 2009–2010, 20. Total applicants accepted 2009–2010, 7. Number full-time enrolled (new admits only) 2009–2010, 7. Total enrolled 2009–2010 full-time, 13. Openings 2010–2011, 6. The median number of years required for completion of a degree in 2008–2009 were 3. The number of students enrolled full- and part-time who were dismissed or voluntarily withdrew from this program

area in 2008–2009 were 0. *School Counseling MA/MS (Master of Arts/Science)*—Applications 2009–2010, 106. Total applicants accepted 2009–2010, 68. Number part-time enrolled (new admits only) 2009–2010, 66. Total enrolled 2009–2010 part-time, 125. Openings 2010–2011, 25. The median number of years required for completion of a degree in 2008–2009 were 3. The number of students enrolled full- and part-time who were dismissed or voluntarily withdrew from this program area in 2008–2009 were 1.

Scores: Entries appear in this order: required test or GPA, minimum score (if required), median score of students entering in 2009–2010. *Combined Clinical/Counseling/School Psychology PhD (Doctor of Philosophy)*: GRE-V no minimum stated, GRE-Q no minimum stated, GRE-Analytical no minimum stated, overall undergraduate GPA no minimum stated, last 2 years GPA no minimum stated; *Experimental and Applied Psychological Science PhD (Doctor of Philosophy)*: GRE-V no minimum stated, GRE-Q no minimum stated, GRE-Analytical no minimum stated, overall undergraduate GPA no minimum stated, last 2 years GPA no minimum stated; *School Psychology EdS (School Psychology)*: GRE-V no minimum stated, GRE-Q no minimum stated, GRE-Analytical no minimum stated, overall undergraduate GPA no minimum stated, last 2 years GPA no minimum stated; *School Counseling MA/MS (Master of Arts/Science)*: overall undergraduate GPA no minimum stated, last 2 years GPA no minimum stated.

Other Criteria: (importance of criteria rated low, medium, or high): GRE scores—medium, research experience—medium, work experience—medium, extracurricular activity—low, clinically related public service—medium, GPA—high, letters of recommendation—medium, interview—medium, statement of goals and objectives—high, undergraduate major in psychology—medium, specific undergraduate psychology courses taken—medium. The different graduate programs weight the above criteria in different ways. For example, research experience is much more important for the two PhD programs. For additional information on admission requirements, go to http://www.usu.edu/psychology/.

Student Characteristics: The following represents characteristics of students in 2009–2010 in all graduate psychology programs in the department: Female—full-time 36, part-time 103; Male—full-time 45, part-time 22; African American/Black—full-time 1, part-time 0; Hispanic/Latino(a)—full-time 5, part-time 2; Asian/Pacific Islander—full-time 2, part-time 0; American Indian/Alaska Native—full-time 4, part-time 0; Caucasian/White—full-time 68, part-time 121; Multi-ethnic—full-time 1, part-time 2; students subject to the Americans With Disabilities Act—full-time 1, part-time 0; Unknown ethnicity—full-time 0, part-time 0; International students who hold an F-1 or J-1 Visa—full-time 1, part-time 0.

Financial Information/Assistance:
Tuition for Full-Time Study: *Master's:* State residents: per academic year $4,502, $225 per credit hour; Nonstate residents: per academic year $13,970, $699 per credit hour. *Doctoral:* State residents: per academic year $4,502, $225 per credit hour; Nonstate residents: per academic year $13,970, $699 per credit hour. Tuition is subject to change. See the following Web site for updates and changes in tuition costs: http://www.usu.edu/registrar/payment/.

Financial Assistance:
First-Year Students: Teaching assistantships available for first year. Average amount paid per academic year: $10,000. Average number of hours worked per week: 20. Apply by March 1. Research assistantships available for first year. Average amount paid per academic year: $10,000. Average number of hours worked per week: 20. Fellowships and scholarships available for first year. Average amount paid per academic year: $12,000. Apply by January 15.

Advanced Students: Teaching assistantships available for advanced students. Average amount paid per academic year: $10,000. Average number of hours worked per week: 20. Apply by March 1. Research assistantships available for advanced students. Average amount paid per academic year: $10,000. Average number of hours worked per week: 20.

Additional Information: Of all students currently enrolled full time, 90% benefited from one or more of the listed financial assistance programs.

Internships/Practica: Doctoral Degree (PhD Combined Clinical/Counseling/School Psychology): For those doctoral students for whom a professional internship was required in this program prior to graduation, (6) students applied for an internship in 2008–2009, with (6) students obtaining an internship. Of those students who obtained an internship, (6) were paid internships. Of those students who obtained an internship, (6) students placed in APA/CPA accredited internships, (0) students placed in internships not APA/CPA accredited, but listed with the Association of Psychology Postdoctoral and Internship Programs (APPIC), (0) students placed in internships conforming to guidelines of the Council of Directors of School Psychology Programs (CDSPP), (0) students placed in internships that were not APA/CPA accredited, APPIC or CDSPP listed. Master's Degree (EdS School Psychology): An internship experience, such as a final research project or "capstone" experience is required of graduates. Master's Degree (MA/MS School Counseling): An internship experience, such as a final research project or "capstone" experience is required of graduates. Students in the Combined PhD program are placed in a variety of sites for practicum training including community mental health centers, the USU Counseling Center, the Center for Persons with Disabilities (a University Center for Excellence), residential eating disorders treatment facility, and medical facilities in the area. Students from the Combined program accept internships across the country. Students in the School Psychology and School Counseling programs complete practica and internships in school districts. Internship experiences can be in Utah or completed out-of-state.

Housing and Day Care: On-campus housing is available. See the following Web site for more information: http://www.housing.usu.edu. On-campus day care facilities are available. See the following Web site for more information: http://www.childrenshouse.usu.edu/.

Employment of Department Graduates:
Master's Degree Graduates: Of those who graduated in the academic year 2008–2009, the following categories and numbers represent the postgraduate activities and employment of master's degree graduates: Enrolled in a psychology doctoral program (0), enrolled in another graduate/professional program (0), enrolled in a postdoctoral residency/fellowship (n/a), employed in independent practice (n/a), employed in an academic position at a univer-

sity (0), employed in an academic position at a 2-year/4-year college (0), employed in other positions at a higher education institution (0), employed in a professional position in a school system (8), employed in business or industry (0), employed in government agency (0), employed in a community mental health/counseling center (0), employed in a hospital/medical center (0), still seeking employment (0), other employment position (0), total from the above (master's) (8).

Doctoral Degree Graduates: Of those who graduated in the academic year 2008–2009, the following categories and numbers represent the postgraduate activities and employment of doctoral degree graduates: Enrolled in a psychology doctoral program (n/a), enrolled in another graduate/professional program (0), enrolled in a postdoctoral residency/fellowship (3), employed in independent practice (0), employed in an academic position at a university (2), employed in an academic position at a 2-year/4-year college (0), employed in other positions at a higher education institution (0), employed in a professional position in a school system (1), employed in business or industry (0), employed in government agency (0), employed in a community mental health/counseling center (1), employed in a hospital/medical center (0), still seeking employment (0), not seeking employment (0), other employment position (0), do not know (0), total from the above (doctoral) (7).

Additional Information:
Orientation, Objectives, and Emphasis of Department: The Utah State University Department of Psychology offers two graduate PhD programs. The Experimental and Applied Psychological Sciences program offers training in a number of areas including behavior analysis, social/cognition, and research methods. The combined Clinical/Counseling/School Psychology offers integrated training across clinical, counseling, and school psychology (accredited by the American Psychological Association since 1975). Emphasis areas within this program include: child/school psychology, rural/multicultural psychology, and health/neuropsychology. The department also offers an EdS program in School Psychology and an MS program in School Counseling. The School Counseling program is a part-time, distance-based program. The two graduate PhD programs share a common core of doctoral courses intended to provide an advanced overview of several major areas of psychology. All doctoral programs offer extensive training within their specific areas; however, the common core is designed to ensure that no student will complete the PhD without being exposed to the diverse theoretical and methodological perspectives in the field of psychology. The common core also provides students the opportunity to become aware of the scholarly interests of faculty members in all programs, thus broadening students' choices of faculty advisors and dissertation chairpersons. Full tuition waivers are available to PhD students for 70 semester hours of academic credit.

Special Facilities or Resources: Students in the School Psychology and Combined programs benefit from the department's Psychology Community Clinic for supervised experience in actual therapy. In addition, the department has cooperative relations with other campus and off-campus facilities that provide excellent settings for student training, including the Bear River Mental Health Center, the USU Center for Persons with Disabilities, and the USU Counseling Center. Students in the EAPS program may work in animal (rat and pigeon) labs of their faculty supervisors.

Information for Students With Physical Disabilities: See the following Web site for more information: http://www.usu.edu/drc/.

Application Information:
Send to Utah State University, School of Graduate Studies, Logan, UT 84322-0900. Application available online. URL of online application: http://www.usu.edu/graduateschool/. Students are admitted in the Fall, application deadline January 15. Combined Clinical/Counseling/School Psychology Program deadline is January 15, Experimental and Applied Psychological Science begins reviewing applications January 31, School Psychology deadline is February 1, and School Counseling deadline is May 1. *Fee:* $55.

Utah, University of
Department of Educational Psychology, Counseling Psychology and School Psychology Programs
College of Education
1705 East Campus Center Drive, Room 327
Salt Lake City, UT 84112-9255
Telephone: (801) 581-7148
Fax: (801) 581-5566
E-mail: *clark@ed.utah.edu*
Web: *http://www.ed.utah.edu/edps/*

Department Information:
1949. Chairperson: Elaine Clark. Number of faculty: total—full-time 15, part-time 4; women—full-time 7, part-time 3; total—minority—full-time 2, part-time 1; women minority—part-time 1.

Programs and Degrees Offered:
Listed in the following order: Program area, degree type (T if terminal Master's), number awarded 7/08–6/09. Counseling Psychology PhD (Doctor of Philosophy) 4, School Psychology PhD (Doctor of Philosophy) 7, Learning Sciences PhD (Doctor of Philosophy) 3, Instructional Design and Educational Technology Other 14, Reading and Literacy PhD (Doctor of Philosophy) 3, Reading and Literacy MEd (Education) 14, Statistics MA/MS (Master of Arts/Science) (T) 1, Professional Counseling MA/MS (Master of Arts/Science) (T) 15, School Counseling MEd (Education) 11.

APA Accreditation: Counseling PhD (Doctor of Philosophy). School PhD (Doctor of Philosophy).

Student Applications/Admissions:
Student Applications
Counseling Psychology PhD (Doctor of Philosophy)—Applications 2009–2010, 80. Total applicants accepted 2009–2010, 4. Number full-time enrolled (new admits only) 2009–2010, 4. Total enrolled 2009–2010 full-time, 44, part-time, 2. Openings 2010–2011, 6. The median number of years required for completion of a degree in 2008–2009 were 6. The number of students enrolled full- and part-time who were dismissed or voluntarily withdrew from this program area in 2008–2009 were 1. *School Psychology PhD (Doctor of Philosophy)*—Applications 2009–2010, 27. Total applicants accepted 2009–2010, 8. Number full-time enrolled (new admits only) 2009–2010, 8. Number part-time enrolled (new admits only) 2009–2010, 3. Total enrolled 2009–2010 full-time, 28, part-time, 19.

Openings 2010–2011, 8. The median number of years required for completion of a degree in 2008–2009 were 6. The number of students enrolled full- and part-time who were dismissed or voluntarily withdrew from this program area in 2008–2009 were 0. *Learning Sciences PhD (Doctor of Philosophy)*—Applications 2009–2010, 7. Total applicants accepted 2009–2010, 5. Number full-time enrolled (new admits only) 2009–2010, 5. Total enrolled 2009–2010 full-time, 6, part-time, 8. Openings 2010–2011, 5. The median number of years required for completion of a degree in 2008–2009 were 5. The number of students enrolled full- and part-time who were dismissed or voluntarily withdrew from this program area in 2008–2009 were 0. *Instructional Design and Educational Technology Other*—Applications 2009–2010, 16. Total applicants accepted 2009–2010, 15. Number full-time enrolled (new admits only) 2009–2010, 15. Total enrolled 2009–2010 full-time, 19, part-time, 18. Openings 2010–2011, 20. The median number of years required for completion of a degree in 2008–2009 were 2. The number of students enrolled full- and part-time who were dismissed or voluntarily withdrew from this program area in 2008–2009 were 0. *Reading and Literacy PhD (Doctor of Philosophy)*—Applications 2009–2010, 2. Total applicants accepted 2009–2010, 1. Number full-time enrolled (new admits only) 2009–2010, 1. Total enrolled 2009–2010 full-time, 3. Openings 2010–2011, 4. The median number of years required for completion of a degree in 2008–2009 were 4. The number of students enrolled full- and part-time who were dismissed or voluntarily withdrew from this program area in 2008–2009 were 0. *Reading and Literacy MEd (Education)*—Applications 2009–2010, 35. Total applicants accepted 2009–2010, 25. Number full-time enrolled (new admits only) 2009–2010, 25. Total enrolled 2009–2010 full-time, 32. Openings 2010–2011, 30. The median number of years required for completion of a degree in 2008–2009 were 2. The number of students enrolled full- and part-time who were dismissed or voluntarily withdrew from this program area in 2008–2009 were 0. *Statistics MA/MS (Master of Arts/Science)*—Applications 2009–2010, 3. Total applicants accepted 2009–2010, 3. Number full-time enrolled (new admits only) 2009–2010, 3. Total enrolled 2009–2010 full-time, 6. The number of students enrolled full- and part-time who were dismissed or voluntarily withdrew from this program area in 2008–2009 were 0. *Professional Counseling MA/MS (Master of Arts/Science)*—Applications 2009–2010, 37. Total applicants accepted 2009–2010, 0. Number full-time enrolled (new admits only) 2009–2010, 0. Total enrolled 2009–2010 full-time, 16, part-time, 8. Openings 2010–2011, 10. The median number of years required for completion of a degree in 2008–2009 were 3. The number of students enrolled full- and part-time who were dismissed or voluntarily withdrew from this program area in 2008–2009 were 0. *School Counseling MEd (Education)*—Applications 2009–2010, 47. Total applicants accepted 2009–2010, 20. Number full-time enrolled (new admits only) 2009–2010, 20. Number part-time enrolled (new admits only) 2009–2010, 0. Total enrolled 2009–2010 full-time, 27, part-time, 13. Openings 2010–2011, 20. The median number of years required for completion of a degree in 2008–2009 were 2. The number of students enrolled full- and part-time who were dismissed or voluntarily withdrew from this program area in 2008–2009 were 0.

Scores: Entries appear in this order: required test or GPA, minimum score (if required), median score of students entering in 2009–2010. *Counseling Psychology PhD (Doctor of Philosophy)*: GRE-V no minimum stated, GRE-Q no minimum stated, GRE-Analytical no minimum stated, overall undergraduate GPA no minimum stated; *School Psychology PhD (Doctor of Philosophy)*: GRE-V no minimum stated, GRE-Q no minimum stated, GRE-Analytical no minimum stated, overall undergraduate GPA no minimum stated; *Learning Sciences PhD (Doctor of Philosophy)*: GRE-V no minimum stated, GRE-Q no minimum stated, GRE-Analytical no minimum stated, overall undergraduate GPA no minimum stated; *Instructional Design and Educational Technology Other*: overall undergraduate GPA no minimum stated; *Reading and Literacy PhD (Doctor of Philosophy)*: GRE-V no minimum stated, GRE-Q no minimum stated, GRE-Analytical no minimum stated, overall undergraduate GPA no minimum stated; *Reading and Literacy MEd (Education)*: GRE-Analytical no minimum stated, overall undergraduate GPA no minimum stated; *Statistics MA/MS (Master of Arts/Science)*: GRE-V no minimum stated, GRE-Q no minimum stated, GRE-Analytical no minimum stated, overall undergraduate GPA no minimum stated; *Professional Counseling MA/MS (Master of Arts/Science)*: GRE-V no minimum stated, GRE-Q no minimum stated, GRE-Analytical no minimum stated, overall undergraduate GPA no minimum stated; *School Counseling MEd (Education)*: GRE-V no minimum stated, GRE-Q no minimum stated, GRE-Analytical no minimum stated, overall undergraduate GPA no minimum stated.

Other Criteria: (importance of criteria rated low, medium, or high): GRE scores—high, research experience—high, work experience—high, extracurricular activity—medium, clinically related public service—medium, GPA—high, letters of recommendation—high, interview—high, statement of goals and objectives—high, undergraduate major in psychology—medium. Each program reviews and rates its own applicants.

Student Characteristics: The following represents characteristics of students in 2009–2010 in all graduate psychology programs in the department: Female—full-time 197, part-time 0; Male—full-time 87, part-time 0; African American/Black—full-time 1, part-time 0; Hispanic/Latino(a)—full-time 14, part-time 0; Asian/Pacific Islander—full-time 7, part-time 0; American Indian/Alaska Native—full-time 1, part-time 0; Caucasian/White—full-time 210, part-time 0; Multi-ethnic—full-time 5, part-time 0; students subject to the Americans With Disabilities Act—full-time 0, part-time 0; Unknown ethnicity—full-time 48, part-time 0; International students who hold an F-1 or J-1 Visa—full-time 0, part-time 0.

Financial Information/Assistance:
Tuition for Full-Time Study: *Master's:* State residents: per academic year $4,302; Nonstate residents: per academic year $14,834. *Doctoral:* State residents: per academic year $4,302; Nonstate residents: per academic year $14,834. Tuition is subject to change. See the following Web site for updates and changes in tuition costs: http://www.ed.utah.edu.

Financial Assistance:
First-Year Students: Teaching assistantships available for first year. Average amount paid per academic year: $11,500. Average number of hours worked per week: 20. Apply by April. Research assistantships available for first year. Average amount paid per academic year: $11,500. Average number of hours worked per week: 20.

Advanced Students: Teaching assistantships available for advanced students. Average amount paid per academic year: $11,500. Average number of hours worked per week: 20. Apply by April. Research assistantships available for advanced students. Average amount paid per academic year: $11,500. Average number of hours worked per week: 20. Traineeships available for advanced students. Fellowships and scholarships available for advanced students. Average amount paid per academic year: $11,500. Average number of hours worked per week: 20. Apply by March.

Additional Information: Of all students currently enrolled full time, 75% benefited from one or more of the listed financial assistance programs.

Internships/Practica: Doctoral Degree (PhD Counseling Psychology): For those doctoral students for whom a professional internship was required in this program prior to graduation, (8) students applied for an internship in 2008–2009, with (7) students obtaining an internship. Of those students who obtained an internship, (7) were paid internships. Of those students who obtained an internship, (7) students placed in APA/CPA accredited internships, (0) students placed in internships not APA/CPA accredited, but listed with the Association of Psychology Postdoctoral and Internship Programs (APPIC), (0) students placed in internships conforming to guidelines of the Council of Directors of School Psychology Programs (CDSPP), (0) students placed in internships that were not APA/CPA accredited, APPIC or CDSPP listed. Doctoral Degree (PhD School Psychology): For those doctoral students for whom a professional internship was required in this program prior to graduation, (7) students applied for an internship in 2008–2009, with (7) students obtaining an internship. Of those students who obtained an internship, (7) were paid internships. Of those students who obtained an internship, (0) students placed in APA/CPA accredited internships, (0) students placed in internships not APA/CPA accredited, but listed with the Association of Psychology Postdoctoral and Internship Programs (APPIC), (0) students placed in internships conforming to guidelines of the Council of Directors of School Psychology Programs (CDSPP), (7) students placed in internships that were not APA/CPA accredited, APPIC or CDSPP listed. Practica for counseling psychology doctoral students vary and include such settings as U of U counseling center and other campus services, community mental health settings, hospital settings, and private practice. Predoctoral internships are typically taken nationally in university counseling centers, community mental health settings, veterans hospitals, and specialty settings. School Psychology practica initially focus on participation in an on campus clinic and gradually move into field based settings appropriate to the field of school psychology. Specialized practica also allow for supervised experiences in early childhood settings, "stand alone" community based clinics and specialized treatment programs. Predoctoral internships are completed in local school districts or in other approved settings.

Housing and Day Care: On-campus housing is available. See the following Web site for more information: Residential Living: http://www.orl.utah.edu/. On-campus day care facilities are available. See the following Web site for more information: Child Care: http://www.childcare.utah.edu/.

Employment of Department Graduates:
Master's Degree Graduates: Of those who graduated in the academic year 2008–2009, the following categories and numbers represent the postgraduate activities and employment of master's degree graduates: Enrolled in a postdoctoral residency/fellowship (n/a), employed in independent practice (n/a), employed in an academic position at a 2-year/4-year college (0), employed in a professional position in a school system (4), employed in a community mental health/counseling center (12), employed in a hospital/medical center (0), still seeking employment (1), not seeking employment (2), other employment position (1), total from the above (master's) (20).

Doctoral Degree Graduates: Of those who graduated in the academic year 2008–2009, the following categories and numbers represent the postgraduate activities and employment of doctoral degree graduates: Enrolled in a psychology doctoral program (n/a), employed in an academic position at a university (5), employed in an academic position at a 2-year/4-year college (0), employed in other positions at a higher education institution (3), employed in a professional position in a school system (2), employed in business or industry (1), employed in government agency (0), employed in a community mental health/counseling center (1), still seeking employment (3), other employment position (0), do not know (0), total from the above (doctoral) (15).

Additional Information:
Orientation, Objectives, and Emphasis of Department: The Department of Educational Psychology at the University of Utah is characterized by an emphasis on the application of behavioral sciences to educational and psychological processes. The department is organized into 3 program areas: Counseling and Counseling Psychology (MS, MEd, PhD), School Psychology (MS, MEd, PhD), Learning Sciences with three subprograms: Learning and Cognition (PhD), Reading and Literacy (MEd and PhD), a master's level program in Instructional Design and Educational Technology, IDET (MEd), and an interdepartmental program which leads to a Master's in Statistics (MSTAT). The basic master's level program includes one to two years of academic work (and in some cases an additional year of internship). Doctoral programs include Counseling Psychology (APA accredited since 1957), School Psychology (APA accredited since 1986), and Learning Sciences: Learning and Cognition area. The emphasis of the department is on the application of psychological principles in educational and human service settings. In addition, doctoral programs represent a scientist–practitioner model with considerable emphasis on the development of research as well as professional skills.

Special Facilities or Resources: A variety of research and training opportunities are available to students through relationships the department has developed with various university and community facilities. Included are the university counseling center, medical center, computer center, and the adjacent regional Veterans Administration Medical Center. Community facilities include local school districts, community mental health centers, children's hospital, general hospitals, child guidance clinics, and various state social service agencies. The department maintains its own statistics laboratory. Students have access to computer stations and use of the college computer network.

Information for Students With Physical Disabilities: See the following Web site for more information: http://disability.utah.edu/.

GRADUATE STUDY IN PSYCHOLOGY

Application Information:
Send to Admission, University of Utah, Department of Educational Psychology, 1705 E Campus Ctr Dr., Rm 327, Salt Lake City, Utah 84112-9255. Application available online. URL of online application: http://edps.ed.utah.edu/. Students are admitted in the Fall, application deadline December 15. *Fee:* $55.

Utah, University of
Department of Psychology
Social and Behavioral Science
380 South 1530 East, Room 502
Salt Lake City, UT 84112
Telephone: (801) 581-6124
Fax: (801) 581-5841
E-mail: *nancy.seegmiller@psych.utah.edu*
Web: *http://www.psych.utah.edu*

Department Information:
1925. Chairperson: Cynthia A. Berg. Number of faculty: total—full-time 28, part-time 3; women—full-time 14, part-time 1; total—minority—full-time 5; women minority—full-time 2.

Programs and Degrees Offered:
Listed in the following order: Program area, degree type (T if terminal Master's), number awarded 7/08–6/09. Developmental Psychology PhD (Doctor of Philosophy) 3, Social Psychology PhD (Doctor of Philosophy) 5, Clinical Psychology PhD (Doctor of Philosophy) 1, Cognition and Neuroscience PhD (Doctor of Philosophy) 2.

APA Accreditation: Clinical PhD (Doctor of Philosophy).

Student Applications/Admissions:
Student Applications
Developmental Psychology PhD (Doctor of Philosophy)—Applications 2009–2010, 16. Total applicants accepted 2009–2010, 2. Number full-time enrolled (new admits only) 2009–2010, 1. Number part-time enrolled (new admits only) 2009–2010, 0. Openings 2010–2011, 3. The median number of years required for completion of a degree in 2008–2009 were 7. The number of students enrolled full- and part-time who were dismissed or voluntarily withdrew from this program area in 2008–2009 were 0. Social Psychology PhD (Doctor of Philosophy)—Applications 2009–2010, 30. Total applicants accepted 2009–2010, 2. Number full-time enrolled (new admits only) 2009–2010, 2. Number part-time enrolled (new admits only) 2009–2010, 0. Openings 2010–2011, 4. The median number of years required for completion of a degree in 2008–2009 were 6. The number of students enrolled full- and part-time who were dismissed or voluntarily withdrew from this program area in 2008–2009 were 1. Clinical Psychology PhD (Doctor of Philosophy)—Applications 2009–2010, 122. Total applicants accepted 2009–2010, 5. Number full-time enrolled (new admits only) 2009–2010, 5. Number part-time enrolled (new admits only) 2009–2010, 0. Openings 2010–2011, 5. The median number of years required for completion of a degree in 2008–2009 were 7. The number of students enrolled full- and part-time who were dismissed or voluntarily withdrew from this program area in 2008–2009 were 2. Cognition and Neuroscience PhD (Doctor of Philosophy)—Applications 2009–2010, 19. Total applicants accepted 2009–2010, 2. Number full-time enrolled (new admits only) 2009–2010, 2. Number part-time enrolled (new admits only) 2009–2010, 0. Openings 2010–2011, 4. The median number of years required for completion of a degree in 2008–2009 were 6. The number of students enrolled full- and part-time who were dismissed or voluntarily withdrew from this program area in 2008–2009 were 0.

Other Criteria: (importance of criteria rated low, medium, or high): GRE scores—medium, research experience—high, work experience—medium, extracurricular activity—medium, clinically related public service—medium, GPA—medium, letters of recommendation—high, interview—high, statement of goals and objectives—high, undergraduate major in psychology—medium, specific undergraduate psychology courses taken—medium.

Student Characteristics: The following represents characteristics of students in 2009–2010 in all graduate psychology programs in the department: Female—full-time 39, part-time 0; Male—full-time 21, part-time 0; African American/Black—full-time 0, part-time 0; Hispanic/Latino(a)—full-time 2, part-time 0; Asian/Pacific Islander—full-time 4, part-time 0; American Indian/Alaska Native—full-time 0, part-time 0; Caucasian/White—full-time 54, part-time 0; Multi-ethnic—full-time 0, part-time 0; students subject to the Americans With Disabilities Act—full-time 0, part-time 0; Unknown ethnicity—full-time 0, part-time 0; International students who hold an F-1 or J-1 Visa—full-time 4, part-time 0.

Financial Information/Assistance:
Financial Assistance:
First-Year Students: Teaching assistantships available for first year. Average amount paid per academic year: $12,000. Average number of hours worked per week: 20. Research assistantships available for first year. Average amount paid per academic year: $12,000. Average number of hours worked per week: 20. Fellowships and scholarships available for first year. Average amount paid per academic year: $12,000.

Advanced Students: Teaching assistantships available for advanced students. Average amount paid per academic year: $12,000. Average number of hours worked per week: 20. Research assistantships available for advanced students. Average amount paid per academic year: $12,000. Average number of hours worked per week: 20. Fellowships and scholarships available for advanced students. Average amount paid per academic year: $12,000.

Additional Information: Of all students currently enrolled full time, 95% benefited from one or more of the listed financial assistance programs. Application and information available online at: http://www.psych.utah.edu.

Internships/Practica: Doctoral Degree (PhD Clinical Psychology): For those doctoral students for whom a professional internship was required in this program prior to graduation, (5) students applied for an internship in 2008–2009, with (5) students obtaining an internship. Of those students who obtained an internship, (5) were paid internships. Of those students who obtained an internship, (5) students placed in APA/CPA accredited internships, (0) students placed in internships not APA/CPA accredited, but listed with the Association of Psychology Postdoctoral and Internship Programs (APPIC), (0) students placed in internships conforming to guidelines of the Council of Directors of

School Psychology Programs (CDSPP), (0) students placed in internships that were not APA/CPA accredited, APPIC or CDSPP listed. Extensive clinical training experiences are available through close ties with facilities in the community. A sample of these include the Veteran's Administration Hospital, the University Medical Center, Primary Children's Hospital, the Children's Behavioral Therapy Unit, the Juvenile Detention Center, the University Neuropsychiatric Institute, the University Counseling Center, and local community health centers. There are four APA-approved internships in the local community.

Housing and Day Care: On-campus housing is available. See the following Web site for more information: http://www.housing.utah.edu. On-campus day care facilities are available.

Employment of Department Graduates:

Master's Degree Graduates: Of those who graduated in the academic year 2008–2009, the following categories and numbers represent the postgraduate activities and employment of master's degree graduates: Enrolled in a postdoctoral residency/fellowship (n/a), employed in independent practice (n/a), total from the above (master's) (0).

Doctoral Degree Graduates: Of those who graduated in the academic year 2008–2009, the following categories and numbers represent the postgraduate activities and employment of doctoral degree graduates: Enrolled in a psychology doctoral program (n/a), enrolled in another graduate/professional program (0), enrolled in a postdoctoral residency/fellowship (1), employed in independent practice (0), employed in an academic position at a university (6), employed in an academic position at a 2-year/4-year college (0), employed in other positions at a higher education institution (1), employed in a professional position in a school system (0), employed in business or industry (2), employed in government agency (0), employed in a community mental health/counseling center (0), employed in a hospital/medical center (0), still seeking employment (0), not seeking employment (0), other employment position (0), do not know (0), total from the above (doctoral) (10).

Additional Information:

Orientation, Objectives, and Emphasis of Department: We offer comprehensive training in psychology, including Clinical (general, child-family, health, & neuropsychology emphases), Developmental, Experimental-Physiological, and Social. Students generally receive support throughout their training. Students are selected for area programs with individual faculty advisers. They do research in their areas, and clinical students also receive applied training. Graduates accept jobs in academic departments, research centers, and applied settings.

Special Facilities or Resources: Special facilities include the Early Childhood Education Center and 3 on-campus hospitals.

Application Information:

Send to Graduate Admissions Secretary, Psychology Department, 380 S. 1530 East, Room 502, Salt Lake City, UT 84112. Application available online. URL of online application: http://www.psych.utah.edu/graduate/index.html. Students are admitted in the Fall, application deadline December 15. *Fee:* $55.

VERMONT

Goddard College
MA Psychology and Counseling Program
123 Pitkin Road
Plainfield, VT 05667
Telephone: (802) 454-8311, (800) 468-4888
Fax: (802) 454-1029
E-mail: *Steven.James@goddard.edu*
Web: *http://www.goddard.edu*

Department Information:
1988. Chairperson: Steven E. James, PhD. Number of faculty: total—full-time 1, part-time 6; women—part-time 5; total—minority—full-time 1, part-time 3; women minority—part-time 3.

Programs and Degrees Offered:
Listed in the following order: Program area, degree type (T if terminal Master's), number awarded 7/08–6/09. Organizational Development MA/MS (Master of Arts/Science) (T) 1, Sexual Orientation MA/MS (Master of Arts/Science) (T) 4, Psychology MA/MS (Master of Arts/Science) (T) 0, Counseling MA/MS (Master of Arts/Science) (T) 17.

Student Applications/Admissions:
Student Applications
Organizational Development MA/MS (Master of Arts/Science)—Applications 2009–2010, 4. Total applicants accepted 2009–2010, 1. Number full-time enrolled (new admits only) 2009–2010, 1. Number part-time enrolled (new admits only) 2009–2010, 0. Openings 2010–2011, 2. The median number of years required for completion of a degree in 2008–2009 were 3. The number of students enrolled full- and part-time who were dismissed or voluntarily withdrew from this program area in 2008–2009 were 0. *Sexual Orientation MA/MS (Master of Arts/Science)*—Applications 2009–2010, 5. Total applicants accepted 2009–2010, 5. Number full-time enrolled (new admits only) 2009–2010, 4. Number part-time enrolled (new admits only) 2009–2010, 1. Total enrolled 2009–2010 full-time, 9, part-time, 6. Openings 2010–2011, 15. The median number of years required for completion of a degree in 2008–2009 were 2. The number of students enrolled full- and part-time who were dismissed or voluntarily withdrew from this program area in 2008–2009 were 2. *Psychology MA/MS (Master of Arts/Science)*—Applications 2009–2010, 0. Total applicants accepted 2009–2010, 0. Number full-time enrolled (new admits only) 2009–2010, 0. Number part-time enrolled (new admits only) 2009–2010, 0. Openings 2010–2011, 1. The median number of years required for completion of a degree in 2008–2009 were 2. The number of students enrolled full- and part-time who were dismissed or voluntarily withdrew from this program area in 2008–2009 were 0. *Counseling MA/MS (Master of Arts/Science)*—Applications 2009–2010, 30. Total applicants accepted 2009–2010, 27. Number full-time enrolled (new admits only) 2009–2010, 10. Number part-time enrolled (new admits only) 2009–2010, 6. Total enrolled 2009–2010 full-time, 27, part-time, 11. Openings 2010–2011, 20. The median number of years required for completion of a degree in 2008–2009 were 2. The number of students enrolled full- and part-time who were dismissed or voluntarily withdrew from this program area in 2008–2009 were 4.

Other Criteria: (importance of criteria rated low, medium, or high): research experience—low, work experience—high, extracurricular activity—medium, clinically related public service—high, GPA—medium, letters of recommendation—high, interview—low, statement of goals and objectives—high, iconoclastic intent—high, undergraduate major in psychology—high, specific undergraduate psychology courses taken—medium. For additional information on admission requirements, go to http://www.goddard.edu.

Student Characteristics: The following represents characteristics of students in 2009–2010 in all graduate psychology programs in the department: Female—full-time 27, part-time 12; Male—full-time 10, part-time 5; African American/Black—full-time 1, part-time 0; Hispanic/Latino(a)—full-time 1, part-time 0; Asian/Pacific Islander—part-time 0; American Indian/Alaska Native—part-time 0; Caucasian/White—full-time 33, part-time 17; Multi-ethnic—full-time 2, part-time 0; students subject to the Americans With Disabilities Act—full-time 3, part-time 0; Unknown ethnicity—full-time 0, part-time 0; International students who hold an F-1 or J-1 Visa—full-time 0, part-time 1.

Financial Information/Assistance:
Tuition for Full-Time Study: *Master's:* State residents: per academic year $15,000, $625 per credit hour; Nonstate residents: per academic year $15,000, $625 per credit hour. Tuition is subject to change. See the following Web site for updates and changes in tuition costs: http://www.goddard.edu.

Financial Assistance:
First-Year Students: Fellowships and scholarships available for first year. Average amount paid per academic year: $1,445. Average number of hours worked per week: 0.
Advanced Students: Fellowships and scholarships available for advanced students. Average amount paid per academic year: $1,445. Average number of hours worked per week: 0.
Additional Information: Of all students currently enrolled full time, 0% benefited from one or more of the listed financial assistance programs. Application and information available online at: www.goddard.edu.

Internships/Practica: Master's Degree (MA/MS Organizational Development): An internship experience, such as a final research project or "capstone" experience is required of graduates. Master's Degree (MA/MS Sexual Orientation): An internship experience, such as a final research project or "capstone" experience is required of graduates. Master's Degree (MA/MS Psychology): An internship experience, such as a final research project or "capstone" experience is required of graduates. Master's Degree (MA/MS Counseling): An internship experience, such as a final research project or "capstone" experience is required of graduates. Students are required to complete a minimum of 300 hours of supervised practicum during the program. This practicum takes place at a location convenient to the student that has been reviewed and evaluated by the program faculty as appropriate to the student's plan of study, providing appropriate licensed supervision and offering direct counseling experience. Students propose sites at which they would like to work to the faculty for review and approval.

Housing and Day Care: On-campus housing is available. Contact: Paul.Shper@goddard.edu. No on-campus day care facilities are available.

Employment of Department Graduates:
Master's Degree Graduates: Of those who graduated in the academic year 2008–2009, the following categories and numbers represent the postgraduate activities and employment of master's degree graduates: Enrolled in a psychology doctoral program (8), enrolled in another graduate/professional program (0), enrolled in a postdoctoral residency/fellowship (n/a), employed in independent practice (n/a), employed in an academic position at a university (4), employed in an academic position at a 2-year/4-year college (0), employed in other positions at a higher education institution (1), employed in a professional position in a school system (2), employed in business or industry (3), employed in government agency (2), employed in a community mental health/counseling center (2), employed in a hospital/medical center (1), still seeking employment (0), not seeking employment (1), other employment position (1), total from the above (master's) (25).
Doctoral Degree Graduates: Of those who graduated in the academic year 2008–2009, the following categories and numbers represent the postgraduate activities and employment of doctoral degree graduates: Enrolled in a psychology doctoral program (n/a), total from the above (doctoral) (0).

Additional Information:
Orientation, Objectives, and Emphasis of Department: Graduate study in Psychology & Counseling consists of a unique combination of intensive campus residencies and directed, independent study off campus. Students design their own emphasis of study or enter into the defined concentrations in organizational development or sexual orientation studies. The primary goal of the program is to develop skills in individual, family and/or community psychology, grounded in theory and research, personal experience and self-knowledge, and relevant to current social complexities. While pursuing their own specialized interests, students gain mastery in the broad range of subjects necessary for the effective and ethical practice of counseling. Study begins each semester with a week-long residency at the college, a time of planning for the ensuing semester and attending seminars. Returning home, the student begins implementation of the detailed study plan based upon the student's particular interests and needs and mastery of relevant theory and research and completion of a supervised practicum with a minimum of 300 hours. Through appropriate design of their study plan, students may meet the educational requirements for master's level licensure or certification in their state. The program is approved by the Council of Applied Master's Programs in Psychology.

Application Information:
Send to Admissions Office. Application available online. URL of online application: http://www.goddard.edu/admissions/. Students are admitted in the Fall, application deadline 9/15; Spring, application deadline 3/15. *Fee:* $40. Waiver by written petition.

Saint Michael's College
Psychology Department/Graduate Program in Clinical Psychology
Saint Michael's College
One Winooski Park
Colchester, VT 05439
Telephone: (802) 654-2206
Fax: (802) 654-2697
E-mail: *rmiller@smcvt.edu*
Web: *http://www.smcvt.edu/graduate/psych/default.asp*

Department Information:
1984. Director: Ronald B. Miller. Number of faculty: total—full-time 4, part-time 7; women—full-time 1, part-time 4.

Programs and Degrees Offered:
Listed in the following order: Program area, degree type (T if terminal Master's), number awarded 7/08–6/09. Clinical Psychology MA/MS (Master of Arts/Science) (T) 17.

Student Applications/Admissions:
Student Applications
Clinical Psychology MA/MS (*Master of Arts/Science*)—Applications 2009–2010, 23. Total applicants accepted 2009–2010, 19. Number full-time enrolled (new admits only) 2009–2010, 9. Number part-time enrolled (new admits only) 2009–2010, 6. Total enrolled 2009–2010 full-time, 27, part-time, 29. Openings 2010–2011, 17. The median number of years required for completion of a degree in 2008–2009 were 4. The number of students enrolled full- and part-time who were dismissed or voluntarily withdrew from this program area in 2008–2009 were 2.
Scores: Entries appear in this order: required test or GPA, minimum score (if required), median score of students entering in 2009–2010. Clinical Psychology MA/MS (*Master of Arts/Science*): overall undergraduate GPA 3.0, psychology GPA 3.25.
Other Criteria: (importance of criteria rated low, medium, or high): research experience—low, work experience—high, extracurricular activity—medium, clinically related public service—high, GPA—high, letters of recommendation—high, interview—high, statement of goals and objectives—high, undergraduate major in psychology—medium, specific undergraduate psychology courses taken—high.

Student Characteristics: The following represents characteristics of students in 2009–2010 in all graduate psychology programs in the department: Female—full-time 18, part-time 20; Male—full-time 9, part-time 9; African American/Black—full-time 0, part-time 1; Hispanic/Latino(a)—full-time 1, part-time 1; Asian/Pacific Islander—full-time 0, part-time 0; American Indian/Alaska Native—full-time 0, part-time 0; Caucasian/White—full-time 23, part-time 23; Multi-ethnic—full-time 2, part-time 1; students subject to the Americans With Disabilities Act—full-time 1, part-time 0; Unknown ethnicity—full-time 1, part-time 3; International students who hold an F-1 or J-1 Visa—full-time 1, part-time 0.

Financial Information/Assistance:
Tuition for Full-Time Study: *Master's:* State residents: $510 per credit hour; Nonstate residents: $510 per credit hour. Tuition is

subject to change. See the following Web site for updates and changes in tuition costs: http://www.smcvt.edu/graduate/courses/tuition.asp.

Financial Assistance:
First-Year Students: Teaching assistantships available for first year. Average number of hours worked per week: 20. Apply by July 1.
Advanced Students: No information provided.
Additional Information: Of all students currently enrolled full time, 5% benefited from one or more of the listed financial assistance programs. Application and information available online at: http://www.smcvt.edu/graduate/admission/finaid.asp.

Internships/Practica: Master's Degree (MA/MS Clinical Psychology): An internship experience, such as a final research project or "capstone" experience is required of graduates. We have practice and internship sites in the following settings: schools, college counseling centers, teaching hospitals, correctional centers, Visiting Nurses Association, community mental health outpatient and residential offices, drug and alcohol treatment center, adolescent day treatment program.

Housing and Day Care: No on-campus housing is available. On-campus day care facilities are available. See the following Web site for more information: Child Care is available on campus, information can be obtained from the Web site, http://www.smcvt.edu/elc/default.asp.

Employment of Department Graduates:
Master's Degree Graduates: Of those who graduated in the academic year 2008–2009, the following categories and numbers represent the postgraduate activities and employment of master's degree graduates: Enrolled in a psychology doctoral program (1), enrolled in another graduate/professional program (0), enrolled in a postdoctoral residency/fellowship (n/a), employed in independent practice (n/a), employed in an academic position at a university (0), employed in an academic position at a 2-year/4-year college (0), employed in other positions at a higher education institution (0), employed in a professional position in a school system (1), employed in business or industry (0), employed in government agency (1), employed in a community mental health/counseling center (5), employed in a hospital/medical center (1), still seeking employment (0), other employment position (6), do not know (2), total from the above (master's) (17).
Doctoral Degree Graduates: Of those who graduated in the academic year 2008–2009, the following categories and numbers represent the postgraduate activities and employment of doctoral degree graduates: Enrolled in a psychology doctoral program (n/a), total from the above (doctoral) (0).

Additional Information:
Orientation, Objectives, and Emphasis of Department: The focus of the MA program in clinical psychology is on the integration of theory, research, and practice in the preparation of professional psychologists. Our goal is to provide an educational milieu that respects the individual educational goals of the student, and fosters intellectual, personal, and professional development. The program is eclectic in orientation and the faculty offer a diversity of interests, orientations, and experiences within the framework of our curriculum. We see ourselves as preparing students for professional practice in community agencies, schools, hospitals, and public and private clinics. Cross-registration in courses offered by the college's other master's degree programs in education, administration, and theology is available for those wishing an interdisciplinary emphasis. The curriculum is also designed with two further objectives in mind: (1) the preparation of students for state licensing examinations, and (2) further doctoral study in professional psychology at another institution. All classes are held in the evening, permitting full- or part-time study. The program seeks to integrate a psychodynamic understanding of the therapeutic relationship with humanistic values, and a social systems perspective.

Special Facilities or Resources: St. Michael's College offers the graduate student a faculty committed to teaching and professional training in a non-bureaucratic learning environment. All clinical courses are taught by highly experienced clinical practitioners who serve as part-time faculty. The full-time faculty teach core courses in general, developmental, and social psychology, as well as research methods. The college has excellent computing facilities for the support of social science research.

Application Information:
Send to Graduate Admission, Saint Michael's College, One Winooski Park, Box 286, Colchester, VT 05439. Application available online. URL of online application: http://www.smcvt.edu/graduate/admission/. Fall enrollment is recommended, and applications for Fall are encouraged by July 1, in order to be eligible for TA positions. *Fee:* $35.

Vermont, University of
Department of Psychology
Arts and Sciences
2 Colchester Avenue; John Dewey Hall
Burlington, VT 05405-0134
Telephone: (802) 656-2670
Fax: (802) 656-8783
E-mail: *psychology@uvm.edu*
Web: *http://www.uvm.edu/psychology*

Department Information:
1937. Chairperson: William Falls, PhD Number of faculty: total—full-time 25, part-time 2; women—full-time 13, part-time 1; total—minority—full-time 2; women minority—full-time 1; faculty subject to the Americans With Disabilities Act 1.

Programs and Degrees Offered:
Listed in the following order: Program area, degree type (T if terminal Master's), number awarded 7/08–6/09. General/Experimental Psychology PhD (Doctor of Philosophy) 2, Clinical Psychology PhD (Doctor of Philosophy) 3.

APA Accreditation: Clinical PhD (Doctor of Philosophy). Student Outcome Data Website: http://www.uvm.edu/psychology/?Page=programs/graduate/clinical/clinical_applicant_data.html&SM=gradmenu.html.

Student Applications/Admissions:
Student Applications
General/Experimental Psychology PhD (Doctor of Philosophy)—Applications 2009–2010, 36. Total applicants accepted 2009–

2010, 4. Number full-time enrolled (new admits only) 2009–2010, 4. Number part-time enrolled (new admits only) 2009–2010, 0. Openings 2010–2011, 8. The median number of years required for completion of a degree in 2008–2009 were 6. The number of students enrolled full- and part-time who were dismissed or voluntarily withdrew from this program area in 2008–2009 were 0. *Clinical Psychology PhD (Doctor of Philosophy)*—Applications 2009–2010, 157. Total applicants accepted 2009–2010, 4. Number full-time enrolled (new admits only) 2009–2010, 3. Number part-time enrolled (new admits only) 2009–2010, 0. Openings 2010–2011, 8. The median number of years required for completion of a degree in 2008–2009 were 6. The number of students enrolled full- and part-time who were dismissed or voluntarily withdrew from this program area in 2008–2009 were 0.

Scores: Entries appear in this order: required test or GPA, minimum score (if required), median score of students entering in 2009–2010. *Clinical Psychology PhD (Doctor of Philosophy):* GRE-V no minimum stated, 600, GRE-Q no minimum stated, 685, overall undergraduate GPA no minimum stated, 3.79.

Other Criteria: (importance of criteria rated low, medium, or high): GRE scores—high, research experience—high, work experience—medium, extracurricular activity—low, clinically related public service—medium, GPA—high, letters of recommendation—high, interview—high, statement of goals and objectives—high, undergraduate major in psychology—high, specific undergraduate psychology courses taken—medium. Clinically related public service is of importance for clinical program only. For additional information on admission requirements, go to http://www.uvm.edu/psychology/?Page=programs/graduate/application.html&SM=gradmenu.html.

Student Characteristics: The following represents characteristics of students in 2009–2010 in all graduate psychology programs in the department: Female—full-time 50, part-time 0; Male—full-time 10, part-time 0; African American/Black—full-time 1, part-time 0; Hispanic/Latino(a)—full-time 5, part-time 0; Asian/Pacific Islander—full-time 0, part-time 0; American Indian/Alaska Native—full-time 0, part-time 0; Caucasian/White—full-time 54, part-time 0; Multi-ethnic—full-time 0, part-time 0; students subject to the Americans With Disabilities Act—full-time 0, part-time 0; Unknown ethnicity—full-time 0, part-time 0; International students who hold an F-1 or J-1 Visa—full-time 0, part-time 0.

Financial Information/Assistance:
Tuition for Full-Time Study: *Doctoral:* State residents: $488 per credit hour; Nonstate residents: $1,162 per credit hour. Tuition is subject to change. See the following Web site for updates and changes in tuition costs: http://www.uvm.edu/~stdfinsv/?Page=graduate-tuition.html&SM=tuitionsubmenu.html.

Financial Assistance:
First-Year Students: Teaching assistantships available for first year. Average amount paid per academic year: $15,000. Average number of hours worked per week: 20. Research assistantships available for first year. Average amount paid per academic year: $23,000. Average number of hours worked per week: 20. Traineeships available for first year. Average amount paid per academic year: $15,000. Average number of hours worked per week: 20.

Advanced Students: Teaching assistantships available for advanced students. Average amount paid per academic year: $15,000. Average number of hours worked per week: 20. Research assistantships available for advanced students. Average amount paid per academic year: $23,000. Average number of hours worked per week: 20. Traineeships available for advanced students. Average amount paid per academic year: $15,000. Average number of hours worked per week: 20.

Additional Information: Of all students currently enrolled full time, 100% benefited from one or more of the listed financial assistance programs. Application and information available online at: http://www.uvm.edu/psychology/.

Internships/Practica: Doctoral Degree (PhD Clinical Psychology): For those doctoral students for whom a professional internship was required in this program prior to graduation, (4) students applied for an internship in 2008–2009, with (4) students obtaining an internship. Of those students who obtained an internship, (4) were paid internships. Of those students who obtained an internship, (4) students placed in APA/CPA accredited internships, (0) students placed in internships not APA/CPA accredited, but listed with the Association of Psychology Postdoctoral and Internship Programs (APPIC), (0) students placed in internships conforming to guidelines of the Council of Directors of School Psychology Programs (CDSPP), (0) students placed in internships that were not APA/CPA accredited, APPIC or CDSPP listed. Multiple clinical practica are available, including outpatient and inpatient adult assessment and psychotherapy, outpatient child and adolescent assessment and psychotherapy, community mental health centers, and medical centers/hospitals. All practica are funded for 20 hours per week.

Housing and Day Care: On-campus housing is available. See the following Web site for more information: http://reslife.uvm.edu/~rlweb/graduate_students/. On-campus day care facilities are available. See the following Web site for more information: http://www.uvm.edu/~ips1/ccc/.

Employment of Department Graduates:
Master's Degree Graduates: Of those who graduated in the academic year 2008–2009, the following categories and numbers represent the postgraduate activities and employment of master's degree graduates: Enrolled in a psychology doctoral program (0), enrolled in another graduate/professional program (0), enrolled in a postdoctoral residency/fellowship (n/a), employed in independent practice (n/a), employed in an academic position at a university (0), employed in an academic position at a 2-year/4-year college (0), employed in other positions at a higher education institution (0), employed in a professional position in a school system (0), employed in business or industry (0), employed in government agency (0), employed in a community mental health/counseling center (0), employed in a hospital/medical center (0), still seeking employment (0), other employment position (0), total from the above (master's) (0).

Doctoral Degree Graduates: Of those who graduated in the academic year 2008–2009, the following categories and numbers represent the postgraduate activities and employment of doctoral degree graduates: Enrolled in a psychology doctoral program (n/a), enrolled in a postdoctoral residency/fellowship (1), employed in independent practice (0), employed in an academic position at a university (0), employed in an academic position at a 2-year/4-year college (0), employed in other positions at a higher education institution (2), employed in a professional position in a school system (0), employed in business or industry (0), employed in government agency (0), employed in a community mental health/counseling center (0), employed in a hospital/medical center (1), still seeking employment (0), other employment position (0), do not know (1), total from the above (doctoral) (5).

Additional Information:

Orientation, Objectives, and Emphasis of Department: The clinical psychology program is based upon a scientist–practitioner model and is designed to develop competent professional psychologists who can function in applied academic or research positions. Training stresses early placement in a variety of nearby clinical facilities and simultaneous research training relevant to clinical problems. Clinical orientations are primarily cognitive-behavioral. The general/experimental program admits students in three broad specialty areas: (1) basic and applied developmental and social psychology that includes research on ways in which people simultaneously influence and are influenced by social situations and cultural contexts; (2) biobehavioral psychology that focuses on behavioral and neurobiological approaches to learning, memory, emotion, and drug abuse; and (3) human behavioral pharmacology and substance abuse treatment. Students must fulfill general/experimental program requirements as well as requirements for the specialty area in which they are accepted. Applicants should be as specific as possible about their program interest areas.

Special Facilities or Resources: The department has excellent laboratories in behavioral neuroscience, group dynamics, developmental, human psychophysiology, and general human testing. Excellent computer facilities and an in-house psychology clinic with clinical research equipment are available.

Information for Students With Physical Disabilities: See the following Web site for more information: http://www.uvm.edu/~access/.

Application Information:
Send to Graduate College, Admissions Office, Waterman Building, University of Vermont, Burlington, VT 05405. Application available online. URL of online application: http://www.uvm.edu/~gradcoll/?Page=admissions.html. Students are admitted in the Fall, application deadline December 1. Deadline is December 1 for Clinical program and January 2 for General/Experimental program. *Fee:* $40. Possibility of waiver for minority applicants.

VIRGINIA

Argosy University/Washington, DC
Clinical Psychology
American School of Professional Psychology
1550 Wilson Boulevard, Suite 600
Arlington, VA 22209
Telephone: (703) 526-5800
Fax: (571) 480-7402
E-mail: *rbarrett@argosy.edu*
Web: *http://www.argosy.edu*

Department Information:
1994. Chair, Clinical Psychology Programs: Robert F. Barrett, PhD. Number of faculty: total—full-time 26, part-time 4; women—full-time 16, part-time 3; total—minority—full-time 9, part-time 1; women minority—full-time 7, part-time 1.

Programs and Degrees Offered:
Listed in the following order: Program area, degree type (T if terminal Master's), number awarded 7/08–6/09. Clinical Psychology MA/MS (Master of Arts/Science) (T) 33, Clinical Psychology PsyD (Doctor of Psychology) 55.

APA Accreditation: Clinical PsyD (Doctor of Psychology). Student Outcome Data Website: http://www.argosy.edu/colleges/ProgramDetail.aspx?ID=887&section=outcomes.

Student Applications/Admissions:
Student Applications
Clinical Psychology MA/MS (Master of Arts/Science)—Applications 2009–2010, 31. Total applicants accepted 2009–2010, 19. Number full-time enrolled (new admits only) 2009–2010, 24. Number part-time enrolled (new admits only) 2009–2010, 3. Total enrolled 2009–2010 full-time, 34, part-time, 9. Openings 2010–2011, 20. The median number of years required for completion of a degree in 2008–2009 were 2. The number of students enrolled full- and part-time who were dismissed or voluntarily withdrew from this program area in 2008–2009 were 0. Clinical Psychology PsyD (Doctor of Psychology)—Applications 2009–2010, 212. Total applicants accepted 2009–2010, 73. Number full-time enrolled (new admits only) 2009–2010, 62. Number part-time enrolled (new admits only) 2009–2010, 15. Total enrolled 2009–2010 full-time, 364, part-time, 26. Openings 2010–2011, 90. The median number of years required for completion of a degree in 2008–2009 were 5. The number of students enrolled full- and part-time who were dismissed or voluntarily withdrew from this program area in 2008–2009 were 22.
Scores: Entries appear in this order: required test or GPA, minimum score (if required), median score of students entering in 2009–2010. Clinical Psychology MA/MS (Master of Arts/Science): overall undergraduate GPA 3.0, last 2 years GPA 3.0; Clinical Psychology PsyD (Doctor of Psychology): overall undergraduate GPA 3.25, Masters GPA 3.25.
Other Criteria: (importance of criteria rated low, medium, or high): research experience—low, work experience—low, extracurricular activity—low, clinically related public service—medium, GPA—high, letters of recommendation—high, interview—high, statement of goals and objectives—high, specific undergraduate psychology courses taken—high. Clinical experience is less important for applicants to MA program.

Student Characteristics: The following represents characteristics of students in 2009–2010 in all graduate psychology programs in the department: Female—full-time 337, part-time 30; Male—full-time 61, part-time 5; African American/Black—full-time 92, part-time 16; Hispanic/Latino(a)—full-time 19, part-time 4; Asian/Pacific Islander—full-time 20, part-time 1; American Indian/Alaska Native—full-time 1, part-time 0; Caucasian/White—full-time 243, part-time 13; Multi-ethnic—full-time 0, part-time 0; students subject to the Americans With Disabilities Act—full-time 16, part-time 0; Unknown ethnicity—full-time 23, part-time 1; International students who hold an F-1 or J-1 Visa—full-time 8, part-time 0.

Financial Information/Assistance:
Tuition for Full-Time Study: *Master's:* State residents: per academic year $23,952, $998 per credit hour; Nonstate residents: per academic year $23,952, $998 per credit hour. *Doctoral:* State residents: per academic year $23,952, $998 per credit hour; Nonstate residents: per academic year $23,952, $998 per credit hour. Tuition is subject to change. See the following Web site for updates and changes in tuition costs: http://www.argosy.edu.

Financial Assistance:
First-Year Students: Fellowships and scholarships available for first year. Average amount paid per academic year: $500.
Advanced Students: Teaching assistantships available for advanced students. Average amount paid per academic year: $1,827. Average number of hours worked per week: 5. Research assistantships available for advanced students. Average amount paid per academic year: $1,425. Average number of hours worked per week: 4. Fellowships and scholarships available for advanced students. Average amount paid per academic year: $2,850. Average number of hours worked per week: 8.
Additional Information: Of all students currently enrolled full time, 33% benefited from one or more of the listed financial assistance programs.

Internships/Practica: Doctoral Degree (PsyD Clinical Psychology): For those doctoral students for whom a professional internship was required in this program prior to graduation, (87) students applied for an internship in 2008–2009, with (76) students obtaining an internship. Of those students who obtained an internship, (73) were paid internships. Of those students who obtained an internship, (29) students placed in APA/CPA accredited internships, (38) students placed in internships not APA/CPA accredited, but listed with the Association of Psychology Postdoctoral and Internship Programs (APPIC), (0) students placed in internships conforming to guidelines of the Council of Directors of School Psychology Programs (CDSPP), (9) students placed in internships that were not APA/CPA accredited, APPIC or CDSPP listed. Master's Degree (MA/MS Clinical Psychology): An internship experience, such as a final research project or "capstone" experience is required of graduates. Practicum training is designed to give students the opportunity to work under supervision with a clinical population within a mental health delivery system. Students learn to apply their theoretical knowledge; implement, develop, and assess the efficacy of clinical techniques; and develop the professional attitudes important for the identity of a professional psychologist. Doctoral students complete two training practicum sequences (600 hours each) focusing on assessment or psychotherapy skills or integrating the two. Master's students are required to complete one practicum (600 hours). All doctoral students are required to complete a one year (12 month) internship as a condition for graduation. This intensive and supervised contact with clients is essential for giving greater breadth and depth to the student's overall academic experience. Typically, students will begin the internship during their fourth or fifth year, depending on the student's progress through the curriculum.

Housing and Day Care: No on-campus housing is available. No on-campus day care facilities are available.

Employment of Department Graduates:
Master's Degree Graduates: Of those who graduated in the academic year 2008–2009, the following categories and numbers represent the postgraduate activities and employment of master's degree graduates: Enrolled in a psychology doctoral program (9), enrolled in a postdoctoral residency/fellowship (n/a), employed in independent practice (n/a), employed in a professional position in a school system (1), employed in business or industry (1), employed in a community mental health/counseling center (2), not seeking employment (1), other employment position (1), do not know (18), total from the above (master's) (33).

Doctoral Degree Graduates: Of those who graduated in the academic year 2008–2009, the following categories and numbers represent the postgraduate activities and employment of doctoral degree graduates: Enrolled in a psychology doctoral program (n/a), enrolled in a postdoctoral residency/fellowship (7), employed in independent practice (8), employed in an academic position at a university (6), employed in an academic position at a 2-year/4-year college (1), employed in other positions at a higher education institution (2), employed in a professional position in a school system (3), employed in business or industry (1), employed in government agency (2), employed in a community mental health/counseling center (1), other employment position (7), do not know (17), total from the above (doctoral) (55).

Additional Information:
Orientation, Objectives, and Emphasis of Department: The doctoral program in clinical psychology (PsyD) is designed to educate and train students to function effectively in diverse professional roles. The program emphasizes the development of attitudes, knowledge, and skills essential in the formation of professional psychologists who are committed to the ethical provision of quality services. The school offers a broad-based curriculum, providing a meaningful integration of diverse theoretical perspectives, scholarship, and practice. The program offers concentrations in forensic psychology, health and neuropsychology, child and family, and diversity. Opportunities are available for students to develop expertise in a number of areas including the provision of services to specific populations such as children and families; theoretical perspectives such as cognitive-behavioral, family systems, psychodynamic, and client centered; and areas of application such as forensics and health psychology. The Master's degree (MA) in clinical psychology is designed to meet the needs of both those students seeking a terminal degree for work in the mental health field and those who eventually plan to pursue a doctoral degree. The program provides a solid core of basic psychology, as well as a strong clinical orientation with an emphasis in psychological assessment.

Special Facilities or Resources: Argosy University is conveniently located minutes from downtown Washington, DC. The on-site library has developed a focused psychology collection consisting of reference titles and books, journals, diagnostic assessment instruments, and audiovisual equipment. There are two computer labs and students have full access to both computerized literature searches and electronic text of most journals. In addition, students have access to the rich library resources of the Washington, DC, area including the National Library of Medicine and the Library of Congress.

Application Information:
Send to Admissions Department, Argosy University/Washington, DC, 1550 Wilson Boulevard, Ste. 600, Arlington, VA 22209. Students are admitted in the Fall, application deadline January 15. *Fee:* $50.

College of William and Mary
Department of Psychology/Predoctoral MA Program
P.O. Box 8795
Williamsburg, VA 23187-8795
Telephone: (757) 221-3870
Fax: (757) 221-3896
E-mail: *tlcoates@wm.edu*
Web: *http://www.wm.edu/as/psychology/*

Department Information:
1946. Chairperson: Constance J. Pilkington, PhD. Number of faculty: total—full-time 21, part-time 7; women—full-time 8, part-time 3.

Programs and Degrees Offered:
Listed in the following order: Program area, degree type (T if terminal Master's), number awarded 7/08–6/09. General Psychology MA/MS (Master of Arts/Science) (T) 6.

Student Applications/Admissions:
Student Applications
General Psychology MA/MS (Master of Arts/Science)—Applications 2009–2010, 86. Total applicants accepted 2009–2010, 15. Number full-time enrolled (new admits only) 2009–2010, 7. Number part-time enrolled (new admits only) 2009–2010, 0. Openings 2010–2011, 7. The median number of years required for completion of a degree in 2008–2009 were 2. The number of students enrolled full- and part-time who were dismissed or voluntarily withdrew from this program area in 2008–2009 were 0.

Scores: Entries appear in this order: required test or GPA, minimum score (if required), median score of students entering in 2009–2010. *General Psychology MA/MS (Master of Arts/Science):* GRE-V no minimum stated, 550, GRE-Q no minimum stated, 670, GRE-Analytical no minimum stated.

Other Criteria: (importance of criteria rated low, medium, or high): GRE scores—medium, research experience—high, work experience—medium, extracurricular activity—low, clinically related public service—low, GPA—medium, letters of recommendation—high, statement of goals and objectives—high. For additional information on admission requirements, go to http://www.wm.edu/as/psychology/gradprogram/maprogram/Index.php.

Student Characteristics: The following represents characteristics of students in 2009–2010 in all graduate psychology programs in the department: Female—full-time 7, part-time 0; Male—full-time 7, part-time 0; African American/Black—full-time 0, part-time 0; Hispanic/Latino(a)—full-time 0, part-time 0; Asian/Pacific Islander—full-time 0, part-time 0; American Indian/Alaska Native—full-time 0, part-time 0; Caucasian/White—full-time 14, part-time 0; Multi-ethnic—full-time 0, part-time 0; students subject to the Americans With Disabilities Act—full-time 0, part-time 0; Unknown ethnicity—full-time 0, part-time 0; International students who hold an F-1 or J-1 Visa—full-time 1, part-time 0.

Financial Information/Assistance:
Tuition for Full-Time Study: *Master's:* State residents: per academic year $10,514, $315 per credit hour; Nonstate residents: per academic year $24,204, $840 per credit hour. Tuition is subject to change. See the following Web site for updates and changes in tuition costs: http://www.wm.edu/admission/financialaid/tuition/.

Financial Assistance:
First-Year Students: Teaching assistantships available for first year. Average amount paid per academic year: $9,000. Average number of hours worked per week: 20. Apply by February 15. Research assistantships available for first year. Average amount paid per academic year: $9,000. Average number of hours worked per week: 20. Apply by February 15. Fellowships and scholarships available for first year. Average amount paid per academic year: $9,000. Average number of hours worked per week: 20. Apply by February 15.

Advanced Students: Teaching assistantships available for advanced students. Average amount paid per academic year: $9,000. Average number of hours worked per week: 20. Apply by February 15. Research assistantships available for advanced students. Average amount paid per academic year: $9,000. Average number of hours worked per week: 20. Apply by February 15. Fellowships and scholarships available for advanced students. Average amount paid per academic year: $9,000. Average number of hours worked per week: 20. Apply by February 15.

Additional Information: Of all students currently enrolled full time, 100% benefited from one or more of the listed financial assistance programs. Application and information available online at: http://www.wm.edu/admission/financialaid/.

Housing and Day Care: On-campus housing is available. See the following Web site for more information: http://www.wm.edu/offices/residencelife/oncampus/residencehalls/graduate/index.php. On-campus day care facilities are available. See the following Web site for more information: http://www.wm.edu/offices/wccc/.

Employment of Department Graduates:
Master's Degree Graduates: Of those who graduated in the academic year 2008–2009, the following categories and numbers represent the postgraduate activities and employment of master's degree graduates: Enrolled in a psychology doctoral program (5), enrolled in a postdoctoral residency/fellowship (n/a), employed in independent practice (n/a), employed in other positions at a higher education institution (1), do not know (1), total from the above (master's) (7).

Doctoral Degree Graduates: Of those who graduated in the academic year 2008–2009, the following categories and numbers represent the postgraduate activities and employment of doctoral degree graduates: Enrolled in a psychology doctoral program (n/a), total from the above (doctoral) (0).

Additional Information:
Orientation, Objectives, and Emphasis of Department: The general psychology MA program is designed to prepare students for admission to PhD programs. Students are not admitted if they are not planning to further their education. There is a heavy research emphasis throughout both years of the program.

Special Facilities or Resources: Our faculty members develop and work with the MA students to design, conduct, and analyze research data. These studies are often published in professional journals. Subjects accessible for research include individuals from the community, college students, and rats. Computer facilities are available in the department that are strictly for MA students.

Information for Students With Physical Disabilities: See the following Web site for more information: http://www.wm.edu/offices/deanofstudents/services/disabilityservices/.

Application Information:
Send to Director of Graduate Admissions, Psychology Department, The College of William and Mary, P.O. Box 8795, Williamsburg, VA 23187-8795. Application available online. URL of online application: http://www.applyweb.com/apply/wmgrad/. Students are admitted in the Fall, application deadline February 15. *Fee:* $45.

George Mason University
Department of Psychology
Humanities and Social Sciences
4400 University Drive, MSN 3F5
Fairfax, VA 22030-4444
Telephone: (703) 993-1342
Fax: (703) 993-1359
E-mail: *dwiggin3@gmu.edu*
Web: *http://psychology.gmu.edu/*

Department Information:
1966. Chairperson: Deborah Boehm-Davis. Number of faculty: total—full-time 46, part-time 17; women—full-time 18, part-time 9; total—minority—full-time 4; women minority—full-time 1.

Programs and Degrees Offered:
Listed in the following order: Program area, degree type (T if terminal Master's), number awarded 7/08–6/09. Clinical Psychology PhD (Doctor of Philosophy) 5, Industrial/Organizational PhD (Doctor of Philosophy) 5, Biopsychology PhD (Doctor of Philosophy) 4, School Psychology MA/MS (Master of Arts/Science) (T)

10, Industrial/Organizational MA/MS (Master of Arts/Science) (T) 22, Human Factors and Applied Cognition MA/MS (Master of Arts/Science) (T) 8, Biopsychology MA/MS (Master of Arts/Science) (T) 3, Applied Developmental MA/MS (Master of Arts/Science) (T) 11, Human Factors and Applied Cognition PhD (Doctor of Philosophy) 6, Applied Developmental PhD (Doctor of Philosophy) 4.

APA Accreditation: Clinical PhD (Doctor of Philosophy). Student Outcome Data Website: http://psychology.gmu.edu/clinical/stats.htm.

Student Applications/Admissions:
Student Applications
Clinical Psychology PhD (Doctor of Philosophy)—Applications 2009–2010, 176. Total applicants accepted 2009–2010, 11. Number full-time enrolled (new admits only) 2009–2010, 5. Number part-time enrolled (new admits only) 2009–2010, 0. Total enrolled 2009–2010 full-time, 37, part-time, 3. Openings 2010–2011, 8. The median number of years required for completion of a degree in 2008–2009 were 5. The number of students enrolled full- and part-time who were dismissed or voluntarily withdrew from this program area in 2008–2009 were 1. *Industrial/Organizational PhD (Doctor of Philosophy)*—Applications 2009–2010, 108. Total applicants accepted 2009–2010, 16. Number full-time enrolled (new admits only) 2009–2010, 6. Number part-time enrolled (new admits only) 2009–2010, 0. Total enrolled 2009–2010 full-time, 25, part-time, 6. Openings 2010–2011, 7. The median number of years required for completion of a degree in 2008–2009 were 6. The number of students enrolled full- and part-time who were dismissed or voluntarily withdrew from this program area in 2008–2009 were 1. *Biopsychology PhD (Doctor of Philosophy)*—Applications 2009–2010, 13. Total applicants accepted 2009–2010, 4. Number full-time enrolled (new admits only) 2009–2010, 2. Number part-time enrolled (new admits only) 2009–2010, 0. Openings 2010–2011, 4. The median number of years required for completion of a degree in 2008–2009 were 6. The number of students enrolled full- and part-time who were dismissed or voluntarily withdrew from this program area in 2008–2009 were 0. *School Psychology MA/MS (Master of Arts/Science)*—Applications 2009–2010, 53. Total applicants accepted 2009–2010, 19. Number full-time enrolled (new admits only) 2009–2010, 7. Number part-time enrolled (new admits only) 2009–2010, 0. Openings 2010–2011, 10. The median number of years required for completion of a degree in 2008–2009 were 3. The number of students enrolled full- and part-time who were dismissed or voluntarily withdrew from this program area in 2008–2009 were 2. *Industrial/Organizational MA/MS (Master of Arts/Science)*—Applications 2009–2010, 143. Total applicants accepted 2009–2010, 22. Number full-time enrolled (new admits only) 2009–2010, 12. Number part-time enrolled (new admits only) 2009–2010, 3. Total enrolled 2009–2010 full-time, 21, part-time, 10. Openings 2010–2011, 15. The median number of years required for completion of a degree in 2008–2009 were 2. The number of students enrolled full- and part-time who were dismissed or voluntarily withdrew from this program area in 2008–2009 were 0. *Human Factors and Applied Cognition MA/MS (Master of Arts/Science)*—Applications 2009–2010, 35. Total applicants accepted 2009–2010, 17. Number full-time enrolled (new admits only) 2009–2010, 5. Number part-time enrolled (new admits only) 2009–2010, 2. Total enrolled 2009–2010 full-time, 17, part-time, 5. Openings 2010–2011, 20. The median number of years required for completion of a degree in 2008–2009 were 2. The number of students enrolled full- and part-time who were dismissed or voluntarily withdrew from this program area in 2008–2009 were 0. *Biopsychology MA/MS (Master of Arts/Science)*—Applications 2009–2010, 6. Total applicants accepted 2009–2010, 5. Number full-time enrolled (new admits only) 2009–2010, 2. Number part-time enrolled (new admits only) 2009–2010, 1. Total enrolled 2009–2010 full-time, 9, part-time, 12. Openings 2010–2011, 6. The median number of years required for completion of a degree in 2008–2009 were 3. The number of students enrolled full- and part-time who were dismissed or voluntarily withdrew from this program area in 2008–2009 were 0. *Applied Developmental MA/MS (Master of Arts/Science)*—Applications 2009–2010, 37. Total applicants accepted 2009–2010, 11. Number full-time enrolled (new admits only) 2009–2010, 5. Number part-time enrolled (new admits only) 2009–2010, 6. Total enrolled 2009–2010 full-time, 18, part-time, 15. Openings 2010–2011, 11. The median number of years required for completion of a degree in 2008–2009 were 3. The number of students enrolled full- and part-time who were dismissed or voluntarily withdrew from this program area in 2008–2009 were 0. *Human Factors and Applied Cognition PhD (Doctor of Philosophy)*—Applications 2009–2010, 20. Total applicants accepted 2009–2010, 9. Number full-time enrolled (new admits only) 2009–2010, 6. Number part-time enrolled (new admits only) 2009–2010, 0. Total enrolled 2009–2010 full-time, 16, part-time, 1. Openings 2010–2011, 7. The median number of years required for completion of a degree in 2008–2009 were 5. The number of students enrolled full- and part-time who were dismissed or voluntarily withdrew from this program area in 2008–2009 were 0. *Applied Developmental PhD (Doctor of Philosophy)*—Applications 2009–2010, 20. Total applicants accepted 2009–2010, 10. Number full-time enrolled (new admits only) 2009–2010, 5. Number part-time enrolled (new admits only) 2009–2010, 0. Total enrolled 2009–2010 full-time, 25, part-time, 2. Openings 2010–2011, 5. The median number of years required for completion of a degree in 2008–2009 were 5. The number of students enrolled full- and part-time who were dismissed or voluntarily withdrew from this program area in 2008–2009 were 1.

Scores: Entries appear in this order: required test or GPA, minimum score (if required), median score of students entering in 2009–2010. *Clinical Psychology PhD (Doctor of Philosophy)*: GRE-V no minimum stated, GRE-Q no minimum stated, overall undergraduate GPA no minimum stated, last 2 years GPA 3.0, psychology GPA 3.25; *Industrial/Organizational PhD (Doctor of Philosophy)*: GRE-V no minimum stated, GRE-Q no minimum stated, overall undergraduate GPA no minimum stated, last 2 years GPA 3.0, psychology GPA 3.25; *Biopsychology PhD (Doctor of Philosophy)*: GRE-V no minimum stated, GRE-Q no minimum stated, last 2 years GPA 3.0, psychology GPA 3.25; *School Psychology MA/MS (Master of Arts/Science)*: GRE-V no minimum stated, GRE-Q no minimum stated, overall undergraduate GPA no minimum stated, last 2 years GPA 3.0, psychology GPA 3.25; *Industrial/Organizational MA/MS (Master of Arts/Science)*: GRE-V no minimum stated, GRE-Q no minimum stated, overall undergraduate GPA no minimum stated, last 2 years GPA 3.0, psychology GPA 3.25; *Biopsychology MA/MS (Master of Arts/Science)*: GRE-V no minimum stated, GRE-Q no minimum stated, overall undergraduate

GPA no minimum stated, last 2 years GPA 3.0, psychology GPA 3.25.

Other Criteria: (importance of criteria rated low, medium, or high): GRE scores—high, research experience—medium, work experience—medium, extracurricular activity—low, clinically related public service—medium, GPA—high, letters of recommendation—high, interview—high, statement of goals and objectives—high, undergraduate major in psychology—medium, specific undergraduate psychology courses taken—high. The Clinical and School programs interview a select group by invitation only. The Biopsychology, Developmental, Human Factors/Applied Cognition, and Industrial/Organizational programs do not require an interview but hold an open house for selected students to attend. Clinical and Applied Developmental PhD are are required to submit the PhD Departmental Form where they select two faculty they wish to work with. This is strongly recommended but not required for other concentrations. For additional information on admission requirements, go to http://psychology.gmu.edu/.

Student Characteristics: The following represents characteristics of students in 2009–2010 in all graduate psychology programs in the department: Female—full-time 141, part-time 33; Male—full-time 60, part-time 21; African American/Black—full-time 9, part-time 0; Hispanic/Latino(a)—full-time 6, part-time 1; Asian/Pacific Islander—full-time 12, part-time 5; American Indian/Alaska Native—full-time 2, part-time 0; Caucasian/White—full-time 125, part-time 37; Multi-ethnic—full-time 14, part-time 4; students subject to the Americans With Disabilities Act—full-time 0, part-time 0; Unknown ethnicity—full-time 33, part-time 7; International students who hold an F-1 or J-1 Visa—full-time 1, part-time 0.

Financial Information/Assistance:
Tuition for Full-Time Study: Master's: State residents: per academic year $9,552, $398 per credit hour; Nonstate residents: per academic year $23,688, $987 per credit hour. *Doctoral:* State residents: per academic year $9,552, $398 per credit hour; Nonstate residents: per academic year $23,688, $987 per credit hour. Tuition is subject to change. See the following Web site for updates and changes in tuition costs: http://studentaccounts.gmu.edu/.

Financial Assistance:
First-Year Students: Teaching assistantships available for first year. Average amount paid per academic year: $14,000. Apply by January 1. Research assistantships available for first year. Average amount paid per academic year: $14,000. Apply by January 1. Fellowships and scholarships available for first year. Average amount paid per academic year: $1,000. Apply by January 1.

Advanced Students: Teaching assistantships available for advanced students. Average amount paid per academic year: $14,000. Apply by February 15. Research assistantships available for advanced students. Average amount paid per academic year: $14,000. Apply by February 15.

Additional Information: Of all students currently enrolled full time, 40% benefited from one or more of the listed financial assistance programs. Application and information available online at: http://psychology.gmu.edu/.

Internships/Practica: Doctoral Degree (PhD Clinical Psychology): For those doctoral students for whom a professional internship was required in this program prior to graduation, (7) students applied for an internship in 2008–2009, with (7) students obtaining an internship. Of those students who obtained an internship, (7) were paid internships. Of those students who obtained an internship, (7) students placed in APA/CPA accredited internships, (0) students placed in internships not APA/CPA accredited, but listed with the Association of Psychology Postdoctoral and Internship Programs (APPIC), (0) students placed in internships conforming to guidelines of the Council of Directors of School Psychology Programs (CDSPP), (0) students placed in internships that were not APA/CPA accredited, APPIC or CDSPP listed. Master's Degree (MA/MS School Psychology): An internship experience, such as a final research project or "capstone" experience is required of graduates. Master's Degree (MA/MS Biopsychology): An internship experience, such as a final research project or "capstone" experience is required of graduates. All programs either require or offer practicum placements in a wide variety of settings, including mental health treatment facilities, medical facilities, schools, government agencies, the military, and businesses and organizations.

Housing and Day Care: On-campus housing is available. See the following Web site for more information: http://housing.gmu.edu/. On-campus day care facilities are available. See the following Web site for more information: http://www.gmu.edu/depts/cdc/.

Employment of Department Graduates:
Master's Degree Graduates: Of those who graduated in the academic year 2008–2009, the following categories and numbers represent the postgraduate activities and employment of master's degree graduates: Enrolled in a postdoctoral residency/fellowship (n/a), employed in independent practice (n/a), total from the above (master's) (0).

Doctoral Degree Graduates: Of those who graduated in the academic year 2008–2009, the following categories and numbers represent the postgraduate activities and employment of doctoral degree graduates: Enrolled in a psychology doctoral program (n/a), total from the above (doctoral) (0).

Additional Information:
Orientation, Objectives, and Emphasis of Department: All graduate programs emphasize both basic research and the application of research to solving problems in families, schools, industry, government, and health care settings.

Special Facilities or Resources: The Developmental research area includes individual test rooms, a family interaction room, and a number of faculty research areas; some of the test rooms are equipped with video and computers. Biopsychology includes a rodent colony, modern facilities for behavior testing (including drug self-administration), a Neurolucida system for neuroanatomical evaluation, and extensive histological capability. Biopsychology also has collaborative relationships with the Center for Biomedical Genomics and Informatics for gene microarray work, and the Krasnow Institute for Advanced Study for neuroanatomy, neurophysiology, and neural modeling work. The Human Factors/Applied Cognitive labs include numerous workstations for computer display and data collection, several eyetrackers, several simulators (including a cockpit simulator) and human electrophysiology; a Near Infrared Imaging System is planned for the very near future. Industrial/Organizational research space includes laboratory space for work on groups, teamwork, and leadership. Clinical facilities include a professional Clinic, and research/interview space in faculty labs. The Center for Cognitive Development, housed in the same building as the Clinic, works with local school systems, and the School and Clinical programs, on issues related to child development. Some students use nearby resources for research, such as the National Institutes of Health.

Information for Students With Physical Disabilities: See the following Web site for more information: http://www.gmu.edu/depts/unilife/ods/.

Application Information:
Send to College of Humanities and Social Sciences Graduate Admissions, George Mason University, 4400 University Drive, MSN 2D2, Fairfax, VA 22030-4444. Application available online. URL of online application: http://admissions.gmu.edu/grad/applynow/. Students are admitted in the Fall, application deadline December 1. December 1 for Clinical PhD; Applied Developmental PhD; December 15 for Industrial/Organizational PhD; January 1 for Biopsychology PhD; Human Factors/Applied Cognition PhD; January 15 for School MA; February 1 for Applied Developmental MA; Biopsychology MA; Industrial/Organizational MA; Human Factors/Applied Cognition MA. *Fee:* $60.

Institute for the Psychological Sciences
Department of Psychology
2001 Jefferson Davis Highway Suite 511
Arlington, VA 22202
Telephone: (703) 416-1441
E-mail: *wnordling@ipsciences.edu*
Web: *http://www.ipsciences.edu*

Department Information:
1999. Chairperson: William Nordling, PhD. Number of faculty: total—full-time 10, part-time 3; women—full-time 2; total—minority—full-time 1; women minority—full-time 1.

Programs and Degrees Offered:
Listed in the following order: Program area, degree type (T if terminal Master's), number awarded 7/08–6/09. General Psychology MA/MS (Master of Arts/Science) (T) 0, Clinical Psychology PsyD (Doctor of Psychology) 3, Clinical Psychology MA/MS (Master of Arts/Science) (T) 10.

Student Applications/Admissions:
Student Applications
General Psychology MA/MS (*Master of Arts/Science*)—Applications 2009–2010, 0. Total applicants accepted 2009–2010, 0. Number full-time enrolled (new admits only) 2009–2010, 0. Openings 2010–2011, 10. The median number of years required for completion of a degree in 2008–2009 were 2. The number of students enrolled full- and part-time who were dismissed or voluntarily withdrew from this program area in 2008–2009 were 0. *Clinical Psychology PsyD (Doctor of Psychology)*—Applications 2009–2010, 29. Total applicants accepted 2009–2010, 17. Number full-time enrolled (new admits only) 2009–2010, 16. Total enrolled 2009–2010 full-time, 28. Openings 2010–2011, 8. The median number of years required for completion of a degree in 2008–2009 were 6. The number of students enrolled full- and part-time who were dismissed or voluntarily withdrew from this program area in 2008–2009 were 1. *Clinical Psychology MA/MS (Master of Arts/Science)*—Applications 2009–2010, 62. Total applicants accepted 2009–2010, 49. Number full-time enrolled (new admits only) 2009–2010, 29. Number part-time enrolled (new admits only) 2009–2010, 1. Total enrolled 2009–2010 full-time, 41, part-time, 5. Openings 2010–2011, 35. The median number of years required for completion of a degree in 2008–2009 were 2. The number of students enrolled full- and part-time who were dismissed or voluntarily withdrew from this program area in 2008–2009 were 3.

Scores: Entries appear in this order: required test or GPA, minimum score (if required), median score of students entering in 2009–2010. *General Psychology MA/MS (Master of Arts/Science):* overall undergraduate GPA 3.0, last 2 years GPA 3.0, psychology GPA 3.0; *Clinical Psychology PsyD (Doctor of Psychology):* overall undergraduate GPA 3.0, last 2 years GPA 3.0, psychology GPA 3.0, Masters GPA 3.5; *Clinical Psychology MA/MS (Master of Arts/Science):* overall undergraduate GPA 3.0, last 2 years GPA 3.0, psychology GPA 3.0.

Other Criteria: (importance of criteria rated low, medium, or high): GRE scores—medium, research experience—medium, work experience—high, extracurricular activity—medium, clinically related public service—high, GPA—high, letters of recommendation—high, interview—high, statement of goals and objectives—high, essays on application—high, undergraduate major in psychology—medium, specific undergraduate psychology courses taken—medium. For additional information on admission requirements, go to http://www.ipsciences.edu.

Student Characteristics: The following represents characteristics of students in 2009–2010 in all graduate psychology programs in the department: Female—full-time 46, part-time 6; Male—full-time 19, part-time 2; African American/Black—full-time 3, part-time 1; Hispanic/Latino(a)—full-time 7, part-time 1; Asian/Pacific Islander—full-time 3, part-time 0; American Indian/Alaska Native—full-time 0, part-time 0; Caucasian/White—full-time 52, part-time 6; Multi-ethnic—full-time 0, part-time 0; students subject to the Americans With Disabilities Act—full-time 0, part-time 0; Unknown ethnicity—full-time 0, part-time 0; International students who hold an F-1 or J-1 Visa—full-time 10, part-time 1.

Financial Information/Assistance:
Tuition for Full-Time Study: Master's: State residents: per academic year $18,000, $775 per credit hour; Nonstate residents: per academic year $18,000, $775 per credit hour. *Doctoral:* State residents: per academic year $20,000, $785 per credit hour; Nonstate residents: per academic year $20,000, $785 per credit hour. Tuition is subject to change. Additional fees are assessed to students beyond the costs of tuition for the following: library, student activities, graduation, transcript requests, practicum fee. Tuition costs vary by program. See the following Web site for updates and changes in tuition costs: http://www.ipsciences.edu.

Financial Assistance:
First-Year Students: Fellowships and scholarships available for first year. Average amount paid per academic year: $2,500. Average number of hours worked per week: 0. Apply by March 15.

Advanced Students: Teaching assistantships available for advanced students. Average number of hours worked per week: 10. Apply by March 15. Research assistantships available for advanced students. Average number of hours worked per week: 10. Apply by March 15. Traineeships available for advanced students. Average number of hours worked per week: 10. Apply by March 15. Fellowships and scholarships available for advanced students. Average amount paid per academic year: $6,250. Apply by March 15.

Additional Information: Of all students currently enrolled full time, 47% benefited from one or more of the listed financial assistance programs. Application and information available online at: http://ipsciences.edu/pages/financial-aid.php.

Internships/Practica: Doctoral Degree (PsyD Clinical Psychology): For those doctoral students for whom a professional internship was required in this program prior to graduation, (4) students applied for an internship in 2008–2009, with (4) students obtaining an internship. Of those students who obtained an internship, (4) were paid internships. Of those students who obtained an internship, (4) students placed in APA/CPA accredited internships, (0) students placed in internships not APA/CPA accredited, but listed with the Association of Psychology Postdoctoral and Internship Programs (APPIC), (0) students placed in internships conforming to guidelines of the Council of Directors of School Psychology Programs (CDSPP), (0) students placed in internships that were not APA/CPA accredited, APPIC or CDSPP listed. Master's Degree (MA/MS General Psychology): An internship experience, such as a final research project or "capstone" experience is required of graduates. In their third year of training, PsyD students participate in a year long practicum in the IPS training clinic. PsyD students in their fourth year of training and MS students in an optional third year of training have access to a wide variety of externship/practicum sites given that the Institute is located in the Washington, DC Metro Area.

Housing and Day Care: No on-campus housing is available. No on-campus day care facilities are available.

Employment of Department Graduates:
Master's Degree Graduates: Of those who graduated in the academic year 2008–2009, the following categories and numbers represent the postgraduate activities and employment of master's degree graduates: Enrolled in a psychology doctoral program (6), enrolled in another graduate/professional program (3), enrolled in a postdoctoral residency/fellowship (n/a), employed in independent practice (n/a), employed in an academic position at a university (0), employed in an academic position at a 2-year/4-year college (0), employed in other positions at a higher education institution (1), employed in a professional position in a school system (2), employed in business or industry (0), employed in government agency (0), employed in a community mental health/counseling center (3), employed in a hospital/medical center (0), still seeking employment (0), not seeking employment (10), other employment position (3), do not know (0), total from the above (master's) (28).
Doctoral Degree Graduates: Of those who graduated in the academic year 2008–2009, the following categories and numbers represent the postgraduate activities and employment of doctoral degree graduates: Enrolled in a psychology doctoral program (n/a), enrolled in another graduate/professional program (1), enrolled in a postdoctoral residency/fellowship (4), employed in independent practice (0), employed in an academic position at a university (0), employed in an academic position at a 2-year/4-year college (0), employed in other positions at a higher education institution (2), employed in a professional position in a school system (0), employed in business or industry (0), employed in government agency (0), employed in a community mental health/counseling center (4), employed in a hospital/medical center (0), still seeking employment (0), not seeking employment (4), other employment position (0), do not know (0), total from the above (doctoral) (15).

Additional Information:
Orientation, Objectives, and Emphasis of Department: The Department adopts a practitioner-scholar model of training and education of psychologists. In doing so, the degree programs form students who can practice scientific psychology integrated with a Catholic worldview.

Special Facilities or Resources: The Washington, DC Metro Area is an environment rich in educational and cultural resources for students. In addition to the IPS library, students have access to the libraries of other universities and centers of learning within the area. The IPS also has a chapel and a chaplain who provide students with opportunities for spiritual development.

Application Information:
Send to The Institute for the Psychological Sciences, Attn: Admissions, 2001 Jefferson Davis Highway, Suite 511 Arlington, VA 22202. Application available online. URL of online application: http://www.ipsciences.edu. Students are admitted in the Fall, application deadline February 15. Interviews must be completed by March 15th. Space permitting, applications will be accepted until May 1. *Fee:* $50.

Marymount University
Department of Forensic Psychology
School of Education and Human Services
2807 North Glebe Road
Arlington, VA 22207
Telephone: (703) 284-5705
Fax: (703) 284-5708
E-mail: *grad.admissions@marymount.edu*
Web: *http://www.marymount.edu/academic/sehs/fp/fphome.htm*

Department Information:
2000. Chairperson: Dr. Jason Doll. Number of faculty: total—full-time 3, part-time 11; women—full-time 2, part-time 8; minority—part-time 4; women minority—part-time 4.

Programs and Degrees Offered:
Listed in the following order: Program area, degree type (T if terminal Master's), number awarded 7/08–6/09. Forensic Psychology MA/MS (Master of Arts/Science) (T) 95.

Student Applications/Admissions:
Student Applications
Forensic Psychology MA/MS *(Master of Arts/Science)*—Applications 2009–2010, 236. Total applicants accepted 2009–2010, 105. Number full-time enrolled (new admits only) 2009–2010,

95. Total enrolled 2009–2010 full-time, 134, part-time, 43. Openings 2010–2011, 92. The median number of years required for completion of a degree in 2008–2009 were 2. The number of students enrolled full- and part-time who were dismissed or voluntarily withdrew from this program area in 2008–2009 were 0.

Scores: Entries appear in this order: required test or GPA, minimum score (if required), median score of students entering in 2009–2010. *Forensic Psychology MA/MS (Master of Arts/Science):* GRE-V 450, GRE-Q 450, GRE-Analytical 4.0, overall undergraduate GPA 3.0.

Other Criteria: (importance of criteria rated low, medium, or high): GRE scores—medium, research experience—low, work experience—medium, extracurricular activity—medium, clinically related public service—low, GPA—high, letters of recommendation—medium, statement of goals and objectives—medium, undergraduate major in psychology—low, specific undergraduate psychology courses taken—low. For additional information on admission requirements, go to http://www.marymount.edu/academic/sehs/fp/fpadmiss.htm.

Student Characteristics: The following represents characteristics of students in 2009–2010 in all graduate psychology programs in the department: Female—full-time 99, part-time 86; Male—full-time 16, part-time 14; African American/Black—full-time 14, part-time 12; Hispanic/Latino(a)—full-time 4, part-time 3; Asian/Pacific Islander—full-time 1, part-time 1; American Indian/Alaska Native—full-time 1, part-time 1; Caucasian/White—full-time 95, part-time 83; Multi-ethnic—full-time 0, part-time 0; students subject to the Americans With Disabilities Act—full-time 0, part-time 0; Unknown ethnicity—full-time 0, part-time 0; International students who hold an F-1 or J-1 Visa—full-time 0, part-time 0.

Financial Information/Assistance:
Tuition for Full-Time Study: *Master's:* State residents: $725 per credit hour; Nonstate residents: $725 per credit hour. Tuition is subject to change. Additional fees are assessed to students beyond the costs of tuition for the following: $7/credit hr-tech fee; new student fee $40 (one-time); $55 internship application fee. See the following Web site for updates and changes in tuition costs: http://www.marymount.edu/financialinfo/tuition.html.

Financial Assistance:
First-Year Students: Research assistantships available for first year. Average amount paid per academic year: $2,500. Average number of hours worked per week: 20.
Advanced Students: Research assistantships available for advanced students. Average amount paid per academic year: $2,500. Average number of hours worked per week: 20.
Additional Information: Application and information available online at: http://www.marymount.edu/financialaid/graduate.html.

Internships/Practica: Master's Degree (MA/MS Forensic Psychology): An internship experience, such as a final research project or "capstone" experience is required of graduates. Forensic psychology students may choose an internship in a wide variety of settings, including local and state correctional facilities, local community mental health treatment centers, victim witness programs, domestic violence programs and shelters, national and local mental health advocacy organizations, child welfare agencies and advocacy organizations, adult services agencies (serving incapacitated and incompetent adults), juvenile court services, state and local law enforcement, federal law enforcement and justice agencies, and any and all areas in which psychological expertise and psychological services (including counseling) would be applied in a legal setting (criminal, civil, and juvenile justice).

Housing and Day Care: On-campus housing is available. See the following Web site for more information: http://www.marymount.edu/studentlife/residence/. No on-campus day care facilities are available.

Employment of Department Graduates:
Master's Degree Graduates: Of those who graduated in the academic year 2008–2009, the following categories and numbers represent the postgraduate activities and employment of master's degree graduates: Enrolled in a postdoctoral residency/fellowship (n/a), employed in independent practice (n/a), total from the above (master's) (0).
Doctoral Degree Graduates: Of those who graduated in the academic year 2008–2009, the following categories and numbers represent the postgraduate activities and employment of doctoral degree graduates: Enrolled in a psychology doctoral program (n/a), total from the above (doctoral) (0).

Additional Information:
Orientation, Objectives, and Emphasis of Department: The Department of Forensic Psychology offers a Master of Arts in Forensic Psychology. This degree provides graduates with the skills and knowledge they need to provide effective, high quality services in a variety of forensic settings. These settings include probation and parole, victim assistance, law enforcement, and other arenas within the juvenile, civil, and criminal justice systems. To accomplish this goal, the program balances the acquisition of traditional psychological knowledge and skills with a specialized understanding of the justice system.

Special Facilities or Resources: The location of Marymount in suburban Washington provides our students with a large number of opportunities for internships and employment in the area, especially with federal agencies. The university is a member of the Washington Consortium of College and Universities, which gives the students access to the library facilities and classes of most of the major universities in the area. In addition, the Department of Forensic Psychology has a joint research project with the FBI's Behavioral Science Unit. Selected students have the opportunity to work on research projects with faculty using closed criminal case files provided by the FBI. Also, approximately every other summer, students have the opportunity to learn about and experience forensic psychology in the English justice system via a collaborative relationship with the Forensic Psychology Program at London Metropolitan University.

Information for Students With Physical Disabilities: See the following Web site for more information: http://www.marymount.edu/studentlife/disability/index.html.

Application Information:
Send to Office of Graduate Admissions, Marymount University, 2807 N. Glebe Road, Arlington, VA 22207. Application available online. URL of online application: http://www.marymount.edu/admissions/

undergrad/applications.html. Students are admitted in the Fall, application deadline February 15. *Fee:* $40.

Old Dominion University
Department of Psychology
College of Sciences
Mills Godwin Building—Room 250
Norfolk, VA 23529-0267
Telephone: (757) 683-4439
Fax: (757) 683-5087
E-mail: *bwinstea@odu.edu*
Web: *http://www.sci.odu.edu/psychology/*

Department Information:
1954. Chairperson: Barbara Winstead. Number of faculty: total—full-time 24, part-time 6; women—full-time 11, part-time 4; total—minority—full-time 3; women minority—full-time 2.

Programs and Degrees Offered:
Listed in the following order: Program area, degree type (T if terminal Master's), number awarded 7/08–6/09. General Psychology MA/MS (Master of Arts/Science) (T) 5, Industrial/Organizational Psychology PhD (Doctor of Philosophy) 3, Human Factors PhD (Doctor of Philosophy) 0, Applied Experimental Psychology PhD (Doctor of Philosophy) 1, Clinical Psychology PsyD (Doctor of Psychology) 5.

APA Accreditation: Clinical PsyD (Doctor of Psychology). Student Outcome Data Website: http://sci.odu.edu/vcpcp/program/Program_Data.shtml.

Student Applications/Admissions:
Student Applications
General Psychology MA/MS (Master of Arts/Science)—Applications 2009–2010, 45. Total applicants accepted 2009–2010, 10. Number full-time enrolled (new admits only) 2009–2010, 6. Total enrolled 2009–2010 full-time, 13, part-time, 5. Openings 2010–2011, 4. The median number of years required for completion of a degree in 2008–2009 were 2. The number of students enrolled full- and part-time who were dismissed or voluntarily withdrew from this program area in 2008–2009 were 1. *Industrial/Organizational Psychology PhD (Doctor of Philosophy)*—Applications 2009–2010, 43. Total applicants accepted 2009–2010, 6. Number full-time enrolled (new admits only) 2009–2010, 4. Total enrolled 2009–2010 full-time, 10, part-time, 8. Openings 2010–2011, 3. The median number of years required for completion of a degree in 2008–2009 were 5. The number of students enrolled full- and part-time who were dismissed or voluntarily withdrew from this program area in 2008–2009 were 1. *Human Factors PhD (Doctor of Philosophy)*—Applications 2009–2010, 7. Total applicants accepted 2009–2010, 3. Number full-time enrolled (new admits only) 2009–2010, 2. Total enrolled 2009–2010 full-time, 4, part-time, 5. Openings 2010–2011, 3. The number of students enrolled full- and part-time who were dismissed or voluntarily withdrew from this program area in 2008–2009 were 0. *Applied Experimental Psychology PhD (Doctor of Philosophy)*—Applications 2009–2010, 10. Total applicants accepted 2009–2010, 3. Number full-time enrolled (new admits only) 2009–2010, 3. Total enrolled 2009–2010 full-time, 8, part-time, 4. Openings 2010–2011, 3. The median number of years required for completion of a degree in 2008–2009 were 5. The number of students enrolled full- and part-time who were dismissed or voluntarily withdrew from this program area in 2008–2009 were 0. *Clinical Psychology PsyD (Doctor of Psychology)*—Applications 2009–2010, 214. Total applicants accepted 2009–2010, 10. Number full-time enrolled (new admits only) 2009–2010, 6. Total enrolled 2009–2010 full-time, 49. Openings 2010–2011, 6. The median number of years required for completion of a degree in 2008–2009 were 4. The number of students enrolled full- and part-time who were dismissed or voluntarily withdrew from this program area in 2008–2009 were 0.

Other Criteria: (importance of criteria rated low, medium, or high): GRE scores—high, research experience—high, work experience—medium, extracurricular activity—medium, clinically related public service—low, GPA—high, letters of recommendation—high, interview—medium, statement of goals and objectives—medium.

Student Characteristics: The following represents characteristics of students in 2009–2010 in all graduate psychology programs in the department: Female—full-time 24, part-time 15; Male—full-time 11, part-time 7; African American/Black—full-time 1, part-time 1; Hispanic/Latino(a)—full-time 0, part-time 0; Asian/Pacific Islander—full-time 1, part-time 0; American Indian/Alaska Native—full-time 0, part-time 0; Caucasian/White—full-time 32, part-time 21; Multi-ethnic—full-time 1, part-time 0; students subject to the Americans With Disabilities Act—full-time 0, part-time 0; Unknown ethnicity—full-time 0, part-time 0; International students who hold an F-1 or J-1 Visa—full-time 2, part-time 0.

Financial Information/Assistance:
Tuition for Full-Time Study: *Master's:* State residents: $338 per credit hour; Nonstate residents: $844 per credit hour. *Doctoral:* State residents: $338 per credit hour; Nonstate residents: $844 per credit hour. Tuition is subject to change.

Financial Assistance:
First-Year Students: Teaching assistantships available for first year. Average amount paid per academic year: $12,000. Average number of hours worked per week: 20. Apply by January 5. Research assistantships available for first year. Average amount paid per academic year: $12,000. Average number of hours worked per week: 20. Apply by January 5. Fellowships and scholarships available for first year. Average amount paid per academic year: $15,000. Apply by January 5.

Advanced Students: Teaching assistantships available for advanced students. Average amount paid per academic year: $12,000. Average number of hours worked per week: 20. Research assistantships available for advanced students. Average amount paid per academic year: $12,000. Average number of hours worked per week: 20. Fellowships and scholarships available for advanced students. Average amount paid per academic year: $15,000.

Additional Information: Of all students currently enrolled full time, 80% benefited from one or more of the listed financial assistance programs.

Internships/Practica: Doctoral Degree (PsyD Clinical Psychology): For those doctoral students for whom a professional internship was required in this program prior to graduation, (12) students applied for an internship in 2008–2009, with (10) students obtaining an internship. Of those students who obtained an internship, (10) were paid internships. Of those students who obtained an internship, (9) students placed in APA/CPA accredited internships, (1) students placed in internships not APA/CPA accredited, but listed with the Association of Psychology Postdoctoral and Internship Programs (APPIC), (0) students placed in internships conforming to guidelines of the Council of Directors of School Psychology Programs (CDSPP), (0) students placed in internships that were not APA/CPA accredited, APPIC or CDSPP listed. Internships are highly encouraged for those enrolled in all three PhD programs and are required for the PsyD program and are available at local businesses, hospitals, and military and government agencies, as well as out-of-state. Practicum and internship experiences are also available for all graduate students.

Housing and Day Care: On-campus housing is available. See the following Web site for more information: http://studentaffairs.odu.edu/housing/communities/sophomore/powhatan.shtml. On-campus day care facilities are available. See the following Web site for more information: http://education.odu.edu/esse/academics/specprog/cdc.shtml.

Employment of Department Graduates:
Master's Degree Graduates: Of those who graduated in the academic year 2008–2009, the following categories and numbers represent the postgraduate activities and employment of master's degree graduates: Enrolled in a psychology doctoral program (5), enrolled in another graduate/professional program (0), enrolled in a postdoctoral residency/fellowship (n/a), employed in independent practice (n/a), employed in other positions at a higher education institution (1), employed in government agency (1), do not know (0), total from the above (master's) (7).
Doctoral Degree Graduates: Of those who graduated in the academic year 2008–2009, the following categories and numbers represent the postgraduate activities and employment of doctoral degree graduates: Enrolled in a psychology doctoral program (n/a), employed in an academic position at a 2-year/4-year college (1), employed in other positions at a higher education institution (1), employed in business or industry (2), total from the above (doctoral) (4).

Additional Information:
Orientation, Objectives, and Emphasis of Department: The department offers PhD programs in Applied Experimental, Human Factors, and Industrial/Organizational psychology. Concentrations within Applied Experimental include health, community, developmental, cognition, and quantitative. Concentrations within Human Factors include aviation, cognitive processes, and modeling and simulation. Concentrations within Industrial/Organizational include organizational and personnel. A program of graduate study leading to the degree of Master of Science with a concentration in general psychology is also offered by the department. The department participates in the Virginia Consortium Program in Clinical Psychology, which in collaboration with Eastern Virginia Medical School and Norfolk State University, offers the PsyD in Clinical Psychology.

Special Facilities or Resources: The department has a new Human Computer Interaction and Usability Analysis lab, a driving simulator, eyetrack recording equipment, computer labs for data collection and other research facilities. A close collaboration with the Virginia Modeling, Analysis and Simulation Center provides students with opportunities to engage in command and control simulation, surgical simulation, and virtual reality research. The psychology faculty and graduate students also maintain active collaborations with NASA Langley Research Center, Eastern Virginia Medical School, the Center for Pediatric Research, Children's Hospital of the King's Daughters, and community and government groups, such as Virginia Department of Motor Vehicles, Department of Public Health, and Tidewater AIDS Crisis Taskforce.

Information for Students With Physical Disabilities: See the following Web site for more information: http://studentaffairs.odu.edu/disabilityservices/.

Application Information:
Send to Old Dominion University, Office of Graduate Admissions, 105 Rollins Hall, Norfolk, VA 23529-0050. Application available online. URL of online application: http://admissions.odu.edu/graduate.php. Students are admitted in the Fall, application deadline January 5. January 5 for PhD, May 15 for MS. *Fee:* $50. The fee is waived or deferred if the applicant is an ODU graduate.

Radford University
Department of Psychology
Humanities and Behavioral Sciences
P.O. Box 6946
Radford, VA 24142-6946
Telephone: (540) 831-5361
Fax: (540) 831-6113
E-mail: *hlips@radford.edu*
Web: *http://www.radford.edu/psyc-web*

Department Information:
1937. Chairperson: Hilary M. Lips. Number of faculty: total—full-time 22, part-time 3; women—full-time 9, part-time 3.

Programs and Degrees Offered:
Listed in the following order: Program area, degree type (T if terminal Master's), number awarded 7/08–6/09. Counseling Psychology PsyD (Doctor of Psychology) 0, Clinical Psychology MA/MS (Master of Arts/Science) (T) 6, Experimental Psychology MA/MS (Master of Arts/Science) (T) 3, Industrial/Organizational Psychology MA/MS (Master of Arts/Science) (T) 13, School Psychology EdS (School Psychology) 7.

Student Applications/Admissions:
Student Applications
Counseling Psychology PsyD (Doctor of Psychology)—Applications 2009–2010, 7. Total applicants accepted 2009–2010, 4. Number full-time enrolled (new admits only) 2009–2010, 3. Openings 2010–2011, 5. The number of students enrolled full- and part-time who were dismissed or voluntarily withdrew from this program area in 2008–2009 were 0. *Clinical Psychology MA/MS (Master of Arts/Science)*—Applications 2009–2010, 42. Total applicants accepted 2009–2010, 26. Number full-time enrolled (new admits only) 2009–2010, 8. Number part-

time enrolled (new admits only) 2009–2010, 0. Openings 2010–2011, 8. The median number of years required for completion of a degree in 2008–2009 were 2. The number of students enrolled full- and part-time who were dismissed or voluntarily withdrew from this program area in 2008–2009 were 0. *Experimental Psychology MA/MS (Master of Arts/Science)*—Applications 2009–2010, 22. Total applicants accepted 2009–2010, 10. Number full-time enrolled (new admits only) 2009–2010, 6. Openings 2010–2011, 8. The median number of years required for completion of a degree in 2008–2009 were 2. The number of students enrolled full- and part-time who were dismissed or voluntarily withdrew from this program area in 2008–2009 were 0. *Industrial/Organizational Psychology MA/MS (Master of Arts/Science)*—Applications 2009–2010, 45. Total applicants accepted 2009–2010, 27. Number full-time enrolled (new admits only) 2009–2010, 10. Openings 2010–2011, 13. The median number of years required for completion of a degree in 2008–2009 were 2. The number of students enrolled full- and part-time who were dismissed or voluntarily withdrew from this program area in 2008–2009 were 0. *School Psychology EdS (School Psychology)*—Applications 2009–2010, 28. Total applicants accepted 2009–2010, 19. Number full-time enrolled (new admits only) 2009–2010, 13. Openings 2010–2011, 12. The median number of years required for completion of a degree in 2008–2009 were 3. The number of students enrolled full- and part-time who were dismissed or voluntarily withdrew from this program area in 2008–2009 were 1.

Scores: Entries appear in this order: required test or GPA, minimum score (if required), median score of students entering in 2009–2010. *Counseling Psychology PsyD (Doctor of Psychology):* GRE-V no minimum stated, 523, GRE-Q no minimum stated, 518, overall undergraduate GPA no minimum stated, 3.11, Masters GPA no minimum stated, 3.88; *Clinical Psychology MA/MS (Master of Arts/Science):* GRE-V no minimum stated, 497, GRE-Q no minimum stated, 544, overall undergraduate GPA no minimum stated, 3.5; *Experimental Psychology MA/MS (Master of Arts/Science):* GRE-V no minimum stated, 598, GRE-Q no minimum stated, 518, overall undergraduate GPA no minimum stated; *Industrial/Organizational Psychology MA/MS (Master of Arts/Science):* GRE-V no minimum stated, 479, GRE-Q no minimum stated, 590, overall undergraduate GPA no minimum stated, 3.55; *School Psychology EdS (School Psychology):* GRE-V no minimum stated, 484, GRE-Q no minimum stated, 545, overall undergraduate GPA no minimum stated, 3.10.

Other Criteria: (importance of criteria rated low, medium, or high): GRE scores—medium, research experience—high, work experience—high, extracurricular activity—medium, clinically related public service—high, GPA—high, letters of recommendation—high, interview—high, statement of goals and objectives—medium, undergraduate major in psychology—medium, specific undergraduate psychology courses taken—low. Interview required for doctoral program but not for masters' programs. For additional information on admission requirements, go to http://www.radford.edu/psyc-web/.

Student Characteristics: The following represents characteristics of students in 2009–2010 in all graduate psychology programs in the department: Female—full-time 83, part-time 0; Male—full-time 4, part-time 0; African American/Black—full-time 6, part-time 0; Hispanic/Latino(a)—full-time 0, part-time 0; Asian/Pacific Islander—full-time 2, part-time 0; American Indian/Alaska Native—full-time 0, part-time 0; Caucasian/White—full-time 79, part-time 0; Multi-ethnic—full-time 0, part-time 0; students subject to the Americans With Disabilities Act—full-time 0, part-time 0; Unknown ethnicity—full-time 0, part-time 0; International students who hold an F-1 or J-1 Visa—full-time 0, part-time 0.

Financial Information/Assistance:
Tuition for Full-Time Study: *Master's:* State residents: per academic year $5,688, $316 per credit hour; Nonstate residents: per academic year $11,340, $630 per credit hour. Tuition is subject to change. Tuition costs vary by program. See the following Web site for updates and changes in tuition costs: http://finaid.asp.radford.edu/grfs99.html.

Financial Assistance:
First-Year Students: Teaching assistantships available for first year. Average amount paid per academic year: $8,000. Average number of hours worked per week: 20. Apply by March 1. Research assistantships available for first year. Average amount paid per academic year: $4,000. Average number of hours worked per week: 10. Apply by March 1. Traineeships available for first year. Average amount paid per academic year: $13,500. Average number of hours worked per week: 20. Fellowships and scholarships available for first year. Average amount paid per academic year: $1,000. Apply by March 1.

Advanced Students: Teaching assistantships available for advanced students. Average amount paid per academic year: $8,700. Average number of hours worked per week: 20. Apply by February 15. Research assistantships available for advanced students. Average amount paid per academic year: $3,100. Average number of hours worked per week: 10. Apply by February 15. Traineeships available for advanced students. Average amount paid per academic year: $13,500. Average number of hours worked per week: 20. Fellowships and scholarships available for advanced students. Average amount paid per academic year: $600. Apply by April 1.

Additional Information: Of all students currently enrolled full time, 60% benefited from one or more of the listed financial assistance programs. Application and information available online at: http://finaid.asp.radford.edu/grprog.html.

Internships/Practica: Master's Degree (MA/MS Industrial/Organizational Psychology): An internship experience, such as a final research project or "capstone" experience is required of graduates. Internships and/or practica are required for all programs.

Housing and Day Care: On-campus housing is available. See the following Web site for more information: http://www.radford.edu/~res-life/. No on-campus day care facilities are available.

Employment of Department Graduates:
Master's Degree Graduates: Of those who graduated in the academic year 2008–2009, the following categories and numbers represent the postgraduate activities and employment of master's degree graduates: Enrolled in a psychology doctoral program (3), enrolled in a postdoctoral residency/fellowship (n/a), employed in independent practice (n/a), employed in other positions at a higher education institution (2), employed in a professional position in a school system (7), employed in business or industry (11), employed in a community mental health/counseling center (9),

other employment position (3), total from the above (master's) (35).

Doctoral Degree Graduates: Of those who graduated in the academic year 2008–2009, the following categories and numbers represent the postgraduate activities and employment of doctoral degree graduates: Enrolled in a psychology doctoral program (n/a), total from the above (doctoral) (0).

Additional Information:
Orientation, Objectives, and Emphasis of Department: The department aims to train psychologists who are well versed in both the theoretical and applied aspects of the discipline. The emphasis of the department is eclectic: school, clinical, experimental, industrial/organizational and counseling options are available at the graduate level. The School program is an EdS program that also provides preparation for certification and licensing as a school psychologist in Virginia. The Psy.D program in Counseling Psychology, with an emphasis on rural mental health, started in the Fall of 2008.

Special Facilities or Resources: We have computer laboratories and some research space for use by graduate students. We have good animal lab facilities. The department has established a center for gender studies and a laboratory for brain research.

Information for Students With Physical Disabilities: See the following Web site for more information: http://www.radford.edu/~dro/.

Application Information:
Send to College of Graduate and Professional Studies, P.O. Box 6928, Radford University, Radford, VA 24142. Application available online. URL of online application: http://gradcollege.asp.radford.edu/admissions.html. Students are admitted in the Fall, application deadline February 15. Applications for the PsyD program in Counseling Psychology are due January 15. *Fee:* $50.

Regent University
Doctoral Program in Clinical Psychology
School of Psychology and Counseling
1000 Regent University Drive
Virginia Beach, VA 23464
Telephone: (757) 352-4828
Fax: (757) 352-4304
E-mail: *judijo2@regent.edu*
Web: *http://www.regent.edu/psyd*

Department Information:
1996. Chairperson: Judith L. Johnson, PhD. Number of faculty: total—full-time 10, part-time 8; women—full-time 6, part-time 6; total—minority—full-time 2, part-time 3; women minority—full-time 2, part-time 3; faculty subject to the Americans With Disabilities Act 1.

Programs and Degrees Offered:
Listed in the following order: Program area, degree type (T if terminal Master's), number awarded 7/08–6/09. Clinical Psychology PsyD (Doctor of Psychology) 17.

APA Accreditation: Clinical PsyD (Doctor of Psychology).

Student Applications/Admissions:
Student Applications
Clinical Psychology PsyD (Doctor of Psychology)—Applications 2009–2010, 88. Total applicants accepted 2009–2010, 37. Number full-time enrolled (new admits only) 2009–2010, 17. Number part-time enrolled (new admits only) 2009–2010, 0. Openings 2010–2011, 22. The median number of years required for completion of a degree in 2008–2009 were 5. The number of students enrolled full- and part-time who were dismissed or voluntarily withdrew from this program area in 2008–2009 were 0.

Other Criteria: (importance of criteria rated low, medium, or high): GRE scores—high, research experience—medium, work experience—medium, extracurricular activity—medium, clinically related public service—medium, GPA—high, letters of recommendation—medium, interview—medium, statement of goals and objectives—medium, leadership experiences—medium, undergraduate major in psychology—medium, specific undergraduate psychology courses taken—medium. For additional information on admission requirements, go to: http://www.regent.edu/acad/schcou/admissions/index.htm.

Student Characteristics: The following represents characteristics of students in 2009–2010 in all graduate psychology programs in the department: Female—full-time 76, part-time 12; Male—full-time 26, part-time 2; African American/Black—full-time 11, part-time 6; Hispanic/Latino(a)—full-time 5, part-time 1; Asian/Pacific Islander—full-time 2, part-time 1; American Indian/Alaska Native—full-time 2, part-time 0; Caucasian/White—full-time 75, part-time 11; Multi-ethnic—full-time 1, part-time 0; students subject to the Americans With Disabilities Act—full-time 1, part-time 0; Unknown ethnicity—full-time 3, part-time 1; International students who hold an F-1 or J-1 Visa—full-time 3, part-time 0.

Financial Information/Assistance:
Tuition for Full-Time Study: Doctoral: State residents: $755 per credit hour; Nonstate residents: $755 per credit hour. Tuition is subject to change.

Financial Assistance:
First-Year Students: Fellowships and scholarships available for first year. Average amount paid per academic year: $3,700. Apply by August 1.

Advanced Students: Teaching assistantships available for advanced students. Average amount paid per academic year: $7,500. Average number of hours worked per week: 12. Apply by April 1. Research assistantships available for advanced students. Average amount paid per academic year: $7,500. Average number of hours worked per week: 12. Apply by April 1. Fellowships and scholarships available for advanced students. Average amount paid per academic year: $3,700. Apply by April 1.

Additional Information: Of all students currently enrolled full time, 98% benefited from one or more of the listed financial assistance programs.

Internships/Practica: Doctoral Degree (PsyD Clinical Psychology): For those doctoral students for whom a professional internship was required in this program prior to graduation, (24) students applied for an internship in 2008–2009, with (21) students obtaining an internship. Of those students who obtained an internship, (21) were paid internships. Of those students who obtained an internship, (19) students placed in APA/CPA accredited internships, (2) students placed in internships not APA/CPA accredited, but listed with the Association of Psychology Postdoctoral and Internship Programs (APPIC), (0) students placed in internships conforming to guidelines of the Council of Directors of School Psychology Programs (CDSPP), (0) students placed in internships that were not APA/CPA accredited, APPIC or CDSPP listed. All PsyD students complete a three semester placement in the campus training clinic, the Psychological Services Center, during their second year. A three semester practicum placement is completed during the third year at any of a wide variety of community practicum sites such as military and VA clinics, inpatient brain injury units, psychiatric hospitals, group practices, community mental health agencies, Christian outpatient practices, or correctional settings.

Housing and Day Care: On-campus housing is available. See the following Web site for more information: http://www.regent.edu/campus/housing. No on-campus day care facilities are available.

Employment of Department Graduates:

Master's Degree Graduates: Of those who graduated in the academic year 2008–2009, the following categories and numbers represent the postgraduate activities and employment of master's degree graduates: Enrolled in a postdoctoral residency/fellowship (n/a), employed in independent practice (n/a), total from the above (master's) (0).

Doctoral Degree Graduates: Of those who graduated in the academic year 2008–2009, the following categories and numbers represent the postgraduate activities and employment of doctoral degree graduates: Enrolled in a psychology doctoral program (n/a), enrolled in a postdoctoral residency/fellowship (2), employed in an academic position at a university (1), employed in other positions at a higher education institution (1), employed in government agency (3), employed in a community mental health/counseling center (4), employed in a hospital/medical center (6), total from the above (doctoral) (17).

Additional Information:

Orientation, Objectives, and Emphasis of Department: The Doctoral Program in Clinical Psychology adopts a practitioner-scholar model of clinical training within an educational context committed to the integration of scientific psychology and a Christian worldview. The clinical training is broad and general, however, marital and family therapy, consulting psychology, clinical child psychology, and health psychology are emphases among the faculty and in the curriculum.

Personal Behavior Statement: The Community Life form is contained in the application.

Special Facilities or Resources: Regent is located in Virginia Beach, Virginia which is part of Tidewater, the largest urban area in Virginia. There are numerous community resources for practica. The campus also houses the Psychological Services Center, our doctoral training clinic that provides services to the campus and surrounding community. The PSC includes state of the art technology for videotaping and observation of clinical activities.

Application Information:
Send to Central Enrollment, SC218, 1000 Regent University Drive, Virginia Beach, Virginia 23464. Application available online. URL of online application: http://www.regent.edu/psychology/apply. Students are admitted in the Fall, application deadline January 15. *Fee:* $50.

Virginia Commonwealth University
Department of Psychology
Humanities and Sciences
806 West Franklin Street, Box 842018
Richmond, VA 23284-2018
Telephone: (804) 828-1193
Fax: (804) 828-2237
E-mail: *wkliewer@vcu.edu*
Web: *http://www.has.vcu.edu/psy/*

Department Information:
1969. Chairperson: Wendy Kliewer. Number of faculty: total—full-time 37; women—full-time 20; total—minority—full-time 7; women minority—full-time 4; faculty subject to the Americans With Disabilities Act 1.

Programs and Degrees Offered:
Listed in the following order: Program area, degree type (T if terminal Master's), number awarded 7/08–6/09. Clinical Psychology PhD (Doctor of Philosophy) 6, Counseling Psychology PhD (Doctor of Philosophy) 8, Social Psychology PhD (Doctor of Philosophy) 1, Biopsychology PhD (Doctor of Philosophy) 1, Developmental Psychology PhD (Doctor of Philosophy) 1, Health Psychology PhD (Doctor of Philosophy) 0.

APA Accreditation: Clinical PhD (Doctor of Philosophy). Student Outcome Data Website: http://www.has.vcu.edu/psy/clinical/admissions.html. Counseling PhD (Doctor of Philosophy).

Student Applications/Admissions:
Student Applications

Clinical Psychology PhD (Doctor of Philosophy)—Applications 2009–2010, 176. Total applicants accepted 2009–2010, 13. Number full-time enrolled (new admits only) 2009–2010, 7. Number part-time enrolled (new admits only) 2009–2010, 0. Total enrolled 2009–2010 full-time, 49, part-time, 6. Openings 2010–2011, 7. The median number of years required for completion of a degree in 2008–2009 were 6. The number of students enrolled full- and part-time who were dismissed or voluntarily withdrew from this program area in 2008–2009 were 1. Counseling Psychology PhD (Doctor of Philosophy)—Applications 2009–2010, 132. Total applicants accepted 2009–2010, 13. Number full-time enrolled (new admits only) 2009–2010, 6. Total enrolled 2009–2010 full-time, 39, part-time, 5. Openings 2010–2011, 6. The median number of years required for completion of a degree in 2008–2009 were 6. The number of students enrolled full- and part-time who were dismissed or voluntarily withdrew from this program area in 2008–2009 were 0. Social Psychology PhD (Doctor of Philosophy)—Applications 2009–2010, 24. Total applicants accepted 2009–2010, 4. Number full-time enrolled (new admits only) 2009–2010, 2. Number part-time enrolled (new admits only) 2009–2010, 0. Total enrolled 2009–2010 full-time, 12, part-time, 4. Openings 2010–2011, 3. The median number of years required for completion of a degree in 2008–2009 were 5. The number of students enrolled full- and part-time who were dismissed or voluntarily withdrew from this program area in 2008–2009 were 0. *Biopsychology PhD (Doctor of Philosophy)*—Applications 2009–2010, 22. Total applicants accepted 2009–2010, 2. Number full-time enrolled (new admits only) 2009–2010, 1. Number part-time enrolled (new admits only) 2009–2010, 0. Total enrolled 2009–2010 full-time, 6, part-time, 4. Openings 2010–2011, 1. The median number of years required for completion of a degree in 2008–2009 were 5. The number of students enrolled full- and part-time who were dismissed or voluntarily withdrew from this program area in 2008–2009 were 0. *Developmental Psychology PhD (Doctor of Philosophy)*—Applications 2009–2010, 15. Total applicants accepted 2009–2010, 4. Number full-time enrolled (new admits only) 2009–2010, 2. Number part-time enrolled (new admits only) 2009–2010, 1. Total enrolled 2009–2010 full-time, 7, part-time, 1. Openings 2010–2011, 2. The median number of years required for completion of a degree in 2008–2009 were 4. The number of students enrolled full- and part-time who were dismissed or voluntarily withdrew from this program area in 2008–2009 were 0. *Health Psychology PhD (Doctor of Philosophy)*—Applications 2009–2010, 20. Total applicants accepted 2009–2010, 0. Number full-time enrolled (new admits only) 2009–2010, 0. Number part-time enrolled (new admits only) 2009–2010, 0. Openings 2010–2011, 2. The number of students enrolled full- and part-time who were dismissed or voluntarily withdrew from this program area in 2008–2009 were 0.

Scores: Entries appear in this order: required test or GPA, minimum score (if required), median score of students entering in 2009–2010. *Clinical Psychology PhD (Doctor of Philosophy)*: GRE-V no minimum stated, GRE-Q no minimum stated, GRE-Analytical no minimum stated, overall undergraduate GPA no minimum stated, last 2 years GPA no minimum stated, psychology GPA no minimum stated; *Counseling Psychology PhD (Doctor of Philosophy)*: GRE-V no minimum stated, GRE-Q no minimum stated, GRE-Analytical no minimum stated, overall undergraduate GPA no minimum stated, last 2 years GPA no minimum stated, psychology GPA no minimum stated; *Social Psychology PhD (Doctor of Philosophy)*: GRE-V no minimum stated, GRE-Q no minimum stated, GRE-Analytical no minimum stated, overall undergraduate GPA no minimum stated, last 2 years GPA no minimum stated, psychology GPA no minimum stated; *Biopsychology PhD (Doctor of Philosophy)*: GRE-V no minimum stated, GRE-Q no minimum stated, GRE-Analytical no minimum stated, overall undergraduate GPA no minimum stated, last 2 years GPA no minimum stated, psychology GPA no minimum stated; *Developmental Psychology PhD (Doctor of Philosophy)*: GRE-V no minimum stated, GRE-Q no minimum stated, GRE-Analytical no minimum stated, overall undergraduate GPA no minimum stated, last 2 years GPA no minimum stated, psychology GPA no minimum stated; *Health Psychology PhD (Doctor of Philosophy)*: GRE-V no minimum stated, GRE-Q no minimum stated, GRE-Analytical no minimum stated, overall undergraduate GPA no minimum stated, last 2 years GPA no minimum stated, psychology GPA no minimum stated.

Other Criteria: (importance of criteria rated low, medium, or high): GRE scores—high, research experience—high, work experience—high, extracurricular activity—medium, clinically related public service—medium, GPA—high, letters of recommendation—high, interview—medium, statement of goals and objectives—medium. The experimental programs stress research experience, GPA, letters of recommendation, and GREs more than the clinical and counseling programs. The clinical and counseling programs stress match between student interests and faculty interests. This match is important, but not as highly stressed by the Experimental programs. Clinical and counseling programs stress importance of clinically related public service, interviews, and statement of goals and objectives. For additional information on admission requirements, go to http://www.has.vcu.edu/psy/.

Student Characteristics: The following represents characteristics of students in 2009–2010 in all graduate psychology programs in the department: Female—full-time 90, part-time 15; Male—full-time 23, part-time 5; African American/Black—full-time 12, part-time 3; Hispanic/Latino(a)—full-time 7, part-time 1; Asian/Pacific Islander—full-time 4, part-time 1; American Indian/Alaska Native—full-time 0, part-time 0; Caucasian/White—full-time 90, part-time 15; Multi-ethnic—full-time 0, part-time 0; students subject to the Americans With Disabilities Act—full-time 1, part-time 0; Unknown ethnicity—full-time 0, part-time 0; International students who hold an F-1 or J-1 Visa—full-time 3, part-time 0.

Financial Information/Assistance:
Tuition for Full-Time Study: *Master's:* State residents: per academic year $7,224; Nonstate residents: per academic year $15,904. *Doctoral:* State residents: per academic year $7,224; Nonstate residents: per academic year $15,904. Tuition is subject to change.

Financial Assistance:
   First-Year Students: Teaching assistantships available for first year. Average amount paid per academic year: $13,520. Average number of hours worked per week: 20. Research assistantships available for first year. Average amount paid per academic year: $13,520. Average number of hours worked per week: 20. Fellowships and scholarships available for first year.
   Advanced Students: Teaching assistantships available for advanced students. Average amount paid per academic year: $13,520. Average number of hours worked per week: 20. Research assistantships available for advanced students. Average amount paid per academic year: $13,520. Average number of hours worked per week: 20. Fellowships and scholarships available for advanced students.
   Additional Information: Of all students currently enrolled full time, 98% benefited from one or more of the listed financial assistance programs.

Internships/Practica: Doctoral Degree (PhD Clinical Psychology): For those doctoral students for whom a professional internship was required in this program prior to graduation, (8) students applied for an internship in 2008–2009, with (7) students obtaining an internship. Of those students who obtained an internship, (7) were paid internships. Of those students who obtained an internship, (6) students placed in APA/CPA accredited internships, (0) students placed in internships not APA/CPA accredited, but listed with the Association of Psychology Postdoctoral and Internship Programs (APPIC), (0) students placed in internships conforming to guidelines of the Council of Directors of School Psychology Programs (CDSPP), (1) students placed in internships that were not APA/CPA accredited, APPIC or CDSPP listed. Doctoral Degree (PhD Counseling Psychology): For those doctoral students for whom a professional internship was required in this program prior to graduation, (11) students applied for an internship in 2008–2009, with (11) students obtaining an internship. Of those students who obtained an internship, (10) were paid internships. Of those students who obtained an internship, (11) students placed in APA/CPA accredited internships, (0) students placed in internships not APA/CPA accredited, but listed with the Association of Psychology Postdoctoral and Internship Programs (APPIC), (0) students placed in internships conforming to guidelines of the Council of Directors of School Psychology Programs (CDSPP), (0) students placed in internships that were not APA/CPA accredited, APPIC or CDSPP listed. Practicum (external) and internship required for clinical and counseling programs. Sites include the following: VA hospitals, federal prisons, counseling centers, medical campus opportunities, Children's Hospitals, and juvenile facilities.

Housing and Day Care: On-campus housing is available. See the following Web site for more information: http://www.housing.vcu.edu. On-campus day care facilities are available. See the following Web site for more information: http://www.soe.vcu.edu/cdc.

Employment of Department Graduates:
Master's Degree Graduates: Of those who graduated in the academic year 2008–2009, the following categories and numbers represent the postgraduate activities and employment of master's degree graduates: Enrolled in a postdoctoral residency/fellowship (n/a), employed in independent practice (n/a), total from the above (master's) (0).
Doctoral Degree Graduates: Of those who graduated in the academic year 2008–2009, the following categories and numbers represent the postgraduate activities and employment of doctoral degree graduates: Enrolled in a psychology doctoral program (n/a), enrolled in another graduate/professional program (0), do not know (9), total from the above (doctoral) (9).

Additional Information:
Orientation, Objectives, and Emphasis of Department: The graduate programs in psychology are designed to provide a core education in the basic science of psychology and to enable students to develop skills specific to their area of interest. Students are educated first as psychologists, and are then helped to develop competence in a more specialized area relevant to their scholarly and professional objectives. In addition to formal research requirements for the thesis and dissertation, students in the graduate programs are encouraged to conduct independent research, participate in research teams, or collaborate with faculty conducting research on an ongoing basis. The clinical and counseling psychology programs strongly emphasize the scientist–practitioner model. Students in the clinical program may elect to develop specialized competency in one of several different tracks, including behavior therapy/cognitive behavior therapy, behavioral medicine, clinical child, and adult psychotherapy process. The counseling psychology program prepares students to function in a variety of research and applied settings and to work with people experiencing a broad range of emotional, social, or behavioral problems. The experimental program stresses the acquisition of experimental skills as well as advanced training in one of three specialty areas: biopsychology, developmental psychology, and social psychology. We currently are developing an experimentally-oriented doctoral program in Health Psychology.

Special Facilities or Resources: The department maintains laboratories for research in the areas of health, biopsychology, developmental, social, psychophysiology, behavioral assessment, and psychotherapy process. The department also operates the Center for Psychological Services and Development, which provides mental health services for clients referred from throughout the Richmond metropolitan area. Students in the clinical and counseling programs complete practica in the Center and in a variety of off-campus practicum facilities located in the community. Cooperation with a variety of programs and departments on the University's medical campus, the Medical College of Virginia, is extensive for both research and training.

Information for Students With Physical Disabilities: See the following Web site for more information: http://www.students.vcu.edu/dss/.

Application Information:
Send to School of Graduate Studies - VCU Box 843051, Richmond, VA 23284. Application available online. URL of online application: http://www.graduate.vcu.edu/admission. Students are admitted in the Fall, application deadline. Deadlines are December 1 for Counseling Psychology, December 10 for Clinical Psychology, December 15 for Social Psychology, January 10 for Health Psychology, Developmental Psychology, and Biopsychology. Students applying to the Experimental Program should clearly indicate the division to which they are seeking admission. *Fee:* $50.

Virginia Consortium Program in Clinical Psychology
Program in Clinical Psychology
EVMS, NSU & ODU
Virginia Beach Higher Education Center, 1881 University Drive/Suite 239
Virginia Beach, VA 23453
Telephone: (757) 368-1820
Fax: (757) 368-1823
E-mail: *exoneill@odu.edu*
Web: *http://www.sci.odu.edu/vcpcp/*

Department Information:
1978. Chairperson: Michael L. Stutts, PhD Number of faculty: total—full-time 33; women—full-time 18; total—minority—full-time 9; women minority—full-time 7.

Programs and Degrees Offered:
Listed in the following order: Program area, degree type (T if terminal Master's), number awarded 7/08–6/09. Virginia Consortium Program in Clinical Psychology PsyD (Doctor of Psychology) 5.

APA Accreditation: Clinical PsyD (Doctor of Psychology). Student Outcome Data Website: http://www.sci.odu.edu/vcpcp/program/Program_Data.shtml.

Student Applications/Admissions:
Student Applications
Virginia Consortium Program in Clinical Psychology PsyD (Doctor of Psychology)—Applications 2009–2010, 214. Total applicants accepted 2009–2010, 10. Number full-time enrolled (new admits only) 2009–2010, 6. Number part-time enrolled

(new admits only) 2009–2010, 0. Openings 2010–2011, 6. The median number of years required for completion of a degree in 2008–2009 were 4. The number of students enrolled full- and part-time who were dismissed or voluntarily withdrew from this program area in 2008–2009 were 0.

Scores: Entries appear in this order: required test or GPA, minimum score (if required), median score of students entering in 2009–2010. *Virginia Consortium Program in Clinical Psychology PsyD (Doctor of Psychology):* GRE-V no minimum stated, 575, GRE-Q no minimum stated, 680, overall undergraduate GPA 2.5, last 2 years GPA 3.0, psychology GPA 3.0, Masters GPA 3.0.

Other Criteria: (importance of criteria rated low, medium, or high): GRE scores—medium, research experience—medium, work experience—medium, extracurricular activity—low, clinically related public service—medium, GPA—medium, letters of recommendation—medium, interview—high, statement of goals and objectives—high, undergraduate major in psychology—medium, specific undergraduate psychology courses taken—medium. For additional information on admission requirements, go to http://www.sci.odu.edu/vcpcp/application/admission.shtml.

Student Characteristics: The following represents characteristics of students in 2009–2010 in all graduate psychology programs in the department: Female—full-time 37, part-time 0; Male—full-time 12, part-time 0; African American/Black—full-time 5, part-time 0; Hispanic/Latino(a)—full-time 3, part-time 0; Asian/Pacific Islander—full-time 7, part-time 0; American Indian/Alaska Native—full-time 0, part-time 0; Caucasian/White—full-time 34, part-time 0; Multi-ethnic—full-time 0, part-time 0; students subject to the Americans With Disabilities Act—full-time 0, part-time 0; Unknown ethnicity—full-time 0, part-time 0; International students who hold an F-1 or J-1 Visa—full-time 0, part-time 0.

Financial Information/Assistance:
Tuition for Full-Time Study: *Doctoral:* State residents: per academic year $15,000; Nonstate residents: per academic year $15,000. Tuition is subject to change. Additional fees are assessed to students beyond the costs of tuition for the following: dissertation binding & microfilming; a $150 graduation fee. See the following Web site for updates and changes in tuition costs: http://www.sci.odu.edu/vcpcp/application/financial_aid.shtml.

Financial Assistance:
First-Year Students: Teaching assistantships available for first year. Average amount paid per academic year: $8,000. Average number of hours worked per week: 10. Apply by January 2. Research assistantships available for first year. Average amount paid per academic year: $7,000. Average number of hours worked per week: 8. Apply by January 2.

Advanced Students: Teaching assistantships available for advanced students. Average amount paid per academic year: $8,250. Average number of hours worked per week: 10. Apply by March 15. Research assistantships available for advanced students. Average amount paid per academic year: $7,500. Average number of hours worked per week: 8. Apply by March 15. Traineeships available for advanced students. Average amount paid per academic year: $8,000. Average number of hours worked per week: 20. Apply by March 15.

Additional Information: Of all students currently enrolled full time, 100% benefited from one or more of the listed financial assistance programs. Application and information available online at: http://www.sci.odu.edu/vcpcp/application/financial_aid.shtml.

Internships/Practica: Doctoral Degree (PsyD Virginia Consortium Program in Clinical Psychology): For those doctoral students for whom a professional internship was required in this program prior to graduation, (12) students applied for an internship in 2008–2009, with (10) students obtaining an internship. Of those students who obtained an internship, (10) were paid internships. Of those students who obtained an internship, (9) students placed in APA/CPA accredited internships, (1) students placed in internships not APA/CPA accredited, but listed with the Association of Psychology Postdoctoral and Internship Programs (APPIC), (0) students placed in internships conforming to guidelines of the Council of Directors of School Psychology Programs (CDSPP), (0) students placed in internships that were not APA/CPA accredited, APPIC or CDSPP listed. Practicum training is offered in a variety of diverse settings: mental health centers, medical hospitals, children's residential treatment facilities, public school systems, university counseling centers, social services clinics, private practices, and rehabilitation units. Settings include inpatient, partial hospitalization, residential, and outpatient. Populations include infants, children, adolescents, adults, and the elderly from most socioeconomic levels and ethnic groups. Services include most forms of assessment; individual, group, and family intervention modalities; and consultative and other indirect services. Placements are arranged to ensure that each student is exposed to several settings and populations.

Housing and Day Care: On-campus housing is available. Graduate housing is available at some of the sponsoring schools. However, the program operates on a calendar year and the schools on an academic year, so students must vacate graduate housing at the end of the spring semester while still in classes. This leaves them looking for housing and moving during the summer semester. No on-campus day care facilities are available.

Employment of Department Graduates:
Master's Degree Graduates: Of those who graduated in the academic year 2008–2009, the following categories and numbers represent the postgraduate activities and employment of master's degree graduates: Enrolled in a postdoctoral residency/fellowship (n/a), employed in independent practice (n/a), total from the above (master's) (0).

Doctoral Degree Graduates: Of those who graduated in the academic year 2008–2009, the following categories and numbers represent the postgraduate activities and employment of doctoral degree graduates: Enrolled in a psychology doctoral program (n/a), enrolled in a postdoctoral residency/fellowship (1), employed in independent practice (1), employed in a hospital/medical center (2), not seeking employment (1), total from the above (doctoral) (5).

Additional Information:
Orientation, Objectives, and Emphasis of Department: The Virginia Consortium is a single, unified program co-sponsored now by three institutions: Eastern Virginia Medical School, Norfolk State University, and Old Dominion University. Its mission is to produce practicing clinical psychologists who are competent in individual and cultural diversity, educated in the basic subjects

and methods of psychological science, capable of critically assimilating and generating new knowledge, proficient in the delivery and evaluation of clinical services, and able to assume leadership positions in health service delivery organizations. The curriculum is generalist in content and in theoretical orientation. Knowledge acquired in the classroom is applied in an orderly sequence of supervised practica providing exposure to multiple settings, populations, and intervention modalities. Practicum objectives are integrated with the goals of classroom education to facilitate systematic and cumulative acquisition of clinical skills. In the third year, the student pursues individual interests by integrating individualized coursework with advanced practica and a clinical dissertation. In the fourth year, the student continues advanced practica and competes for a full-time clinical internship to be taken in year five. Dissertation defense is expected to occur prior to internship.

Special Facilities or Resources: Students are considered full-time in all three sponsoring schools. This permits access to three libraries with several computerized literature search databases and 400 periodicals in psychology; three computing centers; multiple health services; and a variety of athletic facilities. Research may be conducted at practicum placement facilities.

Information for Students With Physical Disabilities: See the following Web site for more information: http://www.sci.odu.edu/vcpcp/schools.shtml.

Application Information:
Send to Program Office, Virginia Consortium Program in Clinical Psychology, Virginia Beach Higher Education Center, 1881 University Drive/Suite 239, Virginia Beach, VA 23453. Application available online. URL of online application: http://www.sci.odu.edu/vcpcp/application/application.shtml. Students are admitted in the Fall, application deadline January 2. *Fee:* $50.

Virginia Polytechnic Institute and State University
Department of Psychology
College of Science
109 Williams Hall
Blacksburg, VA 24061
Telephone: (540) 231-6581
Fax: (540) 231-3652
E-mail: *kirbydd@vt.edu*
Web: *http://www.psyc.vt.edu/*

Department Information:
1965. Chairperson: Robert S. Stephens. Number of faculty: total—full-time 25; women—full-time 8; total—minority—full-time 2; women minority—full-time 1.

Programs and Degrees Offered:
Listed in the following order: Program area, degree type (T if terminal Master's), number awarded 7/08–6/09. Clinical Psychology PhD (Doctor of Philosophy) 8, Industrial/Organizational Psychology PhD (Doctor of Philosophy) 3, Developmental and Biological Psychology PhD (Doctor of Philosophy) 3.

APA Accreditation: Clinical PhD (Doctor of Philosophy). Student Outcome Data Website: http://www.psyc.vt.edu/graduate/clinical/.

Student Applications/Admissions:
Student Applications
Clinical Psychology PhD (Doctor of Philosophy)—Applications 2009–2010, 140. Total applicants accepted 2009–2010, 10. Number full-time enrolled (new admits only) 2009–2010, 7. Number part-time enrolled (new admits only) 2009–2010, 0. Openings 2010–2011, 6. The median number of years required for completion of a degree in 2008–2009 were 5. The number of students enrolled full- and part-time who were dismissed or voluntarily withdrew from this program area in 2008–2009 were 0. *Industrial/Organizational Psychology PhD (Doctor of Philosophy)*—Applications 2009–2010, 57. Total applicants accepted 2009–2010, 7. Number full-time enrolled (new admits only) 2009–2010, 3. Number part-time enrolled (new admits only) 2009–2010, 0. Total enrolled 2009–2010 full-time, 12. Openings 2010–2011, 4. The median number of years required for completion of a degree in 2008–2009 were 4. The number of students enrolled full- and part-time who were dismissed or voluntarily withdrew from this program area in 2008–2009 were 1. *Developmental and Biological Psychology PhD (Doctor of Philosophy)*—Applications 2009–2010, 29. Total applicants accepted 2009–2010, 11. Number full-time enrolled (new admits only) 2009–2010, 5. Number part-time enrolled (new admits only) 2009–2010, 0. Total enrolled 2009–2010 full-time, 19. Openings 2010–2011, 6. The median number of years required for completion of a degree in 2008–2009 were 4. The number of students enrolled full- and part-time who were dismissed or voluntarily withdrew from this program area in 2008–2009 were 1.

Scores: Entries appear in this order: required test or GPA, minimum score (if required), median score of students entering in 2009–2010. Clinical Psychology PhD (Doctor of Philosophy): GRE-V no minimum stated, GRE-Q no minimum stated.

Other Criteria: (importance of criteria rated low, medium, or high): GRE scores—high, research experience—high, work experience—low, clinically related public service—medium, GPA—high, letters of recommendation—high, interview—medium, statement of goals and objectives—medium, undergraduate major in psychology—low, specific undergraduate psychology courses taken—low, congruence of applicant's goals with program objectives and faculty research - high. For additional information on admission requirements, go to http://www.psyc.vt.edu/graduate/.

Student Characteristics: The following represents characteristics of students in 2009–2010 in all graduate psychology programs in the department: Female—full-time 47, part-time 0; Male—full-time 29, part-time 0; African American/Black—full-time 7, part-time 0; Hispanic/Latino(a)—full-time 3, part-time 0; Asian/Pacific Islander—full-time 6, part-time 1; American Indian/Alaska Native—full-time 0, part-time 0; Caucasian/White—full-time 60, part-time 3; Multi-ethnic—full-time 0, part-time 0; students subject to the Americans With Disabilities Act—full-time 0, part-time 0; Unknown ethnicity—full-time 0, part-time 0; International students who hold an F-1 or J-1 Visa—full-time 4, part-time 0.

Financial Information/Assistance:
Tuition for Full-Time Study: *Doctoral:* State residents: per academic year $10,228; Nonstate residents: per academic year

$17,928. Tuition is subject to change. See the following Web site for updates and changes in tuition costs: http://www.vt.edu/tuition/.

Financial Assistance:
First-Year Students: Teaching assistantships available for first year. Average amount paid per academic year: $14,049. Average number of hours worked per week: 20. Research assistantships available for first year. Average amount paid per academic year: $15,318. Average number of hours worked per week: 20.
Advanced Students: Teaching assistantships available for advanced students. Average amount paid per academic year: $14,895. Average number of hours worked per week: 20. Research assistantships available for advanced students. Average amount paid per academic year: $16,173. Average number of hours worked per week: 20.
Additional Information: Of all students currently enrolled full time, 95% benefited from one or more of the listed financial assistance programs. Application and information available online at: http://www.psyc.vt.edu/graduate.

Internships/Practica: Doctoral Degree (PhD Clinical Psychology): For those doctoral students for whom a professional internship was required in this program prior to graduation, (6) students applied for an internship in 2008–2009, with (4) students obtaining an internship. Of those students who obtained an internship, (4) were paid internships. Of those students who obtained an internship, (3) students placed in APA/CPA accredited internships, (0) students placed in internships not APA/CPA accredited, but listed with the Association of Psychology Postdoctoral and Internship Programs (APPIC), (0) students placed in internships conforming to guidelines of the Council of Directors of School Psychology Programs (CDSPP), (1) students placed in internships that were not APA/CPA accredited, APPIC or CDSPP listed. Students in clinical psychology complete practica in department-run, off-campus clinics serving adults and children from the community. They also complete an externship in one of a variety of local agency and hospital settings. They also are required to complete a predoctoral clinical internship as part of the PhD. Students in industrial/organizational psychology are encouraged to pursue summer internships.

Housing and Day Care: On-campus housing is available. See the following Web site for more information: http://www.studentprograms.vt.edu/housing/. No on-campus day care facilities are available.

Employment of Department Graduates:
Master's Degree Graduates: Of those who graduated in the academic year 2008–2009, the following categories and numbers represent the postgraduate activities and employment of master's degree graduates: Enrolled in a postdoctoral residency/fellowship (n/a), employed in independent practice (n/a), total from the above (master's) (0).
Doctoral Degree Graduates: Of those who graduated in the academic year 2008–2009, the following categories and numbers represent the postgraduate activities and employment of doctoral degree graduates: Enrolled in a psychology doctoral program (n/a), enrolled in a postdoctoral residency/fellowship (4), employed in an academic position at a university (1), employed in other positions at a higher education institution (1), employed in business or industry (3), employed in government agency (4), still seeking employment (1), total from the above (doctoral) (14).

Additional Information:
Orientation, Objectives, and Emphasis of Department: The graduate programs are designed to ensure that students receive excellent preparation in research methods and psychological theory in order to be successful in either academic or applied settings. Training and experience in the teaching of psychology is available. The Clinical Psychology program is based on the clinical scientist model and emphasizes research methods and theory in understanding, preventing, and treating health and mental health problems in adults and children. Clinical concentrations include child, adult, and health psychology. The Industrial/Organizational psychology program prepares students for research and teaching positions as well as for the solution of individual, group, and organizational problems in applied work settings. Psychometrics, research design, and statistics are emphasized. The Developmental and Biological Psychology program trains students in experimental psychology with a focus on preparing psychologists for teaching and research settings. Students may concentrate their studies in developmental or psychobiological research areas or both.

Special Facilities or Resources: The Psychological Services Center and Child Study Center are located off-campus and provide the foundation for practicum and research training in Clinical Psychology. The Center for Research in Health Behavior is also located off-campus and is primarily involved in prevention research supported by the National Institutes of Health. Virginia Tech Community Partners is another off-campus research facility, located in downtown Roanoke. Faculty, students, and staff benefit from Virginia Tech's state-of-the-art communications system that links every dormitory room, laboratory, office, and classroom to computing capabilities, audio and video data, and the World Wide Web. The entire campus has easy access to supercomputers across the country, worldwide libraries and data systems. Department resources also include two state-of-the-art laboratories that are dedicated to undergraduate and graduate teaching and research. The psychophysiological laboratory includes eight computer workstations, five EEG/Evoked Potential work stations (32 channel Neuroscan; Neurosearch-24), eye tracker equipment, Coulbourn physiological units, and extensive perception equipment. The other computer laboratory includes 25 computer workstations with cognitive and neurophysiological experiments, SAS and SPSS statistical packages, Bilog and Multilog programs. Graduate students also have ready access to PC and Macintosh computers for word processing and Internet access.

Information for Students With Physical Disabilities: See the following Web site for more information: http://www.ssd.vt.edu/.

Application Information:
Send to Graduate School Admissions, Graduate Life Center (Mail code 0325), Virginia Polytechnic Institute and State University, Blacksburg, VA 24061, and Graduate Admissions Coordinator, 109 Williams Hall, Department of Psychology 0436, Virginia Tech, Blacksburg, VA 24061. Application available online. URL of online application: https://www.applyweb.com/apply/vtechg/index.html. Students are admitted in the Fall, application deadline December 5. Application deadline for Clinical program is December 5; for Developmental and Biological Psychol-

ogy is January 5; and for Industrial/Organizational Psychology is January 15. *Fee:* $65.

Virginia State University
Department of Psychology
School of Engineering, Science, and Technology
1 Hayden Drive Box 9079 Hunter-McDaniel 102S
Petersburg, VA 23806
Telephone: (804) 524-5938
Fax: (804) 524-5460
E-mail: *ohill@vsu.edu*
Web: *http://www.vsu.edu/pages/783.asp*

Department Information:
1883. Chairperson: Oliver W. Hill, Jr., PhD Number of faculty: total—full-time 14, part-time 7; women—full-time 9, part-time 5; total—minority—full-time 13, part-time 5; women minority—full-time 9, part-time 4.

Programs and Degrees Offered:
Listed in the following order: Program area, degree type (T if terminal Master's), number awarded 7/08–6/09. Psychology MA/MS (Master of Arts/Science) (T) 25, Health Psychology PhD (Doctor of Philosophy) 0.

Student Applications/Admissions:
Student Applications
Psychology MA/MS (Master of Arts/Science)—Applications 2009–2010, 30. Total applicants accepted 2009–2010, 24. Number full-time enrolled (new admits only) 2009–2010, 22. Number part-time enrolled (new admits only) 2009–2010, 2. Total enrolled 2009–2010 full-time, 54, part-time, 8. Openings 2010–2011, 15. The median number of years required for completion of a degree in 2008–2009 were 3. The number of students enrolled full- and part-time who were dismissed or voluntarily withdrew from this program area in 2008–2009 were 4. Health Psychology PhD (Doctor of Philosophy)—Applications 2009–2010, 20. Total applicants accepted 2009–2010, 4. Number full-time enrolled (new admits only) 2009–2010, 4. Number part-time enrolled (new admits only) 2009–2010, 0. Openings 2010–2011, 4. The number of students enrolled full- and part-time who were dismissed or voluntarily withdrew from this program area in 2008–2009 were 0.
Scores: Entries appear in this order: required test or GPA, minimum score (if required), median score of students entering in 2009–2010. Psychology MA/MS (Master of Arts/Science): GRE-V no minimum stated, GRE-Q no minimum stated; Health Psychology PhD (Doctor of Philosophy): GRE-V no minimum stated, GRE-Q no minimum stated.
Other Criteria: (importance of criteria rated low, medium, or high): GRE scores—medium, research experience—medium, work experience—low, extracurricular activity—low, clinically related public service—low, GPA—high, letters of recommendation—high, interview—high, statement of goals and objectives—medium, undergraduate major in psychology—medium, specific undergraduate psychology courses taken—high.

Student Characteristics: The following represents characteristics of students in 2009–2010 in all graduate psychology programs in the department: Female—full-time 35, part-time 7; Male—full-time 7, part-time 5; African American/Black—full-time 39, part-time 12; Hispanic/Latino(a)—full-time 0, part-time 0; Asian/Pacific Islander—full-time 1, part-time 0; American Indian/Alaska Native—full-time 0, part-time 0; Caucasian/White—full-time 2, part-time 0; Multi-ethnic—full-time 0, part-time 0; students subject to the Americans With Disabilities Act—full-time 0, part-time 0; Unknown ethnicity—full-time 0, part-time 0; International students who hold an F-1 or J-1 Visa—full-time 1, part-time 0.

Financial Information/Assistance:
Tuition for Full-Time Study: *Master's:* State residents: per academic year $5,677; Nonstate residents: per academic year $12,142. *Doctoral:* State residents: per academic year $5,677; Nonstate residents: per academic year $12,142. Tuition is subject to change. See the following Web site for updates and changes in tuition costs: http://www.vsu.edu/pages/448.asp.

Financial Assistance:
First-Year Students: Research assistantships available for first year. Average amount paid per academic year: $6,000. Average number of hours worked per week: 20. Apply by March 31.
Advanced Students: Research assistantships available for advanced students. Average amount paid per academic year: $6,000. Apply by March 31. Fellowships and scholarships available for advanced students. Average amount paid per academic year: $6,000. Average number of hours worked per week: 0. Apply by March 31.
Additional Information: Of all students currently enrolled full time, 75% benefited from one or more of the listed financial assistance programs.

Internships/Practica: Master's Degree (MA/MS Psychology): An internship experience, such as a final research project or "capstone" experience is required of graduates. Clinical students must complete three sections of practicum. Placements usually match the student's career goals and the characteristics of the practicum site. PhD students in the clinical health track must complete a 1-year internship.

Housing and Day Care: On-campus housing is available. See the following Web site for more information: http://www.vsu.edu/pages/326.asp. No on-campus day care facilities are available.

Employment of Department Graduates:
Master's Degree Graduates: Of those who graduated in the academic year 2008–2009, the following categories and numbers represent the postgraduate activities and employment of master's degree graduates: Enrolled in a psychology doctoral program (13), enrolled in another graduate/professional program (7), enrolled in a postdoctoral residency/fellowship (n/a), employed in independent practice (n/a), employed in a professional position in a school system (2), employed in business or industry (15), employed in government agency (13), employed in a community mental health/counseling center (2), employed in a hospital/medical center (4), total from the above (master's) (56).
Doctoral Degree Graduates: Of those who graduated in the academic year 2008–2009, the following categories and numbers represent the postgraduate activities and employment of doctoral

degree graduates: Enrolled in a psychology doctoral program (n/a), total from the above (doctoral) (0).

Additional Information:
Orientation, Objectives, and Emphasis of Department: Students who select the General Psychology master's program usually plan to apply to doctoral programs. Students who select the Clinical program either have aspirations to attend a doctoral program or have a goal to obtain state licensure and practice with their Master's degree in private or public agencies. Students who have been admitted to doctoral programs after completion of any concentration -General or Clinical- of our master's program usually matriculated successfully. Students in the Clinical Master's programs learn diagnostic and evaluation skills, and are placed in practicum sites. All students must complete a thesis. Our PhD program in Health Psychology has two tracks: a clinical health track that requires a year-long internship, and a behavioral community health track. This PhD program started in Fall 2008.

Special Facilities or Resources: The psychology department recently renovated its clinical lab to expand its test library, add videotaping capability, and provide electronic report writing capability. The psychology experimental computer lab was updated in Fall 2006. Current faculty research projects include studies of cardiovascular response to stress in African-Americans, STD/HIV prevention and health care seeking behavior in African-Americans, religiosity and health, stress and burnout among healthcare workers, cognitive variables in mathematics performance, and psychoepistemology.

Information for Students With Physical Disabilities: See the following Web site for more information: http://www.vsu.edu/pages/323.asp.

Application Information:
Send to School of Graduate Studies, Research and Outreach, 1 Hayden Drive, Box 9080, VSU, Petersburg, VA 23806-0001. Application available online. URL of online application: http://www.vsu.edu/pages/4542.asp. Students are admitted in the Fall, application deadline January 15. PhD applicants have a deadline of January 15; Master's applicants have a deadline of April 1. *Fee:* $25.

Virginia, University of
Curry Programs in Clinical and School Psychology
Curry School of Education
P.O. Box 400270
Charlottesville, VA 22904-4270
Telephone: (434) 924-7472
Fax: (434) 924-1433
E-mail: *rer5r@virginia.edu*
Web: *http://curry.edschool.virginia.edu/clinpsych*

Department Information:
1976. Director: Ronald E. Reeve. Number of faculty: total—full-time 6, part-time 2; women—full-time 3, part-time 1; minority—part-time 1; women minority—part-time 1.

Programs and Degrees Offered:
Listed in the following order: Program area, degree type (T if terminal Master's), number awarded 7/08–6/09. Clinical Psychology PhD (Doctor of Philosophy) 6.

APA Accreditation: Clinical PhD (Doctor of Philosophy).

Student Applications/Admissions:
Student Applications

Clinical Psychology PhD (Doctor of Philosophy)—Applications 2009–2010, 131. Total applicants accepted 2009–2010, 8. Number full-time enrolled (new admits only) 2009–2010, 5. Number part-time enrolled (new admits only) 2009–2010, 0. Openings 2010–2011, 6. The median number of years required for completion of a degree in 2008–2009 were 5. The number of students enrolled full- and part-time who were dismissed or voluntarily withdrew from this program area in 2008–2009 were 0.

Other Criteria: (importance of criteria rated low, medium, or high): GRE scores—medium, research experience—medium, work experience—medium, extracurricular activity—low, clinically related public service—medium, GPA—high, letters of recommendation—high, interview—high, statement of goals and objectives—high, undergraduate major in psychology—medium, specific undergraduate psychology courses taken—medium. For additional information on admission requirements, go to http://curry.edschool.virginia.edu/clinpsych/.

Student Characteristics: The following represents characteristics of students in 2009–2010 in all graduate psychology programs in the department: Female—full-time 26, part-time 0; Male—full-time 4, part-time 0; African American/Black—full-time 5, part-time 0; Hispanic/Latino(a)—full-time 1, part-time 0; Asian/Pacific Islander—full-time 2, part-time 0; American Indian/Alaska Native—full-time 0, part-time 0; Caucasian/White—full-time 22, part-time 0; Multi-ethnic—full-time 0, part-time 0; students subject to the Americans With Disabilities Act—full-time 0, part-time 0; Unknown ethnicity—full-time 0, part-time 0; International students who hold an F-1 or J-1 Visa—full-time 0, part-time 0.

Financial Information/Assistance:
Tuition for Full-Time Study: Doctoral: State residents: per academic year $12,093; Nonstate residents: per academic year $22,093. See the following Web site for updates and changes in tuition costs: http://www.virginia.edu/studentaccounts/tuition_and_fee.html.

Financial Assistance:
First-Year Students: Teaching assistantships available for first year. Average amount paid per academic year: $2,000. Average number of hours worked per week: 10. Apply by March 1. Research assistantships available for first year. Average amount paid per academic year: $5,000. Average number of hours worked per week: 10. Apply by March 1. Fellowships and scholarships

available for first year. Average amount paid per academic year: $13,000. Average number of hours worked per week: 10. Apply by March 1.

Advanced Students: Teaching assistantships available for advanced students. Average amount paid per academic year: $2,000. Average number of hours worked per week: 10. Apply by March 1. Research assistantships available for advanced students. Average amount paid per academic year: $5,000. Average number of hours worked per week: 10. Apply by March 1. Fellowships and scholarships available for advanced students. Average amount paid per academic year: $6,000. Average number of hours worked per week: 10. Apply by March 1.

Additional Information: Of all students currently enrolled full time, 100% benefited from one or more of the listed financial assistance programs. Application and information available online at: http://www.virginia.edu/financialaid/gradstudents.php.

Internships/Practica: Doctoral Degree (PhD Clinical Psychology): For those doctoral students for whom a professional internship was required in this program prior to graduation, (6) students applied for an internship in 2008–2009, with (6) students obtaining an internship. Of those students who obtained an internship, (6) were paid internships. Of those students who obtained an internship, (6) students placed in APA/CPA accredited internships, (0) students placed in internships not APA/CPA accredited, but listed with the Association of Psychology Postdoctoral and Internship Programs (APPIC), (0) students placed in internships conforming to guidelines of the Council of Directors of School Psychology Programs (CDSPP), (0) students placed in internships that were not APA/CPA accredited, APPIC or CDSPP listed. Students undertake external clinical practica and school internships in area public and private schools, state mental hospitals/residential treatment centers for children or adults, a regional medically affiliated children's rehabilitation center, a family stress clinic, and other mental health settings in the university and community. During the fifth year of training, students complete a full-time one-year internship in clinical psychology.

Housing and Day Care: On-campus housing is available. See the following Web site for more information: http://www.virginia.edu/housing/. On-campus day care facilities are available. See the following Web site for more information: http://www.virginia.edu/childdevelopmentcenter/.

Employment of Department Graduates:
Master's Degree Graduates: Of those who graduated in the academic year 2008–2009, the following categories and numbers represent the postgraduate activities and employment of master's degree graduates: Enrolled in a postdoctoral residency/fellowship (n/a), employed in independent practice (n/a), total from the above (master's) (0).
Doctoral Degree Graduates: Of those who graduated in the academic year 2008–2009, the following categories and numbers represent the postgraduate activities and employment of doctoral degree graduates: Enrolled in a psychology doctoral program (n/a), enrolled in a postdoctoral residency/fellowship (6), total from the above (doctoral) (6).

Additional Information:
Orientation, Objectives, and Emphasis of Department: The primary goal of the training program in the Curry Programs in Clinical and School Psychology is to produce clinical and school psychologists who will make substantial contributions to the field in a variety of professional and scientific roles. The majority of graduates seek leadership positions in settings such as medical centers, schools, and mental health agencies, while others pursue academic and research careers. All students complete a common core of coursework and practica in both basic science and professional skills. Students have the opportunity for specialized training and research in concentration areas such as family therapy, forensic psychology, and school interventions, among others. The predominant theoretical and practice orientations of the faculty are cognitive behavioral, psychodynamic, and family systems. All students are expected to develop clinical and research skills, and the integration of clinical, classroom, and research experiences is emphasized. Many students in the PhD program pursue training in both clinical and school psychology through the clinical-school track. A separate Ed.D. program in school psychology admits experienced school psychologists who are prepared for leadership positions in school and university settings.

Special Facilities or Resources: The Curry Program operates a comprehensive psychological clinic, the Center for Clinical Psychology Services, serving families, couples, and individuals of all ages and diverse backgrounds, within the Sheila Johnson Center for Human Services. The new Sheila Johnson Center is well equipped for live and videotaped supervision and conveniently located in the new Bavaro Hall, with faculty and student offices nearby. In addition, the Program has close working relationships with numerous community agencies, schools, clinics, and hospitals that permit training and research in many different mental health and educational settings. Our students have research and consultation opportunities with numerous projects, including the Center for Positive Youth Development, Young Women Leaders Program, Virginia Youth Violence Project, Center for the Advanced Study of Teaching and Learning, and the Prisoners and Their Families Project. The Curry School of Education is a national leader in instructional technology, with outstanding computing facilities and technology support, smart classrooms, and its own library. Students enjoy easy access to the extensive University of Virginia Library system, which includes a collection of nearly 5 million volumes and has state-of-the-art electronic library resources.

Information for Students With Physical Disabilities: See the following Web site for more information: http://www.virginia.edu/accessibility/.

Application Information:
Send to Admissions Office, Curry School of Education, P.O. Box 400261, University of Virginia, Charlottesville, VA 22904-4261. Application available online. URL of online application: http://curry.edschool.virginia.edu/admissions/. Students are admitted in the Fall, application deadline January 5. *Fee:* $60. If fee imposes economic hardship, it may be waived. Request information from Curry School Admissions office at address above.

GRADUATE STUDY IN PSYCHOLOGY

Virginia, University of
Department of Psychology
102 Gilmer Hall, P.O. Box 400400
Charlottesville, VA 22904-4400
Telephone: (434) 982-4750
Fax: (434) 982-4766
E-mail: *psychology@virginia.edu*
Web: *http://www.virginia.edu/psychology/*

Department Information:
1929. Chairperson: Dennis Proffitt. Number of faculty: total—full-time 36; women—full-time 10; total—minority—full-time 6; women minority—full-time 1.

Programs and Degrees Offered:
Listed in the following order: Program area, degree type (T if terminal Master's), number awarded 7/08–6/09. Quantitative Psychology PhD (Doctor of Philosophy) 2, Social Psychology PhD (Doctor of Philosophy) 2, Clinical Psychology PhD (Doctor of Philosophy) 5, Cognitive Psychology PhD (Doctor of Philosophy) 4, Community Psychology PhD (Doctor of Philosophy) 0, Developmental Psychology PhD (Doctor of Philosophy) 3, Neuroscience and Behavior PhD (Doctor of Philosophy) 1.

APA Accreditation: Clinical PhD (Doctor of Philosophy).

Student Applications/Admissions:
Student Applications
Quantitative Psychology PhD (Doctor of Philosophy)—Applications 2009–2010, 11. Total applicants accepted 2009–2010, 4. Number full-time enrolled (new admits only) 2009–2010, 2. Number part-time enrolled (new admits only) 2009–2010, 0. Openings 2010–2011, 2. The median number of years required for completion of a degree in 2008–2009 were 6. The number of students enrolled full- and part-time who were dismissed or voluntarily withdrew from this program area in 2008–2009 were 0. *Social Psychology PhD (Doctor of Philosophy)*—Applications 2009–2010, 109. Total applicants accepted 2009–2010, 6. Number full-time enrolled (new admits only) 2009–2010, 5. Number part-time enrolled (new admits only) 2009–2010, 0. Openings 2010–2011, 3. The median number of years required for completion of a degree in 2008–2009 were 7. The number of students enrolled full- and part-time who were dismissed or voluntarily withdrew from this program area in 2008–2009 were 0. *Clinical Psychology PhD (Doctor of Philosophy)*—Applications 2009–2010, 284. Total applicants accepted 2009–2010, 8. Number full-time enrolled (new admits only) 2009–2010, 5. Number part-time enrolled (new admits only) 2009–2010, 0. Openings 2010–2011, 6. The median number of years required for completion of a degree in 2008–2009 were 8. The number of students enrolled full- and part-time who were dismissed or voluntarily withdrew from this program area in 2008–2009 were 0. *Cognitive Psychology PhD (Doctor of Philosophy)*—Applications 2009–2010, 46. Total applicants accepted 2009–2010, 4. Number full-time enrolled (new admits only) 2009–2010, 2. Number part-time enrolled (new admits only) 2009–2010, 0. Openings 2010–2011, 3. The median number of years required for completion of a degree in 2008–2009 were 7. The number of students enrolled full- and part-time who were dismissed or voluntarily withdrew from this program area in 2008–2009 were 0. *Community Psychology PhD (Doctor of Philosophy)*—Applications 2009–2010, 35. Total applicants accepted 2009–2010, 3. Number full-time enrolled (new admits only) 2009–2010, 1. Number part-time enrolled (new admits only) 2009–2010, 0. Openings 2010–2011, 2. The number of students enrolled full- and part-time who were dismissed or voluntarily withdrew from this program area in 2008–2009 were 0. *Developmental Psychology PhD (Doctor of Philosophy)*—Applications 2009–2010, 50. Total applicants accepted 2009–2010, 3. Number full-time enrolled (new admits only) 2009–2010, 1. Number part-time enrolled (new admits only) 2009–2010, 0. Openings 2010–2011, 4. The number of students enrolled full- and part-time who were dismissed or voluntarily withdrew from this program area in 2008–2009 were 0. *Neuroscience and Behavior PhD (Doctor of Philosophy)*—Applications 2009–2010, 12. Total applicants accepted 2009–2010, 4. Number full-time enrolled (new admits only) 2009–2010, 1. Number part-time enrolled (new admits only) 2009–2010, 0. Openings 2010–2011, 1. The median number of years required for completion of a degree in 2008–2009 were 7. The number of students enrolled full- and part-time who were dismissed or voluntarily withdrew from this program area in 2008–2009 were 0.

Scores: Entries appear in this order: required test or GPA, minimum score (if required), median score of students entering in 2009–2010. *Quantitative Psychology PhD (Doctor of Philosophy)*: GRE-V no minimum stated, GRE-Q no minimum stated, GRE-Analytical no minimum stated, overall undergraduate GPA no minimum stated, last 2 years GPA no minimum stated, psychology GPA no minimum stated, Masters GPA no minimum stated; *Social Psychology PhD (Doctor of Philosophy)*: GRE-V no minimum stated, GRE-Q no minimum stated, GRE-Analytical no minimum stated, overall undergraduate GPA no minimum stated, last 2 years GPA no minimum stated, psychology GPA no minimum stated, Masters GPA no minimum stated; *Clinical Psychology PhD (Doctor of Philosophy)*: GRE-V no minimum stated, GRE-Q no minimum stated, GRE-Analytical no minimum stated, overall undergraduate GPA no minimum stated, last 2 years GPA no minimum stated, psychology GPA no minimum stated, Masters GPA no minimum stated; *Cognitive Psychology PhD (Doctor of Philosophy)*: GRE-V no minimum stated, GRE-Q no minimum stated, GRE-Analytical no minimum stated, overall undergraduate GPA no minimum stated, last 2 years GPA no minimum stated, psychology GPA no minimum stated, Masters GPA no minimum stated; *Community Psychology PhD (Doctor of Philosophy)*: GRE-V no minimum stated, GRE-Q no minimum stated, GRE-Analytical no minimum stated, overall undergraduate GPA no minimum stated, last 2 years GPA no minimum stated, psychology GPA no minimum stated, Masters GPA no minimum stated; *Developmental Psychology PhD (Doctor of Philosophy)*: GRE-V no minimum stated, GRE-Q no minimum stated, GRE-Analytical no minimum stated, overall undergraduate GPA no minimum stated, last 2 years GPA no minimum stated, psychology GPA no minimum stated, Masters GPA no minimum stated; *Neuroscience and Behavior PhD (Doctor of Philosophy)*: GRE-V no minimum stated, GRE-Q no minimum stated, GRE-Analytical no minimum stated, overall undergraduate GPA no minimum stated, last 2 years GPA no minimum stated, psychology GPA no minimum stated, Masters GPA no minimum stated.

Other Criteria: (importance of criteria rated low, medium, or high): GRE scores—medium, research experience—high, work experience—medium, extracurricular activity—low, clinically related public service—low, GPA—high, letters of recommendation—high, interview—medium, statement of goals and objectives—high, Publications and presentations at conferences are valued as actual work experience in an area related to the degree sought.

Student Characteristics: The following represents characteristics of students in 2009–2010 in all graduate psychology programs in the department: Female—full-time 62, part-time 0; Male—full-time 28, part-time 0; African American/Black—full-time 7, part-time 0; Hispanic/Latino(a)—full-time 0, part-time 0; Asian/Pacific Islander—full-time 5, part-time 0; American Indian/Alaska Native—full-time 1, part-time 0; Caucasian/White—full-time 76, part-time 0; Multi-ethnic—full-time 1, part-time 0; students subject to the Americans With Disabilities Act—full-time 0, part-time 0; Unknown ethnicity—full-time 0, part-time 0; International students who hold an F-1 or J-1 Visa—full-time 6, part-time 0.

Financial Information/Assistance:

Tuition for Full-Time Study: *Doctoral:* State residents: per academic year $12,584; Nonstate residents: per academic year $22,584. Tuition is subject to change.

Financial Assistance:

First-Year Students: Teaching assistantships available for first year. Average amount paid per academic year: $9,250. Average number of hours worked per week: 10. Research assistantships available for first year. Average amount paid per academic year: $17,000. Average number of hours worked per week: 20. Fellowships and scholarships available for first year. Average amount paid per academic year: $6,750. Average number of hours worked per week: 0.

Advanced Students: Teaching assistantships available for advanced students. Average amount paid per academic year: $9,250. Average number of hours worked per week: 10. Research assistantships available for advanced students. Average amount paid per academic year: $17,000. Average number of hours worked per week: 20. Fellowships and scholarships available for advanced students. Average amount paid per academic year: $6,750. Average number of hours worked per week: 0.

Additional Information: Of all students currently enrolled full time, 100% benefited from one or more of the listed financial assistance programs.

Internships/Practica: Doctoral Degree (PhD Clinical Psychology): For those doctoral students for whom a professional internship was required in this program prior to graduation, (6) students applied for an internship in 2008–2009, with (6) students obtaining an internship. Of those students who obtained an internship, (6) were paid internships. Of those students who obtained an internship, (6) students placed in APA/CPA accredited internships, (0) students placed in internships not APA/CPA accredited, but listed with the Association of Psychology Postdoctoral and Internship Programs (APPIC), (0) students placed in internships conforming to guidelines of the Council of Directors of School Psychology Programs (CDSPP), (0) students placed in internships that were not APA/CPA accredited, APPIC or CDSPP listed. For clinical program: Multiple practica at University Hospital, state mental hospital for children and adults, Kluge Children's Center; community mental health center; Law and Psychiatry Unit; Department Clinic and other places as connections and student interest suggest.

Housing and Day Care: On-campus housing is available. See the following Web site for more information: http://www.virginia.edu/housing/. On-campus day care facilities are available. See the following Web site for more information: http://www.virginia.edu/childdevelopmentcenter/.

Employment of Department Graduates:

Master's Degree Graduates: Of those who graduated in the academic year 2008–2009, the following categories and numbers represent the postgraduate activities and employment of master's degree graduates: Enrolled in a psychology doctoral program (13), enrolled in a postdoctoral residency/fellowship (n/a), employed in independent practice (n/a), employed in an academic position at a university (13), employed in government agency (1), employed in a community mental health/counseling center (1), still seeking employment (2), total from the above (master's) (30).

Doctoral Degree Graduates: Of those who graduated in the academic year 2008–2009, the following categories and numbers represent the postgraduate activities and employment of doctoral degree graduates: Enrolled in a psychology doctoral program (n/a), total from the above (doctoral) (0).

Additional Information:

Orientation, Objectives, and Emphasis of Department: The department emphasizes research on a wide spectrum of psychological issues with clinical, developmental, social, cognitive, neuroscience and behavior, quantitative, and community specialties. In addition, new tracks are being developed, such as social ecology and development, law and psychology, family, and minority issues.

Special Facilities or Resources: The department has in excess of 50,000 square feet for offices, laboratories, seminar rooms, and classrooms. Special facilities include rooms for psychophysical investigations, a suite of rooms devoted to developmental, clinical, and social laboratories, and specialized research facilities for the study of animal behavior and psychobiology. Sound-attenuated rooms, electrically shielded rooms, numerous one-way vision rooms, surgery and vivarium rooms, and a darkroom are all available. There is also a library for psychology and biology housed in the same building. There are ample computer facilities. All labs are connected to a local area network and a university-wide local area network. This allows the labs to connect to other available University machines such as IBM RS/6000 Unix machines.

Information for Students With Physical Disabilities: See the following Web site for more information: http://www.virginia.edu/accessibility.

Application Information:

Send to Dean of the Graduate School, The University of Virginia, P.O. Box 400775, 437 Cabell Hall, Charlottesville, VA 22904-4775. Application available online. URL of online application: http://www.virginia.edu/psychology/graduate/. Students are admitted in the Fall, application deadline December 1. *Fee:* $60.

WASHINGTON

Antioch University, Seattle
PsyD in Psychology
School of Applied Psychology, Counseling and Family Therapy
2326 6th Avenue
Seattle, WA 98121-1814
Telephone: (206) 441-5352
Fax: (206) 441-3307
E-mail: asuarez@antioch.edu
Web: http://www.antiochsea.edu/

Department Information:
2004. Dean of the School of Applied Psychology: Carol Stanley PhD. Number of faculty: total—full-time 10; women—full-time 7; total—minority—full-time 2; women minority—full-time 2; faculty subject to the Americans With Disabilities Act 1.

Programs and Degrees Offered:
Listed in the following order: Program area, degree type (T if terminal Master's), number awarded 7/08–6/09. Clinical Psychology PsyD (Doctor of Psychology) 14.

Student Applications/Admissions:

Student Applications
Clinical Psychology PsyD (Doctor of Psychology)—Applications 2009–2010, 56. Total applicants accepted 2009–2010, 21. Number full-time enrolled (new admits only) 2009–2010, 16. Number part-time enrolled (new admits only) 2009–2010, 1. Total enrolled 2009–2010 full-time, 28, part-time, 32. Openings 2010–2011, 20. The median number of years required for completion of a degree in 2008–2009 were 4. The number of students enrolled full- and part-time who were dismissed or voluntarily withdrew from this program area in 2008–2009 were 2.

Scores: Entries appear in this order: required test or GPA, minimum score (if required), median score of students entering in 2009–2010. Clinical Psychology PsyD (Doctor of Psychology): overall undergraduate GPA 3.0, 3.6.

Other Criteria: (importance of criteria rated low, medium, or high): research experience—low, work experience—low, extracurricular activity—medium, clinically related public service—high, GPA—high, letters of recommendation—high, interview—high, statement of goals and objectives—high, undergraduate major in psychology—low, specific undergraduate psychology courses taken—high. For additional information on admission requirements, go to http://www.antiochsea.edu/academics/psychology/psyd-overview.html.

Student Characteristics: The following represents characteristics of students in 2009–2010 in all graduate psychology programs in the department: Female—full-time 37, part-time 0; Male—full-time 23, part-time 0; African American/Black—full-time 3, part-time 0; Hispanic/Latino(a)—full-time 4, part-time 0; Asian/Pacific Islander—full-time 9, part-time 0; American Indian/Alaska Native—full-time 1, part-time 0; Caucasian/White—full-time 24, part-time 0; Multi-ethnic—full-time 19, part-time 0; students subject to the Americans With Disabilities Act—full-time 3, part-time 0; Unknown ethnicity—full-time 0, part-time 0; International students who hold an F-1 or J-1 Visa—full-time 7, part-time 0.

Financial Information/Assistance:
Tuition for Full-Time Study: *Master's:* State residents: $600 per credit hour; Nonstate residents: $600 per credit hour. *Doctoral:* State residents: $690 per credit hour; Nonstate residents: $690 per credit hour. Additional fees are assessed to students beyond the costs of tuition for the following: Quarterly student service fee and technology fee. See the following Web site for updates and changes in tuition costs: http://www.antiochsea.edu/currentstudents/classes.html.

Financial Assistance:
First-Year Students: Fellowships and scholarships available for first year. Average amount paid per academic year: $15,080. Average number of hours worked per week: 15.
Advanced Students: No information provided.
Additional Information: Of all students currently enrolled full time, 10% benefited from one or more of the listed financial assistance programs. Application and information available online at: http://www.antiochsea.edu/currentstudents/classes.html.

Internships/Practica: Doctoral Degree (PsyD Clinical Psychology): For those doctoral students for whom a professional internship was required in this program prior to graduation, (17) students applied for an internship in 2008–2009, with (15) students obtaining an internship. Of those students who obtained an internship, (2) were paid internships. Of those students who obtained an internship, (0) students placed in APA/CPA accredited internships, (6) students placed in internships not APA/CPA accredited, but listed with the Association of Psychology Postdoctoral and Internship Programs (APPIC), (0) students placed in internships conforming to guidelines of the Council of Directors of School Psychology Programs (CDSPP), (9) students placed in internships that were not APA/CPA accredited, APPIC or CDSPP listed. Practical experience is integrated throughout the program, starting with a first year Social Justice Project. The program includes two years of supervised practicum experience by a licensed psychologist in preparation for internship. Internship takes one year if done full time or two years if done part time.

Housing and Day Care: No on-campus housing is available. No on-campus day care facilities are available.

Employment of Department Graduates:
Master's Degree Graduates: Of those who graduated in the academic year 2008–2009, the following categories and numbers represent the postgraduate activities and employment of master's degree graduates: Enrolled in a postdoctoral residency/fellowship (n/a), employed in independent practice (n/a), total from the above (master's) (0).
Doctoral Degree Graduates: Of those who graduated in the academic year 2008–2009, the following categories and numbers represent the postgraduate activities and employment of doctoral degree graduates: Enrolled in a psychology doctoral program (n/a), enrolled in another graduate/professional program (1), enrolled in

a postdoctoral residency/fellowship (1), employed in independent practice (14), employed in an academic position at a university (3), employed in an academic position at a 2-year/4-year college (1), employed in a community mental health/counseling center (2), employed in a hospital/medical center (3), other employment position (2), total from the above (doctoral) (27).

Additional Information:
Orientation, Objectives, and Emphasis of Department: The PsyD program follows a practitioner/scholar model: theory and application of clinical assessment, diagnosis and treatment are emphasized. It offers several concentrations including: adult psychotherapy, art therapy, and child and family systems. In addition, there are two concentrations offered in rotation every other year: Forensic psychology (2010-11) and Health psychology (2009-10). You have the flexibility to pursue your PsyD in clinical psychology full time or part time.

Information for Students With Physical Disabilities: See the following Web site for more information: http://www.antiochseattle.edu/studentservices/disability.html.

Application Information:
Send to Admissions Office, 2326 6th Avenue, Seattle, WA 98121-1814. Application available online. URL of online application: http://antiochsea.edu/futurestudents/admissions/graduate_psyd.html. Students are admitted in the Fall, application deadline January 15. *Fee:* $75.

Argosy University/Seattle
Clinical Psychology
American School of Professional Psychology
2601-A Elliott Avenue
Seattle, WA 98121
Telephone: (206) 283-4500
Fax: (206) 283-5777
E-mail: *fparks@argosy.edu*
Web: *http://www.argosy.edu*

Department Information:
1997. Chairperson: Frances M. Parks, PhD, ABPP. Number of faculty: total—full-time 10, part-time 2; women—full-time 5; total—minority—full-time 2; faculty subject to the Americans With Disabilities Act 1.

Programs and Degrees Offered:
Listed in the following order: Program area, degree type (T if terminal Master's), number awarded 7/08–6/09. Clinical Psychology MA/MS (Master of Arts/Science) 16, Clinical Psychology PsyD (Doctor of Psychology) 16.

Student Applications/Admissions:
Student Applications
Clinical Psychology MA/MS (Master of Arts/Science)—Number full-time enrolled (new admits only) 2009–2010, 12. Number part-time enrolled (new admits only) 2009–2010, 2. Total enrolled 2009–2010 full-time, 20, part-time, 10. Openings 2010–2011, 28. The median number of years required for completion of a degree in 2008–2009 were 2. *Clinical Psychology PsyD (Doctor of Psychology)*—Number full-time enrolled (new admits only) 2009–2010, 6. Number part-time enrolled (new admits only) 2009–2010, 0. Total enrolled 2009–2010 full-time, 77, part-time, 14. Openings 2010–2011, 14. The median number of years required for completion of a degree in 2008–2009 were 6.

Other Criteria: (importance of criteria rated low, medium, or high): research experience—low, work experience—medium, extracurricular activity—medium, clinically related public service—high, GPA—high, letters of recommendation—high, interview—high, statement of goals and objectives—high, undergraduate major in psychology—low, specific undergraduate psychology courses taken—medium. For entry into master's-level programs, work experience is not expected. For additional information on admission requirements, go to http://www.argosy.edu/admissions/.

Student Characteristics: The following represents characteristics of students in 2009–2010 in all graduate psychology programs in the department: Female—full-time 78, part-time 19; Male—full-time 19, part-time 5; African American/Black—full-time 4, part-time 1; Hispanic/Latino(a)—full-time 2, part-time 0; Asian/Pacific Islander—full-time 4, part-time 2; American Indian/Alaska Native—full-time 1, part-time 0; Caucasian/White—full-time 70, part-time 19; Multi-ethnic—full-time 3, part-time 1; students subject to the Americans With Disabilities Act—full-time 4, part-time 0; Unknown ethnicity—full-time 13, part-time 1; International students who hold an F-1 or J-1 Visa—full-time 0, part-time 0.

Financial Information/Assistance:
Financial Assistance:
First-Year Students: Fellowships and scholarships available for first year. Average amount paid per academic year: $3,000.
Advanced Students: Teaching assistantships available for advanced students. Research assistantships available for advanced students. Fellowships and scholarships available for advanced students. Average amount paid per academic year: $3,000.
Additional Information: Of all students currently enrolled full time, 10% benefited from one or more of the listed financial assistance programs.

Internships/Practica: The Argosy, Seattle clinical program's current list of approved practicum sites for master's and doctoral level students includes state and community mental health facilities, state correctional facilities from minimum to maximum security, juvenile detention centers, outpatient clinics, private psychiatric hospitals, psychiatric units and community hospitals, treatment centers for the developmentally disabled and behavior disordered, and chemical dependence treatment programs. We also have practicum placements in multicultural or diverse practicum settings, including mental health agencies serving Native Americans, Asian-Americans, and African-Americans. An onsite clinic, the Psychology Center, offers training in assessment and psychotherapy; it serves a diverse population with an emphasis on providing services for the underserved.

Housing and Day Care: No on-campus housing is available. No on-campus day care facilities are available.

GRADUATE STUDY IN PSYCHOLOGY

Employment of Department Graduates:
Master's Degree Graduates: Of those who graduated in the academic year 2008–2009, the following categories and numbers represent the postgraduate activities and employment of master's degree graduates: Enrolled in a postdoctoral residency/fellowship (n/a), employed in independent practice (n/a), total from the above (master's) (0).
Doctoral Degree Graduates: Of those who graduated in the academic year 2008–2009, the following categories and numbers represent the postgraduate activities and employment of doctoral degree graduates: Enrolled in a psychology doctoral program (n/a), total from the above (doctoral) (0).

Additional Information:
Orientation, Objectives, and Emphasis of Department: The primary purpose of the program is to educate and train students in the major aspects of clinical psychology. To ensure that students are prepared adequately, the curriculum integrates theory, training, research and practice, preparing students to work with a wide range of populations in need of psychological services and in a broad range of roles.

Special Facilities or Resources: The Clinical and Counseling Psychology Departments have developed an onsite clinic, the Psychology Center. Clinical students may receive training in psychological assessment and in psychotherapy through this site. It also provides opportunities for research.

Application Information:
Send to Admissions Office, Argosy University/Seattle, 2601-A Elliott Avenue, Seattle, WA 98121. Application available online. URL of online application: http://www.argosy.edu/admissions/. Students are admitted in the Fall, application deadline April 15; Spring, application deadline November 1; Summer, application deadline March 1. The above deadline dates are recommended dates. *Fee:* $50.

Central Washington University
Department of Psychology
College of the Sciences
400 East University Way
Ellensburg, WA 98926-7575
Telephone: (509) 963-2381
Fax: (509) 963-2307
E-mail: *steins@cwu.edu*
Web: *http://www.cwu.edu/~psych/*

Department Information:
1965. Chairperson: Stephanie Stein. Number of faculty: total—full-time 20, part-time 31; women—full-time 10, part-time 19; minority—part-time 1; women minority—part-time 1.

Programs and Degrees Offered:
Listed in the following order: Program area, degree type (T if terminal Master's), number awarded 7/08–6/09. Mental Health Counseling MA/MS (Master of Arts/Science) (T) 6, School Counseling MEd (Education) 2, Experimental Psychology MA/MS (Master of Arts/Science) (T) 5, School Psychology MEd (Education) 10, Experimental Psychology (ABA Specialization) MA/MS (Master of Arts/Science) (T) 0.

Student Applications/Admissions:
Student Applications
Mental Health Counseling MA/MS (Master of Arts/Science)—Applications 2009–2010, 38. Total applicants accepted 2009–2010, 15. Number full-time enrolled (new admits only) 2009–2010, 15. Number part-time enrolled (new admits only) 2009–2010, 0. Total enrolled 2009–2010 full-time, 27, part-time, 3. Openings 2010–2011, 10. The median number of years required for completion of a degree in 2008–2009 were 2. The number of students enrolled full- and part-time who were dismissed or voluntarily withdrew from this program area in 2008–2009 were 0. *School Counseling MEd (Education)*—Applications 2009–2010, 17. Total applicants accepted 2009–2010, 9. Number full-time enrolled (new admits only) 2009–2010, 5. Number part-time enrolled (new admits only) 2009–2010, 0. Total enrolled 2009–2010 full-time, 14, part-time, 1. Openings 2010–2011, 5. The median number of years required for completion of a degree in 2008–2009 were 2. The number of students enrolled full- and part-time who were dismissed or voluntarily withdrew from this program area in 2008–2009 were 0. *Experimental Psychology MA/MS (Master of Arts/Science)*—Applications 2009–2010, 17. Total applicants accepted 2009–2010, 14. Number full-time enrolled (new admits only) 2009–2010, 5. Number part-time enrolled (new admits only) 2009–2010, 0. Total enrolled 2009–2010 full-time, 23, part-time, 2. Openings 2010–2011, 12. The median number of years required for completion of a degree in 2008–2009 were 2. The number of students enrolled full- and part-time who were dismissed or voluntarily withdrew from this program area in 2008–2009 were 1. *School Psychology MEd (Education)*—Applications 2009–2010, 14. Total applicants accepted 2009–2010, 13. Number full-time enrolled (new admits only) 2009–2010, 6. Number part-time enrolled (new admits only) 2009–2010, 0. Total enrolled 2009–2010 full-time, 15, part-time, 3. Openings 2010–2011, 11. The median number of years required for completion of a degree in 2008–2009 were 3. The number of students enrolled full- and part-time who were dismissed or voluntarily withdrew from this program area in 2008–2009 were 0. *Experimental Psychology (ABA Specialization) MA/MS (Master of Arts/Science)*—Applications 2009–2010, 4. Total applicants accepted 2009–2010, 4. Number full-time enrolled (new admits only) 2009–2010, 4. Number part-time enrolled (new admits only) 2009–2010, 0. Openings 2010–2011, 5. The number of students enrolled full- and part-time who were dismissed or voluntarily withdrew from this program area in 2008–2009 were 0.

Other Criteria: (importance of criteria rated low, medium, or high): GRE scores—medium, research experience—medium, work experience—medium, extracurricular activity—low, clinically related public service—medium, GPA—high, letters of recommendation—high, statement of goals and objectives—high, undergraduate major in psychology—medium, specific undergraduate psychology courses taken—medium. For additional information on admission requirements, go to http://www.cwu.edu/~masters/new_index.html.

Student Characteristics: The following represents characteristics of students in 2009–2010 in all graduate psychology programs in the department: Female—full-time 51, part-time 6; Male—full-time 33, part-time 3; African American/Black—full-time 0, part-time 0; Hispanic/Latino(a)—full-time 6, part-time 0; Asian/Pacific Islander—full-time 3, part-time 0; American Indian/Alaska Native—full-time 1, part-time 0; Caucasian/White—full-time 63, part-time 9; Multi-ethnic—full-time 11, part-time 0; students subject to the Americans With Disabilities Act—full-time 0, part-time 0; Unknown ethnicity—full-time 0, part-time 0; International students who hold an F-1 or J-1 Visa—full-time 0, part-time 0.

Financial Information/Assistance:
Tuition for Full-Time Study: *Master's:* State residents: per academic year $6,618, $245 per credit hour; Nonstate residents: per academic year $14,742, $546 per credit hour. Tuition is subject to change. See the following Web site for updates and changes in tuition costs: http://www.cwu.edu/~regi/tuition.html.

Financial Assistance:
First-Year Students: Teaching assistantships available for first year. Average amount paid per academic year: $16,565. Average number of hours worked per week: 20. Apply by February 1. Research assistantships available for first year. Average amount paid per academic year: $16,565. Average number of hours worked per week: 20. Apply by February 1.
Advanced Students: Teaching assistantships available for advanced students. Average amount paid per academic year: $16,565. Average number of hours worked per week: 20. Apply by February 1. Research assistantships available for advanced students. Average amount paid per academic year: $16,565. Average number of hours worked per week: 20. Apply by February 1.
Additional Information: Of all students currently enrolled full time, 15% benefited from one or more of the listed financial assistance programs. Application and information available online at: http://www.cwu.edu/~masters/student_funding.html.

Internships/Practica: Master's Degree (MA/MS Mental Health Counseling): An internship experience, such as a final research project or "capstone" experience is required of graduates. Master's Degree (MA/MS Experimental Psychology): An internship experience, such as a final research project or "capstone" experience is required of graduates. The Mental Health Counseling Psychology program requires four quarters of practica and a 900 hour internship. School Counseling program requires four quarters of practica and a 400 hour internship. School Psychology program requires two quarters of practica and a one-year internship. Recent school psychology internships have been paid positions. Practica in applied experimental psychology are offered. Students enrolled in the Experimental Psychology-Applied Behavior Analysis specialization are required to complete 1500 hours of supervised practicum (as required by the Behavior Analysis Certification Board) in partial fulfillment of the requirements to sit for the Board Certified Behavior Analyst certification exam.

Housing and Day Care: On-campus housing is available. See the following Web site for more information: http://www.cwu.edu/~housing/. On-campus day care facilities are available. See the following Web site for more information: http://www.cwu.edu/~ecenter/eclc/.

Employment of Department Graduates:
Master's Degree Graduates: Of those who graduated in the academic year 2008–2009, the following categories and numbers represent the postgraduate activities and employment of master's degree graduates: Enrolled in a postdoctoral residency/fellowship (n/a), employed in independent practice (n/a), employed in an academic position at a university (1), employed in other positions at a higher education institution (0), employed in a professional position in a school system (13), employed in business or industry (0), employed in government agency (4), employed in a community mental health/counseling center (2), do not know (1), total from the above (master's) (21).
Doctoral Degree Graduates: Of those who graduated in the academic year 2008–2009, the following categories and numbers represent the postgraduate activities and employment of doctoral degree graduates: Enrolled in a psychology doctoral program (n/a), total from the above (doctoral) (0).

Additional Information:
Orientation, Objectives, and Emphasis of Department: Central Washington University's graduate program in psychology prepares students for professional employment in a variety of settings, including mental health agencies, public schools, community colleges, and business or industry. We also prepare students for successful completion of doctoral degree programs in psychology. The programs include extensive supervision in practicum and internship settings and research partnerships with faculty mentors. Our School Psychology program is NASP approved. Our Mental Health Counseling program is CACREP accredited. The educational requirements of the Animal Behavior Society's Associate Applied Animal Behaviorist Certificate can be met by completing the MS Experimental degree program with an appropriate selection of core and elective courses. Additionally, a specialization in Applied Behavior Analysis is offered through the MS Experimental degree program. Completion of this track will allow individuals to sit for the Board Certified Behavior Analyst certification exam.

Special Facilities or Resources: Our facilities include an on-site community counseling and psychological assessment center for training in counseling and testing; animal research laboratories, including a laboratory for the study of language learning in chimpanzees; a human behavior laboratory; a computer lab; and a complete mechanical and electrical instrumentation services center.

Information for Students With Physical Disabilities: See the following Web site for more information: http://www.cwu.edu/~dss/cms/.

Application Information:
Send to Office of Graduate Studies, Central Washington University, 400 E. University Way, Ellensburg, WA 98926-7510. Application available online. URL of online application: http://www.cwu.edu/~masters/new_apply.html. Students are admitted in the Fall, application deadline April 1. *Fee:* $50. Application fee may be waived by demonstration of financial need.

Eastern Washington University
Department of Psychology
College of Social and Behavioral Sciences
151 Martin Hall
Cheney, WA 99004-6325
Telephone: (509) 359-2478
Fax: (509) 359-6325
E-mail: *psychology@ewu.edu*
Web: *http://www.ewu.edu/psychology/*

Department Information:
1934. Chairperson: Theresa Martin, PhD Number of faculty: total—full-time 14, part-time 1; women—full-time 6; total—minority—full-time 1; women minority—full-time 1; faculty subject to the Americans With Disabilities Act 1.

Programs and Degrees Offered:
Listed in the following order: Program area, degree type (T if terminal Master's), number awarded 7/08–6/09. School Psychology MA/MS (Master of Arts/Science) (T) 8, Psychology MA/MS (Master of Arts/Science) (T) 20, School Psychology Respecialization Diploma 9.

Student Applications/Admissions:
Student Applications
School Psychology MA/MS (Master of Arts/Science)—Applications 2009–2010, 17. Total applicants accepted 2009–2010, 12. Number full-time enrolled (new admits only) 2009–2010, 12. Total enrolled 2009–2010 full-time, 31. Openings 2010–2011, 12. The median number of years required for completion of a degree in 2008–2009 were 3. The number of students enrolled full- and part-time who were dismissed or voluntarily withdrew from this program area in 2008–2009 were 0. Psychology MA/MS (Master of Arts/Science)—Applications 2009–2010, 60. Total applicants accepted 2009–2010, 11. Number full-time enrolled (new admits only) 2009–2010, 11. Number part-time enrolled (new admits only) 2009–2010, 0. Total enrolled 2009–2010 full-time, 21, part-time, 2. Openings 2010–2011, 12. The median number of years required for completion of a degree in 2008–2009 were 2. The number of students enrolled full- and part-time who were dismissed or voluntarily withdrew from this program area in 2008–2009 were 0. School Psychology Respecialization Diploma—The median number of years required for completion of a degree in 2008–2009 were 2.
Scores: Entries appear in this order: required test or GPA, minimum score (if required), median score of students entering in 2009–2010. School Psychology MA/MS (Master of Arts/Science): GRE-V no minimum stated, GRE-Q no minimum stated, GRE-Analytical no minimum stated, last 2 years GPA 3.00; Psychology MA/MS (Master of Arts/Science): GRE-V no minimum stated, GRE-Q no minimum stated, GRE-Analytical no minimum stated, last 2 years GPA 3.00.
Other Criteria: (importance of criteria rated low, medium, or high): GRE scores—medium, research experience—medium, work experience—medium, extracurricular activity—medium, clinically related public service—medium, GPA—medium, letters of recommendation—medium, interview—medium, statement of goals and objectives—medium, undergraduate major in psychology—medium, specific undergraduate psychology courses taken—medium. For additional information on admission requirements, go to http://www.ewu.edu/x5980.xml.

Student Characteristics: The following represents characteristics of students in 2009–2010 in all graduate psychology programs in the department: African American/Black—full-time 0, part-time 0; Hispanic/Latino(a)—full-time 0, part-time 0; Asian/Pacific Islander—full-time 0, part-time 0; American Indian/Alaska Native—full-time 0, part-time 0; Caucasian/White—full-time 0, part-time 0; Multi-ethnic—full-time 0, part-time 0; students subject to the Americans With Disabilities Act—full-time 0, part-time 0; Unknown ethnicity—full-time 0, part-time 0; International students who hold an F-1 or J-1 Visa—full-time 0, part-time 0.

Financial Information/Assistance:
Tuition for Full-Time Study: *Master's:* State residents: per academic year $7,476; Nonstate residents: per academic year $18,030. Tuition is subject to change. Tuition costs vary by program. See the following Web site for updates and changes in tuition costs: http://www.ewu.edu/x7032.xml.

Financial Assistance:
First-Year Students: Teaching assistantships available for first year. Average number of hours worked per week: 20. Apply by March 1. Fellowships and scholarships available for first year. Apply by March 1.
Advanced Students: No information provided.
Additional Information: Of all students currently enrolled full time, 50% benefited from one or more of the listed financial assistance programs. Application and information available online at: http://www.ewu.edu/x27032.xml.

Internships/Practica: Master's Degree (MA/MS School Psychology): An internship experience, such as a final research project or "capstone" experience is required of graduates. Master's Degree (MA/MS Psychology): An internship experience, such as a final research project or "capstone" experience is required of graduates.

Housing and Day Care: On-campus housing is available. See the following Web site for more information: http://www.ewu.edu/x4739.xml. On-campus day care facilities are available. See the following Web site for more information: http://www.ewu.edu/x4346.xml.

Employment of Department Graduates:
Master's Degree Graduates: Of those who graduated in the academic year 2008–2009, the following categories and numbers represent the postgraduate activities and employment of master's degree graduates: Enrolled in a postdoctoral residency/fellowship (n/a), employed in independent practice (n/a), total from the above (master's) (0).
Doctoral Degree Graduates: Of those who graduated in the academic year 2008–2009, the following categories and numbers represent the postgraduate activities and employment of doctoral degree graduates: Enrolled in a psychology doctoral program (n/a), total from the above (doctoral) (0).

Additional Information:
Orientation, Objectives, and Emphasis of Department: Master's level graduate study in psychology provides the student with ad-

vanced preparation for practice in the field or for entering doctoral-level programs in psychology. Two programs are offered by the department: an MS in psychology with a concentration in either clinical or general/experimental psychology and an MS in school psychology.

Information for Students With Physical Disabilities: See the following Web site for more information: http://www.ewu.edu/x2336.xml.

Application Information:
Send to Eastern Washington University, Department of Psychology, Cheney, WA 99004, 509-359-2478. Application available online. URL of online application: http://www.ewu.edu/x5980.xml. Students are admitted in the Fall, application deadline March 1. *Fee:* $50.

Gonzaga University
Department of Counselor Education
School of Education
East 501 Boone Avenue
Spokane, WA 99258-0025
Telephone: (509) 313-3512
Fax: (509) 313-5964
E-mail: *bennette@gonzaga.edu*
Web: *http://www.gonzaga.edu/Academics/
    Colleges+and+Schools/School+of+Education/
    Counselor+Education/default.asp*

Department Information:
1960. Chairperson: Elisabeth Bennett. Number of faculty: total—full-time 4, part-time 9; women—full-time 1, part-time 6; minority—part-time 2; women minority—part-time 1.

Programs and Degrees Offered:
Listed in the following order: Program area, degree type (T if terminal Master's), number awarded 7/08–6/09. School Counseling MA/MS (Master of Arts/Science) (T) 9, Community Counseling MA/MS (Master of Arts/Science) (T) 15, Marriage and Family Counseling MA/MS (Master of Arts/Science) (T) 0.

Student Applications/Admissions:
Student Applications
School Counseling MA/MS (Master of Arts/Science)—Applications 2009–2010, 48. Total applicants accepted 2009–2010, 12. Number full-time enrolled (new admits only) 2009–2010, 11. Number part-time enrolled (new admits only) 2009–2010, 1. Total enrolled 2009–2010 full-time, 20, part-time, 2. Openings 2010–2011, 10. The median number of years required for completion of a degree in 2008–2009 were 2. The number of students enrolled full- and part-time who were dismissed or voluntarily withdrew from this program area in 2008–2009 were 1. Community Counseling MA/MS (Master of Arts/Science)—Applications 2009–2010, 80. Total applicants accepted 2009–2010, 26. Number full-time enrolled (new admits only) 2009–2010, 25. Number part-time enrolled (new admits only) 2009–2010, 2. Total enrolled 2009–2010 full-time, 41, part-time, 4. Openings 2010–2011, 20. The median number of years required for completion of a degree in 2008–2009 were 2. The number of students enrolled full- and part-time who were dismissed or voluntarily withdrew from this program area in 2008–2009 were 2. Marriage and Family Counseling MA/MS (Master of Arts/Science)—Applications 2009–2010, 0. Total applicants accepted 2009–2010, 0. Number full-time enrolled (new admits only) 2009–2010, 0. Openings 2010–2011, 10. The median number of years required for completion of a degree in 2008–2009 were 2. The number of students enrolled full- and part-time who were dismissed or voluntarily withdrew from this program area in 2008–2009 were 0.

Scores: Entries appear in this order: required test or GPA, minimum score (if required), median score of students entering in 2009–2010. School Counseling MA/MS (Master of Arts/Science): overall undergraduate GPA 3.0; Community Counseling MA/MS (Master of Arts/Science): overall undergraduate GPA 3.0; Marriage and Family Counseling MA/MS (Master of Arts/Science): overall undergraduate GPA 3.0.

Other Criteria: (importance of criteria rated low, medium, or high): GRE scores—low, work experience—medium, extracurricular activity—medium, clinically related public service—medium, GPA—medium, letters of recommendation—high, interview—high, statement of goals and objectives—high, emotional intelligence—high, undergraduate major in psychology—low, specific undergraduate psychology courses taken—low.

Student Characteristics: The following represents characteristics of students in 2009–2010 in all graduate psychology programs in the department: Female—full-time 81, part-time 1; Male—full-time 21, part-time 12; African American/Black—full-time 1, part-time 0; Hispanic/Latino(a)—full-time 1, part-time 0; Asian/Pacific Islander—full-time 2, part-time 1; American Indian/Alaska Native—full-time 3, part-time 0; Caucasian/White—full-time 82, part-time 11; Multi-ethnic—full-time 1, part-time 0; students subject to the Americans With Disabilities Act—full-time 1, part-time 0; Unknown ethnicity—full-time 12, part-time 0; International students who hold an F-1 or J-1 Visa—full-time 1, part-time 1.

Financial Information/Assistance:
Tuition for Full-Time Study: *Master's:* State residents: $745 per credit hour; Nonstate residents: $745 per credit hour. Tuition is subject to change. Additional fees are assessed to students beyond the costs of tuition for the following: Regular university fees, specialty fees for particular courses such as assessment and clinicals. Tuition costs vary by program. See the following Web site for updates and changes in tuition costs: http://www.gonzaga.edu/.

Financial Assistance:
First-Year Students: Teaching assistantships available for first year. Average amount paid per academic year: $2,700. Average number of hours worked per week: 6. Apply by April 15. Research assistantships available for first year. Average amount paid per academic year: $2,700. Average number of hours worked per week: 6. Apply by April 15.

Advanced Students: Teaching assistantships available for advanced students. Average amount paid per academic year: $2,800. Average number of hours worked per week: 6. Apply by April 15. Research assistantships available for advanced students. Average amount paid per academic year: $2,800. Average number of hours worked per week: 6. Apply by April 15.

Additional Information: Of all students currently enrolled full time, 35% benefited from one or more of the listed financial assistance programs.

Internships/Practica: Master's Degree (MA/MS School Counseling): An internship experience, such as a final research project or "capstone" experience is required of graduates. Master's Degree (MA/MS Community Counseling): An internship experience, such as a final research project or "capstone" experience is required of graduates. Master's Degree (MA/MS Marriage and Family Counseling): An internship experience, such as a final research project or "capstone" experience is required of graduates. Students complete a 100-hour practicum and a 600-hour internship at a site chosen by the student to meet his or her professional interests. School track students currently are placed in schools at elementary, junior high, high school, and alternative settings. Agency track students are placed at sites including but not limited to geriatric, hospital, community mental health, adolescent, marriage and family, child, community college, career, and life-skills settings. A strong reputation within our community has enabled students to select quality placements in diverse settings of the student's choosing.

Housing and Day Care: On-campus housing is available. See the following Web site for more information: http://www.gonzaga.edu/Academics/Colleges-and-Schools/School-of-Education/Graduate-Admissions/Graduate-Housing.asp. No on-campus day care facilities are available.

Employment of Department Graduates:
Master's Degree Graduates: Of those who graduated in the academic year 2008–2009, the following categories and numbers represent the postgraduate activities and employment of master's degree graduates: Enrolled in a psychology doctoral program (4), enrolled in another graduate/professional program (1), enrolled in a postdoctoral residency/fellowship (n/a), employed in independent practice (n/a), employed in an academic position at a 2-year/4-year college (1), employed in other positions at a higher education institution (3), employed in a professional position in a school system (10), employed in business or industry (1), employed in government agency (1), employed in a community mental health/counseling center (7), employed in a hospital/medical center (1), still seeking employment (1), other employment position (2), total from the above (master's) (32).
Doctoral Degree Graduates: Of those who graduated in the academic year 2008–2009, the following categories and numbers represent the postgraduate activities and employment of doctoral degree graduates: Enrolled in a psychology doctoral program (n/a), total from the above (doctoral) (0).

Additional Information:
Orientation, Objectives, and Emphasis of Department: The philosophical theme running throughout the university is humanism. A realistic, balanced attitude is a necessary prerequisite for assisting others professionally. Careful selection of students helps to insure the inclusion of healthy individuals with the highest potential for success, as does faculty modeling, encouragement of trust, and communication of clear expectations. Indicators of counselor success are demonstration of skills and conflict resolution, consistent interpersonal behaviors, recognition of strengths and weaknesses, a clear grasp of goals, and self-knowledge of one's impact on others, as well as a strong academic performance. Acquisition of counseling competence comes through both personal and professional growth. Immersion in an intensive course of study with a closely linked group of peers encourages open and honest processing, which in turn contributes to personal growth. The department believes that students must possess insight and awareness, and clarity about the boundaries between their personal issues and those of the client. Students training to become professionals must be treated as professionals. Faculty practice collegiality with students, maintain high standards of performance, and furnish an atmosphere of professionalism. Students share cases, exchanging professional advice and input. In addition to the presentation of major theories of counseling, students must develop a personal theory of counseling and demonstrate competence in its use. Faculty are humanistic, but eclectic, disseminating information about effective techniques without imposing any one approach on the students. Students are closely observed in the classroom, practicum and internship and receive critical monitoring and evaluation from faculty, field supervisor, and peers. School and Community Programs are CACREP accredited. The Community Counseling Program now hosts a Marriage and Family Program. Our theme statement is "We are practitioners who are intentional in the development of relationships that honor the strengths of all individuals and the promotion of transformational growth."

Special Facilities or Resources: The Department of Counselor Education is proud to offer a modern and complete clinic training center, with four practicum rooms, a departmental library, and conference room. The clinic has two-way glass, and is equipped with audio-video technological equipment which can be operated in the clinic room by either the student (for taping and reviewing personal work) or by any department faculty member from faculty offices (for viewing and/or taping).

Application Information:
Send to Graduate Admissions, School of Education, Gonzaga University, 502 East Boone, Spokane, WA 99258-0025. Application available online. URL of online application: http://www.gonzaga.edu/Academics/Colleges-and-Schools/School-of-Education/Graduate-Admissions/GraduateAdmissionsForms/Requirements.asp. Students are admitted in the Fall, application deadline January 15. We have two applications deadlines. The first in January is for early admittance. The second, March 15, is regular admittance. *Fee:* $50.

Puget Sound, University of
School of Education
1500 North Warner #1051
Tacoma, WA 98416
Telephone: (253) 879-3344
Fax: (253) 879-3926
E-mail: *kirchner@pugetsound.edu*
Web: *http://www.pugetsound.edu*

Department Information:
Director: Grace L. Kirchner. Number of faculty: total—full-time 2, part-time 4; women—full-time 2, part-time 1.

Programs and Degrees Offered:
Listed in the following order: Program area, degree type (T if terminal Master's), number awarded 7/08–6/09. Agency Counseling MEd (Education) 2, School Counseling MEd (Education) 7.

Student Applications/Admissions:
Student Applications
Agency Counseling MEd (Education)—Applications 2009–2010, 3. Total applicants accepted 2009–2010, 3. Number full-time enrolled (new admits only) 2009–2010, 0. Number part-time enrolled (new admits only) 2009–2010, 3. Openings 2010–2011, 5. The median number of years required for completion of a degree in 2008–2009 were 2. The number of students enrolled full- and part-time who were dismissed or voluntarily withdrew from this program area in 2008–2009 were 0. School Counseling MEd (Education)—Applications 2009–2010, 21. Total applicants accepted 2009–2010, 20. Number full-time enrolled (new admits only) 2009–2010, 0. Number part-time enrolled (new admits only) 2009–2010, 9. Openings 2010–2011, 12. The median number of years required for completion of a degree in 2008–2009 were 3. The number of students enrolled full- and part-time who were dismissed or voluntarily withdrew from this program area in 2008–2009 were 1.

Other Criteria: (importance of criteria rated low, medium, or high): GRE scores—medium, work experience—medium, extracurricular activity—low, clinically related public service—medium, GPA—medium, letters of recommendation—medium, interview—medium, statement of goals and objectives—medium.

Student Characteristics: The following represents characteristics of students in 2009–2010 in all graduate psychology programs in the department: Female—full-time 0, part-time 21; Male—full-time 0, part-time 6; African American/Black—full-time 0, part-time 1; Hispanic/Latino(a)—full-time 0, part-time 2; Asian/Pacific Islander—full-time 0, part-time 0; American Indian/Alaska Native—full-time 0, part-time 1; Caucasian/White—full-time 0, part-time 11; Multi-ethnic—full-time 0, part-time 0; students subject to the Americans With Disabilities Act—full-time 0, part-time 0; Unknown ethnicity—full-time 0, part-time 12; International students who hold an F-1 or J-1 Visa—full-time 0, part-time 0.

Financial Information/Assistance:
Tuition for Full-Time Study: *Master's:* State residents: $727 per credit hour; Nonstate residents: $727 per credit hour. Tuition is subject to change. See the following Web site for updates and changes in tuition costs: http://www.pugetsound.edu/admission/financing-your-education/graduate-students/.

Financial Assistance:
First-Year Students: No information provided.
Advanced Students: No information provided.
Additional Information: Of all students currently enrolled full time, 90% benefited from one or more of the listed financial assistance programs. Application and information available online at: http://www.pugetsound.edu/admission/apply/graduate-students/.

Internships/Practica: We require a 400-hour internship in a school or agency setting. These 400 hours are in addition to an on-campus practicum that meets once per week for the academic year.

Housing and Day Care: On-campus housing is available. Students must carry 2 units per semester to qualify for on campus housing. No on-campus day care facilities are available.

Employment of Department Graduates:
Master's Degree Graduates: Of those who graduated in the academic year 2008–2009, the following categories and numbers represent the postgraduate activities and employment of master's degree graduates: Enrolled in a psychology doctoral program (0), enrolled in a postdoctoral residency/fellowship (n/a), employed in independent practice (n/a), employed in an academic position at a university (0), employed in an academic position at a 2-year/4-year college (0), employed in other positions at a higher education institution (0), employed in a professional position in a school system (4), employed in business or industry (0), employed in government agency (0), employed in a community mental health/counseling center (0), employed in a hospital/medical center (0), not seeking employment (2), other employment position (0), do not know (4), total from the above (master's) (10).
Doctoral Degree Graduates: Of those who graduated in the academic year 2008–2009, the following categories and numbers represent the postgraduate activities and employment of doctoral degree graduates: Enrolled in a psychology doctoral program (n/a), total from the above (doctoral) (0).

Additional Information:
Orientation, Objectives, and Emphasis of Department: We are housed in the School of Education and our primary mission is to train school counselors; however, many of our graduates find employment in social service settings.

Information for Students With Physical Disabilities: See the following Web site for more information: http://www.pugetsound.edu/academics/academic-resources/disabilities-service.

Application Information:
Send to Office of Admission. Application available online. URL of online application: http://www.pugetsound.edu/admission/apply/. Students are admitted in the Fall, application deadline March 1. *Fee:* $65. $25 if previously admitted to University.

Seattle Pacific University
Clinical Psychology Department
School of Psychology, Family and Community
3307 Third Avenue, West
Seattle, WA 98119
Telephone: (206) 281-2839
Fax: (206) 281-2695
E-mail: *clinicalpsyc@spu.edu*
Web: http://www.spu.edu/depts/spfc/clinicalpsych

Department Information:
1995. Chairperson: Jay R. Skidmore, PhD. Number of faculty: total—full-time 7, part-time 7; women—full-time 4, part-time 4; total—minority—full-time 1.

Programs and Degrees Offered:
Listed in the following order: Program area, degree type (T if terminal Master's), number awarded 7/08–6/09. Clinical Psychology PhD (Doctor of Philosophy) 16.

APA Accreditation: Clinical PhD (Doctor of Philosophy).

Student Applications/Admissions:

Student Applications

Clinical Psychology PhD (Doctor of Philosophy)—Applications 2009–2010, 126. Total applicants accepted 2009–2010, 16. Number full-time enrolled (new admits only) 2009–2010, 15. Number part-time enrolled (new admits only) 2009–2010, 0. Total enrolled 2009–2010 full-time, 63, part-time, 11. Openings 2010–2011, 16. The median number of years required for completion of a degree in 2008–2009 were 6. The number of students enrolled full- and part-time who were dismissed or voluntarily withdrew from this program area in 2008–2009 were 2.

Other Criteria: (importance of criteria rated low, medium, or high): GRE scores—high, research experience—medium, work experience—low, extracurricular activity—low, clinically related public service—medium, GPA—high, letters of recommendation—medium, interview—high, statement of goals and objectives—high, match with program—high, undergraduate major in psychology—medium, specific undergraduate psychology courses taken—medium. For additional information on admission requirements, go to http://www.spu.edu/depts/spfc/clinicalpsych/.

Student Characteristics: The following represents characteristics of students in 2009–2010 in all graduate psychology programs in the department: Female—full-time 51, part-time 9; Male—full-time 12, part-time 2; African American/Black—full-time 1, part-time 0; Hispanic/Latino(a)—full-time 3, part-time 0; Asian/Pacific Islander—full-time 4, part-time 1; American Indian/Alaska Native—full-time 1, part-time 0; Caucasian/White—full-time 60, part-time 10; Multi-ethnic—full-time 4, part-time 0; students subject to the Americans With Disabilities Act—full-time 0, part-time 0; Unknown ethnicity—full-time 0, part-time 0; International students who hold an F-1 or J-1 Visa—full-time 0, part-time 0.

Financial Information/Assistance:

Tuition for Full-Time Study: *Doctoral:* State residents: $634 per credit hour; Nonstate residents: $634 per credit hour. Tuition is subject to change.

Financial Assistance:

First-Year Students: No information provided.

Advanced Students: Teaching assistantships available for advanced students. Average amount paid per academic year: $8,000. Average number of hours worked per week: 15. Research assistantships available for advanced students. Average amount paid per academic year: $4,000. Average number of hours worked per week: 8. Fellowships and scholarships available for advanced students. Average amount paid per academic year: $8,000.

Additional Information: Of all students currently enrolled full time, 30% benefited from one or more of the listed financial assistance programs.

Internships/Practica: Doctoral Degree (PhD Clinical Psychology): For those doctoral students for whom a professional internship was required in this program prior to graduation, (16) students applied for an internship in 2008–2009, with (12) students obtaining an internship. Of those students who obtained an internship, (12) were paid internships. Of those students who obtained an internship, (11) students placed in APA/CPA accredited internships, (1) students placed in internships not APA/CPA accredited, but listed with the Association of Psychology Postdoctoral and Internship Programs (APPIC), (0) students placed in internships conforming to guidelines of the Council of Directors of School Psychology Programs (CDSPP), (0) students placed in internships that were not APA/CPA accredited, APPIC or CDSPP listed. Clinical training requirements include two one-year practicum placements during the 3rd and 4th years of the program (part-time, averaging 16 hours/week, resulting in average total practicum experience of approximately 1200 hours), as well as a full-time one-year (2000 hours) clinical psychology internship during the 5th year of the PhD program. Practicum placements are external to the university in a variety of mental health centers, hospitals, medical/dental clinics, and rehabilitation facilities in the greater Puget Sound area. Students apply for their internship in the APPIC Match and each year most obtain placements at competitive mental health and medical centers around the country. Theoretical models and orientations among the faculty include cognitive behavioral, psychodynamic, interpersonal, family systems, and humanistic approaches. Faculty tend to integrate more than one perspective in theories, teaching and professional practices. We incorporate and contribute to evidence-based research, and expect our students to utilize clinical science as well as theory in their clinical work.

Housing and Day Care: No on-campus housing is available. On-campus day care facilities are available at First Free Methodist Church, across the street from SPU campus.

Employment of Department Graduates:

Master's Degree Graduates: Of those who graduated in the academic year 2008–2009, the following categories and numbers represent the postgraduate activities and employment of master's degree graduates: Enrolled in a postdoctoral residency/fellowship (n/a), employed in independent practice (n/a), total from the above (master's) (0).

Doctoral Degree Graduates: Of those who graduated in the academic year 2008–2009, the following categories and numbers represent the postgraduate activities and employment of doctoral degree graduates: Enrolled in a psychology doctoral program (n/a), enrolled in a postdoctoral residency/fellowship (3), employed in independent practice (4), employed in an academic position at a university (2), employed in an academic position at a 2-year/4-year college (1), employed in other positions at a higher education institution (1), employed in a community mental health/counseling center (2), employed in a hospital/medical center (1), do not know (2), total from the above (doctoral) (16).

Additional Information:

Orientation, Objectives, and Emphasis of Department: The Clinical Psychology PhD program at SPU is designed to provide training in professional psychology in accordance with the Local Clinical Scientist (LCS) model of doctoral education, described in the article, "The local clinical scientist: a bridge between science and practice" published in American Psychologist (Stricker & Trierweiler, 1995). The Local Clinical Scientist extends the scientific and professional ideals in the original Boulder Scientist-Practitioner (BSP) model of clinical psychology. At the same time, we try to encompass broader concepts of science and more explicitly integrate the art of clinical practice. We also endorse the core competencies outlined by the National Council of Schools and Programs of Professional Psychology (NCSPP), and are committed to helping students achieve mastery of the core competencies of clinical skills. Our doctoral program typically requires four years of graduate coursework, during which clinical practicum training as well as dissertation research are also completed, followed by a one-year full-time internship (elsewhere) in the fifth year. We are an APA-accredited program in clinical psychology, and also a "designated doctoral program" with ASPPB/NR, which verifies that our curriculum meets the educational requirements for licensing psychologists in the United States.

Personal Behavior Statement: Refer to the student application.

Special Facilities or Resources: The School maintains a fully-equipped suite of psychology research laboratories, including a psycho-physiological lab, child developmental lab, and social psychology lab. The University's newly-opened Science Building has wet labs, animal learning facilities, and a psycho-physiological demonstration classroom. The Department is housed in Marston Hall, which was completely renovated for us in 2001. The University Library is a 4-story structure with conference rooms, private study rooms and group meeting rooms. The library contains approximately 10,000 volumes relevant to the field of psychology, including books, media, a test file, and over 500 journals available in paper, microfilm, and full-text online. In addition to traditional inter-library loan services, Seattle Pacific University is a member of the Orbis Cascade Alliance, a consortium of 26 public and private academic libraries in Washington and Oregon which provides access to a combined collection of over 22 million volumes of books and other materials. Students have access to several computer labs on campus, which have SPSS installed. Student are given an SPU e-mail account and have 24/7 access to our online Blackboard where program forms, syllabi, schedules, etc. are posted for students to download.

Information for Students With Physical Disabilities: See the following Web site for more information: http://www.spu.edu/depts/cfl/dss/.

Application Information:
Send to Graduate Center, Seattle Pacific University. Application available online. URL of online application: https://app.applyyourself.com/?id=spu-grad. Students are admitted in the Fall, application deadline December 15. *Fee:* $75.

Seattle University
Graduate Psychology Program
Arts and Sciences
901 12th Avenue, P.O. Box 222000
Seattle, WA 98122-1090
Telephone: (206) 296-5400
Fax: (206) 296-2141
E-mail: *krycka@seattleu.edu*
Web: *http://www.seattleu.edu/artsci/map/default.aspx*

Department Information:
1981. Director, Graduate Program: Kevin Krycka, PsyD. Number of faculty: total—full-time 4, part-time 6; women—full-time 2, part-time 3.

Programs and Degrees Offered:
Listed in the following order: Program area, degree type (T if terminal Master's), number awarded 7/08–6/09. Existential-Phenomenological Psychology MA/MS (Master of Arts/Science) (T) 19.

Student Applications/Admissions:
Student Applications
Existential-Phenomenological Psychology MA/MS (*Master of Arts/Science*)—Applications 2009–2010, 65. Total applicants accepted 2009–2010, 29. Number full-time enrolled (new admits only) 2009–2010, 25. Number part-time enrolled (new admits only) 2009–2010, 0. Total enrolled 2009–2010 full-time, 42, part-time, 5. Openings 2010–2011, 22. The median number of years required for completion of a degree in 2008–2009 were 2. The number of students enrolled full- and part-time who were dismissed or voluntarily withdrew from this program area in 2008–2009 were 0.

Scores: Entries appear in this order: required test or GPA, minimum score (if required), median score of students entering in 2009–2010. Existential-Phenomenological Psychology MA/MS (*Master of Arts/Science*): overall undergraduate GPA 3.0.

Other Criteria: (importance of criteria rated low, medium, or high): research experience—low, work experience—medium, extracurricular activity—medium, clinically related public service—high, GPA—high, letters of recommendation—high, interview—high, Bio/writing sample—high, undergraduate major in psychology—medium, specific undergraduate psychology courses taken—high. Some awareness of existential-phenomenological perspective in psychology and philosophy. For additional information on admission requirements, go to http://www.seattleu.edu/artsci/map/Inner.aspx?id=19170.

Student Characteristics: The following represents characteristics of students in 2009–2010 in all graduate psychology programs in the department: Female—full-time 34, part-time 4; Male—full-time 8, part-time 1; African American/Black—full-time 3, part-time 1; Hispanic/Latino(a)—full-time 2, part-time 0; Asian/Pacific Islander—full-time 3, part-time 0; American Indian/Alaska Native—full-time 0, part-time 0; Caucasian/White—full-time 34, part-time 4; Multi-ethnic—full-time 0, part-time 0; students subject to the Americans With Disabilities Act—full-time 0, part-time 0; Unknown ethnicity—full-time 0, part-time 0; International students who hold an F-1 or J-1 Visa—full-time 4, part-time 0.

Financial Information/Assistance:
Tuition for Full-Time Study: Master's: State residents: per academic year $15,270, $590 per credit hour; Nonstate residents: per academic year $15,270, $590 per credit hour. Tuition is subject to change. See the following Web site for updates and changes in tuition costs: http://www.seattleu.edu/sfs/.

Financial Assistance:
First-Year Students: Fellowships and scholarships available for first year. Average amount paid per academic year: $2,500. Apply by January 15.

Advanced Students: Fellowships and scholarships available for advanced students. Average amount paid per academic year: $2,500. Apply by January 15.

Additional Information: Of all students currently enrolled full time, 40% benefited from one or more of the listed financial

assistance programs. Application and information available online at: http://www.seattleu.edu/sfs/.

Internships/Practica: Master's Degree (MA/MS Existential-Phenomenological Psychology): An internship experience, such as a final research project or "capstone" experience is required of graduates. A variety of supervised internships (typically about 20 hrs/week during second year) in a wide variety of community agencies, hospitals, shelters and clinics.

Housing and Day Care: On-campus housing is available. See the following Web site for more information: http://www.seattleu.edu/housing/. No on-campus day care facilities are available.

Employment of Department Graduates:
Master's Degree Graduates: Of those who graduated in the academic year 2008–2009, the following categories and numbers represent the postgraduate activities and employment of master's degree graduates: Enrolled in a psychology doctoral program (4), enrolled in a postdoctoral residency/fellowship (n/a), employed in independent practice (n/a), employed in a professional position in a school system (2), employed in business or industry (5), employed in a community mental health/counseling center (14), employed in a hospital/medical center (2), still seeking employment (1), other employment position (4), total from the above (master's) (32).
Doctoral Degree Graduates: Of those who graduated in the academic year 2008–2009, the following categories and numbers represent the postgraduate activities and employment of doctoral degree graduates: Enrolled in a psychology doctoral program (n/a), total from the above (doctoral) (0).

Additional Information:
Orientation, Objectives, and Emphasis of Department: With an emphasis on existential-phenomenological psychology, this master's degree is designed to offer an interdisciplinary program focusing on the qualitative, experiential study of psychological events in the context of the person's life. By laying the foundations for a therapeutic attitude, the program prepares students for entrance into the helping professions or for further study of the psychological world. It is humanistic in that it intends to deepen the appreciation for the human condition by rigorous reflection on immediate psychological experiences and on the wisdom accumulated by the long tradition of the humanities. It is phenomenological in that it develops an attitude of openness and wonder toward psychological reality without holding theoretical prejudgments. It is therapeutic in that it focuses on the psychological conditions that help people deal with the difficulties of life.

Special Facilities or Resources: The Program has a tradition of involving selected students in qualitative research projects.

Information for Students With Physical Disabilities: See the following Web site for more information: http://www.seattleu.edu/sas/DisabilityServices/.

Application Information:
Send to Graduate Admissions Office, Seattle University, PO Box 222000, Seattle, WA 98122-1090. Application available online. URL of online application: http://www.seattleu.edu/admission/graduate/Default.aspx. Students are admitted in the Fall, application deadline January 15. *Fee:* $55.

Walla Walla University
School of Education and Psychology
204 South College Avenue
College Place, WA 99324
Telephone: (509) 527-2211, (800) 541-8900
Fax: (509) 527-2248
E-mail: *lee.stough@wallawalla.edu*
Web: *http://www.wallawalla.edu/counseling*

Department Information:
1965. Dean: Julian Melgosa. Number of faculty: total—full-time 5; women—full-time 2; total—minority—full-time 1.

Programs and Degrees Offered:
Listed in the following order: Program area, degree type (T if terminal Master's), number awarded 7/08–6/09. Counseling Psychology MA/MS (Master of Arts/Science) (T) 8.

Student Applications/Admissions:
Student Applications
Counseling Psychology MA/MS (Master of Arts/Science)—Applications 2009–2010, 15. Total applicants accepted 2009–2010, 12. Number full-time enrolled (new admits only) 2009–2010, 12. Total enrolled 2009–2010 full-time, 17, part-time, 1. Openings 2010–2011, 12. The median number of years required for completion of a degree in 2008–2009 were 2. The number of students enrolled full- and part-time who were dismissed or voluntarily withdrew from this program area in 2008–2009 were 2.
Scores: Entries appear in this order: required test or GPA, minimum score (if required), median score of students entering in 2009–2010. *Counseling Psychology MA/MS (Master of Arts/Science)*: GRE-V no minimum stated, 460, GRE-Q no minimum stated, 540, GRE-Analytical no minimum stated, 3, overall undergraduate GPA 2.75.
Other Criteria: (importance of criteria rated low, medium, or high): GRE scores—medium, research experience—low, work experience—medium, extracurricular activity—low, clinically related public service—medium, GPA—high, letters of recommendation—high, interview—high, statement of goals and objectives—high, undergraduate major in psychology—low, specific undergraduate psychology courses taken—low.

Student Characteristics: The following represents characteristics of students in 2009–2010 in all graduate psychology programs in the department: Female—full-time 9, part-time 1; Male—full-time 8, part-time 0; African American/Black—full-time 0, part-time 0; Hispanic/Latino(a)—full-time 1, part-time 0; Asian/Pacific Islander—full-time 0, part-time 0; American Indian/Alaska Native—full-time 0, part-time 0; Caucasian/White—full-time 15, part-time 1; Multi-ethnic—full-time 1, part-time 0; students subject to the Americans With Disabilities Act—full-time 0, part-time 0; Unknown ethnicity—full-time 0, part-time 0; International students who hold an F-1 or J-1 Visa—full-time 0, part-time 0.

Financial Information/Assistance:
Tuition for Full-Time Study: *Master's:* State residents: $492 per credit hour; Nonstate residents: $492 per credit hour. Tuition is subject to change.

Financial Assistance:

First-Year Students: Fellowships and scholarships available for first year. Average amount paid per academic year: $2,340. Average number of hours worked per week: 0.

Advanced Students: Fellowships and scholarships available for advanced students. Average amount paid per academic year: $2,340. Average number of hours worked per week: 0.

Additional Information: Of all students currently enrolled full time, 100% benefited from one or more of the listed financial assistance programs. Application and information available online at: http://www.wallawalla.edu/finaid.

Internships/Practica: Master's Degree (MA/MS Counseling Psychology): An internship experience, such as a final research project or "capstone" experience is required of graduates. The School of Education and Psychology operates a free counseling center for the community on site. The counseling center, comprised of four private counseling rooms and a group room, is equipped with one-way mirrors and video-cameras. During the second year of their program, students begin working in the center and have the opportunity to develop their clinical skills counseling individuals, couples, and families presenting with a variety of concerns. Program faculty provide individual and group supervision in either live or videotaped formats on a regular basis. After successfully completing the supervised practica, students complete a 400-600 hour internship at an approved site in the community. The School has developed relationships with various agencies where students will receive quality internship experiences that fit their interests.

Housing and Day Care: On-campus housing is available. Student Administration Walla Walla University 204 South College Avenue College Place, WA 99324. On-campus day care facilities are available. Child Development Center Walla Walla University 204 South College Avenue College Place, WA 99324.

Employment of Department Graduates:

Master's Degree Graduates: Of those who graduated in the academic year 2008–2009, the following categories and numbers represent the postgraduate activities and employment of master's degree graduates: Enrolled in a postdoctoral residency/fellowship (n/a), employed in independent practice (n/a), employed in a professional position in a school system (1), employed in a community mental health/counseling center (5), still seeking employment (1), other employment position (1), total from the above (master's) (8).

Doctoral Degree Graduates: Of those who graduated in the academic year 2008–2009, the following categories and numbers represent the postgraduate activities and employment of doctoral degree graduates: Enrolled in a psychology doctoral program (n/a), total from the above (doctoral) (0).

Additional Information:

Orientation, Objectives, and Emphasis of Department: The School of Education and Psychology offers thesis and non-thesis Master of Arts degrees in counseling psychology. Our program is designed to promote clinical, theoretical, academic, and personal growth through study, supervision, and service. Students are expected to attain a broad range of competence in the core areas of counseling psychology including human development and learning, individual and group counseling, career development, assessment, ethics, research, and statistics. Faculty present an integrative approach to treatment that focuses on the core principles, core processes, and a variety of strategies for working with emotion, cognition, and interpersonal and systemic factors. Students acquire a range of clinical skills they can use in working with diverse clients and learn to apply theory to practice through supervised practica and internship experiences. In a supportive yet challenging environment, students are encouraged to build upon life experiences and personal strengths, and take advantage of the opportunities to expand their awareness of self and others. If students desire, faculty assist them in the development and application of a philosophy of Christian service. All graduates are prepared to take the National Counselor's Exam and to become Licensed Mental Health Counselors, or to continue their training in doctoral programs.

Special Facilities or Resources: The School of Education and Psychology operates a free counseling center for the community where ongoing outcome research is being conducted. An enriched preschool program for children ages 3-5 is located in the on-site child development center.

Application Information:
Send to Graduate Studies, Walla Walla University, 204 South College Avenue, College Place, WA 99324. Application available online. URL of online application: http://www.wallawalla.edu/academics/graduate/checklist.html. Students are admitted in the Fall, application deadline. Qualified students are admitted throughout the spring and summer until the cohort is full. *Fee:* $50.

Washington State University
Department of Psychology
Liberal Arts
P.O. Box 644820
Pullman, WA 99164-4820
Telephone: (509) 335-2631
Fax: (509) 335-5043
E-mail: *psych@wsu.edu*
Web: *http://www.wsu.edu/psychology*

Department Information:
1946. Chairperson: John Hinson. Number of faculty: total—full-time 17, part-time 2; women—full-time 6, part-time 2; total—minority—full-time 2; women minority—full-time 1.

Programs and Degrees Offered:
Listed in the following order: Program area, degree type (T if terminal Master's), number awarded 7/08–6/09. Experimental PhD (Doctor of Philosophy) 4, Clinical PhD (Doctor of Philosophy) 6.

APA Accreditation: Clinical PhD (Doctor of Philosophy).

Student Applications/Admissions:
Student Applications
Experimental PhD (Doctor of Philosophy)—Applications 2009–2010, 62. Total applicants accepted 2009–2010, 6. Number full-time enrolled (new admits only) 2009–2010, 6. Number part-time enrolled (new admits only) 2009–2010, 0. Openings 2010–2011, 7. The median number of years required for com-

pletion of a degree in 2008–2009 were 5. The number of students enrolled full- and part-time who were dismissed or voluntarily withdrew from this program area in 2008–2009 were 0. *Clinical PhD (Doctor of Philosophy)*—Applications 2009–2010, 185. Total applicants accepted 2009–2010, 7. Number full-time enrolled (new admits only) 2009–2010, 7. Number part-time enrolled (new admits only) 2009–2010, 0. Openings 2010–2011, 7. The median number of years required for completion of a degree in 2008–2009 were 6. The number of students enrolled full- and part-time who were dismissed or voluntarily withdrew from this program area in 2008–2009 were 0.

Other Criteria: (importance of criteria rated low, medium, or high): GRE scores—high, research experience—high, work experience—medium, extracurricular activity—low, clinically related public service—high, GPA—high, letters of recommendation—high, interview—high, statement of goals and objectives—high. Applicants to the Experimental Psychology program are not expected to demonstrate any clinically-related public service. Applicants to the Experimental Psychology program are not required to have an interview, but a visit is encouraged.

Student Characteristics: The following represents characteristics of students in 2009–2010 in all graduate psychology programs in the department: Female—full-time 28, part-time 0; Male—full-time 16, part-time 0; African American/Black—full-time 1, part-time 0; Hispanic/Latino(a)—full-time 2, part-time 0; Asian/Pacific Islander—full-time 6, part-time 0; American Indian/Alaska Native—full-time 1, part-time 0; Caucasian/White—full-time 34, part-time 0; Multi-ethnic—full-time 0, part-time 0; students subject to the Americans With Disabilities Act—full-time 0, part-time 0; Unknown ethnicity—full-time 0, part-time 0; International students who hold an F-1 or J-1 Visa—full-time 0, part-time 0.

Financial Information/Assistance:
Tuition for Full-Time Study: *Doctoral:* State residents: per academic year $8,602, $478 per credit hour; Nonstate residents: per academic year $19,644, $1,091 per credit hour. Tuition is subject to change. See the following Web site for updates and changes in tuition costs: http://www.gradsch.wsu.edu/future-students/financingforfuturestudents/.

Financial Assistance:
First-Year Students: Teaching assistantships available for first year. Average amount paid per academic year: $13,500. Average number of hours worked per week: 20. Apply by December 15.

Advanced Students: Teaching assistantships available for advanced students. Average amount paid per academic year: $14,500. Average number of hours worked per week: 20. Apply by December 15.

Additional Information: Of all students currently enrolled full time, 100% benefited from one or more of the listed financial assistance programs.

Internships/Practica: Doctoral Degree (PhD Clinical): For those doctoral students for whom a professional internship was required in this program prior to graduation, (10) students applied for an internship in 2008–2009, with (10) students obtaining an internship. Of those students who obtained an internship, (10) were paid internships. Of those students who obtained an internship, (10) students placed in APA/CPA accredited internships, (0) students placed in internships not APA/CPA accredited, but listed with the Association of Psychology Postdoctoral and Internship Programs (APPIC), (0) students placed in internships conforming to guidelines of the Council of Directors of School Psychology Programs (CDSPP), (0) students placed in internships that were not APA/CPA accredited, APPIC or CDSPP listed. Psychology Clinic Practicum; Counseling Services Practicum; Medical Psychology Practicum at University Hospital.

Housing and Day Care: On-campus housing is available. See the following Web site for more information: http://www.livingat.wsu.edu/hdrl/FutureStudents/FS_Main.htm. On-campus day care facilities are available. See the following Web site for more information: http://www.gradsch.wsu.edu/future-students/resourcesforgradsstudents/.

Employment of Department Graduates:
Master's Degree Graduates: Of those who graduated in the academic year 2008–2009, the following categories and numbers represent the postgraduate activities and employment of master's degree graduates: Enrolled in a postdoctoral residency/fellowship (n/a), employed in independent practice (n/a), total from the above (master's) (0).

Doctoral Degree Graduates: Of those who graduated in the academic year 2008–2009, the following categories and numbers represent the postgraduate activities and employment of doctoral degree graduates: Enrolled in a psychology doctoral program (n/a), enrolled in a postdoctoral residency/fellowship (6), employed in independent practice (0), employed in an academic position at a university (1), employed in an academic position at a 2-year/4-year college (1), employed in business or industry (1), employed in government agency (1), employed in a community mental health/counseling center (0), total from the above (doctoral) (10).

Additional Information:
Orientation, Objectives, and Emphasis of Department: The objectives of the graduate programs are to prepare individuals to make contributions and hold leadership positions in basic and applied research, teaching, clinical psychology, public service, or some combination of these areas. The clinical program is a broad, general one requiring student commitment to both research and clinical work. The emphases within the experimental program are cognitive, behavior analysis, physiological psychology, social, and visual perception.

Special Facilities or Resources: The Department of Psychology is located in Johnson Tower, near the center of campus. Fully equipped laboratories and shop facilities are available for research in social behavior, cognition, perception, human and animal learning, the experimental and applied analysis of behavior, and physiological and sensory psychology. The Psychology Clinic is operated as a training facility within the department.

Information for Students With Physical Disabilities: See the following Web site for more information: http://drc.wsu.edu/.

Application Information:
Send to Must apply to the WSU Graduate School (online application at http://www.gradsch.wsu.edu) and the Psychology Department (online aplication instructions at http://www.wsu.edu/psychology/apply). Application available online. URL of online application: http://www.gradsch.wsu.edu. Students are admitted in the Fall, application deadline December 15. *Fee:* $50.

Washington State University
Educational Leadership and Counseling Psychology
Education
P.O. Box 642136
Pullman, WA 99164-2136
Telephone: (509) 335-7016
Fax: (509) 335-2097
E-mail: *church@mail.wsu.edu*
Web: *http://www.education.wsu.edu/graduate/specializations/ counselingpsych*

Department Information:
Chairperson: Dr. Phyllis Erdman. Number of faculty: total—full-time 12; women—full-time 5; total—minority—full-time 3; women minority—full-time 2.

Programs and Degrees Offered:
Listed in the following order: Program area, degree type (T if terminal Master's), number awarded 7/08–6/09. Counseling Psychology PhD (Doctor of Philosophy) 0, Educational Psychology PhD (Doctor of Philosophy) 0, Counseling MEd (Education) 7, Educational Psychology MEd (Education) 1.

APA Accreditation: Counseling PhD (Doctor of Philosophy). Student Outcome Data Website: http://education.wsu.edu/graduate/specializations/counselingpsych/phd/.

Student Applications/Admissions:
Student Applications
  Counseling Psychology PhD (Doctor of Philosophy)—Applications 2009–2010, 119. Total applicants accepted 2009–2010, 13. Number full-time enrolled (new admits only) 2009–2010, 5. Total enrolled 2009–2010 full-time, 31, part-time, 10. Openings 2010–2011, 7. The number of students enrolled full- and part-time who were dismissed or voluntarily withdrew from this program area in 2008–2009 were 0. *Educational Psychology PhD (Doctor of Philosophy)*—Applications 2009–2010, 9. Total applicants accepted 2009–2010, 7. Number full-time enrolled (new admits only) 2009–2010, 4. Number part-time enrolled (new admits only) 2009–2010, 0. Total enrolled 2009–2010 full-time, 8, part-time, 3. Openings 2010–2011, 4. The number of students enrolled full- and part-time who were dismissed or voluntarily withdrew from this program area in 2008–2009 were 0. *Counseling MEd (Education)*—Applications 2009–2010, 37. Total applicants accepted 2009–2010, 16. Number full-time enrolled (new admits only) 2009–2010, 16. Number part-time enrolled (new admits only) 2009–2010, 0. Total enrolled 2009–2010 full-time, 35, part-time, 24. Openings 2010–2011, 20. The median number of years required for completion of a degree in 2008–2009 were 2. The number of students enrolled full- and part-time who were dismissed or voluntarily withdrew from this program area in 2008–2009 were 1. *Educational Psychology MEd (Education)*—Applications 2009–2010, 9. Total applicants accepted 2009–2010, 3. Number full-time enrolled (new admits only) 2009–2010, 1. Number part-time enrolled (new admits only) 2009–2010, 0. Openings 2010–2011, 3. The median number of years required for completion of a degree in 2008–2009 were 2. The number of students enrolled full- and part-time who were dismissed or voluntarily withdrew from this program area in 2008–2009 were 0.

Scores: Entries appear in this order: required test or GPA, minimum score (if required), median score of students entering in 2009–2010. *Counseling Psychology PhD (Doctor of Philosophy)*: GRE-V no minimum stated, 500, GRE-Q no minimum stated, 555, overall undergraduate GPA no minimum stated, 3.49; *Counseling MEd (Education)*: GRE-V no minimum stated, 450, GRE-Q no minimum stated, 550, GRE-Analytical no minimum stated, 4.5, overall undergraduate GPA no minimum stated, 3.53.

Other Criteria: (importance of criteria rated low, medium, or high): GRE scores—medium, research experience—medium, work experience—medium, extracurricular activity—medium, clinically related public service—medium, GPA—high, letters of recommendation—high, statement of goals and objectives—high. For additional information on admission requirements, go to http://education.wsu.edu/graduate/specializations/counselingpsych.

Student Characteristics: The following represents characteristics of students in 2009–2010 in all graduate psychology programs in the department: Female—full-time 57, part-time 33; Male—full-time 14, part-time 9; African American/Black—full-time 4, part-time 2; Hispanic/Latino(a)—full-time 12, part-time 6; Asian/Pacific Islander—full-time 12, part-time 5; American Indian/Alaska Native—full-time 2, part-time 1; Caucasian/White—full-time 30, part-time 25; Multi-ethnic—full-time 1, part-time 0; students subject to the Americans With Disabilities Act—full-time 0, part-time 0; Unknown ethnicity—full-time 10, part-time 3; International students who hold an F-1 or J-1 Visa—full-time 0, part-time 0.

Financial Information/Assistance:
Tuition for Full-Time Study: *Master's:* State residents: per academic year $8,862, $443 per credit hour; Nonstate residents: per academic year $21,660, $1,083 per credit hour. *Doctoral:* State residents: per academic year $8,862, $443 per credit hour; Nonstate residents: per academic year $21,660, $1,083 per credit hour. Tuition is subject to change. See the following Web site for updates and changes in tuition costs: http://www.finaid.wsu.edu/coa.html.

Financial Assistance:
  First-Year Students: Teaching assistantships available for first year. Average amount paid per academic year: $12,865. Average number of hours worked per week: 20. Research assistantships available for first year. Average amount paid per academic year:

$12,865. Average number of hours worked per week: 20. Fellowships and scholarships available for first year.

Advanced Students: Teaching assistantships available for advanced students. Average amount paid per academic year: $13,653. Average number of hours worked per week: 20. Research assistantships available for advanced students. Average amount paid per academic year: $13,653. Average number of hours worked per week: 20. Fellowships and scholarships available for advanced students.

Additional Information: Of all students currently enrolled full time, 75% benefited from one or more of the listed financial assistance programs. Application and information available online at: http://www.finaid.wsu.edu/.

Internships/Practica: Doctoral Degree (PhD Counseling Psychology): For those doctoral students for whom a professional internship was required in this program prior to graduation, (4) students applied for an internship in 2008–2009, with (3) students obtaining an internship. Of those students who obtained an internship, (3) were paid internships. Of those students who obtained an internship, (3) students placed in APA/CPA accredited internships, (0) students placed in internships not APA/CPA accredited, but listed with the Association of Psychology Postdoctoral and Internship Programs (APPIC), (0) students placed in internships conforming to guidelines of the Council of Directors of School Psychology Programs (CDSPP), (0) students placed in internships that were not APA/CPA accredited, APPIC or CDSPP listed.

Housing and Day Care: On-campus housing is available. See the following Web site for more information: http://housing.wsu.edu/. On-campus day care facilities are available. See the following Web site for more information: http://www.childrenscenter.wsu.edu.

Employment of Department Graduates:
Master's Degree Graduates: Of those who graduated in the academic year 2008–2009, the following categories and numbers represent the postgraduate activities and employment of master's degree graduates: Enrolled in a postdoctoral residency/fellowship (n/a), employed in independent practice (n/a), total from the above (master's) (0).
Doctoral Degree Graduates: Of those who graduated in the academic year 2008–2009, the following categories and numbers represent the postgraduate activities and employment of doctoral degree graduates: Enrolled in a psychology doctoral program (n/a), total from the above (doctoral) (0).

Additional Information:

Information for Students With Physical Disabilities: See the following Web site for more information: http://drc.wsu.edu/.

Application Information:
Send to College of Education, Office of Graduate Studies, 252 Cleveland Hall, P O Box 642114, Pullman, WA 99164-2114. Application available online. URL of online application: http://gradsch.wsu.edu/FutureStudents/Admission/Apply.aspx. Students are admitted in the Fall, application deadline January 10. *Fee:* $50.

Washington, University of
Department of Psychology
Arts and Sciences
Box 351525
Seattle, WA 98195-1525
Telephone: (206) 543-8687
Fax: (206) 685-3157
E-mail: *mizumori@u.washington.edu*
Web: *http://www.web.psych.washington.edu/*

Department Information:
1917. Chairperson: Sheri J.Y. Mizumori, PhD Number of faculty: total—full-time 45, part-time 5; women—full-time 17, part-time 4; total—minority—full-time 10; women minority—full-time 3.

Programs and Degrees Offered:
Listed in the following order: Program area, degree type (T if terminal Master's), number awarded 7/08–6/09. Animal Behavior PhD (Doctor of Philosophy) 3, Clinical Psychology PhD (Doctor of Philosophy) 5, Child Clinical PhD (Doctor of Philosophy) 1, Cognition and Perception PhD (Doctor of Philosophy) 3, Developmental Psychology PhD (Doctor of Philosophy) 0, Behavioral Neuroscience PhD (Doctor of Philosophy) 4, Social and Personality Psychology PhD (Doctor of Philosophy) 2.

APA Accreditation: Clinical PhD (Doctor of Philosophy). Student Outcome Data Website: http://web.psych.washington.edu/areas/admissionsdata/clinical.html.

Student Applications/Admissions:
Student Applications
Animal Behavior PhD (Doctor of Philosophy)—Applications 2009–2010, 32. Total applicants accepted 2009–2010, 3. Number full-time enrolled (new admits only) 2009–2010, 1. Number part-time enrolled (new admits only) 2009–2010, 0. Openings 2010–2011, 3. The median number of years required for completion of a degree in 2008–2009 were 7. The number of students enrolled full- and part-time who were dismissed or voluntarily withdrew from this program area in 2008–2009 were 0. *Clinical Psychology PhD (Doctor of Philosophy)*—Applications 2009–2010, 244. Total applicants accepted 2009–2010, 5. Number full-time enrolled (new admits only) 2009–2010, 4. Number part-time enrolled (new admits only) 2009–2010, 0. Total enrolled 2009–2010 full-time, 34, part-time, 5. Openings 2010–2011, 2. The median number of years required for completion of a degree in 2008–2009 were 7. The number of students enrolled full- and part-time who were dismissed or voluntarily withdrew from this program area in 2008–2009 were 0. *Child Clinical PhD (Doctor of Philosophy)*—Applications 2009–2010, 195. Total applicants accepted 2009–2010, 6. Number full-time enrolled (new admits only) 2009–2010, 4. Number part-time enrolled (new admits only) 2009–2010, 0. Total enrolled 2009–2010 full-time, 24, part-time, 8. Openings 2010–2011, 3. The median number of years required for completion of a degree in 2008–2009 were 7. The number of students enrolled full- and part-time who were dismissed or voluntarily withdrew from this program area in 2008–2009 were 2. *Cognition and Perception PhD (Doctor of Philosophy)*—Applications 2009–2010, 49. Total applicants accepted 2009–2010, 3. Number full-time enrolled (new admits only) 2009–

2010, 1. Number part-time enrolled (new admits only) 2009–2010, 1. Total enrolled 2009–2010 full-time, 12, part-time, 6. Openings 2010–2011, 3. The median number of years required for completion of a degree in 2008–2009 were 9. The number of students enrolled full- and part-time who were dismissed or voluntarily withdrew from this program area in 2008–2009 were 3. *Developmental Psychology PhD (Doctor of Philosophy)*—Applications 2009–2010, 43. Total applicants accepted 2009–2010, 4. Number full-time enrolled (new admits only) 2009–2010, 2. Number part-time enrolled (new admits only) 2009–2010, 0. Total enrolled 2009–2010 full-time, 11, part-time, 2. Openings 2010–2011, 1. The number of students enrolled full- and part-time who were dismissed or voluntarily withdrew from this program area in 2008–2009 were 1. *Behavioral Neuroscience PhD (Doctor of Philosophy)*—Applications 2009–2010, 35. Total applicants accepted 2009–2010, 2. Number full-time enrolled (new admits only) 2009–2010, 2. Number part-time enrolled (new admits only) 2009–2010, 0. Total enrolled 2009–2010 full-time, 10, part-time, 2. Openings 2010–2011, 3. The median number of years required for completion of a degree in 2008–2009 were 7. The number of students enrolled full- and part-time who were dismissed or voluntarily withdrew from this program area in 2008–2009 were 0. *Social and Personality Psychology PhD (Doctor of Philosophy)*—Applications 2009–2010, 103. Total applicants accepted 2009–2010, 3. Number full-time enrolled (new admits only) 2009–2010, 2. Number part-time enrolled (new admits only) 2009–2010, 0. Total enrolled 2009–2010 full-time, 12, part-time, 3. Openings 2010–2011, 2. The median number of years required for completion of a degree in 2008–2009 were 6. The number of students enrolled full- and part-time who were dismissed or voluntarily withdrew from this program area in 2008–2009 were 1.

Scores: Entries appear in this order: required test or GPA, minimum score (if required), median score of students entering in 2009–2010. *Clinical Psychology PhD (Doctor of Philosophy)*: GRE-V no minimum stated, 625, GRE-Q no minimum stated, 745, overall undergraduate GPA no minimum stated, 3.67; *Child Clinical PhD (Doctor of Philosophy)*: GRE-V no minimum stated, 625, GRE-Q no minimum stated, 745, overall undergraduate GPA no minimum stated, 3.67.

Other Criteria: (importance of criteria rated low, medium, or high): GRE scores—high, research experience—high, work experience—medium, extracurricular activity—low, clinically related public service—low, GPA—medium, letters of recommendation—high, interview—high, statement of goals and objectives—high, Individual areas evaluate applications differently, but all require a strong background in research and/or statistics. For additional information on admission requirements, go to http://web.psych.washington.edu/graduate/apply.html.

Student Characteristics: The following represents characteristics of students in 2009–2010 in all graduate psychology programs in the department: Female—full-time 69, part-time 18; Male—full-time 40, part-time 8; African American/Black—full-time 5, part-time 0; Hispanic/Latino(a)—full-time 5, part-time 3; Asian/Pacific Islander—full-time 24, part-time 3; American Indian/Alaska Native—full-time 0, part-time 0; Caucasian/White—full-time 73, part-time 19; Multi-ethnic—full-time 2, part-time 1; students subject to the Americans With Disabilities Act—full-time 1, part-time 0; Unknown ethnicity—full-time 0, part-time 0; International students who hold an F-1 or J-1 Visa—full-time 11, part-time 1.

Financial Information/Assistance:

Tuition for Full-Time Study: *Doctoral:* State residents: per academic year $10,727; Nonstate residents: per academic year $24,067. Tuition is subject to change. See the following Web site for updates and changes in tuition costs: http://www.washington.edu/admin/pb/home/opb-tuition.htm.

Financial Assistance:

First-Year Students: Teaching assistantships available for first year. Average amount paid per academic year: $15,669. Average number of hours worked per week: 20. Research assistantships available for first year. Average amount paid per academic year: $15,669. Average number of hours worked per week: 20. Traineeships available for first year. Average amount paid per academic year: $15,669. Average number of hours worked per week: 20.

Advanced Students: Teaching assistantships available for advanced students. Average amount paid per academic year: $16,848. Average number of hours worked per week: 20. Research assistantships available for advanced students. Average amount paid per academic year: $16,848. Average number of hours worked per week: 20. Traineeships available for advanced students. Average amount paid per academic year: $16,848. Average number of hours worked per week: 20.

Additional Information: Of all students currently enrolled full time, 95% benefited from one or more of the listed financial assistance programs. Application and information available online at: http://web.psych.washington.edu/graduate/apply.html.

Internships/Practica: Doctoral Degree (PhD Clinical Psychology): For those doctoral students for whom a professional internship was required in this program prior to graduation, (8) students applied for an internship in 2008–2009, with (7) students obtaining an internship. Of those students who obtained an internship, (7) were paid internships. Of those students who obtained an internship, (7) students placed in APA/CPA accredited internships, (0) students placed in internships not APA/CPA accredited, but listed with the Association of Psychology Postdoctoral and Internship Programs (APPIC), (0) students placed in internships conforming to guidelines of the Council of Directors of School Psychology Programs (CDSPP), (0) students placed in internships that were not APA/CPA accredited, APPIC or CDSPP listed. Doctoral Degree (PhD Child Clinical): For those doctoral students for whom a professional internship was required in this program prior to graduation, (6) students applied for an internship in 2008–2009, with (5) students obtaining an internship. Of those students who obtained an internship, (5) were paid internships. Of those students who obtained an internship, (5) students placed in APA/CPA accredited internships, (0) students placed in internships not APA/CPA accredited, but listed with the Association of Psychology Postdoctoral and Internship Programs (APPIC), (0) students placed in internships conforming to guidelines of the Council of Directors of School Psychology Programs (CDSPP), (0) students placed in internships that were not APA/CPA accredited, APPIC or CDSPP listed. A variety of local and national predoctoral internships are available in clinical psychology.

Housing and Day Care: On-campus housing is available. See the following Web site for more information: http://hfs.washington.

edu/. On-campus day care facilities are available. See the following Web site for more information: http://www.washington.edu/admin/hr/benefits/worklife/childcare/children-centers.html.

Employment of Department Graduates:
Master's Degree Graduates: Of those who graduated in the academic year 2008–2009, the following categories and numbers represent the postgraduate activities and employment of master's degree graduates: Enrolled in a postdoctoral residency/fellowship (n/a), employed in independent practice (n/a), total from the above (master's) (0).
Doctoral Degree Graduates: Of those who graduated in the academic year 2008–2009, the following categories and numbers represent the postgraduate activities and employment of doctoral degree graduates: Enrolled in a psychology doctoral program (n/a), enrolled in a postdoctoral residency/fellowship (4), employed in an academic position at a university (4), employed in other positions at a higher education institution (1), employed in business or industry (2), employed in a community mental health/counseling center (1), do not know (6), total from the above (doctoral) (18).

Additional Information:
Orientation, Objectives, and Emphasis of Department: The program is committed to research-oriented scientific psychology. No degree programs are available in counseling or humanistic psychology. The clinical program emphasizes both clinical and research competencies and has areas of specialization in child clinical, and subspecialties in behavioral medicine, health psychology, and community psychology. Diversity science and quantitative psychology minors are now available to students in our program.

Special Facilities or Resources: University and urban settings provide many resources, including the University of Washington Medical Center, UW Autism Center, Addictive Behaviors Research Center, Psychological Services and Training Center, Behavioral Research & Therapy Clinics, Institute for Learning and Brain Sciences, UW Center for Anxiety and Traumatic Stress, Washington National Primate Research Center, Children's Hospital and Regional Medical Center; nearby Veterans Administration facilities, and Sound Mental Health.

Information for Students With Physical Disabilities: See the following Web site for more information: http://www.washington.edu/admin/dso/.

Application Information:
Send to Graduate Selections Committee, Department of Psychology, Box 351525, University of Washington, Seattle, WA 98195-1525. Application available online. URL of online application: http://web.psych.washington.edu/graduate/apply.html. Students are admitted in the Fall, application deadline December 15. *Fee:* $65. The fee waiver application is only available to U.S. citizens and those holding permanent resident status. These applicants may be qualified to apply for an application fee waiver, based upon their financial profiles.

WEST VIRGINIA

Marshall University
Department of Psychology
Liberal Arts
One John Marshall Drive
Huntington, WV 25755-2672
Telephone: (304) 696-6446
Fax: (304) 696-2784
E-mail: *mewaldt@marshall.edu*
Web: *http://www.marshall.edu/psych/*

Department Information:
Chairperson: Steven Mewaldt. Number of faculty: total—full-time 19, part-time 7; women—full-time 6, part-time 3; total—minority—full-time 1.

Programs and Degrees Offered:
Listed in the following order: Program area, degree type (T if terminal Master's), number awarded 7/08–6/09. Clinical Psychology PsyD (Doctor of Psychology) 2, Psychology MA/MS (Master of Arts/Science) (T) 28.

APA Accreditation: Clinical PsyD (Doctor of Psychology).

Student Applications/Admissions:

Student Applications

Clinical Psychology PsyD (Doctor of Psychology)—Applications 2009–2010, 60. Total applicants accepted 2009–2010, 10. Number full-time enrolled (new admits only) 2009–2010, 9. Number part-time enrolled (new admits only) 2009–2010, 1. Total enrolled 2009–2010 full-time, 39, part-time, 6. Openings 2010–2011, 10. The median number of years required for completion of a degree in 2008–2009 were 5. The number of students enrolled full- and part-time who were dismissed or voluntarily withdrew from this program area in 2008–2009 were 0. *Psychology MA/MS (Master of Arts/Science)*—Applications 2009–2010, 32. Total applicants accepted 2009–2010, 21. Number full-time enrolled (new admits only) 2009–2010, 11. Number part-time enrolled (new admits only) 2009–2010, 6. Total enrolled 2009–2010 full-time, 23, part-time, 34. Openings 2010–2011, 25. The median number of years required for completion of a degree in 2008–2009 were 3. The number of students enrolled full- and part-time who were dismissed or voluntarily withdrew from this program area in 2008–2009 were 2.

Scores: Entries appear in this order: required test or GPA, minimum score (if required), median score of students entering in 2009–2010. *Clinical Psychology PsyD (Doctor of Psychology)*: GRE-V 450, 500, GRE-Q 450, 500.

Other Criteria: (importance of criteria rated low, medium, or high): GRE scores—medium, research experience—medium, work experience—medium, extracurricular activity—medium, clinically related public service—medium, GPA—high, letters of recommendation—medium, interview—medium, statement of goals and objectives—high, undergraduate major in psychology—medium, specific undergraduate psychology courses taken—high, MA program admission is based primarily on GPA and GRE scores; PsyD program considers these, plus statement of professional goals, clinical and research experience, commitment to and understanding of rural psychological service delivery, and letters of recommendation. An interview may be required of PsyD applicants. For additional information on admission requirements, go to http://www.marshall.edu/psych/.

Student Characteristics: The following represents characteristics of students in 2009–2010 in all graduate psychology programs in the department: Female—full-time 39, part-time 45; Male—full-time 13, part-time 14; African American/Black—full-time 0, part-time 0; Hispanic/Latino(a)—full-time 0, part-time 0; Asian/Pacific Islander—full-time 0, part-time 1; American Indian/Alaska Native—full-time 1, part-time 1; Caucasian/White—full-time 45, part-time 52; Multi-ethnic—full-time 0, part-time 0; students subject to the Americans With Disabilities Act—full-time 0, part-time 0; Unknown ethnicity—full-time 0, part-time 0; International students who hold an F-1 or J-1 Visa—full-time 0, part-time 0.

Financial Information/Assistance:

Tuition for Full-Time Study: *Master's:* State residents: per academic year $5,516, $307 per credit hour; Nonstate residents: per academic year $13,836, $769 per credit hour. *Doctoral:* State residents: $1,068 per credit hour; Nonstate residents: $1,449 per credit hour. Tuition is subject to change. Tuition costs vary by program. See the following Web site for updates and changes in tuition costs: http://www.marshall.edu/bursar.

Financial Assistance:

First-Year Students: Teaching assistantships available for first year. Research assistantships available for first year. Average amount paid per academic year: $3,000. Average number of hours worked per week: 10.

Advanced Students: Teaching assistantships available for advanced students. Average amount paid per academic year: $3,000. Average number of hours worked per week: 10. Apply by April 15. Research assistantships available for advanced students. Average amount paid per academic year: $3,000. Average number of hours worked per week: 10. Traineeships available for advanced students. Average amount paid per academic year: $3,000. Average number of hours worked per week: 10.

Additional Information: Of all students currently enrolled full time, 50% benefited from one or more of the listed financial assistance programs. Application and information available online at: http://www.marshall.edu/sfa/.

Internships/Practica: Doctoral Degree (PsyD Clinical Psychology): For those doctoral students for whom a professional internship was required in this program prior to graduation, (11) students applied for an internship in 2008–2009, with (10) students obtaining an internship. Of those students who obtained an internship, (10) were paid internships. Of those students who obtained an internship, (6) students placed in APA/CPA accredited internships, (0) students placed in internships not APA/CPA accredited, but listed with the Association of Psychology Postdoctoral and Internship Programs (APPIC), (0) students placed in internships conforming to guidelines of the Council of Directors of School Psychology Programs (CDSPP), (4) students placed in internships that were not APA/CPA accredited, APPIC or CDSPP listed. PsyD program: 2nd year students work in department's clinic in Huntington; 3rd year students work at variety of sites in the Huntington community; 4th year students work at rural placements. Some are in collaboration with primary medical facilities; some may require an overnight stay. Students must complete a full-year, full-time or 2 year, part-time predoctoral internship in order to graduate. Clinical MA: Practicum students work in Marshall's community clinic in Dunbar, WV; master's level interns work in area mental health agencies. MA level students interested in I/O have access to a variety of business and organizational field placements.

Housing and Day Care: On-campus housing is available. See the following Web site for more information: http://www.marshall.edu/residence-services/. On-campus day care facilities are available. See the following Web site for more information: http://www.marshall.edu/cda.

Employment of Department Graduates:
Master's Degree Graduates: Of those who graduated in the academic year 2008–2009, the following categories and numbers represent the postgraduate activities and employment of master's degree graduates: Enrolled in a psychology doctoral program (2), enrolled in another graduate/professional program (1), enrolled in a postdoctoral residency/fellowship (n/a), employed in independent practice (n/a), employed in an academic position at a 2-year/4-year college (1), employed in government agency (1), employed in a community mental health/counseling center (4), total from the above (master's) (9).
Doctoral Degree Graduates: Of those who graduated in the academic year 2008–2009, the following categories and numbers represent the postgraduate activities and employment of doctoral degree graduates: Enrolled in a psychology doctoral program (n/a), enrolled in another graduate/professional program (0), enrolled in a postdoctoral residency/fellowship (0), employed in independent practice (1), employed in an academic position at a university (0), employed in an academic position at a 2-year/4-year college (0), employed in other positions at a higher education institution (0), employed in a professional position in a school system (0), employed in business or industry (0), employed in government agency (0), employed in a community mental health/counseling center (0), employed in a hospital/medical center (1), still seeking employment (0), not seeking employment (0), other employment position (0), do not know (0), total from the above (doctoral) (2).

Additional Information:
Orientation, Objectives, and Emphasis of Department: Our PsyD program in Clinical Psychology (offered on our Huntington WV campus) accepted its first students in Fall 2002 and received APA accreditation in the spring of 2006. The program is also recognized as a designated program by the National Register/ASPPC Designation project. The program's emphasis is on preparing scholar-practitioners for rural/underserved populations in Appalachia and other rural areas. Particular foci of the doctoral program include understanding the needs and challenges of working in rural communities, preparing doctoral level psychologists to work within these communities, and provision of services to those areas through the training program itself. A wide range of theoretical perspectives are represented on our faculty. The MA program can be individualized to address a variety of academic and professional objectives for students. There is an "area of emphasis" available in clinical psychology (based in our S. Charleston, WV campus) which prepares students for entry level clinical work at the MA level. Students can also take coursework, do research, and obtain field placements in interest areas such as I/O psychology and a variety of disciplinary areas such as developmental, cognitive, social, etc. The MA program is a popular foundation program for students intending to complete Marshall's EdS program in School Psychology.

Special Facilities or Resources: Departmental and university computer facilities are available to students for clinical work and for research projects in all programs. Online library resources are excellent. Through department clinics, clinical students are afforded the opportunity to work, under supervision, with clients from the community and university. Placements for Psy D students are available at nearby community mental health centers, state hospitals, and the VA, as well as at a variety of more rural sites for advanced training. MA-level students interested in I/O have access to a variety of business and organizational field placements. Faculty have a variety of active, ongoing research projects available for student collaboration.

Information for Students With Physical Disabilities: See the following Web site for more information: http://www.marshall.edu/disabled/.

Application Information:
Send to MA Program: Admissions Office, Marshall University Graduate College, 100 Angus Peyton Dr., S. Charleston, WV 25303-1600. Application available online. URL of online application: http://www.marshall.edu/psych/ Students are admitted in the Fall, application deadline January 15. January 15 deadline for Psy D program (all new Psy D students start in subsequent Fall semester); MA program has ongoing review of applicants; new MA students can begin in any semester. *Fee:* $40.

West Virginia University
Department of Counseling, Rehabilitation Counseling and Counseling Psychology
Human Resources and Education
502 Allen Hall, P.O. Box 6122
Morgantown, WV 26506-6122
Telephone: (304) 293-2227
Fax: (304) 293-4082
E-mail: *James.Bartee@mail.wvu.edu*
Web: *http://counseling.wvu.edu*

Department Information:
1948. Chairperson: Margaret K. Glenn. Number of faculty: total—full-time 12; women—full-time 6; total—minority—full-time 2; women minority—full-time 1; faculty subject to the Americans With Disabilities Act 1.

Programs and Degrees Offered:
Listed in the following order: Program area, degree type (T if terminal Master's), number awarded 7/08–6/09. Counseling Psychology PhD (Doctor of Philosophy) 2.

APA Accreditation: Counseling PhD (Doctor of Philosophy). Student Outcome Data Website: http://counseling.wvu.edu/counseling_psychology/future_students/program_data.

Student Applications/Admissions:
Student Applications
Counseling Psychology PhD (Doctor of Philosophy)—Applications 2009–2010, 29. Total applicants accepted 2009–2010, 6. Number full-time enrolled (new admits only) 2009–2010, 6. Number part-time enrolled (new admits only) 2009–2010, 0. Total enrolled 2009–2010 full-time, 26, part-time, 15. Openings 2010–2011, 6. The median number of years required for completion of a degree in 2008–2009 were 6. The number of students enrolled full- and part-time who were dismissed or voluntarily withdrew from this program area in 2008–2009 were 1.

Scores: Entries appear in this order: required test or GPA, minimum score (if required), median score of students entering in 2009–2010. Counseling Psychology PhD (Doctor of Philosophy): GRE-V 500, GRE-Q 500, GRE-Analytical no minimum stated, Masters GPA 3.5.

Other Criteria: (importance of criteria rated low, medium, or high): GRE scores—medium, research experience—medium, work experience—high, extracurricular activity—medium, clinically related public service—medium, GPA—medium, letters of recommendation—high, interview—high, statement of goals and objectives—high, goodness of fit—high. For additional information on admission requirements, go to http://counseling.wvu.edu/counseling_psychology/future_students/admissions.

Student Characteristics: The following represents characteristics of students in 2009–2010 in all graduate psychology programs in the department: Female—full-time 17, part-time 10; Male—full-time 9, part-time 5; African American/Black—full-time 3, part-time 1; Hispanic/Latino(a)—full-time 0, part-time 1; Asian/Pacific Islander—full-time 1, part-time 0; American Indian/Alaska Native—full-time 0, part-time 1; Caucasian/White—full-time 22, part-time 12; Multi-ethnic—full-time 0, part-time 0; students subject to the Americans With Disabilities Act—full-time 0, part-time 1; Unknown ethnicity—full-time 0, part-time 0; International students who hold an F-1 or J-1 Visa—full-time 1, part-time 0.

Financial Information/Assistance:
Tuition for Full-Time Study: *Doctoral:* State residents: per academic year $6,074, $341 per credit hour; Nonstate residents: per academic year $17,274, $963 per credit hour. Tuition is subject to change. Additional fees are assessed to students beyond the costs of tuition for the following: $586 mandatory fees per semester. See the following Web site for updates and changes in tuition costs: http://adm.wvu.edu/home/cost_of_attendance.

Financial Assistance:
First-Year Students: Teaching assistantships available for first year. Average amount paid per academic year: $10,000. Average number of hours worked per week: 20. Research assistantships available for first year. Average amount paid per academic year: $10,000. Average number of hours worked per week: 20. Fellowships and scholarships available for first year. Average amount paid per academic year: $15,000. Average number of hours worked per week: 0.

Advanced Students: Teaching assistantships available for advanced students. Average amount paid per academic year: $10,000. Average number of hours worked per week: 20. Research assistantships available for advanced students. Average amount paid per academic year: $10,000. Average number of hours worked per week: 20. Fellowships and scholarships available for advanced students. Average amount paid per academic year: $15,000. Average number of hours worked per week: 0.

Additional Information: Of all students currently enrolled full time, 88% benefited from one or more of the listed financial assistance programs. Application and information available online at: http://www.finaid.wvu.edu/.

Internships/Practica: Doctoral Degree (PhD Counseling Psychology): For those doctoral students for whom a professional internship was required in this program prior to graduation, (6) students applied for an internship in 2008–2009, with (5) students obtaining an internship. Of those students who obtained an internship, (5) were paid internships. Of those students who obtained an internship, (4) students placed in APA/CPA accredited internships, (0) students placed in internships not APA/CPA accredited, but listed with the Association of Psychology Postdoctoral and Internship Programs (APPIC), (0) students placed in internships conforming to guidelines of the Council of Directors of School Psychology Programs (CDSPP), (1) students placed in internships that were not APA/CPA accredited, APPIC or CDSPP listed. The doctoral program offers a variety of opportunities for internship and practicum experience. Some of the placement sites include: the federal prison system, mental health agencies, employee assistant programs, private practices, VA hospitals, local school systems, university counseling center, and others.

Housing and Day Care: On-campus housing is available. See the following Web site for more information: http://housing.wvu.edu/. On-campus day care facilities are available. See the following Web site for more information: http://childlearningcenter.wvu.edu/.

Employment of Department Graduates:
Master's Degree Graduates: Of those who graduated in the academic year 2008–2009, the following categories and numbers represent the postgraduate activities and employment of master's degree graduates: Enrolled in a postdoctoral residency/fellowship (n/a), employed in independent practice (n/a), total from the above (master's) (0).

Doctoral Degree Graduates: Of those who graduated in the academic year 2008–2009, the following categories and numbers represent the postgraduate activities and employment of doctoral degree graduates: Enrolled in a psychology doctoral program (n/a), enrolled in a postdoctoral residency/fellowship (1), employed in an academic position at a 2-year/4-year college (1), total from the above (doctoral) (2).

Additional Information:
Orientation, Objectives, and Emphasis of Department: The department represents a variety of theoretical orientations. The objective of the department is to train professionals to serve primarily clients who are relatively normal but who are experiencing difficulties related to personal adjustment, interpersonal relationships, developmental problems, crises, academic or career stress, or decisions. The employment settings for our graduates typically include college and university counseling and testing

services, community mental health agencies, clinics, hospitals, schools, rehabilitation centers, correctional centers, the United States Armed Services, and private practice.

Special Facilities or Resources: Facilities include an extensive medical center, including video equipment and computer terminals; training and observation rooms; and practicum and internship sites in a variety of settings for master's and doctoral students.

Information for Students With Physical Disabilities: See the following Web site for more information: http://socialjustice.wvu.edu/office_of_disability_services.

Application Information:
Send to Admissions Coordinator, Department of Counseling, Rehabilitation Counseling and Counseling Psychology, West Virginia University, P.O. Box 6122, Morgantown, WV 25606-6122. Application available online. URL of online application: http://counseling.wvu.edu/counseling_psychology/future_students/admissions. Students are admitted in the Fall, application deadline December 1. *Fee:* $50.

West Virginia University
Department of Psychology
Eberly College of Arts and Sciences
P.O. Box 6040
Morgantown, WV 26506-6040
Telephone: (304) 293-2001, ext. 31628
Fax: (304) 293-6606
E-mail: *Debra.Swinney@mail.wvu.edu*
Web: *http://www.psychology.wvu.edu*

Department Information:
1929. Chairperson: Michael Perone. Number of faculty: total—full-time 24; women—full-time 16.

Programs and Degrees Offered:
Listed in the following order: Program area, degree type (T if terminal Master's), number awarded 7/08–6/09. Life-Span Developmental Psychology PhD (Doctor of Philosophy) 0, Clinical Psychology PhD (Doctor of Philosophy) 5, Behavioral Neuroscience PhD (Doctor of Philosophy) 0, Behavior Analysis PhD (Doctor of Philosophy) 5, Clinical Psychology MA/MS (Master of Arts/Science) (T) 0, Applied Behavior Analysis MA/MS (Master of Arts/Science) (T) 0.

APA Accreditation: Clinical PhD (Doctor of Philosophy). Student Outcome Data Website: http://community.wvu.edu/~ktl000/StudentData.html.

Student Applications/Admissions:
Student Applications
Life-Span Developmental Psychology PhD (Doctor of Philosophy)—Applications 2009–2010, 16. Total applicants accepted 2009–2010, 5. Number full-time enrolled (new admits only) 2009–2010, 4. Number part-time enrolled (new admits only) 2009–2010, 0. Openings 2010–2011, 5. The number of students enrolled full- and part-time who were dismissed or voluntarily withdrew from this program area in 2008–2009 were 1. *Clinical Psychology PhD (Doctor of Philosophy)*—Applications 2009–2010, 121. Total applicants accepted 2009–2010, 10. Number full-time enrolled (new admits only) 2009–2010, 10. Number part-time enrolled (new admits only) 2009–2010, 0. Openings 2010–2011, 6. The median number of years required for completion of a degree in 2008–2009 were 5. The number of students enrolled full- and part-time who were dismissed or voluntarily withdrew from this program area in 2008–2009 were 0. *Behavioral Neuroscience PhD (Doctor of Philosophy)*—Applications 2009–2010, 0. Total applicants accepted 2009–2010, 0. Number full-time enrolled (new admits only) 2009–2010, 0. Number part-time enrolled (new admits only) 2009–2010, 0. Openings 2010–2011, 3. The number of students enrolled full- and part-time who were dismissed or voluntarily withdrew from this program area in 2008–2009 were 0. *Behavior Analysis PhD (Doctor of Philosophy)*—Applications 2009–2010, 32. Total applicants accepted 2009–2010, 4. Number full-time enrolled (new admits only) 2009–2010, 4. Number part-time enrolled (new admits only) 2009–2010, 0. Openings 2010–2011, 5. The median number of years required for completion of a degree in 2008–2009 were 5. The number of students enrolled full- and part-time who were dismissed or voluntarily withdrew from this program area in 2008–2009 were 1. *Clinical Psychology MA/MS (Master of Arts/Science)*—Applications 2009–2010, 7. Total applicants accepted 2009–2010, 2. Number full-time enrolled (new admits only) 2009–2010, 2. Number part-time enrolled (new admits only) 2009–2010, 0. Openings 2010–2011, 2. The number of students enrolled full- and part-time who were dismissed or voluntarily withdrew from this program area in 2008–2009 were 0. *Applied Behavior Analysis MA/MS (Master of Arts/Science)*—Applications 2009–2010, 18. Total applicants accepted 2009–2010, 2. Number full-time enrolled (new admits only) 2009–2010, 2. Number part-time enrolled (new admits only) 2009–2010, 0. Openings 2010–2011, 5. The number of students enrolled full- and part-time who were dismissed or voluntarily withdrew from this program area in 2008–2009 were 0.

Scores: Entries appear in this order: required test or GPA, minimum score (if required), median score of students entering in 2009–2010. *Life-span Developmental Psychology PhD (Doctor of Philosophy)*: GRE-V 500, 465, GRE-Q 500, 605, GRE-Analytical no minimum stated, 4.5, overall undergraduate GPA 3.00, 3.72, last 2 years GPA no minimum stated, psychology GPA no minimum stated; *Clinical Psychology PhD (Doctor of Philosophy)*: GRE-V 500, 585, GRE-Q 500, 645, GRE-Analytical no minimum stated, 4.5, GRE-Subject (Psychology) no minimum stated, 690, overall undergraduate GPA 3.00, 3.61, last 2 years GPA no minimum stated, psychology GPA no minimum stated; *Behavioral Neuroscience PhD (Doctor of Philosophy)*: GRE-V 500, GRE-Q 500, GRE-Analytical no minimum stated, overall undergraduate GPA 3.00, last 2 years GPA no minimum stated, psychology GPA no minimum stated; *Behavior Analysis PhD (Doctor of Philosophy)*: GRE-V 500, 540, GRE-Q 500, 645, GRE-Analytical no minimum stated, 5.25, overall undergraduate GPA 3.00, 3.83, last 2 years GPA no minimum stated, psychology GPA no minimum stated; *Clinical Psychology MA/MS (Master of Arts/Science)*: GRE-V 500, 665, GRE-Q 500, 625, GRE-Analytical no minimum stated, 4.5, GRE-Subject (Psychology) no minimum stated, 670, overall undergraduate GPA 3.00, 3.83, last 2 years GPA no minimum stated, psychology GPA no minimum stated; *Applied Behavior Analysis MA/MS (Master of Arts/Science)*: GRE-V 500, 455,

GRE-Q 500, 640, GRE-Analytical no minimum stated, 4.25, overall undergraduate GPA 3.00, 3.37, last 2 years GPA no minimum stated, psychology GPA no minimum stated.

Other Criteria: (importance of criteria rated low, medium, or high): GRE scores—high, research experience—high, work experience—medium, extracurricular activity—medium, clinically related public service—medium, GPA—high, letters of recommendation—high, interview—high, statement of goals and objectives—high, specific undergraduate psychology courses taken—medium, Match between faculty and student interests is of high importance. Only clinical programs give high value to clinically related public service. Research experience is of medium importance for the Master's program. For additional information on admission requirements, go to http://psychology.wvu.edu/future_students/graduate_programs.

Student Characteristics: The following represents characteristics of students in 2009–2010 in all graduate psychology programs in the department: Female—full-time 63, part-time 0; Male—full-time 26, part-time 0; African American/Black—full-time 2, part-time 0; Hispanic/Latino(a)—full-time 2, part-time 0; Asian/Pacific Islander—full-time 2, part-time 0; American Indian/Alaska Native—full-time 0, part-time 0; Caucasian/White—full-time 79, part-time 0; Multi-ethnic—full-time 0, part-time 0; students subject to the Americans With Disabilities Act—full-time 0, part-time 0; Unknown ethnicity—full-time 4, part-time 0; International students who hold an F-1 or J-1 Visa—full-time 7, part-time 0.

Financial Information/Assistance:

Tuition for Full-Time Study: *Master's:* State residents: per academic year $5,838, $327 per credit hour; Nonstate residents: per academic year $16,920, $943 per credit hour. *Doctoral:* State residents: per academic year $5,838, $327 per credit hour; Nonstate residents: per academic year $16,920, $943 per credit hour. Tuition is subject to change. See the following Web site for updates and changes in tuition costs: http://adm.wvu.edu/home/cost_of_attendance.

Financial Assistance:

First-Year Students: Teaching assistantships available for first year. Average amount paid per academic year: $11,086. Average number of hours worked per week: 20. Apply by December 15. Research assistantships available for first year. Average amount paid per academic year: $11,086. Average number of hours worked per week: 20. Apply by December 15. Traineeships available for first year. Average amount paid per academic year: $11,086. Average number of hours worked per week: 20. Apply by December 15. Fellowships and scholarships available for first year. Average amount paid per academic year: $17,500. Average number of hours worked per week: 0. Apply by December 15.

Advanced Students: Teaching assistantships available for advanced students. Average amount paid per academic year: $11,635. Average number of hours worked per week: 20. Apply by December 15. Research assistantships available for advanced students. Average amount paid per academic year: $11,635. Average number of hours worked per week: 20. Apply by December 15. Traineeships available for advanced students. Average amount paid per academic year: $11,635. Average number of hours worked per week: 20. Apply by December 15. Fellowships and scholarships available for advanced students. Average amount paid per academic year: $17,500. Average number of hours worked per week: 0. Apply by December 15.

Additional Information: Of all students currently enrolled full time, 93% benefited from one or more of the listed financial assistance programs. Application and information available online at: http://psychology.wvu.edu/future_students/graduate_programs.

Internships/Practica: Doctoral Degree (PhD Clinical Psychology): For those doctoral students for whom a professional internship was required in this program prior to graduation, (8) students applied for an internship in 2008–2009, with (7) students obtaining an internship. Of those students who obtained an internship, (7) were paid internships. Of those students who obtained an internship, (7) students placed in APA/CPA accredited internships, (0) students placed in internships not APA/CPA accredited, but listed with the Association of Psychology Postdoctoral and Internship Programs (APPIC), (0) students placed in internships conforming to guidelines of the Council of Directors of School Psychology Programs (CDSPP), (0) students placed in internships that were not APA/CPA accredited, APPIC or CDSPP listed. Master's Degree (MA/MS Clinical Psychology): An internship experience, such as, a final research project or "capstone" experience is required of graduates. Paid clinical placements at out-of-department sites are available for doctoral clinical students who have earned master's degrees. These out-of-department practicum sites include WVU Carruth Counseling Center, Kennedy Federal Correctional Institution, Hopemont Hospital, Sharpe Hospital, the Robert C. Byrd Health Sciences Center, a private practice, various behavioral/community mental health agencies, and children and youth services agencies. These sites are located in Morgantown, and across the state and region. Stipends for practicum range from $13,000 to $16,000, require 16 hours of work per week, and virtually all last 12 months.

Housing and Day Care: On-campus housing is available. See the following Web site for more information: http://housing.wvu.edu/. On-campus day care facilities are available. See the following Web site for more information: http://childlearningcenter.wvu.edu/.

Employment of Department Graduates:

Master's Degree Graduates: Of those who graduated in the academic year 2008–2009, the following categories and numbers represent the postgraduate activities and employment of master's degree graduates: Enrolled in a postdoctoral residency/fellowship (n/a), employed in independent practice (n/a), total from the above (master's) (0).

Doctoral Degree Graduates: Of those who graduated in the academic year 2008–2009, the following categories and numbers represent the postgraduate activities and employment of doctoral degree graduates: Enrolled in a psychology doctoral program (n/a), enrolled in a postdoctoral residency/fellowship (4), employed in an academic position at a university (4), employed in business or industry (1), employed in a community mental health/counseling center (1), total from the above (doctoral) (10).

Additional Information:

Orientation, Objectives, and Emphasis of Department: The Psychology Department offers the Doctor of Philosophy degree in Behavior Analysis and Life-Span Developmental, Clinical Child, and Clinical Psychology, and terminal Professional Master's degrees in Applied Behavior Analysis and Clinical Psychology. The Department employs a junior colleague model of training, in which graduate students participate fully in research, teaching, and service activities. The Behavior Analysis doctoral program trains students in basic research, theory, and applications of behavioral psychology. These three areas of study are integrated in the Behavior Analysis curriculum; however, a student may emphasize either basic or applied research. The Master's degree program in Applied Behavior Analysis trains students in the applications of behavior principles and concepts in situations of daily life. The Life-Span Developmental program emphasizes cognitive and social/personality development across the life span. It combines breadth of exposure across a variety of perspectives on the life span with depth and rigor in research training and the opportunity to specialize in an age period such as infancy, childhood, adolescence, or adulthood and old age. The Master's and PhD Clinical programs have a behavioral/cognitive behavioral orientation. The Clinical Doctoral programs train scientist–practitioners who function effectively in academic, medical center, or clinical applied settings. Specializations in developmental psychology, behavior analysis, and health psychology are available. The Clinical Professional Master's Program is designed to train practitioners with a terminal Master's degree to work with adults in rural areas.

Special Facilities or Resources: The Department moved into the new Life Sciences Building in July 2002. This building has modern animal research quarters for work with rats, pigeons, and other species. There are several computer-based laboratories and other laboratories for studies of learning in humans and animals, behavioral pharmacology, and neurosciences. There are additional facilities for human research in learning, cognition, small group processes, developmental psychology, social behavior, and psychophysiology. Clinical practicum opportunities are available through the Department's Quin Curtis Center for Psychological Service, Training, and Research, as well as in numerous mental health agencies throughout the state. Videotaping and direct observation equipment and facilities are available. The West Virginia University Medical Center provides facilities for research and training in such departments and areas as behavioral medicine and psychiatry, pediatrics, neurology, and dentistry. Local preschools and public schools have been cooperative in providing access to children and facilities for child development research; local businesses and other agencies offer sites for practice and research in applied behavior analysis, local senior centers and homes provide access to older adult populations, and the University's Center on Aging-Education Unit and Center for Women's Studies facilitate research related to their purviews. The University maintains an extensive network of computer facilities, and the Department provides an office and a computer for every graduate student.

Information for Students With Physical Disabilities: See the following Web site for more information: http://socialjustice.wvu.edu/office_of_disability_services.

Application Information:
Send to Departmental Admissions Committee, Department of Psychology, West Virginia University, P.O. Box 6040, Morgantown, WV 26506-6040. Application available online. URL of online application: http://psychology.wvu.edu/future_students/graduate_programs/doctoral_programs/how_to_apply. Students are admitted in the Fall, application deadline December 15. Professional MA in Clinical Psychology and MA in Applied Behavior Analysis application deadline is March 1. *Fee:* $50.

WISCONSIN

Marquette University
Department of Counselor Education and Counseling Psychology
College of Education
561 North 15th Street 146 Schroeder Complex
Milwaukee, WI 53201-1881
Telephone: (414) 288-5790
Fax: (414) 288-6100
E-mail: *alan.burkard@marquette.edu*
Web: *http://www.marquette.edu/education/grad/cecp.shtml*

Department Information:
1996. Chairperson: Alan W. Burkard. Number of faculty: total—full-time 7; women—full-time 3; total—minority—full-time 1; women minority—full-time 1.

Programs and Degrees Offered:
Listed in the following order: Program area, degree type (T if terminal Master's), number awarded 7/08–6/09. Counseling MA/MS (Master of Arts/Science) (T) 34, Counseling Psychology PhD (Doctor of Philosophy) 5.

APA Accreditation: Counseling PhD (Doctor of Philosophy). Student Outcome Data Website: http://www.marquette.edu/education/grad/cecp_doctorate_disclosure.shtml.

Student Applications/Admissions:

Student Applications

Counseling MA/MS (Master of Arts/Science)—Applications 2009–2010, 104. Total applicants accepted 2009–2010, 30. Number full-time enrolled (new admits only) 2009–2010, 30. Number part-time enrolled (new admits only) 2009–2010, 6. Total enrolled 2009–2010 full-time, 61, part-time, 20. Openings 2010–2011, 40. The median number of years required for completion of a degree in 2008–2009 were 2. The number of students enrolled full- and part-time who were dismissed or voluntarily withdrew from this program area in 2008–2009 were 3. *Counseling Psychology PhD (Doctor of Philosophy)*—Applications 2009–2010, 72. Total applicants accepted 2009–2010, 4. Number full-time enrolled (new admits only) 2009–2010, 4. Number part-time enrolled (new admits only) 2009–2010, 0. Total enrolled 2009–2010 full-time, 26, part-time, 10. Openings 2010–2011, 4. The median number of years required for completion of a degree in 2008–2009 were 6. The number of students enrolled full- and part-time who were dismissed or voluntarily withdrew from this program area in 2008–2009 were 0.

Scores: Entries appear in this order: required test or GPA, minimum score (if required), median score of students entering in 2009–2010. *Counseling MA/MS (Master of Arts/Science):* GRE-V no minimum stated, 463, GRE-Q no minimum stated, 554, GRE-Analytical no minimum stated, 4.44, overall undergraduate GPA no minimum stated, 3.35; *Counseling Psychology PhD (Doctor of Philosophy):* GRE-V no minimum stated, 470, GRE-Q no minimum stated, 553, GRE-Analytical no minimum stated, 4.5, overall undergraduate GPA no minimum stated, 3.33, Masters GPA no minimum stated, 3.64.

Other Criteria: (importance of criteria rated low, medium, or high): GRE scores—medium, research experience—medium, work experience—medium, extracurricular activity—medium, clinically related public service—medium, GPA—high, letters of recommendation—high, interview—high, statement of goals and objectives—high, undergraduate major in psychology—low, specific undergraduate psychology courses taken—medium. Applicants' goals and objectives, interviews, and letters of recommendation are important for admission into all our master's and doctoral programs. Research experience is much more important for admission into our PhD program. For additional information on admission requirements, go to http://www.marquette.edu/education/grad/cecp_grad_admissions.shtml.

Student Characteristics: The following represents characteristics of students in 2009–2010 in all graduate psychology programs in the department: Female—full-time 73, part-time 14; Male—full-time 18, part-time 6; African American/Black—full-time 5, part-time 1; Hispanic/Latino(a)—full-time 2, part-time 1; Asian/Pacific Islander—full-time 5, part-time 1; American Indian/Alaska Native—full-time 0, part-time 0; Caucasian/White—full-time 65, part-time 17; Multi-ethnic—full-time 0, part-time 0; students subject to the Americans With Disabilities Act—full-time 2, part-time 1; Unknown ethnicity—full-time 14, part-time 0; International students who hold an F-1 or J-1 Visa—full-time 2, part-time 0.

Financial Information/Assistance:

Tuition for Full-Time Study: *Master's:* State residents: $645 per credit hour; Nonstate residents: $645 per credit hour. *Doctoral:* State residents: $645 per credit hour; Nonstate residents: $645 per credit hour. See the following Web site for updates and changes in tuition costs: http://www.marquette.edu/grad/future_tuition.shtml.

Financial Assistance:

First-Year Students: Teaching assistantships available for first year. Average amount paid per academic year: $3,000. Average number of hours worked per week: 10. Apply by February 15. Research assistantships available for first year. Average amount paid per academic year: $6,600. Average number of hours worked per week: 10. Apply by February 15. Fellowships and scholarships available for first year. Average amount paid per academic year: $0. Average number of hours worked per week: 0. Apply by February 15.

Advanced Students: Teaching assistantships available for advanced students. Average amount paid per academic year: $3,000. Average number of hours worked per week: 10. Apply by February 15. Research assistantships available for advanced students. Average amount paid per academic year: $6,600. Average number of hours worked per week: 10. Apply by February 15. Traineeships available for advanced students. Fellowships and scholarships available for advanced students. Average amount paid per academic year: $13,000. Average number of hours worked per week: 0.

Additional Information: Of all students currently enrolled full time, 100% benefited from one or more of the listed financial assistance programs. Application and information available online at: http://www.marquette.edu/grad/finaid_index.shtml.

Internships/Practica: Doctoral Degree (PhD Counseling Psychology): For those doctoral students for whom a professional internship was required in this program prior to graduation, (7) students applied for an internship in 2008–2009, with (6) students obtaining an internship. Of those students who obtained an internship, (6) were paid internships. Of those students who obtained an internship, (6) students placed in APA/CPA accredited internships, (0) students placed in internships not APA/CPA accredited, but listed with the Association of Psychology Postdoctoral and Internship Programs (APPIC), (0) students placed in internships conforming to guidelines of the Council of Directors of School Psychology Programs (CDSPP), (0) students placed in internships that were not APA/CPA accredited, APPIC or CDSPP listed. We work with a wide range of inpatient and outpatient agencies and educational institutions serving a broad range of clients from children to seniors and from relatively minor adjustment issues to serious psychopathology. We currently work with approximately 60 agencies and schools and continually try to find additional sites which offer superior clinical experience and supervision.

Housing and Day Care: On-campus housing is available. See the following Web site for more information: http://www.marquette.edu/orl/. On-campus day care facilities are available. Child care information is available by calling (414) 288-5655.

Employment of Department Graduates:
Master's Degree Graduates: Of those who graduated in the academic year 2008–2009, the following categories and numbers represent the postgraduate activities and employment of master's degree graduates: Enrolled in a psychology doctoral program (6), enrolled in another graduate/professional program (2), enrolled in a postdoctoral residency/fellowship (n/a), employed in independent practice (n/a), employed in other positions at a higher education institution (3), employed in a professional position in a school system (11), employed in business or industry (1), employed in a community mental health/counseling center (19), employed in a hospital/medical center (2), total from the above (master's) (44).
Doctoral Degree Graduates: Of those who graduated in the academic year 2008–2009, the following categories and numbers represent the postgraduate activities and employment of doctoral degree graduates: Enrolled in a psychology doctoral program (n/a), enrolled in a postdoctoral residency/fellowship (2), employed in an academic position at a university (4), employed in other positions at a higher education institution (1), employed in a community mental health/counseling center (1), employed in a hospital/medical center (5), other employment position (1), total from the above (doctoral) (14).

Additional Information:
Orientation, Objectives, and Emphasis of Department: Our Master's in Counseling and PhD in Counseling Psychology programs are based on a comprehensive biopsychosocial approach to understanding human behavior. We believe that a sensitivity to biological, psychological, social, multicultural, and developmental influences on behavior increases students' effectiveness both as practitioners and as researchers. We use a generalist approach that includes broad preparation in the diverse areas needed to practice competently as psychological scientists and practitioners in today's health care systems. The masters program in counseling includes school counseling and community counseling (3 focus areas: addiction-mental health, adult, child/adolescent).

Special Facilities or Resources: Our faculty, and Marquette University as a whole, are committed to offering high quality education. Our coursework, practica, research activities, and other training opportunities are all designed to provide very current and comprehensive preparation. Our student body is small, so students receive substantial individual attention. We are also committed to developing students' competencies to work with diverse multicultural groups, and we welcome applications from individuals with diverse backgrounds. All of the full-time faculty are engaged in a variety of research projects with which students may become involved. In addition, department faculty are associated with two research centers that provide a variety of excellent opportunities for research and professional training: the Center for Addiction and Behavioral Health Research, and the Integrative Neuroscience Research Center. Furthermore, our close affiliation with the Behavior Clinic, a community-based facility focusing on children 0-5 years of age and their parents, provides counseling and research opportunities for our students.

Information for Students With Physical Disabilities: See the following Web site for more information: http://www.marquette.edu/oses/disabilityservices/.

Application Information:
Send to Graduate School, P.O. Box 1881, Milwaukee, WI 53201. Application available online. URL of online application: http://www.marquette.edu/grad/future_apply.shtml. Students are admitted in the Fall, application deadline December 1. The application deadline for the PhD program is December 1, and February 1 for the master's programs. *Fee:* $50. Fee waived for Marquette Alumni.

Marquette University
Department of Psychology
Arts and Sciences
P.O. Box 1881
Milwaukee, WI 53201-1881
Telephone: (414) 288-7218
Fax: (414) 288-5333
E-mail: *kristy.nielson@marquette.edu*
Web: *http://www.marquette.edu/psyc*

Department Information:
1952. Chairperson: Kristy A. Nielson. Number of faculty: total—full-time 17; women—full-time 8; total—minority—full-time 1; women minority—full-time 1.

Programs and Degrees Offered:
Listed in the following order: Program area, degree type (T if terminal Master's), number awarded 7/08–6/09. Clinical Psychology PhD (Doctor of Philosophy) 11.

APA Accreditation: Clinical PhD (Doctor of Philosophy).

Student Applications/Admissions:
Student Applications
Clinical Psychology PhD (Doctor of Philosophy)—Applications 2009–2010, 118. Total applicants accepted 2009–2010, 10. Number full-time enrolled (new admits only) 2009–2010, 8. Number part-time enrolled (new admits only) 2009–2010, 0. Total enrolled 2009–2010 full-time, 32, part-time, 18. Openings 2010–2011, 6. The median number of years required for completion of a degree in 2008–2009 were 7. The number of students enrolled full- and part-time who were dismissed or voluntarily withdrew from this program area in 2008–2009 were 0.
Scores: Entries appear in this order: required test or GPA, minimum score (if required), median score of students entering in 2009–2010. Clinical Psychology PhD (Doctor of Philosophy): GRE-V 430, 550, GRE-Q 470, 690, GRE-Analytical no minimum stated, overall undergraduate GPA 3.0, 3.6.
Other Criteria: (importance of criteria rated low, medium, or high): GRE scores—high, research experience—high, work experience—low, clinically related public service—medium, GPA—medium, letters of recommendation—high, interview—high, statement of goals and objectives—high, undergraduate major in psychology—medium, specific undergraduate psychology courses taken—high. For additional information on admission requirements, go to http://www.mu.edu/psyc.

Student Characteristics: The following represents characteristics of students in 2009–2010 in all graduate psychology programs in the department: Female—full-time 23, part-time 11; Male—full-time 9, part-time 7; African American/Black—full-time 1, part-time 0; Hispanic/Latino(a)—full-time 2, part-time 0; Asian/Pacific Islander—full-time 1, part-time 1; American Indian/Alaska Native—part-time 1; Caucasian/White—full-time 28, part-time 15; Multi-ethnic—part-time 1; students subject to the Americans With Disabilities Act—full-time 0, part-time 0; Unknown ethnicity—full-time 0, part-time 0; International students who hold an F-1 or J-1 Visa—full-time 0, part-time 0.

Financial Information/Assistance:
Tuition for Full-Time Study: *Doctoral:* State residents: $926 per credit hour; Nonstate residents: $926 per credit hour. Tuition is subject to change. See the following Web site for updates and changes in tuition costs: http://www.grad.mu.edu.

Financial Assistance:
First-Year Students: Teaching assistantships available for first year. Average amount paid per academic year: $14,750. Average number of hours worked per week: 20. Apply by December 15. Research assistantships available for first year. Average amount paid per academic year: $14,750. Average number of hours worked per week: 20. Apply by December 15. Fellowships and scholarships available for first year. Average amount paid per academic year: $16,000. Average number of hours worked per week: 0. Apply by December 15.
Advanced Students: Teaching assistantships available for advanced students. Average amount paid per academic year: $14,750. Average number of hours worked per week: 20. Apply by December 15. Research assistantships available for advanced students. Average amount paid per academic year: $14,750. Average number of hours worked per week: 20. Apply by December 15. Traineeships available for advanced students. Average number of hours worked per week: 8. Apply by December 15. Fellowships and scholarships available for advanced students. Average amount paid per academic year: $16,000. Average number of hours worked per week: 0. Apply by December 15.

Additional Information: Of all students currently enrolled full time, 45% benefited from one or more of the listed financial assistance programs. Application and information available online at: http://www.grad.mu.edu.

Internships/Practica: Doctoral Degree (PhD Clinical Psychology): For those doctoral students for whom a professional internship was required in this program prior to graduation, (4) students applied for an internship in 2008–2009, with (3) students obtaining an internship. Of those students who obtained an internship, (3) were paid internships. Of those students who obtained an internship, (3) students placed in APA/CPA accredited internships, (0) students placed in internships not APA/CPA accredited, but listed with the Association of Psychology Postdoctoral and Internship Programs (APPIC), (0) students placed in internships conforming to guidelines of the Council of Directors of School Psychology Programs (CDSPP), (0) students placed in internships that were not APA/CPA accredited, APPIC or CDSPP listed. Doctoral students obtain supervised clinical experience throughout their training. Practica are offered both in the Department's training clinic (the Center for Psychological Services) and in community agencies. The Department's training clinic provides assessment and intervention services to members of the general community under the supervision of licensed clinical faculty members. Students have averaged 750 hours in the clinic, and typically acquire 1,500 to 2,000 hours in pre-internship practicum experiences. Marquette University's urban location provides a wealth of training opportunities in the community. Recent practicum experiences have included placements in agencies that provide training in neuropsychological assessment, geropsychology, behavioral medicine, pediatric health, and family therapy. Doctoral students are required to complete a 2,000 hour internship. To date, students have completed APA-approved internships in settings located in the Milwaukee area as well as eight different states.

Housing and Day Care: On-campus housing is available. See the following Web site for more information: http://www.mu.edu/or/. On-campus day care facilities are available.

Employment of Department Graduates:
Master's Degree Graduates: Of those who graduated in the academic year 2008–2009, the following categories and numbers represent the postgraduate activities and employment of master's degree graduates: Enrolled in a psychology doctoral program (1), enrolled in a postdoctoral residency/fellowship (n/a), employed in independent practice (n/a), total from the above (master's) (1).
Doctoral Degree Graduates: Of those who graduated in the academic year 2008–2009, the following categories and numbers represent the postgraduate activities and employment of doctoral degree graduates: Enrolled in a psychology doctoral program (n/a), enrolled in another graduate/professional program (0), enrolled in a postdoctoral residency/fellowship (6), employed in independent practice (2), employed in an academic position at a university (1), employed in an academic position at a 2-year/4-year college (0), employed in other positions at a higher education institution (0), employed in a professional position in a school system (0), employed in business or industry (0), employed in government

agency (1), employed in a community mental health/counseling center (0), employed in a hospital/medical center (0), still seeking employment (0), not seeking employment (0), other employment position (1), total from the above (doctoral) (11).

Additional Information:
Orientation, Objectives, and Emphasis of Department: The Clinical Psychology program offers courses and training leading to the degree of Doctor of Philosophy (PhD) in Clinical Psychology. All doctoral students acquire a Master of Science degree as they progress toward the doctoral degree. The doctoral program is approved by the American Psychological Association to train scientist-professionals. Students receive a solid foundation in scientific areas of psychology and in the historical foundations of psychology. Training in research skills such as statistics, measurement, and research methods ensures competence in conducting empirical research and in critically evaluating one's own and others' clinical and empirical work. Students become competent in professional practice skills such as assessment, interventions, and consultation. Supervised clinical experiences are planned throughout the curriculum. Graduates of the doctoral program are prepared for employment as academics, researchers, clinical psychologists, consultants, teachers, and administrators.

Special Facilities or Resources: The department is located in completely refurbished and modern quarters that include a psychology clinic, an undergraduate teaching laboratory, and ample space for both faculty and student research. A full range of computer services is available at no charge to students. Located in a large metropolitan area, Marquette University is within easy commuting distance to a variety of hospitals and agencies in which training and research opportunities may be available.

Information for Students With Physical Disabilities: See the following Web site for more information: http://www.mu.edu/oses/disabilityservices.

Application Information:
Send to Graduate School, 305 Holthusen Hall, Marquette University, 1324 W. Wisconsin Avenue, Milwaukee, WI 53201-1881. Application available online. URL of online application: http://www.marquette.edu/grad/apply. Students are admitted in the Fall, application deadline December 15. *Fee:* $50. Waived for Marquette University alumni. Waived for evidence of financial need.

Wisconsin School of Professional Psychology
Professional School
9120 West Hampton Avenue, Suite 212
Milwaukee, WI 53225
Telephone: (414) 464-9777
Fax: (414) 358-5590
E-mail: *kathleenrusch@sbcglobal.net*
Web: *http://www.wspp.edu*

Department Information:
1980. President: Kathleen M. Rusch, PhD Number of faculty: total—full-time 7, part-time 24; women—full-time 5, part-time 10; minority—part-time 2; women minority—part-time 1.

Programs and Degrees Offered:
Listed in the following order: Program area, degree type (T if terminal Master's), number awarded 7/08–6/09. Clinical Psychology PsyD (Doctor of Psychology) 6.

APA Accreditation: Clinical PsyD (Doctor of Psychology). Student Outcome Data Website: http://www.wspp.edu/wacompl.html.

Student Applications/Admissions:
Student Applications
Clinical Psychology PsyD (Doctor of Psychology)—Applications 2009–2010, 20. Total applicants accepted 2009–2010, 15. Number full-time enrolled (new admits only) 2009–2010, 8. Number part-time enrolled (new admits only) 2009–2010, 7. Total enrolled 2009–2010 full-time, 22, part-time, 55. Openings 2010–2011, 15. The median number of years required for completion of a degree in 2008–2009 were 6. The number of students enrolled full- and part-time who were dismissed or voluntarily withdrew from this program area in 2008–2009 were 0.
Scores: Entries appear in this order: required test or GPA, minimum score (if required), median score of students entering in 2009–2010. *Clinical Psychology PsyD (Doctor of Psychology):* GRE-V 500, 500, GRE-Q 500, 500, GRE-Analytical 4.5, 4.5, overall undergraduate GPA 3.0, 3.0, last 2 years GPA no minimum stated, psychology GPA 3.5, 3.5, Masters GPA 3.75, 3.75.
Other Criteria: (importance of criteria rated low, medium, or high): GRE scores—medium, research experience—low, work experience—high, extracurricular activity—medium, clinically related public service—high, GPA—medium, letters of recommendation—high, interview—high, statement of goals and objectives—high, Essay—high, undergraduate major in psychology—medium, specific undergraduate psychology courses taken—high. For additional information on admission requirements, go to http://www.wspp.edu/admissions.html.

Student Characteristics: The following represents characteristics of students in 2009–2010 in all graduate psychology programs in the department: Female—full-time 21, part-time 43; Male—full-time 1, part-time 12; African American/Black—full-time 0, part-time 4; Hispanic/Latino(a)—full-time 0, part-time 0; Asian/Pacific Islander—full-time 1, part-time 1; American Indian/Alaska Native—full-time 0, part-time 0; Caucasian/White—full-time 21, part-time 50; Multi-ethnic—full-time 0, part-time 0; students subject to the Americans With Disabilities Act—full-time 0, part-time 2; Unknown ethnicity—full-time 0, part-time 0; International students who hold an F-1 or J-1 Visa—full-time 0, part-time 0.

Financial Information/Assistance:
Tuition for Full-Time Study: *Master's:* State residents: $700 per credit hour; Nonstate residents: $700 per credit hour. *Doctoral:* State residents: $700 per credit hour; Nonstate residents: $700 per credit hour. Tuition is subject to change. Additional fees are assessed to students beyond the costs of tuition for the following: $50 materials fee for all assessment courses.

Financial Assistance:
First-Year Students: Fellowships and scholarships available for first year. Average amount paid per academic year: $3,000.

Average number of hours worked per week: 0. Apply by February 15.

Advanced Students: Traineeships available for advanced students. Average number of hours worked per week: 12. Fellowships and scholarships available for advanced students. Average amount paid per academic year: $1,000. Average number of hours worked per week: 0. Apply by February 15.

Additional Information: Of all students currently enrolled full time, 4% benefited from one or more of the listed financial assistance programs. Application and information available online at: http://www.wspp.edu/FAWSPP.html.

Internships/Practica: Doctoral Degree (PsyD Clinical Psychology): For those doctoral students for whom a professional internship was required in this program prior to graduation, (12) students applied for an internship in 2008–2009, with (12) students obtaining an internship. Of those students who obtained an internship, (11) were paid internships. Of those students who obtained an internship, (1) students placed in APA/CPA accredited internships, (11) students placed in internships not APA/CPA accredited, but listed with the Association of Psychology Postdoctoral and Internship Programs (APPIC), (0) students placed in internships conforming to guidelines of the Council of Directors of School Psychology Programs (CDSPP), (0) students placed in internships that were not APA/CPA accredited, APPIC or CDSPP listed. WSPP has an on-site training clinic, the Psychology Center, which is designed to serve two purposes: to provide supervised training to students and to provide quality clinical services to an inner-city, multicultural, disadvantaged population. The Center also maintains contracts and affiliations with a number of local service agencies to provide on-site services. Regardless of whether on- or off-site, all practica are supervised by WSPP faculty to ensure quality of supervision and communication with our DCT. Some 40 supervisors, all licensed and most National Register listed, are readily available. For assessment practica, WSPP maintains a library of psychological tests available for student use free of charge. Thus, all students are guaranteed ample practicum opportunities (the program requires 2,000 hours) without having to search for sites or supervisors. This high level of clinical training has led to our 100% internship placement rate to date.

Housing and Day Care: No on-campus housing is available. No on-campus day care facilities are available.

Employment of Department Graduates:

Master's Degree Graduates: Of those who graduated in the academic year 2008–2009, the following categories and numbers represent the postgraduate activities and employment of master's degree graduates: Enrolled in a psychology doctoral program (0), enrolled in another graduate/professional program (0), enrolled in a postdoctoral residency/fellowship (n/a), employed in independent practice (n/a), employed in an academic position at a university (0), employed in an academic position at a 2-year/4-year college (0), employed in other positions at a higher education institution (0), employed in a professional position in a school system (0), employed in business or industry (0), employed in government agency (0), employed in a community mental health/counseling center (0), employed in a hospital/medical center (0), still seeking employment (0), not seeking employment (0), other employment position (0), do not know (0), total from the above (master's) (0).

Doctoral Degree Graduates: Of those who graduated in the academic year 2008–2009, the following categories and numbers represent the postgraduate activities and employment of doctoral degree graduates: Enrolled in a psychology doctoral program (n/a), enrolled in a postdoctoral residency/fellowship (0), employed in independent practice (0), employed in an academic position at a university (0), employed in an academic position at a 2-year/4-year college (0), employed in other positions at a higher education institution (0), employed in a professional position in a school system (1), employed in business or industry (0), employed in government agency (3), employed in a community mental health/counseling center (0), employed in a hospital/medical center (2), still seeking employment (0), not seeking employment (0), other employment position (0), do not know (0), total from the above (doctoral) (6).

Additional Information:

Orientation, Objectives, and Emphasis of Department: The Wisconsin School of Professional Psychology has as its goal the provision of a doctoral level education that emphasizes the acquisition of the traditional skills which defined the professional in the past, while staying open to new developments as they emerge. Our APA-accredited program balances theoretical and practical coursework, taking its impetus from the American Psychological Association's Vail Conference. The school's curriculum was developed in accordance with APA norms and is continually evaluated to assure compliance with the requirements of that body. WSPP trains students toward competence in the following areas: self-awareness, assessment, research and evaluation, ethics and professional standards, management and supervision, relationship, intervention, respect for diversity, consultation, social responsibility and community service. In its training philosophy, the school emphasizes clarity of verbal expression in written and oral communication, the development of clinical acumen, and an appreciation of the link between scientific data and clinical practice. Our program's small size and large faculty create abundant opportunities for mentorship with practicing psychologists in an apprentice-like setting.

Special Facilities or Resources: The Wisconsin School of Professional Psychology maintains a Training Clinic which includes facilities for research and practicum work associated with clinical courses. The Training Center houses an outpatient mental health clinic which serves a primarily inner city culturally diverse population, as well as provides opportunities for supervised experience with a wide range of clinical problems and populations. The center offers services to the community on a sliding fee basis. Supervision is provided by faculty.

Application Information:

Send to Wisconsin School of Professional Psychology, 9120 W. Hampton Avenue, Milwaukee, WI 53225. Application available online. URL of online application: http://www.wspp.edu/admissions.html. Students are admitted in the Fall, application deadline January 15; Spring, application deadline October 15. *Fee:* $75.

Wisconsin, University of, Eau Claire
Department of Psychology
Arts and Sciences
University of Wisconsin-Eau Claire
Eau Claire, WI 54702
Telephone: (715) 836-5733
Fax: (715) 836-2214
E-mail: *lozarb@uwec.edu*
Web: *http://www.uwec.edu/psyc*

Department Information:
1965. Chairperson: Lori Bica. Number of faculty: total—full-time 16, part-time 4; women—full-time 9, part-time 3.

Programs and Degrees Offered:
Listed in the following order: Program area, degree type (T if terminal Master's), number awarded 7/08–6/09. School Psychology EdS (School Psychology) 7.

Student Applications/Admissions:
Student Applications
School Psychology EdS (School Psychology)—Applications 2009–2010, 40. Total applicants accepted 2009–2010, 13. Number full-time enrolled (new admits only) 2009–2010, 8. Number part-time enrolled (new admits only) 2009–2010, 1. Total enrolled 2009–2010 full-time, 25, part-time, 1. Openings 2010–2011, 8. The median number of years required for completion of a degree in 2008–2009 were 3. The number of students enrolled full- and part-time who were dismissed or voluntarily withdrew from this program area in 2008–2009 were 0.
Scores: Entries appear in this order: required test or GPA, minimum score (if required), median score of students entering in 2009–2010. School Psychology EdS (School Psychology): GRE-V 400, 450, overall undergraduate GPA 3.0, 3.51.
Other Criteria: (importance of criteria rated low, medium, or high): GRE scores—high, research experience—medium, work experience—medium, extracurricular activity—medium, clinically related public service—medium, GPA—high, letters of recommendation—high, interview—high, statement of goals and objectives—high. For additional information on admission requirements, go to www.uwec.edu/psyc/graduate.htm.

Student Characteristics: The following represents characteristics of students in 2009–2010 in all graduate psychology programs in the department: Female—full-time 20, part-time 0; Male—full-time 5, part-time 1; African American/Black—full-time 0, part-time 0; Hispanic/Latino(a)—full-time 0, part-time 0; Asian/Pacific Islander—full-time 1, part-time 1; American Indian/Alaska Native—full-time 0, part-time 0; Caucasian/White—full-time 24, part-time 0; Multi-ethnic—full-time 0, part-time 0; students subject to the Americans With Disabilities Act—full-time 1, part-time 0; Unknown ethnicity—full-time 0, part-time 0; International students who hold an F-1 or J-1 Visa—full-time 1, part-time 1.

Financial Information/Assistance:
Tuition for Full-Time Study: Master's: State residents: per academic year $7,722, $429 per credit hour; Nonstate residents: per academic year $18,688, $1,038 per credit hour. Tuition is subject to change. See the following Web site for updates and changes in tuition costs: http://www.uwec.edu/admissions/graduate.

Financial Assistance:
First-Year Students: Teaching assistantships available for first year. Average amount paid per academic year: $7,013. Average number of hours worked per week: 13. Apply by March 1. Fellowships and scholarships available for first year. Average amount paid per academic year: $500. Apply by March 1.
Advanced Students: Teaching assistantships available for advanced students. Average amount paid per academic year: $7,013. Average number of hours worked per week: 13. Apply by March 1. Fellowships and scholarships available for advanced students. Average amount paid per academic year: $500. Apply by March 1.
Additional Information: Of all students currently enrolled full time, 80% benefited from one or more of the listed financial assistance programs. Application and information available online at: http://www.uwec.edu/admissions/graduate/fininfo.htm.

Internships/Practica: Internships are required for the Educational Specialist degree and comprise the third year of training. Students must complete a year of full-time practice as school psychologists under the supervision of an appropriately credentialed school psychologist. Students may enroll in the internship upon completion of all requirements except the thesis.

Housing and Day Care: No on-campus housing is available. On-campus day care facilities are available. See the following Web site for more information: http://www.uwec.edu/children.

Employment of Department Graduates:
Master's Degree Graduates: Of those who graduated in the academic year 2008–2009, the following categories and numbers represent the postgraduate activities and employment of master's degree graduates: Enrolled in a postdoctoral residency/fellowship (n/a), employed in independent practice (n/a), employed in a professional position in a school system (8), total from the above (master's) (8).
Doctoral Degree Graduates: Of those who graduated in the academic year 2008–2009, the following categories and numbers represent the postgraduate activities and employment of doctoral degree graduates: Enrolled in a psychology doctoral program (n/a), total from the above (doctoral) (0).

Additional Information:
Orientation, Objectives, and Emphasis of Department: The School Psychology program is offered by the Department of Psychology in cooperation with the College of Education and Human Services. The School Psychology program is based on the scientist–practitioner model. As scientists, students develop a strong data- and research-based orientation as problem solvers in the practice of school psychology. As practitioners, students develop a high level of competence in skills required of school psychologists: assessment, intervention, and evaluation at the individual, group,

and systems levels. Two values guide all aspects of the school psychologist's activities and the training program: 1) sensitivity to and respect for individual differences and diversity; and 2) high standards of ethical and professional conduct. The program has two unique features: the Human Development Center and an ongoing collaborative relationship with the Lac du Flambeau American Indian community.

Special Facilities or Resources: Extensive on-campus and field site training opportunities are available. Two interdisciplinary clinics—the Human Development Center (Psychology-School Psychology; Special Education-Learning Disabilities and Early Childhood; Communication Sciences and Disorders; and Elementary Education-Reading) and the Psychological Services Center (Psychology-School Psychology and Nursing)—provide on-campus training in diagnostics and intervention services. Area schools, residential facilities for developmentally disabled, emotionally disturbed youth and adults, and clinics offer an extensive array of additional supervised training settings. In addition, the program has a continuing collaborative relationship with the Lac du Flambeau American Indian community which offers opportunities for short-term or semester-long practica.

Information for Students With Physical Disabilities: See the following Web site for more information: www.uwec.edu/ssd.

Application Information:
Send to Office of Admissions, UW-Eau Claire, Eau Claire, WI 54702-4004. Application available online. URL of online application: http://apply.wisconsin.edu/. Students are admitted in the Fall, application deadline March 1. *Fee:* $56.

Wisconsin, University of, La Crosse
Department of Psychology/School Psychology
College of Liberal Studies
1725 State Street, 341 Graff Main Hall
La Crosse, WI 54601
Telephone: (608) 785-8441
Fax: (608) 785-8443
E-mail: *dixon.robe@uwlax.edu*
Web: *http://www.uwlax.edu/schoolpsych/*

Department Information:
1967. Chairperson: Emily J. Johnson. Number of faculty: total—full-time 18, part-time 4; women—full-time 13, part-time 2; total—minority—full-time 1.

Programs and Degrees Offered:
Listed in the following order: Program area, degree type (T if terminal Master's), number awarded 7/08–6/09. School Psychology EdS (School Psychology) 15.

Student Applications/Admissions:
Student Applications
School Psychology EdS (*School Psychology*)—Applications 2009–2010, 54. Total applicants accepted 2009–2010, 23. Number full-time enrolled (new admits only) 2009–2010, 12. Total enrolled 2009–2010 full-time, 24, part-time, 29. Openings 2010–2011, 12. The median number of years required for completion of a degree in 2008–2009 were 3. The number of students enrolled full- and part-time who were dismissed or voluntarily withdrew from this program area in 2008–2009 were 0.

Scores: Entries appear in this order: required test or GPA, minimum score (if required), median score of students entering in 2009–2010. *School Psychology EdS (School Psychology):* GRE-V no minimum stated, 450, GRE-Q no minimum stated, 560, GRE-Analytical no minimum stated, 4.4, overall undergraduate GPA no minimum stated, 3.52, last 2 years GPA no minimum stated, 3.7, psychology GPA no minimum stated, 3.67.

Other Criteria: (importance of criteria rated low, medium, or high): GRE scores—medium, research experience—medium, work experience—medium, extracurricular activity—medium, clinically related public service—high, GPA—high, letters of recommendation—high, interview—high, statement of goals and objectives—high, undergraduate major in psychology—low, specific undergraduate psychology courses taken—low.

Student Characteristics: The following represents characteristics of students in 2009–2010 in all graduate psychology programs in the department: Female—full-time 24, part-time 0; Male—full-time 0, part-time 0; African American/Black—full-time 0, part-time 0; Hispanic/Latino(a)—full-time 1, part-time 0; Asian/Pacific Islander—full-time 0, part-time 0; American Indian/Alaska Native—full-time 0, part-time 0; Caucasian/White—full-time 23, part-time 0; Multi-ethnic—full-time 0, part-time 0; students subject to the Americans With Disabilities Act—full-time 1, part-time 0; Unknown ethnicity—full-time 0, part-time 0; International students who hold an F-1 or J-1 Visa—full-time 0, part-time 0.

Financial Information/Assistance:
Tuition for Full-Time Study: Master's: State residents: per academic year $7,671, $426 per credit hour; Nonstate residents: per academic year $17,736, $985 per credit hour. Tuition is subject to change. Additional fees are assessed to students beyond the costs of tuition for the following: special course fees may be assessed for certain courses for supplemental materials and/or equipment. See the following Web site for updates and changes in tuition costs: http://www.uwlax.edu/cashiers/tuitionfeeschedule.htm.

Financial Assistance:
First-Year Students: Research assistantships available for first year. Average amount paid per academic year: $6,648. Average number of hours worked per week: 14. Apply by March 1.

Advanced Students: Research assistantships available for advanced students. Average amount paid per academic year: $6,648. Average number of hours worked per week: 14. Apply by March 1.

Additional Information: Of all students currently enrolled full time, 17% benefited from one or more of the listed financial assistance programs. Application and information available online at: http://www.uwlax.edu/schoolpsych/Graduate-Assistantships.htm.

Internships/Practica: The School Psychology program prepares graduate students for certification as School Psychologists through academic coursework, 700 hours of supervised school practica, and a one year, 1200-hour school internship. Graduate students are placed in local schools as early and intensively as possible. During their second, third and fourth semesters students spend two days per week working in local schools under the direct supervision of experienced school psychologists. During these school practica, students develop professional skills in assessment, consultation, intervention, counseling, and case management. Many of the core courses require projects which are completed in the schools during practica.

Housing and Day Care: On-campus housing is available. See the following Web site for more information: http://www.uwlax.edu/ResLife/. On-campus day care facilities are available. See the following Web site for more information: http://www.uwlax.edu/childcare/.

Employment of Department Graduates:
Master's Degree Graduates: Of those who graduated in the academic year 2008–2009, the following categories and numbers represent the postgraduate activities and employment of master's degree graduates: Enrolled in a postdoctoral residency/fellowship (n/a), employed in independent practice (n/a), employed in a professional position in a school system (7), total from the above (master's) (7).
Doctoral Degree Graduates: Of those who graduated in the academic year 2008–2009, the following categories and numbers represent the postgraduate activities and employment of doctoral degree graduates: Enrolled in a psychology doctoral program (n/a), total from the above (doctoral) (0).

Additional Information:
Orientation, Objectives, and Emphasis of Department: The emphasis of this program is to train school psychologists who are effective teacher, parent and school consultants. The program also emphasizes a pupil services model which addresses the educational and mental health needs of all children. The School Psychology knowledge base includes areas of Professional School Psychology, Educational Psychology, Psychological Foundations, Educational Foundations, and Mental Health. To provide psychological services in education, graduates of the School Psychology program must also have considerable knowledge of curriculum, special education and pupil services. Graduates of the program are employed in public schools or educational agencies which serve public schools.

Special Facilities or Resources: Extensive fieldwork in local schools is a key to professional training. Faculty work closely with field supervisors and observe student performance in the field.

Information for Students With Physical Disabilities: See the following Web site for more information: http://www.uwlax.edu/drs/.

Application Information:
Send to School Psychology Admissions, 341 Graff Main Hall, University of Wisconsin-La Crosse, 1725 State Street, La Crosse, WI 54601. Application available online. URL of online application: http://www.uwlax.edu/schoolpsych/. Students are admitted in the Fall, application deadline January 15. *Fee:* $56.

Wisconsin, University of, Madison
Department of Counseling Psychology, Counseling Psychology Program
School of Education
115 North Orchard Street
Madison, WI 53715-1150
Telephone: (608) 262-4708
Fax: (608) 265-3347
E-mail: *mgarity@education.wisc.edu*
Web: *http://www.education.wisc.edu/cp*

Department Information:
1964. Chairperson: Bruce E. Wampold. Number of faculty: total—full-time 8, part-time 1; women—full-time 5, part-time 1; total—minority—full-time 3; women minority—full-time 2; faculty subject to the Americans With Disabilities Act 1.

Programs and Degrees Offered:
Listed in the following order: Program area, degree type (T if terminal Master's), number awarded 7/08–6/09. Counseling MA/MS (Master of Arts/Science) (T) 20, Counseling Psychology PhD (Doctor of Philosophy) 7.

APA Accreditation: Counseling PhD (Doctor of Philosophy).

Student Applications/Admissions:
Student Applications
Counseling MA/MS (Master of Arts/Science)—Applications 2009–2010, 151. Total applicants accepted 2009–2010, 24. Number full-time enrolled (new admits only) 2009–2010, 15. Total enrolled 2009–2010 full-time, 29, part-time, 1. Openings 2010–2011, 18. The median number of years required for completion of a degree in 2008–2009 were 2. The number of students enrolled full- and part-time who were dismissed or voluntarily withdrew from this program area in 2008–2009 were 0. Counseling Psychology PhD (Doctor of Philosophy)—Applications 2009–2010, 77. Total applicants accepted 2009–2010, 6. Number full-time enrolled (new admits only) 2009–2010, 6. Number part-time enrolled (new admits only) 2009–2010, 0. Total enrolled 2009–2010 full-time, 49. Openings 2010–2011, 8. The median number of years required for completion of a degree in 2008–2009 were 8. The number of students enrolled full- and part-time who were dismissed or voluntarily withdrew from this program area in 2008–2009 were 2.

Scores: Entries appear in this order: required test or GPA, minimum score (if required), median score of students entering in 2009–2010. Counseling MA/MS (Master of Arts/Science): GRE-V no minimum stated, GRE-Q no minimum stated, GRE-Analytical no minimum stated, last 2 years GPA 3.0; Counseling Psychology PhD (Doctor of Philosophy): GRE-V no minimum stated, GRE-Q no minimum stated, GRE-Analytical no minimum stated, last 2 years GPA 3.0.

Other Criteria: (importance of criteria rated low, medium, or high): GRE scores—medium, research experience—high, work experience—medium, extracurricular activity—high, clinically related public service—high, GPA—medium, letters of recommendation—high, interview—high, statement of goals and objectives—high. For Master's, no interview required.

Student Characteristics: The following represents characteristics of students in 2009–2010 in all graduate psychology programs in the department: Female—full-time 52, part-time 0; Male—full-time 26, part-time 1; African American/Black—full-time 8, part-time 0; Hispanic/Latino(a)—full-time 11, part-time 0; Asian/Pacific Islander—full-time 8, part-time 0; American Indian/Alaska Native—full-time 1, part-time 0; Caucasian/White—full-time 47, part-time 1; Multi-ethnic—full-time 3, part-time 0; students subject to the Americans With Disabilities Act—full-time 0, part-time 0; Unknown ethnicity—full-time 0, part-time 0; International students who hold an F-1 or J-1 Visa—full-time 0, part-time 0.

Financial Information/Assistance:

Tuition for Full-Time Study: *Master's:* State residents: per academic year $5,517, $659 per credit hour; Nonstate residents: per academic year $25,073, $1,568 per credit hour. *Doctoral:* State residents: per academic year $5,517, $659 per credit hour; Nonstate residents: per academic year $25,042, $1,568 per credit hour. Tuition is subject to change. See the following Web site for updates and changes in tuition costs: http://registrar.wisc.edu.

Financial Assistance:

First-Year Students: Teaching assistantships available for first year. Average amount paid per academic year: $14,000. Average number of hours worked per week: 13. Apply by January 5. Research assistantships available for first year. Average amount paid per academic year: $14,000. Average number of hours worked per week: 13. Apply by January 5. Fellowships and scholarships available for first year. Average amount paid per academic year: $14,000. Average number of hours worked per week: 13. Apply by January 5.

Advanced Students: Teaching assistantships available for advanced students. Average amount paid per academic year: $14,000. Average number of hours worked per week: 13. Research assistantships available for advanced students. Average amount paid per academic year: $14,000. Average number of hours worked per week: 13. Fellowships and scholarships available for advanced students. Average amount paid per academic year: $14,000. Average number of hours worked per week: 13.

Additional Information: Of all students currently enrolled full time, 35% benefited from one or more of the listed financial assistance programs.

Internships/Practica: Doctoral Degree (PhD Counseling Psychology): For those doctoral students for whom a professional internship was required in this program prior to graduation, (9) students applied for an internship in 2008–2009, with (7) students obtaining an internship. Of those students who obtained an internship, (7) were paid internships. Of those students who obtained an internship, (7) students placed in APA/CPA accredited internships, (0) students placed in internships not APA/CPA accredited, but listed with the Association of Psychology Postdoctoral and Internship Programs (APPIC), (0) students placed in internships conforming to guidelines of the Council of Directors of School Psychology Programs (CDSPP), (0) students placed in internships that were not APA/CPA accredited, APPIC or CDSPP listed. Both master's and doctoral students are required to take at least two semesters of practica. For doctoral students (and some master's students), local sites include Dane County Community Mental Health Agency, Mendota Mental Health Institute, University of Wisconsin Counseling and Consultation Services, Veteran's Administration Hospital, and Family Therapy, Inc. Master's students may pursue practica in three types of settings: public schools, student services offices and counseling centers in higher education and community mental health agencies and private clinics. The majority of practicum placements are in the Madison area but some are placed in nearby metropolitan areas in Wisconsin such as Milwaukee and Green Bay, as well as in rural communities served by regional mental health clinics.

Housing and Day Care: On-campus housing is available. See the following Web site for more information: http://www.housing.wisc.edu/. On-campus day care facilities are available.

Employment of Department Graduates:

Master's Degree Graduates: Of those who graduated in the academic year 2008–2009, the following categories and numbers represent the postgraduate activities and employment of master's degree graduates: Enrolled in a psychology doctoral program (6), enrolled in a postdoctoral residency/fellowship (n/a), employed in independent practice (n/a), total from the above (master's) (6).

Doctoral Degree Graduates: Of those who graduated in the academic year 2008–2009, the following categories and numbers represent the postgraduate activities and employment of doctoral degree graduates: Enrolled in a psychology doctoral program (n/a), enrolled in a postdoctoral residency/fellowship (2), employed in an academic position at a university (2), still seeking employment (1), do not know (1), total from the above (doctoral) (6).

Additional Information:

Orientation, Objectives, and Emphasis of Department: The master's and doctoral programs are intended to provide a closely integrated didactic experimental curriculum for the preparation of counseling professionals. The master's degree strongly emphasizes service delivery, and its practica/internship components reflect that emphasis. The doctoral degree emphasizes the integration of counseling and psychological theory and practice with substantive development of research skills in the domains encompassed by counseling psychology. The PhD program in counseling psychology is APA-accredited utilizing the scientist–practitioner model. Students are prepared for academic, service-delivery, research, and administrative positions in professional psychology. The Department infuses principles of multiculturalism throughout the curriculum.

Special Facilities or Resources: The department possesses excellent computer facilities including multimedia production. Also, two counseling psychologists employed at the University Counseling Service are adjunct professors in the department and provide us with on-going linkage with that service for practica and internships. We also have very up-to-date computer software assessment resources. The department, together with departments of Rehabilitation Psychology, Special Education, and School Psychology, utilizes an interdisciplinary training center that provides professional training practices.

Information for Students With Physical Disabilities: See the following Web site for more information: http://www.mcburney.wisc.edu.

Application Information:

Send to Department of Counseling Psychology, Graduate Admissions, UW-Madison, 115 North Orchard Street, Rust-Schreiner Hall, Madison, WI 53715. Application available online. URL of online application: https://www.gradsch.wisc.edu/eapp/eapp.pl. Students are admitted in the Fall, application deadline; Summer, application deadline. For the Fall, application deadline is PhD- December 15, Master's- February 1. For the Summer, application deadlines are the same. *Fee:* $56.

Wisconsin, University of, Madison
Department of Educational Psychology, School Psychology Program
1025 West Johnson Street
Madison, WI 53706-1796
Telephone: (608) 262-3432
Fax: (608) 262-0843
E-mail: *edpsych@wisc.edu*
Web: *http://www.education.wisc.edu/edpsych/*

Department Information:
1960. Chairperson: Charles W. Kalish. Number of faculty: total—full-time 9; women—full-time 4; total—minority—full-time 1; women minority—full-time 1.

Programs and Degrees Offered:
Listed in the following order: Program area, degree type (T if terminal Master's), number awarded 7/08–6/09. School Psychology PhD (Doctor of Philosophy) 3, Quantitative Psychology PhD (Doctor of Philosophy) 1, Learning Science PhD (Doctor of Philosophy) 0, Human Development PhD (Doctor of Philosophy).

APA Accreditation: School PhD (Doctor of Philosophy).

Student Applications/Admissions:
Student Applications
School Psychology PhD (Doctor of Philosophy)—Applications 2009–2010, 70. Total applicants accepted 2009–2010, 9. Number full-time enrolled (new admits only) 2009–2010, 4. Openings 2010–2011, 8. The median number of years required for completion of a degree in 2008–2009 were 6. The number of students enrolled full- and part-time who were dismissed or voluntarily withdrew from this program area in 2008–2009 were 0. *Quantitative Psychology PhD (Doctor of Philosophy)*—Applications 2009–2010, 14. Total applicants accepted 2009–2010, 6. Number full-time enrolled (new admits only) 2009–2010, 2. Total enrolled 2009–2010 full-time, 11. Openings 2010–2011, 3. The median number of years required for completion of a degree in 2008–2009 were 6. The number of students enrolled full- and part-time who were dismissed or voluntarily withdrew from this program area in 2008–2009 were 0. *Learning Science PhD (Doctor of Philosophy)*—*Human Development PhD (Doctor of Philosophy)*—
Scores: Entries appear in this order: required test or GPA, minimum score (if required), median score of students entering in 2009–2010. *School Psychology PhD (Doctor of Philosophy):* overall undergraduate GPA 3.0, 3.61; *Quantitative Psychology PhD (Doctor of Philosophy):* overall undergraduate GPA 3.0, 3.52.
Other Criteria: (importance of criteria rated low, medium, or high): GRE scores—medium, research experience—medium, work experience—medium, extracurricular activity—low, clinically related public service—medium, GPA—medium, letters of recommendation—high, interview—high, statement of goals and objectives—high.

Student Characteristics: The following represents characteristics of students in 2009–2010 in all graduate psychology programs in the department: Female—full-time 33, part-time 0; Male—full-time 8, part-time 0; African American/Black—full-time 2, part-time 0; Hispanic/Latino(a)—full-time 2, part-time 0; Asian/Pacific Islander—full-time 4, part-time 0; American Indian/Alaska Native—full-time 1, part-time 0; Caucasian/White—full-time 32, part-time 0; Multi-ethnic—full-time 0, part-time 0; students subject to the Americans With Disabilities Act—full-time 0, part-time 0; Unknown ethnicity—full-time 0, part-time 0; International students who hold an F-1 or J-1 Visa—full-time 0, part-time 0.

Financial Information/Assistance:
Tuition for Full-Time Study: Master's: State residents: per academic year $10,518, $659 per credit hour; Nonstate residents: per academic year $25,072, $1,569 per credit hour. *Doctoral:* State residents: per academic year $10,518, $659 per credit hour; Nonstate residents: per academic year $25,072, $1,569 per credit hour. Tuition is subject to change. See the following Web site for updates and changes in tuition costs: http://www.registrar.wisc.edu/.

Financial Assistance:
First-Year Students: Teaching assistantships available for first year. Average amount paid per academic year: $14,087. Average number of hours worked per week: 20. Apply by December 1. Research assistantships available for first year. Average amount paid per academic year: $16,506. Average number of hours worked per week: 20. Apply by December 1. Traineeships available for first year. Apply by December 1. Fellowships and scholarships available for first year. Average amount paid per academic year: $18,756. Average number of hours worked per week: 0. Apply by December 1.

Advanced Students: Teaching assistantships available for advanced students. Average amount paid per academic year: $16,264. Average number of hours worked per week: 20. Apply by December 1. Research assistantships available for advanced students. Average amount paid per academic year: $16,506. Average number of hours worked per week: 20. Apply by December 1. Traineeships available for advanced students. Apply by December 1. Fellowships and scholarships available for advanced students. Average amount paid per academic year: $18,756. Average number of hours worked per week: 0. Apply by December 1.

Additional Information: Of all students currently enrolled full time, 76% benefited from one or more of the listed financial assistance programs. Application and information available online at: http://www.grad.wisc.edu/education/funding.

Internships/Practica: Doctoral Degree (PhD School Psychology): For those doctoral students for whom a professional internship was required in this program prior to graduation, (5) students applied for an internship in 2008–2009, with (5) students obtaining an internship. Of those students who obtained an internship, (5) were paid internships. Of those students who obtained an internship, (0) students placed in APA/CPA accredited internships, (5) students placed in internships not APA/CPA accredited, but listed with the Association of Psychology Postdoctoral and Internship Programs (APPIC), (0) students placed in internships conforming to guidelines of the Council of Directors of School Psychology Programs (CDSPP), (0) students placed in internships that were not APA/CPA accredited, APPIC or CDSPP listed. The School Psychology program admits students interested in obtaining a PhD. Students working toward this goal complete a two-semester clinical practicum experience during year two (200-hour minimum) and a two-semester field practicum during year three (400-hour minimum). This practicum experience is provided by the department. After the master's, students are required to complete either an APA approved internship or establish one of their own in a school (public or private), clinic, or hospital, that is approved by the program (minimum 200 hours) to complete their PhD requirements. The Wisconsin Internship Consortium in Professional School Psychology (WICPSP) is also administered through the School Psychology Program. The primary focus of the predoctoral internship program is to provide advanced training for graduate students from a wide variety of cooperating sites where an internship is provided over several rotations. This internship is implemented according to Ethical Principles of Psychologists (APA, 1992), and the criteria published by the National Register of Health Service Providers and the National Association of School Psychologists are also followed. Criteria endorsed by the Council of Directors of School Psychology are also met.

Housing and Day Care: On-campus housing is available. See the following Web site for more information: http://www.housing.wisc.edu. On-campus day care facilities are available. http://occfr.wisc.edu.

Employment of Department Graduates:

Master's Degree Graduates: Of those who graduated in the academic year 2008–2009, the following categories and numbers represent the postgraduate activities and employment of master's degree graduates: Enrolled in a psychology doctoral program (5), enrolled in a postdoctoral residency/fellowship (n/a), employed in independent practice (n/a), total from the above (master's) (5).
Doctoral Degree Graduates: Of those who graduated in the academic year 2008–2009, the following categories and numbers represent the postgraduate activities and employment of doctoral degree graduates: Enrolled in a psychology doctoral program (n/a), enrolled in another graduate/professional program (0), enrolled in a postdoctoral residency/fellowship (1), employed in an academic position at a university (1), employed in a professional position in a school system (3), employed in business or industry (1), total from the above (doctoral) (6).

Additional Information:

Orientation, Objectives, and Emphasis of Department: The School Psychology program, within the Department of Educational Psychology, prepares professional psychologists to use knowledge of the behavioral sciences in ways that enhance the learning and adjustment of both normal and exceptional children, their families, and their teachers. A balanced emphasis is placed on developing competencies necessary for functioning in both applied settings such as schools and community agencies, and in research positions in institutions of higher education. The program focus is the study of psychological and educational principles which influence the adjustment of individuals from birth to 21 years. Students are required to demonstrate competencies in the substantive content areas of psychological and educational theory and practice.

Special Facilities or Resources: The Educational and Psychological Training Center serves advanced graduate students in educational psychology. It provides diagnostic and treatment services for children and adolescents experiencing a variety of learning and behavior problems. The Laboratory of Experimental Design provides assistance to students and faculty in the design and analysis of research. Members of the laboratory include graduate students and faculty in the quantitative area.

Information for Students With Physical Disabilities: See the following Web site for more information: http://www.mcburney.wisc.edu.

Application Information:
Send to Graduate Admissions Coordinator, Educational Psychology, 1025 W. Johnson Street, Madison, WI 53706-1796. Application available online. URL of online application: http://www.grad.wisc.edu/education/admissions. Students are admitted in the Fall, application deadline December 1. *Fee:* $56.

Wisconsin, University of, Madison
Department of Psychology
College of Letters and Science
W. J. Brogden Psychology Building, 1202 West Johnson Street
Madison, WI 53706
Telephone: (608) 262-2079
Fax: (608) 262-4029
E-mail: *gradinfo@psych.wisc.edu*
Web: *http://www.psych.wisc.edu/*

Department Information:
1888. Chairperson: Patricia G. Devine. Number of faculty: total—full-time 31; women—full-time 16; total—minority—full-time 3; women minority—full-time 2.

Programs and Degrees Offered:
Listed in the following order: Program area, degree type (T if terminal Master's), number awarded 7/08–6/09. Individualized Graduate Major PhD (Doctor of Philosophy) 3, Biology of Brain & Behavior PhD (Doctor of Philosophy) 2, Clinical Psychology PhD (Doctor of Philosophy) 5, Cognitive and Cognitive Neurosciences PhD (Doctor of Philosophy) 1, Developmental Psychology PhD (Doctor of Philosophy) 0, Social Psychology and Personality PhD (Doctor of Philosophy) 2, Perception PhD (Doctor of Philosophy) 0.

APA Accreditation: Clinical PhD (Doctor of Philosophy).

Student Applications/Admissions:
Student Applications
Individualized Graduate Major PhD (Doctor of Philosophy)—Applications 2009–2010, 22. Total applicants accepted 2009–2010, 0. Number full-time enrolled (new admits only) 2009–2010, 2. Number part-time enrolled (new admits only) 2009–

2010, 0. The median number of years required for completion of a degree in 2008–2009 were 7. The number of students enrolled full- and part-time who were dismissed or voluntarily withdrew from this program area in 2008–2009 were 0. *Biology Of Brain & Behavior PhD (Doctor of Philosophy)*—Applications 2009–2010, 29. Total applicants accepted 2009–2010, 2. Number full-time enrolled (new admits only) 2009–2010, 1. Number part-time enrolled (new admits only) 2009–2010, 0. The median number of years required for completion of a degree in 2008–2009 were 5. The number of students enrolled full- and part-time who were dismissed or voluntarily withdrew from this program area in 2008–2009 were 0. *Clinical Psychology PhD (Doctor of Philosophy)*—Applications 2009–2010, 198. Total applicants accepted 2009–2010, 6. Number full-time enrolled (new admits only) 2009–2010, 4. Number part-time enrolled (new admits only) 2009–2010, 0. The median number of years required for completion of a degree in 2008–2009 were 7. The number of students enrolled full- and part-time who were dismissed or voluntarily withdrew from this program area in 2008–2009 were 2. *Cognitive and Cognitive Neurosciences PhD (Doctor of Philosophy)*—Applications 2009–2010, 63. Total applicants accepted 2009–2010, 4. Number full-time enrolled (new admits only) 2009–2010, 3. Number part-time enrolled (new admits only) 2009–2010, 0. The median number of years required for completion of a degree in 2008–2009 were 6. *Developmental Psychology PhD (Doctor of Philosophy)*—Applications 2009–2010, 39. Total applicants accepted 2009–2010, 4. Number full-time enrolled (new admits only) 2009–2010, 1. Total enrolled 2009–2010 full-time, 9. The number of students enrolled full- and part-time who were dismissed or voluntarily withdrew from this program area in 2008–2009 were 0. *Social Psychology and Personality PhD (Doctor of Philosophy)*—Applications 2009–2010, 66. Total applicants accepted 2009–2010, 2. Number full-time enrolled (new admits only) 2009–2010, 2. Number part-time enrolled (new admits only) 2009–2010, 0. The median number of years required for completion of a degree in 2008–2009 were 7. The number of students enrolled full- and part-time who were dismissed or voluntarily withdrew from this program area in 2008–2009 were 1. *Perception PhD (Doctor of Philosophy)*—Applications 2009–2010, 1. Total applicants accepted 2009–2010, 0. Number full-time enrolled (new admits only) 2009–2010, 0. Number part-time enrolled (new admits only) 2009–2010, 0. The number of students enrolled full- and part-time who were dismissed or voluntarily withdrew from this program area in 2008–2009 were 0.

Scores: Entries appear in this order: required test or GPA, minimum score (if required), median score of students entering in 2009–2010. *Individualized Graduate Major PhD (Doctor of Philosophy)*: GRE-V no minimum stated, GRE-Q no minimum stated, GRE-Analytical no minimum stated, overall undergraduate GPA 3.0, last 2 years GPA 3.0; *Biology of Brain & Behavior PhD (Doctor of Philosophy)*: GRE-V no minimum stated, GRE-Q no minimum stated, GRE-Analytical no minimum stated, overall undergraduate GPA 3.0, last 2 years GPA 3.0; *Clinical Psychology PhD (Doctor of Philosophy)*: GRE-V no minimum stated, GRE-Q no minimum stated, GRE-Analytical no minimum stated, overall undergraduate GPA 3.0, last 2 years GPA 3.0; *Cognitive and Cognitive Neurosciences PhD (Doctor of Philosophy)*: GRE-V no minimum stated, GRE-Q no minimum stated, GRE-Analytical no minimum stated, overall undergraduate GPA 3.0, last 2 years GPA 3.0; *Developmental Psychology PhD (Doctor of Philosophy)*: GRE-V no minimum stated, GRE-Q no minimum stated, GRE-Analytical no minimum stated, overall undergraduate GPA 3.0, last 2 years GPA 3.0; *Social Psychology and Personality PhD (Doctor of Philosophy)*: GRE-V no minimum stated, GRE-Q no minimum stated, GRE-Analytical no minimum stated, overall undergraduate GPA 3.0, last 2 years GPA 3.0; *Perception PhD (Doctor of Philosophy)*: GRE-V no minimum stated, GRE-Q no minimum stated, GRE-Analytical no minimum stated, overall undergraduate GPA 3.0, last 2 years GPA 3.0.

Other Criteria: (importance of criteria rated low, medium, or high): GRE scores—high, research experience—high, GPA—high, letters of recommendation—high, interview—high, statement of goals and objectives—high. For additional information on admission requirements, go to http://glial.psych.wisc.edu/index.php/psychgradprospective.

Student Characteristics: The following represents characteristics of students in 2009–2010 in all graduate psychology programs in the department: Female—full-time 55, part-time 0; Male—full-time 36, part-time 0; African American/Black—full-time 3, part-time 0; Hispanic/Latino(a)—full-time 0, part-time 0; Asian/Pacific Islander—full-time 9, part-time 0; American Indian/Alaska Native—full-time 4, part-time 0; Caucasian/White—full-time 60, part-time 0; Multi-ethnic—full-time 0, part-time 0; students subject to the Americans With Disabilities Act—full-time 0, part-time 0; Unknown ethnicity—full-time 15, part-time 0; International students who hold an F-1 or J-1 Visa—full-time 8, part-time 0.

Financial Information/Assistance:

Tuition for Full-Time Study: *Doctoral:* State residents: per academic year $5,258, $657 per credit hour; Nonstate residents: per academic year $12,536, $1,567 per credit hour. Tuition is subject to change. Additional fees are assessed to students beyond the costs of tuition for the following: Segregated Fees. See the following Web site for updates and changes in tuition costs: http://registrar.wisc.edu/.

Financial Assistance:

First-Year Students: Teaching assistantships available for first year. Average amount paid per academic year: $14,088. Average number of hours worked per week: 20. Apply by December 15. Research assistantships available for first year. Average amount paid per academic year: $16,668. Average number of hours worked per week: 20. Apply by December 15. Traineeships available for first year. Average amount paid per academic year: $21,180. Average number of hours worked per week: 20. Apply by December 15. Fellowships and scholarships available for first year. Average amount paid per academic year: $18,567. Average number of hours worked per week: 0. Apply by December 15.

Advanced Students: Teaching assistantships available for advanced students. Average amount paid per academic year: $16,264. Average number of hours worked per week: 20. Research assistantships available for advanced students. Average amount paid per academic year: $16,668. Average number of hours worked per week: 20. Traineeships available for advanced students. Average amount paid per academic year: $21,180. Average number of hours worked per week: 20. Fellowships and scholarships available for advanced students. Average amount paid per academic year: $12,375. Average number of hours worked per week: 0.

Additional Information: Of all students currently enrolled full time, 100% benefited from one or more of the listed financial assistance programs. Application and information available online at: http://info.gradsch.wisc.edu/admin/admissions/appinstr.html.

Internships/Practica: Doctoral Degree (PhD Clinical Psychology): For those doctoral students for whom a professional internship was required in this program prior to graduation, (1) students applied for an internship in 2008–2009, with (1) students obtaining an internship. Of those students who obtained an internship, (1) were paid internships. Of those students who obtained an internship, (1) students placed in APA/CPA accredited internships, (0) students placed in internships not APA/CPA accredited, but listed with the Association of Psychology Postdoctoral and Internship Programs (APPIC), (0) students placed in internships conforming to guidelines of the Council of Directors of School Psychology Programs (CDSPP), (0) students placed in internships that were not APA/CPA accredited, APPIC or CDSPP listed. Clinical psychology graduate students are required to complete a minimum of 400 hours of practicum experience, of which at least 150 hours are in direct service experience and at least 75 hours are in formally scheduled supervision. Each student will complete a 160-hour clerkship at a preapproved site which is designed to expose students to diverse clinical populations and the practice of clinical psychology in an applied setting. Also, a one-year internship is required.

Housing and Day Care: On-campus housing is available. See the following Web site for more information: http://www.housing.wisc.edu. On-campus day care facilities are available. See the following Web site for more information: http://www.housing.wisc.edu/occfr.

Employment of Department Graduates:
Master's Degree Graduates: Of those who graduated in the academic year 2008–2009, the following categories and numbers represent the postgraduate activities and employment of master's degree graduates: Enrolled in a postdoctoral residency/fellowship (n/a), employed in independent practice (n/a), total from the above (master's) (0).
Doctoral Degree Graduates: Of those who graduated in the academic year 2008–2009, the following categories and numbers represent the postgraduate activities and employment of doctoral degree graduates: Enrolled in a psychology doctoral program (n/a), total from the above (doctoral) (0).

Additional Information:
Orientation, Objectives, and Emphasis of Department: The psychology PhD program is characterized by the following goals: emphasis both on extensive academic training in general psychology and on intensive research training in the student's particular area of concentration, a wide offering of content courses and seminars permitting the student considerable freedom in working out a program of study in collaboration with the major professor, and early and continuing commitment to research. Students are expected to become competent scholars and creative scientists in their own areas of concentration.

Special Facilities or Resources: The department has an extraordinary array of research facilities. Virtually all laboratories are fully computer controlled, and the department's general-purpose facilities are freely available to all graduate students. The Brogden and the Harlow Primate Laboratory have special facilities for housing animals, as well as for behavioral, pharmacological, anatomical, immunological, and physiological studies. We are well-equipped for studies of visual, auditory, and language perception and other areas of cognitive psychology. In addition, the Psychology Department Research and Training Clinic is housed in the Brogden Building. Many of the faculty and graduate students are affiliated with the Institute of Aging, the Waisman Center on Mental Retardation and Human Development, the Wisconsin Regional Primate Research Center, the Health Emotions Center, the Neuroscience Training Program, the Keck Neuroimaging Center, the Hearing Training Program, the Institute for Research on Poverty, the NSF National Consortium on Violence Research, and the Women's Studies Research Center. There are strong ties to the departments of Anatomy, Anthropology, Communicative Disorders, Educational Psychology, Entomology, Immunology, Industrial Engineering, Ophthalmology, Psychiatry, Sociology, Wildlife Ecology, Zoology, the Mass Communication Research Center, the Institute for Research on Poverty, and the Survey Research Laboratory.

Information for Students With Physical Disabilities: See the following Web site for more information: http://www.mcburney.wisc.edu/.

Application Information:
Send to Graduate Admissions Department of Psychology University of Wisconsin 1202 W Johnson Street, Madison, WI 53706. Application available online. URL of online application: http://info.gradsch.wisc.edu/admin/admissions/appinstr.html. Students are admitted in the Fall, application deadline December 15. For complete application instructions, including supplemental departmental application, please visit: http://glial.psych.wisc.edu/index.php/psychgradprospective/psychgradapplicationprocess. Fee: $56. For application fee grants: http://info.gradsch.wisc.edu/education/diversity/funding.html Fee grants not available to international applicants.

Wisconsin, University of, Madison
Human Development and Family Studies
School of Human Ecology
3rd Floor Middleton Building, 1305 Linden Drive
Madison, WI 53706
Telephone: (608) 263-2381
Fax: (608) 265-6048
E-mail: *hdfs@mail.sohe.wisc.edu*
Web: *http://www.sohe.wisc.edu/hdfs/*

Department Information:
1903. Chairperson: Linda J. Roberts. Number of faculty: total—full-time 10, part-time 1; women—full-time 7, part-time 1; total—minority—full-time 2; women minority—full-time 2.

Programs and Degrees Offered:
Listed in the following order: Program area, degree type (T if terminal Master's), number awarded 7/08–6/09. Human Development & Family Studies PhD (Doctor of Philosophy) 3, Human Development & Family Studies MA/MS (Master of Arts/Science) 2.

GRADUATE STUDY IN PSYCHOLOGY

Student Applications/Admissions:
Student Applications
Human Development & Family Studies PhD (Doctor of Philosophy)—Applications 2009–2010, 19. Total applicants accepted 2009–2010, 4. Number full-time enrolled (new admits only) 2009–2010, 1. Number part-time enrolled (new admits only) 2009–2010, 0. Openings 2010–2011, 5. The median number of years required for completion of a degree in 2008–2009 were 5. The number of students enrolled full- and part-time who were dismissed or voluntarily withdrew from this program area in 2008–2009 were 0. Human Development & Family Studies MA/MS (Master of Arts/Science)—Applications 2009–2010, 22. Total applicants accepted 2009–2010, 13. Number full-time enrolled (new admits only) 2009–2010, 3. Number part-time enrolled (new admits only) 2009–2010, 0. Total enrolled 2009–2010 full-time, 10, part-time, 1. Openings 2010–2011, 5. The median number of years required for completion of a degree in 2008–2009 were 3. The number of students enrolled full- and part-time who were dismissed or voluntarily withdrew from this program area in 2008–2009 were 0.

Scores: Entries appear in this order: required test or GPA, minimum score (if required), median score of students entering in 2009–2010. Human Development & Family Studies PhD (Doctor of Philosophy): GRE-V no minimum stated, 528, GRE-Q no minimum stated, 555, GRE-Analytical no minimum stated, 5.1, overall undergraduate GPA 3.0, 3.62; Human Development & Family Studies MA/MS (Master of Arts/Science): GRE-V no minimum stated, 525, GRE-Q no minimum stated, 597, GRE-Analytical no minimum stated, 4.3, overall undergraduate GPA 3.0, 3.61.

Other Criteria: (importance of criteria rated low, medium, or high): GRE scores—medium, research experience—medium, work experience—low, GPA—high, letters of recommendation—high, statement of goals and objectives—high, Fit w/ faculty interests—high. For additional information on admission requirements, go to http://www.grad.wisc.edu/education/admissions/index.html.

Student Characteristics: The following represents characteristics of students in 2009–2010 in all graduate psychology programs in the department: Female—full-time 24, part-time 1; Male—full-time 3, part-time 0; African American/Black—full-time 1, part-time 0; Hispanic/Latino(a)—full-time 1, part-time 1; Asian/Pacific Islander—full-time 7, part-time 0; American Indian/Alaska Native—full-time 0, part-time 0; Caucasian/White—full-time 18, part-time 0; Multi-ethnic—full-time 0, part-time 0; students subject to the Americans With Disabilities Act—full-time 0, part-time 0; Unknown ethnicity—full-time 0, part-time 0; International students who hold an F-1 or J-1 Visa—full-time 6, part-time 0.

Financial Information/Assistance:
Tuition for Full-Time Study: Master's: State residents: per academic year $10,517, $659 per credit hour; Nonstate residents: per academic year $25,072, $1,568 per credit hour. Doctoral: State residents: per academic year $10,517, $659 per credit hour; Nonstate residents: per academic year $25,072, $1,568 per credit hour. Tuition is subject to change. See the following Web site for updates and changes in tuition costs: http://registrar.wisc.edu/tuition_&_fees.htm.

Financial Assistance:
First-Year Students: Teaching assistantships available for first year. Average amount paid per academic year: $9,392. Average number of hours worked per week: 13. Apply by January 10. Research assistantships available for first year. Average number of hours worked per week: 13. Fellowships and scholarships available for first year. Apply by January 10.

Advanced Students: Teaching assistantships available for advanced students. Average amount paid per academic year: $10,843. Average number of hours worked per week: 13. Apply by January 10. Research assistantships available for advanced students. Average number of hours worked per week: 13. Fellowships and scholarships available for advanced students. Apply by January 10.

Additional Information: Of all students currently enrolled full time, 80% benefited from one or more of the listed financial assistance programs. Application and information available online at: http://www.grad.wisc.edu/education/funding/index.html.

Housing and Day Care: On-campus housing is available. See the following Web site for more information: http://www.housing.wisc.edu/. On-campus day care facilities are available. See the following Web site for more information: http://occfr.wisc.edu/child_care/campus_centers.htm.

Employment of Department Graduates:
Master's Degree Graduates: Of those who graduated in the academic year 2008–2009, the following categories and numbers represent the postgraduate activities and employment of master's degree graduates: Enrolled in a psychology doctoral program (1), enrolled in a postdoctoral residency/fellowship (n/a), employed in independent practice (n/a), employed in other positions at a higher education institution (1), total from the above (master's) (2).

Doctoral Degree Graduates: Of those who graduated in the academic year 2008–2009, the following categories and numbers represent the postgraduate activities and employment of doctoral degree graduates: Enrolled in a psychology doctoral program (n/a), enrolled in a postdoctoral residency/fellowship (1), employed in other positions at a higher education institution (2), total from the above (doctoral) (3).

Additional Information:
Orientation, Objectives, and Emphasis of Department: The UW Human Development and Family Studies Graduate Program provides opportunities for advanced study and research on human development and families across the life span. Two assumptions are basic to the philosophy and organization of the program. First, we can only understand individual development within its social context, and families are an essential component of this context. Second, we can only understand families within their larger social context—historical change, social class, ethnicity, and public policy. The program offers courses on development in infancy, childhood, adolescence, adulthood, and old age. Other courses focus on family relationships, process, and diversity. The faculty bring the perspectives of many different disciplines and methodologies to their work. Faculty and students never lose sight, however, of the connections among human development, family life, and the broader sociohistorical context.

Special Facilities or Resources: Because the department has joint faculty in UW-Extension, students often work in the community doing community based research and outreach projects. Departmental faculty have affiliated appointments with research centers and other programs on campus, which students have access to. The Family Interaction Lab in the department provides a naturalistic, home-like setting for unobtrusive videotaping of interactions. A control room is located adjacent to the interaction room for camera control, taping, editing, dubbing and coding of videotapes. The department is also affiliated with the Center for Excellence in Family Studies.

Information for Students With Physical Disabilities: See the following Web site for more information: http://www.mcburney.wisc.edu/services/.

Application Information:
Send to Graduate Admissions Human Development & Family Studies Graduate Program, University of Wisconsin—Madison, 3rd Fl Middleton Bldg., 1305 Linden Drive Madison, WI 53706. Application available online. URL of online application: https://www.gradsch.wisc.edu/eapp/eapp.pl. Students are admitted in the Fall, application deadline January 10. *Fee:* $56.

Wisconsin, University of, Milwaukee
Department of Psychology
College of Letters and Science
P.O. Box 413
Milwaukee, WI 53201-0413
Telephone: (414) 229-4747
Fax: (414) 229-5219
E-mail: *suelima@uwm.edu*
Web: *http://psychology.uwm.edu*

Department Information:
1956. Chairperson: David Osmon. Number of faculty: total—full-time 23; women—full-time 7; total—minority—full-time 2.

Programs and Degrees Offered:
Listed in the following order: Program area, degree type (T if terminal Master's), number awarded 7/08–6/09. Experimental Health Psychology MA/MS (Master of Arts/Science) (T) 2, Experimental Behavior Analysis MA/MS (Master of Arts/Science) (T) 1, Clinical Psychology PhD (Doctor of Philosophy) 7, Experimental PhD (Doctor of Philosophy) 7.

APA Accreditation: Clinical PhD (Doctor of Philosophy). Student Outcome Data Website: http://www4.uwm.edu/letsci/psychology/graduate/phdprograms/clinical/index.cfm.

Student Applications/Admissions:
Student Applications
Experimental Health Psychology MA/MS (*Master of Arts/Science*)—Applications 2009–2010, 12. Total applicants accepted 2009–2010, 4. Number full-time enrolled (new admits only) 2009–2010, 2. Number part-time enrolled (new admits only) 2009–2010, 0. Openings 2010–2011, 2. The median number of years required for completion of a degree in 2008–2009 were 6. The number of students enrolled full- and part-time who were dismissed or voluntarily withdrew from this program area in 2008–2009 were 0. *Experimental Behavior Analysis MA/MS (Master of Arts/Science)*—Applications 2009–2010, 10. Total applicants accepted 2009–2010, 2. Number full-time enrolled (new admits only) 2009–2010, 2. Number part-time enrolled (new admits only) 2009–2010, 0. Total enrolled 2009–2010 full-time, 4, part-time, 2. Openings 2010–2011, 2. The median number of years required for completion of a degree in 2008–2009 were 4. The number of students enrolled full- and part-time who were dismissed or voluntarily withdrew from this program area in 2008–2009 were 0. *Clinical Psychology PhD (Doctor of Philosophy)*—Applications 2009–2010, 104. Total applicants accepted 2009–2010, 8. Number full-time enrolled (new admits only) 2009–2010, 6. Number part-time enrolled (new admits only) 2009–2010, 0. Openings 2010–2011, 6. The median number of years required for completion of a degree in 2008–2009 were 6. The number of students enrolled full- and part-time who were dismissed or voluntarily withdrew from this program area in 2008–2009 were 0. *Experimental PhD (Doctor of Philosophy)*—Applications 2009–2010, 19. Total applicants accepted 2009–2010, 9. Number full-time enrolled (new admits only) 2009–2010, 5. Number part-time enrolled (new admits only) 2009–2010, 0. Openings 2010–2011, 5. The median number of years required for completion of a degree in 2008–2009 were 6. The number of students enrolled full- and part-time who were dismissed or voluntarily withdrew from this program area in 2008–2009 were 0.

Scores: Entries appear in this order: required test or GPA, minimum score (if required), median score of students entering in 2009–2010. Experimental Health Psychology MA/MS (*Master of Arts/Science*): GRE-V no minimum stated, GRE-Q no minimum stated, GRE-Analytical no minimum stated, GRE-Subject (Psychology) no minimum stated, overall undergraduate GPA no minimum stated, last 2 years GPA no minimum stated, psychology GPA no minimum stated; *Experimental Behavior Analysis MA/MS (Master of Arts/Science)*: GRE-V no minimum stated, GRE-Q no minimum stated, GRE-Analytical no minimum stated, GRE-Subject (Psychology) no minimum stated, overall undergraduate GPA no minimum stated, last 2 years GPA no minimum stated, psychology GPA no minimum stated; *Clinical Psychology PhD (Doctor of Philosophy)*: GRE-V no minimum stated, 563, GRE-Q no minimum stated, 657, GRE-Analytical no minimum stated, 4.3, overall undergraduate GPA no minimum stated, 3.8, last 2 years GPA no minimum stated, psychology GPA no minimum stated; *Experimental PhD (Doctor of Philosophy)*: GRE-V no minimum stated, 524, GRE-Q no minimum stated, 690, GRE-Analytical no minimum stated, 4.0, GRE-Subject (Psychology) no minimum stated, 655, overall undergraduate GPA no minimum stated, 3.4, last 2 years GPA no minimum stated, psychology GPA no minimum stated.

Other Criteria: (importance of criteria rated low, medium, or high): GRE scores—high, research experience—high, work experience—low, extracurricular activity—low, clinically related public service—medium, GPA—high, letters of recommendation—high, interview—high, statement of goals and objectives—high, undergraduate major in psychology—medium, specific undergraduate psychology courses taken—medium, No interview is required for admission to the PhD Program in Experimental Psychology, but an interview is required for admission to the PhD Program in Clinical Psychology. For additional information on admission requirements, go to http://www4.uwm.edu/letsci/psychology/graduate/gradapp.cfm.

Student Characteristics: The following represents characteristics of students in 2009–2010 in all graduate psychology programs in the department: Female—full-time 40, part-time 2; Male—full-time 27, part-time 0; African American/Black—full-time 2, part-time 0; Hispanic/Latino(a)—full-time 6, part-time 0; Asian/Pacific Islander—full-time 6, part-time 0; American Indian/Alaska Native—full-time 0, part-time 0; Caucasian/White—full-time 53, part-time 2; Multi-ethnic—full-time 0, part-time 0; students subject to the Americans With Disabilities Act—full-time 0, part-time 0; Unknown ethnicity—full-time 0, part-time 0; International students who hold an F-1 or J-1 Visa—full-time 5, part-time 0.

Financial Information/Assistance:
Tuition for Full-Time Study: Master's: State residents: per academic year $9,997, $839 per credit hour; Nonstate residents: per academic year $23,664, $1,693 per credit hour. *Doctoral:* State residents: per academic year $9,997, $839 per credit hour; Nonstate residents: per academic year $23,664, $1,693 per credit hour. Tuition is subject to change. Additional fees are assessed to students beyond the costs of tuition for the following: additional student fees vary from $490 to $812 per year. See the following Web site for updates and changes in tuition costs: http://www.bfs.uwm.edu/fees/.

Financial Assistance:
First-Year Students: Teaching assistantships available for first year. Average amount paid per academic year: $11,605. Average number of hours worked per week: 20. Apply by December 3 or 31. Research assistantships available for first year. Average amount paid per academic year: $17,000. Average number of hours worked per week: 20. Apply by December 3 or 31. Fellowships and scholarships available for first year. Average amount paid per academic year: $14,000. Average number of hours worked per week: 0. Apply by December 3 or 31.

Advanced Students: Teaching assistantships available for advanced students. Average amount paid per academic year: $13,453. Average number of hours worked per week: 20. Apply by December 3 or 31. Research assistantships available for advanced students. Average amount paid per academic year: $17,000. Average number of hours worked per week: 20. Apply by December 3 or 31. Fellowships and scholarships available for advanced students. Average amount paid per academic year: $14,000. Average number of hours worked per week: 0. Apply by December 3 or 31.

Additional Information: Of all students currently enrolled full time, 86% benefited from one or more of the listed financial assistance programs. Application and information available online at: http://www4.uwm.edu/letsci/psychology/graduate/gradapp.cfm.

Internships/Practica: Doctoral Degree (PhD Clinical Psychology): For those doctoral students for whom a professional internship was required in this program prior to graduation, (4) students applied for an internship in 2008–2009, with (3) students obtaining an internship. Of those students who obtained an internship, (3) were paid internships. Of those students who obtained an internship, (3) students placed in APA/CPA accredited internships, (0) students placed in internships not APA/CPA accredited, but listed with the Association of Psychology Postdoctoral and Internship Programs (APPIC), (0) students placed in internships conforming to guidelines of the Council of Directors of School Psychology Programs (CDSPP), (0) students placed in internships that were not APA/CPA accredited, APPIC or CDSPP listed. Master's Degree (MA/MS Experimental Health Psychology): An internship experience, such as, a final research project or "capstone" experience is required of graduates. Master's Degree (MA/MS Experimental Behavior Analysis): An internship experience, such as a final research project or "capstone" experience is required of graduates. Numerous training sites in the greater Milwaukee area are used for clinical training practica, providing students with excellent training in clinical psychology, including neuropsychology and health psychology. These training experiences equip clinical doctoral students to compete for nationally recognized predoctoral internships.

Housing and Day Care: On-campus housing is available. See the following Web site for more information: http://www4.uwm.edu/housing/. On-campus day care facilities are available. See the following Web site for more information: http://www4.uwm.edu/ccc/.

Employment of Department Graduates:
Master's Degree Graduates: Of those who graduated in the academic year 2008–2009, the following categories and numbers represent the postgraduate activities and employment of master's degree graduates: Enrolled in a postdoctoral residency/fellowship (n/a), employed in independent practice (n/a), employed in business or industry (2), employed in a hospital/medical center (1), total from the above (master's) (3).
Doctoral Degree Graduates: Of those who graduated in the academic year 2008–2009, the following categories and numbers represent the postgraduate activities and employment of doctoral degree graduates: Enrolled in a psychology doctoral program (n/a), enrolled in a postdoctoral residency/fellowship (11), employed in an academic position at a 2-year/4-year college (3), total from the above (doctoral) (14).

Additional Information:
Orientation, Objectives, and Emphasis of Department: The department has a PhD program in clinical psychology (which includes earning the MS), a PhD program in experimental psychology (which includes earning the MS), and terminal MS programs in experimental health psychology and experimental behavior analysis. The experimental PhD program offers specializations in behavior analysis, health psychology, and neuroscience. Regardless of the specialization area, the goal of the program is to provide the students with an understanding of psychology as a scientific discipline and to prepare them for careers in research and teaching. The clinical PhD program follows the Boulder model, in which students are trained as both scientists and practitioners through integration of research, practical experience, and coursework in psychopathology, assessment, and psychotherapy. A predoctoral clinical internship is required. Although a clinical student may emphasize either the basic or applied aspect of psychology, the goal of the program is excellence in both areas. Students in the clinical as well as the experimental program are directly involved in research under the direction of their major professor. Most of the students in the clinical and experimental doctoral programs are funded via teaching assistantships (or, sometimes, research assistantships or project assistantships), which require approximately 20 hours of work per week. Due to insufficient funds, the department does not offer teaching assistantships or other financial support to students in the terminal master's programs.

Special Facilities or Resources: The department moved to a completely remodeled building in 1985, which contains a separate research laboratory for each member of the faculty and specifically designed quarters for teaching laboratory courses. Special construction, air conditioning, and ventilation were included in the teaching and research laboratories to accommodate work with animal subjects and human participants. There is also a mechanical and woodworking shop and an electronics shop, supervised by a full-time technician. The department training clinic is housed in a separate wing of the building with its own offices, clerical staff, research space, clinic rooms, and full-time director.

Information for Students With Physical Disabilities: See the following Web site for more information: http://www4.uwm.edu/sac/.

Application Information:
Send to Chairperson, Graduate Admissions Committee, Department of Psychology, P.O. Box 413, Milwaukee, WI 53201-0413. Application available online. URL of online application: http://www4.uwm.edu/letsci/psychology/graduate/gradapp.cfm. Students are admitted in the Fall, application deadline December 3. The application deadline is December 3 for the PhD program in Clinical Psychology and December 31 for the other programs. Note that two separate applications are required: one to the psychology department and one to the Graduate School. *Fee:* $56. Application fee for foreign students is $96.

Wisconsin, University of, Milwaukee
Educational Psychology
Education
2400 East Hartford IP0413
Milwaukee, WI 53211
Telephone: (414) 229-4767
Fax: (414) 229-4939
E-mail: *nadya@uwm.edu*
Web: *http://www.uwm.edu/Dept/EdPsych*

Department Information:
1965. Chairperson: Nadya A. Fouad. Number of faculty: total—full-time 22, part-time 7; women—full-time 14, part-time 6; total—minority—full-time 12; women minority—full-time 10.

Programs and Degrees Offered:
Listed in the following order: Program area, degree type (T if terminal Master's), number awarded 7/08–6/09. Counseling MA/MS (Master of Arts/Science) 118, School Psychology EdS (School Psychology) 7, Counseling Psychology PhD (Doctor of Philosophy) 2, School Psychology PhD (Doctor of Philosophy) 4, Learning and Development PhD (Doctor of Philosophy) 1, Research Methodology MA/MS (Master of Arts/Science) 0, Learning and Development MA/MS (Master of Arts/Science) (T) 1, Research Methodology PhD (Doctor of Philosophy) 1.

APA Accreditation: Counseling PhD (Doctor of Philosophy). School PhD (Doctor of Philosophy).

Student Applications/Admissions:
Student Applications
Counseling MA/MS (Master of Arts/Science)—Applications 2009–2010, 100. Total applicants accepted 2009–2010, 80. Number full-time enrolled (new admits only) 2009–2010, 40. Number part-time enrolled (new admits only) 2009–2010, 24. Total enrolled 2009–2010 full-time, 80, part-time, 63. Openings 2010–2011, 65. The median number of years required for completion of a degree in 2008–2009 were 4. The number of students enrolled full- and part-time who were dismissed or voluntarily withdrew from this program area in 2008–2009 were 0. *School Psychology EdS (School Psychology)*—Applications 2009–2010, 30. Total applicants accepted 2009–2010, 8. Number full-time enrolled (new admits only) 2009–2010, 6. Number part-time enrolled (new admits only) 2009–2010, 2. Total enrolled 2009–2010 full-time, 14, part-time, 28. Openings 2010–2011, 10. The median number of years required for completion of a degree in 2008–2009 were 4. The number of students enrolled full- and part-time who were dismissed or voluntarily withdrew from this program area in 2008–2009 were 0. *Counseling Psychology PhD (Doctor of Philosophy)*—Applications 2009–2010, 80. Total applicants accepted 2009–2010, 7. Number full-time enrolled (new admits only) 2009–2010, 5. Number part-time enrolled (new admits only) 2009–2010, 0. Openings 2010–2011, 6. The median number of years required for completion of a degree in 2008–2009 were 5. The number of students enrolled full- and part-time who were dismissed or voluntarily withdrew from this program area in 2008–2009 were 0. *School Psychology PhD (Doctor of Philosophy)*—Applications 2009–2010, 22. Total applicants accepted 2009–2010, 6. Number full-time enrolled (new admits only) 2009–2010, 6. Number part-time enrolled (new admits only) 2009–2010, 0. Openings 2010–2011, 5. The median number of years required for completion of a degree in 2008–2009 were 5. The number of students enrolled full- and part-time who were dismissed or voluntarily withdrew from this program area in 2008–2009 were 0. *Learning and Development PhD (Doctor of Philosophy)*—Applications 2009–2010, 3. Total applicants accepted 2009–2010, 2. Number full-time enrolled (new admits only) 2009–2010, 1. Number part-time enrolled (new admits only) 2009–2010, 1. Total enrolled 2009–2010 full-time, 5, part-time, 2. Openings 2010–2011, 2. The median number of years required for completion of a degree in 2008–2009 were 4. The number of students enrolled full- and part-time who were dismissed or voluntarily withdrew from this program area in 2008–2009 were 0. *Research Methodology MA/MS (Master of Arts/Science)*—Applications 2009–2010, 1. Total applicants accepted 2009–2010, 1. Number full-time enrolled (new admits only) 2009–2010, 1. Number part-time enrolled (new admits only) 2009–2010, 0. Openings 2010–2011, 5. The median number of years required for completion of a degree in 2008–2009 were 2. The number of students enrolled full- and part-time who were dismissed or voluntarily withdrew from this program area in 2008–2009 were 0. *Learning and Development MA/MS (Master of Arts/Science)*—Applications 2009–2010, 3. Total applicants accepted 2009–2010, 1. Number full-time enrolled (new admits only) 2009–2010, 0. Number part-time enrolled (new admits only) 2009–2010, 1. Openings 2010–2011, 5. The median number of years required for completion of a degree in 2008–2009 were 2. The number of students enrolled full- and part-time who were dismissed or voluntarily withdrew from this program area in 2008–2009 were 0. *Research Methodology PhD (Doctor of Philosophy)*—Applications 2009–2010, 7. Total applicants accepted 2009–2010, 2. Number full-time enrolled (new admits only) 2009–2010, 1. Number part-time enrolled

(new admits only) 2009–2010, 0. Total enrolled 2009–2010 full-time, 3, part-time, 5. Openings 2010–2011, 2. The median number of years required for completion of a degree in 2008–2009 were 4. The number of students enrolled full- and part-time who were dismissed or voluntarily withdrew from this program area in 2008–2009 were 0.

Scores: Entries appear in this order: required test or GPA, minimum score (if required), median score of students entering in 2009–2010. *Counseling MA/MS (Master of Arts/Science):* overall undergraduate GPA 3.0, last 2 years GPA 3.0; *School Psychology EdS (School Psychology):* overall undergraduate GPA 3.0, last 2 years GPA 3.0; *Counseling Psychology PhD (Doctor of Philosophy):* GRE-V 300, 510, GRE-Q 280, 450, GRE-Analytical 3, 5, overall undergraduate GPA no minimum stated; *School Psychology PhD (Doctor of Philosophy):* GRE-V 510, 645, GRE-Q 380, 540, GRE-Analytical 3, 5, overall undergraduate GPA 3.0, last 2 years GPA 3.0, Masters GPA 3.0; *Learning and Development PhD (Doctor of Philosophy):* overall undergraduate GPA 3.0, last 2 years GPA 3.0, Masters GPA 3.0; *Research Methodology MA/MS (Master of Arts/Science):* overall undergraduate GPA 3.0, last 2 years GPA 3.0; *Learning and Development MA/MS (Master of Arts/Science):* overall undergraduate GPA 3.0, last 2 years GPA no minimum stated, psychology GPA no minimum stated; *Research Methodology PhD (Doctor of Philosophy):* GRE-V 390, 640, GRE-Q 300, 530, GRE-Analytical 4, 5, overall undergraduate GPA 3.0, last 2 years GPA 3.0, Masters GPA 3.0.

Other Criteria: (importance of criteria rated low, medium, or high): GRE scores—medium, research experience—high, work experience—low, clinically related public service—medium, GPA—high, letters of recommendation—high, interview—high, statement of goals and objectives—high, research interests—high, undergraduate major in psychology—medium, specific undergraduate psychology courses taken—low, Clinical experiences not required for Research Methodology or Learning/Development. For additional information on admission requirements, go to http://www4.uwm.edu/soe/departments/ed_psychology/.

Student Characteristics: The following represents characteristics of students in 2009–2010 in all graduate psychology programs in the department: Female—full-time 137, part-time 82; Male—full-time 33, part-time 17; African American/Black—full-time 11, part-time 8; Hispanic/Latino(a)—full-time 10, part-time 3; Asian/Pacific Islander—full-time 7, part-time 0; American Indian/Alaska Native—full-time 0, part-time 0; Caucasian/White—full-time 142, part-time 88; Multi-ethnic—full-time 0, part-time 0; students subject to the Americans With Disabilities Act—full-time 0, part-time 0; Unknown ethnicity—full-time 0, part-time 0; International students who hold an F-1 or J-1 Visa—full-time 7, part-time 2.

Financial Information/Assistance:
  Tuition for Full-Time Study: Master's: State residents: per academic year $12,864, $804 per credit hour; Nonstate residents: per academic year $26,896, $1,681 per credit hour. Doctoral: State residents: per academic year $12,864, $804 per credit hour; Nonstate residents: per academic year $26,896, $1,681 per credit hour. Tuition is subject to change. Additional fees are assessed to students beyond the costs of tuition for the following: assessment courses have additional course fees. See the following Web site for updates and changes in tuition costs: http://www.bfs.uwm.edu/fees.

Financial Assistance:
  First-Year Students: Teaching assistantships available for first year. Average amount paid per academic year: $13,200. Average number of hours worked per week: 20. Research assistantships available for first year. Average amount paid per academic year: $17,000. Average number of hours worked per week: 20. Fellowships and scholarships available for first year. Average amount paid per academic year: $13,200. Average number of hours worked per week: 20.

  Advanced Students: Teaching assistantships available for advanced students. Average amount paid per academic year: $15,950. Average number of hours worked per week: 20. Research assistantships available for advanced students. Average amount paid per academic year: $17,000. Average number of hours worked per week: 20. Fellowships and scholarships available for advanced students. Average amount paid per academic year: $15,950. Average number of hours worked per week: 20.

  Additional Information: Of all students currently enrolled full time, 65% benefited from one or more of the listed financial assistance programs. Application and information available online at: http://www4.uwm.edu/soe/departments/ed_psychology/.

Internships/Practica: Doctoral Degree (PhD Counseling Psychology): For those doctoral students for whom a professional internship was required in this program prior to graduation, (11) students applied for an internship in 2008–2009, with (11) students obtaining an internship. Of those students who obtained an internship, (10) were paid internships. Of those students who obtained an internship, (10) students placed in APA/CPA accredited internships, (0) students placed in internships not APA/CPA accredited, but listed with the Association of Psychology Postdoctoral and Internship Programs (APPIC), (0) students placed in internships conforming to guidelines of the Council of Directors of School Psychology Programs (CDSPP), (1) students placed in internships that were not APA/CPA accredited, APPIC or CDSPP listed. Doctoral Degree (PhD School Psychology): For those doctoral students for whom a professional internship was required in this program prior to graduation, (2) students applied for an internship in 2008–2009, with (2) students obtaining an internship. Of those students who obtained an internship, (2) were paid internships. Of those students who obtained an internship, (2) students placed in APA/CPA accredited internships, (0) students placed in internships not APA/CPA accredited, but listed with the Association of Psychology Postdoctoral and Internship Programs (APPIC), (0) students placed in internships conforming to guidelines of the Council of Directors of School Psychology Programs (CDSPP), (0) students placed in internships that were not APA/CPA accredited, APPIC or CDSPP listed. Students are placed in a variety of educational, business, and community settings as part of their graduate training.

Housing and Day Care: On-campus housing is available. See the following Web site for more information: Housing: http://www4.uwm.edu/future_students/future_student_life/housing.cfm. On-campus day care facilities are available. See the following Web site for more information: http://www.uwm.edu/ccc.

Employment of Department Graduates:
  Master's Degree Graduates: Of those who graduated in the academic year 2008–2009, the following categories and numbers

represent the postgraduate activities and employment of master's degree graduates: Enrolled in a psychology doctoral program (6), enrolled in another graduate/professional program (1), enrolled in a postdoctoral residency/fellowship (n/a), employed in independent practice (n/a), employed in an academic position at a university (0), employed in an academic position at a 2-year/4-year college (0), employed in other positions at a higher education institution (7), employed in a professional position in a school system (27), employed in business or industry (8), employed in government agency (4), employed in a community mental health/counseling center (17), employed in a hospital/medical center (9), still seeking employment (18), other employment position (27), do not know (2), total from the above (master's) (126).

Doctoral Degree Graduates: Of those who graduated in the academic year 2008–2009, the following categories and numbers represent the postgraduate activities and employment of doctoral degree graduates: Enrolled in a psychology doctoral program (n/a), employed in independent practice (1), employed in an academic position at a university (1), employed in other positions at a higher education institution (1), employed in a professional position in a school system (2), employed in a community mental health/counseling center (1), employed in a hospital/medical center (1), other employment position (1), total from the above (doctoral) (8).

Additional Information:

Orientation, Objectives, and Emphasis of Department: The department has one MS program with majors in Community Counseling, School Counseling, School Psychology (also EdS), Research Methods, as well as Learning and Development. The PhD program in Educational Psychology includes Research Methods, Learning & Development, School Psychology and Counseling Psychology. The PhD programs in School Psychology and Counseling Psychology follow the model of training outlined by the American Psychological Association. The programs are based on the scientist–practitioner model, in which students are trained as psychological scientists with specializations in school or counseling psychology. A strong, multicultural perspective undergirds the programs, with an emphasis on the contextual factors in student's work, and both provide unique training in the psychological, social, and educational needs of multiethnic populations within an urban psychosocial context. Students gain the knowledge, skills, and attitudes to work in a heterogeneous environment. Students are prepared to work in academic, service delivery, research and administrative positions.

Special Facilities or Resources: The department possesses excellent computer facilities. The department enjoys a strong collaborative relationship with the Department of Psychology, working together in an on-campus psychology clinic. We also have strong linkages to urban community and school partners, which provide students with a diverse set of research and practice opportunities.

Information for Students With Physical Disabilities: See the following Web site for more information: http://www4.uwm.edu/sac/.

Application Information:

Send to Department of Educational Psychology, UW-Milwaukee, P.O. Box 413, Milwaukee, WI 53201. Application available online. URL of online application: http://www.graduateschool.uwm.edu/. Students are admitted in the Fall, application deadline Varies*. *School Psychology: EdS- January 2 *School Psychology: PhD- December 15 *School/Community Counseling: M.S.- March 1 *Counseling Psychology: PhD- December 1 *Learning & Development: M.S., PhD - Rolling admission *Research Methodology: M.S., PhD - Rolling admission Admission once per academic year for Counseling and School Psychology programs. Research Methods and Learning & Development programs have rolling admissions and will consider applications at anytime. Fee: $56. An additional $40 is required for applicants who have non-US college work.

Wisconsin, University of, Stout
Psychology Department / Master of Science in Applied Psychology (MSAP)
College of Education, Health and Human Sciences
McCalmont Hall 304
Menomonie, WI 54751-0790
Telephone: (715) 232-2653
Fax: (715) 232-5303
E-mail: *gorbatenkok@uwstout.edu*
Web: *http://www3.uwstout.edu/programs/msap/index.cfm*

Department Information:

1982. Program Director: Dr. Kristina Gorbatenko-Roth. Number of faculty: total—full-time 14; women—full-time 9; total—minority—full-time 2; women minority—full-time 1.

Programs and Degrees Offered:

Listed in the following order: Program area, degree type (T if terminal Master's), number awarded 7/08–6/09. Applied Psychology MA/MS (Master of Arts/Science) (T) 9.

Student Applications/Admissions:

Student Applications

Applied Psychology MA/MS (Master of Arts/Science)—Applications 2009–2010, 29. Total applicants accepted 2009–2010, 19. Number full-time enrolled (new admits only) 2009–2010, 10. Number part-time enrolled (new admits only) 2009–2010, 0. Total enrolled 2009–2010 full-time, 26, part-time, 1. Openings 2010–2011, 20. The median number of years required for completion of a degree in 2008–2009 were 2. The number of students enrolled full- and part-time who were dismissed or voluntarily withdrew from this program area in 2008–2009 were 0.

Scores: Entries appear in this order: required test or GPA, minimum score (if required), median score of students entering in 2009–2010. *Applied Psychology MA/MS (Master of Arts/Science)*: GRE-V no minimum stated, GRE-Q no minimum stated, overall undergraduate GPA 3.0, 3.5.

Other Criteria: (importance of criteria rated low, medium, or high): GRE scores—medium, research experience—high, work experience—high, extracurricular activity—medium, clinically related public service—low, GPA—high, letters of recommendation—high, statement of goals and objectives—high, applied experience—high, undergraduate major in psychology—low, specific undergraduate psychology courses taken—high. For additional information on admission requirements, go to http://www3.uwstout.edu/programs/msap/apply.cfm.

Student Characteristics: The following represents characteristics of students in 2009–2010 in all graduate psychology programs in the department: Female—full-time 17, part-time 1; Male—full-time 9, part-time 0; African American/Black—full-time 1, part-time 0; Hispanic/Latino(a)—full-time 0, part-time 0; Asian/Pacific Islander—full-time 3, part-time 0; American Indian/Alaska Native—full-time 0, part-time 0; Caucasian/White—full-time 22, part-time 1; Multi-ethnic—full-time 0, part-time 0; students subject to the Americans With Disabilities Act—full-time 0, part-time 0; Unknown ethnicity—full-time 0, part-time 0; International students who hold an F-1 or J-1 Visa—full-time 2, part-time 0.

Financial Information/Assistance:
Tuition for Full-Time Study: *Master's:* State residents: per academic year $8,712, $363 per credit hour; Nonstate residents: per academic year $13,440, $560 per credit hour. Tuition is subject to change. Additional fees are assessed to students beyond the costs of tuition for the following: SPSS and other computer software required; to be purchased by student. See the following Web site for updates and changes in tuition costs: http://www.uwstout.edu/stubus/.

Financial Assistance:
First-Year Students: Teaching assistantships available for first year. Average amount paid per academic year: $6,831. Average number of hours worked per week: 13. Traineeships available for first year. Average amount paid per academic year: $6,831. Average number of hours worked per week: 13.
Advanced Students: Teaching assistantships available for advanced students. Average amount paid per academic year: $10,260. Average number of hours worked per week: 13. Traineeships available for advanced students.
Additional Information: Of all students currently enrolled full time, 50% benefited from one or more of the listed financial assistance programs. Application and information available online at: http://www3.uwstout.edu/grad/finance.cfm.

Internships/Practica: Master's Degree (MA/MS Applied Psychology): An internship experience, such as, a final research project or "capstone" experience is required of graduates. UW-Stout has a reputation for its experiential-based curriculum. Approximately 700 students annually are in co-op or internship placements. The institution has an extensive network of business and industry contacts for the internship experience that is organized through the Placement and Co-op Services office. MSAP students are required to do an internship and are encouraged to seek out placement sites early in their program work. Program evaluation concentration students are also required to do a practicum. 85% of MSAP courses involve 'hands-on' applied learning.

Housing and Day Care: On-campus housing is available. See the following Web site for more information: http://www.uwstout.edu/housing/. On-campus day care facilities are available. For information about child care services, contact the Child and Family Study Center, 715/232-1478 or e-mail cfsc@uwstout.edu.

Employment of Department Graduates:
Master's Degree Graduates: Of those who graduated in the academic year 2008–2009, the following categories and numbers represent the postgraduate activities and employment of master's degree graduates: Enrolled in a psychology doctoral program (0), enrolled in another graduate/professional program (1), enrolled in a postdoctoral residency/fellowship (n/a), employed in independent practice (n/a), employed in an academic position at a 2-year/4-year college (0), employed in other positions at a higher education institution (1), employed in a professional position in a school system (0), employed in business or industry (5), employed in government agency (1), employed in a community mental health/counseling center (0), employed in a hospital/medical center (0), other employment position (0), do not know (1), total from the above (master's) (9).
Doctoral Degree Graduates: Of those who graduated in the academic year 2008–2009, the following categories and numbers represent the postgraduate activities and employment of doctoral degree graduates: Enrolled in a psychology doctoral program (n/a), total from the above (doctoral) (0).

Additional Information:
Orientation, Objectives, and Emphasis of Department: The MS in Applied Psychology (MSAP) is a two-year program designed around a core of psychological theories, principles, and research methods. The program emphasizes experiential learning, as over 85% of the required courses involve applied projects. Students choose from among three concentration areas: industrial/organizational psychology, program evaluation, and applied health psychology. Dual concentrations in industrial/organizational psychology and program evaluation as well as program evaluation and health psychology are common. The MSAP program is designed to provide students with the knowledge, experience, skills, and abilities to apply theories and methods to the identification of and solution to a variety of 21st century, real-world problems in business and industry, health care, and non-profit organizations. A majority of classes incorporate real-world, hands-on learning opportunities that involve extensive group work and communication with external stakeholders. Numerous opportunities exist outside of formal courses for additional applied experience.

Special Facilities or Resources: The university has numerous consulting relationships with local and regional businesses and industries, health related organizations, governmental agencies, and non-profit organizations. MSAP students utilize the latest multimedia hardware and software to perform both quantitative and qualitative analyses. Several facilities and labs within the College of Human Development and the Psychology Department will receive or have received lab modernization funds.

Information for Students With Physical Disabilities: See the following Web site for more information: http://www.uwstout.edu/disability/.

Application Information:
Send to Dr. Kristina Gorbatenko-Roth, Program Director, M.S. Applied Psychology, Psychology Department, University of Wisconsin-Stout, Menomonie, WI 54751-0790. Application available online. URL of online application: http://www3.uwstout.edu/programs/msap/apply.cfm. Students are admitted in the Fall, application deadline February 1. All students applying to the graduate study at UW-Stout must apply to both the university-level Graduate School and also to the MSAP program. The MSAP program and the Graduate School each have separate application materials. Applications are accepted past the deadline, space permitting. *Fee:* $56.

WYOMING

Wyoming, University of
Department of Psychology
Arts and Sciences
Department 3415, 1000 East University Avenue
Laramie, WY 82071
Telephone: (307) 766-6303
Fax: (307) 766-2926
E-mail: *cpepper@uwyo.edu*
Web: *http://www.uwyo.edu/psychology*

Department Information:
1909. Chairperson: Carolyn Pepper. Number of faculty: total—full-time 15; women—full-time 7; total—minority—full-time 1; women minority—full-time 1.

Programs and Degrees Offered:
Listed in the following order: Program area, degree type (T if terminal Master's), number awarded 7/08–6/09. Clinical Psychology PhD (Doctor of Philosophy) 2, Developmental Psychology PhD (Doctor of Philosophy) 0, General Psychology PhD (Doctor of Philosophy) 1, Psychology and Law PhD (Doctor of Philosophy) 1.

APA Accreditation: Clinical PhD (Doctor of Philosophy).

Student Applications/Admissions:
Student Applications
Clinical Psychology PhD (Doctor of Philosophy)—Applications 2009–2010, 69. Total applicants accepted 2009–2010, 8. Number full-time enrolled (new admits only) 2009–2010, 4. Openings 2010–2011, 5. The median number of years required for completion of a degree in 2008–2009 were 8. The number of students enrolled full- and part-time who were dismissed or voluntarily withdrew from this program area in 2008–2009 were 2. *Developmental Psychology PhD (Doctor of Philosophy)*—Applications 2009–2010, 9. Total applicants accepted 2009–2010, 2. Number full-time enrolled (new admits only) 2009–2010, 2. Openings 2010–2011, 2. The number of students enrolled full- and part-time who were dismissed or voluntarily withdrew from this program area in 2008–2009 were 0. *General Psychology PhD (Doctor of Philosophy)*—Applications 2009–2010, 14. Total applicants accepted 2009–2010, 1. Number full-time enrolled (new admits only) 2009–2010, 1. Openings 2010–2011, 2. The median number of years required for completion of a degree in 2008–2009 were 5. The number of students enrolled full- and part-time who were dismissed or voluntarily withdrew from this program area in 2008–2009 were 0. *Psychology and Law PhD (Doctor of Philosophy)*—Applications 2009–2010, 4. Total applicants accepted 2009–2010, 0. Number full-time enrolled (new admits only) 2009–2010, 0. Total enrolled 2009–2010 full-time, 3. Openings 2010–2011, 2. The median number of years required for completion of a degree in 2008–2009 were 5. The number of students enrolled full- and part-time who were dismissed or voluntarily withdrew from this program area in 2008–2009 were 0.

Other Criteria: (importance of criteria rated low, medium, or high): GRE scores—high, research experience—high, work experience—low, extracurricular activity—low, clinically related public service—medium, GPA—medium, letters of recommendation—high, interview—high, statement of goals and objectives—high, Work Experience is relevant to the Clinical Program only. For additional information on admission requirements, go to http://uwadmnweb.uwyo.edu/psychology/grad.asp.

Student Characteristics: The following represents characteristics of students in 2009–2010 in all graduate psychology programs in the department: Female—full-time 28, part-time 0; Male—full-time 13, part-time 0; African American/Black—full-time 0, part-time 0; Hispanic/Latino(a)—full-time 2, part-time 0; Asian/Pacific Islander—full-time 1, part-time 0; American Indian/Alaska Native—full-time 1, part-time 0; Caucasian/White—full-time 35, part-time 0; Multi-ethnic—full-time 1, part-time 0; students subject to the Americans With Disabilities Act—full-time 0, part-time 0; Unknown ethnicity—full-time 1, part-time 0; International students who hold an F-1 or J-1 Visa—full-time 3, part-time 0.

Financial Information/Assistance:
Tuition for Full-Time Study: *Master's:* State residents: per academic year $4,392, $183 per credit hour; Nonstate residents: per academic year $12,552, $523 per credit hour. *Doctoral:* State residents: per academic year $4,392, $183 per credit hour; Nonstate residents: per academic year $12,552, $523 per credit hour. See the following Web site for updates and changes in tuition costs: http://www.uwyo.edu/sfa.

Financial Assistance:
First-Year Students: Teaching assistantships available for first year. Average amount paid per academic year: $11,349. Average number of hours worked per week: 20. Research assistantships available for first year. Average amount paid per academic year: $11,349. Average number of hours worked per week: 20.

Advanced Students: Teaching assistantships available for advanced students. Average amount paid per academic year: $15,795. Average number of hours worked per week: 20. Research assistantships available for advanced students. Average amount paid per academic year: $15,795. Average number of hours worked per week: 20.

Additional Information: Of all students currently enrolled full time, 100% benefited from one or more of the listed financial assistance programs.

Internships/Practica: Doctoral Degree (PhD Clinical Psychology): For those doctoral students for whom a professional internship was required in this program prior to graduation, (7) students applied for an internship in 2008–2009, with (7) students obtaining an internship. Of those students who obtained an internship, (7) were paid internships. Of those students who obtained an internship, (7) students placed in APA/CPA accredited internships, (0) students placed in internships not APA/CPA accredited, but listed with the Association of Psychology Postdoctoral and Internship Programs (APPIC), (0) students placed in internships conforming to guidelines of the Council of Directors of School Psychology Programs (CDSPP), (0) students placed in internships that were not APA/CPA accredited, APPIC or CDSPP listed. Given Wyoming's large geographic area (approximately 100,000 square miles) and small population (approximately 500,000), we arrange practica and clerkships for Clinical students in various settings throughout the state. Clerkships are typically conducted in the summer for extended periods of time. Practica and clerkships include a variety of clinical populations such as children, adolescents, adults, and elderly people. They occur in a range of placements including outpatient mental health centers, inpatient hospitals, VA Medical Centers and residential programs. Specialty experiences include forensic evaluation, substance abuse training, and parent training.

Housing and Day Care: On-campus housing is available. See the following Web site for more information: http://www.uwyo.edu/reslife-dining/. On-campus day care facilities are available. See the following Web site for more information: http://www.uwyo.edu/ecec.

Employment of Department Graduates:
Master's Degree Graduates: Of those who graduated in the academic year 2008–2009, the following categories and numbers represent the postgraduate activities and employment of master's degree graduates: Enrolled in a postdoctoral residency/fellowship (n/a), employed in independent practice (n/a), total from the above (master's) (0).
Doctoral Degree Graduates: Of those who graduated in the academic year 2008–2009, the following categories and numbers represent the postgraduate activities and employment of doctoral degree graduates: Enrolled in a psychology doctoral program (n/a), enrolled in a postdoctoral residency/fellowship (1), employed in a community mental health/counseling center (1), employed in a hospital/medical center (1), total from the above (doctoral) (3).

Additional Information:
Orientation, Objectives, and Emphasis of Department: The University of Wyoming is the only four-year university in the state of Wyoming. The graduate curriculum provides breadth of training in psychology and permits specialization in various content areas. The Clinical Psychology PhD program is based on the scientist–practitioner model. Some clinical students may also pursue a concentration in developmental psychology, psychology and law, or social-personality with experimental graduate program faculty. The goal of the clinical program is to provide students with the knowledge base and broad conceptual skills necessary for professional practice and/or research in a variety of settings. The PhD program in Experimental Psychology provides students with broad training that can be used in a variety of academic and applied settings. Students may concentrate in Developmental Psychology or in Social Psychology. Students in any of the programs may pursue a Psychology and Law concentration. All programs contain opportunities for both applied and basic research training.

Special Facilities or Resources: The department has approximately 24,000 square feet of laboratory, office, and clinic space in a science complex with direct access to the university's science library and various computer labs. Faculty laboratories range from wet laboratories designed for the biological aspects of human behavior to labs designed to assess mock jurors and jury decision-making. The Psychology Clinic has ample space for individual or small group assessment and treatment. These facilities also have observation mirrors and video tape-recording capability.

Information for Students With Physical Disabilities: See the following Web site for more information: http://www.uwyo.edu/udss.

Application Information:
Send to Graduate Admissions Committee, Department of Psychology, University of Wyoming, Dept. 3415, 1000 E. University Avenue, Laramie, WY 82071. Application available online. URL of online application: http://www.uwyo.edu/psychology. Students are admitted in the Fall, application deadline January 15. *Fee:* $50. There is no fee for applying to the program. Only students who are accepted into and are officially entering the program are charged the fee.

CANADA

Acadia University
Department of Psychology
18 University Avenue
Wolfville, NS B4P 2R6
Telephone: (902) 585-1301
Fax: (902) 585-1078
E-mail: *peter.horvath@acadiau.ca*
Web: *http://gradstudies.acadiau.ca/psychology.html*

Department Information:
1926. Head: Dr. Peter McLeod. Number of faculty: total—full-time 12, part-time 4; women—full-time 6, part-time 1; total—minority—full-time 1.

Programs and Degrees Offered:
Listed in the following order: Program area, degree type (T if terminal Master's), number awarded 7/08–6/09. Clinical Psychology MA/MS (Master of Arts/Science) (T) 4.

Student Applications/Admissions:
Student Applications
Clinical Psychology MA/MS (Master of Arts/Science)—Applications 2009–2010, 43. Total applicants accepted 2009–2010, 5. Number full-time enrolled (new admits only) 2009–2010, 5. Total enrolled 2009–2010 full-time, 8. Openings 2010–2011, 5. The median number of years required for completion of a degree in 2008–2009 were 2.
Scores: Entries appear in this order: required test or GPA, minimum score (if required), median score of students entering in 2009–2010. *Clinical Psychology MA/MS (Master of Arts/Science):* GRE-V 500, GRE-Q 500, overall undergraduate GPA 3.0, last 2 years GPA 3.0, psychology GPA 3.0.
Other Criteria: (importance of criteria rated low, medium, or high): GRE scores—high, research experience—high, work experience—medium, extracurricular activity—medium, clinically related public service—medium, GPA—high, letters of recommendation—high, interview—high, statement of goals and objectives—high, undergraduate major in psychology—high. For additional information on admission requirements, go to http://gradstudies.acadiau.ca/psychology.html.

Student Characteristics: The following represents characteristics of students in 2009–2010 in all graduate psychology programs in the department: Female—full-time 7, part-time 0; Male—full-time 1, part-time 0; African American/Black—full-time 0, part-time 0; Hispanic/Latino(a)—full-time 0, part-time 0; Asian/Pacific Islander—full-time 0, part-time 0; American Indian/Alaska Native—full-time 0, part-time 0; Caucasian/White—full-time 8, part-time 0; Multi-ethnic—full-time 0, part-time 0; students subject to the Americans With Disabilities Act—full-time 0, part-time 0; Unknown ethnicity—full-time 0, part-time 0; International students who hold an F-1 or J-1 Visa—full-time 0, part-time 0.

Financial Information/Assistance:
Tuition for Full-Time Study: *Master's:* State residents: per academic year $3,612; Nonstate residents: per academic year $4,635. Tuition is subject to change. See the following Web site for updates and changes in tuition costs: http://gradstudies.acadiau.ca/fees.html.

Financial Assistance:
First-Year Students: Teaching assistantships available for first year. Average amount paid per academic year: $9,000. Average number of hours worked per week: 10. Apply by February 1. Research assistantships available for first year. Average amount paid per academic year: $12,000.
Advanced Students: Teaching assistantships available for advanced students. Average amount paid per academic year: $8,000. Average number of hours worked per week: 10.
Additional Information: Of all students currently enrolled full time, 100% benefited from one or more of the listed financial assistance programs. Application and information available online at: http://financialaid.acadiau.ca/.

Internships/Practica: Master's Degree (MA/MS Clinical Psychology): An internship experience, such as, a final research project or "capstone" experience is required of graduates. Two 250-hour internships are mandatory in intervention and assessment. An internship in community psychology is available.

Housing and Day Care: On-campus housing is available. See the following Web site for more information: http://www.acadiau.ca/studentaffairs/residencelife/. No on-campus day care facilities are available.

Employment of Department Graduates:
Master's Degree Graduates: Of those who graduated in the academic year 2008–2009, the following categories and numbers represent the postgraduate activities and employment of master's degree graduates: Enrolled in another graduate/professional program (1), enrolled in a postdoctoral residency/fellowship (n/a), employed in independent practice (n/a), employed in a community mental health/counseling center (3), total from the above (master's) (4).
Doctoral Degree Graduates: Of those who graduated in the academic year 2008–2009, the following categories and numbers represent the postgraduate activities and employment of doctoral degree graduates: Enrolled in a psychology doctoral program (n/a), total from the above (doctoral) (0).

Additional Information:
Orientation, Objectives, and Emphasis of Department: The department's principle objective is to train MSc students in clinical psychology. The department's orientation is eclectic although there is an emphasis on cognitive approaches to problems in psychology. Master's-level registration as a psychologist is available in all Maritime Provinces in Canada. Our curriculum is also highly respected, and graduates going on to doctoral programs elsewhere have had full recognition of coursework in all instances. We are registered with CAMPP.

Special Facilities or Resources: The department is part of the cooperative clinical PhD program of Dalhousie University.

GRADUATE STUDY IN PSYCHOLOGY

Application Information:
Send to Admissions Office, Acadia University, Wolfville, NS, B4P 2R6. Application available online. URL of online application: http://www.acadiau.ca/admissions/gradPrograms.htm. Students are admitted in the Fall, application deadline February 1. *Fee:* $50. Note: All dollar amounts specified in this entry are Canadian dollars.

Alberta, University of (2009 data)
Department of Psychology
P217 Biological Sciences Building
Edmonton, AB T6G 2E9
Telephone: (708) 492-5216
Fax: (708) 492-1768
E-mail: douglas.grant@ualberta.ca
Web: http://www.psych.ualberta.ca

Department Information:
1961. Chair: Douglas S. Grant. Number of faculty: total—full-time 32; women—full-time 8; total—minority—full-time 2.

Programs and Degrees Offered:
Listed in the following order: Program area, degree type (T if terminal Master's), number awarded 7/08–6/09. Experimental Psychology MA/MS (Master of Arts/Science) 1, Experimental Psychology PhD (Doctor of Philosophy) 6.

Student Applications/Admissions:
Student Applications
Experimental Psychology MA/MS (Master of Arts/Science)—Applications 2009–2010, 31. Total applicants accepted 2009–2010, 9. Number full-time enrolled (new admits only) 2009–2010, 6. Total enrolled 2009–2010 full-time, 27. Openings 2010–2011, 5. The median number of years required for completion of a degree in 2008–2009 were 3. The number of students enrolled full- and part-time who were dismissed or voluntarily withdrew from this program area in 2008–2009 were 0. *Experimental Psychology PhD (Doctor of Philosophy)*—Applications 2009–2010, 22. Total applicants accepted 2009–2010, 12. Number full-time enrolled (new admits only) 2009–2010, 5. Total enrolled 2009–2010 full-time, 33. Openings 2010–2011, 5. The median number of years required for completion of a degree in 2008–2009 were 6. The number of students enrolled full- and part-time who were dismissed or voluntarily withdrew from this program area in 2008–2009 were 1.

Other Criteria: (importance of criteria rated low, medium, or high): GRE scores—high, research experience—high, work experience—low, extracurricular activity—low, GPA—high, letters of recommendation—high, statement of goals and objectives—high. For additional information on admission requirements, go to http://www.psych.ualberta.ca/graduate/appinfo.php.

Student Characteristics: The following represents characteristics of students in 2009–2010 in all graduate psychology programs in the department: Female—full-time 26, part-time 0; Male—full-time 12, part-time 0; African American/Black—full-time 0, part-time 0; Hispanic/Latino(a)—full-time 0, part-time 0; Asian/Pacific Islander—full-time 6, part-time 0; American Indian/Alaska Native—full-time 0, part-time 0; Caucasian/White—full-time 0, part-time 0; Multi-ethnic—full-time 0, part-time 0; students subject to the Americans With Disabilities Act—full-time 0, part-time 0; Unknown ethnicity—full-time 0, part-time 0; International students who hold an F-1 or J-1 Visa—full-time 0, part-time 0.

Financial Information/Assistance:
Tuition for Full-Time Study: Master's: State residents: per academic year $4,249; Nonstate residents: per academic year $7,840. *Doctoral:* State residents: per academic year $4,249; Nonstate residents: per academic year $7,840. Tuition is subject to change. See the following Web site for updates and changes in tuition costs: http://www.gradstudies.ualberta.ca/regfees/index.htm.

Financial Assistance:
First-Year Students: Teaching assistantships available for first year. Average amount paid per academic year: $22,690. Average number of hours worked per week: 12. Apply by January 15. Research assistantships available for first year. Average amount paid per academic year: $22,690. Average number of hours worked per week: 12. Apply by January 15. Fellowships and scholarships available for first year. Average number of hours worked per week: 3. Apply by January 15.

Advanced Students: Teaching assistantships available for advanced students. Average amount paid per academic year: $23,330. Average number of hours worked per week: 12. Apply by January 15. Research assistantships available for advanced students. Average amount paid per academic year: $23,330. Average number of hours worked per week: 12. Apply by January 15. Fellowships and scholarships available for advanced students. Average number of hours worked per week: 3. Apply by January 15.

Additional Information: Of all students currently enrolled full time, 95% benefited from one or more of the listed financial assistance programs. Application and information available online at: http://www.psych.ualberta.ca/graduate/finsupport.php.

Internships/Practica: No information provided.

Housing and Day Care: On-campus housing is available. See the following Web site for more information: housing@ualberta.ca, http://www.uofaweb.ualberta.ca/residences/. On-campus day care facilities are available. There are a number of child care agencies. Please ask the Psychology Graduate Assistant for current telephone numbers for child care on campus.

Employment of Department Graduates:
Master's Degree Graduates: Of those who graduated in the academic year 2008–2009, the following categories and numbers represent the postgraduate activities and employment of master's degree graduates: Enrolled in another graduate/professional program (1), enrolled in a postdoctoral residency/fellowship (n/a), employed in independent practice (n/a), employed in an academic position at a university (1), not seeking employment (1), total from the above (master's) (3).
Doctoral Degree Graduates: Of those who graduated in the academic year 2008–2009, the following categories and numbers represent the postgraduate activities and employment of doctoral degree graduates: Enrolled in a psychology doctoral program (n/a), enrolled in a postdoctoral residency/fellowship (2), employed in

a professional position in a school system (1), employed in a government agency (1), total from the above (doctoral) (4).

Additional Information:
Orientation, Objectives, and Emphasis of Department: The goal of the graduate program is to train competent and independent researchers who will make significant contributions to the discipline of psychology. The program entails early and sustained involvement in research and ensures that students attain expertise in focal and related domains. The program offers training that leads to degrees in a range of research areas, including: Behaviour, Systems and Cognitive Neuroscience; Cognition; Comparative Cognition and Behaviour Developmental Science; and Social and Cultural Psychology. Recent PhD graduates from the Department have successfully found positions in universities and colleges, branches of government, and industry. A reasonably close match between the research interests of prospective students and faculty members is essential because the program involves apprenticeship-style training. Although many faculty members conduct research on problems that have practical and social significance, we do not have programs in clinical, counseling, or industrial/organizational psychology.

Special Facilities or Resources: The department maintains a number of specialized support facilities for staff and student use including an electronics shop, labs for teaching and research use, and an instructional technology lab to support teaching. In addition, the department maintains a psychology reading room and a small facility for photographic needs. Department computing resources include approximately 300 computers used in research and a further 40 computers used for administration and instructional needs. All staff and student computers have network capability on the department and campus networks. Technical assistance for research, teaching, and administrative needs is provided by department technical staff. For research services, the department maintains a fully equipped electronics shop staffed by technicians who design, build, and maintain custom laboratory equipment and data acquisition devices for laboratory applications. The shop contains a variety of professional equipment for electronics and fabrication work and stocks supplies for research and equipment needs. Technical staff also provide a full range of assistance with equipment selection and ordering, equipment repair, and new equipment configuration and setup. Other resources include the University Teaching Program, which improves the teaching skills of graduate students through workshops and practica, and the Community-University Partnership, which facilitates community- and school-based research.

Information for Students With Physical Disabilities: See the following Web site for more information: http://www.uofaweb.ualberta.ca/SSDS/.

Application Information:
Send to Graduate Program Assistant, Department of Psychology, P-217D Biological Sciences, University of Alberta, Edmonton, AB Canada T6G 2E9. Application available online. URL of online application: http://www.psych.ualberta.ca/graduate/appinfo.php. Students are admitted in the Fall, application deadline January 15. The Department admits approximately ten graduate students per year. Students holding an undergraduate degree are admitted either to the Master's Program or directly to the PhD program; upon successful completion of the Master's degree they would normally continue in the PhD program. Students holding a qualifying Master's Degree are admitted directly to the PhD Program. *Fee:* $100. Note: All dollar amounts specified in this entry are Canadian dollars.

British Columbia, University of
Department of Psychology
2136 West Mall, Kenny Psychology Building
Vancouver, BC V6T 1Z4
Telephone: (604) 822-3144
Fax: (604) 822-6923
E-mail: *gradsec@psych.ubc.ca*
Web: *http://www.psych.ubc.ca*

Department Information:
1951. Head: Eric Eich. Number of faculty: total—full-time 48, part-time 27; women—full-time 21, part-time 15.

Programs and Degrees Offered:
Listed in the following order: Program area, degree type (T if terminal Master's), number awarded 7/08–6/09. Behavioral Neuroscience PhD (Doctor of Philosophy) 1, Clinical PhD (Doctor of Philosophy) 3, Forensic PhD (Doctor of Philosophy) 4, Developmental PhD (Doctor of Philosophy) 1, Cognitive Science PhD (Doctor of Philosophy) 4, Social/Personality PhD (Doctor of Philosophy) 4, Quantitative Methods PhD (Doctor of Philosophy) 0, Health PhD (Doctor of Philosophy) 0.

APA Accreditation: Clinical PhD (Doctor of Philosophy). Student Outcome Data Website: http://www.psych.ubc.ca/grad-pgm/areasspec.psy?contid=101306171911.

CPA Accreditation: Clinical PhD (Doctor of Philosophy).

Student Applications/Admissions:
Student Applications
Behavioral Neuroscience PhD (Doctor of Philosophy)—Applications 2009–2010, 8. Total applicants accepted 2009–2010, 2. Number full-time enrolled (new admits only) 2009–2010, 2. Number part-time enrolled (new admits only) 2009–2010, 0. Openings 2010–2011, 6. The median number of years required for completion of a degree in 2008–2009 were 6. The number of students enrolled full- and part-time who were dismissed or voluntarily withdrew from this program area in 2008–2009 were 0. Clinical PhD (Doctor of Philosophy)—Applications 2009–2010, 110. Total applicants accepted 2009–2010, 7. Number full-time enrolled (new admits only) 2009–2010, 5. Number part-time enrolled (new admits only) 2009–2010, 0. Openings 2010–2011, 8. The median number of years required for completion of a degree in 2008–2009 were 7. The number of students enrolled full- and part-time who were dismissed or voluntarily withdrew from this program area in 2008–2009 were 1. Forensic PhD (Doctor of Philosophy)—Applications 2009–2010, 0. Total applicants accepted 2009–2010, 0. Number full-time enrolled (new admits only) 2009–2010, 0. Number part-time enrolled (new admits only) 2009–2010, 0. The median number of years required for completion of a degree in 2008–2009 were 7. The number of students enrolled full- and part-time who were dismissed or voluntarily withdrew from this program area in 2008–2009 were 0. Developmental

PhD (Doctor of Philosophy)—Applications 2009–2010, 21. Total applicants accepted 2009–2010, 1. Number full-time enrolled (new admits only) 2009–2010, 1. Number part-time enrolled (new admits only) 2009–2010, 0. Openings 2010–2011, 6. The median number of years required for completion of a degree in 2008–2009 were 7. The number of students enrolled full- and part-time who were dismissed or voluntarily withdrew from this program area in 2008–2009 were 1. *Cognitive Science PhD (Doctor of Philosophy)*—Applications 2009–2010, 32. Total applicants accepted 2009–2010, 10. Number full-time enrolled (new admits only) 2009–2010, 4. Number part-time enrolled (new admits only) 2009–2010, 0. Openings 2010–2011, 8. The median number of years required for completion of a degree in 2008–2009 were 6. The number of students enrolled full- and part-time who were dismissed or voluntarily withdrew from this program area in 2008–2009 were 0. *Social/Personality PhD (Doctor of Philosophy)*—Applications 2009–2010, 54. Total applicants accepted 2009–2010, 9. Number full-time enrolled (new admits only) 2009–2010, 7. Number part-time enrolled (new admits only) 2009–2010, 0. Openings 2010–2011, 10. The median number of years required for completion of a degree in 2008–2009 were 6. The number of students enrolled full- and part-time who were dismissed or voluntarily withdrew from this program area in 2008–2009 were 2. *Quantitative Methods PhD (Doctor of Philosophy)*—Applications 2009–2010, 8. Total applicants accepted 2009–2010, 2. Number full-time enrolled (new admits only) 2009–2010, 1. Number part-time enrolled (new admits only) 2009–2010, 0. Openings 2010–2011, 4. The number of students enrolled full- and part-time who were dismissed or voluntarily withdrew from this program area in 2008–2009 were 0. *Health PhD (Doctor of Philosophy)*—Applications 2009–2010, 13. Total applicants accepted 2009–2010, 6. Number full-time enrolled (new admits only) 2009–2010, 4. Number part-time enrolled (new admits only) 2009–2010, 0. Openings 2010–2011, 6. The number of students enrolled full- and part-time who were dismissed or voluntarily withdrew from this program area in 2008–2009 were 1.

Scores: Entries appear in this order: required test or GPA, minimum score (if required), median score of students entering in 2009–2010. *Behavioral Neuroscience PhD (Doctor of Philosophy)*: GRE-V 580, 500, GRE-Q 740, 625, GRE-Analytical 5.0, 4.5, last 2 years GPA 76, 81; *Clinical PhD (Doctor of Philosophy)*: GRE-V 580, 630, GRE-Q 740, 740, GRE-Analytical 5.0, 5.0, last 2 years GPA 76, 84; *Developmental PhD (Doctor of Philosophy)*: GRE-V 580, 630, GRE-Q 740, 770, GRE-Analytical 5.0, 5.0, last 2 years GPA 76, 90; *Cognitive Science PhD (Doctor of Philosophy)*: GRE-V 580, 575, GRE-Q 740, 670, GRE-Analytical 5.0, 4.5, last 2 years GPA 76, 87; *Social/Personality PhD (Doctor of Philosophy)*: GRE-V 580, 720, GRE-Q 740, 770, GRE-Analytical 5.0, 5.0, last 2 years GPA 76, 88; *Quantitative Methods PhD (Doctor of Philosophy)*: GRE-V 580, 530, GRE-Q 740, 530, GRE-Analytical 5.0, 6.0, last 2 years GPA 76, 88; *Health PhD (Doctor of Philosophy)*: GRE-V 580, 625, GRE-Q 740, 675, GRE-Analytical 5.0, 4.8, last 2 years GPA 76, 86.

Other Criteria: (importance of criteria rated low, medium, or high): GRE scores—medium, research experience—high, clinically related public service—low, GPA—high, letters of recommendation—high, interview—medium, statement of goals and objectives—high, undergraduate major in psychology—high, specific undergraduate psychology courses taken—medium. For additional information on admission requirements, go to http://www.psych.ubc.ca/grad-pgm/admissions.psy.

Student Characteristics: The following represents characteristics of students in 2009–2010 in all graduate psychology programs in the department: Female—full-time 80, part-time 0; Male—full-time 31, part-time 0; African American/Black—full-time 0, part-time 0; Hispanic/Latino(a)—full-time 0, part-time 0; Asian/Pacific Islander—full-time 0, part-time 0; American Indian/Alaska Native—full-time 0, part-time 0; Caucasian/White—full-time 0, part-time 0; Multi-ethnic—full-time 0, part-time 0; students subject to the Americans With Disabilities Act—full-time 0, part-time 0; Unknown ethnicity—full-time 0, part-time 0; International students who hold an F-1 or J-1 Visa—full-time 0, part-time 0.

Financial Information/Assistance:

Tuition for Full-Time Study: *Master's:* State residents: per academic year $4,018; Nonstate residents: per academic year $4,018. *Doctoral:* State residents: per academic year $4,018; Nonstate residents: per academic year $4,018. Tuition is subject to change. See the following Web site for updates and changes in tuition costs: http://www.grad.ubc.ca/apply/tuition/.

Financial Assistance:

First-Year Students: Teaching assistantships available for first year. Average amount paid per academic year: $10,914. Average number of hours worked per week: 12. Apply by January 15. Research assistantships available for first year. Average amount paid per academic year: $5,000. Apply by January 15. Fellowships and scholarships available for first year. Average amount paid per academic year: $17,500. Apply by January 15.

Advanced Students: Teaching assistantships available for advanced students. Average amount paid per academic year: $11,342. Average number of hours worked per week: 12. Apply by January 15. Research assistantships available for advanced students. Average amount paid per academic year: $5,000. Apply by January 15. Fellowships and scholarships available for advanced students. Average amount paid per academic year: $16,000. Apply by September 15.

Additional Information: Of all students currently enrolled full time, 100% benefited from one or more of the listed financial assistance programs. Application and information available online at: http://www.psych.ubc.ca/grad-pgm/admissions.psy.

Internships/Practica: Doctoral Degree (PhD Clinical): For those doctoral students for whom a professional internship was required in this program prior to graduation, (4) students applied for an internship in 2008–2009, with (4) students obtaining an internship. Of those students who obtained an internship, (4) were paid internships. Of those students who obtained an internship, (4) students placed in APA/CPA accredited internships, (0) students placed in internships not APA/CPA accredited, but listed with the Association of Psychology Postdoctoral and Internship Programs (APPIC), (0) students placed in internships conforming to guidelines of the Council of Directors of School Psychology Programs (CDSPP), (0) students placed in internships that were not APA/CPA accredited, APPIC or CDSPP listed. A 4-month practicum in an approved agency is required of clinical students during the summer after the second or third year of the program or during the third year. A 1-year internship at a mental health agency accredited by CPA or APA is required for the PhD in clinical psychology.

Housing and Day Care: On-campus housing is available. See the following Web site for more information: http://www.grad.ubc.ca/campus-community/residential-graduate-colleges. On-campus day care facilities are available. See the following Web site for more information: http://www.childcare.ubc.ca/.

Employment of Department Graduates:

Master's Degree Graduates: Of those who graduated in the academic year 2008–2009, the following categories and numbers represent the postgraduate activities and employment of master's degree graduates: Enrolled in a postdoctoral residency/fellowship (n/a), employed in independent practice (n/a), total from the above (master's) (0).

Doctoral Degree Graduates: Of those who graduated in the academic year 2008–2009, the following categories and numbers represent the postgraduate activities and employment of doctoral degree graduates: Enrolled in a psychology doctoral program (n/a), enrolled in a postdoctoral residency/fellowship (4), employed in independent practice (1), employed in an academic position at a university (3), employed in an academic position at a 2-year/4-year college (1), employed in business or industry (1), employed in a government agency (4), employed in a hospital/medical center (2), total from the above (doctoral) (17).

Additional Information:

Orientation, Objectives, and Emphasis of Department: The department is organized into seven subject content areas with which faculty and graduate students are affiliated. Graduate training emphasizes a high degree of research competence and, from the beginning of the program, students are involved in increasingly independent research activities.

Special Facilities or Resources: The department is housed in an attractive building of about 90,000 square feet, designed for psychological research. The department has well-equipped research facilities including a psychology clinic, observation galleries, and animal, psychophysiological, perceptual, cognitive, and social/personality laboratories.

Information for Students With Physical Disabilities: See the following Web site for more information: http://www.students.ubc.ca/access/drc.cfm.

Application Information:
Send to Graduate Secretary, Department of Psychology, University of British Columbia, Vancouver, BC, Canada V6T 1Z4. Application available online. URL of online application: http://www.grad.ubc.ca/apply/online/. Students are admitted in the Fall, application deadline January 15. Fee: $90. The application fee for international applicants is $150. The application fee is waived for international applicants whose correspondence address is located in one of the world's 50 least developed countries, as declared by the United Nations. Note: All dollar amounts specified in this entry are Canadian dollars.

Calgary, University of
Department of Psychology
2500 University Drive, Northwest
Calgary, AB T2N 1N4
Telephone: (403) 220-5561
Fax: (403) 282-8249
E-mail: *psycgrad@ucalgary.ca*
Web: *http://psych.ucalgary.ca/*

Department Information:
1964. Head: Dr. Keith Dobson. Number of faculty: total—full-time 31; women—full-time 11; total—minority—full-time 2; women minority—full-time 1.

Programs and Degrees Offered:
Listed in the following order: Program area, degree type (T if terminal Master's), number awarded 7/08–6/09. Psychology PhD (Doctor of Philosophy) 6, Clinical Psychology PhD (Doctor of Philosophy) 4.

CPA Accreditation: Clinical PhD (Doctor of Philosophy).

Student Applications/Admissions:

Student Applications

Psychology PhD (Doctor of Philosophy)—Applications 2009–2010, 36. Total applicants accepted 2009–2010, 9. Number full-time enrolled (new admits only) 2009–2010, 20. Openings 2010–2011, 7. The median number of years required for completion of a degree in 2008–2009 were 3. The number of students enrolled full- and part-time who were dismissed or voluntarily withdrew from this program area in 2008–2009 were 0. *Clinical Psychology PhD (Doctor of Philosophy)*—Applications 2009–2010, 55. Total applicants accepted 2009–2010, 7. Number full-time enrolled (new admits only) 2009–2010, 7. Openings 2010–2011, 7. The median number of years required for completion of a degree in 2008–2009 were 3. The number of students enrolled full- and part-time who were dismissed or voluntarily withdrew from this program area in 2008–2009 were 0.

Scores: Entries appear in this order: required test or GPA, minimum score (if required), median score of students entering in 2009–2010. *Psychology PhD (Doctor of Philosophy)*: GRE-V no minimum stated, GRE-Q no minimum stated, GRE-Analytical no minimum stated, overall undergraduate GPA 3.0, last 2 years GPA 3.4, Masters GPA 3.4; *Clinical Psychology PhD (Doctor of Philosophy)*: GRE-V no minimum stated, GRE-Q no minimum stated, GRE-Analytical no minimum stated, overall undergraduate GPA 3.0, last 2 years GPA 3.6, Masters GPA 3.6.

Other Criteria: (importance of criteria rated low, medium, or high): GRE scores—medium, research experience—high, work experience—medium, extracurricular activity—low, clinically related public service—medium, GPA—high, letters of recommendation—high, interview—medium, statement of goals and objectives—medium, Research proposal—medium, undergraduate major in psychology—high, specific undergraduate psychology courses taken—high. For additional information on admission requirements, go to http://psych.ucalgary.ca/graduate.

Student Characteristics: The following represents characteristics of students in 2009–2010 in all graduate psychology programs in the department: Female—full-time 57, part-time 0; Male—full-time 16, part-time 0; African American/Black—full-time 0, part-time 0; Hispanic/Latino(a)—full-time 0, part-time 0; Asian/Pacific Islander—full-time 7, part-time 0; American Indian/Alaska Native—full-time 0, part-time 0; Caucasian/White—full-time 66, part-time 0; Multi-ethnic—full-time 0, part-time 0; students subject to the Americans With Disabilities Act—full-time 0, part-time 0; Unknown ethnicity—full-time 0, part-time 0; International students who hold an F-1 or J-1 Visa—full-time 0, part-time 0.

Financial Information/Assistance:
   Tuition for Full-Time Study: *Doctoral:* State residents: per academic year $5,359; Nonstate residents: per academic year $12,164. Tuition is subject to change. See the following Web site for updates and changes in tuition costs: http://www.grad.ucalgary.ca/fees.

Financial Assistance:
   First-Year Students: Teaching assistantships available for first year. Average amount paid per academic year: $15,302. Average number of hours worked per week: 12. Fellowships and scholarships available for first year. Average amount paid per academic year: $4,198.
   Advanced Students: Teaching assistantships available for advanced students. Average amount paid per academic year: $15,302. Average number of hours worked per week: 12. Fellowships and scholarships available for advanced students. Average amount paid per academic year: $5,698.
   Additional Information: Of all students currently enrolled full time, 100% benefited from one or more of the listed financial assistance programs. Application and information available online at: http://www.grad.ucalgary.ca/Funding/.

Internships/Practica: Doctoral Degree (PhD Clinical Psychology): For those doctoral students for whom a professional internship was required in this program prior to graduation, (4) students applied for an internship in 2008–2009, with (4) students obtaining an internship. Of those students who obtained an internship, (4) were paid internships. Of those students who obtained an internship, (4) students placed in APA/CPA accredited internships, (0) students placed in internships not APA/CPA accredited, but listed with the Association of Psychology Postdoctoral and Internship Programs (APPIC), (0) students placed in internships conforming to guidelines of the Council of Directors of School Psychology Programs (CDSPP), (0) students placed in internships that were not APA/CPA accredited, APPIC or CDSPP listed. Practica are available at several settings, including Alberta Health Services and other community services.

Housing and Day Care: On-campus housing is available. See the following Web site for more information: http://www.ucalgary.ca/residence/. On-campus day care facilities are available. See the following Web site for more information: http://www.ucalgary.ca/uccc/.

Employment of Department Graduates:
   Master's Degree Graduates: Of those who graduated in the academic year 2008–2009, the following categories and numbers represent the postgraduate activities and employment of master's degree graduates: Enrolled in a postdoctoral residency/fellowship (n/a), employed in independent practice (n/a), total from the above (master's) (0).
   Doctoral Degree Graduates: Of those who graduated in the academic year 2008–2009, the following categories and numbers represent the postgraduate activities and employment of doctoral degree graduates: Enrolled in a psychology doctoral program (n/a), enrolled in a postdoctoral residency/fellowship (1), employed in independent practice (2), employed in an academic position at a university (2), employed in other positions at a higher education institution (1), employed in business or industry (3), employed in a community mental health/counseling center (1), employed in a hospital/medical center (4), total from the above (doctoral) (14).

Additional Information:
   Orientation, Objectives, and Emphasis of Department: This is a research-oriented department with a strong focus on applied problems. We offer both a clinical psychology and a psychology program. Specific research programs in psychology include: behavioral neuroscience, cognition and cognitive development (CCD), industrial/organizational psychology (I/O), social psychology, perception aging and cognitive ergonomics (PACE), and theoretical psychology.

Application Information:
Send to Graduate Programs Administrator, Department of Psychology, 2500 University Drive NW, University of Calgary, Calgary, AB T2N1N4 Canada. Application available online. URL of online application: https://www.gradapplication.ucalgary.ca/account/instructions.asp. Students are admitted in the Fall, application deadline January 7. The deadline for the Clinical Psychology program is January 7, and the deadline for the Industrial/Organizational program is January 15. Fee: $100. International student application fee is $130. Note: All dollar amounts specified in this entry are Canadian dollars.

Carleton University
Department of Psychology
Faculty of Arts and Social Sciences
1125 Colonel By Drive
Ottawa, ON K1S 5B6
Telephone: (613) 520-2647
Fax: (613) 520-3667
E-mail: *psychchair@carleton.ca*
Web: *http://www.carleton.ca/psychology/*

Department Information:
   1952. Chairperson: Janet Mantler. Number of faculty: total—full-time 48; women—full-time 22; total—minority—full-time 4; women minority—full-time 3.

Programs and Degrees Offered:
   Listed in the following order: Program area, degree type (T if terminal Master's), number awarded 7/08–6/09. Psychology MA/MS (Master of Arts/Science) (T) 30, Neuroscience MA/MS (Master of Arts/Science) 6, Psychology PhD (Doctor of Philosophy) 10.

Student Applications/Admissions:
   Student Applications
      Psychology MA/MS (Master of Arts/Science)—Applications 2009–2010, 158. Total applicants accepted 2009–2010, 58.

Number full-time enrolled (new admits only) 2009–2010, 31. Number part-time enrolled (new admits only) 2009–2010, 1. Total enrolled 2009–2010 full-time, 68, part-time, 14. Openings 2010–2011, 35. The median number of years required for completion of a degree in 2008–2009 were 2. The number of students enrolled full- and part-time who were dismissed or voluntarily withdrew from this program area in 2008–2009 were 3. *Neuroscience MA/MS (Master of Arts/Science)*—Applications 2009–2010, 23. Total applicants accepted 2009–2010, 10. Number full-time enrolled (new admits only) 2009–2010, 13. Number part-time enrolled (new admits only) 2009–2010, 0. Openings 2010–2011, 8. The median number of years required for completion of a degree in 2008–2009 were 2. The number of students enrolled full- and part-time who were dismissed or voluntarily withdrew from this program area in 2008–2009 were 4. *Psychology PhD (Doctor of Philosophy)*—Applications 2009–2010, 29. Total applicants accepted 2009–2010, 19. Number full-time enrolled (new admits only) 2009–2010, 20. Number part-time enrolled (new admits only) 2009–2010, 0. Total enrolled 2009–2010 full-time, 70, part-time, 20. Openings 2010–2011, 14. The median number of years required for completion of a degree in 2008–2009 were 4. The number of students enrolled full- and part-time who were dismissed or voluntarily withdrew from this program area in 2008–2009 were 3.

Scores: Entries appear in this order: required test or GPA, minimum score (if required), median score of students entering in 2009–2010. *Psychology MA/MS (Master of Arts/Science)*: overall undergraduate GPA 70, 79, last 2 years GPA 72, 80, psychology GPA 79, 85; *Neuroscience MA/MS (Master of Arts/Science)*: overall undergraduate GPA 70, last 2 years GPA 72, 80, psychology GPA 77, 85; *Psychology PhD (Doctor of Philosophy)*: last 2 years GPA 80, 80, psychology GPA 80, 85, Masters GPA 80, 90.

Other Criteria: (importance of criteria rated low, medium, or high): research experience—high, work experience—medium, extracurricular activity—medium, GPA—high, letters of recommendation—high, statement of goals and objectives—high, undergraduate major in psychology—high, specific undergraduate psychology courses taken—high. For additional information on admission requirements, go to http://www.carleton.ca/psychology/prospective-students/graduate/.

Student Characteristics: The following represents characteristics of students in 2009–2010 in all graduate psychology programs in the department: Female—full-time 111, part-time 29; Male—full-time 52, part-time 5; African American/Black—full-time 2, part-time 0; Asian/Pacific Islander—full-time 1, part-time 0; American Indian/Alaska Native—full-time 1, part-time 0; Caucasian/White—full-time 159, part-time 34; Unknown ethnicity—full-time 0, part-time 0; International students who hold an F-1 or J-1 Visa—full-time 4, part-time 0.

Financial Information/Assistance:
Tuition for Full-Time Study: Master's: State residents: per academic year $6,848; Nonstate residents: per academic year $14,992. *Doctoral:* State residents: per academic year $6,848; Nonstate residents: per academic year $14,992. Tuition is subject to change. See the following Web site for updates and changes in tuition costs: http://www.carleton.ca/fees/.

Financial Assistance:
First-Year Students: Teaching assistantships available for first year. Average amount paid per academic year: $9,638. Average number of hours worked per week: 10. Apply by January 15. Research assistantships available for first year. Average amount paid per academic year: $3,000. Apply by January 15. Fellowships and scholarships available for first year. Average amount paid per academic year: $5,000. Apply by January 15.

Advanced Students: Teaching assistantships available for advanced students. Average amount paid per academic year: $9,638. Average number of hours worked per week: 10. Apply by January 15. Research assistantships available for advanced students. Average amount paid per academic year: $3,500. Apply by January 15. Fellowships and scholarships available for advanced students. Average amount paid per academic year: $8,000. Apply by January 15.

Additional Information: Of all students currently enrolled full time, 62% benefited from one or more of the listed financial assistance programs. Application and information available online at: http://www.carleton.ca/psychology/prospective-students/graduate/scholarships-and-wards/.

Internships/Practica: No information provided.

Housing and Day Care: On-campus housing is available. See the following Web site for more information: http://www.carleton.ca/housing/. On-campus day care facilities are available. See the following Web site for more information: http://www.cbccc.ca/.

Employment of Department Graduates:
Master's Degree Graduates: Of those who graduated in the academic year 2008–2009, the following categories and numbers represent the postgraduate activities and employment of master's degree graduates: Enrolled in a psychology doctoral program (24), enrolled in a postdoctoral residency/fellowship (n/a), employed in independent practice (n/a), employed in a government agency (10), still seeking employment (1), not seeking employment (1), other employment position (2), do not know (2), total from the above (master's) (40).

Doctoral Degree Graduates: Of those who graduated in the academic year 2008–2009, the following categories and numbers represent the postgraduate activities and employment of doctoral degree graduates: Enrolled in a psychology doctoral program (n/a), enrolled in a postdoctoral residency/fellowship (5), employed in an academic position at a university (2), employed in a government agency (2), other employment position (1), total from the above (doctoral) (10).

Additional Information:
Orientation, Objectives, and Emphasis of Department: The program is strongly research-oriented, although practical courses such as quantitative methods, testing and behavior modification are available. This degree however does not offer training in applied areas (e.g. clinical, educational, counseling psychology, etc).

Information for Students With Physical Disabilities: See the following Web site for more information: http://www.carleton.ca/paulmenton/.

Application Information:
Send to Graduate Studies Administrator B-557 Loeb Building 1125 Colonel By Drive Ottawa, ON K1S 5B6. Application available online.

GRADUATE STUDY IN PSYCHOLOGY

URL of online application: http://www.carleton.ca/psychology/prospective-students/graduate/how-to-apply/. Students are admitted in the Fall, application deadline January 15; Winter, application deadline November 1. *Fee:* $100. Note: All dollar amounts specified in this entry are Canadian dollars.

Concordia University
Department of Psychology
7141 Sherbrooke Street West
Montreal, QC H4B 1R6
Telephone: (514) 848-2424, (2205)
Fax: (514) 848-4545
E-mail: *Shirley.Black@concordia.ca*
Web: *http://psychology.concordia.ca*

Department Information:
1963. Chairperson: Jean-Roch Laurence, PhD. Number of faculty: total—full-time 37, part-time 17; women—full-time 12, part-time 4.

Programs and Degrees Offered:
Listed in the following order: Program area, degree type (T if terminal Master's), number awarded 7/08–6/09. Research and Clinical Training PhD (Doctor of Philosophy) 5, Research PhD (Doctor of Philosophy) 3.

APA Accreditation: Clinical PhD (Doctor of Philosophy).

CPA Accreditation: Clinical PhD (Doctor of Philosophy).

Student Applications/Admissions:
Student Applications
Research and Clinical Training PhD (Doctor of Philosophy)—Applications 2009–2010, 178. Total applicants accepted 2009–2010, 13. Number full-time enrolled (new admits only) 2009–2010, 10. Number part-time enrolled (new admits only) 2009–2010, 0. Openings 2010–2011, 11. The median number of years required for completion of a degree in 2008–2009 were 7. The number of students enrolled full- and part-time who were dismissed or voluntarily withdrew from this program area in 2008–2009 were 1. Research PhD (Doctor of Philosophy)—Applications 2009–2010, 52. Total applicants accepted 2009–2010, 10. Number full-time enrolled (new admits only) 2009–2010, 6. Number part-time enrolled (new admits only) 2009–2010, 0. Total enrolled 2009–2010 full-time, 56, part-time, 1. Openings 2010–2011, 11. The median number of years required for completion of a degree in 2008–2009 were 5. The number of students enrolled full- and part-time who were dismissed or voluntarily withdrew from this program area in 2008–2009 were 0.

Other Criteria: (importance of criteria rated low, medium, or high): GRE scores—low, research experience—high, work experience—medium, extracurricular activity—low, clinically related public service—medium, GPA—medium, letters of recommendation—high, interview—medium, statement of goals and objectives—high, undergraduate major in psychology—high, specific undergraduate psychology courses taken—medium. Research Option does not require clinically related service. Thesis Supervisor is required for admission to graduate program. For additional information on admission requirements, go to http://psychology.concordia.ca/graduateprograms/applyingtopsychology/.

Student Characteristics: The following represents characteristics of students in 2009–2010 in all graduate psychology programs in the department: Female—full-time 101, part-time 0; Male—full-time 31, part-time 1; African American/Black—full-time 0, part-time 0; Hispanic/Latino(a)—full-time 0, part-time 0; Asian/Pacific Islander—full-time 0, part-time 0; American Indian/Alaska Native—full-time 0, part-time 0; Caucasian/White—full-time 0, part-time 0; Multi-ethnic—full-time 0, part-time 0; students subject to the Americans With Disabilities Act—full-time 0, part-time 0; Unknown ethnicity—full-time 0, part-time 0; International students who hold an F-1 or J-1 Visa—full-time 0, part-time 0.

Financial Information/Assistance:
Tuition for Full-Time Study: *Master's:* State residents: per academic year $3,466; Nonstate residents: per academic year $16,296. *Doctoral:* State residents: per academic year $3,466; Nonstate residents: per academic year $12,235. Tuition is subject to change. Tuition costs vary by program. See the following Web site for updates and changes in tuition costs: http://tuitionandfees.concordia.ca.

Financial Assistance:
First-Year Students: Teaching assistantships available for first year. Average amount paid per academic year: $3,750. Average number of hours worked per week: 10. Apply by August 1. Research assistantships available for first year. Average amount paid per academic year: $11,250. Average number of hours worked per week: 10. Fellowships and scholarships available for first year. Average amount paid per academic year: $20,000. Apply by October.

Advanced Students: Teaching assistantships available for advanced students. Average amount paid per academic year: $7,500. Average number of hours worked per week: 10. Apply by August 1. Research assistantships available for advanced students. Average amount paid per academic year: $7,500. Average number of hours worked per week: 10. Fellowships and scholarships available for advanced students. Average amount paid per academic year: $21,200. Apply by October.

Additional Information: Of all students currently enrolled full time, 74% benefited from one or more of the listed financial assistance programs. Application and information available online at: http://graduatestudies.concordia.ca/awards.

Internships/Practica: Doctoral Degree (PhD Research and Clinical Training): For those doctoral students for whom a professional internship was required in this program prior to graduation, (10) students applied for an internship in 2008–2009, with (10) students obtaining an internship. Of those students who obtained an internship, (9) were paid internships. Of those students who obtained an internship, (8) students placed in APA/CPA accredited internships, (0) students placed in internships not APA/CPA accredited, but listed with the Association of Psychology Postdoctoral and Internship Programs (APPIC), (0) students placed in internships conforming to guidelines of the Council of Directors of School Psychology Programs (CDSPP), (2) students placed in internships that were not APA/CPA accredited, APPIC or CDSPP listed. Clinical students complete a variety of practica and internships while in program residence. All clinical students receive extensive practicum experience in psychotherapy and assessment in our on-campus training clinic, the Applied Psychology Center (APC). APC clients are seen by graduate students under the supervision of clinical faculty. The types of services offered by the APC reflect the interests of clinical supervisors and students, and may include individual, family, or marital psychotherapy, behavior therapy for sexual or phobic difficulties, and treatment of child disorders. During the summer of their second year, students also complete a full-time practicum at a mental health facility in the Montreal area. During their final year in the program, students complete their full-time, predoctoral clinical internships. Recent students have undertaken predoctoral internships at a variety of mental health facilities across Canada and the United States. All students are encouraged to seek internship positions in settings accredited by either the Canadian or American Psychological Associations.

Housing and Day Care: No on-campus housing is available. On-campus day care facilities are available. See the following Web site for more information: http://deanofstudents.concordia.ca/childcare/.

Employment of Department Graduates:
Master's Degree Graduates: Of those who graduated in the academic year 2008–2009, the following categories and numbers represent the postgraduate activities and employment of master's degree graduates: Enrolled in a psychology doctoral program (16), enrolled in another graduate/professional program (0), enrolled in a postdoctoral residency/fellowship (n/a), employed in independent practice (n/a), employed in an academic position at a university (0), employed in an academic position at a 2-year/4-year college (0), employed in other positions at a higher education institution (0), employed in a professional position in a school system (0), employed in business or industry (0), employed in a government agency (0), employed in a community mental health/counseling center (0), employed in a hospital/medical center (0), still seeking employment (0), not seeking employment (0), other employment position (0), do not know (1), total from the above (master's) (17).
Doctoral Degree Graduates: Of those who graduated in the academic year 2008–2009, the following categories and numbers represent the postgraduate activities and employment of doctoral degree graduates: Enrolled in a psychology doctoral program (n/a), enrolled in another graduate/professional program (0), enrolled in a postdoctoral residency/fellowship (2), employed in independent practice (3), employed in an academic position at a university (1), employed in an academic position at a 2-year/4-year college (0), employed in other positions at a higher education institution (0), employed in a professional position in a school system (0), employed in business or industry (0), employed in a government agency (0), employed in a community mental health/counseling center (3), employed in a hospital/medical center (0), still seeking employment (0), other employment position (0), do not know (0), total from the above (doctoral) (10).

Additional Information:
Orientation, Objectives, and Emphasis of Department: Graduate education in both experimental and clinical psychology is strongly research-oriented and intended for students who are planning to complete the PhD degree. The research program for all students is based on an apprentice-type model. An outstanding feature of graduate education at Concordia is that students pursuing only research studies and students pursuing research and clinical studies may conduct their research in the laboratory of any faculty member. A wide variety of contemporary research areas are represented, ranging from behavioral neurobiology, to cognitive and developmental science, to applied interventions with humans. Research findings from numerous areas are integrated in an effort to solve problems associated with appetitive motivation and drug dependence, memory and aging, human cognition and development, developmental psychobiology, adult and child psychopathology, and sexual dysfunctions, to name several examples. Clinical training is based on the scientist–practitioner model. That is, clinical students meet the same research requirements as other students, and receive extensive professional training in the delivery of psychological services. Students may choose to specialize their clinical training with children or adults.

Special Facilities or Resources: The department has extensive animal and human research facilities that are supported by provincial, federal, and U.S. granting agencies as well as various internal and private sector funds. Research laboratories are well equipped. The department also contains two research centers that are jointly funded by the Government of Quebec and the University, the Center for Studies in Behavioral Neurobiology, and the Center for Research in Human Development. Both centers coordinate multidisciplinary research programs, provide state-of-the-art laboratory equipment, and sponsor colloquia by specialists from other universities in North America and abroad. All graduate students benefit from activities supported by the research centers.

Information for Students With Physical Disabilities: See the following Web site for more information: http://supportservices.concordia.ca/disabilities.

Application Information:
Send to Concordia University, Graduate Admissions Application Centre P.O. Box 2002, Station H, Montréal, Québec H3G 2V4, Canada. Application available online. URL of online application: http://psychology.concordia.ca/graduateprograms/applyingtopsychology/graduateapplication/. Students are admitted in the Fall, application deadline December 15. *Fee:* $90. Note: All dollar amounts specified in this entry are Canadian dollars.

Dalhousie University
Department of Psychology
Life Sciences Centre
Halifax, NS B3H 4J1
Telephone: (902) 494-3839
Fax: (902) 494-6585
E-mail: *Ray.Klein@dal.ca*
Web: *http://psychology.dal.ca/*

Department Information:
1863. Chairperson: Ray Klein. Number of faculty: total—full-time 26, part-time 12; women—full-time 12, part-time 4.

GRADUATE STUDY IN PSYCHOLOGY

Programs and Degrees Offered:
Listed in the following order: Program area, degree type (T if terminal Master's), number awarded 7/08–6/09. Clinical Psychology PhD (Doctor of Philosophy) 3, Experimental-Animal PhD (Doctor of Philosophy) 0, Experimental—Human PhD (Doctor of Philosophy) 2, Neuroscience MA/MS (Master of Arts/Science) 2, Experimental—Animal MA/MS (Master of Arts/Science) 1, Neuroscience PhD (Doctor of Philosophy) 1, Experimental—Human MA/MS (Master of Arts/Science) 6.

CPA Accreditation: Clinical PhD (Doctor of Philosophy).

Student Applications/Admissions:
Student Applications
Clinical Psychology PhD (Doctor of Philosophy)—Applications 2009–2010, 76. Total applicants accepted 2009–2010, 5. Number full-time enrolled (new admits only) 2009–2010, 5. Number part-time enrolled (new admits only) 2009–2010, 0. Openings 2010–2011, 6. The median number of years required for completion of a degree in 2008–2009 were 5. The number of students enrolled full- and part-time who were dismissed or voluntarily withdrew from this program area in 2008–2009 were 0. *Experimental-Animal PhD (Doctor of Philosophy)*—Applications 2009–2010, 6. Total applicants accepted 2009–2010, 0. Number full-time enrolled (new admits only) 2009–2010, 0. Number part-time enrolled (new admits only) 2009–2010, 0. Openings 2010–2011, 6. The median number of years required for completion of a degree in 2008–2009 were 5. The number of students enrolled full- and part-time who were dismissed or voluntarily withdrew from this program area in 2008–2009 were 0. *Experimental—Human PhD (Doctor of Philosophy)*—Applications 2009–2010, 6. Total applicants accepted 2009–2010, 3. Number full-time enrolled (new admits only) 2009–2010, 3. Number part-time enrolled (new admits only) 2009–2010, 0. Openings 2010–2011, 6. The median number of years required for completion of a degree in 2008–2009 were 5. The number of students enrolled full- and part-time who were dismissed or voluntarily withdrew from this program area in 2008–2009 were 1. *Neuroscience MA/MS (Master of Arts/Science)*—Applications 2009–2010, 11. Total applicants accepted 2009–2010, 0. Number full-time enrolled (new admits only) 2009–2010, 0. Number part-time enrolled (new admits only) 2009–2010, 0. Openings 2010–2011, 6. The median number of years required for completion of a degree in 2008–2009 were 2. The number of students enrolled full- and part-time who were dismissed or voluntarily withdrew from this program area in 2008–2009 were 0. *Experimental—Animal MA/MS (Master of Arts/Science)*—Applications 2009–2010, 19. Total applicants accepted 2009–2010, 0. Number full-time enrolled (new admits only) 2009–2010, 0. Number part-time enrolled (new admits only) 2009–2010, 0. Openings 2010–2011, 6. The median number of years required for completion of a degree in 2008–2009 were 2. The number of students enrolled full- and part-time who were dismissed or voluntarily withdrew from this program area in 2008–2009 were 0. *Neuroscience PhD (Doctor of Philosophy)*—Applications 2009–2010, 3. Total applicants accepted 2009–2010, 2. Number full-time enrolled (new admits only) 2009–2010, 2. Number part-time enrolled (new admits only) 2009–2010, 0. Openings 2010–2011, 6. The median number of years required for completion of a degree in 2008–2009 were 5. The number of students enrolled full- and part-time who were dismissed or voluntarily withdrew from this program area in 2008–2009 were 0. *Experimental—Human MA/MS (Master of Arts/Science)*—Applications 2009–2010, 19. Total applicants accepted 2009–2010, 3. Number full-time enrolled (new admits only) 2009–2010, 3. Number part-time enrolled (new admits only) 2009–2010, 0. Openings 2010–2011, 6. The median number of years required for completion of a degree in 2008–2009 were 2. The number of students enrolled full- and part-time who were dismissed or voluntarily withdrew from this program area in 2008–2009 were 0.

Other Criteria: (importance of criteria rated low, medium, or high): GRE scores—medium, research experience—high, work experience—low, extracurricular activity—low, clinically related public service—low, GPA—high, letters of recommendation—high, interview—medium, statement of goals and objectives—high, undergraduate major in psychology—high, specific undergraduate psychology courses taken—high. Clinically related public service is high for clinical program. For additional information on admission requirements, go to http://psychology.dal.ca/Programs/.

Student Characteristics: The following represents characteristics of students in 2009–2010 in all graduate psychology programs in the department: Female—full-time 46, part-time 0; Male—full-time 19, part-time 0; African American/Black—full-time 0, part-time 0; Hispanic/Latino(a)—full-time 0, part-time 0; Asian/Pacific Islander—full-time 2, part-time 0; American Indian/Alaska Native—full-time 1, part-time 0; Caucasian/White—full-time 62, part-time 0; Multi-ethnic—full-time 0, part-time 0; students subject to the Americans With Disabilities Act—full-time 0, part-time 0; Unknown ethnicity—full-time 0, part-time 0; International students who hold an F-1 or J-1 Visa—full-time 1, part-time 0.

Financial Information/Assistance:
Tuition for Full-Time Study: *Master's:* State residents: per academic year $8,260. *Doctoral:* State residents: per academic year $8,587. Tuition is subject to change. See the following Web site for updates and changes in tuition costs: http://www.dal.ca/studentaccounts/.

Financial Assistance:
First-Year Students: Teaching assistantships available for first year. Average amount paid per academic year: $2,614. Average number of hours worked per week: 10. Fellowships and scholarships available for first year.

Advanced Students: Teaching assistantships available for advanced students. Average number of hours worked per week: 10. Fellowships and scholarships available for advanced students.

Additional Information: Of all students currently enrolled full time, 100% benefited from one or more of the listed financial assistance programs. Application and information available online at: http://psychology.dal.ca/.

Internships/Practica: Doctoral Degree (PhD Clinical Psychology): For those doctoral students for whom a professional internship was required in this program prior to graduation, (5) students applied for an internship in 2008–2009, with (5) students obtaining an internship. Of those students who obtained an internship, (5) were paid internships. Of those students who obtained an internship, (5) students placed in APA/CPA accredited internships, (0) students placed in internships not APA/CPA accredited, but listed with the Association of Psychology Postdoctoral and Internship Programs (APPIC), (0) students placed in internships conforming to guidelines of the Council of Directors of School Psychology Programs (CDSPP), (0) students placed in internships that were not APA/CPA accredited, APPIC or CDSPP listed. Practicum training is integrated into the Clinical Psychology PhD curriculum, to complement knowledge and skills developed through coursework, to provide opportunities to master specific assessment and intervention techniques, and to ensure that students meet expectations with regard to core competencies. Brief practica are incorporated into a number of the core clinical courses; however, the majority of practicum hours are accumulated through community placements, under the supervision of registered psychologists. Dalhousie is situated in close proximity to a variety of excellent health care facilities, including the IWK Health Centre, the QEII Health Centre, the Nova Scotia Hospital, the Canadian Forces Hospital at CFB Stadacona, and the East Coast Forensic Hospital. Under the guidance of the Field Placement Coordinator, students select and complete a program of practicum placements designed to meet their individual training needs. Students are required to complete a minimum of 600 hours of formal practicum training, but it is recognized that additional practicum hours (for a total of about 1000-1200 hrs) are often necessary to ensure a competitive internship application.

Housing and Day Care: On-campus housing is available. See the following Web site for more information: http://housing.dal.ca. On-campus day care facilities are available. See the following Web site for more information: http://universitychildrenscentre.dal.ca.

Employment of Department Graduates:
Master's Degree Graduates: Of those who graduated in the academic year 2008–2009, the following categories and numbers represent the postgraduate activities and employment of master's degree graduates: Enrolled in a psychology doctoral program (5), enrolled in another graduate/professional program (0), enrolled in a postdoctoral residency/fellowship (n/a), employed in independent practice (n/a), employed in an academic position at a university (0), employed in an academic position at a 2-year/4-year college (0), employed in other positions at a higher education institution (0), employed in a professional position in a school system (0), employed in business or industry (0), employed in a government agency (0), employed in a community mental health/counseling center (1), employed in a hospital/medical center (1), still seeking employment (0), other employment position (0), do not know (1), total from the above (master's) (8).
Doctoral Degree Graduates: Of those who graduated in the academic year 2008–2009, the following categories and numbers represent the postgraduate activities and employment of doctoral degree graduates: Enrolled in a psychology doctoral program (n/a), enrolled in another graduate/professional program (1), enrolled in a postdoctoral residency/fellowship (2), employed in independent practice (0), employed in an academic position at a university (2), employed in an academic position at a 2-year/4-year college (0), employed in other positions at a higher education institution (0), employed in a professional position in a school system (0), employed in business or industry (0), employed in a government agency (0), employed in a community mental health/counseling center (0), employed in a hospital/medical center (2), still seeking employment (0), other employment position (1), do not know (0), total from the above (doctoral) (8).

Additional Information:
Orientation, Objectives, and Emphasis of Department: The Department of Psychology offers graduate training leading to MSc and PhD degrees in psychology and in psychology/neuroscience, and to a PhD in clinical psychology. Our graduate programs emphasize training for research. They are best described as apprenticeship programs in which students work closely with a faculty member who has agreed to supervise the student's research. Compared with many other graduate programs, we place less emphasis on course work and greater emphasis on research, scholarship, and independent thinking. The graduate program in psychology/neuroscience is coordinated by the Psychology Department and an interdisciplinary Neuroscience Program Committee with representation from the Departments of Anatomy, Biochemistry, Pharmacology, Physiology and Biophysics, and Psychology. Master's level students in psychology and psychology/neuroscience are expected to advance into the corresponding PhD programs. We do not have a terminal Master's program. The PhD program in clinical psychology is cooperatively administered by the Psychology Department and the Clinical Program Committee with representation from Acadia University, Dalhousie University, Mount Saint Vincent University, Saint Mary's University, and professional psychologists from the teaching hospitals. It is a structured five-year program which follows the scientist–practitioner model. During the first four years of the clinical psychology program, students complete required courses, conduct supervised and thesis research, and gain clinical experience through field placements. In the fifth year, students are placed in a full-year clinical internship.

Special Facilities or Resources: The Department of Psychology is located in the Life Sciences Centre which also contains the departments of biology, earth sciences, and oceanography. The psychology building contains very extensive laboratory areas, some with circulating sea-water aquaria, and is designed for research with a range of animal groups (humans, cats, birds, fish, invertebrates) using a range of research techniques in behavior, electrophysiology, neuroanatomy, immunocytochemistry, neurogenetics, and so forth. The department also houses an electronics and woodworking shop, an animal care facility, a surgical facility, a computer lab for word processing, communications, and access to a mainframe; specific neuroscience facilities are in close proximity to hospitals.

Information for Students With Physical Disabilities: See the following Web site for more information: http://studentaccessibility.dal.ca/.

Application Information:
Send to Graduate Program Secretary, Psychology Department, Dalhousie University, Halifax, NS B3H 4J1. Application available online. URL of online application: http://www.registrar.dal.ca/prospective/graduateapp.html. Students are admitted in the Fall, application deadline January 1. *Fee:* $70. Note: All dollar amounts specified in this entry are Canadian dollars.

GRADUATE STUDY IN PSYCHOLOGY

Guelph, University of
Department of Psychology
College of Social and Applied Human Sciences
4th Floor MacKinnon Extension
Guelph, ON N1G 2W1
Telephone: (519) 824-4120 ext. 53508
Fax: (519) 837-8629
E-mail: *marmurek@psy.uoguelph.ca*
Web: *http://www.uoguelph.ca/psychology/*

Department Information:
1966. Chairperson: Harvey H. C. Marmurek. Number of faculty: total—full-time 32; women—full-time 12; total—minority—full-time 4; women minority—full-time 4.

Programs and Degrees Offered:
Listed in the following order: Program area, degree type (T if terminal Master's), number awarded 7/08–6/09. Clinical Psychology:Applied Developmental Emphasis MA/MS (Master of Arts/Science) 3, Industrial/Organizational MA/MS (Master of Arts/Science) 3, Applied Social MA/MS (Master of Arts/Science) 2, Industrial/Organizational PhD (Doctor of Philosophy) 4, Applied Social PhD (Doctor of Philosophy) 1, Clinical Psychology:Applied Developmental Emphasis PhD (Doctor of Philosophy) 1, Neuroscience and Applied Cognitive Science MA/MS (Master of Arts/Science) 3, Neuroscience and Applied Cognitive Science PhD (Doctor of Philosophy) 0.

CPA Accreditation: Clinical PhD (Doctor of Philosophy).

Student Applications/Admissions:
Student Applications
Clinical Psychology:Applied Developmental Emphasis MA/MS (Master of Arts/Science)—Applications 2009–2010, 97. Total applicants accepted 2009–2010, 7. Number full-time enrolled (new admits only) 2009–2010, 7. Number part-time enrolled (new admits only) 2009–2010, 0. Openings 2010–2011, 5. The median number of years required for completion of a degree in 2008–2009 were 2. The number of students enrolled full- and part-time who were dismissed or voluntarily withdrew from this program area in 2008–2009 were 0. *Industrial/Organizational MA/MS (Master of Arts/Science)*—Applications 2009–2010, 28. Total applicants accepted 2009–2010, 2. Number full-time enrolled (new admits only) 2009–2010, 2. Number part-time enrolled (new admits only) 2009–2010, 0. Openings 2010–2011, 4. The median number of years required for completion of a degree in 2008–2009 were 2. The number of students enrolled full- and part-time who were dismissed or voluntarily withdrew from this program area in 2008–2009 were 0. *Applied Social MA/MS (Master of Arts/Science)*—Applications 2009–2010, 16. Total applicants accepted 2009–2010, 3. Number full-time enrolled (new admits only) 2009–2010, 3. Number part-time enrolled (new admits only) 2009–2010, 0. Openings 2010–2011, 4. The median number of years required for completion of a degree in 2008–2009 were 2. The number of students enrolled full- and part-time who were dismissed or voluntarily withdrew from this program area in 2008–2009 were 0. *Industrial/Organizational PhD (Doctor of Philosophy)*—Applications 2009–2010, 1. Total applicants accepted 2009–2010, 1. Number full-time enrolled (new admits only) 2009–2010, 1. Total enrolled 2009–2010 full-time, 6, part-time, 2. Openings 2010–2011, 3. The median number of years required for completion of a degree in 2008–2009 were 5. *Applied Social PhD (Doctor of Philosophy)*—Applications 2009–2010, 3. Total applicants accepted 2009–2010, 1. Number full-time enrolled (new admits only) 2009–2010, 1. Number part-time enrolled (new admits only) 2009–2010, 0. Total enrolled 2009–2010 full-time, 14. Openings 2010–2011, 4. The median number of years required for completion of a degree in 2008–2009 were 5. The number of students enrolled full- and part-time who were dismissed or voluntarily withdrew from this program area in 2008–2009 were 1. *Clinical Psychology:Applied Developmental Emphasis PhD (Doctor of Philosophy)*—Applications 2009–2010, 9. Total applicants accepted 2009–2010, 6. Number full-time enrolled (new admits only) 2009–2010, 6. Number part-time enrolled (new admits only) 2009–2010, 0. Total enrolled 2009–2010 full-time, 28, part-time, 2. Openings 2010–2011, 5. The median number of years required for completion of a degree in 2008–2009 were 7. The number of students enrolled full- and part-time who were dismissed or voluntarily withdrew from this program area in 2008–2009 were 0. *Neuroscience and Applied Cognitive Science MA/MS (Master of Arts/Science)*—Applications 2009–2010, 17. Total applicants accepted 2009–2010, 4. Number full-time enrolled (new admits only) 2009–2010, 4. Number part-time enrolled (new admits only) 2009–2010, 0. Openings 2010–2011, 4. The median number of years required for completion of a degree in 2008–2009 was 1. The number of students enrolled full- and part-time who were dismissed or voluntarily withdrew from this program area in 2008–2009 were 0. *Neuroscience and Applied Cognitive Science PhD (Doctor of Philosophy)*—Applications 2009–2010, 0. Total applicants accepted 2009–2010, 0. Number full-time enrolled (new admits only) 2009–2010, 2. Number part-time enrolled (new admits only) 2009–2010, 0. Openings 2010–2011, 4. The number of students enrolled full- and part-time who were dismissed or voluntarily withdrew from this program area in 2008–2009 were 0.

Scores: Entries appear in this order: required test or GPA, minimum score (if required), median score of students entering in 2009–2010. *Clinical Psychology:Applied Developmental Emphasis MA/MS (Master of Arts/Science)*: GRE-V no minimum stated, GRE-Q no minimum stated, GRE-Analytical no minimum stated, GRE-Subject (Psychology) no minimum stated, overall undergraduate GPA no minimum stated, last 2 years GPA no minimum stated, psychology GPA no minimum stated; *Industrial/Organizational MA/MS (Master of Arts/Science)*: GRE-V no minimum stated, GRE-Q no minimum stated, GRE-Analytical no minimum stated, GRE-Subject (Psychology) no minimum stated, overall undergraduate GPA no minimum stated, last 2 years GPA no minimum stated, psychology GPA no minimum stated; *Applied Social MA/MS (Master of Arts/Science)*: GRE-V no minimum stated, GRE-Q no minimum stated, GRE-Analytical no minimum stated, GRE-Subject (Psychology) no minimum stated, overall undergraduate GPA no minimum stated, last 2 years GPA no minimum stated, psychology GPA no minimum stated; *Industrial/Organizational PhD (Doctor of Philosophy)*: GRE-V no minimum stated, GRE-Q no minimum stated, GRE-Analytical no minimum stated, GRE-Subject (Psychology) no minimum stated, overall undergraduate GPA no minimum stated, last 2 years GPA no minimum stated, psychology GPA no minimum stated, Masters GPA no minimum stated; *Applied Social PhD (Doctor of Philosophy)*: GRE-V no minimum stated, GRE-Q no minimum stated, GRE-Analytical no minimum stated, GRE-Subject (Psychology) no minimum stated, overall undergraduate GPA no minimum stated, last 2 years GPA no minimum stated, psychology GPA no minimum stated, Masters GPA no minimum stated; *Clinical Psychology:Applied Developmental Emphasis PhD (Doctor of Philosophy)*: GRE-V no minimum stated, 558, GRE-Q no minimum stated, 658, GRE-Analytical no minimum stated, 5.7, GRE-Subject (Psychology) no minimum stated, 669, overall undergraduate GPA no minimum stated, last 2 years GPA no minimum stated, psychology GPA no minimum stated, Masters GPA no minimum stated; *Neuroscience and Applied Cognitive Science MA/MS (Master of Arts/Science)*: GRE-V no minimum stated, GRE-Q no minimum stated, GRE-Analytical no minimum stated, overall undergraduate GPA no minimum stated, last 2 years GPA no minimum stated, psychology GPA no minimum stated; *Neuroscience and Applied Cognitive Science PhD (Doctor of Philosophy)*: GRE-V no minimum stated, GRE-Q no minimum stated, GRE-Analytical no minimum stated, overall undergraduate GPA no minimum stated, last 2 years GPA no minimum stated, psychology GPA no minimum stated, Masters GPA no minimum stated.

Other Criteria: (importance of criteria rated low, medium, or high): GRE scores—high, research experience—high, work experience—medium, extracurricular activity—low, clinically related public service—low, GPA—high, letters of recommendation—high, interview—high, statement of goals and objectives—high. For additional information on admission requirements, go to http://www.uoguelph.ca/psychology/.

Student Characteristics: The following represents characteristics of students in 2009–2010 in all graduate psychology programs in the department: Female—full-time 75, part-time 4; Male—full-time 21, part-time 0; African American/Black—full-time 3, part-time 0; Hispanic/Latino(a)—full-time 0, part-time 0; Asian/Pacific Islander—full-time 3, part-time 0; American Indian/Alaska Native—full-time 0, part-time 0; Caucasian/White—full-time 88, part-time 4; Multi-ethnic—full-time 2, part-time 0; students subject to the Americans With Disabilities Act—full-time 0, part-time 0; Unknown ethnicity—full-time 0, part-time 0; International students who hold an F-1 or J-1 Visa—full-time 2, part-time 0.

Financial Information/Assistance:
Tuition for Full-Time Study: *Master's:* State residents: per academic year $8,235; Nonstate residents: per academic year $19,647. *Doctoral:* State residents: per academic year $8,235; Nonstate residents: per academic year $19,647. Tuition is subject to change. See the following Web site for updates and changes in tuition costs: http://www.uoguelph.ca/registrar/studentfinance/index.cfm?fees/index.

Financial Assistance:
First-Year Students: Teaching assistantships available for first year. Average amount paid per academic year: $10,520. Average number of hours worked per week: 10. Research assistantships available for first year. Fellowships and scholarships available for first year.

Advanced Students: Teaching assistantships available for advanced students. Average amount paid per academic year: $10,520. Average number of hours worked per week: 10. Research assistantships available for advanced students. Fellowships and scholarships available for advanced students.

Additional Information: Of all students currently enrolled full time, 100% benefited from one or more of the listed financial assistance programs. Application and information available online at: http://www.uoguelph.ca/psychology/page.cfm?id=2.

Internships/Practica: Doctoral Degree (PhD Clinical Psychology:Applied Developmental Emphasis): For those doctoral students for whom a professional internship was required in this program prior to graduation, (3) students applied for an internship in 2008–2009, with (3) students obtaining an internship. Of those students who obtained an internship, (3) were paid internships. Of those students who obtained an internship, (2) students placed in APA/CPA accredited internships, (1) students placed in internships not APA/CPA accredited, but listed with the Association of Psychology Postdoctoral and Internship Programs (APPIC), (0) students placed in internships conforming to guidelines of the Council of Directors of School Psychology Programs (CDSPP), (0) students placed in internships that were not APA/CPA accredited, APPIC or CDSPP listed. Clinical Psychology: Applied Developmental Emphasis students work two days per week with the psychological services staff at local public school boards. During a later semester, they are placed four days a week in a service facility for atypical children. Applied Social Psychology students select practica in settings that include community health facilities, correctional and medical treatment settings, and private consulting firms. Industrial/Organizational and Applied Cognitive Science practica take place in industrial, governmental, and military settings.

Housing and Day Care: On-campus housing is available. See the following Web site for more information: http://www.housing.uoguelph.ca/page.cfm. On-campus day care facilities are available. See the following Web site for more information: http://www.uoguelph.ca/studentaffairs/childcare/home/index.shtml.

Employment of Department Graduates:
Master's Degree Graduates: Of those who graduated in the academic year 2008–2009, the following categories and numbers represent the postgraduate activities and employment of master's degree graduates: Enrolled in a psychology doctoral program (2), enrolled in another graduate/professional program (1), enrolled in a postdoctoral residency/fellowship (n/a), employed in independent practice (n/a), employed in an academic position at a university (0), employed in an academic position at a 2-year/4-year college (0), employed in other positions at a higher education institution (0), employed in a professional position in a school system (0), employed in business or industry (1), employed in a government agency (1), employed in a community mental health/counseling center (0), employed in a hospital/medical center (0), still seeking employment (1), other employment position (0), do not know (1), total from the above (master's) (7).

GRADUATE STUDY IN PSYCHOLOGY

Doctoral Degree Graduates: Of those who graduated in the academic year 2008–2009, the following categories and numbers represent the postgraduate activities and employment of doctoral degree graduates: Enrolled in a psychology doctoral program (n/a), enrolled in another graduate/professional program (0), enrolled in a postdoctoral residency/fellowship (1), employed in an academic position at a university (0), employed in an academic position at a 2-year/4-year college (0), employed in other positions at a higher education institution (0), employed in business or industry (4), employed in a community mental health/counseling center (1), total from the above (doctoral) (6).

Additional Information:
Orientation, Objectives, and Emphasis of Department: The Department of Psychology offers graduate programs leading to a Master of Arts and a Doctor of Philosophy in four fields: Neuroscience and Applied Cognitive Science, Applied Social Psychology, Clinical Psychology: Applied Developmental Emphasis, and Industrial/Organizational Psychology. The four fields follow a scientist–practitioner model and provide training in both research and professional skills, as well as a firm grounding in theory and research in relevant content areas. The Clinical PhD program is accredited by the Canadian Psychological Association.

Special Facilities or Resources: Faculty offices and laboratories are located mainly in the MacKinnon Building and Blackwood Hall. Graduate students have office space in Blackwood Hall and the MacKinnon Building. The department is well supported with computer facilities. These include a microcomputer laboratory and extensive microcomputer support for research, teaching, data analysis, and word processing. Facilities for animal research include a fully equipped surgery room and physiological recording equipment. For research with human subjects, the department possesses portable video-recording equipment, observation rooms and experimental chambers. All of these facilities are supplemented by excellent workshop and technical support. The Centre for Psychological Services is a non-profit organization associated with the Department of Psychology at the University of Guelph. The Centre provides high quality psychological services at a reasonable cost, working with families and the community. The Centre is involved in training students in Clinical Psychology: Applied Developmental Emphasis and offers workshops and presentations to professionals in the community. Consulting experience is available via coursework to Industrial/Organizational Psychology, allowing them to apply the knowledge gained in their courses.

Information for Students With Physical Disabilities: See the following Web site for more information: http://www.csd.uoguelph.ca/csd/.

Application Information:
Send to Graduate Secretary, Department of Psychology, University of Guelph, Guelph, Ontario N1G 2W1, Canada. Telephone: (519) 824-4120, ext. 53508. Application available online. URL of online application: http://horizon.ouac.on.ca/guelph/grad/. Students are admitted in the Fall, application deadline December 15. All applications are reviewed in January. Interviews to take place in February. Offers to follow in March. Notification of Non-Admission: May - June. *Fee:* $100. Deferral Fee: $100 in Canadian Dollars. Note: All dollar amounts specified in this entry are Canadian dollars.

Manitoba, University of
Psychology Graduate Office
P514 Duff Roblin Building
Winnipeg, MB R3T 2N2
Telephone: (204) 474-6377
Fax: (204) 474-7917
E-mail: *Psyc_Grad_Office@umanitoba.ca*
Web: *http://www.umanitoba.ca/psychology*

Department Information:
1947. Head: Todd A. Mondor. Number of faculty: total—full-time 42, part-time 3; women—full-time 16.

Programs and Degrees Offered:
Listed in the following order: Program area, degree type (T if terminal Master's), number awarded 7/08–6/09. Applied Behavioural Analysis PhD (Doctor of Philosophy) 2, Social/Personality Psychology PhD (Doctor of Philosophy) 1, Brain and Cognitive Sciences PhD (Doctor of Philosophy) 1, Clinical Psychology PhD (Doctor of Philosophy) 5, Developmental Psychology PhD (Doctor of Philosophy) 0, Methodology PhD (Doctor of Philosophy) 0, School Psychology MA/MS (Master of Arts/Science) (T) 10.

APA Accreditation: Clinical PhD (Doctor of Philosophy).

CPA Accreditation: Clinical PhD (Doctor of Philosophy).

Student Applications/Admissions:
Student Applications
Applied Behavioural Analysis PhD (Doctor of Philosophy)—Applications 2009–2010, 7. Total applicants accepted 2009–2010, 0. Number full-time enrolled (new admits only) 2009–2010, 0. Number part-time enrolled (new admits only) 2009–2010, 0. Openings 2010–2011, 4. The median number of years required for completion of a degree in 2008–2009 were 2. The number of students enrolled full- and part-time who were dismissed or voluntarily withdrew from this program area in 2008–2009 were 0. *Social/Personality Psychology PhD (Doctor of Philosophy)*—Applications 2009–2010, 9. Total applicants accepted 2009–2010, 1. Number full-time enrolled (new admits only) 2009–2010, 1. Number part-time enrolled (new admits only) 2009–2010, 0. Openings 2010–2011, 4. The median number of years required for completion of a degree in 2008–2009 were 3. The number of students enrolled full- and part-time who were dismissed or voluntarily withdrew from this program area in 2008–2009 were 0. *Brain and Cognitive Sciences PhD (Doctor of Philosophy)*—Applications 2009–2010, 9. Total applicants accepted 2009–2010, 2. Number full-time enrolled (new admits only) 2009–2010, 2. Number part-time enrolled (new admits only) 2009–2010, 0. Openings 2010–2011, 4. The median number of years required for completion of a degree in 2008–2009 were 2. The number of students enrolled full- and part-time who were dismissed or voluntarily withdrew from this program area in 2008–2009 were 0. *Clinical Psychology PhD (Doctor of Philosophy)*—Applications 2009–2010, 56. Total applicants accepted 2009–2010, 5. Number full-time enrolled (new admits only) 2009–2010, 5. Number part-time enrolled (new admits only) 2009–2010, 0. Total enrolled 2009–2010 full-time, 54, part-time, 1. Openings 2010–2011, 5. The median number of years required for com-

pletion of a degree in 2008–2009 were 3. The number of students enrolled full- and part-time who were dismissed or voluntarily withdrew from this program area in 2008–2009 were 0. *Developmental Psychology PhD (Doctor of Philosophy)*—Applications 2009–2010, 5. Total applicants accepted 2009–2010, 1. Number full-time enrolled (new admits only) 2009–2010, 1. Number part-time enrolled (new admits only) 2009–2010, 0. Openings 2010–2011, 2. The number of students enrolled full- and part-time who were dismissed or voluntarily withdrew from this program area in 2008–2009 were 0. *Methodology PhD (Doctor of Philosophy)*—Applications 2009–2010, 1. Total applicants accepted 2009–2010, 0. Number full-time enrolled (new admits only) 2009–2010, 0. Number part-time enrolled (new admits only) 2009–2010, 0. Openings 2010–2011, 3. The number of students enrolled full- and part-time who were dismissed or voluntarily withdrew from this program area in 2008–2009 were 0. *School Psychology MA/MS (Master of Arts/Science)*—Applications 2009–2010, 19. Total applicants accepted 2009–2010, 11. Number full-time enrolled (new admits only) 2009–2010, 11. Number part-time enrolled (new admits only) 2009–2010, 0. Openings 2010–2011, 8. The median number of years required for completion of a degree in 2008–2009 were 2. The number of students enrolled full- and part-time who were dismissed or voluntarily withdrew from this program area in 2008–2009 were 0.

Scores: Entries appear in this order: required test or GPA, minimum score (if required), median score of students entering in 2009–2010. *Applied Behavioural Analysis PhD (Doctor of Philosophy)*: GRE-V no minimum stated, GRE-Q no minimum stated, last 2 years GPA no minimum stated; *Social/Personality Psychology PhD (Doctor of Philosophy)*: GRE-V 480, 480, GRE-Q 470, 470, last 2 years GPA 3.65, 3.65; *Brain and Cognitive Sciences PhD (Doctor of Philosophy)*: GRE-V 480, 515, GRE-Q 650, 690, last 2 years GPA 3.44, 3.61; *Clinical Psychology PhD (Doctor of Philosophy)*: GRE-V 480, 564, GRE-Q 510, 644, last 2 years GPA 3.99, 4.15; *Developmental Psychology PhD (Doctor of Philosophy)*: GRE-V 460, 460, GRE-Q 550, 550, overall undergraduate GPA 3.58, 3.58; *Methodology PhD (Doctor of Philosophy)*: GRE-V no minimum stated, GRE-Q no minimum stated, last 2 years GPA no minimum stated.

Other Criteria: (importance of criteria rated low, medium, or high): GRE scores—high, research experience—high, work experience—medium, extracurricular activity—low, clinically related public service—medium, GPA—high, letters of recommendation—medium, interview—low, statement of goals and objectives—low, undergraduate major in psychology—high, specific undergraduate psychology courses taken—medium. For additional information on admission requirements, go to http://www.umanitoba.ca/psychology.

Student Characteristics: The following represents characteristics of students in 2009–2010 in all graduate psychology programs in the department: Female—full-time 99, part-time 0; Male—full-time 23, part-time 1; African American/Black—full-time 0, part-time 0; Hispanic/Latino(a)—full-time 0, part-time 0; Asian/Pacific Islander—full-time 0, part-time 0; American Indian/Alaska Native—full-time 0, part-time 0; Caucasian/White—full-time 0, part-time 0; Multi-ethnic—full-time 0, part-time 0; students subject to the Americans With Disabilities Act—full-time 0, part-time 0; Unknown ethnicity—full-time 0, part-time 0; International students who hold an F-1 or J-1 Visa—full-time 0, part-time 0.

Financial Information/Assistance:
   Tuition for Full-Time Study: *Master's:* State residents: per academic year $4,177. *Doctoral:* State residents: per academic year $4,177.

Financial Assistance:
   First-Year Students: Teaching assistantships available for first year. Average number of hours worked per week: 12. Apply by TBA. Research assistantships available for first year. Apply by TBA. Fellowships and scholarships available for first year.
   Advanced Students: Teaching assistantships available for advanced students. Average number of hours worked per week: 12. Apply by TBA. Research assistantships available for advanced students. Apply by TBA. Fellowships and scholarships available for advanced students.
   Additional Information: Of all students currently enrolled full time, 60% benefited from one or more of the listed financial assistance programs. Application and information available online at: http://www.umanitoba.ca/psychology.

Internships/Practica: Doctoral Degree (PhD Clinical Psychology): For those doctoral students for whom a professional internship was required in this program prior to graduation, (7) students applied for an internship in 2008–2009, with (7) students obtaining an internship. Of those students who obtained an internship, (7) were paid internships. Of those students who obtained an internship, (7) students placed in APA/CPA accredited internships, (0) students placed in internships not APA/CPA accredited, but listed with the Association of Psychology Postdoctoral and Internship Programs (APPIC), (0) students placed in internships conforming to guidelines of the Council of Directors of School Psychology Programs (CDSPP), (0) students placed in internships that were not APA/CPA accredited, APPIC or CDSPP listed. Clinical students have access to practica at our Psychological Service Center. A limited number of practica within the community are available for senior graduate students. However, the department does not offer an internship program.

Housing and Day Care: On-campus housing is available. See the following Web site for more information: http://www.umanitoba.ca/student/housing. On-campus day care facilities are available. See the following Web site for more information: http://www.umanitoba.ca/student/resource/playcare.

Employment of Department Graduates:
   Master's Degree Graduates: Of those who graduated in the academic year 2008–2009, the following categories and numbers represent the postgraduate activities and employment of master's degree graduates: Enrolled in a psychology doctoral program (4), enrolled in a postdoctoral residency/fellowship (n/a), employed in independent practice (n/a), employed in a professional position in a school system (10), total from the above (master's) (14).
   Doctoral Degree Graduates: Of those who graduated in the academic year 2008–2009, the following categories and numbers represent the postgraduate activities and employment of doctoral degree graduates: Enrolled in a psychology doctoral program (n/a), employed in an academic position at a university (2), total from the above (doctoral) (2).

Additional Information:
   Orientation, Objectives, and Emphasis of Department: The primary purpose of our program is to provide training in several

specialized areas of psychology for individuals desiring to advance their level of knowledge, their research skills, and their applied capabilities. The MA program is designed to provide a broad foundation, as well as specialized skills, in the scientific approach to psychology. The PhD program provides a higher degree of specialization coupled with more intensive training in research and application. Specialized areas of training within the department include applied behavioral analysis, brain and cognitive sciences, clinical, developmental, methodology, school, and social/personality.

Special Facilities or Resources: Basic research facilities are housed in over 100 dedicated research rooms. We host a large computer lab maintained by a crew of three excellent computer technicians, integrated animal care facilities under the supervision of a dedicated animal care technician, and a field station at which avian behavior may be studied. These resources are augmented by collaborative relationships we have with other university departments, local hospitals, St. Amant Centre, and the National Research Council: Institute for Biodiagnostics.

Information for Students With Physical Disabilities: disability_services@umanitoba.ca.

Application Information:
Send to Faculty of Graduate Studies, 500 University Centre, University of Manitoba, Winnipeg, MB R3T 2N2. Application available online. URL of online application: http://www.umanitoba.ca/faculties/graduate_studies/prospective/admissions/. Students are admitted in the Fall, application deadline January 15. Application fees are subject to change. Note: All dollar amounts specified in this entry are Canadian dollars.

McGill University
Department of Educational and Counselling Psychology
Faculty of Education, Room 614
3700 McTavish Street
Montreal, QC H3A 1Y2
Telephone: (514) 398-4242
Fax: (514) 398-6968
E-mail: *samantha.ryan@mcgill.ca*
Web: *http://www.mcgill.ca/edu-ecp*

Department Information:
1965. Chair: Alenoush Saroyan. Number of faculty: total—full-time 13, part-time 32; women—full-time 11.

Programs and Degrees Offered:
Listed in the following order: Program area, degree type (T if terminal Master's), number awarded 7/08–6/09. Counselling Psychology PhD (Doctor of Philosophy) 3, Educational Psychology PhD (Doctor of Philosophy) 13, School/Applied Child Psychology PhD (Doctor of Philosophy) 2.

APA Accreditation: Counseling PhD (Doctor of Philosophy). Student Outcome Data Website: http://www.mcgill.ca/edu-ecp/prospective/graduate/counselling/. School PhD (Doctor of Philosophy). Student Outcome Data Website: http://www.mcgill.ca/edu-ecp/prospective/graduate/schoolapplied/.

CPA Accreditation: Counseling PhD (Doctor of Philosophy).

Student Applications/Admissions:
Student Applications
Counselling Psychology PhD (Doctor of Philosophy)—Applications 2009–2010, 23. Total applicants accepted 2009–2010, 4. Number full-time enrolled (new admits only) 2009–2010, 4. Number part-time enrolled (new admits only) 2009–2010, 0. Openings 2010–2011, 8. The median number of years required for completion of a degree in 2008–2009 were 7. The number of students enrolled full- and part-time who were dismissed or voluntarily withdrew from this program area in 2008–2009 were 0. *Educational Psychology PhD (Doctor of Philosophy)*—Applications 2009–2010, 13. Total applicants accepted 2009–2010, 10. Number full-time enrolled (new admits only) 2009–2010, 5. Total enrolled 2009–2010 full-time, 35. Openings 2010–2011, 12. The median number of years required for completion of a degree in 2008–2009 were 7. The number of students enrolled full- and part-time who were dismissed or voluntarily withdrew from this program area in 2008–2009 were 0. *School/Applied Child Psychology PhD (Doctor of Philosophy)*—Applications 2009–2010, 10. Total applicants accepted 2009–2010, 7. Number full-time enrolled (new admits only) 2009–2010, 9. Number part-time enrolled (new admits only) 2009–2010, 0. Openings 2010–2011, 15. The median number of years required for completion of a degree in 2008–2009 were 5. The number of students enrolled full- and part-time who were dismissed or voluntarily withdrew from this program area in 2008–2009 were 0.

Other Criteria: (importance of criteria rated low, medium, or high): GRE scores—medium, research experience—medium, work experience—medium, extracurricular activity—medium, clinically related public service—medium, GPA—high, letters of recommendation—high, interview—medium, statement of goals and objectives—high, undergraduate major in psychology—high, specific undergraduate psychology courses taken—medium. For additional information on admission requirements, go to http://www.mcgill.ca/edu-ecp/prospective/graduate/.

Student Characteristics: The following represents characteristics of students in 2009–2010 in all graduate psychology programs in the department: Female—full-time 324, part-time 1; Male—full-time 61, part-time 1; African American/Black—full-time 0, part-time 0; Hispanic/Latino(a)—full-time 0, part-time 0; Asian/Pacific Islander—full-time 0, part-time 0; American Indian/Alaska Native—full-time 0, part-time 0; Caucasian/White—full-time 0, part-time 0; Multi-ethnic—full-time 0, part-time 0; students subject to the Americans With Disabilities Act—full-time 0, part-time 0; Unknown ethnicity—full-time 0, part-time 0; International students who hold an F-1 or J-1 Visa—full-time 0, part-time 0.

Financial Information/Assistance:
Tuition for Full-Time Study: *Master's:* State residents: per academic year $3,500, $117 per credit hour; Nonstate residents: per academic year $12,000, $400 per credit hour. *Doctoral:* State residents: per academic year $3,500, $117 per credit hour; Nonstate residents: per academic year $3,500, $117 per credit hour.

Tuition is subject to change. Tuition costs vary by program. See the following Web site for updates and changes in tuition costs: http://www.mcgill.ca/student-accounts/fees/tuition/gradstud/.

Financial Assistance:

First-Year Students: Research assistantships available for first year. Average amount paid per academic year: $5,000. Fellowships and scholarships available for first -year. Average amount paid per academic year: $5,000.

Advanced Students: Teaching assistantships available for advanced students. Average amount paid per academic year: $2,000. Average number of hours worked per week: 3. Apply by variable. Research assistantships available for advanced students. Average amount paid per academic year: $8,000. Average number of hours worked per week: 10. Fellowships and scholarships available for advanced students.

Additional Information: Of all students currently enrolled full time, 50% benefited from one or more of the listed financial assistance programs. Application and information available online at: http://www.mcgill.ca/edu-ecp/students/financial/.

Internships/Practica: Doctoral Degree (PhD Counselling Psychology): For those doctoral students for whom a professional internship was required in this program prior to graduation, (5) students applied for an internship in 2008–2009, with (5) students obtaining an internship. Of those students who obtained an internship, (5) were paid internships. Of those students who obtained an internship, (4) students placed in APA/CPA accredited internships, (0) students placed in internships not APA/CPA accredited, but listed with the Association of Psychology Postdoctoral and Internship Programs (APPIC), (0) students placed in internships conforming to guidelines of the Council of Directors of School Psychology Programs (CDSPP), (1) students placed in internships that were not APA/CPA accredited, APPIC or CDSPP listed. Doctoral Degree (PhD School/Applied Child Psychology): For those doctoral students for whom a professional internship was required in this program prior to graduation, (5) students applied for an internship in 2008–2009, with (5) students obtaining an internship. Of those students who obtained an internship, (4) were paid internships. Of those students who obtained an internship, (3) students placed in APA/CPA accredited internships, (0) students placed in internships not APA/CPA accredited, but listed with the Association of Psychology Postdoctoral and Internship Programs (APPIC), (2) students placed in internships conforming to guidelines of the Council of Directors of School Psychology Programs (CDSPP), (0) students placed in internships that were not APA/CPA accredited, APPIC or CDSPP listed. All students in the professional psychology programs, the MA (non-thesis) and PhD in Counseling Psychology, the MEd, MA in Educational Psychology and the MA (School/Applied Child Psychology option) and PhD in School/Applied Child Psychology are required to complete internships. According to the program option these may be in mental health facilities, community social service agencies, schools, psychoeducational clinics, etc. In some internships, more than one setting is advised or required. New internship opportunities are regularly added, and students are welcome to seek out those which may especially suit their needs, subject to program approval.

Housing and Day Care: On-campus housing is available. See the following Web site for more information: http://www.mcgill.ca/gradapplicants/housing/. On-campus day care facilities are available. See the following Web site for more information: http://www.mcgill.ca/daycare/.

Employment of Department Graduates:

Master's Degree Graduates: Of those who graduated in the academic year 2008–2009, the following categories and numbers represent the postgraduate activities and employment of master's degree graduates: Enrolled in a postdoctoral residency/fellowship (n/a), employed in independent practice (n/a), total from the above (master's) (0).

Doctoral Degree Graduates: Of those who graduated in the academic year 2008–2009, the following categories and numbers represent the postgraduate activities and employment of doctoral degree graduates: Enrolled in a psychology doctoral program (n/a), total from the above (doctoral) (0).

Additional Information:

Orientation, Objectives, and Emphasis of Department: There are five broad areas of major graduate-level specialization: Counseling Psychology, Human Development, Learning Sciences, Health Professions Education, and School/Applied Child Psychology. A substantial base in research methods and statistics is provided and adjusted to students' entering competence. Graduate students in professional school psychology normally enter the Master's program and are considered for transfer to the PhD (if that is their goal) after 2 years, for a further 4 to 5 years of training. Graduate studies directed toward research, academic, and leadership careers follow a similar enrollment pattern except that the program normally requires one year less at the doctoral level. Students are welcome to take selected courses in other departments and at other Quebec universities.

Special Facilities or Resources: The Department has the Laboratory for Applied Cognitive Science, Teaching and Learning Services, International Centre for Youth Gambling Problems and High Risk Behaviour, Neuroscience Lab for Research and Education in Developmental Disorders, Psychoeducational and Counselling Clinic, Psychoeducational Assessment Library, and educational computer labs.

Information for Students With Physical Disabilities: See the following Web site for more information: http://www.mcgill.ca/osd/.

Application Information:
Send to Alexander Nowak, Graduate Program Advisor, Professional Psychology Graduate Programs (Counselling Psychology and School/Applied Child Psychology); Geri Norton, Graduate Program Coordinator, Professional Educational Psychology Graduate Programs (Educational Psychology). Application available online. URL of online application: www.mcgill.ca/applying/graduate. Students are admitted in the Fall, application deadline December 15; January 15. School/Applied Child Psych Deadline - December 15; Counselling Psychology - December 15; Educational Psychology - January 15; Special circumstances may be examined on an individual basis. *Fee:* $100. Note: All dollar amounts specified in this entry are Canadian dollars.

GRADUATE STUDY IN PSYCHOLOGY

McGill University
Department of Psychology
1205 Avenue Docteur Penfield
Montreal, QC H3A 1B1
Telephone: (514) 398-6124
Fax: (514) 398-4896
E-mail: giovanna.locascio@mcgill.ca
Web: http://www.psych.mcgill.ca

Department Information:
1922. Chairperson: Keith Franklin. Number of faculty: total—full-time 39, part-time 7; women—full-time 14, part-time 4.

Programs and Degrees Offered:
Listed in the following order: Program area, degree type (T if terminal Master's), number awarded 7/08–6/09. Experimental Psychology PhD (Doctor of Philosophy) 5, Clinical Psychology PhD (Doctor of Philosophy) 4.

APA Accreditation: Clinical PhD (Doctor of Philosophy).

CPA Accreditation: Clinical PhD (Doctor of Philosophy).

Student Applications/Admissions:
Student Applications
Experimental Psychology PhD (Doctor of Philosophy)—Applications 2009–2010, 76. Total applicants accepted 2009–2010, 20. Number full-time enrolled (new admits only) 2009–2010, 12. Number part-time enrolled (new admits only) 2009–2010, 0. Openings 2010–2011, 15. The median number of years required for completion of a degree in 2008–2009 were 5. The number of students enrolled full- and part-time who were dismissed or voluntarily withdrew from this program area in 2008–2009 were 0. Clinical Psychology PhD (Doctor of Philosophy)—Applications 2009–2010, 112. Total applicants accepted 2009–2010, 8. Number full-time enrolled (new admits only) 2009–2010, 5. Number part-time enrolled (new admits only) 2009–2010, 0. Openings 2010–2011, 8. The median number of years required for completion of a degree in 2008–2009 were 6. The number of students enrolled full- and part-time who were dismissed or voluntarily withdrew from this program area in 2008–2009 were 0.
Scores: Entries appear in this order: required test or GPA, minimum score (if required), median score of students entering in 2009–2010. Experimental Psychology PhD (Doctor of Philosophy): GRE-V no minimum stated, GRE-Q no minimum stated, GRE-Analytical no minimum stated, GRE-Subject (Psychology) no minimum stated, overall undergraduate GPA no minimum stated, last 2 years GPA no minimum stated, psychology GPA no minimum stated, Masters GPA no minimum stated; Clinical Psychology PhD (Doctor of Philosophy): GRE-V no minimum stated, GRE-Q no minimum stated, GRE-Analytical no minimum stated, GRE-Subject (Psychology) no minimum stated, overall undergraduate GPA no minimum stated, last 2 years GPA no minimum stated, psychology GPA no minimum stated, Masters GPA no minimum stated.

Other Criteria: (importance of criteria rated low, medium, or high): GRE scores—high, research experience—high, work experience—medium, extracurricular activity—low, clinically related public service—medium, GPA—high, letters of recommendation—high, interview—medium, statement of goals and objectives—high, undergraduate major in psychology—medium, specific undergraduate psychology courses taken—high. For additional information on admission requirements, go to http://www.psych.mcgill.ca.

Student Characteristics: The following represents characteristics of students in 2009–2010 in all graduate psychology programs in the department: Female—full-time 77, part-time 0; Male—full-time 31, part-time 0; African American/Black—full-time 0, part-time 0; Hispanic/Latino(a)—full-time 0, part-time 0; Asian/Pacific Islander—full-time 0, part-time 0; American Indian/Alaska Native—full-time 0, part-time 0; Caucasian/White—full-time 0, part-time 0; Multi-ethnic—full-time 0, part-time 0; students subject to the Americans With Disabilities Act—full-time 0, part-time 0; Unknown ethnicity—full-time 0, part-time 0; International students who hold an F-1 or J-1 Visa—full-time 0, part-time 0.

Financial Information/Assistance:
Tuition for Full-Time Study: Master's: State residents: per academic year $3,600; Nonstate residents: per academic year $7,100. *Doctoral:* State residents: per academic year $3,600; Nonstate residents: per academic year $3,600. Tuition is subject to change. See the following Web site for updates and changes in tuition costs: http://www.psych.mcgill.ca. Note: International - Master's is $15,345. International - PhD - $4,200.

Financial Assistance:
First-Year Students: Teaching assistantships available for first year. Fellowships and scholarships available for first year.
Advanced Students: Teaching assistantships available for advanced students. Fellowships and scholarships available for advanced students.
Additional Information: Of all students currently enrolled full time, 100% benefited from one or more of the listed financial assistance programs. Application and information available online at: http://www.mcgill.ca/studentaid/.

Internships/Practica: Doctoral Degree (PhD Clinical Psychology): For those doctoral students for whom a professional internship was required in this program prior to graduation, (9) students applied for an internship in 2008–2009, with (9) students obtaining an internship. Of those students who obtained an internship, (9) were paid internships. Of those students who obtained an internship, (9) students placed in APA/CPA accredited internships, (0) students placed in internships not APA/CPA accredited, but listed with the Association of Psychology Postdoctoral and Internship Programs (APPIC), (0) students placed in internships conforming to guidelines of the Council of Directors of School Psychology Programs (CDSPP), (0) students placed in internships that were not APA/CPA accredited, APPIC or CDSPP listed. The majority of students in our clinical program complete their internships within Montreal, especially at McGill-affiliated hospitals. These include three large and two small general hospitals, a large psychiatric hospital, and a large children's hospital, where a wide range of assessment and treatment skills can be acquired. Specialized, advanced training is provided at other institutions in the areas of neuropsychology, hearing impairments, orthopedic disabilities, and rehabilitation. One advantage of having a local internship is that it facilitates the integration of the student's clinical and research activities. In addition, the department is able to monitor the quality of the training at the placements. All placements have active, ongoing commitments to research. Students have also completed internships at a wide variety of settings in other parts of Canada, the United States, and Europe. Settings outside Montreal must meet with staff approval.

Housing and Day Care: On-campus housing is available. See the following Web site for more information: http://www.mcgill.ca/residences/. On-campus day care facilities are available. See the following Web site for more information: http://www.mcgill.ca/daycare/.

Employment of Department Graduates:
Master's Degree Graduates: Of those who graduated in the academic year 2008–2009, the following categories and numbers represent the postgraduate activities and employment of master's degree graduates: Enrolled in a postdoctoral residency/fellowship (n/a), employed in independent practice (n/a), total from the above (master's) (0).
Doctoral Degree Graduates: Of those who graduated in the academic year 2008–2009, the following categories and numbers represent the postgraduate activities and employment of doctoral degree graduates: Enrolled in a psychology doctoral program (n/a), enrolled in a postdoctoral residency/fellowship (3), employed in an academic position at a university (2), employed in a government agency (1), employed in a hospital/medical center (3), total from the above (doctoral) (9).

Additional Information:
Orientation, Objectives, and Emphasis of Department: McGill University's Department of Psychology offers graduate work leading to the PhD degree. The program in experimental psychology includes the areas of cognitive science (perception, learning, and language), developmental, social, personality, quantitative, and behavioral neuroscience. A program in clinical psychology is also offered. The basic purpose of the graduate program is to provide the student with an environment in which he or she is free to develop skills and expertise that will serve during a professional career in teaching, research, or clinical service as a psychologist. Individually conceived and conducted research in the student's area of interest is the single most important activity of all graduate students in the department.

Application Information:
Send to Giovanna LoCascio, Graduate Program Coordinator, McGill University, Department of Psychology, 1205 Docteur Penfield Avenue, Montreal, Quebec H3A 1B1. Application available online. URL of online application: http://www.psych.mcgill.ca or www.mcgill.ca. Students are admitted in the Fall, application deadline December 1. Note: Students are required to apply online. All supporting documents must be submitted by the deadline to the Psychology Department. *Fee:* $100. Note: All dollar amounts specified in this entry are Canadian dollars.

New Brunswick, University of
Department of Psychology
P.O. Box 4400
Fredericton, NB E3B 5A3
Telephone: (506) 453-4707
Fax: (506) 447-3063
E-mail: *voyer@unb.ca*
Web: *http://www.unbf.ca/psychology*

Department Information:
1966. Chairperson: E. Sandra Byers. Number of faculty: total—full-time 14; women—full-time 8; total—minority—full-time 1; women minority—full-time 1.

Programs and Degrees Offered:
Listed in the following order: Program area, degree type (T if terminal Master's), number awarded 7/08–6/09. Clinical PhD (Doctor of Philosophy) 2, Experimental and Applied PhD (Doctor of Philosophy) 2.

CPA Accreditation: Clinical PhD (Doctor of Philosophy).

Student Applications/Admissions:
Student Applications
Clinical PhD (Doctor of Philosophy)—Applications 2009–2010, 57. Total applicants accepted 2009–2010, 4. Number full-time enrolled (new admits only) 2009–2010, 3. Number part-time enrolled (new admits only) 2009–2010, 0. Openings 2010–2011, 6. The median number of years required for completion of a degree in 2008–2009 were 8. The number of students enrolled full- and part-time who were dismissed or voluntarily withdrew from this program area in 2008–2009 were 0. *Experimental and Applied PhD (Doctor of Philosophy)*—Applications 2009–2010, 8. Total applicants accepted 2009–2010, 2. Number full-time enrolled (new admits only) 2009–2010, 3. Number part-time enrolled (new admits only) 2009–2010, 0. Total enrolled 2009–2010 full-time, 12, part-time, 2. Openings 2010–2011, 6. The median number of years required for completion of a degree in 2008–2009 were 8. The number of students enrolled full- and part-time who were dismissed or voluntarily withdrew from this program area in 2008–2009 were 1.
Scores: Entries appear in this order: required test or GPA, minimum score (if required), median score of students entering in 2009–2010. *Clinical PhD (Doctor of Philosophy)*: GRE-V no minimum stated, GRE-Q no minimum stated, GRE-Analytical no minimum stated, GRE-Subject (Psychology) no minimum stated; *Experimental and Applied PhD (Doctor of Philosophy)*: GRE-V no minimum stated, GRE-Q no minimum stated, GRE-Analytical no minimum stated, GRE-Subject (Psychology) no minimum stated.
Other Criteria: (importance of criteria rated low, medium, or high): GRE scores—medium, research experience—high, work experience—medium, extracurricular activity—low, clinically related public service—low, GPA—high, letters of recommendation—high, interview—high, statement of goals and objectives—high, undergraduate major in psychology—

high, specific undergraduate psychology courses taken—medium, More emphasis is placed on research experience for students admitted to the Experimental & Applied program. A telephone interview is required for applicants to both of our programs. For additional information on admission requirements, go to http://www.unbf.ca/arts//psychology/graduate/grad-admin.html.

Student Characteristics: The following represents characteristics of students in 2009–2010 in all graduate psychology programs in the department: Female—full-time 37, part-time 2; Male—full-time 7, part-time 0; African American/Black—full-time 0, part-time 0; Hispanic/Latino(a)—full-time 1, part-time 0; Asian/Pacific Islander—full-time 0, part-time 0; American Indian/Alaska Native—full-time 0, part-time 0; Caucasian/White—full-time 41, part-time 2; Multi-ethnic—full-time 2, part-time 0; students subject to the Americans With Disabilities Act—full-time 0, part-time 0; Unknown ethnicity—full-time 0, part-time 0; International students who hold an F-1 or J-1 Visa—full-time 0, part-time 0.

Financial Information/Assistance:
Tuition for Full-Time Study: *Doctoral:* State residents: per academic year $6,126; Nonstate residents: per academic year $10,497. Tuition is subject to change.

Financial Assistance:
First-Year Students: Teaching assistantships available for first year. Average amount paid per academic year: $4,000. Average number of hours worked per week: 6. Apply by January 15. Fellowships and scholarships available for first year. Average amount paid per academic year: $9,500. Apply by January 15.
Advanced Students: Teaching assistantships available for advanced students. Average amount paid per academic year: $4,400. Average number of hours worked per week: 6. Apply by January 15. Fellowships and scholarships available for advanced students. Average amount paid per academic year: $11,600. Apply by January 15.
Additional Information: Of all students currently enrolled full time, 30% benefited from one or more of the listed financial assistance programs.

Internships/Practica: Doctoral Degree (PhD Clinical): For those doctoral students for whom a professional internship was required in this program prior to graduation, (1) students applied for an internship in 2008–2009, with (1) students obtaining an internship. Of those students who obtained an internship, (1) were paid internships. Of those students who obtained an internship, (1) students placed in APA/CPA accredited internships, (0) students placed in internships not APA/CPA accredited, but listed with the Association of Psychology Postdoctoral and Internship Programs (APPIC), (0) students placed in internships conforming to guidelines of the Council of Directors of School Psychology Programs (CDSPP), (0) students placed in internships that were not APA/CPA accredited, APPIC or CDSPP listed. Students in the Clinical program have completed practica in the following types of local agencies: mental health clinic, general hospital, university counseling services, psychiatric hospital, or school system.

Housing and Day Care: On-campus housing is available. See the following Web site for more information: http://www.unbf.ca/housing/reslife/index.htm. On-campus day care facilities are available. See the following Web site for more information: http://www.unb.ca/chdc/index.html.

Employment of Department Graduates:
Master's Degree Graduates: Of those who graduated in the academic year 2008–2009, the following categories and numbers represent the postgraduate activities and employment of master's degree graduates: Enrolled in a postdoctoral residency/fellowship (n/a), employed in independent practice (n/a), total from the above (master's) (0).
Doctoral Degree Graduates: Of those who graduated in the academic year 2008–2009, the following categories and numbers represent the postgraduate activities and employment of doctoral degree graduates: Enrolled in a psychology doctoral program (n/a), enrolled in another graduate/professional program (0), enrolled in a postdoctoral residency/fellowship (0), employed in independent practice (1), employed in an academic position at a university (1), employed in an academic position at a 2-year/4-year college (0), employed in other positions at a higher education institution (1), employed in a professional position in a school system (0), employed in business or industry (0), employed in a government agency (1), employed in a community mental health/counseling center (1), employed in a hospital/medical center (2), still seeking employment (0), other employment position (0), do not know (0), total from the above (doctoral) (7).

Additional Information:
Orientation, Objectives, and Emphasis of Department: The Department of Psychology offers an integrated MA/PhD degree designed to provide extensive specialized study in either Clinical Psychology or Experimental and Applied Psychology. The Clinical Program provides graduates with both sufficient skills in assessment, treatment, and outcome evaluation to initiate careers in service settings under appropriate supervision, and with the knowledge and training needed for an academic career. The Experimental and Applied Program emphasizes individual training and the development of skills to equally prepare the student for a research-oriented career in academic or applied settings.

Special Facilities or Resources: The department occupies Keirstead Hall, which is well supplied with research equipment. The facilities include laboratories for research in human learning, cognition and perception, and development, as well as physiological psychology and neuropsychology; a direct line to the computer center; space for research and teaching in clinical, community, behavior therapy, biofeedback, and other areas of applied or clinical psychology.

Application Information:
Send to School of Graduate Studies, University of New Brunswick, P.O. Box 4400, Fredericton, New Brunswick Canada E3B 5A3. Application available online. URL of online application: http://www.unbf.ca/arts//psychology/graduate/gradapp.html. Students are admitted in the Fall, application deadline January 15. *Fee:* $50. The School of Graduate Studies offers fee waivers to selected applicants on the basis of academic merit. Note: All dollar amounts specified in this entry are Canadian dollars.

Ottawa, University of
School of Psychology
Lamoureux Hall, 145 Jean-Jacques Lussier
Ottawa, ON K1N 6N5
Telephone: (613) 562-5800 X4197
Fax: (613) 562-5147
E-mail: mcote@uottawa.ca
Web: http://www.socialsciences.uottawa.ca/psy/eng/index.asp

Department Information:
1941. Director and Associate Dean: Luc Pelletier. Number of faculty: total—full-time 49, part-time 34; women—full-time 19, part-time 34.

Programs and Degrees Offered:
Listed in the following order: Program area, degree type (T if terminal Master's), number awarded 7/08–6/09. Clinical Psychology PhD (Doctor of Philosophy) 6, Experimental Psychology PhD (Doctor of Philosophy) 5.

APA Accreditation: Clinical PhD (Doctor of Philosophy). Student Outcome Data Website: http://www.socialsciences.uottawa.ca/psy/eng/prog2_stats1.asp.

CPA Accreditation: Clinical PhD (Doctor of Philosophy).

Student Applications/Admissions:
Student Applications
Clinical Psychology PhD (Doctor of Philosophy)—Applications 2009–2010, 165. Total applicants accepted 2009–2010, 20. Number full-time enrolled (new admits only) 2009–2010, 18. Number part-time enrolled (new admits only) 2009–2010, 0. Total enrolled 2009–2010 full-time, 101, part-time, 3. Openings 2010–2011, 15. The median number of years required for completion of a degree in 2008–2009 were 6. The number of students enrolled full- and part-time who were dismissed or voluntarily withdrew from this program area in 2008–2009 were 0. Experimental Psychology PhD (Doctor of Philosophy)—Applications 2009–2010, 50. Total applicants accepted 2009–2010, 23. Number full-time enrolled (new admits only) 2009–2010, 16. Number part-time enrolled (new admits only) 2009–2010, 0. Openings 2010–2011, 15. The median number of years required for completion of a degree in 2008–2009 were 5. The number of students enrolled full- and part-time who were dismissed or voluntarily withdrew from this program area in 2008–2009 were 0.
Other Criteria: (importance of criteria rated low, medium, or high): research experience—high, work experience—low, extracurricular activity—low, clinically related public service—medium, GPA—high, letters of recommendation—high, statement of goals and objectives—high, undergraduate major in psychology—high, specific undergraduate psychology courses taken—high. Bilingualism is more important for the clinical program than for the experimental program. For additional information on admission requirements, go to http://www.grad.uottawa.ca/Default.aspx?tabid=1406.

Student Characteristics: The following represents characteristics of students in 2009–2010 in all graduate psychology programs in the department: Female—full-time 142, part-time 6; Male—full-time 23, part-time 4; African American/Black—full-time 1, part-time 0; Hispanic/Latino(a)—full-time 0, part-time 0; Asian/Pacific Islander—full-time 10, part-time 0; American Indian/Alaska Native—full-time 0, part-time 0; Caucasian/White—full-time 153, part-time 0; Multi-ethnic—full-time 1, part-time 0; students subject to the Americans With Disabilities Act—full-time 0, part-time 0; Unknown ethnicity—full-time 0, part-time 0; International students who hold an F-1 or J-1 Visa—full-time 1, part-time 0.

Financial Information/Assistance:
Tuition for Full-Time Study: *Doctoral:* State residents: per academic year $5,941, $226 per credit hour; Nonstate residents: per academic year $14,526, $479 per credit hour. Tuition is subject to change. See the following Web site for updates and changes in tuition costs: http://www.registrar.uottawa.ca/Default.aspx?tabid=2708.

Financial Assistance:
First-Year Students: Teaching assistantships available for first year. Average amount paid per academic year: $9,836. Average number of hours worked per week: 10. Apply by June. Research assistantships available for first year. Average amount paid per academic year: $9,836. Average number of hours worked per week: 10. Apply by June. Fellowships and scholarships available for first-year. Average amount paid per academic year: $9,836. Apply by March.
Advanced Students: Teaching assistantships available for advanced students. Average amount paid per academic year: $9,836. Average number of hours worked per week: 10. Apply by June. Research assistantships available for advanced students. Average amount paid per academic year: $9,836. Average number of hours worked per week: 10. Apply by June. Traineeships available for advanced students. Average amount paid per academic year: $28,000. Average number of hours worked per week: 30. Apply by October. Fellowships and scholarships available for advanced students. Average amount paid per academic year: $9,836. Apply by October.
Additional Information: Of all students currently enrolled full time, 95% benefited from one or more of the listed financial assistance programs. Application and information available online at: http://www.socialsciences.uottawa.ca/psy/eng/graduate_programs.asp.

Internships/Practica: Doctoral Degree (PhD Clinical Psychology): For those doctoral students for whom a professional internship was required in this program prior to graduation, (8) students applied for an internship in 2008–2009, with (7) students obtaining an internship. Of those students who obtained an internship, (6) were paid internships. Of those students who obtained an internship, (6) students placed in APA/CPA accredited internships, (0) students placed in internships not APA/CPA accredited, but listed with the Association of Psychology Postdoctoral and Internship Programs (APPIC), (0) students placed in internships conforming to guidelines of the Council of Directors of School Psychology Programs (CDSPP), (1) students placed in internships that were not APA/CPA accredited, APPIC or CDSPP listed. Internships, required of all clinical program students, take place in accredited external settings in Canada and the USA as well as in local, approved training units. There is one internal training unit: the Centre for Psychological Services. There are twenty external units providing practicum training:

Brockville Mental Health Centre, Canadian Forces Health Services, Catholic School Board of Eastern Ontario, Center for the Treatment of Sexual Abuse and Childhood Trauma, Centre Hospitalier Pierre Janet, Children's Hospital of Eastern Ontario, Centre psycho-social de Vanier, Conseil des écoles catholiques de langue française, Crossroads Children's Centre, Emerging Minds, Montfort Hospital, Ottawa-Carleton Detention Centre, Ottawa Mindfulness Clinic, Royal Ottawa Hospital, Santé Familiale de Clarence-Rockland, The Children's Aid Society of Ottawa-Carleton, The Ottawa Hospital, The Rehabilitation Centre, Ottawa Children's Treatment Center, and Western Quebec School Board. External research internships for the Experimental Program within the University of Ottawa take place in the departments of Sociology, Physiotherapy, Epidemiology, and the Faculties of Education and Administration. External research internships for the Experimental Program are: Canadian Armed Forces, Children's Hospital of Eastern Ontario, Communications Research Center of Canada, Department of Psychology at Carleton University, ENAP, Federal Government of Canada (Animal Care), NORTEL, Ottawa General Hospital, Royal Ottawa Hospital, and The Ministry of Health.

Housing and Day Care: On-campus housing is available. See the following Web site for more information: http://www.uottawa.ca/students/housing/. On-campus day care facilities are available. See the following Web site for more information: http://www.communitylife.uottawa.ca/en/campus-service.php.

Employment of Department Graduates:
Master's Degree Graduates: Of those who graduated in the academic year 2008–2009, the following categories and numbers represent the postgraduate activities and employment of master's degree graduates: Enrolled in a postdoctoral residency/fellowship (n/a), employed in independent practice (n/a), total from the above (master's) (0).
Doctoral Degree Graduates: Of those who graduated in the academic year 2008–2009, the following categories and numbers represent the postgraduate activities and employment of doctoral degree graduates: Enrolled in a psychology doctoral program (n/a), enrolled in a postdoctoral residency/fellowship (3), employed in independent practice (2), employed in a government agency (3), employed in a hospital/medical center (3), do not know (3), total from the above (doctoral) (15).

Additional Information:
Orientation, Objectives, and Emphasis of Department: The objective of the program in Experimental Psychology is to train researchers in one or more of the following areas - neuro-imaging, psychopharmacology, psychoneuroendocrinology, psychophysiology, human and animal cognition, perception, learning, language, sleep and dreams, social, cognitive and emotional development, personality, intergroup relations, motivation, and the social psychology of health, sports and work. Students interested in behavioral neuroscience and its sub-disciplines may also enroll in the Behavioural Neurosciences Specialization Program, which is a collaborative program coordinated by the University of Ottawa and Carleton University. The objective of the Clinical Psychology program is to provide doctoral training in the area of clinical psychology and prepare students to work with adults and youth. Professional training includes cognitive-behavioral, experiential, interpersonal, and community consultation approaches. Thesis supervisors within the clinical program have special expertise in areas such as social development of children, behavior problems and mental health problems throughout the life span, depression, assessment, psychotherapy, marital therapy, family psychology, community psychology, health psychology, and program evaluation. Clinical students may also elect to choose a thesis supervisor from the Experimental program or adjunct professors/clinical professors who are members of the Faculty of Graduate and Postdoctoral Studies.

Special Facilities or Resources: The School of Psychology clinical training unit, the Centre for Psychological Services, offers assessment and treatment for adults, youth, families and couples. The Centre for Research on Educational and Community Services provides program evaluation and consultation services to local social services agencies.

Information for Students With Physical Disabilities: See the following Web site for more information: http://www.sass.uottawa.ca/access/.

Application Information:
Send to Faculty of Social Sciences, 55 Laurier Avenue East, Desmarais Building, Room 3156, Ottawa, Ont., K1N 6N5, Canada. Application available online. URL of online application: http://www.grad.uottawa.ca/apply. Students are admitted in the Fall, application deadline December 15. Experimental program - January 15. *Fee:* $100. Note: All dollar amounts specified in this entry are Canadian dollars.

Queen's University
Department of Psychology
Humphrey Hall, 62 Arch Street
Kingston, ON K7L 3N6
Telephone: (613) 533-2872
Fax: (613) 533-2499
E-mail: *psychead@queensu.ca*
Web: *http://www.queensu.ca/psychology/index.html*

Department Information:
1949. Chairperson: Dr. Rick Beninger. Number of faculty: total—full-time 31; women—full-time 15; total—minority—full-time 3; women minority—full-time 3.

Programs and Degrees Offered:
Listed in the following order: Program area, degree type (T if terminal Master's), number awarded 7/08–6/09. Brain, Behavior, and Cognitive Science PhD (Doctor of Philosophy) 1, Clinical Psychology PhD (Doctor of Philosophy) 3, Developmental Psychology PhD (Doctor of Philosophy) 1, Social-Personality Psychology PhD (Doctor of Philosophy) 5, Clinical Psychology MA/MS (Master of Arts/Science) 4, Developmental Psychology MA/MS (Master of Arts/Science) 2, Social-Personality Psychology MA/MS (Master of Arts/Science) 2, Brain, Behavior, and Cognitive Science MA/MS (Master of Arts/Science) 2.

CPA Accreditation: Clinical PhD (Doctor of Philosophy).

Student Applications/Admissions:
Student Applications
Brain, Behavior, and Cognitive Science PhD *(Doctor of Philosophy)*—Applications 2009–2010, 4. Total applicants accepted

2009–2010, 0. Number full-time enrolled (new admits only) 2009–2010, 3. Number part-time enrolled (new admits only) 2009–2010, 0. Openings 2010–2011, 8. The median number of years required for completion of a degree in 2008–2009 were 4. The number of students enrolled full- and part-time who were dismissed or voluntarily withdrew from this program area in 2008–2009 were 0. *Clinical Psychology PhD (Doctor of Philosophy)*—Applications 2009–2010, 15. Total applicants accepted 2009–2010, 7. Number full-time enrolled (new admits only) 2009–2010, 6. Number part-time enrolled (new admits only) 2009–2010, 0. Total enrolled 2009–2010 full-time, 25, part-time, 1. Openings 2010–2011, 10. The median number of years required for completion of a degree in 2008–2009 were 6. The number of students enrolled full- and part-time who were dismissed or voluntarily withdrew from this program area in 2008–2009 were 0. *Developmental Psychology PhD (Doctor of Philosophy)*—Applications 2009–2010, 2. Total applicants accepted 2009–2010, 1. Number full-time enrolled (new admits only) 2009–2010, 1. Number part-time enrolled (new admits only) 2009–2010, 0. Openings 2010–2011, 6. The median number of years required for completion of a degree in 2008–2009 were 7. The number of students enrolled full- and part-time who were dismissed or voluntarily withdrew from this program area in 2008–2009 were 1. *Social-Personality Psychology PhD (Doctor of Philosophy)*—Applications 2009–2010, 6. Total applicants accepted 2009–2010, 3. Number full-time enrolled (new admits only) 2009–2010, 3. Number part-time enrolled (new admits only) 2009–2010, 0. Openings 2010–2011, 5. The median number of years required for completion of a degree in 2008–2009 were 4. The number of students enrolled full- and part-time who were dismissed or voluntarily withdrew from this program area in 2008–2009 were 0. *Clinical Psychology MA/MS (Master of Arts/Science)*—Applications 2009–2010, 111. Total applicants accepted 2009–2010, 13. Number full-time enrolled (new admits only) 2009–2010, 9. Number part-time enrolled (new admits only) 2009–2010, 0. Openings 2010–2011, 8. The median number of years required for completion of a degree in 2008–2009 were 2. The number of students enrolled full- and part-time who were dismissed or voluntarily withdrew from this program area in 2008–2009 were 0. *Developmental Psychology MA/MS (Master of Arts/Science)*—Applications 2009–2010, 22. Total applicants accepted 2009–2010, 5. Number full-time enrolled (new admits only) 2009–2010, 1. Number part-time enrolled (new admits only) 2009–2010, 0. Openings 2010–2011, 5. The median number of years required for completion of a degree in 2008–2009 were 2. The number of students enrolled full- and part-time who were dismissed or voluntarily withdrew from this program area in 2008–2009 were 0. *Social-Personality Psychology MA/MS (Master of Arts/Science)*—Applications 2009–2010, 26. Total applicants accepted 2009–2010, 5. Number full-time enrolled (new admits only) 2009–2010, 2. Number part-time enrolled (new admits only) 2009–2010, 0. Openings 2010–2011, 7. The median number of years required for completion of a degree in 2008–2009 were 2. The number of students enrolled full- and part-time who were dismissed or voluntarily withdrew from this program area in 2008–2009 were 0. *Brain, Behavior, and Cognitive Science MA/MS (Master of Arts/Science)*—Applications 2009–2010, 17. Total applicants accepted 2009–2010, 3. Number full-time enrolled (new admits only) 2009–2010, 4. Number part-time enrolled (new admits only) 2009–2010, 0. Openings 2010–2011, 4. The median number of years required for completion of a degree in 2008–2009 were 2. The number of students enrolled full- and part-time who were dismissed or voluntarily withdrew from this program area in 2008–2009 were 0.

Scores: Entries appear in this order: required test or GPA, minimum score (if required), median score of students entering in 2009–2010. *Brain, Behavior, and Cognitive Science PhD (Doctor of Philosophy)*: GRE-V no minimum stated, 584, GRE-Q no minimum stated, 704, GRE-Analytical no minimum stated, 5.3, GRE-Subject (Psychology) no minimum stated, 749, last 2 years GPA no minimum stated, psychology GPA no minimum stated, Masters GPA no minimum stated; *Clinical Psychology PhD (Doctor of Philosophy)*: GRE-V no minimum stated, 584, GRE-Q no minimum stated, 704, GRE-Analytical no minimum stated, 5.3, GRE-Subject (Psychology) no minimum stated, 749, last 2 years GPA no minimum stated, psychology GPA no minimum stated, Masters GPA no minimum stated; *Developmental Psychology PhD (Doctor of Philosophy)*: GRE-V no minimum stated, 584, GRE-Q no minimum stated, 704, GRE-Analytical no minimum stated, 5.3, GRE-Subject (Psychology) no minimum stated, 749, last 2 years GPA no minimum stated, psychology GPA no minimum stated, Masters GPA no minimum stated; *Social-Personality Psychology PhD (Doctor of Philosophy)*: GRE-V no minimum stated, 584, GRE-Q no minimum stated, 704, GRE-Analytical no minimum stated, 5.3, GRE-Subject (Psychology) no minimum stated, 749, last 2 years GPA no minimum stated, psychology GPA no minimum stated, Masters GPA no minimum stated; *Clinical Psychology MA/MS (Master of Arts/Science)*: GRE-V no minimum stated, 584, GRE-Q no minimum stated, 704, GRE-Analytical no minimum stated, 5.3, GRE-Subject (Psychology) no minimum stated, 749, overall undergraduate GPA no minimum stated, last 2 years GPA no minimum stated; *Developmental Psychology MA/MS (Master of Arts/Science)*: GRE-V no minimum stated, 584, GRE-Q no minimum stated, 704, GRE-Analytical no minimum stated, 5.3, GRE-Subject (Psychology) no minimum stated, 749, overall undergraduate GPA no minimum stated, last 2 years GPA no minimum stated; *Social-Personality Psychology MA/MS (Master of Arts/Science)*: GRE-V no minimum stated, 584, GRE-Q no minimum stated, 704, GRE-Analytical no minimum stated, 5.3, GRE-Subject (Psychology) no minimum stated, 749, overall undergraduate GPA no minimum stated, last 2 years GPA no minimum stated; *Brain, Behavior, and Cognitive Science MA/MS (Master of Arts/Science)*: GRE-V no minimum stated, 584, GRE-Q no minimum stated, 704, GRE-Analytical no minimum stated, 5.3, GRE-Subject (Psychology) no minimum stated, 749, overall undergraduate GPA no minimum stated, last 2 years GPA no minimum stated.

Other Criteria: (importance of criteria rated low, medium, or high): GRE scores—high, research experience—medium, work experience—low, extracurricular activity—low, clinically related public service—low, GPA—high, letters of recommendation—high, statement of goals and objectives—high, supervisor availability—high, undergraduate major in psychology—high, specific undergraduate psychology courses taken—high. For additional information on admission requirements, go to http://www.queensu.ca/psychology/Graduate/Prospective-Students.html.

Student Characteristics: The following represents characteristics of students in 2009–2010 in all graduate psychology programs in the department: Female—full-time 67, part-time 1; Male—full-time 18, part-time 0; African American/Black—full-time 0, part-time 0; Hispanic/Latino(a)—full-time 0, part-time 0; Asian/Pacific Islander—full-time 10, part-time 0; American Indian/Alaska Native—full-time 1, part-time 0; Caucasian/White—full-time 74, part-time 1; Multi-ethnic—full-time 0, part-time 0; students subject to the Americans With Disabilities Act—full-time 0, part-time 0; Unknown ethnicity—full-time 0, part-time 0; International students who hold an F-1 or J-1 Visa—full-time 3, part-time 0.

Financial Information/Assistance:
Tuition for Full-Time Study: Master's: State residents: per academic year $6,932; Nonstate residents: per academic year $13,280. *Doctoral:* State residents: per academic year $6,932; Nonstate residents: per academic year $13,280. Tuition is subject to change. See the following Web site for updates and changes in tuition costs: http://www.queensu.ca/registrar/currentstudents/fees.html.

Financial Assistance:
First-Year Students: Teaching assistantships available for first year. Average amount paid per academic year: $7,571. Average number of hours worked per week: 10. Fellowships and scholarships available for first year. Average amount paid per academic year: $20,000. Average number of hours worked per week: 0. Apply by October.
Advanced Students: Teaching assistantships available for advanced students. Average amount paid per academic year: $7,571. Average number of hours worked per week: 10. Fellowships and scholarships available for advanced students. Average amount paid per academic year: $20,000. Average number of hours worked per week: 0. Apply by October.
Additional Information: Of all students currently enrolled full time, 60% benefited from one or more of the listed financial assistance programs. Application and information available online at: http://www.queensu.ca/psychology/Graduate/Funding-Opportunities.html.

Internships/Practica: Doctoral Degree (PhD Clinical Psychology): For those doctoral students for whom a professional internship was required in this program prior to graduation, (4) students applied for an internship in 2008–2009, with (4) students obtaining an internship. Of those students who obtained an internship, (4) were paid internships. Of those students who obtained an internship, (4) students placed in APA/CPA accredited internships, (0) students placed in internships not APA/CPA accredited, but listed with the Association of Psychology Postdoctoral and Internship Programs (APPIC), (0) students placed in internships conforming to guidelines of the Council of Directors of School Psychology Programs (CDSPP), (0) students placed in internships that were not APA/CPA accredited, APPIC or CDSPP listed. Clinical program students must complete a predoctoral internship in an approved setting under the primary supervision of a registered psychologist. Students are expected to seek placement in a CPA/APA-approved site.

Housing and Day Care: On-campus housing is available. See the following Web site for more information: http://housing.queensu.ca/residences/. On-campus day care facilities are available. See the following Web site for more information: http://www.queensu.ca/daycare/index.html.

Employment of Department Graduates:
Master's Degree Graduates: Of those who graduated in the academic year 2008–2009, the following categories and numbers represent the postgraduate activities and employment of master's degree graduates: Enrolled in a psychology doctoral program (10), enrolled in a postdoctoral residency/fellowship (n/a), employed in independent practice (n/a), total from the above (master's) (10).
Doctoral Degree Graduates: Of those who graduated in the academic year 2008–2009, the following categories and numbers represent the postgraduate activities and employment of doctoral degree graduates: Enrolled in a psychology doctoral program (n/a), employed in independent practice (3), employed in an academic position at a university (4), do not know (3), total from the above (doctoral) (10).

Additional Information:
Orientation, Objectives, and Emphasis of Department: All programs stress empirical research. The Brain, Behavior, and Cognitive Science program, the Developmental program, and the Social-Personality program emphasize research skills and scholarship, preparing students for either academic positions or for research positions in government, industry, and the like. The Clinical program is based on a scientist–practitioner model of training that emphasizes the integration of research and clinical skills in the understanding, assessment, treatment, and prevention of psychological problems.

Special Facilities or Resources: Extensive computer and laboratory facilities are available to graduate students for research and clinical experience. Financial assistance is available in the form of federal, provincial, and university fellowships, scholarships and bursaries. For 2009-10, incoming Master's students received a minimum of $18,000. PhD students received a minimum of $18,500. A portion of this guaranteed minimum is in the form of a teaching assistantship.

Information for Students With Physical Disabilities: See the following Web site for more information: http://www.queensu.ca/equity/disabilities/.

Application Information:
Send to The Registrar, School of Graduate Studies and Research, Gordon Hall, Queen's University, Kingston, ON Canada K7L 3N6. Application available online. URL of online application: http://www.queensu.ca/futurestudents/apply/. Students are admitted in the Fall, application deadline December 1. *Fee:* $95. Note: All dollar amounts specified in this entry are Canadian dollars.

REGINA, University of
Department of Psychology
3737 Wascana Parkway
Regina, SK S4S 0A2
Telephone: (306) 585-4157
Fax: (306) 585-5429
E-mail: *richard.maclennan@uregina.ca*
Web: *http://www.arts.uregina.ca/psychology*

Department Information:
1965. Department Head: Richard MacLennan. Number of faculty: total—full-time 20; women—full-time 10.

Programs and Degrees Offered:
Listed in the following order: Program area, degree type (T if terminal Master's), number awarded 7/08–6/09. Clinical Psychology MA/MS (Master of Arts/Science) (T) 7, Clinical Psychology PhD (Doctor of Philosophy) 4, Experimental and Applied Psychology MA/MS (Master of Arts/Science) (T) 2, Experimental and Applied Psychology PhD (Doctor of Philosophy) 1.

CPA Accreditation: Clinical PhD (Doctor of Philosophy).

Student Applications/Admissions:
Student Applications
Clinical Psychology MA/MS (Master of Arts/Science)—Applications 2009–2010, 27. Total applicants accepted 2009–2010, 6. Number full-time enrolled (new admits only) 2009–2010, 6. Number part-time enrolled (new admits only) 2009–2010, 0. Total enrolled 2009–2010 full-time, 14, part-time, 2. Openings 2010–2011, 6. The median number of years required for completion of a degree in 2008–2009 were 2. The number of students enrolled full- and part-time who were dismissed or voluntarily withdrew from this program area in 2008–2009 were 0. Clinical Psychology PhD (Doctor of Philosophy)—Applications 2009–2010, 7. Total applicants accepted 2009–2010, 4. Number full-time enrolled (new admits only) 2009–2010, 0. Number part-time enrolled (new admits only) 2009–2010, 0. Openings 2010–2011, 6. The median number of years required for completion of a degree in 2008–2009 were 4. The number of students enrolled full- and part-time who were dismissed or voluntarily withdrew from this program area in 2008–2009 were 0. Experimental and Applied Psychology MA/MS (Master of Arts/Science)—Applications 2009–2010, 4. Total applicants accepted 2009–2010, 1. Number full-time enrolled (new admits only) 2009–2010, 1. Number part-time enrolled (new admits only) 2009–2010, 0. Total enrolled 2009–2010 full-time, 3, part-time, 4. Openings 2010–2011, 2. The median number of years required for completion of a degree in 2008–2009 were 2. The number of students enrolled full- and part-time who were dismissed or voluntarily withdrew from this program area in 2008–2009 were 0. Experimental and Applied Psychology PhD (Doctor of Philosophy)—Applications 2009–2010, 4. Total applicants accepted 2009–2010, 3. Number full-time enrolled (new admits only) 2009–2010, 0. Number part-time enrolled (new admits only) 2009–2010, 0. Openings 2010–2011, 3. The median number of years required for completion of a degree in 2008–2009 were 4. The number of students enrolled full- and part-time who were dismissed or voluntarily withdrew from this program area in 2008–2009 were 0.
Other Criteria: (importance of criteria rated low, medium, or high): GRE scores—high, research experience—medium, work experience—low, extracurricular activity—low, clinically related public service—medium, GPA—high, letters of recommendation—high, statement of goals and objectives—high, undergraduate major in psychology—high, specific undergraduate psychology courses taken—low. For additional information on admission requirements, go to http://www.arts.uregina.ca/psychology.

Student Characteristics: The following represents characteristics of students in 2009–2010 in all graduate psychology programs in the department: Female—full-time 38, part-time 5; Male—full-time 12, part-time 1; African American/Black—full-time 1, part-time 0; Hispanic/Latino(a)—full-time 0, part-time 0; Asian/Pacific Islander—full-time 3, part-time 0; American Indian/Alaska Native—full-time 1, part-time 0; Caucasian/White—full-time 40, part-time 5; Multi-ethnic—full-time 0, part-time 0; students subject to the Americans With Disabilities Act—full-time 0, part-time 0; Unknown ethnicity—full-time 5, part-time 1; International students who hold an F-1 or J-1 Visa—full-time 0, part-time 0.

Financial Information/Assistance:
Tuition for Full-Time Study: *Master's:* State residents: per academic year $3,644, $202 per credit hour; Nonstate residents: per academic year $4,694, $260 per credit hour. *Doctoral:* State residents: per academic year $3,704, $206 per credit hour; Nonstate residents: per academic year $4,754, $264 per credit hour. See the following Web site for updates and changes in tuition costs: http://www.uregina.ca/gradstudies/main/cost_of_study.shtml.

Financial Assistance:
First-Year Students: Teaching assistantships available for first year. Average amount paid per academic year: $2,186. Average number of hours worked per week: 7. Apply by June 15. Research assistantships available for first year. Average amount paid per academic year: $5,500. Average number of hours worked per week: 7. Apply by February 28. Fellowships and scholarships available for first year. Average amount paid per academic year: $6,000. Average number of hours worked per week: 0. Apply by June 15.

Advanced Students: Teaching assistantships available for advanced students. Average amount paid per academic year: $2,292. Average number of hours worked per week: 7. Apply by June 15. Research assistantships available for advanced students. Average amount paid per academic year: $6,000. Average number of hours worked per week: 7. Apply by February 28. Fellowships and scholarships available for advanced students. Average amount paid per academic year: $7,000. Average number of hours worked per week: 0. Apply by June 15.

Additional Information: Of all students currently enrolled full time, 55% benefited from one or more of the listed financial assistance programs. Application and information available online at: http://www.uregina.ca/gradstudies/scholarships/fgsr_funding.jsp.

Internships/Practica: Doctoral Degree (PhD Clinical Psychology): For those doctoral students for whom a professional internship was required in this program prior to graduation, (4) students applied for an internship in 2008–2009, with (3) students obtaining an internship. Of those students who obtained an internship, (3) were paid internships. Of those students who obtained an internship, (3) students placed in APA/CPA accredited internships, (0) students placed in internships not APA/CPA accredited, but listed with the Association of Psychology Postdoctoral and Internship Programs (APPIC), (0) students placed in internships conforming to guidelines of the Council of Directors of School Psychology Programs (CDSPP), (0) students placed in internships that were not APA/CPA accredited, APPIC or CDSPP listed. Master's Degree (MA/MS Clinical Psychology): An internship experience, such as, a final research project or "capstone" experience is required of graduates. Master's Degree (MA/MS Experimental and Applied Psychology): An internship experience, such as, a final research project or "capstone" experience is required of graduates. A wide array of community resources are available and well utilized in providing practicum and internship training. The department cannot guarantee placement in these facilities.

Housing and Day Care: On-campus housing is available. See the following Web site for more information: http://www.uregina.ca/residences/. On-campus day care facilities are available. Wascana Co-operative Day Care (306) 585-5311.

Employment of Department Graduates:
Master's Degree Graduates: Of those who graduated in the academic year 2008–2009, the following categories and numbers represent the postgraduate activities and employment of master's degree graduates: Enrolled in a psychology doctoral program (5), enrolled in another graduate/professional program (0), enrolled in a postdoctoral residency/fellowship (n/a), employed in independent practice (n/a), employed in an academic position at a university (0), employed in an academic position at a 2-year/4-year college (0), employed in other positions at a higher education institution (0), employed in a professional position in a school system (0), employed in business or industry (0), employed in a government agency (0), employed in a community mental health/counseling center (0), employed in a hospital/medical center (0), still seeking employment (0), not seeking employment (0), other employment position (0), do not know (0), total from the above (master's) (5).
Doctoral Degree Graduates: Of those who graduated in the academic year 2008–2009, the following categories and numbers represent the postgraduate activities and employment of doctoral degree graduates: Enrolled in a psychology doctoral program (n/a), enrolled in another graduate/professional program (1), enrolled in a postdoctoral residency/fellowship (0), employed in independent practice (0), employed in an academic position at a university (0), employed in an academic position at a 2-year/4-year college (0), employed in other positions at a higher education institution (0), employed in a professional position in a school system (0), employed in business or industry (0), employed in a government agency (0), employed in a community mental health/counseling center (0), employed in a hospital/medical center (4), still seeking employment (0), other employment position (0), do not know (0), total from the above (doctoral) (5).

Additional Information:
Orientation, Objectives, and Emphasis of Department: Teaching and research are oriented toward clinical, social, and applied approaches. The majority of graduate students are in clinical psychology. Faculty orientation is eclectic. Cognitive behavioral and humanistic approaches are represented. Neuropsychology is also well represented.

Special Facilities or Resources: The department has clinical/counselling rooms for research purposes, a small testing library, permanent space for faculty research, and observation rooms and computer labs.

Information for Students With Physical Disabilities: See the following Web site for more information: http://www.uregina.ca/studserv/disability/index.shtml.

Application Information:
Send to Dean, Faculty of Graduate Studies and Research University of Regina 3737 Wascana Parkway Regina, SK S4S 0A2. Application available online. URL of online application: https://dataware.cc.uregina.ca/app/Misc/introduction.cfm. Students are admitted in the Fall, application deadline February 15. *Fee:* $90. Note: All dollar amounts specified in this entry are Canadian dollars.

Ryerson University
Department of Psychology
350 Victoria Street
Toronto, ON M5B 2K3
Telephone: (416) 979-5000
Fax: (416) 979-5273
E-mail: *mantony@psych.ryerson.ca*
Web: *http://www.ryerson.ca/psychology/*

Department Information:
1974. Chairperson: Jean-Paul Boudreau. Number of faculty: total—full-time 29, part-time 11; women—full-time 17, part-time 8; total—minority—full-time 3; women minority—full-time 3.

Programs and Degrees Offered:
Listed in the following order: Program area, degree type (T if terminal Master's), number awarded 7/08–6/09. Clinical Psychology MA/MS (Master of Arts/Science) 0, Psychological Science MA/MS (Master of Arts/Science) 0, Clinical Psychology PhD (Doctor of Philosophy) 0, Psychological Science PhD (Doctor of Philosophy) 0.

Student Applications/Admissions:
Student Applications
Clinical Psychology MA/MS (Master of Arts/Science)—Applications 2009–2010, 154. Total applicants accepted 2009–2010, 9. Number full-time enrolled (new admits only) 2009–2010, 9. Number part-time enrolled (new admits only) 2009–2010, 0. Openings 2010–2011, 8. The number of students enrolled full- and part-time who were dismissed or voluntarily withdrew from this program area in 2008–2009 were 0. *Psychological Science MA/MS (Master of Arts/Science)*—Applications 2009–2010, 38. Total applicants accepted 2009–2010, 7. Number full-time enrolled (new admits only) 2009–2010, 7. Number part-time enrolled (new admits only) 2009–2010, 0. Openings 2010–2011, 8. The number of students enrolled full- and part-time who were dismissed or voluntarily withdrew from this program area in 2008–2009 were 0. *Clinical Psychology PhD (Doctor of Philosophy)*—Applications 2009–2010, 17. Total applicants accepted 2009–2010, 14. Number full-time enrolled (new admits only) 2009–2010, 14. Number part-time enrolled (new admits only) 2009–2010, 0. Openings 2010–2011, 8. The number of students enrolled full- and part-time who were dismissed or voluntarily withdrew from this program area in 2008–2009 were 0. *Psychological Science PhD (Doctor of Philosophy)*—Applications 2009–2010, 9. Total applicants accepted 2009–2010, 9. Number full-time enrolled (new admits only) 2009–2010, 9. Number part-time enrolled (new admits only) 2009–2010, 0. Openings 2010–2011, 9. The median number of years required for completion of a degree in 2008–2009 were 3. The number of students enrolled full- and part-time who were dismissed or voluntarily withdrew from this program area in 2008–2009 were 0.

Other Criteria: (importance of criteria rated low, medium, or high): GRE scores—medium, research experience—high, work experience—medium, extracurricular activity—low, clinically related public service—low, GPA—high, letters of recommendation—high, interview—high, statement of goals and objectives—high, undergraduate major in psychology—medium, specific undergraduate psychology courses taken—medium, Undergraduate major in psychology is strongly recommended for both fields, and is especially important for the clinical psychology field. For additional information on admission requirements, go to http://www.ryerson.ca/psychology/graduate/admissions/.

Student Characteristics: The following represents characteristics of students in 2009–2010 in all graduate psychology programs in the department: Female—full-time 50, part-time 0; Male—full-time 5, part-time 0; African American/Black—full-time 0, part-time 0; Hispanic/Latino(a)—full-time 0, part-time 0; Asian/Pacific Islander—full-time 12, part-time 0; American Indian/Alaska Native—full-time 0, part-time 0; Caucasian/White—full-time 43, part-time 0; Multi-ethnic—full-time 0, part-time 0; students subject to the Americans With Disabilities Act—full-time 0, part-time 0; Unknown ethnicity—full-time 0, part-time 0; International students who hold an F-1 or J-1 Visa—full-time 0, part-time 0.

Financial Information/Assistance:
Tuition for Full-Time Study: *Master's:* State residents: per academic year $8,313; Nonstate residents: per academic year $17,079. *Doctoral:* State residents: per academic year $8,313; Nonstate residents: per academic year $17,079. Tuition is subject to change. See the following Web site for updates and changes in tuition costs: http://www.ryerson.ca/graduate/fees/.

Financial Assistance:
First-Year Students: Teaching assistantships available for first year. Average amount paid per academic year: $9,750. Average number of hours worked per week: 10. Research assistantships available for first year. Average amount paid per academic year: $9,750. Average number of hours worked per week: 10. Fellowships and scholarships available for first -year. Average amount paid per academic year: $7,000. Average number of hours worked per week: 0.
Advanced Students: Teaching assistantships available for advanced students. Average amount paid per academic year: $10,530. Average number of hours worked per week: 10. Research assistantships available for advanced students. Average amount paid per academic year: $10,530. Average number of hours worked per week: 10. Fellowships and scholarships available for advanced students. Average amount paid per academic year: $7,000. Average number of hours worked per week: 0.
Additional Information: Of all students currently enrolled full time, 100% benefited from one or more of the listed financial assistance programs. Application and information available online at: http://www.ryerson.ca/psychology/graduate/admissions/finances/.

Internships/Practica: Our clinical psychology students have been successful at securing practicum placements at top training centres, including Baycrest, Bellwood Health Services, the Centre for Addiction and Mental Health, Hamilton Health Sciences, Humber River Regional Hospital, North York General Hospital, St. Joseph's Healthcare Hamilton, Toronto General Hospital, Ryerson Centre for Student Development and Counselling, Toronto Rehabilitation Institute, and others. With a focus on breadth and depth training in research methodology, possible practicum placements for the Psychological Science students include both internal sites such as the research labs of faculty in the Ryerson Department of Psychology as well as external sites such as the Centre for Addiction and Mental Health, Defense Research and Development Canada, Health Canada, Hospital for Sick Children, MultiHealth Systems (MHS), Rotman Research Institute, and Transport Canada.

Housing and Day Care: No on-campus housing is available. On-campus day care facilities are available. See the following Web site for more information: http://www.ryerson.ca/ece/researchlabs/elc/.

Employment of Department Graduates:
Master's Degree Graduates: Of those who graduated in the academic year 2008–2009, the following categories and numbers represent the postgraduate activities and employment of master's degree graduates: Enrolled in a postdoctoral residency/fellowship (n/a), employed in independent practice (n/a), total from the above (master's) (0).
Doctoral Degree Graduates: Of those who graduated in the academic year 2008–2009, the following categories and numbers represent the postgraduate activities and employment of doctoral degree graduates: Enrolled in a psychology doctoral program (n/a), total from the above (doctoral) (0).

Additional Information:
Orientation, Objectives, and Emphasis of Department: Launched in the fall of 2007, our program offers students opportunities to study in either Clinical Psychology (CPA accreditation anticipated in the next two years) or Psychological Science. The Psychological Science stream offers opportunities to specialize in research areas that include cognition and perception; neuroscience; history, culture, and individual differences; social, community, and forensic psychology; and developmental psychology. The graduate program in Psychology offers an innovative curriculum that is anchored in research training. Trained at some of the top universities in Canada, the United States, and around the world, the core faculty (including 20 hired since 2005) bring a rigorous and student-centered approach to scientific and clinical training. Based in a department known for excellence in training, the program takes advantage of its downtown Toronto location, with proximity to major sites for practicum training and clinical research, and offers students access to world-class training opportunities.

Special Facilities or Resources: The department has developed a new state-of-the-art lab facility that includes over 10,000 square feet of research space. This new space has been built from the ground up to serve the research and training needs of our psychology graduate students and faculty. We are also developing a fully equipped, in-house training clinic to meet the requirements of our clinical psychology program.

Information for Students With Physical Disabilities: See the following Web site for more information: http://www.ryerson.ca/studentservices/accesscentre/.

GRADUATE STUDY IN PSYCHOLOGY

Application Information:
Send to Graduate Admissions Office School of Graduate Studies, Ryerson University, 350 Victoria Street, Toronto, Ontario M5B 2K3 Canada. Application available online. URL of online application: http://www.ryerson.ca/psychology/graduate/admissions/. Students are admitted in the Fall, application deadline December 3. *Fee:* $100. Note: All dollar amounts specified in this entry are Canadian dollars.

Saint Mary's University
Department of Psychology
923 Robie Street
Halifax, NS B3H 3C3
Telephone: (902) 420-5846
Fax: (902) 496-8287
E-mail: *vic.catano@smu.ca*
Web: *http://www.smu.ca/academic/science/psych/*

Department Information:
1966. Chairperson: Victor Catano. Number of faculty: total—full-time 19, part-time 25; women—full-time 8, part-time 10.

Programs and Degrees Offered:
Listed in the following order: Program area, degree type (T if terminal Master's), number awarded 7/08–6/09. Industrial/Organizational Psychology MA/MS (Master of Arts/Science) (T) 7, Industrial/Organizational Psychology PhD (Doctor of Philosophy) 0.

Student Applications/Admissions:
Student Applications
Industrial/Organizational Psychology MA/MS (Master of Arts/Science)—Applications 2009–2010, 31. Total applicants accepted 2009–2010, 10. Number full-time enrolled (new admits only) 2009–2010, 8. Number part-time enrolled (new admits only) 2009–2010, 0. Total enrolled 2009–2010 full-time, 23, part-time, 3. Openings 2010–2011, 8. The median number of years required for completion of a degree in 2008–2009 were 2. The number of students enrolled full- and part-time who were dismissed or voluntarily withdrew from this program area in 2008–2009 were 0. *Industrial/Organizational Psychology PhD (Doctor of Philosophy)*—Applications 2009–2010, 4. Total applicants accepted 2009–2010, 2. Number full-time enrolled (new admits only) 2009–2010, 1. Number part-time enrolled (new admits only) 2009–2010, 0. Total enrolled 2009–2010 full-time, 10, part-time, 6. Openings 2010–2011, 3. The number of students enrolled full- and part-time who were dismissed or voluntarily withdrew from this program area in 2008–2009 were 0.
Scores: Entries appear in this order: required test or GPA, minimum score (if required), median score of students entering in 2009–2010. *Industrial/Organizational Psychology MA/MS (Master of Arts/Science):* GRE-V no minimum stated, GRE-Q no minimum stated, GRE-Analytical no minimum stated, GRE-Subject (Psychology) no minimum stated, overall undergraduate GPA no minimum stated; *Industrial/Organizational Psychology PhD (Doctor of Philosophy):* GRE-V no minimum stated, GRE-Q no minimum stated, GRE-Analytical no minimum stated, GRE-Subject (Psychology) no minimum stated, overall undergraduate GPA no minimum stated.

Other Criteria: (importance of criteria rated low, medium, or high): GRE scores—high, research experience—high, work experience—low, extracurricular activity—low, GPA—high, letters of recommendation—medium, statement of goals and objectives—high, undergraduate major in psychology—high, specific undergraduate psychology courses taken—low.

Student Characteristics: The following represents characteristics of students in 2009–2010 in all graduate psychology programs in the department: Female—full-time 21, part-time 5; Male—full-time 12, part-time 4; African American/Black—full-time 0, part-time 0; Hispanic/Latino(a)—full-time 0, part-time 0; Asian/Pacific Islander—part-time 0; American Indian/Alaska Native—full-time 0, part-time 0; Caucasian/White—full-time 33, part-time 9; Multi-ethnic—full-time 0, part-time 0; students subject to the Americans With Disabilities Act—full-time 0, part-time 0; Unknown ethnicity—full-time 0, part-time 0; International students who hold an F-1 or J-1 Visa—full-time 1, part-time 0.

Financial Information/Assistance:
Tuition for Full-Time Study: *Master's:* State residents: per academic year $3,700; Nonstate residents: per academic year $7,048. *Doctoral:* State residents: per academic year $5,000; Nonstate residents: per academic year $7,232. Tuition is subject to change. See the following Web site for updates and changes in tuition costs: http://fgsr.smu.ca/grad_pro_fin.html.

Financial Assistance:
First-Year Students: Teaching assistantships available for first year. Average amount paid per academic year: $5,000. Average number of hours worked per week: 13. Apply by February 1. Research assistantships available for first year. Average amount paid per academic year: $7,500. Average number of hours worked per week: 10. Traineeships available for first year. Average amount paid per academic year: $9,000. Average number of hours worked per week: 40. Apply by March. Fellowships and scholarships available for first year. Average amount paid per academic year: $7,200. Average number of hours worked per week: 0. Apply by February 1.
Advanced Students: Teaching assistantships available for advanced students. Average amount paid per academic year: $5,000. Average number of hours worked per week: 13. Apply by June 1. Research assistantships available for advanced students. Average amount paid per academic year: $7,500. Average number of hours worked per week: 10. Traineeships available for advanced students. Average amount paid per academic year: $8,000. Average number of hours worked per week: 10. Fellowships and scholarships available for advanced students. Average amount paid per academic year: $15,000. Average number of hours worked per week: 0. Apply by June 1.
Additional Information: Of all students currently enrolled full time, 90% benefited from one or more of the listed financial assistance programs. Application and information available online at: http://fgsr.smu.ca/grad_pro_app.html.

Internships/Practica: Master's Degree (MA/MS Industrial/Organizational Psychology): An internship experience, such as, a final research project or "capstone" experience is required of graduates. Masters' students are required to complete a supervised, full-time, paid internship (minimum of 500 hours) in the summer following their first year or part-time during their second year. Placements are available in a variety of government agencies, human resource departments, research agencies, and private consulting firms. Salaries range from $6,000 to $13,000 for the four months.

Housing and Day Care: On-campus housing is available. See the following Web site for more information: http://www.smu.ca/administration/resoffic/welcome.html. On-campus day care facilities are available. See the following Web site for more information: http://www.smu.ca/administration/studentservices/daycare.html.

Employment of Department Graduates:
Master's Degree Graduates: Of those who graduated in the academic year 2008–2009, the following categories and numbers represent the postgraduate activities and employment of master's degree graduates: Enrolled in a psychology doctoral program (1), enrolled in another graduate/professional program (0), enrolled in a postdoctoral residency/fellowship (n/a), employed in independent practice (n/a), employed in an academic position at a university (0), employed in an academic position at a 2-year/4-year college (0), employed in other positions at a higher education institution (0), employed in a professional position in a school system (0), employed in business or industry (3), employed in a government agency (2), employed in a community mental health/counseling center (0), employed in a hospital/medical center (0), still seeking employment (0), other employment position (0), do not know (0), total from the above (master's) (6).
Doctoral Degree Graduates: Of those who graduated in the academic year 2008–2009, the following categories and numbers represent the postgraduate activities and employment of doctoral degree graduates: Enrolled in a psychology doctoral program (n/a), total from the above (doctoral) (0).

Additional Information:
Orientation, Objectives, and Emphasis of Department: Masters' students will acquire a background in theory and research that is consistent with the scientist–practitioner model, preparing themselves for employment and/or continued graduate education. Full-time students normally require two years to complete the program. Part-time students may take two to four years longer. Masters' students are normally provided with financial support for two years. PhD students will acquire a background in theory and research that is consistent with the scientist–practitioner model, preparing them for an academic career or a career in consulting and/or industry. Full-time students normally require three years to complete the program, but may complete it in two years. PhD students are normally provided with financial support for three years.

Special Facilities or Resources: General research laboratories, graduate computer lab, small-group research space, graduate student offices, and a tests and measurements library that includes psychological test batteries are available. Support systems include audiovisual equipment, computer facilities, and a technical workshop. Students may be involved in the CN Centre for Occupational Health & Safety, as well as the Centre for Leadership Excellence.

Information for Students With Physical Disabilities: See the following Web site for more information: http://www.smu.ca/administration/atlcentre/welcome.html.

Application Information:
Send to Faculty of Graduate Studies & Research, Saint Mary's University, Halifax, Nova Scotia, Canada B3H 3C3. Application available online. URL of online application: http://fgsr.smu.ca/grad_pro_app.html. Students are admitted in the Fall, application deadline February 1. *Fee:* $70. Note: All dollar amounts specified in this entry are Canadian dollars.

Saskatchewan, University of
Department of Psychology
Arts and Science
9 Campus Drive
Saskatoon, SK S7N 5A5
Telephone: (306) 966-6657
Fax: (306) 966-6630
E-mail: *joni.morman@usask.ca*
Web: *http://www.artsandscience.usask.ca/psychology/*

Department Information:
1946. Head: Valerie Thompson. Number of faculty: total—full-time 24, part-time 3; women—full-time 9, part-time 1; ; women minority—part-time 1.

Programs and Degrees Offered:
Listed in the following order: Program area, degree type (T if terminal Master's), number awarded 7/08–6/09. Clinical PhD (Doctor of Philosophy) 11, Applied Social PhD (Doctor of Philosophy) 1, Basic Behavioural Science PhD (Doctor of Philosophy) 1, Culture and Human Development PhD (Doctor of Philosophy) 0.

APA Accreditation: Clinical PhD (Doctor of Philosophy).

CPA Accreditation: Clinical PhD (Doctor of Philosophy).

Student Applications/Admissions:
Student Applications
Clinical PhD (Doctor of Philosophy)—Applications 2009–2010, 54. Total applicants accepted 2009–2010, 8. Number full-time enrolled (new admits only) 2009–2010, 6. Number part-time enrolled (new admits only) 2009–2010, 0. Openings 2010–2011, 6. The median number of years required for completion of a degree in 2008–2009 were 7. The number of students enrolled full- and part-time who were dismissed or voluntarily withdrew from this program area in 2008–2009 were 0. *Applied Social PhD (Doctor of Philosophy)*—Applications 2009–2010, 10. Total applicants accepted 2009–2010, 6. Number full-time enrolled (new admits only) 2009–2010, 5. Number part-time enrolled (new admits only) 2009–2010, 0. The median number of years required for completion of a degree in 2008–2009 were 7. The number of students enrolled full- and part-time who were dismissed or voluntarily withdrew from this program area in 2008–2009 were 0. *Basic Behavioural Science PhD (Doctor of Philosophy)*—Applications 2009–2010, 11. Total applicants accepted 2009–2010, 4. Number full-time enrolled (new admits only) 2009–2010, 3. Number part-time enrolled (new admits only) 2009–2010, 0. The median number of years required for completion of a degree in 2008–2009 were 4. The number of students enrolled full- and part-time who were dismissed or voluntarily withdrew from this program area in 2008–2009 were 0. *Culture and Human Development PhD (Doctor of Philosophy)*—Applications 2009–2010, 13. Total applicants accepted 2009–2010, 2. Number full-time enrolled (new

admits only) 2009–2010, 2. Total enrolled 2009–2010 full-time, 8. The median number of years required for completion of a degree in 2008–2009 were 4. The number of students enrolled full- and part-time who were dismissed or voluntarily withdrew from this program area in 2008–2009 were 0.

Scores: Entries appear in this order: required test or GPA, minimum score (if required), median score of students entering in 2009–2010. *Clinical PhD (Doctor of Philosophy)*: GRE-V no minimum stated, GRE-Q no minimum stated, GRE-Analytical no minimum stated, GRE-Subject (Psychology) no minimum stated, overall undergraduate GPA 80, 85, last 2 years GPA 80, 85, psychology GPA 80, 85, Masters GPA 80, 85; *Applied Social PhD (Doctor of Philosophy)*: GRE-V no minimum stated, GRE-Q no minimum stated, GRE-Analytical no minimum stated, GRE-Subject (Psychology) no minimum stated, last 2 years GPA no minimum stated, psychology GPA no minimum stated; *Basic Behavioural Science PhD (Doctor of Philosophy)*: Masters GPA no minimum stated; *Culture and Human Development PhD (Doctor of Philosophy)*: last 2 years GPA no minimum stated, psychology GPA no minimum stated.

Other Criteria: (importance of criteria rated low, medium, or high): GRE scores—medium, research experience—high, work experience—medium, extracurricular activity—low, clinically related public service—low, GPA—high, letters of recommendation—high, interview—high, statement of goals and objectives—high, GRE scores are not required for the Basic Behavioural Science (BBS) and Culture and Human Development (C&HD) applications. For additional information on admission requirements, go to http://artsandscience.usask.ca/psychology/files/GradChecklist.pdf.

Student Characteristics: The following represents characteristics of students in 2009–2010 in all graduate psychology programs in the department: Female—full-time 67, part-time 0; Male—full-time 19, part-time 0; Caucasian/White—full-time 0, part-time 0; Unknown ethnicity—full-time 0, part-time 0; International students who hold an F-1 or J-1 Visa—full-time 2, part-time 0.

Financial Information/Assistance:
Tuition for Full-Time Study: *Master's:* State residents: per academic year $3,611; Nonstate residents: per academic year $3,611. *Doctoral:* State residents: per academic year $3,611; Nonstate residents: per academic year $3,611. Tuition is subject to change. See the following Web site for updates and changes in tuition costs: http://www.usask.ca/cgsr/prospective_students/tuition.php.

Financial Assistance:
First-Year Students: Fellowships and scholarships available for first -year. Average amount paid per academic year: $16,000.
Advanced Students: Fellowships and scholarships available for advanced students. Average amount paid per academic year: $16,000.
Additional Information: Of all students currently enrolled full time, 80% benefited from one or more of the listed financial assistance programs. Application and information available online at: http://artsandscience.usask.ca/psychology/.

Internships/Practica: Doctoral Degree (PhD Clinical): For those doctoral students for whom a professional internship was required in this program prior to graduation, (3) students applied for an internship in 2008–2009, with (3) students obtaining an internship. Of those students who obtained an internship, (3) were paid internships. Of those students who obtained an internship, (2) students placed in APA/CPA accredited internships, (1) students placed in internships not APA/CPA accredited, but listed with the Association of Psychology Postdoctoral and Internship Programs (APPIC), (0) students placed in internships conforming to guidelines of the Council of Directors of School Psychology Programs (CDSPP), (0) students placed in internships that were not APA/CPA accredited, APPIC or CDSPP listed. Full-time internships and practicum training concurrent with coursework are required at the MA and PhD levels in both clinical and applied social programs. In the clinical program, four-month MA internship placements are available at a number of hospital and outpatient clinics throughout the province. At the PhD level, 12-month internships have been arranged in larger clinical settings with diversified client populations in Canada and the United States. The applied social program requires four-month applied research internships at both the MA and PhD levels. Practicum and internship placements are arranged in a wide variety of government, institutional, and business settings.

Housing and Day Care: On-campus housing is available. See the following Web site for more information: http://explore.usask.ca/housing/. On-campus day care facilities are available. See the following Web site for more information: http://students.usask.ca/support/childcare/.

Employment of Department Graduates:
Master's Degree Graduates: Of those who graduated in the academic year 2008–2009, the following categories and numbers represent the postgraduate activities and employment of master's degree graduates: Enrolled in a postdoctoral residency/fellowship (n/a), employed in independent practice (n/a), employed in a community mental health/counseling center (1), employed in a hospital/medical center (1), do not know (6), total from the above (master's) (8).
Doctoral Degree Graduates: Of those who graduated in the academic year 2008–2009, the following categories and numbers represent the postgraduate activities and employment of doctoral degree graduates: Enrolled in a psychology doctoral program (n/a), employed in other positions at a higher education institution (1), do not know (7), total from the above (doctoral) (8).

Additional Information:
Orientation, Objectives, and Emphasis of Department: All graduate programs are small and highly selective. The clinical program focuses on PhD training, based on a scientist–practitioner model with an eclectic theoretical perspective. The goal is to train people who will be able to function in a wide variety of community, agency, academic, and research settings. The applied social program attempts to train people at the MA and PhD level for researcher consultant positions in applied (MA) or academic (PhD) settings. Areas of concentration include program development and evaluation, group processes, and organizational development. The basic behavioural science programs are individually structured, admitting a few students to work with active research supervisors, most frequently in behavioral neuroscience, neuropsychology, cognitive psychology or culture and development.

Special Facilities or Resources: The Department has a Psychological Services Centre, an animal lab, and a cognitive science lab with access to fMRI facilities. There are also numerous microcomputers, excellent mainframe computer facilities, and a good research library. The Women's Studies Research Unit promotes scholarly research by, for, and about women, providing a source of support for all women studying, teaching, researching, and working on campus.

Information for Students With Physical Disabilities: See the following Web site for more information: http://students.usask.ca/disability/.

Application Information:
Send to Graduate Chair, University of Saskatchewan, Department of Psychology, 9 Campus Drive, Saskatoon, SK Canada S7N 5A5. Application available online. URL of online application: http://artsandscience.usask.ca/psychology/. Students are admitted in the Fall, application deadline December 15. Fee: $75. Note: All dollar amounts specified in this entry are Canadian dollars.

Simon Fraser University
Department of Psychology
8888 University Drive
Burnaby, BC V5A 1S6
Telephone: (778) 782-3354
Fax: (778) 782-3427
E-mail: *turner@sfu.ca*
Web: *http://www.psyc.sfu.ca/*

Department Information:
1965. Chair, J. Donald Read. Number of faculty: total—full-time 40; women—full-time 12.

Programs and Degrees Offered:
Listed in the following order: Program area, degree type (T if terminal Master's), number awarded 7/08–6/09. Experimental Psychology PhD (Doctor of Philosophy) 3, Clinical Psychology PhD (Doctor of Philosophy) 3.

APA Accreditation: Clinical PhD (Doctor of Philosophy).

CPA Accreditation: Clinical PhD (Doctor of Philosophy).

Student Applications/Admissions:
Student Applications
Experimental Psychology PhD (Doctor of Philosophy)—Applications 2009–2010, 53. Total applicants accepted 2009–2010, 14. Number full-time enrolled (new admits only) 2009–2010, 9. Total enrolled 2009–2010 full-time, 40. Openings 2010–2011, 8. The median number of years required for completion of a degree in 2008–2009 were 6. The number of students enrolled full- and part-time who were dismissed or voluntarily withdrew from this program area in 2008–2009 were 0. Clinical Psychology PhD (Doctor of Philosophy)—Applications 2009–2010, 131. Total applicants accepted 2009–2010, 14. Number full-time enrolled (new admits only) 2009–2010, 6. Total enrolled 2009–2010 full-time, 64. Openings 2010–2011, 8. The median number of years required for completion of a degree in 2008–2009 were 6. The number of students enrolled full- and part-time who were dismissed or voluntarily withdrew from this program area in 2008–2009 were 0.

Scores: Entries appear in this order: required test or GPA, minimum score (if required), median score of students entering in 2009–2010. *Experimental Psychology PhD (Doctor of Philosophy)*: GRE-V no minimum stated, 570, GRE-Q no minimum stated, 630, GRE-Analytical no minimum stated, 4.5, overall undergraduate GPA no minimum stated, 3.58; *Clinical Psychology PhD (Doctor of Philosophy)*: GRE-V no minimum stated, 555, GRE-Q no minimum stated, 650, GRE-Analytical no minimum stated, 5.0, GRE-Subject (Psychology) no minimum stated, 715, overall undergraduate GPA no minimum stated, 3.97.

Other Criteria: (importance of criteria rated low, medium, or high): GRE scores—high, research experience—high, work experience—low, extracurricular activity—low, clinically related public service—low, GPA—high, letters of recommendation—high, interview—high, statement of goals and objectives—high, undergraduate major in psychology—high, specific undergraduate psychology courses taken—medium, Interview is more relevant to admission to clinical program. For additional information on admission requirements, go to http://www.psyc.sfu.ca/grad/.

Student Characteristics: The following represents characteristics of students in 2009–2010 in all graduate psychology programs in the department: Female—full-time 75, part-time 0; Male—full-time 29, part-time 0; African American/Black—full-time 0, part-time 0; Hispanic/Latino(a)—full-time 0, part-time 0; Asian/Pacific Islander—full-time 0, part-time 0; American Indian/Alaska Native—full-time 0, part-time 0; Caucasian/White—full-time 0, part-time 0; Multi-ethnic—full-time 0, part-time 0; students subject to the Americans With Disabilities Act—full-time 0, part-time 0; Unknown ethnicity—full-time 0, part-time 0; International students who hold an F-1 or J-1 Visa—full-time 0, part-time 0.

Financial Information/Assistance:
Tuition for Full-Time Study: *Master's:* State residents: per academic year $4,697; Nonstate residents: per academic year $4,697. *Doctoral:* State residents: per academic year $4,697; Nonstate residents: per academic year $4,697. Tuition is subject to change. See the following Web site for updates and changes in tuition costs: http://students.sfu.ca/fees/gradfees.html.

Financial Assistance:
First-Year Students: Teaching assistantships available for first year. Average amount paid per academic year: $16,422. Average number of hours worked per week: 15. Research assistantships available for first year. Fellowships and scholarships available for first year. Average amount paid per academic year: $6,250. Apply by March 15.

Advanced Students: Teaching assistantships available for advanced students. Average amount paid per academic year: $19,377. Average number of hours worked per week: 15. Research assistantships available for advanced students. Fellowships and scholarships available for advanced students. Average amount paid per academic year: $6,250. Apply by March 15.

Additional Information: Of all students currently enrolled full time, 100% benefited from one or more of the listed financial assistance programs. Application and information available online at: http://www.psyc.sfu.ca/grad.

Internships/Practica: Doctoral Degree (PhD Clinical Psychology): For those doctoral students for whom a professional internship was required in this program prior to graduation, (5) students applied for an internship in 2008–2009, with (5) students obtaining an internship. Of those students who obtained an internship, (5) were paid internships. Of those students who obtained an internship, (5) students placed in APA/CPA accredited internships, (0) students placed in internships not APA/CPA accredited, but listed with the Association of Psychology Postdoctoral and Internship Programs (APPIC), (0) students placed in internships conforming to guidelines of the Council of Directors of School Psychology Programs (CDSPP), (0) students placed in internships that were not APA/CPA accredited, APPIC or CDSPP listed. Students in the Clinical Program are required to complete an MA practicum and a PhD internship. The practica are coordinated by the Director of Clinical Training, and take place primarily in local multi-disciplinary community settings under the overall supervision of psychology personnel. Internships are all external to the program.

Housing and Day Care: On-campus housing is available. See the following Web site for more information: http://students.sfu.ca/residences/. On-campus day care facilities are available. See the following Web site for more information: http://www.sfu.ca/childcare-society/.

Employment of Department Graduates:
Master's Degree Graduates: Of those who graduated in the academic year 2008–2009, the following categories and numbers represent the postgraduate activities and employment of master's degree graduates: Enrolled in a psychology doctoral program (10), enrolled in another graduate/professional program (2), enrolled in a postdoctoral residency/fellowship (n/a), employed in independent practice (n/a), employed in business or industry (1), total from the above (master's) (13).
Doctoral Degree Graduates: Of those who graduated in the academic year 2008–2009, the following categories and numbers represent the postgraduate activities and employment of doctoral degree graduates: Enrolled in a psychology doctoral program (n/a), enrolled in another graduate/professional program (0), enrolled in a postdoctoral residency/fellowship (2), employed in independent practice (1), employed in an academic position at a university (1), employed in an academic position at a 2-year/4-year college (2), employed in other positions at a higher education institution (0), employed in a professional position in a school system (0), employed in business or industry (0), employed in a government agency (0), employed in a community mental health/counseling center (0), employed in a hospital/medical center (0), total from the above (doctoral) (6).

Additional Information:
Orientation, Objectives, and Emphasis of Department: The department has a mainstream, empirical orientation. The department offers graduate work leading to master's and doctoral degrees in psychology or clinical psychology. Within the Psychology Graduate Program, all graduate students work on topics from one of the following research areas: cognitive and biological psychology, developmental psychology, law and forensic psychology, social psychology, or theory and methods. The Clinical Psychology Program subscribes to the scientist–practitioner model, and offers training in General Clinical and specializations in Clinical Child, Clinical Forensic, and Clinical Neuropsychology. In cooperation with the University of British Columbia, Law and Forensic Psychology students are allowed leave from one university to complete degree requirements in the other, in order to obtain both PhD and LL.B. degrees.

Special Facilities or Resources: The Psychology Department has numerous technical resources available to its members. A microcomputer lab houses 18 workstations running Windows XP and hosts a variety of statistical packages (SPSS, SAS, Lisrel, MathCAD, Systat), productivity packages (Microsoft Office, Acrobat, Write-N-Cite), Internet packages (Firefox, Thunderbird, secure file transfer programs), and other utility programs. While the University provides central e-mail service, the Department provides in-house file storage, printing, scanning, photocopying and teleconferencing resources. One conference room with an LCD projector and workstation is available for presentations (colloquia, thesis defences, etc.). Other portable multimedia equipment include LCD projectors, VCRs, and audio recording devices. Students normally receive office space in the research laboratories of their supervisors. Most faculty labs have computers and printers for graduate students. Neuroscience labs for animal studies are equipped for physiological and behavioral research, as well as advanced microscopy and image analysis. The department's array of technical and information technologies are managed and maintained by a five-member IT staff. The Clinical Program operates a separate training clinic with a full-time director, office coordinator, and is staffed by clinical students. It has an extensive test library, audio/video recording capabilities, and presentation projection facilities. The Library has excellent resources including online databases in psychology; inter-library loans of books and journals are readily accessible.

Information for Students With Physical Disabilities: See the following Web site for more information: http://students.sfu.ca/csd/.

Application Information:
Send to Anita Turner, Graduate Program Assistant, Psychology Department, Simon Fraser University, 8888 University Drive, Burnaby, BC V5A 1S6. Application available online. URL of online application: http://www.sfu.ca/gradstudents/applicants/. Students are admitted in the Fall, application deadline December 13. The application materials should be sent in one complete package. Reference forms and letters should be in sealed envelopes and signed by the referee. The graduate application check list must be included with the application materials. *Fee:* $75. Note: All dollar amounts specified in this entry are Canadian dollars.

Toronto, University of
Department of Psychology
100 St. George Street
Toronto, ON M5S 3G3
Telephone: (416) 978-3404
Fax: (416) 976-4811
E-mail: *chair@psych.utoronto.ca*
Web: *http://www.psych.utoronto.ca*

Department Information:
1891. Graduate Chair: Morris Moscovitch. Number of faculty: total—full-time 69, part-time 31; women—full-time 26, part-time 11.

CANADA

Programs and Degrees Offered:
Listed in the following order: Program area, degree type (T if terminal Master's), number awarded 7/08–6/09. Behavioral Neuroscience MA/MS (Master of Arts/Science) 7, Cognition/Perception PhD (Doctor of Philosophy) 4, Developmental Psychology MA/MS (Master of Arts/Science) 9, Behavioral Neuroscience PhD (Doctor of Philosophy) 6, Cognition/Perception MA/MS (Master of Arts/Science) 5, Social/Personality/Abnormal PhD (Doctor of Philosophy) 3, Developmental Psychology PhD (Doctor of Philosophy), Social/Personality/Abnormal MA/MS (Master of Arts/Science) 4.

Student Applications/Admissions:
Student Applications
Behavioral Neuroscience MA/MS (Master of Arts/Science)—Applications 2009–2010, 13. Total applicants accepted 2009–2010, 4. Number full-time enrolled (new admits only) 2009–2010, 4. Total enrolled 2009–2010 full-time, 4. Openings 2010–2011, 10. The median number of years required for completion of a degree in 2008–2009 was 1. The number of students enrolled full- and part-time who were dismissed or voluntarily withdrew from this program area in 2008–2009 were 0. *Cognition/Perception PhD (Doctor of Philosophy)*—Applications 2009–2010, 12. Total applicants accepted 2009–2010, 1. Total enrolled 2009–2010 full-time, 49. Openings 2010–2011, 10. The median number of years required for completion of a degree in 2008–2009 were 5. The number of students enrolled full- and part-time who were dismissed or voluntarily withdrew from this program area in 2008–2009 were 1. *Developmental Psychology MA/MS (Master of Arts/Science)*—Applications 2009–2010, 26. Total applicants accepted 2009–2010, 4. Number full-time enrolled (new admits only) 2009–2010, 2. Total enrolled 2009–2010 full-time, 2. Openings 2010–2011, 10. The median number of years required for completion of a degree in 2008–2009 was 1. The number of students enrolled full- and part-time who were dismissed or voluntarily withdrew from this program area in 2008–2009 were 0. *Behavioral Neuroscience PhD (Doctor of Philosophy)*—Applications 2009–2010, 1. Total applicants accepted 2009–2010, 0. Number full-time enrolled (new admits only) 2009–2010, 0. Total enrolled 2009–2010 full-time, 32. Openings 2010–2011, 10. The median number of years required for completion of a degree in 2008–2009 were 7. The number of students enrolled full- and part-time who were dismissed or voluntarily withdrew from this program area in 2008–2009 were 1. *Cognition/Perception MA/MS (Master of Arts/Science)*—Applications 2009–2010, 78. Total applicants accepted 2009–2010, 18. Number full-time enrolled (new admits only) 2009–2010, 12. Total enrolled 2009–2010 full-time, 12. Openings 2010–2011, 10. The median number of years required for completion of a degree in 2008–2009 was 1. The number of students enrolled full- and part-time who were dismissed or voluntarily withdrew from this program area in 2008–2009 were 0. *Social/Personality/Abnormal PhD (Doctor of Philosophy)*—Applications 2009–2010, 11. Total applicants accepted 2009–2010, 0. Total enrolled 2009–2010 full-time, 25. Openings 2010–2011, 10. The median number of years required for completion of a degree in 2008–2009 were 5. The number of students enrolled full- and part-time who were dismissed or voluntarily withdrew from this program area in 2008–2009 were 0. *Developmental Psychology PhD (Doctor of Philosophy)*—Applications 2009–2010, 6. Total applicants accepted 2009–2010, 2. Number full-time enrolled (new admits only) 2009–2010, 2. Total enrolled 2009–2010 full-time, 13. Openings 2010–2011, 10. The number of students enrolled full- and part-time who were dismissed or voluntarily withdrew from this program area in 2008–2009 were 0. *Social/Personality/Abnormal MA/MS (Master of Arts/Science)*—Applications 2009–2010, 87. Total applicants accepted 2009–2010, 10. Number full-time enrolled (new admits only) 2009–2010, 6. Total enrolled 2009–2010 full-time, 6. Openings 2010–2011, 10. The median number of years required for completion of a degree in 2008–2009 was 1.

Scores: Entries appear in this order: required test or GPA, minimum score (if required), median score of students entering in 2009–2010. *Behavioral Neuroscience MA/MS (Master of Arts/Science):* GRE-V no minimum stated, 520, GRE-Q no minimum stated, 610, GRE-Analytical no minimum stated, 4, last 2 years GPA 3.7, 3.7; *Cognition/Perception PhD (Doctor of Philosophy):* GRE-V no minimum stated, 570, GRE-Q no minimum stated, 710, GRE-Analytical no minimum stated, 4.5, last 2 years GPA 3.7, 3.7, Masters GPA 3.7, 3.7; *Developmental Psychology MA/MS (Master of Arts/Science):* GRE-V no minimum stated, 535, GRE-Q no minimum stated, 690, GRE-Analytical no minimum stated, 4.5, last 2 years GPA 3.7, 4; *Behavioral Neuroscience PhD (Doctor of Philosophy):* GRE-V no minimum stated, 520, GRE-Q no minimum stated, 610, GRE-Analytical no minimum stated, 4, last 2 years GPA 3.7, 3.7, Masters GPA 3.7, 3.7; *Cognition/Perception MA/MS (Master of Arts/Science):* GRE-V no minimum stated, 570, GRE-Q no minimum stated, 710, GRE-Analytical no minimum stated, 4.5, last 2 years GPA 3.7, 3.7; *Social/Personality/Abnormal PhD (Doctor of Philosophy):* GRE-V no minimum stated, 580, GRE-Q no minimum stated, 720, GRE-Analytical no minimum stated, 4.5, last 2 years GPA 3.7, 4, Masters GPA 3.7, 4; *Developmental Psychology PhD (Doctor of Philosophy):* GRE-V no minimum stated, 545, GRE-Q no minimum stated, 745, GRE-Analytical no minimum stated, 5.8, last 2 years GPA 3.7, 4, Masters GPA 3.7, 4; *Social/Personality/Abnormal MA/MS (Master of Arts/Science):* GRE-V no minimum stated, 580, GRE-Q no minimum stated, 720, GRE-Analytical no minimum stated, 4.5, last 2 years GPA 3.7, 4.

Other Criteria: (importance of criteria rated low, medium, or high): GRE scores—high, research experience—high, work experience—low, extracurricular activity—low, GPA—high, letters of recommendation—high, interview—high, statement of goals and objectives—high, undergraduate major in psychology—medium, specific undergraduate psychology courses taken—medium. For additional information on admission requirements, go to http://home.psych.utoronto.ca/graduate/Admission.htm.

Student Characteristics: The following represents characteristics of students in 2009–2010 in all graduate psychology programs in the department: Female—full-time 95, part-time 0; Male—full-time 48, part-time 0; Caucasian/White—full-time 0, part-time 0; Unknown ethnicity—full-time 0, part-time 0.

Financial Information/Assistance:
Tuition for Full-Time Study: *Master's:* State residents: per academic year $7,440; Nonstate residents: per academic year $15,661. *Doctoral:* State residents: per academic year $7,440; Nonstate residents: per academic year $15,661. Tuition is subject to change.

See the following Web site for updates and changes in tuition costs: http://www.fees.utoronto.ca/.

Financial Assistance:
First-Year Students: Teaching assistantships available for first year. Average amount paid per academic year: $6,000. Average number of hours worked per week: 10. Apply by June 1. Traineeships available for first year. Average amount paid per academic year: $6,000. Apply by December 15. Fellowships and scholarships available for first year. Average amount paid per academic year: $10,340. Apply by December 15.

Advanced Students: Teaching assistantships available for advanced students. Average amount paid per academic year: $6,000. Average number of hours worked per week: 10. Apply by June 1. Traineeships available for advanced students. Average amount paid per academic year: $6,000. Apply by December 15. Fellowships and scholarships available for advanced students. Average amount paid per academic year: $10,340. Apply by December 15.

Additional Information: Of all students currently enrolled full time, 100% benefited from one or more of the listed financial assistance programs. Application and information available online at: http://home.psych.utoronto.ca/graduate/Admission.htm.

Internships/Practica: No information provided.

Housing and Day Care: On-campus housing is available. See the following Web site for more information: http://www.housing.utoronto.ca/. On-campus day care facilities are available. See the following Web site for more information: http://www.familycare.utoronto.ca/.

Employment of Department Graduates:
Master's Degree Graduates: Of those who graduated in the academic year 2008–2009, the following categories and numbers represent the postgraduate activities and employment of master's degree graduates: Enrolled in a psychology doctoral program (18), enrolled in another graduate/professional program (0), enrolled in a postdoctoral residency/fellowship (n/a), employed in independent practice (n/a), total from the above (master's) (18).
Doctoral Degree Graduates: Of those who graduated in the academic year 2008–2009, the following categories and numbers represent the postgraduate activities and employment of doctoral degree graduates: Enrolled in a psychology doctoral program (n/a), enrolled in another graduate/professional program (0), enrolled in a postdoctoral residency/fellowship (5), employed in a government agency (1), employed in a hospital/medical center (1), do not know (6), total from the above (doctoral) (13).

Additional Information:
Orientation, Objectives, and Emphasis of Department: The purpose of graduate training at the University of Toronto is to prepare students for careers in teaching and research. Teaching and research apprenticeships, therefore, constitute a large portion of such training. Research training is supplemented by courses and seminars. In some cases the courses are designed to provide up-to-date fundamental background information in psychology. The bulk of instruction, however, takes place in informal seminars; these provide an opportunity for the discussion of theoretical issues, the formulation of research problems, and the review of current developments in specific research areas. In the past, most of our graduates have entered academic careers. More recently, graduates have also taken research and managerial positions in research institutes, hospitals, government agencies, and industrial corporations.

Special Facilities or Resources: The department has modern laboratories at the St. George, Mississauga, and Scarborough campuses, as well as a fully equipped electronic workshop. Students have access to an extensive computer system including the university's central computer, the department's Sun computer, and many advanced microcomputers. The department has close ties to several medical hospitals, as well as the Rotman Research Institute of Baycrest Centre and the Centre for Addiction and Mental Health.

Information for Students With Physical Disabilities: See the following Web site for more information: http://www.accessibility.utoronto.ca/index.htm.

Application Information:
Send to Graduate Studies, Department of Psychology, University of Toronto, 100 St. George Street, Toronto, Ontario, Canada M5S 3G3. Application available online. URL of online application: https://apply.sgs.utoronto.ca/. Students are admitted in the Fall, application deadline December 1. *Fee:* $110. Note: All dollar amounts specified in this entry are Canadian dollars.

Victoria, University of
Department of Psychology
P.O. Box 3050 STN CSC
Victoria, BC V8W 3P5
Telephone: (250) 721-7525
Fax: (250) 721-8929
E-mail: *psychair@uvic.ca*
Web: *http://www.web.uvic.ca/psyc/*

Department Information:
1963. Chairperson: Elizabeth Brimacombe. Number of faculty: total—full-time 32, part-time 2; women—full-time 12, part-time 2; total—minority—full-time 3.

Programs and Degrees Offered:
Listed in the following order: Program area, degree type (T if terminal Master's), number awarded 7/08–6/09. Social Psychology PhD (Doctor of Philosophy) 2, Cognition and Brain Science PhD (Doctor of Philosophy) 2, Experimental Neuropsychology PhD (Doctor of Philosophy) 0, Clinical Neuropsychology PhD (Doctor of Philosophy) 2, Clinical Lifespan Psychology PhD (Doctor of Philosophy) 1, Lifespan Development and Aging PhD (Doctor of Philosophy) 1.

APA Accreditation: Clinical PhD (Doctor of Philosophy).

CPA Accreditation: Clinical PhD (Doctor of Philosophy).

Student Applications/Admissions:
Student Applications
Social Psychology PhD (Doctor of Philosophy)—Applications 2009–2010, 37. Total applicants accepted 2009–2010, 2. Num-

ber full-time enrolled (new admits only) 2009–2010, 2. Openings 2010–2011, 3. The median number of years required for completion of a degree in 2008–2009 were 5. The number of students enrolled full- and part-time who were dismissed or voluntarily withdrew from this program area in 2008–2009 were 0. *Cognition and Brain Science PhD (Doctor of Philosophy)*—Applications 2009–2010, 11. Total applicants accepted 2009–2010, 1. Number full-time enrolled (new admits only) 2009–2010, 3. Openings 2010–2011, 2. The median number of years required for completion of a degree in 2008–2009 were 5. The number of students enrolled full- and part-time who were dismissed or voluntarily withdrew from this program area in 2008–2009 were 0. *Experimental Neuropsychology PhD (Doctor of Philosophy)*—Applications 2009–2010, 9. Total applicants accepted 2009–2010, 2. Number full-time enrolled (new admits only) 2009–2010, 1. Openings 2010–2011, 2. The number of students enrolled full- and part-time who were dismissed or voluntarily withdrew from this program area in 2008–2009 were 0. *Clinical Neuropsychology PhD (Doctor of Philosophy)*—Applications 2009–2010, 39. Total applicants accepted 2009–2010, 4. Openings 2010–2011, 4. The median number of years required for completion of a degree in 2008–2009 were 7. The number of students enrolled full- and part-time who were dismissed or voluntarily withdrew from this program area in 2008–2009 were 0. *Clinical Lifespan Psychology PhD (Doctor of Philosophy)*—Applications 2009–2010, 84. Total applicants accepted 2009–2010, 9. Number full-time enrolled (new admits only) 2009–2010, 3. Total enrolled 2009–2010 full-time, 18. Openings 2010–2011, 6. The median number of years required for completion of a degree in 2008–2009 were 6. The number of students enrolled full- and part-time who were dismissed or voluntarily withdrew from this program area in 2008–2009 were 0. *Lifespan Development and Aging PhD (Doctor of Philosophy)*—Applications 2009–2010, 27. Total applicants accepted 2009–2010, 1. Total enrolled 2009–2010 full-time, 7. Openings 2010–2011, 4. The median number of years required for completion of a degree in 2008–2009 were 6. The number of students enrolled full- and part-time who were dismissed or voluntarily withdrew from this program area in 2008–2009 were 0.

Other Criteria: (importance of criteria rated low, medium, or high): GRE scores—high, research experience—high, work experience—medium, extracurricular activity—medium, clinically related public service—medium, GPA—high, letters of recommendation—high, interview—high, statement of goals and objectives—high, undergraduate major in psychology—high, specific undergraduate psychology courses taken—high. Group interview required for Clinical Programs only. For additional information on admission requirements, go to http://web.uvic.ca/psyc/graduate/admissions.php.

Student Characteristics: The following represents characteristics of students in 2009–2010 in all graduate psychology programs in the department: Female—full-time 58, part-time 0; Male—full-time 14, part-time 0; African American/Black—full-time 1, part-time 0; Hispanic/Latino(a)—full-time 0, part-time 0; Asian/Pacific Islander—full-time 11, part-time 0; American Indian/Alaska Native—full-time 1, part-time 0; Caucasian/White—full-time 47, part-time 0; Multi-ethnic—full-time 12, part-time 0; students subject to the Americans With Disabilities Act—full-time 0, part-time 0; Unknown ethnicity—full-time 0, part-time 0; International students who hold an F-1 or J-1 Visa—full-time 0, part-time 0.

Financial Information/Assistance:
Tuition for Full-Time Study: *Master's:* State residents: per academic year $4,851; Nonstate residents: per academic year $5,774. *Doctoral:* State residents: per academic year $4,851; Nonstate residents: per academic year $5,774. Tuition is subject to change. See the following Web site for updates and changes in tuition costs: http://registrar.uvic.ca/grad/continuing/fees/tuitionandfees.html.

Financial Assistance:
First-Year Students: Teaching assistantships available for first year. Average amount paid per academic year: $4,500. Research assistantships available for first year. Average amount paid per academic year: $4,500. Fellowships and scholarships available for first year. Average amount paid per academic year: $15,000.

Advanced Students: Teaching assistantships available for advanced students. Average amount paid per academic year: $4,500. Research assistantships available for advanced students. Average amount paid per academic year: $4,500. Fellowships and scholarships available for advanced students. Average amount paid per academic year: $15,000.

Additional Information: Of all students currently enrolled full time, 95% benefited from one or more of the listed financial assistance programs. Application and information available online at: http://registrar.uvic.ca/safa/.

Internships/Practica: Internships and practica for students in the clinical program are arranged through the clinical program.

Housing and Day Care: On-campus housing is available. See the following Web site for more information: http://www.hfcs.uvic.ca/. On-campus day care facilities are available. See the following Web site for more information: http://www.stas.uvic.ca/dayc/.

Employment of Department Graduates:
Master's Degree Graduates: Of those who graduated in the academic year 2008–2009, the following categories and numbers represent the postgraduate activities and employment of master's degree graduates: Enrolled in a postdoctoral residency/fellowship (n/a), employed in independent practice (n/a), total from the above (master's) (0).

Doctoral Degree Graduates: Of those who graduated in the academic year 2008–2009, the following categories and numbers represent the postgraduate activities and employment of doctoral degree graduates: Enrolled in a psychology doctoral program (n/a), enrolled in a postdoctoral residency/fellowship (3), employed in independent practice (6), employed in an academic position at a university (4), employed in a community mental health/counseling center (5), employed in a hospital/medical center (6), total from the above (doctoral) (24).

Additional Information:
Orientation, Objectives, and Emphasis of Department: The graduate program in psychology emphasizes the training of research competence, and, in the case of neuropsychology and lifespan, the acquisition of clinical skills. The department's orientation is strongly empirical, and students are expected to develop mastery of appropriate methods and design as well as of specific content areas of psychology. The program is directed toward the

PhD degree, although students must obtain a master's degree as part of the normal requirements. Formal programs of study, involving a coordinated sequence of courses, are offered for both experimental and clinical neuropsychology (up to but not including a clinical internship), lifespan development, clinical lifespan development, social psychology, and cognition and brain sciences. Individual programs of study may be designed according to the interests of individual students and faculty members in such areas as addictions, consumer and industrial psychology, environmental psychology, experimental and applied behavior analysis, psychopathology, and human psychophysiology.

Special Facilities or Resources: Fully equipped facilities include a psychology clinic operating as an outpatient service and teaching clinic; large observation rooms with audio and video recording equipment for the study of group interaction and other social processes; microcomputer-based cognition laboratories; experimental rooms with one-way mirrors; electrophysiological recording rooms; and specialized labs for the study of visual and auditory perception. We have recently constructed a new Brain and Cognition Laboratory featuring two state-of-the-art event-related potential (ERP) systems. The Department enjoys good community contact with local hospitals (general, rehabilitation, and extended care), schools, and private and government agencies, which provide sites for both research and practicum experiences.

Information for Students With Physical Disabilities: See the following Web site for more information: http://rcsd.uvic.ca/.

Application Information:
Send to Graduate Admissions and Records, University of Victoria, PO Box 3025, STN CSC Victoria BC V8W 3P2 Canada. Application available online. URL of online application: http://registrar.uvic.ca/grad/. Students are admitted in the Fall, application deadline January 1. *Fee:* $100. $125 if any post-secondary transcripts come from institutions outside of Canada. Note: All dollar amounts specified in this entry are Canadian dollars.

Waterloo, University of
Department of Psychology
200 University Avenue West
Waterloo, ON N2L 3G1
Telephone: (519) 888-4567
Fax: (519) 746-8631
E-mail: *mzanna@uwaterloo.ca*
Web: *http://www.psychology.uwaterloo.ca/*

Department Information:
1963. Chairperson: Mark Zanna. Number of faculty: total—full-time 38, part-time 1; women—full-time 15, part-time 1.

Programs and Degrees Offered:
Listed in the following order: Program area, degree type (T if terminal Master's), number awarded 7/08–6/09. Industrial/Organizational Psychology PhD (Doctor of Philosophy) 2, Social Psychology PhD (Doctor of Philosophy) 0, Cognitive Psychology PhD (Doctor of Philosophy) 3, Behavioral Neuroscience PhD (Doctor of Philosophy) 2, Clinical Psychology PhD (Doctor of Philosophy) 2, Developmental Psychology PhD (Doctor of Philosophy) 1, Industrial/Organizational Psychology MA/MS (Master of Arts/Science) (T) 5, Developmental Psychology MA/MS (Master of Arts/Science) (T) 1.

APA Accreditation: Clinical PhD (Doctor of Philosophy). Student Outcome Data Website: http://www.psychology.uwaterloo.ca/gradprog/programs/phd/clinical/index.html.

CPA Accreditation: Clinical PhD (Doctor of Philosophy).

Student Applications/Admissions:
Student Applications
Industrial/Organizational Psychology PhD (Doctor of Philosophy)—Applications 2009–2010, 23. Total applicants accepted 2009–2010, 6. Number full-time enrolled (new admits only) 2009–2010, 2. Openings 2010–2011, 4. The number of students enrolled full- and part-time who were dismissed or voluntarily withdrew from this program area in 2008–2009 were 1. *Social Psychology PhD (Doctor of Philosophy)*—Applications 2009–2010, 33. Total applicants accepted 2009–2010, 9. Number full-time enrolled (new admits only) 2009–2010, 5. Total enrolled 2009–2010 full-time, 26, part-time, 1. Openings 2010–2011, 5. *Cognitive Psychology PhD (Doctor of Philosophy)*—Applications 2009–2010, 17. Total applicants accepted 2009–2010, 5. Number full-time enrolled (new admits only) 2009–2010, 4. Total enrolled 2009–2010 full-time, 17, part-time, 1. Openings 2010–2011, 5. *Behavioral Neuroscience PhD (Doctor of Philosophy)*—Applications 2009–2010, 22. Total applicants accepted 2009–2010, 12. Number full-time enrolled (new admits only) 2009–2010, 8. Total enrolled 2009–2010 full-time, 20, part-time, 1. Openings 2010–2011, 6. *Clinical Psychology PhD (Doctor of Philosophy)*—Applications 2009–2010, 123. Total applicants accepted 2009–2010, 7. Number full-time enrolled (new admits only) 2009–2010, 5. Total enrolled 2009–2010 full-time, 24, part-time, 4. Openings 2010–2011, 5. *Developmental Psychology PhD (Doctor of Philosophy)*—Applications 2009–2010, 18. Total applicants accepted 2009–2010, 3. Number full-time enrolled (new admits only) 2009–2010, 2. Openings 2010–2011, 5. The number of students enrolled full- and part-time who were dismissed or voluntarily withdrew from this program area in 2008–2009 were 1. *Industrial/Organizational Psychology MA/MS (Master of Arts/Science)*—Applications 2009–2010, 19. Total applicants accepted 2009–2010, 3. Number full-time enrolled (new admits only) 2009–2010, 2. Total enrolled 2009–2010 full-time, 8. Openings 2010–2011, 4. *Developmental Psychology MA/MS (Master of Arts/Science)*—Applications 2009–2010, 3. Total applicants accepted 2009–2010, 1. Number full-time enrolled (new admits only) 2009–2010, 1. Total enrolled 2009–2010 full-time, 1. Openings 2010–2011, 5.

Scores: Entries appear in this order: required test or GPA, minimum score (if required), median score of students entering in 2009–2010. *Industrial/Organizational Psychology PhD (Doctor of Philosophy)*: GRE-V no minimum stated, GRE-Q no minimum stated, GRE-Analytical no minimum stated, last 2 years GPA no minimum stated, Masters GPA no minimum stated; *Social Psychology PhD (Doctor of Philosophy)*: GRE-V no minimum stated, GRE-Q no minimum stated, GRE-Analytical no minimum stated, last 2 years GPA no minimum stated, Masters GPA no minimum stated; *Cognitive Psychology PhD (Doctor of Philosophy)*: GRE-V no minimum stated, GRE-Q no minimum stated, GRE-Analytical no minimum stated, last 2 years GPA no minimum stated, Masters GPA no minimum stated; *Behavioral Neuroscience PhD (Doctor of Philosophy)*: GRE-V no minimum stated, GRE-Q no minimum stated, GRE-Analytical no minimum stated, last 2 years GPA no minimum stated, Masters GPA no minimum stated; *Clinical Psychology PhD (Doctor of Philosophy)*: GRE-V no minimum stated, GRE-Q no minimum stated, GRE-Analytical no minimum stated, last 2 years GPA no minimum stated, psychology GPA no minimum stated, Masters GPA no minimum stated; *Developmental Psychology PhD (Doctor of Philosophy)*: GRE-V no minimum stated, GRE-Q no minimum stated, GRE-Analytical no minimum stated, last 2 years GPA no minimum stated, Masters GPA no minimum stated; *Industrial/Organizational Psychology MA/MS (Master of Arts/Science)*: GRE-V no minimum stated, GRE-Q no minimum stated, GRE-Analytical no minimum stated, last 2 years GPA no minimum stated; *Developmental Psychology MA/MS (Master of Arts/Science)*: last 2 years GPA no minimum stated.

Other Criteria: (importance of criteria rated low, medium, or high): GRE scores—high, research experience—medium, work experience—low, clinically related public service—medium, GPA—high, letters of recommendation—high, interview—medium, statement of goals and objectives—low, undergraduate major in psychology—high, specific undergraduate psychology courses taken—medium. For additional information on admission requirements, go to http://www.psychology.uwaterloo.ca/gradprog/index.html.

Student Characteristics: The following represents characteristics of students in 2009–2010 in all graduate psychology programs in the department: Female—full-time 74, part-time 2; Male—full-time 35, part-time 5; African American/Black—full-time 0, part-time 0; Hispanic/Latino(a)—full-time 0, part-time 0; Asian/Pacific Islander—full-time 0, part-time 0; American Indian/Alaska Native—full-time 0, part-time 0; Caucasian/White—full-time 0, part-time 0; Multi-ethnic—full-time 0, part-time 0; students subject to the Americans With Disabilities Act—full-time 0, part-time 0; Unknown ethnicity—full-time 0, part-time 0; International students who hold an F-1 or J-1 Visa—full-time 0, part-time 0.

Financial Information/Assistance:
Tuition for Full-Time Study: *Master's:* State residents: per academic year $7,190; Nonstate residents: per academic year $17,228. *Doctoral:* State residents: per academic year $7,190; Nonstate residents: per academic year $17,228. Tuition is subject to change. See the following Web site for updates and changes in tuition costs: http://www.adm.uwaterloo.ca/infofin/students/stdfees.htm.

Financial Assistance:
First-Year Students: Teaching assistantships available for first year. Research assistantships available for first year. Fellowships and scholarships available for first year.
Advanced Students: Teaching assistantships available for advanced students. Research assistantships available for advanced students. Fellowships and scholarships available for advanced students.
Additional Information: Of all students currently enrolled full time, 100% benefited from one or more of the listed financial assistance programs. Application and information available online at: http://www.psychology.uwaterloo.ca/gradprog/scholarships.html.

Internships/Practica: Doctoral Degree (PhD Clinical Psychology): For those doctoral students for whom a professional internship was required in this program prior to graduation, (4) students applied for an internship in 2008–2009, with (4) students obtaining an internship. Of those students who obtained an internship, (4) were paid internships. Of those students who obtained an internship, (4) students placed in APA/CPA accredited internships, (0) students placed in internships not APA/CPA accredited, but listed with the Association of Psychology Postdoctoral and Internship Programs (APPIC), (0) students placed in internships conforming to guidelines of the Council of Directors of School Psychology Programs (CDSPP), (0) students placed in internships that were not APA/CPA accredited, APPIC or CDSPP listed. Master's Degree (MA/MS Industrial/Organizational Psychology): An internship experience, such as, a final research project or "capstone" experience is required of graduates. Master's Degree (MA/MS Developmental Psychology): An internship experience, such as, a final research project or "capstone" experience is required of graduates. The Applied Master's program requires a 4-month supervised internship. The Clinical program requires a 4-month practicum during the program of study and a 12-month internship at the conclusion of the academic program. Most practicum placements are with local hospitals, schools or industries.

Housing and Day Care: On-campus housing is available. See the following Web site for more information: http://www.housing.uwaterloo.ca. On-campus day care facilities are available. See the following Web site for more information: http://www.studentservices.uwaterloo.ca/childcare/.

Employment of Department Graduates:
Master's Degree Graduates: Of those who graduated in the academic year 2008–2009, the following categories and numbers represent the postgraduate activities and employment of master's degree graduates: Enrolled in a psychology doctoral program (1), enrolled in a postdoctoral residency/fellowship (n/a), employed in independent practice (n/a), employed in business or industry (2), employed in a government agency (1), employed in a community mental health/counseling center (1), still seeking employment (1), total from the above (master's) (6).
Doctoral Degree Graduates: Of those who graduated in the academic year 2008–2009, the following categories and numbers represent the postgraduate activities and employment of doctoral degree graduates: Enrolled in a psychology doctoral program (n/a), enrolled in a postdoctoral residency/fellowship (5), employed in an academic position at a university (1), employed in a professional position in a school system (1), employed in a government agency (1), employed in a hospital/medical center (2), total from the above (doctoral) (10).

Additional Information:
Orientation, Objectives, and Emphasis of Department: There is a strong emphasis on research in all six divisions of the PhD program, and MASc students are prepared for careers in applied psychology in a variety of areas. Students are involved either through participation in ongoing faculty research or through development of their own ideas; coursework is intended to provide students with general knowledge and intensive preparation in

their area of concentration. For some of the programs, the blending of theory and practice is experienced in internship and practicum arrangements.

Special Facilities or Resources: Within a large 4-story building, extensive laboratory facilities are available for animal and human research. Additional educational and resource centers operate in conjunction with academic and research programs. Research requiring special populations is often carried out at community institutions under the supervision of faculty members. Considerable investment has been made to technical services including excellent computer facilities and consulting personnel who are available for student research and courses.

Information for Students With Physical Disabilities: See the following Web site for more information: http://www.studentservices.uwaterloo.ca/disabilities/.

Application Information:
Send to Graduate Studies Office, University of Waterloo, 200 University Avenue West, Waterloo, ON N2L 3G1. Application available online. URL of online application: http://www.grad.uwaterloo.ca/students/applyingonline.asp. Students are admitted in the Fall, application deadline December 15. The December 15 deadline applies to the Clinical and Social programs only. All other programs have a deadline of January 15. *Fee:* $100. Note: All dollar amounts specified in this entry are Canadian dollars.

Western Ontario, The University of
Department of Psychology
Room 7406 Social Science Centre, 1151 Richmond Street North
London, ON N6A 5C2
Telephone: (519) 661-2064
Fax: (519) 661-3961
E-mail: *psych-grad@uwo.ca*
Web: *http://www.psychology.uwo.ca*

Department Information:
1931. Chairperson: Albert Katz. Number of faculty: total—full-time 54, part-time 29; women—full-time 10, part-time 11.

Programs and Degrees Offered:
Listed in the following order: Program area, degree type (T if terminal Master's), number awarded 7/08–6/09. Cognition and Perception PhD (Doctor of Philosophy) 3, Developmental Psychology PhD (Doctor of Philosophy) 1, Industrial/Organizational Psychology PhD (Doctor of Philosophy) 4, Clinical Psychology PhD (Doctor of Philosophy) 5, Personality and Measurement PhD (Doctor of Philosophy) 0, Behavioural and Cognitive Neuroscience PhD (Doctor of Philosophy) 3, Social Psychology PhD (Doctor of Philosophy) 1.

CPA Accreditation: Clinical PhD (Doctor of Philosophy).

Student Applications/Admissions:
Student Applications
Cognition and Perception PhD (Doctor of Philosophy)—Applications 2009–2010, 13. Total applicants accepted 2009–2010, 3. Number full-time enrolled (new admits only) 2009–2010, 3. Number part-time enrolled (new admits only) 2009–2010, 0. Openings 2010–2011, 3. The median number of years required for completion of a degree in 2008–2009 were 4. The number of students enrolled full- and part-time who were dismissed or voluntarily withdrew from this program area in 2008–2009 were 0. *Developmental Psychology PhD (Doctor of Philosophy)*—Applications 2009–2010, 21. Total applicants accepted 2009–2010, 8. Number full-time enrolled (new admits only) 2009–2010, 5. Number part-time enrolled (new admits only) 2009–2010, 0. Openings 2010–2011, 2. The median number of years required for completion of a degree in 2008–2009 were 5. The number of students enrolled full- and part-time who were dismissed or voluntarily withdrew from this program area in 2008–2009 were 1. *Industrial/Organizational Psychology PhD (Doctor of Philosophy)*—Applications 2009–2010, 30. Total applicants accepted 2009–2010, 4. Number full-time enrolled (new admits only) 2009–2010, 4. Number part-time enrolled (new admits only) 2009–2010, 0. Openings 2010–2011, 5. The median number of years required for completion of a degree in 2008–2009 were 4. The number of students enrolled full- and part-time who were dismissed or voluntarily withdrew from this program area in 2008–2009 were 2. *Clinical Psychology PhD (Doctor of Philosophy)*—Applications 2009–2010, 119. Total applicants accepted 2009–2010, 6. Number full-time enrolled (new admits only) 2009–2010, 4. Number part-time enrolled (new admits only) 2009–2010, 0. Openings 2010–2011, 4. The median number of years required for completion of a degree in 2008–2009 were 6. The number of students enrolled full- and part-time who were dismissed or voluntarily withdrew from this program area in 2008–2009 were 1. *Personality and Measurement PhD (Doctor of Philosophy)*—Applications 2009–2010, 7. Total applicants accepted 2009–2010, 4. Number full-time enrolled (new admits only) 2009–2010, 2. Number part-time enrolled (new admits only) 2009–2010, 0. Openings 2010–2011, 1. The number of students enrolled full- and part-time who were dismissed or voluntarily withdrew from this program area in 2008–2009 were 0. *Behavioural and Cognitive Neuroscience PhD (Doctor of Philosophy)*—Applications 2009–2010, 13. Total applicants accepted 2009–2010, 6. Number full-time enrolled (new admits only) 2009–2010, 4. Number part-time enrolled (new admits only) 2009–2010, 0. Openings 2010–2011, 5. The median number of years required for completion of a degree in 2008–2009 were 4. The number of students enrolled full- and part-time who were dismissed or voluntarily withdrew from this program area in 2008–2009 were 2. *Social Psychology PhD (Doctor of Philosophy)*—Applications 2009–2010, 41. Total applicants accepted 2009–2010, 7. Number full-time enrolled (new admits only) 2009–2010, 3. Number part-time enrolled (new admits only) 2009–2010, 0. Openings 2010–2011, 3. The median number of years required for completion of a degree in 2008–2009 were 4. The number of students enrolled full- and part-time who were dismissed or voluntarily withdrew from this program area in 2008–2009 were 1.

Other Criteria: (importance of criteria rated low, medium, or high): GRE scores—medium, research experience—high, work experience—low, extracurricular activity—low, clinically related public service—low, GPA—high, letters of recommendation—high, interview—medium, statement of goals and objectives—high. An applicant is accepted into our program to work with individual faculty members. The Department gives preference to applicants who have a high potential for success in graduate school and who also share research interests with prospective faculty supervisors. Whereas most of our applicants have an Honour's degree in Psychology, we give full consideration to applicants with an undergraduate Honour's degree (or its equivalent) in other relevant areas. An Honour's degree in Psychology (or its equivalent) is required for admission into the Clinical MSc. A Master's degree in Psychology (with content that is primarily Clinical) is required for admission into the Clinical PhD.

Student Characteristics: The following represents characteristics of students in 2009–2010 in all graduate psychology programs in the department: Female—full-time 79, part-time 0; Male—full-time 50, part-time 0; African American/Black—full-time 0, part-time 0; Hispanic/Latino(a)—full-time 0, part-time 0; Asian/Pacific Islander—full-time 0, part-time 0; American Indian/Alaska Native—full-time 0, part-time 0; Caucasian/White—full-time 0, part-time 0; Multi-ethnic—full-time 0, part-time 0; students subject to the Americans With Disabilities Act—full-time 0, part-time 0; Unknown ethnicity—full-time 0, part-time 0; International students who hold an F-1 or J-1 Visa—full-time 0, part-time 0.

Financial Information/Assistance:
Tuition for Full-Time Study: *Doctoral:* State residents: per academic year $7,200; Nonstate residents: per academic year $15,000. Tuition is subject to change. See the following Web site for updates and changes in tuition costs: http://wwww.registrar.uwo.ca.

Financial Assistance:
First-Year Students: Teaching assistantships available for first year. Average amount paid per academic year: $11,194. Average number of hours worked per week: 10. Fellowships and scholarships available for first -year. Average amount paid per academic year: $9,000.

Advanced Students: Teaching assistantships available for advanced students. Average amount paid per academic year: $11,194. Average number of hours worked per week: 10. Fellowships and scholarships available for advanced students. Average amount paid per academic year: $12,000.

Additional Information: Of all students currently enrolled full time, 85% benefited from one or more of the listed financial assistance programs. Application and information available online at: http://www.psychology.uwo.ca.

Internships/Practica: Doctoral Degree (PhD Clinical Psychology): For those doctoral students for whom a professional internship was required in this program prior to graduation, (1) students applied for an internship in 2008–2009, with (1) students obtaining an internship. Of those students who obtained an internship, (1) were paid internships. Of those students who obtained an internship, (1) students placed in APA/CPA accredited internships, (0) students placed in internships not APA/CPA accredited, but listed with the Association of Psychology Postdoctoral and Internship Programs (APPIC), (0) students placed in internships conforming to guidelines of the Council of Directors of School Psychology Programs (CDSPP), (0) students placed in internships that were not APA/CPA accredited, APPIC or CDSPP listed. Clinical psychology students complete a one-year internship (CPA accredited) near the end of their doctoral training. Students in industrial/organizational psychology typically meet professional training requirements through a combination of practicum courses and placements.

Housing and Day Care: On-campus housing is available. See the following Web site for more information: www.uwo.ca/hfs/. On-campus day care facilities are available. See the following Web site for more information: Western Y Child Care Centre: http://www.westerndaycare.com/. Mary J. Wright University Laboratory Preschool: http://www.thelabschool.uwo.ca/.

Employment of Department Graduates:
Master's Degree Graduates: Of those who graduated in the academic year 2008–2009, the following categories and numbers represent the postgraduate activities and employment of master's degree graduates: Enrolled in a postdoctoral residency/fellowship (n/a), employed in independent practice (n/a), total from the above (master's) (0).

Doctoral Degree Graduates: Of those who graduated in the academic year 2008–2009, the following categories and numbers represent the postgraduate activities and employment of doctoral degree graduates: Enrolled in a psychology doctoral program (n/a), enrolled in another graduate/professional program (1), enrolled in a postdoctoral residency/fellowship (3), employed in independent practice (0), employed in an academic position at a university (3), employed in an academic position at a 2-year/4-year college (1), employed in other positions at a higher education institution (3), employed in a professional position in a school system (0), employed in business or industry (2), employed in a government agency (0), employed in a community mental health/counseling center (1), employed in a hospital/medical center (1), other employment position (2), total from the above (doctoral) (17).

Additional Information:
Orientation, Objectives, and Emphasis of Department: The department is organized into seven subject content areas, with initial graduate selection procedures administered by area faculty and area committees. Applicants must indicate an area of interest. The department is research-intensive and is oriented toward training researchers. Graduate students are expected to be continuously involved in research as well as to complete required courses and comprehensive exams. The clinical psychology program adopts the scientist–practitioner model, where both research and professional skills are developed.

Special Facilities or Resources: UWO is a beautiful campus located near the downtown core of London, Ontario. Western's campus has a number of facilities that benefit the research and academic aspects of students' lives, as well as the other aspects of everyday life. UWO has a great library system (6 major libraries), which includes electronic access to the vast majority of relevant journals. The computer facilities are first-rate in a number of respects. ITS (Information Technology Services) provides computing resources on a campus-wide basis, including web-based email and technical assistance for your home and office computers. The Faculty of Social Science is unique in that it provides its own additional computing facilities and access to software that is important for your research as well as technical support. For the more advanced, there are multiple clusters of Sparc Workstations and Linux machines for computational work conducted either using regular or parallel programming. The Department of Psychology has a large undergraduate participant pool plus affiliations with a number of researchers in various hospital and clinical settings. There is access to numerous types of advanced technology used for studying psychological processes of various sorts, such as a research-only 4-tesla fMRI set-up housed at Robarts Research Institute.

Information for Students With Physical Disabilities: See the following Web site for more information: Student Development Centre: http://www.sdc.uwo.ca/ssd.

Application Information:
Send to The Graduate Office, Department of Psychology, Social Science Centre, The University of Western Ontario, 1151 Richmond Street, London, Ontario, Canada N6A 5C2. Application available online. URL of online application: http://grad.uwo.ca/. Students are admitted in the Fall, application deadline January 7. *Fee:* $95. Note: All dollar amounts specified in this entry are Canadian dollars.

Wilfrid Laurier University
Department of Psychology
75 University Avenue, West
Waterloo, ON N2L 3C5
Telephone: (519) 884-1970, Ext. 3371
Fax: (519) 746-7605
E-mail: *rsharkey@wlu.ca*
Web: *http://www.wlu.ca/homepage.php?grp_id=44*

Department Information:
1956. Chairperson: Dr. Rudy Eikelboom. Number of faculty: total—full-time 31, part-time 14; women—full-time 11, part-time 10; total—minority—full-time 2, part-time 1; women minority—full-time 1, part-time 1.

Programs and Degrees Offered:
Listed in the following order: Program area, degree type (T if terminal Master's), number awarded 7/08–6/09. Community Psychology PhD (Doctor of Philosophy), Developmental Psychology PhD (Doctor of Philosophy) 2, Social Psychology PhD (Doctor of Philosophy) 2, Behavioural Neuroscience MA/MS (Master of Arts/Science) (T) 1, Cognitive Neuroscience MA/MS (Master of Arts/Science) (T) 3, Community Psychology MA/MS (Master of Arts/Science) 1, Social Psychology MA/MS (Master of Arts/Science) (T) 2, Developmental Psychology MA/MS (Master of Arts/Science) 2, Behavioural Neuroscience PhD (Doctor of Philosophy) 1, Cognitive Neuroscience PhD (Doctor of Philosophy) 1.

Student Applications/Admissions:
Student Applications
Community Psychology PhD (Doctor of Philosophy)—Applications 2009–2010, 10. Total applicants accepted 2009–2010, 2. Number full-time enrolled (new admits only) 2009–2010, 2. Number part-time enrolled (new admits only) 2009–2010, 0. Total enrolled 2009–2010 full-time, 7, part-time, 2. Openings 2010–2011, 3. The number of students enrolled full- and part-time who were dismissed or voluntarily withdrew from this program area in 2008–2009 were 0. *Developmental Psychology PhD (Doctor of Philosophy)*—Applications 2009–2010, 34. Total applicants accepted 2009–2010, 8. Number full-time enrolled (new admits only) 2009–2010, 2. Number part-time enrolled (new admits only) 2009–2010, 1. Total enrolled 2009–2010 full-time, 8, part-time, 1. Openings 2010–2011, 6. The median number of years required for completion of a degree in 2008–2009 were 2. The number of students enrolled full- and part-time who were dismissed or voluntarily withdrew from this program area in 2008–2009 were 0. *Social Psychology PhD (Doctor of Philosophy)*—Applications 2009–2010, 34. Total applicants accepted 2009–2010, 3. Number full-time enrolled (new admits only) 2009–2010, 0. Number part-time enrolled (new admits only) 2009–2010, 0. Openings 2010–2011, 6. The median number of years required for completion of a degree in 2008–2009 were 2. The number of students enrolled full- and part-time who were dismissed or voluntarily withdrew from this program area in 2008–2009 were 0. *Behavioural Neuroscience MA/MS (Master of Arts/Science)*—Applications 2009–2010, 6. Total applicants accepted 2009–2010, 2. Number full-time enrolled (new admits only) 2009–2010, 2. Number part-time enrolled (new admits only) 2009–2010, 0. Openings 2010–2011, 3. The median number of years required for completion of a degree in 2008–2009 were 2. The number of students enrolled full- and part-time who were dismissed or voluntarily withdrew from this program area in 2008–2009 were 0. *Cognitive Neuroscience MA/MS (Master of Arts/Science)*—Applications 2009–2010, 10. Total applicants accepted 2009–2010, 5. Number full-time enrolled (new admits only) 2009–2010, 5. Number part-time enrolled (new admits only) 2009–2010, 0. Openings 2010–2011, 3. The median number of years required for completion of a degree in 2008–2009 was 1. The number of students enrolled full- and part-time who were dismissed or voluntarily withdrew from this program area in 2008–2009 were 0. *Community Psychology MA/MS (Master of Arts/Science)*—Applications 2009–2010, 33. Total applicants accepted 2009–2010, 6. Number full-time enrolled (new admits only) 2009–2010, 6. Number part-time enrolled (new admits only) 2009–2010, 0. Total enrolled 2009–2010 full-time, 16, part-time, 2. Openings 2010–2011, 6. The median number of years required for completion of a degree in 2008–2009 were 2. The number of students enrolled full- and part-time who were dismissed or voluntarily withdrew from this program area in 2008–2009 were 0. *Social Psychology MA/MS (Master of Arts/Science)*—Applications 2009–2010, 34. Total applicants accepted 2009–2010, 3. Number full-time enrolled (new admits only) 2009–2010, 3. Total enrolled 2009–2010 full-time, 7. Openings 2010–2011, 6. The median number of years required for completion of a degree in 2008–2009 were 2. The number of students enrolled full- and part-time who were dismissed or voluntarily withdrew from this program area in 2008–2009 were 0. *Developmental Psychology MA/MS (Master of Arts/Science)*—Applications 2009–2010, 34. Total applicants accepted 2009–2010, 8. Number full-time enrolled (new admits only) 2009–2010, 8. Total enrolled 2009–2010 full-time, 15. Openings 2010–2011, 6. The median number of years required for completion of a degree in 2008–2009 were 2. The number of students enrolled full- and part-time who

were dismissed or voluntarily withdrew from this program area in 2008–2009 were 0. *Behavioural Neuroscience PhD (Doctor of Philosophy)*—Applications 2009–2010, 2. Total applicants accepted 2009–2010, 1. Number full-time enrolled (new admits only) 2009–2010, 1. Total enrolled 2009–2010 full-time, 2. Openings 2010–2011, 1. The median number of years required for completion of a degree in 2008–2009 were 5. The number of students enrolled full- and part-time who were dismissed or voluntarily withdrew from this program area in 2008–2009 were 0. *Cognitive Neuroscience PhD (Doctor of Philosophy)*—Applications 2009–2010, 4. Total applicants accepted 2009–2010, 1. Number full-time enrolled (new admits only) 2009–2010, 1. Number part-time enrolled (new admits only) 2009–2010, 0. Openings 2010–2011, 1. The median number of years required for completion of a degree in 2008–2009 were 4. The number of students enrolled full- and part-time who were dismissed or voluntarily withdrew from this program area in 2008–2009 were 0.

Other Criteria: (importance of criteria rated low, medium, or high): research experience—medium, work experience—low, extracurricular activity—low, clinically related public service—low, GPA—high, letters of recommendation—high, interview—medium, statement of goals and objectives—high.

Student Characteristics: The following represents characteristics of students in 2009–2010 in all graduate psychology programs in the department: Female—full-time 52, part-time 5; Male—full-time 20, part-time 0; African American/Black—full-time 2, part-time 0; Hispanic/Latino(a)—full-time 0, part-time 0; Asian/Pacific Islander—full-time 2, part-time 0; American Indian/Alaska Native—full-time 0, part-time 0; Caucasian/White—full-time 68, part-time 0; Multi-ethnic—full-time 0, part-time 0; students subject to the Americans With Disabilities Act—full-time 0, part-time 0; Unknown ethnicity—full-time 0, part-time 0; International students who hold an F-1 or J-1 Visa—full-time 0, part-time 0.

Financial Information/Assistance:
Tuition for Full-Time Study: *Master's:* State residents: per academic year $6,519; Nonstate residents: per academic year $14,654. *Doctoral:* State residents: per academic year $6,519; Nonstate residents: per academic year $14,654. Tuition is subject to change. See the following Web site for updates and changes in tuition costs: http://www.wlu.ca/page.php?grp_id=36&p=654.

Financial Assistance:
First-Year Students: No information provided.
Advanced Students: No information provided.
Additional Information: Of all students currently enrolled full time, 0% benefited from one or more of the listed financial assistance programs. Application and information available online at: http://www.wlu.ca/page.php?grp_id=36&p=600.

Internships/Practica: No information provided.

Housing and Day Care: On-campus housing is available. See the following Web site for more information: http://www.mylaurier.ca/residence. On-campus day care facilities are available. Contact the Abwunza Child Care Centre at abwunzacc@kwymca.org for more information.

Employment of Department Graduates:
Master's Degree Graduates: Of those who graduated in the academic year 2008–2009, the following categories and numbers represent the postgraduate activities and employment of master's degree graduates: Enrolled in a postdoctoral residency/fellowship (n/a), employed in independent practice (n/a), total from the above (master's) (0).
Doctoral Degree Graduates: Of those who graduated in the academic year 2008–2009, the following categories and numbers represent the postgraduate activities and employment of doctoral degree graduates: Enrolled in a psychology doctoral program (n/a), total from the above (doctoral) (0).

Additional Information:
Orientation, Objectives, and Emphasis of Department: Graduate students can obtain an MA, MSc or PhD in one of the five fields of: 1) Behavioural Neuroscience, 2) Cognitive Neuroscience, 3) Community Psychology, 4) Social, and 5) Developmental. The objective of the MA, MSc and PhD programs in the fields of Behavioural, Cognitive, Social and Developmental Psychology is to develop competence in designing, conducting, and evaluating research. Five half-credit courses and a thesis constitute the degree requirements in these MA/MSc programs. The purpose of these programs is to prepare students for doctoral studies, or for employment in an environment requiring research skills. Students in good standing can be considered for admission to the PhD programs in these areas, which involve 7 half-credit courses, 2 comprehensive papers and a dissertation. In the field of Community Psychology, the objective is to train scientist–practitioners with skills in community collaboration. Students receive training in theory, research, and practice that will enable them to analyze the implications of social change for the delivery of community services. Six half-credit courses and a thesis are required for the MA degree. Students who complete this program are prepared for either doctoral level training or for employment in community research and service. Students in good standing can be considered for admission to the PhD program in this area, which involves 6 half-credit courses, 2 comprehensive papers and a dissertation.

Special Facilities or Resources: The department has free unlimited access to the university computers, microprocessors, extensive electromechanical equipment, full-time electronics research associate, full-time field supervisor, and access to a wide variety of field settings for research and consultation.

Information for Students With Physical Disabilities: See the following Web site for more information: http://www.mylaurier.ca/accessible/.

Application Information:
Send to Rita Sharkey, Graduate Program Assistant, Psychology Department, Wilfrid Laurier University, 75 University Avenue West, Waterloo, ON N2L 3C5. Application available online. URL of online application: http://www.wlu.ca/page.php?grp_id=36&p=600. Students are admitted in the Fall, application deadline January 15. *Fee:* $75. Note: All dollar amounts specified in this entry are Canadian dollars.

Windsor, University of

Psychology
Faculty of Arts and Social Sciences
401 Sunset Avenue
Windsor, ON N9B 3P4
Telephone: (519) 253-3000, x 2232
Fax: (519) 973-7021
E-mail: *paivio@uwindsor.ca*
Web: *http://www.uwindsor.ca/psychology*

Department Information:
1944. Head: Sandra Paivio. Number of faculty: total—full-time 31; women—full-time 18; total—minority—full-time 2.

Programs and Degrees Offered:
Listed in the following order: Program area, degree type (T if terminal Master's), number awarded 7/08–6/09. Applied Social Psychology PhD (Doctor of Philosophy) 1, Clinical Psychology PhD (Doctor of Philosophy) 10.

APA Accreditation: Clinical PhD (Doctor of Philosophy).

CPA Accreditation: Clinical PhD (Doctor of Philosophy).

Student Applications/Admissions:
Student Applications
Applied Social Psychology PhD (Doctor of Philosophy)—Applications 2009–2010, 26. Total applicants accepted 2009–2010, 11. Number full-time enrolled (new admits only) 2009–2010, 6. Number part-time enrolled (new admits only) 2009–2010, 0. Openings 2010–2011, 5. The median number of years required for completion of a degree in 2008–2009 were 7. The number of students enrolled full- and part-time who were dismissed or voluntarily withdrew from this program area in 2008–2009 were 0. *Clinical Psychology PhD (Doctor of Philosophy)*—Applications 2009–2010, 159. Total applicants accepted 2009–2010, 24. Number full-time enrolled (new admits only) 2009–2010, 12. Number part-time enrolled (new admits only) 2009–2010, 0. Openings 2010–2011, 12. The median number of years required for completion of a degree in 2008–2009 were 7. The number of students enrolled full- and part-time who were dismissed or voluntarily withdrew from this program area in 2008–2009 were 0.
Scores: Entries appear in this order: required test or GPA, minimum score (if required), median score of students entering in 2009–2010. *Applied Social Psychology PhD (Doctor of Philosophy)*: GRE-V no minimum stated, GRE-Q no minimum stated, GRE-Analytical no minimum stated, GRE-Subject (Psychology) no minimum stated, overall undergraduate GPA no minimum stated, last 2 years GPA no minimum stated, psychology GPA no minimum stated; *Clinical Psychology PhD (Doctor of Philosophy)*: GRE-V no minimum stated, GRE-Q no minimum stated, GRE-Analytical no minimum stated, GRE-Subject (Psychology) no minimum stated, overall undergraduate GPA no minimum stated, last 2 years GPA no minimum stated.
Other Criteria: (importance of criteria rated low, medium, or high): GRE scores—high, research experience—medium, work experience—low, extracurricular activity—low, clinically related public service—medium, GPA—high, letters of recommendation—high, interview—medium, statement of goals and objectives—medium, Honours Thesis—high, undergraduate major in psychology—high, specific undergraduate psychology courses taken—high. For additional information on admission requirements, go to http://www.uwindsor.ca/psychology.

Student Characteristics: The following represents characteristics of students in 2009–2010 in all graduate psychology programs in the department: Female—full-time 96, part-time 0; Male—full-time 21, part-time 0; African American/Black—full-time 0, part-time 0; Hispanic/Latino(a)—full-time 0, part-time 0; Asian/Pacific Islander—full-time 0, part-time 0; American Indian/Alaska Native—full-time 0, part-time 0; Caucasian/White—full-time 0, part-time 0; Multi-ethnic—full-time 0, part-time 0; students subject to the Americans With Disabilities Act—full-time 0, part-time 0; Unknown ethnicity—full-time 0, part-time 0; International students who hold an F-1 or J-1 Visa—full-time 0, part-time 0.

Financial Information/Assistance:
Tuition for Full-Time Study: *Doctoral:* State residents: per academic year $6,720; Nonstate residents: per academic year $15,510. Tuition is subject to change. See the following Web site for updates and changes in tuition costs: http://www.uwindsor.ca/units/cashiers/main.nsf.

Financial Assistance:
First-Year Students: Teaching assistantships available for first year. Average amount paid per academic year: $9,260. Average number of hours worked per week: 10. Apply by January 15. Research assistantships available for first year. Average number of hours worked per week: 10. Fellowships and scholarships available for first year. Average amount paid per academic year: $6,000. Apply by January 15.
Advanced Students: Teaching assistantships available for advanced students. Average amount paid per academic year: $10,316. Average number of hours worked per week: 10. Research assistantships available for advanced students. Average number of hours worked per week: 10. Fellowships and scholarships available for advanced students. Average amount paid per academic year: $6,000.
Additional Information: Of all students currently enrolled full time, 90% benefited from one or more of the listed financial assistance programs.

Internships/Practica: Doctoral Degree (PhD Clinical Psychology): For those doctoral students for whom a professional internship was required in this program prior to graduation, (8) students applied for an internship in 2008–2009, with (8) students obtaining an internship. Of those students who obtained an internship, (8) were paid internships. Of those students who obtained an internship, (7) students placed in APA/CPA accredited internships, (0) students placed in internships not APA/CPA accredited, but listed with the Association of Psychology Postdoctoral and Internship Programs (APPIC), (0) students placed in internships conforming to guidelines of the Council of Directors of School Psychology Programs (CDSPP), (1) students placed in internships that were not APA/CPA accredited, APPIC or CDSPP listed. A wide variety of clinical practica are available in the Windsor-Detroit area, and clinical students obtain additional summer practicum positions across the country. Students are placed in predoctoral internships throughout Canada and the

U.S. Applied Social students obtain practica and internships in business and industry, community and health-related agencies.

Housing and Day Care: On-campus housing is available. See the following Web site for more information: http://www.uwindsor.ca/residence. No on-campus day care facilities are available.

Employment of Department Graduates:
Master's Degree Graduates: Of those who graduated in the academic year 2008–2009, the following categories and numbers represent the postgraduate activities and employment of master's degree graduates: Enrolled in a psychology doctoral program (15), enrolled in a postdoctoral residency/fellowship (n/a), employed in independent practice (n/a), total from the above (master's) (15). *Doctoral Degree Graduates:* Of those who graduated in the academic year 2008–2009, the following categories and numbers represent the postgraduate activities and employment of doctoral degree graduates: Enrolled in a psychology doctoral program (n/a), enrolled in a postdoctoral residency/fellowship (1), employed in independent practice (3), employed in an academic position at a university (1), employed in business or industry (1), employed in a community mental health/counseling center (4), employed in a hospital/medical center (4), total from the above (doctoral) (14).

Additional Information:
Orientation, Objectives, and Emphasis of Department: The mission of the graduate programs in the Department of Psychology is to provide graduate students with a foundation of theory, research, and practice to enable them to conduct research and/or apply psychology in a variety of settings including universities, private practice, schools, health/medical organizations, social service agencies, businesses, and basic/applied research firms. Graduate offerings are divided into two areas: clinical and applied social. Students applying for the clinical program apply directly into specialty tracks of adult clinical, child clinical, or clinical neuropsychology. Each of the areas combines theoretical, substantive, and methodological coursework with a variety of applied training experiences.

Special Facilities or Resources: The Department of Psychology's PhD program is unique in that all areas of specialization (Applied Social, Clinical Neuropsychology, Adult Clinical and Child Clinical) have an applied focus. Applied training and research resources include the Psychological Services & Research Centre, the Child Study Centre, the Emotion-Cognition Research Laboratory, Health Research Centre for the Study of Violence against Women, Health & Well-being Laboratory, the Student Counselling Centre, and the Psycholinguistics and Neurolinguistics Laboratory. There are faculty-student research groups in the areas of eating disorders, trauma and psychotherapy, problem gambling, computer-mediated communication, feminist research, emotional competence, culture and diversity, health psychology, neuro-psychoanalysis, aging, forgiveness, applied memory, multicultural and counselling research, and autism. The department is affiliated with the Summit Centre for Preschool Children with Autism. The university campus has wireless computer access throughout. Researchers have access to a participant pool and web-based participant recruitment as well as systems that allow for web-based data collection.

Information for Students With Physical Disabilities: See the following Web site for more information: http://www.uwindsor.ca/disability/.

Application Information:
Send to Office of the Registrar, Graduate Studies Division, University of Windsor, 401 Sunset Avenue, Windsor, Ontario, Canada N9B 3P4. Application available online. URL of online application: http://www.uwindsor.ca/registrar. Students are admitted in the Fall, application deadline January 15. *Fee:* $85. Note: All dollar amounts specified in this entry are Canadian dollars.

York University
Graduate Program in Psychology
4700 Keele Street, Room 297, Behavioural Science Building
Toronto, ON M3J 1P3
Telephone: (416) 736-5290
Fax: (416) 736-5814
E-mail: *schuller@yorku.ca*
Web: *http://www.yorku.ca/gradpsyc/index.html*

Department Information:
1963. Director, Graduate Program in Psychology: Dr. Regina Schuller. Number of faculty: total—full-time 80; women—full-time 40.

Programs and Degrees Offered:
Listed in the following order: Program area, degree type (T if terminal Master's), number awarded 7/08–6/09. Clinical-Developmental PhD (Doctor of Philosophy) 14, Brain, Behaviour and Cognitive Sciences PhD (Doctor of Philosophy) 8, Clinical PhD (Doctor of Philosophy) 18, Developmental and Cognitive Processes PhD (Doctor of Philosophy) 7, History and Theory Of Psychology PhD (Doctor of Philosophy) 1, Social and Personality Psychology PhD (Doctor of Philosophy) 7, Quantitative Methods PhD (Doctor of Philosophy).

APA Accreditation: Clinical PhD (Doctor of Philosophy). Student Outcome Data Website: http://www.yorku.ca/gradpsyc/prospectiveclinicalpsychologygradstudents.html.

CPA Accreditation: Clinical PhD (Doctor of Philosophy). Clinical PhD (Doctor of Philosophy).

Student Applications/Admissions:
Student Applications
Clinical-Developmental PhD (Doctor of Philosophy)—Applications 2009–2010, 103. Total applicants accepted 2009–2010, 11. Number full-time enrolled (new admits only) 2009–2010, 11. Number part-time enrolled (new admits only) 2009–2010, 0. Total enrolled 2009–2010 full-time, 65, part-time, 12. Openings 2010–2011, 12. The median number of years required for completion of a degree in 2008–2009 were 6. The number of students enrolled full- and part-time who were dismissed or voluntarily withdrew from this program area in 2008–2009 were 2. *Brain, Behaviour and Cognitive Sciences PhD (Doctor of Philosophy)*—Applications 2009–2010, 22. Total applicants accepted 2009–2010, 9. Number full-time enrolled (new admits only) 2009–2010, 9. Number part-time enrolled (new admits only) 2009–2010, 0. Total enrolled 2009–2010 full-time, 31, part-time, 5. Openings 2010–2011, 5. The median number of years required for completion of a degree in 2008–2009 were 6. The number of students enrolled full- and

part-time who were dismissed or voluntarily withdrew from this program area in 2008–2009 were 2. *Clinical PhD (Doctor of Philosophy)*—Applications 2009–2010, 128. Total applicants accepted 2009–2010, 9. Number full-time enrolled (new admits only) 2009–2010, 9. Number part-time enrolled (new admits only) 2009–2010, 0. Total enrolled 2009–2010 full-time, 56, part-time, 11. Openings 2010–2011, 8. The median number of years required for completion of a degree in 2008–2009 were 6. The number of students enrolled full- and part-time who were dismissed or voluntarily withdrew from this program area in 2008–2009 were 2. *Developmental and Cognitive Processes PhD (Doctor of Philosophy)*—Applications 2009–2010, 23. Total applicants accepted 2009–2010, 7. Number full-time enrolled (new admits only) 2009–2010, 6. Number part-time enrolled (new admits only) 2009–2010, 0. Total enrolled 2009–2010 full-time, 25, part-time, 5. Openings 2010–2011, 4. The median number of years required for completion of a degree in 2008–2009 were 6. The number of students enrolled full- and part-time who were dismissed or voluntarily withdrew from this program area in 2008–2009 were 2. *History and Theory Of Psychology PhD (Doctor of Philosophy)*—Applications 2009–2010, 9. Total applicants accepted 2009–2010, 3. Number full-time enrolled (new admits only) 2009–2010, 3. Number part-time enrolled (new admits only) 2009–2010, 0. Openings 2010–2011, 2. The median number of years required for completion of a degree in 2008–2009 were 6. The number of students enrolled full- and part-time who were dismissed or voluntarily withdrew from this program area in 2008–2009 were 0. *Social and Personality Psychology PhD (Doctor of Philosophy)*—Applications 2009–2010, 44. Total applicants accepted 2009–2010, 5. Number full-time enrolled (new admits only) 2009–2010, 5. Number part-time enrolled (new admits only) 2009–2010, 0. Total enrolled 2009–2010 full-time, 28, part-time, 5. Openings 2010–2011, 5. The median number of years required for completion of a degree in 2008–2009 were 6. The number of students enrolled full- and part-time who were dismissed or voluntarily withdrew from this program area in 2008–2009 were 0. *Quantitative Methods PhD (Doctor of Philosophy)*—Openings 2010–2011, 2.

Scores: Entries appear in this order: required test or GPA, minimum score (if required), median score of students entering in 2009–2010. *Clinical-Developmental PhD (Doctor of Philosophy)*: GRE-V no minimum stated, GRE-Q no minimum stated, GRE-Analytical no minimum stated, GRE-Subject (Psychology) no minimum stated; *Brain, Behaviour and Cognitive Sciences PhD (Doctor of Philosophy)*: GRE-V no minimum stated, GRE-Q no minimum stated, GRE-Analytical no minimum stated; *Clinical PhD (Doctor of Philosophy)*: GRE-V no minimum stated, GRE-Q no minimum stated, GRE-Analytical no minimum stated, GRE-Subject (Psychology) no minimum stated; *Developmental and Cognitive Processes PhD (Doctor of Philosophy)*: GRE-V no minimum stated, GRE-Q no minimum stated, GRE-Analytical no minimum stated; *History and Theory of Psychology PhD (Doctor of Philosophy)*: GRE-V no minimum stated, GRE-Q no minimum stated, GRE-Analytical no minimum stated; *Social and Personality Psychology PhD (Doctor of Philosophy)*: GRE-V no minimum stated, GRE-Q no minimum stated, GRE-Analytical no minimum stated; *Quantitative Methods PhD (Doctor of Philosophy)*: GRE-V no minimum stated, GRE-Q no minimum stated, GRE-Analytical no minimum stated.

Other Criteria: (importance of criteria rated low, medium, or high): GRE scores—high, research experience—high, work experience—medium, clinically related public service—low, GPA—high, letters of recommendation—high, statement of goals and objectives—medium, undergraduate major in psychology—medium, specific undergraduate psychology courses taken—low. The nonclinical areas place no weight on clinically related public service. For additional information on admission requirements, go to http://www.yorku.ca/gradpsyc/howtoapply.html.

Student Characteristics: The following represents characteristics of students in 2009–2010 in all graduate psychology programs in the department: Female—full-time 182, part-time 32; Male—full-time 34, part-time 3; African American/Black—full-time 0, part-time 0; Hispanic/Latino(a)—full-time 0, part-time 0; Asian/Pacific Islander—full-time 0, part-time 0; American Indian/Alaska Native—full-time 0, part-time 0; Caucasian/White—full-time 0, part-time 0; Multi-ethnic—full-time 0, part-time 0; students subject to the Americans With Disabilities Act—full-time 0, part-time 0; Unknown ethnicity—full-time 0, part-time 0; International students who hold an F-1 or J-1 Visa—full-time 0, part-time 0.

Financial Information/Assistance:
Tuition for Full-Time Study: *Master's:* State residents: per academic year $5,501; Nonstate residents: per academic year $11,989. *Doctoral:* State residents: per academic year $5,501; Nonstate residents: per academic year $11,989. Tuition is subject to change. See the following Web site for updates and changes in tuition costs: http://sfs.yorku.ca/fees/courses/index.php.

Financial Assistance:
First-Year Students: Teaching assistantships available for first year. Average amount paid per academic year: $6,000. Average number of hours worked per week: 10. Research assistantships available for first year. Average amount paid per academic year: $9,000. Average number of hours worked per week: 10. Traineeships available for first year. Fellowships and scholarships available for first year. Average amount paid per academic year: $6,000.

Advanced Students: Teaching assistantships available for advanced students. Average amount paid per academic year: $14,400. Average number of hours worked per week: 10. Research assistantships available for advanced students. Average amount paid per academic year: $8,000. Average number of hours worked per week: 10. Fellowships and scholarships available for advanced students.

Additional Information: Of all students currently enrolled full time, 100% benefited from one or more of the listed financial assistance programs. Application and information available online at: http://futurestudents.yorku.ca/graduate/fees_and_funding.

Internships/Practica: Doctoral internships are available; practicum work is done on a half-time basis during the academic year and, when possible, full-time during the summer. Research practica, and a clinical practicum as part of the Clinical Area's programme, are done on campus. Clinical internships are available in the York University Psychology Clinic (newly opened) and a variety of hospitals, clinics, and counseling centers in the city and elsewhere.

Housing and Day Care: On-campus housing is available. See the following Web site for more information: http://www.yorku.ca/

stuhouse/yorkapts/rates.htm. On-campus day care facilities are available. See the following Web site for more information: http://www.yorku.ca/daycare/; http://www.yorku.ca/children/.

Employment of Department Graduates:
Master's Degree Graduates: Of those who graduated in the academic year 2008–2009, the following categories and numbers represent the postgraduate activities and employment of master's degree graduates: Enrolled in a psychology doctoral program (28), enrolled in another graduate/professional program (4), enrolled in a postdoctoral residency/fellowship (n/a), employed in independent practice (n/a), do not know (8), total from the above (master's) (40).
Doctoral Degree Graduates: Of those who graduated in the academic year 2008–2009, the following categories and numbers represent the postgraduate activities and employment of doctoral degree graduates: Enrolled in a psychology doctoral program (n/a), enrolled in another graduate/professional program (0), enrolled in a postdoctoral residency/fellowship (2), employed in independent practice (1), employed in an academic position at a university (2), employed in an academic position at a 2-year/4-year college (1), employed in other positions at a higher education institution (0), employed in a professional position in a school system (1), employed in business or industry (0), employed in a government agency (0), employed in a community mental health/counseling center (1), employed in a hospital/medical center (1), still seeking employment (0), other employment position (6), do not know (0), total from the above (doctoral) (15).

Additional Information:
Orientation, Objectives, and Emphasis of Department: Strength and depth are emphasized in the areas of brain, behaviour and cognitive science (learning, perception, physiological, psychometrics); clinical; clinical-development; developmental cognitive processes; history and theory; quantitative methods; and social-personality. The department prepares students as researchers and practitioners in a given area. Most students admitted to the MA are accepted on the assumption that they will continue into PhD studies.

Special Facilities or Resources: The department has a vivarium; substantial computing facilities; audiovisual equipment including VCRs; and observational laboratories with two-way mirrors.

Information for Students With Physical Disabilities: See the following Web site for more information: http://www.yorku.ca/dshub/.

Application Information:
Send to Mailing Address: Office of Graduate Admissions, P.O. Box GA2300, York University, 4700 Keele Street, Toronto, Ontario M3J 1P3, Canada or Courier Address: Office of Graduate Admissions, Bennett Centre for Student Services, York University, 4700 Keele Street, Toronto, Ontario, M3J 1P3, Canada. Application available online. URL of online application: http://futurestudents.yorku.ca/graduate/apply_now. Students are admitted in the Fall, application deadline December 15. *Fee:* $90. Note: All dollar amounts specified in this entry are Canadian dollars.

INDEX OF PROGRAMS BY AREA OF STUDY OFFERED

B

Behavioral Psychology
American University (PhD)
Appalachian State University (MA/MS—terminal)
Auburn University (MA/MS—terminal)
Boston College (PhD)
Boston University (MA/MS—terminal)
California State University, Sacramento (MA/MS—terminal)
California, University of, Berkeley (PhD)
California, University of, Davis (PhD)
California, University of, Los Angeles (PhD)
Carnegie Mellon University (PhD)
Cincinnati, University of (PhD)
City University of New York (PhD)
City University of New York: Graduate Center (PhD)
City University of New York: Graduate School and University Center (PhD)
Claremont Graduate University (MA/MS—terminal, PhD)
Colorado, University of, Boulder (PhD)
Cornell University (PhD)
Drexel University (MA/MS—terminal)
Eastern Michigan University (MA/MS—terminal)
Florida Institute of Technology (MA/MS, MA/MS—terminal, PhD)
Florida International University (MA/MS—terminal)
Florida State University (MA/MS—terminal)
Florida, University of (PhD)
Georgia Southern University (PsyD)
Georgia State University (PhD)
Hofstra University (PhD)
Illinois State University (MA/MS—terminal)
Indiana University (PhD)
Iowa, University of (PhD)
Jacksonville State University (MA/MS—terminal)
Kansas, University of (MA/MS, PhD)
Long Island University (Other)
Manitoba, University of (PhD)
Maryland, University of, Baltimore County (MA/MS—terminal)
Massachusetts, University of, Dartmouth (MA/MS—terminal, Other)
Michigan State University (PhD)
Middle Tennessee State University (MA/MS—terminal)
Minnesota State University—Mankato (MA/MS)
Minnesota, University of (PhD)
Mississippi State University (PhD)
Missouri, University of, St. Louis (PhD)
Nebraska, University of, Omaha (MA/MS)
Nevada, University of, Reno (PhD)
North Carolina, University of, Wilmington (MA/MS—terminal)
Northeastern University (MA/MS—terminal, PhD)
Ohio State University, The (PhD)
Pacific, University of the (MA/MS—terminal)
Saskatchewan, University of (PhD)
Southern California, University of, Keck School of Medicine (PhD)
State University of New York, Binghamton University (PhD)
Syracuse University (PhD)
Tennessee, University of, Knoxville (PhD)
Texas, University of, Austin (PhD)
Texas, University of, Pan American (MA/MS)
The Chicago School of Professional Psychology (MA/MS—terminal, PsyD, Respecialization Diploma)
The College at Brockport - State University of New York (MA/MS—terminal)
Toronto, University of (MA/MS, PhD)
University at Buffalo, State University of New York (PhD)
Utah State University (PhD)
Washington University in St. Louis (PhD)
Washington, University of (PhD)
West Virginia University (MA/MS—terminal, PhD)
Wilfrid Laurier University (MA/MS—terminal, PhD)
Wisconsin, University of, Milwaukee (MA/MS—terminal)

Biological Psychology
Arizona, The University of (PhD)
Brandeis University (PhD)
British Columbia, University of (PhD)
California, University of, Berkeley (PhD)
City University of New York: Graduate School and University Center (PhD)
Colorado, University of, Boulder (PhD)
Delaware, University of (PhD)
George Mason University (MA/MS—terminal, PhD)
Illinois, University of, Chicago (PhD)
Illinois, University of, Urbana–Champaign (PhD)
Indiana University-Purdue University Indianapolis (PhD)
Johns Hopkins University (PhD)
Maine, University of (PhD)
Miami University of Ohio (PhD)
Michigan, University of (PhD)
Minnesota, University of (PhD)
Nebraska, University of, Lincoln (PhD)
Nebraska, University of, Omaha (MA/MS)
Nevada, University of, Reno (PhD)
New Orleans, University of (PhD)
North Carolina, University of, Chapel Hill (PhD)
Pittsburgh, University of (PhD)
Rutgers University—New Brunswick (PhD)
Stony Brook University (PhD)
Texas, University of, Austin (PhD)
Virginia Commonwealth University (PhD)
Virginia Polytechnic Institute and State University (PhD)
Virginia, University of (PhD)
Washington State University (PhD)
Washington, University of (PhD)
Wayne State University (PhD)
Western Ontario, The University of (PhD)
Wisconsin, University of, Madison (PhD)

C

Child and Adolescent Psychology
Alabama, University of, at Birmingham (PhD)
Alfred University (EdS, PsyD)
Alliant International University: Irvine (MA/MS—terminal, PsyD)
Arcadia University (MA/MS—terminal)
Argosy University/Orange County (PsyD)
Bowling Green State University (PhD)
Central Florida, University of (PhD)
Clark University (PhD)
Delaware, University of (PhD)
Denver, University of (EdS, MA/MS, PhD)
DePaul University (PhD)
Duke University (PhD)
Duquesne University (MEd)
Florida International University (PhD)
Georgia, University of (PhD)
Illinois State University (MA/MS—terminal)
Illinois, University of, Urbana–Champaign (PhD)
John F. Kennedy University (MA/MS—terminal)
Lewis University (MA/MS)
Loyola University of Chicago (PhD)
Maine, University of (PhD)
Maryland, University of (PhD)
McGill University (PhD)
Memphis, University of (PhD)
Minnesota, University of (PhD)
New Orleans, University of (PhD)
Ohio State University, The (PhD)
Ohio University (PhD)
Oklahoma State University (PhD)
Oklahoma, University of (PhD)
Pennsylvania State University (PhD)
Rhode Island, University of, Chafee Social Sciences Center (MA/MS—terminal, PhD)
Seattle Pacific University (PhD)
Southern Illinois University Carbondale (PhD)
Temple University (PhD)
Texas A&M University (PhD)
Texas, University of, Austin (PhD)

INDEX OF PROGRAMS BY AREA OF STUDY OFFERED

Tufts University (MA/MS, MA/MS—terminal, Other, PhD)
Tulane University (PhD)
University at Buffalo, State University of New York (MA/MS—terminal, MEd)
Utah State University (PhD)
Utah, University of (PhD)
Victoria, University of (PhD)
Virginia Commonwealth University (PhD)
Washington State University (PhD)
Washington, University of (PhD)
West Virginia University (PhD)
Wheaton College (PsyD)
Wisconsin, University of, Milwaukee (PhD)
Yeshiva University (PsyD)
York University (PhD)

Clinical Psychology
Acadia University (MA/MS—terminal)
Adelphi University (PhD)
Adler School of Professional Psychology (PsyD)
Alabama, University of (PhD)
Alabama, University of, at Birmingham (PhD)
Alaska, University of, Fairbanks/Anchorage (PhD)
Alliant International University: Fresno/Sacramento (PhD, PsyD)
Alliant International University: Los Angeles (PhD, PsyD)
Alliant International University: San Diego (PhD, PsyD, Respecialization Diploma)
Alliant International University: San Francisco (PhD, PsyD, Respecialization Diploma)
American International College (MA/MS—terminal)
American University (PhD)
Antioch University New England (PsyD)
Antioch University, Santa Barbara (PsyD)
Antioch University, Seattle (PsyD)
Appalachian State University (MA/MS—terminal)
Argosy University/Atlanta (MA/MS—terminal, PsyD)
Argosy University/Chicago (formerly the Illinois School of Professional Psychology) (PsyD)
Argosy University/Orange County (MA/MS—terminal, PsyD)
Argosy University/San Francisco Bay Area (MA/MS—terminal, PsyD)
Argosy University/Schaumburg (MA/MS—terminal, PsyD)
Argosy University/Seattle (MA/MS, PsyD)
Argosy University/Washington, D.C. (MA/MS—terminal, PsyD)
Arizona State University (PhD)
Arizona, The University of (PhD)
Arkansas, University of (PhD)
Auburn University (PhD)
Augusta State University (MA/MS—terminal)
Azusa Pacific University (MA/MS, MA/MS—terminal, PsyD)
Ball State University (MA/MS—terminal)
Barry University (MA/MS—terminal)

Baylor University (PsyD)
Benedictine University (MA/MS—terminal)
Boston University (PhD)
Bowling Green State University (PhD)
Brenau University (MA/MS—terminal)
Brigham Young University (PhD)
British Columbia, University of (PhD)
Bryn Mawr College (PhD)
Calgary, University of (PhD)
California Institute of Integral Studies (PsyD)
California Lutheran University (MA/MS—terminal, PsyD)
California State University, Dominguez Hills (MA/MS—terminal)
California State University, Fullerton (MA/MS—terminal)
California State University, Northridge (MA/MS—terminal)
California, University of, Berkeley (PhD)
California, University of, Los Angeles (PhD)
California, University of, Santa Barbara (PhD)
Case Western Reserve University (PhD)
Central Florida, University of (MA/MS—terminal, PhD)
Central Michigan University (PhD)
Chestnut Hill College (MA/MS—terminal, PsyD)
Cincinnati, University of (PhD)
Citadel, The (MA/MS—terminal)
City University of New York: Graduate Center (PhD)
City University of New York: Graduate School and University Center (PhD)
Clark University (PhD)
Colorado, University of, at Colorado Springs (MA/MS—terminal, PhD)
Colorado, University of, Boulder (PhD)
Colorado, University of, Denver (MA/MS—terminal, PhD)
Concordia University (PhD)
Connecticut, University of (PhD)
Dalhousie University (PhD)
Dayton, University of (MA/MS—terminal)
Delaware, University of (PhD)
Denver, University of (MA/MS—terminal, PhD, PsyD)
Duke University (PhD)
Duquesne University (PhD)
East Carolina University (PhD)
East Tennessee State University (PhD)
Eastern Illinois University (MA/MS—terminal)
Eastern Kentucky University (MA/MS—terminal)
Eastern Michigan University (MA/MS—terminal, PhD)
Eastern Washington University (MA/MS—terminal)
Emory University (PhD)
Emporia State University (MA/MS—terminal)
Fairleigh Dickinson University, Metropolitan Campus (PhD)
Fielding Graduate University (PhD, Respecialization Diploma)

Florida Institute of Technology (PsyD)
Florida International University (PhD)
Florida State University (PhD)
Florida, University of (PhD)
Fordham University (PhD)
Fort Hays State University (MA/MS—terminal)
Francis Marion University (MA/MS—terminal)
Fuller Theological Seminary (PhD, PsyD)
Gallaudet University (PhD)
George Fox University (PsyD)
George Mason University (PhD)
George Washington University (PhD)
Georgia Southern University (MA/MS—terminal, PsyD)
Georgia State University (PhD)
Georgia, University of (PhD)
Guelph, University of (MA/MS, PhD)
Hartford, University of (MA/MS—terminal, PsyD)
Harvard University (PhD)
Hawaii, University of, Manoa (PhD)
Hofstra University (PhD)
Houston, University of (PhD)
Idaho State University (PhD)
Illinois Institute of Technology (PhD)
Illinois State University (MA/MS—terminal)
Illinois, University of, Chicago (PhD)
Illinois, University of, Urbana–Champaign (PhD)
Immaculata University (PsyD)
Indiana State University (PsyD)
Indiana University (PhD)
Indiana University of Pennsylvania (PsyD)
Indiana University-Purdue University Indianapolis (MA/MS—terminal, PhD)
Indianapolis, University of (MA/MS, PsyD)
Institute for the Psychological Sciences (MA/MS—terminal, PsyD)
Iowa, University of (PhD)
John F. Kennedy University (PsyD)
Kansas, University of (PhD)
Kean University (PsyD)
Kent State University (PhD)
Kentucky, University of (PhD)
La Verne, University of (PsyD)
Lamar University-Beaumont (MA/MS—terminal)
Loma Linda University (PhD, PsyD)
Long Island University (MA/MS—terminal, PhD, PsyD)
Louisiana, University of, Monroe (MA/MS)
Louisville, University of (PhD)
Loyola University Maryland (MA/MS—terminal, PsyD)
Loyola University of Chicago (PhD)
Maine, University of (PhD)
Manitoba, University of (PhD)
Marquette University (PhD)
Marshall University (MA/MS—terminal, PsyD)
Maryland, University of (PhD)
Maryland, University of, Baltimore County (PhD)
Marywood University (PsyD)

INDEX OF PROGRAMS BY AREA OF STUDY OFFERED

Massachusetts School of Professional Psychology (PsyD, Respecialization Diploma)
Massachusetts, University of (PhD)
Massachusetts, University of, Dartmouth (MA/MS—terminal)
McGill University (PhD)
Miami University of Ohio (PhD)
Michigan School of Professional Psychology (PsyD)
Michigan State University (PhD)
Michigan, University of (PhD)
Middle Tennessee State University (MA/MS—terminal)
Midwestern State University (MA/MS—terminal)
Midwestern University (MA/MS, PsyD)
Millersville University (MA/MS—terminal)
Minnesota State University—Mankato (MA/MS)
Minnesota, University of (PhD)
Mississippi State University (MA/MS—terminal)
Mississippi, University of (PhD)
Missouri State University (MA/MS—terminal)
Missouri, University of (PhD)
Missouri, University of, Kansas City (PhD)
Missouri, University of, St. Louis (PhD)
Montana State University Billings (MA/MS—terminal)
Montana, The University of (PhD)
Morehead State University (Kentucky) (MA/MS—terminal)
Murray State University (MA/MS—terminal)
Nebraska, University of, Lincoln (PhD)
Nevada, University of, Las Vegas (PhD)
Nevada, University of, Reno (PhD)
New Brunswick, University of (PhD)
New Mexico Highlands University (MA/MS—terminal)
New Mexico, University of (PhD)
New York University (MA/MS—terminal, PhD)
North Carolina, University of, Chapel Hill (PhD)
North Carolina, University of, Charlotte (MA/MS—terminal, PhD)
North Carolina, University of, Wilmington (MA/MS—terminal)
North Dakota State University (MA/MS—terminal)
North Dakota, University of (PhD)
North Texas, University of (PhD)
Northern Illinois University (PhD)
Northern Iowa, University of (MA/MS—terminal)
Northwestern University (PhD)
Northwestern University, Feinberg School of Medicine (PhD)
Nova Southeastern University (PhD, PsyD)
Ohio State University, The (PhD)
Ohio University (PhD)
Oklahoma State University (PhD)
Old Dominion University (PsyD)
Oregon, University of (PhD)
Ottawa, University of (PhD)

Pace University (PsyD)
Pacific Graduate School of Psychology & Stanford University School of Medicine, Department of Psychiatry and Behavioral Sciences (PsyD)
Pacific University (PsyD)
Pacific, University of the (MA/MS—terminal)
Pacifica Graduate Institute (PhD)
Palo Alto University (Other, PhD)
Penn State Harrisburg (MA/MS—terminal)
Pennsylvania State University (PhD)
Pennsylvania, University of (PhD)
Philadelphia College of Osteopathic Medicine (MA/MS—terminal, Other, PsyD, Respecialization Diploma)
Phillips Graduate Institute (PsyD)
Pittsburg State University (MA/MS—terminal)
Pittsburgh, University of (PhD)
Puerto Rico, University of (PhD)
Purdue University (PhD)
Queen's University (MA/MS, PhD)
Radford University (MA/MS—terminal)
Regent University (PsyD)
Regina, University of (MA/MS—terminal, PhD)
Rhode Island, University of, Chafee Social Sciences Center (PhD)
Roger Williams University (MA/MS—terminal)
Roosevelt University (MA/MS—terminal, PsyD)
Rosalind Franklin University of Medicine and Science (PhD)
Rutgers University—New Brunswick (PhD)
Rutgers—The State University of New Jersey (PsyD)
Ryerson University (MA/MS, PhD)
Saint Michael's College (MA/MS—terminal)
Sam Houston State University (MA/MS—terminal, PhD)
San Diego State University/University of California, San Diego Joint Doctoral Program in Clinical Psychology (PhD)
San Jose State University (MA/MS—terminal)
Saskatchewan, University of (PhD)
Saybrook University (PhD, PsyD)
Seattle University (MA/MS—terminal)
Simon Fraser University (PhD)
South Alabama, University of (MA/MS—terminal, PhD)
South Carolina, University of (PhD)
South Carolina, University of, Aiken (MA/MS—terminal)
South Dakota, University of (PhD)
South Florida, University of (PhD)
Southern California, University of (PhD)
Southern Illinois University Carbondale (PhD)
Southern Illinois University Edwardsville (MA/MS—terminal)
Southern Methodist University (PhD)
Southern Oregon University (MA/MS—terminal)
Spalding University (PsyD)

State University of New York, Binghamton University (PhD)
Stony Brook University (PhD)
Suffolk University (PhD, Respecialization Diploma)
Syracuse University (PhD)
Teachers College, Columbia University (MA/MS—terminal, PhD)
Temple University (PhD)
Tennessee, University of, Knoxville (PhD)
Texas A&M University (PhD)
Texas A&M University-Commerce (MA/MS—terminal)
Texas of the Permian Basin, The University of (MA/MS—terminal)
Texas Southwestern Medical Center at Dallas, The University of (PhD)
Texas Tech University (PhD)
Texas, University of, Austin (PhD)
Texas, University of, El Paso (MA/MS—terminal)
Texas, University of, Pan American (MA/MS—terminal)
Texas, University of, Tyler (MA/MS—terminal)
The Chicago School of Professional Psychology (MA/MS—terminal, PsyD, Respecialization Diploma)
The College at Brockport - State University of New York (MA/MS—terminal)
The New School for Social Research (PhD)
The School of Professional Psychology at Forest Institute (MA/MS—terminal, PsyD)
Toledo, University of (PhD)
Towson University (MA/MS—terminal)
Tulsa, University of (MA/MS—terminal, PhD)
Uniformed Services University of the Health Sciences (PhD)
University at Albany, State University of New York (PhD)
University at Buffalo, State University of New York (PhD)
University of the Rockies (PsyD)
Utah, University of (PhD)
Vanderbilt University (PhD)
Vanguard University of Southern California (MA/MS—terminal)
Vermont, University of (PhD)
Victoria, University of (PhD)
Virginia Consortium Program in Clinical Psychology (PsyD)
Virginia Polytechnic Institute and State University (PhD)
Virginia State University (MA/MS—terminal)
Virginia, University of (PhD)
Walden University (PhD)
Washburn University (MA/MS—terminal)
Washington University in St. Louis (PhD)
Washington, University of (PhD)
Waterloo, University of (PhD)
Wayne State University (PhD)
West Chester University of Pennsylvania (MA/MS—terminal)
West Virginia University (MA/MS—terminal, PhD)

INDEX OF PROGRAMS BY AREA OF STUDY OFFERED

Western Illinois University (MA/MS—terminal)
Western Ontario, The University of (PhD)
Wheaton College (MA/MS—terminal, PsyD)
Wichita State University (PhD)
Widener University (PsyD)
William Paterson University (MA/MS—terminal)
Windsor, University of (PhD)
Wisconsin School of Professional Psychology (PsyD)
Wisconsin, University of, Madison (PhD)
Wisconsin, University of, Milwaukee (PhD)
Wright Institute (PsyD)
Wright State University (PsyD)
Wyoming, University of (PhD)
Xavier University (PsyD)
Yale University (PhD)
York University (PhD)

Cognitive Psychology
Alabama, University of (PhD)
Arizona State University (PhD)
Arizona, The University of (PhD)
Ball State University (MA/MS—terminal)
Boston College (PhD)
Boston University (PhD)
Bowling Green State University (PhD)
Brandeis University (PhD)
British Columbia, University of (PhD)
Calgary, University of (PhD)
California, University of, Berkeley (PhD)
California, University of, Davis (PhD)
California, University of, Irvine (PhD)
California, University of, Los Angeles (PhD)
California, University of, Riverside (PhD)
California, University of, Santa Cruz (PhD)
Carleton University (MA/MS)
Carnegie Mellon University (PhD)
Chicago, University of (PhD)
City University of New York: Brooklyn College (MA/MS—terminal, PhD)
City University of New York: Graduate School and University Center (PhD)
Claremont Graduate University (MA/MS—terminal, PhD)
Colorado State University (PhD)
Colorado, University of, Boulder (PhD)
Columbia University (MEd, PhD)
Connecticut, University of (PhD)
Cornell University (PhD)
Delaware, University of (PhD)
Denver, University of (PhD)
Drexel University (PhD)
Duke University (PhD)
Emory University (PhD)
Florida State University (PhD)
Florida, University of (PhD)
George Mason University (MA/MS—terminal, PhD)
Georgia State University (PhD)
Georgia, University of (PhD)
Guelph, University of (MA/MS, PhD)
Harvard University (PhD)
Hawaii, University of, Manoa (PhD)
Houston, University of (PhD)

Illinois State University (MA/MS—terminal)
Illinois, University of, Chicago (PhD)
Illinois, University of, Urbana–Champaign (PhD)
Illinois, University of, Urbana–Champaign (PhD)
Indiana University (PhD)
Iowa State University (PhD)
Iowa, University of (PhD)
Johns Hopkins University (PhD)
Kansas State University (PhD)
Kansas, University of (PhD)
Lehigh University (PhD)
Manitoba, University of (PhD)
Maryland, University of (PhD)
Massachusetts, University of (PhD)
Miami University of Ohio (PhD)
Michigan State University (PhD)
Michigan, University of (PhD)
Middle Tennessee State University (MA/MS—terminal)
Minnesota, University of (PhD)
Mississippi State University (PhD)
Missouri, University of (PhD)
Montana State University (MA/MS)
Nebraska, University of, Lincoln (PhD)
Nebraska, University of, Omaha (MA/MS)
Nevada, University of, Las Vegas (PhD)
New Hampshire, University of (PhD)
New Mexico State University (MA/MS, PhD)
New Mexico, University of (PhD)
New York University, Graduate School of Arts and Science (PhD)
North Carolina, University of, Chapel Hill (PhD)
North Dakota State University (PhD)
Northeastern University (PhD)
Northern Illinois University (PhD)
Northwestern University (PhD)
Notre Dame, University of (PhD)
Ohio State University, The (PhD)
Ohio University (PhD)
Oklahoma, University of (PhD)
Oregon, University of (MA/MS—terminal, PhD)
Pennsylvania State University (PhD)
Pittsburgh, University of (PhD)
Purdue University (PhD)
Queen's University (PhD)
Rensselaer Polytechnic Institute (PhD)
Rice University (PhD)
Rutgers University—New Brunswick (PhD)
Saskatchewan, University of (PhD)
South Florida, University of (PhD)
Southern California, University of (PhD)
Southern Illinois University Carbondale (PhD)
Stanford University (PhD)
State University of New York, Binghamton University (PhD)
Stony Brook University (PhD)
Syracuse University (PhD)
Temple University (PhD)
Texas A&M University (PhD)
Texas A&M University-Commerce (MA/MS—terminal, PhD)

Texas Tech University (PhD)
Texas, University of, Austin (PhD)
Texas, University of, Dallas (PhD)
Texas, University of, El Paso (PhD)
Toledo, University of (PhD)
Toronto, University of (MA/MS, PhD)
University at Albany, State University of New York (PhD)
University at Buffalo, State University of New York (PhD)
Utah, University of (PhD)
Vanderbilt University (PhD)
Victoria, University of (PhD)
Virginia, University of (PhD)
Washington State University (PhD)
Washington University in St. Louis (PhD)
Washington, University of (PhD)
Waterloo, University of (PhD)
Western Ontario, The University of (PhD)
Wilfrid Laurier University (MA/MS—terminal, PhD)
Wisconsin, University of, Madison (PhD)
Yale University (PhD)
Yeshiva University (PsyD)
York University (PhD)

Community Counseling
Arcadia University (MA/MS—terminal), MA/MS—terminal)
Arizona State University (MA/MS—terminal)
Austin Peay State University (MA/MS—terminal)
Cleveland State University (MEd)
Gonzaga University (MA/MS—terminal)
Houston Baptist University (MA/MS—terminal)
Kean University (MA/MS—terminal)
Lewis & Clark College, Graduate School of Education and Counseling (MA/MS—terminal)
Louisiana, University of, Lafayette (MA/MS—terminal)
Loyola University of Chicago (MA/MS—terminal)
Marquette University (MA/MS—terminal)
Massachusetts, University of, Boston (MA/MS—terminal)
Northeastern University (MA/MS—terminal)
Northern Arizona University (MA/MS—terminal)
Oklahoma, University of (MEd)
Philadelphia College of Osteopathic Medicine (MA/MS—terminal, Other)
University at Buffalo, State University of New York (MA/MS—terminal)
University of the Rockies (MA/MS—terminal)
Washington State University (MEd)
Wisconsin, University of, Milwaukee (MA/MS)

Community Psychology
Alaska, University of, Fairbanks/Anchorage (PhD)
California, University of, Berkeley (PhD)
Central Connecticut State University (MA/MS—terminal)

INDEX OF PROGRAMS BY AREA OF STUDY OFFERED

DePaul University (PhD)
George Mason University (PhD)
George Washington University (PhD)
Georgia State University (PhD)
Hawaii, University of, Manoa (PhD)
Illinois, University of, Chicago (PhD)
Illinois, University of, Urbana–Champaign (PhD)
La Verne, University of (PsyD)
Lamar University-Beaumont (MA/MS—terminal)
Maryland, University of, Baltimore County (PhD)
Marywood University (MA/MS—terminal)
Massachusetts, University of, Lowell (MA/MS—terminal)
Metropolitan State University (MA/MS—terminal)
Michigan State University (PhD)
New Haven, University of (MA/MS)
North Carolina State University (PhD)
North Carolina, University of, Charlotte (MA/MS—terminal)
Portland State University (PhD)
Puerto Rico, University of (PhD)
Sage Colleges, The (MA/MS—terminal)
Seton Hall University (EdS)
South Carolina, University of (PhD)
Temple University (MA/MS—terminal)
Texas A&M International University (MA/MS—terminal)
Vanderbilt University (MA/MS—terminal, MEd, PhD)
Virginia, University of (PhD)
West Virginia University (MA/MS—terminal)
Western Illinois University (MA/MS—terminal)
Wichita State University (PhD)
Wilfrid Laurier University (MA/MS, PhD)

Comparative Psychology
California, University of, Davis (PhD)
Oklahoma, University of (PhD)
York University (PhD)

Consulting Psychology
Alliant International University: San Diego (PhD)
Alliant International University: San Francisco (PhD)
New Haven, University of (MA/MS—terminal)
The Chicago School of Professional Psychology (PsyD)
Wayne State University (MA/MS—terminal, PhD)

Counseling Psychology
Adelphi University (MA/MS—terminal)
Adler School of Professional Psychology (MA/MS—terminal)
Akron, University of (PhD)
Angelo State University (MA/MS—terminal)
Arcadia University (MA/MS—terminal)
Argosy University/Orange County (EdD, MA/MS—terminal)
Arizona State University (MA/MS—terminal, PhD)
Assumption College (MA/MS—terminal)
Auburn University (PhD)
Augusta State University (MA/MS—terminal)
Ball State University (MA/MS—terminal, PhD)
Baltimore, University of (MA/MS—terminal)
Boston College (PhD)
Brenau University (MA/MS—terminal)
Brigham Young University (PhD)
California Institute of Integral Studies (MA/MS—terminal)
California Lutheran University (MA/MS—terminal)
California Polytechnic State University (MA/MS—terminal)
California State University, Sacramento (MA/MS—terminal)
Central Arkansas, University of (MA/MS—terminal, PhD)
Central Oklahoma, University of (MA/MS—terminal)
Central Washington University (MA/MS—terminal, MEd)
Chestnut Hill College (MA/MS—terminal)
Citadel, The (MA/MS—terminal)
Cleveland State University (PhD)
Colorado State University (PhD)
Denver, University of (MA/MS—terminal, PhD)
Florida International University (MA/MS—terminal)
Florida State University (MA/MS, PhD)
Florida, University of (PhD)
Fordham University (PhD)
Francis Marion University (MA/MS—terminal)
Frostburg State University (MA/MS—terminal)
Georgia, University of (PhD)
Goddard College (MA/MS—terminal)
Houston Baptist University (MA/MS—terminal)
Houston, University of (PhD)
Humboldt State University (MA/MS—terminal)
Illinois State University (MA/MS—terminal)
Illinois, University of, Urbana–Champaign (PhD)
Immaculata University (MA/MS, MA/MS—terminal)
Indiana State University (MA/MS, PhD)
Indiana University (PhD)
Iowa State University (PhD)
Iowa, University of (PhD)
John F. Kennedy University (MA/MS—terminal)
Kansas, University of (MA/MS—terminal, PhD)
Kentucky, University of (EdS, MA/MS, PhD)
La Salle University (MA/MS)
Lehigh University (MEd, PhD)
Lewis & Clark College, Graduate School of Education and Counseling (MA/MS—terminal)
Lewis University (MA/MS)
Louisiana State University Shreveport (MA/MS—terminal)
Louisiana Tech University (PhD)
Louisville, University of (PhD)
Loyola University Maryland (MA/MS—terminal)
Loyola University of Chicago (PhD)
Marquette University (PhD)
Maryland, University of (PhD)
Massachusetts School of Professional Psychology (MA/MS—terminal)
McGill University (PhD)
Memphis, University of (PhD)
Miami, University of (MA/MS—terminal, PhD)
Midwestern State University (MA/MS—terminal)
Millersville University (MA/MS—terminal, MEd)
Minnesota, University of (MA/MS—terminal, PhD)
Missouri, University of, Kansas City (PhD)
Morehead State University (Kentucky) (MA/MS—terminal)
Nebraska, University of, Lincoln (PhD)
New Mexico State University (PhD)
New York University (MA/MS—terminal, PhD)
North Florida, University of (MA/MS—terminal)
North Texas, University of (PhD)
Northeastern University (MA/MS—terminal, PhD)
Northern Arizona University (PhD)
Northern Colorado, University of (PhD)
Notre Dame, University of (PhD)
Nova Southeastern University (MA/MS—terminal)
Ohio State University, The (PhD)
Oklahoma State University (PhD)
Oklahoma, University of (PhD)
Oregon, University of (PhD)
Our Lady of the Lake University (MA/MS—terminal, PsyD)
Pacific University (MA/MS—terminal)
Pennsylvania State University (PhD)
Pennsylvania, University of (Other)
Puget Sound, University of (MEd)
Radford University (PsyD)
Roosevelt University (MA/MS—terminal)
Rosalind Franklin University of Medicine and Science (MA/MS—terminal)
Rutgers—The State University of New Jersey, New Brunswick (MEd)
Sage Colleges, The (MA/MS—terminal, Other)
Saint Francis, University of (MA/MS, MA/MS—terminal, MEd, Other)
Saint Mary's University of Minnesota (MA/MS—terminal)
Santa Clara University (MA/MS, MA/MS—terminal)
Seton Hall University (EdS, MA/MS, MEd, PhD)

INDEX OF PROGRAMS BY AREA OF STUDY OFFERED

South Alabama, University of (PhD)
Southern Illinois University Carbondale (PhD)
Southern Oregon University (MA/MS—terminal)
Springfield College (MA/MS—terminal)
St. Thomas, University of (MA/MS—terminal, PsyD)
State University of New York at New Paltz (MA/MS—terminal)
Teachers College, Columbia University (Other, PhD)
Temple University (MA/MS—terminal)
Tennessee, University of, Knoxville (PhD)
Texas A&M International University (MA/MS—terminal)
Texas A&M University (PhD)
Texas Tech University (PhD)
Texas Woman's University (MA/MS—terminal, PhD)
Texas, University of, Austin (MEd, PhD)
Texas, University of, Tyler (MA/MS—terminal)
The Chicago School of Professional Psychology (MA/MS—terminal)
The New School for Social Research (MA/MS—terminal)
The School of Professional Psychology at Forest Institute (MA/MS—terminal)
Towson University (MA/MS—terminal)
University at Buffalo, State University of New York (PhD)
University of the Rockies (MA/MS—terminal)
Utah, University of (MA/MS—terminal, PhD)
Virginia Commonwealth University (PhD)
Walden University (PhD)
Walla Walla University (MA/MS—terminal)
Washington State University (PhD)
West Florida, The University of (MA/MS—terminal)
West Georgia, University of (MA/MS—terminal)
West Virginia University (PhD)
Western Michigan University (MA/MS—terminal, PhD)
Wheaton College (MA/MS—terminal)
William Paterson University (MA/MS—terminal)
Wisconsin, University of, Madison (MA/MS—terminal, PhD)
Wisconsin, University of, Milwaukee (PhD)
Yeshiva University (MA/MS—terminal)

D

Developmental Psychology
Akron, University of (PhD)
Alabama, University of (PhD)
Alabama, University of, at Birmingham (PhD)
American International College (EdD)
Arizona State University (PhD)
Ball State University (MA/MS—terminal, PhD)
Boston College (MA/MS—terminal, PhD)
Boston University (PhD)
Bowling Green State University (PhD)
Brandeis University (PhD)
British Columbia, University of (PhD)
Bryn Mawr College (PhD)
California State University, Northridge (MA/MS—terminal)
California, University of, Berkeley (PhD)
California, University of, Davis (MA/MS—terminal, PhD)
California, University of, Los Angeles (PhD)
California, University of, Merced (PhD)
California, University of, Riverside (PhD)
California, University of, Santa Cruz (PhD)
Carnegie Mellon University (PhD)
Chicago, University of (PhD)
City University of New York: Graduate School and University Center (PhD)
Claremont Graduate University (MA/MS—terminal, PhD)
Clark University (PhD)
Connecticut, University of (PhD)
Cornell University (PhD)
Denver, University of (PhD)
DePaul University (PhD)
Duke University (PhD)
Florida International University (PhD)
Florida State University (PhD)
Florida, University of (PhD)
Fordham University (PhD)
George Mason University (MA/MS—terminal, PhD)
Georgia State University (PhD)
Georgia, University of (PhD)
Guelph, University of (MA/MS, PhD)
Harvard University (PhD)
Hawaii, University of, Manoa (PhD)
Humboldt State University (MA/MS—terminal)
Illinois State University (MA/MS—terminal)
Illinois, University of, Urbana–Champaign (PhD)
Illinois, University of, Urbana–Champaign (PhD)
Indiana University (MA/MS, PhD)
Iowa, University of (PhD)
Johns Hopkins University (PhD)
Kansas, University of (PhD)
Loyola University of Chicago (PhD)
Maine, University of (PhD)
Manitoba, University of (PhD)
Maryland, University of (PhD)
Maryland, University of, Baltimore County (PhD)
Massachusetts, University of (PhD)
Miami, University of (PhD)
Michigan, University of (PhD)
Millersville University (MA/MS, MEd)
Minnesota, University of (PhD)
Missouri, University of (PhD)
Montana, The University of (PhD)
Nebraska, University of, Lincoln (PhD)
Nebraska, University of, Omaha (MA/MS, MA/MS—terminal, PhD)
New Hampshire, University of (PhD)
New Mexico, University of (PhD)
New Orleans, University of (PhD)
New York University (PhD)
North Carolina State University (PhD)
North Carolina, University of, Chapel Hill (PhD)
North Florida, University of (MA/MS—terminal)
Northern Illinois University (PhD)
Northwestern University (PhD)
Notre Dame, University of (PhD)
Ohio State University, The (PhD)
Oklahoma State University (PhD)
Oklahoma, University of (PhD)
Oregon, University of (PhD)
Pennsylvania State University (PhD)
Pennsylvania, University of (MA/MS, PhD)
Pittsburgh, University of (MA/MS, PhD)
Portland State University (PhD)
Purdue University (PhD)
Queen's University (MA/MS, PhD)
Rutgers University—New Brunswick (PhD)
Southern California, University of (PhD)
Stanford University (PhD)
Temple University (PhD)
Texas A&M University (PhD)
Texas of the Permian Basin, The University of (MA/MS—terminal)
Texas, University of, Austin (PhD)
Texas, University of, Dallas (MA/MS—terminal, PhD)
The New School for Social Research (PhD)
Toronto, University of (MA/MS, PhD)
Tufts University (MA/MS, Other, PhD)
Tulane University (PhD)
Utah, University of (PhD)
Vanderbilt University (PhD)
Victoria, University of (PhD)
Virginia Commonwealth University (PhD)
Virginia Polytechnic Institute and State University (PhD)
Virginia, University of (PhD)
Washington University in St. Louis (PhD)
Washington, University of (PhD)
Waterloo, University of (MA/MS—terminal, PhD)
West Virginia University (PhD)
Western Ontario, The University of (PhD)
Wilfrid Laurier University (MA/MS, PhD)
Wisconsin, University of, Madison (PhD)
Wisconsin, University of, Milwaukee (MA/MS—terminal, PhD)
Wyoming, University of (PhD)
Yale University (PhD)
York University (PhD)

E

Educational Psychology
Alliant International University: Irvine (MA/MS—terminal, PsyD)
Alliant International University: Los Angeles (MA/MS—terminal, PsyD)
Alliant International University: San Diego (MA/MS—terminal, PsyD)
Alliant International University: San Francisco (MA/MS—terminal, PsyD)

INDEX OF PROGRAMS BY AREA OF STUDY OFFERED

American International College (EdD, MA/MS)
Arizona State University (MEd, PhD)
Ball State University (MA/MS—terminal, PhD)
City University of New York: Graduate School and University Center (PhD)
East Carolina University (MA/MS—terminal)
Fordham University (MEd, PhD)
Hawaii, University of (MEd, PhD)
Houston, University of (MEd, PhD)
Illinois, University of, Urbana–Champaign (MEd)
Indiana University (MA/MS, PhD)
Iowa, University of (PhD)
Kansas, University of (EdS, MA/MS—terminal, MEd, PhD)
Kean University (MA/MS—terminal)
Kentucky, University of (MA/MS—terminal, PhD)
Marist College (MEd)
Maryland, University of (PhD)
McGill University (PhD)
Michigan, University of (PhD)
Mississippi State University (PhD)
New York University (MA/MS—terminal)
Northern Arizona University (PhD)
Northern Colorado, University of (MA/MS—terminal, PhD)
Oklahoma State University (PhD)
Oklahoma, University of (MEd, PhD)
Rutgers—The State University of New Jersey, New Brunswick (MEd, PhD)
Springfield College (MA/MS—terminal)
Temple University (PhD)
Tennessee, University of, Knoxville (PhD)
Texas A&M International University (MA/MS—terminal)
Texas A&M University (PhD)
Texas A&M University-Commerce (PhD)
Texas Tech University (MA/MS, PhD)
Texas, University of, Austin (MA/MS—terminal, MEd, PhD)
University at Buffalo, State University of New York (MA/MS—terminal, PhD)
Utah, University of (MA/MS—terminal, MEd, Other, PhD)
Walden University (PhD)
Washington State University (MEd, PhD)
Wayne State University (PhD)
Wisconsin, University of, Madison (PhD)
Wisconsin, University of, Milwaukee (PhD)

Environmental Psychology
City University of New York: Graduate School and University Center (PhD)
Humboldt State University (MA/MS—terminal)
Victoria, University of (PhD)

Experimental Psychology (Applied)
Akron, University of (PhD)
Angelo State University (MA/MS—terminal)
Arizona State University (MA/MS—terminal)
Auburn University (MA/MS—terminal, PhD)
Augusta State University (MA/MS—terminal)
California State University, Long Beach (MA/MS—terminal)
Central Florida, University of (PhD)
Central Michigan University (PhD)
Central Washington University (MA/MS—terminal)
Cincinnati, University of (PhD)
Clemson University (PhD)
DePaul University (PhD)
Florida International University (PhD)
Florida, University of (PhD)
Fordham University (PhD)
Fort Hays State University (MA/MS—terminal)
Hawaii, University of, Manoa (PhD)
Idaho, University of (MA/MS—terminal)
Louisiana, University of, Lafayette (MA/MS—terminal)
Louisiana, University of, Monroe (MA/MS—terminal)
Marietta College (MA/MS—terminal)
Memphis, University of (PhD)
Mississippi State University (MA/MS—terminal)
Missouri State University (MA/MS—terminal)
New Brunswick, University of (PhD)
New Mexico State University (PhD)
North Carolina, University of, Wilmington (MA/MS—terminal)
North Texas, University of (PhD)
Oklahoma, University of (PhD)
Old Dominion University (PhD)
Penn State Harrisburg (MA/MS—terminal)
Regina, University of (MA/MS—terminal, PhD)
Rice University (PhD)
Ryerson University (MA/MS, PhD)
Saint Joseph's University (MA/MS—terminal)
Southeastern Louisiana University (MA/MS—terminal)
Tennessee, University of, Chattanooga (MA/MS—terminal)
Texas, University of, Arlington (PhD)
Texas, University of, Pan American (MA/MS)
University at Albany, State University of New York (PhD)
Vanderbilt University (MA/MS—terminal, PhD)
Washington College (MA/MS—terminal)
West Virginia University (PhD)
Wichita State University (PhD)
Wyoming, University of (PhD)

Experimental Psychology (General)
Alabama, University of, at Huntsville (MA/MS—terminal)
Alberta, University of (MA/MS, PhD)
American University (MA/MS—terminal)
Appalachian State University (MA/MS—terminal)
Arkansas, University of (PhD)
California State University, Fullerton (MA/MS—terminal)
California State University, Long Beach (MA/MS—terminal)
California State University, Northridge (MA/MS)
California, University of, San Diego (PhD)
Carnegie Mellon University (PhD)
Case Western Reserve University (PhD)
Central Connecticut State University (MA/MS—terminal)
Central Michigan University (MA/MS—terminal)
Central Oklahoma, University of (MA/MS)
Central Washington University (MA/MS—terminal)
Chicago, University of (PhD)
City University of New York: Brooklyn College (MA/MS—terminal)
Claremont Graduate University (PhD)
College of William and Mary (MA/MS—terminal)
Colorado, University of, at Colorado Springs (MA/MS—terminal)
Dalhousie University (MA/MS, PhD)
East Tennessee State University (MA/MS—terminal)
Eastern Kentucky University (MA/MS—terminal)
Eastern Michigan University (MA/MS—terminal)
Eastern Washington University (MA/MS—terminal)
Emporia State University (MA/MS—terminal)
Florida Atlantic University (MA/MS—terminal, PhD)
Fort Hays State University (MA/MS—terminal)
Georgia Southern University (MA/MS—terminal)
Harvard University (PhD)
Idaho State University (MA/MS—terminal)
Idaho, University of (MA/MS—terminal)
Indiana State University (MA/MS—terminal)
Iona College (MA/MS—terminal)
Kent State University (PhD)
Kentucky, University of (PhD)
Long Island University (MA/MS—terminal)
Louisiana, University of, Lafayette (MA/MS—terminal)
Louisiana, University of, Monroe (MA/MS—terminal)
Louisville, University of (PhD)
Maine, University of (MA/MS)
Marietta College (MA/MS—terminal)
Marist College (MA/MS—terminal)
Massachusetts, University of, Dartmouth (MA/MS—terminal)
McGill University (PhD)
Memphis, University of (MA/MS—terminal)
Miami, University of (MA/MS—terminal)
Middle Tennessee State University (MA/MS—terminal)
Mississippi State University (MA/MS—terminal)
Mississippi, University of (PhD)

891

INDEX OF PROGRAMS BY AREA OF STUDY OFFERED

Missouri State University (MA/MS—terminal)
Montana State University Billings (MA/MS—terminal)
Montana, The University of (PhD)
Morehead State University (Kentucky) (MA/MS—terminal)
Murray State University (MA/MS—terminal)
Nebraska, University of, Lincoln (PhD)
New York University, Graduate School of Arts and Science (PhD)
North Carolina, University of, Wilmington (MA/MS—terminal)
North Dakota, University of (PhD)
Northern Michigan University (MA/MS)
Old Dominion University (MA/MS—terminal)
Ottawa, University of (PhD)
Queen's University (MA/MS, PhD)
Radford University (MA/MS—terminal)
Regina, University of (PhD)
Rhode Island College (MA/MS—terminal)
Ryerson University (MA/MS, PhD)
Saint Joseph's University (MA/MS—terminal)
Sam Houston State University (MA/MS—terminal)
San Jose State University (MA/MS—terminal)
Seton Hall University (MA/MS—terminal)
Simon Fraser University (PhD)
South Alabama, University of (MA/MS—terminal)
South Carolina, University of (PhD)
Southeastern Louisiana University (MA/MS—terminal)
Southern Connecticut State University (MA/MS—terminal)
State University of New York at New Paltz (MA/MS—terminal)
Stony Brook University (PhD)
Syracuse University (PhD)
Tennessee, University of, Knoxville (MA/MS—terminal, PhD)
Texas A&M International University (MA/MS—terminal)
Texas A&M University-Commerce (MA/MS—terminal)
Texas Tech University (PhD)
Texas, University of, Arlington (PhD)
Texas, University of, Austin (PhD)
Texas, University of, Pan American (MA/MS—terminal)
Towson University (MA/MS—terminal)
Tufts University (PhD)
Utah State University (PhD)
Utah, University of (PhD)
Vermont, University of (PhD)
Victoria, University of (PhD)
Villanova University (MA/MS—terminal)
Wake Forest University (MA/MS—terminal)
Walden University (PhD)
Washington College (MA/MS—terminal)
Wayne State University (PhD)
West Chester University of Pennsylvania (MA/MS—terminal)
West Florida, The University of (MA/MS—terminal)
Western Illinois University (MA/MS—terminal)
Wisconsin, University of, Madison (PhD)
Wyoming, University of (PhD)
Xavier University (MA/MS—terminal)

F

Family Psychology
Alliant International University: San Diego (PhD, PsyD)
Antioch University, Santa Barbara (PsyD)
Argosy University/Orange County (EdD)
Azusa Pacific University (MA/MS, PsyD)
California, University of, Riverside (PhD)
Fuller Theological Seminary (PhD, PsyD)
Lewis & Clark College, Graduate School of Education and Counseling (MA/MS—terminal)
North Carolina State University (PhD)
Pennsylvania State University (PhD)
Portland State University (PhD)
Texas, University of, Tyler (MA/MS—terminal)
The Chicago School of Professional Psychology (MA/MS—terminal, PsyD)
University of the Rockies (MA/MS—terminal)
Vanguard University of Southern California (MA/MS—terminal)
Wayne State University (MA/MS)
Wheaton College (MA/MS—terminal)

Forensic Psychology
Adler School of Professional Psychology (MA/MS—terminal)
Alliant International University: Fresno (PhD, PsyD)
Alliant International University: Irvine (PsyD)
Alliant International University: Los Angeles (PsyD)
Alliant International University: Sacramento (PsyD)
Alliant International University: San Diego (PsyD)
American International College (MA/MS—terminal)
Argosy University/Orange County (MA/MS—terminal)
Arizona State University (PhD)
Arizona, The University of (PhD)
Baltimore, University of (MA/MS—terminal)
British Columbia, University of (PhD)
Carleton University (MA/MS—terminal, PhD)
City University of New York: John Jay College of Criminal Justice (MA/MS—terminal)
Denver, University of (MA/MS—terminal)
Drexel University (PhD)
Fairleigh Dickinson University, Metropolitan Campus (MA/MS—terminal)
Florida International University (PhD)
Marymount University (MA/MS—terminal)
Massachusetts School of Professional Psychology (MA/MS—terminal, PsyD)
Missouri State University (MA/MS—terminal)
Nebraska, University of, Lincoln (PhD)
Palo Alto University (Other)
Roger Williams University (MA/MS—terminal)
Sage Colleges, The (Other)
Saskatchewan, University of (PhD)
The Chicago School of Professional Psychology (MA/MS—terminal, Other, PsyD)
Tulsa, University of (MA/MS, MA/MS—terminal)
Widener University (Other)
Wisconsin School of Professional Psychology (PsyD)

G

Gender Psychology
Goddard College (MA/MS—terminal)
Hawaii, University of, Manoa (PhD)
Texas Woman's University (MA/MS—terminal, PhD)

General Psychology (Theory, History, and Philosophy)
Adelphi University (MA/MS—terminal)
Angelo State University (MA/MS—terminal)
Arizona, The University of (PhD)
Boston University (MA/MS—terminal)
Brandeis University (MA/MS—terminal)
Brigham Young University (MA/MS—terminal, PhD)
California State University, Sacramento (MA/MS—terminal)
Central Oklahoma, University of (MA/MS—terminal)
Dayton, University of (MA/MS—terminal)
DePaul University (MA/MS—terminal)
Drexel University (MA/MS—terminal)
Fairleigh Dickinson University, Metropolitan Campus (MA/MS—terminal)
Goddard College (MA/MS—terminal)
Hartford, University of (MA/MS—terminal)
Indiana University-Purdue University Indianapolis (PhD)
Institute for the Psychological Sciences (MA/MS—terminal)
Long Island University (MA/MS—terminal)
Marist College (MA/MS—terminal)
Marshall University (MA/MS—terminal)
Marywood University (MA/MS—terminal)
Memphis, University of (MA/MS—terminal)
New Mexico Highlands University (MA/MS—terminal)
New York University, Graduate School of Arts and Science (MA/MS—terminal)
North Florida, University of (MA/MS—terminal)

INDEX OF PROGRAMS BY AREA OF STUDY OFFERED

Northcentral University (MA/MS, PhD)
Northern Arizona University (MA/MS—terminal)
Northern Iowa, University of (MA/MS)
Pace University (MA/MS—terminal)
Palo Alto University (MA/MS—terminal)
Pennsylvania, University of (PhD)
Pittsburg State University (MA/MS—terminal)
Saint Francis, University of (MA/MS—terminal)
Sam Houston State University (MA/MS—terminal)
Seton Hall University (MA/MS, MEd)
Southern Connecticut State University (MA/MS—terminal)
State University of New York at New Paltz (MA/MS—terminal)
Stephen F. Austin State University (MA/MS—terminal)
The Chicago School of Professional Psychology (MA/MS—terminal, PsyD)
The New School for Social Research (MA/MS—terminal)
University at Buffalo, State University of New York (MA/MS—terminal)
University of the Rockies (MA/MS)
Virginia State University (MA/MS—terminal)
Walden University (MA/MS—terminal)
Washburn University (MA/MS—terminal)
West Chester University of Pennsylvania (MA/MS—terminal)
West Florida, The University of (MA/MS—terminal)
Yeshiva University (MA/MS—terminal)
York University (PhD)

Geropsychology
Adler School of Professional Psychology (MA/MS—terminal)
Akron, University of (PhD)
Brenau University (MA/MS—terminal)
Colorado, University of, at Colorado Springs (PhD)
Florida, University of (PhD)
North Carolina State University (PhD)
Washington University in St. Louis (PhD)
West Virginia University (PhD)
Yeshiva University (PsyD)

H

Health Psychology
Alabama, University of, at Birmingham (PhD)
Antioch University, Seattle (PsyD)
Appalachian State University (MA/MS—terminal)
Brandeis University (PhD)
British Columbia, University of (PhD)
California, University of, Irvine (PhD)
California, University of, Los Angeles (PhD)
California, University of, Merced (PhD)
California, University of, Riverside (PhD)
Carleton University (MA/MS—terminal, PhD)
Carnegie Mellon University (PhD)
Central Connecticut State University (MA/MS—terminal)
City University of New York: Graduate School and University Center (PhD)
Claremont Graduate University (MA/MS—terminal)
Clemson University (PhD)
Colorado, University of, Boulder (PhD)
Colorado, University of, Denver (PhD)
Connecticut, University of (PhD)
Drexel University (PhD)
Duke University (MA/MS, PhD)
East Tennessee State University (PhD)
George Fox University (PsyD)
George Washington University (PhD)
Guelph, University of (MA/MS, PhD)
Houston, University of (PhD)
Indiana University-Purdue University Indianapolis (MA/MS—terminal, PhD)
Indianapolis, University of (PsyD)
Iowa, University of (PhD)
Kansas State University (Other)
Kansas, University of (PhD)
Kent State University (PhD)
Kentucky, University of (PhD)
Memphis, University of (PhD)
Midwestern University (PsyD)
Missouri, University of, Kansas City (PhD)
New Mexico State University (PhD)
New Mexico, University of (PhD)
North Carolina State University (PhD)
North Carolina, University of, Charlotte (PhD)
North Dakota State University (PhD)
North Texas, University of (PhD)
Northern Arizona University (MA/MS—terminal)
Ohio State University, The (PhD)
Ohio University (PhD)
Old Dominion University (PhD)
Our Lady of the Lake University (PsyD)
Philadelphia College of Osteopathic Medicine (Other)
Pittsburgh, University of (PhD)
Rhode Island, University of, Chafee Social Sciences Center (PhD)
Rosalind Franklin University of Medicine and Science (PhD)
Rutgers University—New Brunswick (PhD)
Seattle Pacific University (PhD)
Southern California, University of, Keck School of Medicine (PhD)
Stony Brook University (PhD)
Syracuse University (PhD)
Texas State University-San Marcos (MA/MS—terminal)
Texas, University of, Arlington (PhD)
The New School for Social Research (MA/MS—terminal)
Uniformed Services University of the Health Sciences (PhD)
Utah, University of (PhD)
Virginia Commonwealth University (PhD)
Virginia State University (PhD)
Walden University (PhD)
Wisconsin, University of, Milwaukee (MA/MS—terminal, PhD)
Wisconsin, University of, Stout (MA/MS—terminal)
Yeshiva University (PhD)

Human Development and Family Studies
Concordia University (PhD)
Cornell University (PhD)
Illinois, University of, Urbana–Champaign (MA/MS—terminal, PhD)
Pennsylvania State University, The (PhD)
Texas, University of, Austin (PhD)
Wisconsin, University of, Madison (MA/MS, PhD)

Human Factors
Arizona State University (MA/MS—terminal)
California State University, Long Beach (MA/MS—terminal)
California State University, Northridge (MA/MS—terminal)
Central Florida, University of (PhD)
Cincinnati, University of (PhD)
Clemson University (PhD)
Connecticut, University of (PhD)
George Mason University (MA/MS—terminal, PhD)
Idaho, University of (MA/MS—terminal)
Kansas State University (PhD)
New Mexico State University (PhD)
North Carolina State University (PhD)
Old Dominion University (PhD)
Rice University (PhD)
South Dakota, University of (PhD)
Texas Tech University (PhD)
Wichita State University (PhD)
Wright State University (PhD)

Humanistic Psychology
Saybrook University (MA/MS), MA/MS, PhD)
West Georgia, University of (MA/MS—terminal, PsyD)

I

Industrial/Organizational Psychology
Adler School of Professional Psychology (MA/MS—terminal)
Akron, University of (MA/MS—terminal, PhD)
Alliant International University: Fresno/Sacramento (MA/MS—terminal, PsyD)
Alliant International University: Los Angeles (MA/MS—terminal, PhD, Respecialization Diploma)
Alliant International University: San Diego (MA/MS—terminal, PhD, Respecialization Diploma)
Alliant International University: San Francisco (MA/MS—terminal, PhD, Respecialization Diploma)
Angelo State University (MA/MS—terminal)

INDEX OF PROGRAMS BY AREA OF STUDY OFFERED

Appalachian State University (MA/MS—terminal)
Auburn University (PhD)
Austin Peay State University (MA/MS—terminal)
Baltimore, University of (MA/MS—terminal)
Bowling Green State University (PhD)
Calgary, University of (PhD)
California State University, Long Beach (MA/MS—terminal)
California State University, Sacramento (MA/MS—terminal)
Carnegie Mellon University (PhD)
Central Florida, University of (MA/MS—terminal, PhD)
Central Michigan University (MA/MS—terminal, PhD)
City University of New York: Brooklyn College (MA/MS—terminal)
City University of New York: Graduate School and University Center (PhD)
Claremont Graduate University (MA/MS—terminal, PhD)
Clemson University (PhD)
Colorado State University (PhD)
Connecticut, University of (PhD)
DePaul University (PhD)
East Carolina University (MA/MS—terminal)
Eastern Kentucky University (MA/MS—terminal)
Emporia State University (MA/MS—terminal)
Florida Institute of Technology (MA/MS, MA/MS—terminal, PhD)
Florida International University (PhD)
George Mason University (MA/MS—terminal, PhD)
Georgia, University of (PhD)
Goddard College (MA/MS—terminal)
Guelph, University of (MA/MS, PhD)
Hartford, University of (MA/MS—terminal)
Harvard University (PhD)
Hofstra University (MA/MS—terminal, PhD)
Houston, University of (PhD)
Idaho, University of (MA/MS—terminal)
Illinois Institute of Technology (MA/MS—terminal, PhD)
Illinois State University (MA/MS—terminal)
Illinois, University of, Urbana–Champaign (MA/MS—terminal, PhD)
Indiana University-Purdue University Indianapolis (MA/MS—terminal)
Iona College (MA/MS—terminal)
Kansas State University (MA/MS—terminal, Other, PhD)
Kean University (MA/MS—terminal)
Lamar University-Beaumont (MA/MS—terminal)
Louisiana Tech University (MA/MS—terminal, PhD)
Maryland, University of (PhD)
Massachusetts School of Professional Psychology (MA/MS—terminal, Other)
Michigan State University (PhD)
Middle Tennessee State University (MA/MS—terminal)
Minnesota State University—Mankato (MA/MS—terminal)
Minnesota, University of (PhD)
Missouri State University (MA/MS—terminal)
Missouri, University of, St. Louis (PhD)
Nebraska, University of, Omaha (MA/MS, MA/MS—terminal, PhD)
Nevada, University of, Reno (PhD)
New Haven, University of (MA/MS—terminal)
New York University, Graduate School of Arts and Science (MA/MS—terminal)
North Carolina State University (PhD)
North Carolina, University of, Charlotte (MA/MS—terminal, PhD)
Northern Arizona University (MA/MS—terminal, MEd)
Northern Illinois University (PhD)
Northern Iowa, University of (MA/MS—terminal)
Northern Kentucky University (MA/MS—terminal)
Northern Michigan University (MA/MS—terminal)
Ohio University (PhD)
Oklahoma, University of (MA/MS—terminal, PhD)
Old Dominion University (PhD)
Palo Alto University (Other)
Pennsylvania State University (PhD)
Philadelphia College of Osteopathic Medicine (MA/MS—terminal)
Portland State University (PhD)
Puerto Rico, University of (PhD)
Purdue University (PhD)
Radford University (MA/MS—terminal)
Rice University (PhD)
Roosevelt University (MA/MS—terminal)
Saint Mary's University (MA/MS—terminal, PhD)
San Diego State University (MA/MS—terminal)
San Jose State University (MA/MS—terminal)
Saybrook University (MA/MS, PhD)
Sonoma State University (MA/MS)
South Florida, University of (PhD)
Southeastern Louisiana University (Other)
Southern Illinois University Carbondale (PhD)
Southern Illinois University Edwardsville (MA/MS—terminal)
Springfield College (MA/MS—terminal)
St. Cloud State University (MA/MS—terminal)
Temple University (MA/MS—terminal)
Tennessee, University of, Chattanooga (MA/MS—terminal)
Tennessee, University of, Knoxville (PhD)
Texas A&M University (PhD)
Texas, University of, Arlington (MA/MS—terminal)
The Chicago School of Professional Psychology (MA/MS—terminal, Other, PhD, PsyD)
Towson University (MA/MS)
Tulsa, University of (MA/MS, MA/MS—terminal, PhD)
University at Albany, State University of New York (MA/MS—terminal, PhD)
Virginia Polytechnic Institute and State University (PhD)
Walden University (MA/MS—terminal, PhD)
Waterloo, University of (MA/MS—terminal, PhD)
Wayne State University (MA/MS—terminal, PhD)
West Chester University of Pennsylvania (MA/MS—terminal)
West Florida, The University of (MA/MS—terminal)
Western Ontario, The University of (PhD)
Windsor, University of (PhD)
Wisconsin, University of, Stout (MA/MS—terminal)
Wright State University (PhD)
Xavier University (MA/MS—terminal)

M

Marriage and Family Therapy
Adler School of Professional Psychology (MA/MS—terminal)
Alliant International University: Irvine (MA/MS—terminal, PsyD)
Alliant International University: Los Angeles (MA/MS—terminal)
Alliant International University: Sacramento (MA/MS—terminal, PsyD)
Alliant International University: San Diego (MA/MS—terminal, PsyD)
Argosy University/Orange County (MA/MS—terminal)
Azusa Pacific University (MA/MS—terminal)
California Lutheran University (MA/MS—terminal)
California Polytechnic State University (MA/MS—terminal)
Geneva College (MA/MS)
Gonzaga University (MA/MS—terminal)
Kean University (Other)
La Salle University (MA/MS)
Lewis & Clark College, Graduate School of Education and Counseling (MA/MS—terminal)
Massachusetts, University of, Boston (MA/MS—terminal)
Miami, University of (MA/MS—terminal)
Northcentral University (MA/MS, PhD)
Oklahoma, University of (PhD)
Our Lady of the Lake University (MA/MS—terminal)
Saint Mary's University of Minnesota (MA/MS—terminal, Other)
Seton Hall University (EdS, MA/MS)
Springfield College (MA/MS—terminal)
The Chicago School of Professional Psychology (MA/MS—terminal, PsyD)

University of the Rockies (MA/MS—terminal)
Wayne State University (MA/MS)

Mental Health Counseling
Boston College (MA/MS—terminal)
Central Washington University (MA/MS—terminal)
City University of New York: Brooklyn College (MA/MS—terminal)
City University of New York: John Jay College of Criminal Justice (MA/MS—terminal)
Florida State University (MA/MS—terminal)
Fordham University (MEd)
Geneva College (MA/MS)
Indiana State University (MA/MS)
Indianapolis, University of (MA/MS—terminal)
Iona College (MA/MS—terminal)
Marist College (MA/MS—terminal)
Marquette University (MA/MS—terminal)
Marywood University (MA/MS—terminal)
Massachusetts, University of, Boston (MA/MS—terminal)
Miami, University of (MA/MS—terminal)
Michigan School of Professional Psychology (MA/MS—terminal)
Middle Tennessee State University (MEd)
Missouri, University of, Kansas City (EdS, MA/MS—terminal)
New Mexico State University (MA/MS—terminal)
Northeastern University (MA/MS—terminal)
Nova Southeastern University (MA/MS—terminal)
Pennsylvania, University of (MEd)
Rosalind Franklin University of Medicine and Science (MA/MS—terminal)
Rowan University (MA/MS—terminal)
Saint Francis, University of (MA/MS—terminal)
Saybrook University (MA/MS)
Seton Hall University (EdS)
Springfield College (MA/MS—terminal)
State University of New York at New Paltz (MA/MS—terminal)
University at Buffalo, State University of New York (MA/MS—terminal)
Vanderbilt University (MEd)
West Florida, The University of (MA/MS—terminal)

Multicultural Psychology
Alliant International University: Los Angeles (PhD, PsyD)
Alliant International University: San Francisco (PhD, PsyD)
Denver, University of (PsyD)
Fordham University (Other)
Goddard College (MA/MS—terminal)
Hawaii, University of, Manoa (PhD)
John F. Kennedy University (PsyD)
Massachusetts, University of, Lowell (MA/MS—terminal)
Memphis, University of (PhD)

New Mexico State University (EdS)
Pennsylvania, University of (PhD)
The Chicago School of Professional Psychology (PhD)
Utah State University (PhD)

N

Neuropsychology
Arizona, The University of (PhD)
Boston University (PhD)
Brigham Young University (PhD)
Chicago, University of (PhD)
Cincinnati, University of (PhD)
City University of New York: Graduate Center (PhD)
City University of New York: Graduate School and University Center (PhD)
Colorado State University (PhD)
Concordia University (PhD)
Connecticut, University of (PhD)
Delaware, University of (PhD)
Drexel University (PhD)
Duke University (PhD)
Fielding Graduate University (Other)
George Washington University (PhD)
Georgia State University (PhD)
Houston, University of (PhD)
Idaho, University of (PhD)
Michigan State University (PhD)
New Mexico, University of (PhD)
Old Dominion University (PsyD)
Philadelphia College of Osteopathic Medicine (Other)
Purdue University (PhD)
Rice University (PhD)
San Diego State University (MA/MS)
Saskatchewan, University of (PhD)
South Florida, University of (PhD)
Temple University (PhD)
Texas Woman's University (PhD)
Utah, University of (PhD)
Victoria, University of (PhD)
Virginia Consortium Program in Clinical Psychology (PsyD)
Washington State University (PhD)
Wayne State University (PhD)
Yale University (PhD)
Yeshiva University (PhD, PsyD)

Neuroscience
Alabama, University of, at Birmingham (PhD)
American University (PhD)
Arizona State University (PhD)
Arizona, The University of (PhD)
Baylor University (PhD)
Boston College (PhD)
Bowling Green State University (PhD)
Brandeis University (PhD)
British Columbia, University of (PhD)
California, University of, Berkeley (PhD)
California, University of, Davis (PhD)
California, University of, Irvine (PhD)
California, University of, Los Angeles (PhD)
California, University of, Riverside (PhD)

Carleton University (MA/MS)
City University of New York (PhD)
City University of New York: Brooklyn College (PhD)
City University of New York: Graduate Center (PhD)
City University of New York: Graduate School and University Center (PhD)
Colorado, University of, Boulder (PhD)
Concordia University (PhD)
Connecticut, University of (PhD)
Cornell University (PhD)
Dalhousie University (MA/MS, PhD)
Delaware, University of (PhD)
Denver, University of (PhD)
Drexel University (PhD)
Duke University (PhD)
Emory University (PhD)
Florida State University (PhD)
Florida, University of (PhD)
George Washington University (PhD)
Georgia, University of (PhD)
Guelph, University of (MA/MS, PhD)
Hawaii, University of, Manoa (PhD)
Houston, University of (PhD)
Idaho, University of (PhD)
Illinois, University of, Urbana–Champaign (PhD)
Indiana University (PhD)
Iowa, University of (PhD)
Johns Hopkins University (PhD)
Kansas State University (PhD)
Kansas, University of (PhD)
Manitoba, University of (PhD)
Maryland, University of (PhD)
Massachusetts, University of (PhD)
Miami, University of (PhD)
Michigan, University of (PhD)
Missouri, University of (PhD)
Missouri, University of, St. Louis (PhD)
Nebraska, University of, Omaha (MA/MS, PhD)
Nevada, University of, Las Vegas (PhD)
Nevada, University of, Reno (PhD)
New Hampshire, University of (PhD)
North Dakota State University (PhD)
Northeastern University (PhD)
Northern Illinois University (PhD)
Northwestern University (PhD)
Ohio State University, The (PhD)
Oregon, University of (PhD)
Pittsburgh, University of (PhD)
Rice University (PhD)
Rutgers University—New Brunswick (PhD)
Seton Hall University (MA/MS—terminal)
South Carolina, University of (PhD)
Southern California, University of (PhD)
Southern Illinois University Carbondale (PhD)
Stanford University (PhD)
State University of New York, Binghamton University (PhD)
Stony Brook University (PhD)
Texas A&M University (PhD)
Texas Christian University (PhD)
Texas, University of, Austin (PhD)
Toronto, University of (MA/MS, PhD)
Tulane University (PhD)

INDEX OF PROGRAMS BY AREA OF STUDY OFFERED

University at Buffalo, State University of New York (PhD)
Vanderbilt University (PhD)
Victoria, University of (PhD)
Virginia, University of (PhD)
Washington, University of (PhD)
Waterloo, University of (PhD)
Wayne State University (PhD)
West Virginia University (PhD)
Western Ontario, The University of (PhD)
Wilfrid Laurier University (MA/MS—terminal, PhD)
Wisconsin, University of, Madison (PhD)
Wisconsin, University of, Milwaukee (PhD)
Yale University (PhD)
York University (PhD)

O

Other
Adelphi University (MA/MS—terminal)
Central Arkansas, University of (MA/MS—terminal)
City University of New York: Graduate School and University Center (PhD)
Denver, University of (MA/MS—terminal)
Fielding Graduate University (MA/MS—terminal, PhD)
Houston, University of (MEd)
Miami, University of (PhD)
Mississippi State University (PhD)
Northeastern University (MA/MS—terminal, Other)
Pittsburg State University (MA/MS, MA/MS—terminal)
Pittsburgh, University of (PhD)
Puerto Rico, University of (PhD)
Temple University (MA/MS—terminal)
Wisconsin, University of, Madison (PhD)

P

Personality Psychology
Boston College (PhD)
British Columbia, University of (PhD)
California, University of, Berkeley (PhD)
California, University of, Davis (PhD)
Cornell University (PhD)
Florida State University (PhD)
Illinois, University of, Chicago (PhD)
Illinois, University of, Urbana–Champaign (PhD)
Iowa, University of (PhD)
Kansas State University (PhD)
Manitoba, University of (PhD)
Michigan State University (PhD)
Michigan, University of (PhD)
Minnesota, University of (PhD)
Missouri, University of (PhD)
Nebraska, University of, Lincoln (PhD)
New Hampshire, University of (PhD)
Northeastern University (PhD)
Northwestern University (PhD)
Oklahoma, University of (PhD)
Oregon, University of (PhD)

Queen's University (MA/MS, PhD)
Stanford University (PhD)
Texas Tech University (PhD)
Toronto, University of (MA/MS, PhD)
Washington University in St. Louis (PhD)
Washington, University of (PhD)
Western Ontario, The University of (PhD)
Wisconsin, University of, Madison (PhD)
York University (PhD)

Physiological Psychology
Alabama, University of, at Birmingham (PhD)
Boston University (PhD)
Denver, University of (PhD)
Hawaii, University of, Manoa (PhD)
Nebraska, University of, Lincoln (PhD)
Nebraska, University of, Omaha (PhD)
New Mexico, University of (PhD)
New Orleans, University of (PhD)
Northeastern University (PhD)
Northwestern University (PhD)
Ohio University (PhD)
Oklahoma, University of (PhD)
Purdue University (PhD)
Texas A&M University (PhD)
Tulane University (PhD)
West Virginia University (PhD)
Widener University (PsyD)

Psychoanalytic Psychology
Adelphi University (Other)
City University of New York: Graduate School and University Center (PhD)
Sonoma State University (MA/MS)
The New School for Social Research (PhD)

Psycholinguistics
Delaware, University of (PhD)
Denver, University of (PhD)
Illinois, University of, Urbana–Champaign (PhD)
Illinois, University of, Urbana–Champaign (PhD)
Iowa, University of (PhD)
Northeastern University (PhD)

Psychopharmacology
Alliant International University: San Francisco (MA/MS—terminal)
Auburn University (PhD)
Fairleigh Dickinson University, Metropolitan Campus (MA/MS—terminal)
Iowa, University of (PhD)
Nova Southeastern University (MA/MS—terminal)
State University of New York, Binghamton University (PhD)

Q

Quantitative Psychology
Arizona State University (PhD)
Boston College (PhD)
British Columbia, University of (PhD)
California, University of, Davis (PhD)

California, University of, Los Angeles (PhD)
California, University of, Merced (PhD)
Claremont Graduate University (MA/MS—terminal, PhD)
Fordham University (PhD)
Hawaii, University of, Manoa (PhD)
Houston, University of (MEd, PhD)
Illinois State University (MA/MS—terminal)
Illinois, University of, Urbana–Champaign (PhD)
Illinois, University of, Urbana–Champaign (MA/MS—terminal, PhD)
Iowa, University of (MA/MS, PhD)
Kansas, University of (MEd, PhD)
Manitoba, University of (PhD)
Middle Tennessee State University (MA/MS—terminal)
Minnesota, University of (PhD)
Missouri, University of (PhD)
Nebraska, University of, Lincoln (PhD)
North Carolina State University (PhD)
North Carolina, University of, Chapel Hill (PhD)
Notre Dame, University of (PhD)
Ohio State University, The (PhD)
Ohio University (PhD)
Oklahoma, University of (PhD)
Penn State Harrisburg (MA/MS—terminal)
Purdue University (PhD)
Rhode Island, University of, Chafee Social Sciences Center (PhD)
Southern California, University of (PhD)
Tennessee, University of, Knoxville (PhD)
Texas of the Permian Basin, The University of (MA/MS—terminal)
Texas, University of, Austin (PhD)
Utah, University of (PhD)
Vanderbilt University (PhD)
Virginia, University of (PhD)
Wisconsin, University of, Madison (PhD)
Wisconsin, University of, Milwaukee (MA/MS, PhD)
York University (PhD)

R

Rehabilitation Psychology
Adler School of Professional Psychology (MA/MS—terminal)
Ball State University (MA/MS—terminal)
Florida State University (MA/MS—terminal)
Illinois Institute of Technology (MA/MS—terminal, PhD)
Massachusetts, University of, Boston (MA/MS—terminal)
University at Buffalo, State University of New York (MA/MS—terminal)

S

School Counseling
Arcadia University (MA/MS—terminal)
Austin Peay State University (MA/MS—terminal)

INDEX OF PROGRAMS BY AREA OF STUDY OFFERED

Boston College (MA/MS—terminal)
Cleveland State University (MEd)
Fordham University (MEd)
Geneva College (MA/MS)
Gonzaga University (MA/MS—terminal)
Houston, University of (MEd)
Immaculata University (MA/MS, MA/MS—terminal)
Lehigh University (MEd)
Lewis University (MA/MS—terminal)
Louisiana Tech University (MA/MS—terminal)
Louisiana, University of, Lafayette (MA/MS—terminal)
Loyola University of Chicago (MEd)
Marywood University (MA/MS—terminal)
Massachusetts, University of, Boston (MA/MS—terminal)
Middle Tennessee State University (MEd)
Millersville University (MEd)
Missouri, University of, Kansas City (EdS)
Northeastern University (MA/MS—terminal)
Northern Arizona University (MEd)
Nova Southeastern University (MA/MS—terminal)
Pennsylvania, University of (MEd, Other)
Puget Sound, University of (MEd)
Roberts Wesleyan College (MA/MS—terminal)
Rutgers—The State University of New Jersey, New Brunswick (MEd)
Saint Francis, University of (MEd)
Seton Hall University (MA/MS, MEd)
Springfield College (EdS)
State University of New York at New Paltz (MA/MS—terminal)
Texas, University of, Austin (MEd)
Texas, University of, Tyler (MA/MS—terminal)
University at Buffalo, State University of New York (MEd)
Utah State University (MA/MS—terminal)
Utah, University of (MEd)
Vanderbilt University (MEd)
Washington State University (MEd)
Wisconsin, University of, Milwaukee (MA/MS)

School Psychology

Adelphi University (MA/MS—terminal)
Alfred University (EdS, PsyD)
Alliant International University: Irvine (MA/MS—terminal, PsyD)
Alliant International University: Los Angeles (MA/MS—terminal, PsyD)
Alliant International University: San Diego (MA/MS—terminal, PsyD)
Alliant International University: San Francisco (MA/MS—terminal, PsyD)
Appalachian State University (EdS)
Arizona State University (PhD)
Ball State University (EdS, MA/MS, PhD)
Brigham Young University (EdS)
California, University of, Berkeley (PhD)
California, University of, Santa Barbara (MEd, PhD)
Central Arkansas, University of (MA/MS—terminal, PhD)
Central Michigan University (Other, PhD)
Central Washington University (MEd)
Cincinnati, University of (EdS, PhD)
Citadel, The (EdS)
City University of New York: Brooklyn College (MA/MS)
Columbia University (MEd, PhD)
Connecticut, University of (MA/MS, PhD)
Denver, University of (EdS, MA/MS, PhD)
Duquesne University (Other, PhD)
East Carolina University (MA/MS—terminal, PhD)
Eastern Illinois University (Other)
Eastern Kentucky University (Other)
Eastern Washington University (MA/MS—terminal, Respecialization Diploma)
Emporia State University (EdS)
Fairleigh Dickinson University, Metropolitan Campus (MA/MS—terminal, PsyD)
Florida State University (EdS, PhD)
Fordham University (Other, PhD)
Fort Hays State University (EdS)
Francis Marion University (MA/MS—terminal)
Gallaudet University (Other)
George Mason University (MA/MS—terminal)
Georgia, University of (PhD)
Hartford, University of (MA/MS—terminal)
Hofstra University (PsyD)
Houston, University of (PhD)
Humboldt State University (MA/MS—terminal)
Illinois State University (Other, PhD)
Immaculata University (MA/MS—terminal, PsyD)
Indiana State University (EdS, MEd, PhD)
Indiana University (EdS, PhD)
Iona College (MA/MS—terminal)
Iowa, University of (PhD)
Kansas, University of (EdS, PhD)
Kean University (Other, PsyD)
Kent State University (EdS, PhD)
Kentucky, University of (EdS, MA/MS, PhD)
Lehigh University (EdS, PhD)
Lewis & Clark College, Graduate School of Education and Counseling (EdS)
Louisiana State University Shreveport (Other)
Manitoba, University of (MA/MS—terminal)
Marist College (MA/MS—terminal)
Maryland, University of (PhD)
Marywood University (EdS)
Massachusetts School of Professional Psychology (MA/MS—terminal, PsyD)
Massachusetts, University of, Boston (EdS)
McGill University (PhD)
Memphis, University of (MA/MS—terminal, PhD)
Middle Tennessee State University (EdS)
Millersville University (MA/MS)
Minnesota State University—Mankato (PsyD)
Minnesota State University—Moorhead (EdS)
Minnesota, University of (EdS, PhD)
Mississippi State University (PhD)
Montana, The University of (MA/MS, PhD)
Nebraska, University of, Lincoln (PhD)
Nebraska, University of, Omaha (EdS, MA/MS)
New Mexico State University (EdS)
North Carolina State University (PhD)
Northeastern University (MA/MS—terminal, PhD)
Northern Arizona University (Other, PhD)
Northern Colorado, University of (EdS, Other, PhD)
Northern Illinois University (PhD)
Nova Southeastern University (Other)
Ohio State University (MA/MS—terminal, PhD)
Oklahoma State University (EdS, PhD)
Our Lady of the Lake University (MA/MS—terminal)
Pace University (EdS, PsyD)
Pennsylvania State University (PhD)
Philadelphia College of Osteopathic Medicine (EdS, MA/MS—terminal, PsyD, Respecialization Diploma)
Pittsburg State University (EdS)
Radford University (EdS)
Rhode Island, University of, Chafee Social Sciences Center (MA/MS—terminal, PhD)
Roberts Wesleyan College (MA/MS—terminal)
Rutgers—The State University of New Jersey (PsyD)
Sam Houston State University (MA/MS—terminal)
Seton Hall University (EdS)
South Carolina, University of (PhD)
South Florida, University of (EdS, PhD)
Southern Illinois University Edwardsville (EdS, MA/MS—terminal)
State University of New York, College at Plattsburgh (MA/MS—terminal)
Syracuse University (PhD)
Temple University (MA/MS, PhD)
Tennessee, University of, Knoxville (PhD)
Texas A&M University (PhD)
Texas A&M University-Commerce (EdS)
Texas Woman's University (EdS, PhD)
Texas, University of, Austin (PhD)
Texas, University of, Tyler (MA/MS—terminal)
The Chicago School of Professional Psychology (EdS)
Towson University (MA/MS)
Tufts University (EdS)
Tulane University (PhD)
University at Buffalo, State University of New York (MA/MS—terminal, PhD)
Utah State University (EdS)
Utah, University of (PhD)
Virginia, University of (PhD)
Walden University (PhD)
Wayne State University (MA/MS)
Western Illinois University (Other)

INDEX OF PROGRAMS BY AREA OF STUDY OFFERED

Winthrop University (Other)
Wisconsin, University of, Eau Claire (EdS)
Wisconsin, University of, La Crosse (EdS)
Wisconsin, University of, Madison (PhD)
Wisconsin, University of, Milwaukee (EdS, PhD)

Social Psychology
Alabama, University of (PhD)
American University (MA/MS—terminal)
Arizona State University (PhD)
Arizona, The University of (PhD)
Ball State University (MA/MS—terminal)
Baylor University (PhD)
Boston College (PhD)
Brandeis University (PhD)
Brigham Young University (PhD)
British Columbia, University of (PhD)
California, University of, Berkeley (PhD)
California, University of, Davis (PhD)
California, University of, Irvine (PhD)
California, University of, Los Angeles (PhD)
California, University of, Riverside (PhD)
California, University of, Santa Cruz (PhD)
Carnegie Mellon University (PhD)
Chicago, University of (PhD)
City University of New York: Graduate School and University Center (PhD)
Claremont Graduate University (MA/MS—terminal, PhD)
Clark University (PhD)
Colorado State University (PhD)
Colorado, University of, Boulder (PhD)
Connecticut, University of (PhD)
Cornell University (PhD)
Dayton, University of (MA/MS—terminal)
Delaware, University of (PhD)
Denver, University of (PhD)
Duke University (PhD)
Florida State University (PhD)
Florida, University of (PhD)
George Washington University (PhD)
Georgia State University (PhD)
Georgia, University of (PhD)
Guelph, University of (MA/MS, PhD)
Harvard University (PhD)
Hawaii, University of, Manoa (PhD)
Houston, University of (PhD)
Illinois State University (MA/MS—terminal)
Illinois, University of, Chicago (PhD)
Illinois, University of, Urbana–Champaign (PhD)
Indiana University (PhD)
Iowa State University (PhD)
Iowa, University of (PhD)
Kansas State University (PhD)
Kansas, University of (PhD)
Lehigh University (PhD)
Loyola University of Chicago (MA/MS—terminal, PhD)
Maine, University of (PhD)
Manitoba, University of (PhD)
Maryland, University of (PhD)
Massachusetts, University of (PhD)
Miami University of Ohio (PhD)
Michigan State University (PhD)
Michigan, University of (PhD)
Minnesota, University of (PhD)
Missouri, University of (PhD)
Montana State University (MA/MS)
Nebraska, University of, Lincoln (PhD)
Nebraska, University of, Omaha (MA/MS)
New Hampshire, University of (PhD)
New Mexico State University (MA/MS, PhD)
New York University, Graduate School of Arts and Science (PhD)
North Carolina, University of, Chapel Hill (PhD)
North Dakota State University (PhD)
Northeastern University (PhD)
Northern Illinois University (PhD)
Northern Iowa, University of (MA/MS—terminal)
Northwestern University (PhD)
Ohio State University, The (PhD)
Ohio University (PhD)
Oklahoma, University of (PhD)
Oregon, University of (MA/MS—terminal, PhD)
Pennsylvania State University (PhD)
Pittsburgh, University of (PhD)
Portland State University (PhD)
Puerto Rico, University of (PhD)
Purdue University (PhD)
Queen's University (MA/MS, PhD)
Rutgers University—New Brunswick (PhD)
San Diego State University (MA/MS)
Saskatchewan, University of (PhD)
Southern California, University of (PhD)
Southern Illinois University Carbondale (PhD)
Stanford University (PhD)
Stony Brook University (PhD)
Syracuse University (PhD)
Temple University (PhD)
Texas A&M University (PhD)
Texas Christian University (PhD)
Texas Tech University (PhD)
Texas, University of, Austin (PhD)
Texas, University of, Dallas (MA/MS—terminal)
Texas, University of, El Paso (PhD)
The New School for Social Research (MA/MS—terminal, PhD)
Toledo, University of (PhD)
Toronto, University of (MA/MS, PhD)
Tulane University (PhD)
University at Albany, State University of New York (PhD)
University at Buffalo, State University of New York (PhD)
Utah, University of (PhD)
Victoria, University of (PhD)
Virginia Commonwealth University (PhD)
Virginia, University of (PhD)
Washington University in St. Louis (PhD)
Washington, University of (PhD)
Waterloo, University of (PhD)
Western Ontario, The University of (PhD)
Wichita State University (PhD)
Wilfrid Laurier University (MA/MS—terminal, PhD)
Windsor, University of (PhD)
Wisconsin, University of, Madison (PhD)
Wyoming, University of (PhD)
Yale University (PhD)
York University (PhD)

Sport Psychology
Adler School of Professional Psychology (MA/MS—terminal)
Denver, University of (MA/MS—terminal)
John F. Kennedy University (MA/MS—terminal)
Springfield College (MA/MS—terminal)
University of the Rockies (MA/MS, PsyD)

ALPHABETICAL INDEX OF INSTITUTIONS

Acadia University
  Department of Psychology, 839
Adelphi University
  The Derner Institute of Advanced Psychological Studies, School of Professional Psychology, 485
Adler School of Professional Psychology
  Professional School, 225
Akron, University of
  Department of Counseling, Collaborative Program in Counseling Psychology, 563
  Department of Psychology, 564
Alabama, University of
  Department of Psychology, 1
Alabama, University of, at Birmingham
  Department of Psychology, 3
Alabama, University of, at Huntsville
  Department of Psychology, 4
Alaska, University of, Fairbanks/Anchorage
  Department of Psychology/Joint PhD Program in Clinical-Community Psychology, 13
Alberta, University of
  Department of Psychology, 840
Alfred University
  Division of School Psychology, 486
Alliant International University: Fresno
  Forensic Psychology Programs, 33
Alliant International University: Fresno/Sacramento
  Programs in Clinical Psychology, 34
  Programs in Organizational Psychology, 36
Alliant International University: Irvine
  Forensic Psychology Program, 37
  Marital and Family Therapy Program, 38
  Programs in Educational and School Psychology, 40
Alliant International University: Los Angeles
  Forensic Psychology Programs, 41
  Programs in Clinical Psychology and Marital and Family Therapy, 42
  Programs in Educational and School Psychology, 44
  Programs in Organizational Psychology, 45
Alliant International University: Sacramento
  Forensic Psychology Program, 47
  Marital and Family Therapy Program, 48
Alliant International University: San Diego
  Forensic Psychology Programs, 49
  Programs in Clinical Psychology and Marital and Family Therapy, 50
  Programs in Educational and School Psychology, 53
  Programs in Organizational Psychology, 54
Alliant International University: San Francisco
  Programs in Clinical Psychology and Clinical Psychopharmacology, 56

Programs in Educational and School Psychology, 58
  Programs in Organizational Psychology, 59
American International College
  Department of Graduate Psychology, 362
American University
  Department of Psychology, 167
Angelo State University
  Department of Psychology, Sociology, and Social Work, 704
Antioch University New England
  Clinical Psychology, 460
Antioch University, Santa Barbara
  Graduate Psychology Programs, 60
Antioch University, Seattle
  PsyD in Psychology, 794
Appalachian State University
  Department of Psychology, 546
Arcadia University
  Department of Psychology, 616
Argosy University/Atlanta
  Clinical Psychology, 202
Argosy University/Chicago (formerly the Illinois School of Professional Psychology)
  Clinical Psychology Programs, 227
Argosy University/Orange County
  Psychology, 62
Argosy University/San Francisco Bay Area
  Clinical Psychology, 63
Argosy University/Schaumburg
  Clinical Psychology, 229
Argosy University/Seattle
  Clinical Psychology, 795
Argosy University/Washington, D.C.
  Clinical Psychology, 771
Arizona State University
  Applied Psychology, 15
  Department of Psychology, 16
  Division of Psychology in Education, 17
Arizona, The University of
  Department of Psychology, 20
Arkansas, University of
  Department of Psychology, 29
Assumption College
  Division of Counseling Psychology, 363
Auburn University
  Department of Psychology, 5
  Special Education, Rehabilitation, Counseling/School Psychology, 7
Augusta State University
  Department of Psychology, 203
Austin Peay State University
  Department of Psychology, 686
Azusa Pacific University
  Department of Graduate Psychology, 65
Ball State University
  Department of Counseling Psychology and Guidance Services, 271
  Department of Educational Psychology, 273
  Department of Psychological Science, 274

Baltimore, University of
  Division of Applied Behavioral Sciences, 344
Barry University
  Department of Psychology, 173
Baylor University
  Department of Psychology and Neuroscience, PhD Program in Psychology, 705
Benedictine University
  Graduate Department of Clinical Psychology, 230
Boston College
  Department of Counseling, Developmental, and Educational Psychology, 364
  Department of Psychology, 366
Boston University
  Department of Psychology, 367
  Division of Graduate Medical Sciences, Program in Mental Health Counseling and Behavioral Medicine, 369
Bowling Green State University
  Department of Psychology, 566
Brandeis University
  Department of Psychology, 370
Brenau University
  Psychology/ M.S. in Clinical Counseling Psychology, 204
Brigham Young University
  Department of Counseling Psychology and Special Education, 756
  Department of Psychology, 757
British Columbia, University of
  Department of Psychology, 841
Bryn Mawr College
  Department of Psychology, 617
Calgary, University of
  Department of Psychology, 843
California Institute of Integral Studies
  PsyD Program, 67
California Lutheran University
  Psychology Department, 68
California Polytechnic State University
  Psychology and Child Development, 70
California State University, Dominguez Hills
  Department of Psychology, 71
California State University, Fullerton
  Department of Psychology, 72
California State University, Long Beach
  Department of Psychology, 73
California State University, Northridge
  Department of Psychology, 75
California State University, Sacramento
  Department of Psychology, 77
California, University of, Berkeley
  Psychology Department, 79
  School Psychology Program, 81
California, University of, Davis
  Department of Psychology, 82
  Human Development, 84

ALPHABETICAL INDEX

California, University of, Irvine
- Department of Cognitive Sciences, 85
- Department of Psychology and Social Behavior, 86

California, University of, Los Angeles
- Department of Psychology, 88

California, University of, Merced
- Psychological Sciences, 90

California, University of, Riverside
- Department of Psychology, 91

California, University of, San Diego
- Department of Psychology, 92

California, University of, Santa Barbara
- Counseling, Clinical, and School Psychology, 94

California, University of, Santa Cruz
- Psychology Department, 95

Carleton University
- Department of Psychology, 844

Carnegie Mellon University
- Department of Psychology, 618
- Tepper School of Business at Carnegie Mellon, 619

Case Western Reserve University
- Department of Psychology, 568

Central Arkansas, University of
- Department of Psychology and Counseling, 30

Central Connecticut State University
- Department of Psychology, 152

Central Florida, University of
- Department of Psychology, 174

Central Michigan University
- Department of Psychology, 395

Central Oklahoma, University of
- Department of Psychology, 594

Central Washington University
- Department of Psychology, 796

Chestnut Hill College
- Department of Professional Psychology, 620

Chicago, University of
- Department of Psychology, 231

Cincinnati, University of
- Department of Psychology, 569
- Human Services/School Psychology, 571

Citadel, The
- Department of Psychology, 674

City University of New York
- Department of Psychology/Biopsychology and Behavioral Neuroscience PhD Subprogram, 488

City University of New York: Brooklyn College
- Department of Psychology, 490
- School Psychologist Graduate Program, School of Education, 491

City University of New York: Graduate Center
- Learning Processes and Behavior Analysis Doctoral Subprogram, 493
- Neuropsychology Doctoral Program, 494

City University of New York: Graduate School and University Center
- PhD Program in Educational Psychology, 495
- PhD Program in Psychology, 497

City University of New York: John Jay College of Criminal Justice
- Department of Psychology, 498

Claremont Graduate University
- Graduate Department of Psychology, 97

Clark University
- Frances L. Hiatt School of Psychology, 372

Clemson University
- Department of Psychology, 675

Cleveland State University
- Counseling Psychology Specialization of Urban Education Doctoral Program, 573

College of William and Mary
- Department of Psychology/Predoctoral MA Program, 772

Colorado State University
- Department of Psychology, 133

Colorado, University of, at Colorado Springs
- Department of Psychology, 135

Colorado, University of, Boulder
- Department of Psychology and Neuroscience, 136

Colorado, University of, Denver
- Department of Psychology, 138

Columbia University
- Health and Behavior Studies/School Psychology, 500

Concordia University
- Department of Psychology, 846

Connecticut, University of
- Department of Psychology, 153
- School Psychology Program, 155

Cornell University
- Department of Human Development, 501
- Graduate Field of Psychology, 503

Dalhousie University
- Department of Psychology, 847

Dayton, University of
- Department of Psychology, 574

Delaware, University of
- Department of Psychology, 165

Denver, University of
- Child, Family, and School Psychology Program, 139
- Counseling Psychology, 141
- Department of Psychology, 142
- Graduate School of Professional Psychology, 145

DePaul University
- Department of Psychology, 233

Drexel University
- Department of Psychology, 622

Duke University
- Department of Psychology and Neuroscience, 547

Duquesne University
- Department of Counseling, Psychology and Special Education, School Psychology Program, 624
- Department of Psychology, 625

East Carolina University
- Department of Psychology, 549

East Tennessee State University
- Department of Psychology, 687

Eastern Illinois University
- Department of Psychology, 235

Eastern Kentucky University
- Department of Psychology, 317

Eastern Michigan University
- Department of Psychology, 397

Eastern Washington University
- Department of Psychology, 798

Emory University
- Department of Psychology, 206

Emporia State University
- Department of Psychology, Art Therapy, Rehabilitation, and Mental Health Counseling, 302

Fairleigh Dickinson University, Metropolitan Campus
- School of Psychology, 463

Fielding Graduate University
- School of Psychology, 100

Florida Atlantic University
- Psychology, 176

Florida Institute of Technology
- School of Psychology, 177

Florida International University
- Psychology, 179

Florida State University
- Department of Psychology, 181
- Psychological Services in Education: PhD Combined Counseling/School Psychology, 183

Florida, University of
- Department of Clinical and Health Psychology, 185
- Department of Psychology, 187

Fordham University
- Department of Psychology, 504
- Division of Psychological and Educational Services, 505

Fort Hays State University
- Department of Psychology, 303

Francis Marion University
- Master's of Science in Applied Psychology, 677

Frostburg State University
- MS in Counseling Psychology Program, 345

Fuller Theological Seminary
- Department of Clinical Psychology, 101

Gallaudet University
- Department of Psychology, 169

Geneva College
- Master of Arts in Counseling, 626

George Fox University
- Graduate Department of Clinical Psychology, 605

George Mason University
- Department of Psychology, 773

George Washington University
- Department of Psychology, 171

Georgia Southern University
- Department of Psychology, 207

Georgia State University
- Department of Psychology, 209

Georgia, University of
- Department of Counseling and Human Development Services, 210
- Department of Psychology, 212
- School Psychology Program, 213

ALPHABETICAL INDEX

Goddard College
  MA Psychology & Counseling Program, 766
Gonzaga University
  Department of Counselor Education, 799
Guelph, University of
  Department of Psychology, 850
Hartford, University of
  Department of Psychology, 157
  Department of Psychology: Graduate Institute of Professional Psychology, 158
Harvard University
  Department of Psychology, 373
Hawaii, University of
  Department of Educational Psychology, 217
Hawaii, University of, Manoa
  Department of Psychology, 218
Hofstra University
  Department of Psychology, 507
Houston Baptist University
  Psychology Department, 706
Houston, University of
  Department of Educational Psychology, 708
  Department of Psychology, 710
Humboldt State University
  Department of Psychology, 103
Idaho State University
  Department of Psychology, 221
Idaho, University of
  Department of Psychology and Communication Studies, 222
Illinois Institute of Technology
  Institute of Psychology, 236
Illinois State University
  Department of Psychology, 238
Illinois, University of, Chicago
  Department of Psychology (M/C 285), 240
Illinois, University of, Urbana–Champaign
  Department of Educational Psychology, 242
  Department of Human and Community Development, 244
Illinois, University of, Urbana–Champaign
  Department of Psychology, 246
Immaculata University
  Department of Graduate Psychology, 628
Indiana State University
  Department of Communication Disorders & Counseling, School, & Educational Psychology, 276
  Department of Communication Disorders, Counseling, School, and Educational Psychology, 277
  Department of Psychology, 279
Indiana University
  Department of Counseling and Educational Psychology, 280
  Department of Psychological and Brain Sciences, 282
Indiana University of Pennsylvania
  Department of Psychology/Clinical Psychology Doctoral Program, 630

Indiana University-Purdue University Indianapolis
  Department of Psychology, 284
Indianapolis, University of
  Graduate Psychology Program, 286
Institute for the Psychological Sciences
  Department of Psychology, 776
Iona College
  Department of Psychology/Masters of Arts in Psychology, 509
Iowa State University
  Department of Psychology, 294
Iowa, University of
  Department of Psychological and Quantitative Foundations, 295
  Department of Psychology, 297
Jacksonville State University
  Department of Psychology, 9
John F. Kennedy University
  College of Professional Studies, 104
Johns Hopkins University
  Department of Psychological and Brain Sciences, 346
Kansas State University
  Department of Psychology, 305
Kansas, University of
  Department of Applied Behavioral Science (formerly Human Development), 306
  Department of Psychology, 307
  Psychology and Research in Education, 309
Kean University
  Department of Psychology; Department of Doctoral Programs in Psychology, 465
Kent State University
  Department of Psychology, 575
  School Psychology Program, 577
Kentucky, University of
  Department of Educational, School, and Counseling Psychology, 318
  Department of Psychology, 321
La Salle University
  Department of Psychology, 631
La Verne, University of
  Psychology Department, 106
Lamar University-Beaumont
  Department of Psychology, 712
Lehigh University
  Department of Education and Human Services, 632
  Department of Psychology, 634
Lewis & Clark College, Graduate School of Education and Counseling
  Counseling Psychology Department, 606
Lewis University
  Department of Psychology, 248
Loma Linda University
  Department of Psychology, 107
Long Island University
  Department of Psychology, 511
  Psychology/Clinical Psychology, 512
Louisiana State University Shreveport
  Department of Psychology, 332
Louisiana Tech University
  Department of Psychology and Behavioral Sciences, 333

Louisiana, University of, Lafayette
  Department of Psychology, 335
Louisiana, University of, Monroe
  Department of Psychology, 336
Louisville, University of
  Department of Educational & Counseling Psychology, 322
  Psychological and Brain Sciences, 324
Loyola University Maryland
  Department of Psychology, 348
Loyola University of Chicago
  Counseling Psychology, 249
  Department of Psychology, 250
Maine, University of
  Department of Psychology, 342
Manitoba, University of
  Psychology Graduate Office, 852
Marietta College
  Department of Psychology, 578
Marist College
  Department of Psychology, 514
Marquette University
  Department of Counselor Education and Counseling Psychology, 817
  Department of Psychology, 818
Marshall University
  Department of Psychology, 811
Maryland, University of
  Department of Counseling and Personnel Services, School and Counseling Psychology Programs, 349
  Department of Psychology, 351
  Institute for Child Study/Department of Human Development, 353
Maryland, University of, Baltimore County
  Department of Psychology, 354
Marymount University
  Department of Forensic Psychology, 777
Marywood University
  Department of Psychology and Counseling, 636
Massachusetts School of Professional Psychology
  Professional School, 375
Massachusetts, University of
  Department of Psychology, 377
Massachusetts, University of, Boston
  Counseling and School Psychology, 378
Massachusetts, University of, Dartmouth
  Psychology Department, 380
Massachusetts, University of, Lowell
  Community Social Psychology Master's Program, 382
McGill University
  Department of Educational and Counselling Psychology, 854
  Department of Psychology, 856
Memphis, University of
  Department of Counseling, Educational Psychology and Research, Program in Counseling Psychology, 688
  Department of Psychology, 690
Metropolitan State University
  Psychology/MA in Psychology Program, 412

ALPHABETICAL INDEX

Miami University of Ohio
  Department of Psychology, 580
Miami, University of
  Department of Educational & Psychological Studies/Area of Counseling Psychology, 189
  Department of Psychology, 190
Michigan School of Professional Psychology, 399
Michigan State University
  Department of Psychology, 400
Michigan, University of
  Combined Program in Education and Psychology, 402
  Department of Psychology, 403
Middle Tennessee State University
  Department of Psychology, 692
Midwestern State University
  Department of Psychology, 713
Midwestern University
  Clinical Psychology, 22
  Department of Behavioral Medicine/Clinical Psychology Program, 252
Millersville University
  Department of Psychology, 638
Minnesota State University—Mankato
  Department of Psychology, 413
Minnesota State University—Moorhead
  School Psychology Program, 414
Minnesota, University of
  Department of Educational Psychology: Counseling and Student Personnel; School Psychology, 415
  Department of Psychology, 417
  Institute of Child Development, 420
Mississippi State University
  Department of Counseling and Educational Psychology, 428
  Department of Psychology, 429
Mississippi, University of
  Department of Psychology, 431
Missouri State University
  Psychology Department, 433
Missouri, University of
  Department of Psychological Sciences, 434
Missouri, University of, Kansas City
  Department of Psychology, 436
  Division of Counseling and Educational Psychology, 437
Missouri, University of, St. Louis
  Department of Psychology, 439
Montana State University
  Department of Psychology, 445
Montana State University Billings
  Department of Psychology, 446
Montana, The University of
  Department of Psychology, 447
Morehead State University (Kentucky)
  Department of Psychology, 325
Murray State University
  Department of Psychology, 327
Nebraska, University of, Lincoln
  Department of Educational Psychology, 450
  Department of Psychology, 451

Nebraska, University of, Omaha
  Department of Psychology, 453
Nevada, University of, Las Vegas
  Department of Psychology, 456
Nevada, University of, Reno
  Department of Psychology/296, 457
New Brunswick, University of
  Department of Psychology, 857
New Hampshire, University of
  Department of Psychology, 461
New Haven, University of
  Graduate Psychology, 160
New Mexico Highlands University
  Department of Social and Behavioral Sciences, 478
New Mexico State University
  Counseling and Educational Psychology, 479
  Department of Psychology, 481
New Mexico, University of
  Department of Psychology, 482
New Orleans, University of
  Department of Psychology, 337
New York University
  Department of Applied Psychology, 515
New York University, Graduate School of Arts and Science
  Department of Psychology, 517
North Carolina State University
  Department of Psychology, 551
North Carolina, University of, Chapel Hill
  Department of Psychology, 552
North Carolina, University of, Charlotte
  Department of Psychology, 554
North Carolina, University of, Wilmington
  Psychology, 556
North Dakota State University
  Department of Psychology, 559
North Dakota, University of
  Department of Psychology, 560
North Florida, University of
  Department of Psychology, 192
North Texas, University of
  Department of Psychology, 714
Northcentral University
  School of Psychology, 23
Northeastern University
  Department of Counseling & Applied Educational Psychology, 383
  Department of Psychology, 385
Northern Arizona University
  Department of Psychology, 24
  Educational Psychology, 26
Northern Colorado, University of
  School of Applied Psychology and Counselor Education, 146
  School of Psychological Sciences, 148
Northern Illinois University
  Department of Psychology, 253
Northern Iowa, University of
  Department of Psychology, 299
Northern Kentucky University
  Department of Psychological Science, 328
Northern Michigan University
  Department of Psychology, 405
Northwestern University
  Department of Psychology, 255

Northwestern University, Feinberg School of Medicine
  Department of Psychiatry and Behavioral Sciences, Division of Psychology, 257
Notre Dame, University of
  Department of Psychology, 288
Nova Southeastern University
  Center for Psychological Studies, 193
Ohio State University
  School of Physical Activity and Educational Services, 581
Ohio State University, The
  Department of Psychology, 583
Ohio University
  Department of Psychology, 585
Oklahoma State University
  Department of Psychology, 595
  School of Applied Health and Educational Psychology, 596
Oklahoma, University of
  Department of Educational Psychology, 598
  Department of Psychology, 600
Old Dominion University
  Department of Psychology, 779
Oregon, University of
  Counseling Psychology, 608
  Department of Psychology, 609
Ottawa, University of
  School of Psychology, 859
Our Lady of the Lake University
  Psychology, 716
Pace University
  Department of Psychology, 519
Pacific Graduate School of Psychology & Stanford University School of Medicine, Department of Psychiatry and Behavioral Sciences
  PGSP-Stanford PsyD Consortium, 109
Pacific University
  School of Professional Psychology, 611
Pacific, University of the
  Department of Psychology, 111
Pacifica Graduate Institute
  PhD in Clinical Psychology with emphasis in Depth Psychology, 112
Palo Alto University
  Clinical Psychology Program, 113
Penn State Harrisburg
  Psychology Program, 639
Pennsylvania State University
  Counseling Psychology Program, 641
  Department of Psychology, 642
  Program in School Psychology, 644
Pennsylvania State University, The
  Department of Human Development and Family Studies, Graduate Program in Human Development and Family Studies, 645
Pennsylvania, University of
  Applied Psychology-Human Development Division, 647
  Department of Psychology, 649
Philadelphia College of Osteopathic Medicine
  Psychology Department, 650
Phillips Graduate Institute
  Clinical Psychology Doctoral Program, 115

ALPHABETICAL INDEX

Pittsburg State University
  Department of Psychology and Counseling, 311
Pittsburgh, University of
  Department of Psychology in Education, 653
  Psychology, 654
Portland State University
  Psychology Department, 612
Puerto Rico, University of
  Department of Psychology, 666
Puget Sound, University of
  School of Education, 800
Purdue University
  Department of Psychological Sciences, 289
Queen's University
  Department of Psychology, 860
Radford University
  Department of Psychology, 780
Regent University
  Doctoral Program in Clinical Psychology, 782
Regina, University of
  Department of Psychology, 862
Rensselaer Polytechnic Institute
  Cognitive Science, 520
Rhode Island College
  Psychology Department, 669
Rhode Island, University of, Chafee Social Sciences Center
  Department of Psychology, 670
Rice University
  Department of Psychology, 718
Roberts Wesleyan College
  Social Science Division/Graduate Psychology Program, 521
Roger Williams University
  Department of Psychology, 672
Roosevelt University
  Department of Psychology, 258
Rosalind Franklin University of Medicine and Science
  Department of Psychology, 260
Rowan University
  Department of Psychology, 466
Rutgers University—New Brunswick
  Graduate Program in Psychology, 467
Rutgers—The State University of New Jersey
  Department of Applied Psychology, 469
  Department of Clinical Psychology, 470
Rutgers—The State University of New Jersey, New Brunswick
  Department of Educational Psychology, 472
Ryerson University
  Department of Psychology, 864
Sage Colleges, The
  Department of Psychology, 523
Saint Francis, University of
  Psychology and Counseling, 291
Saint Joseph's University
  Department of Psychology, 655
Saint Mary's University
  Department of Psychology, 866
Saint Mary's University of Minnesota
  Counseling and Psychological Services, 421

Saint Michael's College
  Psychology Department/Graduate Program in Clinical Psychology, 767
Sam Houston State University
  Department of Psychology, 720
San Diego State University
  Department of Psychology, 116
San Diego State University/University of California, San Diego Joint Doctoral Program in Clinical Psychology
  SDSU Department of Psychology/UCSD Department of Psychiatry, 118
San Jose State University
  Department of Psychology, 119
Santa Clara University
  Department of Counseling Psychology, 121
Saskatchewan, University of
  Department of Psychology, 867
Saybrook University
  Graduate School, 122
Seattle Pacific University
  Clinical Psychology Department, 801
Seattle University
  Graduate Psychology Program, 803
Seton Hall University
  Professional Psychology and Family Therapy, 473
  Psychology/Experimental Psychology, 475
Simon Fraser University
  Department of Psychology, 869
Sonoma State University
  Department of Psychology, 124
South Alabama, University of
  Department of Psychology, 10
South Carolina, University of
  Department of Psychology, 678
South Carolina, University of, Aiken
  Department of Psychology/Applied Clinical Psychology Graduate Program, 680
South Dakota, University of
  Department of Psychology, 684
South Florida, University of
  Department of Psychological and Social Foundations, 196
  Department of Psychology, 198
Southeastern Louisiana University
  Department of Psychology, 338
Southern California, University of
  Department of Psychology, 125
Southern California, University of, Keck School of Medicine
  Department of Preventive Medicine, Division of Health Behavior Research, 127
Southern Connecticut State University
  Department of Psychology, 161
Southern Illinois University Carbondale
  Department of Psychology, 262
Southern Illinois University Edwardsville
  Department of Psychology, 263
Southern Methodist University
  Department of Psychology, 722
Southern Oregon University
  Master in Mental Health Counseling, 614
Spalding University
  School of Professional Psychology, 330
Springfield College
  Department of Psychology, 386

St. Cloud State University
  Department of Psychology, 422
St. Thomas, University of
  Graduate School of Professional Psychology, 424
Stanford University
  Department of Psychology, 128
State University of New York at New Paltz
  Department of Psychology, 524
State University of New York, Binghamton University
  Psychology, 526
State University of New York, College at Plattsburgh
  Psychology Department, 527
Stephen F. Austin State University
  Department of Psychology, 723
Stony Brook University
  Department of Psychology, 528
Suffolk University
  Department of Psychology, 388
Syracuse University
  Department of Psychology, 530
Teachers College, Columbia University
  Department of Counseling and Clinical Psychology/Program in Clinical Psychology, 532
Temple University
  Department of Psychological Studies in Education, 657
  Department of Psychology, 658
Tennessee, University of, Chattanooga
  Department of Psychology, 694
Tennessee, University of, Knoxville
  Department of Educational Psychology and Counseling, 695
  Department of Psychology, 697
  Industrial and Organizational Psychology Program, 698
Texas A&M International University
  Department of Behavioral, Applied Sciences & Criminal Justice, 724
Texas A&M University
  Department of Psychology, 726
  Educational Psychology, 727
Texas A&M University-Commerce
  Department of Psychology and Special Education, 729
Texas Christian University
  Department of Psychology, 731
Texas of the Permian Basin, The University of
  Psychology Department, 732
Texas Southwestern Medical Center at Dallas, The University of
  Division of Psychology, Graduate Program in Clinical Psychology, 733
Texas State University-San Marcos
  Psychology Department/Master of Arts in Health Psychology Program, 735
Texas Tech University
  Department of Psychology, 736
  Educational Psychology and Leadership/Educational Psychology, 738
Texas Woman's University
  Department of Psychology and Philosophy, 739

ALPHABETICAL INDEX

Texas, University of, Arlington
   Department of Psychology, 741
Texas, University of, Austin
   Department of Educational Psychology, 743
   Department of Human Development and Family Sciences, 746
   Department of Psychology, 747
Texas, University of, Dallas
   Psychological Sciences, 749
Texas, University of, El Paso
   Department of Psychology, 751
Texas, University of, Pan American
   Department of Psychology and Anthropology, 752
Texas, University of, Tyler
   Department of Psychology, 753
The Chicago School of Professional Psychology
   Professional School, 265
The College at Brockport, State University of New York
   Department of Psychology, 534
The New School for Social Research
   Department of Psychology, 535
The School of Professional Psychology at Forest Institute
   Clinical Psychology, 441
Toledo, University of
   Department of Psychology, 587
Toronto, University of
   Department of Psychology, 870
Towson University
   Department of Psychology, 356
Tufts University
   Department of Education; School Psychology Program, 390
   Department of Psychology, 391
   Eliot-Pearson Department of Child Development, 392
Tulane University
   Department of Psychology, 339
Tulsa, University of
   Department of Psychology, 602
Uniformed Services University of the Health Sciences
   Medical and Clinical Psychology, 358
University at Albany, State University of New York
   Department of Psychology, 537
University at Buffalo, State University of New York
   Department of Counseling, School, and Educational Psychology, 539
   Department of Psychology, 541
University of the Rockies
   Psychology, 150
Utah State University
   Department of Psychology, 759
Utah, University of
   Department of Educational Psychology, Counseling Psychology and School Psychology Programs, 761
   Department of Psychology, 764
Vanderbilt University
   Human & Organizational Development, 699
   Psychological Sciences, 701

Vanguard University of Southern California
   Graduate Program in Clinical Psychology, 130
Vermont, University of
   Department of Psychology, 768
Victoria, University of
   Department of Psychology, 872
Villanova University
   Department of Psychology, 660
Virginia Commonwealth University
   Department of Psychology, 783
Virginia Consortium Program in Clinical Psychology
   Program in Clinical Psychology, 785
Virginia Polytechnic Institute and State University
   Department of Psychology, 787
Virginia State University
   Department of Psychology, 789
Virginia, University of
   Curry Programs in Clinical and School Psychology, 790
   Department of Psychology, 792
Wake Forest University
   Department of Psychology, 557
Walden University
   Psychology, 425
Walla Walla University
   School of Education and Psychology, 804
Washburn University
   Department of Psychology, 313
Washington College
   Department of Psychology, 360
Washington State University
   Department of Psychology, 805
   Educational Leadership and Counseling Psychology, 807
Washington University in St. Louis
   Department of Psychology, 442
Washington, University of
   Department of Psychology, 808
Waterloo, University of
   Department of Psychology, 874
Wayne State University
   Department of Psychology, 406
   Division of Theoretical and Behavioral Foundations-Educational Psychology, 408
West Chester University of Pennsylvania
   Department of Psychology, 661
West Florida, The University of
   Department of Psychology, 199
West Georgia, University of
   Department of Psychology, 215
West Virginia University
   Department of Counseling, Rehabilitation Counseling and Counseling Psychology, 812
   Department of Psychology, 814
Western Illinois University
   Department of Psychology, 267
Western Michigan University
   Counselor Education & Counseling Psychology, 409
Western Ontario, The University of
   Department of Psychology, 876
Wheaton College
   Department of Psychology, 268

Wichita State University
   Department of Psychology, 314
Widener University
   Institute for Graduate Clinical Psychology, 662
   Law-Psychology (JD-PsyD) Graduate Training Program, 664
Wilfrid Laurier University
   Department of Psychology, 878
William Paterson University
   Psychology/MA in Clinical and Counseling Psychology, 476
Windsor, University of
   Psychology, 880
Winthrop University
   Department of Psychology, 681
Wisconsin School of Professional Psychology
   Professional School, 820
Wisconsin, University of, Eau Claire
   Department of Psychology, 822
Wisconsin, University of, La Crosse
   Department of Psychology/School Psychology, 823
Wisconsin, University of, Madison
   Department of Counseling Psychology, Counseling Psychology Program, 824
   Department of Educational Psychology, School Psychology Program, 826
   Department of Psychology, 827
   Human Development & Family Studies, 829
Wisconsin, University of, Milwaukee
   Department of Psychology, 831
   Educational Psychology, 833
Wisconsin, University of, Stout
   Psychology Department / Master of Science in Applied Psychology (MSAP), 835
Wright Institute
   Graduate School of Psychology, 131
Wright State University
   Department of Psychology, 588
   School of Professional Psychology, 590
Wyoming, University of
   Department of Psychology, 837
Xavier University
   Department of Psychology, 591
Yale University
   Department of Psychology, 162
Yeshiva University
   Ferkauf Graduate School of Psychology, 543
York University
   Graduate Program in Psychology, 881